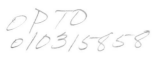

Editor: Darlene Barela Cooke
Managing Editor: Victoria M. Vaughn
Editorial Assistant: Robert J. Sharp
Marketing Manager: Diane M. Harnish
Production Coordinator: Felecia R. Weber
Project Editor: Jeffrey S. Myers
Freelance Copyeditors: Judith Fruchter Minkove, Christine A. Hajewski
Illustration Planner: Wayne Hubbel
Cover Designer: Mario Fernandez
Typesetter: Maryland Composition Co., Inc.
Printer and Binder: RR Donnelley & Sons Company

Copyright © 1998 Williams & Wilkins

351 West Camden Street
Baltimore, Maryland 21201-2436 USA

Rose Tree Corporate Center
1400 North Providence Road
Building II, Suite 5025
Media, Pennsylvania 19063-2043 USA

Accurate indications, adverse reactions and dosage schedules for drugs are provided in this book, but it is possible that they may change. The reader is urged to review the package information data of the manufacturers of the medications mentioned.

Printed in the United States of America

Fourth Edition, 1982

Library of Congress Cataloging-in-Publication Data

Walsh and Hoyt's clinical neuro-ophthalmology.—5th ed. / edited by
    Neil R. Miller, Nancy J. Newman.
         p.   cm.
      Includes bibliographical references and indexes.
      ISBN 0-683-30230-2 (vol. 1).—ISBN 0-683-30231-0 (vol. 2).—
    ISBN 0-683-30232-9 (vol. 3).—ISBN 0-683-30233-7 (vol. 4).—
    ISBN 0-683-30234-5 (vol. 5).
      1. Neuroophthalmology.   2. Eye Diseases.   I. Miller, Neil R.
    II. Newman, Nancy J.   III. Hoyt, William Fletcher, 1926–   .
    IV. Walsh, Frank Burton, 1896–   Clinical neuro-ophthalmology.
      [DNLM: 1. Neurologic Manifestations.   WW 140 W223   1997]
    RE725.W33   1997
    617.7—dc21
    DNLM/DLC
    for Library of Congress   96-50372
                                                                          CIP

The publishers have made every effort to trace the copyright holders for borrowed material. If they have inadvertently overlooked any, they will be pleased to make the necessary arrangements at the first opportunity.

To purchase additional copies of this book, call our customer service department at **(800) 638-0672** or fax orders to **(800) 447-8438.** For other book services, including chapter reprints and large quantity sales, ask for the Special Sales department.

Canadian customers should call **(800) 665-1148,** or fax **(800) 665-0103.** For all other calls originating outside of the United States, please call **(410) 528-4223** or fax us at **(410) 528-8550.**

Visit *Williams & Wilkins on the Internet:* **http://www.wwilkins.com** or contact our customer service department at custserv@wwilkins.com. Williams & Wilkins customer service representatives are available from 8:30 am to 6:00 pm, EST, Monday through Friday, for telephone access.

                                                                              98 99 00
                                                                    1 2 3 4 5 6 7 8 9 10

Walsh and Hoyt's
Clinical
Neuro-Ophthalmology

VOLUME THREE

Fifth Editi

To Vicki Vaughn, who always thought that this edition should, could, and would see the light of day.

NRM

To my parents, Edna B. Newman and the late Dr. Abraham B. Newman, for their commitment to education and their children.

NJN

*To Vicki Vaughn, who always thought that this edition should, could, and would
see the light of day.*

NRM

*To my parents, Edna B. Newman and the late Dr. Abraham B. Newman, for
their commitment to education and their children.*

NJN

Walsh and Hoyt's
Clinical
Neuro-Ophthalmology

VOLUME THREE   Fifth Edition

Editor: Darlene Barela Cooke
Managing Editor: Victoria M. Vaughn
Editorial Assistant: Robert J. Sharp
Marketing Manager: Diane M. Harnish
Production Coordinator: Felecia R. Weber
Project Editor: Jeffrey S. Myers
Freelance Copyeditors: Judith Fruchter Minkove, Christine A. Hajewski
Illustration Planner: Wayne Hubbel
Cover Designer: Mario Fernandez
Typesetter: Maryland Composition Co., Inc.
Printer and Binder: RR Donnelley & Sons Company

Copyright © 1998 Williams & Wilkins

351 West Camden Street
Baltimore, Maryland 21201-2436 USA

Rose Tree Corporate Center
1400 North Providence Road
Building II, Suite 5025
Media, Pennsylvania 19063-2043 USA

Accurate indications, adverse reactions and dosage schedules for drugs are provided in this book, but it is possible that they may change. The reader is urged to review the package information data of the manufacturers of the medications mentioned.

Printed in the United States of America

Fourth Edition, 1982

Library of Congress Cataloging-in-Publication Data

Walsh and Hoyt's clinical neuro-ophthalmology.—5th ed. / edited by
  Neil R. Miller, Nancy J. Newman.
     p.   cm.
   Includes bibliographical references and indexes.
    ISBN 0-683-30230-2 (vol. 1).—ISBN 0-683-30231-0 (vol. 2).—
  ISBN 0-683-30232-9 (vol. 3).—ISBN 0-683-30233-7 (vol. 4).—
ISBN 0-683-30234-5 (vol. 5).
    1. Neuroophthalmology. 2. Eye Diseases. I. Miller, Neil R.
  II. Newman, Nancy J. III. Hoyt, William Fletcher, 1926–   .
  IV. Walsh, Frank Burton, 1896–   Clinical neuro-ophthalmology.
   [DNLM: 1. Neurologic Manifestations.   WW 140 W223   1997]
  RE725.W33   1997
  617.7—dc21
  DNLM/DLC
  for Library of Congress   96-50372
                                  CIP

The publishers have made every effort to trace the copyright holders for borrowed material. If they have inadvertently overlooked any, they will be pleased to make the necessary arrangements at the first opportunity.

To purchase additional copies of this book, call our customer service department at **(800) 638-0672** or fax orders to **(800) 447-8438.** For other book services, including chapter reprints and large quantity sales, ask for the Special Sales department.

Canadian customers should call **(800) 665-1148,** or fax **(800) 665-0103.** For all other calls originating outside of the United States, please call **(410) 528-4223** or fax us at **(410) 528-8550.**

Visit Williams & Wilkins on the Internet: **http://www.wwilkins.com** or contact our customer service department at **custserv@wwilkins.com.** Williams & Wilkins customer service representatives are available from 8:30 am to 6:00 pm, EST, Monday through Friday, for telephone access.

                                                        98 99 00
                  1 2 3 4 5 6 7 8 9 10

Preface

In 1947, Frank Walsh wrote the first truly comprehensive textbook of neuro-ophthalmology. He published a second edition 10 years later. In 1969, Dr. Walsh enlisted the aid of a recent fellow, Dr. William Hoyt, in the writing of a new edition of this text. The third edition of Walsh and Hoyt's Clinical Neuro-Ophthalmology became the standard reference source for ophthalmologists, neurologists and other physicians with specialties overlapping the field of neuro-ophthalmology. In 1980, the baton was passed from Dr. Hoyt to one of us (NRM), who authored the 4th edition of Walsh and Hoyt's Clinical Neuro-Ophthalmology, a multi-volume textbook of nearly 5,000 pages. This edition took 14 years to produce, with the volumes published sequentially. Inevitably, the material was destined to become outdated, especially the first two volumes, which were published in 1982 and 1985. Thus, upon completion of the 4th edition, the question arose as to whether or not to write a new edition. It was not an easy decision. Clearly, it was no longer feasible for a single author to produce a current and comprehensive textbook in a timely manner. The information explosion that had occurred in medicine in general and in neuro-ophthalmology in particular, made a single- or dual-authored multi-volume comprehensive textbook impractical.

In January, 1995, a survey was distributed to the known buyers of the 4th edition of Walsh and Hoyt's Clinical Neuro-Ophthalmology. Approximately one-half of the respondents were ophthalmologists, and a third of the respondents considered themselves specialists in neuro-ophthalmology. The comments were surprisingly consistent. People simply wanted a comprehensive, authoritative textbook of neuro-ophthalmology. Also considered important were extensive illustrations, a cumulative index, and detailed reference listing. The idea of multiple authors was embraced by the majority of respondents.

The two of us subsequently agreed to organize, edit, and rewrite several of the chapters for a 5th edition. We invited 60 international experts in various aspects of neuro-ophthalmology to each write a chapter. These contributors have in some cases updated the material from the 4th edition and in other cases completely written or rewritten their chapters. They have brought a depth of understanding and a wealth of knowledge to the 5th edition that could not possibly be accomplished with single or dual authorship. Furthermore, the publication of this 5-volume work has occurred in the nearly record time of two years.

The 5th edition consists of five volumes. We have continued the overall organization of the 4th edition; namely, an anatomic approach to the physiology and pathophysiology of the neuro-ophthalmologic afferent and efferent systems, followed by volumes dedicated to specific systemic and neurologic disease processes that may involve the visual sensory and ocular motor pathways. Volume 1 contains subject matter previously included in the first and second volumes of the 4th edition. This includes the visual sensory system and the optic nerve, as well as the ocular motor system, the autonomic nervous system, and the sensory innervation of the eye and orbit. This volume has been extensively reorganized and rewritten with emphasis on disease pathogenesis. We have added chapters specifically covering the techniques of examination of the various systems, as well as a chapter on traumatic optic neuropathies. We conclude Volume 1 with a review of the neuro-ophthalmologic manifestations of nonorganic disease. Volume 2 contains chapters on central and peripheral nervous system neoplasms and their neuro-ophthalmologic manifestations. Additional chapters include the related topics of complications of cancer therapies, the paraneoplastic disorders, and the phacomatoses. This volume concludes with new chapters on the degenerative and metabolic diseases of adults and children. Volume 3 is devoted to vascular disease. Volumes 4 and 5 cover infectious and inflammatory diseases of the nervous system, including demyelinating disorders. Hundreds of new illustrations and tables have been added. Each volume has its own index corresponding to the pages in that volume, and a cumulative index for all five volumes is provided as a separate book. To help readers peruse chapters for content, we have added a summary of major and minor headings at the beginning of each chapter.

In response to the changing aspects of neuro-ophthalmology as a specialty, in this edition we have tried to emphasize patient management. There is less historic background and more information on current therapeutic strategies. Individual illustrative case histories are still included, some from previous editions of the textbook, others new. For the most part, old references have been maintained and new ones added. However, as was true with the 4th edition, there will be times when the previous editions provide further insight into a topic and not merely historical perspective. As is the case with all multi-authored texts, the chapters may vary in their individual approach to the topics, but as editors, we have tried to maintain a consistent emphasis and style.

We hope that our readers will find in this 5th edition the things they liked about the previous editions as well as new aspects unique to these volumes. We trust that it will be used frequently and easily in the day-to-day practice of ophthalmologists, neurologists, neurosurgeons, and neuro-ophthalmologists. We believe this 5th edition of Walsh and Hoyt's Clinical Neuro-Ophthalmology carries on the tradition of the first four editions by being a comprehensive textbook of neuro-ophthalmology that provides the most current information available. It is a mark of our times and of the growth of our specialty that it would now take more than 60 authors to do it right.

Acknowledgments

There are many persons who have played major roles in the development and publication of this multivolume text. First and foremost, we wish to thank our contributors. Without their tireless efforts, there would be no book. Gary Lees and Juan Garcia from the Department of Medical Art of the Johns Hopkins Hospital provided superb illustrations, often in an inordinately short period of time. The Wilmer photography service, particularly Terry George, David Emmert, Mark Herring, and Ben Kilburg, performed above and beyond the call of duty to photograph illustrations for numerous chapters, not just those written by NRM. Kurt Simons, a computer "guru" if there ever was one, was always available to convert files from one format to another, retrieve lost files, etc. Our copyediting staff, led by Judy Minkove, and our compositor, Chris Hajewski, kept the project on target by burning the midnight oil. Our team at Williams & Wilkins, namely Darlene Cooke, Rob Sharp, Felecia Weber, and Diane Harnish, were a delight to work with, and it was Vicki Vaughn who kept the whole project together. Without her, this project would have failed.

NRM would like to personally thank Elizabeth Farr Bradley, MD; Jennie Hunnewell, MD; David Klink, MD; Christopher Girkin, MD; and J. D. Perry, MD for critically reviewing nearly every chapter in the book. Their suggestions made good chapters even better. He also would like to thank Carol, Elizabeth, and Penny for once again putting up with the demands of the project.

NJN would like to personally thank those colleagues who reviewed portions of the text, including Alexander P. Auchus, MD; Valerie Biousse, MD; Donald Bliwise, PhD; Louis R. Caplan, MD; C. Michael Cawley III, MD; Mark R. Gilbert, MD; David A. Hafler, MD, PhD; Steven M. Hersch, MD, PhD; Jorge L. Juncos, MD; Jeffrey J. Olson, MD; Nelson M. Oyesiku, MD, PhD; Susan Brothers Peterman, MD; and Krish Sathian, MD, PhD, as well as Wendy Wiley, who provided expert editorial assistance. She would also like to thank Thomas M. Aaberg, MD, for his unflagging support of the academic mission of the Department of Ophthalmology at Emory University and the Emory residents and fellows from whom much time and energy were diverted. She acknowledges her teachers in neurology and neuro-ophthalmology, including C. Miller Fisher, MD; Raymond D. Adams, MD; E.P. Richardson, MD; Norman J. Schatz, MD; Ronald M. Burde, MD; Joel S. Glaser, MD; and William F. Hoyt, MD. In addition, special mention must be made of three extraordinary individuals: Steven A. Newman, MD, who introduced his sister to the wonderful world of neuro-ophthalmology; Simmons Lessell, MD, who mentored and fathered the neuro-ophthalmologist she was to become; and Neil R. Miller, MD, her mentor, colleague, partner, and friend.

Contributors

Anthony C. Arnold, MD
Associate Professor of Ophthalmology
Chief, Neuro-Ophthalmology Division
Jules Stein Eye Institute
Department of Ophthalmology
UCLA School of Medicine
Los Angeles, California

Lea Averbuch-Heller, MD
Assistant Professor
Department of Neurology
University Hospitals of Cleveland
Case Western Reserve University
Cleveland, Ohio

Robert S. Baker, MD, FRCP, FRCS
Professor and Chairman of Ophthalmology
Professor of Neurosurgery, Neurology, and Pediatrics
Kentucky Clinic
Lexington, Kentucky

Jason J.S. Barton, MD
Beth Israel Deaconess Medical Center
Harvard Medical School
Boston, Massachusetts

Roy W. Beck, MD, PhD
Director, Jaeb Center for Health Research
Clinical Professor of Ophthalmology and
Adjunct Professor of Epidemiology and Biostatistics
University of South Florida
Tampa, Florida

Mark S. Borchert, MD
Associate Professor of Clinical Ophthalmology and
  Neurology
Children's Hospital Los Angeles
School of Medicine, University of Southern California
Los Angeles, California

Paul W. Brazis, MD
Associate Professor of Neurology
Mayo Medical School
Consultant in Neurology and Neuro-Ophthalmology
Mayo Clinic, Jacksonville
Jacksonville, Florida

Michael C. Brodsky, MD
Professor of Ophthalmology and Pediatrics
University of Arkansas for Medical Sciences
Chief of Pediatric Ophthalmology
Arkansas Children's Hospital
Little Rock, Arkansas

Wayne T. Cornblath, MD
Kellogg Eye Institute
Assistant Professor of Ophthalmology and Neurology
University of Michigan
Ann Arbor, Michigan

Shelley Ann Cross, MD
Consultant in Neurology
Mayo Clinic
Assistant Professor of Neurology
Mayo Medical School
Rochester, Minnesota

Jon N. Currie, MBBS, FRACP
Director, Drug and Alcohol Services
Western Sydney Area Health Services
Head, Neuro-Ophthalmology Service
Westmead Hospital
Sydney, New South Wales, Australia

Kathleen B. Digre, MD
Associate Professor of Neurology and Ophthalmology
Director of Neuro-Ophthalmology Clinic
Moran Eye Center
University of Utah
Salt Lake City, Utah

Dominic E. Dwyer, BSc, MBBS, FRACP, FRCPA
Department of Virology
Center for Infectious Diseases and Microbiology
  Laboratory Services
ICPMR, Westmead Hospital
Westmead, New South Wales, Australia

Eric R. Eggenberger, DO
Michigan State University Clinical Center
Assistant Professor
Michigan State University
East Lansing, Michigan

Craig Evinger, PhD
Professor, Department of Neurology and Behavior
Associate Professor, Department of Ophthalmology
University Hospital and Medical Center at Stony Brook
SUNY Stony Brook
Stony Brook, New York

Warren L. Felton III, MD
Associate Professor
Departments of Neurology and Ophthalmology
Chairman, Division of Neuro-Ophthalmology
Medical College of Virginia—Virginia Commonwealth
  University
Richmond, Virginia

William A. Fletcher, MD
Foothills Hospital
Associate Professor
Department of Clinical Neurosciences Division of
  Ophthalmology
University of Calgary
Calgary, Alberta, Canada

Benjamin M. Frishberg, MD
Clinical Professor of Ophthalmology
Assistant Clinical Professor of Neurology
Howard University School of Medicine
Assistant Clinical Professor of Neurology
Georgetown University Medical Center
Director of Neuro-Ophthalmology
Howard University Hospital
Washington, D.C.
North County Neurology Associates
La Jolla, California

Steven L. Galetta, MD
Professor of Neurology and Ophthalmology
Director, Neuro-Ophthalmology Service
University of Pennsylvania School of Medicine
Philadelphia, Pennsylvania

James A. Garrity, MD
Associate Professor of Ophthalmology
Mayo Medical School
Consultant, Department of Ophthalmology
Mayo Clinic
Rochester, Minnesota

John W. Gittinger, Jr., MD
Professor and Chair, Department of Ophthalmology
  Professor of Neurology
University of Massachusetts Medical School
Worcester, Massachusetts

Robert A. Goldberg, MD
Chief, Orbital and Ophthalmic Plastic Surgery Division
Jules Stein Eye Institute
Associate Professor of Ophthalmology
UCLA School of Medicine
Los Angeles, California

Karl C. Golnik, MD
Assistant Professor of Ophthalmology and Neurosurgery
University of Cincinnati
The Cincinnati Eye Institute
Cincinnati, Ohio

Steven R. Hamilton, MD
Eye Associates Northwest
Assistant Clinical Professor of Neurology and
  Ophthalmology
University of Washington School of Medicine
Seattle, Washington

Thomas R. Hedges III, MD
Professor of Ophthalmology
Associate Professor of Neurology
Tufts University School of Medicine
Director of Neuro-Ophthalmology, New England Eye
  Center
Boston, Massachusetts

Paul N. Hoffman, MD, PhD
Associate Professor of Ophthalmology and Neurology
Johns Hopkins School of Medicine
Baltimore, Maryland

Saunders L. Hupp, MD
Professor, Ophthalmology and Neuro-Ophthalmology
Department of Ophthalmology
University of South Alabama College of Medicine
Mobile, Alabama

Daniel M. Jacobson, MD
Director, Neuro-Ophthalmology Service
Departments of Neurology and Ophthalmology
Marshfield Clinic
Marshfield, Wisconsin
Clinical Associate Professor
Departments of Ophthalmology and Visual Sciences, and
  Neurology
University of Wisconsin Medical School
Madison, Wisconsin

Chris A. Johnson, PhD
Professor, Department of Ophthalmology
Director, Optics and Visual Assessment Lab (OVAL)
UC Davis Medical Center
Sacramento, California

Randy H. Kardon, MD, PhD
Director of Neuro-Ophthalmology
Associate Professor
University of Iowa Hospitals and Clinics
Veterans Administration Medical Center
Iowa City, Iowa

Barrett J. Katz, MD
Professor of Ophthalmology, Neurology, and
  Neurosurgery
University of Rochester School of Medicine
Strong Memorial Hospital
Rochester, New York

David I. Kaufman, DO
Director, Clinical Neurosciences Unit
Michigan State University
Sparrow Hospital
Professor, Neuro-Ophthalmology
East Lansing, Michigan

James R. Keane, MD
Professor of Neurology
University of Southern California
Los Angeles, California

Shalom E. Kelman, MD
Associate Professor of Ophthalmology
University of Maryland School of Medicine
Baltimore, Maryland

John L. Keltner, MD
Chairman, Department of Ophthalmology
Professor of Ophthalmology, Neurology, and Neurological
  Surgery
UC Davis Medical Center
Sacramento, California

**Christopher Kennard, PhD, BSc, MBBS, FRCP,
  FRCOphth**
Chairman and Head of the Neuroscience and
  Psychological Medicine Divisions
Imperial College School of Medicine
Charing Cross Hospital
London, United Kingdom

John S. Kennerdell, MD
Chairman, Department of Ophthalmology
Professor, Allegheny University Health Sciences at
  Allegheny General Hospital
Adjunct Professor of Ophthalmology
University of Pittsburgh
Pittsburgh, Pennsylvania

Lanning B. Kline, MD
Professor of Clinical Ophthalmology
Combined Program in Ophthalmology Eye Foundation
  Hospital, University of Alabama School of Medicine
Birmingham, Alabama

Gregory S. Kosmorsky, DO
Head, Section of Neuro-Ophthalmology
Division of Ophthalmology
The Cleveland Clinic Foundation
Cleveland, Ohio

Ralph W. Kuncl, MD, PhD
Professor of Neurology
Neuromuscular Division
Johns Hopkins Hospital
Baltimore, Maryland

Andrew G. Lee, MD
Cullen Eye Institute
Assistant Professor of Ophthalmology, Neurology and
  Neurosurgery
Baylor College of Medicine
Neuro-Ophthalmology Consultant
Division of Neurosurgery
M.D. Anderson Cancer Center
Houston, Texas

R. John Leigh, MD
Staff Neurologist
Cleveland Veterans Affairs Medical Center Professor,
  Department of Neurology, Neurosciences,
  Otolaryngology, and Biomedical Engineering
Case Western Reserve University
Cleveland, Ohio

Simmons Lessell, MD
Massachusetts Eye and Ear Infirmary
Professor of Ophthalmology
Harvard Medical School
Boston, Massachusetts

Robert L. Lesser, MD
Associate Clinical Professor of Ophthalmology
Department of Ophthalmology and Visual Science
Yale University School of Medicine
New Haven, Connecticut
Clinical Professor of Neurology and Neurosurgery
University of Connecticut School of Medicine
Farmington, Connecticut

Grant T. Liu, MD
Assistant Professor of Neurology and Ophthalmology
Division of Neuro-Ophthalmology
Departments of Neurology and Ophthalmology
Hospital of the University of Pennsylvania
Children's Hospital of Philadelphia
Scheie Eye Institute
Philadelphia, Pennsylvania

Joseph C. Maroon, MD
Professor and Chairman, Division of Neurosurgery
Allegheny University of the Health Sciences
Allegheny Campus
Pittsburgh, Pennsylvania

Linda Kirschen McLoon, PhD
Associate Professor, Department of Ophthalmology
University of Minnesota
Minneapolis, Minnesota

Neil R. Miller, MD
Professor of Ophthalmology, Neurology, and
  Neurosurgery
Frank B. Walsh Professor of Neuro-Ophthalmology
Johns Hopkins Medical Institutions
Baltimore, Maryland

Mark L. Moster, MD
Professor and Senior Associate Chairman
Department of Neurology
Temple University School of Medicine
Chairman, Department of Neurosensory Sciences
Albert Einstein Medical Center
Philadelphia, Pennsylvania

Golnaz Moazami, MD
Instructor in Clinical Ophthalmology
Edward S. Harkness Eye Institute
Columbia-Presbyterian Medical Center
New York, New York

Nancy J. Newman, MD
Cyrus H. Stoner Professor of Ophthalmology
Associate Professor of Ophthalmology and Neurology
Instructor in Neurological Surgery
Emory University School of Medicine
Atlanta, Georgia
Lecturer in Ophthalmology
Harvard Medical School
Boston, Massachusetts

Steven A. Newman, MD
Associate Professor of Ophthalmology and Neurological
    Surgery
Department of Ophthalmology
University of Virginia Medical Center
Charlottesville, Virginia

Jeffrey G. Odel, MD
Associate Clinical Professor of Ophthalmology
Edward S. Harkness Eye Institute
Columbia-Presbyterian Medical Center
New York, New York

Kimberly Peele Cockerham, MD
Director, Oculoplastics, Orbital Disease, and
    Reconstruction
Staff, Neuro-Ophthalmology
Walter Reed Army Medical Hospital
Washington, District of Columbia

Stephen C. Pollock, MD
Associate Professor of Ophthalmology
Duke University Eye Center
Durham, North Carolina

Jonathan D. Porter, PhD
Departments of Anatomy and Neurobiology
Professor of Anatomy, Neurobiology, and Ophthalmology
University of Kentucky Medical Center
Lexington, Kentucky

Valerie A. Purvin, MD
Chief, Neuro-Ophthalmology Section
Midwest Eye Institute
Associate Clinical Professor of Ophthalmology and
    Neurology
Indiana University Medical Center
Indianapolis, Indiana

Michael X. Repka, MD
Wilmer Eye Institute
Johns Hopkins Hospital
Associate Professor
Johns Hopkins University School of Medicine
Baltimore, Maryland

Joseph F. Rizzo, III, MD
Massachusetts Eye and Ear Infirmary
Assistant Professor
Department of Ophthalmology
Harvard Medical School
Boston, Massachusetts

Matthew Rizzo, MD
University of Iowa
Professor of Neurology and Public Policy
Adjunct Professor of Engineering
Director of the Visual Function Laboratory
Division of Behavioral Neurology and Cognitive
    Neuroscience
Iowa City, Iowa

Alfredo A. Sadun, MD, PhD
Professor, Departments of Ophthalmology and
    Neurological Surgery
Doheny Eye Institute, University of Southern California
    School of Medicine
Los Angeles, California

John B. Selhorst, MD
Professor and Chairman
Department of Neurology
Saint Louis University
St. Louis, Missouri

James A. Sharpe, MD, FRCPC
Professor of Neurology and Head, Division of Neurology
University of Toronto
Head of Neurology, The Toronto Hospital
Toronto, Ontario, Canada

William T. Shults, MD
Chief of Neuro-Ophthalmology
Devers Eye Institute
Department of Ophthalmology
Portland, Oregon

Patrick A. Sibony, MD
Professor, Department of Ophthalmology
University Hospital and Medical Center at Stony Brook
SUNY Stony Brook
Stony Brook, New York

Barry Skarf, MD, PhD
Director, Neuro-Ophthalmology Unit
Departments of Eye Care Services, Neurology and
    Neurosurgery
Henry Ford Health Sciences Center
Detroit, Michigan

Thomas L. Slamovits, MD
Montefiore Medical Center
Professor of Ophthalmology, Neurology, and
   Neurosurgery
Albert Einstein College of Medicine
Bronx, New York

Craig H. Smith, MD
Director, Neuro-Ophthalmology Research Unit
Swedish Hospital Medical Center
Clinical Professor of Medicine, Neurology and
   Ophthalmology
University of Washington
Seattle, Washington

Kenneth D. Steinsapir, MD
Assistant Clinical Professor
Jules Stein Eye Institute
UCLA School of Medicine
Los Angeles, California

H. Stanley Thompson, MD
University of Iowa Hospitals and Clinics
Professor of Ophthalmology
University of Iowa
Iowa City, Iowa

B. Todd Troost, MD
Professor of Neurology and Anesthesia
Chairman, Department of Neurology
Bowman Gray School of Medicine
Wake Forest University
Winston-Salem, North Carolina

Michael Wall, MD
Professor of Neurology and Ophthalmology
University of Iowa College of Medicine
Veterans Administration Hospital
Iowa City, Iowa

Joel M. Weinstein, MD
Associate Clinical Professor of Ophthalmology,
   Neurology, and Neurosurgery
University of Wisconsin School of Medicine
Madison, Wisconsin

Jacqueline M.S. Winterkorn, MD, PhD
Clinical Professor
Departments of Ophthalmology, Neurology and
   Neuroscience
Cornell University Medical College
Attending in Ophthalmology and Neurology
The New York Hospital Cornell Medical Center
New York, New York

Jonathan D. Wirtschafter, MD
Professor of Ophthalmology, Neurology, and
   Neurosurgery
University of Minnesota Medical School
Minneapolis, Minnesota

Rochelle S. Zak, MD
New York Hospital, Westchester Division
White Plains, New York

David S. Zee, MD
Professor, Departments of Neurology and Ophthalmology
Johns Hopkins Hospital
Baltimore, Maryland

Contents

VOLUME THREE

SECTION XI: Vascular Anatomy and Pathology

SECTION XI:
Vascular Anatomy and Pathology

Vascular diseases of the brain are major causes of neuro-ophthalmologic manifestations. These diseases are characterized pathologically by impaired blood flow through normal or damaged blood vessels or by leakage of blood or its components through the walls of such vessels. Impaired circulation or leakage, in turn, causes ischemia, infarction, hemorrhage, or a combination of these processes, thus damaging cerebral, orbital, or ocular tissue and causing disturbances that affect the visual sensory, ocular motor, or pupillary systems. The chapters that follow are concerned with the anatomy of the vcerebral vascular system and the major categories of vascular disease that produce neuro-ophthalmologic manifestations.

CHAPTER 52

Anatomy and Physiology of the Cerebral Vascular System

Neil R. Miller

In this chapter, we consider the anatomy of the cerebral vascular system and the physiology of cerebral blood flow (CBF). The reader interested in pursuing these subjects in more detail should obtain the excellent books *Cerebral Blood Flow*, edited by James H. Wood (1987) and *Neurovascular Neuro-ophthalmology*, written by Mark Kupersmith (1993).

ARTERIAL SYSTEM OF THE BRAIN

ORIGIN OF THE CEREBRAL ARTERIAL BLOOD SUPPLY FROM THE AORTIC ARCH

The cerebral arterial blood supply is derived from the aortic arch through three major vessels: the innominate (brachiocephalic) artery, the left common carotid artery, and the left subclavian artery (Fig. 52.1).

The **innominate** artery arises at the level of the upper border of the right second costal cartilage as the largest trunk of the aortic arch. It ascends the short distance to the level of the upper border of the right sternoclavicular articulation, where it gives off the **right common carotid artery** (Fig. 52.1). At this point, the innominate artery becomes the right subclavian artery. The right common carotid artery ascends to the upper level of the thyroid cartilage, where it bifurcates into the **right internal and external carotid arteries** (Fig. 52.1).

The **left common carotid artery** arises from the apex of the aortic arch and runs for a short distance through the thorax before entering the base of the neck and ascending to the level of the hyoid bone, where it divides into the **left internal and external carotid arteries** (Fig. 52.1).

Although the right subclavian artery originates as the innominate artery, the **left subclavian artery** arises directly from the aortic arch. The first branch of each subclavian artery is the **vertebral artery**, although occasionally the left vertebral artery arises directly from the aortic arch rather than from the left subclavian artery. The two vertebral arteries ascend from the base of the neck through the foramina in the transverse processes of the upper six vertebrae and wind behind the upper articular processes of the atlas before entering the cranial cavity through the foramen magnum (Fig. 52.1).

INTERNAL CAROTID ARTERY AND ITS BRANCHES

Several classifications have been proposed to describe the course and segments of the internal carotid artery (Fischer, 1938; Gibo, 1981a; Lasjaunias and Berenstein, 1987). Although we recognize the merits of these classifications, we

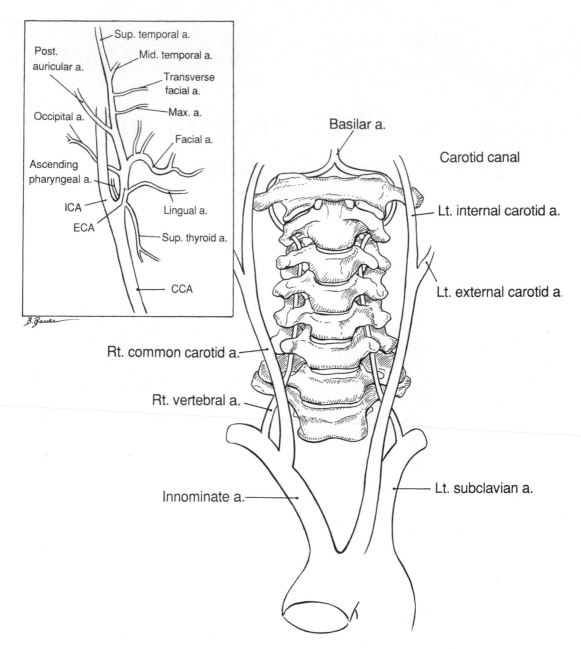

Figure 52.1. Schematic drawing of the origin of the cerebral blood vessels from the aortic arch. *Inset* shows the main branches of the external carotid artery.

prefer and have chosen to use in this section the classification described by Bouthillier et al. (1996) that separates the vessel into seven segments, C1–C7, numbered in the direction of blood flow (Fig. 52.2).

Cervical Segment (C1)

The **cervical segment** (C1) of the internal carotid artery begins at the level of the bifurcation of the common carotid artery. This segment runs inside the carotid sheath with the internal jugular vein lateral to the artery and the vagus nerve usually posterolateral. Inside the sheath, the artery is sur-

rounded by fat, a venous plexus, and postganglionic sympathetic nerves. The carotid sheath is a duplication of the prevertebral fascia (Casberg, 1950) and divides into two layers at the extracranial entrance of the carotid canal. The inner layer continues as the periosteum of the carotid canal, whereas the outer layer continues as the periosteum of the extracranial surface of the skull base.

The cervical segment of the internal carotid artery ascends behind the tonsillar fossa to the base of the skull. This portion of the artery usually has no branches, although exceptions do occur. The **primitive hypoglossal artery** is an anomalous vessel that originates from the extracranial portion of the

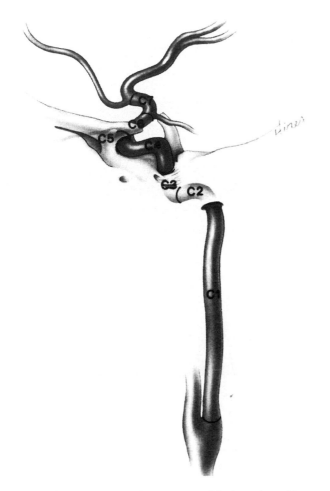

Figure 52.2. Classification of the segments of the internal carotid artery. The classification includes the entire artery and uses a numerical scale in the direction of blood flow. *C1,* cervical segment; *C2,* petrous segment; *C3,* lacerum segment; *C4,* cavernous segment; *C5,* clinoid segment; *C6,* ophthalmic segment; *C7,* communicating segment. (From Bouthillier A, van Loveren HR, Keller JT. Segments of the internal carotid artery: A new classification. Neurosurgery *38:*425–433, 1996.)

internal carotid artery and anastomoses with the basilar artery and its terminal branches (Batujeff, 1889—see below). The **occipital artery,** usually a branch of the external carotid artery, may originate at the bifurcation of the common carotid artery or from the proximal portion of the internal carotid artery (Adachi and Hasebe, 1928). In some persons, the extracranial portion of the internal carotid artery gives rise to small arteries that contribute to the blood supply of the sympathetic nerve plexus (Havelius and Hindfelt, 1985). Damage to these vessels may produce Horner's syndrome. The cervical segment of the internal carotid artery ends where the vessel enters the carotid canal of the petrous bone anterior to the jugular foramen.

The internal carotid artery enters the cranial cavity by passing through the carotid canal. This canal is lined by periosteum and is located in the petrous portion of the temporal bone. The anterior or interior orifice of the canal opens onto the posterior wall of the **foramen lacerum** and is just anterior to the jugular foramen. The posterior orifice of the canal is located at the petrous apex.

Petrous Segment (C2)

The segment of the internal carotid artery within the carotid canal is called the **petrous segment** (C2) (Figs. 52.2–52.4). Like the cervical segment, the petrous segment is surrounded by fat, a venous plexus, and postganglionic sympathetic nerves. The petrous segment is usually separated into two parts: a vertical or ascending portion and a horizontal portion (Paullus et al., 1977) (Fig. 52.4), although some authors consider the bend in this segment between the two parts as a third part (Bouthillier et al., 1996). In any event, both parts of the vessel have predictable courses and relationships to surrounding structures.

The **vertical** part is the proximal part of the petrous segment of the internal carotid artery. It passes directly upward after entering the carotid canal to lie adjacent to the jugular fossa posteriorly, the eustachian tube anteriorly, and the tympanic bone anterolaterally. Its length varies from 6.0 to 15.0 mm. The vessel then turns anteromedially to form a genu and becomes the horizontal segment (Fig. 52.4).

The **horizontal** part of the petrous segment of the internal carotid artery begins at the genu and passes anteromedially within the petrous bone to emerge near its apex (Fig. 52.4). During its course, this portion of the vessel lies just anterior to both the cochlea and the trigeminal ganglion, separated from them by thin plates of bone. The length of the horizontal part of the petrous segment of the internal carotid artery ranges from 15.0 to 25.1 mm (Paullus et al., 1977).

Two main branches may arise from the petrous segment of the internal carotid artery. The **caroticotympanic artery** is a small vessel that enters the tympanic cavity through a foramen in the wall of the vertical portion of the carotid canal to supply the tympanic membrane. It seems to be a rare structure, because it was not found in any of the 50 specimens examined by Paullus et al. (1977). The **vidian (pterygoid) artery** usually arises from the internal maxillary artery, but it may arise from the horizontal segment of the internal carotid artery and enter the pterygoid canal along with the pterygoid nerve. This artery is somewhat more common than the caroticotympanic artery, but it was still seen in only 15 (30%) of 50 specimens examined by Paullus et al. (1977).

In addition to the caroticotympanic and vidian arteries, the petrous segment of the internal carotid artery gives rise to several much smaller arteries (Havelius and Hindfelt, 1995). These vessels probably are vasa nervorum for the sympathetic nerves.

Lacerum Segment (C3)

The internal carotid artery exits from the petrous bone superiorly to enter the cavernous sinus (Figs. 52.2 and 52.5). Before it does so, however, there is a brief portion of the vessel, the **lacerum segment** (C3), that begins where the carotid canal ends and that ascends in the vertical canal of the foramen lacerum toward the posterior aspect of the cavernous sinus, ending at the superior margin of the petrolin-

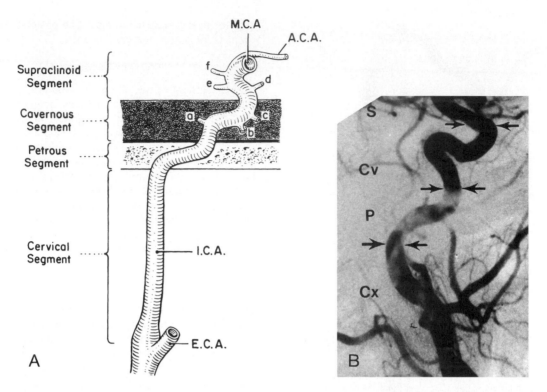

Figure 52.3.   The main segments of the internal carotid artery. *A,* schematic drawing of the internal carotid artery (*I.C.A.*), showing the major intracavernous and intracranial branches. In this illustration, the artery is divided into only four segments: cervical, petrous, cavernous, and supraclinoid. *A.C.A.,* anterior cerebral artery; *E.C.A.,* external carotid artery; *M.C.A.,* middle cerebral artery; *a,* meningohypophyseal trunk; *b,* artery of the inferior cavernous sinus; *c,* capsular artery (of McConnell); *d,* ophthalmic artery; *e,* posterior communicating artery; *f,* anterior choroidal artery. (From Day AL. Arterial distributions and variants. In Cerebral Blood Flow. Editor, Wood JH, p 22. New York, McGraw-Hill, 1987.) *B,* cerebral arteriogram showing the same four segments (*arrows*) of the internal carotid artery as seen in *A. Cx,* cervical segment; *P,* petrous segment; *Cv,* cavernous segment; *S,* supraclinoid segment.

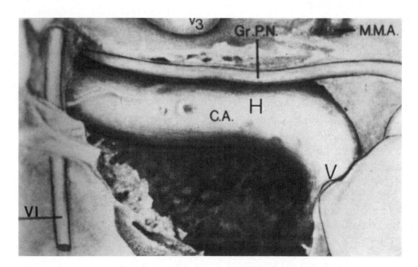

Figure 52.4.   The petrous segment of the internal carotid artery. View through right posterior fossa showing the vertical (*V*) and horizontal (*H*) portions of this segment. *C.A.,* internal carotid artery; *Gr.P.N.,* greater superficial petrosal nerve; *M.M.A.,* middle meningeal artery; *V3,* mandibular division of the trigeminal nerve; *VI,* abducens nerve. (From Paullus WS, Pait TG, Rhoton AL Jr. Microsurgic exposure of the petrous portion of the cartid artery. J Neurosurg *47*:713–726, 1977.)

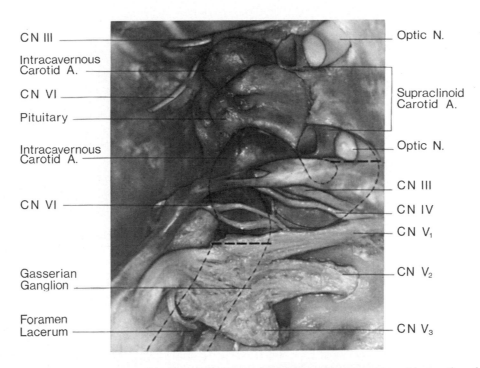

Figure 52.5.   The lacerum and cavernous segments of the internal carotid artery. The pathway of the internal carotid artery through the foramen lacerum and the cavernous sinus are outlined by *dotted lines*. The lacerum segment of the artery extends from the foramen lacerum to the first *horizontal dotted line*. The cavernous segment of the artery begins at the first *horizontal dotted line* and ends at the second *horizontal dotted line*. Note that the artery continues superiorly for several millimeters after entering the cavernous sinus. It then turns anteriorly, inferiorly and, finally, superiorly again at which time it exits the cavernous sinus *(second horizontal dotted line)*. *CN III,* oculomotor nerve; *CN IV,* trochlear nerve; *CN V₁,* ophthalmic division of trigeminal nerve; *CN V₂,* maxillary division of trigeminal nerve; *CN V₃,* mandibular division of trigeminal nerve; *CN VI,* abducens nerve. (From Harris FS, Rhoton AL Jr. Anatomy of the cavernous sinus: A microsurgic study. J Neurosurg *45:*169–180, 1976.)

gual ligament, a continuation of the periosteum of the carotid canal that runs between the lingula of the sphenoid bone anteriorly and the petrous apex posteriorly (Fig. 52.5). The lacerum segment of the internal carotid artery is completely surrounded by periosteum, a thin layer of fat, a venous plexus, and postganglionic sympathetic nerves.

Cavernous Segment (C4)

The **cavernous segment** (C4) of the internal carotid artery begins at the superior margin of the petrolingual ligament at the posterior aspect of the cavernous sinus. Within the sinus, the artery may turn immediately and course anteriorly for several millimeters, or it may continue superiorly for a few millimeters before turning anteriorly (Figs. 52.2, 52.3, 52.5, and 52.6). It then abruptly bends back superiorly and posteriorly, at which point it pierces a portion of the dura mater called the proximal dural ring that is formed by the junction of the medial and inferior periosteum of the anterior clinoid process.

The cavernous segment of the internal carotid artery was separated into four smaller segments by Teufel (1964) (Fig. 52.7). The most proximal part, designated C4 in this classification, is that portion of the vessel that begins at the base of the cavernous sinus and travels superiorly and slightly anteriorly. The next part, C3, is the part of the cavernous segment that bends anteriorly. The third part, C2, is the part of the cavernous segment that travels anteriorly. The most

distal part of the cavernous portion of the internal carotid artery, C1, is that part that bends upward and exits the cavernous sinus.

Three groups of branches arise from the cavernous segment of the internal carotid artery (Stattin, 1961; Parkinson, 1964; Rhoton et al., 1979a; Day, 1987; Tran-Dinh, 1987; Inoue et al., 1990). The **meningohypophyseal trunk** (posterior trunk of Tran-Dinh, 1987) is the most proximal branch and is almost always present (Figs. 52.8–52.11). It was identified in 100% of specimens examined by Parkinson (1964), by Rhoton et al. (1979a), and by Tran-Dinh (1987). Inoue et al. (1990) identified it in 88% of their specimens. It usually arises below the level of the dorsum sellae near the apex of the curve between the lacerum and cavernous segments of the artery. The meningohypophyseal trunk gives rise to three smaller branches, any of which may occasionally arise directly from the internal carotid artery (Lasjaunias, 1984; Inoue et al., 1990; Krisht et al., 1994a):

1. The **tentorial artery** (the artery of Bernasconi-Cassinari) supplies the intracavernous portions of the oculomotor and trochlear nerves before it terminates in the free edge of the tentorium cerebelli (Ono et al., 1984a; Lang, 1991);
2. The **inferior hypophyseal artery** courses medially to supply the posterior part of the capsule of the pituitary gland and a large portion of the gland itself (Cahill et al., 1996); and

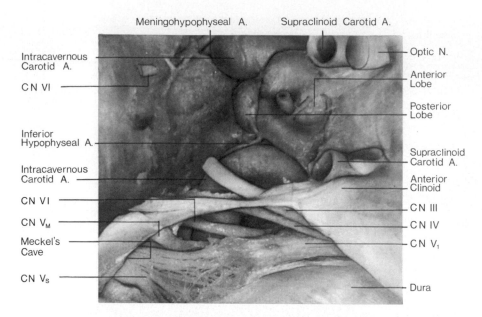

Figure 52.6. Cavernous segment of internal carotid artery. The lateral wall of the cavernous sinus has been removed. The tortuous carotid artery enters the cavernous sinus and continues superiorly before turning anteriorly. *CN III*, oculomotor nerve; *CN IV*, trochlear nerve; *CN VI*, ophthalmic division of trigeminal nerve; *CN V$_M$*, motor root of trigeminal nerve; *CN V$_s$*, sensory root of trigeminal nerve; *CN VI*, abducens nerve. (From Harris FS, Rhoton AL Jr. Anatomy of the cavernous sinus: A microsurgic study. J Neurosurg *45:*169–180, 1976.)

3. The **dorsal meningeal artery** perforates the dura mater of the posterior wall of the cavernous sinus to supply the tip of the petrous bone, the upper clivus, and the abducens nerve (Lang, 1991).

The **artery of the inferior cavernous sinus** (the lateral trunk of Tran-Dinh, 1987) originates from the lateral aspect of the horizontal segment of the cavernous portion of the

internal carotid artery distal to the origin of the meningohypophyseal trunk (Fig. 52.12). It curves over the abducens nerve, then usually divides into three branches that supply the dura and cranial nerves within the cavernous sinus (Lasjaunias et al., 1977; Inoue et al., 1990; Lang, 1991; Krisht et al., 1994a; Cahill et al., 1996). A superior (tentorial) ramus supplies the roof of the cavernous sinus and the oculomotor and trochlear nerves as they enter the sinus. This branch may

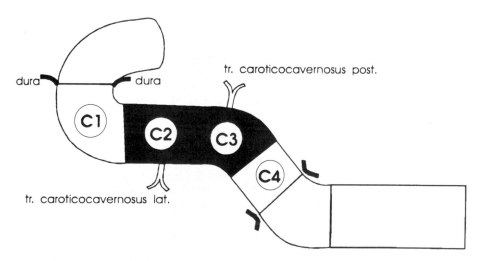

Figure 52.7. The portions of the cavernous segment of the internal carotid artery. The most proximal part of the segment, *C4,* is that portion of the vessel that begins at the base of the cavernous sinus and travels superiorly and slightly anteriorly. *C3* is the next part of the cavernous segment that bends anteriorly. *C2* is the part of the cavernous segment that travels anteriorly. The most distal part of the cavernous segment of the internal carotid artery, *C1,* is that part that bends upward and exits the cavernous sinus. *tr. caroticocavernosus lat.,* small arterial branches that arise from the lateral wall of C2; *tr. caroticocavernosus post.,* small arterial branches that arise from the superior aspect of the posterior curvature of C3. (From Helmke K, Krüger O, Laas R. Acta Neurochir *127:*1–5, 1994.)

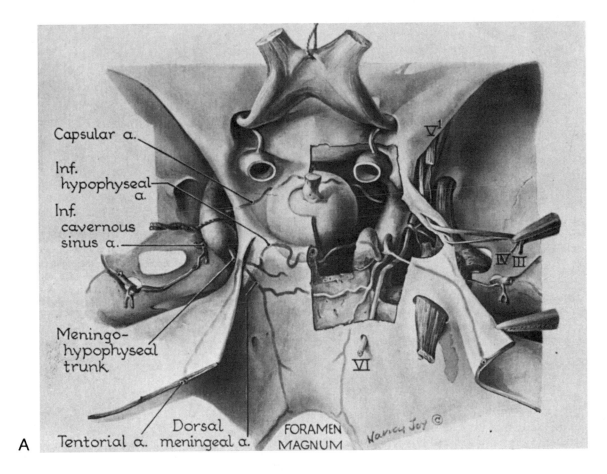

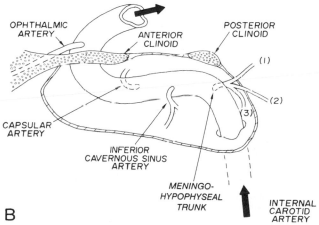

Figure 52.8. Schematic drawings of the intracavernous branches of the internal carotid artery. Note the courses of the capsular, inferior hypophyseal, inferior cavernous sinus, and tentorial arteries. *A,* View from above. (From Parkinson D. Can J Surg *7:*251–268, 1964.) *B,* Lateral view. *1,* tentorial artery; *2,* dorsal meningeal artery; *3,* inferior hypophyseal artery. (From Grove AS Jr. The dural shunt syndrome: Pathophysiology and clinical course. Ophthalmology *91:*31–44, 1984.)

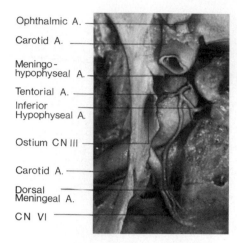

Figure 52.9. The meningohypophyseal trunk and its branches. Superior view of the right cavernous sinus shows a portion of the cavernous segment of the internal carotid artery from which arises the meningohypophyseal trunk and its three branches: (1) the tentorial artery, (2), the dorsal meningeal artery, and (3) the inferior hypophyseal artery (which then divides into two branches). (From Harris FS, Rhoton AL Jr. Anatomy of the cavernous sinus: A microsurgic study. J Neurosurg *45:*169–180, 1976.)

occasionally give rise to the tentorial artery. An anterior ramus usually divides into a medial and a lateral branch. The medial branch supplies the dura of the superior orbital fissure and the oculomotor, trochlear, and abducens nerves as they enter the orbit (Natori and Rhoton, 1995). This branch may anastomose with the ophthalmic artery. The lateral branch courses to the foramen rotundum, supplies the dura in this region of the temporal fossa, and terminates as the artery of the foramen rotundum. It may anastomose with the middle meningeal branch of the internal maxillary artery and thus provide a collateral pathway between the internal

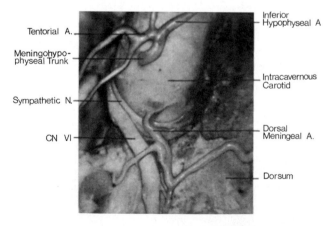

Figure 52.10. The meningohypophyseal trunk and its branches. In this specimen, the meningohypophyseal trunk gives off only two main branches: (1) a tentorial artery and (2) an inferior hypophyseal artery. The dorsal meningeal artery originates as a separate branch directly from the internal carotid artery. *CN VI,* abducens nerve. (From Harris FS, Rhoton AL Jr. Anatomy fo the cavernous sinus: A microsurgic study. J Neurosurg *45:* 169–180, 1976.)

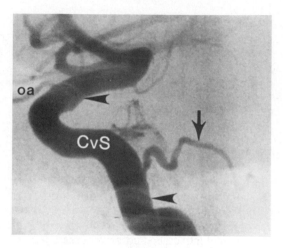

Figure 52.11. Cerebral arteriogram, lateral view, shows the cavernous segment of the internal carotid artery (*CvS*) between *arrowheads.* Note an enlarged meningohypophyseal artery (*arrow*) arising from this segment. *oa,* ophthalmic artery.

and external carotid arteries (Parkinson, 1964; Margolis and Newton, 1969—see below).

The posterior ramus of the artery of the inferior cavernous sinus also divides into a medial and a lateral branch. The medial branch courses to the region of the foramen ovale and supplies the abducens nerve, the gasserian ganglion, and the motor root of the trigeminal nerve (Lang, 1991). It may anastomose with the accessory meningeal artery of the proximal internal maxillary artery. The lateral branch supplies the gasserian ganglion and adjacent dura. It may anastomose with the cavernous branch of the middle meningeal artery as that artery emerges from the foramen spinosum. The artery of the inferior cavernous sinus is present in 65–84% of normal persons (Harris and Rhoton, 1976; Lasjaunias et al., 1987; Rhoton et al., 1979a; Tran-Dinh, 1987). In rare persons, it arises as a branch of the meningohypophyseal trunk (Rhoton et al., 1979a).

The **capsular arteries** (McConnell's arteries, McConnell,

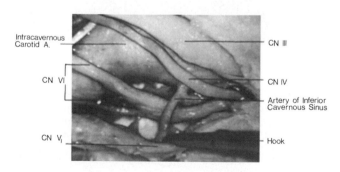

Figure 52.12. Anatomy of the artery of the inferior cavernous sinus. Lateral view of the right internal carotid artery within the cavernous sinus shows the artery of the inferior cavernous sinus originating from the lateral aspect of the horizontal segment of the internal carotid artery. (From Harris FS, Rhoton AL Jr. Anatomy of the cavernous sinus: A microsurgic study. J Neurosurg *45:*169–180, 1976.)

1953; medial group, Tran-Dinh, 1987) arise from the medial side of the cavernous portion of the internal carotid artery between the artery and the pituitary gland, distal to the point of origin of the artery of the inferior cavernous sinus (Fig. 52.8). They are inconstant vessels, being present in only 28% of specimens examined by Harris and Rhoton (1976) and by Tran-Dinh (1987), and in only 8% of specimens examined by Inoue et al. (1990).

The internal carotid artery pierces the dura medial to the anterior clinoid process and exits the cavernous sinus just beneath and lateral to the optic nerve (Fig. 52.8). It continues posteriorly for a short distance before curving superiorly and slightly anteriorly once again, where it is just inferior and lateral to the intracranial portion of the optic nerve and the anterior optic chiasm. The shape formed by the cavernous and the proximal intracranial portions of the internal carotid artery together is a somewhat elongated "S." These two segments are thus often called the **carotid siphon** (Paullus et al., 1977; Rhoton et al., 1979a).

Clinoid Segment (C5)

When the internal carotid artery exits the cavernous sinus to form the anterior portion of the carotid siphon, it does not immediately become intradural. Rather, there is a small transdural segment of the artery between the cavernous segment and the distal intradural segments that is tightly attached to surrounding osseous structures by dense connective tissue (Figs. 52.2 and 52.13). This tissue begins with the proximal dural ring described above and ends with the distal dural ring that is continuous with the adjacent dura of the falciform ligament, the anterior clinoid process, and the roof of the cavernous sinus. This transdural segment of the internal carotid artery is called the **dural transition region** of the artery by Knosp et al. (1988) and the **clinoid segment** (C5) by Bouthillier et al. (1996). The segment is located adjacent or just inferior to the anterior clinoid process, in a region that has also been called the paraclinoid area.

Ophthalmic Segment (C6)

The **ophthalmic segment** (C6) of the internal carotid artery begins at the distal dural ring and ends just proximal to the origin of the posterior communicating artery. This segment gives rise to the ophthalmic artery (see below) and to one or more superior hypophyseal arteries that supply the infundibulum of the pituitary gland, the intracranial portion of the ipsilateral optic nerve, and the anteroventral portion of the optic chiasm (Marinković et al., 1990; Krisht et al., 1994b) (Figs. 52.14–52.19). The superior hypophyseal arteries may also supply the premammillary portion of the floor of the 3rd ventricle and even the proximal portion of the ipsilateral optic tract (Lang, 1991). A few small vessels that arise from the ophthalmic segment of the internal carotid artery terminate in the dura mater covering the anterior clinoid process, sella turcica, and tuberculum sellae.

Ophthalmic Artery and Its Branches

The ophthalmic artery is the most proximal major intradural branch of the internal carotid artery. It usually arises from the anterior wall of the ophthalmic segment of the artery as that vessel emerges from the distal dural ring just beneath the ipsilateral optic nerve (Hayreh and Dass, 1962a; Lombardi and Passerini, 1969) (Figs. 52.16 and 52.19). The origin of the ophthalmic artery is intradural in about 90% of persons, but about 10% of the time, the ophthalmic artery originates extradurally, from either the cavernous or the clinoid segment of the internal carotid artery (Punt, 1979). Rarely, the ophthalmic artery originates either as two trunks, one from the internal carotid artery and the other from the middle meningeal artery (the latter trunk being more prominent), or as a single trunk from the middle meningeal artery (Hayreh and Dass, 1962a).

When the ophthalmic artery arises from the internal carotid artery, as it does in most people, it courses anterolaterally below the optic nerve and enters the optic canal. The

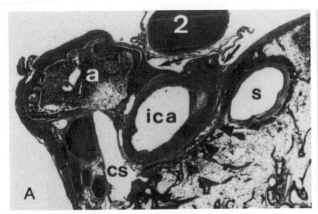 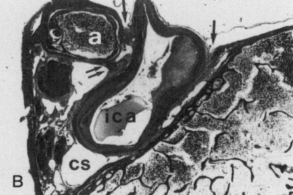

Figure 52.13.   The clinoid segment of the internal carotid artery. Histologic section through the left paraclinoid region. *A,* Anterior section shows dural strands (*arrows*) that fix the clinoid portion of the internal carotid artery (*ica*) to the anterior clinoid process (*a*) and to the sphenoid bone. *2,* optic nerve; *cs,* cavernous sinus; *s,* sphenoid sinus. *Arrowheads* indicate the boundaries of the carotid sulcus. *B,* Posterior section shows strong strands of connective tissue (*single and double arrows*) that fix the clinoid segment of the internal carotid artery (*ica*) to the anterior clinoid process (*a*) and to the sphenoid bone. *cs,* cavernous sinus. (From Knosp E, Müller G, Perneczky A. The paraclinoid carotid artery: Anatomical aspects of a microsurgic approach. Neurosurgery 22:896–901, 1988.)

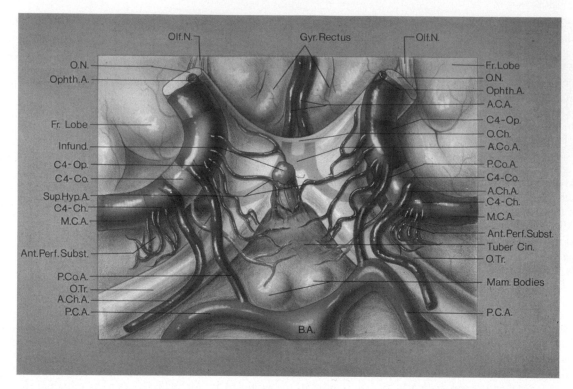

Figure 52.14. Inferior view of the perforating branches of the supraclinoid portion of the internal carotid artery. In this illustration, this portion of the artery is divided into three smaller segments that are named for the main arterial branch that arises from them. The ophthalmic segment (*C4-Op.*) is named for the ophthalmic artery (*Ophth.A.*), the communicating segment (*C4-Co.*) is named for the posterior communicating artery (*P.Co.A.*), and the choroidal segment (*C4-Ch.*), named for the anterior choroidal artery (*A.Ch.A.*). Note that the main perforating branches that supply the optic nerves (*O.N.*) and the optic chiasm (*O.Ch.*) arise from the ophthalmic segment, whereas the branches that supply the optic tracts (*O.Tr.*) arise from the communicating and choroidal segments. *A.C.A.*, anterior cerebral artery; *A.Co.A.*, anterior communicating artery; *M.C.A.*, middle cerebral artery; *P.C.A.*, posterior cerebral artery; *Sup.Hyp.A.*, superior hypophyseal artery; *Ant.Perf. Subst.*, anterior perforated substance; *Fr.Lobe*, frontal lobe; *Gyr. Rectus*, gyrus rectus; *Olf. N.*, olfactory nerve; *Mam.Bodies*, mammillary bodies; *Infund.*, infundibulum; *Tuber. Cin.*, tuber cinereum. (From Gibo H, Lenkey C, Rhoton AL Jr. Microsurgic anatomy of the supraclinoid portion of the internal carotid artery. J Neurosurg *55:*560–574, 1981.)

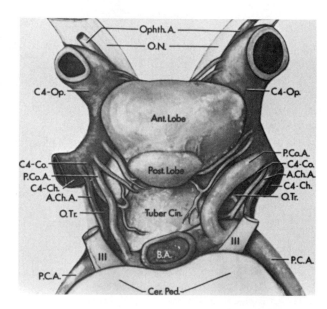

Figure 52.15. Inferior view of the perforating branches of the supraclinoid portion of the internal carotid artery. Note multiple branches to the posterior lobe of the pituitary gland and to the tuber cinereum. These branches arise from the ophthalmic (*C4-Op.*), communicating (*C4-Co.*), and choroidal (*C4-Ch.*) segments of the artery. *A.Ch.A.*, anterior choroidal artery; *P.Co.A.*, posterior communicating artery; *O.N.*, optic nerve; *O.Tr.*, optic tract; *P.C.A.*, posterior cerebral artery; *B.A.*, basilar artery; *III*, oculomotor nerve; *Cer. Ped.*, cerebral peduncle. (From Gibo H, Lenkey C, Rhoton AL Jr. Microsurgic anatomy of the supraclinoid portion of the internal carotid artery. J Neurosurg *55:*560–574, 1981.)

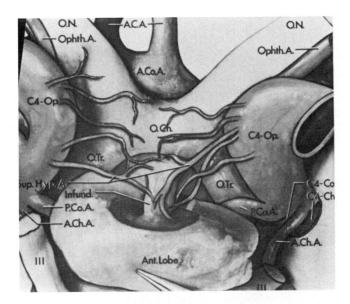

Figure 52.16. Inferior view of the perforating branches of the supraclinoid portion of the internal carotid artery. The anterior lobe of the pituitary is reflected backward to show the numerous branches that originate from the ophthalmic segment of the internal carotid artery (*C4-Op.*) and supply the optic chiasm (*O.Ch.*), distal portions of the optic nerves (*O.N.*), and the infundibulum (*Infund.*). Among this group of vessels are the paired superior hypophyseal arteries *(Sup.Hyp.A.). A.Ch.A.,* anterior choroidal artery; *P.Co.A.,* posterior communicating artery; *Ophth.A.,* ophthalmic artery; *A.C.A.,* anterior cerebral artery; *A.Co.A.,* anterior communicating artery; *C4-Co.,* communicating segment of the internal carotid artery; *C4-Ch.,* choroidal segment of the internal carotid artery; *O.Tr.,* optic tract; *III,* oculomotor nerve. (From Gibo H, Lenkey C, Rhoton AL Jr. Microsurgic anatomy of the supraclinoid portion of the internal carotid artery. J Neurosurg *55:*560–574, 1981.)

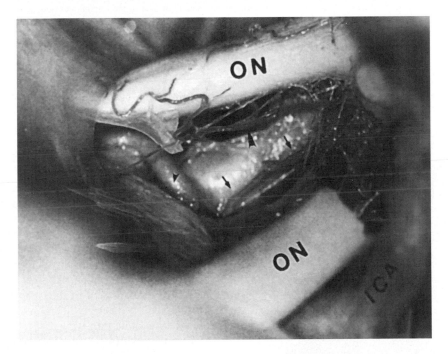

Figure 52.17. Anatomy of the superior hypophyseal artery. Dorsal view from a left subfrontal approach shows a superior hypophyseal artery (*arrows*) originating from the medial aspect of the right internal carotid artery just distal to the origin of the ophthalmic artery (*small arrowhead*). The artery courses posterosuperiorly, branches in a candelabra-like fashion, and gives off a recurrent anterior branch (*large arrowhead*) that provides the main blood supply to the right optic nerve (*ON*). *ICA,* internal carotid artery. (From Krisht AF, Barrow DL, Barnett DW, et al. The microsurgic anatomy of the superior hypophyseal artery. Neurosurgery *35:*899–903, 1994.)

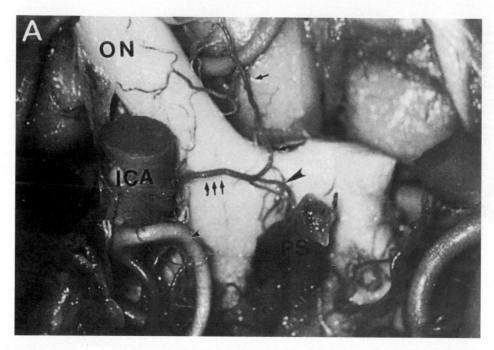

Figure 52.18.   Anatomy of the superior hypophyseal artery. Inferior view of the suprasellar region shows a right superior hypophyseal artery (*three small arrows*) arising from the right internal carotid artery (*ICA*). The superior hypophyseal artery courses medially across the ventral surface of the optic chiasm for a short distance before bifurcating into an anterior branch that supplies the ventral surface of the intracranial portion of the right optic nerve (*single small arrow*) and a posterior branch that supplies the ventral surface of the chiasm (*large arrowhead*). The *small arrowhead* points to the posterior communicating artery. (From Krisht AF, Barrow DL, Barnett DW, et al. The microsurgic anatomy of the superior hypophyseal artery. Neurosurgery *35:* 899–903, 1994.)

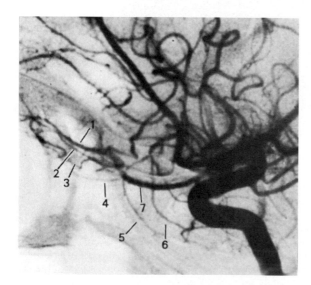

Figure 52.19.   Cerebral arteriogram, lateral view, showing the origin and course of the ophthalmic artery (*7* and *1*) and several of its branches, including the supraorbital artery (*2*), lacrimal artery (*3*), and central retinal artery (*4*). *5* and *6,* branches of the middle cerebral artery. (From Taveras JM, Wood EH. Diagnostic Neuroradiology, Vol 2. Baltimore, Williams & Wilkins, 1976.)

length of the intracranial segment of the ophthalmic artery is usually about 3 mm, but it may be as much as 7 mm. It infrequently gives off intracranial perforating branches that run posteriorly to supply the ventral aspect of the ipsilateral optic nerve, the optic chiasm, and the pituitary stalk (Dawson, 1958; Gibo et al., 1981a; Lang, 1991).

As the ophthalmic artery enters the optic canal, it pierces the dural sheath of the optic nerve, usually inferolateral but sometimes directly below the nerve (Fig. 52.20). Once it pierces the dura, the ophthalmic artery is surrounded, or at least covered, by dura, and it is thus separated from the substance of the nerve throughout its course within the optic canal until it emerges at the apex of the orbit. Its course generally parallels that of the optic nerve, although it may deviate slightly laterally. This intracanalicular segment of the artery is quite thin-walled.

The **intraorbital portion** of the ophthalmic artery may be divided into three segments (Hayreh and Dass, 1962b) (Fig. 52.21). The first part extends from where the ophthalmic artery enters the orbit to where the artery crosses under or over the optic nerve. The second part of the artery is the segment that crosses the nerve. In almost all cases, the ophthalmic artery crosses the nerve from lateral to medial, with the artery crossing beneath the nerve in about 80% of persons and above the nerve in the remaining 20%. The third part of the intraorbital portion of the ophthalmic artery, lying medial to the nerve, extends from the point at which the

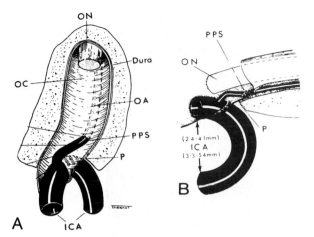

Figure 52.20. The origin of the ophthalmic artery and its entrance into the optic canal. *A,* View from above of the right internal carotid artery (*ICA*) and ophthalmic artery (*OA*). The ophthalmic artery originates from the undersurface of the internal carotid artery. It then runs anteriorly beneath the optic nerve (*ON*). Just inside the optic canal (*OC*), the artery pierces the dura lining the canal (*PPS*), thus acquiring its own dural sheath that separates it from the intracanalicular portion of the optic nerve. *P,* optic foramen. *B,* Lateral view of origin of the ophthalmic artery and its entrance into the optic canal. Note that the ophthalmic artery penetrates the dura inferiorly (*PPS*) just after it enters the canal (P). Also note that the internal carotid artery (*ICA*) narrows slightly as it exits the cavernous sinus to become intradural. (From Hayreh SS. Arteries of the orbit in the human being. Br J Surg *50:*938–953, 1963.)

artery has crossed under or over the optic nerve to its termination.

The course of the ophthalmic artery within the orbit is quite variable, as are its branches (Hayreh, 1962; Ducasse et al., 1986a; Zhao and Li, 1987). Major variations depend on whether the artery has crossed over or under the optic nerve (Hayreh, 1962) (Fig. 52.22). When the ophthalmic artery crosses over the nerve, its first major branch is usually the central retinal artery, followed by the lateral posterior ciliary artery, lacrimal artery, various muscular arteries, medial posterior ciliary arteries, posterior ethmoid artery, supraorbital artery, anterior ethmoid artery, and medial palpebral artery. When the ophthalmic artery crosses beneath the optic nerve, it usually sends small perforating branches to the optic nerve, followed by the lateral posterior ciliary artery, central retinal artery, medial muscular arteries, medial posterior ciliary artery, lacrimal artery, posterior ethmoid artery, supraorbital artery, anterior ethmoid artery, and medial palpebral arteries. Minor branches from the intraorbital portion of the ophthalmic artery supply the loose areolar tissue within the

orbit, the lacrimal sac, and the periosteum of the orbital walls (periorbita). The ophthalmic artery also gives rise to a number of small meningeal branches (Kuru, 1967). One of these branches, the anterior falx artery, arises from the anterior ethmoid artery and supplies the anterior portion of the falx cerebri (Kuru, 1967; Pollock and Newton, 1968). Whether it has crossed over or under the optic nerve, the ophthalmic artery terminates by bifurcating into a supratrochlear (or frontal) artery and a dorsal nasal (or nasal) artery.

The number of posterior ciliary arteries varies. There are usually two or three major trunks that immediately subdivide into many small, tortuous branches that pierce the sclera medially, laterally, and superiorly adjacent to the optic nerve where they form an anastomotic ring, the circle of Zinn and Haller (Hayreh, 1962; Risco et al., 1981; Zhao and Li, 1987; Olver et al., 1990) (Figs. 52.23–52.25). These branches are called **short posterior ciliary arteries**, and they often give rise to one or more **cilioretinal arteries** that supply the retina in the region of the optic disc (Randall, 1887; Jackson, 1911) (Figs. 52.26–52.28). Cilioretinal arteries are present in about

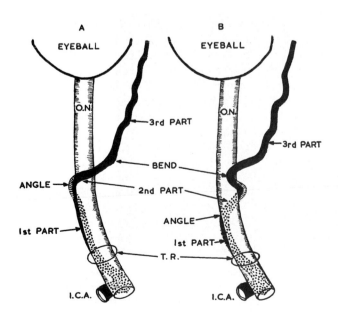

Figure 52.21. Schematic drawing of the three segments of the intraorbital ophthalmic artery. The first part extends from the point of entrance of the artery into the orbit (*T.R.*) to the point at which the artery crosses over (*left side of illustration*) or under (*right side of illustration*) the optic nerve (O.N.). The second part is the segment that crosses the nerve. The third part of the ophthalmic artery extends from the point at which the artery has crossed over or under the nerve to its termination. *I.C.A.,* internal carotid artery. (From Hayreh SS, Dass R. The ophthalmic artery. II. Intra-orbital course. Br J Ophthalmol *46:* 165–185, 1962.)

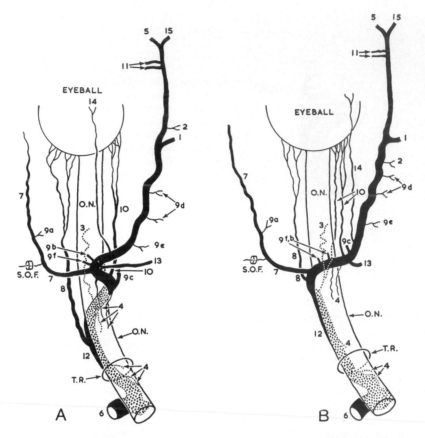

Figure 52.22. Branches of the ophthalmic artery. *A*, Pattern of branches when the artery crosses beneath the nerve. *B*, Pattern of branches when the artery crosses over the nerve. *1*, anterior ethmoid artery; *2*, areolar branch; *3*, central retinal artery; *4*, collateral branch; *5*, dorsal nasal branch; *6*, internal carotid artery; *7*, lacrimal artery; *8*, lateral posterior ciliary artery; *9*, muscular artery (*a*, branch to lateral rectus; *b*, branch to levator palpebrae superioris; *c*, branch to medial rectus; *d*, branch to superior oblique; *e*, branch to superior rectus); *10*, medial posterior ciliary artery; *11*, medial palpebral artery; *12*, ophthalmic artery; *13*, posterior ethmoid artery; *14*, supraorbital artery; *15*, supratrochlear artery; *O.N.*, optic nerve; *S.O.F.*, superior orbital fissure; *T.R.*, tendinous ring. (From Hayreh SS. The ophthalmic artery. III. Branches. Br J Ophthalmol *46*:212–247, 1962.)

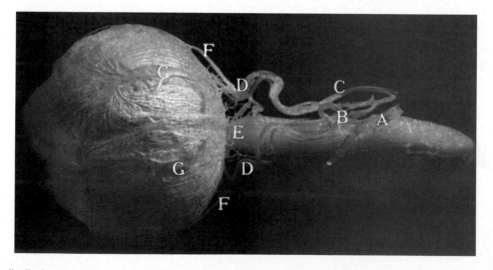

Figure 52.23. The distribution of the long and short ciliary arteries. *A*, ophthalmic artery; *B*, nasal posterior ciliary artery; *C*, temporal posterior ciliary artery; *D*, nasal and temporal short posterior ciliary arteries; *E*, circle of Zinn; *F*, nasal and temporal long porterior temporal arteries; *G*, vortex veins. (From Zhao Y, Li F. Microangioarchitecture of the ciliary artery circulation of the posterior pole. Jpn J Ophthalmol *31*:147–159, 1987.)

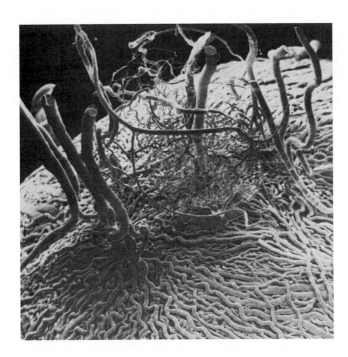

Figure 52.24. Low power scanning electron micrograph showing the vasculature of the globe viewed from behind the globe. The long and short posterior ciliary arteries are seen, as are their branches to the choroid and optic disc. (From Risco JM, Grimson BS, Johnson PT. Angioarchitecture of the ciliary artery circulation of the posterior pole. Arch Ophthalmol *99:*864–868, 1981.)

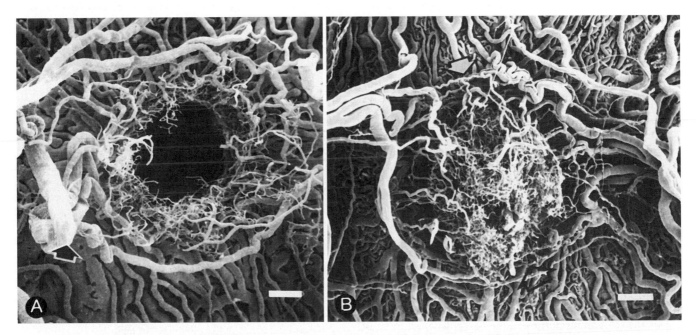

Figure 52.25. Low power scanning electron micrographs showing the circle of Zinn and Haller. *A,* Micrograph shows anastomoses between medial and lateral short posterior ciliary arteries forming a complete circle of Zinn and Haller. Note double supply (*solid arrow*) that forms an incomplete anastomosis from which pial vessels also arise. Bar = 400 microns. *B,* Micrograph shows anastomoses between medial and lateral short posterior ciliary arteries forming a complete circle of Zinn and Haller. Note that some of the circle is composed of very small arteries (*arrows*). Bar = 500 microns. (From Olver JM, Spalton DJ, McCartney ACE. Microvascular study of the retroliminar optic nerve in man: The possible significance in anterior ischaemic neuropathy. Eye *4:*7–24, 1990.)

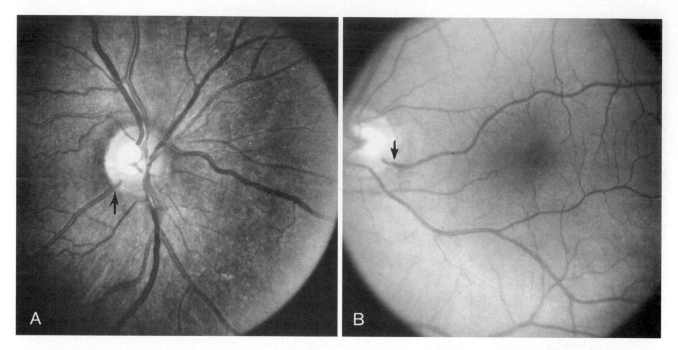

Figure 52.26. *A* and *B,* Ophthalmoscopic appearance of cilioretinal artery (*arrow*). Note that it arises separately from the rest of the retinal arteries.

50% of normal patients (Justice and Lehmann, 1976). Between two and four posterior ciliary arteries pierce the sclera medially and laterally somewhat farther from the optic nerve and pass around the globe within the sclera. These vessels are called **long posterior ciliary arteries** (Ducasse et al., 1986b) (Figs. 52.22 and 52.23). They supply internal structures of the anterior portion of the eye.

The **central retinal artery** has a tortuous course along the inferior surface of the optic nerve before it pierces the optic nerve sheaths 10–15 mm posterior to the globe (Fig. 52.29). For 1–3 mm, the artery runs within the subarachnoid space of the optic nerve. It then gives off numerous branches that anastomose with surface branches of the pial vascular network surrounding the nerve (Zhao and Li, 1987). These branches and the branches passing anteriorly from the short posterior ciliary arteries constitute a dense vascular network. Within the optic nerve, the central retinal artery gives off numerous branches that supply the axial portion of the nerve (Figs. 52.29 and 52.30). As these branches pass peripherally, becoming smaller in caliber until they become capillaries, they often anastomose with penetrating branches of the pial vascular network. The central retinal artery passes though the retrolaminar and laminar portions of the optic nerve to reach the prelaminar portion of the nerve, where it gives off its terminal branches that supply the inner layers of the retina (Hayreh, 1963a) (Fig. 52.31).

A number of branches of the ophthalmic artery anastomose with small arteries that originate from larger branches of the external carotid artery, thus forming an important collateral circulation to the eye and orbit. The main arteries that anastomose in this manner are the anterior and posterior ethmoid arteries and the lacrimal artery. This anastomotic network is probably responsible for maintenance of blood supply to the eye when the optic nerve is removed to treat a meningioma or glioma (see Chapters 39 and 40). The ophthalmic artery may also be an important collateral pathway in patients with occlusive disease of the ipsilateral internal carotid artery and may contribute to cerebral perfusion in such cases (Kerty et al., 1996).

Communicating Segment (C7)

The most distal segment of the internal carotid artery is the **communicating segment** (C7). This segment begins just proximal to the origin of the posterior communicating artery and ends at the bifurcation of the internal carotid artery. Two major branches arise from this segment: the posterior communicating artery and the anterior choroidal artery. These arteries and their branches are discussed below. In addition, the communicating segment of the internal carotid artery gives rise to numerous small perforating vessels. Those that arise from the more proximal portion of the segment terminate in the ipsilateral optic tract, the premammillary portion of the floor of the 3rd ventricle, the optic chiasm, the pituitary stalk, and the anterior and posterior perforated substance (Fig. 52.16) (Rosner et al., 1984). Such vessels apparently are not present in all persons. Since they were seen in only 60% of the specimens examined by Gibo et al. (1981a). Perforating arteries that arise from the more distal portion of the communicating segment (called the choroidal segment by some authors) terminate in the anterior perforated substance, the ipsilateral optic tract, and the uncus (Rosner et al., 1984; Marinković et al., 1990) (Fig. 52.16).

Posterior Communicating Artery and Its Branches

The **posterior communicating artery** arises from the posterior wall of the communicating segment of the internal

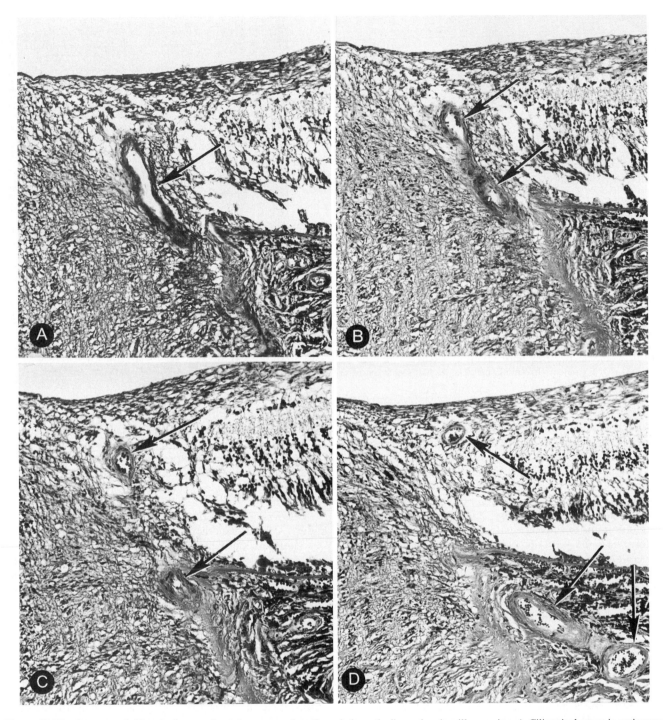

Figure 52.27. Anatomy of cilioretinal artery shown in cross-sections through the optic disc and peripapillary region. *A,* Cilioretinal artery in optic nerve head (*arrow*). *B* and *C,* The cilioretinal artery (*arrows*) extends toward retina and sclera at two different levels. *D,* The cilioretinal artery extends into peripapillary retina and peripapillary sclera. (From Vaghefi HA, Green WR, Kelley JS, et al. Correlation of clinicopathologic findings in a patient with congenital night blindness, branch retinal vein occlusion, cilioretinal artery, drusen of the optic nerve head, and intraretinal pigmented lesion. Arch Ophthalmol *96:*2097–2104, 1978.)

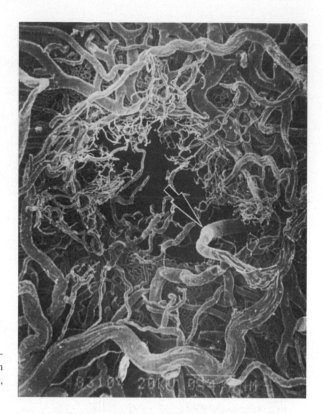

Figure 52.28. Scanning electron micrograph of vascular cast showing the cilioretinal artery (*arrow*). The artery enters the eye at the edge of the optic disc. (From Zhao Y, Li F. Microangioarchitecture of optic papilla. Jpn J Ophthalmol *31:*147–159, 1987.)

carotid artery, 6–15 mm distal to the origin of the ophthalmic artery (Gibo et al., 1981a) (Figs. 52.2, 52.14–52.16, 52.32, and 52.33). This vessel then passes posteromedially below the tuber cinereum and above the sella turcica and oculomotor nerve to join the posterior cerebral artery. During embryogenesis, the posterior communicating artery continues as the posterior cerebral artery, but by birth, the posterior cerebral artery usually arises from the basilar system (see below), and the posterior communicating artery is one of the components of the circle of Willis (Fig. 52.32). In about 20% of persons, however, the posterior communicating artery remains the origin of the posterior cerebral artery (''fetal configuration'') (Pedroza et al., 1987) (Fig. 52.34). When the posterior communicating artery is small or of normal size, it courses posteromedially to join the posterior cerebral artery medial to the oculomotor nerve. In the fetal configuration, however, it passes posterolaterally above or lateral to the oculomotor nerve. The posterior communicating artery ranges in length from 5–22 mm, with the majority of posterior communicating arteries being 12–16 mm long (Lang, 1985; Vincentelli et al., 1990).

Between 4 and 14 perforating arteries originate from the posterior communicating artery (Gibo et al., 1981a; Pedroza et al., 1987; Vincentelli et al., 1990). These branches course superiorly and terminate in the premammillary part of the floor of the 3rd ventricle, the posterior perforated substance and interpeduncular fossa, the ipsilateral optic tract, the pituitary stalk, and the optic chiasm (see Table 2 in Pedroza et al., 1987). They also supply parts of the thalamus, hypothalamus, subthalamus, and internal capsule (Saeki and Rhoton, 1977; Rhoton et al., 1979b; Vincentelli et al., 1990).

The largest and most constant branch that arises from the posterior communicating artery is the **premammillary** or **anterior thalamoperforating artery** (Rhoton et al., 1979b; Pedroza et al., 1987) (Fig. 52.32*A*). This artery enters the floor of the 3rd ventricle anterior to or beside the mammillary bodies.

Dilations of the origin of the posterior communicating artery, called ''junctional dilations'' (Epstein et al., 1970) or ''infundibular widenings'' (Hassler and Saltzman, 1963), occur in some persons. Although some authors regard these dilations as an early stage of aneurysm formation (Hassler and Saltzman, 1963), others (Epstein et al., 1970) consider them to be simple anomalies that are neither aneurysmal nor preaneurysmal.

Anterior Choroidal Artery and Its Branches

The **anterior choroidal artery** is the most distal major artery that arises from the internal carotid artery prior to its bifurcation. It arises from the posterior wall of the distal portion of the communicating segment of the internal carotid artery, 7.5–24 mm distal to the origin of the ophthalmic artery and 2.5–10 mm proximal to the terminal bifurcation of the internal carotid artery (Otomo, 1965; Saeki and Rhoton, 1977; Gibo et al., 1981a; Lang, 1985; Gomes et al., 1986) (Figs. 52.2, 52.14–52.16, 52.35). In about 25% of persons, however, it originates from the middle cerebral, posterior cerebral, or posterior communicating artery (Carpenter et al., 1954; Herman et al., 1966; Rhoton et al., 1979c). It courses posteriorly below the optic tract but above the posterior communicating artery, eventually terminating after passing

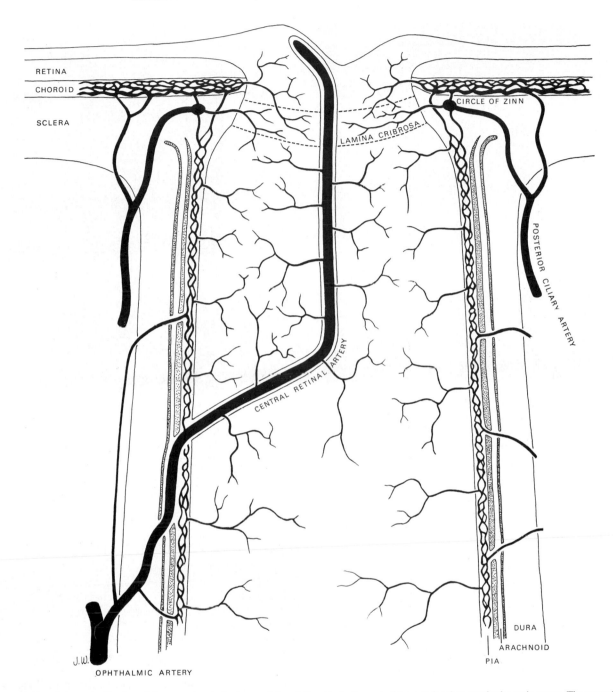

Figure 52.29. Schematic drawing of the central retinal artery and its relationship to the rest of the arteries that supply the optic nerve. The central retinal artery pierces the dura of the nerve about 10–15 mm posterior to the globe. It sends branches to the pial vascular network and then travels within the nerve to the globe. Within the nerve, the artery gives off numerous branches that supply the axial portion of the nerve and anastomose with penetrating branches of the pial vessel network. The artery gives off terminal branches that supply the inner layers of the retina. (From Hogan MJ, Alvarado JA, Weddell JE. Histology of the Human Eye. An Atlas and Textbook, p 534. Philadelphia, WB Saunders, 1971.)

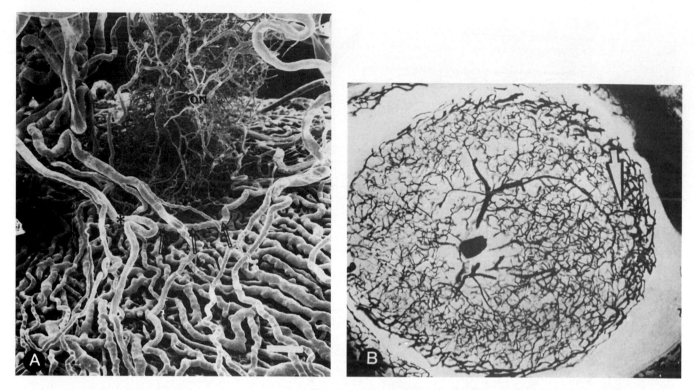

Figure 52.30. Vascular network of the retrolaminar portion of the optic nerve. *A,* Low-power electron micrograph shows longitudinal appearance of the vasculature of a portion of the intraorbital optic nerve (*ON*). Note extensive vascular network within the nerve. Also note circle of Zinn and Haller surrounding nerve *(arrows). asterisk,* short posterior ciliary artery. (From Olver JM, Spalton DJ, McCartney ACE. Microvascular study of the retiolaminar optic nerve in man: The possible significance in anterior ischaemic optic neuropathy. Eye *4:*7–24, 1990.) *B,* Transverse view of injected optic nerve shows that central retinal artery gives off radial branches that anastomose with branches of the pial vascular network. (Vascular ink injection and tissue section method, × 41.) (From Zhao Y, Li F. Microangioarchitecture of optic papilla. Jpn J Ophthalmol *31:*147–159, 1987.)

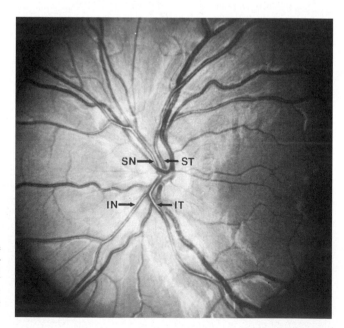

Figure 52.31. Ophthalmoscopic appearance of the terminal branches of the central retinal artery. The artery usually gives off four main branches: superior temporal (*ST*), superior nasal (*SN*), inferior temporal (*IT*), and inferior nasal (*IN*). A single trunk may give rise to the superior vessels, inferior vessels, or both sets of vessels. In this eye, the superior retinal arteries arise as separate vessels, whereas the inferior retinal arteries arise from a single trunk.

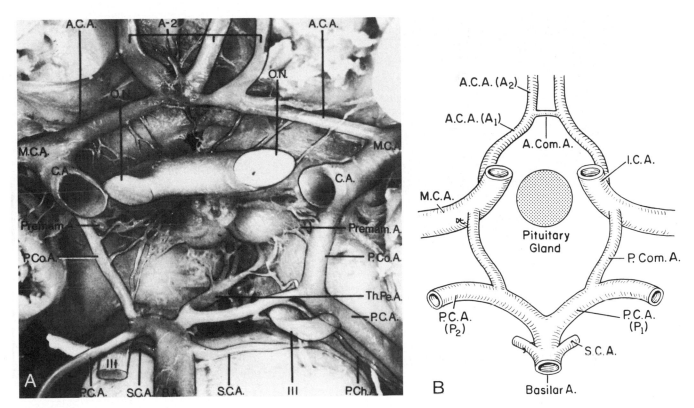

Figure 52.32. The posterior communicating artery and the circle of Willis. *A,* Each posterior communicating artery (*P.Co.A.*) arises from the posterior wall of the supraclinoid portion of the ipsilateral internal carotid artery, passes posteromedially, and joins the ipsilateral posterior cerebral artery (*P.C.A.*). A prominent premammillary artery (*Premam.A.*) originates from each posterior communicating artery. This vessel supplies the mammillary bodies and the floor of the 3rd ventricle. Also shown in this photograph are the other arteries that make up the circle of Willis. *A.C.A.,* anterior cerebral artery; *A-2,* second portion of the anterior cerebral artery; *B.A.,* basilar artery; *C.A.,* internal carotid artery; *M.C.A.,* middle cerebral artery; *O.N.,* optic nerve; *P.Ch.A.,* posterior choroidal artery; *S.C.A.,* superior cerebellar artery; *Th.Pe.A.,* posterior thalamoperforating artery; *III* oculomotor nerve. (From Rhoton AL Jr, Hardy DG, Chambers SM. Microsurgic anatomy and dissection of the sphenoid bone, cavernous sinus and sellar region. Surg Neurol *12*:63-104, 1979.) *B,* Schematic drawing of the the relationships of the arteries that comprise the circle of Willis. The supraclinoid portion of the internal carotid artery (*I.C.A.*) is shown with three of its major branches: the posterior communicating artery *P.Com.A.,* the middle cerebral artery (*M.C.A.*), and the anterior cerebral artery (*A.C.A.*). Two segments of the anterior cerebral artery are shown: the A-1 segment (*A.C.A.(A₁)*), the portion between the internal carotid artery and the anterior communicating artery (*A.Com.A.*), and the A-2 segment (*A.C.A.(A₂)*), a 5-mm segment distal to the anterior communicating artery that extends to the genu of the corpus callosum. The distal end of the basilar artery is shown with its two most distal branches: the superior cerebellar artery (*S.C.A.*) and the posterior cerebral artery (*P.C.A.*). Two segments of the posterior cerebral artery are shown. The P-1 segment (*P.C.A.(P₁)*) of the posterior cerebral artery begins at its origin from the basilar artery and ends where the artery joins with the posterior communicating artery. The P-2 segment (*P.C.A.(P₂)*) is the portion of the vessel distal to the posterior communicating artery. (From Day AL. In Cerebral Blood Flow. Editor, Wood JH, pp 19–36. New York, McGraw-Hill, 1987.)

through the choroidal fissure to reach the choroid plexus in the temporal horn and trigone (atrium) of the lateral ventricle (Fujii et al., 1980a; Gibo et al., 1981a). The anterior choroidal artery provides the main blood supply to the ipsilateral optic tract. It also sends branches to the hilum and anterolateral aspect of the ipsilateral lateral geniculate body, and to the cerebral peduncle, uncus, and temporal lobe. These branches usually are fairly small and terminate in the optic radiation, globus pallidus, mesencephalon, thalamus, and the retrolenticular and posterior portion of the posterior limb of the internal capsule. Occasionally, however, one or more of the branches is quite large and may supply a larger region than normally expected (Marinković et al., 1994). The

course and location of the branches of the anterior choroidal artery were described beautifully by Rhoton et al. (1979c) and by Fujii et al. (1980a).

Terminal Branches of the Internal Carotid Artery: Anterior and Middle Cerebral Arteries

After giving off the anterior choroidal artery, the internal carotid artery terminates as a bifurcation in the area below the anterior perforated substance at the medial end of the sylvian fissure. This bifurcation produces two major arteries: the anterior cerebral and middle cerebral arteries. These arteries and their branches supply major areas of the brain,

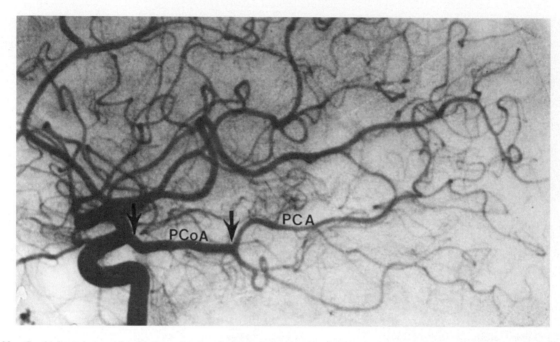

Figure 52.33. Cerebral arteriogram, lateral view, showing the posterior communicating artery (*PCoA*) from its origin from the internal carotid artery (*left arrow*) to its junction (*right arrow*) with the posterior cerebral artery (*PCA*).

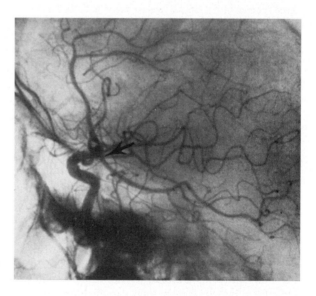

Figure 52.34. Origin of the posterior cerebral artery from the internal carotid artery (*arrow*).

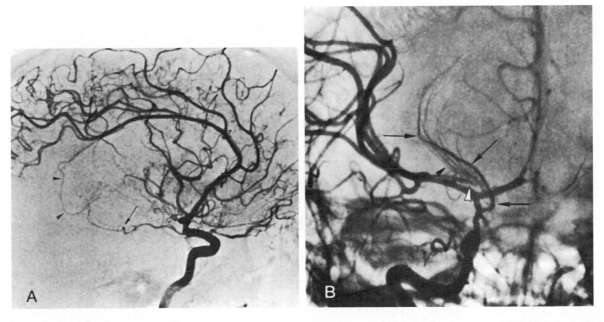

Figure 52.35. Cerebral arteriogram showing course of anterior choroidal artery. *A*, Lateral view shows anterior choroidal artery (*arrow*) arising from internal carotid artery and extending posteriorly. The artery is not obscured because the middle cerebral artery is occluded. Note course of distal segment of pericallosal artery around the splenium of the corpus callosum (*arrowheads*). *B*, Anteroposterior view. Note the proximity of the anterior choroidal artery (*arrows*) to lenticulostriate arteries *(black arrowhead)* that arise from a single trunk *(white arrowhead)*.

including portions of the ocular motor and visual sensory pathways (Figs. 52.3A and 52.36).

Anterior Cerebral Artery, Anterior Communicating Artery, and Their Branches

ANTERIOR CEREBRAL ARTERY AND ITS BRANCHES

The **anterior cerebral artery** originates as the medial and smaller of the two terminal branches of the internal carotid artery (Lin and Kricheff, 1974; Perlmutter and Rhoton, 1976) (Figs. 52.2, 52.14, 52.16, 52.32, 52.37, and 52.38). It courses anteromedially to the hemispheric fissure, passing over the optic chiasm or the distal portion of the optic nerves and below the medial olfactory stria with a slightly posterior, convex curve (Figs. 52.32, 52.37, and 52.38). In the interhemispheric fissure, it is joined to the opposite anterior cerebral artery by the **anterior communicating artery** (Figs. 52.14, 52.16, 52.32, 52.39–52.43). The segment of the anterior cerebral artery between the internal carotid and anterior communicating arteries is called the **A-1** or precommunicating segment. The segment of the anterior cerebral artery distal to the anterior communicating artery is usually separated into four smaller segments (A-2 to A-5) (Fischer, 1938; Perlmutter and Rhoton, 1978).

The length of the A-1 segment of the anterior cerebral artery ranges from 7–22 mm, but it is usually 12–15 mm long (Perlmutter and Rhoton, 1976; Lang, 1985; Gomes et al., 1986). This segment, particularly its proximal portion, gives rise to a large number of branches that terminate in the anterior perforated substance, the distal portion of the optic nerve, the optic chiasm, and the proximal portion of

the optic tract (Wollschlaeger et al., 1971; Perlmutter and Rhoton, 1976; Rosner et al., 1984; Gomes et al., 1986) (Figs. 52.32A and 52.40–52.43). In addition, the recurrent artery of Heubner (see below) may occasionally arise from the distal portion of this segment (Gomes et al., 1984, 1986).

The portion of the anterior cerebral artery distal to its junction with the anterior communicating artery ascends in front of the lamina terminalis, passes between the cerebral hemispheres in the longitudinal fissure, makes a smooth curve around the genu of the corpus callosum, and passes posteriorly above the corpus callosum in the pericallosal cistern (Perlmutter and Rhoton, 1978) (Figs. 52.37, 52.38, and 52.44). As noted above, this portion of the anterior cerebral artery may be divided into four segments. The **A-2** segment is about 5 mm long and extends from the anterior communicating artery junction to the genu of the corpus callosum. The remaining three segments are often referred to together as the **pericallosal artery** (Figs. 52.37, 52.38, and 52.44). The **A-3** segment corresponds to the portion of the pericallosal artery that courses around the genu of the corpus callosum. The **A-4** and **A-5** segments are portions of the distal pericallosal artery separated by a line parallel to and just behind the coronal suture. The distal portion of the anterior cerebral artery (segments A-2 to A-5) gives rise to a number of important branches (Perlmutter and Rhoton, 1978; Gomes et al., 1986).

The first major branch of the distal anterior cerebral artery is the **recurrent artery of Heubner** (Heubner, 1872; Shellshear, 1920; Perlmutter and Rhoton, 1976; Gomes et al., 1984, 1986). This vessel usually originates from the most proximal portion of the A-2 segment, almost always within

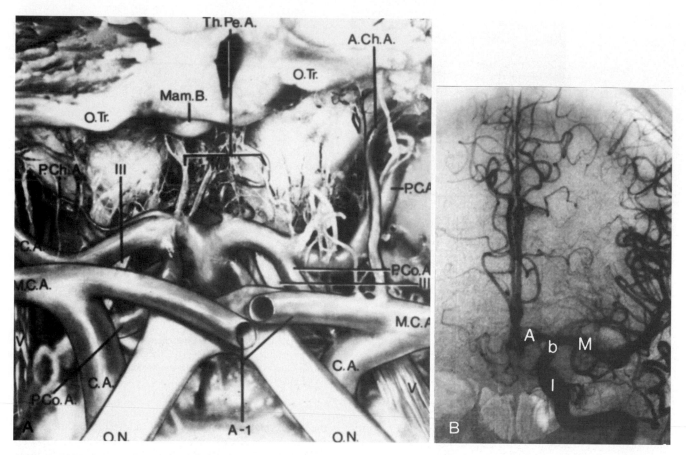

Figure 52.36. The terminal bifurcation of the internal carotid artery. *A,* Coronal view of the bifurcation of each internal carotid artery (*C.A.*) into a middle cerebral artery (*M.C.A.*) and an anterior cerebral artery (*A-1*). Note that the bifurcation occurs just distal to the origin of the posterior communicating artery (*P.Co.A.*) and that the left anterior choroidal artery (*A.Ch.A.*) seems to originate right at the bifurcation. *O.N.,* optic nerve; *O.Tr.,* optic tract; *Mam.B.,* mammillary body; *Th.Pe.A.,* thalamoperforating arteries; *P.Ch.A.,* posterior choroidal artery; *P.C.A.,* posterior cerebral artery; *III,* oculomotor nerve; *V,* trigeminal nerve. (From Rhoton AL Jr, Hardy DG, Chambers SM. Microsurgic anatomy and dissection of the sphenoid bone, cavernous sinus and sellar region. Surg Neurol *12:*63–104, 1979.) *B,* Cerebral arteriogram, anteroposterior view, showing bifurcation (*b*) of internal carotid artery (*I*) into anterior (*A*) and middle (*M*) cerebral arteries.

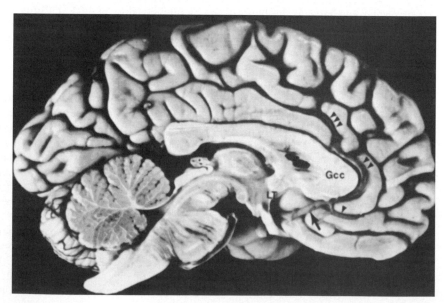

Figure 52.37. Sagittal section of brain showing portions of the anterior cerebral artery. The A-2 segment ascends in front of the lamina terminalis (*LT*), passes between the cerebral hemispheres in the longitudinal fissure, and makes a smooth curve around the genu of the corpus callosum (*Gcc*). The artery then passes above the corpus callosum in the pericallosal cistern. *Single arrow,* the A-2 segment of the anterior cerebral artery; *single arrowhead,* the frontopolar artery; *double arrowhead,* the pericallosal artery; *triple arrowhead,* the callosomarginal artery. (From Gluhbegovic N, Williams TH. The Human Brain. A Photographic Guide, p 47. Hagerstown, MD, Harper & Row, 1980.)

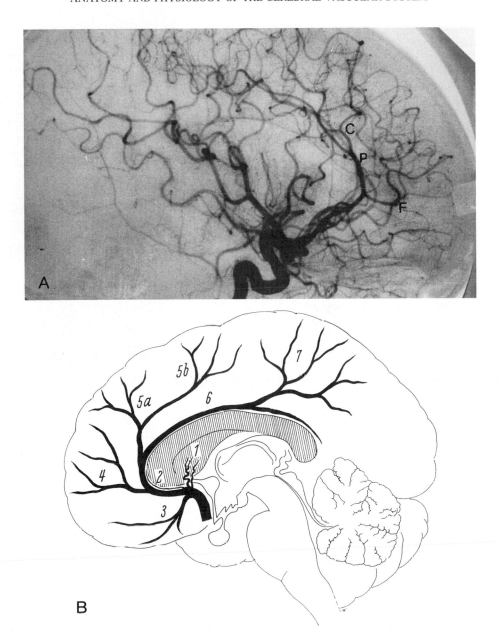

Figure 52.38.   The course and branches of the anterior cerebral artery. *A,* Cerebral arteriogram, lateral view, showing course of the anterior cerebral artery. Branches of the artery that are visible on the arteriogram include the frontopolar artery (*F*), the callosomarginal artery (*C*), and the pericallosal artery (*P*). *B,* Schematic drawing of the anterior cerebral artery in sagittal section, showing several of its major branches. *1,* anterior striate arteries; *2,* proximal A-2 segment; *3,* orbital (orbitofrontal) artery; *4,* frontopolar artery; *5a,* callosomarginal artery–prefrontal branch; *5b,* callosomarginal artery–cingular branch; *6,* pericallosal artery; *7,* posterior frontal artery. (From Krayenbuhl HA, Yaşargil MG. Cerebral Angiography. 2nd edition, p 44. Philadelphia, JB Lippincott, 1968.)

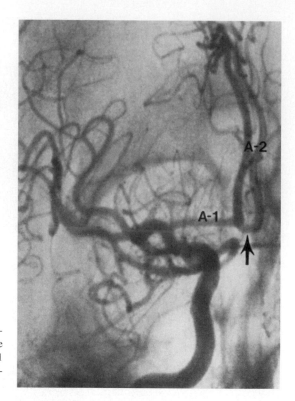

Figure 52.39. Cerebral arteriogram, anteroposterior view, showing the anterior communicating artery (*arrow*) connecting the two anterior cerebral arteries. The segment of the anterior cerebral artery proximal to the anterior communicating artery is called the A-1 segment (*A-1*). The segment of the anterior cerebral artery distal to the anterior communicating artery is called the A-2 segment (*A-2*).

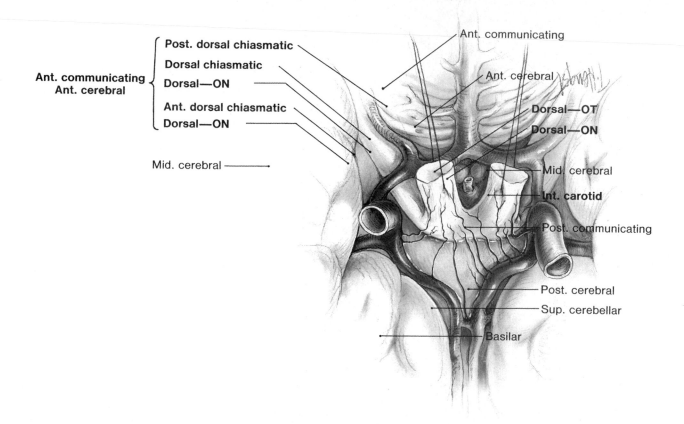

Figure 52.40. Schematic representation of the blood supply to the dorsal portions of the intracranial optic nerves and the optic chiasm from the A-1 segments of the anterior cerebral and anterior communicating arteries. (Redrawn from Wollschlaeger PB, Ide C, Hart W. Arterial blood supply of the human optic chiasm and surrounding structures. Ann Ophthalmol *3:*862–869, 1971.)

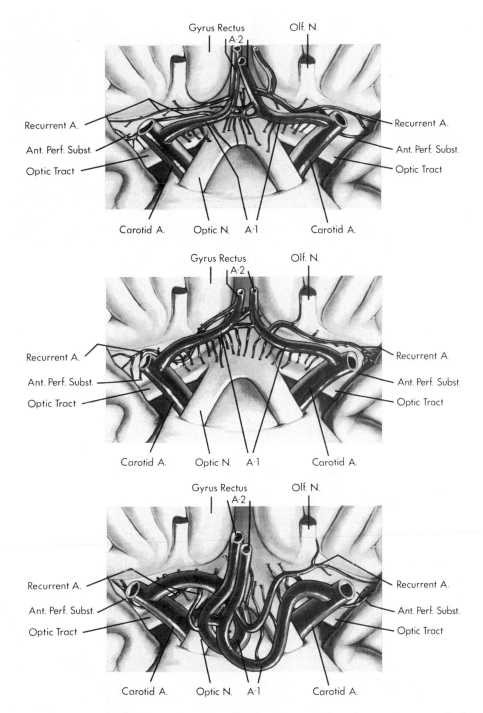

Figure 52.41. Anterior views of the A-1 and proximal A-2 segments of the anterior cerebral arteries, anterior communicating arteries, and recurrent arteries of Heubner, showing variations in the blood supply to the intracranial optic nerves and optic chiasm. Gyrus recti and olfactory nerves are located superiorly. (From Perlmutter D, Rhoton AL Jr. Microsurgic anatomy of the anterior cerebral-anterior communicating-recurrent artery complex. J Neurosurg *45:*259–272, 1976.)

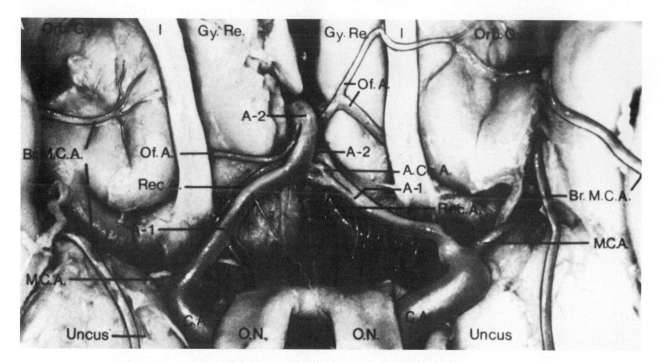

Figure 52.42. Anterior-subfrontal view of the perforating branches of the A-1 segments of the anterior cerebral arteries (*A-1*) that supply the intracranial portions of the optic nerves and the optic chiasm. *A-2,* A-2 segment of the anterior cerebral artery; *A.Co.A.,* anterior communicating artery; *M.C.A.,* middle cerebral artery; *Of.A.,* orbitofrontal arteries; *Orb. Gy.,* orbital gyri; *O.N.,* optic nerve; *Gy.Re.,* gyrus rectus; *Rec.A.,* recurrent artery of Heubner. (From Perlmutter D, Rhoton AL Jr. Microsurgic anatomy of the anterior cerebral-anterior communicating-recurrent artery complex. J Neurosurg *49:*204–228, 1978.)

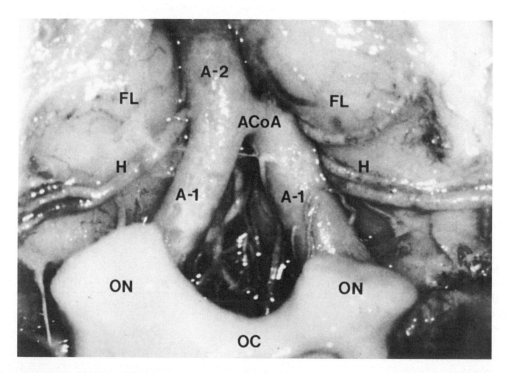

Figure 52.43. Recurrent artery of Heubner (*H*) seen from beneath the frontal lobes. The artery arises from the A-2 segment of the anterior cerebral artery (*A-2*). On the left side of the photograph, the artery arises as a single vessel. On the right side, there are two separate arteries. Note multiple perforating branches to the optic nerves and optic chiasm from the A-1 segment of the anterior cerebral artery (*A-1*). *ACoA,* anterior communicating artery; *OC,* optic chiasm; *ON,* optic nerve; *FL,* undersurface of frontal lobe. (From Gomes F, Dujovny M, Umansky F, et al. Microsurgic anatomy of the recurrent artery of Heubner. J Neurosurg *60:*130–139, 1984.)

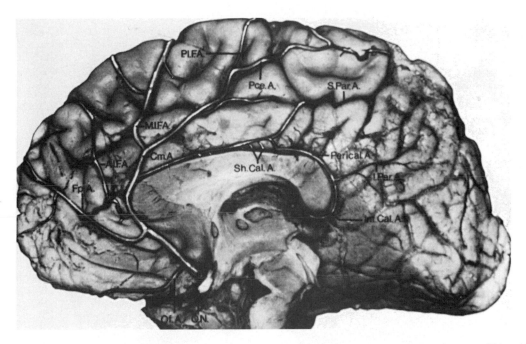

Figure 52.44. Medial surface of cerebral hemisphere, showing cortical branches of anterior cerebral artery. *O.N.,* optic nerve; *Of.A.,* orbitofrontal artery; *Fp.A.,* frontopolar artery; *A.I.F.A.,* anterior internal frontal artery; *M.I.F.A.,* middle internal frontal artery; *P.I.F.A.,* posterior internal frontal artery; *Cm.A.,* callosomarginal artery; *Sh.Cal.A.,* short callosal arteries; *Perical.A.,* pericallosal artery; *Pce.A.,* paracentral artery; *S.Par.A.,* superior parietal artery; *I.Par.A.,* inferior parietal artery; *Inf.Cal.A.,* inferior callosal artery. (From Perlmutter D, Rhoton AL Jr. Microsurgic anatomy of the anterior cerebral-anterior communicating-recurrent artery complex. J Neurosurg *49:*204–228, 1978.)

4 mm of the anterior communicating artery (Figs. 52.41 and 52.43). Less commonly, it arises from the distal portion of the A-1 segment or from the junction of the anterior cerebral and anterior communicating arteries. It supplies branches to the olfactory region, the undersurface of the frontal lobe, the anterior perforated substance, and the sylvian fissure (Gomes et al., 1984; Rosner et al., 1984). Although there is usually one recurrent artery of Heubner on each side, there occasionally may be two such vessels on one or both sides (Fig. 52.43), and in some patients the vessel is absent (see Table 1 in Gomes et al., 1984).

The A-2 segment of the anterior cerebral artery not only is the origin of the recurrent artery of Heubner but also gives off numerous branches that supply the optic nerves, optic chiasm, optic tract, and suprachiasmatic area. These branches are not as numerous as those that arise from the A-1 segment (Perlmutter and Rhoton, 1976). The A-2 segment also supplies branches to the anterior perforated substance (Rosner et al., 1984).

The **orbital (orbitofrontal) artery** arises either directly from the infracallosal portion of the A-2 segment or from a common trunk that also gives rise to the frontopolar artery. Coursing anteriorly on the medial surface of the hemisphere or on the inferior surface of the frontal lobe, the orbital artery supplies the medial basal region of the frontal lobe, including the gyrus rectus, the medial part of the orbital gyri, and the olfactory bulb and tract (Figs. 52.38, 52.42, 52.44, and 52.45).

The **frontopolar artery** usually arises from the infracallosal portion of the A-2 segment of the anterior cerebral artery,

but it occasionally originates from a common trunk with the orbital artery or from the callosomarginal artery when the latter has a proximal origin. The frontopolar artery passes anteriorly along the medial surface of the cerebral hemisphere in a gentle, bow-like curve toward the frontal pole (Figs. 52.38, 52.44, and 52.45). It supplies the anterior portion of the medial and lateral surfaces of the superior frontal gyrus.

The **callosomarginal artery** courses over the cingulate gyrus, runs in the cingulate sulcus, and terminates in the paracentral lobule (Figs. 52.37, 52.38, and 52.44). It usually arises from the A-3 segment as a distinct vessel, but it may consist of a group of several ascending vessels arising from the A-2 segment, and it may even originate from the A-4 segment (Gomes et al., 1986). The branches of the callosomarginal artery ascend on the medial surface of the hemisphere and continue on to the lateral convexity for a distance of about 2 cm. These branches are called the anterior, middle, and posterior **internal frontal arteries** and the **paracentral artery**. They supply portions of the premotor, motor, and sensory cortex (Lin and Kricheff, 1974; Moscow et al., 1974; Gomes et al., 1986). These arteries, particularly the paracentral artery, arise from the A-4 or A-5 segments of the anterior cerebral artery in some persons.

The **superior parietal** and **inferior parietal** arteries are terminal branches of the anterior cerebral artery. They arise from the A-5 segment and supply portions of the superior and inferior surfaces of the parietal lobe, respectively (Figs. 52.44 and 52.45).

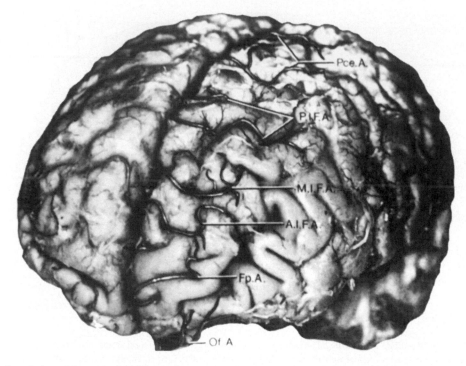

Figure 52.45. Anterolateral view of the cerebral hemispheres showing cortical branches of the anterior cerebral artery as they pass from the longitudinal fissure over the superior frontal gyrus to the cerebral convexity. From anterior to posterior, the branches are the orbitofrontal (*Of.A.*), frontopolar (*Fp.A.*), anterior (*A.I.F.A.*), middle (*M.I.F.A.*), and posterior (*P.I.F.A.*) internal frontal, and paracentral (*Pce.A.*) arteries. (From Perlmutter D, Rhoton AL Jr. J Neurosurg *49:*204–228, 1978.)

ANTERIOR COMMUNICATING ARTERY AND ITS BRANCHES

The **anterior communicating artery** ranges in length from less than 1 mm to 7 mm, but it is usually 2–3 mm long (Fisher, 1965; Perlmutter and Rhoton, 1976; Gomes et al., 1986). It completes the anterior portion of the circle of Willis by joining the two anterior cerebral arteries in the interhemispheric fissure (Figs. 52.14, 52.16, 52.32, 52.39–52.43). The diameter of the anterior communicating artery seems to be related to the difference in size between the A-1 segments of the right and left anterior cerebral arteries (Tindall et al., 1970). As the difference in diameter between the two A-1 segments increases, so does the size of the anterior communicating artery. Most persons have only a single anterior communicating artery, but the vessel may have many anatomic variations (Serizawa et al., 1994), and two or even three anterior communicating arteries may be present in up to 40% of normal persons (Critchley, 1930; Fisher, 1965; Perlmutter and Rhoton, 1976; Gomes et al., 1986) (Figs. 52.41 and 52.46).

Like the A-1 and A-2 segments of the anterior cerebral arteries, the anterior communicating artery supplies arterial branches to the dorsal surface of both optic nerves and the optic chiasm (Perlmutter and Rhoton, 1976; Crowell and Morawetz, 1977; Tulleken, 1978; Gomes et al., 1986; Serizawa et al., 1994) (Figs. 52.32*A*, 52.40, 52.41, and 52.47). It also supplies branches to the suprachiasmatic hypothalamic region, the anterior perforated substance, and the frontal lobe (Rosner et al., 1984; Serizawa et al., 1994).

Middle Cerebral Artery and Its Branches

The **middle cerebral artery** is the largest and most complex of the cerebral arteries. It is the larger of the two terminal branches of the internal carotid artery, originating at the medial end of the sylvian fissure, lateral to the optic chiasm, below the anterior perforated substance, and posterior to the division of the olfactory tract into its medial and lateral olfactory stria (Figs. 52.2, 52.32, 52.36, 52.42, 52.48, 52.49). From its origin, it courses laterally below the anterior perforated substance, parallel with and about 1 cm posterior to the sphenoid ridge. Within the sylvian fissure, it turns sharply in a posterosuperior direction (the genu) to reach the surface of the insula. At the periphery of the insula, branches from the middle cerebral artery supply the medial surface of the opercula of the frontal, temporal, and parietal lobes (Fig. 52.50). Other branches pass around the opercula to reach the lateral cortical surface and some of the inferior surface of the cerebral hemisphere (Gibo et al., 1981b) (Figs. 52.48–52.50).

The middle cerebral artery and its branches are usually separated into four parts: the **M-1 (sphenoidal, horizontal) segment**, the **M-2 (insular) segments**, the **M-3 (opercular) segments**, and the **M-4 (cortical) segments** (Fischer, 1938; Krayenbühl and Yaşargil, 1968, 1973; Gibo et al., 1981b; Umansky et al., 1984; Artero et al., 1985).

The M-1 segment begins at the origin of the middle cerebral artery and consists of the portion of the vessel that extends laterally within the sylvian fissure, below the anterior perforated substance and parallel to the sphenoid ridge. This

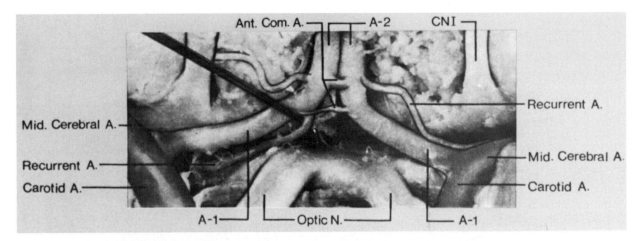

Figure 52.46. Double anterior communicating arteries (*Ant. Com. A.*). *A-1,* A-1 segment of the anterior cerebral artery; *A-2,* A-2 segment of the anterior cerebral artery; *Recurrent A.,* recurrent artery of Heubner; *CNI,* olfactory nerve. (From Perlmutter D, Rhoton AL Jr. J Neurosurg *45:*259–272, 1976.)

segment usually bifurcates to form a superior and an inferior trunk (Figs. 52.48 and 52.51), but it may trifurcate to form a superior, a middle, and an inferior trunk, or even divide into four or more trunks in about 10% of persons (Gibo et al., 1981b; Artero et al., 1985). The segment terminates at the genu.

The M-2 segments include the portions of the two or more trunks of the middle cerebral artery that overlie and supply the insula (Figs. 52.48*B* and 52.51). These segments begin at the genu of the middle cerebral artery and terminate at the circular sulcus of the insula.

The M-3 segments begin at the circular sulcus of the insula and end at the surface of the sylvian fissure (Fig. 52.51). These branches are closely adherent to, and course over, the surface of the frontoparietal and temporal opercula to reach the superficial part of the sylvian fissure.

The arterial trunks that make up the M-4 segments begin at the surface of the sylvian fissure and extend over the lateral surface of the cerebral hemisphere. The more anterior branches of these trunks turn sharply upward or downward after leaving the sylvian fissure. Intermediate branches follow a gradual posterior incline from the fissure, and posterior

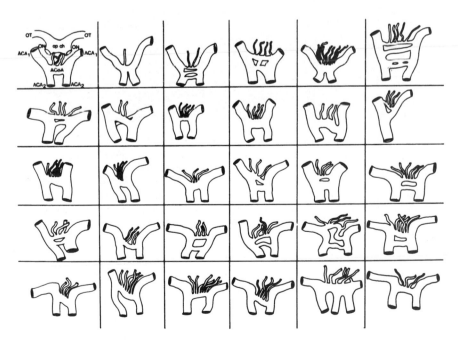

Figure 52.47. Different anatomic patterns of the anterior communicating artery (*ACoA*), showing variations in the number of perforating vessels supplying the distal optic nerves (*ON*) and the optic chiasm (*op ch*). *OT,* optic tract. (From Gomes F, Dujovny M, Umansky F, et al. Microsurgic anatomy of the recurrent artery of Heubner. J Neurosurg *60:*130–139, 1984.)

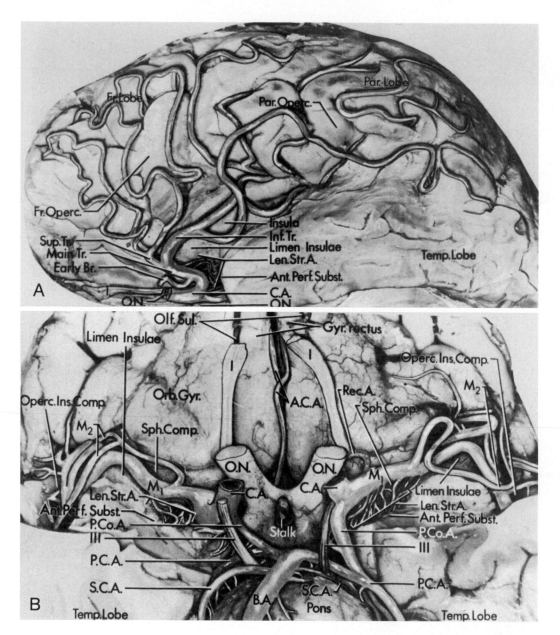

Figure 52.48. Origin of the middle cerebral artery from the internal carotid artery (*C.A.*). *A*, Lateral view shows division of the main trunk (*Main Tr.*) into a small superior trunk (*Sup. Tr.*) and a large inferior trunk *(Inf. Tr.)*. *Ant.Perf. Subst.*, anterior perforated substance; *Len.Str.A.*, lenticulostriate arteries; *O.N.*, optic nerve. *B*, Basal view shows relationship of initial segment of middle cerebral artery (M_1) to surrounding structures. Note origin of the lenticulostriate arteries (*Len.Str.A.*) from this segment and their supply of the anterior perforated substance *(Ant. Perf. Subst.)*. *A.C.A.*, anterior cerebral artery; *B.A.*, basilar artery; M_2, distal segment of middle cerebral artery; *P.C.A.*, posterior cerebral artery; *P.Co.A.*, posterior communicating artery; *Rec.A.*, recurrent artery of Heubner; *S.C.A.*, superior cerebellar artery; *I*, olfactory nerve; *III*, oculomotor nerve; *O.N.*, optic nerve. (From Gibo H, Carver CC, Rhoton AL Jr, et al. Microsurgic anatomy of the middle cerebral artery. J Neurosurg *54*:151–169, 1981.)

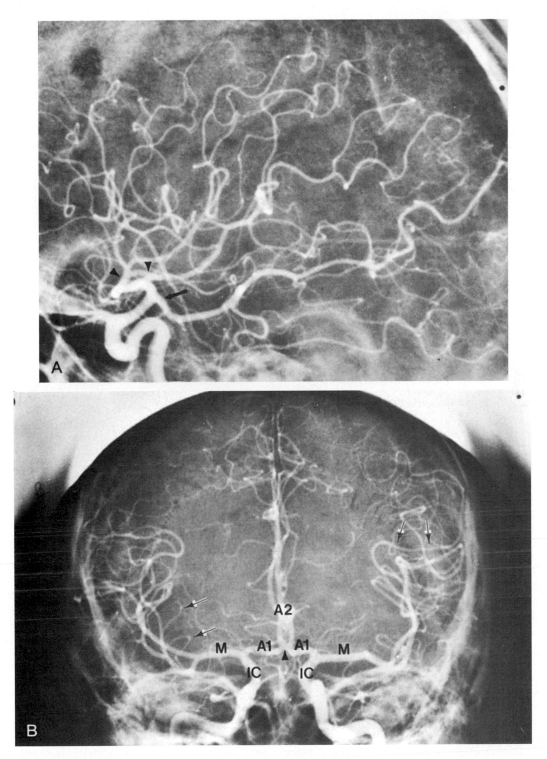

Figure 52.49. Cerebral arteriogram showing origin and course of the middle cerebral artery. *A,* Lateral view shows origin and branches of middle cerebral artery. In this case, the artery arises as two separate branches (*arrowheads*). The view is unobscured by branches of the anterior cerebral artery because this vessel was hypoplastic and did not fill during the arteriogram. Note origin of the posterior cerebral artery directly from the internal carotid artery (*arrow*). *B,* anteroposterior view shows simultaneous filling of both middle cerebral arteries (*M*). Note their relationship to the internal carotid (*IC*), A-1 (*A1*) and A-2 (*A2*) segments of the anterior cerebral artery, and the anterior communicating artery (*arrowhead*). Arrows point to anterior branches in the sylvian fissure on the right and to posterior branches on the left.

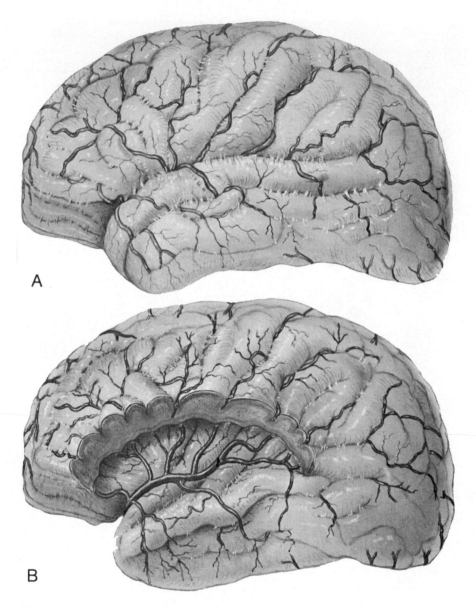

Figure 52.50.   Lateral surface of the brain and its relationship to branches of the middle cerebral artery. *A,* The frontoparietal operculum is intact. *B,* The frontoparietal operculum has been cut, and the temporal lobe is pulled downward. (From Taveras JM, Wood EH. Diagnostic Neuroradiology. 2nd edition, Vol 2. Baltimore, Williams & Wilkins, 1976.)

branches pass backward in nearly the same direction as the long axis of the fissure.

Perforating branches of the middle cerebral artery supply several subcortical regions of the brain (Ring, 1974; Gibo et al., 1981b; Rosner et al., 1984; Umansky et al., 1984; Artero et al., 1985; Marinković et al., 1985; Umansky et al., 1985). Medial, intermediate, and lateral **lenticulostriate arteries** and other deep perforating vessels supply portions of the globus pallidus, caudate nucleus, internal capsule, and the anterior portion of the optic radiations (Fig. 52.48). The majority of these vessels originate from the proximal 17 mm of the middle cerebral artery (Umansky et al., 1985).

The cortical territory supplied by the middle cerebral ar-

tery is extensive and includes most of the lateral surface of the hemisphere, all of the insular and opercular surfaces, the lateral part of the orbital surface of the frontal lobe, the temporal pole, and the lateral part of the inferior surface of the temporal lobe (Fig. 52.52). Twelve cortical arteries are usually described (Gibo et al., 1981b). The **orbitofrontal**, **prefrontal**, **precentral**, and **central** arteries supply portions of the frontal lobe. The **anterior parietal**, **posterior parietal**, and **angular** arteries supply portions of the parietal and occipital lobes. Portions of the temporal and occipital lobes are supplied by the **temporo-occipital**, **posterior temporal**, **middle temporal**, **anterior temporal**, and **temporopolar** arteries. Penetrating arterioles from these cortical branches

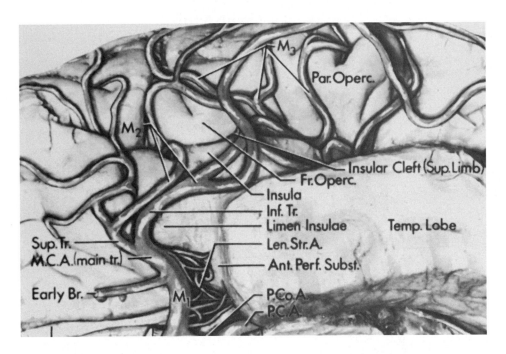

Figure 52.51. Medial surface of the cerebral hemisphere showing M-1, M-2, and M-3 segments of the middle cerebral artery. Note that the artery arises as a single vessel (*M.C.A.* (*main tr.*)) and divides into a small superior artery (*Sup. Tr.*) and a large inferior artery (*Inf. Tr.*). The proximal portions of these trunks are the M-2 segments and the more distal portions that reach the surface of the insula are the M-3 segments. *Len.Str.A.,* lenticulostriate arteries; *P.C.A.,* posterior cerebral artery; *P.Co.A.,* posterior communicating artery; *Ant. Perf. Subst.,* anterior perforated substance. (From Gibo H, Carver CC, Rhoton AL Jr, et al. Microsurgic anatomy of the middle cerebral artery. J Neurosurg *54:*151–169, 1981.)

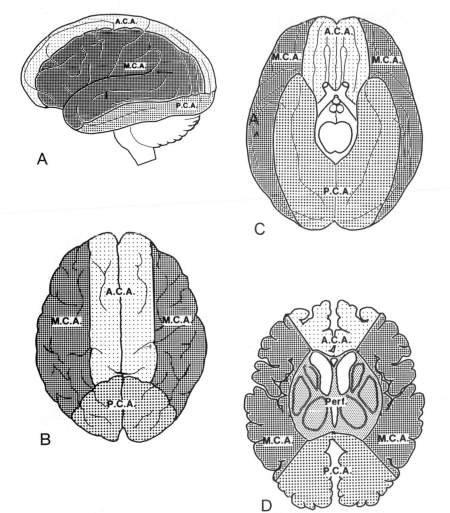

Figure 52.52. Cortical and subcortical supply of the cerebral hemispheres by the anterior (*A.C.A.*), middle (*M.C.A.*), and posterior (*P.C.A.*) cerebral arteries and their perforating branches (*Perf.*). *A,* Lateral surface; *B,* Basal surface; *C,* Superior surface; *D,* Axial section through basal ganglia. (From Day AL. Arterial distributions and variants. In Cerebral Blood Flow. Editor, Wood JH, p 22. New York, McGraw-Hill, 1987.)

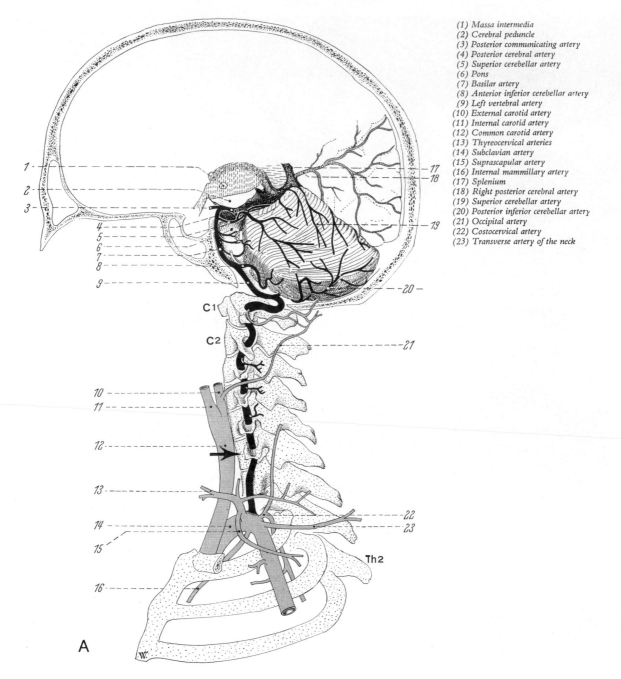

(1) Massa intermedia
(2) Cerebral peduncle
(3) Posterior communicating artery
(4) Posterior cerebral artery
(5) Superior cerebellar artery
(6) Pons
(7) Basilar artery
(8) Anterior inferior cerebellar artery
(9) Left vertebral artery
(10) External carotid artery
(11) Internal carotid artery
(12) Common carotid artery
(13) Thyreocervical arteries
(14) Subclavian artery
(15) Suprascapular artery
(16) Internal mammillary artery
(17) Splenium
(18) Right posterior cerebral artery
(19) Superior cerebellar artery
(20) Posterior inferior cerebellar artery
(21) Occipital artery
(22) Costocervical artery
(23) Transverse artery of the neck

Figure 52.53.   The course of the vertebral artery. *A,* Schematic drawing showing the extracranial and intracranial course of the left vertebral artery and its branches. Note that the vessel enters the vertebral processes at C6 (*arrow*). (From Krayenbühl HA, Yaşargil MG. Cerebral Angiography, 2nd edition. Philadelphia, JB Lippincott, 1968.)

also supply subcortical white matter, including the paraventricular portions of the optic radiations.

VERTEBROBASILAR ARTERIAL SYSTEM AND ITS BRANCHES

The two vertebral arteries, the basilar artery, and the two posterior cerebral arteries, constitute the posterior circulatory system of the brain. This system supplies the cervical portion of the spinal cord, the brainstem, the cerebellum, and portions of the occipital lobes (Gillilan, 1964; Hassler, 1967). It thus supports most of the principal ocular motor and cerebral visual sensory areas of the brain.

Vertebral Artery and Its Branches

In most normal persons, one vertebral artery arises on each side as the first branch of the subclavian artery (Figs.

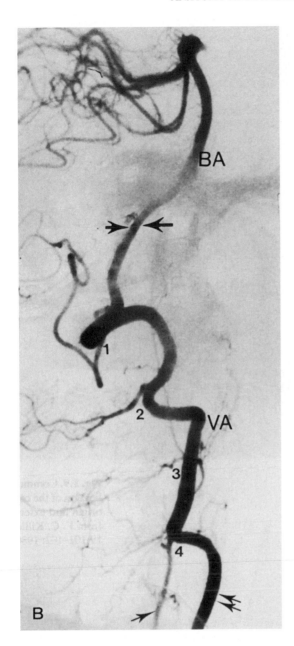

Figure 52.53. *(continued) B,* Arteriogram resulting from selective injection of the right vertebral artery. *Double arrows* show the origin of the vessel just above the aortic arch. The termination of the vertebral artery (*VA*) is marked by *large arrows* on each side of the vessel. This vertebral artery enters the vertebral canal at the C4 level (*4*). Note that the contralateral vertebral artery, which is hypoplastic, fills by retrograde fashion (*single arrow*). Note collaterals at the C1 (*1*), C2 (*2*), and C3 (*3*) disk spaces. *BA,* basilar artery. (From Huber P. Cerebral Angiography, 2nd edition. New York, Georg Thieme Verlag, 1982.)

52.1 and 52.53). The vertebral artery usually arises from the medial dorsal aspect of the parent vessel. Occasionally, however, the right vertebral artery originates directly from the aortic arch or from a common innominate trunk, and, in about 8% of persons, the left vertebral artery arises from the aortic arch before the origin of the subclavian artery.

The extradural portions of the vertebral arteries are often of different caliber (Hutchinson and Yates, 1956), with the left artery usually being larger than the right. One vertebral artery may even be aplastic or anomalous (Fig. 52.53*B*), leaving the basilar artery and its branches dependent on only one vessel.

Each vertebral artery usually enters the ipsilateral transverse process of the 6th cervical vertebra (Fig. 52.53*A*). Occasionally, however, both vessels enter the transverse pro-

cesses of the 7th, 5th, or even the 4th cervical vertebrae (Bell et al., 1950) (Fig. 52.53*B*). The vertebral arteries then ascend through the transverse processes of the cervical vertebrae, pass behind the lateral masses of the axis, enter the dura mater behind the occipital condyles, and ascend through the foramen magnum to the ventral surface of the medulla where they join to form the basilar artery at the pontomedullary junction (Fig. 52.54). Each vertebral artery may be divided into an extradural and an intradural segment.

The **extradural** portion of the vertebral artery may be further divided into three segments (Oliveira et al., 1985; Abd El-Bary et al., 1995) (Fig. 52.53*A*). The first segment extends from the origin of the artery to its entrance into the lowest transverse foramen. The second segment ascends through the transverse foramina of the upper cervical verte-

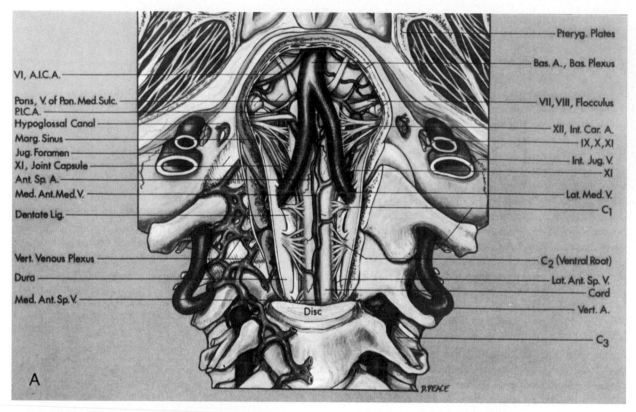

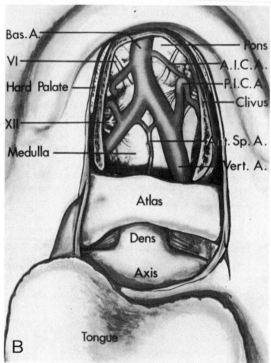

Figure 52.54. Junction of the vertebral arteries to form the the basilar artery. *A,* Each vertebral artery ascends through the transverse processes of the cervical vertebrae, passes behind the lateral masses of the axis, enters the dura mater behind the occipital condyles, and ascends through the foramen magnum to the ventral surface of the medulla, where they join to form the basilar artery at the pontomedullary junction. Note the origin of the anterior spinal artery from the anterior ventral spinal arteries that originate just inferior to the junction of the vertebral arteries to form the basilar artery. *B,* Posterior view of the junction of the two vertebral arteries (*Vert.A.*) to form the basilar artery (*Bas.A.*) at the pontomedullary junction. Note the origins and initial courses of the anterior spinal artery (*Ant.Sp.A.*), the posterior inferior cerebellar artery (*P.I.C.A.*), and the anterior inferior cerebellar artery (*A.I.C.A.*). *VI,* abducens nerve; *XII,* hypoglossal nerve. (From de Oliveira E, Rhoton AL Jr, Peace D. Microsurgic anatomy of the region of the foramen magnum. Surg Neurol *24:*293–352, 1985.)

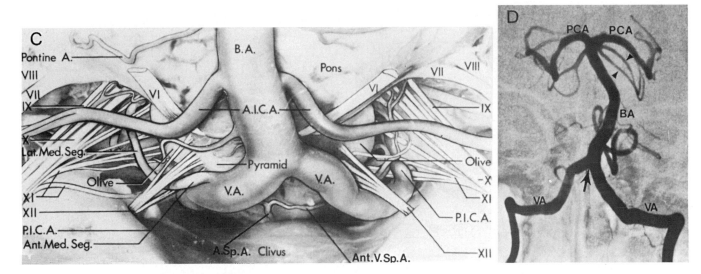

Figure 52.54. *(continued) C,* Another view of the two vertebral arteries (*V.A.*) joining together at the level of the caudal medulla. Note the origin of the posterior inferior cerebellar artery (*P.I.C.A.*) just before the termination of each vertebral artery. *A.I.C.A.,* anterior inferior cerebellar artery; *A.Sp.A.,* anterior spinal artery; *Ant.V.Sp.A.,* anterior ventral spinal artery; *B.A.,* basilar artery. *VI,* abducens nerve; *VII,* facial nerve; *VIII,* vestibulocochlear nerve; *IX,* glossopharyngeal nerve; *X,* vagus nerve; *XI,* spinal accessory nerve; *XII,* hypoglossal nerve. (From Lister JR, Rhoton AL Jr, Matsushima T., et al. Microsurgical anatomy of the posterior inferior cerebellar artery. Neurosurgery *10:*170–199, 1982.) *D,* Cerebral arteriogram, anteroposterior view, shows both vertebral arteries (*VA*) joining (*arrow*) to form the basilar artery (*BA*). Note a double superior cerebellar artery on the left side (*double arrows*). *PCA,* posterior cerebral artery.

brae in front of the cervical nerve roots. This segment deviates laterally just above the axis in order to reach the laterally located transverse foramen of the atlas. The third segment, the one most intimately related to the foramen magnum, extends from the foramen in the transverse process of the atlas to the site of passage through the dura mater. This segment passes medially behind the lateral mass of the atlas, across the groove on the upper surface of the lateral part of the posterior arch of the atlas, and enters the vertebral canal by passing anterior to the lateral border of the atlanto-occipital membrane. The third segment is partially covered by the posterior atlanto-occipital membrane, the rectus capitis posterior major muscle, and the superior and inferior oblique muscles of the neck. It is surrounded by a venous plexus composed of anastomoses between the deep cervical and epidural veins. The terminal extradural segment of the vertebral artery gives rise to the posterior meningeal and posterior spinal arteries, branches to the deep cervical muscles, and, occasionally, the posterior inferior cerebellar artery (see below).

The **intradural** portion of the vertebral artery begins at the dural foramen just inferior to the lateral edge of the foramen magnum. The dura in this region, much thicker than in other areas, forms a funnel-shaped foramen around a 4–6-mm length of the artery (Lazorthes et al., 1954). The first cervical nerve exits the spinal canal, and the posterior spinal artery enters the canal through this dural foramen with the vertebral artery. These three structures are bound together at the foramen by fibrous dural bands.

Once it has penetrated the dura mater, each vertebral artery ascends from the lower lateral to the upper anterior surface of the medulla. This portion of the artery may be separated into two segments (Lister et al., 1982; Oliveira et al., 1985). The lateral medullary segment begins at the dural foramen and passes anterior and superior along the lateral medullary surface to the preolivary sulcus. The anterior medullary segment begins at the preolivary sulcus, courses in front of, or between, the hypoglossal rootlets, and crosses the pyramid to join with the opposite vertebral artery to form the origin of the basilar artery at or near the pontomedullary sulcus (Fig. 52.54).

Anomalies of the distal end of the vertebral arteries are not rare. A hypoplastic vertebral artery (usually on the right side) may terminate in a posterior inferior cerebellar artery (PICA). The segment between the origin of the PICA and the basilar artery may be hypoplastic (Fields et al., 1965). In some persons, one or both vertebral arteries terminate in muscular branches between the 1st and 2nd cervical vertebrae. In such persons, the basilar artery originates from the anterior spinal artery or from the carotid system.

The branches that arise from the intradural portion of the vertebral artery are the posterior spinal, posterior inferior cerebellar, anterior spinal, and anterior and posterior meningeal arteries.

Posterior Spinal Artery

The paired posterior spinal arteries usually arise from the posteromedial aspect of the vertebral arteries just outside the dura mater, but they may also arise from the initial intradural part of the vertebral arteries or rarely from the posterior inferior cerebellar arteries. In the subarachnoid space, each posterior spinal artery divides into an ascending and a de-

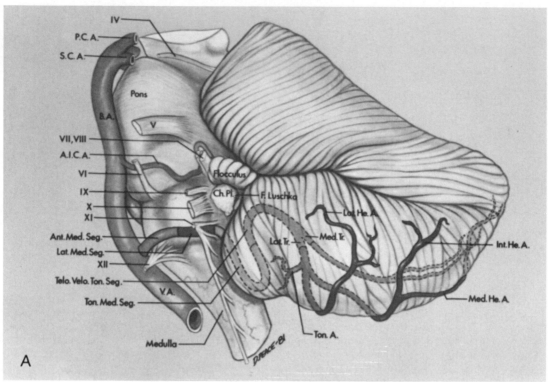

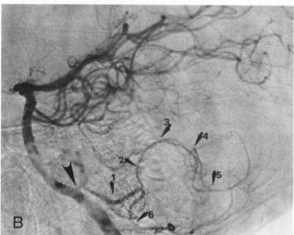

Figure 52.55. The posterior inferior cerebellar artery. *A*, Schematic drawing of the posterior inferior cerebellar artery in lateral view, showing its anterior (*Ant.Med. Seg.*), lateral (*Lat.Med. Seg.*), and tonsillar (*Ton.Med.Seg.*) median segments and its lateral (*Lat.Tr.*) and medial (*Med.Tr.*) trunks. Note the various terminal arteries, including the lateral (*Lat.He.A.*), medial (*Med.He.A.*), and internal (*Int.He.A.*) hemisphere arteries and the tonsillar artery (*Ton.A.*). *A.I.C.A.*, anterior inferior cerebellar artery; *B.A.*, basilar artery; *P.C.A.*, posterior cerebral artery; *S.C.A.*, superior cerebellar artery; *V.A.*, vertebral artery. *Roman numerals* refer to specific cranial nerves. (From Lister JR, Rhoton AL Jr, Matsushima T, et al. Microsurgic anatomy of the posterior inferior cerebellar artery. Neurosurgery *10:*170–199, 1982.) *B*, Cerebral arteriogram, lateral view, showing origin (*arrowhead*) and course of the posterior inferior cerebellar artery. Numbers refer to segments of the vessel: *1*, perimedullary segment; *2*, caudal curve; *3*, retromedullary segment; *4*, superior retrotonsillar segment *5*, retrotonsillar branch; *6*, tonsillohemispheric branch. (From Taveras JM, Wood EH. Diagnostic Neuroradiology, 2nd edition, Vol 2. Baltimore, Williams & Wilkins, 1976.)

scending branch. The ascending branch supplies portions of the brainstem, including the inferior cerebellar peduncle, as well as the choroid plexus near the foramen of Magendie. It may also give rise to branches that anastomose with branches of the posterior inferior cerebellar artery. The descending branch passes downward to supply the superficial part of the dorsal half of the cervical spinal cord.

Posterior Inferior Cerebellar Artery

The PICA is the largest branch of the vertebral artery (Lister et al., 1982; Oliveira et al., 1985; Heimans et al., 1985; Amarenco and Hauw, 1989) (Figs. 52.53–52.56). It usually originates from the intradural portion of the vertebral artery, but, as noted above, it may occasionally originate

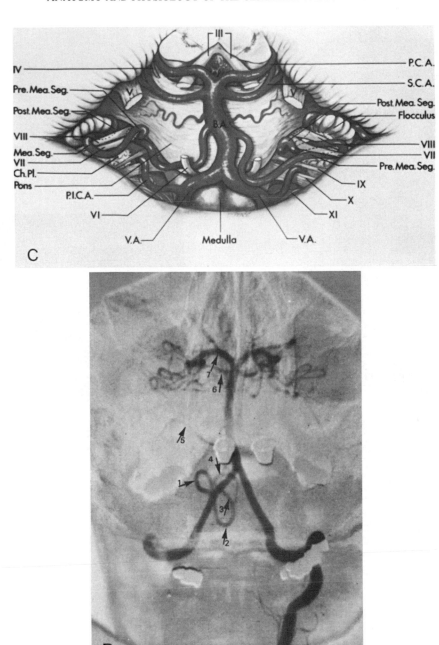

Figure 52.55. *C,* Schematic drawing of vertebrobasilar arterial system in posteroanterior view, showing the origin and initial course of the posterior inferior cerebellar artery (*P.I.C.A.*). Note the relationships of this vessel and of the anterior inferior cerebellar artery to the lower cranial nerves (*VI-XI*). *B.A.,* basilar artery; *P.C.A.,* posterior cerebral artery; *S.C.A.,* superior cerebellar artery; *V.A.,* vertebral artery; *III,* oculomotor nerve. (From Lister JR, Rhoton AL Jr, Matsushima T, et al. Microsurgic anatomy of the posterior inferior cerebellar artery. Neurosurgery *10:*170–199, 1982.) *D,* Cerebral arteriogram, posteroanterior view shows segments of the posterior inferior cerebellar artery. Numbers *1–4* correspond to those in *part B* of figure; however, *5* is anterior inferior cerebellar artery, *is* superior cerebellar artery, and *7* is posterior cerebral artery. (From Taveras JM, Wood EH. Diagnostic Neuroradiology, 2nd edition, Vol 2. Baltimore, Williams & Wilkins, 1976.)

from the terminal extradural part of the vertebral artery. Although there are substantial variations in the course and area of supply of this vessel, it usually courses around the anterolateral surface of the medulla, passing near the rootlets of the glossopharyngeal, vagus, accessory, and hypoglossal cranial nerves (Sunderland, 1948). It then passes around the cerebellar tonsil near the caudal half of the roof of the 4th ventricle, where it usually bifurcates into a medial and a lateral trunk. These trunks in turn give rise to perforating, choroidal, and cortical terminal branches.

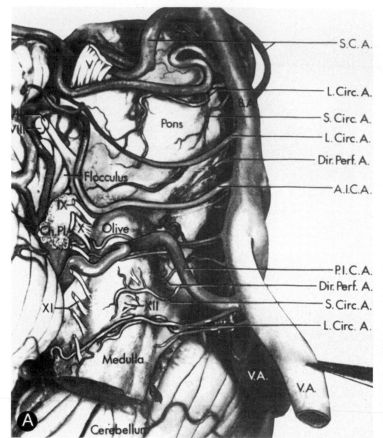

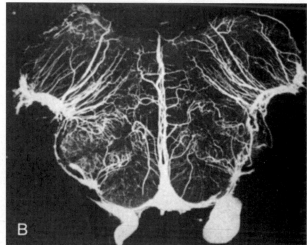

Figure 52.56. Brainstem perforating arteries of the posterior inferior cerebellar artery. *A,* Lateral view of the brainstem showing the posterior inferior cerebellar artery (*P.I.C.A.*) as it arises from the vertebral artery (*V.A.*) and begins its course around the medulla. Note the direct perforating arteries (*Dir.Perf.A.*) and the long (*L.Circ.A.*) and short (*S.Circ.A.*) circumflex arteries that arise from it and supply the lower brainstem. Similar perforating arteries arise from the basilar artery (*B.A.*). *A.I.C.A.,* anterior inferior cerebellar artery; *S.C.A.,* superior cerebellar artery. *Roman numerals* refer to specific cranial nerves. (From Lister JR, Rhoton AL Jr, Matsushima T, et al. Microsurgic anatomy of the posterior inferior cerebellar artery. Neurosurgery *10:* 170–199, 1982.) *B,* Vascular injection of upper medulla showing direct and circumflex penetrating arteries. At least some of these vessels arise from the posterior inferior cerebellar arteries. (From Hassler O. Deep cerebral venous system in man: A microangiographic study on its areas of drainage and its anastomoses with the superficial cerebral brain. Neurology *17:*368–375, 1967.)

The perforating arteries that arise from the PICA terminate in the brainstem and are similar to those that arise from the basilar, anterior inferior cerebellar, and superior cerebellar arteries (see below). These arteries are of two types: direct and circumflex (Fig. 52.56).

Direct perforating arteries pursue a direct course to enter the brainstem. **Circumflex perforating arteries** pass around the brainstem before entering it. The lengths of the circumflex perforating arteries are variable. Some travel less than 90 around the circumference of the brainstem before entering it (short circumflex arteries), whereas others travel almost 180 to enter the dorsal portion of the brainstem (long circumflex arteries). Both long and short circumflex types of perforating arteries send branches into the brainstem along their course.

The choroidal arteries that arise from the PICA supply the tela choroidea and choroid plexus in the roof and the medial part of the lateral recess of the 4th ventricle (Fujii et al., 1980b; Lister et al., 1982). The number of these vessels

varies considerably. In the study performed by Lister et al., the maximum number was 11, with an average of 6.

The most constant area supplied by the PICA is most of the ipsilateral half of the suboccipital surface of the cerebellum, including the suboccipital surface of the hemisphere and tonsil, the ipsilateral half of the vermis, and the anterior aspect of the tonsil (Amarenco and Hauw, 1989). The cortical branches of the PICA therefore include hemispheric, vermian, and tonsillar branches (Fig. 52.55A). The vermian branches usually arise from the medial trunk, whereas the hemispheric and tonsillar branches most often arise from the lateral trunk.

Anterior Spinal Artery

The anterior spinal artery is formed by the union of the paired anterior ventral spinal arteries, each of which originates from the anterior medullary segment of the ipsilateral vertebral artery near the origin of the basilar artery (Figs.

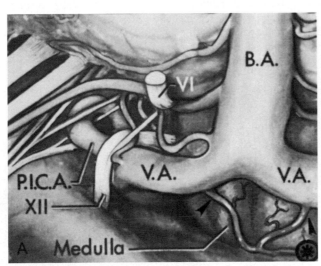 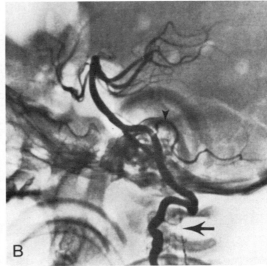

Figure 52.57. The anterior spinal artery. *A,* Origin of the anterior spinal artery (*circled asterisk*) from the paired anterior ventral spinal arteries (*arrowheads*) that arise from the vertebral artery (*V.A.*). *B.A.,* basilar artery; *P.I.C.A.,* posterior inferior cerebellar artery; *VI,* abducens nerve; *XII,* hypoglossal nerve. (From Lister JR, Rhoton AL Jr, Matsushima T, et al. Microsurgic anatomy of the posterior inferior cerebellar artery. Neurosurgery *10:*170–199, 1982.) *B,* Vertebral arteriogram, lateral view, showing anterior spinal artery (*arrow*) descending down the spinal cord. The posterior inferior cerebellar artery is marked with an *arrowhead.*

52.54 and 52.56). The junction of the anterior ventral spinal arteries is almost always near the lower end of the inferior olivary nuclei.

The anterior spinal artery descends through the foramen magnum on the anterior surface of the medulla and the spinal cord in or near the anterior median fissure (Fig. 52.57). At the level of the medulla, it supplies the pyramids and their decussation, the hypoglossal nuclei, fascicles, and nerves, and the posterior longitudinal fasciculus (Margaretten et al., 1954).

Meningeal Arteries

The dura mater around the foramen magnum is supplied by the anterior and posterior meningeal branches of each vertebral artery, meningeal branches of the ascending pharyngeal artery, and the occipital arteries (Newton, 1968). In fact, these arteries, along with the dorsal meningeal branch of the meningohypophyseal trunk which arises from the intracavernous segment of the internal carotid artery (see above), supply all of the dura lining the posterior cranial fossa (Oliveira et al., 1985).

Basilar Artery and Its Branches

The basilar artery is an unpaired vessel that originates from the fusion of the two vertebral arteries at the pontomedullary junction (Figs. 52.53–52.55 and 52.57). In the infant, the basilar artery is short and straight, but it elongates, widens, and becomes tortuous with advancing age (Sunderland, 1948). It is almost always a single vessel, but a basilar artery fenestration, i.e., a duplication of a segment of the vessel, is observed angiographically in 0.6–1% of the population and is found in 5% of some autopsy studies (Wollschlaeger

et al., 1967; Takahashi et al., 1973) (Fig. 52.58). The most common site of a basilar artery fenestration is the proximal trunk, near the junction of the vertebral arteries (Nakasu et al., 1982; De Caro et al., 1991, 1996).

The length of the basilar artery in an adult ranges from 15–40 mm, with an average of 32–34 mm (Saeki and Rhoton, 1977; Hardy et al., 1980). It is normally a midline vessel, but in 11 specimens examined by Hardy et al. (1980), the

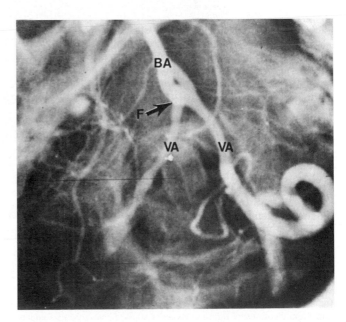

Figure 52.58. Fenestration (*F*) of the basilar artery (*BA*) near its origin from the junction of the vertebral arteries (*VA*).

artery deviated as far laterally as the origin of the abducens nerve.

The basilar artery ascends along the ventral aspect of the brainstem and eventually terminates by dividing into the two posterior cerebral arteries (Tulleken and Luiten, 1986) (Figs. 52.14, 52.15, 52.32, 52.36, 52.48*B,* and 52.54*D*). This bifurcation may occur as far caudally as 1.3 mm below the pon-

tomesencephalic junction or as far rostrally as the mammillary bodies (Saeki and Rhoton, 1977). In most cases, however, the bifurcation occurs at the upper border of the pons (Stopford, 1916a; Saeki and Rhoton, 1977).

Numerous important arteries originate from the basilar artery, and these supply specific areas of the brainstem and cerebellum (Amarenco and Hauw, 1989). These branches

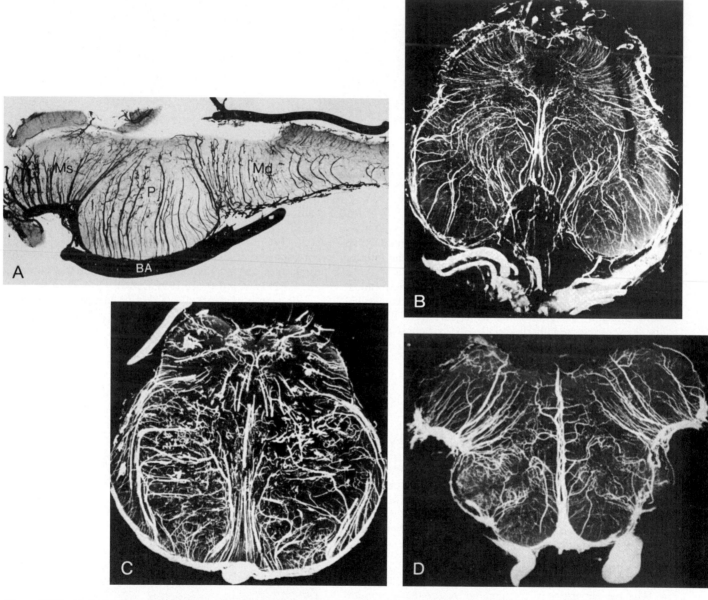

Figure 52.59. Brainstem perforating arteries arising from the basilar artery. *A,* Injected brainstem sectioned longitudinally. Note numerous perforating arteries, both direct and circumflex, arising from the basilar artery (*BA*) and supplying the mesencephalon (*Ms*), pons (*P*), and medulla (*Md*). *B,* Cross-section through the mesencephalon showing both direct and circumflex perforating arteries. Although some of these vessels may originate from the superior cerebellar and posterior cerebral arteries, many undoubtedly arise from the basilar artery. *C,* Cross-section through the pons showing both direct and circumflex perforating arteries. Although some of these arteries may originate from the anterior inferior cerebellar artery, the majority originate directly from the basilar artery. *D,* Cross-section through the medulla showing both direct and circumflex perforating arteries. Many of these arteries probably arise from the posterior inferior cerebellar artery; however, others undoubtedly originate directly from the basilar artery. (From Hassler O. Deep cerebral venous system in man: A microangiographic study on its areas of drainage and its anastomoses with the superficial cerebral brain. Neurology *17:*368–375, 1967.)

are often separated into two groups: perforating arteries and superficial arteries.

Perforating Branches of the Basilar Artery

The perforating arteries that originate from the basilar artery, like those that originate from other major vessels that supply the brainstem, are small in caliber. They arise in vertically oriented clusters from the posterior and lateral surfaces of the upper centimeter of the vessel, and they supply structures within the medulla, pons, and mesencephalon (Figs. 52.56*B* and 52.59). Like the perforating vessels that arise from the posterior inferior cerebellar artery (see above), the anterior inferior cerebellar artery, and the superior cerebellar artery (see below), the perforating vessels that arise from the basilar artery have constant and predictable courses (Tulleken and Luiten, 1987). There are two main types of perforating vessels: direct (median, paramedian) and circumflex (tranverse, circumferential) (Busch, 1966).

The **direct** arteries enter the brainstem immediately after originating from the basilar artery to supply median and paramedian structures (Figs. 52.59–52.61). These vessels sup-

ply all of the midline and paramedian nuclei of the cranial nerves, including the ocular motor nerves (Fig. 52.61).

The **circumflex** arteries travel for some distance around the brainstem before entering it, occasionally contacting or even compressing a cranial nerve near its junction with the brainstem (Klun and Prestor, 1986). Short circumflex arteries travel less than 90 around the brainstem before entering it, whereas long circumflex arteries travel as much as 180 around the brainstem before their termination (Figs. 52.59 and 52.60). Both types of circumflex arteries send branches into the brainstem along their course. Shrontz et al. (1986) examined 27 human brains with no evidence of intracranial pathology. These investigators found an average of 11 short and 8 long circumflex arteries originating from the basilar artery. The circumflex arteries primarily supply the lateral and dorsal regions of the brainstem, which are also supplied by similar branches from the posterior and anterior inferior cerebellar, and superior cerebellar arteries (see below). Located in the area supplied by these penetrating arteries are the main sensory and motor nuclei of the trigeminal nerve and its spinal root, the facial nuclei, portions of the vestibular

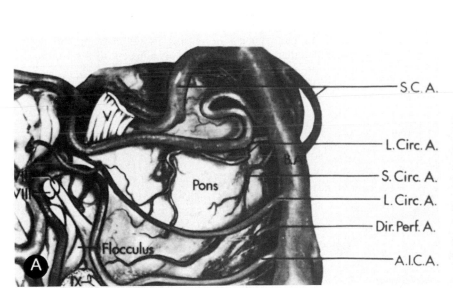
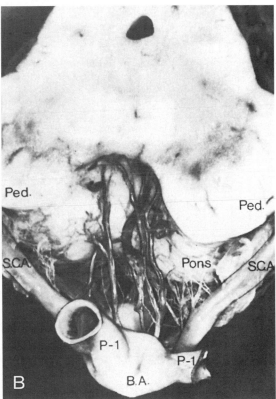

Figure 52.60. Brainstem perforating arteries arising from the basilar artery. *A,* Side view of the proximal and middle segments of the basilar artery (*B.A.*). Note that direct perforating arteries (*Dir.Perf.A.*) enter the brainstem immediately, whereas circumflex arteries travel some distance around the brainstem before entering it. Short circumflex arteries (*S.Circ.A.*) travel less than 90 around the brainstem before entering, whereas long circumflex arteries (*L.Circ.A.*) travel as much as 180 around the brainstem before they perforate it. *A.I.C.A.,* anterior inferior cerebellar artery; *S.C.A.,* superior cerebellar artery; *Roman numerals* refer to specific cranial nerves. (From Lister JR, Rhoton AL Jr, Matsushima T, et al. Microsurgic anatomy of the posterior inferior cerebellar artery. Neurosurgery *10:*170–199, 1982.) *B,* View of tip of the basilar artery shows multiple direct perforating vessels entering the ventral surface of the brainstem. Note also direct perforating vessels originating from the superior cerebellar artery (*S.C.A.*). *Ped.,* cerebral peduncle; *P-1,* P-1 segment of the posterior cerebral artery. (From Saeki N, Rhoton AL Jr. Microsurgic anatomy of the upper basilar artery and the posterior circle of Willis. J Neurosurg *46:*563–578, 1977.)

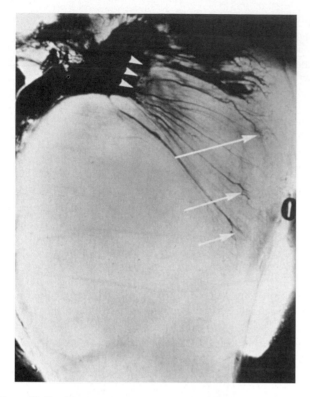

Figure 52.61. Blood supply to ocular motor nuclei and the medial longitudinal fasciculus. Sagittal section of brainstem with mesencephalon above and pons below. Perforating arteries (*arrowheads*) begin ventrally and course dorsally to supply the oculomotor nuclei (*long arrow*), trochlear nuclei (*medium arrow*), and the medial longitudinal fasciculus (*short white arrow*). India ink injection. (Courtesy of Dr. S. Shafey. University of Miami School of Medicine.)

nuclear complex, and all of the structures of the upper pontine tegmentum (Lang, 1991).

Superficial Branches of the Basilar Artery

The superficial arteries that arise from the basilar artery are unpredictable in number and location. Nevertheless, the main branches are the anterior inferior cerebellar arteries (AICA), the internal auditory arteries, the trigeminal arteries, the superior cerebellar arteries, and the terminal posterior cerebral arteries.

ANTERIOR INFERIOR CEREBELLAR ARTERY (AICA)

Each AICA usually arises as a single vessel, but in some persons, there may be two or even three such vessels on one or both sides (Stopford, 1916a and b; Sunderland, 1948; Naidich et al., 1976a and b; Salamon and Huang, 1976; Martin et al., 1980; Heimans et al., 1985) (Figs. 52.53*A*, 52.54*C*, 52.55*A* and *C*, 52.56*A*, and 52.62). In rare patients, the AICA may be absent on one or both sides (Salamon and Huang, 1976).

The AICA usually originates from the proximal third of the basilar artery and then courses around the pons toward the cerebellopontine angle (Fig. 52.63). Its proximal portion occasionally is in contact with the trigeminal nerve and may even distort it (Klun and Prestor, 1986). More often, however, the proximal portion of the AICA passes caudal to the trigeminal nerve and lies in contact with the ***abducens nerve*** (Cushing, 1910; Martin et al., 1980; Perneczky, 1981; Shrontz et al., 1986) (Figs. 52.62*A*, 52.63, and 52.64). The precise relationship of the AICA to the abducens nerve depends on the distance between the pontomedullary sulcus and the point at which the artery crosses the nerve (Naidich et al., 1976a). When the crossing is within 6 mm of the pontomedullary sulcus, the artery is adjacent to the ventral

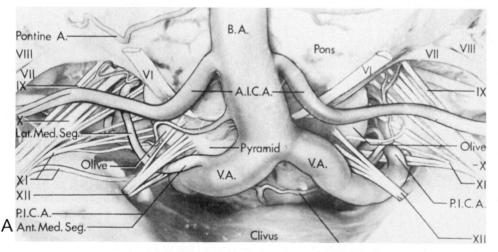

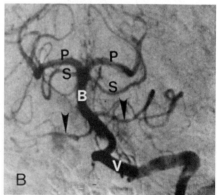

Figure 52.62. Origin of the anterior inferior cerebellar artery. *A,* The anterior inferior cerebellar arteries (*A.I.C.A.*) arise from the proximal third of the basilar artery (*B.A.*) and course under the abducens nerves (*VI*) around the pons toward the cerebellopontine angle. *P.I.C.A.,* posterior inferior cerebellar artery. *Roman numerals* refer to specific cranial nerves. (From Lister JR, Rhoton AL Jr, Matsushima T, et al. Microsurgic anatomy of the posterior inferior cerebellar artery. Neurosurgery *10:*170–199, 1982.) *B,* Cerebral arteriogram, anteroposterior view, showing origin of the anterior inferior cerebellar arteries (*arrowheads*) from the proximal third of the basilar artery (*B*). Note that the left anterior inferior cerebellar artery is larger and more developed than is the right artery. *P,* Posterior cerebral artery; *S,* Superior cerebellar artery; *V,* Vertebral artery.

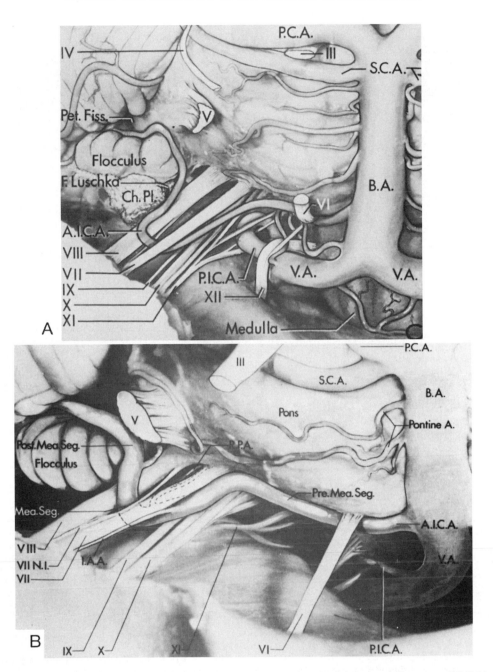

Figure 52.63. Course of anterior inferior cerebellar artery around brainstem. *A,* The anterior inferior cerebellar artery (*A.I.C.A.*) originates from the proximal third of the basilar artery (*B.A.*), passes under the abducens nerve (*VI*), and courses around the pons, passing between the facial (*VII*) and vestibulocochlear (*VIII*) nerves on its way to the cerebellopontine angle. *P.C.A.,* posterior cerebral artery; *S.C.A.,* superior cerebellar artery; *V.A.,* vertebral artery. *Roman numerals* refer to specific cranial nerves. (From Lister JR, Rhoton AL Jr, Matsushima T, et al. Microsurgic anatomy of the posterior inferior cerebellar artery. Neurosurgery *10:*170–199, 1982.) *B,* The anterior inferior cerebellar artery (*A.I.C.A.*) originates at the junction between the vertebral (*V.A.*) and basilar (*B.A.*) arteries. It passes under the abducens nerve, courses around the pons, and passes into the cerebellopontine angle with the facial nerve (*VII*) and the nervus intermedius (*VII N.I.*) on one side and the vestibulocochlear nerve (*VIII*) on the other. *P.C.A.,* posterior cerebral artery; *P.I.C.A.,* posterior inferior cerebellar artery; *R.P.A.,* recurrent perforating arteries; *S.C.A.,* superior cerebellar artery. *Roman numerals* refer to specific cranial nerves. (From Martin RG, Grant JL, Peace D, et al. Microsurgic relationship, of the anterior inferior cerebellar artery and the facial-vestibulocochlear nerve complex. Neurosurgery *6:*483–507, 1980.)

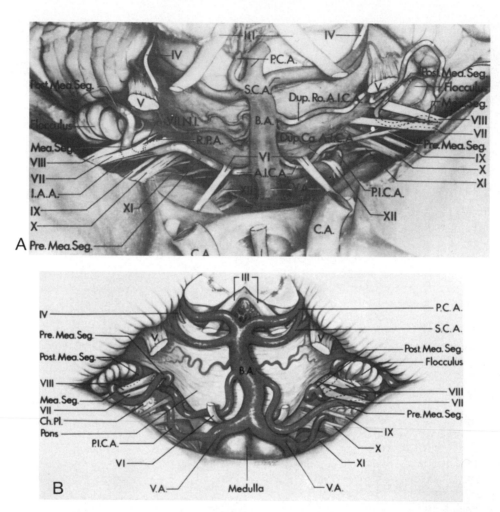

Figure 52.64. Relationships of anterior inferior cerebellar artery to abducens nerve. *A,* View of ventral brainstem shows right anterior inferior cerebellar artery (*A.I.C.A.*) passing caudal to abducens nerve (*VI*). The left anterior inferior cerebellar artery exists as two vessels, a rostral artery (*Dup.Ro.A.I.C.A.*), which passes just beneath the trigeminal nerve (*V*), and a caudal artery (*Dup.Ca.A.I.C.A.*) that passes just beneath the left abducens nerve. *B,* Drawing of the vertebrobasilar arterial system and its primary superficial branches. The anterior inferior cerebellar artery is separated into premeatal (*Pre.Mea.Seg.*), meatal (*Mea.Seg.*), and postmeatal (*Post.Mea.Seg.*) segments. Note that the premeatal segment of the right anterior inferior cerebellar artery passes rostral to the abducens nerve (*VI*), whereas the premeatal segment of the left anterior inferior cerebellar artery passes caudal to the nerve. *B.A.,* basilar artery; *C.A.,* internal carotid artery; *I.A.A.,* internal auditory artery; *P.C.A.,* posterior cerebral artery; *P.I.C.A.,* posterior inferior cerebellar artery; *R.P.A.,* recurrent perforating arteries; *S.C.A.,* superior cerebellar artery; *Roman numerals* refer to specific cranial nerves. (From Martin RG, Grant JL, Peace D, et al. Microsurgic relationships of the anterior inferior cerebellar artery and the facial-vestibulocochlear nerve complex. Neurosurgery *6:*483–507, 1980.)

aspect of the nerve. When the crossing is 6–8 mm from the sulcus, the artery may be in contact with either the ventral or the dorsal aspect of the nerve. When the crossing is 8–11 mm from the sulcus, the artery is always adjacent to the dorsal aspect of the nerve, and when the AICA is more than 11 mm rostral to the sulcus, it does not come in contact with the nerve. In rare cases, the nerve is actually perforated by the artery (Cushing, 1910; von Mitterwallner, 1955).

After crossing the abducens nerve, the AICA passes toward the cerebellopontine angle, where it usually divides into a rostral and a caudal trunk. One or both of these trunks is usually in contact with the facial nerve, the vestibulocochlear nerve, or both (Figs. 52.63 and 52.64). Before, during, or after coming in contact with the facial-vestibulocochlear nerve complex, one or both of the trunks forms a loop on or adjacent to the surface of the pons or the cerebellar floccu-

lus. The trunks eventually terminate by penetrating the brainstem and cerebellum.

Many smaller vessels originate from the AICA and its main trunks, including one or more internal auditory (or labyrinthine) arteries, several recurrent perforating arteries (including the trigeminal arteries), choroidal arteries, a subarcuate artery, and, rarely, a cerebellosubarcuate artery (Martin et al., 1980; Heimans et al., 1985; Amarenco and Hauw, 1989; Marinković and Gibo, 1995; Brunsteins and Ferreri, 1995).

Internal Auditory (Labyrinthine) Arteries. These vessels may arise directly from the basilar artery (Cavatorti, 1908; Sunderland, 1945; Nager, 1954; Brunsteins and Ferreri, 1995), the AICA (Martin et al., 1980; Brunsteins and Ferreri, 1995), or both. Regardless of their origin, they enter the internal auditory canal to supply the bone and dura lining the canal and the nerves within the canal (Figs. 52.63*B* and 52.64*A*). They terminate by giving rise to small anterior vestibular, cochlear, and vestibulocochlear arteries that supply the organs of the inner ear (Nager, 1954; Fisch, 1968; Lang, 1991; Brunsteins and Ferreri, 1995).

Recurrent Perforating Arteries. These arteries send branches to the facial and vestibulocochlear nerves and to the portion of the brainstem surrounding the entry zone of these nerves (Lang, 1991) (Figs. 52.63*B* and 52.64*A*). They also send branches to: (*a*) the middle cerebellar peduncle and the adjacent part of the pons; (*b*) the region of the pons around the entry zone of the trigeminal nerve; (*c*) the choroid plexus of the cerebellopontine angle; (*d*) the dorsolateral medulla; and (*e*) the glossopharyngeal (9th) and vagus (10th) nerves (Lang, 1991). Some of these vessels penetrate the brainstem immediately after originating from the AICA (direct branches), whereas others travel for a variable distance around the brainstem before they enter it (circumflex branches). Some authors refer to the branches of the AICA that supply the trigeminal nerve root as "the trigeminal arteries" (Watt and McKillop, 1935; Marinković and Gibo, 1995). These vessels commonly originate directly from the basilar artery (see below). Rarely, they arise from the superior cerebellar artery (Marinković and Gibo, 1995).

Choroidal Arteries. These vessels usually arise from the main trunk of the AICA or from its caudal trunk (Fujii et al., 1980a and b). They supply the portion of the choroid plexus in the cerebellopontine angle and the adjacent part of the lateral recess of the 4th ventricle.

Subarcuate Artery. The subarcuate artery usually originates from a branch of the AICA medial to the porus acusticus internus. It then penetrates the dura covering the subarcuate fossa and enters the subarcuate canal, where it supplies the mastoid in the region of the semicircular canals.

Cerebellosubarcuate Artery. In some persons, a small branch of the AICA divides into two smaller branches. One of the branches supplies the subarcuate fossa, and the other branch supplies the cerebellar flocculus and the adjacent inferior cerebellar cortex.

Internal Auditory Arteries. As noted above, the AICA gives rise to one or more vessels that enter the internal auditory canal and therefore were named internal auditory arteries by Martin et al. (1980). Nevertheless, larger arteries that enter the canal to supply its bone and dura, as well as the neural structures within, may directly originate from the basilar artery (Cavatorti, 1908; Stopford, 1916a and b).

Trigeminal Arteries. The trigeminal arteries are small vessels that supply the trigeminal nerve root. They arise most often from the superolateral pontine branch of the basilar artery and from the peduncular cerebellar branch of the anterior inferior cerebellar artery (Marinković and Gibo, 1995). The number of trigeminal arteries varies from two to six, and they often form a vascular ring around the nerve root.

SUPERIOR CEREBELLAR ARTERY

The superior cerebellar artery arises from the basilar artery near its apex (Figs. 52.32, 52.48*B*, 52.53, 52.55, 52.56*A*, 52.60, 52.62*B*, 52.63–52.65). The course of the superior cer-

ebellar artery is the most constant of all the major and minor branches of the vertebrobasilar arterial system, usually following a line around the upper pons in a horizontal plane (Heimans et al., 1985; Shrontz et al., 1986; Amarenco and Hauw, 1989) (Fig. 52.65). Although it usually arises as a single vessel, the superior cerebellar artery may arise as a double vessel on one or both sides (Tulleken and Luiten, 1987) (Fig. 52.54*D*), and it almost always divides into a rostral and a caudal trunk (Hardy et al., 1980; Shrontz et al., 1986) (Fig. 52.65*A* and *C*). The bifurcation may occur at any point along the course of the vessel, but it occurs most often near the point of maximum descent of the artery on the lateral side of the brainstem. Salamon and Huang (1976) found that the bifurcation was ventral to the brainstem in 30% of cases and lateral to it in 70%.

Either as one or two vessels, the superior cerebellar artery encircles the brainstem near the pontomesencephalic junction, passing below the oculomotor and trochlear nerves and above the trigeminal nerve (Saeki and Rhoton, 1977; Hardy et al., 1980; Amarenco and Hauw, 1989) (Fig. 52.66). In many persons, the trigeminal nerve is in contact with the main artery or one of its trunks, but it is uncommon for such contact to distort the nerve (Hardy and Rhoton, 1978; Klun and Prestor, 1986). Although the superior cerebellar artery is rarely in contact with either the oculomotor or trochlear nerves, Milisavljevic et al. (1986a) described a case in which the right trochlear nerve exited the brainstem as two bundles separated by the main trunk of the superior cerebellar artery (Fig. 52.67). Proximally, the main artery and its rostral and caudal trunks are usually medial to the free edge of the tentorium cerebelli, although Blinkov et al. (1992) described a mediolateral variant in which the main trunk or a lateral secondary trunk crossed beneath the free edge of the tentorium in the medial incisural space and then proceeded in a lateral direction. Distally, the superior cerebellar artery and its branches pass below the tentorium.

After passing the trigeminal nerve, the superior cerebellar artery, either as one or two vessels, enters the precerebellar fissure (cerebellomesencephalic groove), between the dorsal surface of the mesencephalon and the anterosuperior part of the cerebellum (Figs. 52.65 and 52.66). It then divides into numerous terminal branches that supply the superior cerebellar cortex (Hardy et al., 1980; Amarenco and Hauw, 1989).

The superior cerebellar artery and its trunks give rise to a number of smaller arteries that supply the brainstem and cerebellum (Amarenco and Hauw, 1989). These smaller arteries are usually classified as perforating, cortical, or precerebellar arteries (Hardy et al., 1980).

Like the perforating arteries that arise from the basilar, posterior inferior cerebellar, and anterior inferior cerebellar arteries, the perforating arteries that originate from the superior cerebellar artery may be separated into direct and circumflex types. Direct perforating arteries have a straight course and immediately penetrate the brainstem. Circumflex arteries course around the brainstem before terminating within it (Figs. 52.65*C* and 52.66). Short circumflex arteries travel less than 90 around the circumference of the brainstem, whereas long circumflex arteries may reach the dorsal surface of the brainstem before they terminate. Both types

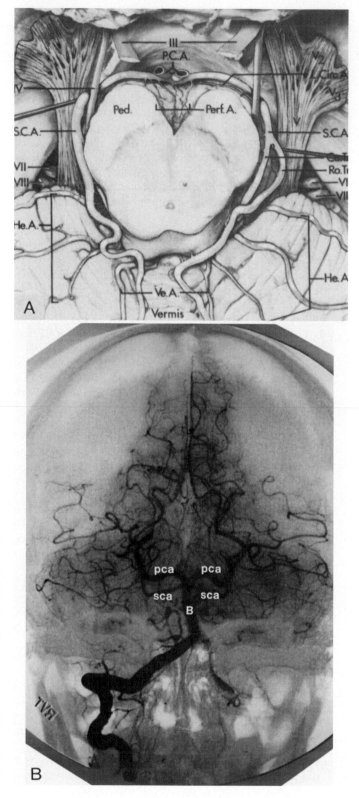

Figure 52.65. The origin and course of the superior cerebellar arteries. *A,* The superior cerebellar arteries (*S.C.A.*) originate from the basilar artery just below its terminal division into the two posterior cerebral arteries (*P.C.A.*). The arteries course directly around the mesencephalon passing caudal to the oculomotor (*III*) trochear (*IV*) nerves. About halfway around the brainstem, each artery usually divides into two trunks, called the rostral (*Ro.Tr.*) and caudal (*Ca.Tr.*) trunks. They then continue around to the dorsal aspect of the brainstem, at which point they enter the precerebellar fissure (cerebello-mesencephalic groove), between the dorsal surface of the mesencephalon and the anterosuperior part of the cerebellum. Both arteries then divide into numerous terminal branches that supply the superior surface and vermis of the cerebellum. These terminal vessels include the hemispheric arteries (*He.A.*) and the vermian arteries (*Ve.A.*). *V,* trigeminal nerve; *V₁,* ophthalmic division of the trigeminal nerve; *V₂,* maxillary division of the trigeminal nerve; *V₃,* mandibular division of the trigeminal nerve; *VII,* facial nerve; *VIII,* vestibulocochlear nerve. (From Hardy DG, Peace DA, Rhoton AL Jr. Microsurgic anatomy of the superior cerebellar artery. Neurosurgery 6:10–28, 1980.) *B,* Vertebral arteriogram, anteroposterior view, shows origin and initial course of the superior cerebellar arteries (*sca*). Note that these vessels arise from the basilar artery (*B*) just inferior to its terminal division into the two posterior cerebral arteries (*pca*).

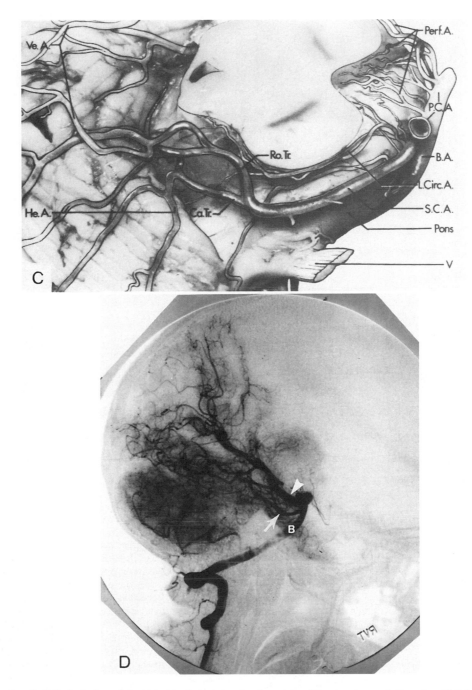

Figure 52.65. *(continued) C,* Sagittal view of the rostral brainstem showing the origin of the superior cerebellar artery (*S.C.A.*) from the basilar artery (*B.A.*) just below its division into the two posterior cerebral arteries (*P.C.A.*). Note the horizontal course of the superior cerebellar artery around the mesencephalon and its division into a rostral (*Ro.Tr.*) and a caudal (*Ca.Tr.*) trunk. Terminal branches of the superior cerebellar artery include the vermian (*Ve.A.*) and hemispheric (*He.A.*) arteries. This illustration shows several long circumflex arteries (*L.Circ.A.*) originating from the superior cerebellar artery. It also shows numerous perforating arteries (*Perf.A.*) originating from the tip of the basilar artery and the proximal segments of the posterior cerebral arteries. *V,* trigeminal nerve. (From Hardy DG, Peace DA, Rhoton AL Jr. Microsurgic anatomy of the superior cerebellar artery. Neurosurgery *6:*10–28, 1980.) *D,* Vertebral arteriogram, lateral view, shows origin of the superior cerebellar artery (*arrow*) from the basilar artery just below the origin of the posterior cerebral arteries (*arrowhead*). Note the horizontal course of the vessel as it passes posteriorly around the brainstem.

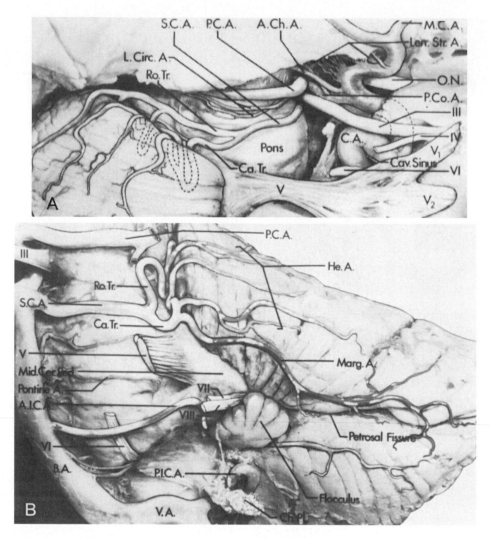

Figure 52.66. The origin and course of the superior cerebellar artery. *A,* Lateral view of the pontomesencephalic junction shows that the course of the superior cerebellar artery (*S.C.A.*) is roughly parallel to that of the posterior cerebral artery (*P.C.A.*). It passes caudal to the oculomotor nerve (*III*), and its caudal trunk (*Ca.Tr.*) is in contact with the trigeminal nerve (*V*). *A.Ch.A.,* anterior choroidal artery; *C.A.,* internal carotid artery; *L.Circ.A.,* long circumflex arteries; *Len.Str.A.,* lenticulostriate arteries; *M.C.A.,* middle cerebral artery; *P.Co.A.,* posterior communicating artery; *Ro.Tr.,* rostral trunk of the superior cerebellar artery; *O.N.,* optic nerve; *V₁,* ophthalmic division of the trigeminal nerve; *V₂,* maxillary division of the trigeminal nerve; *IV,* trochlear nerve. *B,* Lateral view of the pons shows the origin of the superior cerebellar artery (*S.C.A.*) from the basilar artery (*B.A.*). The artery continues around the brainstem for a short distance before dividing into a rostral trunk (*Ro.Tr.*) and a caudal trunk (*Ca.Tr.*), both of which give rise to terminal hemispheric arteries (*He.A.*), marginal arteries (*Marg.A.*), and vermian arteries (not shown). Note that the course of this artery parallels the courses of the posterior cerebral (*P.C.A.*) and anterior inferior cerebellar (*A.I.C.A.*) arteries. *P.I.C.A.,* posterior inferior cerebellar artery; *V.A.,* vertebral artery; *Mid.Cer.Ped.,* middle cerebellar peduncle; *Ch.Pl.,* choroid plexus; *Roman numerals* refer to specific cranial nerves. (From Hardy DG, Peace DA, Rhoton AL Jr. Microsurgic anatomy of the superior cerebellar artery. Neurosurgery 6:10–28, 1980.)

of circumflex arteries send branches into the brainstem along their course.

According to Hardy et al. (1980), the main superior cerebellar artery gives off up to six perforating branches. These branches are usually of the long circumflex type, but they also may be direct or short circumflex. Over half of these vessels terminate in the tegmentum near the junction between the superior and middle cerebellar peduncles, whereas the remainder terminate in the interpeduncular fossa (usually the direct type), the cerebral peduncle, and the collicular region.

Perforating branches from the rostral and caudal trunks of the superior cerebellar artery are most often circumflex. As many as 10 branches may arise from the rostral trunk, and up to 6 branches may arise from the caudal trunk. These vessels course around the brainstem to reach two main areas: the region of the junction of the superior and middle cerebellar peduncles and the quadrigeminal area.

The cortical branches of the superior cerebellar artery are divided into hemispheric, vermian, and marginal arteries (Figs. 52.65 and 52.66). The hemispheric arteries arise from the rostral and caudal trunks in the depths of the precerebel-

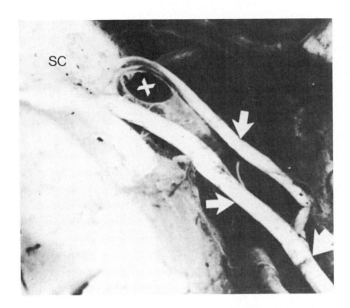

Figure 52.67. Caudal view of right trochlear nerve (*large arrow*) that arises as two separate bundles (*small arrows*) between which runs the superior cerebellar artery (*x*). *SC,* right inferior colliculus. (From Milisavljević M, Marinković S, Lolić-Draganić V, et al. Oculomotor, trochlear, and abducens nerves penetrated by cerebral vessels: Microanatomy and possible clinical significance. Arch Neurol *43:*58–61, 1986.)

lar fissure. They give rise to the precerebellar arteries (see below) and then supply a portion of the tentorium cerebelli and the tentorial surface of the cerebellar hemispheres lateral to the vermis (Ono et al., 1984a). The vermian arteries arise from the rostral trunk of the superior cerebellar artery within the precerebellar fissure. They supply the cerebellar vermis. The marginal artery is found in about half of normal persons. It arises from the proximal superior cerebellar artery as the first cortical branch and supplies the region of the horizontal cerebellar fissure. The cortical arteries are the terminal branches of the superior cerebellar artery. They anastomose with branches of the anterior and posterior inferior cerebellar arteries of both ipsilateral and contralateral sides. Krayenbühl and Yaşargil (1957) called this vascular network the "hemispherical plexus."

Precerebellar arteries arise from the hemispheric and vermian arteries within the precerebellar fissure. They supply the deep cerebellar nuclei, the inferior colliculi, and the superior medullary velum. Rarely, the superior cerebellar artery gives rise to a choroidal artery that supplies a portion of the choroid plexus in the 4th ventricle. Fujii et al. (1980b) found such a vessel in only one of 25 brains that they examined.

POSTERIOR CEREBRAL ARTERY AND ITS BRANCHES

Each of the two posterior cerebral arteries supplies not only the posterior part of the ipsilateral cerebral hemisphere, as its name implies, but also sends important branches to the thalamus, mesencephalon, and other deep structures, including the splenium of the corpus callosum and the walls and choroid plexus of the lateral and 3rd ventricles (Margolis et al., 1974; Zeal and Rhoton, 1978; Hebel and von Cramon,

1987; Marinković et al., 1987). The posterior cerebral artery arises in the embryo as a branch of the ipsilateral internal carotid artery, but by birth, its most frequent origin is from the basilar artery as its terminal branch (Williams, 1936; Padget, 1948). Nevertheless, in about 20% of normal patients, the posterior cerebral artery retains its origin from the internal carotid artery (von Mitterwallner, 1955) (Figs. 52.34 and 52.68). Although most persons have well-developed, symmetric posterior cerebral arteries, in about 25% of cases, one or both vessels is abnormally thin or rudimentary (Tulleken and Luiten, 1987).

Several different classifications of the parts of the posterior cerebral artery have been proposed (Percheron, 1976a; Zeal and Rhoton, 1978). The initial segment of the vessel between its origin and the posterior communicating artery is usually called the **P-1** segment (Krayenbühl and Yaşargil, 1968, 1973; Saeki and Rhoton, 1977), the basilar communicating artery (Percheron, 1976a), or the mesencephalic artery (Kaplan and Ford, 1966) (Fig. 52.69). This vessel is usually 3–9 mm long (Lang, 1985). The remainder of the posterior cerebral artery, which may be separated into two or three segments (called the P-2–P-4 segments), initially lies within the peduncular and ambient cisterns superior to the tentorium cerebelli as it courses around the mesencephalon (Blinkov et al., 1992) (Figs. 52.70 and 52.71). It then proceeds posteriorly from the pulvinar in the lateral aspect of the quadrigeminal cistern to the anterior limit of the calcarine fissure (Figs. 52.70–52.73). This course is usually straight, although the vessel occasionally has a looping cephalic course that causes it to pass high under the medial temporal lobe (Shrontz et al., 1986).

The posterior cerebral artery gives rise to three types of branches (Milisavljevic et al., 1986b):

1. Central branches to the brainstem;
2. Ventricular branches to the choroid plexus and walls of the lateral and third ventricles and adjacent structures; and
3. Terminal branches to the cerebral cortex and splenium of the corpus callosum. These branches form an extensive anastomotic network among themselves and with terminal vessels from other major intracranial arteries.

Central Branches. The central branches that arise from the posterior cerebral artery and enter the brainstem are divided into two groups as are similar branches from other major arteries in the vertebrobasilar system: direct and circumflex. The direct perforating branches arise from the parent trunk and pass directly into the brainstem. This group includes the **thalamoperforating** or **interpeduncular arteries**, the **thalamogeniculate arteries**, and the **peduncular perforating arteries**.

Thalamoperforating arteries arise from both the posterior communicating artery and the posterior cerebral artery (Figs. 52.32, 52.36, and 52.69). As noted above, thalamoperforating arteries that arise from the posterior communicating artery are called **anterior** thalamoperforating arteries, the largest of which is the **premammillary artery** (Figs. 52.32*A*

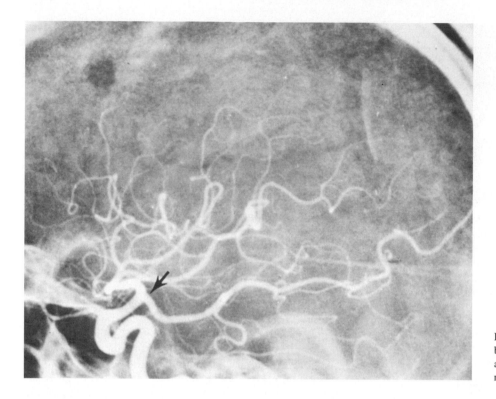

Figure 52.68. Origin of the posterior cerebral artery (*arrow*) from the internal carotid artery in a patient with occlusion of the anterior cerebral artery.

and 52.69*B*). One of these arteries, the **anterior thalamo-subthalamic paramedian artery**, supplies the anterior region of the thalamus, including the ventral anterior nucleus and part of the ventral lateral nucleus. This vessel is often called the polar artery of Percheron (Percheron, 1973, 1976b) (Fig. 52.74). Similar vessels that arise from the posterior cerebral artery are called by a variety of names, including **posterior thalamoperforating arteries**, **paramedian thalamic arteries**, and **interpeduncular arteries** (Percheron, 1973, 1976a and b, 1977; Zeal and Rhoton, 1978; Marinković et al., 1986a; Pedroza et al., 1986). Almost all of these arteries arise from the P-1 segment of the posterior cerebral artery (Zeal and Rhoton, 1978; Marinković et al., 1986a; Pedroza et al., 1986; Tulleken and Luiten, 1987) (Fig. 52.75). The most important of these arteries, the posterior thalamosubthalamic paramedian artery, supplies the paramedian part of the rostral mesencephalon and thalamus, including the intralaminar nuclear group and most of the dorsomedial nucleus (Percheron, 1976a) (Fig. 52.74).

All of the **thalamoperforating arteries**, regardless of the major artery from which they arise, enter the brain through the posterior perforated substance, interpeduncular fossa, and medial surface of the cerebral peduncles. They supply all of the anterior and part of the posterior thalamus. They also supply the hypothalamus, subthalamus, substantia nigra, red nucleus, oculomotor and trochlear nuclei, proximal part of the oculomotor nerve, mesencephalic reticular formation, pretectum, rostromedial floor of the 4th ventricle, and the posterior portion of the internal capsule (Plets et al., 1970; Percheron, 1973, 1976a and b, 1977; Marinković et al., 1986a; Pedroza et al., 1986; Lang, 1991; Cahill et al., 1996).

Marinković et al. (1986b) observed extensive intraparen-

chymal anastomoses among (*a*)branches of a single thalamoperforating artery, (*b*) thalamoperforating arteries from the same posterior cerebral artery, (*c*) thalamoperforating arteries and branches of the basilar and superior cerebellar arteries on the same side, and (*d*) thalamoperforating arteries on one side and various contralateral arteries (Fig. 52.76).

From two to 12 **thalamogeniculate arteries** arise either individually or from a common stem directly from the posterior cerebral artery (usually from the P-2 segment) beneath the lateral thalamus. They perforate the inferior surface of the geniculate bodies to supply the posterior half of the lateral thalamus, the posterior limb of the internal capsule, and the optic tract (Milisavljević et al., 1991) (Fig. 52.77). These vessels typically anastomose with the posterior thalamoperforating arteries, and they may also anastomose with the medial posterior choroidal artery, mesencephalothalamic artery, or both.

Peduncular perforating branches of the posterior cerebral artery arise from the segment of the artery just distal to its junction with the posterior communicating artery. As many as six vessels (Zeal and Rhoton, 1978) supply the corticospinal tract and corticobulbar pathways as well as the substantia nigra, red nucleus, and other structures of the mesencephalic tegmentum. Anastomoses among these vessels are common (Milisavljevic et al., 1986b). These branches may supply the interpeduncular portion of the oculomotor nerve (Dreyfus et al., 1957; Lang, 1991) and may even perforate it (Milisavljevic et al., 1986a) (Fig. 52.78).

The circumflex arteries that arise from the posterior cerebral artery, like those from other arteries in the vertebrobasilar arterial system, are divided into short and long types (Figs. 52.75*A* and 52.76). Short circumflex arteries pass only

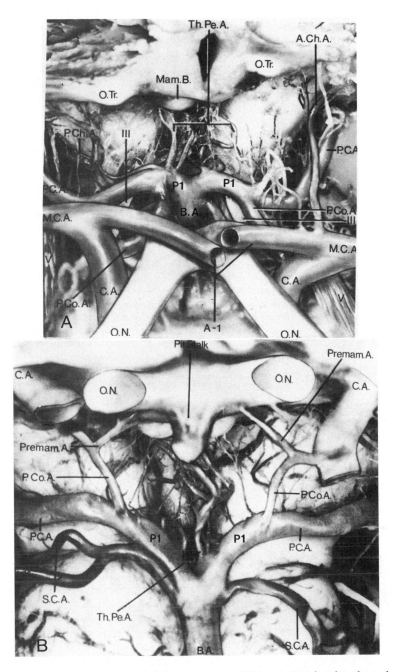

Figure 52.69. Two views of the P-1 segment (*P1*) of the posterior cerebral artery (*P.C.A.*). *A,* Anterior view shows the two posterior cerebral arteries arising from the basilar artery (*B.A.*). The left P-1 segment is longer than the right. Note the thalamoperforating arteries (*Th.Pe.A.*) that arise from these segments. Also note the right posterior choroidal artery (*P.Ch.A.*) arising from the right P-1 segment near its junction with the posterior communicating artery (*P.Co.A.*). *B,* Posterior view shows the two posterior cerebral arteries arising as the terminal bifurcation of the basilar artery. Note the relationship of the P-1 segments to the superior cerebellar arteries (*S.C.A.*). Again note perforating arteries arising from the P-1 segments, including the thalamoperforating arteries. *A-1,* A-1 segments of the anterior cerebral arteries; *A.Ch.A.,* anterior choroidal artery; *C.A.,* internal carotid artery; *M.C.A.,* middle cerebral artery; *Premam.A.,* premammillary artery; *Mam.B.,* mammillary body; *O.N.,* optic nerve; *O.Tr.,* optic tract; *III,* oculomotor nerve; *V,* trigeminal nerve. (From Rhoton AL Jr, Hardy DG, Chambers SM. Microsurgic anatomy and dissection of the sphenoid bone, cavernous sinus, and sellar region. Surg Neurol *12:* 63–104, 1979.)

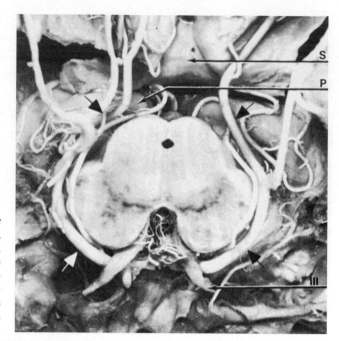

Figure 52.70. Cisternal segments of the posterior cerebral artery. The *short arrows* indicate the approximate site of junction of the peduncular, ambient, and quadrigeminal segments. *S,* splenium of the corpus callosum; *P,* pulvinar; *III,* oculomotor nerve. (From Margolis MT, Newton TH, Hoyt WF. The posterior cerebral artery. Anatomic, neuroradiologic, and neuro-ophthalmologic considerations. Part I. Gross and roentgenologic anatomy. In Neuro-Ophthalmology Symposium of the University of Miami and the Bascom Palmer Eye Institute. Editor, Smith JL, pp 162–192. Hallandale, FL, Huffman Publishing Co., 1970.)

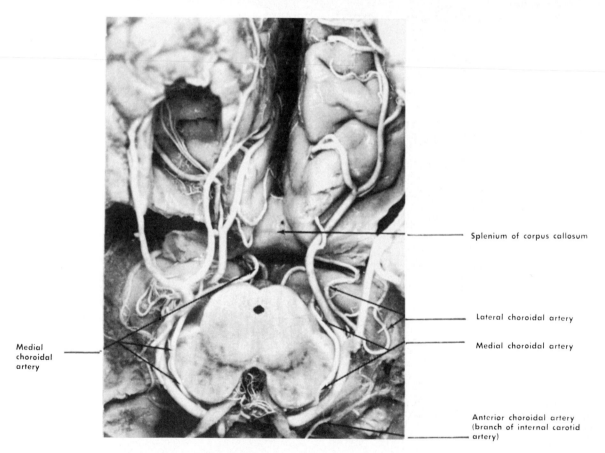

Figure 52.71. Origin and course of the posterior cerebral artery. The artery is viewed from beneath the brain in a posteroanterior direction. Note the courses of the medial and lateral choroidal arteries that arise from the posterior cerebral artery and their relationship to the anterior choroidal artery that arises from the internal carotid artery. (From Margolis MT, Newton TH, Hoyt WF. The posterior cerebral artery. Anatomic, neuroradiologic, and neuro-ophthalmologic considerations. Part 1. Gross and roentgenologic anatomy. In Neuro-Ophthalmology Symposium of the University of Miami and the Bascom Palmer Eye Institute. Editor, Smith JL, pp 162–192. Hallandale, FL, Huffman Publishing Co., 1970.)

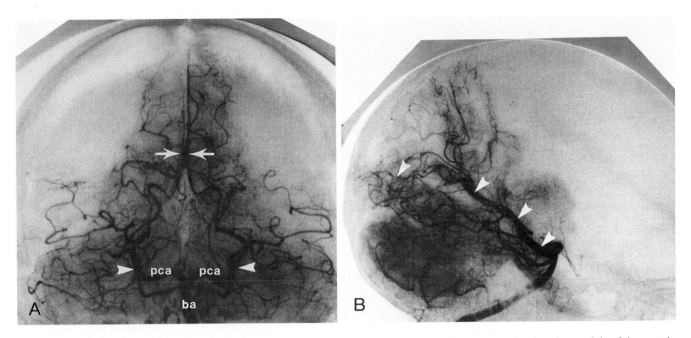

Figure 52.72. Cerebral arteriogram showing origin and course of the posterior cerebral arteries. *A,* Posteroanterior view shows origin of the posterior cerebral arteries *(pca)* from the basilar artery *(ba),* their course around the brainstem in the ambient cistern *(arrowheads),* and their termination in the cerebral cortex *(arrows). B,* Lateral view shows ascending course of the posterior cerebral artery *(arrowheads).*

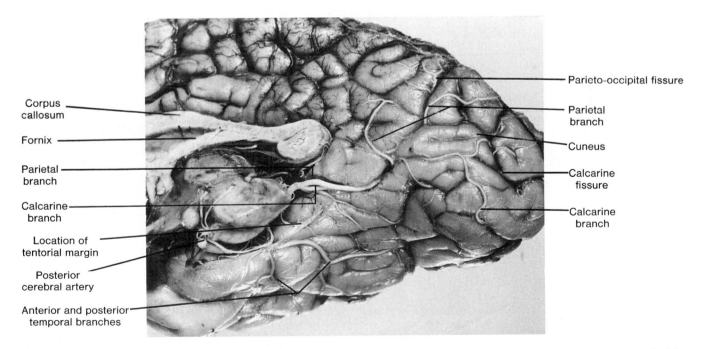

Figure 52.73. Lateral view of the posterior cerebral artery and its branches that supply the striate cortex. (From Lindenberg R, Walsh FB, Sacks JG. Neuropathology of Vision. Philadelphia, Lea & Febiger, 1973.)

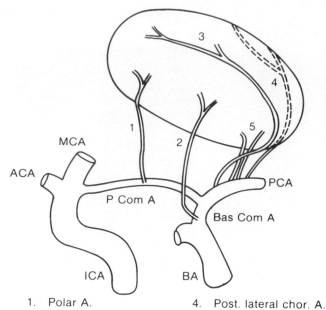

Figure 52.74. Blood supply of the thalamus, showing the contributions from the posterior communicating artery (*P Com A*) and the posterior cerebral artery (*PCA*). *Polar A*, polar artery; *Paramedian A*, paramedian artery; *Post. medial chor. A.*, posterior medial choroidal artery; *Post. lateral chor. A.*, posterior lateral choroidal artery; *ACA*, anterior cerebral artery; *BA*, basilar artery; *Bas Com A*, basilar communicating artery; *ICA*, internal carotid artery; *MCA*, middle cerebral artery. (From Biller J, Sand JJ, Corbett JJ, et al. Syndrome of the paramedian thalamic arteries: Clinical and neuroimaging correlation. J Clin Neuroophthalmol *5:*217–223, 1985.)

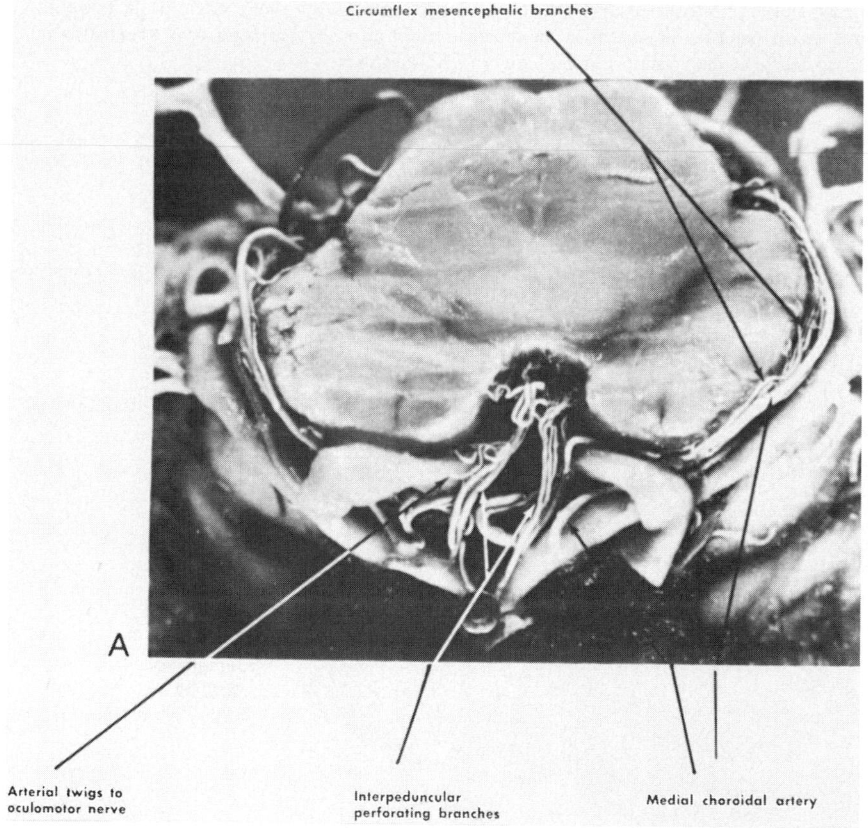

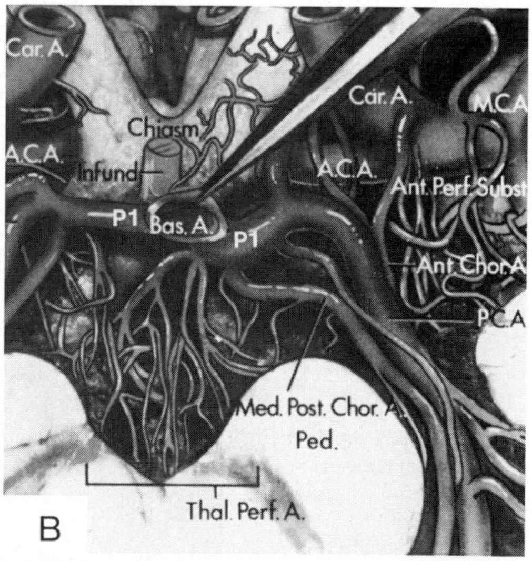

1. Polar A.
2. Paramedian A.
3. Post. medial chor. A.
4. Post. lateral chor. A.
5. Thalamogeniculate pedicle

Figure 52.75. Four views of the perforating arteries that originate from the P-1 (mesencephalic) segment of the posterior cerebral artery. *A,* In this photograph, both direct interpeduncular and circumflex perforating branches of the posterior cerebral artery are evident. Note arterial twigs to the interpeduncular portion of the oculomotor nerve. (From Margolis MT, Newton TH, Hoyt WF. The posterior cerebral artery. Anatomic, neuroradiologic, and neuro-ophthalmologic considerations. Part I. Gross and roentgenologic anatomy. In Neuro-Ophthalmology Symposium of the University of Miami and the Bascom Palmer Eye Institute. Editor, Smith JL, pp 162–192. Hallandale, FL., Huffman Publishing Co., 1970.) *B,* Photograph shows large number of thalamoperforating arteries (*Thal.Perf.A.*) originating from the P-1 segments (P1) of the posterior cerebral arteries (*P.C.A.*). Note the origin of the medial posterior choroidal artery (*Med.-Post.Chor.A.*). *A.C.A.,* anterior cerebral artery; *Ant.Chor.A.;* anterior choroidal artery; *Ant.Perf.Subst.,* anterior perforated substance; *Car.A.,* internal carotid artery; *Infund.,* infundibulum; *M.C.A.,* middle cerebral artery; *Ped.,* cerebral peduncle. (From Ono M, Ono M, Rhoton AL Jr, et al. Microsurgic anatomy of the region of the tentorial incisura. J Neurosurg *60:*365–399, 1984.)

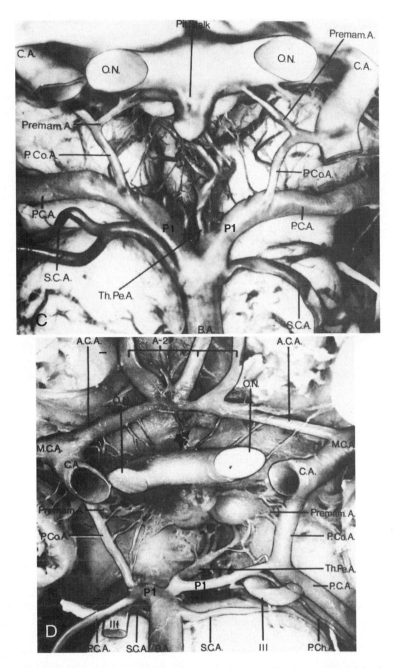

Figure 52.75. *(continued) C,* Posteroinferior view of the circle of Willis shows thalamoperforating arteries originating from the P-1 segments *(P1)* of the posterior cerebral arteries *(P.C.A.)*. Also note the origin of the premammillary arteries *(Premam.A.)* from the posterior communicating arteries *(P.Co.A.)*. These vessels supply the ventral surface of the optic nerves *(O.N.)*, optic chiasm, and optic tracts. *D,* View of the circle of Willis in another specimen shows that the right P-1 segment *(P1)* of the posterior cerebral artery *(P.C.A.)* gives rise to a single large thalamoperforating artery *(Th.Pe.A.)* that subsequently gives rise to numerous arteries that supply the thalamus and mammillary bodies. *A.C.A.,* anterior cerebral artery; *A-2,* A-2 segments of the anterior cerebral arteries; *B.A.,* basilar artery; *C.A.,* internal carotid artery; *M.C.A.,* middle cerebral artery; *P.Ch.A.,* posterior choroidal artery; *S.C.A.,* superior cerebellar artery. (From Saeki N, Rhoton AL Jr. Microsurgic anatomy of the upper basilar artery and the posterior circle of Willis. J Neurosurg *46:*563–578, 1977.)

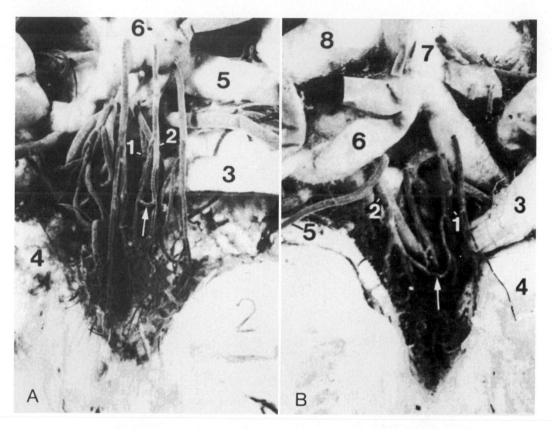

Figure 52.76.   Anastomoses among thalamoperforating arteries. *A,* Anastomosis (*arrow*) between thalamoperforating artery (*1*) arising from left posterior cerebral artery (*5*) and direct perforating mesencephalic branch (*2*) arising from the tip of the basilar artery (*6*). *3,* oculomotor nerve; *4,* cerebral peduncle. *B,* Anastomosis (*arrow*) between thalamoperforating branches from the right (*6*) and left posterior cerebral arteries. *1,* thalamoperforating artery arising from left posterior cerebral artery; *2,* thalamoperforating artery arising from right posterior cerebral artery; *3,* left oculomotor nerve; *4,* left cerebral peduncle; *5,* peduncular artery arising directly from P-1 segment of the right posterior cerebral artery; *7,* basilar artery; *8,* right optic tract. (From Marinković SV, Milisavljević MM, Kocacević MS. Anastomoses among the thalamoperforating branches of the posterior cerebral artery. Arch Neurol *43:*811–814, 1986.)

a short distance around the brainstem before entering it. They do not pass beyond the geniculate bodies. These vessels have also been called ''peduncular,'' ''mesencephalic,'' ''tegmental thalamoperforating,'' and ''perforating thalamic'' arteries (Zeal and Rhoton, 1978). Long circumflex arteries pass around the brainstem to supply the superior and inferior colliculi and surrounding structures. They have therefore been called the ''quadrigeminal arteries.'' They encircle the mesencephalon medial to the posterior cerebral artery and send five or more small rami to the ipsilateral cerebral peduncle, geniculate bodies, and, occasionally, the mesencephalic tegmentum. At least one of these vessels supplies the free edge of the tentorium cerebelli (Ono et al., 1984a). The terminal branches of the long circumflex arteries form an extensive network of vessels over the colliculi, where they anastomose with each other and with terminal branches of the superior cerebellar artery (Milisavljevic et al., 1986b).

Ventricular and Plexus Branches.   The two groups of branches from the posterior cerebral artery that enter the lateral and 3rd ventricles to supply the choroid plexus and ventricular walls are the medial and lateral posterior choroidal arteries (Margolis et al., 1969; Fujii et al., 1980a) (Figs. 52.71, 52.75, 52.77, 52.79, and 52.80). Extensive anastomo-

ses exist: (*a*) between branches from medial posterior choroidal arteries, lateral posterior choroidal arteries, or both on the same side; (*b*) between branches from the medial and lateral posterior choroidal arteries on the same side; and (*c*) between branches from the right and left medial posterior choroidal arteries, the lateral posterior choroidal arteries, or both (Milisavljevic et al., 1986b).

One or two **medial** posterior choroidal arteries arise from the posteromedial aspect of one of the segments of the posterior cerebral artery (usually the P-1 segment) or occasionally from one of its terminal branches, encircle the mesencephalon medial to the main trunk of the posterior cerebral artery, enter the roof of the 3rd ventricle between the thalami, and course through the foramen of Monro to enter the lateral ventricle (Figs. 52.71, 52.75, 52.77, 52.79, and 52.80). These vessels supply the choroid plexus in the roof of the 3rd ventricle and part of the choroid plexus in the body of the lateral ventricle (Fujii et al., 1980a; Tulleken and Luiten, 1987). Along their course, they also send branches to the cerebral peduncle, tegmentum of the mesencephalon, medial and lateral geniculate bodies, superior and inferior colliculi, pulvinar, pineal gland, and medial thalamus.

One to nine **lateral** posterior choroidal arteries also arise

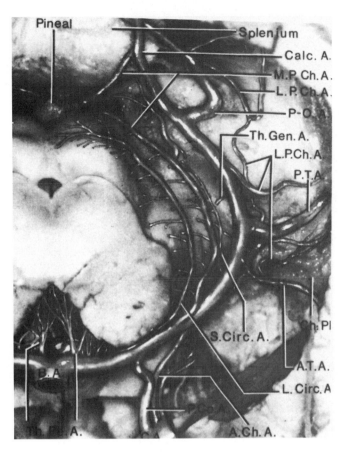

Figure 52.77. Inferior view of the origin of the right posterior cerebral artery from the basilar artery (*B.A.*) and its course around the mesencephalon. The medial part of the temporal lobe has been removed to expose the pulvinar and choroid plexus (*Ch.Pl.*) of the temporal horn. The central branches of the posterior cerebral artery include the thalamoperforating arteries (*Th.Pe.A.*), long circumflex (*L.Circ.A.*) and short circumflex (*S.Circ.A.*) arteries. The right anterior choroidal artery (*A.Ch.A.*) passes above the posterior cerebral artery to the choroidal plexus of the temporal horn. The thalamogeniculate arteries (*Th.Gen.A.*) penetrate the brain in the region of the geniculate bodies. The lateral posterior choroidal arteries (*L.P.Ch.A.*) can be traced into the temporal horn of the ventricle. Two medial posterior choroidal arteries (*M.P.Ch.A.*) are seen. One arises from the posterior cerebral artery, whereas the other arises from the calcarine artery (*Calc.A.*). An anterior temporal artery (*A.T.A.*) and a posterior temporal artery (*P.T.A.*) supply the temporal lobe. The terminal posterior cerebral artery bifurcates into the the parieto-occipital artery (*P-O.A.*) and the calcarine artery. *C.A.*, internal carotid artery; *P.Co.A.*, posterior communicating artery. (From Zeal AA, Rhoton AL Jr. Microsurgic anatomy of the posterior cerebral artery. J Neurosurg *48*:534–559, 1978.)

directly from the posterior cerebral artery but, just as often, they arise from one of its cortical branches (see below). These vessels pass laterally through the choroidal fissure and then upward over the pulvinar to enter the temporal horn, trigone, and body of the lateral ventricle, where they supply the choroid plexus in these areas (Figs. 52.71, 52.75, 52.77, 52.79, and 52.80). Some lateral posterior choroidal

arteries send branches to the ipsilateral cerebral peduncle, the posterior commissure, part of the body and anterior portion of the column of the fornix, the lateral geniculate body, the pulvinar, and the body of the caudate nucleus. Some of these arteries also anastomose with terminal branches of the anterior choroidal artery (Carpenter et al., 1954; Galatius-Jensen and Ringberg, 1963).

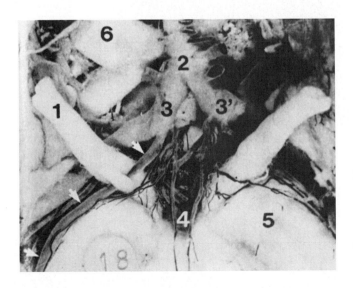

Figure 52.78. Ventral view of right oculomotor nerve (*1*) penetrated by long circumflex mesencephalic artery (*arrows*) originating from the right posterior cerebral artery (*3*). Note other direct and circumflex perforating branches (*4*) arising from the right and left (*3*) posterior cerebral arteries. *2*, basilar artery; *5*, left cerebral peduncle; *6*, right optic nerve. (From Milisavljević M, Marinković S, Lolić-Draganić V, et al. Oculomotor, trochlear, and abducens nerves penetrated by cerebral vessels: Microanatomy and possible clinical significance. Arch Neurol *43*:58–61, 1986.)

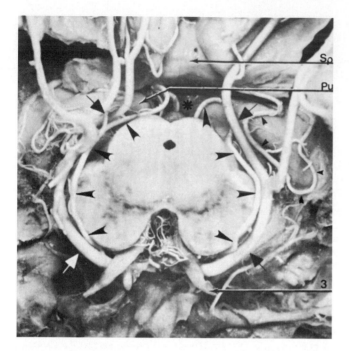

Figure 52.79. The origins and courses of the medial and lateral posterior choroidal arteries. Each medial posterior choroidal artery (*large arrowheads*) arises from the proximal segment of the posterior cerebral artery (*black and white arrows*) and encircles the mesencephalon medial to the main trunk of the posterior cerebral artery. The medial posterior choroidal artery then enters the roof of the 3rd ventricle between the thalami (*asterisk*), courses through the foramen of Monro, and enters the lateral ventricle. Each lateral posterior choroidal artery (*small arrowheads*) arises from a distal segment of the posterior cerebral artery, passes laterally over the choroidal fissure and then upward over the pulvinar (*Pu*) to enter the temporal horn, trigone, and body of the lateral ventricle. *Sp*, splenium of the corpus callosum; *3*, oculomotor nerve. (From Margolis MT, Newton TH, Hoyt WF. The posterior cerebral artery. Anatomic, neuroradiologic, and neuro-ophthalmologic considerations. Part I. Gross and roentgenologic anatomy. In Neuro-Ophthalmology Symposium of the University of Miami and the Bascom Palmer Eye Institute. Editor, Smith JL, pp 162–192. Hallandale, FL, Huffman Publishing Co., 1970.)

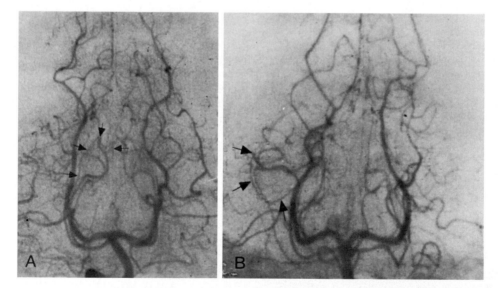

Figure 52.80. Cerebral arteriogram (Towne projection) showing course of the posterior choroidal arteries *(arrows)*. *A*, Course of the medial posterior choroidal artery is medial to the main trunk of the posterior cerebral artery. *B*, Course of the lateral posterior choroidal artery is lateral to the main trunk of the posterior cerebral artery.

CORTICAL BRANCHES OF POSTERIOR CEREBRAL A.
- COMMON VARIATIONS -

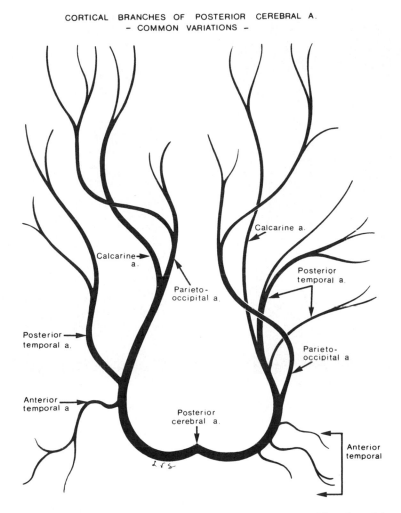

Figure 52.81. Schematic drawing of the common variations in the origin and course of the cortical branches of the posterior cerebral artery. (From Margolis MT, Newton TH, Hoyt WF. The posterior cerebral artery. Anatomic, neuroradiologic, and neuro-ophthalmologic considerations. Part I. Gross and roentgenologic anatomy. In Neuro-Ophthalmology Symposium of the University of Miami and the Bascom Palmer Eye Institute. Editor, Smith JL, pp 162–192. Hallandale, FL, Huffman Publishing Co., 1970.)

Cerebral Branches. The main cerebral branches of the posterior cerebral artery are the inferior temporal group of arteries, the parieto-occipital artery, and the calcarine artery (Margolis et al., 1974; Zeal and Rhoton, 1978; Marinković et al., 1987) (Figs. 52.73 and 52.81–52.83). Together these arteries supply most of the occipital lobe and portions of the parietal and temporal lobes (Figs. 52.84–52.87).

The **inferior temporal arteries** include the hippocampal artery and the anterior, middle, posterior, and common temporal arteries. These arteries supply mainly the inferior parts of the temporal lobe (Figs. 52.84 and 52.85). The posterior temporal artery also supplies the inferior surface of the occipital lobe as far posteriorly as the occipital pole (Zeal and Rhoton, 1978; Marinković et al., 1987). The common temporal artery (also called the lateral occipital or temporo to occipital artery) is present in 20–40% of normal brains and also supplies the inferior surface of the occipital lobe.

The **parieto-occipital artery**, one of the two main terminal branches of the posterior cerebral artery, usually arises in the calcarine sulcus and is almost always singular (Marinković et al., 1987) (Figs. 52.81–52.83). It enters the rostral portion of the calcarine sulcus and then continues along the parieto-occipital sulcus. During its course, it divides into two to four terminal stems, the branches of which are distributed to the medial and sometimes the lateral surface of the occipital and parietal lobes (Figs. 52.84 and 52.86). When the artery is large, it also supplies portions of the mesencephalon, thalamus, pulvinar, lateral geniculate bodies, and the splenium of the corpus callosum.

The **calcarine artery**, the second major terminal branch of the posterior cerebral artery, arises in the ambient or quadrigeminal cistern or in the proximal part of the calcarine sulcus (Figs. 52.81–52.83). It then enters the calcarine sulcus and runs along it, supplying its floor as well as its dorsal

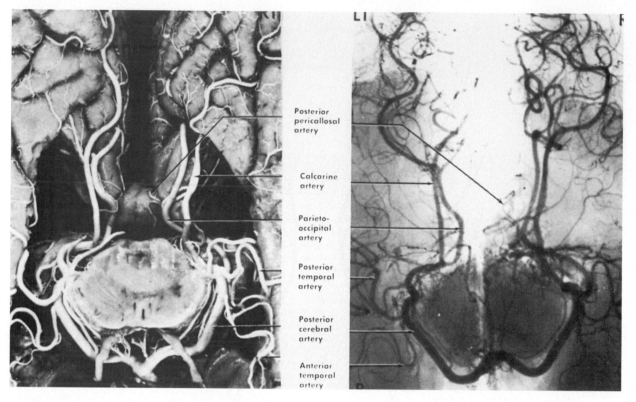

Figure 52.82. Cortical branches of the posterior cerebral artery. (From Margolis MT, Newton TH, Hoyt WF. The posterior cerebral artery. Anatomic, neuroradiologic, and neuro-ophthalmologic considerations. Part I. Gross and roentgenologic anatomy. In Neuro-Ophthalmology Symposium of the University of Miami and the Bascom Palmer Eye Institute. Editor, Smith JL, pp 162–192. Hallandale, FL, Huffman Publishing Co., 1970.)

and ventral banks (Figs. 52.84 and 52.87). It also supplies a variable portion of the cuneus and the lingual gyrus. In some persons, the calcarine artery supplies not only the medial surface, but also a small part of the lateral surface of the occipital lobe. Furuno et al. (1995) described a patient in whom the calcarine artery arose from the internal carotid artery.

LEPTOMENINGEAL ARTERIOLES

A leptomeningeal plexus of arterioles is interlaced over the entire surface of each cerebral hemisphere. This pial arteriolar plexus interconnects the supply areas of all the major cerebral arteries (Clark and Wentsler, 1938; Florey, 1925) (Fig. 52.88).

There are no capillaries in the pia mater. Penetrating arterioles from the pial plexus and from larger cortical arteries are 15–16 microns in diameter (Hyde, 1959). The smaller, shorter vessels provide a rich blood supply to the gray matter, whereas the larger, longer penetrating vessels supply the white matter. As might be expected, the gray matter, which has a higher metabolic rate, also has greater vascularity.

CIRCLE OF WILLIS

The basal arterial circle, first completely illustrated by Thomas Willis in 1664, forms a system of communications

between branches of the internal carotid and basilar arteries (Figs. 52.32, 52.75D, and 52.89). This circle is closed anteriorly by the anterior communicating artery and the proximal segments of both anterior cerebral arteries. Posteriorly, the circle is completed by the two posterior communicating arteries and the proximal segments of both posterior cerebral arteries. Under normal conditions, blood flow through the internal carotid arteries is so rapid that blood from each carotid system supplies each hemisphere without cross-flow from the opposite side. Similarly, the posterior cerebral circulation is normally maintained exclusively by the vertebrobasilar system.

There is substantial evidence that the circle of Willis is normally a potential rather than an actual source of collateral blood flow. Kramer (1912) injected methylene blue into the carotid and vertebral arteries of experimental animals and demonstrated that the dye did not pass from one arterial system into the other unless there was obstruction or reduced pressure on the side of the circle opposite the injection. Rogers (1947) suggested that flow around the circle of Willis is potential rather than actual because, like all anastomoses, it is capable of opening and providing a bypass if one of the main channels that it joins becomes occluded.

The circle of Willis usually is not symmetric. There is great variability in the length and diameter of the vessels that compose it, and anomalous circles are the rule rather than the exception (Padget, 1944; Alpers et al., 1959; Riggs

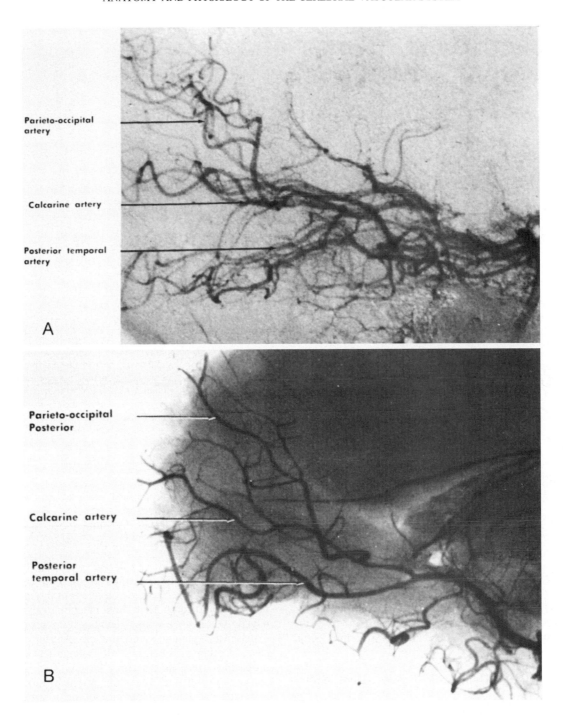

Figure 52.83.   Cerebral arteriogram, lateral view, showing cortical branches of the posterior cerebral artery. *A,* Normal patient. *B,* Injected specimen. (Compare with Figure 52.73.) (From Margolis MT, Newton TH, Hoyt WF. The posterior cerebral artery. Anatomic, neuroradiologic, and neuro-ophthalmologic considerations. Part I. Gross and roentgenologic anatomy. In Neuro-Ophthalmology Symposium of the University of Miami and the Bascom Palmer Eye Institute. Editor, Smith JL, pp 162–192. Hallandale, FL, Huffman Publishing Co., 1970.)

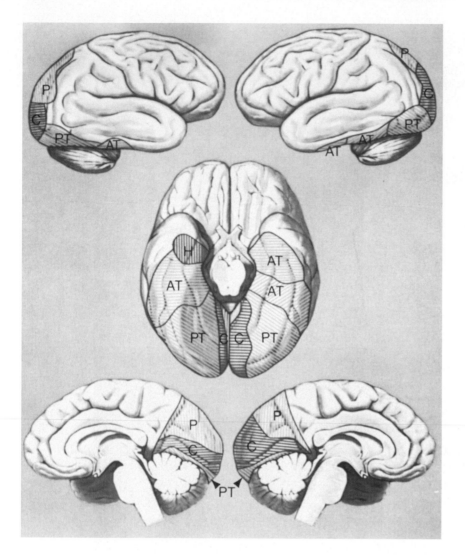

Figure 52.84. Lateral, medial, and basal views of the brain showing the distribution of the cortical branches of the posterior cerebral artery. The most common pattern of distribution is shown on the right cerebral hemisphere (*upper* and *lower left* and left half of basal view, *center*). The second most common pattern is shown on the left cerebral hemisphere (*upper* and *lower right* and right half of basal view, *center*). *AT,* distribution of anterior temporal artery; *C,* Distribution of calcarine artery; *H,* distribution of hippocampal artery; *P,* distribution of parieto-occipital artery; *PT,* distribution of posterior temporal artery. (From Zeal AA, Rhoton AL Jr. Microsurgic anatomy of the posterior cerebral artery. J Neurosurg *48:*534–559, 1978.)

and Rupp, 1963; Perlmutter and Rhoton, 1976; Saeki and Rhoton, 1977; Kamath, 1981; El Khamlichi et al., 1986; Hillen, 1987) (Fig. 52.90). The most common anomaly is hypoplasia of one or more of the arterial components of the circle, but aplasia of one or more arteries also may occur (McCullough, 1962).

INTERNAL CAROTID-BASILAR ANASTOMOSES

There are three primary arteries that connect the carotid and basilar arteries during development. These anastomotic vessels usually disappear by birth, but one or more of them may occasionally persist after birth, providing an anastomotic channel between the carotid and basilar artery systems in addition to that which normally exists (the posterior communicating artery).

Internal carotid-basilar artery anastomoses are of importance in several respects. First, they are often associated with other vascular abnormalities, particularly intracranial aneurysms and arteriovenous malformations (AVMs). These vascular lesions are particularly difficult to treat when they arise from, or are located adjacent to, the anastomotic vessel that is

providing a major portion of the blood supply to the posterior fossa. Second, they provide an aberrant blood supply to the brainstem and cerebellum. Patients with disease of the internal carotid artery in whom such anastomoses exist may thus experience signs and symptoms of posterior circulation disease. In other patients, neurologic manifestations of vertebrobasilar artery disease may be modified by a persistent anastomotic channel from the internal carotid artery that maintains circulation to a region of the brainstem or cerebellum that would normally be damaged. Finally, these anastomoses may preclude certain types of surgery for disease of the internal carotid artery (e.g., ligation of the artery for treatment of aneurysm), because manipulation of that artery would adversely affect the blood supply to the brainstem and cerebellum.

The three primary anastomoses that may persist in life are:

1. The primitive trigeminal artery;
2. The primitive acoustic (otic) artery; and
3. The primitive hypoglossal artery (Fig. 52.91).
   Other anastomoses may occur but are much less common.

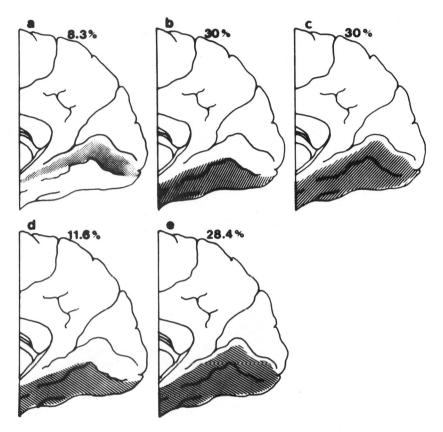

Figure 52.85.   Variation in areas supplied by *a,* the lingual artery (no variation); *b* and *c,* the posterior temporal artery; and *d* and *e,* the common temporal artery. (From Marinković SV, Milisavljević MM, Lolić-Draganić V, et al. Distribution of the occipital branches of the posterior cerebral artery: Correlation with occipital lobe infarcts. Stroke *18:*728–732, 1987.)

Persistent Primitive Trigeminal Artery

A primitive trigeminal artery is the most common persistent carotid-basilar anastomotic channel (Fig. 52.92). This vessel is the main source of blood to the hindbrain during the development of the basilar arterial circulation (Padget, 1948). When it persists after birth, it is usually of large caliber and normally connects the portion of the internal carotid artery just proximal to the cavernous sinus with the rostral portion of the basilar artery (Fig. 52.92). In this setting, the segment of the basilar artery proximal to the trigeminal artery is hypoplastic, as is the ipsilateral posterior communicating artery. Harrison and Luttrell (1953) emphasized that the persistent primitive trigeminal artery is invariably adjacent to the ipsilateral oculomotor and trochlear nerves.

Three forms of persistent trigeminal artery may exist (Saltzman, 1959; Lie, 1968). In type I, the artery supplies blood to both posterior cerebral and superior cerebellar arteries and to the rostral part of the basilar artery. In type II, the artery provides the blood supply to both superior cerebellar arteries, to the rostral part of the basilar artery, and to one or both of the posterior cerebral arteries. The other posterior cerebral artery receives its blood supply from the ipsilateral posterior communicating artery. In type III, both posterior cerebral arteries receive blood from the posterior communicating arteries. The persistent primitive trigeminal artery

supplies only the rostral part of the basilar artery and both superior cerebellar arteries. In rare instances, the persistent primitive trigeminal artery communicates directly with a branch of the basilar artery rather than with the artery itself (Teal et al., 1973.)

A substantial number of patients with a persistent trigeminal artery also have one or more intracranial aneurysms, AVMs, or both (Agnoli, 1982). These abnormalities are usually anatomically related to the persistent vessel. Such patients usually become symptomatic when they experience acute subarachnoid hemorrhage. In other patients, a persistent trigeminal artery may compress surrounding neural structures, producing various neurologic deficits, including ocular motor nerve pareses and trigeminal neuralgia (Jackson and Garza-Mercado, 1960; Campbell and Dyken, 1961; Madonick and Ruskin, 1962; Ikezaki et al., 1989). In still other cases, the anomalous vessel allows a diseased internal carotid artery to affect the portion of the brain normally supplied by the basilar artery and its branches. Heeney and Koo (1980) described a 65-year-old woman who experienced three episodes of complete blindness and dizziness. She was found to have high-grade stenosis of the left internal carotid artery and a persistent trigeminal artery. It was thought that the persistent trigeminal artery allowed emboli from the ulcerated left internal carotid artery to pass to the basilar artery and thus to affect the visual cortex bilaterally.

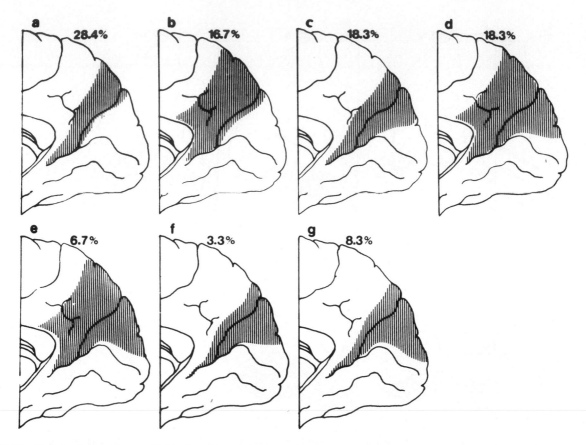

Figure 52.86.   Variation in the areas supplied by branching of the terminal stems of the parieto-occipital artery. (From Marinković SV, Milisavljević MM, Lolić-Draganić V, et al. Distribution of the occipital branches of the posterior cerebral artery: Correlation with occipital lobe infarcts. Stroke *18:* 728–732, 1987.)

Persistent Primitive Acoustic (Otic) Artery

This artery is in a slightly lower position than the trigeminal artery (Fig. 52.91). It usually connects the intrapetrosal portion of the internal carotid artery with the portion of the basilar artery just proximal to the origin of the anterior inferior cerebellar arteries (Kempe and Smith, 1969; Reynolds et al., 1980) (Fig. 52.93). It is a rare anomaly, and it is usually asymptomatic, although the patient described by Kempe and Smith had ipsilateral trigeminal neuralgia, hemifacial spasm, and glossopharyngeal neuralgia, all of which were thought to have been caused by a persistent acoustic artery.

Persistent Primitive Hypoglossal Artery

This vessel, initially the principal source of blood to the caudal end of the basilar artery, usually undergoes involution before the embryo reaches 6 mm in length. When an abnormal fusion occurs at the caudal end of the basilar artery, the primitive hypoglossal artery persists as an anomalous, extracranial, carotid-basilar anastomosis. This vessel courses adjacent to its homologous cranial nerve. It arises from the cervical portion of the internal carotid artery, enters the skull via the hypoglossal canal, and joins the basilar artery at or near its origin from the junction of the two vertebral arteries

(Morris and Moffat, 1956; Bruetman and Fields, 1963; De Caro et al., 1995) (Figs. 52.91 and 52.94). When this vessel is present, one of the vertebral arteries (usually the contralateral one) is always hypoplastic. The entire cerebral hemisphere and the supply area of the contralateral occipital lobe are thus dependent upon one carotid artery (De Caro et al., 1995). Patients with a persistent hypoglossal artery have an extremely high prevalence of aneurysms in the territory of the basilar artery or at the site of origin of the artery itself (Weir, 1987) (Fig. 52.95). This condition is extremely rare.

Other Anterior-Posterior Circulation Anastomoses

Anastomoses between the anterior and posterior cerebral circulations may occasionally exist in addition to the three types described above. Sunderland (1941) described an artery that branched from the basilar artery about midway up the pons at the level of the trigeminal nerve roots. The artery coursed laterally over the abducens nerve, entered Meckel's cave, and then entered the cavernous sinus, where it joined the lateral aspect of the internal carotid artery just after that vessel had entered the sinus.

A **proatlantal intersegmental artery** may connect the internal or external carotid artery with the ipsilateral vertebral artery before the latter vessel passes through the foramen

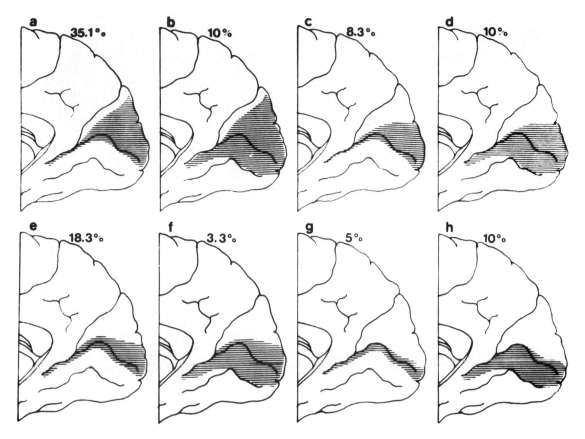

Figure 52.87. Variation in areas supplied by the calcarine artery. (From Marinković SV, Milisavljević MM, Lolić-Draganić V, et al. Distribution of the occipital branches of the posterior cerebral artery: Correlation with occipital lobe infarcts. Stroke *18:*728–732, 1987.)

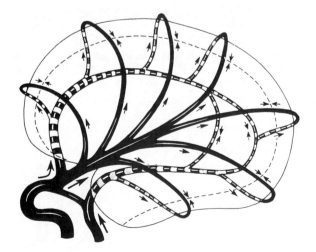

Figure 52.88. Schematic illustration of the border zone leptomeningeal anastomoses among the three major cerebral arteries (*dashed lines*). (From Zülch KJ. Neurologische Diagnostik bei Endokraniellen Komplikationen von oto-rhinologischen Erkrankungen. Arch Ohr Nas Kehlkopfheilk *183:*79–85, 1964.)

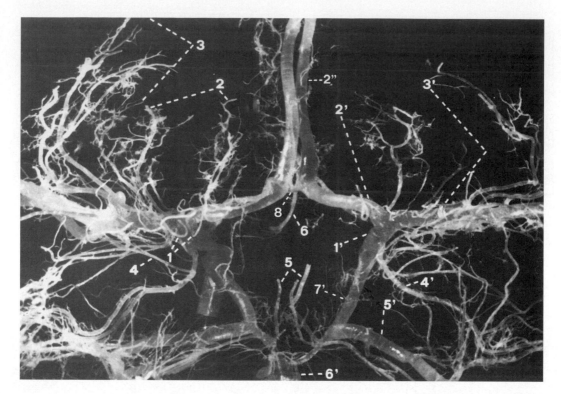

Figure 52.89. The arteries that comprise the circle of Willis. The plastic cast is viewed dorsally and slightly rostrally. *1'*, internal carotid artery; *2'*, anterior cerebral artery (A-1 segment); *2''*, anterior cerebral artery (A-2 segment); *3'*, middle cerebral artery; *4'*, anterior choroidal artery; *5'*, posterior cerebral artery; *6'*, basilar artery; *7'*, posterior communicating artery. Note extensive branches of these vessels *(numbers 1–6)*. (From Marinković SV, Milisavljević MM, Marinković ZD. The perforating branches of the internal carotid artery: The microsurgic anatomy of their extracerebral segments. Neurosurgery *26:*472–479, 1990).

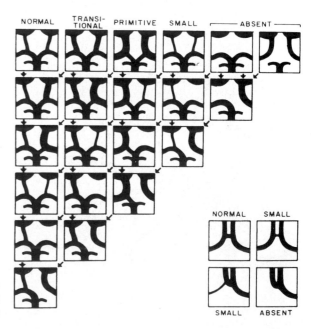

Figure 52.90. Schematic illustration of variations in the circle of Willis, posterior portion (*top left*) and anterior portion (*bottom right*). (From Padget DH. Intracranial Aneurysms. Editor, Dandy WE. Ithaca, New York, Comstock Publishing Co., 1944.)

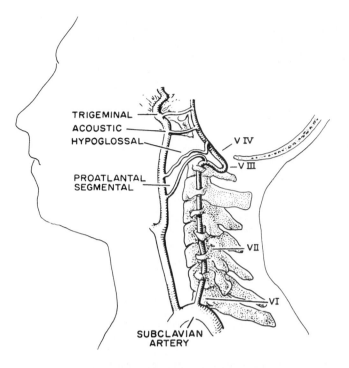

Figure 52.91. Persistent primitive arteries interconnecting the internal carotid and basilar arterial systems.

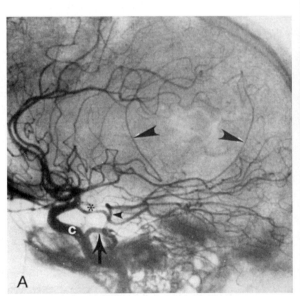

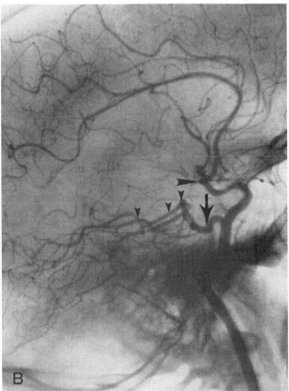

Figure 52.92. Cerebral arteriograms showing persistent primitive trigeminal arteries. *A,* In a patient with an oligodendroglioma that has widened the branches of the middle cerebral artery (*large arrowheads*), the basilar artery (*small arrowhead*) is filled via a persistent trigeminal artery (*arrow*). The contralateral posterior cerebral artery originates from the basilar artery, whereas the ipsilateral posterior cerebral artery (*asterisk*) originates from the internal carotid artery (*c*). *B,* In a patient with occlusion of the middle cerebral artery (*arrowhead*), there is a large primitive trigeminal artery (*arrow*) that supplies the basilar artery and both posterior cerebral arteries (*small arrowheads*).

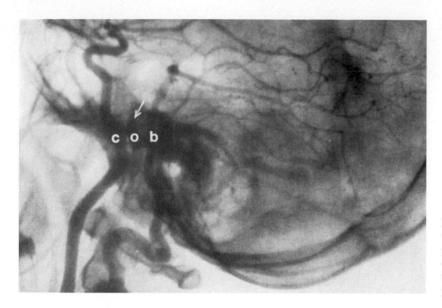

Figure 52.93. Persistent primitive acoustic (otic) artery (*o* and *arrow*) is shown connecting the intrapetrosal portion of the internal carotid artery (*c*) with the portion of the basilar artery (*b*) just proximal to the origin of the anterior inferior cerebellar arteries (not visible in this photograph).

magnum (Gottschau, 1885; Suzuki et al., 1979) (Fig. 52.96). This anomaly is extremely rare.

The superior and the anterior inferior cerebellar arteries may rarely arise from the internal carotid artery rather than from the basilar artery (Teal et al., 1972; Scotti, 1975; Matsuda et al., 1979; Cobb et al., 1983). When they do so, they are often associated with adjacent aneurysms or AVMs.

Parkinson et al. (1979) described a congenital anastomosis between the cervical portions of the internal carotid and vertebral arteries.

EXTERNAL CAROTID ARTERY

The **external carotid artery** originates from the common carotid artery opposite the upper border of the thyroid cartilage (Fig. 52.1). It takes a slightly curved course, passing upward and forward, and then inclining backward to the space behind the neck of the mandible, where it divides into its two terminal branches: the superficial temporal and internal maxillary arteries. It rapidly diminishes in size throughout its course in the neck as it gives off its many branches. Medial to the external carotid artery are the hyoid bone, the wall of the pharynx, the superior laryngeal nerve, and a portion of the parotid gland. Lateral to it, in the lower part of its course, is the internal carotid artery. Posterior to it, near its origin, is the superior laryngeal nerve. Superiorly, it is separated from the internal carotid artery by the styloglossus and stylopharyngeus muscles, the glossopharyngeal nerve, the pharyngeal branch of the vagus nerve, and part of the parotid gland.

The branches of the external carotid artery are usually divided into four sets: anterior, posterior, ascending, and terminal (Figs. 52.1 and 52.97). The anterior set is composed of the superior thyroid artery, the lingual artery, and the external maxillary or facial artery. The posterior arteries are the occipital and the posterior auricular. The only ascending artery is the ascending pharyngeal, and the terminal branches, as noted above, are the superficial temporal and internal maxillary arteries.

Anterior Branches of the External Carotid Artery

The **superior thyroid artery** arises from the external carotid artery just below the level of the greater cornu of the hyoid bone and ends in the thyroid gland. Along its course, it gives rise to branches that supply adjacent muscles, the superior laryngeal nerve, and the larynx.

The **lingual artery** arises from the external carotid artery opposite the tip of the greater cornu of the hyoid bone, between the superior thyroid and external maxillary arteries. Initially it runs obliquely upward and medially above the hyoid bone. It then curves downward and forward, forming a loop that is crossed by the hypoglossal nerve, before passing beneath the digastric and stylohyoid muscles. It next runs horizontally forward beneath the hyoglossus muscle. After passing the hyoglossus, it ascends almost perpendicular to the level of the tongue, where it turns forward to run along the lower surface of the tongue to its tip. Along its course, the lingual artery gives off branches to the muscles attached to the hyoid bone, the sublingual gland, the mucous membrane of the mouth and gums, and the tongue.

The **external maxillary artery** (facial artery) arises in the carotid triangle just distal to the origin of the lingual artery. It courses obliquely beneath the digastric and stylohyoid muscles, over which it arches to enter a groove on the posterior surface of the submaxillary gland. It then curves upward over the body of the mandible at the anteroinferior angle of the masseter. The artery next passes forward and upward across the cheek to the angle of the mouth, then ascends along the side of the nose, and ends beneath the medial canthal ligament of the eye as the **angular artery**. This vessel is remarkably tortuous, both in the neck and in the face. It is therefore able to accommodate itself to the movements of the pharynx, mandible, lips, and cheeks.

The branches of the external maxillary artery may be divided into two sets: those given off in the neck (cervical branches), and those given off to the face (facial branches). The cervical branches are the ascending palatine, tonsillar,

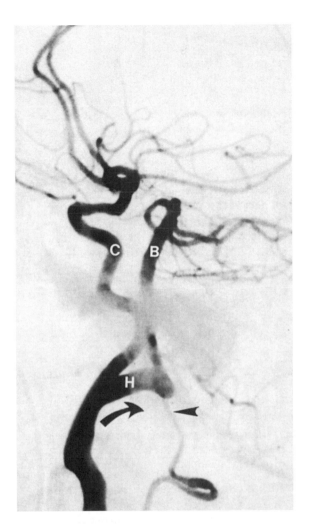

Figure 52.94. Persistent primitive hypoglossal artery (*H* and *curved arrow*) connects the cervical portion of the internal carotid artery (*C*) with the basilar artery (*B*) near the latter's origin. Note that the contralateral vertebral artery is hypoplastic (*arrowhead*).

glandular, submental, and muscular arteries. These vessels supply the soft palate, palatine glands, palatine tonsil, submaxillary gland, and the mylohyoid and digastric muscles. The facial branches are the inferior and superior labial, lateral nasal, muscular, and angular arteries. These vessels supply the labial glands, mucous membrane and muscles of the upper and lower lip, the nasal septum portions of the nose, the lacrimal sac, and various superficial facial muscles, including the orbicularis oculi.

Posterior Branches of the External Carotid Artery

The occipital and posterior auricular arteries are the only two branches that originate from the posterior aspect of the external carotid artery.

The **occipital artery** arises from the posterior aspect of the external carotid artery opposite the origin of the external maxillary artery near the lower margin of the posterior belly of the digastric muscle and ends in the posterior part of the scalp. At its origin it is covered by the stylohyoid muscle and by the posterior belly of the digastric muscle, and the hypoglossal nerve winds around it. It then crosses the internal carotid artery, internal jugular vein, and the vagus and spinal accessory nerves. It next ascends to the space between the transverse process of the atlas and the mastoid process of the temporal bone, covered by the posterior neck muscles. Then it changes course and runs vertically upward, pierces the fascia connecting the cranial attachment of the trapezius muscle with the sternocleidomastoid muscle, and ascends in a tortuous course in the superficial fascia of the scalp, where it divides into numerous branches that reach as high as the vertex of the skull and anastomose with branches of the posterior auricular and superficial temporal arteries (see below). Its terminal portion is accompanied by the greater occipital nerve.

The occipital artery provides branches to the digastric, stylohyoid, splenius capitis, and sternocleidomastoid muscles. It also provides: (*a*) an auricular branch that enters the skull through the mastoid foramen and supplies the dura mater, diploë, and mastoid air cells; (*b*) a meningeal branch that ascends with the internal jugular vein, enters the skull through the jugular foramen, and supplies the dura mater in the posterior fossa; and (*c*) a descending branch (the largest branch of the occipital artery) that descends on the back of the neck and divides into a superficial and a deep vessel. The superficial vessel runs beneath the splenius muscle, giving off branches that pierce that muscle to supply the trapezius, whereas the deep vessel runs between the two semispinalis muscles to anastomose with the vertebral artery on that side.

The terminal branches of each occipital artery are very tortuous. They are distributed to the back of the head, where they anastomose with similar branches from the contralateral occipital artery, and supply the occipitalis muscle, and the pericranium, subcutaneous tissue, and skin overlying the occiput.

The **posterior auricular artery** is a small vessel that arises from the posterior aspect of the external carotid artery opposite the apex of the styloid process. It ascends under the parotid gland but over the styloid process to the groove between the cartilage of the ear and the mastoid process, immediately above which it divides into its terminal branches.

The posterior auricular artery provides small branches to the digastric, stylohyoid, and sternocleidomastoid muscles, and to the parotid gland. One of its larger branches, the stylomastoid artery, enters the stylomastoid foramen and supplies the tympanic cavity, tympanic membrane, semicircular canals, and mastoid air cells. A second branch supplies the auricle of the ear, and a third branch, which anastomoses with the occipital artery (see above), supplies the occipitalis muscle and the scalp.

Ascending Branch of the External Carotid Artery: Ascending Pharyngeal Artery

The **ascending pharyngeal artery** is the smallest major branch of the external carotid artery. It arises near the origin of the artery and ascends vertically between the internal ca-

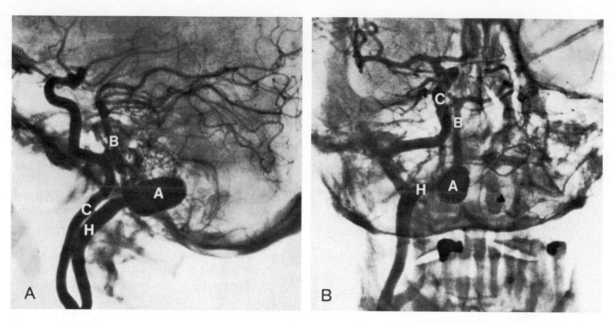

Figure 52.95.   Large saccular aneurysm (*A*) at the junction of a primitive hypoglossal artery (*H*) with the basilar artery (*B*). *C,* internal carotid artery. *A,* Lateral view. *B,* Anteroposterior view.

rotid artery and the side of the pharynx to the undersurface of the base of the skull, where it lies on the capitus longus muscle. This artery gives off: (*a*) three or four pharyngeal branches that supply the pharyngeal muscles; (*b*) a palatine branch that supplies the soft palate, tonsil, and auditory canal; (*c*) prevertebral branches that supply the cervical sympathetic trunk, the hypoglossal and vagus nerves, and the cervical lymph nodes; (*d*) the inferior tympanic artery that supplies the medial wall of the tympanic cavity; and (*e*) meningeal branches that supply the dura mater.

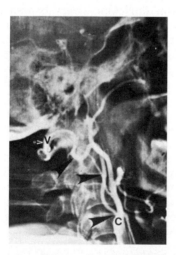

Figure 52.96.   In a patient with internal carotid artery occlusion, a large proatlantal artery (*arrowheads*) connects the occluded internal carotid artery (*c*) with the ipsilateral vertebral artery (*v* and *white arrow*). (From Taveras JM, Wood EH. Diagnostic Neuroradiology, 2nd edition, Vol 2. Baltimore, Williams & Wilkins, 1976.)

Terminal Branches of the External Carotid Artery

The terminal branches of the external carotid artery are the superficial temporal artery and the internal maxillary artery. These vessels are extremely important from a neuro-ophthalmologic standpoint.

Superficial Temporal Artery

The **superficial temporal artery** is the smaller of the two terminal branches of the external carotid artery, and it appears to be the continuation of that vessel (Fig. 52.97). It begins in the substance of the parotid gland behind the neck of the mandible. Although still within the substance of the gland, it gives off the transverse facial artery, which supplies the parotid gland, the parotid duct, and the masseter muscle. The artery then crosses over the posterior root of the zygomatic process of the temporal bone to ascend anterior to the ear, deep to the subcutaneous tissue and superficial to the temporalis fascia. Immediately above the zygomatic arch, the superfical temporal artery gives off the middle temporal artery that supplies the temporalis muscle, a zygomatico-orbital artery that supplies the orbicularis oculi muscle and perforates the zygoma to enter the lateral orbit, and anterior auricular branches that are distributed to the anterior portion of the auricle, lobule, and external meatus.

Between 2 and 5 cm above the zygomatic process, over 90% of superficial temporal arteries divide into two terminal branches: the frontal (or anterior) and the parietal (or posterior) (Romanes, 1967; Gray and Goss, 1973; Stock et al., 1980; Marano et al., 1985; Daumann et al., 1989) (Fig. 52.98). The frontal branch runs tortuously upward and forward to the forehead, supplying the facial muscles, skin, and pericranium in this region. It anastomoses with the supraorbital artery. The parietal branch is larger than the frontal. It

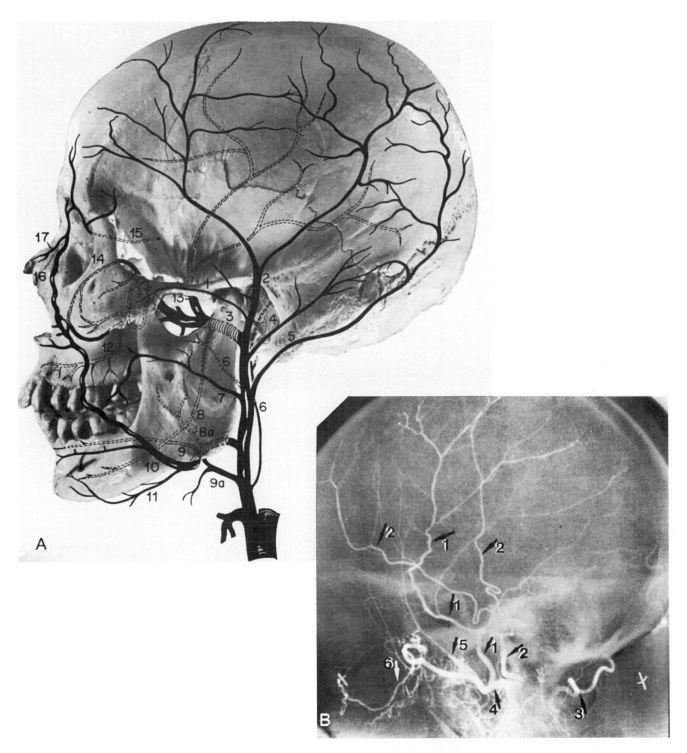

Figure 52.97. Branches of the external carotid artery. *A,* Schematic representation of the external carotid artery. *1,* zygomatico-orbital artery; *2,* superficial temporal artery; *3,* internal maxillary artery; *4,* posterior auricular artery; *5,* occipital artery; *6,* ascending pharyngeal artery; *7,* transverse facial artery; *8,* inferior alveolar artery; *8a,* ascending pharyngeal artery; *9,* deep lingual artery; *9a,* lingual artery; *10,* facial artery; *11,* submental artery; *12,* palatine artery; *13,* middle meningeal artery; *14,* infraorbital artery; *15,* ophthalmic artery (filling retrograde); *16,* angular artery; *17,* dorsal nasal artery. *B,* Normal external carotid arteriogram, lateral view, shows middle meningeal artery (*1*), superficial temporal artery (*2*), occipital artery (*3*), internal maxillary artery (*4*), deep temporal artery (*5*), and palatine artery (*6*). (From Taveras JM, Wood EH. Diagnostic Neuroradiology, 2nd edition, Vol 2. Baltimore, Williams & Wilkins, 1976.)

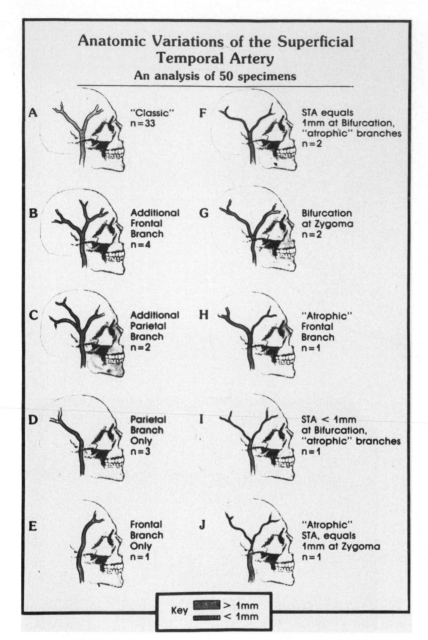

Figure 52.98. Anatomic variations of the superficial temporal artery. Note that in most cases, the artery divides just above the zygomatic arch into two main branches: a frontal (anterior) branch and a parietal (posterior) branch. (From Marano SR, Fischer DW, Gaines C, et al. Anatomic study of the superficial temporal artery. Neurosurgery *16:*786–789, 1985.)

curves upward and backward on the side of the head, lying superficial to the temporalis fascia, and anastomoses with the posterior auricular and occipital arteries.

In about 10% of persons, the superficial temporal artery has an anomalous branching pattern (Marano et al., 1985; Daumann et al., 1989) (Fig. 52.98). The most common anomaly is an additional frontal branch. Other anomalies include two parietal branches, bifurcation at the zygoma rather than above it, and no branching at all. When the artery does not branch, it simply continues its course in either the normal frontal or the normal parietal direction.

Internal Maxillary Artery

The **internal maxillary artery**, the larger of the two terminal branches of the external carotid artery, arises behind the neck of the mandible (Fig. 52.97). Like the superficial temporal artery, it initially is embedded in the parotid gland. It then passes forward between the ramus of the mandible and the sphenomandibular ligament to run either superficial or deep to the external pterygoid muscle. It terminates in the pterygopalatine fossa. This vessel supplies the deep structures of the face, and is usually considered to consist of three portions (Allen et al., 1973).

The first or **mandibular portion** passes horizontally forward between the ramus of the mandible and the insertion of the sphenomandibular ligament, where it lies parallel to, and a little below, the auriculotemporal nerve (Fig. 52.99). During its short course, it gives off several branches: the anterior tympanic artery, the deep auricular artery, the middle meningeal artery, and the inferior alveolar artery.

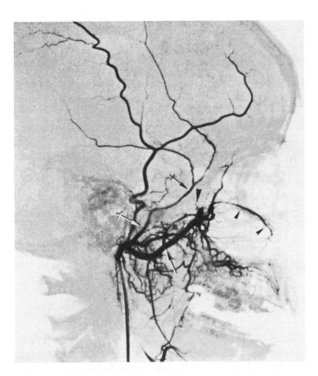

Figure 52.99. External carotid arteriogram, lateral view, shows the course of the internal maxillary artery. The mandibular and pterygoid segments are easily followed (*arrow*), whereas pterygopalatine segment is seen head on (*large arrowhead*). The course of the middle meningeal artery is shown by *crossed arrows*, and the infraorbital artery is identified by *small arrowheads*). (From Huber P. Cerebral Angiography, 2nd edition. New York, Georg Thieme Verlag, 1982.)

The **anterior tympanic artery** passes upward behind the temporomandibular articulation, enters the tympanic cavity through the pterygotympanic fissure, and ramifies upon the tympanic membrane. It forms a vascular circle around the membrane with the stylomastoid branch of the posterior auricular artery (see above).

The **deep auricular artery** arises near the anterior tympanic artery. It ascends in the substance of the parotid gland behind the temporomandibular articulation, pierces the cartilaginous or bony wall of the external acoustic meatus, and supplies this region.

The **middle meningeal artery** is the largest artery that supplies the dura mater. It ascends between the sphenomandibular ligament and the external pterygoid muscle, entering the cranium through the foramen spinosum in the sphenoid bone (Figs. 52.97 and 52.99). On entering the cranium, this artery gives off several small branches. These branches supply the gasserian ganglion and surrounding dura, the portion of the facial nerve within the facial canal, and the tensor tympani muscle and lining of the tympanic canal. One or more of these branches may also anastomose with branches of the meningohypophyseal trunk (particularly the artery to the inferior cavernous sinus), providing collateral pathways between the cavernous portion of the internal and external carotid arteries (Parkinson, 1964, 1965; Pribram et al., 1966; Wallace et al., 1967; Margolis and Newton, 1969). In addi-

tion, orbital branches pass through the superior orbital fissure (Natori and Rhoton, 1995) or through separate canals in the greater wing of the sphenoid to anastomose with the lacrimal artery or other branches of the ophthalmic artery (Ducasse et al., 1985, 1986c). The middle meningeal artery then runs forward in a groove on the greater wing of the sphenoid bone, dividing into a large anterior and a small posterior branch. The anterior branch crosses the greater wing of the sphenoid to a groove in the sphenoidal angle of the parietal bone, and finally divides into numerous branches that spread out between the dura mater and the internal surface of the cranium. Some of these branches pass upward as far as the vertex, whereas others pass backward to the occipital region. The posterior branch of the middle meningeal artery curves backward on the squama of the temporal bone to reach the parietal bone, where it divides into several branches. The terminal branches of the middle meningeal artery supply the inner table of the adjacent bone of the skull and, to some extent, the adjacent dura mater. In addition, an **accessory meningeal artery** sometimes branches from the middle meningeal artery before it enters the skull. This vessel enters the skull through the foramen ovale and supplies the gasserian ganglion and surrounding dura.

The **inferior alveolar artery** descends with the inferior alveolar nerve to the mandibular foramen on the medial surface of the ramus of the mandible. Accompanied by the nerve, it runs along the mandibular canal in the substance of the bone. Opposite the first premolar tooth, it divides into two branches, the incisor and the mental.

The second or **pterygoid portion** of the internal maxillary artery runs obliquely forward and upward on the surface of the external pterygoid muscle and under cover of the ramus of the mandible and the insertion of the temporalis muscle (Fig. 52.99). It then passes between the two heads of origin of the external pterygoid muscle muscle to enter the pterygoid fossa. This portion of the internal maxillary artery gives off several branches that supply the pterygoid, masseter, and buccinator muscles. It also gives off two deep temporal branches, the anterior and posterior deep temporal arteries. These vessels ascend between the temporalis muscle and the pericranium. Both vessels supply the temporalis muscle and anastomose with the middle temporal branch of the superficial temporal artery. In addition, the anterior branch anastomoses with the lacrimal artery in the orbit by means of small branches that perforate the zygomatic bone and greater wing of the sphenoid (Ducasse et al., 1985, 1986c).

The third or **pterygopalatine portion** of the internal maxillary artery lies in the pterygopalatine fossa adjacent to the sphenopalatine ganglion (Fig. 52.99). It gives off six major branches: the posterior superior alveolar artery, the infraorbital artery, the descending palatine artery, the artery of the pterygoid canal, a pharyngeal branch, and the sphenopalatine artery.

The **posterior superior alveolar artery** supplies the molar and premolar teeth, the gums, and the lining of the maxillary sinus.

The **infraorbital artery** appears to be the normal continuation of the internal maxillary artery. It runs along the infraorbital groove and canal with the infraorbital nerve. During this course, the artery gives off an orbital branch with anastomotic connections to the arteries of the inferior oblique and inferior rectus muscles and to the lacrimal and dorsal nasal arteries (Hayreh, 1963a; Ducasse et al., 1985; Coulter et al., 1990). It also gives off anterior superior alveolar branches that supply the upper incisor and canine teeth and the mucous membrane of the maxillary sinus. The infraorbital artery then emerges on the face after passing through the infraorbital foramen. On the face, some branches pass upward to the medial canthal region where they anastomose with the angular branch of the external maxillary artery (see above). Others run toward the nose, where they anastomose with terminal branches of the ophthalmic artery. Still others descend to anastomose with terminal branches of the external maxillary, transverse facial, and buccinator arteries.

The **descending palatine artery** anastomoses with the sphenopalatine artery, which also originates from the internal maxillary artery, and with the ascending palatine artery which originates from the external maxillary artery. This vessel supplies the gums, mucous membrane of the roof of the mouth, soft palate, and palatine tonsil.

The **artery of the pterygoid canal** passes backward along the pterygoid canal with the corresponding nerve. It supplies the upper part of the pharynx, the internal auditory canal, and the tympanic cavity.

The **pharyngeal branch** of the pterygoid portion of the internal maxillary artery is a small vessel that runs backward through the pharyngeal canal with the pharyngeal nerve. Like the artery of the pterygoid canal, this artery supplies the upper part of the pharynx and the internal auditory canal.

The **sphenopalatine artery** passes through the sphenopalatine foramen into the cavity of the nose. It supplies the conchae and meatuses as well as the bone and mucous membrane of parts of the frontal, maxillary, ethmoid, and sphenoid sinuses.

VENOUS SYSTEM OF THE BRAIN

The system of vessels that drains venous blood from the cranium includes cerebral and posterior fossa veins, diploic veins, meningeal veins, dural sinuses, orbital veins, and the internal and external jugular veins (Kapp and Schmidek, 1984; Capra and Kapp, 1987; Andeweg, 1996).

VEINS OF THE BRAIN: CEREBRAL AND POSTERIOR FOSSA VEINS

The veins of the brain possess no valves, and their walls are extremely thin because they have no muscularis. These vessels pierce the arachnoid and the inner or meningeal layer of the dura mater to drain into the cranial venous sinuses (see below). The veins of the brain are usually separated into those that drain the cerebral hemispheres and those that drain the posterior fossa.

Cerebral Veins

The cerebral veins are of two types: superficial and deep (Ono et al., 1984b; Oka et al., 1985; Curé et al., 1994; Meder et al., 1994). **Superficial cerebral veins** collect blood from large and small **pial veins** that cover the surface of the cerebral hemispheres, anastomosing extensively with each other (Duvernoy, 1983) (Fig. 52.100). The superficial cerebral veins have an extremely variable pattern over the hemispheres, but some of them are consistent enough to be given names. **Deep cerebral veins** drain the subcortical structures of the telencephalon and diencephalon (Fig. 52.101). These vessels vary considerably in number, but they are more consistent in size, shape, and location than are the superficial cerebral veins with which they anastomose extensively (Hassler, 1966; Ono et al., 1984; Smith and Sanford, 1984; Oka et al., 1985; Curé et al., 1994; Meder et al., 1994).

Superficial Cerebral Veins

Most investigators describe the main superficial cerebral veins as the superior, middle, and inferior cerebral veins (Meder et al., 1994). Oka et al. (1985) devised a much more elaborate nomenclature, naming the veins for the lobe of the cerebrum that they drain and further dividing the veins on each lobe on the basis of whether they drain: (*a*) the lateral (convexity) surface, (*b*) the medial (falcine) surface, or (*c*) the inferior (basal) surface. A final subdivision of these veins is based on the direction in which they course. Some of these veins receive contributions from deep structures, but all of them receive major contributions from the cerebral cortex. We have chosen to use the standard nomenclature for the superficial cerebral veins in this text, rather than that used by Oka et al., because of the complexity of the latter naming system and the substantial variability in the location of these veins.

Ten to 20 **superior cerebral veins** drain the superior regions of the cerebral cortex, including the medial surface and the convexity of the frontal, parietal, and occipital lobes (Piffer et al., 1985). These veins run upward to open in the superior sagittal (longitudinal) sinus (Figs. 52.102 and 52.103). In a study of 10 unfixed human brains, Andrews et al. (1989) found that about six to seven of these veins drain the anterior frontal region, three veins drain each posterior frontal region, four veins drain each parietal region, and one vein drains each occipital region. The majority of these vessels initially ascend upward and backward. However, as they reach the superior convexity of the brain, they turn rostrally and enter the superior sinus against the flow of blood (Sargent, 1911; Oka et al., 1985) (Fig. 52.103). Only one or two of the superior cerebral veins, the anterior frontal veins, join the superior sagittal sinus in the direction of the flow of blood.

Some authors have named individual superior cerebral veins based on their relative position to underlying cerebral structures; e.g., precentral vein, postcentral vein, occipital vein, occipitotemporal vein (Oka et al., 1985; Sener, 1994). One of the largest of these named veins usually travels in or near the central sulcus and is called the **rolandic (or central) vein** (Merwarth, 1942; Oka et al., 1985). This vein drains the region of the primary motor and somesthetic sensory cortex (Fig. 52.102).

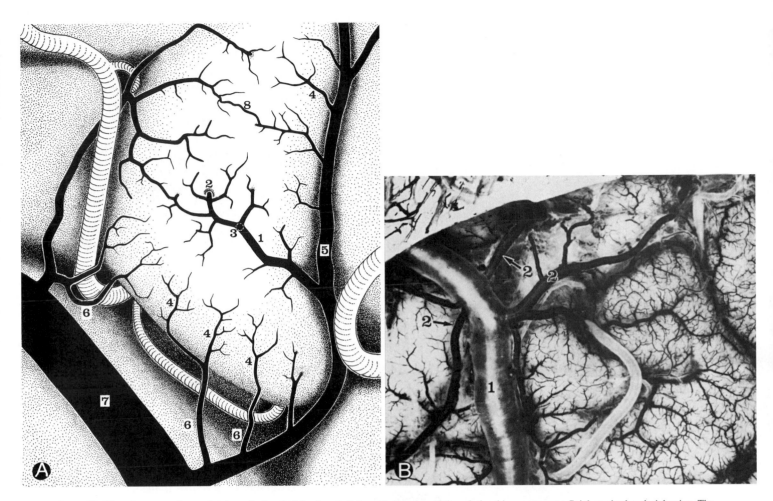

Figure 52.100. Anatomy of superficial cerebral and pial veins. *A*, Schematic drawing of the relationship among superficial cerebral and pial veins. The pial arteries have been removed. *1*, central vein of the gyrus; note its angular path; *2*, junction point of an intracortical vein at the pial vein extremity; *3*, junction point of an intracortical vein but the vein is not visible; *4*, small peripheral superficial veins; *5*, marginal vein; *6*, collecting veins of the pial network crossing over the arteries to flow into the main superficial cerebral vein (*7*); *8*, pial venous anastomoses. *B*, Surface of parietal lobe in which the veins have been injected with India ink. Numerous pial veins can be seen on the surface of the hemisphere, many of which anastomose with each other. The pial veins drain into collecting veins (*2*) that in turn cross over the sulci to flow into the superficial cerebral vein (*1*). (From Duvernoy HM. Cortical veins of the human brain. In The Cerebral Veins. An Experimental and Clinical Update. Editors, Auer LM, Loew F, pp 3–38. New York, Springer-Verlag, 1983.)

Piffer et al. (1986) studied the anatomy of the walls of the superior cerebral veins. These investigators found that at the junction of the veins with the superior sagittal sinus, their walls contain an increased amount of collagen fascicles and elastic fibers, compared with the composition of the walls along the rest of the vein. This increased amount of connective tissue is continuous with that of the sinus itself. It is believed that this fibrous structure helps to maintain the structural integrity of these vessels and therefore plays a role in the regulation of blood flow within them.

Most of the lateral surface of each cerebral hemisphere is drained by a descending vein, the **superficial middle cerebral (sylvian) vein** (Fig. 52.102). According to Wolf et al. (1963), this vessel shows the greatest variation in size and course of all the superficial cerebral veins.

The superficial middle cerebral vein (of which there may be two) originates near the horizontal or posterior limb of the Sylvian fissure. Each vein runs downward and forward within the fissure toward the pterion and then medially along the sphenoid ridge to end in the sphenoparietal or cavernous sinuses.

The superficial middle cerebral vein is connected with the superior sagittal sinus via the **vein of Trolard** (the greater anastomotic vein) and with the lateral sinus through the **vein of Labbé** (the lesser or inferior anastomotic vein) (Figs. 52.102 and 52.103). There is considerable variation in the size and exact location of these collateral channels (Meder et al., 1994).

The **inferior cerebral veins** drain the undersurface of the cerebral hemisphere. Those veins under the temporal lobe

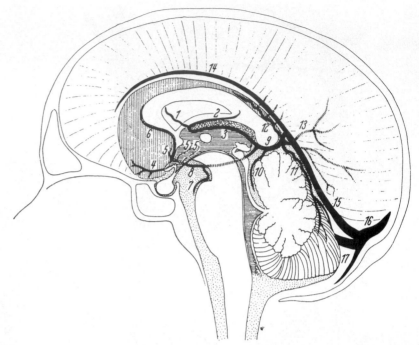

Figure 52.101. The deep cerebral veins, basal veins, and cerebellar veins. *1,* anterior caudate vein; *2,* terminal vein; *3,* internal cerebral vein; *4,* anterior cerebral vein; *5,* lenticulostriate veins; *6,* anterior vein of the corpus callosum; *7,* prepontine vein; *8,* basal vein (of Rosenthal); *9,* great vein of Galen; *10,* inferior cerebellar veins; *11,* superior cerebellar veins; *12,* pericallosal vein; *13,* internal occipital veins; *14,* inferior sagittal sinus; *15,* straight sinus; *16,* torcular herophili; *17,* occipital sinus. (From Krayenbühl H, Yaşargil MG. Cerebral Angiography, 2nd edition. Philadelphia, JB Lippincott, 1968.)

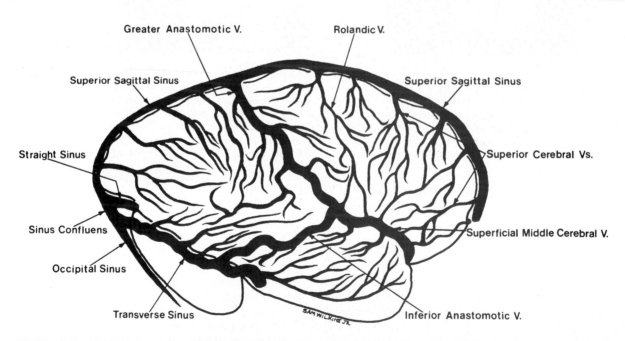

Figure 52.102. Schematic illustration of the superficial cerebral veins. (From Capra NF, Kapp JP. Anatomic and physiologic aspects of venous system. In Cerebral Blood Flow. Physiologic and Clinical Aspects. Editor, Wood JH, pp 37–58. New York, McGraw-Hill, 1987.)

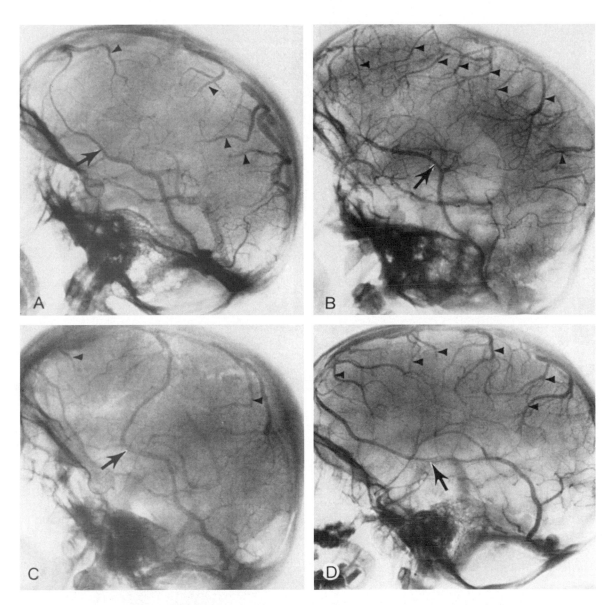

Figure 52.103.   Drainage pattern and anastomoses of superficial cerebral veins. *A,* Anastomosis between vein of Labbé and frontal ascending vein (*arrow*); *B,* Anastomosis between vein of Labbé and sylvian vein (*arrow*); *C,* Anastomosis between vein of Labbé and vein of Trolard (*arrow*); *D,* Anastomosis between vein of Labbé and ascending frontal vein (*arrow*). Note that in all four photographs, superior superficial veins (*arrowheads*) are seen draining upward into the superior sagittal sinus. Most of these veins turn rostrally before entering the sinus, thus entering it against the flow of draining blood. (From Krayenbühl HA, Yaşargil MG. Cerebral Angiography, 2nd edition. Philadelphia, JB Lippincott, 1968.)

anastomose with the middle cerebral and basal veins and eventually drain into the cavernous, sphenoparietal, and superior petrosal sinuses, whereas those on the orbital surface of the frontal lobe join the superficial frontal veins and empty into the superior sagittal sinus.

Deep Cerebral Veins

The principal deep cerebral veins are the insular and striate veins, the subependymal veins, the medullary veins, the basal vein (of Rosenthal), and the great cerebral vein (of Galen) (Fig. 52.101). These vessels have been studied in

detail by a number of investigators, particularly Rhoton and his colleagues (Matsushima et al., 1983; Ono et al., 1984b; Oka et al., 1985).

INSULAR AND STRIATE VEINS

A variable number of veins over the surface of the insula have a configuration similar to the branches of the middle cerebral artery (Fig. 52.104). These veins usually drain into the deep middle cerebral vein, which in turn empties into the basal cerebral vein or, occasionally, into the sphenoparietal sinus (see below). In addition to the insular veins, the

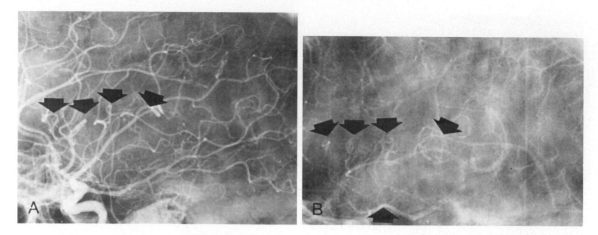

Figure 52.104. Insular and striate veins. *A,* Cerebral arteriogram, arterial phase, shows loops made by branches of the middle cerebral artery in the sylvian fissure (*arrows*). *B,* Cerebral arteriogram, venous phase, shows similar loops (*arrows*) made by insular and striate veins. Fine veins are seen converging downward over the insular surface (*single arrow*). (From Taveras JM, Wood EH. Diagnostic Neuroradiology, 2nd edition, Vol 2. Baltimore, Williams & Wilkins, 1976.)

deep middle cerebral vein receives the striate veins and veins from the inferior aspect of the frontal lobe. Wolf and Huang (1963) identified an **uncal vein** that runs along the medial aspect of the temporal lobe. This vessel drains either into the sphenoparietal venous sinus anterior to the uncus or directly into the cavernous sinus.

SUBEPENDYMAL VEINS

As their name implies, these vessels are located just beneath the ependymal surface of the ventricles. The main subependymal veins are the two internal cerebral veins, the thalamostriate (terminal) veins, and the septal veins, but there are many others as well.

The **internal cerebral veins** are paired vessels that are situated just off the midline. They are adjacent to each other in the tela choroidea of the roof of the 3rd ventricle for most of their course. Their configuration is therefore that of the roof of the 3rd ventricle (Figs. 52.101, 52.105, and 52.106). These veins begin at the foramen of Monro. They initially extend slightly upward and backward and then downward and backward, forming a fairly regular, semicircular or elliptical curve, the anterior slope of which is about equal in length and arc to the posterior slope. They leave the roof of the 3rd ventricle at the velum interpositum just above the suprapineal recess and enter the upper portion of the quadrigeminal cistern, where they join to form a short trunk, the

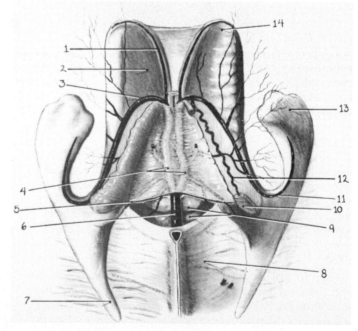

Figure 52.105. Schematic illustration of the deep cerebral veins seen from above. On each side, a septal vein (*1*) joins with a thalamostriate vein (*2*) to form the internal cerebral vein (*4*). The internal cerebral veins are located within the velum interpositum (*5*). They join posteriorly to from the great vein of Galen (*6*). In this illustration, the choroid plexus has been removed on the right side to show the choroid vein (*12*). *2,* anterior horn at its junction with the body of the lateral ventricle; *7,* occipital horn of the lateral ventricle; *8,* tentorium cerebelli; *9,* superior and inferior colliculi; *10,* choroid plexus; *11,* initial segment of the thalamostriate vein; *13,* temporal horn of the lateral ventricle; *14,* frontal horn of the lateral ventricle. (From Taveras JM, Wood EH. Diagnostic Neuroradiology, 2nd edition, Vol 2. Baltimore, Williams & Wilkins, 1976.)

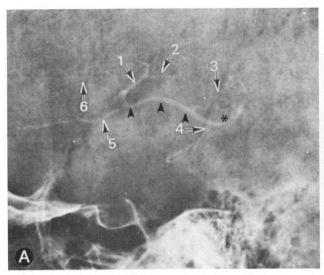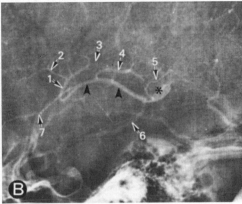

Figure 52.106. Angiographic appearance of the internal cerebral vein. *A,* The internal cerebral vein (*arrowheads*) is formed from the junction of the thalamostriate vein (*1*) and the septal vein (*5*). The internal cerebral vein then drains into the great vein of Galen (*asterisk*). *2,* posterior caudate vein; *3,* medial atrial vein; *4,* inferior ventricular vein; *6,* anterior caudate veins. *B,* the internal cerebral vein (*arrowheads*) is formed from the junction of the thalamostriate (*1*) and septal (*7*) veins. It drains into the great vein of Galen (*asterisk*), which also receives blood from the basal vein of Rosenthal (*6*). *2,* anterior caudate vein; *3,* posterior caudate vein; *4,* medial subependymal vein perforating the roof of the 3rd ventricle to join the internal cerebral vein; *5,* medial atrial vein. (From Taveras JM, Wood EH. Diagnostic Neuroradiology, 2nd edition, Vol 2. Baltimore, Williams & Wilkins, 1976.)

great cerebral vein (of Galen—see below), in the posterior incisural space.

The main tributary of the internal cerebral vein on each side is the **thalamostriate** (or **terminal**) **vein**. This vein is formed by tributaries running on the wall of the lateral ventricle, and it also receives the **choroid vein**, which runs along the choroid plexus of the lateral ventricle (Fig. 52.105). The thalamostriate vein courses posteromedially with the stria terminalis in the body of the lateral ventricle in a groove between the head of the caudate nucleus and the thalamus. This vein is, therefore, situated on the inferolateral aspect of the ventricular wall and actually outlines the approximate size of the lateral ventricle.

Near the posterior edge of the foramen of Monro, the thalamostriate vein turns abruptly and terminates in the internal cerebral vein (Figs. 52.105 and 52.106). The junction of the internal cerebral and thalamostriate veins is called the **venous angle** (Krayenbühl and Yaşargil, 1968, 1973; Ono et al., 1984b). Here, the **septal vein**, extending backward from the frontal horn of the lateral ventricle on each side, also usually joins the internal cerebral vein (Figs. 52.105 and 52.106).

The **posterior callosal vein** is a small vessel that extends around the splenium of the corpus callosum. It then empties into the anterior portion of the vein of Galen (great cerebral vein) just behind its junction with the two internal cerebral veins.

MEDULLARY VEINS

There are numerous veins that are distributed radially in the depths of the cerebral hemispheres. These are the **medullary veins**. The deeper veins drain into other deep cerebral veins, whereas the more superficial medullary veins drain into the superficial cerebral veins. There are, however, anastomoses between the two groups.

BASAL VEIN (OF ROSENTHAL)

The **basal vein** (Rosenthal, 1824) originates on the medial aspect of the anterior portion of the temporal lobe, near the optic chiasm. It is formed from tributaries arising on the medial surface and temporal horn of the temporal lobe, from a small anterior cerebral vein that runs adjacent to the anterior cerebral artery, and from the large, deep middle cerebral vein (Padget, 1956; Meder et al., 1994) (Fig. 52.107).

The basal vein passes around the mesencephalon beneath the uncus and hippocampal gyrus. Its course parallels, but is slightly rostral to, the course of the posterior cerebral artery. Just superior and posterior to the pineal gland in the posterior incisural space, it usually unites with the two internal cerebral veins and the contralateral basal vein to form the vein of Galen (Rosenthal, 1824; Ono et al., 1984b) (Figs. 52.105–52.107). Variations from this classic confluence are common, however. The basal vein may empty into the vein of Galen after that vein has already formed but before it enters the straight sinus, or the basal vein may empty directly into the straight sinus, into the lateral sinus, or via the lateral mesencephalic vein into the superior petrosal sinus (Wolf et al., 1963).

Along its course, the basal vein receives blood from veins coming from the hippocampal gyrus, the interpeduncular fossa, and the mesencephalon (Meder et al., 1994). Inferior striate veins, which drain the corpus striatum and the anterior perforated substance, also empty into the basal vein.

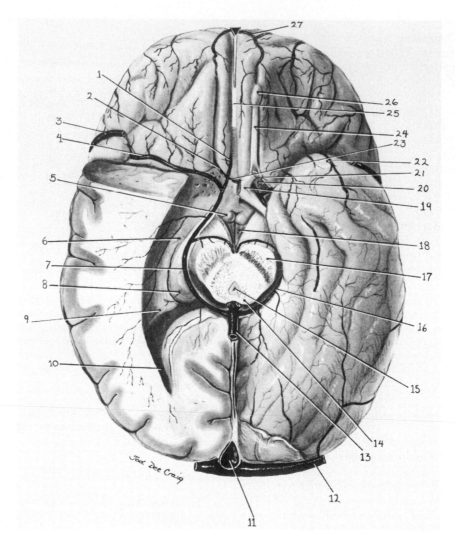

Figure 52.107.   Schematic illustration of the origin and course of the basal vein (of Rosenthal). The tip of the temporal lobe on the right side has been removed, and a horizontal cross cut through the right temporal and occipital lobes that exposes the temporal horn, occipital horn, and atrium of the right lateral ventricle is shown. The right basal vein (*7*) is fed by a number of veins, including the anterior cerebral vein (*1*), the olfactory vein (*2*), and the deep middle cerebral vein (*4*). The two basal veins join with the two internal cerebral veins (shown cut) to form the vein of Galen (*13*). *3,* superficial middle vein; *5,* mammillary body; *6,* temporal horn of the lateral ventricle; *8,* hippocampus; *9,* collateral eminence; *10,* posterior horn of the lateral ventricle; *11,* superior sagittal sinus; *12,* lateral (transverse) sinus; *14,* quadrigeminal plate; *15,* cerebral aqueduct; *16,* left basal vein; *17,* cerebral peduncle; *18,* posterior perforated substance; *19,* optic chiasm; *20,* anterior perforated substance; *21,* lateral olfactory striae; *22,* anterior tip of left temporal lobe; *23,* anterior communicating vein; *24,* olfactory tract; *25,* longitudinal (interhemispheric) fissure; *26,* olfactory bulb; *27,* superficial cerebral vein. (From Taveras JM, Wood EH. Diagnostic Neuroradiology, 2nd edition, Vol 2. Baltimore, Williams & Wilkins, 1976.)

GREAT CEREBRAL VEIN (OF GALEN)

As noted above, the great cerebral vein of Galen, often called either the ''great cerebral vein'' or the ''vein of Galen,'' usually arises from the confluence of the two internal cerebral veins and the two basal veins in the posterior incisural space just posterior and superior to the pineal gland (Ono et al., 1984b; Lasjaunias et al., 1987) (Figs. 52.101 and 52.105–52.107). This short vessel, about 2 cm in length, runs upward and backward around the splenium of the corpus callosum to end in the straight sinus at the junction of the falx cerebri and the tentorium cerebelli (Fig. 52.101). Along its course, the vein of Galen receives blood from

a number of supratentorial and infratentorial veins. These include the pericallosal veins, the internal occipital veins, and the veins draining the tentorial surface of the cerebellum, the cerebellomesencephalic fissure, and the superior half of the roof of the fourth ventricle (Ono et al., 1984b; Lasjaunias et al.).

Posterior Fossa Veins

The veins of the posterior fossa may be divided into four groups: (*a*) superficial, (*b*) deep, (*c*) brainstem, and (*d*) bridging veins. Matsushima et al. (1983) provided a nomenclature for these veins that is based on their relationship to the three cortical surfaces of the cerebellum, the three deep fissures between the brainstem and cerebellum, and the three subdivisions of the brainstem in the posterior fossa.

The **superficial veins** of the posterior fossa are named for the three cortical surfaces of the cerebellum they drain (Matsushima et al., 1983). The superior hemispheric and vermian veins drain the tentorial surface, which faces the tentorium cerebelli. The inferior hemispheric and inferior vermian veins drain the suboccipital surface, which is below and between the lateral and sigmoid sinuses. The anterior hemispheric veins drain the petrosal surface, which faces forward toward the posterior surface of the petrous bone.

The **deep veins** of the posterior fossa are located in the fissures between the cerebellum and the brainstem and on the three cerebellar peduncles. The major deep veins in the fissures, named after those fissures, are called the cerebellomesencephalic, cerebellopontine, and cerebellomedullary veins. Similarly, those deep veins located on the peduncles are simply called the veins of the superior, middle, and inferior peduncles, respectively.

The **brainstem veins** may be separated into two groups, longitudinal and lateral, based on their course. The veins in each group are further separated both by their location with respect to the brainstem (e.g., median, lateral, or anterolateral) and by the portion of the brainstem that they drain (e.g., mesencephalon, pons, or medulla).

The veins of the posterior fossa terminate as **bridging veins**. These veins collect into three groups:

1. A galenic group drains into the great cerebral vein of Galen;
2. A petrosal group drains into the superior and inferior petrosal sinuses; and
3. A tentorial group drains into the tentorial sinuses near the torcular herophili (from the Latin, meaning "winepress of Herophilus").

DIPLOIC VEINS

The **diploic veins** occupy channels in the diploë of the cranial bones (Fig. 52.108). They are large and contain pouch-like dilations at irregular intervals. Their walls are thin and formed of endothelium resting upon a layer of elastic tissue. These vessels communicate with the meningeal veins, with the sinuses of the dura mater, and with the veins of the pericranium. The four major diploic veins are:

1. The frontal, which drains into the superior sagittal sinus;
2. The anterior temporal, which is confined chiefly to the frontal bone and empties into the sphenoparietal sinus and into one of the deep temporal veins through an opening in the greater wing of the sphenoid;
3. The posterior temporal, which is located in the parietal bone and ends in the lateral sinus; and
4. The occipital, the largest of the four, which is confined to the occipital bone and which opens either externally into the occipital vein or internally into the lateral sinus or into the continence of sinuses (torcular herophili).

MENINGEAL VEINS

The small venous channels that drain the dura mater covering the brain are the **meningeal veins**. They are actually small sinuses that accompany the meningeal arteries, usually in pairs (venae comitantes). The largest meningeal veins accompany the middle meningeal artery (Oka et al., 1985). The meningeal veins are responsible for the grooves on the inner table of the skull.

The meningeal veins receive blood from the diploic veins of the calvarium and from some of the cortical veins. Depending on their location, the meningeal veins drain into the large dural sinuses at the base of the skull or into the superior sagittal sinus and its venous lacunae (Crosby et al., 1962; Oka et al., 1985).

DURAL SINUSES

The sinuses of the dura mater are venous channels that drain blood from the brain, dura, and diploë (Figs. 52.109 and 52.110). Situated between the two layers of the dura mater, they are devoid of valves and are lined by endothelial cells and by connective tissue that is continuous with that of the veins that drain into them (Piffer et al., 1986). They are often divided into two groups: (a) the **posterosuperior group**, which are located at the upper and back parts of the skull; and (b) the **anteroinferior group**, which are located at the base of the skull.

Posterosuperior Dural Sinuses

The posterosuperior group of dural sinuses is composed of the superior sagittal, inferior sagittal, straight, lateral (transverse), sigmoid, tentorial, and occipital sinuses. The superior sagittal, inferior sagittal, straight, and occipital sinuses are single, unpaired structures, whereas the lateral, sigmoid, and tentorial sinuses are paired structures.

Superior Sagittal Sinus

The **superior sagittal (longitudinal) sinus** begins at or near the foramen cecum ossis frontalis and extends posteriorly in the **attached margin** of the falx cerebri, becoming larger as it receives more venous outflow (Figs. 52.109, 52.111, and 52.112). Near the internal occipital protuberance, it usually deviates to the right to drain into the right lateral (transverse) sinus, although it may drain completely to the left sinus or equally into both lateral sinuses (Kaplan et al., 1972, 1974; Oka et al., 1985). In the same region, it joins with the straight sinus and the occipital sinus to form the confluence of sinuses (torcular herophili).

The superior sagittal sinus has the shape of an inverted triangle when viewed in cross-section (Fig. 52.113). Although it does not contain valves per se, the middle 12–14 cm of the sinus contain a complex of bands, bridges, cusps, and chords, often called collectively *chordae willisii* (Willis, 1664; Browder et al., 1972). The openings of cortical veins into the lateral walls of the sinus are usually lined by these structures, which may protect the cerebral veins from the effects of sudden increases in intracranial pressure.

As noted above, the superior sagittal sinus receives the

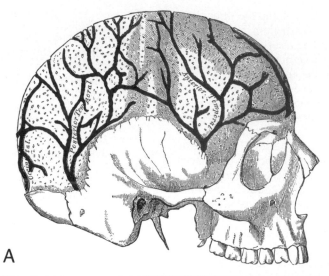

A

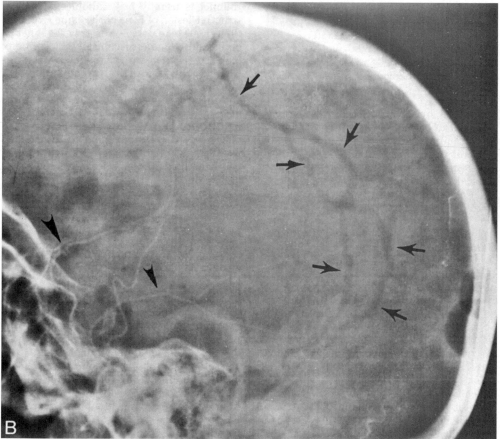

B

Figure 52.108.   Diploic veins. *A,* The diploic veins are visualized by removal of the outer table of the skull. (From Lewis WH. Gray's Anatomy of the Human Body, 23rd edition. Philadelphia, Lea & Febiger, 1936.) *B,* Skull x-ray shows clearly visible posterior temporal diploic veins *(posterior arrows)* in a patient who has undergone an external carotid arteriogram that shows the anterior *(large arrowhead)* and posterior *(small arrowhead)* branches of the middle meningeal artery. (From Taveras JM, Wood EH. Diagnostic Neuroradiology, 2nd edition, Vol 1. Baltimore, Williams & Wilkins, 1976.)

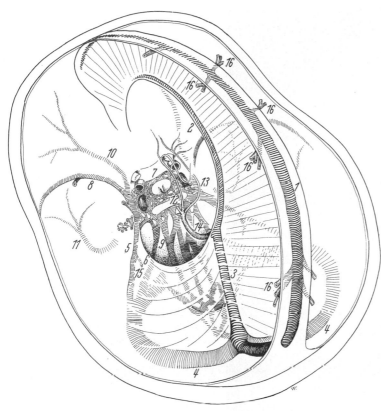

Figure 52.109. Schematic illustration of dural sinuses and their relationship to the deep internal veins. *1,* superior sagittal sinus; *2,* inferior sagittal sinus; *3,* straight sinus; *4,* lateral (transverse) sinus; *5,* superior petrosal sinus; *6,* inferior petrosal sinus; *7,* cavernous sinus; *8,* sphenoparietal sinus; *9,* basilar plexus; *10,* superior ophthalmic vein; *11,* middle meningeal vein; *12,* internal cerebral vein; *13,* basal vein of Rosenthal; *14,* great vein of Galen; *15,* petrosal vein; *16,* ascending cerebral veins. (From Krayenbühl HA, Yaşargil MG. Cerebral Angiography, 2nd edition. Philadelphia, JB Lippincott, 1968.)

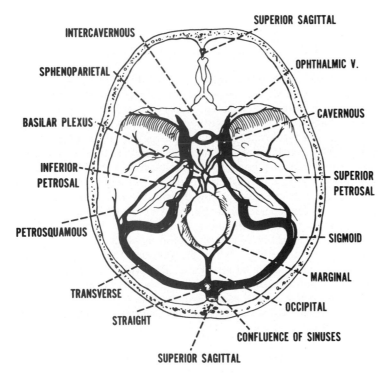

Figure 52.110. View of the base of the brain showing dural sinuses. (From Capra NF, Kapp JP. Anatomic and physiologic aspects of venous system. In Cerebral Blood Flow. Physiologic and Clinical Aspects. Editor, Wood JH, pp 37–58. New York, McGraw-Hill, 1987.)

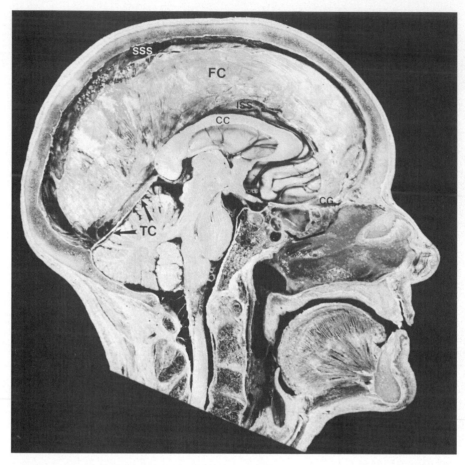

Figure 52.111. The superior sagittal sinus. In a cadaver specimen, the superior sagittal sinus (*SSS*) is seen within the falx cerebri (*FC*). The sinus becomes larger as it extends inferiorly. The inferior border of the falx cerebri arches over the corpus callosum (*CC*) and contains the inferior sagittal sinus (*ISS*). *CG,* crista galli; *TC,* tentorium cerebelli. (From Gluhbegovic N, Williams TH. The Human Brain: A Photographic Guide. Hagerstown, MD, Harper & Row, 1980.)

superior cerebral veins, the vein of Trolard, some of the inferior cerebral veins on the orbital surface of the frontal lobe, veins from the diploë and dura mater, and, near the posterior extent of the sagittal suture, veins from the pericranium (Andrews et al., 1989; Curé et al., 1994; Meder et al., 1994). Most of the cortical veins empty directly into the sinus, although some join the meningeal veins, which then empty into the sinus.

Enlarged venous spaces called **lacunae** are contained in the dura mater adjoining the superior sagittal sinus. The lacunae are largest and most constant in the parietal and posterior frontal regions. Smaller lacunae are found in the occipital and anterior frontal regions. The lacunae receive drainage of the meningeal veins that accompany the meningeal arteries in the dura mater (Oka et al., 1985). The cortical veins that empty into the superior sagittal sinus usually do so directly after passing beneath the lacunae, although some veins occasionally empty into the lacunae rather than directly into the sinus (Oka et al., 1985).

Small projections, the **arachnoid villi**, invaginate the dura mater to project into the lacunae and into the superior sagittal sinus (Figs. 52.113–52.116). Collections of these villi, forming cauliflower-like clumps, are called **arachnoid granulations** (Figs. 52.113–52.116). The arachnoid villi and granulations are responsible for transport of cerebrospinal fluid (CSF) from the subarachnoid space to the cerebral venous sinuses. Upton and Weller (1985) studied the pathways for CSF drainage in human arachnoid granulations. They found that at the base of each granulation, a thin neck of arachnoid projects through an aperture in the dural lining of the sinus and expands to form a core of collagenous trabeculae and interwoven channels. An apical cap of arachnoid cells surmounts the collagenous core, and channels extend through the cap to reach subendothelial regions of the granulation. These channels within the granulation are lined by compact collagen, and they may contain macrophages. Following recent subarachnoid hemorrhage, erythrocytes can be found in the channels, suggesting that the channels are in continuity with the subarachnoid space and are the CSF drainage pathways. Other investigators, however, have demonstrated cytochemical evidence of sodium-potassium-adenosine triphosphatase activity in the outermost cell layer of the arachnoid granulations (Go et al., 1986). This latter finding supports the theory that these granulations have a capacity for *active* as well as passive transport of CSF from the subarachnoid space to the superior sagittal and other dural sinuses.

Inferior Sagittal Sinus

The **inferior sagittal (longitudinal) sinus** travels in the **free margin** of the falx cerebri (Figs. 52.101 and 52.109).

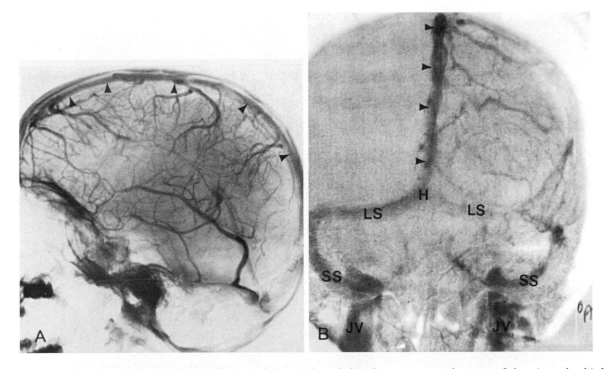

Figure 52.112. Angiographic appearance of the superior sagittal sinus. *A,* Lateral view shows anteroposterior extent of sinus (*arrowheads*). Note the superior superficial veins that drain upward and then turn rostrally to enter the sinus against the flow of blood. *B,* Anteroposterior view in a patient in whom the superior sagittal sinus (*arrowheads*) primarily drains the left hemisphere. The sinus ends at the torcular herophili (*H*) from which venous blood is drained via the lateral (transverse) (*LS*) and sigmoid (*SS*) sinuses into the internal jugular jugular veins (*JV*).

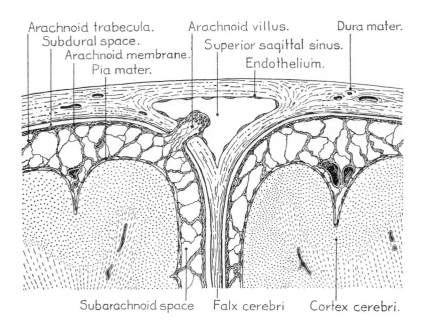

Figure 52.113. Schematic illustration of cross section of the superior sagittal sinus. Note that the sinus has the shape of an inverted triangle. (From Weed LH. The absorption of cerebrospinal fluid into the venous system. Am J Anat *31:* 191–221, 1923.)

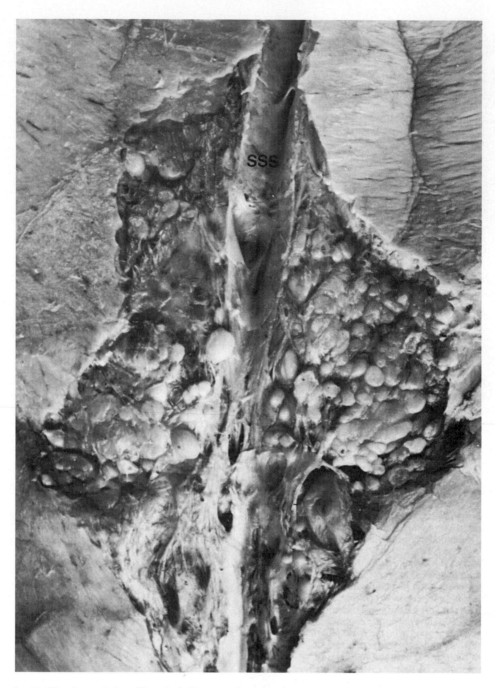

Figure 52.114.   Arachnoid villi and granulations. These bulb-like protrusions show considerable variation in size and shape. Mostly arranged in clusters, they project into the lateral lacunae and the superior sagittal sinus (*SSS*). (From Gluhbegovic N, Williams TH. The Human Brain: A Photographic Guide. Hagerstown, MD, Harper & Row, 1980.)

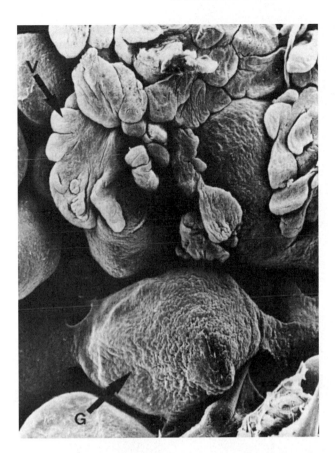

Figure 52.115. Scanning electron microscopic view of the surface of arachnoid villi (*V*) and granulations (*G*) that project into the superior sagittal sinus. Venous openings are present at the bases of the granulations. (From Upton ML, Weller RO. The morphology of cerebrospinal fluid drainage pathways in human arachnoid granulations. J Neurosurg *63:*867–875, 1985.)

It begins as a small vessel formed by the convergence of the falcial plexus of veins anterior to the middle of the falx (McCord et al., 1972). As it proceeds posteriorly, the inferior sagittal sinus receives veins that drain the roof of the corpus callosum, the cingulate gyrus, and the adjacent medial hemisphere (Oka et al., 1985; Capra and Kapp, 1987; Curé et al., 1994; Meder et al., 1994).

The inferior sagittal sinus is continuous posteriorly with the **straight sinus**, which also receives the vein of Galen before joining with the superior sagittal and occipital sinuses to form the torcular herophili (Figs. 52.101, 52.109, 52.110, and 52.117). Most of the venous blood carried by the inferior sagittal sinus drains via the straight sinus into the left lateral sinus, and for this reason, the inferior sagittal sinus is often described as ''forming'' the left lateral sinus. In fact, either or both lateral sinuses may originate from the torcular herophili.

Straight Sinus (Tentorial Sinus, Sinus Rectus)

The **straight sinus** is located in the junction of the falx cerebri with the tentorium cerebelli, just behind the splenium

of of the corpus callosum (Figs. 52.101, 52.109, and 52.117). It is formed chiefly by the union of the inferior sagittal sinus and the great cerebral vein of Galen (Curé et al., 1994). It runs downward and backward from the end of the inferior sagittal sinus to the lateral sinus of the side opposite to that into which the superior sagittal sinus drains (usually the left). The terminal portion of the straight sinus communicates by a cross-branch with the confluence of sinuses. Numerous tributaries from the tentorium and the posterior falx cerebri, near its attachment to the ridge of the tentorium, empty into the posterior portion of the straight sinus.

Lateral (Transverse) Sinuses

The **lateral sinus** on each side commences at the occipital protuberance. Each sinus passes laterally and forward in the attached margin of the tentorium cerebelli to the base of the petrous portion of the temporal bone (Figs. 52.109, 52.110, 52.112*B,* 52.117, and 52.118). It then leaves the tentorium and curves downward and medially to reach the jugular foramen, where it ends in the **internal jugular vein**.

The lateral sinuses receive blood from the superior sagittal and straight sinuses. Each lateral sinus also receives blood from cortical veins draining the lateral and basal surfaces of the ipsilateral temporal lobe (including the vein of Labbé) and the basal surface of the ipsilateral occipital lobe (Curé et al., 1994; Meder et al., 1994). Both sinuses also receive blood from the superior petrosal sinuses at the base of the petrous portion of the temporal bone, and from some of the inferior cerebellar veins, diploic veins, and pericranial veins.

It has already been noted that although the superior sagittal sinus may drain equally to the left and right lateral sinuses, it usually drains predominantly or completely to one of them. The *right* lateral sinus usually is larger and receives most of the drainage from the superior sagittal sinus (Zouaoui, 1988). The *left* lateral sinus usually is smaller and receives predominantly the drainage of the straight sinus. Thus, the right lateral sinus, right sigmoid sinus, and right jugular vein contain blood from the superficial parts of the brain, whereas the left lateral sinus, left sigmoid sinus, and left jugular vein contain blood mainly from the deep parts of the brain drained by the internal cerebral, basal, and great veins (see below).

Sigmoid Sinuses

The **sigmoid sinuses** originate at the posterior aspect of the petrous portion of the temporal bone. They follow a sinuous course before traversing the jugular foramen, where they become continuous with the internal jugular veins (Figs. 52.109, 52.110, 52.112*B,* and 52.118). Throughout its course, each sigmoid sinus receives inconstant veins from the cerebellum, the lateral pons, and the medulla. They communicate with the extracranial circulation via condyloid emissary veins.

Although some investigators consider the sigmoid sinuses to be a portion of the lateral sinuses, Waltner (1944) observed that variations in the lateral and sigmoid sinuses can occur independent of each other and that they seem to develop from separate anlagen. His argument is supported by documented cases in which a well-formed sigmoid sinus

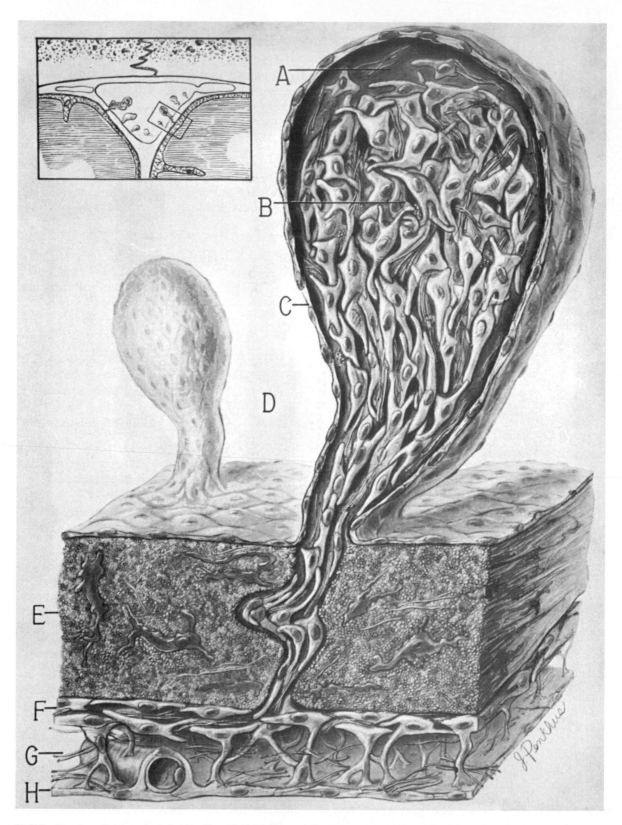

Figure 52.116. Drawing of a normal arachnoid villus. The inset (*upper left*) shows the superior sagittal sinus in cross-section (see also *Fig. 52.113*). The large drawing shows the area within the small rectangle in the inset. *A,* Loosely organized endothelial space in arachnoid villus. *B,* Meshwork of arachnoid cells and collagen that forms core of the villus. *C,* Endothelium of the sinus reflected over the villus and separating it from the sinus lumen. *D,* Lumen of the superior sagittal sinus. *E,* Dural wall of sinus. *F,* Arachnoid cells lining the inner aspect of the arachnoid membrane. *G,* Subarachnoid space containing arachnoid cells, fibrous trabeculae, and a large blood vessel. *H,* pia mater. (From Shabo AL, Maxwell DS. The morphology of the arachnoid villi: A light and electron microscopic study in the monkey. J Neurosurg *29:*451–463, 1968.)

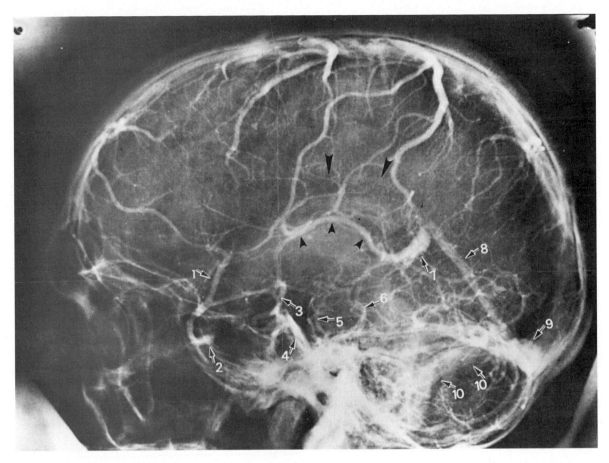

Figure 52.117.   Angiographic appearance of straight sinus. Cerebral arteriogram, lateral view, venous phase, shows faint staining of inferior sagittal sinus (*large arrowheads*) draining into the straight sinus (*8*) which also receives venous blood from the vein of Galen (*7*). The straight sinus drains directly into the torcular herophili (*9*) from which the blood travels to the lateral (transverse sinus) (*10*), the sigmoid sinus, and the internal jugular vein. *1,* superficial middle cerebral vein draining into the sphenoparietal sinus (*2*). *3,* uncal vein; *4,* inferior petrosal sinus; *5,* anterior pontomesencephalic veins; *6,* lateral anastomotic mesencephalic vein; *small arrowheads,* internal cerebral vein. (From Taveras JM, Wood EH. Diagnostic Neuroradiology, 2nd edition, Vol 2. Baltimore, Williams & Wilkins, 1976.)

drains the ipsilateral superior petrosal sinus in the absence of a lateral sinus (Capra and Kapp, 1987).

Tentorial Sinuses

The **tentorial sinuses** course through the tentorium cerebelli (Gibbs and Gibbs, 1934; Browder et al., 1975; Bisaria, 1985). They were classified by Matsushima et al. (1989) into four groups according to their drainage. Group I sinuses receive venous blood from the cerebral hemispheres through bridging veins. Group II sinuses are both drained and formed by the terminal portions of the cerebellar hemispheric or vermian veins. Group III sinuses originate as small veins within the tentorium itself. Group IV sinuses are formed by a bridging vein from the cerebral hemisphere or brainstem to the free edge of the tentorium. They may be remnants of the embryonic tentorial sinus (Padget, 1956).

Occipital Sinus

The **occipital sinus** is the smallest of the cranial sinuses (Figs. 52.101, 52.110, and 52.118). It is situated in the at-

tached margin of the falx cerebelli and is generally a single structure, although two such vessels are occasionally present. The occipital sinus is formed by several small venous channels in the region of the foramen magnum. It ends in the confluence of sinuses.

Confluence of Sinuses (Torcular Herophili)

The superior sagittal sinus, straight sinus, lateral sinuses, and occipital sinus typically have substantial communications near the internal occipital protuberance. The junction of these sinuses is called the **confluence of sinuses** or the **torcular Herophili** (Figs. 52.101, 52.109, 52.110, 52.112, 52.117, and 52.118). Four major configurations of the sinuses forming the torcular were described by Woodhall (1936):

1. A common pool configuration in which the superior sagittal sinus and the straight sinus course together into a single channel from which the lateral sinuses originate (9%);

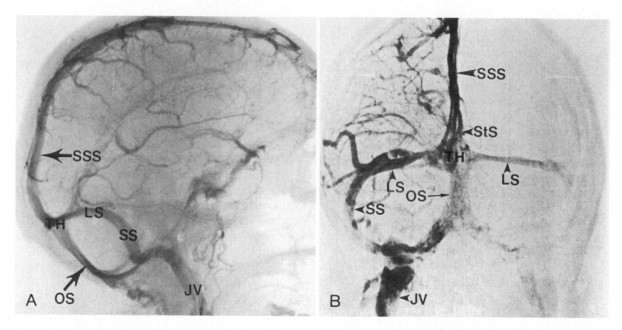

Figure 52.118.   Angiographic appearance of the basal dural sinuses. *A*, Lateral view shows the superior sagittal (*SSS*) and occipital (*OS*) sinuses draining into the torcular herophili (*TH*). The torcular drains into the lateral (transverse) sinus (*LS*). The lateral sinus drains into the sigmoid sinus (*SS*) and both sigmoid sinuses drain into the internal jugular vein (*JV*). *B*, Anteroposterior view of the same region as the photograph on the *left*. *StS*, straight sinus.

2. A plexiform configuration in which either the superior sagittal sinus, the straight sinus, or both branch to form the lateral sinus(es) and then enter the confluence as smaller vessels (56%);
3. An ipsilateral configuration in which the superior sagittal sinus supplies one lateral sinus and the straight sinus supplies the other lateral sinus (31%); and
4. A unilateral configuration in which both the superior sagittal sinus and the straight sinus contribute to one large lateral sinus (4%). In this last configuration, the opposite lateral sinus is absent.

Anteroinferior Group of Sinuses

This group of sinuses includes the cavernous sinuses, intercavernous sinuses, basilar sinus, sphenoparietal sinuses, and the superior and inferior petrosal sinuses. As is the case with the posterosuperior group of sinuses, the anteroinferior group of sinuses may be separated into paired and unpaired sinuses. There is only one basilar sinus, but there are two cavernous, intercavernous, sphenoparietal, superior petrosal, and inferior petrosal sinuses.

Cavernous Sinuses

Each **cavernous sinus** is situated at the side of the body of the sphenoid bone (Fig. 52.110) and extends from the superior orbital fissure to the tip of the petrous portion of the temporal bone, a distance of slightly more than 2 cm (Natori and Rhoton, 1995). The sphenoid sinus and the pituitary gland are medial to the cavernous sinus, and the middle cranial fossa and temporal lobe are lateral to it.

The cavernous sinus is not a large venous cavern. Rather,

it may be considered either a plexus of various-sized veins that divide, coalesce, and completely surround the cavernous segment of the carotid artery (Bonnet, 1955; Parkinson, 1965, 1973) or an unbroken, trabeculated, venous channel (Bedford, 1966; Harris and Rhoton, 1976; Inoue et al., 1990; Spinelli et al., 1994) (Figs. 52.119 and 52.120). Rhoton and his colleagues (Harris and Rhoton, 1976; Rhoton et al., 1979a, 1984; Oka et al., 1985; Inoue et al., 1990) separate the cavernous sinus into four main venous spaces relative to the cavernous segment of the internal carotid artery: the medial, anteroinferior, posterosuperior, and lateral compartments.

The medial compartment of the cavernous sinus lies between the pituitary gland and the internal carotid artery. It may be as wide as 7 mm, but may be obliterated when the artery is tortuous. The anteroinferior compartment is located in the concavity below the first curve of the intracavernous portion of the carotid artery. The abducens nerve enters this space after passing laterally around the artery. The posterosuperior compartment is located between the carotid artery and the posterior half of the roof of the cavernous sinus. The meningohypophyseal artery arises within this space. These three venous compartments are substantially larger than the space between the carotid artery and the lateral wall of the cavernous sinus. The lateral compartment is so narrow that when the abducens nerve passes through it, the nerve is **adherent to the carotid artery medially** and to the lateral sinus wall laterally (Bedford, 1966).

As noted above, the cavernous segment of the internal carotid artery and the abducens nerve are located within the body of the cavernous sinus, as is the oculosympathetic trunk. In the lateral wall of the cavernous sinus are the intra-

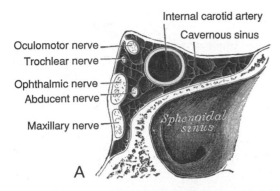

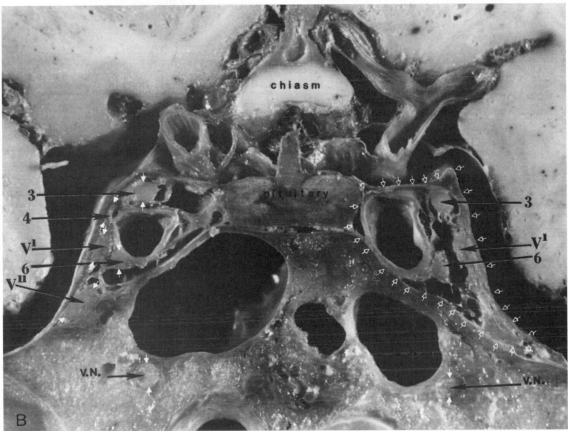

Figure 52.119. The cavernous sinus. *A,* Slightly oblique view showing that the sinus is a plexus of veins that surround the internal carotid artery and the abducens nerve. The oculomotor, trochlear, ophthalmic, and maxillary nerves are located in the deep layer of the lateral wall of the sinus. (From Lewis WH. Gray's Anatomy of the Human Body, 23rd edition. Philadelphia, Lea & Febiger, 1936.) *B,* Transverse section through the cavernous sinuses in a cadaver. *White hollow arrows (right side of photograph)* indicate the boundaries of the cavernous sinus. *White solid arrows (left side of photograph)* outline boundaries of cranial nerves. Note the trabeculated nature of the cavernous sinuses. *3,* oculomotor nerve; *4,* trochlear nerve; *V_1,* ophthalmic nerve; *V_{11},* maxillary nerve; *6,* abducens nerve; *V.N.,* vidian nerve. (Courtesy of W.F. Hoyt.)

cavernous portions of the oculomotor and trochlear nerves, and the intracavernous portions of the ophthalmic, maxillary, and, rarely, the mandibular divisions of the trigeminal nerve (Umansky and Nathan, 1982; Kawase et al., 1996).

Anteriorly, the cavernous sinus receives the sphenoparietal sinus, the superior ophthalmic vein, and the middle cerebral vein (Harris and Rhoton, 1976; Rhoton et al., 1979a, 1984; Oka et al., 1985; Inoue et al., 1990; Spinelli et al., 1994) (Fig. 52.110). Through communications with the precentral and postcentral veins that empty into the superior sagittal sinus, the middle cerebral veins establish communications between the superior sagittal and the cavernous sinuses. The cavernous sinus also communicates with the pterygoid plexus through emissary veins, and with the internal jugular vein through the carotid plexus (Spinelli et al., 1994). Each cavernous sinus communicates with its counterpart on

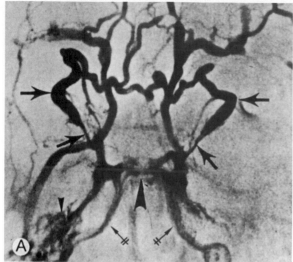

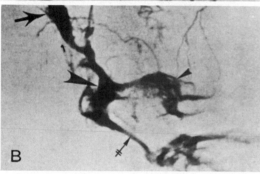

Figure 52.120. Angiographic appearance of the cavernous sinus. *A,* Venogram, submentovertical view, shows filling of both cavernous sinuses from the superior ophthalmic veins (*arrows*). There is opacification of the intercavernous sinus (*large arrowhead*). The cavernous sinuses drain to the pterygoid plexus (*small arrowhead*) and to the inferior petrosal sinuses (*cross-hatched arrows*). *B,* Lateral view of same venogram shows drainage of superior ophthalmic vein (*arrow*) to cavernous sinus (*large arrowhead*) which drains to pterygoid plexus (*small arrowhead*) and to inferior petrosal sinus (*cross-hatched arrow*). (From Huber P. Cerebral Angiography, 2nd edition. New York, Georg Thieme Verlag, 1982.)

the opposite side through the intercavernous and basilar sinuses (see below) (Fig. 52.110).

Intercavernous Sinuses

The intercavernous sinuses are located within the sella turcica (Figs. 52.110 and 52.120*A*). They join the cavernous sinuses on each side and are usually named based on their relationship to the pituitary gland. The anterior intercavernous sinus passes anterior to the pituitary gland, and the posterior intercavernous sinus passes posterior to the gland. In fact, these intercavernous connections can occur at any site along the anterior, inferior, or posterior surface of the gland (Renn and Rhoton, 1975; Harris and Rhoton, 1976; Rhoton et al., 1979, 1984). The anterior intercavernous sinus is usually larger than the posterior, but they may be equal in size, and either or both may be absent (Renn and Rhoton, 1975).

Basilar Sinus

This venous structure is a multiloculated cavity located posterior to the clivus and within the dura on the posterior aspect of the dorsum sellae (Fig. 52.110). The largest and most constant connection across the midline between the cavernous sinuses (Renn and Rhoton, 1975), the basilar sinus also receives the superior and inferior petrosal sinuses. The abducens nerve often enters the posterior margin of the cavernous sinus by passing through the basilar sinus (Harris and Rhoton, 1976).

Sphenoparietal Sinuses

The sphenoparietal sinuses (of Breschet) are the largest of the venous channels coursing with the meningeal arteries (Oka et al., 1985). They accompany the anterior branches of the middle meningeal arteries above the level of the pterion.

Each sphenoparietal sinus forms near the lateral edge of the lesser wing of the sphenoid bone (Fig. 52.110). It usually receives contributions from the middle meningeal veins and the superficial sylvian veins, but it may develop as the direct communication of a major branch from either (Wolf et al., 1963).

The sphenoparietal sinus courses in the inferoposterior ridge of the lesser wing of the sphenoid bone and normally ends in the anteroinferior angle of the cavernous sinus (Fig. 52.110). The size of the sinus varies considerably in direct proportion to the size and number of the contributing vessels.

The sphenoparietal sinus has access to the superior sagittal sinus via communications with superficial sylvian veins, in addition to having frequent communications with the basal vein of Rosenthal and branches of the orbitofrontal veins. Blood in the sphenoparietal sinus may flow in either direction.

Superior and Inferior Petrosal Sinuses

The cavernous sinuses and the basilar sinus are continuous posteriorly with the superior and inferior petrosal sinuses (Fig. 52.110, 52.121, and 52.122). The **superior petrosal sinus** runs in the attached margin of the tentorium cerebelli above or below Meckel's cave. It usually terminates in the proximal part of the sigmoid sinus, but it may terminate in the lateral sinus (Oka et al., 1985) (Figs. 52.109, 52.110, and 52.121). This sinus drains part of the inferior surface of the cerebral hemisphere and the superior surface of the cerebellum.

The **inferior petrosal sinus**, shorter but larger than the superior petrosal sinus, passes with the abducens nerve beneath the petroclinoid ligament (Gebarski and Gebarski, 1995; Rubinstein et al., 1995) (Figs. 52.109, 52.110, and 52.120–52.122). It receives contributions from the lower surface of the cerebellum, from the brainstem, and from the internal auditory veins. It communicates with the basilar sinus. The inferior petrosal sinus usually drains into the internal jugular vein, but it may empty into the distal portion of the sigmoid sinus.

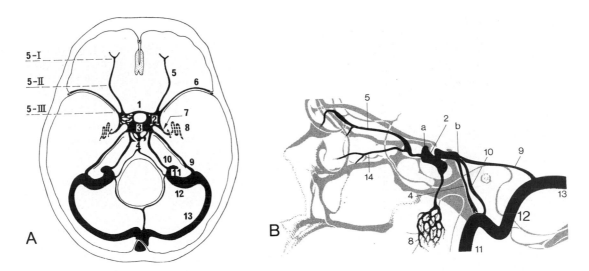

Figure 52.121. The superior and inferior petrosal sinuses and their relationship to the rest of the basal sinuses. *A*, Schematic illustration of the basal sinuses seen from above. Note that the superior petrosal sinus (*9*) begins at the cavernous sinus and drains into the proximal sigmoid (*12*) or distal lateral (*13*) sinus. The inferior petrosal sinus (*10*) originates in the same region but drains inferiorly into the internal jugular vein (*11*) or the distal sigmoid sinus. *1*, anterior intercavernous sinus; *3*, posterior intercavernous sinus; *4*, basilar sinus; *5*, superior ophthalmic vein; *5-I*, first segment of the superior ophthalmic vein; *5-II*, second segment of the superior ophthalmic vein; *5-III*, third segment of the superior ophthalmic vein; *6*, sphenoparietal sinus; *7*, foramen ovale plexus; *8*, pterygoid plexus. *B*, Lateral view of the same sinuses. Note that the superior petrosal sinus (*9*) courses horizontally from the posterior aspect of the cavernous sinus (*2*) to the proximal sigmoid (*12*) or distal lateral (*13*) sinus, whereas the inferior petrosal sinus (*10*) courses posteroinferiorly to drain into internal jugular vein (*11*) or the distal sigmoid sinus. *a*, anterior intercavernous sinus; *b*, posterior intercavernous sinus; *4*, basilar sinus; *5*, superior ophthalmic vein; *8*, pterygoid plexus; *14*, inferior ophthalmic vein. (From Huber P. Cerebral Angiography, 2nd edition. New York, Georg Thieme Verlag, 1982.)

ORBITAL VEINS

The orbital venous system is composed of a freely anastomosing, valveless, and variable network of vessels that includes three principal veins: the superior ophthalmic vein, the inferior ophthalmic vein, and the central retinal vein (Spinelli et al., 1994).

Superior Ophthalmic Vein

The **superior ophthalmic vein**, the principal vein of the orbit, begins in the upper medial corner of the orbital margin. It is formed by the union of the supraorbital veins of the forehead and the angular veins of the medial canthal area. It initially passes near the trochlea and then turns upward to lie just underneath the periosteum of the roof of the orbit (Figs. 52.120, 52.121, and 52.123). It then takes a downward loop and assumes a position just beneath the superior rectus muscle. In this position, it courses posterolaterally within the muscle cone. When it reaches the junction of the middle and posterior thirds of the orbit, it makes a distinct bend inferiorly, briefly runs alongside

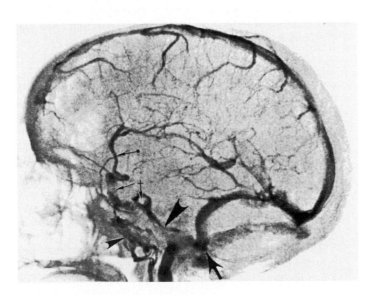

Figure 52.122. Lateral angiographic view of the inferior petrosal sinus. Note its posteroinferior course (*large arrowhead*) from the region of the cavernous sinus (*crossed arrow*) to the region of the junction between the sigmoid sinus and the internal jugular vein (*arrow*). *Small arrowhead,* pterygoid plexus; *thin arrow,* anterior intercavernous sinus; *dot-tipped arrow,* deep middle cerebral vein. (From Krayenbühl HA, Yaşargil MG. Cerebral Angiography. Philadelphia, JB Lippincott, 1968.)

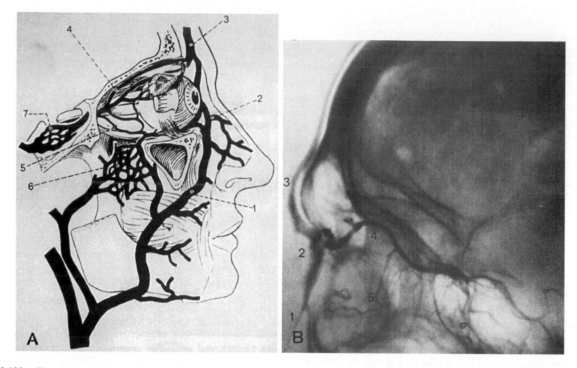

Figure 52.123. The course of the superior ophthalmic vein. *A,* Diagram of orbital veins and their ways of drainage. *1,* facial vein; *2,* angular vein; *3,* frontal vein; *4,* superior ophthalmic vein; *5,* inferior ophthalmic vein; *6,* pterygoid plexus; *7,* cavernous sinus. *B,* Normal orbital venogram in lateral view. *1,* injection needle; *2,* angular vein; *3,* frontal vein; *4,* superior ophthalmic vein; *5,* inferior ophthalmic vein. (From Krayenbühl HA, Yaşargil MG. Cerebral Angiography, 2nd edition. Philadelphia, JB Lippincott, 1968.)

the ophthalmic artery lateral to the optic nerve, and then enters the superior orbital fissure through the annulus of Zinn (Natori and Rhoton, 1995). As it passes through the superior orbital fissure, the superior ophthalmic vein bends downward to enter the cavernous sinus (Lombardi and Passerini, 1967; Spinelli et al., 1994). The superior ophthalmic vein receives blood from two large ethmoidal veins, the four vortex veins of the eye, and a large lacrimal vein (which may occasionally enter the cavernous sinus independently).

Inferior Ophthalmic Vein

The **inferior ophthalmic vein** is an inconstant structure that arises from a venous plexus on the orbital floor (Fig. 52.123). When present, it receives branches from the lower eyelid, the area of the lacrimal sac, the inferior extraocular muscles, and the two inferior vortex veins of the eye. It may join with the superior ophthalmic vein, anastomose with the superior ophthalmic vein via small emissary channels, or pass through the superior orbital fissure to enter the cavernous sinus separate from the superior ophthalmic vein (Spinelli et al., 1994; Natori and Rhoton, 1995).

Central Retinal Vein

The **central retinal vein** drains the retina and the intraorbital parts of the optic nerve. Formed by the union of various

retinal veins at the level of the lamina cribrosa, it runs through the core of the optic nerve in company with the central retinal artery, and the two vessels share a common wall during their course (Fig. 52.124). Within the lamina cribrosa, the central retinal vein anastomoses through lateral twigs with the choroidal venous plexus. These small anastomotic channels may enlarge to become **optociliary veins** that shunt blood from the retinal to the choroidal circulation in patients with central retinal vein occlusion or chronic compression of the central retinal vein (Anderson, 1970; see Chapters 8, 13, and 40).

The central retinal vein exits from the optic nerve about 10 mm posterior to the globe, usually in company with the central retinal artery (Fig. 52.124). The vein normally courses for 4–8 mm through the vaginal spaces surrounding the nerve before it pierces the dura to exit the nerve. It then joins a plexus of veins in the orbital fat, receives numerous tributaries from the optic nerve, exits the orbit through the annulus of Zinn and the superior orbital fissure, and finally enters the cavernous sinus (Hayreh, 1963b; Spinelli et al., 1994; Natori and Rhoton, 1995).

EXTRACRANIAL CEREBRAL VEINS

The **internal jugular vein** is the most important drainage channel in the craniocervical region. It collects blood from the brain, the superficial parts of the face, and the neck. The

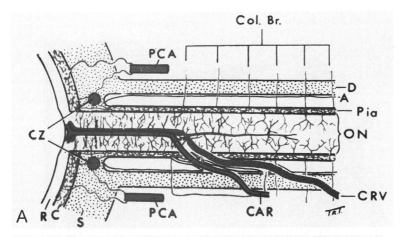

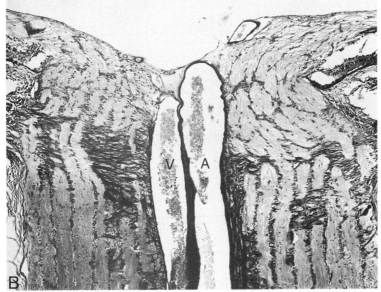

Figure 52.124. The central retinal vein. *A,* Schematic illustration of the course of the central retinal vein (*CRV*) and its relationship to the central retinal artery (*CAR*). Note that the vessels are adjacent to each other within the optic nerve (*ON*) and that they exit the nerve in the same general area. *A,* arachnoid; *C,* choroid; *Col. Br.,* collateral branches supplying the peripheral optic nerve; *CZ,* circle of Zinn and Haller; *D,* dura; *PCA,* posterior ciliary artery; *R,* retina; *S,* sclera. (From Hayreh SS. Pathogenesis of oedema of the optic disc (papilloedema): A preliminary report. Br J Ophthalmol *48:*522–543, 1964.) *B,* Histologic appearance of normal central retinal artery (*A*) and central retinal vein (*V*) showing that they share a common wall. This anatomic feature probably explains why atherosclerotic disease that affects the central retinal artery may also obstruct the central retinal vein. (Courtesy of W. Richard Green).

internal jugular vein originates in the posterior compartment of the jugular foramen from the sigmoid sinuses, which themselves receive blood from the sinuses that form the torcular herophili (Figs. 52.112*B,* 52.118, 52.121*B,* 52.122, and 52.125).

At its origin, the internal jugular vein is somewhat dilated, and this dilation is called the **jugular bulb** (Fig. 52.125). The vein then runs vertically down the side of the neck, lying at first lateral to the internal carotid artery and then lateral to the common carotid artery. At the base of the neck, it unites with the subclavian vein to form the innominate vein.

In addition to receiving blood from the lateral sinuses, the internal jugular vein is joined by the inferior petrosal sinus and the facial, lingual, pharyngeal, superior thyroid, and middle thyroid veins. The occipital vein may also occasionally empty into the internal jugular vein. The thoracic duct on the left side and the right lymphatic duct open into the angle formed by the union of the internal jugular and subclavian veins.

The **vertebral vein** is formed on both sides by the confluence of the anterior and posterior venous roots (Braun and Tournade, 1977). The anterior root of the vertebral vein originates at the level of the junction of the anterior and middle thirds of the occipital venous plexus from the anterior condylar vein. It follows an oblique downward, outward, and forward course, crossing the anterior condylar canal before it joins the posterior root of the vertebral vein. The posterior root originates at the level of the posterior third of the occipital venous plexus, crosses the atlanto-occipital membrane, and terminates by joining the anterior root to form the vertebral vein.

The **external jugular vein** receives the greater part of the blood from the exterior of the cranium and the deep parts of the face. It is formed by the junction of the posterior division of the posterior facial vein and the posterior auricular vein. This vessel originates in the substance of the parotid gland at the level of the angle of the mandible and runs perpendicularly down the neck to end in the subclavian vein.

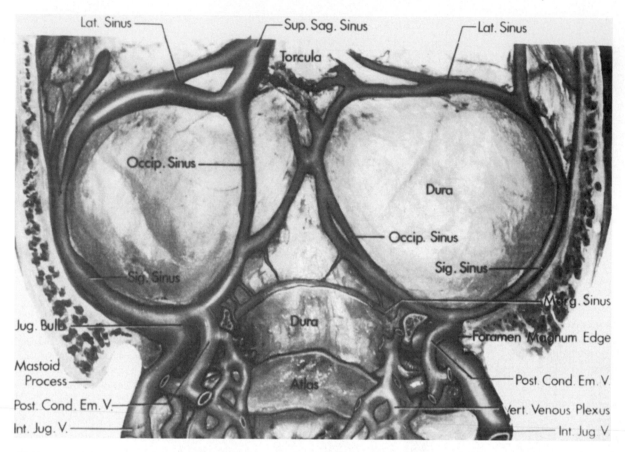

Figure 52.125. The origin and initial course of the internal jugular vein. The internal jugular vein (*Int.Jug.V.*) is formed primarily by the sigmoid and occipital sinuses. It also receives drainage from the posterior condylar emissary veins (*Post.Cond.Em.V.*). The confluence of these vessels is called the jugular bulb. (From de Oliveira E, Rhoton AL Jr, Peace D. Microsurgic anatomy of the region of the foramen magnum. Surg Neurol *24*:293–352, 1985.)

PHYSIOLOGY OF CEREBRAL BLOOD FLOW

CBF may be measured by a number of different techniques, including nitrous oxide washout (Kety and Schmidt, 1945), xenon-133 (Hoed et al., 1966; Obrist et al., 1975) and krypton-85 (Lassen and Munck, 1955) clearance, electromagnetic flowmetry (Greenfield and Tindall, 1965), oxygen-15 steady-state inhalation combined with positron emission tomography (Cone, 1985; Leenders et al., 1990), and duplex ultrasound scanning (B-mode imaging and pulsed Doppler shift analysis—Leopold et al., 1987). The currently accepted standard for measurement of CBF is by intra-arterial injection of xenon, although the xenon and oxygen inhalation methods, duplex scanning, and other noninvasive techniques are favored by many investigators (Leopold et al., 1987; Leenders et al., 1990).

The magnitude of CBF is dependent on a number of factors, including the size of the lumen of the vessels composing the cerebral arterial tree, perfusion pressure, cerebral metabolism, and blood viscosity (Kee and Wood, 1987; Miller and Bell, 1987; Pickard, 1987). Mean CBF remains remarkably constant at about 50–52 ml/100 g brain tissue/min over the wide range of mean arterial blood presssure of 60–170 mm Hg in the normal adult (Lassen, 1964). For the entire brain

of the average adult, this is about 750 ml/min, or 15% of the total resting cardiac output. A system of *autoregulation* maintains constant CBF despite substantial variations in blood pressure (Lassen, 1959).

AUTOREGULATION OF CEREBRAL BLOOD FLOW

If the cerebral vascular bed were a system of branching, rigid pipes, CBF would be a simple function of the perfusion pressure (the difference between cerebral vascular inflow and outflow pressures) divided by the parallel resistance to flow along these pipes. The pressure-flow relationship could therefore be expressed in the same form as Ohm's law:

$$F = P/R$$

where F is flow, P is pressure, and R is resistance. Resistance to flow is governed by the caliber of the tubing, its length, and the nature of the fluid that flows within it. If it is assumed that the system of rigid tubes is being perfused at a steady rate by a newtonian fluid that has a laminar flow pattern, then the flow can be expressed in terms of the Poiseuille equation:

$$F = \pi r^4 (P_{in} - P_{out})/8nL$$

where F is flow, r is vessel radius, P is pressure, n is viscosity, and L is length. The limitations of such analogies are clear: blood is a non-newtonian fluid; the effective length of the vascular bed may vary as precapillary vessels open and close, exposing different parts of the network to blood; the perfusing intravascular pressure is pulsatile; and the vessels are not rigid but are both distensible and actively contractile. Nevertheless, the fundamental relationships between flow, perfusion, pressure, and resistance in the intact human cerebrovascular bed can be reasonably well described by these equations (Green and Rapela, 1984).

The cerebrovascular bed is at all times subject to the combined influence of a number of physical and chemical stimuli that adjust vascular caliber so as to alter the blood supply to different parts of the brain. These stimuli may be of local or systemic origin and activate different mechanisms that change cerebrovascular resistance. The end points of these processes provide a precise and rapid matching of local CBF to changes in local neuronal metabolic requirements, ensuring an adequate supply of blood, oxygen, and glucose even under conditions of stress.

Three mechanisms that control the caliber of arterial vessels play a role in the autoregulation of CBF (Gotoh et al., 1972; Meyer et al., 1973; Strandgaard and Paulson, 1984):

1. Arterial smooth muscle responds directly to variations of blood pressure by constricting or dilating, thus changing the diameter of the vessel lumen.
2. Local concentrations of metabolites directly affect vascular tone. Because any change in blood flow causes cellular metabolites to be carried away at a different rate, vascular tone changes, and the size of the vascular lumen is altered accordingly.
3. Autonomic neural influences of local or remote origin may control vascular tone, changing the size of the arterial lumen.

Autoregulation is, unfortunately, not perfect. Vasoconstriction, vascular occlusion, or a drop in mean arterial pressure below 60 mm Hg may cause CBF to fall. Neuronal activity does not become impaired, however, until mean flow is reduced to about 20 ml/100 g/min, and neuronal death does not occur until flow falls to 5 ml/100 g/min for a prolonged period (Lassen, 1978). Similarly, when mean arterial pressure exceeds 170 mm Hg, autoregulation is overridden, and CBF rises. This is called the "breakthrough phenomenon," because the arterioles are unable to contain the pressure sufficiently to protect the capillaries (Skinhoj and Strandgaard, 1973). Indeed, the arterioles are forcibly expanded, the capillary pressure rises, and hypertensive encephalopathy may develop from edema, hemorrhage, and focal vascular spasm (Arnold, 1981).

FACTORS OTHER THAN AUTOREGULATION AFFECTING CEREBRAL BLOOD FLOW

As noted above, autoregulation of CBF is far from perfect. A number of factors can increase or decrease CBF independent of the size of the arteries.

Blood Viscosity and Cerebral Blood Flow

Although CBF depends on cerebral perfusion pressure and the resistance of the cerebrovascular tree, even when perfusion pressure and vessel caliber remain constant, flow can vary with changes in the viscosity of the blood, in accordance with Poiseuille's equation. Blood viscosity rises exponentially when the hematocrit increases and also is raised when the γ-globulin and fibrinogen concentrations in plasma are elevated.

When the hematocrit rises, flow falls because the oxygen-carrying capacity of the blood is increased and less blood is required to deliver oxygen. Reduced flow itself raises viscosity higher, and a vicious cycle can ensue until stasis occurs (Thomas, 1982). Although autoregulation can compensate for an increase in blood viscosity by vasodilation, this mechanism does not suffice.

Metabolism and Cerebral Blood Flow

The neuronal mass of the brain comprises about 40% of its volume and has a rather high energy requirement. Most neurons have long axons and many dendrites. Energy is therefore needed to transport intracellular material peripherally and centrally, to maintain the structure of the large area of cell membrane, and to create ionic gradients across the membrane. When interneuronal communication occurs, additional energy is required for the release of excitatory and inhibitory neurotransmitters, for their subsequent degradation, and for the restoration of membrane polarization. Thus, CBF is intimately coupled with brain metabolism and brain function (Sokoloff, 1983). Studies using a number of different methods have shown a direct relationship between specific mental or motor activity and changes in blood flow in regions of the cerebral cortex in human subjects (Lassen et al., 1978; Berne et al., 1981; Meyer et al., 1981; Aaslid, 1987).

Cell metabolism comprises the consumption of adenosine triphosphate (ATP) during work and the ensuing consumption of energy to resynthesize ATP from adenosine diphosphate (ADP). Glucose is the sole energy substrate of the brain, unless there is ketosis, and 95% of the normal brain's energy requirement comes from the oxidation of glucose to water and carbon dioxide. Only limited reserves of glucose and glycogen are available within the astrocytes of the brain. The brain is therefore constantly dependent on a blood supply to provide the oxygen and glucose it requires. If the oxygen supply is interrupted, tissue ATP falls to zero within 7 minutes (Siesjo, 1984).

In view of the dependence of the brain on a consistent supply of glucose, it is not surprising that CBF is markedly sensitive to substances that affect cellular metabolism. The most potent of these substances is **carbon dioxide**. An increase in carbon dioxide concentration in the arterial blood perfusing the brain greatly increases CBF. In fact, inhalation of 5% carbon dioxide can produce a 75% rise in CBF in young subjects (Deshmukh and Meyer, 1978).

Carbon dioxide increases CBF by combining with water in the body fluids to form carbonic acid, with subsequent dissociation to form hydrogen ions. The hydrogen ions then cause dilation of the cerebral vessels that is almost directly proportional to the increase in hydrogen ion concentration. Any other substances that increase the acidity of the brain tissue, and which therefore also increase the hydrogen ion concentration, increase CBF. Such substances include lactic acid, pyruvic acid, and other acids formed during metabolism. The increase in regional CBF that occurs during increased regional neuronal activity (e.g., the rise in flow through Broca's area during speech) is thought to be mediated by increased production of carbon dioxide, lactic acid, and pyruvic acid (Ingvar and Schwartz, 1974).

Although an increase in **hydrogen ion** concentration increases CBF, it also greatly **depresses** neuronal activity. Fortunately, the increased CBF carries both carbon dioxide and other acidic substances away from the brain. Loss of carbon dioxide removes carbonic acid from the tissues, and this, along with the removal of other acids, reduces the hydrogen ion concentration toward normal. This mechanism helps to maintain a constant hydrogen ion concentration in the cerebral extracellular fluid and thereby also maintains a normal level of neuronal activity.

Oxygen has almost as potent an effect on CBF as carbon dioxide and hydrogen ion concentration (Brown et al., 1985). Except during periods of intense brain activity, the use of oxygen by the brain tissue remains within a few percent of 3.5 ml of oxygen/100 g of brain tissue/min (Guyton, 1986). If CBF becomes insufficient to supply this amount of oxygen, however, the oxygen deficiency mechanism for vasodilation, which functions in all tissues of the body, immediately causes cerebral vasodilation. This returns blood flow and the transport of oxygen to nearly normal. CBF begins to increase when the partial pressure of oxygen in arterial blood falls below 50 mm Hg (Miller and Bell, 1987). Similarly, a decrease in the partial pressure of oxygen in cerebral *tissue* below 30 mm Hg (normal is 35–40 mm Hg) results in increased CBF.

A number of neuropeptides, including substance P, neuropeptide Y, cholecystokinin, 5-hydroxytryptophan, and norepinephrine, have effects on CBF that are almost as potent as those of carbon dioxide, hydrogen ion, and oxygen (Raichle et al., 1975; Edvinsson et al., 1981, 1983; Griffith et al., 1982; Hendry et al., 1983). Some of these peptides apparently alter neuronal and glial metabolism, whereas others seem to act solely on cerebral resistance (see below).

Sympathetic Nervous System and Cerebral Blood Flow

The cerebral circulatory system has a strong sympathetic innervation that passes upward from the superior cervical sympathetic ganglia along with the cerebral arteries. This innervation supplies both large superficial arteries and the small arteries that penetrate the substance of the brain. Neither transection nor stimulation of these sympathetic nerves normally causes a significant change in CBF, because the local blood flow autoregulatory mechanism is so powerful that it normally compensates almost entirely for the effects of sympathetic dysfunction. Nevertheless, in those conditions in which autoregulation fails to compensate (e.g., when arterial pressure rises significantly during strenuous exer-

cise), the sympathetic nervous system constricts the large and intermediate-sized arteries and prevents the high pressure from ever reaching the smaller blood vessels.

Age and Cerebral Blood Flow

CBF declines sharply in the first two decades of life to the normal adult value (Arnold, 1981), and there is evidence that it decreases further during normal aging (Shenkin et al., 1953; Kety, 1956; Dastur et al., 1963; Naritomi et al., 1979; Melamed et al., 1980; Yamamoto et al., 1980; Mamo et al., 1983; MacInnes et al., 1984; Matsuda et al., 1984; Shaw et al., 1984; Gur et al., 1987; Leenders et al., 1990). Although a reduction of CBF may be caused by decreased neuronal density with age, it is unclear whether or not such reduction occurs during aging (Bowen and Davison, 1978; Leenders et al., 1990). There is no doubt, however, that patients with hypertension, diabetes mellitus, hyperlipidemia, or atherosclerosis experience a significant reduction in CBF as they age (Deshmukh and Meyer, 1978). In addition, defective autoregulation was found in otherwise healthy elderly patients (Wollner et al., 1979). This may be related to a decreased response of the vascular system of such persons to hypercapnia (Deshmukh and Meyer, 1978) or to the development of atherosclerosis (Arnold, 1981).

REFERENCES

Aaslid R. Visually evoked dynamic blood flow response of the human cerebral circulation. Stroke *18*:771–775, 1987.

Abd El-Bary TH, Dujovny M, Ausman JI. Microsurgical anatomy of the atlantal part of the vertebral artery. Surg Neurol *44*:392–401, 1995.

Adachi B, Hasebe K. Das Arteriensystem der Japaner, Vol 1. Kyoto, Maruzen Co., Ltd., 1928.

Agnoli AL. Vascular anomalies and subarachnoid haemorrhage associated with persisting embryonic vessels. Acta Neurochir *60*:183–199, 1982.

Allen WE, Kier EL, Rothman SLG. The maxillary artery: normal arteriographic anatomy. AJR *118*:517–527, 1973.

Alpers BJ, Berry RG, Paddison RM. Anatomical studies of the circle of Willis in normal brain. Arch Neurol Psychiatry *81*:409–418, 1959.

Amarenco P, Hauw J-J. Anatomie des artères cérébelleuses. Rev Neurol *145*:267–276, 1989.

Anderson DR. Vascular supply to the optic nerve of primates. Am J Ophthalmol *70*: 341–351, 1970.

Andeweg J. The anatomy of collateral venous flow from the brain and its value in aetiological interpretation of intracranial pathology. Neuroradiology *38*:621–628, 1996.

Andrews BT, Dujovny M, Mirchandani HG, et al. Microsurgical anatomy of the venous drainage into the superior sagittal sinus. Neurosurgery *24*:514–520, 1989.

Arnold KG. Cerebral blood flow in geriatrics: A review. Age Aging *10*:5–9, 1981.

Artero JC, Ausman JI, Dujovny M, et al. Middle cerebral artery reconstruction. Surg Neurol *24*:5–11, 1985.

Batujeff N. Eine Seltene Arterienanomalie: Ursprung der A. basilaris aus der A. carotis interna. Anat Anz *4*:282, 1889.

Bedford MA. The "cavernous" sinus. Br J Ophthalmol *50*:41–46, 1966.

Bell RH, Swigart LL, Anson BJ. The relation of the vertebral artery to the cervical vertebrae based upon the study of 200 specimens. Quarterly Bulletin Northwestern University Medical School *24*:184–185, 1950.

Berne RM, Winn HR, Rubio R. The local regulation of cerebral blood flow. Prog Cardiovasc Dis *24*:243–260, 1981.

Bisaria KK. Anatomic variations of venous sinuses in the region of the torcular herophili. J Neurosurg *62*:90–95, 1985.

Blinkov SM, Gabibov GA, Tanyashin SV. Variations in the location of the arteries coursing between the brainstem and the free edge of the tentorium. J Neurosurg *76*:973–978, 1992.

Bonnet P. La loge caverneuse et les syndromes de la loge caverneuse. Arch Ophtalmol *15*:357–372, 1955.

Bouthillier A, van Loveren HR, Keller JT. Segments of the internal carotid artery: A new classification. Neurosurgery *38*:425–433, 1996.

Bowen DM, Davison AN. Biochemical changes in the normal ageing brain and in dementia. In Recent Advances in Geriatric Medicine. Editor, Isaacs B, pp 32–45. Edinburgh, Churchill Livingstone, 1978.

Braun JP, Tournade A. Venous drainage in the craniocervical region. Neuroradiology *13*:155–158, 1977.

Browder J, Browder A, Kaplan HA. The venous sinuses of the cerebral dura mater: Anatomical structures within the superior sagittal sinus. Arch Neurol *26*: 175–180, 1972.

Browder J, Kaplan HA, Krieger AJ. Venous channels in the tentorium cerebelli: surgical significance. Surg Neurol *3*:37–39, 1975.

Brown MM, Wade JPH, Marshall J. Fundamental importance of arterial oxygen content in the regulation of cerebral blood flow in man. Brain *108*:81–93, 1985.

Bruetman ME, Fields WS. Persistent hypoglossal artery (arteria hypoglossica primitiva). Arch Neurol *8*:369–372, 1963.

Brunsteins DB, Ferreri AJM. Microsurgical anatomy of the arteries related to the internal acoustic meatus. Acta Anat *152*:143–150, 1995.

Busch W. Beitrag zur Morphologie und Pathologie der Arteria basilaris (Untersuchungsergebnisse bei 1000 Gerhirnen). Arch Psychiatr Nervenkr *208*:326–344, 1966.

Cahill M, Bannigan J, Eustace P. Anatomy of the extraneural blood supply to the intracranial oculomotor nerve. Br J Ophthalmol *80*:177–181, 1996.

Campbell RL, Dyken ML. Four cases of carotid-basilar anastomosis associated with central nervous system dysfunction. J Neurol Neurosurg Psychiatry *24*:250–253, 1961.

Capra NF, Kapp JP. Anatomic and physiologic aspects of venous system. In Cerebral Blood Flow: Physiologic and Clinical Aspects. Editor, Wood JH, pp 37–58. New York, McGraw-Hill, 1987.

Carpenter MB, Noback CR, Moss ML. The anterior choroidal artery: Its origins, course, distribution, and variations. Arch Neurol Psychiatry *71*:714–722, 1954.

Casberg MA. The clinical significance of the cervical fascial planes. Surg Clin North Am *30*:1415–1434, 1950.

Cavatorti P. Il tipo normale e le variazione delle arterie della base dell'encephalo. Monit Zool Ital *10*:248–259, 1908.

Clark SL, Wentsler NE. Pial circulation studied by long-continued direct inspection. Res Publ Assoc Res Nerv Ment Dis *18*:218–228, 1938.

Cobb SR, Hieshima GB, Mehringer CM, et al. Persistent trigeminal artery variant: Carotid-anterior inferior cerebellar artery anastomosis. Surg Neurol *19*:263–266, 1983.

Cone JB. Positron emission tomography: New analytical tool for vascular disease. J Vasc Surg *2*:360, 1985.

Coulter VL, Holds JB, Anderson RL. Avoiding complications of orbital surgery: The orbital branches of the infraorbital artery. Ophthalmic Surg *21*:141–143, 1990.

Critchley M. The anterior cerebral artery and its syndromes. Brain *53*:120–165, 1930.

Crosby EC, Humphrey T, Lauer EW, editors. Correlative Anatomy of the Nervous System, pp 565–571. New York, MacMillan, 1962.

Crowell RM, Morawetz RB. The anterior communicating artery has significant branches. Stroke *8*:272–273, 1977.

Curé JK, Van Tassel P, Smith MT. Normal and variant anatomy of the dural venous sinuses. Semin Ultrasound CT MRI *15*:499–519, 1994.

Cushing H. Strangulation of the nervi abducentes by lateral branches of the basilar artery in cases of brain tumor. Brain *33*:204–235, 1910.

Dastur DK, Lane MH, Hansen DB, et al. Effects of aging on cerebral circulation and metabolism in man. In Human Aging: A Biological and Behavioral Study. Public Health Service Publication 986, pp 59–76. Washington, DC, U.S. Government Printing Office, 1963.

Daumann C, Putz R, Schmidt D. Der Verlauf der Arteria temporalis superficialis. Klin Monatsbl Augenheilkd *194*:37–41, 1989.

Dawson BH. The blood vessels of the human optic chiasma and their relation to those of the hypophysis and hypothalamus. Brain *81*:207–217, 1958.

Day AL. Arterial distributions and variants. In Cerebral Blood Flow: Physiologic and Clinical Aspects. Editor, Wood JH, pp 19–36. New York, McGraw-Hill, 1987.

De Caro R, Parenti A, Munari PF. Fenestration of the vertebrobasilar junction. Acta Neurochir *108*:85–87, 1991.

De Caro R, Parenti A, Munari PF. The persistent primitive hypoglossal artery: A rare anatomic variation with frequent clinical implications. Anat Anz *177*:193–198, 1995.

De Caro R, Parenti A, Munari PF. Persistent primitive lateral vertebrobasilar anastomosis. Acta Neurochir *138*:592–594, 1996.

Deshmukh VD, Meyer JS. Noninvasive Measurement of Regional Blood Flow in Man. New York, Spectrum, 1978.

Dreyfus PM, Hakim S, Adams RD. Diabetic ophthalmoplegia: Report of a case with postmortem study and comments on vascular supply of human oculomotor nerve. Arch Neurol Psychiatry *77*:337–349, 1957.

Ducasse A, Segal A, Delattre JF, et al. La participation de l'artère carotide externe à la vascularisation orbitaire. J Fr Ophtalmol *8*:333–339, 1985.

Ducasse A, Segal A, Delattre J-F, et al. Les principales variations de l'artère ophtalmique. Bull Soc Ophtalmol Fr *86*:603–609, 1986a.

Ducasse A, Segal A, Delattre J-F. Aspects macroscopiques des artères ciliaires longues postérieures. Bull Soc Ophtalmol Fr *86*:845–848, 1986b.

Ducasse A, Segal A, Delattre J-F, et al. L'artère lacrymale: Variations. Bull Soc Ophtalmol Fr *86*:377–385, 1986c.

Duvernoy HM. Cortical veins of the human brain. In The Cerebral Veins: An Experimental and Clinical Update. Editors, Auer LM, Loew F, pp 3–38. New York, Springer-Verlag, 1983.

Edvinsson L, McCulloch J, Uddman R. Substance P: Immunohistochemical localiza-

tion and effect upon cat pial arteries *in vitro* and *in situ*. J Physiol *318*:251–258, 1981.

Edvinsson L, Emson P, McCulloch J, et al. Neuropeptide Y: Cerebrovascular innervation and vasomotor effects in the cat. Neurosci Lett *43*:79–84, 1983.

El Khamlichi A, El Azouzi M, Bellakhdar R, et al. L'apport des techniques d'injection par les résines synthétiques dans l'étude anatomique du polygone artériel de Willis: A propos de 250 cerveaux injectés. Neurochirurgie *32*:333–336, 1986.

Epstein F, Ransohoff J, Budzilovich GN. The clinical significance of junctional dilatation of the posterior communicating artery. J Neurosurg *33*:529–531, 1970.

Fields WS, Breutman ME, Weibel J. Collateral circulation of the brain. Monogr Surg Sci *2*:183–259, 1965.

Fisch U. The surgical anatomy of the so-called internal auditory artery. In Proceedings of the Tenth Nobel Symposium on Disorders of the Skull Base, pp 121–130. Stockholm, Almqvist and Wiksell, 1968.

Fischer E. Die Lageabweichungen der vorderen hirnarterie im gefässbild. Zentralbl Neurochir *3*:300–312, 1938.

Fisher CM. The circle of Willis: Anatomical variations. Vasc Dis *2*:99, 1965.

Florey H. Microscopical observations on the circulation of the blood in the cerebral cortex. Brain *48*:43–61, 1925.

Fujii K, Lenkey C, Rhoton AL Jr. Microsurgical anatomy of the choroidal arteries: Lateral and third ventricles. J Neurosurg *52*:165–188, 1980a.

Fujii K, Lenkey C, Rhoton AL Jr. Microsurgical anatomy of the choroidal arteries: Fourth ventricle and cerebellopontine angles. J Neurosurg *52*:504–524, 1980b.

Furuno M, Yamakawa N, Okada M, et al. Anomalous origin of the calcarine artery. Neuroradiology *37*:658, 1995.

Galatius-Jensen F, Ringberg V. Anastomosis between the anterior choroidal artery and the posterior cerebral artery demonstrated by arteriography. Radiology *81*: 942–944, 1963.

Gebarski SS, Gebarski KS. Inferior petrosal sinus: Imaging-anatomic correlation. Radiology *194*:239–247, 1995.

Gibbs EL, Gibbs FA. The cross section areas of the vessels that form the torcular and the manner in which flow is distributed to the right and to the left lateral sinus. Anat Rec *59*:419–426, 1934.

Gibo H, Lenkey C, Rhoton AL Jr. Microsurgical anatomy of the supraclinoid portion of the internal carotid artery. J Neurosurg *55*:560–574, 1981a.

Gibo H, Carver CC, Rhoton AL Jr, et al. Microsurgical anatomy of the middle cerebral artery. J Neurosurg *54*:151–169, 1981b.

Gillilan L. The correlation of the blood supply to the human brain stem with clinical brain stem lesions. J Neuropathol Exp Neurol *23*:78–108, 1964.

Go KG, Houthoff H-J, Hartsuiker J, et al. Fluid secretion in arachnoid cysts as a clue to cerebrospinal fluid absorption at the arachnoid granulations. J Neurosurg *65*: 642–648, 1986.

Gomes F, Dujovny M, Umansky F, et al. Microsurgical anatomy of the recurrent artery of Heubner. J Neurosurg *60*:130–139, 1984.

Gomes FB, Dujovny M, Umansky F, et al. Microanatomy of the anterior cerebral artery. Surg Neurol *26*:129–141, 1986.

Gotoh F, Ebihara SI, Toyoda M, Shinoara Y. Role of autonomic nervous system in autoregulation of human cerebral circulation. Eur Neurol *6*:203–207, 1972.

Gottschau M. Zwei seltene Varietäten der Stämme des Aortenbogens. Arch Anat Entwickl-Gesch *69*:245–252, 1885.

Gray H, Goss CM, editors. Gray's Anatomy 29th ed., Philadelphia, Lea & Febiger, 1973.

Green HD, Rapela CE. Blood flow in passive and active vascular beds. Circ Res *15* (Suppl 1):11–16, 1984.

Greenfield JC, Tindall GT. Effect of acute increase in intracranial pressure on blood flow in the internal carotid artery of man. J Clin Invest *44*:1343–1351, 1965.

Griffith SG, Lincoln J, Burnstock G. Serotonin as a neurotransmitter in cerebral arteries. Brain Res *247*:388–392, 1982.

Gur RC, Gur RE, Obrist WD, et al. Age and regional cerebral blood flow at rest and during cognitive activity. Arch Gen Psychiatry *44*:617–621, 1987.

Guyton AC. Textbook of Medical Physiology, 7th ed., pp 338–340. Philadelphia, WB Saunders, 1986.

Hardy DG, Rhoton AL Jr. Microsurgical relationships of the superior cerebellar artery and the trigeminal nerve. J Neurosurg *49*:669–678, 1978.

Hardy DG, Peace DA, Rhoton AL Jr. Microsurgical anatomy of the superior cerebellar artery. Neurosurgery *6*:10–28, 1980.

Harris FS, Rhoton AL Jr. Anatomy of the cavernous sinus: A microsurgical study. J Neurosurg *45*:169–180, 1976.

Harrison CR, Luttrell C. Persistent carotid-basilar anastomosis: Three arteriographically demonstrated cases with one anatomical specimen. J Neurosurg *10*: 205–215, 1953.

Hassler O. Deep cerebral venous system in man: A microangiographic study on its areas of drainage and its anastomoses with the superficial cerebral brain. Neurology *16*:505–511, 1966.

Hassler O. Arterial pattern of human brainstem: Normal appearance and deformation in expanding supratentorial conditions. Neurology *17*:368–275, 1967.

Hassler O, Saltzman GF. Angiographic and histologic changes in infundibular widening of the posterior communicating artery. Acta Radiol *1*:321–327, 1963.

Havelius U, Hindfelt B. Minor vessels leaving the extracranial internal carotid artery: Possible clinical implications. Neuro-ophthalmology *5*:51–56, 1985.

Havelius U, Hindfelt B. Minor arteries from the intrapetrosal internal carotid artery:

Possible clinical implications. An anatomical study. Neuro-ophthalmology 15: 203–210, 1995.

Hayreh SS. The ophthalmic artery. III. Branches Br J Ophthalmol 46:212–247, 1962.

Hayreh SS. Arteries of the orbit in the human being. Br J Surg 50:938–953, 1963a.

Hayreh SS. Blood supply and vascular disorders of the optic nerve. Ann Inst Barraquer 4:7–109, 1963b.

Hayreh SS, Dass R. The ophthalmic artery. I. Origin and intra-cranial and intra-canalicular course. Br J Ophthalmol 46:65–98, 1962a.

Hayreh SS, Dass R. The ophthalmic artery. II. Intra-orbital course. Br J Ophthalmol 46:165–185, 1962b.

Hebel N, von Cramon DY. On the posterior infarct. Fortschr Neurol Psychiatr 55: 37–53, 1987.

Heeney DJ, Koo AH. Bilateral cortical blindness associated with carotid stenosis in a patient with a persistent trigeminal artery: Case report. J Neurosurg 52: 709–711, 1980.

Heimans JJ, Valk J, Lohman AHM. Angiographic anatomy of the anterior inferior cerebellar artery. Adv Embryol Cell Biol 92:1–91, 1985.

Hendry SHC, Jones EG, Beinfeld MC. Cholecystokinin-immunoreactive neurons in rat and monkey cerebral cortex make symmetric synapses and have intimate associations with blood vessels. Proc Natl Acad Sci USA 80:2400–2404, 1983.

Herman LH, Fernando OU, Gurdjian ES. The anterior choroidal artery: An anatomical study of its area of distribution. Anat Rec 154:95–102, 1966.

Heubner O. Zur Topographie der Ernanrungsgebiete der einzelnen Hirnarterien. Zentralbl Med Wiss 10:817–821, 1872.

Hillen B. The variability of the Circulus arteriosus (Willisii): Order or anarchy? Acta Anat 129:74–80, 1987.

Hoed T, Rasmussen K, Sveinsdotter E, et al. Regional cerebral blood flow in man determined by intraarterial injection of radioactive inert gas. Circ Res 18: 237–247, 1966.

Hutchinson EC, Yates PO. Cervical portion of the vertebral artery: Clinico-pathological study. Brain 79:319–331, 1956.

Hyde JB. Terminal vessels of the pial arterial plexus. Anat Rec 133:290–291, 1959.

Ikezaki K, Fujii K, Kishikawa T. Persistent primitive trigeminal artery: a possible cause of trigeminal and abducens nerve palsy. J Neurol Neurosurg Psychiatry 52:1449–1450, 1989.

Ingvar DH, Schwartz MS. Blood flow patterns induced in the dominant hemisphere by speech and reading. Brain 97:273–288, 1974.

Inoue T, Rhoton AL Jr, Theele D, et al. Surgical approaches to the cavernous sinus: A microsurgical study. Neurosurgery 26:903–932, 1990.

Jackson E. Cilioretinal and other anomalous retinal vessels. Ophthal Rev 30:264–296, 1911.

Jackson IJ, Garza-Mercado R. Persistent carotid-basilar anastomosis: Occasionally a possible cause of tic douloureux. Angiology 11:103–107, 1960.

Justice J Jr, Lehmann RP. Cilioretinal arteries: A study based on review of stereo fundus photographs and fluorescein angiographic findings. Arch Ophthalmol 94: 1355–1358, 1976.

Kamath S. Observations on the length and diameter of vessels forming the circle of Willis. J Anat 133:419–423, 1981.

Kaplan HA, Ford OH. The Brain Vascular System. Amsterdam, Elsevier, 1966.

Kaplan HA, Browder A, Browder J. Atresia of the rostral superior sagittal sinus: Associated cerebral venous patterns. Neuroradiology 4:208–211, 1972.

Kaplan HA, Browder A, Browder J. Nasal venous drainage and the foramen caecum. Laryngoscope 83:327–329, 1974.

Kapp JP, Schmidek HH, editors. The Cerebral Venous System and Its Disorders. Orlando, FL, Grune & Stratton, 1984.

Kawase T, van Loveren H, Keller JT, et al. Meningeal architecture of the cavernous sinus: Clinical and surgical implications. Neurosurgery 39:527–536, 1996.

Kee DB Jr, Wood JH. Influence of blood rheology on cerebral circulation. In Cerebral Blood Flow: Physiologic and Clinical Aspects. Editor, Wood JH, pp 173–185. New York, McGraw-Hill, 1987.

Kempe LG, Smith DR. Trigeminal neuralgia, facial spasm, and glosso-pharyngeal neuralgia with persistent carotid-basilar anastomosis. J Neurosurg 31:445–451, 1969.

Kerty E, Nyberg-Hansen R, Dahl A, et al. Assessment of the ophthalmic artery as a collateral to the cerebral circulation. Acta Neurol Scand 93:374–379, 1996.

Kety SS. Human cerebral blood flow and oxygen consumption as related to aging. J Chron Dis 3:478–486, 1956.

Kety SS, Schmidt CF. The determination of cerebral blood flow in man by the use of nitrous oxide in low concentrations. Am J Physiol 143:53–66, 1945.

Klun B, Prestor B. Microvascular relations of the trigeminal nerve: An anatomical study. Neurosurgery 19:535–539, 1986.

Knosp E, Müller G, Perneczky A. The paraclinoid carotid artery: Anatomical aspects of a microneurosurgical approach. Neurosurgery 22:896–901, 1988.

Kramer SP. On the function of the circle of Willis. J Exp Med 15:348–355, 1912.

Krayenbühl HA, Yaşargil MG. Die vaskulären Erkrankungen im Gebiet der Arteria vertebralis und Arteria basilaris. Stuttgart, Thieme, 1957.

Krayenbühl HA, Yaşargil MG. Cerebral Arteriography. 2nd ed., Philadelphia, JB Lippincott, 1968.

Krayenbühl H, Yaşargil MG. Radiological anatomy and topography of the cerebral arteries. In Handbook of Clinical Neurology. Editors, Vinken PJ, Bruyn GW, Vol 2, p 65. Amsterdam, North Holland, 1973.

Krisht A, Barnett DW, Barrow DL, et al. The blood supply of the intracavernous cranial nerves: An anatomic study. Neurosurgery 34:275–279, 1994a.

Krisht A, Barrow DL, Barnett DW, et al. The microsurgical anatomy of the superior hypophyseal artery. Neurosurgery 35:899–903, 1994b.

Kupersmith MJ. Neurovascular Neuro-ophthalmology. Heidelberg, Springer-Verlag, 1993.

Kuru Y. Meningeal branches of the ophthalmic artery. Acta Radiol 6:241–251, 1967.

Lang J. Anatomy of the midline. Acta Neurochir Suppl 35:6–22, 1985.

Lang J. Anatomical relationships of cranial nerves and cerebral vessels and their medical significance. Zentrlbl Neurochir 52:165–183, 1991.

Lasjaunias PL. Anatomy of the tentorial arteries. J Neurosurg 61:1159–1160, 1984.

Lasjaunias P, Berenstein A. Arterial anatomy: Introduction. In Surgical Neuroangiography: Functional Anatomy of Craniofacial Arteries, Vol 1, pp 1–32. Berlin, Springer-Verlag, 1987.

Lasjaunias P, Moret J, Mink J. The anatomy of the inferolateral trunk (ILT) of the internal carotid artery. Neuroradiology 13:215–220, 1977.

Lasjaunias P, Terbrugge K, Piske R, et al. Dilatation de la veine de Galien: Formes anatomo-cliniques et traitement endovasculaire à propos de 14 cas explorés et/ou traités entre 1983 et 1986. Neurochirurgie 33:315–333, 1987.

Lassen NA. Cerebral blood flow and oxygen consumption in man. Physiol Rev 39: 183–238, 1959.

Lassen NA. Autoregulation of cerebral blood flow. Circ Res 15 (Suppl 1):201–204, 1964.

Lassen NA. Cerebral blood flow in cerebral ischaemia: A review. Eur Neurol 17 (Suppl 1):4–8, 1978.

Lassen NA, Munck O. The cerebral blood flow in man determined by the use of radioactive krypton. Acta Physiol Scand 33:30–49, 1955.

Lassen NA, Ingvar DH, Skinhoj E. Brain function and blood flow. Sci Am 239: 62–71, 1978.

Lazorthes G, Poulhes J, Gaubert J. La dure-mere de la charniere craniorachidienne. CR Assoc Anat 78:168–172, 1954.

Leenders KL, Perani D, Lammertsma AA, et al. Cerebral blood flow, blood volume and oxygen utilization. Normal values and effect of age. Brain 113:27–47, 1990.

Leopold PW, Shandall AA, Feustel P, et al. Duplex scanning of the internal carotid artery: An assessment of cerebral blood flow. Br J Surg 74:630–633, 1987.

Lie TA. Congenital Anomalies of the Carotid Arteries. Amsterdam, Excerpta Medica, 1968.

Lin JP, Kricheff II. The anterior cerebral artery complex: Section I. Normal anterior cerebral artery complex. In Radiology of the Skull and Brain. Editors, Newton TH, Potts DG, Vol 2, pp 1391–1410. St. Louis, CV Mosby, 1974.

Lister JR, Rhoton AL Jr, Matsushima T, et al. Microsurgical anatomy of the posterior inferior cerebellar artery. Neurosurgery 10:170–199, 1982.

Lombardi G, Passerini A. The orbital veins. Am J Ophthalmol 64:440–447, 1967.

Lombardi G, Passerini A. Ophthalmic artery in axial view. Acta Radiol 9:379–382, 1969.

MacInnes WE, Golden CJ, Gillen RW, et al. Aging, regional cerebral blood flow, and neuropsychological functioning. J Am Geriatr Soc 32:712–718, 1984.

Madonick MJ, Ruskin AP. Recurrent oculomotor paresis: Paresis associated with a vascular anomaly, carotid-basilar anastomosis. Arch Neurol 6:353–357, 1962.

Mamo H, Meric P, Luft A, et al. Hyperfrontal pattern of human cerebral circulation: Variations with age and atherosclerotic state. Arch Neurol 40:626–632, 1983.

Marano SR, Fischer DW, Gaines C, et al. Anatomical study of the superficial temporal artery. Neurosurgery 16:786–789, 1985.

Margaretten I. Syndromes of the anterior spinal artery. J Nerv Ment Dis 58:127–133, 1954.

Margolis MT, Newton TH. Collateral pathways between the cavernous portion of the internal carotid and external carotid arteries. Radiology 93:834–836, 1969.

Margolis MT, Newton TH, Hoyt WF. Gross and roentgenologic anatomy of the posterior cerebral artery. In Radiology of the Skull and Brain. Editors, Newton TH, Potts DG, Vol 2, pp 1551–1576. St. Louis, CV Mosby, 1974.

Marinkovic SV, Gibo H. The blood supply of the trigeminal nerve root, with special reference to the trigeminocerebellar artery. Neurosurgery 37:309–317, 1995.

Marinković SV, Kovacević MS, Marinković JM. Perforating branches of the middle cerebral artery: Microsurgical anatomy of their extracerebral segments. J Neurosurg 63:266–271, 1985.

Marinković S, Milisavljević M, Kovacević M. Interpeduncular perforating branches of the posterior cerebral artery: Microsurgical anatomy of their extracerebral and intracerebral segments. Surg Neurol 26:349–359, 1986a.

Marinković S, Milisavljević M, Kovacević MS. Anastomoses among the thalamoperforating branches of the posterior cerebral artery. Arch Neurol 43:811–814, 1986b.

Marinković SV, Milisavljević MM, Lolić-Draganić V, et al. Distribution of the occipital branches of the posterior cerebral artery: Correlation with occipital lobe infarcts. Stroke 18:728–732, 1987.

Marinković SV, Milisavljević MM, Marinković ZD. The perforating branches of the internal carotid artery: The microsurgical anatomy of their extracerebral segments. Neurosurgery 26:472–479, 1990.

Marinković S, Gibo H, Erdem A. Huge uncal branch of the anterior choroidal artery. Neurol Med Chir 34:423–428, 1994.

Martin RG, Grant JL, Peace D, et al. Microsurgical relationships of the anterior inferior cerebellar artery and the facial-vestibulocochlear nerve complex. Neurosurgery 6:483–507, 1980.

Matsuda H, Maeda T, Masato Y, et al. Age-matched normal values and topographic maps for regional cerebral blood flow measurements by Xe-133 inhalation. Stroke 15:336–342, 1984.

Matsuda I, Handa J, Handa H, et al. Carotid-superior cerebellar anastomosis: A variant of persistent trigeminal artery associated with cerebral aneurysms and angiomatous malformation: Case report. Arch Jpn Chir 48:535–541, 1979.

Matsushima T, Rhoton AL Jr, de Oliveira E, et al. Microsurgical anatomy of the veins of the posterior fossa. J Neurosurg 59:63–105, 1983.

Matsushima T, Suzuki SO, Fukui M, et al. Microsurgical anatomy of the tentorial sinuses. J Neurosurg 71:923–928, 1989.

McConnell EM. The arterial blood supply of the human hypophysis cerebri. Anat Rec 115:175–201, 1953.

McCord GM, Goree JA, Jiminez JP. Venous drainage to the inferior sagittal sinus. Radiology 105:583–589, 1972.

McCullough AW. Some anomalies of the cerebral arterial circle (of Willis) and related vessels. Anat Rec 142:537–543, 1962.

Meder J-F, Chiras J, Roland J, et al. Territoires veineux de l'encéphale. J Neuroradiol 21:118–133, 1994.

Melamed E, Lavy S, Bentin S, et al. Reduction in regional cerebral blood flow during normal aging in man. Stroke 11:31–35, 1980.

Merwarth HR. The syndrome of the rolandic vein: Hemiplegia of venous origin. Am J Surg 56:526–544, 1942.

Meyer JS, Shimazu K, Fukuuchi Y, et al. Cerebral dysautoregulation in central neurogenic orthostatic hypotension (Shy-Drager syndrome). Neurology 23:262–273, 1973.

Meyer JS, Hayman LA, Amano T, et al. Mapping of local blood flow of human brain by CT scanning during stable xenon inhalation. Stroke 12:426–436, 1981.

Milisavljević M, Marinković S, Lolić-Draganić V, et al. Oculomotor, trochlear, and abducens nerves penetrated by cerebral vessels: Microanatomy and possible clinical significance. Arch Neurol 43:58–61, 1986a.

Milisavljević M, Marinković S, Lolić-Draganić V, et al. Anastomoses in the territory of the posterior cerebral arteries. Acta Anat 127:221–225, 1986b.

Milisavljević MM, Marinković SV, Gibo H, et al. The thalamogeniculate perforators of the posterior cerebral artery: The microsurgical anatomy. Neurosurgery 28:523–530, 1991.

Miller JD, Bell BA. Cerebral blood flow: Variations with perfusion pressure and metabolism. In Cerebral Blood Flow: Physiologic and Clinical Aspects. Editor, Wood JH, pp 119–130. New York, McGraw-Hill, 1987.

Morris ED, Moffat DB Abnormal origin of the basilar artery from the cervical part of the internal carotid and its embryological significance. Anat Rec 125:701–712, 1956.

Moscow NP, Michotey P, Salamon G. The anterior cerebral artery complex: Section II. Anatomy of the cortical branches of the anterior cerebral artery. In Radiology of the Skull and Brain. Editors, Newton TH, Potts DG, Vol 2, pp 1411–1420. St. Louis, CV Mosby, 1974.

Nager GT. Origins and relations of the internal auditory artery and the subarcuate artery. Ann Otol Rhinol Laryngol 63:51–61, 1954.

Naidich TP, Kricheff II, George AE, et al. The normal anterior inferior cerebellar artery. Radiology 119:355–373, 1976a.

Naidich TP, Kricheff II, George AE, et al. The anterior inferior cerebellar artery in mass lesions. Radiology 119:375–383, 1976b.

Nakasu Y, Nakasu S, Kidooka M, et al. Aneurysm at the fenestration of basilar artery: Case report. Arch Jpn Chir 51:344–348, 1982.

Naritomi H, Meyer JS, Fumihiko S, et al. Effects of advancing age on regional cerebral blood flow. Arch Neurol 36:410–416, 1979.

Natori Y, Rhoton AL Jr. Microsurgical anatomy of the superior orbital fissure. Neurosurgery 36:762–775, 1995.

Newton TH. The anterior and posterior meningeal branches of the vertebral artery. Radiology 91:271–279, 1968.

Obrist WD, Thompson HK, Wang HS, et al. Regional cerebral blood flow estimated by 133-xenon inhalation. Stroke 6:245–256, 1975.

Oka K, Rhoton AL Jr, Barry M, et al. Microsurgical anatomy of the superficial veins of the cerebrum. Neurosurgery 17:711–748, 1985.

Oliveira E, Rhoton AL Jr, Peace D. Microsurgical anatomy of the region of the foramen magnum. Surg Neurol 24:293–352, 1985.

Olver JM, Spalton DJ, McCartney ACE. Microvascular study of the retrolaminar optic nerve in man: the possible significance in anterior ischaemic optic neuropathy. Eye 4:7–24, 1990.

Ono M, Ono M, Rhoton AL Jr, et al. Microsurgical anatomy of the region of the tentorial incisura. J Neurosurg 60:365–399, 1984a.

Ono M, Rhoton AL Jr, Peace D, et al. Microsurgical anatomy of the deep venous system of the brain. Neurosurgery 15:621–656, 1984b.

Otomo E. The anterior choroidal artery. Arch Neurol 13:656–658, 1965.

Padget DH. The circle of Willis: Its embryology and anatomy. In Intracranial Arterial Aneurisms. Editor, Dandy WE, p 67. Ithaca, Comstock Publishing Co., Cornell University Press, 1944.

Padget DH. The development of the cranial arteries in the human embryo. Contrib Embryol 32:205–262, 1948.

Padget DH. The cranial venous system in man in reference to development, adult configuration, and relation to the arteries. Am J Anat 98:307–356, 1956.

Parkinson D. Collateral circulation of cavernous carotid artery: Anatomy Can J Surg 7:251–268, 1964.

Parkinson D. A surgical approach to the cavernous portion of the carotid artery: Anatomical studies and case report. J Neurosurg 23:474–483, 1965.

Parkinson D. Carotid cavernous fistula: Direct repair with preservation of the carotid artery: Technical note. J Neurosurg 38:99–106, 1973.

Parkinson D, Reddy V, Ross RT. Congenital anastomoses between the vertebral artery and internal carotid artery in the neck: Case report. J Neurosurg 51:697–699, 1979.

Paullus WS, Pait TG, Rhoton AL Jr. Microsurgical exposure of the petrous portion of the carotid artery. J Neurosurg 47:713–726, 1977.

Pedroza A, Dujovny M, Ausman JI, et al. Microvascular anatomy of the interpeduncular fossa. J Neurosurg 64:484–493, 1986.

Pedroza A, Dujovny M, Artero JC, et al. Microanatomy of the posterior communicating artery. Neurosurgery 20:228–235, 1987.

Percheron G. The anatomy of the arterial supply of the human thalamus and its use for the interpretation of thalamic vascular pathology. Z Neurol 205:1–13, 1973.

Percheron G. Les artères du thalamus humain. II. Artères et territoire thalamiques paramédians de l'artère basilaire communicante. Rev Neurol 132:309–324, 1976a.

Percheron G. Les artères du thalamus humain. I. Artère et territoire thalamiques polaires de l'artère communicante postérieure. Rev Neurol 132:297–307, 1976b.

Percheron G. Les artères du thalamus humain. Les artères choroidiennes. I. Étude macroscopique des variations individuelles. II. Systématisation. III. Absence de territoire thalamique constitue de l'artère choroidienne antérieure. IV. Artères et territoires thalamiques du système artériel choroidien et thalamique postéro-latéral. Rev Neurol 133:533–545, 547–558, 1977.

Perlmutter D, Rhoton AL Jr. Microsurgical anatomy of the anterior cerebral-anterior communicating-recurrent artery complex. J Neurosurg 45:259–272, 1976.

Perlmutter D, Rhoton AL Jr. Microsurgical anatomy of the distal anterior cerebral artery. J Neurosurg 49:204–228, 1978.

Perneczky A. Die Arteria cerebelli inferior anterior: Anatomie, Klinik, Mikroneurochirurgie. Fortschr Med 99:511–514, 1981.

Pickard JD. Ionic and eicosanoid regulation of cerebrovascular smooth muscle contraction. In Cerebral Blood Flow: Physiologic and Clinical Aspects. Editor, Wood JH, pp 131–144. New York, McGraw-Hill, 1987.

Piffer CR, Horn Y, Hureau J, et al. Étude anatomique des veins cérébrales supérieures. Anat Anz 160:271–283, 1985.

Piffer CR, Horn Y, Hureau J, et al. Étude anatomo-microscopique des parois des veines cérébrales supérieures. Anat Anz 162:331–350, 1986.

Plets C, De Reuck J, Vander Eecken H, et al. The vascularization of the human thalamus. Acta Neurol Belg 70:687–770, 1970.

Pollock JA, Newton TH. The anterior falx artery: Normal and pathologic anatomy. Radiology 91:1089–1095, 1968.

Pribram HFW, Boulter TR, McCormick WF. Roentgenology of the meningohypophyseal trunk. AJR 98:583–594, 1966.

Punt J. Some observations on aneurysms of the proximal internal carotid artery. J Neurosurg 51:151–154, 1979.

Raichle ME, Hartman BK, Eichling JO, et al. Central noradrenergic regulation of cerebral blood flow and vascular permeability. Proc Natl Acad Sci USA 72:3726–3730, 1975.

Randall BA. Cilioretinal or aberrant vessels. Trans Am Ophthalmol Soc 4:511–517, 1887.

Renn WH, Rhoton AL Jr. Microsurgical anatomy of the sellar region. J Neurosurg 43:288–298, 1975.

Reynolds AF Jr, Stovring J, Turner PT. Persistent otic artery. Surg Neurol 13:115–117, 1980.

Rhoton AL Jr, Hardy DG, Chambers SM. Microsurgical anatomy and dissection of the sphenoid bone, cavernous sinus and sellar region. Surg Neurol 12:63–104, 1979a.

Rhoton AL Jr, Saeki N, Perlmutter D, et al. Microsurgical anatomy of common aneurysm sites. Clin Neurosurg 26:248–306, 1979b.

Rhoton AL Jr, Fujii K, Fradd B. Microsurgical anatomy of the anterior choroidal artery. Surg Neurol 12:171–187, 1979c.

Rhoton AL Jr, Harris FS, Fujii K. Anatomy of the cavernous sinus. In The Cerebral Venous System and its Disorders. Editors, Kapp JP, Schmidek HH, pp 61–91. Orlando, FL, Grune & Stratton, 1984.

Riggs HE, Rupp C. Variation in form of the circle of Willis. The relation of the variations to collateral circulation: Anatomic analysis. Arch Neurol 8:24–30, 1963.

Ring BA. The middle cerebral artery: Section I. Normal middle cerebral artery. In Radiology of the Skull and Brain. Editors, Newton TH, Potts DG, Vol 2, pp 1442–1470. St. Louis, CV Mosby, 1974.

Risco JM, Grimson BS, Johnson PT. Angioarchitecture of the ciliary artery circulation of the posterior pole. Arch Ophthalmol 99:864–868, 1981.

Rogers L. The significance of the circulus arteriosus of Willis. Brain 70:171–178, 1947.

Romanes GJ. Cunningham's Manual of Practical Anatomy. 13th ed., Vol 3, Head and Neck, p 8. London, Oxford University Press, 1967.

Rosenthal F. De intimis cerebri venous seu de venae magnae gelni ramis. Nova Acta

Physiocomedica Academinae Caesareae Leopoldina-Carolinae Naturae Curiosorium *12*:302–312, 1824.

Rosner SS, Rhoton AL Jr, Ono M, et al. Microsurgical anatomy of the anterior perforating arteries. J Neurosurg *61*:468–485, 1984.

Rubinstein D, Burton BS, Walker AL. The anatomy of the inferior petrosal sinus, glossopharyngeal nerve, vagus nerve, and accessory nerve in the jugular foramen. AJNR *16*:185–194, 1995.

Saeki N, Rhoton AL Jr. Microsurgical anatomy of the upper basilar artery and the posterior circle of Willis. J Neurosurg *46*:563–578, 1977.

Salamon G, Huang YP. Radiologic Anatomy of the Brain, pp 303–331. Berlin, Springer-Verlag, 1976.

Saltzmann GF. Patent primitive trigeminal artery studied by cerebral angiography. Acta Radiol *51*:329–336, 1959.

Sargent P. Some points in the anatomy of the intra-cranial blood sinuses. J Anat Physiol *45*:69–72, 1911.

Scotti G. Anterior inferior cerebellar artery originating from the cavernous portion of the internal carotid artery. Radiology *116*:93–94, 1975.

Sener RN. The occipitotemporal vein: A cadaver, MRI and CT study. Neuroradiology *36*:117–120, 1994.

Serizawa T, Saeki N, Fukuda K, et al. Microsurgical anatomy of the anterior communicating artery and its perforating arteries important for interhemispheric translamina terminalis approach: Analysis based on cadaver brains. No Shinkaei Geka *22*:447–454, 1994.

Shaw TG, Mortel KF, Meyer JS, et al. Cerebral blood flow changes in benign aging and cerebrovascular disease. Neurology *34*:855–862, 1984.

Shellshear JL. The basal arteries of the forebrain and their functional significance. J Anat *55*:27–35, 1920.

Shenkin HA, Novack P, Goluboff B, et al. Effects of aging, arteriosclerosis and hypertension upon the cerebral circulation. J Clin Invest *32*:459–465, 1953.

Shrontz C, Dujovny M, Ausman JI, et al. Surgical anatomy of the arteries of the posterior fossa. J Neurosurg *65*:540–544, 1986.

Siesjo BK. Cerebral circulation and metabolism. J Neurosurg *60*:883–908, 1984.

Skinhoj E, Strandgaard S. Pathogenesis of hypertensive encephalopathy. Lancet *1*: 461–462, 1973.

Smith RR, Sanford RA. Disorders of the deep cerebral veins. In The Cerebral Venous System and Its Disorders. Editors, Kapp JP, Schmidek HH, pp 547–556. Orlando, FL, Grune & Stratton, 1984.

Sokoloff L. Measurement of local glucose utilization and its use in localization of functional activity in the central nervous system of animals and man. Recent Progr Horm Res *39*:75–126, 1983.

Spinelli HM, Falcone S, Lee G. Orbital venous approach to the cavernous sinus: An analysis of the facial and orbital venous system. Ann Plast Surg *33*:377–384, 1994.

Stattin S. Meningeal vessels of the internal carotid artery and their angiographic significance. Acta Radiol *255*:329–336, 1961.

Stock AL, Collins HP, Davidson TM. Anatomy of the superficial temporal artery. Head Neck Surg *2*:466–469, 1980.

Stopford JSB. The arteries of the pons and medulla oblongata. J Anat Physiol *50*: 131–164, 1916a.

Stopford JSB. The arteries of the pons and medulla: Part II. J Anat Physiol *50*: 255–280, 1916b.

Strandgaard S, Paulson OB. Cerebral autoregulation. Stroke *15*:413–416, 1984.

Sunderland S. An anomalous anastomosis between the internal carotid and basilar arteries. Aust N Z J Surg *11*:140–142, 1941.

Sunderland S. The arterial relations of the internal auditory meatus. Brain *68*:23–27, 1945.

Sunderland S. Neurovascular relations and anomalies at the base of the brain. J Neurol Neurosurg Psychiatry *11*:243–257, 1948.

Suzuki S, Noabechi T, Itoh I, et al. Persistent proatlantal intersegmental artery and occipital artery originating from internal carotid artery. Neuroradiology *17*: 105–109, 1979.

Takahashi M, Tamakawa Y, Kishikawa T, et al. Fenestration of the basilar artery. Radiology *109*:79–82, 1973.

Teal JS, Rumbaugh CL, Bergeron RT, et al. Persistent carotid-superior cerebellar artery anastomosis: A variant of persistent trigeminal artery. Radiology *103*: 335–341, 1972.

Teal JS, Rumbaugh CL, Segall HD, et al. Anomalous branches of the internal carotid artery. Radiology *106*:567–573, 1973.

Teufel J. Einbrau der Arteria carotis interna in den Canalis caroticus unter Berücksichtigung des transbasalen Venenabflusses. Morph Jb *106*:188–274, 1964.

Thomas DJ. Whole blood viscosity and cerebral blood flow. Stroke *13*:285–287, 1982.

Tindall GT, Kapp J, Odom GL, et al. A combined technique for treating certain aneurysms of the anterior communicating artery. J Neurosurg *33*:41–47, 1970.

Tran-Dinh H. Cavernous branches of the internal carotid artery: Anatomy and nomenclature. Neurosurgery *20*:205–210, 1987.

Tulleken CA. A study of the anatomy of the anterior communicating artery with the aid of the operating microscope. Clin Neurol Neurosurg *80*:169–173, 1978.

Tulleken CAF, Luiten MLFB. The basilar artery bifurcation *in situ* approached via the Sylvian route: An anatomical study in human cadavers. Acta Neurochir *80*: 109–115, 1986.

Tulleken CAF, Luiten MLFB. The basilar artery bifurcation: Microscopical anatomy. Acta Neurochir *85*:50–55, 1987.

Umansky F, Nathan H. The lateral wall of the cavernous sinus: With special reference to the nerves related to it. J Neurosurg *56*:228–234, 1982.

Umansky F, Juarez SM, Dujovny M, et al. Microsurgical anatomy of the proximal segments of the middle cerebral artery. J Neurosurg *61*:458–467, 1984.

Umansky F, Gomes FB, Dujovny M, et al. The perforating branches of the middle cerebral artery: A microanatomical study. J Neurosurg *62*:261–268, 1985.

Upton ML, Weller RO. The morphology of cerebrospinal fluid drainage pathways in human arachnoid granulations. J Neurosurg *63*:867–875, 1985.

Vincentelli F, Caruso G, Grisoli F, et al. Microsurgical anatomy of the cisternal course of the perforating branches of the posterior communicating artery. Neurosurgery *26*:824–831, 1990.

von Mitterwallner F. Variationsstatistische Untersuchungen an den basalen Hirngefässen. Acta Anat *24*:51–88, 1955.

Wallace S, Goldberg HI, Leeds NE, et al. Cavernous branches of the internal carotid artery. AJR *101*:34–46, 1967.

Waltner JG. Anatomic variations of the lateral and sigmoid sinuses. Arch Otology *39*:307–312, 1944.

Watt JC, McKillop AN. Relation of arteries to roots of nerves in posterior cranial fossa in man. Arch Surg *30*:336–345, 1935.

Weir B. Aneurysms Affecting the Nervous System. Baltimore, Williams & Wilkins, 1987.

Williams DJ. The origin of the posterior cerebral artery. Brain *59*:175–180, 1936.

Willis T. Cerebri Anatome: cui Accessit Nervorum Descriptio et Usus. Amsterdam, Gerbrandum Schagen, 1664.

Wolf BS, Huang YP. The insula and deep middle cerebral venous drainage system. AJR *90*:472–489, 1963.

Wolf BS, Huang YP, Newman CM. The superficial sylvian venous drainage system. AJR *89*:398–422, 1963.

Wollner L, McCarthy ST, Soper NDW, et al. Failure of cerebral autoregulation as a cause of brain dysfunction in the elderly. Br Med J *1*:1117–1118, 1979.

Wollschlaeger G, Wollschlaeger PB, Lucas FV, et al. Experience and results with postmortem cerebral angiography performed as routine procedure of the autopsy. AJR *101*:68–87, 1967.

Wollschlaeger PB, Ide C, Hart W. Arterial blood supply of the human optic chiasm and surrounding structures. Ann Ophthalmol *3*:862–869, 1971.

Wood JH, editor. Cerebral Blood Flow: Physiologic and Clinical Aspects. New York, McGraw-Hill, 1987.

Woodhall B. Variations of the cranial venous sinuses in the region of the torcular herophili. Arch Surg *33*:297–314, 1936.

Yamamoto M, Meyer JS, Sakai F, et al. Aging and cerebral vasodilator responses to hypercarbia: Responses in normal aging and in persons with risk factors for stroke. Arch Neurol *37*:489–496, 1980.

Zeal AA, Rhoton AL Jr. Microsurgical anatomy of the posterior cerebral artery. J Neurosurg *48*:534–559, 1978.

Zhao Y, Li F. Microangioarchitecture of optic papilla. Jpn J Ophthalmol *31*:147–159, 1987.

Zouaoui A. Cerebral venous sinuses: Anatomical variants or thrombosis? Acta Anat *133*:318–324, 1988.

Aneurysms

Steven A. Newman

HISTORY

Morgagni is generally credited with first describing aneurysmal dilation of the cerebral vessels in the mid-18th century (Morgagni, 1769). Shortly thereafter, Biumi (1765) reported a case of a ruptured aneurysm, and Blackall (1814) subsequently recognized an aneurysm as a cause of subarachnoid hemorrhage (SAH).

In 1907, Cecil F. Beadles delivered a lecture entitled "Aneurisms of the Larger Cerebral Arteries" to the Royal College of Surgeons of England; the lecture was subsequently published in the journal *Brain* (Beadles, 1907). He based his conclusions on a review of 555 postmortem cases in which cerebral aneurysms were confirmed; 441 had been previously reported (209 from Great Britain, 44 from Canada and the United States, and 188 from the "Continent" [mainly France and Germany]). To these, he added 74 cases from museums in and around London, 30 cases from the Colney Hatch Asylum, and 10 cases from colleagues. He chose to divide his cases into those presenting with SAH (46%), those presenting with localizing central nervous system (CNS) signs and symptoms with (21%) or without (16%) subsequent apoplexy, and those in which the aneu-

rysm was discovered incidentally (17%). He also recognized that aneurysms could obtain significant size without producing any symptoms. These concepts were quite modern in approach and even today contain the basic framework of the approach to aneurysms of the cerebral circulation. He was not, however, able to detect a direct correlation between aneurysmal size and risk of rupture.

Several of the cases reviewed by Beadles (1907) had neuro-ophthalmologic symptoms. These included two cases of huge aneurysms, one previously reported by Byrom Bramwell (1886–1887) and the other by Weir Mitchell (1889) (Fig. 53.1), that presented with progressive visual loss and bitemporal visual field defects. Other cases were characterized in part by progressive optic atrophy. Many of these early cases suffered from the lack of sophisticated quantitative assessment of visual function. In a case of a woman with senile dementia later housed at the University College Museum (No. 3795E), pathologic examination revealed that the right optic nerve passing over the fundus of a large right internal carotid artery (ICA) aneurysm was smaller than the opposite optic nerve. Despite the pathologic

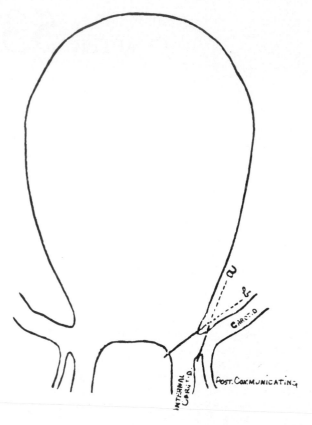

Figure 53.1. Drawing of giant aneurysm that caused a complete bitemporal hemianopia by splitting the optic chiasm. (From Mitchell SW. Aneurysm of an anomolous artery causing anteroposterior division of the chiasm and optic nerves and producing bitemporal hemianopsia. J Nerv Ment Dis *14*:44–62, 1889.)

abnormality, no visual difficulties had been noted prior to death.

Some of the early descriptions of aneurysm cases also suffered from lack of specific diagnosis. For example, a 40-year-old patient was noted to have "double optic neuritis" preceding hemiparesis, a dilated pupil, and episodes suggestive of tonic-clonic seizure activity. This case was later reported to the Pathological Society of London. Vomiting, fits, and coma prior to demise suggested the possibility of increased intracranial pressure (ICP), accounting for the presumed disc swelling (Anderson, 1885). Oculomotor nerve dysfunction, now considered the most frequent neuro-ophthalmologic sign, also occurred in several early cases. Most of these aneurysms were thought to arise from the intracranial ICA; the relationship to the posterior communicating artery was not yet appreciated. Retinal hemorrhages associated with meningeal hemorrhage were assumed to be caused by tracking of subarachnoid blood along the optic nerve sheath. In one case observed by Beadles (1907), retinal hemorrhages accompanied headache, progressive loss of mentation, and "double optic neuritis." Cavernous sinus involvement could produce ophthalmoplegia as well as impairment of trigeminal nerve function. Although originally associated with "dreadful throbbing" in the temple, pain spontaneously resolved along with an audible bruit, leaving the ophthalmoplegia (Hutchinson, 1875).

The modern era of aneurysmal study can be dated to the introduction of cerebral angiography by Moniz (1927). Before this procedure was available, most aneurysms were diagnosed at postmortem examination. As of 1927, cerebral aneurysms could be recognized before they hemorrhaged or at least before the patient died (Moniz, 1933). Norman Dott of Great Britain was the first surgeon to emphasize the importance of this technique (Dott, 1933); Dandy (1944) thought the technique dangerous. In the decade following the introduction of angiography, Dott managed 39 patients with suspected intracranial hemorrhage, establishing fundamental principles of surgical management (Todd et al., 1990).

The first authoritative book on the surgical approach to intracranial aneurysms was written by Dr. Walter Dandy in 1944. He reported his experience of 133 aneurysms in 108 patients. Of 30 patients treated with clipping, 20 were "cured," whereas nine died. Initial approaches included ligation of the parent vessel, wrapping of the aneurysmal wall, and clipping of first the feeding vessel and later the aneurysm itself (Dott, 1933; Dandy, 1938). Dandy (1944) subsequently emphasized six possible methods of treatment: (*a*) clipping the neck of the aneurysmal sac; (*b*) trapping the aneurysm between an intracranial clip and a ligature in the neck; (*c*) trapping the aneurysm between two intracranial clips; (*d*) excising the aneurysm and closing of the entering vessel; (*e*) opening the aneurysm, quickly inserting a piece of muscle large enough to fill the sac, and then thoroughly coagulating the muscle with electrocautery; and (*f*) turning back the aneurysm and coagulating the neck of the sac and the aneurysm itself. With the exception of the last technique and the added ability to perform several of these maneuvers endovascularly, this list still summarizes current potential aneurysm treatments.

Historically, recognition of the importance of vasospasm in producing secondary ischemic changes proved a pivotal point in the treatment of aneurysm patients following rupture (Robertson, 1949; Ecker and Riemenschneider, 1951). Direct surgical approach became increasingly aggressive (Drake, 1984) with the use of the surgical microscope (Lougheed and Marshall, 1969), which supplied both magnification and improved illumination. Since the 1980s, there has been a shift from delayed to earlier surgery, with improvement in overall results (Ljunggren et al., 1981; Kassell and Drake, 1982; Kassell et al., 1990a, 1990b). The addition of endovascular techniques to the armamentarium available for aneurysm treatment has decreased the risks of rebleeding and vasospasm and has contributed to continued improvement in the prognosis for patients with cerebral aneurysms (Debrun et al., 1981; Fox et al., 1987; Barnwell et al., 1989; Higashida et al., 1990; Guglielmi et al., 1991; Higashida et al., 1991; Higashida et al., 1992).

Many excellent references concerning the anatomy, pathogenesis, clinical presentations, and treatment of aneurysms are available to the reader interested in pursuing this subject in more detail. These include the early works by Dandy (1944) and Hamby (1952), the superb monograph by Pertuiset et al. (1987), and the excellent texts by Fox (1983) and by Weir (1987). The advent of endovascular therapy has the potential for major modifications in our diagnostic and therapeutic approach to cerebral aneurysms. Early attempts at endovascular treatment are discussed by Smith et al. (1994). The evolution of concepts in aneurysm surgery is also covered by Ratcheson and Wirth (1994) as part of the *Concepts in Neurosurgery Series*. The Mayo Clinic experience was summarized in 1995 (Meyer et al., 1995), and Schievink (1997a) reviewed medical progress in intracranial aneurysms for the *New England Journal of Medicine*.

DEFINITIONS

Aneurysms are persistent, localized dilations of the wall of a vessel. They may be classified by shape, in which case they are usually described as either **saccular** or nonsaccular. Saccular aneurysms are pouch-like dilations that usually affect only a portion of the vessel wall. Initially called "miliary aneurysms" by Virchow and Charcot, these lesions subsequently were called "berry aneurysms" because of their "shining coats and rounded outlines: They hang like berries on the arterial stalks and are often multiple" (Collier, 1931). In fact, most "berry" aneurysms are neither pedunculated nor polypoid. Instead, they usually have a wide base of origin—an important anatomic point in surgical treatment. Nonsaccular aneurysms are often called **fusiform** or serpentine. When an artery is significantly enlarged and tortuous, the vessel is said to be **dolichoectatic**.

Aneurysms may also be classified by cause. Some seem to result solely from developmental defects in the vessel wall. Others are caused by acquired degenerative change, atherosclerosis, infection and inflammation, neoplasm, and trauma. "True" aneurysms result from a disruption of the internal elastic lamina and subsequent disorganization of the arterial wall. "False" aneurysms, usually traumatic in nature, have a full-thickness disruption in the wall including the media and adventitia. Dissecting aneurysms are caused by a split in the arterial wall that may or may not be continuous with the vessel lumen. These have a significantly different etiology and natural history and are discussed separately in this chapter.

PATHOGENESIS

There are two divergent views regarding the pathogenesis of saccular aneurysms: the congenital hypothesis and the degeneration hypothesis (Weir, 1987; Stehbens, 1989). The **congenital hypothesis** stresses the findings of Eppinger (1887) and Forbus (1930), who described discontinuities or gaps in the media of intracranial arterial bifurcations at sites where saccular aneurysms arise. The congenital hypothesis holds that these abnormalities, which Forbus called "medial defects," are developmental defects in the structure of the wall that predispose that area to aneurysm formation. Late-onset "de novo" development of aneurysms in familial groups argues for a congenital defect of some type (Motuo Fotso et al., 1993; Schievink, 1997b). Similarly, de novo development of "mirror" aneurysms suggests some inherent vessel weakness (van Alphen and Gao, 1991).

The congenital hypothesis is supported by the findings of several groups of investigators of a deficiency of type III collagen in the walls of intracranial arteries in some patients with intracranial aneurysms (Pope et al., 1981; Neil-Dwyer et al., 1983; Ostergaard and Oxlund, 1987; Pope, 1989; Pope et al., 1990; Brega et al., 1996; Mimata et al., 1997). In addition, Chyatte et al. (1990) analyzed elastin and reticular fibers in middle cerebral arteries (MCAs) obtained from patients who died from aneurysmal SAH and from control patients who did not have cerebral aneurysms. Examination of cerebral arteries from normal persons revealed a dense network of fine, reticulated, uniformly distributed fibers composed partly of type III collagen in the arterial media. Reticular fibers in the arterial media of cerebral arteries from patients with aneurysms were significantly decreased, shortened, and irregularly distributed in the media. Elastin appearance and content were identical in both normal patients and patients with aneurysms. Majamaa et al. (1992) found an abnormal thermal denaturation temperature of type III protocollagen in two of six patients with familial aneurysms but not in five sporadic cases. Pope et al. (1991) demonstrated vascular fragility with development of carotid-cavernous aneurysms in five patients with type III collagen mutations, having previously pointed out the possible etiologic role (Pope et al., 1990).

On the other hand, Leblanc et al. (1989a) established fibroblast cell cultures and studied the expression of types I and III collagen in a patient with three intracranial aneurysms whose mother and sister also had intracranial aneurysms. These investigators found no difference in type I and III procollagen in the cells from the aneurysm patient and those from the control cell lines (see also Leblanc et al., 1989b, 1990, 1995). In addition, there was no preponderant human leukocyte antigen (HLA) type (Leblanc et al., 1995). In a case-control study from England, there was no difference in the frequency of polymorphic variations in type III collagen from a consecutive group of 56 aneurysm patients and controls (Adamson et al., 1994). Finally, changes in collagen as well as other components in the vessel wall may be secondary, not primary, to a developing aneurysm (Futami et al., 1995b).

The **degenerative hypothesis** of aneurysm formation views saccular aneurysms as acquired lesions that result from degenerative changes at the arterial junction. This hypothesis is based in part on: (*a*) the age at which aneurysms are found at autopsy; (*b*) the age at which they become symptomatic; (*c*) the histopathologic characteristics of pre-aneurysmal changes in arterial walls and the rarity of such changes in infants or children; (*d*) the increased frequency with which both systemic hypertension and coronary artery disease occur in patients with saccular aneurysms; (*e*) atherosclerotic changes in the walls of intracranial arteries in patients with saccular intracranial aneurysms; (*f*) the development of a new aneurysm in some patients several years after successful clipping of an angiographically isolated aneurysm in a different location; and (g) the production in animals of aneurysms histopathologically similar to those that occur in humans by induction of hemodynamic stress, production of renal hypertension, and ingestion of β-aminopropionitrile (Stehbens, 1983b; Miller et al., 1985; Pelissou et al., 1987; Weir, 1987; Misra et al., 1988; Kim et al., 1989; Stehbens, 1989). Terai et al. (1992) examined the less common aneurysms that occur without an associated branching point. These investigators noted evidence of atherosclerotic changes but no unique structural changes.

According to Stehbens (1983b, 1989), the most plausible explanation for the development of intracranial saccular aneurysms is that they are true acquired lesions caused solely by degenerative and atrophic changes induced by hemodynamic stress on atherosclerotic vessel walls. Most investigators believe, however, that although degenerative changes of the arterial junction play a large part in the pathogenesis of intracranial saccular aneurysms, congenital factors also play a role in some patients. We believe that the process of aneurysm formation is multifactorial and that both acquired and congenital factors play a role. Disruption of collagen and elastic fibers seems to take place throughout the wall of the artery (Austin et al. 1993). Whether this is primary or secondary remains unclear.

The importance of hemodynamic processes in aneurysm formation is supported by the association of aneurysms with vascular anomalies that change flow patterns. Vessel anomalies associated with aneurysms may be congenital. These include persistent primitive vessels, congenital occlusions (Nakai et al., 1992; Guijarro Castro et al., 1994; Ushikoshi et al., 1996), anomalous vessels or collateral flow (Nardi et al., 1990; Hamada et al., 1991; Takeshita et al., 1991b; Moyer and Flamm, 1992; Onishi et al., 1992; Guijarro Castro et al., 1994; Mishima et al., 1994), or vascular fenestrations (Arai et al., 1989; Miyagi et al., 1990; Kalia et al., 1991; Deruty et al., 1992a; Hattori and Kobayashi, 1992; Hoshimaru et al., 1992; San-Galli et al., 1992; Suzuki et al., 1992; Banach and Flamm, 1993; Crivelli et al., 1993; Picard et al., 1993; Finlay and Canham, 1994; Nakamura et al., 1994; De Caro et al., 1995; Okamura et al., 1995; Friedlander and Oglivy, 1996; Graves et al., 1996; Fujimura et al., 1997; Tasker et al., 1997).

Most aneurysms associated with persistent primitive arteries occur with persistent trigeminal arteries (Guglielmi et al., 1990; Miyatake et al. 1990; Tokimura et al., 1991; Chen and Liu, 1993; T. Abe et al., 1994; Ahmad et al., 1994; Hayashi et al., 1994; Nakayama et al., 1994; Ishiguro et al., 1995; Alleyne et al., 1997), where the incidence may be as high as 14%. Less commonly, aneurysms are associated with primitive olfactory (Tsuji et al., 1995), ophthalmic (Islak et al., 1994), or hypoglossal arteries (Tsugu et al., 1990; Yamamoto et al., 1991; Kanai et al., 1992). Abnormal anterior-to-posterior connections clearly predispose to a higher incidence of intracerebral aneurysms (Yilmaz et al., 1995).

Acquired changes in hemodynamics may be related to vascular thrombosis secondary to atherosclerosis or dissection but are often associated with previous vascular surgery. This may be related to previous aneurysm clipping (Koeleveld et al., 1991; van Alphen and Gao, 1991; Striph, 1993;

Latka et al., 1995; Maiuri et al., 1995; Parekh et al., 1995; Kojima et al., 1996) or to large-vessel occlusion (Drapkin and Rose, 1992; Kotwica, 1993; Ladzinski et al., 1994; Hirano et al., 1995; Maiuri et al., 1995; Ogasawara et al., 1995; Timperman et al., 1995). De novo aneurysms also develop following superficial temporal-to-middle cerebral artery (STA-MCA) bypass procedures (Hirano et al., 1995; Ogasawara et al., 1995; Kohno et al., 1996), supporting a role for hemodynamic stress.

Other forms of abnormal hemodynamics associated with an increased incidence of aneurysm development include moyamoya disease and associated arteriovenous malformations (AVMs) (Kawaguchi et al., 1996; Kodama et al., 1996). In moyamoya disease, large-vessel occlusion leads to increased small-vessel collateral flow and potentially greater hemodynamic stress. Increased frequency of aneurysm formation is discussed below.

Saccular aneurysms arise from intracranial arteries more frequently than from arteries in any other location, and they usually occur at the bifurcation of two arteries (Fig. 53.2). This distribution suggests that the intracranial arteries may have unique morphologic characteristics that predispose them to aneurysm formation. Studies of the branch angles of cerebral vessels suggest that the dividing points are positioned normally to minimize hemodynamic stress (Rossitti and Lofgren, 1993).

Grossly, the most notable and perhaps most crucial architectural peculiarities of intracranial arteries are the thinness of their walls and the lack of any perivascular support. Histologically, these vessels are muscular arteries that have three layers: a collagenous adventitia, a muscular media, and an inner intima lined by a layer of endothelial cells. An internal elastic lamina separates the intima from the media. Compared with extracranial arteries of similar size, the internal elastic lamina of intracranial arteries is slightly thicker, but the adventitia and media are slightly thinner. The adventitia lacks an external elastic lamina, and the media is devoid of elastic fibers (Stehbens, 1972; Ostergaard et al., 1987). It seems likely that these architectural features are responsible, at least in part, for the greater frequency of intracranial saccular aneurysms as compared with extracranial aneurysms.

Collagen provides the major load-bearing capability in human connective tissue (Dobrin, 1978; Oxlund and Andreassen, 1980; Dobrin et al., 1984). In vascular tissue, two types of collagen predominate: types I and III (Gay and Miller, 1978). Type I fibers play a major role as supporting elements of high tensile strength, whereas type III collagen is essential for structural stability. Ostergaard and Oxlund (1987) found a deficiency of type III collagen in specimens of MCAs from six of 14 patients who died following rupture of intracranial saccular aneurysms but none in similar specimens from 14 age- and sex-matched patients who died of other causes. The deficiency of collagen in the six specimens was not accompanied by any alteration in the mechanical strength of the artery, but it did result in a significant increase in the extensibility of the artery at stress values corresponding to blood pressures between 100 and 200 mm Hg. These findings, as well as those of other investigators (Pope et al., 1981; Neil-Dwyer et al., 1983; de Paepe et al., 1988; Pope, 1989; ter Berg et al., 1989; Pope et al., 1990), suggest that

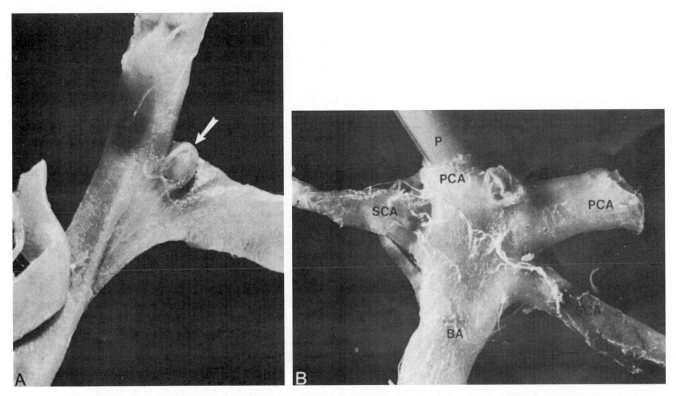

Figure 53.2. Gross pathologic appearance of small aneurysms arising from the bifurcation of intracranial vessels. *A,* Small unruptured aneurysm (*arrow*) arising from the apex of a middle cerebral artery. The texture of the wall is similar to that of the parent vessel. *B,* Small saccular aneurysm with thin, flimsy wall at bifurcation of the basilar artery (*BA*). There is a probe (*P*) in one of the posterior cerebral arteries (*PCA*). *SCA,* superior cerebellar artery. (From Stehbens WE. Etiology and pathogenesis of intracranial berry aneurysms. In Intracranial Aneurysms. Editor, Fox JL, Vol I, pp 358–395. New York, Springer-Verlag, 1983.)

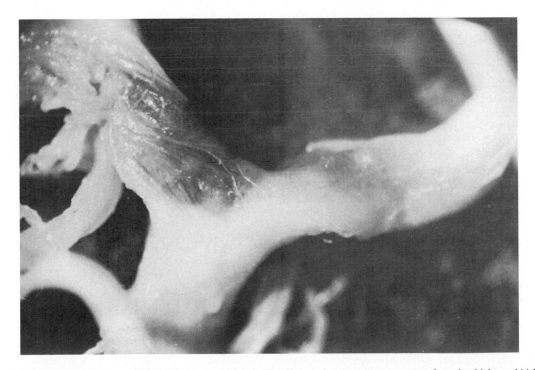

Figure 53.3. Gross appearance of an area of thinning at an arterial fork. The thin area is transparent, a contrast from the thicker, whitish appearance of the rest of the arterial wall. (From Stehbens WE. Pathology of the Cerebral Blood Vessels. St Louis, CV Mosby, 1972.)

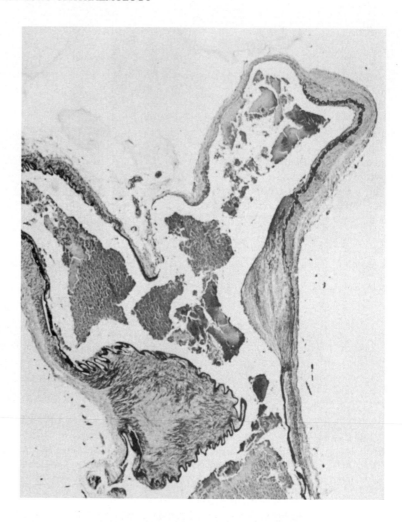

Figure 53.4. Microscopic appearance of an area of thinning at an arterial fork. There is considerable thinning of the media and adventitia with gross loss of internal elastic lamina along the inner or medial aspect of the daughter branch. The media is still visible along most of the wall except for one area where the wall bulges. Verhoeff's elastic stain; ×29. (From Stehbens WE. Histopathology of cerebral aneurysms. Arch Neurol 8: 272–285, 1963.)

there is an abnormality in the biosynthesis of collagen in some patients with intracranial aneurysms (see, however, Leblanc et al., 1989b, 1989c, 1990). In addition, Chyatte and Lewis (1997) reported changes consistent with accelerated degradation of collagen, and other investigators described degradation of elastin and other biochemical abnormalities within aneurysm walls (Skirgaudas et al., 1996; Connolly et al., 1997).

Three types of changes may be seen at the junction between two arteries where an aneurysm develops: (*a*) areas of mural thinning; (*b*) funnel-shaped dilations; and (*c*) evaginations (Stehbens, 1963).

Mural thinning appears grossly as a thin, transparent region at the apex of an arterial fork (Fig. 53.3). The appearance of such a region contrasts sharply with the opacity and atherosclerosis of the adjacent vessel wall. Histologically, an affected segment of the wall exhibits gross thinning as if it had undergone atrophy (Fig. 53.4). The media and adventitia are markedly thinned, and the internal elastic lamina is thin, fragmented, and generally deficient.

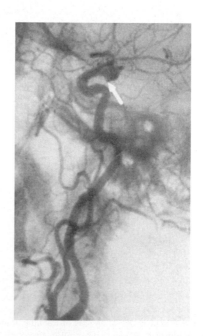

Figure 53.5. Carotid angiogram, lateral view, shows small junctional dilation at the origin of the posterior communicating artery (*arrow*). It is unclear if such a dilation is an early stage of aneurysm formation or is a simple vascular anomaly that does not enlarge or thin with time.

Funnel-shaped dilations occur most frequently at the origin of the posterior communicating artery from the ICA (Hassler and Saltzman, 1959; Stehbens, 1983b), but they also may occur at the origin of other arteries. These abnormalities are called "junctional dilations" (Epstein et al., 1970) or "infundibular widenings" (Hassler and Saltzman, 1963). Although some investigators consider them to be simple anomalies that are neither aneurysmal nor preaneurysmal (Epstein et al., 1970), there is some evidence that they are an early stage of aneurysm formation (Hassler and Saltzman, 1963; Waga and Morikawa, 1979; Sekhar and Heros, 1981). These dilations are curved and look somewhat like a steerhorn (Fig. 53.5). Histologically, the wall of a dilation is thin and attenuated, with the greatest thinning in the region of greatest curvature. The intima is slightly thickened, but the elastic lamina is degenerated, fragmented, and deficient over a large area. Carmichael (1950) thought that these areas were regions of congenital hypoplasia of the vessel wall, but, in fact, funnel-shaped dilations are not seen in infants. They seem instead to result from degenerative or atrophic changes.

Small evaginations in the apical regions of intracranial arterial junctions often do not extend beyond the adventitia and therefore cannot be seen without a microscope (Fig. 53.6). Affected junctions usually form an acute angle, with the apex being slightly blunt. Because the evagination affects only part of the vessel wall, a segment of the parent vessel wall is always intact.

There is remarkable similarity in the ultrastructural appearance of all three types of preaneurysmal abnormalities described above. The lesions all show thickening, lamination, redundancy, and separation of basement membranes, abundant cell debris, and a paucity or absence of elastic lamina (Stehbens, 1975). In many cases, extracellular lipid

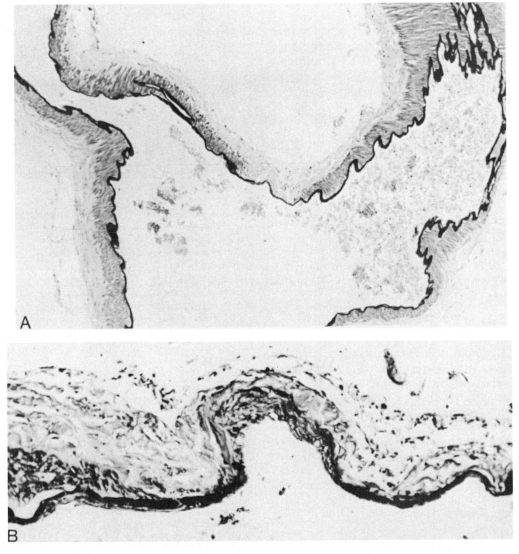

Figure 53.6. Evaginations in the apical regions of intracranial arterial junctions. *A*, Longitudinal section of a cerebral arterial fork shows a microevagination into part of an apical medial raphé. Note loss of the elastica. Verhoeff's elastic stain; ×88. *B*, Small evagination into part of a medial raphé of a blunt apex. Note loss of elastic and thickening of the intima in the region of evagination. Verhoeff's elastic stain; ×294. (From Stehbens WE. Etiology and pathogenesis of intracranial berry aneurysms. In Intracranial Aneurysms. Editor, Fox JL, Vol I. New York, Springer-Verlag, 1983.)

is found adjacent to regions of maximum thinning. Microscopic and immunohistochemical studies of aneurysm walls show full-thickness disruption, disorganization, and changes in fibronectin. This is true both in vivo (Austin et al., 1993) and with experimentally created aneurysms (Futami et al., 1995b).

The increased incidence of aneurysm formation in association with vessel fenestration may be explained by similarities in the orientation of collagen and the structure of the media at fenestration sites and vessel branch points (Finlay and Canham, 1994). It should be noted, however, that this association has been questioned. In a retrospective study of 5190 angiograms, fenestrated arteries were identified in 37 (38 fenestrations). Seven of these patients had a total of 13 aneurysms, but in only one patient did an aneurysm occur at the site of a fenestration. Thus, considering all fenestrations, the incidence of aneurysm formation at a fenestration site was only 3%—no different from the expected incidence of aneurysms at vessel bifurcations (Sanders et al., 1993).

Attempts have been made to correlate the appearance of an aneurysm with its subsequent growth. In a study from Okayama, Japan, aneurysms were classified into five types according to the intraoperative findings: type 1, uniformly thin, smooth surface; type 2, thin neck and thick wall, smooth surface with or without red and/or transparent portions; type 3, uniformly thick wall, smooth surface with or without red portions; type 4, thick neck, bubbled or loculated thin wall at dome with or without red and/or transparent portions; type 5, thick wall in entirety, irregular surface with or without red portions. In this study, these changes correlated with aneurysm size, with types 4 and 5 at greater risk of rupture (Asari and Ohmoto, 1994a).

Studies of the hemodynamics in modeled or in vivo aneurysms suggests maximum stress at the downstream lip of the ostium (Low et al., 1993; Burleson et al., 1995). It is thus likely that growth and rupture occur at this location rather than at the dome. Pulsatility also likely plays an important role in the location of maximal stress and fluid stagnation (Low et al., 1993; Gobin et al., 1994).

CONNECTIVE TISSUE DISEASES

If weakness of the wall of the artery underlies development of an aneurysm, aneurysms should develop with higher frequency in patients with diseases that affect collagen. Indeed, some connective tissue diseases, particularly fibromuscular dysplasia (FMD), Ehlers-Danlos syndrome, Marfan's syndrome, and pseudoxanthoma elasticum (PXE), are thought to be associated with an increased frequency of aneurysm formation (Schievink, 1997b). Although the relationship of the aneurysm to the connective tissue disease may be fortuitous in some cases, in others, the underlying systemic disorder may cause weakening of the supporting connective tissue and adjacent muscle coat in the wall of an intracranial artery, thereby predisposing the area to aneurysm formation (Fox, 1983).

Fibromuscular Dysplasia

FMD is a disorder of medium-diameter arteries (Mettinger, 1982; Mettinger and Ericson, 1982). It is character-

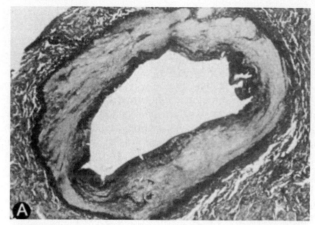

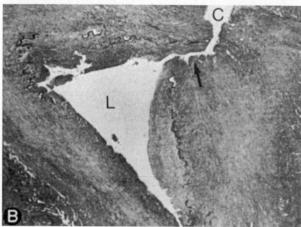

Figure 53.7. Pathology of fibromuscular dysplasia. *A*, Fibromuscular dysplasia affecting the left internal carotid artery. There is irregular intimal thickening, focal fragmentation of the internal elastic lamina, and severe medial fibroplasia. *B*, Higher magnification of a different region of the affected vessel shows partial collapse of the lumen (*L*) with communication through a ruptured arterial wall (*arrow*) with a dissecting channel (*C*). Note asymmetric proliferation in the wall, irregularities and focal absence of the internal elastic lamina, and medial fibroplasia. (From Garcia-Merino JA, Gutierrez JA, Lopez-Lozano JJ, et al. Double lumen dissecting aneurysms of the internal carotid artery in fibromuscular dysplasia: Case report. Stroke *14*:815–818, 1983.)

ized by segmental, nonatheromatous stenoses that can affect any or all three layers (adventitia, media, and intima) of the vessel wall (Fig. 53.7). The most common form of FMD affects the media. Constricting bands in the media are composed of dysplastic fibrous tissue and proliferating smooth muscle cells. These constricting rings alternate with areas of luminal dilation caused by thinning of the media and disruption of the elastic membrane (Sandok, 1983). The arteries most often affected are the renal and vertebral and the common external and internal carotid arteries.

FMD occurs five times more often in women than in men. The average age at presentation is 49 years, and more than 80% of patients are in their 5th decade or older (Reader and Massey, 1980).

Symptoms and signs of FMD are related to the vessel or

vessels affected. When the disease affects the renal arteries, systemic hypertension is common. When the common or internal carotid arteries are affected, patients may experience transient ischemic attacks (TIAs) (including unilateral and homonymous visual field loss, transient monocular visual loss, and diplopia), stroke, or both. Reader and Massey (1980) described a patient with FMD of the right ICA who also had an ipsilateral congenital Horner's syndrome. Extracranial involvement of the carotid arteries may include localized aneurysm formation (Miyauchi and Shionoya, 1991; Auer and Nunnelee, 1996). FMD may also play an etiologic role in patients with multiple extracranial ICA aneurysms (Bour et al., 1992). In one series of 24 extracranial ICA aneurysms in 20 patients, FMD was present in 12 patients (Faggioli et al., 1996). In another series, FMD was associated with an aneurysm of the extracranial ICA in eight of 38 cases (Moreau et al., 1994). A rare extracranial location was noted in a report of aneurysms of the STA associated with

SAH from intracranial vertebral aneurysms in a 39-year-old patient with FMD (Setoyama et al., 1994).

Intracranial aneurysms occasionally occur in patients with FMD (George et al., 1989; Fukazawa et al., 1990) (Fig. 53.8), most frequently in association with simultaneous extracranial involvement of the internal carotid and vertebral arteries (Mandai et al., 1992b). These may also be associated with fusiform intracranial vessel dilation (Belen et al., 1996). About 7% of patients with FMD of the renal arteries harbor one or more intracranial aneurysms (Wylie et al., 1966). Giant intracavernous aneurysms also occur in the setting of FMD (Nishiyama et al., 1992; Lan et al., 1995), but the pathophysiologic role of FMD in such cases is unclear. There are too few cases of intracranial aneurysms associated with FMD affecting the vertebral or internal carotid arteries to provide data for statistical analysis. It therefore is unclear if the occurrence of an intracranial aneurysm in a patient with FMD is coincidental (Lie

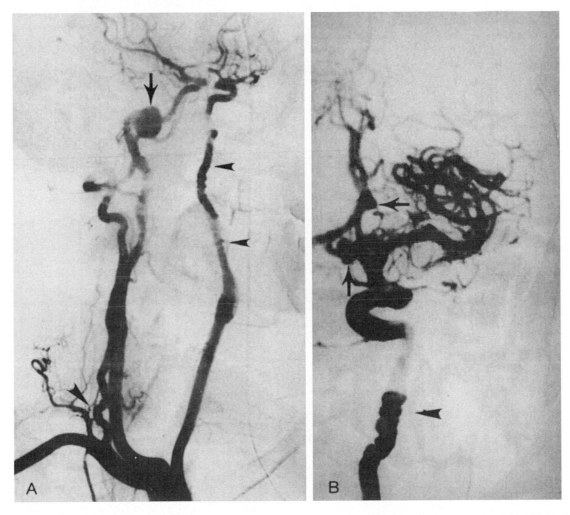

Figure 53.8. Intracranial aneurysms associated with fibromuscular dysplasia. *A,* Typical appearance of fibromuscular dysplasia affecting both internal carotid arteries and the right vertebral artery (*arrowheads*) in a patient with a large, saccular aneurysm of the intracranial portion of the vertebral artery (*arrow*). *B,* Typical "string-of-beads" appearance (*arrowhead*) of fibromuscular dysplasia affecting the internal carotid artery in a patient with an aneurysm of the anterior communicating artery and an aneurysm of the posterior communicating artery (*arrows*). (From George B, Mourier KL, Gelbert F, et al. Vascular abnormalities in the neck associated with intracranial aneurysms. Neurosurgery *24:*499–508, 1989.)

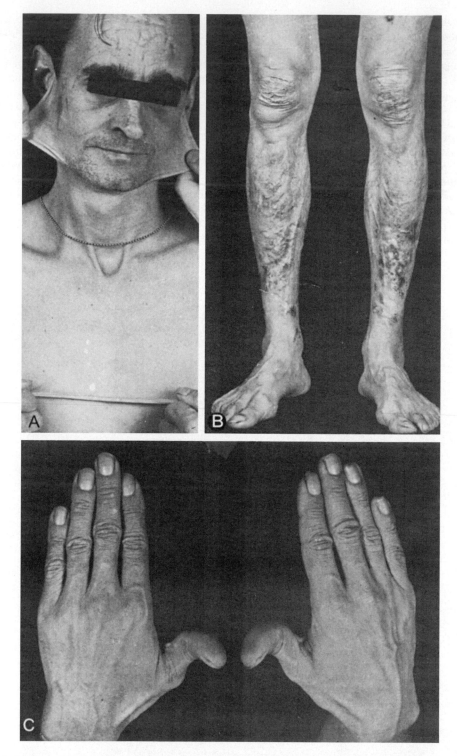

Figure 53.9. The clinical features of Ehlers-Danlos syndrome. *A*, Marked elasticity of skin; *B*, shiny, parchment-thin, hyperpigmented skin overlying the knees and legs (*cigarette paper or papyraceous scars*); *C*, hypermobility of thumbs. (From McKusick VA. Heritable Disorders of Connective Tissue, 4th ed. St. Louis, CV Mosby, 1972.)

and Kim, 1977) or etiologic (George et al., 1989). FMD may also be associated with an increased risk of dissection (see below) and possible SAH if the dissection extends intracranially (Vles et al., 1990).

Ehlers-Danlos Syndrome

Ehlers-Danlos syndrome encompasses a group of inherited disorders of connective tissue, all of which have abnormalities of collagen composition. It is manifested by a wide spectrum of clinical presentations, and at least 10 distinct types can be differentiated on the basis of clinical and genetic differences (Byers and Holbrook, 1985; see Table in Pollack et al., 1997). Type IV Ehlers-Danlos syndrome is character-

ized by a deficiency of type III collagen, resulting in fragility of blood vessels and intestines.

The usual clinical features of Ehlers-Danlos syndrome are hypermobility of joints, and increased elasticity, fragility, bruising, and scarring of the skin (Fig. 53.9). Discontinuities in Bruch's membrane beneath the retinal pigment epithelium of the eye produce the appearance of orange-yellow lines, called **angioid streaks**, radiating from the optic disc. Intraocular hemorrhage from subretinal neovascularization may occur. Complications of defective collagen in patients with Ehlers-Danlos syndrome include spontaneous intestinal rupture, carotid-cavernous sinus fistula, and arterial dissections (Graf, 1965; Schoolman and Kepes, 1967; Julien and De Boucard, 1971; Farley et al., 1983; Guiolet, 1984; Lach et

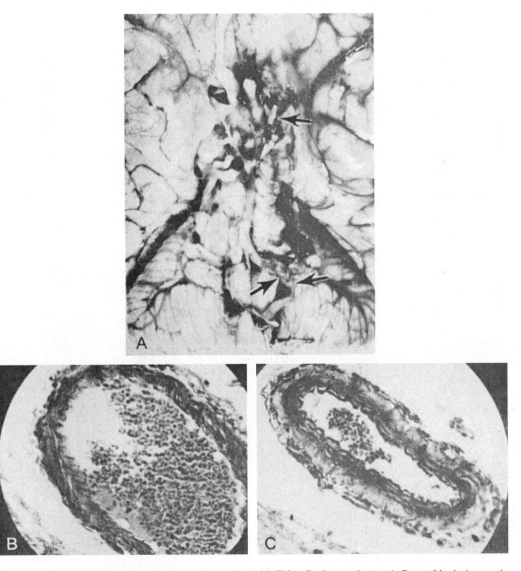

Figure 53.10. Saccular and fusiform intracranial aneurysms in a patient with Ehlers-Danlos syndrome. *A*, Base of brain in a patient who died after clipping of an aneurysm of the internal carotid artery. *Upper arrow* points to clip at site of aneurysm. *Lower arrows* point to fusiform dilations of the left vertebral artery. *B*, Intracranial artery from the same patient shows deficiency of collagenous tissue of adventitial layer. *C*, Histologic appearance of a normal intracranial artery for comparison. (From Rubinstein MK, Cohen NH. Ehlers-Danlos syndrome associated with multiple intracranial aneurysms. Neurology *14*:125–132, 1964.)

al., 1987; Fox et al., 1988; Halbach et al., 1990a; Schievink et al., 1990, 1991a; Kashiwagi et al., 1993; Taki et al., 1994; Debrun et al., 1996; Pollack et al., 1997; Schievink, 1997b). Rubinstein and Cohen (1964) described a patient with Ehlers-Danlos syndrome in whom multiple intracranial aneurysms were present. The adventitia of the intracranial vessels was scanty and loosely organized. The authors attributed the development of the aneurysms to a generalized mesodermal abnormality resulting from defective collagenous support of the affected blood vessels. Similar histopathologic findings were described by Brodribb (1970) in a patient with Ehlers-

Danlos syndrome and an aneurysm of the vertebral artery. de Paepe et al. (1988) described a 55-year-old man with type IV Ehlers-Danlos syndrome who had multiple intracranial aneurysms (Fig. 53.10). One of nine patients reported by de Wazieres et al. (1995) suffered a ruptured cerebral aneurysm, two patients had renal artery dissections, and another patient had a ruptured subclavian artery. In another patient, a vertebral artery rupture into the pleural cavity proved fatal (Minola and Maculotti, 1994). Skin biopsy can confirm the diagnosis of type IV Ehlers-Danlos (Shishkina et al., 1993). Ehlers-Danlos patients, particularly those with type IV, are

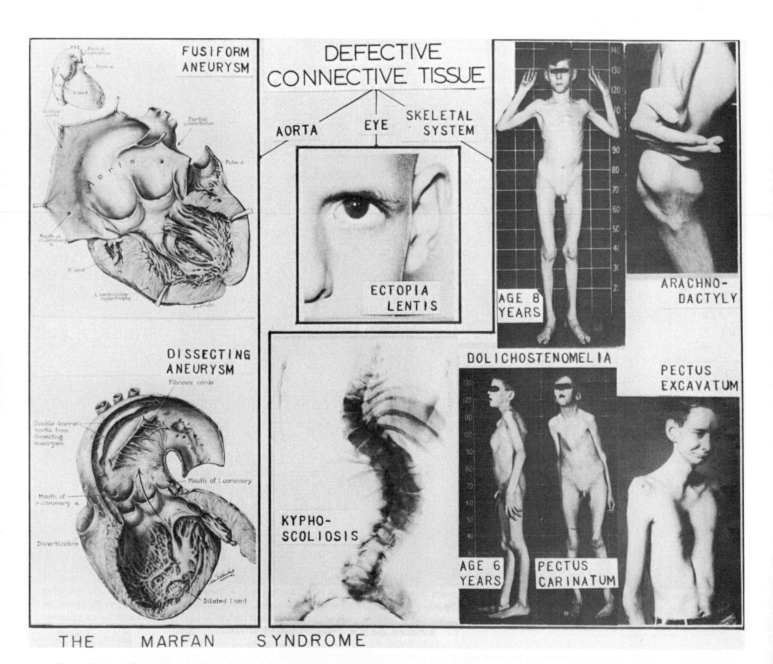

Figure 53.11. Clinical features of Marfan's syndrome. (From MuKusick VA. Heritable Disorders of Connective Tissue, 2nd ed. St. Louis, CV Mosby, 1960.)

at significantly higher risks of complications during endovascular therapy due to vascular fragility (Halbach et al., 1990a; Pollack et al., 1997).

Marfan's Syndrome

Marfan's syndrome is an autosomal-dominant inherited disease with a high degree of penetrance, worldwide occurrence, and equal sex distribution. Patients with Marfan's syndrome may have aortic dilation, dissecting aortic aneurysm, mitral valve prolapse, ectopia lentis, arachnodactyly, loosejointedness, and pectus excavatum (Fig. 53.11).

Marfan's syndrome is thought to result from a biochemical abnormality of connective tissue that causes defective formation of elastic tissue. Vascular changes include diffuse ectasia, thinning, and even aneurysmal dilation of the aorta, pulmonary arteries, and peripheral arteries. The aneurysms that develop in these vessels may eventually rupture or dissect. Histopathologically, the media usually is the only abnormal layer of the affected arterial wall. It shows cystic necrosis with fragmentation and paucity of elastic tissue.

Patients with Marfan's syndrome may have intracranial aneurysms (Speciali et al., 1971; Finney et al., 1976; Matsuda et al., 1979; Resende et al., 1984; Croisile et al., 1988; ter Berg et al., 1989; Hainsworth and Mendelow, 1991; Vandenberg et al., 1996; Schievink, 1997b). In most cases, the aneurysm is large and fusiform rather than saccular (Fig 53.12). Aneurysms of the extracranial portions of the common carotid, internal carotid, and vertebral arteries also occur in patients with Marfan's syndrome (Ohyama et al., 1992). Stehbens et al. (1989) performed a detailed study of cerebral arterial bifurcations by serial sectioning in a 33-year-old woman with Marfan's syndrome who died of septicemia after cardiac surgery. Two bifurcations of the right MCA exhibited atrophic changes associated with early saccular aneurysm formation, suggesting that the mode of development of intracranial saccular aneurysms is similar in patients with and without

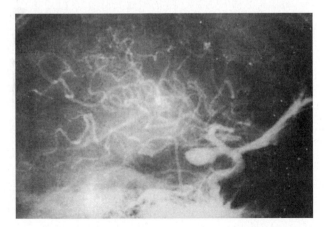

Figure 53.12. Saccular aneurysm arising from the supraclinoid portion of the right internal carotid artery in a patient with Marfan's syndrome. (From Croisile B, Deruty R, Pialat J, et al. Anévrysme de la carotide supraclinoï dienne et méga-dolicho-artères cervicales dans un syndrome de Marfan. Neurochirurgie *34*:342–347, 1988.)

Marfan's syndrome. In a study from the Marfan's clinic in Amsterdam, 129 of 135 patients were followed prospectively for a total of 581 prospective years and further analyzed retrospectively to a total of 2850 years without an SAH (van den Berg et al., 1996). The authors thus concluded that there is insufficient evidence to presume a relationship between symptomatic intracranial aneurysms and Marfan's syndrome on the basis of available data.

Pseudoxanthoma Elasticum (PXE)

PXE is a systemic disorder of connective tissue inherited in an autosomal-recessive fashion. It is characterized by thickening of the skin with elevated yellow areas at skin creases. Patients are at risk for linear breaks in Bruch's membrane within the eye (angioid streaks) and secondary subretinal neovascular membranes, dilation of the aorta, premature calcification of various arteries, and spontaneous gastrointestinal bleeding (Fig. 53.13). The skin and ocular lesions are manifestations of the degenerative changes of the elastic tissue. Patients with PXE may develop intracranial aneurysms (Dixon, 1951; Scheie and Hogan, 1957) (Fig. 53.14). In all of the patients, however, the aneurysm wall is partially calcified, and it is therefore likely that there is no true pathophysiologic connection between the aneurysm and the underlying systemic connective tissue disease.

TUMORS

Internal and external forces in addition to inherent abnormalities in the vessel wall may focally weaken the wall of an artery predisposing to the development of an aneurysm. For example, some patients harbor both an intracranial neoplasm and one or more intracranial aneurysms. The most common tumors associated with aneurysms are pituitary adenomas (Jakubowski and Kendall, 1978; Wakai et al., 1979; see Table 1 in Acqui et al., 1987) and meningiomas (Raskind, 1965; Levin and Gross, 1966; Jimenez et al., 1971).

Most patients with an intracranial tumor and an aneurysm initially develop symptoms and signs of the tumor. Neuroimaging studies are then performed and identify an asymptomatic aneurysm (Handa et al., 1976; Acqui et al., 1987) (Figs. 53.15 and 53.16). In other cases, however, an intracranial or subarachnoid hemorrhage from a ruptured aneurysm leads to neuroimaging studies that identify an asymptomatic intracranial tumor.

Several mechanisms could account for the occurrence of an intracranial neoplasm and aneurysm in the same patient. A vascular neoplasm, such as a meningioma, might increase local cerebral blood flow and thus predispose affected vessels to aneurysm formation. This might be the explanation for the occurrence of an aneurysm on the feeding vessel of a meningioma (O'Neill et al., 1995). In patients with olfactory groove meningiomas and anterior circulation aneurysms, the connection is more tenuous (Simoes et al., 1991; Maiuri et al., 1992). Patients with acromegaly from a growth hormonesecreting pituitary adenoma might have disruption of connective tissue, leading to formation of multiple aneurysms (Schenk and Solleveld, 1968) or ectasia of intracranial arteries (Hatam and Greitz, 1972). The association of an aneu-

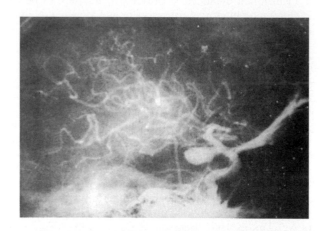

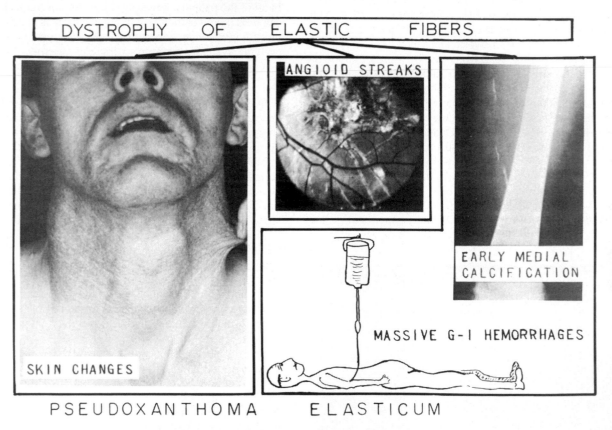

Figure 53.13. Clinical features of pseudoxanthoma elasticum. (From McKusick VA. Heritable Disorders of Connective Tissue, 2nd ed. St. Louis. CV Mosby, 1960.)

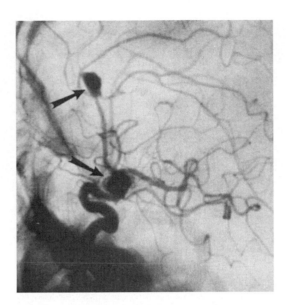

Figure 53.14. Multiple saccular aneurysms in a patient with pseudoxanthoma elasticum. The *lower arrow* indicates an aneurysm of the anterior communicating artery; the *upper arrow* points to an aneurysm at the origin of the pericallosal and callosomarginal arteries.

rysm with a pituitary tumor in the multiple endocrine neoplasia syndrome could be mediated by the endocrine disturbance (Adachi et al., 1993). It seems likely, however, that most, if not all, cases of intracranial aneurysm and neoplasm are coincidental (Taylor, 1961; Pia et al., 1972; Hardy et al., 1991; Shigemori et al., 1991; Stevenson et al., 1994; Pant et al., 1997). Nonetheless, recognizing the presence of

an intracranial aneurysm may well alter the approach to an associated intracranial tumor (Delfini et al., 1990).

TRAUMATIC ANEURYSMS

Trauma is the most obvious extrinsic cause of vascular weakness. In most cases, this leads to development of a "false aneurysm" from disruption of the entire vascular wall or to dissection from a tear in the inner wall permitting access of blood to a split in the media. Occasionally the appearance and the course may resemble that of other saccular aneurysms. The histology of the aneurysm depends on the extent of the initial disruption of the wall (Capanna, 1984; Jakobsson et al., 1984).

Unlike other aneurysms, traumatic aneurysms are more common in children than in adults (Patel and Richardson, 1971; Almeida et al., 1977; Buckingham et al., 1988; Ventureyra and Higgins, 1994; Lam et al., 1996), and they generally occur at a younger age than do nontraumatic aneurysms. Similarly, trauma is a more frequent cause of aneurysms in children than in adults (Herman et al., 1991–1992). This probably reflects the tendency of younger persons to be involved in fights and in motor vehicle and other accidents in which head injury is common. Rarely, an aneurysm may be related to traumatic birth injury (Piatt and Clunie, 1992).

Aneurysms of the cervical portions of the internal carotid and vertebral arteries may develop from the effects of blunt trauma (Fleischer and Guthkelch, 1987; Pretre et al., 1994), but they are much more commonly caused by penetrating injuries, such as puncture wounds sustained during an altercation, surgical radical neck dissection (Minion et al., 1994), surgery for torticollis (Korovessis et al., 1992) or angiography (Lepoire et al., 1964; Adeloye et al., 1970; Oba et al.,

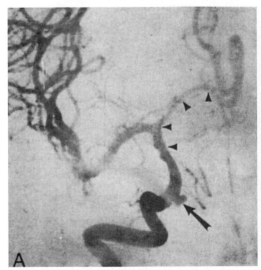
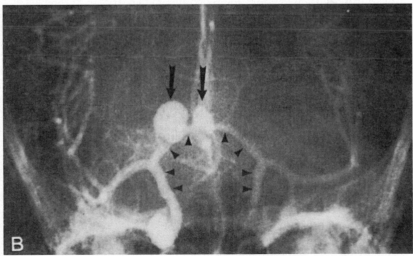

Figure 53.15. Incidental intracranial aneurysms in patients with pituitary adenomas. *A*, The intracavernous and supraclinoid segments of the right internal carotid artery are displaced laterally and the right anterior cerebral artery is elevated by a large pituitary adenoma (*arrowheads*). There is an aneurysm at the junction of the internal carotid and ophthalmic arteries (*arrow*). *B*, The intracavernous and supraclinoid segments of both internal carotid arteries are displaced laterally and both anterior cerebral arteries are elevated by a large pituitary adenoma (*arrowheads*). A bilobed aneurysm of the right anterior cerebral artery projects superiorly and posteriorly (*arrows*). (From Jakubowski J, Kendall B. Coincidental aneurysms with tumours of pituitary origin. J Neurol Neurosurg Psychiatry *41*:972–979, 1978.)

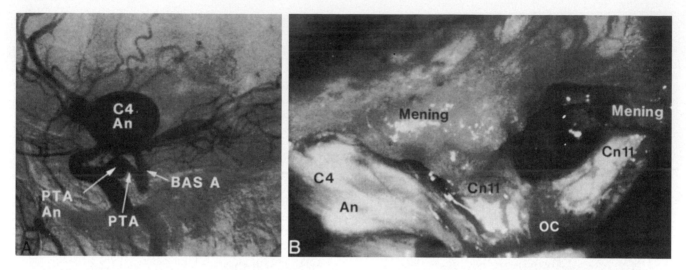

Figure 53.16. Intracranial aneurysms in a patient with bilateral optic canal meningiomas. This 30-year-old man began losing vision in the right eye at age 5. The eye was blind by age 11. Vision in the left eye began to deteriorate at age 28. *A,* Two aneurysms are present. One arises from the supraclinoid portion of the right internal carotid artery *(C4 An)*. The other *(PTA An)* arises from a persistent primitive trigeminal artery *(PTA). BAS A,* Basilar artery. *B,* Operative view shows that both optic nerves *(Cn11)* are encased by separate meningiomas *(Mening)*. The aneurysm arising from the internal carotid artery *(C4 An)* is visible and does not seem to be compressing the right optic nerve. *OC,* optic chiasm. (From Weir B. Aneurysms Affecting the Nervous System. Baltimore, Williams & Wilkins, 1987.)

1983; Vinduska et al., 1993) (Fig. 53.17). There may be an associated fracture of the lower facial bones including the mandible (Cheynet et al., 1992). Traumatic aneurysms may develop after endarterectomy or after dissection (Chaudhary et al., 1979). Murthy and Naidu (1988) described a 40-year-old man who developed swelling of the neck, hoarseness of voice, and a left Horner's syndrome 1–2 hours after neck manipulation by a barber for relief of pain in the neck. The patient was found to have a saccular aneurysm at the origin of the left ICA. These authors suggested that the aneurysm was produced by the neck manipulation, although it is possible that the patient had a long-standing aneurysm producing the neck pain for which he was treated and that the manipulation merely caused further expansion of the aneurysm. Chiropractic neck manipulation clearly has the potential to cause major damage to extracranial vessels, usually dissection with and without associated occlusion (see below and Table 53.1).

Traumatic cervical aneurysms may be asymptomatic or may present as a pulsatile neck mass. Enlargement of such an aneurysm may cause hoarseness, dysphagia, or dyspnea from lower cranial neuropathies or from mechanical compression of neck structures by the mass (Oba et al., 1983; Murthy and Naidu, 1988). Horner's syndrome is frequent (Fleischer and Guthkelch, 1987; Murthy and Naidu). Facial nerve weakness may also result from the surgical approach to traumatic lesions at the skull base (Magnan et al., 1992). In addition, thrombosis of a traumatic cervical aneurysm may produce cerebral ischemic symptoms from the direct effects of the thrombosis or from secondary embolic complications (Clarke and Whittaker, 1980; Pretre et al., 1995). The interval between injury and development of symptoms may be days, weeks, months, or even years (Hardin, 1973). In one remarkable case, a traumatic aneurysm of the cervical

ICA ruptured 40 years after the original injury (Piller et al., 1992).

Trauma that produces an intracranial aneurysm may be of two types (Burton et al., 1968). **Direct** injury to the arterial wall results from bone fragments, missiles, or other foreign bodies that penetrate the cranial or orbital bones (Asari et al., 1977; Kieck and de Villiers, 1984; Braun et al., 1987; Aarabi, 1988). Most of these are associated with intracerebral hematomas and when examined histopathologically are actually false aneurysms characterized by disruption of the entire vessel wall (Haddad et al., 1991). **Indirect** arterial trauma occurs either when a vessel strikes the falx, tentorium, or a bony prominence or from a shearing force produced by acceleration and deceleration of the intracranial contents during blunt trauma (Smith and Bardenheimer, 1968; Handa et al., 1970; Benoit and Wortzman, 1973; Jakobsson et al., 1984).

The majority of traumatic intracranial aneurysms arise directly from the proximal internal carotid and vertebral arteries; however, they may originate from any artery, particularly the major branches of the internal carotid, vertebral, and basilar arteries and their superficial cortical branches (Sadar et al., 1973; Jakobsson et al., 1984; Kieck and de Villiers, 1984; Meguro and Rowed, 1985; Nakstad et al., 1986; Buckingham et al., 1988; Quattrocchi et al., 1990). Vessels are at particular risk of damage when they are in intimate contact with firm structures including the bones of the skull base (Ledic et al., 1992) and dural folds, including the tentorium (Casey and Moore, 1994) and the falx. The ICA is tightly adherent to the periosteum as it exits the petrous carotid canal and then again as it passes through the proximal and distal rings at the anterior clinoid process. Subsequent rupture of an aneurysm in the latter location results in a potentially fatal SAH (Saito et al., 1995).

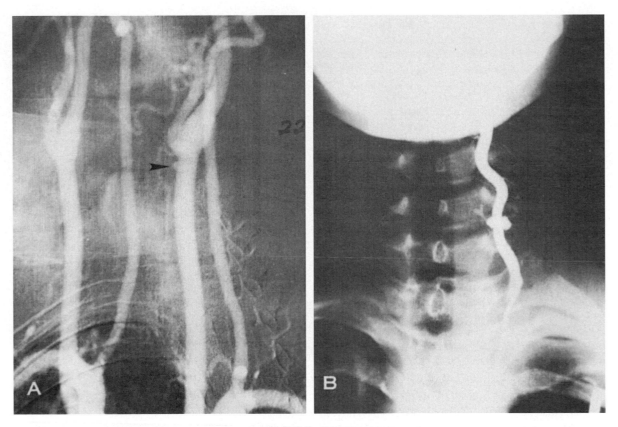

Figure 53.17. Traumatic aneurysms of the cervical portions of the carotid and vertebral arteries. *A,* Small aneurysm at the site of a previous puncture for a percutaneous left carotid angiogram *(arrowhead). B,* Traumatic aneurysm of the left vertebral artery in a patient who suffered a stab wound of the left neck 1 month before the angiogram was performed. (From Taveras JM, Wood EH. Diagnostic Neuroradiology, 2nd ed. Vol 2. Baltimore, Williams & Wilkins, 1976.)

Table 53.1
Dissection Associated with Neck Manipulation

Pratt-Thomas and Berger	1947	Krueger and Okazaki	1980
Kunkle et al.	1952	Schellhas et al.	1980 (2 cases)
Schwarz et al.	1956	Khurana et al.	1980
Ford and Clark	1956	Sherman et al.	1981 (2 cases)
Green and Joynt	1959	Robertson	1981
Smith and Estridge	1962	Simmons et al.	1982
Pribek	1963	Robertson	1982
Kanshepolsky et al.	1972	Horn	1983
Miller and Burton	1974	Braun et al.	1983
Lyness and Wagman	1974	Fritz et al.	1984 (3 cases)
Pratt-Thomas and Berger	1974	Zak and Carmody	1984
Mehalic and Farhat	1974	Cellerier and Georget	1984
Davidson et al.	1974	Amtoft-Nielsen	1984
Okawara and Nibbelink	1975	Daneshmend et al.	1984
Bladin and Merory	1975	Katirji et al.	1985 (2 cases)
Nyberg-Hansen et al.	1976	Sherman et al.	1987
Schmitt	1976	Povlsen et al.	1987
Mueller and Sahs	1976	Mas et al.	1987 (2 cases)
Easton and Sherman	1977	Mas et al.	1989
Beatty	1977	Frumkin and Baloh	1990 (4 cases)
Parkin et al.	1978	Soper et al.	1995
Dumas and Guard	1979	Simnad	1997

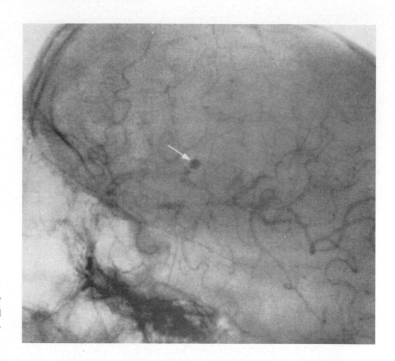

Figure 53.18.   Traumatic aneurysm of the middle meningeal artery *(arrow)* associated with an epidural hematoma. (From Krayenbühl HA, Yaşargil MG. Cerebral Angiography. Philadelphia, JB Lippincott, 1968.)

Traumatic aneurysms originating from the distal portion of an artery are uncommon and likely to be confused with congenital saccular aneurysms (Tokuno et al., 1994). Most of these aneurysms result from severe head injury associated with skull fracture (Burton et al., 1968; Fleischer et al., 1975; Asari et al., 1977; Buckingham et al., 1988). The aneurysm usually develops from a vessel adjacent to the fracture (Fig. 53.18).

Only about 10% of traumatic aneurysms occur in the posterior fossa (Quattrocchi et al., 1990). Such aneurysms are often associated with an occipital bone fracture, usually arise from the posterior inferior cerebellar artery (PICA) (Morard and de Tribolet, 1991), and may be associated with an epidural, subdural, or intraparenchymal hematoma with or without SAH (Aoki et al., 1992). Injuries to the vertebral artery leading to aneurysm formation occur in 46% of cases of cervical vertebral body fractures (Willis et al., 1994). Although most of these injuries are related to minor cervical trauma and result in dissection, a true aneurysm may occasionally develop. Egnor et al. (1991–1992) described a vertebral artery aneurysm in a 15-year-old drummer in a rock band with a habit of head banging. Like the epistaxis that develops in patients with intracavernous traumatic aneurysms (see below), these problems may not develop until days, weeks, or occasionally years after injury (Jakobsson et al., 1984; Steinmetz et al., 1988; Bousquet et al., 1989).

Some traumatic intracranial aneurysms are caused by penetrating missiles, particularly bullet and shell fragments (Salar and Mingrino, 1978; Capanna, 1984; Aarabi, 1988; see Table 2 in Buckingham et al., 1988; Ding, 1988) (Fig. 53.19), whereas others result from seemingly trivial penetrating injury, particularly that resulting from knives, nails, scissors, forks, pencils, and even tree branches (Fleischer et

al., 1975; Braun et al., 1987). Patients suffering such an injury may seem to have a minor superficial wound, when in fact there has been penetration through the skull with damage of superficial or deep intracranial vessels (Fig. 53.20). A self-inflicted pneumatic nail gun injury resulted in a fatal posterior cerebral artery (PCA) aneurysm (Rezai et al., 1994). Among 74 patients with transcranial or transorbital stab wounds, Kieck and de Villiers (1984) identified 26 patients (30%) with traumatic vascular lesions, 11 of which were aneurysms. Neurologic symptoms and signs in these patients were not evident at the time of injury. Instead, they developed from 1 week to several months after injury. The natural history of aneurysms produced by direct penetrating trauma may be more complex than expected. In a prospective study of victims of the Iran-Iraq war, six of 30 traumatically induced aneurysms spontaneously disappeared on follow-up angiography (Amirjamshidi et al., 1996). With the availability of endovascular and microsurgical techniques, treatment of traumatic aneurysms can be tailored to the clinical situation (Aarabi, 1995).

Traumatic intracranial aneurysms may be iatrogenic (Fleischer et al., 1975; Asari et al., 1977; Shigemori et al., 1982; Sekino et al., 1985). Finkemeyer (1955) described a patient in whom an aneurysm of the right MCA developed after removal of a meningioma of the right orbital roof. Two cases of intracranial ICA aneurysms arose following removal of tuberculum sellae meningiomas (Saito et al., 1992). Other cases of intracranial aneurysm formation result from direct arterial injury during surgery for brain tumor (Taylor, 1961; Miyahara et al., 1977; Yamaura et al., 1978; Parkinson and West, 1980; Shigemori et al., 1982) (Fig. 53.21). This may occur more frequently with aggressive attempts to remove craniopharyngiomas because of their propensity to adhere to cerebral vessels (Lakhanpal et al., 1995) (Fig. 53.22).

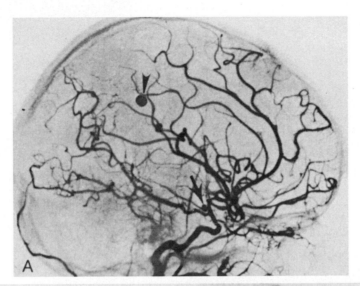

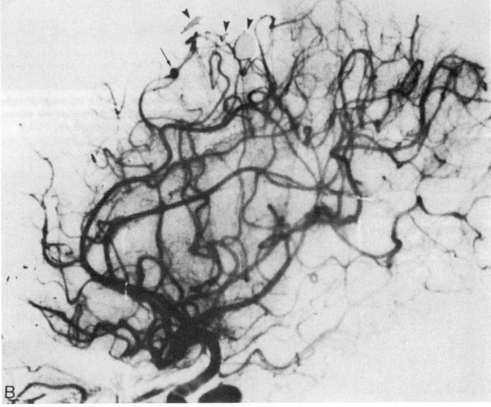

Figure 53.19.   Traumatic intracranial aneurysms caused by penetrating missiles. *A*, Traumatic aneurysm of the anterior choroidal artery caused by a bullet. The bullet entered the skull in the right temporal region, crossed the midline, and eventually lodged in the left parietal lobe *(arrowhead)*. The track of the bullet crossed the origin of the right anterior choroidal artery, where it has produced a traumatic aneurysm *(arrow)*. (From Huber P. Cerebral Angiography, 2nd ed. Stuttgart, Georg Thieme Verlag, 1982.) *B*, Traumatic aneurysm of a cortical branch of the left anterior cerebral artery *(arrow)*. The patient had received a gunshot wound to the head, and the *arrowheads* point to retained fragments of the bullet. (From Fox JL. Intracranial Aneurysms, Vol I. New York, Springer-Verlag, 1983.)

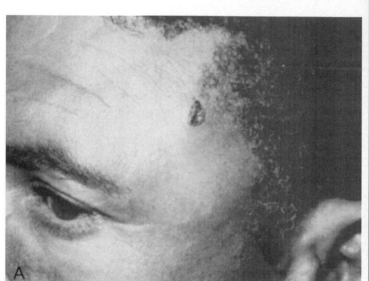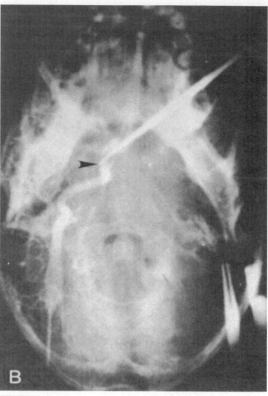

Figure 53.20.   Traumatic aneurysms caused by penetrating injury. *A*, An apparently minor laceration in the left temporal region caused a traumatic aneurysm of the middle meningeal artery. *B*, In another patient, a cerebral angiogram, basal view, shows a knife blade that crosses the midline to injure the contralateral internal carotid artery *(arrowhead)*. (From Kieck CF, de Villiers JC. Vascular lesions due to transcranial stab wounds. J Neurosurg *60*: 42–46, 1984.)

Other surgical procedures that can cause a traumatic aneurysm include subdural tap (Overton and Calverton, 1966), evacuation of subdural hematoma (Eichler et al., 1969), removal of nasal polyps and other rhinologic operations (Sachdev et al., 1977; Yamaura et al., 1978; Wakai et al., 1980; Shigemori et al., 1982), abscess tap (Lassman et al., 1974), ventricular tap (Scharfetter et al., 1976), excision of a colloid cyst (Stoodley et al., 1994), mastoidectomy (Barrett and Lawrence, 1960), middle ear surgery (Welling et al., 1993), transsphenoidal surgery (Paullus et al., 1979; Cabezudo et al., 1981; Awad et al., 1982; Shigemori et al., 1982; Reddy et al., 1990), and aneurysm surgery (Cosgrove et al., 1983; see Table 1 in Sekino et al., 1985; Rowed and Walters, 1994). Transsphenoidal damage to the ICA may be exacerbated by inflammatory or infectious processes that further weaken the wall of the vessel (Takahashi et al., 1991). Endovascular procedures themselves may damage the vascular wall, resulting in subsequent development of a traumatic aneurysm (Kinugasa et al., 1994a). Aggressive skull base surgical procedures may also damage the wall of the ICA leading to aneurysm formation (Sato et al., 1995). Stereotactic biopsy, not surprisingly, may result in aneurysm formation (Sahrakar et al., 1995).

In a most unusual situation, an aneurysm was produced on the STA during arthroscopy of the temporomandibular joint (Carls et al., 1996). This was the only serious complica-

tion in a series of 451 procedures. More commonly, STA aneurysms develop after blunt trauma (Dailey et al., 1994; Merkus et al., 1994). Facial artery aneurysms may be traumatic and seen in association with an AVM (Lutcavage, 1992).

Traumatic aneurysms that arise from the petrous or intracavernous portions of the ICA may produce symptoms from rupture, mass effect, or both. When these aneurysms rupture, they occasionally produce SAH, but more often, they expand medially and inferiorly into the sphenoid sinus and present as progressively severe, and potentially fatal, epistaxis (Seftel et al., 1959; Weaver et al., 1961; Keane and Talalla, 1972; Handa and Handa, 1976; Chambers et al., 1981; Hornibrook and Rhode, 1981; Liu et al., 1985; Ding, 1988; Hamm et al., 1988; Lesoin et al., 1988; Gallina et al., 1990; Hahn et al., 1990; Lee and Wang, 1990; Reiber and Burkey, 1994; Bhatoe et al., 1995). In many cases, epistaxis does not occur immediately after trauma. Instead, it typically occurs 3–12 weeks after injury (Petty, 1969; Wang et al., 1986; Ding, 1988), and rare cases occur 2 years (Ildan et al., 1994) to more than 4 years after trauma (Voris and Basile, 1961; Mahmoud, 1979; Chambers et al., 1981). Simpson et al. (1988) described a patient with a giant traumatic aneurysm of the cavernous portion of the right ICA that produced recurrent, massive epistaxis **30 years** after a head injury. Before epistaxis occurs, the patient may complain of bloody

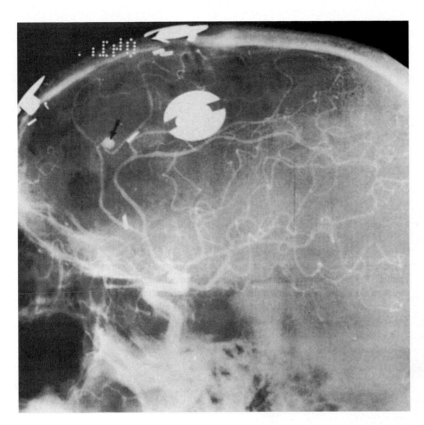

Figure 53.21. Traumatic aneurysm at the junction of the anterior and middle internal frontal branches of the anterior cerebral artery *(arrow)*. The aneurysm developed 13 years after excision of an adjacent astrocytoma. (From Fox JL. Intracranial Aneurysms, Vol I. New York, Springer-Verlag, 1983.)

mucus in the mouth or of swallowing blood. The first episode of epistaxis is rarely fatal, but the likelihood of exsanguination increases with each subsequent hemorrhage. The mortality of posttraumatic aneurysms of the ICA that rupture into the sphenoid sinus is estimated to be 30–50% (Handa and Handa, 1976; Chambers et al., 1981). Inadequate diagnosis and treatment are major contributors to this high mortality.

Some traumatic intracavernous aneurysms are associated with unilateral loss of vision. The loss of vision usually occurs at the time of trauma from direct or indirect damage to the optic nerve (usually within the optic canal) or to the ophthalmic artery (Marmor et al., 1982; Wang et al., 1986; Guest and Schnetler, 1992). The visual loss is almost always ipsilateral to the aneurysm. In rare cases, blindness is not present initially but develops days to weeks after injury (Lee and Wang, 1990).

Keane and Talalla (1972) described a 19-year-old man who began to lose vision in the right eye 3 weeks after a head injury that occurred when the bicycle he was riding was struck by an automobile. Immediately after the accident, the patient had normal visual acuity and normal pupillary responses. At 10 days after the injury, he developed numbness below the left eye and inside the left side of the mouth. At 17 days after the accident, he began to experience left frontal and orbital headaches, and he had a nosebleed that stopped spontaneously. Three weeks after the injury, the patient was watching television when he suddenly noted that although objects seen with the right eye seemed normal,

objects seen with the left eye appeared blue-tinged and surrounded by a blue halo. During the next 10 days, the patient experienced progressive loss of vision in the left eye, intensification of headaches, and increasingly severe recurrent nosebleeds. When examined 10 weeks after injury, the patient had complete blindness in the left eye, a left pupil that did not react to direct light stimulation, and a moderately pale left optic disc. He also had a large soft-tissue mass that filled two-thirds of the nasopharynx. Angiography showed that the mass was a large, multilobulated aneurysm arising from the cavernous portion of the left ICA and extending into the sphenoid sinus. The aneurysm was treated by trapping.

The causes of progressive visual loss in patients with traumatic intracranial aneurysm include hemorrhage and edema within or surrounding the optic nerve and gradual enlargement of the aneurysm with compression of the optic nerve or ophthalmic artery (Maurer et al., 1961; Keane and Talalla, 1972; Teal et al., 1973). Rarely, vision is lost in the contralateral eye because the aneurysm or an associated hematoma compresses the opposite optic nerve or occludes the ophthalmic artery (Araki et al., 1965; Handa et al., 1967). After treatment of the aneurysm, vision in the contralateral eye may improve or or even return to normal (Handa et al., 1967). The prognosis for vision in the ipsilateral eye depends on the pathophysiologic mechanism of its loss and its potential for reversibility (Weinstein et al., 1991).

With progressive enlargment, traumatic intracavernous aneurysms may produce ophthalmoparesis that is frequently painless (Marmor et al., 1982; Braun et al., 1987) but that

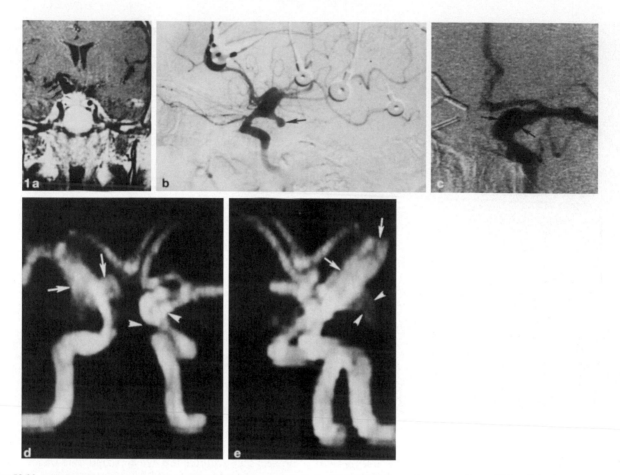

Figure 53.22. Findings in a 14-year-old boy after surgical resection of craniopharyngioma. *A*, Coronal contrast-enhanced T1-weighted magnetic resonance (MR) image shows marked fusiform dilation of the right supraclinoid carotid artery (*black arrows*). *B*, Lateral projection of right common carotid digital subtraction arteriogram confirms the supraclinoid aneurysm and shows extension of the aneurysm into the posterior communicating artery (*black arrow*). *C*, Frontal projection of left carotid digital subtraction arteriogram following surgical repair of the right carotid pseudoaneurysms demonstrates aneurysmal dilation of the left supraclinoid carotid artery (*black arrows*). *D*, Frontal, and *E*, oblique maximum intensity pixel reconstruction images from three-dimensional time-of-flight MR angiogram show extensive fusiform aneurysmal dilation of the right supraclinoid carotid artery (*white arrows*) with extension into the right posterior communicating artery (*E, white arrowheads*). Aneurysmal dilation of the left supraclinoid carotid artery is also present (*D, white arrowheads*). (Images *D* and *E* were reconstructed retrospectively from the original MR angiographic data set using software not available at the time of the original examination). (From Lakhanpal SK, Glasier CM, James CA, et al. MR and CT diagnosis of carotid pseudoaneurysm in children following surgical resection of craniopharyngioma. Ped Radiol 25:249–251, 1995.)

may be associated with mild to severe ipsilateral facial pain (Pecker et al., 1960) or facial hypesthesia (Buckingham et al., 1988). An ipsilateral Horner's syndrome may occur in such cases (Fig. 53.23). Other traumatic intracavernous aneurysms erode into the sphenoid sinus and compress the ipsilateral optic nerve, producing progressive visual loss (see above). Traumatic intracavernous aneurysms thus may produce any form of cavernous sinus syndrome. Patients with a history of head trauma who experience delayed or immediate ophthalmoparesis, progressive visual loss, recurrent epistaxis, or a combination of these, should be considered to have a traumatic intracavernous aneurysm until proven otherwise (Maurer et al., 1961; Araki et al., 1965; Abad et al., 1981). In extremely rare instances, visual loss produced by a traumatic aneurysm is bilateral (Hahn and McLone, 1987). Rarely, delayed rupture of an intracavernous carotid

aneurysm may produce an intracerebral hematoma (Lin, 1995).

Head trauma may occasionally produce a traumatic aneurysm of the ophthalmic artery. When the intracranial portion of the artery is affected, visual acuity in the ipsilateral eye is often impaired (Salmon and Blatt, 1968). Hahn and McLone (1987) described an 8-year-old boy who was hit by a fire truck and sustained multiple injuries, including cerebral contusion, basal skull fracture, fracture of the left humerus, and scalp abrasions. He was comatose for 2 weeks. As he regained consciousness, he was found to have an expressive aphasia, mental confusion, and a memory deficit. The right eye had decreased vision associated with a right inferotemporal quadrantic field defect. The left eye was blind. Neuroimaging revealed bilateral traumatic aneurysms affecting the intracranial portions of the ophthalmic arteries. The patient

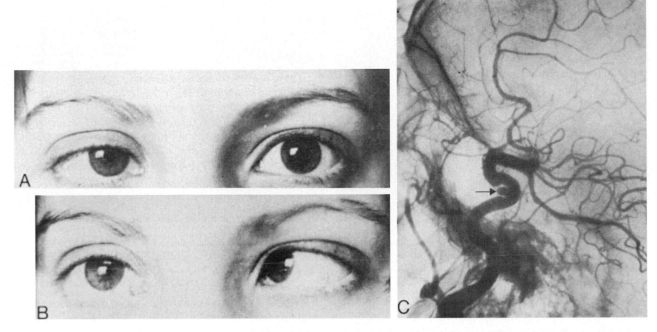

Figure 53.23. Abducens nerve paresis and ipsilateral postganglionic Horner's syndrome from traumatic intracavernous aneurysm. The patient was an 18-year-old woman who suffered severe head trauma in an automobile accident. *A*, The patient fixates with the left eye. The right eye is esotropic, and there is right ptosis. The right pupil is smaller than the left. *B*, On attempted right gaze, the right eye does not abduct beyond the midline. *C*, Carotid angiogram, lateral view, shows a traumatic saccular aneurysm of the intracavernous portion of the right internal carotid artery (*arrow*). (From Abad JM, Alvarez F, Blazquez MG. An unrecognized neurological syndrome: Sixth-nerve palsy and Horner's syndrome due to traumatic intracavernous carotid aneurysm. Surg Neurol *16*:140–144, 1981.)

underwent a bifrontal craniotomy at which time both optic nerves were found to be elevated and thinned from compression by the aneurysms. Fortunately, both aneurysms had necks that allowed them to be clipped. There were no postoperative complications, and the patient experienced a gradual improvement in vision. The authors did not indicate if the visual improvement occurred in one or both eyes.

Trauma to the orbit can produce an aneurysm of the intraorbital portion of the ophthalmic artery (Rahmat et al., 1984). Such an aneurysm may cause pulsating unilateral proptosis. If vision is not damaged from the original injury, subsequent enlargement of the aneurysm may cause progressive loss of vision in the eye and ophthalmoparesis.

The treatment of a traumatic intracranial aneurysm depends on its location. Some aneurysms can be clipped (Hahn and McLone, 1987), but most cannot because they lack a defined neck. Treatment alternatives are therefore limited to excision of the aneurysm combined with reanastomosis of the proximal and distal portions of the affected artery, trapping of the aneurysm, and occlusion of the affected artery (Aarabi, 1988; Rengachary, 1988; Bousquet et al., 1989). The latter two procedures are often combined with some type of bypass procedure designed to provide adequate blood flow to the territory normally supplied by the occluded artery. Endovascular techniques have substantially increased the potential approaches to traumatic aneurysms (see below).

When a traumatic aneurysm arises from the ICA, surgical options include ligation of the artery, trapping the aneurysm

with or without revascularization, direct arteriotomy, intravascular occlusion using a detachable balloon, and thrombosis of the aneurysm using endovascular techniques (Petty, 1969; Salar and Mingrino, 1978; Moore et al., 1979; Dellen, 1980; Parkinson and West, 1980; Hatashita et al., 1983; Capanna, 1984; Wang et al., 1986; Ding, 1988; Simpson et al., 1988) (see below). Traumatic aneurysms that arise from the vertebral and basilar arteries are usually treated with trapping procedures, whereas aneurysms arising from intracerebral vessels are treated by excision and reanastomosis of the affected vessel whenever possible (Weir, 1987). Unfortunately, because of many adhesions to the surrounding parenchyma and a thin wall, intraoperative aneurysm rupture is frequent (Rengachary, 1988).

Not all aneurysms that produce visual or neurologic manifestations after trauma are traumatic in origin. Minor head trauma may precipitate the development of an oculomotor nerve palsy related to a previously unrecognized posterior communicating artery aneurysm (Walter et al., 1994). We saw such a case. The patient was a 32-year-old woman who developed progressive left ptosis and diplopia 24 hours after an altercation with her boyfriend during which she received several blows to the head. When evaluated by us, she had a partial left oculomotor nerve paresis with involvement of the pupil (Fig. 53.24). We did not think the trauma was sufficiently severe to cause the paresis, and we obtained neuroimaging studies that revealed a saccular aneurysm at the junction of the left internal carotid and posterior commu-

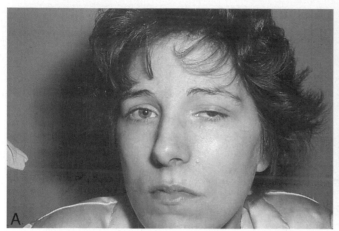
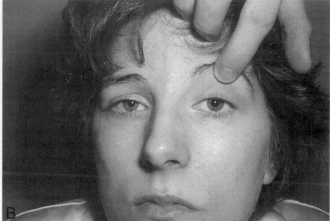

Figure 53.24. Partial left oculomotor nerve palsy that occurred shortly after mild head trauma. *A*, The patient has a partial left ptosis, a minimal exotropia, and a slightly dilated left pupil. *B*, Manual elevation of the left eyelid demonstrates mild anisocoria. (Courtesy of Dr. Neil R. Miller.)

nicating arteries. The aneurysm was successfully clipped, and the patient eventually made a full recovery.

The wall of an artery may be compromised by other forms of trauma, such as radiation therapy. The radiation therapy may be given for treatment of primary or metastatic cancer in the neck and thus predispose to aneurysm development from the common carotid artery or the extracranial portions of the internal carotid or vertebral arteries (Minion et al., 1994; Tanaka et al., 1995), or it may be given to treat an intracranial tumor, such as a pituitary adenoma (Takahashi et al., 1991; Moriyama et al., 1992), glioma (Casey et al., 1993), medulloblastoma (Jensen and Wagner, 1997), or other lesions (Scodary et al., 1990), thus predisposing to intracranial aneurysm formation. John et al. (1993) reported the case of a 55-year-old patient who presented with intermittent profuse bleeding from the ear 5 years after radiotherapy for a nasopharyngeal carcinoma and was found to have an aneurysm of the petrous portion of the ICA within the radiation ports. Intracranial aneurysms may also develop after interstitial radiation (brachytherapy), particularly that used to treat pituitary tumors and skull base malignancies (Thun and Lanfermann, 1991; McConachie and Jacobson, 1994) (Fig. 53.25). In some of these cases, preceding surgery may initially compromise the vessel wall, predisposing to aneurysm formation.

ANEURYSMS CAUSED BY INFECTION ("MYCOTIC" ANEURYSMS)

Inflammatory or infectious processes may weaken the arterial wall and predispose to aneurysm formation. Aneurysms may be caused by a number of different organisms. Bacteria, fungi, and spirochetes all have the potential to produce such lesions. In 1885, Sir William Osler used the term "mycotic" to refer to such aneurysms (Osler, 1885a, 1885b). Although this term is derived from the Greek word *mykes,* which means **fungus,** Osler (1885a, 1885b) was referring to aneurysms caused by bacteria, and the term now is used to describe aneurysms caused by all types of infectious agents.

Mycotic aneurysms account for about 2–7% of all intra-

cranial aneurysms (Roach and Drake, 1965; Olmsted and McGee, 1977; Leipzig and Brown, 1985). These lesions may develop at any age. They occur in infants (Pasqualin et al., 1986; Lee et al., 1990), in young children, and in every subsequent decade of life. They affect men and women equally (Salgado et al., 1987).

Bacterial Aneurysms

Most mycotic aneurysms are caused by bacteria. Such aneurysms tend to be multiple, and they usually arise from peripheral cortical arteries, particularly the MCA (Strang et al., 1961; Bingham, 1977; Bohmfalk et al., 1978; Frazee et al., 1980; Simmons et al., 1980; Bullock et al., 1981; Lee et al., 1990). Involvement of the proximal ICA, unassociated with contiguous infection (Bersani et al., 1992; Krysl et al., 1993; Remy et al., 1994), or of branches of the basilar artery, is less common (Kuki et al., 1994). Distal PCAs may also be involved (Barami and Ko, 1994).

A bacteria-induced aneurysm begins when the organisms become lodged in the lumen of the vessel, often close to a bifurcation. Within 1–14 days, an acute arteritis develops and spreads outward to affect all layers of the vessel wall (Molinari et al., 1973). The wall softens and begins to expand. Bacterial aneurysms are usually less than 1 cm in diameter. Whether saccular or fusiform (Stehbens, 1972), their walls are thin, gray-white, hemorrhagic, and friable. Histopathologically, these aneurysms are associated with severe inflammation characterized by a subendothelial exudate, necrosis of the media and internal elastic lamina, and dense masses of polymorphonuclear leukocytes (Molinari et al., 1973; Weir, 1987). Numerous colonies of bacteria are often present, and the vasculitis may persist despite adequate antibiotic treatment (Takeshita et al., 1991a). Thrombosis may occur and can either occlude the artery or propagate within it. The septic thrombus may undergo subsequent lysis and distal embolization with reestablishment of proximal flow. With rupture, there is a high incidence of secondary intracerebral hematoma (Barami and Ko, 1994).

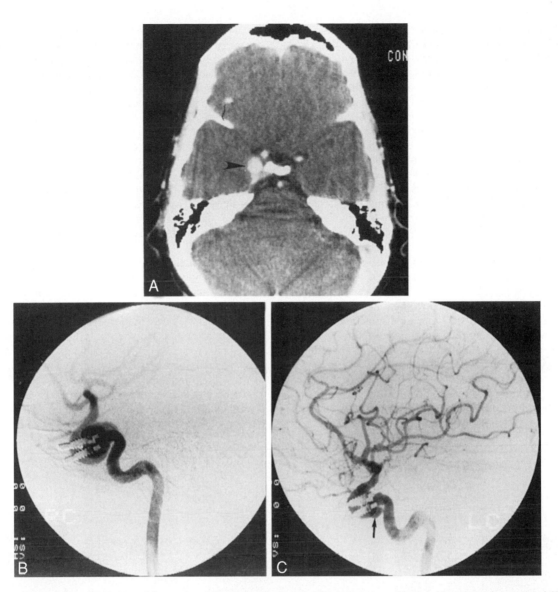

Figure 53.25. Development of an intracranial aneurysm following brachytherapy. The patient was a 51-year-old woman who presented 17 years after transphenoidal implantation of yttrium-90 seeds for treatment of a growth hormone-secreting pituitary adenoma. She complained of episodes of pain in her right eye and intermittent diplopia. *A,* Contrast-enhanced axial computed tomographic scan demonstrates part of a right internal carotid aneurysm (*arrowhead*). *B,* Right internal carotid arteriogram demonstrates the right carotid intracavernous aneurysm arising from an ectatic artery. *C,* Lateral projection of left internal carotid angiogram demonstrates a small aneurysm in intimate relationship to an yttrium-90 seed (*arrow*). (From McConachie NS, Jacobson I. Bilateral aneurysms of the cavernous internal carotid arteries following yttrium-90 implantation. Neuroradiology *36*:611–613, 1994.)

Streptococcus pyogenes and *Staphylococcus aureus* are responsible for the majority of mycotic intracranial aneurysms caused by bacteria (Molinari et al., 1973; Salgado et al., 1987), but nearly every aerobic and anaerobic species of bacteria, even those considered to be of low virulence, can produce such lesions (Weinstein and Schlesinger, 1974; Grossi et al., 1987; Hadley et al., 1988; Brust et al., 1990). These include *Enterococcus faecalis* (Tashima, 1995), *Cardiobacterium hominis* (Lin and Vieco, 1995), *Neisseria mucosa* (Epelbaum et al., 1993), *Salmonella enteritidis* (Lloret et al., 1996), and *Streptococcus milleri* (Perry et al., 1992). In a series of 30 patients, staphylococci were recovered in half of those in whom an organism could be

identified, but the number of negative blood cultures was high (50% of cases) (Hannachi et al., 1991).

The majority of bacterial aneurysms result from organisms carried in emboli from the heart (Patel et al., 1991; Case Records of the Massachusetts General Hospital, 1993). From 70 to 90% of bacteria-induced aneurysms are caused by bacterial endocarditis, although the incidence of clinically identified cerebral aneurysms in patients with bacterial endocarditis is low, ranging from 0.8% (Jones et al., 1969) to 4.7% (Le Cam et al., 1984). Indeed, symptomatic mycotic aneurysms rarely occur in patients with endocarditis (Kanter and Hart, 1990). Neurologic signs and symptoms occurred in 30 of 287 patients (10.4%) with endocarditis reviewed by

Hannachi et al. (1991). Six of these (20%, or 5% of the total number of patients) demonstrated mycotic aneurysms. The findings of Hannachi et al. (1991) are consistent with the findings of others that among patients with infective endocarditis and neurologic symptoms or signs, the frequency of mycotic aneurysm varies from 2–10% (Pankey, 1962; Ziment, 1969; Pruitt et al., 1978; Jones and Siekert, 1989). In a series of 37 patients following valve replacement for endocarditis, two patients experienced rupture of a mycotic aneurysm (Sasaki et al., 1994). In most cases, rupture of a mycotic aneurysm occurs within 4 weeks of the onset of symptoms and signs of endocarditis (McDonald and Korb, 1939; Frazee et al., 1980) (Fig. 53.26), but in some cases, aneurysm rupture is the first manifestation of the underlying condition (Vangelista et al., 1984; Salgado et al., 1987).

It should be emphasized that intracranial hemorrhage that occurs in patients with bacterial endocarditis is often attributed to rupture of a mycotic aneurysm, even when no aneurysm is demonstrable (Pruitt et al., 1978). Walsh and Hoyt (1969a), for example, described two patients with bacterial endocarditis who developed evidence of intracranial hemorrhage. Both patients were thought to have ruptured mycotic aneurysms, although in neither case was there angiographic or pathologic evidence of such a lesion. Most patients with bacterial endocarditis who experience intracranial hemorrhage do so as a result of septic erosion and rupture of the arterial wall without a well-delineated aneurysm. In addition, particularly in patients being anticoagulated, hemorrhagic

transformation of an ischemic brain infarct can result in intracranial hemorrhage that may be massive. Hart et al. (1987) evaluated 17 patients with bacterial endocarditis who experienced intracranial hemorrhage; they were able to document an aneurysm in only two of the patients. In a similar study, Masuda et al. (1992) studied CNS complications of bacterial endocarditis. There was evidence of intracranial hemorrhage in nine patients. Although mycotic aneurysms were found in five of these patients, in only three patients had the aneurysm ruptured. In the other two patients, the aneurysm was occluded by septic emboli. In addition, pyogenic arteritis without aneurysmal dilation around hemorrhage was found in five patients. These observations suggest that rupture of a mycotic aneurysm actually accounts for a minority of patients with endocarditis who experience an intracerebral hemorrhage.

Bacterial aneurysms may develop in patients with diseases other than endocarditis (Barrow and Prats, 1990), including bacterial meningitis (Pospiech et al., 1990; Perry et al., 1992), septicemia (particularly that associated with intravenous drug use), otitis media (Kawakami et al., 1996), and penetrating trauma (Brust et al., 1990). Onishi et al. (1989) described a patient who developed a mycotic aneurysm after transsphenoidal surgery for a pituitary adenoma. The source of the infection was thought to be sinusitis. The aneurysm was treated with systemic antibiotic therapy and disappeared 4 months after surgery. Takahashi et al. (1991) reported a patient who developed an SAH from an anterior temporal

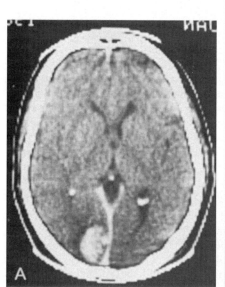
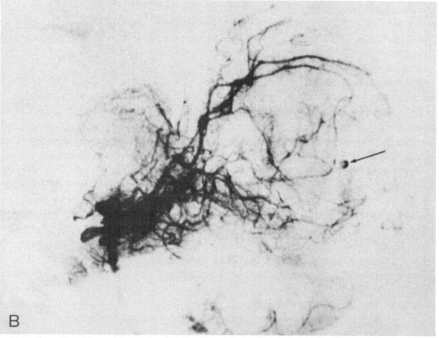

Figure 53.26. Mycotic aneurysm in a patient with bacterial endocarditis. The patient developed bacterial endocarditis after a vasectomy. Two weeks after the onset of signs and symptoms of endocarditis, the patient experienced a severe headache and loss of vision to the left side. He was found to have a stiff neck and a left homonymous hemianopia. *A,* A CT scan shows a density compatible with a hematoma in the right occipital lobe. There is a small area of low density surrounding the hematoma, probably representing cerebral edema. *B,* Vertebral angiogram, lateral view, shows a small aneurysm along a distal branch of the right calcarine artery (*arrow*). (From Fox JL. Intracranial Aneurysms, Vol I. Springer-Verlag, New York, 1983.)

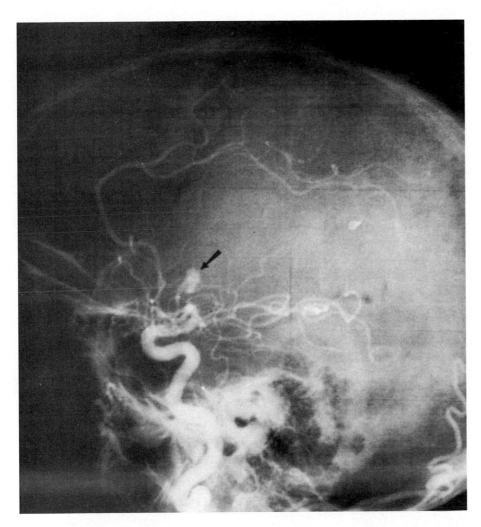

Figure 53.27. Mycotic (bacterial) aneurysm that occurred in a 56-year-old man without an obvious source of infection. A left carotid angiogram, lateral view, shows an aneurysm of the distal middle cerebral artery (*arrow*). Many of the branches of the middle cerebral artery are narrowed or occluded.

mycotic aneurysm following transsphenoidal resection of a craniopharyngioma.

Patients with presumed bacterial mycotic aneurysms are often treated with antibiotics empirically, and thus no organisms are recoverable from the aneurysm wall (Anguita et al. 1991). The finding of a subacute pleomorphic inflammatory cell response in the aneurysm was thought to indicate a resolving infective aneurysm in a child dying of an SAH (Stehbens et al., 1995).

Some patients with proven bacterial mycotic aneurysms seem to have no obvious source for the infection (Brust et al., 1990) (Fig. 53.27). Lee et al. (1990) described a 7-month-old boy in apparently good general health who developed an acute neurologic syndrome associated with a fever. A computed tomographic (CT) scan revealed a large hematoma in the left Sylvian fissure and evidence of SAH. Cerebral angiography demonstrated an aneurysm of the left MCA near its origin and a second aneurysm arising from a distal branch of the same artery. Surgery revealed partial thrombosis of both aneurysms. Treatment consisted of clipping the arterial branches entering the aneurysms, opening the sacs, and removing their contents. Cultures taken from the aneurysm contents and surrounding brain tissue grew *Streptococcus salivarius,* and the patient was treated with penicillin G and cefotaxime. Multiple cultures of the patients blood and cerebrospinal fluid (CSF) were negative, however, and a complete evaluation for a focus of infection was unrevealing as was an evaluation of immunologic function. Engel (1992) reported a 1-year-old who presented with a seizure, was found to have tuberous sclerosis, and subsequently experienced a fatal hemorrhage from a purulent arteritis along with formation of a mycotic aneurysm on the anterior segment of the circle of Willis.

The symptoms and signs in patients with bacterial mycotic aneurysms are usually those of the primary process; e.g., endocarditis, septicemia, meningitis, (Holtzman et al., 1988). Patients with bacterial aneurysms caused by contiguous cavernous sinus thrombosis initially develop painful ophthalmoplegia and proptosis (Shibuya et al., 1976; Micheli et al., 1989). In a case of presumptive bacterial mycotic aneurysm, epistaxis followed complaints of headache, diplopia, fever, and swelling of the right eyelid in a 55-year-old man (Shike et al., 1995).

If left untreated, an estimated 40–80% of bacterial aneurysms eventually rupture, producing catastrophic SAH, intraparenchymal hemorrhage, and even subdural hematoma

(King, 1960; Fox, 1983; Bandoh et al., 1987; Weir, 1987; Holtzman et al., 1988; Takahashi et al., 1990). Although rupture of such an aneurysm may occur days, weeks, or even months after onset of the infection, it may be the first sign that such a disease is present. Prognosis in mycotic aneurysmal rupture is significantly worse than with non-mycotic aneurysms (Clare and Barrow, 1992; Kong and Chan, 1995), with a mortality of up to 80% (Bohmfalk et al., 1978) and a high incidence of residual neurologic deficits in the survivors. Unfortunately, in more than 50% of patients, the aneurysm is completely asymptomatic and unsuspected until it ruptures (Bohmfalk et al., 1978; Salgado et al., 1987; Kanaya et al., 1993). Unexpected rupture may occur months after treatment for endocarditis (Hojer et al., 1993; Terada et al., 1993). About 20–40% of patients experience a neurologic prodrome several days to months before the aneurysm ruptures (Salgado et al., 1987). The prodrome may be a seizure or a slowly progressive neurologic deficit related to the mass effect of the aneurysm. The most common prodrome is a focal neurologic deficit consistent with embolism (Brust et al. 1990). The deficit may be transient and therefore ignored by both the patient and his or her physician. When the deficit is permanent, an evaluation, including neuroimaging studies, may establish the diagnosis before the aneurysm ruptures. In rare cases, bacterial aneurysms are asymptomatic, discovered during neuroimaging studies performed as part of the general management of a patient.

Patients in whom a mycotic aneurysm is suspected on the basis of clinical studies or noninvasive neuroimaging usually undergo conventional angiography to confirm the diagnosis. This procedure is not entirely benign. Based on a retrospective evaluation of published data, van der Meulen et al. (1992) estimated the 12-week survival of patients with a mycotic aneurysm to be 83.75% for patients who did not undergo angiography compared with 83.65% for who underwent angiography. They also concluded that although the mortality of intracranial mycotic aneurysms is relatively small, it increases by 40% (from 0.25% to 0.35%) if angiography is performed. The significance of this retrospective study is unclear. Although we agree that conventional angiography is associated with a definite morbidity and mortality, it is possible that the patients described in this study who underwent angiography had more severe clinical manifestations than those who did not, thus increasing their risk of significant complications and death.

A bacterial aneurysm should be suspected in any patient who experiences a neurologic event, transient or permanent, in the setting of a systemic bacterial infection, particularly endocarditis (Brust et al., 1990). In such cases, magnetic resonance (MR) imaging, MR angiography, spiral CT angiography, or a combination of these techniques often reveal or at least suggest the lesion (Lanfermann et al., 1992). Nevertheless, conventional angiography remains the diagnostic procedure of choice, particularly to determine if more than one aneurysm is present (Salgado et al., 1987).

Optimum therapy for bacteria-induced mycotic aneu-

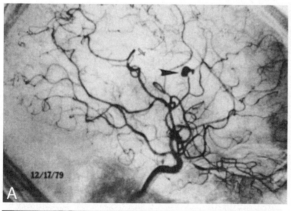

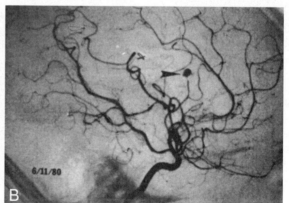

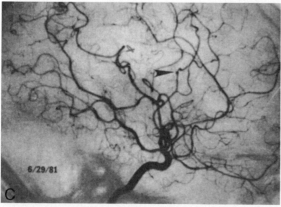

Figure 53.28. Disappearance of a mycotic (bacterial) aneurysm treated with antibiotic therapy. The patient was a 13-year-old boy with bacterial endocarditis caused by *S. aureus* who developed a right hemiplegia and rapidly became comatose. A left intracerebral hematoma was evacuated, an obvious mycotic aneurysm was clipped, and the patient was treated with systemic antibiotics. A series of cerebral angiograms shows the gradual disappearance of a large mycotic aneurysm arising from one of the branches of the left middle cerebral artery (*arrowhead*). (From Morawetz RB, Karp RB. Evolution and resolution of intracranial bacterial (mycotic) aneurysms. Neurosurgery *15*:43–49, 1984.)

rysms is controversial (Jones and Siekert, 1989; Brust et al., 1990). Anecdotal case reports suggest that many unruptured bacterial aneurysms, even those that are quite large, are capable of healing when the patient is treated with systemic antibiotics appropriate for the responsible organism (Cantu et al., 1966; Moskowitz et al., 1974; Bingham, 1977; Bohmfalk et al., 1978; Morawetz and Karp, 1984; Rodesch et al., 1987; Brust et al., 1990; Meyer and Batjer, 1990; Shiraishi et al., 1992; Suzuki et al., 1995b) (Fig. 53.28). Of 28 documented bacterial aneurysms in 17 patients, 20 were assessed angiographically or with CT scanning while the patients were receiving antibiotic therapy (Brust et al., 1990). Of these aneurysms, 10 became smaller or disappeared, and 10 remained unchanged. Eight ruptured aneurysms were operated on with a mortality of 25% and significant residual morbidity in another 25%. Surgery to clip four unruptured aneurysms was uneventful. In another series of 14 patients with 18 bacterial mycotic aneurysms associated with endocarditis seen over a 10-year period, six aneurysms resolved on antibiotics alone (Corr et al., 1995); however, three aneurysms increased in size. Ten patients with residual aneurysms at 6 weeks eventually underwent surgery, of whom six were left with permanent neurologic deficits. It seems reasonable to conclude that nearly all patients require treatment of their underlying infection with antibiotic therapy and careful followup with repeat diagnostic studies (Kojima et al., 1989).

The decision to perform surgery both on ruptured bacterial aneurysms and on unruptured aneurysms located on peripheral branches of the anterior and middle cerebral arteries should be made on an individual basis (Frazee et al., 1980; Morawetz and Karp, 1984; Rodesch et al., 1987; Weir, 1987; Hadley et al., 1988; Holtzman et al., 1988; Brust et al., 1990). When progressive enlargement of an unruptured bacterial aneurysm occurs despite what should be adequate antibiotic therapy, surgical intervention may be of benefit (Yoshida et al., 1990; Tashima et al., 1995). For proximally located aneurysms, carotid ligation or endovascular treatment may be effective (Utoh et al., 1995). Mycotic aneurysms of the cavernous sinus may be occluded using a detachable balloon (Micheli et al., 1989), but this treatment also must be individualized. Obliteration of the parent vessel can occasionally be safely done endovascularly for peripherally located aneurysms (Frizzell et al., 1993), with distally placed microcatheters being used to perfuse amobarbital to pretest for ischemia before permanent occlusion (Khayata et al., 1993).

Because bacterial aneurysms are often located peripherally on intracranial arteries, stereotactic surgery can be used to treat them (Elowiz et al., 1995). The Leksell-Steiner-Lindquist microsurgical guide, with its fiberoptic helium-neon laser, permits rapid isolation of a distal aneurysm with minimal cerebral dissection (Malik et al., 1995). Other localization techniques include the Suetens-Gybels-Vandermeulen angiographic localizer system (D'Angelo et al., 1995). Distal mycotic aneurysms can also be occluded endovascularly, with detachable coils (Kawakami et al., 1996). Patients in whom such surgery is performed may benefit from special anesthetic techniques such as high-dose fentanyl-oxygen anesthesia to preserve intraoperative cardiovascular and cerebrovascular hemodynamics (Shupak et al., 1983).

Fungal Aneurysms

Fungal aneurysms are the "true" mycotic aneurysms. Much less common than bacterial aneurysms, most fungal aneurysms are caused by *Aspergillus* species (Chou et al., 1993; Radhakrishnan et al., 1994, Suzuki et al., 1995a), but Zygomycetes (Tokuda et al. 1995) and *Candida* species are also responsible for some cases (Kikuchi et al., 1985) (Fig. 53.29). Patients with aneurysms caused by *aspergillus fumigatus* or other species often have contiguous paranasal sinus (Suzuki et al., 1995a), orbital, or intracranial disease (e.g., cavernous sinus infection) (Iihara et al., 1990), or they may develop after previous sphenoid sinus surgery (Komatsu et al., 1991). Such patients are often immunosuppressed, either from disease (e.g., leukemia, lymphoma, the acquired immune deficiency syndrome [AIDS]) or from its treatment, including prolonged use of steroids and antibiotics (Piotrowski et al., 1990). Fungi of the Zygomycetes class (e.g., *Rhizopus* species) most often produce an intracranial aneurysm in patients with diabetes mellitus (Shimizu et al., 1991). Candida-induced intracranial aneurysms often occur in patients with endocarditis and in intravenous drug abusers.

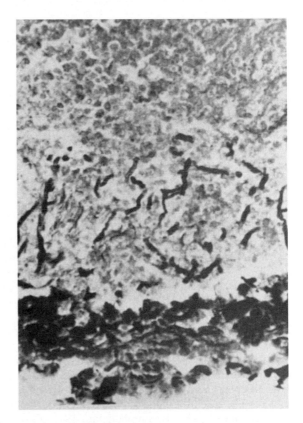

Figure 53.29. Histopathologic appearance of the wall of a mycotic (fungal) intracranial aneurysm that occurred in a 58-year-old diabetic woman who developed unilateral ophthalmoparesis and ipsilateral loss of vision. Angiography showed an intracavernous aneurysm. The patient subsequently died after rupture of a mycotic aneurysm arising from the basilar artery. This specimen, from the wall of the intracavernous aneurysm, shows replacement of the normal anatomy by necrotic tissue containing numerous fungal hyphae. There is widespread intraluminal thrombosis. The organism was *Aspergillus.*

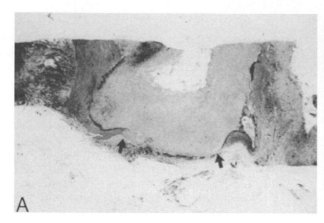
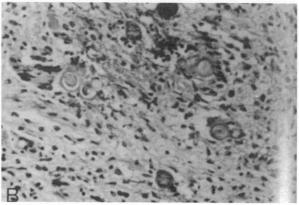

Figure 53.30. Mycotic (fungal) intracranial aneurysm caused by *Coccidioides immitis.* The patient was a 20-year-old woman who developed meningitis that was found to be caused by *Coccidioides immitis.* During treatment with intravenous amphotericin B, she became acutely comatose. Neuroimaging studies demonstrated diffuse subarachnoid hemorrhage, hydrocephalus, and two intracranial aneurysms, one arising from the left internal carotid artery and the other from the distal portion of the basilar artery. The aneurysm arising from the left internal carotid artery was clipped successfully, but the patient died 19 days later after a second intracranial hemorrhage. *A,* Photomicrograph of a portion of the aneurysm arising from the left internal carotid artery shows marked disruption of the internal elastic lamina (*arrows*) and marked fibrous replacement of the media. *B,* High-power photomicrograph of the media of the aneurysm shows numerous spherules of *Coccidioides immitis.* (From Hadley MN, Martin NA, Spetzler RF, et al. Multiple intracranial aneurysms due to *Coccidioides immitis* infection: Case report. J Neurosurg 66:453–456, 1987.)

Fungi other than those described above occasionally may cause an intracranial aneurysm. Mahaley and Spock (1968) described an 11-year-old boy with left orbital and paranasal sinus infection caused by *Penicillium* who experienced an SAH and was found to have an aneurysm at the junction of the left internal carotid and ophthalmic arteries. The aneurysm ruptured during craniotomy, and the patient subsequently died. At autopsy, necrotizing granulomatous inflammation was present in the left maxillary and ethmoid sinuses, the left orbit, and at the base of the brain. Histologic examination revealed a severe inflammatory response within the walls of the anterior, middle, and posterior cerebral arteries and of the basilar artery. Methenamine silver stain of these vessels revealed a fungus morphologically compatible with *Penicillium* (see also Morriss and Spock, 1970). Baudrillard et al. (1985) described a 32-year-old woman who developed a mycotic aneurysm after attempted suicide by drowning. The fungus *Scedosporium apiospermum* was identified and cultured from the lesion. Hadley et al. (1987) described a 20-year-old woman who developed multiple mycotic intracranial aneurysms after recurrent meningitis caused by *Coccidioides immitis* (Fig. 53.30).

Most fungal aneurysms arise from the ICA or the basilar artery (Komatsu et al., 1991; Chou et al., 1993), in contrast to bacterial aneurysms, which usually arise from more peripheral vessels, particularly the middle and anterior cerebral arteries (Bingham, 1977; Bohmfalk et al., 1978; Frazee et al., 1980—see above). Exceptions may occur when fungal mycotic aneurysms are associated with meningitis, however (Takeshita et al., 1992; Kurino et al., 1994). In two cases, peripheral involvement of the superior cerebellar and posterior inferior cerebellar arteries followed meningitis. In another case, an 83-year-old patient died after an SAH secondary to a presumed aspergillus mycotic aneurysm of the MCA, presumably related to a fungal sinusitis (Suzuki et

al., 1995). Masago et al. (1992) described a 75-year-old woman with chronic renal failure from Wegener's granulomatosis who was receiving steroids and immunosuppressive agents when she experienced an SAH. Cerebral angiography showed a fusiform aneurysm arising from an angular branch of the left MCA. Microscopic examination of the aneurysm revealed dense infiltration of hyphae identified as *aspergillus.* The same fungus was found in her lungs.

Thrombosis of adjacent arteries is often associated with fungal aneurysms. These aneurysms take months to develop and rupture, unlike bacterial aneurysms that can develop and rupture within several days to weeks. It is estimated that only about 17% of fungal intracranial aneurysms are multiple (Weir, 1987).

The prognosis of patients with fungal aneurysms is dismal. Most of the patients are in very poor health, being diabetic, immunosuppressed, or on systemic corticosteroids at the time the aneurysm is discovered (Kikuchi et al., 1985). Despite appropriate therapy for local orbital or sinus disease, clipping or trapping of the aneurysm, and use of antifungal agents, there is no recorded case of survival in the literature (Fox, 1983; Weir, 1987).

Spirochetal (Syphilitic) Aneurysms

Syphilis (from the Greek words *syn,* meaning "together," and *philein,* meaning "to love," or from the Greek word *siphlos,* meaning "crippled"), also called lues (from the Latin word for a plague), is caused by the spirochete *Treponema pallidum.* The neuro-ophthalmologic features of syphilis are described in Chapter 67 of this text, but it is appropriate here to emphasize that some intracranial aneurysms are caused by infection of the affected artery by T. pallidum. Although such aneurysms were once thought to be quite common, they are, actually rare. They are usually fusiform rather than saccular. Mitchell and Angrist (1943) described two patients who died from the effects of a ruptured intracranial aneurysm and who both had evidence of systemic syphilis. At autopsy, the aneurysm wall in both patients showed gummatous destruction.

The symptoms and signs produced by syphilitic intracranial aneurysms are nonspecific and usually are caused by rupture of the aneurysm rather than by mass effect (Maass, 1937; Ungerman and Loubeer, 1947; Kopczyński and Drewniak, 1970); however, Scuccimarra et al. (1988) described a 53-year-old man with serologic evidence of syphilis who developed an isolated oculomotor nerve paresis caused by a dolichoectatic basilar artery. The patient also had ectasia of a portion of the left MCA. The arterial abnormalities were thought to have been caused by syphilis, although the authors presented no pathologic data to support this theory.

Miscellaneous "Mycotic" Aneurysms

A unique case of an amoebic intracranial aneurysm was described by Martinez et al. (1980). The patient was a 2-year-old girl who developed encephalitis and died. At autopsy, she had extensive thrombosis of the major intracranial arteries associated with chronic panarteritis, fibrinoid necrosis of vessel walls, and multiple intracranial aneurysms. Histologic examination of affected tissues, including the walls of the aneurysms, showed granulomatous arteritis caused by a free-living amoeba.

Steele et al. (1972) reported the case of a 5-year-old boy who died after rupture of an MCA aneurysm. Within and partly outside the lumen of the aneurysm was a long portion of a plant, which was identified as a spikelet of seeding grass. In this region, there were large masses of polymorphonuclear leukocytes, red blood cells, and fibrin. The infiltrate extended out and around the aneurysm, affecting several adjacent veins.

Soto-Hernandez et al. (1996) reported the case of a 32-year-old man who developed an SAH associated with an aneurysm of the right anterior inferior cerebellar artery (AICA). The CSF had a low concentration of glucose, a high concentration of protein, and a pleocytosis with 5% eosinophils. Enzyme-linked immunosorbent assay and complement fixation reactions for cysticercus were positive in the CSF. At surgery, the aneurysm was found to be surrounded by thickened leptomeninges, which histologically showed dense inflammation and the remains of cysticercus. The aneurysm could not be clipped and was therefore wrapped. Postoperatively, the patient had dizziness and right ear tinnitus. He received prednisone therapy on alternate days and subsequently received albendazole for subarachnoid cysticercosis (see Chapter 62).

Destian et al. (1994) reported a patient with AIDS who presented with intractable epistaxis secondary to rupture of a giant infectious intracavernous carotid artery aneurysm. Culture of the aneurysm grew *Mycobacterium avium intracellulare*. The patient was subsequently treated by excision of the aneurysm and reconstruction of the ICA with a saphenous vein interposition graft.

ARTERITIS

Inflammatory conditions of the arterial wall unassociated with a specific infectious agent may lead to the development of an aneurysm. As noted above, 50% of patients with presumed bacterial mycotic aneurysms are culture-negative (Hannachi et al., 1991). Thus, noninfectious inflammation may play a role in some of these lesions. In the setting of arterial inflammatory disease, a strong argument can be made for an association (Nagayama et al., 1991). Asai et al. (1989) reported a case of multiple saccular aneurysms in a patient with systemic lupus erythematosus (SLE). Examination of the wall of the cerebral artery undergoing clipping revealed evidence of active transmural arteritis. Sakaki et al. (1990) reported two additional cases with similar histopathologic evidence of active arteritis underlying cerebral aneurysms. Dietl et al. (1994) described a patient with Behçet's disease who experienced an SAH associated with bilateral ICA aneurysms, and Ildan et al. (1996) reported a unilateral case. Simultaneous inflammation of other collagen-containing tissue in active SLE also supports the connection (Lerner, 1996). One of the three patients reported by Kawamata et al. (1991) had a negative angiogram 15 years earlier, underscoring the de novo nature of aneurysm development associated with arteritis. The chronic use of steroids in these patients may also play an etiologic role (Kodama et al., 1990). Most of the aneurysms associated with arteritis are proximal, and less than one-third are fusiform (Orita et al., 1992). Prognosis is poor, with mortality in approximately two-thirds of the reported cases. A case of a PCA aneurysm in a patient with relapsing polychondritis was reported by Strobel et al. (1992).

Capone et al. (1994) reported a case of lymphomatoid granulomatosis producing multiple giant fusiform and saccular aneurysms throughout the major intracerebral arteries. MR angiography revealed vascular beading consistent with vasculitis. O'Boynick et al. (1994) reported a case of an MCA aneurysm associated with myxoid degeneration of the wall without another underlying explanation.

Acquired aortitis may also be associated with an increased incidence of aneurysm formation (Nishimura et al., 1994). The role of renal hypertension in such cases may be significant.

NEOPLASTIC ANEURYSMS

Cancerous erosion of an arterial wall can cause formation of an aneurysm. Intracranial neoplastic aneurysms are most often caused by hematogenous emboli from cardiac myxoma or choriocarcinoma (see Table 1 in Ho, 1982; Fox, 1983) (Fig. 53.31). Cerebral metastases of choriocarcinoma occur in 10–20% of patients with metastatic choriocarcinoma, some of whom develop intracranial aneurysms (Gallo et al., 1993). Hematogenous metastasis of other tumors may also produce aneurysms, although much less frequently (Ho, 1982; Kochi et al., 1984). Malignant tumors other than choriocarcinoma that can produce an intracranial aneurysm include malignant fibrous histiocytoma (Maruki et al., 1994) (Fig. 53.32) and small-cell carcinoma of the lung (Murata et al., 1993).

There is a marked female predominance among patients

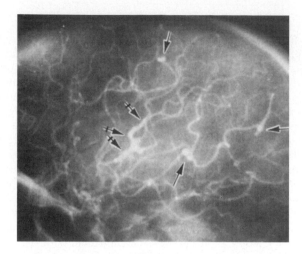

Figure 53.31. Multiple peripheral aneurysms in a patient with cardiac myxoma. The *crossed arrows* point to a lengthy segment of the left middle cerebral artery that shows neoplastic fusiform dilation. The other *arrows* indicate more localized, saccular, neoplastic aneurysms. (Courtesy of Dr. PFJ New.)

with neoplastic intracranial aneurysms, reflecting the tendency for such aneurysms to be caused by emboli from choriocarcinoma. The age range of patients with neoplastic intracranial aneurysms is broad, but most patients are in the 3rd and 4th decades of life, reflecting the tendency for both choriocarcinoma and cardiac myxoma to develop in young adults. Occurrence in childhood is also possible (Hung et al., 1992).

The presenting symptoms and signs of neoplastic intracranial aneurysms are identical with those of mycotic aneurysms. Most become symptomatic when they rupture and produce SAH (Kochi et al., 1984). Others are detected when the patient experiences transient or permanent focal neurologic deficits thought to be of ischemic origin (Komeichi et al., 1996). In an unusual case in a 16-year-old girl, a thrombotic occlusion of the MCA was followed by angiographic evidence of recanalization, subsequent fusiform dilation of the vessel, and rupture. Histopathologic examination of the abnormal vessel after an STA-MCA bypass procedure revealed choriocarcinoma.

Making the correct diagnosis of a neoplastic intracranial aneurysm is obviously critical. One patient suffered a spontaneous splenic rupture associated with the same metastatic choriocarcinoma that caused her metastatic aneurysm and secondary rupture with intracerebral hemorrhage (Giannakopoulos et al., 1992). An even greater imperative to diagnosis

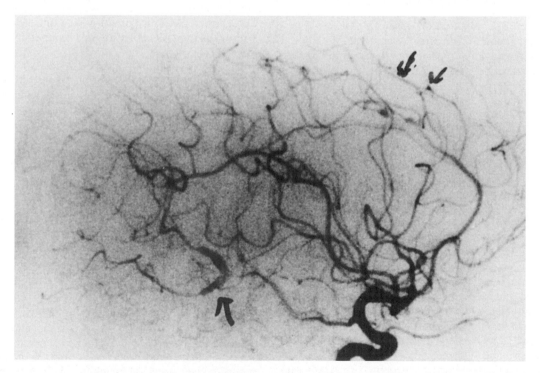

Figure 53.32. Right carotid angiogram in a 44-year-old woman presenting with a 9-month history of periodic scintillating scotomata. The angiogram demonstrates multiple areas of fusiform aneurysmal dilation (*arrows*), including distal branches of the anterior cerebral artery and posterior cerebral artery. Biopsy of posterior lesions demonstrated tumors consisting of polygonally shaped cells containing pale cytoplasm and round to ovoid nuclei tentatively diagnosed as metastatic poorly differentiated sarcoma. Magnetic resonance imaging demonstrated multiple foci of small infarctions. At autopsy, the fusiform aneurysmal dilatations were associated with metastatic malignant fibrous histiocytoma from a cardiac source. (From Maruki C, Suzukawa K, Koike J, et al. Cardiac malignant fibrous histiocytoma metastasizing to the brain: Development of multiple neoplastic cerebral aneurysms. Surg Neurol *41*:40–44, 1994.)

is the potential for response to aneurysm clipping and systemic chemotherapy. Nakahara et al. (1975) described a case of anterior cerebral artery (ACA) aneurysm caused by choriocarcinoma in which the aneurysm disappeared after the patient was treated with chemotherapy. Fujiwara et al. (1992) reported a patient with 6-year follow-up after resolution. The diagnosis may be made on the basis of elevated serum and CSF levels of human chorionic gonadotropin (Mori et al., 1990). If the aneurysm has not ruptured, it may respond to chemotherapy alone (Hove et al., 1990).

Neoplastic aneurysms may be fusiform or saccular (Fig. 53.31). They usually are multiple (Hung et al., 1992), and they often are bilateral (Damasio et al., 1975; Iihara et al., 1991). They most commonly develop on terminal leptomeningeal branches of the cerebral and cerebellar arteries, often near sites of branching. The MCA is affected most often. In many cases, neoplastic aneurysms are located adjacent to areas of stenosis and occlusion that also are caused by tumor emboli (New et al., 1970; Iihara et al., 1991). Neoplastic aneurysms are similar in appearance to mycotic aneurysms, with walls that are thin, gray-white, and quite friable. They usually are less than 5 mm in diameter, but some are 25 mm or more.

The histologic appearance of a neoplastic aneurysm is variable; however, in most cases, neoplastic cells are found in the wall months and even years after surgical removal of the causative tumor (Furuya et al., 1995) (Fig. 53.33). In some aneurysms, cancer cells invade the intima and muscularis, with preservation of the bulging adventitia (Helmer, 1976). In others, the cancer cells invade and replace the entire arterial wall, forming multiple false aneurysms (New et al., 1970). Reina and Seal (1974) described an unusual case in which metastatic carcinoma from an unknown site invaded a portion of the MCA from **outside** the arterial wall.

The treatment of a neoplastic aneurysm depends on whether or not it has ruptured and the cancer that produced it. Suzuki et al. (1994) reported the rapid growth of an aneurysm associated with an atrial myxoma (Fig. 53.34). In another case, a 68-year-old woman developed recurrent occipital hematomas 1 year after resection of an atrial myxoma (Chen et al., 1993). Neuroimaging studies revealed multiple intracranial aneurysms with hemorrhage, and microscopic examination showed invasion of affected vascular walls by tumor cells. Roeltgen et al. (1981) described a case of neoplastic aneurysm caused by cardiac myxoma in which the aneurysm disappeared spontaneously over 6 months as seen on serial angiography. The resolution of the aneurysm was almost certainly caused by thrombotic occlusion of its lumen, because neither the aneurysm nor its branch artery was visible on the cerebral arteriogram. A 37-year-old woman developed multiple infarcts related to myxomatous emboli; angiography also revealed multiple fusiform aneurysms (Iihara et al., 1991). A second angiogram performed 6 months after resection of the myxoma revealed spontaneous resolution or stabilization of most of the aneurysms detected before surgery, but new aneurysms were present at sites that had been normal on the first angiogram. No remarkable changes were seen on a third angiogram except for slight enlargement of one of the aneurysms on a branch of one of

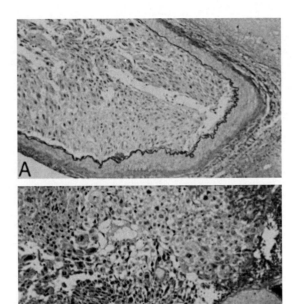

Figure 53.33. Histopathologic appearance of neoplastic intracranial aneurysm. The patient was a 56-year-old man with no known malignancy who developed an acute headache and vomiting. Chest X-ray showed a lung mass, and CT scan showed a mass in the left posterior temporal lobe. A left carotid angiogram showed a small aneurysm arising from a cortical branch of the left posterior temporal artery. The patient underwent a craniotomy, at which time the aneurysm was trapped and excised, and an intracerebral hematoma was evacuated. *A,* Photomicrograph of the affected cortical artery shows that its lumen is filled with tumor cells. *B,* High-power photomicrograph shows tumor cells within the aneurysm. The cells are from an undifferentiated squamous cell carcinoma. (From Kochi N, Tani E, Yokota M, et al. Neoplastic cerebral aneurysm from lung cancer: Case report. J Neurosurg *60:*640–643, 1984.)

the MCAs. At 3 years, the woman was neurologically stable. In another patient, one aneurysm spontaneously resolved following removal of a cardiac myxoma, but a second progressively enlarged and a third appeared (Hayashi et al., 1995). Because the aneurysms were fusiform, and the patient was asymptomatic, no intervention was undertaken. In rare cases, the portion of the affected artery proximal to a neoplastic aneurysm may be clipped, and the aneurysm excised (Kochi et al., 1984). The effect of radiation therapy on neoplastic aneurysms is not known.

ASSOCIATED RISK FACTORS

Progressive aneurysm growth as well as the potential for rupture may be influenced by a number of systemic conditions. Such associations may serve as useful diagnostic markers and may influence management of specific patients.

Hypertension

Animal models of aneurysm formation often utilized induced hypertension to aid in the development of aneurysms

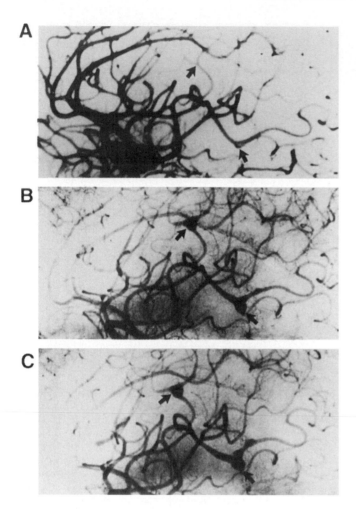

Figure 53.34. Rapid growth of neoplastic aneurysms of the right middle cerebral artery. *A*, Right internal carotid angiogram, lateral view, prior to removal of a cardiac myxoma. *Upper arrow* points to normal bifurcation. *Lower arrow* points to smal aneurysm. *B*, 2 months later, there is a large aneurysm at the originally normal bifurcation (*upper arrow*), and the previously small aneurysm has greatly enlarged (*lower arrow*). *C*, 7 months after surgical removal, both aneurysms are either unchanged or slightly larger (*arrows*). Note that in this patient, the aneurysms continued to develop despite removal of the primary source. (From Suzuki T, Nagai R, Yamazaki T, et al. Rapid growth of intracranial aneurysms secondary to cardiac myxoma. Neurology *44*:570–571, 1994.)

(Futami et al., 1995a, 1995b; Kondo et al., 1977). In addition, systemic hypertension is present in 50–80% of patients with intracranial aneurysms (Black and Hicks, 1952; Walker and Allegre, 1954; Chason and Hindman, 1958; Stehbens, 1962; McCormick and Schmalstieg, 1977; Franks, 1978; Ostergaard and Hog, 1985; Weir, 1987), and it is more common in patients with multiple aneurysms than in patients with a single aneurysm. Retrospective epidemiologic studies strongly support an increased association of aneurysms and hypertension (Juvela, 1996). In Portugal, hypertension increased the risk of aneurysmal SAH eight times (Canhao, 1994). The results of a similar study in Britain were somewhat less impressive but still demonstrated an increased risk associated with hypertension (Adamson et al., 1994). In a

retrospective analysis of Medicare data, the prevalence of hypertension in patients with unruptured aneurysms was 43.2% compared with 34.4% in a random sample (Taylor et al., 1995). For patients with an unruptured cerebral aneurysm as the primary diagnosis, hypertension was a significant risk factor for future SAH (risk ratio: 1.46). In a series of patients with multiple aneurysms, hypertension was present in 50% (Rinne et al., 1994).

The potential role of hypertension in causing aneurysmal rupture is exemplified by the case of a 77-year-old woman who experienced an intracerebral hemorrhage **followed** by rupture of an intracranial aneurysm (Y. Sugita et al., 1995). It was postulated that the intracerebral hemorrhage induced hypertension that led to the rupture of the aneurysm.

Fusiform dilation and dolechiectatic vessel changes are associated with hypertension more often than are saccular aneurysms (see below). In a series of 15 patients with angiographically diagnosed megadolichobasilar anomalies, nine patients had significant hypertension (Okada et al., 1994).

The only two congenital diseases commonly associated with intracranial aneurysm—coarctation of the aorta and polycystic kidney disease (see below)—also are generally accompanied by hypertension. These associations have led many investigators to postulate that hypertension plays a major role in the development of intracranial aneurysms.

One additional point of support for the role of hypertension is the association of cocaine and methamphetamine abuse and aneurysmal rupture (Chadan et al., 1991; Gledhill et al., 1993; Oyesiku et al., 1993; Davis and Swalwell, 1994; Fessler et al., 1997). In a retrospective study of 83 deaths from ruptured aneurysms seen over a 7-year interval in San Diego, California, Davis and Swalwell (1996) found a history of drug abuse in 13 cases. Toxicologic data were available in 39 cases and showed evidence of cocaine use in three and methamphetamine abuse in six (overall incidence of 21%). This contrasted with evidence of methamphetamine in 4.9% and cocaine in 13.6% of unselected autopsies in and around San Diego during the same period of time. The authors concluded that both cocaine and methamphetamine played a significant role in the production and rupture of cerebral aneurysms, and that hypertension was the underlying mechanism in such cases.

Intracranial Arteriovenous Malformations

AVMs may occur in patients with one or more intracranial aneurysms (Fig. 53.35). Walsh and King (1942) wrote the first report of a patient with both an aneurysm and an AVM. Subsequently, other investigators emphasized this association (Paterson and McKissock, 1956; Higashi et al., 1979; Suzuki and Onuma, 1979; Hayashi et al., 1981; Wilkins, 1982; Ostergaard, 1984; Waga et al., 1985; Batjer et al., 1986; Brick and Roberts, 1987; Kaech et al., 1987; Noterman et al., 1987; Mintz and Cosgrove, 1990; Barrow and Reisner, 1993). The significance of this association depends on whether one is viewing it from the standpoint of a patient with a known aneurysm or a known AVM. In a cooperative study (Perret and Nishioka, 1966, 1969), only 37 of 3265 patients with one or more intracranial aneurysms (1.1%) had an intracranial AVM. Fox (1983) reviewed nearly 5000

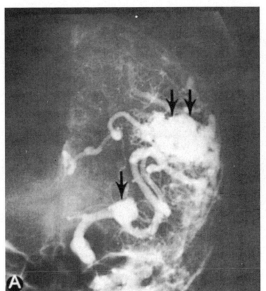
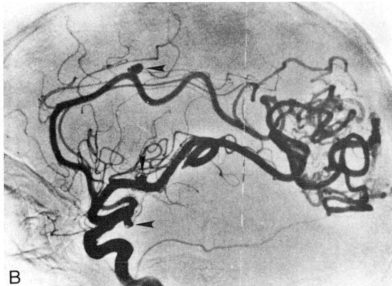

Figure 53.35. Intracranial arteriovenous malformation and aneurysm in the same patient. *A*, There is a large saccular aneurysm arising from the region of the trifurcation of the middle cerebral artery (*arrow*) with an arteriovenous malformation more distally (*double arrows*). *B*, There are three intracranial aneurysms (*arrowheads*) in this patient with an occipital arteriovenous malformation. One of the aneurysms arises from the internal carotid artery at or just above the origin of the anterior choroidal artery. A second aneurysm arises from the middle cerebral artery in the Sylvian fissure, and the third aneurysm arises from the pericallosal artery.

cases of intracranial aneurysm and identified 118 cases in which there was also an intracranial AVM, a prevalence of 2.4%. Some AVMs are too small to appreciate or are obliterated at the time of intracerebral hemorrhage. In three patients with aneurysms examined by Deruty et al. (1992b), the source of intracerebral hemorrhage was a microscopic AVM. Conversely, from 3 to 10% of patients with intracranial AVMs have one or more intracranial aneurysms (Paterson and McKissock, 1956; Perret and Nishioka, 1966, 1969; Higashi et al., 1979; Fox, 1983; Cunha e Sa et al., 1992; Solomon et al., 1994).

Three hypotheses may explain the association of intracranial aneurysms and AVMs: (*a*) the development of the aneurysm is stimulated by increased blood flow to the AVM; (*b*) both the aneurysm and the AVM are congenital anomalies that develop simultaneously in utero; and (*c*) the simultaneous occurrence of an intracranial aneurysm and an AVM is coincidental. It is likely that each of the three hypotheses is correct in specific cases (Deruty et al., 1990).

The blood-flow mechanism (Kikuchi and Kowada, 1994) is particularly likely to be responsible in patients with an aneurysm located on one of the arteries supplying the AVM (T. Abe et al., 1994; Perata et al., 1994; Gobin et al., 1996). This may occur not only with AVMs in the posterior fossa but also with supratentorial AVMs (Mabuchi et al., 1992; McDermott and Sellar, 1994; Pau et al., 1994). The incidence of aneurysms on feeding vessels may be significantly greater than reported. Using superselective catheter techniques, Turjman et al. (1994b) found aneurysms in 58 of 100 patients with AVMs. The aneurysms were multiple in 34 patients (68%). These intranidal aneurysms may be at increased risk

of bleeding (Marks et al., 1992). Thus, it may be appropriate to clip or otherwise treat an asymptomatic aneurysm located on an artery feeding an AVM before performing stereotactic radiosurgery to obliterate the malformation.

Venous aneurysms may also be associated with AVMs, particularly AVMs involving the tentorium. In the study by Lewis et al. (1994), eight of nine patients had one or more venous aneurysms. Two of these patients had more than one venous aneurysm, and two had a vein of Galen aneurysm associated with a tentorial dural AVM.

Some patients with AVMs have intracranial aneurysms unassociated with the malformation. In such cases, a congenital abnormality may be responsible for both lesions (Tamaki et al., 1992).

The coexistence of one or more intracranial aneurysms in a patient with an AVM is of more than academic interest (Barrow and Reisner, 1993). Both aneurysms and AVMs can bleed. When a patient with both lesions experiences an SAH, it is crucial to determine which of the lesions has bled, because the prognosis is considerably different after hemorrhage from an AVM than after hemorrhage from an aneurysm (see below). Although such a determination may be possible from clinical features, neuroimaging studies, or both, the source of bleeding cannot be established with certainty in many cases. Nevertheless, it is thought that among patients with both lesions, it is far more likely that the bleeding is from the aneurysm than from the AVM. For this reason, Batjer et al. (1986) suggested that the safest approach to patients with an SAH and both lesions is treatment of the aneurysm before attempting microsurgical resection of the AVM. Although this approach may be appropriate, Deruty et al. (1990) reported seven patients presenting with SAH with both aneurysms and AVMs in whom the aneurysm was assumed to be the source of bleeding preoperatively in three of the seven. In fact, all six patients who subsequently underwent surgery were found to have bled from the AVM. Distinguishing the source of bleeding may become increasingly important as endovascular techniques allow less invasive treatment of the aneurysm, AVM, or both lesions. In a patient undergoing embolization of an AVM, rupture of an associated aneurysm was thought to have been caused by mechanical stretching and displacement (Abe et al., 1995). Changes in perfusion pressure during embolization may also induce aneurysm rupture.

Congenital Extracranial Disease

The coexistence of congenital abnormalities and intracranial saccular aneurysms is one of the main arguments used to support the hypothesis that aneurysms are congenital in origin. There are, however, only two congenital disorders in which patients have an increased prevalence of intracranial aneurysms compared with the normal population: coarctation of the aorta and polycystic kidney disease (Stehbens, 1962).

Coarctation of the Aorta

Eppinger (1887) described a 15-year-old boy with coarctation of the aorta who collapsed during gymnastics and died 3 days later. SAH from a ruptured aneurysm of the ACA was found at autopsy. Subsequent investigators emphasized that 1–3% of patients with an intracranial aneurysm have coarctation of the aorta (Hacker et al., 1983; Weir, 1987; Gire et al., 1997) and that coarctation of the aorta increases the likelihood of development of an intracranial aneurysm by 400% (Brackett and Morantz, 1982). Coarctation of the aorta also increases the prevalence of multiplicity from 20 to 30% and the mortality rate from SAH from 50 to 75%. It is not clear, however, if this association is related to some underlying abnormality of arteries in such patients or to the hypertension that develops in patients with coarctation of the aorta and that could subsequently induce aneurysm formation. The majority of aneurysmal ruptures in such patients occur in the 2nd decade of life, usually in men.

Polycystic Kidney Disease

Like coarctation of the aorta, polycystic kidney disease is associated with intracranial aneurysm in a higher percentage of patients than expected by coincidence alone (Brown, 1951; Sahs and Meyers, 1951; Bigelow, 1953; Brackett and Morantz, 1982; Kulla et al., 1982; Wakabayashi et al., 1983; Matsumara et al., 1986; van Dijk et al., 1995; Ronkainen et al., 1997; Schievink, 1997b). The prevalence of polycystic kidney disease in patients with intracranial aneurysms is 3–6%, whereas the prevalence of one or more intracranial aneurysms in patients with polycystic kidney disease is 7–16% (Sahs and Meyers, 1951; Bigelow, 1953; Chester et al., 1977; Ruggieri et al., 1994). In an autopsy study of 89 patients with polycystic kidney disease at the Mayo Clinic, aneurysms were found in 22.5% (Schievink et al., 1992a).

There appears to be a definite familial incidence of polycystic kidney disease and intracranial aneurysm (Saifuddin and Dathan, 1987). This is even greater if there is a family history of previous aneurysm rupture (Ruggieri et al., 1994). It is possible, however, that the association is not as strong as previously suspected. In a prospective study, 92 patients with polycystic kidney disease were investigated (Chapman et al., 1992). High-resolution CT scanning was performed in 60 subjects, four-vessel cerebral angiography in 21, and both procedures in 11. Of the 88 patients studied, four had intracranial aneurysms, of which three were multiple. Although greater than in the general population, these numbers are somewhat lower than expected based on previous publications.

Because the majority of patients with polycystic kidney disease and intracranial aneurysms also have systemic hypertension, it is unclear if polycystic kidney disease and intracranial aneurysms occur together because of some biochemical or anatomic defect or because polycystic kidney disease produces systemic hypertension which, in turn, predisposes the patient to the development of the aneurysms. Indeed, intracerebral hemorrhage occurs in patients with polycystic kidney disease who have hypertension and no evidence of an intracranial aneurysm (Ryu, 1990).

Aneurysms associated with polycystic kidney disease have a propensity to involve the MCA (Kuroiwa et al., 1992) and to occur at a younger age than nonfamilial aneurysms (Lozano and Leblanc, 1992; Schievink et al., 1992a; Chauveau et al., 1994). Unsuccessful attempts have been made to look for markers around the PKD1 locus that might predispose to aneurysm formation (Chauveau et al., 1994). Identification of genetic abnormalities, however, does provide a convenient means for screening suspects (Lieske and Toback, 1993). The occurrence of de novo aneurysms in patients with polycystic kidney disease emphasizes the importance of continuous and repetitive monitoring (Tsuruta et al., 1994).

There is substantial literature on screening for aneurysms in patients with polycystic kidney disease and their family members (Wiebers and Torres, 1992; Black, 1994). MR imaging is a reasonably sensitive means of screening such patients (Huston et al., 1993; Ruggieri et al., 1994; Rivera et al., 1995; Ronkainen et al 1995a) (Fig. 53.36), but this technique produces both false-positive and negative-results. Thus, conventional angiography is still required before surgery, and this may be associated with a variety of complications in patients with polycystic kidney disease (Chapman et al., 1992). Alternatives such as MR angiography (Chapman et al., 1993; Huston et al., 1996) and spiral CT angiography (Tampieri et al., 1996) may thus be preferable despite their somewhat reduced sensitivity and specificity to screening using conventional angiography (Fehlings and Gentili, 1991).

Occlusive Disease of the Internal Carotid Artery

Intracranial aneurysms are occasionally found in patients with occlusive disease of the ICA (Fig. 53.37). Stern et al. (1979) described 15 such cases, and Fox (1983) reviewed the literature concerning 33 cases. An additional case was

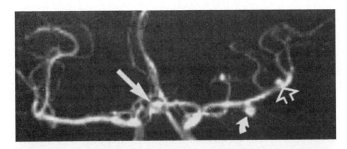

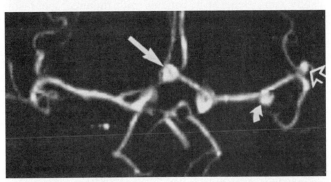

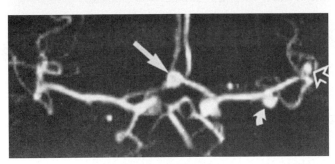

Figure 53.36. Neuroimaging in a patient with a family history of polycystic kidney disease. Magnetic resonance angiogram in a 65-year-old woman with a history of Meniere's disease, a suspected family history of a fatal ruptured aneurysm, and a family history of polycystic kidney disease. Three different projections of the circle of Willis demonstrate saccular aneurysms arising from the anterior communicating artery (*straight solid arrow*), M-1 segment of the left middle cerebral artery (*curved solid arrow*), and bifurcation of the left middle cerebral artery (*open arrow*). (From Ruggieri PM, Poulos N, Masaryk TJ, et al. Occult intracranial aneurysms in polycystic kidney disease: Screening with MR angiography. *Radiology 191*:33–39, 1994.)

contributed by Nakai et al. (1992). In the majority of cases, an asymptomatic aneurysm is identified during angiography performed for symptoms related to the stenosis or occlusion. In a prospective series of 100 patients undergoing angiography for ICA stenosis, nine aneurysms were incidentally discovered (Griffiths et al., 1996). Fox (1983) concluded that there was no consistent relationship between the side or location of the aneurysm and the side of the stenosis. This suggests that disturbance of flow patterns by the stenosis may not be causally related to formation of the aneurysm. However, both problems occur at a similar age, and they may have some relationship to atherosclerosis and its destructive effects. In other cases, unilateral or bilateral hypoplasia of

the ICAs is discovered during an evaluation for a symptomatic aneurysm (El Khamlichi et al., 1989). In such cases, it is possible that both the aneurysm and the hypoplasia are congenital anomalies, that alteration in cerebral blood flow by the hypoplastic arteries induces aneurysm formation, or that the hypoplastic vessels and the aneurysm are unrelated. Even if there is no direct etiologic role, the frequency of aneurysms in these patients raises important questions about the optimum therapy of occlusive disease of the ICAs (Pappada et al., 1996).

Timperman et al. (1995) diagnosed ruptured anterior communicating artery aneurysms in two of 58 patients who had previously undergone balloon occlusion of one ICA for an unclippable giant aneurysm in another location. The results of this study suggest an increased risk of de novo development of distal circulation aneurysms in patients who undergo carotid occlusion for other lesions and strengthen the argument that hemodynamic factors play a role in the development of intracranial aneurysms.

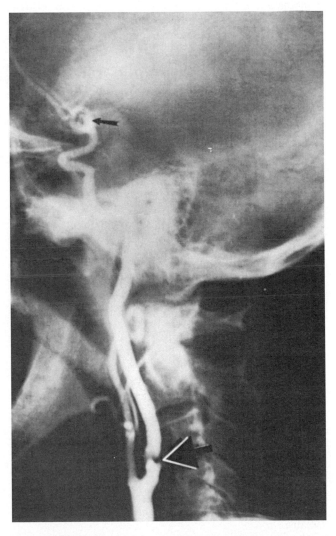

Figure 53.37. Severe stenosis of the internal carotid artery (*large arrow*) in a patient with an asymptomatic aneurysm arising from the origin of the ipsilateral middle cerebral artery (*small arrow*).

Moyamoya Disease

Moyamoya disease is a disorder characterized by: (*a*) a network of fine vessels with a cloud-like or mesh angiographic appearance (moyamoya is the Japanese word for "puff of smoke") located at the base of the brain; (*b*) congenital atresia, acquired stenosis, or occlusion of one or both ICAs; and (*c*) prominent ethmoid and meningeal anastomotic channels (Takeuchi and Shimizu, 1957; Takeuchi, 1961; Nishimoto and Takeuchi, 1968; Suzuki and Takaku, 1969; Suzuki, 1983). The pathologic changes include thinning of the vessel wall, intimal thickening, medial necrosis, discontinuity of the internal elastic membrane of some vessels, and dilation of arterioles.

A variety of neurologic symptoms and signs, usually transient, are the first evidence of moyamoya disease in patients under 21 years of age. In patients over 21 years of age, acute SAH is the most common initial clinical manifestation (Fox, 1983). In some patients, however, a variety of visual deficits caused by occlusion of the ICAs, PCAs, basilar artery, or a combination of these vessels are the initial sign of disease. Visual deficits caused by occlusion of the ICAs include the ocular ischemic syndrome, neovascular glaucoma, central retinal artery occlusion, ischemic optic neuropathy, and the optic chiasmal syndrome (Ahmadi et al., 1984; Chace and Hedges, 1984; Noda et al., 1987). Visual deficits related to posterior circulation (posterior cerebral-basilar artery) occlusion include homonymous visual field defects, concentric constriction of the visual fields, Bálint's syndrome, and cerebral blindness (Morimatsu et al., 1977; Miyamoto et al., 1986; Yoshida et al., 1986; Tashima-Kurita et al., 1989). These conditions are described in detail in Chapter 55 of this text.

It is thought that the primary event in the development of moyamoya disease is early occlusion of the ICA or arteries. Collateral vessels then develop, presumably to compensate for reduced arterial blood flow through the compromised major vessel.

Intracranial aneurysms, almost always saccular, are occasionally found in patients with moyamoya disease (Pool et al., 1967; Nagamine et al., 1981; Kwak et al., 1984a, 1984b; Konishi et al., 1985; Waga and Tochio, 1985; Chen and Liu, 1993; Massoud et al., 1994; Kawaguti et al., 1995; Kawaguchi et al., 1996) (Fig. 53.38). This association occurs with equal frequency in males and females. All ages are affected, and the youngest patients are less than 1 year old (Waga and Tochio, 1985).

The saccular aneurysms that occur in patients with moyamoya disease may arise from network vessels, collateral vessels, or normal vessels of the vertebrobasilar or, less frequently, the carotid circulation. An unusual case of a giant aneurysm of the basilar artery presenting with progressive hemiparesis was reported by Bucciero et al. (1994). Most aneurysms become symptomatic when they rupture (J. Hamada et al., 1994), but they also may produce ischemic or compressive symptoms and signs (Kwak et al., 1984a, 1984b).

The association of intracranial saccular aneurysm and moyamoya disease could be coincidental, particularly in view of the rarity of moyamoya disease compared with the prevalence of intracranial aneurysms in the general population. Stehbens (1983b) and others (Oka et al., 1991; Kageji et al., 1992; Inoue et al., 1994) believe, however, that aneurysm formation in at least some patients with moyamoya disease is related to the hemodynamics of the collateral vessels and thus is acquired.

Smoking

In a study from eastern Finland, **smoking** was significantly more frequent in patients with ruptured aneurysms compared with a population of patients who experienced nonaneurysmal intracerebral hemorrhage, in which diabetes mellitus, anticoagulation, and alcohol consumption occurred more frequently (Juvela et al., 1993a; Juvela, 1996). Smoking was also found to be a significant risk factor for aneurysmal SAH in studies from Portugal (Canhao, 1994) and Great Britain (Morris et al., 1992; Adamson et al., 1994). In an epidemiologic study from Seattle (Longstreth et al., 1994), premenopausal women were at reduced risk for SAH, especially women without a history of smoking or hypertension. Hormone replacement therapy reduced the risk only in postmenopausal women who had never smoked.

Other Risk Factors and Miscellaneous Disorders

Retrospective epidemiologic studies suggest other risk factors in patients with aneurysm and SAH other than those discussed above. For example, aneurysms can enlarge during **pregnancy** (Shutter et al., 1993; Ortiz et al., 1997), but whether this is related to increased blood pressure, hormonal influences, or is entirely fortuitous remains uncertain. **Atherosclerosis** may also play a role in the development of aneurysms. In a retrospective case-control study conducted in Great Britain and Denmark, markers of atherosclerosis, including increased serum cholesterol and apolipoprotein B concentrations as well as reduced concentration of high-density lipoproteins, were significantly more frequent in patients with cerebral aneurysms (Adamson et al., 1994). The association of atherosclerosis and aneurysms is supported histopathologically by the finding of atherosclerotic changes in the walls of cerebral aneurysms (Kosierkiewicz et al., 1994). Recent **alcohol consumption** was noted to play a potential role in subarachnoid bleeds in a retrospective case-control study of hospitalized patients (Juvela et al., 1993b).

Intracranial aneurysms are occasionally discovered in patients with disorders other than those described above. These disorders include neurofibromatosis (NF) (Gomori et al., 1991; Muhonen et al., 1991; Smith and Bowen, 1993; Benatar, 1994; Poli et al., 1994; Sasaki et al., 1995; Uranishi et al., 1995; Kirchhof et al., 1996), tuberous sclerosis (Engel, 1992; Spangler et al., 1997), alkaptonuria (Kaufmann et al., 1990), osteogenesis imperfecta (Okamura et al., 1995), pheochromocytoma, sickle cell anemia (Oyesiku et al., 1991; Diggs and Brookoff, 1993), Klippel-Trénaunay-Weber syndrome (Taira et al., 1991; Spallone and Tcherekayev, 1996), AIDS (Lang et al., 1992), Takayasu's arteritis, Weber-Christian disease (Oyama et al., 1995), the antiphospholipid antibody syndrome (Inoue et al., 1994), and hereditary hemorrhagic telangiectasia (Rendu-Osler-Weber disease) (Fox,

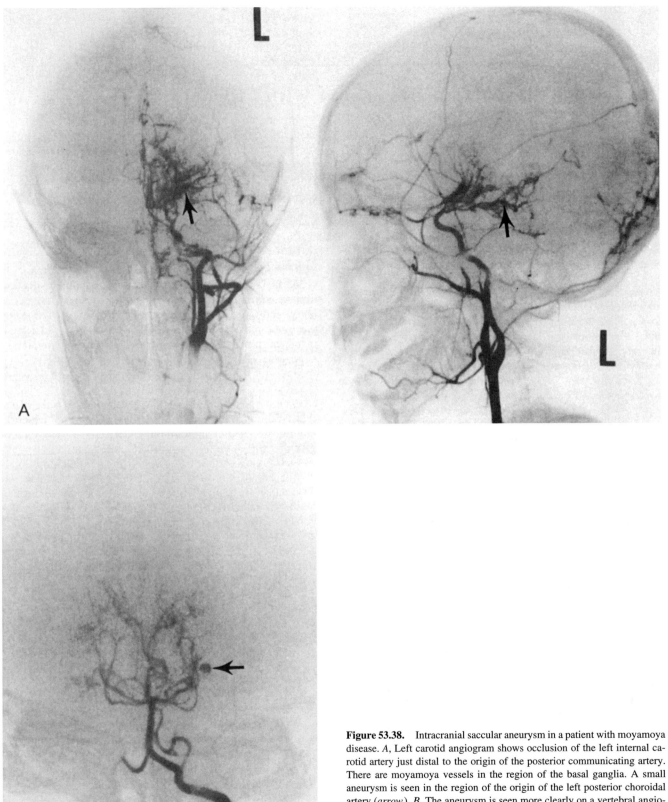

Figure 53.38. Intracranial saccular aneurysm in a patient with moyamoya disease. *A*, Left carotid angiogram shows occlusion of the left internal carotid artery just distal to the origin of the posterior communicating artery. There are moyamoya vessels in the region of the basal ganglia. A small aneurysm is seen in the region of the origin of the left posterior choroidal artery (*arrow*). *B*, The aneurysm is seen more clearly on a vertebral angiogram (*arrow*). (From Waga S, Tochio H. Intracranial aneurysm associated with moyamoya disease in childhood. Surg Neurol *23*:237–243, 1985.)

1983; see Table 1 in Masuzawa et al., 1984; see Table 1 in Brill et al., 1985; DeSouza et al., 1986; Helmchen et al., 1995). Ortiz et al. (1991) reported a patient with a variant of progressive systemic sclerosis characterized by *c*alcinosis, *R*aynaud's phenomenon, *e*sophageal motility abnormalities, *s*clerodactyly, and *t*elangiectatic lesions (CREST syndrome) who had multiple intracranial aneurysms.

Ohkata et al. (1994) reported **extracranial** vertebral artery aneurysms in a patient with NF type 1. A pathologic study of an aneurysm associated with NF demonstrated positive staining with antibodies against desmin and muscle-specific actin, suggesting a smooth muscle origin of abnormal proliferating cells (Malecha and Rubin, 1992). This case parallels reports of abnormal vessel wall proliferation in patients with NF and aneurysms of the renal, mesenteric, and popliteal arteries (Huppman et al., 1996). None the less, it seems likely that the occurrence of aneurysm in patients with these diseases is most often coincidental.

SACCULAR ANEURYSMS

Most neurologic, visual, and neuro-ophthalmologic manifestations of aneurysms result from ruptured or unruptured **saccular** aneurysms. In this section, we consider these aneurysms in detail.

PREVALENCE

The frequency with which ruptured and unruptured saccular aneurysms occur is the subject of numerous studies (Chason and Hindman, 1958; Housepian and Pool, 1958; Stehbens, 1963; Alpers, 1965; McCormick and Nofzinger, 1965; Pakarinen, 1967; Inagawa and Hirano, 1990a, 1990b). Most of these studies are retrospective reviews of autopsy results from a single medical center. Stehbens (1972, 1983a, 1983b) reviewed the results of 14 such studies and found that the prevalence of intracranial saccular aneurysms ranged from 0.2 to 9%, with an average of 2.4%. The variation in prevalence among studies is related to the nature and age distribution of the population studied and to the expertise and enthusiasm of the pathologist. Because most studies were performed retrospectively, it is possible that they underestimated the true prevalence of intracranial arterial aneurysms, particularly if one believes the contention of Hassler (1965) that aneurysms with diameters of 2 mm or less can be found in up to 17% of routine autopsy material and up to 60% in patients dying of SAH from a large aneurysm. On the other hand, angiographic retrospective studies give even lower numbers, with an incidence between 0.5 and 1.1% (Winn et al., 1978; Atkinson et al., 1989). In addition, both autopsy and angiographic series are likely to be biased toward older patients, potentially increasing the apparent frequency. A better estimate of clinically significant unruptured cerebral aneurysms may be in the range of 1% (Inagawa et al., 1990). A correct estimate of the incidence of aneurysms is obviously critical to setting up appropriate life tables (Dell, 1982).

The impact of the presence of aneurysms is directly linked with the incidence of rupture. Cerebrovascular disease remains the third most frequent cause of death in the United States, and SAH may be associated with 5–25% of cases (Crawford and Sarner, 1965).

Most saccular aneurysms occur as isolated, nonhereditary lesions; however, any disorder that affects up to 9% of the population may occasionally be expected to occur in more than one member of some families, particularly if one agrees that hypertension and degenerative vascular disease play a role in the development of aneurysms (see above). In addition, cerebral aneurysms may occur in patients with hereditary connective tissue disorders. It therefore is not surprising that numerous investigators have documented the occurrence of familial intracranial aneurysms, with and without associated systemic diseases (Bannerman et al., 1969; Kak et al., 1970; Maroun et al., 1986; ter Berg et al., 1986; Lozano and Leblanc, 1987; Norrgard et al., 1987; Weir, 1987; Leblanc et al., 1989a; ter Berg et al., 1989; Dierssen et al., 1990; ter Berg et al., 1992; Ronkainen et al., 1993; Schievink et al., 1995a; Schievink, 1997b).

Familial aneurysms have several distinguishing features. Leblanc (1996) noted an increased incidence of women (80% vs 59% in sporadic) and a younger age of rupture, findings that were previously noted by Bromberg et al. (1995b) and Ronkainen et al. (1995b) in families in eastern Finland. These authors also noted that 50% of familial aneurysms were located on the MCA. In a review of seven published series containing at least four siblings, in which at least one underwent angiography, Alberts et al. (1995) demonstrated aneurysms in one-third of patients at risk. The incidence was so high that the authors suggested an autosomal-dominant transmission. Puchner et al. (1994), however, reported a set of monozygotic twins, only one of whom had an intracranial aneurysm.

When aneurysms are familial, rupture in family members tends to occur in the same decade of life (Leblanc et al., 1995), but this may be partially an artifact of their earlier occurrence. It is also suggested that patients with familial SAH have a significantly poorer outcome (52% vs 39% for sporadic aneurysms with hemorrhage) (Bromberg et al., 1995a). Screening for an abnormality in type III collagen has been reported as unrewarding (Leblanc et al., 1995), but Majamaa et al. (1992) reported a difference in the temperature-induced denaturation of type III protocollagen from familial aneurysm patients compared with that from patients with sporadic aneurysms.

Because of the increased risk in family members, it is often suggested that asymptomatic relatives of patients with familial aneurysms should be screened for such lesions at regular intervals (Schievink, 1997b). Leblanc et al. (1994) screened 15 at-risk relatives with angiography and identified one aneurysm and two infundibular dilations. These investigators concluded that intervention produced a benefit of at least 1 year of survival free of sequelae over the natural history in such persons if their life expectancy was 32 years or more. Schievink et al. (1994a) performed a similar prospective screening of at-risk relatives and found a greater frequency in male probands (22%) than in females (9%). In a series of 110 at-risk relatives who underwent MR angiography, 16 aneurysms were detected in 11 persons (Ronkainen et al., 1994).

The diagnosis of an aneurysm usually requires conventional angiography (see below); however, in an attempt to screen individuals at increased risk, less invasive techniques can be employed. These include MR imaging, MR angiography, and spiral CT angiography (see below). An additional screening technique was suggested by Baker et al. (1995a), who assessed serum concentrations of elastase and alpha-1-antitrypsin. The ratio of elastase to alpha-1-antitrypsin was nearly twice as high in patients with unruptured aneurysms as in controls. Leblanc et al. (1995) studied HLA type and concluded that the presence of an aneurysm was not associated with a specific HLA haplotype or antigen. Collagen type III was qualitatively and quantitatively normal. Thus, until a biologic marker for intracranial aneurysms is identified, we believe that MR angiography, spiral CT angiography, or conventional angiography are the only ways to identify patients at risk of harboring a familial cerebral aneurysm. The advantages of screening depend on the frequency of de novo production of aneurysms and their natural history (Obuchowski et al., 1995). More prospective data are obviously necessary.

SEX AND AGE DISTRIBUTION

Overall, saccular intracranial aneurysms occur slightly more often in women than in men, in a ratio of about 1.3 to 1 (McDonald and Korb, 1939; Pakarinen, 1967; Sahs et al., 1969; Stehbens, 1972; Hacker et al., 1983; Kassell and Torner, 1984; Nishimoto et al., 1985). This female predominance does not occur at every age. Aneurysms are actually more common in males during the first 4 decades of life. Indeed, Roche et al. (1988) found that 70% of aneurysms in patients under age 15 occur in males. After the 5th decade, however, women are affected more frequently than men, and this female predominance increases with age (Sahs et al., 1969; Weir, 1987). Interestingly, there is a persistent male predominance in aneurysms of the ACA (Kongable et al., 1996).

Aneurysms may occur in children, even in infants and neonates (McDonald and Korb, 1939; Newcombe and Munns, 1949; Matson, 1965; Pickering et al., 1970; Patel and Richardson, 1971; see Tables 1 and 2 in Becker et al., 1978; see Table 1 in Ventureyra et al., 1980; see Table 1 in Russegger and Grunert, 1987; see Table 1 in Ferrante et al., 1988; Roche et al., 1988; Meyer et al., 1989; Putty et al., 1990; Banna and Lasjaunias, 1991; De Marinis et al., 1991; Herman et al., 1991; Putty et al., 1991; Tanabe et al., 1991; Branley et al., 1992; Herman et al., 1992; Salomao et al., 1992; Scholten et al., 1992; Wolin and Saunders, 1992; Khayata et al., 1994; Milner et al., 1994; Tanaka et al., 1994; Lesser et al., 1997; Tekkok and Ventureyra, 1997). As mentioned above, trauma is a relatively more common cause of aneurysm in childhood (Hahn et al., 1990; Piatt and Clunie, 1992; Ventureyra and Higgins, 1994). Fusiform aneurysms, particularly those that arise from the posterior circulation vessels, may also occur (Greene et al., 1994) and may be associated with systemic pathology (Roy et al., 1990; Taira et al., 1991). Mycotic aneurysms also occur in children (Epelbaum et al., 1993; Stehbens et al., 1995). Nevertheless, aneurysms rarely become symptomatic in patients under 20 years of age. Of 5679 cases from 15 series reviewed by Pakarinen (1967), less than 1% of aneurysms occurred in the 1st decade of life and only 2% in the 2nd. Similar results were reported by other investigators (Sahs et al., 1969; Stehbens, 1972; Hacker et al., 1983; Roche et al., 1988).

The age distribution of symptomatic intracranial aneurysms follows a bell-shaped curve, with the peak incidence of diagnosis occurring in the 5th and 6th decades of life (Pakarinen, 1967; Sahs et al., 1969; Hacker et al., 1983; Nishimoto et al., 1985). Of 4599 cases of intracranial aneurysm reviewed by Nishimoto et al. (1985), 2863 (62%) were diagnosed in the 5th and 6th decades of life. As noted above, men are more commonly affected before about 40 years of age, and women are more commonly affected thereafter. This female predominance in the peak years of diagnosis is responsible for the overall predominance of women among patients with intracranial aneurysms, by a ratio of about 60% to 40% (Kassell and Torner, 1984).

LOCATION AND LATERALITY

Aneurysms may originate from any of the intracranial arteries. Although there is some discrepancy not only between clinical (angiographic) and autopsy studies but also among individual clinical or autopsy studies (see Table 11.6 in Stehbens, 1983a), it is clear that about 85% of all intracranial aneurysms originate from the ICA or one of its branches (Fig. 53.39). The most frequent site of origin is the ICA itself. About 25–40% of all intracranial aneurysms arise from the main trunk of this vessel, usually at the origin of the posterior communicating artery, but also at its terminal bifurcation, at the origin of the ophthalmic artery, or within the cavernous sinus (Locksley, 1966; Hacker et al., 1983; Nishimoto et al., 1985; Weir, 1987) (Fig. 53.40). Another 25–30% of aneurysms originate from the anterior communicating artery. The MCA is the site of origin of about 13–30% of all intracranial aneurysms (Fig. 53.41). Thus, nearly all intracranial aneurysms originate from the internal carotid, anterior communicating, or middle cerebral arteries (Locksley, 1969; Stehbens, 1972; Yoshimoto et al., 1978; Hacker et al., 1983; Kassell and Torner, 1983a; Nishimoto et al., 1985; Weir, 1987). The remaining vessels from which a significant number of aneurysms arise are the basilar artery (3–9%), the ACA (5%), and the vertebral artery (4–5%). In most series, aneurysms that occur on paired vessels are randomly distributed on the right or left side (Yoshimoto et al., 1978; Weir, 1987).

SIZE

Saccular intracranial aneurysms vary in size from less than 2 mm to more than 60 mm in diameter. The size of newly diagnosed aneurysms tends to increase with the age of the patient (Locksley, 1966; Sato et al., 1978). This finding is consistent with serial angiographic studies that show progressive enlargement of aneurysms during intervals ranging

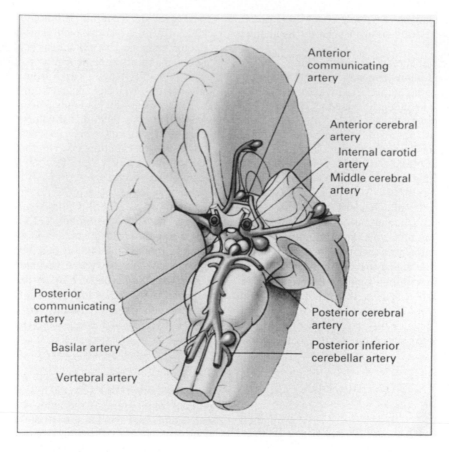

Figure 53.39. Illustration of common sites of intracranial aneurysms on the circle of Willis at the base of the brain (From Schievink WI. Intracranial aneurysms. N Engl J Med *336*:28–40, 1997.)

from 2 weeks to 10 years (Af Björkesten and Troupp, 1962; Piek et al., 1983; Shutter et al., 1993; Miller et al., 1995) (Fig. 53.42). Such enlargement probably reflects two mechanisms. First, there may be thinning of the wall of the aneurysm, thus allowing slow expansion of the sac (Crawford, 1959). Second, there may be recurrent, clinically silent leaks from the aneurysm. During each leak, there is a mesenchymal reaction at the site of bleeding that walls off the blood. Repeated episodes of bleeding thus result in formation of a ''pseudoaneurysm'' within the wall of the true aneurysm (Sarwar et al., 1976). Small aneurysms nevertheless occur in elderly patients, a phenomenon that argues against all of them being developmental and present at birth (Stehbens, 1983b—see above).

Saccular aneurysms less than 3 mm in diameter almost never produce symptoms unless they rupture. Such aneurysms account for less than 2% of ruptured symptomatic aneurysms in most series (Weir, 1987). Nevertheless, small aneurysms may rupture and produce the same catastrophic manifestations as larger aneurysms (Schievink et al., 1992b). Aneurysms 3–10 mm in diameter accounted for approximately 60% of ruptured symptomatic, 70% of unruptured symptomatic, and 75% of unruptured asymptomatic aneurysms in series reported by Weir (1987) and by Wiebers et al. (1987). Orz et al. (1997) reported that of 1248 ruptured

intracranial aneurysms managed at their neurosurgical center at the Shinshu University School of Medicine in Matsumoto, Japan, 475 (38%) were less than 6 mm in diameter. Aneurysms with diameters larger than 25 mm are almost always symptomatic, but they produce symptoms as often by mass effect as by rupture. Such aneurysms account for 3–13% of unruptured, and 3–26% of ruptured, symptomatic aneurysms (Weir, 1987; Wiebers et al., 1987).

MULTIPLE ANEURYSMS

The majority of intracranial aneurysms are solitary lesions. In two large clinical studies that reviewed data on 8071 patients with intracranial saccular aneurysm, 6819 patients (84.5%) had single lesions (Locksley, 1969; Nishimoto et al., 1985). Nevertheless, about 15% of patients with one aneurysm harbor at least one other aneurysm at another site. The first reports of multiple intracranial aneurysms were published in 1842, when Thomson described a 42-year-old man who died after an SAH and was found to have three intracranial aneurysms. Two of the aneurysms arose from the ICA on one side, and the third aneurysm arose from the ICA on the opposite side. In the same year, Kingston described a 14-year-old boy with one aneurysm arising from the ICA and a second aneurysm originating from the basilar ber found (Nehls et al., 1985; Ostergaard and Hog, 1985; Weir, 1987).

Location affects multiplicity (Proust et al., 1994). When the MCA harbors an aneurysm, the incidence of multiplicity increases to 39% (Rinne et al., 1996). This is particularly true of the M-1 segment (Hosoda et al., 1995). Distal ACA aneurysms (Ohno et al., 1990; Hernesniemi et al., 1992) and ophthalmic segment aneurysms (Day, 1990b) also seem to be associated with a high incidence of multiplicity.

Patients with multiple aneurysms tend to have a higher prevalence of systemic hypertension and more pronounced atherosclerosis than do patients with single aneurysms (Ostergaard and Hog, 1985; Weir, 1987), but the prevalence of other systemic disorders that might predispose to aneurysm formation (e.g., connective tissue disease) is no higher in these patients than in patients with single aneurysms. That

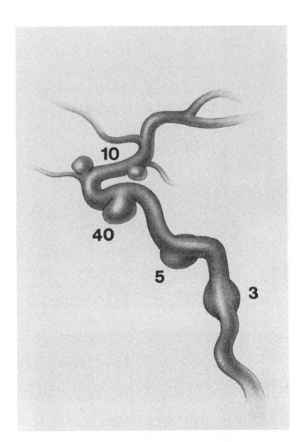

Figure 53.40. Illustration indicating location of 58 internal carotid artery aneurysms treated by intravascular balloon occlusion. Three were in the cervical region, five were in the petrous region, 40 were intracavernous, and 10 were located along the ophthalmic segment. (From Larson JJ, Tew JM Jr, Tomsick TA, et al. Treatment of aneurysms of the internal carotid artery by intravascular balloon occlusion: Long-term follow-up of 58 patients. Neurosurgery *36*:23–30, 1995.)

artery. Numerous angiographic and autopsy studies subsequently documented the occurrence of multiple aneurysms in both adults and children (Hacker et al., 1983; Nehls et al., 1985; Weir, 1987) (Fig. 53.43). The reported prevalence of multiple intracranial aneurysms varies considerably from 3 to 50% (see Table 11.4 in Stehbens, 1983a), but the most reliable figures are probably about 20% for adults (Locksley, 1966; Hacker et al., 1983; Ostergaard and Hog, 1985; Weir, 1987) and 6% for children under 20 years of age (Shucart and Wolpert, 1974; Hacker et al., 1983). Kongable et al. (1996) found that multiple aneurysms leading to SAH occurred more frequently in women than men (32.4% versus 17.6%).

From 50 to 83% of patients with multiple intracranial aneurysms have two aneurysms (Nehls et al., 1985; Ostergaard and Hog, 1985; Weir, 1987; Proust et al., 1994). In about half of these cases, one aneurysm is on each side. In the remaining cases, both aneurysms are on one side or one or both are in the midline. Rarely are more than three aneurysms found in any one patient, but any number can occur, with the frequency being inversely proportional to the num-

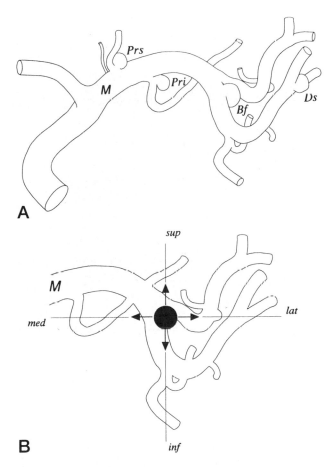

Figure 53.41. Distribution and frequency of middle cerebral artery aneurysms. *A,* Distribution of 690 middle cerebral aneurysms at proximal superior (*Prs*)and proximal inferior (*Pri*) (108), bifurcation (*Bf*) (557), and distal (*Ds*) (25) sites. *B,* Frequencies of the directions of bifurcation middle cerebral artery aneurysms in an anteroposterior angiogram. *Med,* medial (2%); *Sup,* superior (15%); *Lat,* lateral (45%); *Inf,* inferior (38%); *M,* middle cerebral artery. (From Rinne J, Hernesniemi J, Niskanen M, et al. Analysis of 561 patients with 690 middle cerebral artery aneurysms: Anatomic and clinical features as correlated to management outcome. Neurosurgery *38*: 2–11, 1996.)

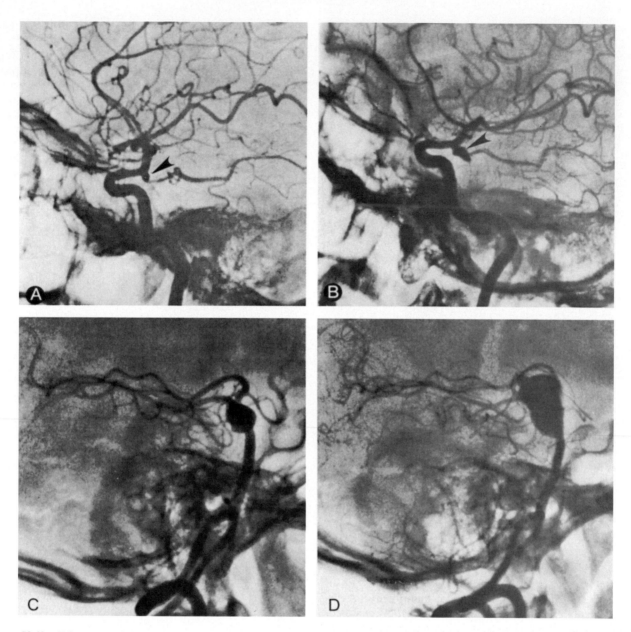

Figure 53.42. Enlargement of saccular aneurysms over time. *A*, Initial angiogram performed shortly after a subarachnoid hemorrhage shows a small aneurysm at the junction of the internal carotid and posterior communicating arteries. The patient refused surgical treatment. *B*, Second angiogram after another hemorrhage 2 years later shows enlargement of the aneurysm. *C*, Cerebral angiogram in another patient shows an aneurysm located at the bifurcation of the basilar artery. The patient did not undergo treatment for this lesion. *D*, Repeat angiogram performed 1 year later shows a substantial increase in the size of the aneurysm.

does not seem to be the case with mycotic aneurysms, which have a significant incidence of multiplicity (Corr et al. 1995). As might be expected, prognosis is affected by multiplicity, with patients with more than one aneurysm faring less well than patients with only one aneurysm (Rinne et al., 1995).

Other interesting observations in patients with multiple aneurysms include the increased incidence of asymmetry in the circle of Willis (74%) (Milenkovic et al., 1995). Multiplicity may further increase the risk of hemorrhage when one of the aneurysms arises from the anterior communicating artery (Proust et al., 1994).

GENERAL CLINICAL MANIFESTATIONS

As recognized by Beadles (1907), aneurysms may cause symptoms in one of three ways. First, large aneurysms can produce symptoms from mass effect, in which case the symptoms depend on the function of the adjacent neural tissue. The frequency of mass effect also depends on the location of the aneurysm. Cavernous sinus aneurysms have a high incidence of locally produced symptoms, whereas distal intradural aneurysms are usually silent unless they bleed or become large (>25 mm). Second, aneurysms may

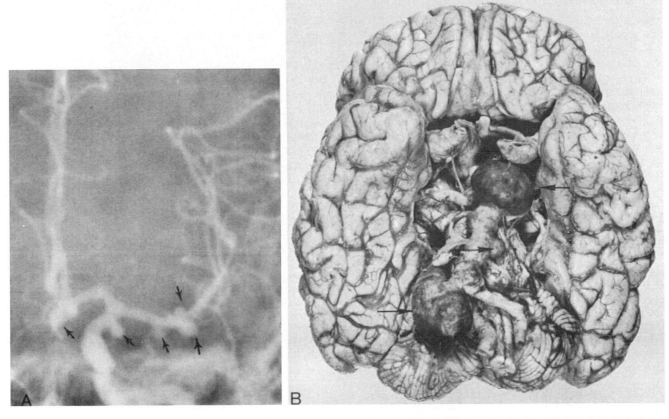

Figure 53.43. Multiple intracranial aneurysms. *A*, Left carotid angiogram shows five aneurysms (*arrows*). One is at the site of the anterior communicating artery, one is at the junction of the internal carotid and posterior communicating arteries, and three arise from branches of the middle cerebral artery. (From Taveras JM, Wood EH. Diagnostic Radiology, 2nd ed, Vol 2. Baltimore, Williams & Wilkins, 1976.) *B*, Autopsy specimen from a patient with severe atherosclerosis shows three large saccular aneurysms arising from the basilar artery (*arrows*). The two larger aneurysms arise from the origin and termination of the basilar artery, respectively. The smallest aneurysm arises from the junction of the basilar and left anterior inferior cerebellar arteries. (From Stehbens WE. The pathology of intracranial arterial aneurysms and their complications. In Intracranial Aneurysms. Editor, Fox JL, Vol I, pp 272–357. Springer-Verlag, New York, 1983.)

alter the distal circulation of their parent vessels or distal branches from those vessels. They may cause vascular compromise (stenosis or thrombosis), distal embolization (artery-artery embolization), or steal phenomena from alterations in the overall hemodynamics of the system. Finally, and most frequently, aneurysms cause symptoms when they rupture. Immediate effects include local loss of perfusion pressure and increased ICP that alters cerebral blood flow. Later effects are caused by spasm of the intracranial vessels mediated through exposure to subarachnoid blood and disturbances in CSF dynamics leading to hydrocephalus.

Unruptured aneurysms may produce: (*a*) progressive cranial nerve, brainstem, or hemisphere dysfunction; (*b*) TIAs or cerebral infarction; (*c*) progressive dementia with or without features of diencephalic amnesia; or (*d*) recurrent grand mal, focal, or psychomotor seizures (Whittle et al., 1985; Przelomski et al., 1986; Provenzale et al., 1996). Aneurysmal rupture causes symptoms and signs of acute SAH, intraparenchymal hemorrhage, or both. The onset of mass effect is related to sudden enlargement of the aneurysm, which is sometimes associated with a limited rupture. Thus, an aneurysm may cause symptoms and signs from the effects of both the mass itself and from SAH.

Visual system involvement with symptomatic aneurysms is common. Brenner and Pendl (1974) found ocular or visual signs or symptoms in 24% of a series of 491 aneurysm cases. Neuro-ophthalmologic signs occurred in 10% of patients without evidence of SAH. Such signs are even more common in patients with ruptured aneurysms (see below).

MANIFESTATIONS OF RUPTURED SACCULAR ANEURYSMS

General Considerations

Few events in human disease can be so sudden and potentially catastrophic as the spontaneous rupture of a major intracranial artery (Fig. 53.44). Depending on the size and nature of the mural defect, the escaping blood may dissect within the vessel wall, ooze slowly around the site, or gush forth under high pressure into the subarachnoid space, the substance of the adjacent brain, or both (Inagawa and Hirano, 1990a). Pressure within the enclosed cranial vault may rise

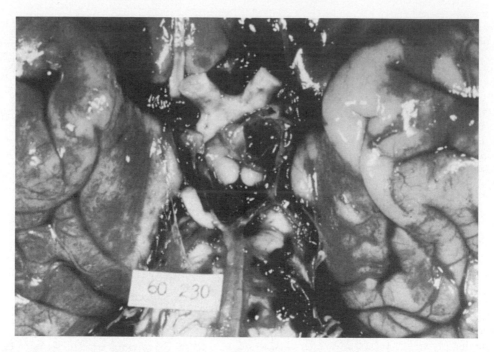

Figure 53.44. Massive subarachnoid hemorrhage from rupture of an internal carotid-posterior communicating artery aneurysm. View of the base of the brain shows that the basal cisterns are filled with blood. There is blood staining and hemorrhage of the temporal and frontal lobes, the brainstem, and the anterior visual sensory apparatus, including the optic nerves, optic chiasm, and optic tracts.

precipitously until it equals the pressure within the leaking vessel. At the same time, the damaged artery contracts, unless sclerotic changes in its wall prevent it from doing so, and the bleeding stops. Clinically, the patient, often without warning, suddenly experiences an excruciating pain in the head as if it were about to explode from within. Directly thereafter, the patient collapses and may experience a generalized or focal seizure. Depending on the location and extent of the hemorrhage, the patient may die immediately or within a few hours, remain in coma for days, or regain consciousness after minutes or hours. The patient may ultimately recover completely, have a persistent major or minor neurologic deficit, or die of a recurrent hemorrhage (Ogden et al., 1997).

The two major causes of spontaneous subarachnoid and intracranial hemorrhage in patients of all ages are saccular aneurysms and AVMs (Bonita and Thomson, 1985; Bevan et al., 1990). Other causes include acute and chronic hypertensive vascular disease, migraine, trauma, neoplasm, vasculitis amyloid angiopathy and anticoagulation (Caplan, 1988). The clinical determination of the source of hemorrhage is usually achieved by a careful history, examination, and neuroimaging studies, particularly CT scanning, MR imaging (including MR angiography), and conventional arteriography (see below and Chapter 55). The source of bleeding and the amount of hemorrhage, especially when acute, may be quantitated best by CT scanning.

Subarachnoid hemorrhage, particularly from rupture of an intracranial aneurysm, may develop at any time and may be related to almost any activity. Mayer and Awad (1994) reported three patients who presented with SAH after singing in a church choir. Schievink et al. (1989) studied a group of 500 consecutive patients with aneurysmal SAH and concluded that about 43% of the patients experienced the hemorrhage during a stressful or exertional event, such as defecation, urination, sexual intercourse (Chang and Ahn, 1996), heavy work, and exercise (Haykowsky et al., 1996). The SAH occurred during a nonstrenuous event such as sitting, standing, and watching television in 34% of patients. In 11.8% of patients, the hemorrhage occurred during rest or sleep. In this study, men were more likely than women to have experienced the SAH during a stressful or strenuous event. Similar findings were reported by other investigators (See Table 3 in Schievink et al. 1989). SAH may also occur during pregnancy (Kriplani et al., 1995), but the frequency of this occurrence is not as high as one might suspect.

In a retrospective study of 120 of 273 patients with aneurysmal SAHs for whom a specific time could be ascribed to the event, a rupture peak occurred between 9 and 10 A.M. with a possible secondary peak in the afternoon hours (Kleinpeter et al., 1995). Most seem to occur during working hours (Vermeer et al., 1997). When these patients were segregated on the basis of blood pressure, only the hypertensive patients had this chronorisk, suggesting a possible dual trigger mechanism. Chyatte et al. (1994) attempted to correlate aneurysmal rupture with climatic conditions. In a retrospective study of 1487 patients with aneurysmal rupture in Connecticut, women were found to have a peak incidence in the Spring whereas men bled more frequently in the late Fall. These authors were able to show a correlation between weather changes and aneurysmal rupture in men but not in women; they concluded that factors that lead to aneurysm rupture in women may be different from those in men.

Warning Signs and Symptoms Before Major Rupture of Intracranial Aneurysm

Many patients develop minor neurologic symptoms and signs days to weeks before they experience a major subarachnoid or intracranial hemorrhage from rupture of an intracranial aneurysm (Gillingham, 1958, 1967; Okawara, 1973; King and Saba, 1974; Ball, 1975; Waga et al., 1975; Duffy, 1983; Huige et al., 1988; Schievink et al., 1988; Juvela, 1992a; Jakobsson et al., 1996; Regli et al., 1997). These manifestations apparently occur from leakage of a small amount of blood from the aneurysm. They occurred in 100 of 273 (37%) patients who subsequently experienced an aneurysmal SAH, usually within 14 days of the hemorrhage (Juvela, 1992a).

The most common warning symptom is an acute, often generalized headache that may be described by the patient as "the worst headache of my life." The headache may be associated with nausea, vomiting, neck pain, photophobia, or a combination of these features. It is often mistaken for an attack of common migraine. Other warning symptoms include facial or eye pain, dizziness, lethargy, and diplopia. Patients with these disturbances may be thought to be suffering from mental exhaustion, sinusitis, a viral illness, psychiatric disease, or other disorders (see Table 4 in Schievink et al., 1988).

Of course, not all sudden severe headaches are caused by SAH. In a study by Strittmatter et al. (1996), 84 patients with severe "thunderclap headaches" (see Chapter 36) who had no evidence of SAH on CT scanning or lumbar puncture had no neurologic deficits over the subsequent 1–6 years (Strittmatter et al., 1996), suggesting that such headaches are not always a predictor of future SAH. Nevertheless, when 562 patients who presented with a severe headache but no evidence of SAH on standard (nonspiral) CT scanning or lumbar puncture underwent a more extensive evaluation, 52 (9.3%) were found to harbor at least one intracranial aneurysm (Takeuchi et al., 1996). Of 46 of these 52 patients who subsequently underwent surgery, eight had evidence of previous localized "minor leak." This study suggests that it is reasonable to perform a more extensive evaluation for an intracranial aneurysm in a patient who experiences a severe "thunderclap headache," even when CT scanning and lumbar puncture give negative results. Whether or not such patients or patients in whom MR angiography, spiral CT angiography, or both are negative, should undergo conventional angiography is less clear (Takeuchi et al., 1994). This point was raised in a study by Sugai et al. (1994) in which 605 angiograms performed between May 1985 and December 1992 were retrospectively reviewed. Unruptured aneurysms were observed in 43 patients (7.1%), but aneurysms were present in 11 of 72 headache patients (15.3%).

Prodromal symptoms and signs may occur days, weeks, or even months before a major subarachnoid or intracerebral hemorrhage. In some cases, the patient may not seek medical attention, preferring to ignore the difficulties he or she has experienced. In most cases, however, the patient is evaluated by a physician, only to be misdiagnosed (Schievink et al., 1988). Concern about misdiagnosis was also raised by Hauerberg et al. (1991), who noted a variety of symptoms consistent with a warning leak (sudden episode of headache, vomiting, nuchal pain, dizziness, or drowsiness) in 166 Danish patients (15.4%), 99 of whom were initially misdiagnosed. Although most symptoms and signs that precede rupture of an intracranial aneurysm are nonspecific, the recognition that a particular neurologic or systemic disturbance is the initial manifestation of an intracranial aneurysm that has not undergone a major rupture may have a significant effect on the patient's ultimate outcome.

The percentage of patients who experience a "warning leak" headache may be fairly low. Linn et al. (1994) retrospectively reviewed the cases of 148 Dutch patients who experienced a severe headache and who were subsequently evaluated by general practioners. SAH had occurred in 37 of the patients (25%) and was associated with an aneurysm in 21 (negative angiogram in six, no angiogram done in six, and death in four). Among the 37 patients with a proven SAH, only two (5.4%) had experienced a previous headache.

Neurologic and Neuro-Ophthalmologic Manifestations of Ruptured Intracranial Aneurysms

A number of neurologic and neuro-ophthalmologic signs can accompany subarachnoid or intracranial hemorrhage from rupture of an intracranial aneurysm (Brenner and Pendl, 1974; McKinna, 1983). Although these signs may occur in patients with intracranial hemorrhage from other causes, they are described here because of the frequency of subarachnoid and intracranial hemorrhage produced by a ruptured intracranial aneurysm. These signs reflect damage to the nervous system from the direct effects of hemorrhage on adjacent cerebral tissue or from peripheral ischemia caused by increased ICP, failure of peripheral circulation associated with thrombosis or, most often, vasospasm. Some of these signs assist in lateralization or localization of the aneurysm, others serve as critical indicators of secondary events such as herniation of the hippocampal gyrus, and still others indicate the severity of the rise in ICP (Fisher et al., 1965).

SAH from rupture of an intracranial aneurysm usually produces violent headache and abrupt but transient loss of consciousness. Lateralizing motor and sensory signs are uncommon, but there may be an initial transient hemiparesis or monoparesis from spasm of the affected vessel. A seizure may occur at the onset. Neuro-ophthalmologic signs include focal visual, sensory, and ocular motor deficits. Rupture of carotid-ophthalmic, anterior cerebral, or anterior communicating artery aneurysms may be associated with loss of central vision in one or both eyes or homonymous or, less commonly, bitemporal field defects from damage to one or both optic nerves, the optic chiasm, or the optic tracts (Ruben and Afshar, 1991). Rupture of an internal carotid-anterior choroidal or PCA aneurysm may produce a homonymous visual field defect. Diplopia may result from damage to one or more of the ocular motor nerves within the subarachnoid space or to the ocular motor control mechanisms within the brainstem after rupture of an aneurysm arising from any point along the supraclinoid portion of the ICA (especially near the origin of the posterior communicating artery) or after rupture of a posterior communicating, posterior cerebral, superior cerebellar, anterior inferior cerebellar, posterior inferior cerebellar, basilar, or vertebral aneurysm (McKinna, 1983). An aneurysm remains one of the most frequent and certainly most important causes of acute oculomotor nerve dysfunction (Shih, 1993; Leng et al., 1994). The critical aspects of this neuro-ophthalmologic sign cannot be overemphasized.

It is estimated that cranial nerve dysfunction is caused by local effects of the aneurysm and rupture in approximately 50% of cases and the effects of subarachnoid blood in the other 50% (Hyland and Barnett, 1953). Abducens nerve paresis that occurs after rupture of an intracranial aneurysm may be directly related to the aneurysm (Michael, 1974; Dumas and Shults, 1982), or it may be a nonlocalizing sign of increased ICP (see Chapter 38). This is the presumptive mechanism for patients who develop abducens nerve palsies in the setting of anterior circulation aneurysmal rupture (Nathal et al., 1992). Unilateral pupillary dilation occurs most frequently after SAH in association with ipsilateral ptosis and ophthalmoparesis from damage to the oculomotor nerve from the aneurysm itself, from blood, from ischemia, or from compression by the hippocampal gyrus. Oculomotor nerve dysfunction may also occur in association with remote aneurysmal rupture, either related to the effects of increased ICP or to the direct irritation of subarachnoid blood (Shih, 1993; Coyne and Wallace, 1994). On rare occasions, isolated pupillary dilation may be the only sign of a ruptured aneurysm, usually one that arises from the basilar artery (Walsh and Hoyt, 1969b; Crompton and Moore, 1981; Gale and Crockard, 1982). Horner's syndrome may occasionally occur after rupture of an aneurysm arising from the vertebrobasilar system (Hudgins et al., 1983). The Horner's syndrome in such cases is caused by damage to oculosympathetic fibers within the brainstem and is therefore central in nature (see Chapter 24). It is almost always associated with other signs of brainstem dysfunction and can thus be distinguished clinically (and pharmacologically) from the post-ganglionic Horner's syndrome caused by both ruptured and unruptured aneurysms arising from the petrous and intracavernous portions of the ICA.

Although rupture of an intracranial aneurysm most often produces SAH, some patients develop a localized intraparenchymal hemorrhage that is related to the location of the aneurysm and the direction of rupture. **Putaminal** hemorrhage is always characterized by abrupt loss of consciousness and hemiplegia (Matsumoto et al., 1992) that affects the face, arm, and leg. Hemisensory deficits, aphasia, or nondominant lobe symptoms and signs may become evident as the patient recovers. There is often conjugate deviation of the eyes to the side of the lesion (Merwarth and Fiering, 1939; Cogan, 1965; Mohr et al., 1984). Patients with such lesions may be unable to direct the eyes voluntarily toward the side of the intact hemisphere. Nevertheless, vestibular stimulation (oculocephalic maneuver; caloric testing) usually elicits a full range of horizontal eye movement. In some instances, instead of a steady deviation of the eyes toward the side of the lesion, there is nystagmus with ipsilaterally-directed quick phases. Homonymous hemianopia ipsilateral to the hemiplegia occurs when the hemorrhage extends posteriorly to affect the optic radiation. Dilation of the pupil of the eye on the side of the hemorrhage (contralateral to the hemiplegia and hemianopia) occurs when there is hippocampal herniation affecting the course of the oculomotor nerve.

Thalamic-subthalamic hemorrhage produces lateralized long tract motor and sensory signs. Neuro-ophthalmologic signs include: (*a*) vertical gaze paresis; (*b*) spastic downward and inward deviation of one or both eyes; (*c*) skew deviation; (*d*) pseudo-abducens nerve paresis (abduction weakness that can be improved by oculocephalic maneuver or caloric testing); and (*e*) small, nonreactive pupils that are usually, but not always, of equal size (Fisher, 1959). The thalamic syndrome (central dysesthesia) may rarely be seen with an unruptured aneurysm (Stoodley et al., 1995). Medial thalamic hemorrhage may cause spastic lateral deviation of the eyes to the side opposite the hemorrhage (ipsilateral to

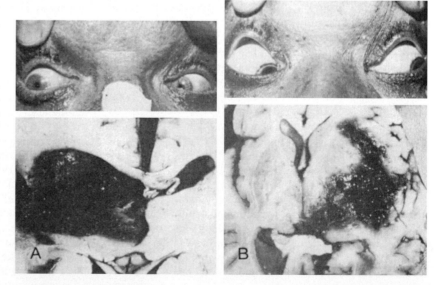

Figure 53.45. Contralateral (''*wrong-way*'') deviation of the eyes caused by thalamic-basal ganglia hemorrhage. *A, above,* The patient's eyes are deviated to the right. *Below,* coronal section immediately posterior to the mammillary bodies shows a left intracerebral hemorrhage affecting the thalamus, internal capsule, and basal ganglia. *B, above,* In another patient with intracranial hemorrhage, the eyes are deviated down and left. *Below,* Horizontal section through the middiencephalon shows a right intracerebral hemorrhage affecting the pretectum, thalamus, posterior limb of the internal capsule, globus pallidus, and putamen. (From Keane JR. Contralateral gaze deviation with supratentorial hemorrhage: Three pathologically verified cases. *Arch Neurol 32:*119–122, 1975.)

the hemiplegia) (Fig. 53.45). This phenomenon is called **wrong-way deviation** (Fisher, 1967; Keane, 1975; Walshe et al., 1977—see Chapter 29).

Pontine hemorrhage from rupture of an aneurysm of the vertebral-basilar arterial system usually is so catastrophic that the patient is deeply comatose in a matter of seconds or minutes. Milder bleeding causes asymmetric quadriplegia or hemiplegia with multiple cranial neuropathies primarily affecting the trigeminal, abducens, and facial nerves. Other ocular signs include unilateral or bilateral conjugate gaze paresis that is not improved by oculocephalic or caloric test-

ing, internuclear ophthalmoplegia (INO), the one-and-a-half syndrome, and a variety of spontaneous vertical eye movements such as ocular bobbing, inverse ocular bobbing (ocular dipping), reverse ocular bobbing, and inverse-reverse ocular bobbing (Fisher, 1964; Susac et al., 1970; Sherman and Salmon, 1977; Osenbach et al., 1986; Rosenberg, 1986; Rosa et al., 1987; Mehler, 1988; Titer and Laureno, 1988—see Chapter 31) (Fig. 53.46). Pupils are characteristically pinpoint.

Intracerebral hemorrhage into the **frontal lobe** causes coma or transient mental confusion. Hall and Young (1992)

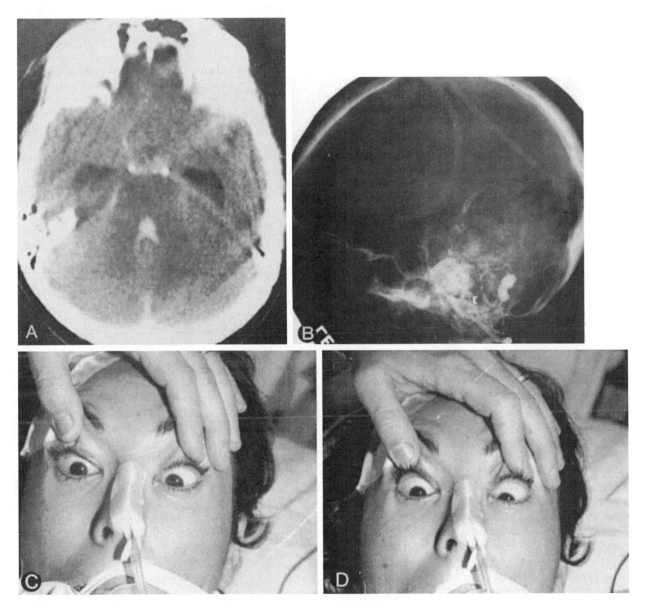

Figure 53.46. Ocular bobbing after rupture of a giant distal posterior inferior cerebellar artery aneurysm. The patient was a 37-year-old woman who became comatose after experiencing the worst headache of her life associated with protracted vomiting. *A,* Unenhanced CT scan shows subarachnoid and intraventricular hemorrhage. *B,* Vertebral angiogram, lateral view, shows a lobulated aneurysm that arises from a distal segment of the right posterior inferior cerebellar artery. *C,* Still photograph demonstrates the approximate resting position of the eyes. *D,* A photograph taken seconds later shows spontaneous downward deviation of both eyes. (From Osenbach RK, Blumenkopf B, McComb B, et al. Ocular bobbing with ruptured giant distal posterior inferior cerebellar artery aneurysm. Surg Neurol 25:149–152, 1986.)

reported a 23-year-old man with acute onset of blunted affect, looseness of associations, and auditory hallucinations related to rupture of an ACA aneurysm into the frontal lobe. Signs can include both grasping and sucking reflexes. A mild hemiparesis may be present and associated with aphasia if the hemorrhage is in the dominant frontal lobe. In rare cases, rupture of an anterior communicating aneurysm causes acute paraparesis or paraplegia from insufficient blood perfusion of both paracentral areas (Maiuri et al., 1986). In other cases, rupture of an anterior cerebral aneurysm is associated with a hemispheric disconnection syndrome caused by hemorrhagic destruction of the anterior portion of the corpus callosum (Levin et al., 1987). Ocular signs are often absent unless the hematoma is quite large, in which case there may be ipsilateral pupillary dilation and conjugate deviation of the eyes toward the side of the lesion. Acute unilateral or bilateral visual loss may accompany the rupture of an A-1 or anterior communicating artery aneurysm (Ruben and Afshar, 1991).

One additional syndrome most commonly seen after rupture of aneurysms of the anterior cerebral or anterior communicating artery is acquired amnesia. Most amnestic syndromes are caused by damage to the medial temporal lobe, but significant memory disturbances may occur after rupture of anterior circulation aneurysms (Tarel et al., 1990; DeLuca and Cicerone, 1991; Stenhouse et al., 1991; DeLuca, 1992; Van der Linden and Bruyer, 1992; DeLuca and Diamond, 1995). DeLuca (1992) reported that following anterior communicating artery aneurysm rupture, 11 patients performed significantly worse than 13 control subjects with intracerebral hemorrhage on tests of delayed verbal memory and on the Wisconsin Card Sorting Test. Greene et al. (1995) emphasized that when associated with paraparesis, amnesia localizes the damage to the territory of the ACA. Tidswell et al. (1995) questioned the specificity of the anterior cerebral ''amnestic syndrome.'' In a study of 37 patients 6 months or more after surgery for ruptured aneurysms, these investigators found no difference in the cognitive outcome (tests of intelligence, attention, executive functions sensitive to frontal lobe lesions, memory, neglect, and mood) between patients with ruptured anterior communicating artery aneurysms and patients with ruptured aneurysms located on other branches of the ICA. However, patients with aneurysmal SAH were significantly more disturbed in focal cognitive functions such as short- and long-term memory and word-finding capacity when compared with patients with SAH of unknown origin. The latter group scored significantly worse on neuropsychological tests related to attention, which can be regarded as a more diffuse cognitive function (Hutter et al., 1994).

Hanley et al. (1990) reported a case of recent visual memory impairment in a woman with to the right cerebral hemisphere from rupture of an MCA aneurysm. Her ability to remember unfamiliar faces was severely impaired, as was her ability to identify the faces of celebrities who had become famous since the time of her illness. By contrast, she performed well on tests of recognition memory for words and had no problem in identifying celebrities from their names or from their faces if they were famous before her ictus.

Acute **cerebellar** hemorrhage from a ruptured aneurysm often begins with headache, dizziness, and inability to stand. Coma may not occur for an hour or two. In most cases, there is initial, bilateral sparing of motor function and sensation. Cerebellar signs include truncal ataxia, unilateral or bilateral limb ataxia, and vestibular nystagmus. The patient may prefer to lie on one side and may become nauseated if moved. Ocular signs include: (a) incomplete horizontal gaze paresis, often with forced deviation of the eyes **away** from the side of the hematoma; (b) minimal ocular response to vestibular stimulation; (c) peripheral facial weakness; (d) central Horner's syndrome; (e) small, reactive pupils; and (f) skew deviation (Ott et al., 1974; Brennan and Bergland, 1977).

Orbital and Intraocular Effects of Subarachnoid and Intracranial Hemorrhage

Massive hemorrhage into the intracranial cavity produces an immediate and precipitous rise in ICP. This pressure may approach or equal systolic arterial pressure at the level of the head. Cerebral blood flow is immediately reduced. The resultant ischemia stimulates the vasomotor center in the brainstem, and systemic blood pressure rises. Over a considerable range, the rise in systolic blood pressure is proportional to the rise in ICP. Eventually a point is reached at which ICP equals arterial pressure, and cerebral blood flow ceases. At some point in the development of these events, the pressure surrounding a leaking cerebral vessel equals the intraluminal pressure, and bleeding stops. The hematoma surrounding the point of rupture then clots and limits further hemorrhage. ICP remains extremely high, because the mass of the hematoma and the blockage of arachnoid villi by blood in the subarachnoid space impair drainage of CSF.

These dramatic pathophysiologic events produce profound changes in the orbital circulation. The radical increase in ICP impairs cerebral blood flow. Carotid arterial blood is shunted into the ophthalmic artery at elevated pressure, causing a corresponding increase in blood flow through the orbital and ocular vessels. If the venous drainage from the orbital and ocular capillary bed is inadequate to cope with this increase in blood flow, venous capillaries become distended and rupture, producing scattered hemorrhages in a number of the tissues within the orbit and inside the eye (Manschot, 1954).

Small **orbital hemorrhages** are a common autopsy finding in patients who die after massive intracranial hemorrhage (Ballantyne, 1943; Walsh and Hedges, 1951) (Fig. 53.47). Only occasionally are such hemorrhages clinically significant. Bisland and Topilow (1952) described a patient who developed preretinal hemorrhages, papilledema, and unilateral proptosis after intraventricular rupture of an intracranial aneurysm during toxemia of pregnancy. The patient died, and a large orbital hemorrhage was found at autopsy.

The prevalence of **intraocular hemorrhages** after rupture of an intracranial aneurysm is unknown. Various series quote figures of 1–40% (Manschot, 1944; Hamby, 1952; Timberlake and Kubik, 1952; Manschot, 1954; Henderson, 1955;

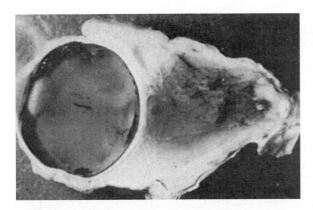

Figure 53.47. Orbital and intraocular hemorrhages caused by a fatal subarachnoid hemorrhage. A longitudinal section through the eye and orbit shows diffuse hemorrhage within the orbit and several retinal and preretinal intraocular hemorrhages. The vaginal sheaths of the optic nerve were filled with blood.

Sarner and Rose, 1967; Fahmy et al., 1969; Fahmy, 1972a, 1973a, 1973b; Fisher, 1975; Charamis et al., 1976; Shinoda et al., 1983; Frizzel et al., 1997). In a series of 250 patients admitted to a neurosurgical service with SAH, 26 (10.5%) had intraocular hemorrhage (Roux et al., 1991). The actual prevalence may be higher, however, because most investigators have not approached the problem systematically using wide pupillary dilation, direct and indirect ophthalmoscopy, and repeated ophthalmoscopic examinations. Nevertheless, intraocular hemorrhages may be seen within hours to days after aneurysm rupture and SAH. Children seem to be affected less often than adults, but even infants may develop such hemorrhages (McLellan et al., 1986).

Intraocular hemorrhages may be intrarctinal, preretinal, or intravitreal. They result from the secondary effects of increased ICP rather than from extravasation of subarachnoid blood into the eye (see below).

Intraretinal hemorrhages are usually seen within a few hours after acute rupture of an aneurysm, but they also may not appear until several days later (Dandy, 1944; Manschot, 1954; Pool and Potts, 1965; Fahmy, 1972a, 1973a, 1973b; Rácz et al., 1977). They are usually small and located in the nerve fiber layer in the macula and near the margin of the optic disc (Figs. 53.48–53.50). Some of these hemorrhages have white centers, a finding that in the past was thought to be restricted to hemorrhages associated with sepsis, anemia, or blood dyscrasia (Litten, 1880; Doherty and Trubek, 1931; Kennedy and Wise, 1965; Holt and Gordon-Smith, 1969). In fact, such white-centered hemorrhages, often called **Roth spots**, can be a nonspecific sign of intracranial and SAH (Phelps, 1971; Van Uitert and Solomon, 1979).

Preretinal hemorrhages may be small or quite extensive, covering areas of the retina 2–3 disc diameters in size (Figs. 53.48–53.50). They usually are located in the posterior pole, but they may occur in the periphery in children. When a preretinal hemorrhage is located in the macula, the patient will have reduced central vision (Fig. 53.49); however, the visual deficit may not be noticed by the patient until the sensorium clears sufficiently several days or even weeks after rupture of the aneurysm. Preretinal hemorrhage occasionally may break into the vitreous cavity. This usually occurs several days after the SAH. It may be spontaneous, or it may coincide with recurrent aneurysmal hemorrhage or with arteriography.

Vitreous hemorrhage associated with SAH is called **Terson's syndrome** (Terson, 1900, 1926; Castrén, 1963; Fox, 1983; Weingeist et al., 1986; Toosi and Malton, 1987; Espinasse-Berrod et al., 1988; Huber et al., 1988; Meier nd Widermann, 1996; Ohkubo et al., 1996; Frizzel et al., 1997). It may occur in one or both eyes and be so severe that it

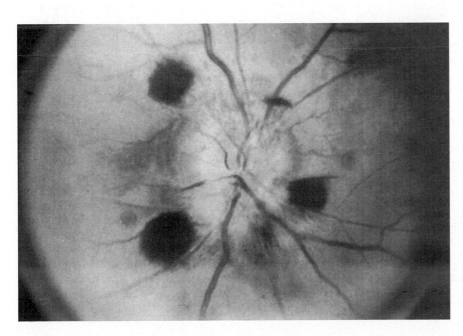

Figure 53.48. Retinal and preretinal hemorrhages in patients with acute subarachnoid hemorrhage from rupture of an intracranial aneurysm. Note that the hemorrhages tend to occur in the posterior pole and to surround the swollen optic disc.

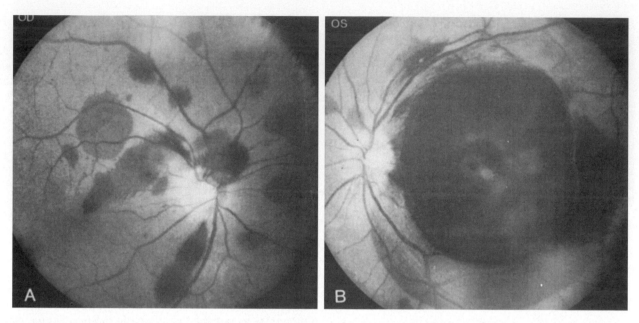

Figure 53.49.   Retinal and preretinal hemorrhages in a 57-year-old man with subarachnoid hemorrhage from rupture of a left anterior communicating artery aneurysm. *A,* The right ocular fundus shows numerous flame-shaped and circular retinal hemorrhages scattered around the optic disc and posterior pole. *B,* The left fundus shows an extensive preretinal hemorrhage obscuring the macula. Superficial retinal hemorrhages also are present. Visual acuity in this eye was hand motions. (From Toosi SH, Malton M. Terson's syndrome: Significance of ocular findings. Ann Ophthalmol *19*:7–12, 1987.)

obscures all fundus detail (Fig. 53.51). As noted above, vitreous hemorrhage may develop at the time of initial SAH, several days later from spontaneous extension of a pre-existing preretinal hemorrhage, following repeat rupture of the aneurysm, or after arteriography. Because of the debilitated state of many patients with ruptured aneurysms, vitreous hemorrhage may not be suspected until several days or weeks after the SAH when the patient is sufficiently alert

to complain of decreased vision. Miller (1991a) reported having seen a 65-year-old woman who was referred because of blurred vision after an SAH from a right internal carotid-posterior communicating aneurysm. On admission to the hospital, she had been somnolent and had a complete right oculomotor nerve paresis. Clipping of the aneurysm was performed within 48 hours after admission. Over the next few days, the patient's sensorium cleared, and she began to

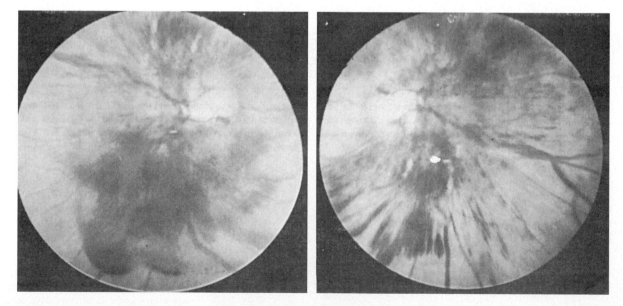

Figure 53.50.   Retinal and preretinal hemorrhages caused by a massive subarachnoid hemorrhage from an anterior cerebral artery aneurysm. Note the presence of soft exudates in some areas.

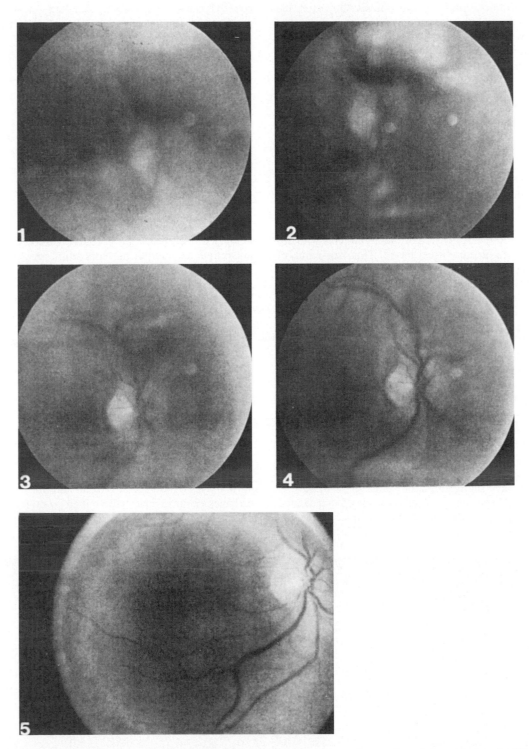

Figure 53.51. Vitreous hemorrhage (*Terson's syndrome*). The patient was a 66-year-old man who experienced an acute subarachnoid hemorrhage from rupture of an aneurysm arising from the supraclinoid portion of the left internal carotid artery. The series of five photographs of the right ocular fundus shows gradual clearing of the hemorrhage. *1*, 24 days after hemorrhage; *2*, 42 days after hemorrhage; *3*, 77 days after hemorrhage; *4*, 98 days after hemorrhage; *5*, 7 months after hemorrhage. (From Fahmy JA. Vitreous hemorrhage in subarachnoid hemorrhage: Terson's syndrome. Report of a case with macular degeneration. Acta Ophthalmol *50*:137–143, 1972.)

complain of difficulty seeing. This initially was thought to be related to the oculomotor nerve paresis; however, the patient eventually convinced her physicians that it was her left eye that was the problem. On examination, the patient had visual acuity of 20/20 OD when the eyelid was raised. Left eye vision was hand motions at about 1 foot. There was no relative afferent pupillary defect (RAPD). A complete right oculomotor nerve paresis with dilation of the pupil was present, but the left eye had full ductions. Ophthalmoscopy was normal on the right, but there was a diffuse vitreous hemorrhage that obscured all fundus detail in the left eye.

Not all patients with SAH develop Terson's syndrome. In a prospective study, Pfausler et al. (1996) found that only 16.7% (10 of 60 consecutive patients) had evidence of vitreous blood following SAH. They did, however, note that vitreous hemorrhage was of prognostic significance. Seven of the 10 patients with Terson's syndrome rebled, and nine of 10 died, compared with only five of the 50 patients who did not have evidence of intravitreal blood. This worsening of prognosis had previously been appreciated. Manschot (1944) reported that the mortality rate in patients with intraocular hemorrhage after SAH was **twice** that in patients without intraocular hemorrhage, and other investigators reported similar findings (Richardson and Hyland, 1941; Walsh and Hedges, 1951; Fahmy, 1973b; Rácz et al., 1977; Shaw et al., 1977; Shinoda et al., 1983).

In almost all cases of Terson's syndrome, the vitreous hemorrhage clears spontaneously with time (Meier and Wiedermann, 1996), but this may take many months and occasionally more than a year. In the series reported by Roux et al. (1991), only four of 26 patients with intraocular hemorrhage associated with a subarachnoid bleed required a vitrectomy, and only one was left with ocular sequelae. In some patients, however, particularly those with severe, bilateral hemorrhage or in visually immature children with severe, unilateral hemorrhage, early vitrectomy may be indicated to provide vision to the patient during recovery from the neurologic event, or, in the case of a child, to prevent amblyopia (Oyakawa et al., 1983; van Rens et al., 1983; Werry and Brewitt, 1983; Turss, 1984; Turut et al., 1984; Weingeist et al., 1986; Espinasse-Berrod et al., 1988; Huber et al., 1988; Ohkubo et al., 1996). Even when vitreous hemorrhage clears completely, some patients are left with poor central vision because of macular damage. Macular abnormalities seen after clearing of vitreous hemorrhage include pigmentary disturbance, scarring, hole, retinoschisis, and epiretinal membrane (Fahmy, 1972b; Shaw and Landers, 1975; Carruthers and Blach, 1976; Clarkson et al., 1980; Sourdille et al., 1980; van Rens et al., 1983; Weingeist et al., 1986; Ohkubo et al., 1996) (Fig. 53.52). Proliferative vitreoretinopathy with associated retinal detachment may also occur in such patients. Daus et al. (1992) described three patients with Terson's syndrome. Failure to clear and rebleed at 5 months lead to bilateral vitrectomies. The patients then developed bilateral focal proliferative vitreoretinopathy (PVR) and retinal tears requiring reoperation for detachment. Velikay et al. (1994) reported PVR in five eyes of four patients following vitreous hemorrhage associated with aneurysmal bleeds, and Ohkubo et al. (1996) reported one case of PVR among eight eyes of seven patients with Terson's syndrome who underwent vitrectomy.

The mechanism by which subarachnoid and intracranial hemorrhage produce intraocular (and particularly vitreous) hemorrhage is somewhat controversial. One of the earliest beliefs was that blood from the subarachnoid space was forced through the optic nerve sheath until it passed through the lamina cribrosa into the eye (Doubler and Marlow, 1917; Symonds, 1923; Riddoch and Goulden, 1925; Robertson, 1936; Vanderlinden and Chisholm, 1974). Pathologic studies do not support this concept. There is no direct connection between the subarachnoid space and the vitreous cavity in normal eyes (Anderson, 1970). In addition, intraocular hemorrhages occur in cases where there is no blood in the optic nerve sheaths (Walsh and Hedges, 1951—see below).

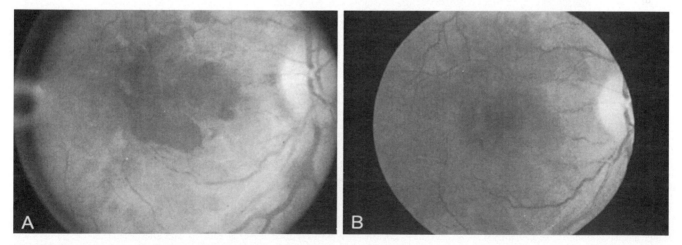

Figure 53.52. Permanent macular damage after macular hemorrhage caused by aneurysmal subarachnoid hemorrhage. *A*, Immediately after the subarachnoid hemorrhage, there is extensive hemorrhage in the posterior pole of the right eye. The macula is obscured by intraretinal hemorrhage, and visual acuity is 20/200. *B*, After clearing of the hemorrhage, visual acuity improved to only 20/80 because of macular pigmentary changes and scarring related to the hemorrhage.

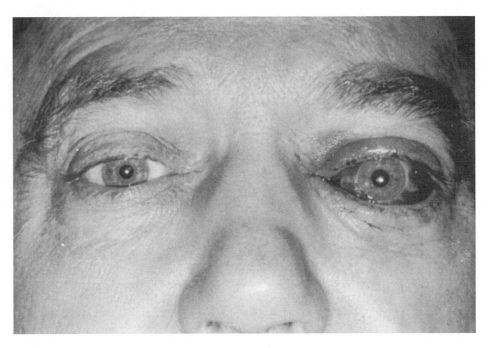

Figure 53.53. Orbital and diffuse subconjunctival hemorrhage in a patient with an acute subarachnoid hemorrhage from an internal carotid-posterior communicating artery aneurysm. Note that the left eye is proptotic, the left eyelid is slightly swollen, and the left pupil is larger than the right.

A second hypothesis is that intraocular hemorrhage results from sudden retinal venous hypertension consequent to transmission of increased ICP to the orbital veins; however, Hayreh (1964) was unable to produce hemorrhagic retinopathy by simply ligating the central retinal vein at its exit from the optic nerve. It therefore is likely that for retinal venous hypertension and intraocular hemorrhage to occur, the central retinal vein must be obstructed before it communicates with the superior ophthalmic vein and with retinochoroidal anastomoses (Muller and Deck, 1974; Kahn and Frenkel, 1975).

A third hypothesis, which most investigators favor, is that the massive and rapid increase in ICP that occurs when an aneurysm ruptures and SAH occurs is transmitted along the optic nerve sheaths. This pressure exceeds the pressure within the central retinal vein, occluding the vein where it traverses the intraorbital portion of the subarachnoid space after exiting the optic nerve about 10 mm behind the eye. The increased pressure also occludes normal retinochoroidal anastomotic channels within the eye. Occlusion of the retinochoroidal channels and the central retinal vein reduces venous drainage from the eye. This reduced venous drainage stresses the intraocular veins, causing them to rupture (Miller and Cuttino, 1948; Manschot and Hampe, 1950; Fox, 1983; Weingeist et al., 1986; Toosi and Malton, 1987).

A **hyphema** (hemorrhage into the anterior chamber of the eye) occasionally occurs in patients who experience an SAH. In such cases, deposition of hemosiderin in the iris stroma may turn its color to brown, resulting in hyperchromia iridis.

Subconjunctival hemorrhage occasionally occurs in patients after SAH (Cucco, 1951; Bisland and Topilow, 1952). According to Heck (1961), subconjunctival hemorrhages that occur in the setting of acute SAH generally are small and punctate, but they can be diffuse on one or both sides of the bulbar conjunctiva usually near the limbus (Fig. 53.53).

Optic nerve sheath hemorrhage may occur in association with SAH (Figs. 53.54–53.58). Although it cannot be identified with the ophthalmoscope, it may be as common as, or more common than, intraocular hemorrhage. White (1895) thought that the blood found within the optic nerve sheaths after SAH had extended from the subarachnoid space through the optic canal. Riddoch and Goulden (1925) agreed that this could occur; however, Ballantyne (1943) thought that hemorrhages in the optic nerve sheaths were independent phenomena related to sudden increased ICP. Walsh and Hedges (1951) serially sectioned the optic nerves in eight cases of spontaneous intracranial hemorrhage and demonstrated that **blood in the sheaths was not continuous with blood in the intracranial subarachnoid space** (see also Huber et al., 1988). They also noted that optic nerve sheath hemorrhages may be subdural, subarachnoid, or both (Fig. 53.57). Subdural hemorrhage was seen more commonly around the proximal portion of the optic nerve adjacent to the eye, whereas SAH seemed to occur more frequently around the portion of the optic nerve near the orbital end of the optic canal. Walsh and Hedges (1951) concluded that **rupture of veins, not transmission of subarachnoid blood, is the predominant source of optic nerve sheath blood,** both in the optic canal and in the orbit. They and others postulated that rupture results from transmission of increased venous pressure from intracranial veins to orbital veins. The small veins of the optic nerve sheaths seem to be particularly vulnerable to rapid increases in orbital venous pressure be-

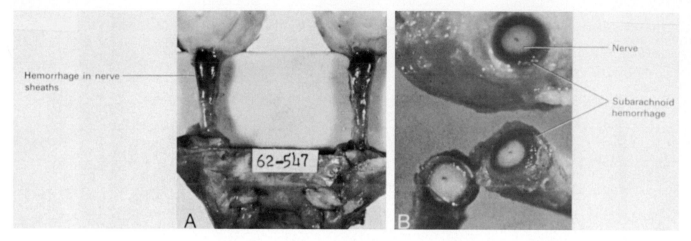

Figure 53.54. Hemorrhage into the optic nerve sheaths in a patient with an acute subarachnoid hemorrhage. *A,* Gross appearance of the intraorbital segments of both optic nerves shows swollen, hemorrhagic nerve sheaths. *B,* Cross-section of one of these nerves shows diffuse subarachnoid hemorrhage surrounding the nerve. (From Lindenberg R, Walsh FB, Sacks JG. Neuropathology of Vision: An Atlas. Philadelphia, Lea & Febiger, 1973.)

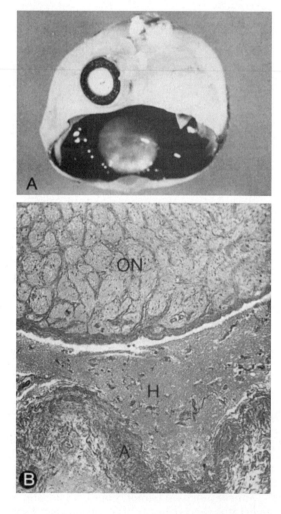

Figure 53.55. Diffuse subarachnoid hemorrhage surrounding the optic nerve in a patient with acute aneurysmal subarachnoid hemorrhage. *A,* Optic nerve cut in cross-section reveals dilated trabeculae of the subarachnoid space filled with hemorrhage. *B,* Histopathologic appearance of nerve shows hemorrhage in the subarachnoid space. *ON,* optic nerve; *A,* thickened arachnoid and dura; *H,* hemorrhage.

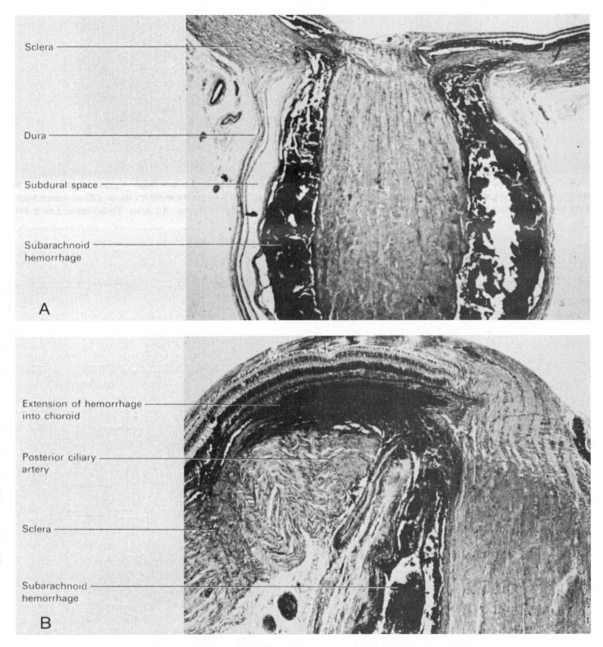

Figure 53.56. Histopathologic appearance of optic nerve sheath hemorrhage. *A,* Longitudinal section through the orbital portion of the optic nerve in a patient with acute subarachnoid hemorrhage shows extensive hemorrhage in the subarachnoid space surrounding the optic nerve. The subdural space is free of blood. *B,* In another section from the same eye, hemorrhage can be seen to extend into the choroid. (From Lindenberg R, Walsh FB, Sacks JG. Neuropathology of Vision: An Atlas. Philadelphia, Lea & Febiger, 1973.)

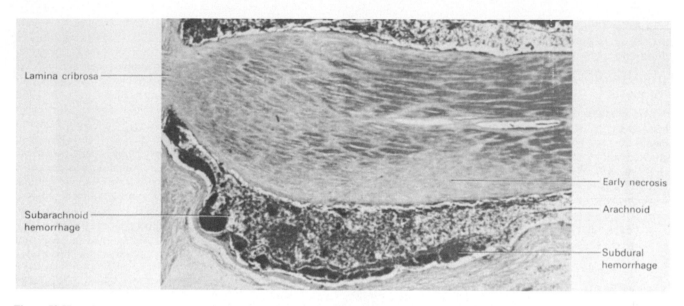

Figure 53.57. Histopathologic appearance of optic nerve sheath hemorrhage. There is both subarachnoid and subdural hemorrhage, and there is early necrosis of the optic nerve. (From Lindenberg R, Walsh FB, Sacks JG. Neuropathology of Vision: An Atlas. Philadelphia, Lea & Febiger, 1973.)

cause their walls within the vaginal spaces are relatively unsupported (Ikui and Mimatsu, 1961; Ikui et al., 1967).

Hemorrhage within the optic nerve may occur in the form of pial, septal, or interfascicular hemorrhage after SAH (Ballantyne, 1943; Walsh and Hedges, 1951; Ikui and Mimatsu, 1961; Huber et al., 1988) (Fig. 53.59). Nerve fibers adjacent to the hemorrhages may subsequently undergo demyelination. Some of these hemorrhages may be responsible for the sudden monocular blurring of vision experienced by some patients with acute SAH from a ruptured intracranial aneurysm.

Papilledema occurs in many, but not all, cases of increased ICP, regardless of cause (see Chapter 10). It not infrequently develops in patients after rupture of an intracranial aneurysm (Figs. 53.48 and 53.60). Riise (1969) observed

papilledema in 18 of 100 patients (18%) who experienced SAH from rupture of an intracranial aneurysm. Fahmy (1972c) studied 192 patients with ruptured intracranial aneurysm and found papilledema in 32 (16%). The papilledema did not vary significantly by age, sex, or site of the aneurysm. In seven patients, the disc swelling was unilateral. It was on the same side as the aneurysm in six of these patients. Other investigators reported a 10–24% prevalence of papilledema in patients with ruptured intracranial aneurysm (Griffith et al., 1938; Dandy, 1944; Manschot, 1944; Krayenbühl and Yaşargil, 1958). According to Uhthoff (1914) and to Tureen (1939), papilledema may develop within hours after the onset of SAH, although in many cases it appears only after several days to weeks (Paton, 1924; Hamby, 1952). In almost all cases, SAH produces papilledema either by blocking CSF

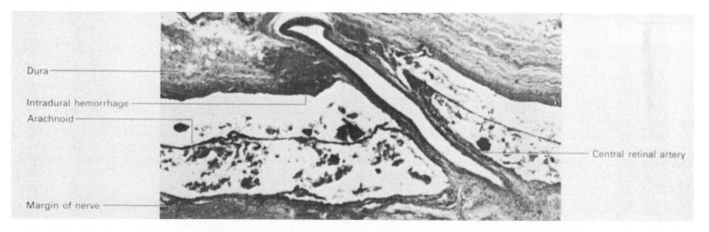

Figure 53.58. Compression of the central retinal artery by subarachnoid and subdural hemorrhage surrounding the optic nerve. The artery is compressed as it crosses the subarachnoid space to become intraneural. Damage to the vessel at this point may produce permanent visual loss from retinal ischemia. (From Lindenberg R, Walsh FB, Sacks JG. Neuropathology of Vision: An Atlas. Philadelphia, Lea & Febiger, 1973.)

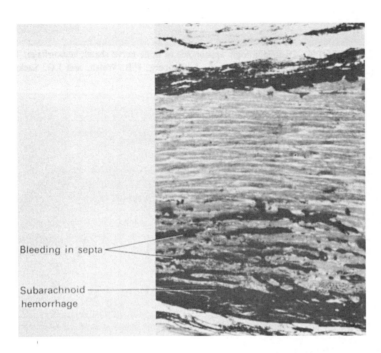

Bleeding in septa

Subarachnoid
hemorrhage

Figure 53.59. Hemorrhage within the optic nerve in the setting of acute subarachnoid hemorrhage. Longitudinal section through the optic nerve in a patient with acute subarachnoid hemorrhage shows not only subarachnoid hemorrhage surrounding the optic nerve but also hemorrhage within the optic nerve itself. (From Lindenberg R, Walsh FB, Sacks JG. Neuropathology of Vision: An Atlas. Philadelphia, Lea & Febiger, 1973.)

flow within the ventricular system or by impeding CSF absorption at the arachnoid villi. It is most likely to occur when there is intraventricular hemorrhage, coexistent systemic hypertension, venous sinus thrombosis, or a large aneurysm that, in addition to rupturing, exerts a mass effect (Griffith et al., 1938). Mori et al. (1990) reported a 55-year-old woman with the sudden onset of motor aphasia and right hemiparesis. Neurologic examination on admission revealed a drowsy state, bilateral papilledema, motor aphasia, and right hemiparesis. CT scanning showed a subcortical hematoma in the left frontoparietal region associated with perifocal edema. Left carotid angiography revealed a fusiform aneurysm at a peripheral branch of the central artery. Surgery demonstrated the aneurysm to be due to metastatic choriocarcinoma.

Intracerebral Hemorrhage Associated with Aneurysmal Rupture

Approximately 20% of all massive nontraumatic intracerebral hemorrhages are caused by ruptured intracranial aneurysms (Masson and Day, 1992). In a study of 512 patients with aneurysmal SAH, Tokuda et al. (1995) documented intracerebral hemorrhage in 98 (19%). The incidence was higher with aneurysms of the distal anterior and middle cerebral arteries. These patients also had a poorer prognosis. There was a 22% incidence of rebleed, compared with 14% in the patients without an intracerebral hematoma. In addition, patients with an intracerebral hematoma had a worse clinical grade at the time of admission (see Table 53.2). The size of the intracerebral bleed correlated with poorer

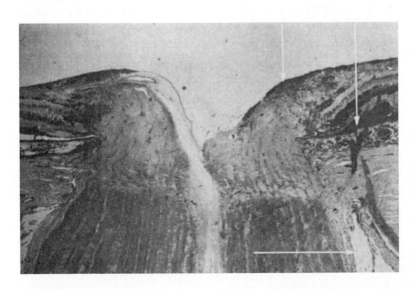

Figure 53.60. Papilledema with both intraretinal and subretinal hemorrhage after a fatal subarachnoid hemorrhage. Note blood on the surface of the optic disc (*short vertical arrow*) and in the subretinal space (*long vertical arrow*). In this specimen, no blood is present in the subarachnoid or subdural spaces surrounding the optic nerve (*horizontal arrow*). (Courtesy of Dr. Richard Lindenberg.)

Table 53.2
Clinical Grading Scales for Subarachnoid Hemorrhage

Grade	Botterell and Colleagues	Hunt and Hess	World Federation of Neurologic Surgeons Glasgow Coma Scale	World Federation of Neurologic Surgeons Motor Deficit
1	Conscious with or without signs of blood in the subarachnoid space	Asymptomatic or minimal headache and slight nuchal rigidity	15	No
2	Drowsy without significant neurologic deficit	Moderate to severe headache, nuchal rigidity, no neurologic deficit other than cranial nerve palsy	13 to 14	No
3	Drowsy with neurologic deficit and probably intracerebral clot	Drowsiness, confusion, or mild focal deficit	13 to 14	Yes
4	Major neurologic deficit and deteriorating due to large intracerebral clot or older patients with less severe neurologic deficit but pre-existing cerebrovascular disease	Stupor, moderate to severe hemiparesis, possible early decerebrate rigidity and vegetative disturbances	7 to 12	No or Yes
5	Moribund or near moribund with failing vital centers and extensor rigidity	Deep coma, decerebrate rigidity, moribund appearance	3 to 6	No or Yes

outcome. Larger aneurysms were associated with a higher incidence of intracerebral hemorrhage (Rosenorn and Eskesen, 1994). The higher frequency of rebleeds in patients with ICH was also noted by Fujii et al. (1996). Intracerebral hematoma did not, however, carry the same ominous prognosis as intraventricular hemorrhage (see below). Only two of 13 patients reported by Schievink et al. (1995a) who experienced sudden death had evidence of an intracerebral hemorrhage, compared with 12 of 13 who had evidence of intraventricular hemorrhage.

The increased incidence of intracerebral hematoma (42%) associated with MCA aneurysms was confirmed by Rinne et al. (1996). The position of the aneurysm on the wall of the artery often determines the location of the intracerebral hematoma (Hosoda et al., 1995). Of aneurysms on the M-1 segment, for example, superior wall aneurysms tend to produce frontal lobe hematomas, whereas aneurysms arising from the inferior wall rupture into the temporal lobe.

Fujii et al. (1995a) noted a higher concentration of thrombin-antithrombin complex formation in patients with intracerebral hemorrhages. Whether or not this plays a pathophysiologic role is unclear, but it may well serve as an additional marker.

Intracerebral hemorrhage is also associated with ruptured dissecting aneurysms (Guridi et al., 1993) (see below). Miscellaneous conditions increase the risk of rupture and secondary intracerebral hemorrhage, including metastatic choriocarcinoma (Giannakopoulos et al., 1992; Gallo et al., 1993), SLE (Orita et al., 1992), and mycotic aneurysms associated with endocarditis (Yoshida et al., 1990; Masuda et al., 1992). Intracerebral hemorrhage may result in an increased risk of seizure activity (Bidzinski et al., 1995).

Intraventricular Hemorrhage Associated with Aneurysmal Rupture

Isolated intraventricular hemorrhage only rarely occurs after rupture of an intracranial aneurysm (Irikura et al.,

1990); however, when an intracranial aneurysm is located within or adjacent to the ventricular system, rupture may lead to both subarachnoid and intraventricular hemorrhage. This is particularly true of aneurysms in the posterior fossa, especially those arising from the vertebral artery (Andoh et al., 1992a) and the PICA (Uranishi et al., 1994; Urbach et al., 1995; Kojima et al., 1996), which often rupture into the 4th ventricle. PCA aneurysms can also cause intraventricular hemorrhage (Orita et al., 1992). Among anterior circulation aneurysms, aneurysms of the anterior choroidal artery are most likely to rupture produce intraventricular hemorrhage (Caram et al., 1960; Butler et al., 1972; Papo et al., 1973; Nishihara et al., 1993). Rupture of an aneurysm on a thalamostriate artery may also lead to an intraventricular hemorrhage (Bergsneider et al., 1994), potentially within the 3rd ventricle, intraventricular blood also occurs in association with moyamoya disease (Chen et al., 1993; J. Hamada et al., 1994). Toxemia of pregnancy (Bisland and Topilow, 1952) may predispose to aneurysmal intraventricular blood; however, because hypertension is one of the leading causes of intraventricular hemorrhage (Stula and Sigstein, 1993), the true pathophysiology in this setting is unclear.

Patients with intraventricular hemorrhage have a guarded prognosis. This is particularly true when aneurysmal rupture is associated with blood within the 4th ventricle. Shapiro et al. (1994) reported that all 28 patients who had a dilated 4th ventricle following hemorrhage eventually died. Prognosis was slightly better if the 4th ventricle was not dilated, although the mortality was still 41%. Among 200 patients with intraventricular hemorrhage, survival when associated with aneurysmal rupture was 35%, compared with 76% survival when associated with angioma and 8% when no cause could be determined (Donauer et al., 1993). In reviewing population records, Schievink et al. (1995a) were able to identify 13 of 113 patients who died before receiving medical attention. Intraventicular hemorrhage was present in 12 of these 13 patients (92%).

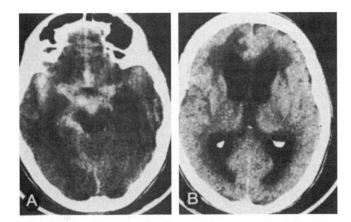

Figure 53.61. Hydrocephalus after aneurysmal subarachnoid hemorrhage. The patient was a 69-year-old woman who experienced an acute subarachnoid hemorrhage from rupture of an internal carotid-posterior communicating artery aneurysm. The aneurysm was clipped 2 days after the hemorrhage. She initially began to recover but subsequently became confused and lethargic. *A*, Unenhanced CT scan performed before surgery shows diffuse hemorrhage in the basal cisterns. Both temporal horns are dilated, indicating acute hydrocephalus. *B*, CT scan performed about 4 weeks after hemorrhage shows complete clearing of subarachnoid blood, but there is diffuse ventricular enlargement. Note periventricular lucenies and rounding of the frontal horns indicating interstitial edema. The patient improved after a ventriculoperitoneal shunt.

Hydrocephalus After Rupture of Intracranial Aneurysm

Non-communicating (obstructive) hydrocephalus, unrelated to the acute rise in ICP that accompanies rupture of an intracranial aneurysm, may develop days to weeks after a massive SAH (Fig. 53.61). When it develops within several days of the hemorrhage, it seems to be related to the presence of intraventricular blood, rather than to the extent of cisternal hemorrhage (van Gijn et al., 1985; Milhorat, 1987). Hydrocephalus that develops 1–6 weeks after SAH is usually caused by arachnoid adhesions at the base of the brain as a result of the inflammatory response to extravasated blood (Schutz et al., 1980) (Fig. 53.62). The adhesions block the CSF pathways sufficiently to cause increased ICP with ventricular dilation. Blockage of arachnoid villi by extravasated blood may be a contributing factor in such cases (Shulman et al., 1963).

In a retrospective study of 105 patients following SAH, Mehta et al. (1996) noted hydrocephalus in 31%. Hydrocephalus was diagnosed when the bicaudate index was greater than the 95th percentile for age on a CT scan within 72 hours of the ictus. The grade of SAH (and therefore the amount of subarachnoid blood) (see Table 53.1) was a significant factor for the development of acute hydrocephalus. Of patients with acute hydrocephalus, 87% (29/32) presented with at least Hunt and Hess grade III (Hunt and Hess, 1968) SAH. In addition, posterior circulation aneurysms were more often associated with acute hydrocephalus. Both premorbid hypertension and intraventricular blood were predictors for acute hydrocephalus, whereas intracisternal blood, age, and

sex were not. External ventricular drainage was not associated with any instances of rebleeding. Ten of twenty-seven (37%) patients with acute hydrocephalus who survived were improved by preoperative external ventricular drainage.

Deterioration associated with hydrocephalus occurred in 22% of patients (143 of 660) followed for 28 days after the initial hemorrhage (Vermeij et al., 1994). In a multivariate analysis, cisternal blood, ventricular blood, and hydrocephalus on initial CT scanning, as well as long-term treatment with tranexamic acid were significantly related to the development and progression of hydrocephalus. The incidence of hydrocephalus requiring shunt procedures increased with cisternal drainage (Moriyama et al., 1995c). Rajshekhar and Harbaugh (1992) found a hydrocephalus incidence of 27% (52 of 194 consecutive patients). All patients were treated with ventriculostomy. Within 24 hours of CSF drainage, 26 patients improved. Seventeen of these patients subsequently underwent surgery, nine of whom did well. All 18 patients who did not improve within this period, including one who worsened, died. In eight patients, the response to ventriculos-

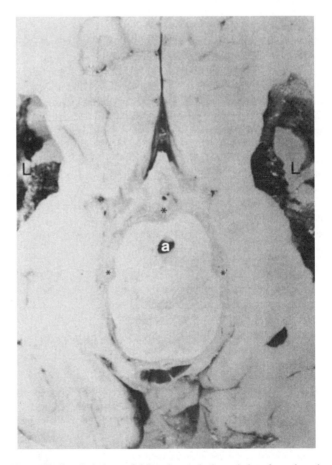

Figure 53.62. Pathology of delayed onset hydrocephalus after subarachnoid hemorrhage. The ambient cistern is obliterated by dense fibrous tissue (*asterisks*). Despite ventriculoperitoneal shunting, the lateral ventricles (*L*) and cerebral aqueduct (*a*) remain dilated. (From Schutz H, Fleming JFR, Humphreys RP, et al. Normal pressure hydrocephalus—High pressure normocephalus. Can J Neurosci 7:211–219, 1980.)

tomy was considered as undetermined because of the proximity of the drain insertion to a definitive surgical procedure. Nevertheless, all of these patients had an excellent outcome. More aggressive use of ventricular drainage can, however, be associated with a higher risk of aneurysmal rebleed (Pare et al., 1992). Rebleed during drainage occurred in seven patients (14%) in the series reported by Rajshekhar and Harbaugh (1992).

The importance of hydrocephalus in the late prognosis of a patient who experiences an aneurysmal SAH cannot be overemphasized. Miller (1991b) described a 63-year-old woman who experienced an acute SAH from rupture of an internal carotid-posterior communicating aneurysm. When the patient was examined in the hospital about 1 week after clipping of the aneurysm, her examination was normal except for a complete oculomotor nerve paresis. She was alert, and her mental status seemed entirely normal. She was discharged from the hospital about 1 week later. About 6 weeks later (8 weeks after hemorrhage), the patient returned for an examination. At that time, she seemed unusually quiet and somewhat confused. Her daughter agreed and stated that this change in personality had begun several weeks earlier and seemed to be worsening. The patient was not eating well, nor did she seem to be concerned about her appearance. Her neurosurgeon thought she was "depressed." A CT scan showed mildly enlarged ventricles unchanged from those seen on a scan that was performed just before discharge from the hospital. Nevertheless, after the patient's condition was discussed at length with her neurosurgeon, the neurosurgeon agreed to tap her ventricular system and to perform a shunt procedure if necessary. The patient's ICP was found to be markedly elevated, and a ventriculoperitoneal shunt was performed. Within 1 week after the shunt, the patient's mental status returned to normal and remained so over the next 5 years.

Patients with this type of hydrocephalus usually do not develop papilledema. When they do, however, it may be sufficiently severe to cause secondary optic atrophy with irreversible visual loss if the increased ICP is not treated immediately.

Hydrocephalus may arise from aneurysmal or intracerebral hematoma obstructing ventricular outflow. This may occur at the foramen of Monro (Goetz et al., 1990), at the cerebral aqueduct, or at the foramina of Luschka and Magendie. Smith et al. (1994) reported a giant posterior communicating artery aneurysm that obstructed the 3rd ventricle, although more commonly, the aneurysms that obstruct the 3rd ventricle arise from the basilar artery or one of its branches (Goetz et al., 1990).

Subdural Hematoma from Ruptured Intracranial Aneurysm

Most intracranial aneurysms rupture into the subarachnoid space, into the substance of the brain, or both. In rare cases, however, an aneurysm ruptures into the subdural space (Bassett and Lemmen, 1950; Clarke and Walton, 1953; Strang et al., 1961; Reichenthal et al., 1986; Jaksche et al., 1988; Kondziolka et al., 1988; Watanabe et al., 1991; Kamiya et al., 1991; Ranganadham et al., 1992; Rusyniak et al., 1992; Ragland et al., 1993; Hatayama et al., 1994; Hubert, 1994; O'Sullivan et al., 1994b; Sanchez et al., 1994; Smith and Castillo, 1995; McLaughlin et al., 1996) (Fig. 53.63) with little or no subarachnoid blood. Kamiya et al. (1991) recognized subdural hematoma in 15 of 484 cases of aneurysmal SAH. Sanchez et al. (1994) postulated that prior local hemorrhage led to scarring and adhesions that permitted access to the subdural space. Aneurysms that produce subdural hemorrhage most often arise from the distal segment of the ACA (Kamiya et al., 1991; Watanabe et al., 1991; Hatayama et al., 1994); however, they may arise from any vessel, particularly those at the base of the skull (McLaughlin et al., 1996). Ranjan and Joseph (1994) reported the unusual case of a giant aneurysm of the anterior ethmoid artery that produced a frontal intraparenchymal and subdural hemorrhage. Aoki et al. (1992) published the case of a posttraumatic subdural hematoma related to the rupture of a false aneurysm of the middle menin-

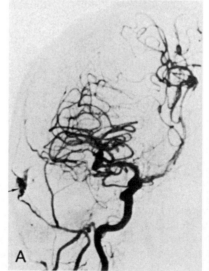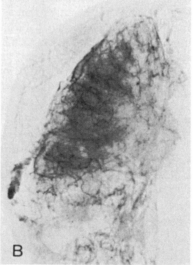

Figure 53.63. Acute subdural hematoma from rupture of an intracranial aneurysm. *A*, Common carotid angiogram, anteroposterior view, shows an aneurysm of the middle meningeal artery (*arrow*) and an associated acute subdural hematoma that compresses the peripheral branches of the middle cerebral artery and causes a right to left shift of the middle and anterior cerebral arteries. *B*, The late arterial phase of the angiogram shows displacement of the cerebral vessels away from the inner table of the skull, indicating that the surface of the hemisphere is displaced by the hematoma. The aneurysm remains opacified. (From Huber P. Cerebral Angiography, 2nd ed. New York, Georg Thieme Verlag, 1982.)

geal artery. The rupture occurred 28 days after the injury. One of two patients reported with SLE and intracranial aneurysms by Sakaki et al. (1990) had a subdural hematoma at the time of her bleed. Kanaya et al. (1993) described a subdural hematoma associated with rupture of a mycotic aneurysm in a patient with endocarditis following mitral valve replacement. The patient was anticoagulated at the time of the hemorrhage. In addition, Kohno et al. (1996) described a patient who experienced a subdural hemorrhage from an aneurysm that developed at the site of an EC-IC bypass.

The clinical picture of an aneurysmal subdural hematoma is usually one of acute, rapidly progressive neurologic deterioration associated with signs of uncal herniation. When treatment of both the hematoma and the aneurysm is undertaken rapidly (within a few hours of signs of uncal herniation), the outcome may be excellent (Reichenthal et al., 1986). Failure to intervene has dire consequences (Watanabe et al., 1991). All eight patients who were not operated in the series reported by Kamiya et al. (1991) died. In rare cases, the clinical picture is that of a typical chronic subdural hematoma and is characterized by slowly progressive mental deterioration and neurologic dysfunction (Hirashima et al., 1981; Sonobe et al., 1981; Koga, 1985; Jaksche et al., 1988). Such patients have an excellent prognosis if the correct diagnosis is made and both the hematoma and the aneurysm are successfully treated.

It is possible for a subdural hematoma that occurs in a patient with a ruptured intracranial aneurysm to be secondarily related. Mori et al. (1995) reported the case of a 52-year-old man with a subarachnoid and subdural hemorrhage associated with a ruptured MCA aneurysm. The subdural hemorrhage was found to be associated with a fracture in the region of the lambdoid suture. It was postulated that the patient experienced an acute SAH from rupture of the MCA aneurysm. He lost consciousness and fell, striking his head and sustaining the fracture, which led to the subdural hematoma.

CLINICAL MANIFESTATIONS ACCORDING TO SITE

The natural history of an aneurysm is related to its location. For example, aneurysms of the anterior communicating artery almost always become symptomatic when they rupture and only occasionally produce signs of a mass lesion. Aneurysms of the cavernous portion of the ICA, however, routinely produce ocular motor nerve pareses and rarely bleed. When they do, a carotid-cavernous fistula is more common than SAH. Aneurysms located at the junction of the internal carotid and posterior communicating arteries are just as likely to rupture and produce SAH as they are to enlarge and produce an oculomotor nerve paresis.

In the section that follows, we discuss the clinical manifestations of unruptured aneurysms that originate from the carotid and vertebrobasilar arterial systems. It should be noted that it is often impossible to identify a single artery of origin of a saccular aneurysm, because most of these lesions arise at the junction of two arteries. Therefore, we identify as originating from a specific artery only those aneurysms that arise from a nonjunctional location. All other aneurysms are designated as originating from a specific junctional location; e.g., the junction between the internal carotid and ophthalmic arteries (carotid-ophthalmic artery aneurysms).

Aneurysms Arising from the Internal Carotid Artery and its Branches

Aneurysms Arising from the Extracranial Portion of the Internal Carotid Artery

Although this chapter is mainly concerned with intracranial aneurysms, extracranial aneurysms may arise from any of the major arteries in the neck and produce neuro-ophthalmologic manifestations. Saccular aneurysms originating from the extracranial portion of the ICA usually present as a mass in the neck (Unal et al., 1992; Kindl et al., 1993; Tertel et al., 1993; Weissman et al., 1994; Halloul et al., 1995) or lateral nasopharynx (Fig. 53.64). Although these may be pulsatile, that is not always the case. Most do not produce neurologic symptoms or signs (Ambler et al., 1967; Margolis et al., 1972; McCollum et al., 1979; Schechter, 1979a, 1979b; Mokri et al., 1982; Trippel et al., 1982; Weir, 1987). Liapis et al. (1994), however, reported a history of TIAs in 11 of 12 patients with extracranial ICA aneurysms, Rosset et al. (1994) reported focal neurologic symptoms in nine of 13 patients (including two with ocular symptoms), and Moreau et al. (1994) documented signs of cerebral ischemia in 26 of 38 (74%) patients. TIAs occurred in five of 18 patients reported by Sahlman et al. (1991) and in nine of 24 patients (37%) in a series reported by Faggioli et al. (1996).

Symptoms and signs produced by saccular aneurysms of the extracranial portion of the ICA include pain in the ipsilateral throat, face, or neck, bruit, difficulty swallowing, and paresis of the lower cranial nerves, particularly the glossopharyngeal, vagus, and accessory nerves. Additionally, Horner's syndrome, usually postganglionic, may occur (Margolis et al., 1972; Schechter 1979a, 1979b; Murthy and Naidu, 1988). Davis et al. (1968) described a patient with a left Horner's syndrome and ipsilateral hemicranial headache who was found to have an extracranial saccular aneurysm arising from the left ICA near the base of the skull. It is unclear if the aneurysm was responsible for the patient's symptoms and signs or was an asymptomatic, coincidental lesion in a patient with Raeder's syndrome (Raeder, 1924; see Chapters 24 and 36). Rarely, hypoglossal dysfunction may be associated with an aneurysm affecting the cervical portion of the ICA (Nusynowitz and Stricof, 1990).

TIAs or stroke may result from emboli originating from an ICA aneurysm or from thrombosis of the ICA at the site of the aneurysm (Gros et al., 1970; Margolis et al., 1972; Mokri et al., 1982). Insight into the possible source of emboli in these patients was provided by Spiegel et al. (1994), who demonstrated a free-floating thrombus by ultrasound in a 90-year-old woman with such an aneurysm. Such patients may also experience transient or permanent visual loss from retinal or optic nerve ischemia (Mokri and Piepgras, 1981) (Fig. 53.65). Dr. William Hoyt (Walsh and Hoyt, 1969c) examined an 8-year-old boy who had a 2 × 4 cm aneurysm of the extracranial portion of the ICA associated with congenital absence of the basilar artery. The child had suddenly become comatose and quadriparetic. When he recovered consciousness, he had spasticity of all extremities, right peripheral facial paresis, right one-and-a-half syndrome (com-

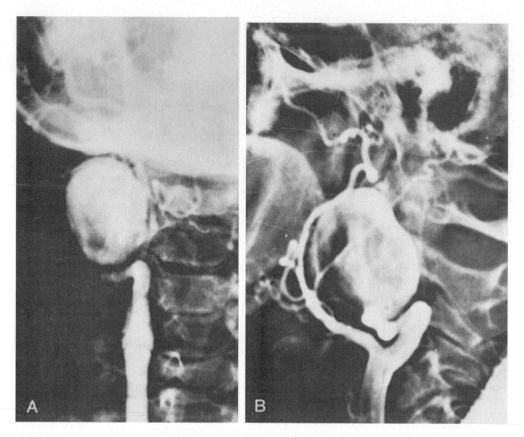

Figure 53.64.   Saccular aneurysms of the cervical portion of the internal carotid artery. *A*, A large oval sac fills with contrast material from the internal carotid artery at the level of C3. The artery deviates laterally around the aneurysm as it courses cranially. The patient had been aware of a fullness in the neck for many years, but only shortly before admission for the angiogram had she appreciated a mass in the neck. *B*, In another case, a very large saccular aneurysm arises from the distal cervical internal carotid artery at the C2 and C3 vertebral levels. The patient had noted a slowly enlarging, pulsatile mass in the neck for many years but had no other symptoms. (From Taveras JM, Wood EH. Diagnostic Radiology, 2nd ed, Vol 2. Baltimore, Williams & Wilkins, 1976.)

plete right horizontal gaze paralysis and right INO—see Chapter 29), and vestibular nystagmus on left or upward gaze. Thrombosis within the aneurysm was thought to have reduced the blood flow to the brainstem, which was being supplied by the carotid vessels in the absence of a basilar artery.

Otolaryngologic symptoms and signs may occur in patients with saccular aneurysms of the extracranial portion of the ICA, because these aneurysms tend to compress or erode into the oropharynx, nasopharynx, or external auditory canal. Patients in whom this occurs may complain of difficulty swallowing (Rowe and Hosni, 1994), hearing, or breathing. They may hear a popping sound when they swallow, and they may experience otorrhagia, epistaxis, and recurrent or chronic otitis (Alexander et al. 1966). Extracranial carotid artery aneurysms may rarely be associated with intracranial aneurysms (Kubo et al., 1992; Tokimura et al., 1992).

Extracranial pseudoaneurysms of the carotid may be related to trauma, or they may occur following surgery or radiation therapy (Minion et al., 1994; Tanaka et al., 1995). They may also develop in patients with FMD (Miyauchi and Shionoya, 1991; Bour et al., 1992; Manninen et al., 1997)

and Ehlers-Danlos syndrome. Bilateral extracranial carotid artery aneurysms can occur (Y. Hamada et al., 1994), and aneurysms in the neck may occasionally arise from branches of the external carotid artery (Anand et al., 1993; Lewis and Lampe, 1993; Minion et al., 1994). Such aneurysms cause some of the same manifestations as ICA aneurysms.

Aneurysms Arising from the Petrous Portion of the Internal Carotid Artery

Most of these aneurysms arise from the lateral aspect of the ICA within the petrous portion of the temporal bone (Anderson et al., 1972; Halbach et al., 1990b) (Fig. 53.66). Aneurysms involving the petrous may also originate below the skull base (Hazarika et al., 1993). Aneurysms within the petrous bone produce a variety of rhinologic, ophthalmologic, and neurologic disturbances that are indistinguishable from those caused by tumors at the base of the skull, particularly paragangliomas of the glomus jugulare (Glassock et al., 1983; Mann et al., 1988) (see Chapter 46). When the aneurysm is relatively small, it may produce hearing loss, tinnitus, or both. There may be otorrhagia (Umezu et al., 1993) or otorrhea. With continued enlargement of the aneu-

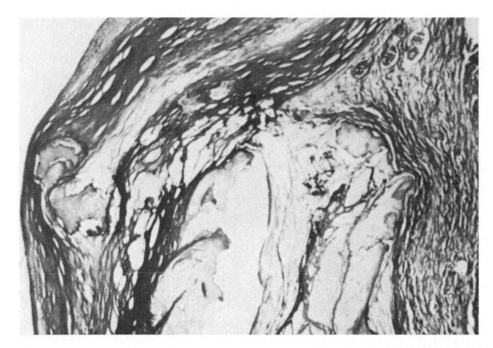

Figure 53.65. Part of the wall of an aneurysm of the extracranial portion of the internal carotid artery. Atherosclerotic changes with large deposits of lipid and calcium can be seen. The patient presented with loss of vision in the ipsilateral eye and had a calcific embolus in the inferior temporal retinal branch artery. (From Mokri B, Piepgras DG. Cervical internal carotid artery aneurysm with calcific embolism to the retina. Neurology *31*:211–214, 1981.)

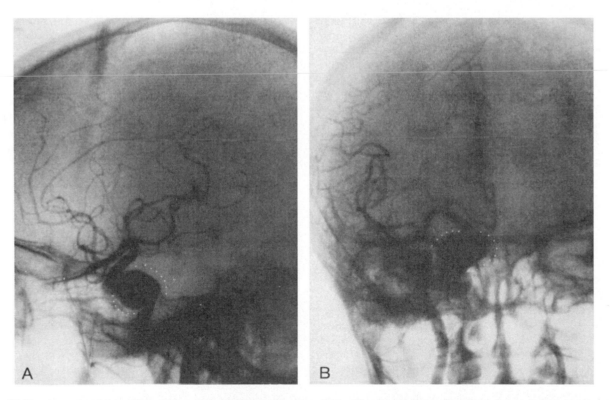

Figure 53.66. Aneurysm of the petrous portion of the internal carotid artery arising within the carotid canal. *A*, Lateral view; *B*, Anteroposterior view.

rysm, both the vestibulocochlear and facial nerves may become compromised, and patients may have both conductive and sensorineural hearing loss, tinnitus, and peripheral facial weakness. Continued enlargement of the aneurysm produces further cranial nerve dysfunction, including ear pain, facial pain or dysesthesia, vertigo, peripheral vestibular nystagmus, loss of pharyngeal sensation, dysphagia, hoarseness, loss of the pharyngeal reflex, weakness of the sternocleidomastoid and trapezius muscles, deviation of the tongue to the opposite side, weakness of abduction of the eye on the side of the aneurysm, and Horner's syndrome (Pecker et al., 1960; Guirguis and Tadros, 1961; Hiranandani et al., 1962; Harrison et al., 1963; Busby et al., 1968; Stallings and McCabe, 1969; Ishikawa et al., 1975; Gupta et al., 1979; Halbach et al., 1990b). Facial pain associated with ipsilateral Horner's syndrome is called **Raeder's paratrigeminal neuralgia** (Raeder, 1924; Grimson and Thompson, 1980) (see Chapter 36). Almost all patients with Raeder's paratrigeminal neuralgia caused by an aneurysm of the petrous portion of the ICA have other neurologic symptoms and signs (Wemple and Smith, 1966), but this is not invariably the case (Walsh and Hoyt, 1969d). Indeed, Wisoff and Flamm (1987) described a patient in whom an isolated Horner's syndrome was caused by an unruptured petrous aneurysm. Similarly, although abducens nerve paresis produced by aneurysm of the petrous portion of the ICA is usually associated with other neurologic symptoms and signs, several authors described patients in whom abducens nerve paresis was the only clinical manifestation of the aneurysm, which was located in the medial portion of the carotid canal (Pecker et al., 1960; Sarwar, 1977).

Conventional angiography remains the gold standard for detection of aneurysms arising from the petrous portion of the ICA. Nevertheless, MR angiography and spiral CT angiography are particularly well suited to identifying these aneurysms (Patrick, 1996).

Aneurysms originating in the intrapetrous segment may grow to giant proportions (Cahill, 1992) at which time they may be very difficult to treat. Rupture of aneurysms of the intrapetrous portion of the ICA may not cause subarachnoid or intracranial hemorrhage. Instead, affected patients may develop acute facial pain and epistaxis (Mann et al., 1988; Banfield et al., 1995). Intrapetrous aneurysms may be readily occluded by balloons (Larson et al., 1995), but the late risks of embolization have led some authors to suggest that revascularization should be performed in such cases (Lawton et al., 1996).

Aneurysms Arising from the Cavernous Portion of the Internal Carotid Artery (Intracavernous Aneurysms)

Aneurysms that arise from the portion of the ICA within the cavernous sinus behave differently from aneurysms originating in any other location within the skull. These aneurysms arise from a large artery as it traverses a venous sinus.

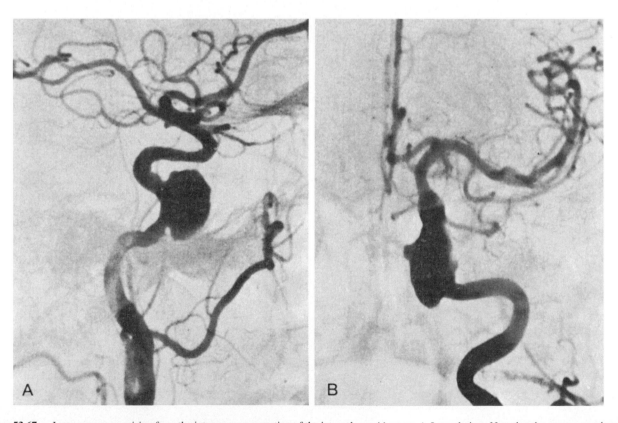

Figure 53.67.   Large aneurysm arising from the intracavernous portion of the internal carotid artery. *A*, Lateral view. Note that the aneurysm arises from the anterior wall of the artery and has a broad neck. *B*, Anteroposterior view.

Such aneurysms may become quite large without rupturing (Fig. 53.67) and indeed without producing any symptoms or signs (Linskey et al., 1990a, 1990b). When they do rupture, they usually rupture into the cavernous sinus, producing a carotid-cavernous sinus fistula (Higashida et al., 1990; Guglielmi et al., 1992a) (see Chapter 54), rather than into the subarachnoid space and basal cistern. Nevertheless, aneurysms that originate from the cavernous sinus may project in such a manner that rupture is associated with SAH (Linskey et al., 1990b; Nishioka et al., 1990; Hayashi et al., 1994; Hamada et al., 1996; Lee et al., 1996), intracerebral hemorrhage (Lin, 1995), or massive subdural hematoma (McLaughlin et al., 1996) followed by transtentorial herniation and death (Barr et al., 1971; Hodes et al., 1988). Cavernous aneurysms that project intradurally were called ''transitional cavernous aneurysms'' by al-Rodhan et al. (1993). Of 23 patients with such aneurysms, 13 (57%) had SAH.

Intracavernous aneurysms comprise only 2–6% of all intracranial aneurysms (Locksley, 1966, 1969; Newton and Potts, 1974; Linskey et al., 1990b) and 3–14% of all aneurysms originating from the ICA or its branches (Pool and Potts, 1965; Sahs et al., 1969). They occur mainly in women over 50 years of age (Meadows, 1959; Cogan and Mount, 1963; Kupersmith et al., 1984; Little et al., 1989; Linskey et al., 1990b). Almost all of these aneurysms actually arise within the cavernous sinus, although some aneurysms that arise from the petrous portion of the ICA or from the origin of the ophthalmic artery may eventually erode into the cavernous sinus (Dandy, 1939).

Aneurysms that arise within the cavernous sinus initially may be quite small (Fig. 53.68), but they gradually enlarge to fill the sinus and thus acquire an added dural coat (the dural lining of the sinus). Once the aneurysm fills the sinus, rupture is extremely unusual, although further expansion may occur over months to years. The aneurysm may kink or even occlude the cavernous portion of the ICA (Terada et al., 1994), and it may eventually elevate the dura of the middle fossa, forming a huge mass that stretches from one side of the fossa to the other (Figs. 53.69 and 53.70). Anterior expansion erodes the optic foramen and superior orbital fissure, resulting in compressive optic neuropathy, ocular motor nerve paresis, and proptosis. Expansion posteriorly may erode the petrous portion of the temporal bone. Inferior expansion is associated with erosion of the aneurysm into the sphenoid sinus or rarely into the nasopharynx. Rupture of such an aneurysm causes dramatic, often fatal, epistaxis (Gallina et al., 1990; Hahn et al., 1990; Lee and Wang, 1990; Linskey et al., 1990b; Romaniuk et al., 1993; Destian et al., 1994; Ildan et al., 1994; Reiber and Burkey, 1994; Bhatoe et al., 1995; Shike et al., 1995; Teitelbaum et al., 1995a; Yang et al., 1995). Medial expansion may cause destruction of the sella turcica and the pituitary gland, producing hypopituitarism with hyperprolactinemia (White and Ballantine, 1961; Kahana et al., 1962; Hancock, 1963; Huber, 1977; Fernandez-Real et al., 1994). The appearance of the sellar region on skull X-ray or with CT scanning may suggest a primary intrasellar neoplasm; however, MR imaging can clearly distinguish an aneurysm from a tumor (Holemans and Cox, 1995) (Fig. 53.71).

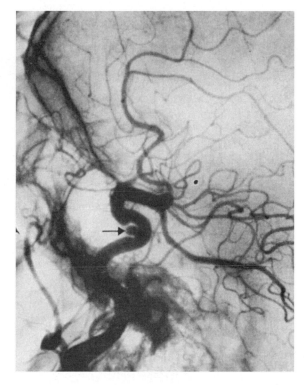

Figure 53.68. Small intracavernous aneurysm (*arrow*) projecting posteriorly in a patient with mild facial pain and an ipsilateral abducens nerve paresis.

The majority of intracavernous aneurysms produce symptoms by local mass effect usually involving the cranial nerves (Larson et al., 1995; Matsumoto et al., 1996). These aneurysms are often partly filled by a laminated clot (Barr et al., 1971), and this clot can produce emboli that cause TIAs (Przelomski et al., 1986; Little et al., 1989). Complete thrombosis also may occur, resulting in spontaneous cure but leaving permanent neurologic and visual deficits (Meadows, 1959; Rapport and Murtagh, 1981; Whittle et al., 1982; Gautier et al., 1986). The thrombosis may not be limited to the aneurysm but may extend to the ICA itself. If this occurs, the artery may become occluded, resulting in contralateral hemiplegia and other signs of hemisphere ischemia (Gautier et al., 1986).

Bilateral intracavernous aneurysms occur in many patients (Alpers et al., 1951; Wilson and Myers, 1963; Maki et al., 1970; Nukui et al., 1977; Johnston, 1979; Faria et al., 1980; Haberbeck-Modesto et al., 1981; Sano et al., 1988). In most cases, only one of the aneurysms is symptomatic (Seltzer and Hurteau, 1957; Odom, 1964; Maki et al., 1970; Rapport and Murtagh, 1981). The symptoms may result from compression of structures within the cavernous sinus (see below) or from rupture of the aneurysm, producing a carotid-cavernous sinus fistula (Alpers et al., 1951; Florin, 1958; Maki et al., 1970; Nukui et al., 1971).

The main symptoms and signs in patients with unruptured intracavernous aneurysms reflect damage to the ocular motor nerves, the oculosympathetic pathway, and the first and second divisions of the trigeminal nerve (Meadows, 1959;

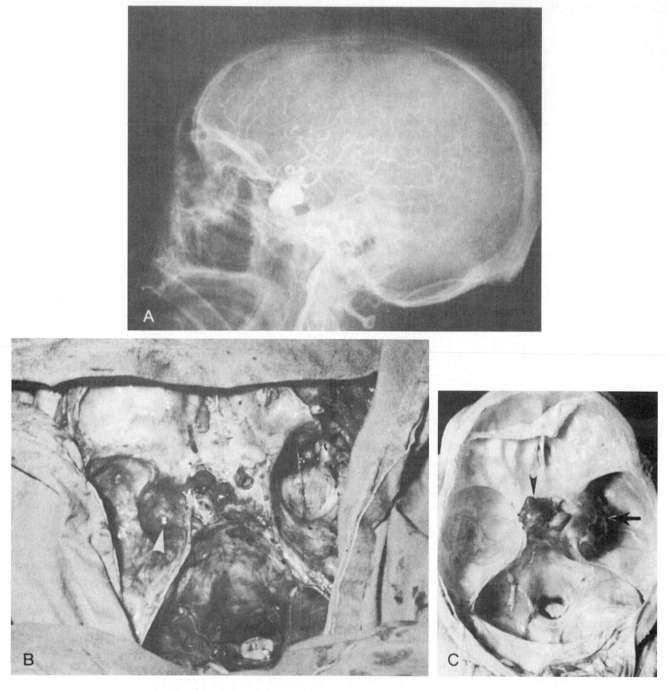

Figure 53.69. Intracavernous aneurysms. *A,* Carotid angiogram shows large aneurysm of the right internal carotid artery within the cavernous sinus. *B,* The patient died after ligation of the artery. Postmortem view of the base of the skull shows expansion of the completely extradural aneurysm (*arrowhead*) into the right middle fossa. *C,* View of the base of the skull in another patient with a large left intracavernous aneurysm shows that the aneurysm has expanded not only into the left middle fossa (*arrow*) but also into the sella turcica and suprasellar cistern (*arrowhead*). (*C,* From Huber A. Eye signs and symptoms of intracranial aneurysm. Neuro-ophthalmology 2:203–216, 1982.)

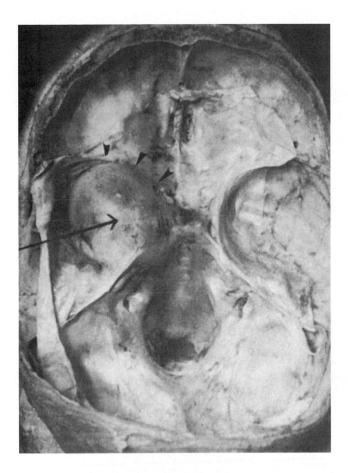

Figure 53.70. Large intracavernous aneurysm (*arrow*) fills much of the right middle fossa. Note that the aneurysm has eroded and expanded the inner sphenoid ridge (*arrowheads*). (From Meadows SP. Intracavernous aneurysms of the internal carotid artery: Their clinical features and natural history. Arch Ophthalmol 62:566–574, 1959.)

Huber, 1982; Kupersmith et al., 1984; Little et al., 1989; Linskey et al., 1990a, 1990b; Vazquez Anon et al., 1992). The visual sensory apparatus may also be affected. The onset of symptoms is occasionally abrupt. More often, it is slow and progressive with bursts of activity during which there may be severe ocular or periocular pain, increased diplopia, and worse ophthalmoparesis.

Paresis of one or more ocular motor nerves is the cardinal feature of an intracavernous aneurysm. The abducens nerve, being situated within the cavernous sinus between the ICA and the lateral wall of the sinus, usually is affected first and may be the only nerve affected at the time of diagnosis (Meadows, 1959; Weintraub and Sananman, 1971; Vukov, 1975; Trobe et al., 1978a; Little et al., 1989; Linskey et al., 1990b). We have seen numerous patients in whom painless diplopia associated with an esotropia and weakness of abduction of one eye was the only clinical manifestation of an ipsilateral intracavernous aneurysm (Fig. 53.72), and Sano et al. (1988) described a 74-year-old woman with systemic hypertension and bilateral intracavernous aneurysms who initially developed a painless right abducens paresis followed 4 years later by a painless left abducens paresis. Only when she began to experience headache and right-sided facial pain was an evaluation performed that revealed the aneurysms.

Some patients with intracavernous aneurysms experience the simultaneous onset of abducens nerve paresis and ipsi-

lateral facial pain from damage to both the abducens and trigeminal nerves (Henderson, 1955; Meadows, 1959; Markwalder and Meienberg, 1983; Kupersmith et al., 1984). In other patients with an intracavernous aneurysm, an apparently isolated abducens nerve paresis (with or without pain) is, in fact, accompanied by an ipsilateral, **postganglionic Horner's syndrome** that may not be appreciated unless a careful examination is performed (Abad et al., 1981; Kupersmith et al., 1984; Gutman et al., 1986; Striph and Burde, 1988) (Fig. 53.73). These signs occur together because the abducens nerve and the oculosympathetic pathway are joined for a short distance within the cavernous sinus (Johnston and Parkinson, 1974; Parkinson et al., 1978; Parkinson, 1979).

Trochlear nerve paresis is rarely the only sign of an intracavernous aneurysm. Nevertheless, Rush and Younge (1981) described a patient who developed an isolated trochlear nerve paresis as the first sign of an intracavernous aneurysm. The patient later developed a complete ophthalmoplegia on the side of the aneurysm. Maurice-Williams and Harvey (1989) also described a patient with an isolated trochlear nerve paresis as the only sign of an intracavernous aneurysm. The patient was treated with atenolol (50 mg twice a day), and her double vision gradually disappeared. She had no neurologic or visual symptoms or signs when she was examined 6 months later. Slavin (1990b) and Arruga

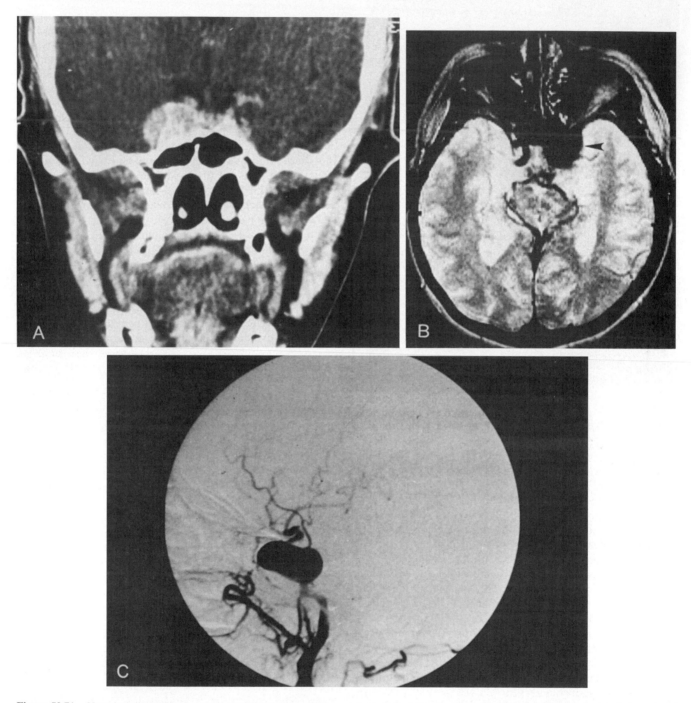

Figure 53.71. Neuroimaging studies in a patient with an intracavernous aneurysm that produced panhypopituitarism. *A*, CT scan, coronal view, shows a lesion of the anterior sellar and parasellar region. The appearance suggests either a meningioma or pituitary adenoma. *B*, Axial MR image shows flow void typical of aneurysm (*arrowhead*). *C*, Anteroposterior view, shows intracavernous aneurysm.

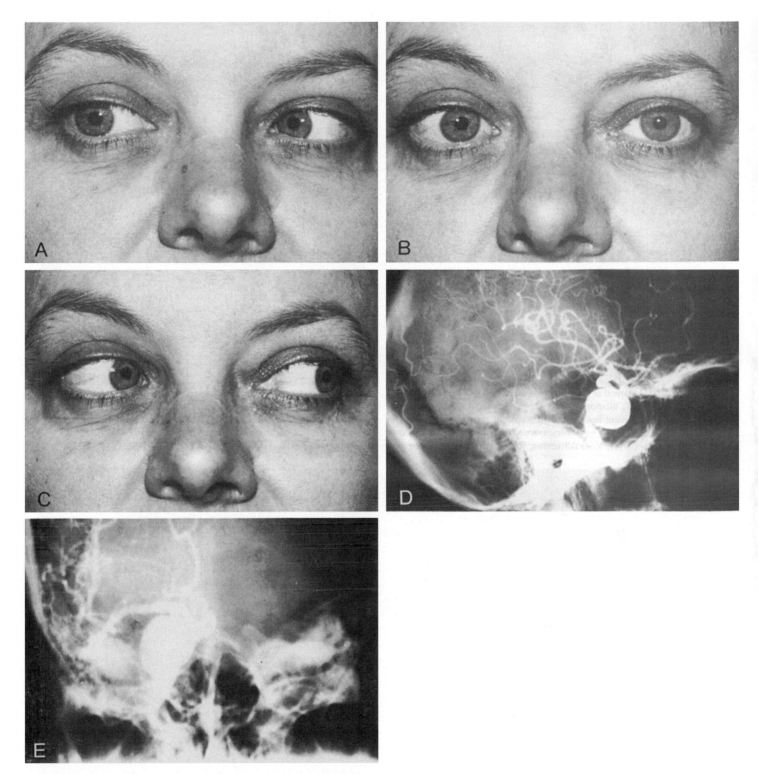

Figure 53.72.   Isolated abducens nerve paresis in a 35-year-old woman with a saccular aneurysm of the intracavernous portion of the ipsilateral internal carotid artery. *A–C*, patient has right abducens nerve paresis. *D* and *E*, right carotid angiogram shows intracavernous aneurysm.

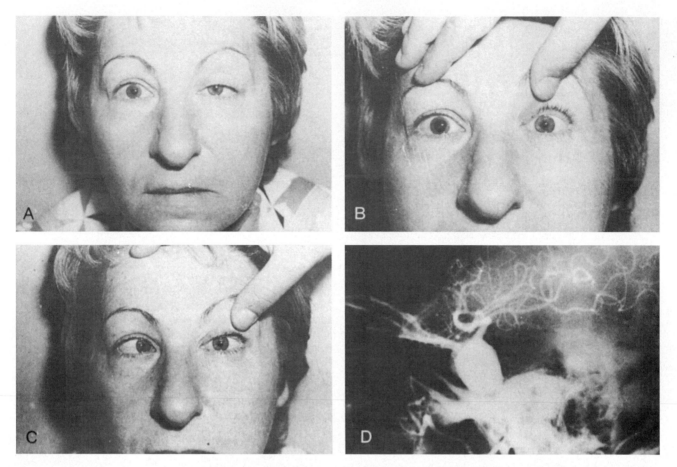

Figure 53.73. Unilateral abducens nerve paresis and ipsilateral postganglionic Horner's syndrome in a patient with an intracavernous aneurysm. *A*, Left ptosis and miosis; *B*, Dilation of the right pupil without dilation of the left pupil after instillation of a 4% cocaine solution confirms a left Horner's syndrome. *C*, The patient has marked limitation of abduction of the left eye consistent with a left abducens nerve paresis. *D*, Left carotid angiogram, lateral view, demonstrates huge intracavernous aneurysm. The aneurysm was treated by gradual occlusion of the left internal carotid artery. (From Gutman I, Levartovski S, Goldhammer Y, et al. Sixth nerve palsy and unilateral Horner's syndrome. Ophthalmology *93*:913–916, 1986.)

et al. (1991) also reported patients with an isolated trochlear nerve palsy associated with an intracavernous aneurysm.

An isolated oculomotor nerve paresis occasionally occurs in patients with an intracavernous aneurysm (Linskey et al., 1990b). Patients in whom the paresis is incomplete may have variable ptosis, ophthalmoparesis, or both. The ophthalmoparesis may affect only one of the extraocular muscles innervated by the oculomotor nerve, all of the muscles innervated by the nerve but incompletely, or even one of the divisions (superior versus inferior) of the nerve (Trobe et al., 1978a; Feder and Camp, 1979; Guy and Day, 1989). The pupil may be dilated or normal, but it is most often nonreactive and either about the same size as, or smaller than, the pupil on the opposite side because of associated damage to the oculosympathetic pathway (Jefferson, 1938; Meadows, 1959; Trobe et al., 1978a) (Fig. 53.74). Walsh and King (1942) described a 38-year-old woman with a right intracavernous aneurysm who developed right ptosis several months before experiencing severe pain in the right eye. She eventually developed a complete right oculomotor nerve paresis, unassociated with dysfunction of either the trochlear or the abducens nerve.

Of 17 patients with intracavernous aneurysms described by Kupersmith et al. (1984), three had oculomotor nerve paresis without evidence of abducens or trochlear damage. All three patients had an incomplete paresis. One of the patients had only a 3-mm ptosis; the other two had ptosis and ophthalmoparesis. All three patients had facial pain in the distribution of the ophthalmic division of the trigeminal nerve. Miller (1991d) examined a 75-year-old woman who developed a mild right ptosis without diplopia or pain. The patient was initially thought to have age-related ptosis caused by dehiscence of the tendon of the levator palpebrae superioris. No treatment was recommended. Over the next 6 months, the patient developed diplopia and was found to have an incomplete right oculomotor nerve paresis. The right pupil was smaller than the left and did not dilate when a solution of 10% cocaine was instilled in the conjunctival sac. Neuroimaging studies revealed an intracavernous aneurysm. The patient denied facial or orbital discomfort. She refused treatment.

Many patients develop simultaneous paresis of more than one ocular motor nerve (Figs. 53.75 and 53.76). The onset of the ophthalmoplegia may be accompanied by severe pain

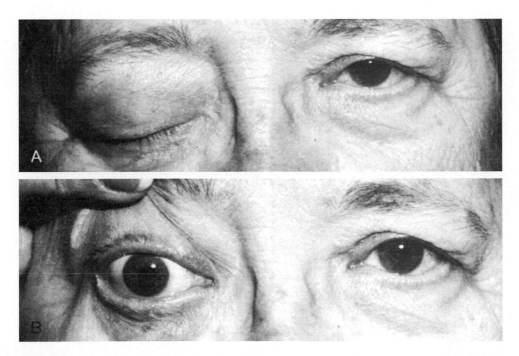

Figure 53.74. Right oculomotor nerve paresis associated with oculosympathetic dysfunction in a patient with an intracavernous aneurysm. *A*, There is a complete right ptosis. *B*, When the right eyelid is held open, the left pupil can be seen to be **smaller** than the right because of concomitant damage to the oculosympathetic pathway on that side.

in the distribution of the ophthalmic division of the trigeminal nerve, numbness of the ipsilateral side of the face, weakness of the jaw and deviation of the jaw toward the side of the lesion, or a combination of these symptoms and signs (Trobe et al., 1978a; Harr and Quencer, 1981; Markwalder and Meienberg, 1983; Kupersmith et al., 1984; Little et al., 1989; Linskey et al., 1990b). The cause of the acute ophthalmoplegia may be sudden expansion of, leakage of blood from, or even thrombosis of the aneurysm (Rapport and Murtagh, 1981; Whittle et al., 1982; Gautier et al., 1986).

Most patients who develop an acute oculomotor nerve paresis, whether isolated or in combination with other ocular motor nerve pareses, are left with a permanent disorder of ocular motility whether or not the aneurysm is treated (Hepler and Cantu, 1967). In some patients, the deficit is caused by a stable oculomotor nerve paresis. In others, the paresis partially resolves, but there is residual strabismus. In still others, **secondary oculomotor nerve synkinesis** (see Chapter 28) develops as the paresis resolves (Walsh and King, 1942; Walsh, 1957; Dailey et al., 1964; Hepler and Cantu, 1967) (Fig. 53.77).

An intracavernous aneurysm may also produce **primary oculomotor nerve synkinesis** (Cox et al., 1979; Lepore and Glaser, 1980). Patients with this syndrome have evidence of aberrant regeneration of the oculomotor nerve (pseudo-Graefe sign, light-near dissociation of the pupil) despite never having experienced acute oculomotor nerve dysfunction (Fig. 53.78). Primary oculomotor nerve synkinesis can also occur with other slowly growing lesions within the cavernous sinus, such as meningiomas and schwannomas, as well as from slow-growing lesions in the subarachnoid

space, including aneurysms (Varma and Miller, 1994) (see below). It probably results from damage to the oculomotor nerve that is sufficiently slow and mild to allow regeneration to occur without causing noticeable symptoms of oculomotor nerve dysfunction (Sibony et al., 1984).

In addition to ocular motor nerve paresis, **trigeminal nerve dysfunction** is a classic manifestation of intracavernous aneurysm (Jefferson, 1938). The first division of the nerve is particularly vulnerable, but all three divisions, including the motor portion of the third division, may be affected (Henderson, 1955; Little et al., 1989) (Fig. 53.76). Ocular and forehead pain is often a prominent symptom in patients with intracavernous aneurysm (Vazquez Anon et al., 1992). It may occur in association with ocular motor neuropathy or in isolation. Of 17 patients with intracavernous aneurysm reported by Kupersmith et al. (1984), 14 experienced pain in the distribution of the first division of the trigeminal nerve. Second division trigeminal pain was present in only two patients and was not severe. All but one of these patients had ophthalmoparesis. All five of the patients with intracavernous aneurysm reported by Henderson (1955) had ipsilateral facial pain and ophthalmoparesis.

Trigeminal pain that occurs in patients with an intracavernous aneurysm is usually constant, lancinating, and severe; however, it may be episodic, and the patient may be asymptomatic between attacks. Such episodic pain may resemble trigeminal neuralgia (Harrison et al., 1963) (see Chapter 36).

Pain in the distribution of the first division of the trigeminal nerve associated with an ipsilateral, postganglionic Horner's syndrome constitutes **Raeder's syndrome** (Raeder, 1924; Grimson and Thompson, 1980). Although Raeder's

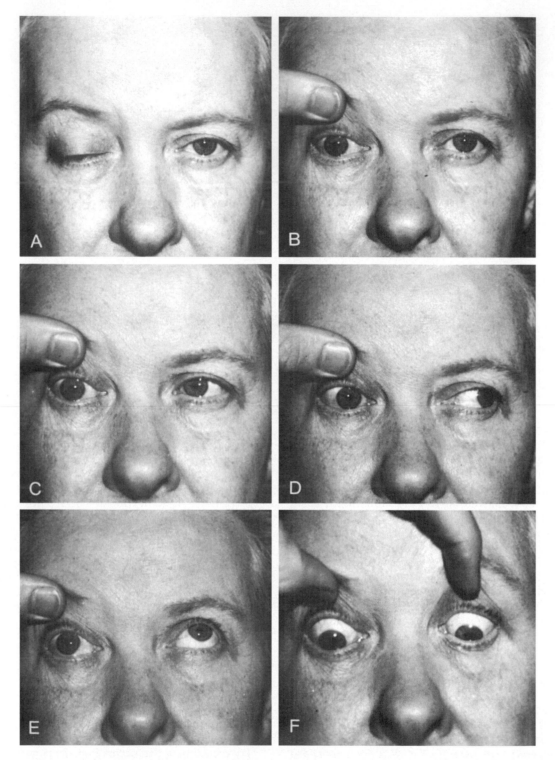

Figure 53.75. Combined pupil-sparing right oculomotor nerve paresis and right abducens nerve paresis in a patient with a large right intracavernous aneurysm. *A*, Patient has almost complete right ptosis. *B*, When right upper eyelid is elevated manually, right eye is seen to be exotropic. *C*, On attempted right gaze, right eye does not abduct fully, indicating weakness of right abducens nerve. *D*, On attempted left gaze, right eye does not adduct fully. *E* and *F*, The patient does not elevate or depress the right eye fully. Note that pupils are of equal size.

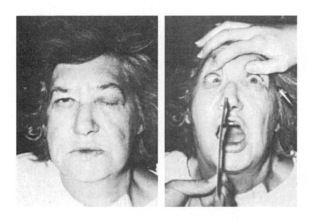

Figure 53.76. Total left-sided ophthalmoplegia from an intracavernous aneurysm. *A,* The patient has a complete ptosis. *B,* The patient is attempting to look to the left and to open her mouth widely. The jaw deviates to the left because of damage to the motor branch of the left trigeminal nerve. The left eye is completely immobile. The left pupil does not react to direct or consensual light stimulation, but it is not dilated because of concomitant damage to the oculosympathetic pathway.

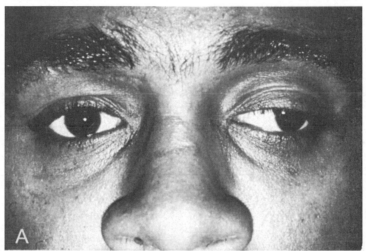

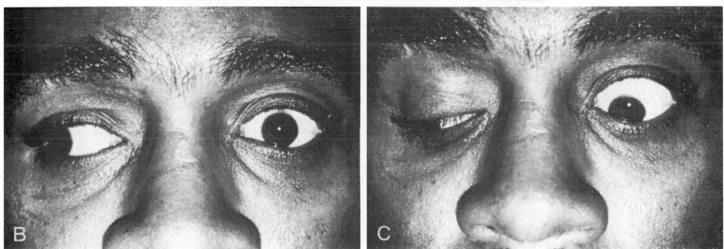

Figure 53.77. Secondary aberrant regeneration in a 34-year-old man who developed an acute oculomotor nerve paresis associated with facial pain and was found to have an ipsilateral intracavernous aneurysm. The patient initially refused treatment. He eventually was treated with occlusion of the left internal carotid artery using a detachable balloon. At 6 months after treatment, the patient has secondary aberrant regeneration of the left oculomotor nerve. *A,* The patient has moderate left ptosis and a left exotropia when he fixes with the nonparetic right eye. *B,* When the patient attempts to adduct the left eye (i.e., when he attempts to look to the right), there is elevation of the left upper eyelid. *C,* The eyelid retraction becomes extreme when the patient attempts to adduct and depress the left eye (i.e., when he attempts to look down and right).

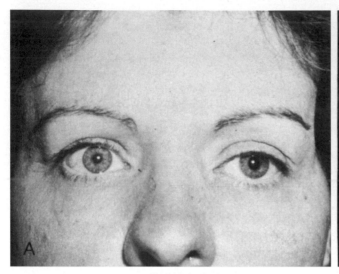
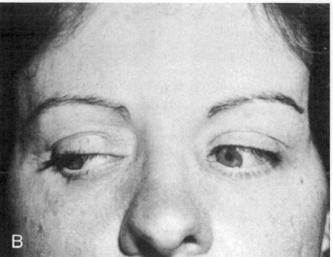

Figure 53.78. Primary aberrant regeneration of the oculomotor nerve in a patient with an intracavernous aneurysm. The patient noted gradual oblique diplopia and left ptosis associated with intermittent left facial pain. She had never experienced an acute oculomotor nerve paresis. *A,* In primary position, there is a moderate left ptosis, a mild left exotropia, and a slightly dilated left pupil. *B,* When the patient attempts to look down and to the right, there is mild elevation of the left upper eyelid and mild constriction of the left pupil.

syndrome may be caused by an aneurysm arising from the petrous portion of the ICA and extending upward to affect the trigeminal nerve, it also occurs in patients with intracavernous aneurysms (Law and Nelson, 1968; Jain et al., 1981; Kashihara et al., 1987). Such patients usually have associated paresis of one or more ocular motor nerves and decreased corneal sensation. Pain misdiagnosed as cluster headache may be caused by an intracavernous pseudoaneurysm (Koenigsberg et al., 1994).

By no means do all patients with intracavernous aneurysms experience severe facial pain. In some cases, pain is a relatively minor complaint. Such patients may complain only of an uncomfortable aching or pressure sensation in and around the orbit. Other patients with intracavernous aneurysms, even patients with severe ophthalmoplegia, never experience pain or discomfort (Meadows, 1959).

Although pain in the distribution of the trigeminal nerve is common in patients with intracavernous aneurysm, trigeminal sensory loss is rare, usually occurring late in the course of the disease (Meadows, 1959). When sensory loss does occur, it is usually mild and asymptomatic. Nakazima et al. (1991) found sensory loss in only one of seven patients with intracavernous aneurysms.

Unilateral or bilateral loss of visual acuity, visual field, or both from **compression of the anterior visual sensory pathway** (optic nerves, optic chiasm, optic tracts) is not a characteristic symptom of patients with intracavernous aneurysm as it is of patients with aneurysms that originate from the supraclinoid portion of the ICA (see below). Visual loss was found, however, in 20% of the 40 patients reported by Vazquez Anon et al. (1992). It usually occurs when an aneurysm arises from the most distal portion of the intracavernous carotid artery, so that the bulk of the lesion is supraclinoid. In such cases, loss of vision usually is unassociated

with ocular motor nerve paresis, may be the only symptom of the aneurysm, and is indistinguishable from that produced by other suprasellar masses that compress the intracranial portions of the optic nerves or the optic chiasm (Meadows, 1959; Huber, 1977; Peiris and Ross Russell, 1980; Norwood et al., 1986) (see Chapter 8) (Figs. 53.79 and 53.80). This type of aneurysm technically should be considered intracavernous, particularly in view of the type of treatment required to obliterate it (see above), but its clinical manifestations are those of a supraclinoid mass. In other cases, loss of vision occurs when an aneurysm located mainly within the cavernous sinus expands anteriorly or superiorly. In these cases, visual loss occurs in the setting of diplopia from paresis of one or more ocular motor nerves (Jefferson, 1937, 1938; Cogan and Mount, 1963; Dailey et al., 1964; Huber, 1976, 1982; Takahashi et al., 1983; Kupersmith et al., 1984; Little et al., 1989). When the aneurysm expands anteriorly, it may compress the intracranial or intracanalicular portion of the optic nerve. When it expands superiorly, it may compress the optic nerve, the optic chiasm, or even the optic tract (Fig. 53.81).

Proptosis, like visual loss, only occurs in patients with an intracavernous aneurysm when the aneurysm is quite large (Walsh and King, 1942; Dandy, 1944; Meadows, 1959; Banna and Lasjaunias, 1991). It results either from erosion of the aneurysm through the superior orbital fissure (Fig. 53.82) or from obstruction of venous outflow from the orbit into the cavernous sinus (Figs. 53.83 and 53.84).

A **bruit** is rarely heard in (or by) patients with an intracavernous aneurysm (Dandy, 1939; Werner et al., 1941; Meadows, 1959). When a bruit is present, it is usually best heard with the bell of the stethoscope over the eye or the temple on the side of the aneurysm.

Endocrine dysfunction may occur in patients with intracavernous aneurysms that expand into the sella turcica and

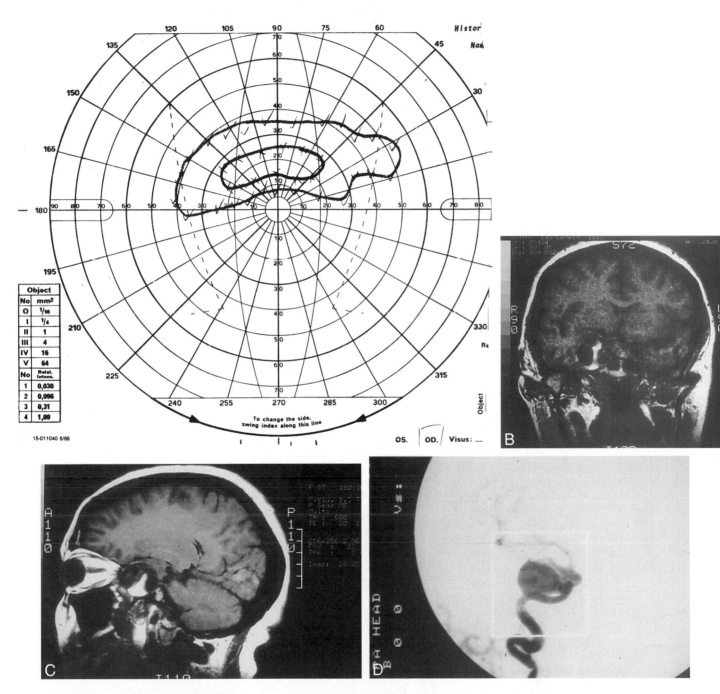

Figure 53.79. Large right-sided intracavernous aneurysm in a 57-year-old woman with progressive visual loss in the right eye. The patient's visual acuity was hand motions at 6 feet in the right eye. *A,* The visual field of the right eye is limited to a superior island. *B,* Coronal T1-weighted magnetic resonance (MR) image shows a large, partially clotted, intracavernous aneurysm with intradural extension into the suprasellar cistern. The aneurysm elevates and compresses the intracranial portion of the right optic nerve. *C,* Sagittal T1-weighted MR image shows marked elevation of the right optic nerve by the aneurysm (*arrowhead*). *D,* Cerebral angiogram shows the appearance of the large aneurysm, which arises from the distal aspect of the intracavernous portion of the right internal carotid artery.

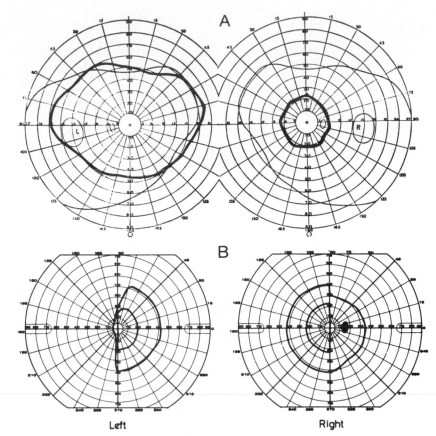

Figure 53.80. Visual field defects in two patients with intracavernous aneurysms that extended superiorly. *A*, The left visual field is full; the right visual field is generally constricted. Visual acuity in the right eye is counting fingers. The aneurysm had expanded superiorly to compress the intracranial portion of the right optic nerve. *B*, There is a bitemporal hemianopia associated with vision of about 20/30 OU. The aneurysm was bilobed and extended upward and medially from the right cavernous sinus to compress the optic chiasm from below and behind. (From Peiris JB, Ross Russell WR. Giant aneurysms of the carotid system presenting as visual field defect. J Neurol Neurosurg Psychiatry *43*:1053–1064, 1980.)

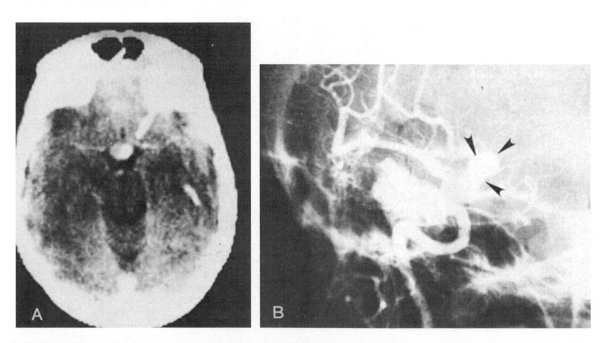

Figure 53.81. Appearance of the intracavernous aneurysm that produced the bitemporal hemianopia depicted in Figure 53.80*B*. *A*, CT scan shows midline position of aneurysm. *B*, Cerebral angiogram, lateral view, shows upward and posterior expansion of aneurysm (*arrowheads*). (From Peiris JB, Ross Russell RW. Giant aneurysms of the carotid system presenting as visual field defect. J Neurol Neurosurg Psychiatry *43*:1053–1064, 1980.)

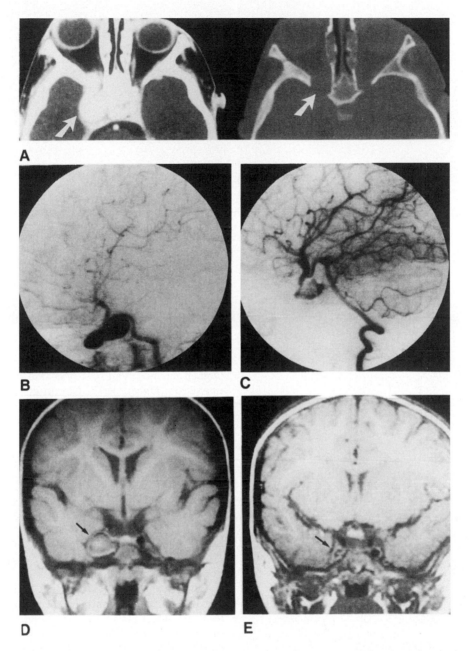

Figure 53.82. Progressive proptosis from an intracavernous aneurysm. The patient was a 13-month-old girl with progressive proptosis of the right eye over a 4-month period. *A Left,* Enhanced, axial computed tomographic (CT) scan shows relative proptosis on the right side and expansion of the area of the right cavernous sinus (*arrow*). *A Right,* CT scan using bone window settings demonstrates enlargement of the superior orbital fissure (*arrow*). *B,* Right carotid angiogram, lateral view, demonstrates a large dumbbell-shaped aneurysm arising from the carotid siphon within the cavernous sinus and extending anteriorly. *C,* Left vertebral angiogram, lateral view, shows filling of the right internal carotid artery through the posterior communicating artery. *D,* Coronal T1-weighted magnetic resonance (MR) image 5 days after balloon embolization shows complete thrombosis of the aneurysm (*arrow*). *E,* Follow-up coronal MR scan 4 months after embolization demonstrates progressive shrinkage of the aneurysm (*arrow*) (From Banna M, Lasjaunias P. Intracavernous carotid aneurysm associated with proptosis in a 13-month-old girl. AJNR *12:*969–970, 1991.)

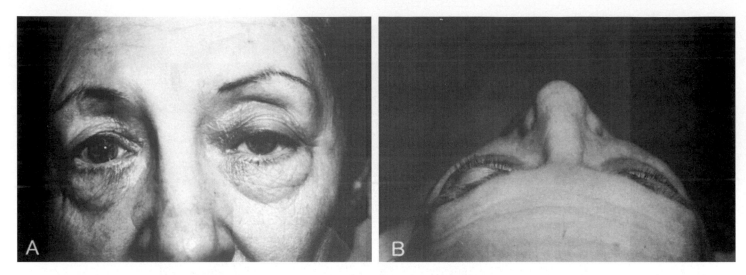

Figure 53.83. Left proptosis and incomplete left oculomotor nerve paresis in a 71-year-old woman with an intracavernous aneurysm. *A*, The patient has mild left ptosis. *B*, View from behind and above the head shows mild left proptosis that resulted from erosion of the aneurysm through the left superior orbital fissure.

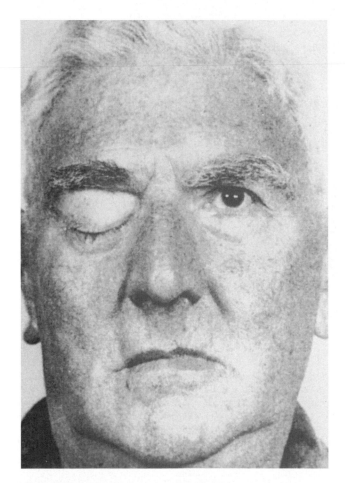

Figure 53.84. Right proptosis and complete right oculomotor nerve paresis in a man with an intracavernous aneurysm. (From Meadows SP. Intracavernous aneurysms of the internal carotid artery: Their clinical features and natural history. Arch Ophthalmol 62:566–574, 1959.)

compress the pituitary gland, but this is rare. The symptoms and signs in such patients are nonspecific, although there is a high incidence of simultaneous visual function disturbance (acuity loss or field defects). Symptoms include amenorrhea in women and decreased libido and hypothyroidism in both women and men (Van 'T Hoff et al., 1961; White and Ballantine, 1961; Huber, 1977, Kayath et al., 1991). Headaches are common. Rare patients develop diabetes insipidus from damage to the pituitary stalk, posterior lobe of the pituitary gland, or both (Huber, 1977).

Aneurysms Arising from the Intradural Portion of the Internal Carotid Artery and its Branches

It is often difficult to be certain if an aneurysm originating from the ICA is arising from its cavernous portion or its most proximal intradural portion. In many cases, the neck of the aneurysm is both extradural and intradural. For this reason, many investigators prefer to classify such aneurysms as infraclinoid or supraclinoid aneurysms. This classification has the advantage of separating ICA aneurysms into those that usually can be approached directly (supraclinoid) and those for which an indirect treatment such as occlusion of the carotid artery (infraclinoid) is required. Although this classification has merit from a surgical standpoint, it does not permit the differentiation of intradural aneurysms that cause progressive visual loss because of their proximity to the optic nerves, chiasm, and tract, from aneurysms that produce diplopia because of their proximity to the ocular motor nerves. For example, Höök and Norlén (1964a) recorded visual field defects in only eight of 79 patients with "supraclinoid" aneurysms (11%). Had these investigators excluded aneurysms arising from the junction of the internal carotid and posterior communicating arteries, the prevalence of visual loss would have been higher. In the sections that follow, we have attempted to correlate clinical manifestations closely with the site of origin of aneurysms of the intradural

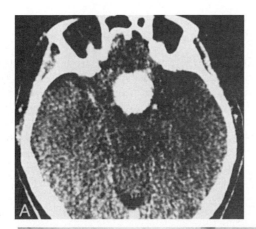

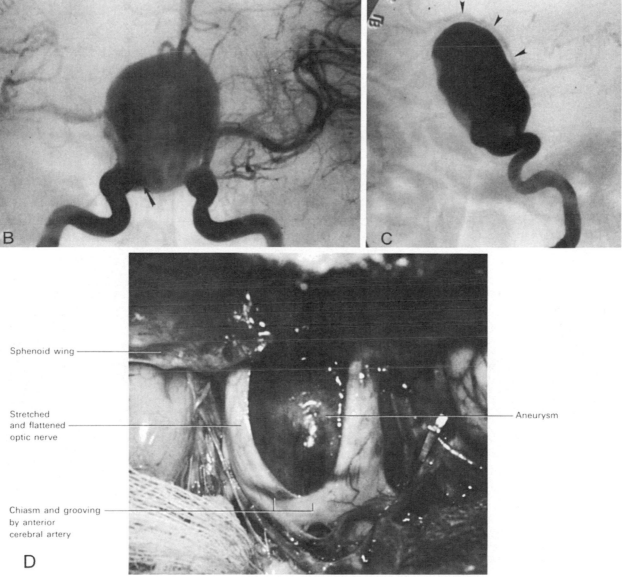

Figure 53.85. Compression of both optic nerves and the optic chiasm from a giant suprasellar (supraclinoid, paraclinoid, paraophthalmic) aneurysm. *A,* Axial computed tomographic scan after intravenous contrast shows well-circumscribed, enhancing lesion filling the suprasellar cistern. *B,* Cerebral angiogram, anteroposterior view after simultaneous injection of both internal carotid arteries, shows the midline location of the aneurysm which seems to arise from the proximal intradural segment of the right internal carotid artery *(arrow).* The A-1 segments of both anterior cerebral arteries and the anterior communicating artery are markedly elevated by the aneurysm. *C,* Right carotid arteriogram shows origin of the aneurysm from the proximal intradural segment of the right internal carotid artery. Note marked elevation of the two anterior cerebral arteries by the aneurysm *(arrowheads). D,* In a similar case examined at autopsy, both optic nerves and the optic chiasm are stretched and flattened by the giant aneurysm. (From Lindenberg R, Walsh FB, Sacks JG. Neuropathology of Vision: An Atlas. Philadelphia, Lea & Febiger, 1973.)

Sphenoid wing

Stretched and flattened optic nerve

Chiasm and grooving by anterior cerebral artery

Aneurysm

portion of the ICA. We are aware that in some cases, the precise origin of an intradural, intracranial aneurysm is impossible to identify. In such cases, it is appropriate to describe the aneurysm as arising from the proximal intradural segment of the ICA (Nutik, 1988b). Although this classification also has inherent weaknesses, it nevertheless allows an appreciation of the importance of location and direction of projection when comparing symptoms and signs produced by aneurysms of the intradural portion of the ICA.

Aneurysms Arising from the Clinoid Segment of the Internal Carotid Artery (Paraclinoid Aneurysms)

When the ICA exits the cavernous sinus to form the anterior portion of the carotid siphon, it does not immediately become intradural. Rather, there is a small transdural segment of the artery between the cavernous segment and the distal intradural segments that is tightly attached to surrounding osseous structures by dense connective tissue, the anat-

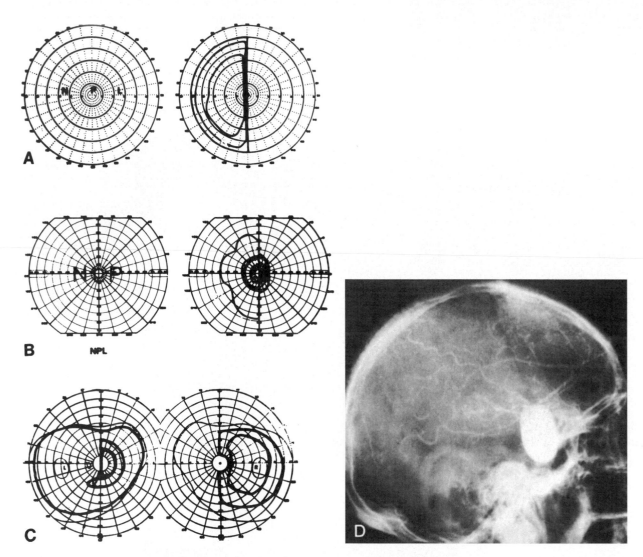

Figure 53.86. Visual loss from supraclinoid aneurysms. *A,* Visual field defects in a 62-year-old woman with a supraclinoid aneurysm arising from the right internal carotid artery. The aneurysm compressed the left optic nerve and the lateral aspect of the optic chiasm. Visual acuity in the right eye is 20/70, and there is a complete temporal field defect. The left eye is blind. *B,* Visual field defects in a 62-year-old man with a supraclinoid aneurysm arising from the left internal carotid artery. The aneurysm stretched both optic nerves and compressed the optic chiasm. Visual acuity in the right eye is counting fingers. The visual field in this eye shows a dense central scotoma and a complete temporal hemianopia. The left eye is blind. *C,* Visual field defects in a 43-year-old woman with a supraclinoid aneurysm arising from the right internal carotid artery. The aneurysm compressed the lateral aspect of the right optic nerve and the optic chiasm. Visual acuity in the right eye is finger counting. The visual field in that eye shows a dense central scotoma and a complete nasal hemianopia. Visual acuity in the left eye is 20/30 and is associated with a relative temporal hemianopia. *D,* A huge aneurysm arises from the supraclinoid portion of the right internal carotid artery. The aneurysm has expanded both downward and upward. It occupies an enlarged sella turcica, and it has compressed the right optic nerve and chiasm, causing blindness of the right eye and a temporal field defect in the visual field of the left eye. (*A–C,* From Peiris JB, Ross Russell RW. Giant aneurysms of the carotid system presenting as visual field defect. J Neurol Neurosurg Psychiatry *43:* 1053–1064, 1980. *D,* Courtesy of Dr. William F. Hoyt.)

omy of which is described in Chapter 52 of this text. The segment is located adjacent or just inferior to the anterior clinoid process, in a region that is also called the paraclinoid area, and it is from this segment that some aneurysms arise (DeJesús et al., 1997). Such aneurysms are called ''paraclinoid,'' ''paraophthalmic,'' or ''ventral'' ICA aneurysms (Yaşargil and Fox, 1975; Nutik, 1978; Pia, 1978; Fox, 1988; Knosp et al., 1988; Nutik, 1988a; Strother et al., 1989). These aneurysms were called ''carotid cave aneurysms'' by Kobayashi et al. (1989), because they are located intradurally at the dural penetration of the ICA on the ventromedial side and seem to be buried in the dural pouch covering the artery. We prefer to call these lesions **paraclinoid aneurysms.** Day (1990b) believed that most paraclinoid aneurysms actually arise from the junction of the internal carotid and superior hypophyseal arteries. He therefore called such lesions ''superior hypophyseal aneurysms.'' Batjer et al. (1994) further divided paraclinoid aneurysms into those that project superiorly or superomedially and those proximal posterior carotid artery wall aneurysms that project posteriorly or posterolaterally.

Regardless of what these aneurysms are called, many become symptomatic when they rupture, causing SAH (Nakagawa et al., 1986; Fox, 1988; Nutik, 1988a; Day, 1990b). Of 89 patients reported by Batjer et al. (1994), 39 (44%) presented with SAH. Others produce transient neurologic defects, presumably from emboli originating within or adjacent to the aneurysm (Przelomski et al., 1986; Kobayashi et al., 1989). Still others are asymptomatic and are identified during an evaluation for unrelated neurologic symptoms (Nutik, 1988a; Kobayashi et al., 1989). Finally, some paraclinoid aneurysms gradually enlarge until they compress adjacent neural structures. Their expansion is usually directed toward the midline, and visual loss is therefore more common than is diplopia (Day, 1990b). They usually displace the chiasm laterally, but they also elevate it (Fig. 53.85), producing symptoms similar to those caused by carotid-ophthalmic aneurysms (Golding et al., 1980; Peiris and Ross Russell, 1980; Farris et al., 1986; Strother et al., 1989). Most patients who experience visual loss from supraclinoid or paraclinoid aneurysms develop slowly progressive, monocular loss of vision from compression of the ipsilateral optic nerve or binocular visual loss from compression of the optic chiasm (Figs. 53.86–53.89).

Some paraclinoid aneurysms that cross the midline somehow produce visual loss only in the contralateral eye, even though they clearly compress both optic nerves and the optic chiasm. Cullen et al. (1966) reported such a case. The patient was a 58-year-old woman who experienced progressive visual loss in the left eye and was found to have a dense temporal field defect in that eye. The visual acuity and visual field in the right eye were said to be normal. An evaluation revealed a giant aneurysm arising from the paraclinoid portion of the right ICA 1.5 cm from its bifurcation. An attempt to clip the aneurysm was unsuccessful, so the right common carotid was slowly occluded in the neck. The patient died about 2 months later after experiencing a massive pulmonary embolus. At autopsy, the aneurysm was found to be deeply embedded in the 3rd ventricle. Both optic nerves and the optic chiasm were stretched, flattened, and displaced up-

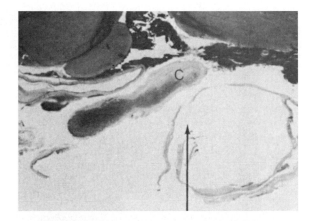

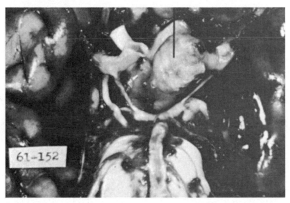

Figure 53.87. Ruptured aneurysm that arose from the supraclinoid portion of the left internal carotid artery. The aneurysm had compressed the left optic nerve and the left side of the optic chiasm. The histologic section (*top*) through the chiasm (*C*) shows demyelination of the visual axons adjacent to the aneurysm (*arrow*). The gross specimen (*bottom*) shows the aneurysm (*vertical line*) compressing the left optic nerve and chiasm. (Courtesy of Dr. Richard Lindenberg.)

wards and backwards over the superior surface of the aneurysm. It is unclear why such obvious damage to these structures produced only monocular contralateral visual loss. We suspect that contrast sensitivity testing and static perimetry would have shown some disorder of visual sensory function in the apparently asymptomatic right eye in this patient, but the fact remains that the only obvious clinical findings were related to the left eye. In rare patients with a prefixed chiasm (see Chapter 4), an enlarging paraclinoid aneurysm compresses the ipsilateral optic tract, producing a complete or an incomplete and incongruous hemianopic field defect.

The destructive effect of paraclinoid aneurysms is not confined to the visual pathways. The orbital portion of the frontal lobe, the olfactory tracts, the hypothalamus, the pituitary stalk, and even the pituitary gland may be compressed. At least nine of the 12 intrasellar aneurysms reviewed by White and Ballantine (1961) were of this type. All nine of the patients had ipsilateral blindness, and six of the nine had a temporal field defect in the contralateral eye. In all cases, the aneurysm was located beneath the ipsilateral optic nerve and the optic chiasm, causing sellar erosion. Other investiga-

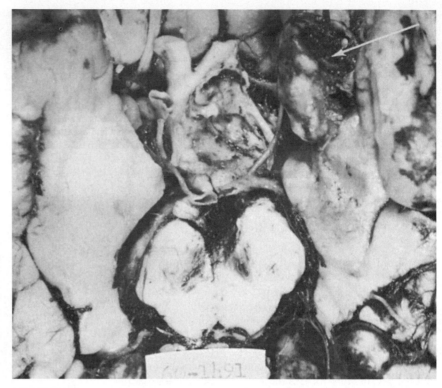

Figure 53.88. Damage to the optic chiasm and optic tract produced by a supraclinoid internal carotid aneurysm (*arrow*). The aneurysm has been moved laterally to expose the changes it had caused to midline structures at the base of the brain. Note the deep depression where the aneurysm was located. The tissue at the base of this depression has been severely damaged and includes the intraorbital portion of the left optic nerve, the left half of the optic chiasm, and the left optic tract. (Courtesy of Dr. Richard Lindenberg.)

tors reported similar cases (Jefferson, 1937; Rhonheimer, 1959; Walsh and Hoyt, 1969f). Several of these patients were thought to have nonorganic visual loss, presumably because they had somewhat fluctuating vision and normal-appearing fundi. In addition, some paraclinoid aneurysms expand inferiorly and compress the structures in the cavernous sinus, producing single or multiple ocular motor nerve pareses, sometimes associated with ipsilateral facial pain or numbness from involvement of the first and second divisions of the trigeminal nerve. The availability of spiral CT angiography, with its multidimensional capability, may prove particularly helpful in the assessment of paraclinoid aneurysms, especially as regards localization of their neck (Tampieri et al., 1995).

The treatment of paraclinoid aneurysms is often somewhat more difficult than the treatment of other intradural aneu-

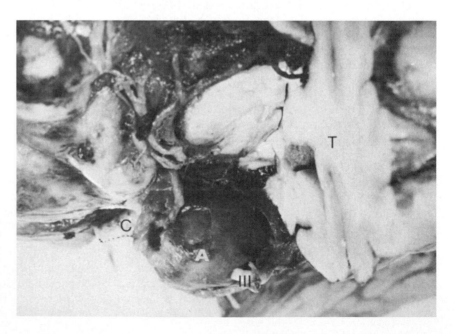

Figure 53.89. Lateral view of a large aneurysm (*A*) that has arisen from the supraclinoid portion of the left internal carotid artery. The aneurysm has displaced the left optic nerve and the optic chiasm (*C*) upward and the left oculomotor nerve (*3rd*) downward. The temporal lobe (*T*) has been cut away to expose the lesion. (Courtesy of Dr. Richard Lindenberg.)

rysms because of the origin of the neck. Clipping may require extensive dissection of the connective tissue that surrounds the ICA in this location, and placement of the clip may be associated with visual loss in the ipsilateral eye from ischemia or compression of the ipsilateral optic nerve or an homonymous visual field defect from inadvertent occlusion of the adjacent anterior choroidal artery (Suzuki et al., 1992).

Aneurysms Arising from the Junction of the Internal Carotid and Superior Hypophyseal Arteries

Day (1990b) suggested that not all aneurysms that arise in the vicinity of the origin of the ophthalmic artery from the ICA actually originate at the bifurcation of these two vessels. He emphasized that the superior hypophyseal artery may arise from the inferomedial surface of the ophthalmic segment of the ICA and that some aneurysms arise from this junction rather than from the junction of the internal carotid and ophthalmic arteries (see also Sugar, 1992). Day (1990b) further separated superior hypophyseal aneurysms into those that project primarily inferiorly or inferomedially toward and behind the anterior clinoid process (paraclinoid variant; see above) and those that project medially or superomedially (suprasellar variant). He emphasized that although aneurysms that arise from the junction of the ophthalmic and internal carotid arteries often compress one or both optic nerves, aneurysms that arise from the junction of the superior hypophyseal and internal carotid arteries do not cause visual loss unless they extend superomedially. Batjer et al. (1994)

also separated superior hypophyseal aneurysms with a medial or inferomedial projection (26 cases) from proximal posterior carotid artery wall aneurysms projecting posteriorly or posterolaterally (19 cases) and from carotid-ophthalmic artery aneurysms with a superior or superomedial projection (44 cases).

The manifestations produced by superior hypophyseal aneurysms are identical with those produced by paraclinoid and carotid-ophthalmic aneurysms.

Aneurysms Arising from the Junction of the Internal Carotid and Ophthalmic Arteries (Carotid-Ophthalmic Aneurysms)

Carotid-ophthalmic aneurysms arise from the anteromedial wall of the ICA adjacent to the origin of the ophthalmic artery (Drake et al., 1968a; Sengupta et al., 1976; Day, 1990a, 1990b) (Figs. 53.90 and 53.91). Because the origin of the ophthalmic artery is intradural in 90% of persons (Punt, 1979), the majority of carotid-ophthalmic aneurysms originate intradurally. In about 10% of persons, however, the origin of the ophthalmic artery is within the cavernous sinus and is thus extradural. In such persons, aneurysms arising at this site also may originate extradurally and require treatment different from that of intradural aneurysms (see above). In addition to differences in treatment, rupture of an intradural carotid-ophthalmic aneurysm results in SAH, whereas rupture of an extradural carotid-ophthalmic aneurysm may

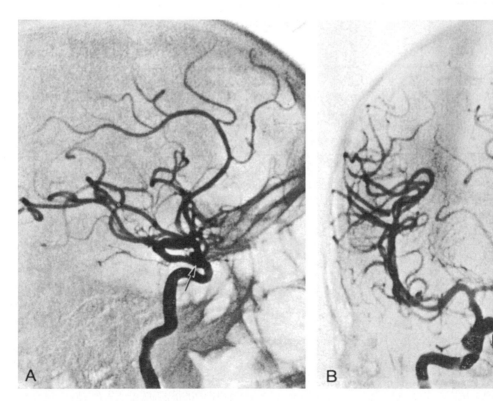

Figure 53.90. Cerebral angiogram showing carotid-ophthalmic aneurysm. *A*, The aneurysm is not well seen on the lateral view (*arrow*). *B*, Anteroposterior view shows aneurysm arising from junction of internal carotid and ophthalmic arteries.

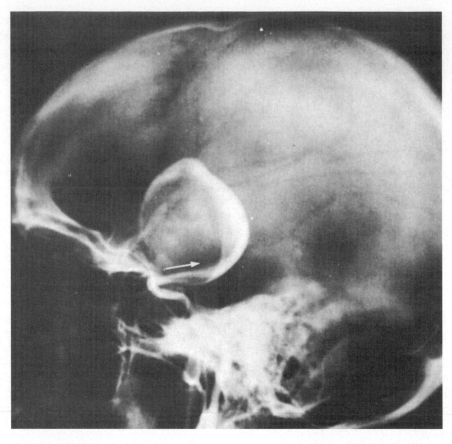

Figure 53.91. Jet effect in huge, left carotid-ophthalmic aneurysm. Note the jet of contrast material as it squirts into the lumen of the aneurysm (*arrow*). The patient had progressive loss of vision in the left eye over a 2-year period. Central and nasal defects were present in the visual field of the left eye. The visual field of the right eye showed a relative superior temporal defect, indicating damage to Wilbrand's knee in the distal portion of the left optic nerve just anterior to the optic chiasm.

produce a carotid-cavernous sinus fistula or a subdural hematoma (Sanchez et al., 1994).

Carotid-ophthalmic aneurysms are rare. Krayenbühl and Yaşargil (1958) found only seven such aneurysms among 290 intracranial aneurysms (2.4%). In the first cooperative study of 2695 intracranial aneurysms (Locksley, 1966), only 5.4% were carotid-ophthalmic aneurysms. Carotid-ophthalmic aneurysms are more common in women, more frequent on the left side, and often associated with other intracranial aneurysms (Drake et al., 1968a; Sengupta et al., 1976). Most of these aneurysms are diagnosed in patients between the 30 and 70 years of age.

Carotid-ophthalmic aneurysms produce neuro-ophthalmologic manifestations by several mechanisms. Some, particularly those that are small, rupture, causing SAH. The hemorrhage may damage surrounding neural structures, including the ipsilateral optic nerve (Guidetti and La Torre, 1970, 1975; Sengupta et al., 1976; Nabawi et al., 1983; Dolenc, 1985). Others cause transient or permanent visual loss from emboli that originate within the aneurysm (Przelomski et al., 1986; Beiran et al., 1995) (Fig. 53.92). Most often, however, carotid-ophthalmic aneurysms produce symptoms by enlarging sufficiently to compress the adjacent anterior

visual sensory apparatus (Huber, 1977; Ferguson and Drake, 1981; Day, 1990a, 1990b; Miller et al., 1995).

Carotid-ophthalmic aneurysms may arise beneath, above, or adjacent to the optic nerves and chiasm depending on the location of the origin of the ophthalmic artery (Kothandaram et al., 1971; Day, 1990a, 1990b). Most of the aneurysms that produce unilateral visual loss are located beneath the optic nerve as it exits from the optic canal (Yaşargil and Smith, 1982) (Figs. 53.93 and 53.94). Such lesions produce an optic neuropathy when they exceed a few millimeters in diameter (Drake et al., 1968a; Guidetti and La Torre, 1970). The visual field defect produced by such aneurysms may be superior, from direct damage to inferior nerve fibers, or inferior, from superior displacement of the nerve such that it is compressed against the superior dural shelf of the optic canal (also called the falciform ligament) (Day, 1990a, 1990b). Some carotid-ophthalmic aneurysms expand anteriorly, widen the optic canal, compress the optic nerve, and produce a painless, progressive, unilateral optic neuropathy (Goldin and Silver, 1957) (Fig. 53.95). Others expand superiorly, compressing the optic nerve and producing monocular visual loss that may be either insidious in onset and slowly progressive (Raymond and Tew, 1978) or acute, painful, and associ-

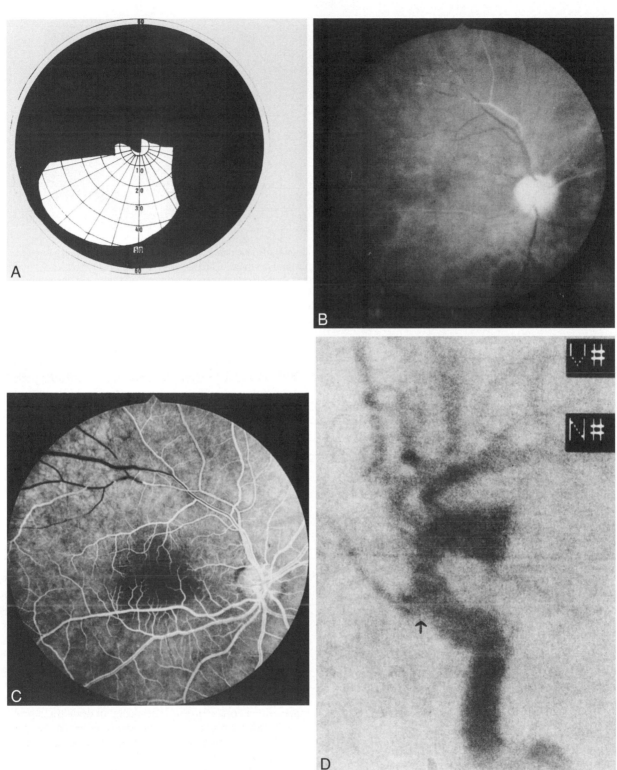

Figure 53.92. Visual loss from emboli related to a carotid-ophthalmic aneurysm. *A*, Visual field of the right eye of a 25-year-old man who complained of progressive loss of vision in the right eye associated with episodes of transient monocular visual loss in the eye 14 months after severe head trauma. The visual field is limited to a small inferior island. *B*, Fundus photograph shows multiple arterial occlusions and optic atrophy. *C*, Fluorescein angiogram in the right eye shows embolic occlusion of the superior temporal branch artery with secondary obstruction of flow in the superior temporal vein. *D*, Right carotid digital subtraction angiogram, lateral view, shows an aneurysm arising from the junction of the internal carotid and ophthalmic arteries (*arrow*). (From Beiran I, Dori D, Pikkel J, et al. Recurrent retinal artery obstruction as a presenting symptom of ophthalmic artery aneurysm: A case report. Graefes Arch Clin Exp Ophthalmol *233*:444–447, 1995.)

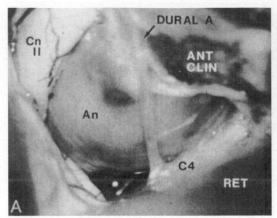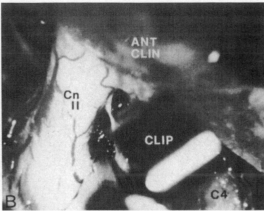

Figure 53.93. Appearance of a right carotid-ophthalmic aneurysm and its relationship to the right optic nerve before and after clipping of the aneurysm. The patient was a 53-year-old woman with progressive loss of vision in the right eye associated with headache. *A*, A large aneurysm (*An*) originating in the region of the origin of the ophthalmic artery from the internal carotid artery (*C4*) displaces the right optic nerve (*Cn II*) medially and superiorly. *Dural A*, dural artery; *ANT CLIN*, anterior clinoid process; *RET*, retractor. *B*, After a clip has been used to obliterate the fundus of the aneurysm, the optic nerve has returned to a normal position. The patient had excellent recovery of vision. (From Weir B. Aneurysms Affecting the Nervous System. Baltimore, Williams & Wilkins, 1987.)

ated with a central scotoma and an ipsilateral RAPD, thus mimicking an attack of retrobulbar optic neuritis (Kuzniecky et al., 1987). If the origin of the ophthalmic artery is above the visual pathways, the aneurysm may be asymptomatic (Diraz et al., 1992); however, if it projects inferiorly, it may compress the superior surface of the ipsilateral optic nerve or anterior chiasm, producing a unilateral or bilateral inferior field defect with or without decreased visual acuity and abnormal color vision.

In rare cases, an aneurysm compresses the optic nerve to such an extent that the nerve is divided longitudinally with part of the nerve on each side of the aneurysm (Beatty, 1986) (Fig. 53.96). In such cases, the optic neuropathy may be surprisingly minimal. A 35-year-old woman underwent a CT scan because of intermittent headache (Miller, 1991e). The scan showed a suprasellar mass on the left side, and an arteriogram showed a carotid-ophthalmic aneurysm. The patient

had no visual complaints. Visual acuity was 20/15 OD and 20/20 OS. Color vision using Hardy-Rand-Rittler pseudoisochromatic plates was 10/10 OD and 8/10 OS, with definite red desaturation in the left eye. Visual field testing showed a subtle central scotoma to red in the left visual field. There was a left RAPD. Ophthalmoscopic examination showed minimal pallor of the left optic disc and slight loss of visibility of the nerve fiber layer in the papillomacular bundle. The patient underwent craniotomy, at which time the left optic nerve was found to be divided longitudinally for about 5 mm by the neck of a 12 mm diameter aneurysm. The optic nerve was gently dissected away from the aneurysm, the neck of the aneurysm was clipped, and the aneurysm sac was resected. Postoperatively, the patient had no change in vision.

Carotid-ophthalmic aneurysms may produce an optic chiasmal or tract syndrome when they expand posteriorly and superiorly (Day, 1990a, 1990b). Medial expansion may be associated with bilateral loss of visual acuity from compression of the contralateral optic nerve. Loss of vision in this setting may be slowly progressive or acute, and one eye may be affected before the other (Berson et al., 1966; Cullen et al., 1966; Miller et al., 1995). When a carotid-ophthalmic aneurysm expands laterally, it may compress the lateral aspect of the optic nerve, optic chiasm, or optic tract, producing a nasal hemianopia or hemianopic scotoma in the ipsilateral eye. This may be associated with a central or temporal defect in the contralateral eye (see Tables 1 and 2 in Farris et al., 1986). Inferior expansion may produce diplopia from paresis of one or more of the ocular motor nerves.

The loss of visual acuity and visual field that occurs in patients with carotid-ophthalmic aneurysms is nonspecific. Loss of visual acuity may be insidious in onset and slowly progressive (Berson et al., 1966), it may be acute and stable (Cullen et al., 1966; Huber, 1976), or it may fluctuate, with marked variations in visual acuity and visual field loss (Klin-

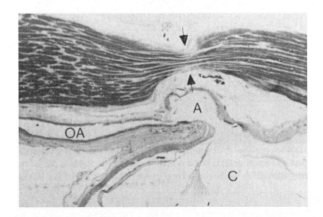

Figure 53.94. Compression of an optic nerve (*arrows*) at the optic foramen by an aneurysm (*A*) at the origin of the ophthalmic artery (*OA*) from the internal carotid artery (*C*). (Courtesy of Dr. Richard Lindenberg.)

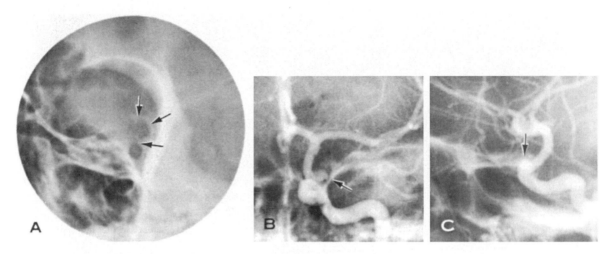

Figure 53.95.   Carotid-ophthalmic aneurysm producing progressive visual loss associated with widening of the optic canal. *A*, Skull x-ray obtained to show appearance of the optic canal shows bone erosion of the roof of the canal and of the anterior clinoid process (*arrows*). *B*, Cerebral angiogram, anteroposterior view, shows lateral expansion of the aneurysm (*arrow*). *C*, Cerebral angiogram, lateral view, shows superior and slight anterior expansion of the aneurysm (*arrow*) (From Taveras JM, Wood EH. Diagnostic Neuroradiology, 2nd ed, Vol 2. Baltimore, Williams & Wilkins, 1976.)

gler, 1951; Norwood et al., 1986). Some patients complain of photopsia (Kothandaram et al., 1971; Ringel and Brick, 1986). When visual loss is acute (and occasionally when it is not), the patient may be thought to have experienced an attack of retrobulbar ischemic optic neuropathy; when the associated visual field defect is a central or cecocentral scotoma and there is associated ocular or orbital pain, a diagnosis of retrobulbar optic neuritis may initially be made (Goldin and Silver, 1957; Walsh and Hoyt, 1969e; Bird et al., 1970; Stern and Ernest, 1975; Huber, 1976; Peiris and Ross Russell, 1980; Takahashi et al., 1983; Ringel and Brick, 1986; Miller et al., 1995). Other patients may be thought to have nonorganic visual loss (Norwood et al., 1986).

Intraocular causes of visual loss such as macular degeneration or optic disc drusen may be suspected in some cases of visual loss caused by carotid-ophthalmic aneurysms. Cunningham and Sewell (1971) described a patient with intermittent blurred vision in both eyes who was found to have decreased vision in the left eye, bilateral constricted visual fields with arcuate scotomas, and optic discs that were pale and contained numerous drusen. The patient's visual difficulties were thought to be caused by the drusen, but neuroimaging studies revealed a left carotid-ophthalmic aneurysm. After ligation of the left ICA, visual acuity in the left eye improved, but the visual field defects did not. It is likely that the field defects were indeed related to the drusen, but that the loss of visual acuity in the left eye was caused by compression of the left optic nerve by the aneurysm, because drusen of the optic disc almost never cause loss of central vision (see Chapter 18).

Visual field defects in patients with carotid-ophthalmic aneurysm are nonspecific (Fig. 53.97). They may be central (suggesting, as noted above, an inflammatory or ischemic process), cecocentral, temporal, altitudinal, or arcuate (Fig. 53.98*A*). Nasal field defects are especially common because of the lateral location of the intradural portion of the ICA

relative to the ipsilateral optic nerve (Peiris and Ross Russell, 1980; Farris et al., 1986; Norwood et al., 1986) (Fig. 53.98*B*). All visual field defects gradually expand, however, until the affected eye is completely blind (Huber, 1976, 1982).

If a carotid-ophthalmic aneurysm compresses the optic nerve near its junction with the optic chiasm, the patient may have, in addition to evidence of a unilateral optic neuropathy (loss of visual acuity, visual field defect, decreased color vision with desaturation of red when compared to the opposite eye, RAPD), a superior temporal field defect in the opposite eye from damage to the presumptive Wilbrand's knee (Berson et al., 1966) (the syndrome of the distal optic nerve; the anterior chiasmal syndrome) (see Chapter 8). A temporal field defect in the eye contralateral to the aneurysm may also be produced when the aneurysm compresses the optic chiasm or ipsilateral optic tract (Huber, 1977; Farris et al., 1986). In almost all cases, however, such a defect is associated with severe visual loss in the ipsilateral eye.

Patients with compression of the optic nerve or chiasm from a carotid-ophthalmic aneurysm eventually develop retinal nerve fiber layer and optic nerve atrophy, which may be associated with increased cupping of the optic disc (Portney and Roth, 1977; Kupersmith and Krohn, 1984). The appearance of the optic disc in such cases should not be mistaken for glaucoma, even when cupping is substantial, because in such cases, any rim tissue that remains is invariably pale compared with the normal-appearing rim tissue in patients with glaucomatous cupping (Trobe et al., 1980) (see Chapter 8).

Most patients in whom a carotid-ophthalmic aneurysm compresses the intracranial or intracanalicular portions of the optic nerve have a normal appearing retina and optic disc until atrophy develops, but this is not always the case. In some cases, the optic disc becomes swollen. Tomsak et al. (1979) described a 60-year-old woman who developed

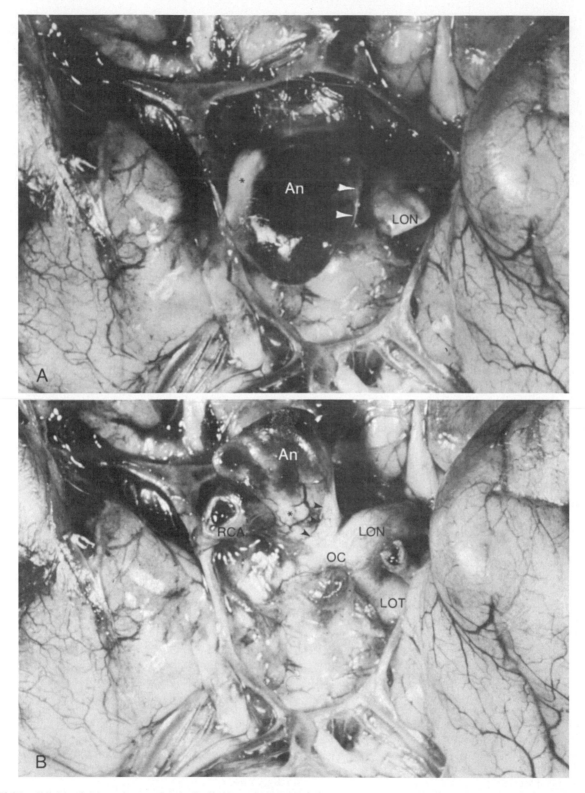

Figure 53.96.   Splitting of right optic nerve longitudinally by a carotid-ophthalmic artery aneurysm. *A*, Basal view shows intact left optic nerve (*LON*). The aneurysm (*An*) has divided the right optic nerve into a lateral and a medial segment. The lateral segment is well seen (*asterisk*). The medial segment is almost hidden by the aneurysm *(arrowheads)*. *B*, After the aneurysm is deflated, both the lateral and medial segments of the divided right optic nerve are visible. *OC,* optic chiasm; *LOT,* left optic tract; *RCA,* right internal carotid artery.

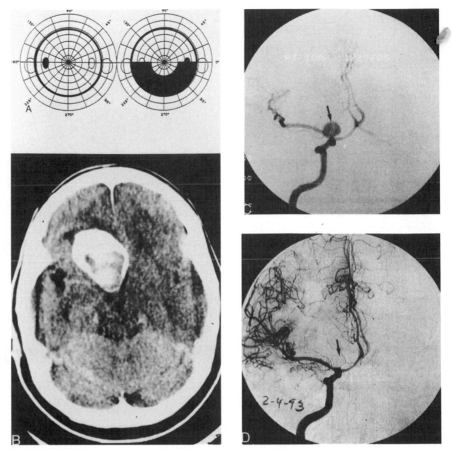

Figure 53.97. Visual field defect caused by a carotid-ophthalmic aneurysm. *A,* Tangent perimetry performed at 1 meter demonstrates an inferior arcuate visual field defect in the right eye compatible with a right optic neuropathy. *B,* Enhanced axial computed tomographic scan demonstrates an irregular mass with central enhancement. Peripheral calcification indicates a likely giant, partially thrombosed, aneurysm. *C,* Coronal digital subtraction angiogram demonstrates an aneurysm arising from the proximal supraclinoid internal carotid artery. The comparison of the size confirms the presence of substantial clot within the aneurysm cavity. *D,* Repeat angiogram following embolization of the aneurysm with Guglielmi detachable electrocoil. Note there is no further filling of the aneurysm cavity with complete sparing of the parent artery (From Vargas ME, Kupersmith MJ, Setton A, et al. Endovascular treatment of giant aneurysms which cause visual loss. Ophthalmology *101*:1091–1098, 1994.)

blurred vision in the left eye associated with mild left supraorbital discomfort and pain on movement of the left eye. Examination revealed a normal right eye. The left eye had visual acuity of 20/25, the left visual field showed an inferotemporal defect, and there was a left RAPD. The left optic disc was mildly swollen, there were hard exudates in the papillomacular area, and choroidal folds were present. The patient was thought to have an anterior optic neuritis (papillitis), but neuroimaging studies revealed a carotid-ophthalmic aneurysm located inferotemporal to the left optic nerve and compressing it against the optic canal. The aneurysm was clipped, and within 48 hours, optic disc swelling began to resolve. Within 1 month after surgery, visual acuity in the left eye had returned to normal.

Jain (1970) described a 44-year-old man who developed decreased vision in the right eye associated with optic disc swelling. Neuroimaging studies revealed an aneurysm arising from the ophthalmic artery 3 mm distal to its origin. The aneurysm projected into the optic canal where it compressed the optic nerve. The optic canal was unroofed, and the ophthalmic artery was clipped proximal to the aneurysm. Postoperatively, the patient's visual acuity improved to 20/25, and the optic disc swelling resolved. Although this aneurysm did not arise from the junction of the internal carotid and ophthalmic arteries and cannot therefore be considered a true carotid-ophthalmic aneurysm, it nevertheless produced findings similar to those described by Tomsak et al. (1979). Optic neuropathy associated with optic disc swelling can also be caused by purely intracranial (Smith, 1979) or intracanalicular (Kennerdell and Maroon, 1975) compressive lesions other than aneurysm, but we believe that this phenomenon is exceptionally rare.

Ocular symptoms other than those of visual sensory dysfunction are rare in patients with carotid-ophthalmic aneurysms. Some aneurysms reach sufficient size that they erode the sphenoid ridge, compressing the optic nerve and the ocular motor nerves passing through the superior orbital fissure. Patients in whom such compression occurs develop ipsilateral blindness, proptosis (Gupta et al., 1990), and ophthalmoparesis (Fig. 53.99). Other aneurysms extend inferomedially and compress or invade the cavernous sinus. Although such aneurysms do not always produce symptoms and signs of a cavernous sinus syndrome (Nutik, 1978), some patients develop ipsilateral ophthalmoparesis from damage to one or more of the ocular motor nerves within the sinus. The ophthalmoparesis may be unassociated with diplopia if visual loss in the affected eye is profound. It may be associated, however, with pain in the distribution of the first (and occasionally the second) division of the trigeminal nerve. Such pain is rare in the absence of ophthalmoparesis.

As is the case with intracavernous aneurysms, endocrine dysfunction is extremely rare in patients with carotid-oph-

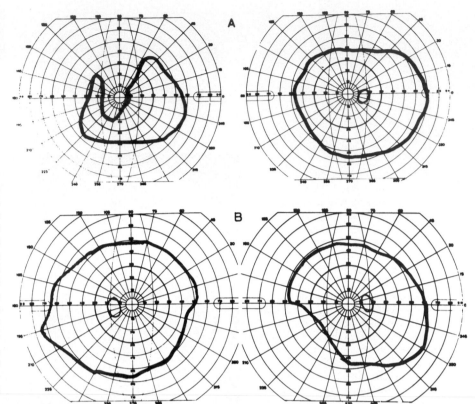

Figure 53.98. Visual field defects in two patients with a carotid-ophthalmic aneurysm. *A,* In a patient with a left carotid-ophthalmic aneurysm and progressive visual loss in the left eye, there is a dense central scotoma that breaks out to the superior periphery in the visual field of that eye. The right visual field is normal. Such a patient may be thought to have experienced a retrobulbar optic neuritis because of the central field defect. *B,* In a patient with a right carotid-ophthalmic aneurysm, there is an inferonasal defect in the visual field of the right eye (From Peiris JB, Ross Russell RW. Giant aneurysms of the carotid system presenting as visual field defect. J Neurol Neurosurg Psychiatry *43:* 1053–1064, 1980.)

thalmic aneurysms. Van 'T Hoff et al. (1961) described a 32-year-old woman who developed amenorrhea when she was 19 years old. Three years later, she discovered that she could see nothing but light with the left eye. Two years after this, she experienced a severe occipital headache associated with vomiting and visual loss in the right eye. Within 1 week, she was blind in both eyes. She was found to have right optic disc swelling, left optic atrophy, a complete right oculomotor nerve paresis, bilateral trochlear paresis, and left abducens paresis. Endocrine evaluation revealed evidence of panhypopituitarism. Angiography showed a large aneurysm originating from the left ICA just above the sella turcica. Although it is not clear that the aneurysm was of the carotid-ophthalmic type, this seems likely, because the initial symptoms were amenorrhea and visual loss in the left eye, and because the aneurysm was located above the sella turcica. A similar case was reported by Krauss et al. (1982), who described a patient with a large carotid-ophthalmic aneurysm arising intradurally but expanding downward and medially into the sella turcica and suprasellar space. The patient had decreased vision in one eye, bilateral visual field defects, and hypopituitarism with hyperprolactinemia of 147–173 ng/ml from compression of the pituitary stalk by the aneurysm. The patient's endocrine dysfunction improved after clipping of the aneurysm. Similar cases were reported by Arseni et al. (1970) and by Verbalis et al. (1982).

Visual loss may occur not only from a carotid-ophthalmic aneurysm but also from its treatment (Litofsky et al., 1994). Direct damage to the optic nerve may occur during removal

of the anterior clinoid process (Nagasawa et al., 1996), dissection of the aneurysm, or from the clip used to occlude the aneurysm. In addition, the blood supply to the nerve may be interrupted by the clip, by coils or balloons used to occlude the aneurysm or its parent artery, or by postoperative vasospasm.

Aneurysms Arising from the Ophthalmic Artery

Most "ophthalmic artery aneurysms" actually arise from the junction of the internal carotid and ophthalmic arteries and not from the more distal portion of the ophthalmic artery itself (Goldin and Silver, 1957; Cunningham and Sewell, 1971; Stern and Ernest, 1975). True ophthalmic artery aneurysms arise from the distal portion of the ophthalmic artery and are extremely rare (Lange-Cosack, 1966; Tönnis and Walter, 1966; Carter and Montgomery 1989; Ogawa et al., 1992) (Fig. 53.100). Nevertheless, such aneurysms may arise from the intracranial, intracanalicular, or intraorbital portion of the vessel. When they arise intracranially or within the optic canal, they enlarge the canal and cause ipsilateral loss of vision from compression of the optic nerve (Parkinson et al., 1961; Raitta, 1968) (Fig. 53.101). In most cases, such aneurysms produce progressive optic atrophy. As noted above, however, Jain (1970) described a 44-year-old man who developed decreased vision in the right eye associated with swelling of the right optic disc swelling from an aneurysm arising from the ophthalmic artery 3 mm distal to its origin. The aneurysm projected into the optic canal where it compressed the optic nerve. The optic canal was unroofed,

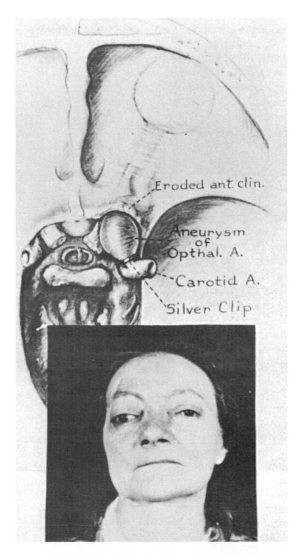

Figure 53.99. Appearance of a patient in whom a large right carotid-ophthalmic aneurysm eroded the inner third of the sphenoid ridge and the optic canal, producing ipsilateral blindness, proptosis, and ophthalmoparesis. (Courtesy of Dr. Lyle French.)

and the ophthalmic artery was clipped proximal to the aneurysm. Postoperatively, the patient's visual acuity improved to 20/25, and the optic disc swelling resolved.

When ophthalmic artery aneurysms occur within the orbit, they may be asymptomatic (Kikuchi and Kowada, 1994) (Fig. 53.102) and identified only during neuroimaging studies performed for other reasons (e.g., headache) or during a postmortem examination (Duke-Elder, 1952). Other aneurysms of the intraorbital portion of the ophthalmic artery may project in such a way as to compress the adjacent optic nerve and cause monocular visual loss (Rubinstein et al., 1968) (Fig. 53.103). The loss of vision may be sudden and stable, sudden and fluctuating, or slowly progressive. Carter and Montgomery (1989) described a 44-year-old woman who developed progressive visual loss in the right eye associated with swelling of the right optic disc from an aneurysm

of the ophthalmic artery at the orbital end of the optic canal. In some cases, an intraorbital ophthalmic artery aneurysm ruptures, causing an acute intraorbital hemorrhage with proptosis and loss of vision (Meyerson and Lazar, 1971) (Fig. 53.104). This clinical picture can also result from rupture of aneurysms arising from the anterior or posterior ethmoid arteries (Ranjan and Joseph, 1994).

Aneurysms Arising from Retinal Arteries

Aneurysms do not usually arise from the central retinal artery; however, aneurysms may arise from retinal vessels. Such lesions may be microaneurysms or macroaneurysms.

Most retinal aneurysms arise from capillaries. Such **retinal microaneurysms** are frequently associated with capillary dropout and are seen in many pathologic states, including diabetes mellitus, sickle cell disease, monoclonal gammopathy, and radiation retinopathy (Robertson, 1973) (Figs. 53.105 and 53.106). In addition, microaneurysms may occur as congenital anomalies and in association primary

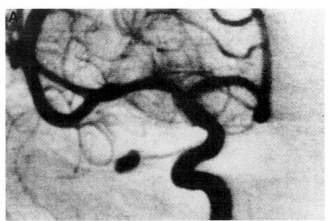

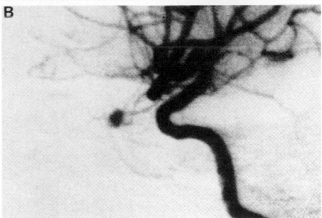

Figure 53.100. Angiographic appearance of an aneurysm arising from the intraorbital segment of the right ophthalmic artery. The patient was a 63-year-old woman with exophthalmos and a 2-week history of worsening visual acuity. Visual acuity was 20/200 OD and 20/20 OS. *A*, Anterior/posterior projection; *B*, Lateral projection. (From Ogawa A, Tominaga T, Yoshimoto T, et al. Intraorbital ophthalmic artery aneurysm: Case report. *Neurosurgery 31*:1102–1104, 1992.)

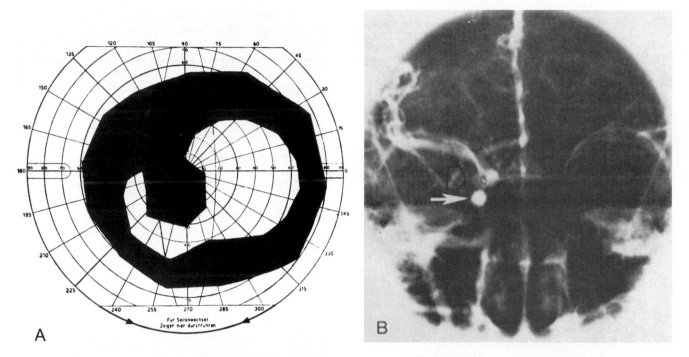

Figure 53.101. Aneurysm of the proximal, right ophthalmic artery producing a unilateral optic neuropathy. *A*, Visual field defect in the right eye shows a dense central scotoma that breaks out to the superior nasal periphery. The vision in this eye was counting fingers. The right optic disc was pale. *B*, Cerebral angiogram, anteroposterior view, shows the aneurysm just distal to the origin of the right ophthalmic artery (*arrow*). (From Raitta C. Ophthalmic artery aneurysm: Causing optic atrophy and enlargement of the optic foramen. Br J Ophthalmol *52*:707–709, 1968.)

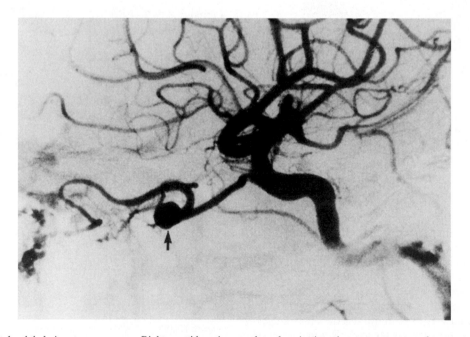

Figure 53.102. Distal ophthalmic artery aneurysm. Right carotid angiogram, lateral projection, demonstrates a saccular aneurysm 15 mm anterior to the origin to the ophthalmic artery (*arrow*) in a patient who also has an arteriovenous malformation fed by branches of the same artery. (From Kikuchi K, Kowada M. Case report: Saccular aneurysm of the intraorbital ophthalmic artery. Br J Radiol *67*:1134–1135, 1994.)

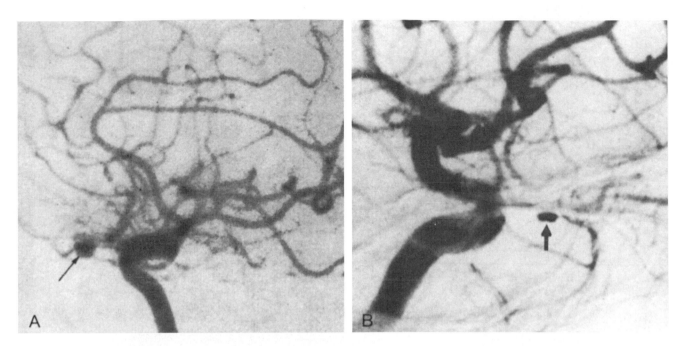

Figure 53.103. Aneurysms arising from the intraorbital portion of the ophthalmic artery. *A*, In a 36-year-old man with progressive loss of visual acuity in the right eye and a dense central scotoma (*arrow*). (From Rubinstein MK, Wilson G, Levin DC. Intraorbital aneurysms of the ophthalmic artery: Report of a unique case and review of the literature. Arch Ophthalmol *80*:42–44, 1968.) *B*, In a 44-year-old woman with progressive visual loss in the right eye and irregular constriction of the right visual field (*arrow*). (From Carter JE, Montgomery RJ. The impossible aneurysm: Canalicular and orbital apex aneurysms of the ophthalmic artery. Neuro-ophthalmology *9*:103–110, 1989.) Arch Ophthalmol *80*:42–44, 1968.) *B*, In a 44-year-old woman with progressive visual loss in the right eye and irregular constriction of the right visual field (*arrow*). (From Carter JE, Montgomery RJ. Neuro-ophthalmology *9*: 103–110, 1989.)

ocular diseases, such as Eales' disease, Coats' disease, and Leber's hereditary miliary aneurysms. The pathogenesis of microaneurysms is obscure. It is speculated that loss of pericytes leads either to weakness in the vascular wall or to endothelial proliferation.

Retinal microaneurysms almost never bleed, and they usually pose no threat to vision. They are, however, useful markers of disease. For example, although microaneurysms tend to increase with increased duration of diabetes mellitus (Feman, 1994), Klein et al. (1995) found a 5-fold increase in the risk of proliferative diabetic retinopathy and a 9-fold increase in the risk of clinically significant macular edema over a 10-year period when there was an increase in the number of retinal microaneurysms by 16 or more. Retinal microaneurysms may also serve as a marker for certain toxic exposures. Vanhoorne et al. (1996) found a correlation between deficiencies in color vision as tested using the Farnsworth-Munsell 100-Hue test and the number of microaneurysms in rayon workers exposed to carbon disulfide. The more microaneurysms present, the more abnormal the color vision and, presumably, the more significant the toxic exposure. An automated method of counting microaneurysms is available (Spencer et al., 1992).

Retinal macroaneurysms are acquired dilations, usually saccular, of the first three orders of retinal arteries (Robertson, 1973; Shirai et al., 1988; Chew and Murphy, 1994) (Fig. 53.107). They often originate at a bifurcation, but they may be located at any point along the vessel (Abdel-Khalek

and Richardson, 1986), and they even occur on the optic disc (Brown and Weinstock, 1985) (Fig. 53.108). They almost always arise on branches of the central retinal artery (Robertson, 1973), although Giuffrè et al. (1987) described a case in which a retinal macroaneurysm arose from a cilioretinal artery, a direct branch from one of the posterior ciliary arteries. They most often arise from the superotemporal branch retinal artery (Tezel et al., 1994a, 1994b), but they may originate from any of the branches of the central retinal artery (Asdourian et al., 1977; François, 1979; Khalil and Lorenzetti, 1979; Dewachter and De Laey, 1982; Palestine et al., 1982; Attali et al., 1984; Abdel-Khalek and Richardson, 1986). Most retinal macroaneurysms are nonpulsatile, but pulsating macroaneurysms occur (Shults and Swan, 1974; Bleckmann, 1983).

Retinal macroaneurysms occur most often in patients with systemic vasculopathies, particularly hypertension and arteriosclerosis (Robertson, 1973; Cleary et al., 1975; Nadel and Gupta, 1976; Dewachter and De Laey, 1982; Attali et al., 1984; Abdel-Khalek and Richardson, 1986; Shirai et al., 1988; Yasui et al., 1988). They are more common in women than in men, and they usually become symptomatic after 60 years of age (Robertson, 1973; Lewis et al., 1976; Spalter, 1982; Abdel-Khalek and Richardson, 1986; Yasui et al., 1988). They usually are single lesions limited to one eye. When multiple macroaneurysms are present in an eye, they all may be located on a single vessel, or they may affect several different vessels (Spalter,

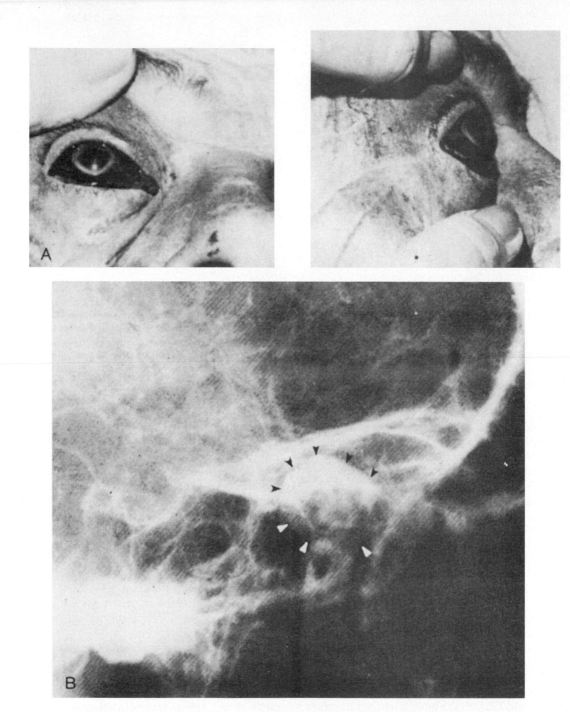

Figure 53.104.   Intraorbital hemorrhage from rupture of a large aneurysm arising from the intraorbital portion of the right ophthalmic artery. The patient was a 55-year-old man who developed acute proptosis of the right eye and diffuse subconjunctival hemorrhage after coughing. *A,* External appearance of the patient. The pupil was fixed and dilated. The eye was blind. *B,* Cerebral angiogram, lateral view of venous phase, shows large intraorbital aneurysm (*arrowheads*). (From Meyerson L, Lazar SJ. Intraorbital aneurysm of the ophthalmic artery. Br J Ophthalmol *55*:199–204, 1971.)

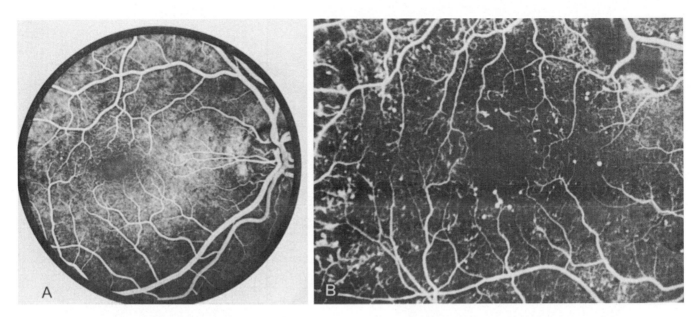

Figure 53.105. Retinal microaneurysms. *A,* Fluorescein angiography in a patient with diabetes mellitus shows numerous microaneurysms that appear as tiny white dots, most of which are temporal to the fovea. *B,* In another patient with diabetes, fluorescein angiography (*magnified view*) shows numerous microaneurysms surrounding the fovea.

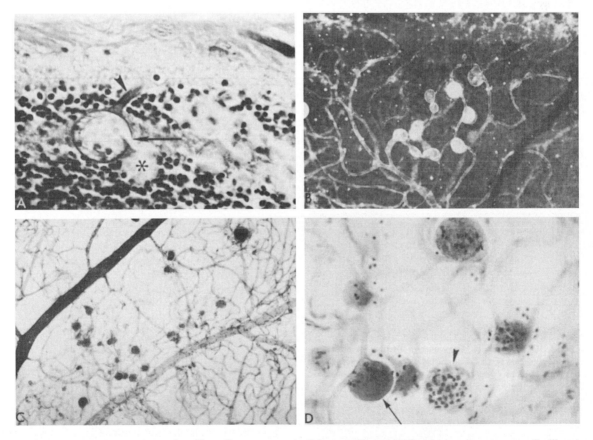

Figure 53.106. Histopathologic appearance of capillary microaneurysms in diabetes mellitus. *A,* Light microscopic appearance. Capillary (*arrowhead*) is continuous with a microaneurysm that is distrupted (*arrow*) and has produced slight hemorrhage (*asterisk*). PAS, × 575. *B,* Flat preparation of the retina shows numerous microaneurysms. AFIP Acc. 219548. (From Friedenwald JS. Am J Ophthalmol *32*:487–498, 1949.) *C,* Trypsin digest preparation of retina shows microaneurysms between a retinal artery and vein. *D,* Higher-power of this region shows some aneurysms that stain deeply (*arrow*) and others that contain polymorphonuclear leukocytes (*arrowhead*). (From Green WR. Retina. In Ophthalmic Pathology: An Atlas and Textbook, 3rd ed, Vol 2, pp 589–1291. Philadelphia, WB Saunders, 1985.)

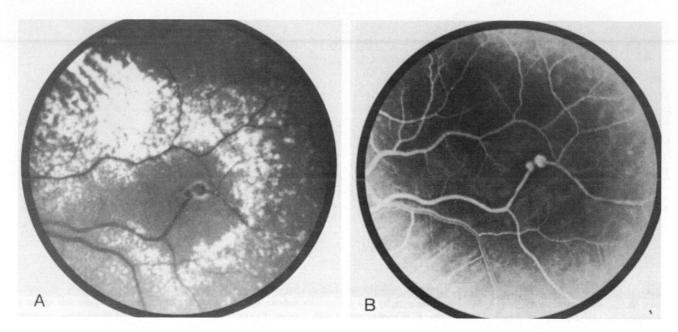

Figure 53.107. Ophthalmoscopic appearance of a retinal artery macroaneurysm. *A*, The aneurysm is surrounded by a ring of hard (lipid) exudate. *B*, Fluorescein angiogram of the aneurysm shows its relationship to the artery from which it originates. Note that there is a small kink in the artery just proximal to the aneurysm.

1982; Bigar and Witmer, 1983). Both eyes are affected in some patients (Godel et al., 1977; François, 1979; Kayazawa, 1980; Shirai et al., 1988).

The histopathology of retinal macroaneurysms is well described (Gold et al., 1976; Perry et al., 1977; Fichte et al., 1978; Green, 1996). The arteries from which the aneurysms arise often contain atheroma. The walls of the aneurysms are thickened by fibroglial proliferation, hemosiderin deposits, lipoidal and proteinaceous exudates, and some extravasated blood (Fig. 53.109). Dilated capillaries often surround the aneurysm, and fresh or organized thrombus may partially or completely fill the aneurysmal lumen.

The cause of retinal macroaneurysms is unknown. Leishman (1957) showed that retinal arteries of older patients with arteriosclerosis show thickening of the vessel wall and replacement of contractile elements by collagen. Arteries affected in such a manner might dilate when subjected to increased pressure (e.g., in systemic hypertension), thus pro-

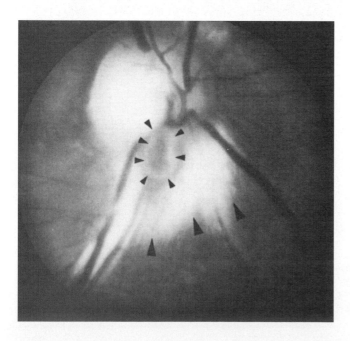

Figure 53.108. Ophthalmoscopic appearance of a retinal arterial macroaneurysm that presented as a mass on the optic disc. The macroaneurysm is seen as an oval lesion (*small arrowheads*) that has a white border and a dark center that may indicate thrombosis within the aneurysm. The patient also has myelinated retinal nerve fibers in this area (*large arrowheads*). (From Brown GC, Weinstock F. Arterial macroaneurysm on the optic disk presenting as a mass lesion. Ann Ophthalmol *17*:519–520, 1985.)

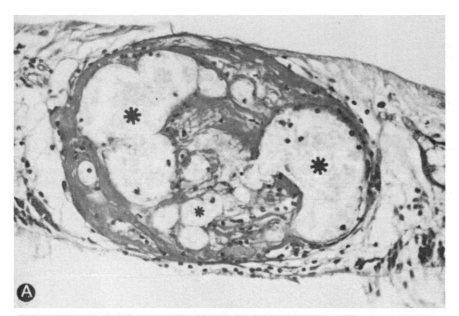

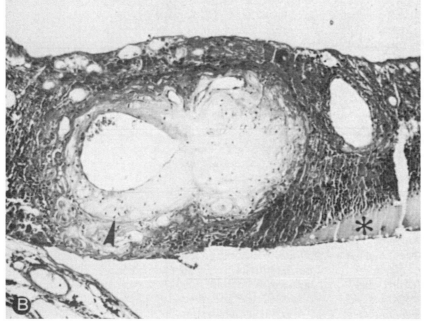

Figure 53.109. Histopathologic appearance of retinal arterial macroaneurysms. *A,* A thrombosed macroaneurysm shows channels of recanalization *(asterisks). B,* Another macroaneurysm has a markedly thickened wall *(arrowhead).* The surrounding retina and subretinal space contain a dense proteinaceous exudate. (From Gold D, LaPiana F, Zimmerman LE. Isolated retinal arterial aneurysms. Am J Ophthalmol *82:*848–857, 1976.)

ducing a macroaneurysm. This hypothesis does not explain why retinal macroaneurysms tend to be single unilateral lesions, however. An alternative hypothesis was proposed by Lewis et al. (1976), who suggested that a retinal macroaneurysm might result from focal damage to the vessel wall, especially at points where emboli lodge. The histopathologic findings described by Gold et al. (1976) and by Fichte et al. (1978) would seem to substantiate this hypothesis.

The appearance of and symptoms produced by a retinal macroaneurysm depend on its location (Tezel et al., 1994a, 1994b). Tezel et al. (1994a) suggested that symptoms depended on whether or not the macroaneurysm was within or outside a 3 mm "critical distance" from the foveola. These authors emphasized that retinal macroaneurysms out-

side this critical distance were usually asymptomatic, but that aneurysms within it often produced visual loss which could be sudden or gradual.

Sudden loss of vision usually results from retinal, preretinal, subretinal, or vitreous hemorrhage (Nadel and Gupta, 1976; Brent et al., 1993). The hemorrhage may occur spontaneously or after a Valsalva maneuver (Avins and Krummenacher, 1983). When the hemorrhage is subretinal, the ophthalmoscopic appearance may mimic that of a malignant melanoma (Perry et al., 1977), and the eye might be mistakenly enucleated for this reason (Fig. 53.110). Most of these hemorrhages are reabsorbed without sequela, but subretinal hemorrhage can produce disciform scarring in the macula associated with permanent central visual loss.

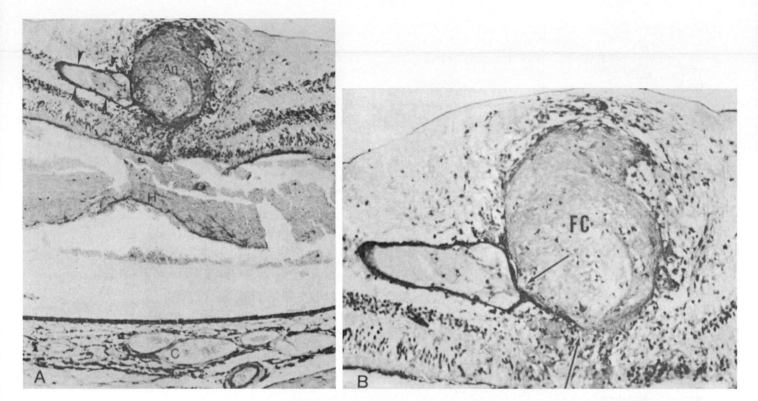

Figure 53.110. Histopathologic appearance of an isolated retinal macroaneurysm that produced a marked subretinal and vitreous hemorrhage. The eye was enucleated because the lesion was thought to be a malignant melanoma. *A*, The aneurysm (*An*) and the retinal artery from which it arises (*arrowheads*) are seen. The aneurysm has ruptured, resulting in hemorrhage into the deep retina and the subretinal space (*H*). The choroid (*C*) is normal in appearance. *B*, Section through the aneurysm shows the ends of the ruptured wall (*arrows*). A laminated fibrin clot (*FC*) is present and seems to have originated from the site of rupture. (From Perry HD, Zimmerman LE, Benson WE. Hemorrhage from isolated aneurysm of a retinal artery: Report of two cases simulating malignant melanoma. Arch Ophthalmol 95:281–283, 1977.)

Gradual distortion and loss of vision related to a retinal macroaneurysm may be caused by retinal edema, nonrhegmatogenous serous retinal detachment, and formation of hard exudates. These complications ultimately may produce cystoid degeneration of the macula with persistent damage to central vision.

The evolution of a macroaneurysm from the time that it becomes symptomatic is, like the histopathology, well described (Cleary et al., 1975; Godel et al., 1977; François, 1979; Palestine et al., 1982; Spalter, 1982; Castier et al., 1984; Holland, 1984; Noble, 1984; Abdel-Khalek and Richardson, 1986). Over time, the walls sclerose, and the lumen becomes occluded. In addition, the artery from which the macroaneurysm arises may become narrow or even occluded. As these changes occur, hemorrhage and exudate resolve, and vision, if previously reduced, often improves.

The treatment of a retinal macroaneurysm depends on whether or not it is symptomatic or likely to become so. Asymptomatic aneurysms probably do not require therapy. Laser photocoagulation of the aneurysm may be appropriate for patients with recurrent hemorrhage or macular exudation (Hudomel and Imre, 1973; Lewis et al., 1976; Amalric et al., 1979; François, 1979; Nouhuys and Deutman, 1980; Constantanides and Hochart, 1981; Makabe, 1981; Abdel-Khalek and Richardson, 1986; François et al., 1987; Shirai

et al., 1988; Joondeph et al., 1989; Psinakis et al., 1989), although this remains controversial. Photocoagulation seals the aneurysm, and also increases the rate of absorption of perianeurysmal exudate. Some investigators recommend that macroaneurysms be treated with photocoagulation before they affect visual function (Yasui et al., 1988). In a long-term follow-up study, however, Brown et al. (1994) questioned the usefulness of photocoagulation. In their study, patients with retinal macroaneurysms who were followed without treatment had a higher incidence of 2-line improvement in vision and a lower incidence of visual deterioration than patients who were treated with photocoagulation. Patients in whom vitreous hemorrhage occurs may benefit from a vitrectomy if the hemorrhage does not clear spontaneously within an appropriate period of time (Brent et al., 1993). Whether or not drainage of subretinal hemorrhage associated with a retinal macroaneurysm is useful is unclear (Hoh and Palmowski, 1992).

Aneurysms Arising from Conjunctival Arteries

Conjunctival aneurysms are extremely rare. They seem to occur most often in patients with glaucoma. Orgul and Flammer (1995) examined 20 patients with low-tension glaucoma and 20 patients with chronic open-angle glaucoma and compared the findings with a control population of 60 normal subjects. Six or more perilimbal aneurysms were found significantly more frequently in the low-tension glaucoma group than in patients with open-angle glaucoma or controls. The implications of this observation are unclear.

Aneurysms Arising from the Proximal Supraclinoid Portion of the Internal Carotid Artery (Supraclinoid Aneurysms)

A saccular aneurysm arising from the proximal, intradural portion of the ICA may have such a large neck or may itself be so large that its origin cannot accurately be determined except that it seems to arise from the 6- to 15-mm segment of artery between the origin of the ophthalmic and posterior communicating arteries (Golding et al., 1980; Gibo et al., 1981; Tateiwa et al., 1997). Such an aneurysm is, of necessity, often described as "suprasellar" or "supraclinoid."

The symptoms and signs produced by supraclinoid aneurysms are identical with those produced by paraclinoid aneurysms. When they rupture, they produce SAH with its associated manifestations. When they act as mass lesions, they compress adjacent structures, including the optic nerves and optic chiasm. Tateiwa et al. (1997) reported the case of a 62-year-old woman who developed progressive visual loss and was found to have evidence of bilateral optic neuropathies. Although the patient's intraocular pressure was normal in both eyes, both optic discs were cupped and pale, initially suggesting a diagnosis of "low-tension" glaucoma (see below). Neuroimaging studies, however, revealed compression of the optic nerves by bilateral supraclinoid ICA aneurysms.

Aneurysms Arising from the Junction of the Internal Carotid and Posterior Communicating Arteries (Internal Carotid-Posterior Communicating Aneurysms)

One of the most common sites of origin of saccular, intracranial aneurysms is the junction of the internal carotid and posterior communicating arteries (Figs. 53.111 and 53.112). It is misleading to refer to aneurysms arising at this location as "posterior communicating" aneurysms. This term should be reserved for aneurysms arising from the distal segment of the posterior communicating artery occasionally do occur (see below).

Aneurysms arising from the junction of the internal carotid and posterior communicating arteries are of particular interest to the ophthalmologist, because they are an important and not uncommon cause of **oculomotor nerve paresis**. From 13 to 30% of acquired oculomotor nerve pareses are caused by aneurysms at this location (Rucker, 1958; Green et al., 1964; Rucker, 1966; Rush and Younge, 1981; Vassiliou et al., 1982; Renowden et al., 1993).

About 35–40% of internal carotid-posterior communicating aneurysms eventually cause an oculomotor nerve paresis (Harris and Udvarhelyi, 1957; Höök and Norlén, 1964a; Odom, 1964; Soni, 1974; Huige et al., 1988). The paresis may result from damage to the nerve at the time the aneurysm ruptures (Hyland and Barnett, 1953; Harris and Udvar-

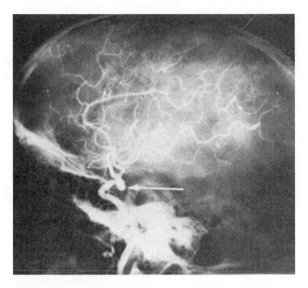

Figure 53.111. Left internal carotid-posterior communicating aneurysm (*arrow*). The aneurysm produced a left oculomotor nerve paresis 5 years before the angiogram was performed.

helyi, 1957; Huber, 1976, 1982; Huige et al., 1988). It also may be caused by an unruptured, expanding aneurysm that compresses or even fenestrates the adjacent oculomotor nerve (Horiuchi et al., 1997). In such cases, the paresis may develop spontaneously or after seemingly trivial head trauma that further damages an already compromised oculomotor nerve (Walter et al., 1994) (Fig. 53.24). Almost 90% of symptomatic, unruptured internal carotid-posterior communicating aneurysms present with signs of oculomotor nerve paresis (Locksley, 1969). Such aneurysms are almost always greater than 4 mm in diameter. Thus, they can be detected by such noninvasive neuroimaging studies as MR angiography and spiral CT angiography (Teasdale et al., 1989).

Any discussion of oculomotor nerve paresis caused by an internal carotid-posterior communicating aneurysm must consider three major issues: (*a*) the occurrence of ipsilateral facial, orbital, or eye pain; (*b*) the degree of dysfunction of

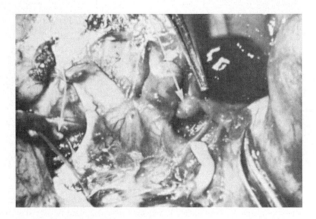

Figure 53.112. Bilateral internal carotid-posterior communicating aneurysms (*arrows*) viewed from below.

the extraocular muscles and the levator palpebrae superioris; and (c) involvement of the pupillary sphincter.

Ipsilateral frontal head **pain**, usually located behind the eye, above the brow, or both, occurs in almost all patients who develop oculomotor nerve paresis after aneurysm rup-

ture and in most patients who develop oculomotor nerve paresis from an unruptured aneurysm (Harris and Udvar-helyi, 1957; Soni, 1974). In patients with ruptured aneu-rysms, the pain occurs at the time of rupture. It is typically sharp and throbbing, and it tends to radiate posteriorly (De-

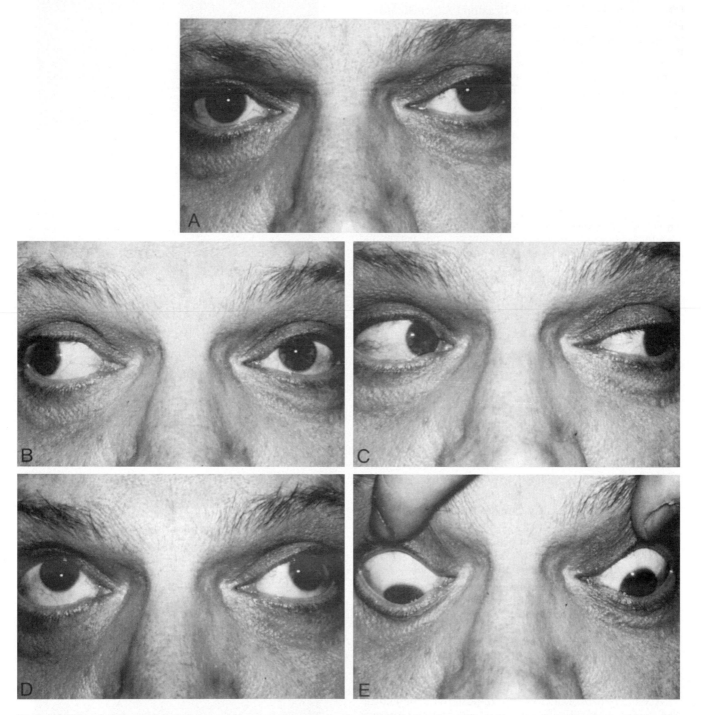

Figure 53.113. *A–E,* Partial left oculomotor nerve paresis in a patient with a left-sided internal carotid-posterior communicating artery aneurysm. The patient initially developed mild left ptosis associated with left-sided forehead pain. He then noted binocular diplopia that was both vertical and horizontal. He was examined 12 hours after the onset of ptosis. Note that he has moderate left ptosis and is using his frontalis to elevate the left upper eyelid. The left eye is exotropic, but the left pupil is about the same size as the right pupil. Within several hours, the left pupil became dilated and poorly reactive, and the oculomotor nerve paresis became complete.

mierre and Safran, 1981). It is often associated with neck pain and stiffness. The oculomotor nerve paresis may also occur at this time, or it may not develop for hours to days. In patients with unruptured aneurysms, head and eye pain may occur intermittently for several years before the aneurysm ruptures or an oculomotor nerve paresis develops. The pain may last for a day or so and then not recur for weeks or months. In some cases, the pain is so severe that it is misinterpreted as trigeminal neuralgia (Höök and Norlén, 1964a).

The pain produced by an unruptured internal carotid-posterior communicating aneurysm seems to be referred pain that is produced by traction or pressure of the aneurysm on the adjacent edge of the tentorium which, like the forehead and eyes, is innervated by the first division of the trigeminal nerve (Feindel et al., 1960). In a study of autopsy material, Lanzino et al. (1993a) demonstrated sensory fibers tracking to the trigeminal nucleus from cells along the oculomotor nerve. They postulated that these fibers originate from the ophthalmic division of the trigeminal nerve and join the oculomotor nerve at the level of the lateral wall of the cavernous sinus. It is also possible that the pain is vascular in origin, because it follows the same distribution when either the internal carotid or the posterior communicating artery is stimulated mechanically (Ray and Wolff, 1940; Pool, 1958).

Pain is not present in every patient who develops an oculomotor nerve paresis from an internal carotid-posterior communicating aneurysm, particularly when the aneurysm has not ruptured. Harris and Udvarhelyi (1957) described four patients in whom painless oculomotor nerve paresis was the only sign of an aneurysm. A young woman examined by Dr. Michael Slavin absolutely denied headache or eye pain during an evaluation for a complete oculomotor nerve paresis. While undergoing a CT scan, she experienced an acute SAH and died shortly thereafter. The scans obtained at the time of the hemorrhage seemed to demonstrate an internal carotid-posterior communicating aneurysm that had ruptured (Slavin, 1990a). The patient's family refused postmortem examination.

Dysfunction of the extraocular muscles and the levator palpebrae superioris in oculomotor nerve paresis caused by internal carotid-posterior communicating aneurysm is extremely variable. The earliest sign is often an isolated, mild ptosis that usually progresses over several hours to days, during which time the extraocular muscles innervated by the oculomotor nerve and the pupillary sphincter become affected (Hamer, 1982; Bartleson et al., 1986) (Figs. 53.113–53.117). In rare cases, the ptosis remains stable for several weeks, during which time it is unassociated with diplopia, limitation of eye movement, or anisocoria (Good, 1990). In other cases, diplopia, mydriasis, or both occur before ptosis becomes apparent (Bartleson et al., 1986; Jones and Mendelson, 1986; Ebner, 1990). Evidence of progressive oculomotor nerve dysfunction develops in nearly all patients over time, regardless of the initial symptoms and signs of the dysfunction; however, Greenspan and Reeves (1990) reported the case of a 38-year-old woman who developed a partial right oculomotor nerve paresis characterized by ptosis, mild weakness of the superior rectus muscle, and a slightly dilated pupil, that **spontaneously resolved** over a 2-week period. The patient was subsequently found to have an aneurysm at the junction of the right internal carotid and posterior communicating arteries (Fig. 53.118).

Damage to the parasympathetic nerves innervating the iris sphincter causes a **dilated and fixed or poorly reactive pupil** occurs in most patients who develop an oculomotor nerve paresis from an internal carotid-posterior communicating aneurysm (Rucker, 1958; Green et al., 1964) (Figs. 53.114 and 53.115). Pupillary dilation may occur shortly before, at the same time as, or shortly after ptosis and ophthalmoparesis develop. Patients in whom damage to parasympathetic fibers occurs may complain of blurred near vision because of reduced or absent accommodation. Rare patients develop unilateral accommodation weakness hours or even days before the pupil becomes dilated.

Because the pupillomotor fibers are located superficially in the superomedial portion of the oculomotor nerve within the subarachnoid space (Sunderland and Hughes, 1946; Kerr

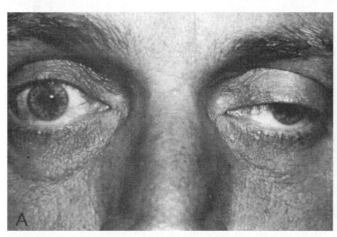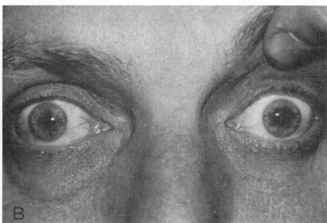

Figure 53.114. Partial left oculomotor nerve paresis in a patient with a left-sided internal carotid-posterior communicating artery aneurysm. *A,* This patient has an incomplete ptosis and ophthalmoparesis; however, the left pupil is moderately dilated and does not react to light (*B*).

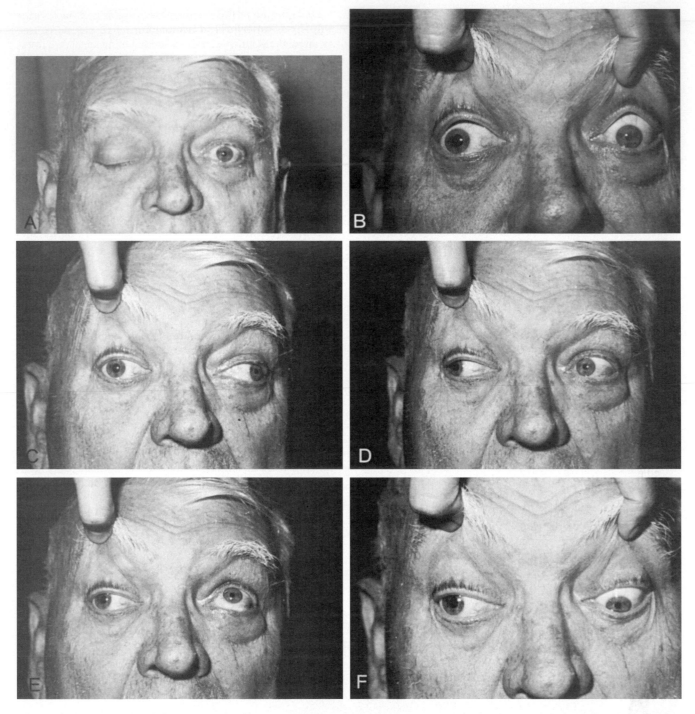

Figure 53.115. *A–F*, Complete right oculomotor nerve paresis with involvement of the pupil. The patient also complained of severe right-sided retrobulbar pain. He was found to have right internal carotid-posterior communicating artery aneurysm.

and Hollowell, 1964) (see Chapter 20), an aneurysm that compresses only the superomedial aspect of the nerve can cause isolated pupillary dilation that appears days to weeks before any other signs of oculomotor nerve damage. In fact, this a phenomenon is exceptionally rare. Basilar artery aneurysms can cause a dilated pupil without other evidence of oculomotor nerve damage (Walsh and Hoyt, 1969b; Cromp-

ton and Moore, 1981; Gale and Crockard, 1982; Bartleson et al., 1986) (see below), but there are almost no reports of internal carotid-posterior communicating aneurysms causing such a finding. Harris and Udvarhelyi (1957) stated that five of 90 patients with internal carotid-posterior communicating aneurysms had "only dilation of the pupil, suggesting a slight oculomotor nerve palsy," but these investigators pro-

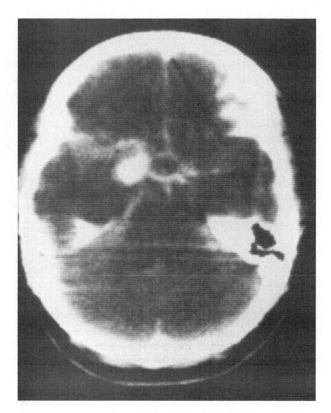

Figure 53.116. Computed tomographic scan of the patient seen in Figure 53.115 shows a well-circumscribed, enhancing lesion at the junction of the right internal carotid and posterior communicating arteries.

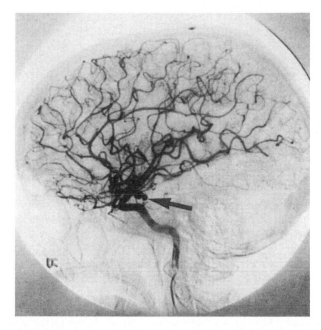

Figure 53.118. Right carotid angiogram shows a bilobed internal carotid-posterior communicating artery aneurysm in a patient who developed a partial right oculomotor nerve paresis that **spontaneously resolved** about 3 weeks after onset.

vided no other details of the examinations. It is possible that their patients had physiologic anisocoria (see Chapters 20 and 24) and not parasympathetic dysfunction from compression of the oculomotor nerve by the aneurysm. It is also possible that the authors overlooked minimal ptosis or oph-

thalmoparesis that was present at about the same time that the pupil became affected.

Payne and Adamkiewicz (1969) described a 35-year-old woman who developed a fixed, dilated pupil in association with an aneurysm located at the junction of the internal carotid and posterior communicating arteries. Although the dilated pupil was the ''principal'' sign exhibited by the patient and emphasized by the authors, she also had an intermittent exotropia and a variable ipsilateral ptosis. The dilated

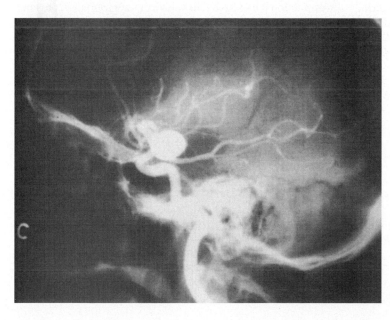

Figure 53.117. Selective right internal carotid arteriogram in the patient whose appearance is seen in Figure 53.115 and whose CT scan is seen in Figure 53.116. The angiogram shows a large aneurysm at the junction of the right internal carotid and posterior communicating arteries. A, Lateral view; B, Anteroposterior view.

pupil overshadowed other signs of oculomotor nerve paresis, but those signs nevertheless **were present.** Wilson and Barmatz (1980) described a 57-year-old woman who experienced an attack of angle closure glaucoma related to pupillary dilation that was part of an aneurysm-induced oculomotor nerve paresis (see below). At the time the pupil became dilated and fixed (with an intraocular pressure of only 35 mm Hg), the movements of the eye were normal, and she reported no diplopia. There was, however, 3 mm of ipsilateral ptosis. As a general rule, therefore, **a fixed, dilated pupil that is unassociated with ptosis or ophthalmoparesis is almost never caused by an internal carotid-posterior communicating aneurysm.**

When pupillary dilation occurs simultaneously with other evidence of ipsilateral oculomotor nerve paresis, particularly when ipsilateral facial or eye pain is present, every effort should be made to exclude an aneurysm, particularly one located at the junction of the internal carotid and posterior communicating arteries (Jefferson, 1947; Soni, 1974). Even children who present in such a manner may harbor such an aneurysm (Branley et al., 1992; Wolin and Saunders, 1992), and they deserve a similar evaluation, even though the incidence of intracranial aneurysms presenting as oculomotor nerve paresis in young children is low (Fox, 1989; Gabianelli et al., 1989). Oculomotor nerve pareses that occur in this setting are often incomplete initially, and partial pupillary involvement often accompanies incomplete ophthalmoparesis (Keane, 1983; Kissel et al., 1983) (Fig. 53.114).

The pupillary dilation that occurs in patients with an oculomotor nerve paresis can occasionally produce chronic angle-closure glaucoma. Wilson and Barmatz (1980) described a 57-year-old woman who experienced sudden pain behind and above the left eye associated with a feeling of faintness and nausea. When initially examined, she had a 3 mm left ptosis. The left conjunctiva was slightly injected and chemotic, and the left pupil was dilated and fixed. Ocular motility was full, the eyes were orthotropic, and the patient denied diplopia. Intraocular pressure was 16 mm Hg in the right eye and 35 mm Hg in the left eye. The right anterior chamber angle was narrow, whereas the left was closed over 75% of its circumference. The patient was treated with 2% pilocarpine to the left eye. As the left pupil constricted, the patient's pain became less severe, and the intraocular pressure in the left eye returned to normal. Over the next 12 hours, the oculomotor nerve paresis became complete, and an evaluation revealed an aneurysm at the junction of the left internal carotid and posterior communicating arteries that was successfully clipped.

Internal carotid-posterior communicating aneurysms may occasionally produce oculomotor nerve paresis in which the pupil does not seem to be affected (Henderson, 1955; Cogan and Mount, 1963; Dailey et al., 1964; Kasoff and Kelly, 1975; Román-Campos and Edwards, 1979; Hamer, 1981a, 1981b; Kissel et al., 1983; Nadeau and Trobe, 1983; O'Connor et al., 1983; Susac, 1984; Ebner, 1990; Ranganadham et al., 1992) at least initially (Fig. 53.113). Such pareses are **almost never complete** (Boghen, 1983; Keane, 1983). Thus, a patient who has a complete oculomotor nerve paresis except for a normal pupil is extraordinarily unlikely to harbor

an internal carotid-posterior communicating artery aneurysm (Teuscher and Meienberg, 1985), whereas a patient with an incomplete paresis and a normal pupil may have an aneurysm that, within hours to days, progresses to become a complete paresis with pupillary involvement. Such a progression always requires an evaluation.

In a previous section on intracavernous aneurysm, we emphasized the tendency of such lesions to produce an oculomotor nerve paresis accompanied by a pupil that is **smaller** than the contralateral pupil because of associated damage to the oculosympathetic pathway in the cavernous sinus. Serdaru et al. (1983) described this phenomenon in a 65-year-old woman with an internal carotid-posterior communicating aneurysm. In this case, the aneurysm expanded inferiorly into the cavernous sinus, where it damaged both the oculomotor nerve and the oculosympathetic pathway, without affecting any of the other cranial nerves. We do not take issue with this case report but emphasize that the syndrome of oculomotor nerve paresis combined with oculosympathetic hypofunction results primarily from **cavernous sinus** lesions and is therefore exceptionally rare in patients with internal carotid-posterior communicating aneurysm.

An oculomotor nerve paresis may occur after treatment of an internal carotid-posterior communicating aneurysm rather than from the effects of the aneurysm itself. In most cases, the paresis is caused by direct injury to the nerve during operation or by compression of the nerve by hematoma, cerebral edema, hydrocephalus, or temporal lobe herniation (Grayson et al., 1974; Soni, 1974; Fox, 1983). In other cases, the clip used to occlude the neck of the aneurysm slips and rotates, resulting in either direct compression of the oculomotor nerve by the clip or compression of the edge of the tentorium by the clip resulting in indirect compression of the oculomotor nerve by the edge of the tentorium. Vasospasm affecting the posterior communicating artery can produce an oculomotor nerve paresis after successful clipping of an internal carotid-posterior communicating artery aneurysm. Kudo (1986) reported such a case. Oculomotor nerve dysfunction may also occur following angiography, presumably from iatrogenic thrombosis of vasa nervorum supplying the oculomotor nerve (Griffiths et al., 1994). Continued improvements in preoperative, intraoperative, and postoperative care of aneurysm patients have resulted in a substantial reduction in the frequency of postoperative oculomotor nerve pareses and an increase in the rate of complete recovery of such pareses.

Some recovery of oculomotor nerve function occurs in almost all patients with aneurysm-induced oculomotor nerve paresis, unless the nerve is transected by the aneurysm or at surgery. Recovery may occur spontaneously or after treatment of the aneurysm, whether or not it has ruptured. In some cases, recovery begins within several days and may be complete within several weeks. This pattern of recovery is most likely to occur when there is an incomplete paresis, when the aneurysm has not ruptured, and when successful clipping of the aneurysm is performed within 1–2 weeks after onset of the paresis (Botterell et al., 1962; Soni, 1974; Perneczky and Czech, 1984; Feely and Kapoor, 1987; Leivo et al., 1996). In a retrospective survey of the literature, Leivo

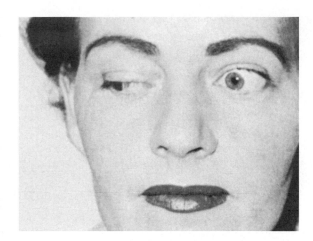

Figure 53.119. Secondary aberrant regeneration of the left oculomotor nerve after a complete left oculomotor nerve paresis caused by a left-sided internal carotid-posterior communicating artery aneurysm. The patient is attempting to look down and to the right. Note incomplete adduction and depression of the left eye associated with left upper eyelid retraction (pseudo-Graefe sign). Aberrant regeneration was first observed about 3 months after the onset of the paresis and clipping of the aneurysm.

et al. (1996) suggested earlier surgery was associated with a better prognosis.

Although Grayson et al. (1974) suggested that complete recovery of an oculomotor nerve paresis can take up to 3 years, it is likely that any recovery that is not complete within several months will be associated with secondary oculomotor nerve synkinesis (aberrant regeneration of the oculomotor nerve) (see Chapter 28) (Walsh, 1957; Hepler and Cantu, 1967; Soni, 1974) (Fig. 53.119). Some patients with secondary oculomotor nerve synkinesis have minimal or no functional deficit; others have disabling diplopia that may not be correctable with surgery or prism therapy.

Primary synkinesis of the oculomotor nerve, most often a consequence of slow-growing lesions located within the cavernous sinus (see above and Chapter 28), was described by Varma and Miller (1994) in a patient with an internal carotid-posterior communicating artery aneurysm. This case emphasizes the importance of evaluating patients with this condition in a timely fashion, rather than assuming that they have a cavernous sinus lesion that does not require urgent treatment.

Some patients, particularly those with long-standing complete oculomotor nerve paresis, severe SAH, or delayed or unsuccessful clipping of the aneurysm, have a persistent, complete oculomotor nerve paresis. Such patients cannot hope to achieve useful binocular single vision regardless of therapy.

An oculomotor nerve paresis is the most common but not the only neurologic sign produced by an unruptured internal carotid-posterior communicating aneurysm. If the aneurysm is extremely large and projects posteriorly, it may produce a dorsal midbrain syndrome, characterized by paralysis of upward gaze, upper eyelid retraction, and pupillary abnormalities including anisocoria and light-near dissociation (Parinaud, 1883; Coppeto and Lessell, 1983; Keane, 1990). In this setting, the syndrome is caused by aneurysmal compression and kinking of the brainstem at the level of the tentorial incisura.

In rare patients, internal carotid-posterior communicating aneurysms cause unilateral or bilateral visual loss (Raymond and Tew, 1978; Peiris and Ross Russell, 1980). In some of these cases, the visual loss results from compression of the ipsilateral optic nerve, the optic chiasm, or the ipsilateral optic tract by the unruptured aneurysm (Figs. 53.120 and 53.121). Walsh and Hoyt (1969g) described a 40-year-old woman who developed a painful right oculomotor nerve paresis that was initially thought to be caused by sinusitis. Visual acuity was 20/40 OD and 20/20 OS. There was a hemianopic paracentral scotoma for small white objects in the visual field of the right eye. The visual field of the left eye was full. There was a right RAPD and an almost complete right oculomotor nerve paresis. The fundi were normal. The patient was eventually found to have a saccular aneurysm at or near the origin

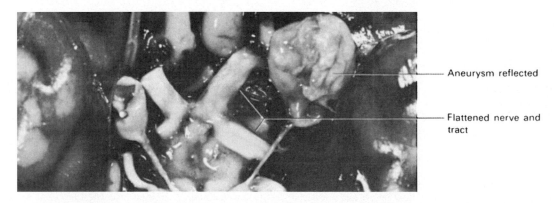

Aneurysm reflected

Flattened nerve and tract

Figure 53.120. Compression of the left optic nerve, left portion of the optic chiasm, and left optic tract by a large internal carotid-posterior communicating artery aneurysm. The aneurysm has been reflected laterally to show the flattened left optic nerve, lateral chiasm, and left optic tract. Although this aneurysm ruptured, it may have produced blindness or a nasal visual field defect in the left eye combined with a temporal visual field defect in the right eye. (From Lindenberg R, Walsh FB, Sacks JG. Neuropathology of Vision: An Atlas. Philadelphia, Lea & Febiger, 1973.)

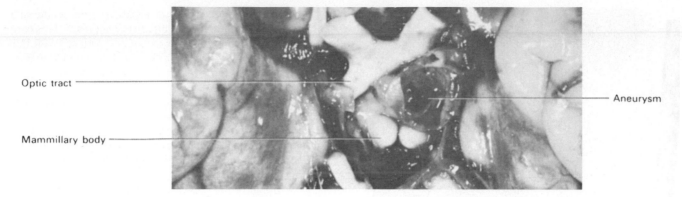

Figure 53.121. Compression of the optic tract by an internal carotid-posterior communicating artery aneurysm. The aneurysm, which arises from the junction of the left internal carotid and posterior communicating arteries projects posteromedially, thus compressing the left optic tract, which is hidden from view by the aneurysm. The optic chiasm and both optic nerves seem unaffected by the aneurysm. Although this aneurysm ruptured, it probably produced a contralateral hemianopia before it did so. (From Lindenberg R, Walsh FB, Sacks JG. Neuropathology of Vision: An Atlas. Philadelphia, Lea & Febiger, 1973.)

of the right posterior communicating artery, projecting toward the right cavernous sinus, and compressing the intracranial portion of the right optic nerve.

Raymond and Tew (1978) described a 59-year-old woman who lost temporal vision in the left eye and was thought to have retrobulbar optic neuritis. She subsequently lost almost all vision in the eye and also developed loss of vision and a temporal field defect in the right eye. Five years later, she began to experience difficulty walking and weakness in the upper extremities. An examination at this time revealed a bitemporal hemianopia associated with visual acuity of 20/40 OD and counting fingers at 4 feet OS (Fig. 53.122A).

The left optic disc was pale. The patient also had mild right central facial weakness, bilateral spasticity of gait, hyperactive deep-tendon reflexes, and bilateral extensor plantar responses. Angiography revealed a giant (30 × 30 × 30 mm) suprasellar aneurysm originating near the origin of the left posterior communicating artery. The aneurysm was treated by gradual occlusion of the cervical portions of the left internal and external carotid arteries combined with ligation of the left ICA distal to the aneurysm and aneurysmorrhaphy. Following this treatment, the patient's visual acuity and visual field returned to normal in the right eye, and left eye vision improved to 20/20 with improvement in the field in

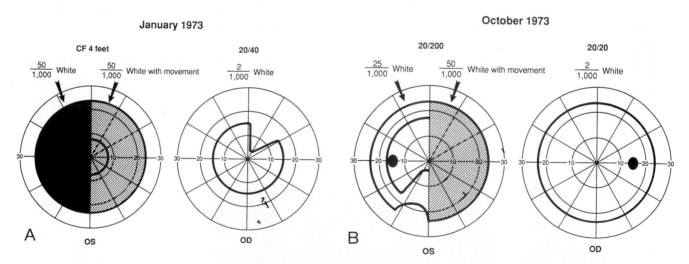

Figure 53.122. Optic chiasmal syndrome with bilateral optic neuropathy in a patient with a left internal carotid-posterior communicating artery aneurysm. *A,* When the patient was initially examined, the right eye had visual acuity of 20/40 with a superior temporal field defect that came within 5 degrees of fixation, and the left eye had visual acuity of counting fingers at 4 feet with complete loss of the temporal field and significant loss of the nasal field. *B,* After trapping of the aneurysm and aneurysmorraphy, the patient's visual acuity improved to 20/20 in the right eye with a full visual field and to 20/200 in the left eye with a relative inferotemporal defect and a relative nasal defect. (From Raymond LA, Tew J. Large suprasellar aneurysms imitating pituitary tumour. J Neurol Neurosurg Psychiatry *41*:83–87, 1978.)

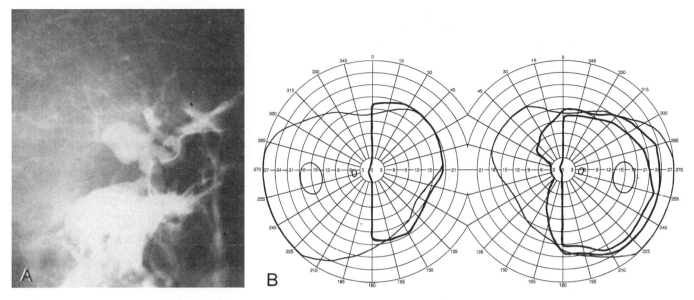

Figure 53.123. Compression of the optic tract by an internal carotid-posterior communicating artery aneurysm. *A*, Cerebral angiogram shows giant aneurysm originating from the junction of the right internal carotid and posterior communicating arteries. *B*, Visual field defect produced by the aneurysm consists of a left incongruous homonymous hemianopia consistent with damage to the right optic tract. (From Peiris JB, Ross Russell RW. Giant aneurysms of the carotid system presenting as visual field defect. J Neurol Neurosurg Psychiatry *43*:1053–1064, 1980.)

that eye (Fig. 53.122*B*). In this case, a giant aneurysm originated from the junction of the internal carotid and posterior communicating arteries and compressed both optic nerves and the optic chiasm.

Peiris and Ross Russell (1980) described a 61-year-old woman with a right internal carotid-posterior communicating aneurysm that projected medially to compress the right optic tract. The patient had visual acuity of 20/40 OD and 20/30 OS. There was an incongruous left homonymous hemianopia from compression of the right optic tract by the aneurysm (Fig. 53.123).

Patients with a complete homonymous hemianopia caused by compression of the optic tract by an aneurysm have an RAPD contralateral to the lesion (on the side of the hemianopia). With time, homonymous hemianopic optic and retinal nerve fiber layer atrophy develop (see Chapter 8).

Sudden expansion and rupture of an internal carotid-posterior communicating aneurysm may cause spasm of distal arterial branches or intracerebral bleeding. Hemiplegia and corresponding homonymous hemianopia may result. An additional rare complication of an aneurysm in this location is a carotid-cavernous sinus fistula (Tytle et al., 1995). This phenomenon occurs when the origin of the posterior communicating artery is within the cavernous sinus rather than intradural.

Mental dysfunction may result when internal carotid-posterior communicating aneurysms compress the mammillary bodies or interfere with the blood supply to the hypothalamus and diencephalon. Walsh and Hoyt (1969h) described a patient with this type of aneurysm who had headaches, oculomotor nerve paresis, and Korsakoff's syndrome. Smith et al. (1994) reported the case of a patient with a giant internal carotid-posterior communicating artery aneurysm who

presented in coma from hydrocephalus caused by obstruction of the 3rd ventricle by the aneurysm.

Aneurysms Arising from the Posterior Communicating Artery

Aneurysms that arise from the posterior communicating artery rather than from its junction with the ICA are rare. They occur with a frequency of 0.1–0.5% in most series (Yoshida et al., 1979; Kamiyama et al., 1980; Abiko and Orita, 1981; Miyazawa et al., 1983; Waga et al., 1984). These aneurysms usually present with SAH, and, because of their proximity to the oculomotor nerve, they can produce an oculomotor nerve paresis at the time of rupture (Ogasawara et al., 1995). A posterior communicating artery aneurysm can also cause an oculomotor nerve paresis by expansion and compression of the nerve rather than from the effects of rupture (Fig. 53.124). Kudo (1990) reported the development of an oculomotor nerve palsy after clipping of a posterior communicating artery aneurysm that was adherent to the oculomotor nerve. The palsy probably occurred because the aneurysm had to be dissected off the nerve in order to clip it.

Posterior communicating artery aneurysms may produce manifestations other than oculomotor nerve pareses. Merva et al. (1985) described a 57-year-old man who developed partial complex seizures and was found to have a giant aneurysm originating from the right posterior communicating artery. At operation, the aneurysm was seen to compress the mesial aspect of the right temporal lobe. There was a moderate amount of scarring with hemosiderin staining in this region, indicating previous leakage from or minimal rupture of the aneurysm.

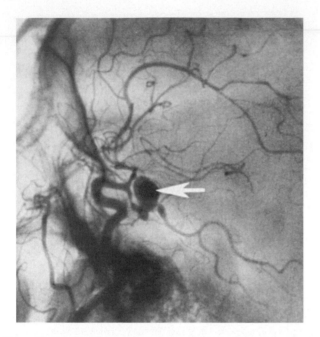

Figure 53.124. Aneurysm of the distal posterior communicating artery. The angiogram shows a large aneurysm (*arrow*) that arises not from the origin of the posterior communicating artery but from the artery itself. The aneurysm compressed the ipsilateral oculomotor nerve and produced a complete oculomotor nerve paresis that resolved after the aneurysm was clipped.

Aneurysms Arising from the Junction of the Internal Carotid and Anterior Choroidal Arteries (Carotid-Choroidal Aneurysms)

Aneurysms arising near the junction of the internal carotid and anterior choroidal arteries are rare (Fig. 53.125). In a cooperative study (Locksley, 1969), 121 of 2672 aneurysms (4.5%) originated from the ICA between the posterior communicating artery and the terminal bifurcation. According to the text of the study, "most" of these aneurysms arose near the anterior choroidal artery. Internal carotid-anterior choroidal artery aneurysms occur twice as often in women as in men and are most often diagnosed in patients over 30 years of age. Most originate spontaneously, but alterations in flow dynamics associated with occlusion of the basilar artery and an STA-MCA bypass were thought to be responsible for the de novo development of an aneurysm at the junction of the anterior choroidal artery in a 61-year-old woman (Hirano et al., 1995).

Internal carotid-anterior choroidal aneurysms usually are asymptomatic unless they rupture. At the time of rupture, they may produce ipsilateral eye pain, oculomotor nerve paresis, or both, in addition to symptoms and signs of SAH (Drake et al., 1968b; Perria et al., 1969, 1971; Yaşargil et al., 1978; Viale and Pau, 1979). Pollard (1988) described a 15-year-old boy who presented with a 4-day history of complete ptosis of the left upper eyelid. He had been experiencing severe headaches for 1 week, associated with two episodes of vomiting. When initially examined, the patient had a complete left oculomotor nerve paresis with involvement of the pupil. A CT scan with intravenous contrast enhance-

ment suggested a vascular lesion, and cerebral angiography disclosed a saccular aneurysm at the junction of the left internal carotid and anterior choroidal arteries. A lumbar puncture showed xanthochromic CSF. At surgery, the aneurysm was found to be compressing the left oculomotor nerve. Although this presentation is similar to that of internal carotid-posterior communicating aneurysms, the potential for an internal carotid-anterior choroidal artery aneurysm to produce an oculomotor nerve paresis generally is not appreciated.

Oculomotor nerve paresis also may develop after clipping of an internal carotid-anterior choroidal aneurysm. Manipulation of the nerve at the time of surgery is responsible for the paresis in most cases, but Wakai et al. (1981) reported a postoperative oculomotor nerve paresis that was caused by compression of the oculomotor nerve by the edge of the tentorium cerebelli that itself was compressed by a long aneurysm clip (Fig. 53.126). The paresis resolved after the clip was replaced with a shorter clip that did not distort the tentorium.

Internal carotid-anterior choroidal aneurysms may produce a contralateral hemiparesis from damage to the ipsilateral corticospinal tract and a contralateral homonymous visual field defect from damage to the ipsilateral optic tract, lateral geniculate body, or both. This damage probably results in most cases from interruption of the blood supply from the anterior choroidal artery to these structures, and, in fact, such signs may develop postoperatively in patients who were neurologically intact before surgery when the anterior choroidal artery is occluded during attempted clipping of the aneurysm (Viale and Pau, 1979). One of the patients described by Perria et al. (1969, 1971) developed a right oculomotor nerve paresis and a right trochlear nerve paresis when his aneurysm ruptured.

Most internal carotid-anterior choroidal artery aneurysms can be clipped without difficulty; however, Komiyama et al. (1994) described a patient with both a carotid-choroidal aneurysm and an ipsilateral internal carotid-posterior communicating artery aneurysm. It may be extremely difficult to separate and clip such "kissing aneurysms" and still preserve flow in their parent arteries.

Aneurysms Arising from the Anterior Choroidal Artery

Aneurysms that arise from the distal anterior choroidal artery, like those that arise from the posterior communicating artery, are exceptionally rare (Fig. 53.127). Knuckey et al. (1988) found only five well-documented cases and added one of their own. Five of these aneurysms ruptured and produced an intraventricular or intracerebral hematoma and hydrocephalus (Caram et al., 1960; Butler et al., 1972; Papo et al., 1973; Tanaka et al., 1980; Knuckey et al., 1988). Strully (1955) described a 27-year-old woman who developed headaches, nausea, vomiting, and blurred vision and was found to have bilateral papilledema. She had no localizing neurologic signs. She was thought to have a tumor of the 3rd or 4th ventricle, but at surgery, a large, thrombosed aneurysm arising from the distal portion of the anterior choroidal artery was found within the posterior portion of the left lateral ventricle. The neck of the aneurysm ruptured at surgery, but it was possible to remove the aneurysm and clip

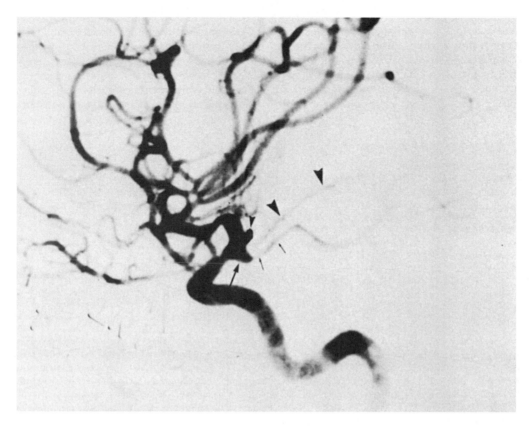

Figure 53.125.   Carotid-choroidal aneurysm. The cerebral angiogram shows a small aneurysm (*small arrowhead*) arising near the origin of the anterior choroidal artery (*large arrowheads*). The angiogram also shows that the anterior choroidal artery originates from the internal carotid artery distal to the origin of the posterior communicating artery (*small arrows*), although their respective courses seem similar on this lateral view. The *large arrow* points to an infundibular widening (*junctional dilation*) at the origin of the posterior communicating artery. Such anatomic abnormalities are thought by some investigators to be preaneurysmal (see text). (From Fox JL. Intracranial Aneurysms, Vol, 1. New York, Springer-Verlag, 1983.)

the artery. Postoperatively, the patient had moderate aphasia, a right hemiplegia, and a right homonymous hemianopia. Inagawa et al. (1990) reported a 75-year-old woman who presented with nausea, vomiting, and headache caused by a ruptured distal anterior choroidal aneurysm associated with a hematoma in the lateral ventricle. A similar case was reported by Nishihara et al. (1993). Hung et al. (1996) emphasized that aneurysms of the anterior choroidal artery can cause manifestations similar to those caused by carotid bifurcation aneurysms, and Morgenstern et al. (1996) described a movement disorder in a patient with a distal anterior choroidal aneurysm.

Aneurysms Arising from the Bifurcation of the Internal Carotid Artery (Carotid Bifurcation Aneurysms)

Aneurysms arising in the region of the terminal bifurcation of the ICA are often called proximal ACA aneurysms or proximal MCA aneurysms (Fig. 53.128). In fact, it is often impossible to determine the precise origin of these aneurysms, particularly when they are large. Thus, we prefer to call them **carotid bifurcation aneurysms**.

Carotid bifurcation aneurysms are about as common as aneurysms arising from the junction of the internal carotid

and anterior choroidal artery. Bull (1962) found 110 such aneurysms among 1769 angiographically verified intracranial aneurysms (6.2%), and they accounted for 4.4% of all single intracranial aneurysms in a large cooperative study (Locksley, 1969). They occur more frequently in women than in men.

Most carotid bifurcation aneurysms become symptomatic only when they bleed. In a cooperative study (Locksley, 1969), 90% of carotid bifurcation aneurysms presented with SAH. All but one of the 14 bifurcation aneurysms encountered by Brihaye et al. (1976) had ruptured at the time of presentation, and all 10 of the bifurcation aneurysms reported by Reynier et al. (1989) presented with SAH. Bifurcation aneurysms nevertheless may become quite large without rupturing (Barth and de Tribolet, 1994), and such aneurysms often produce visual symptoms and signs.

Carotid bifurcation aneurysms that expand **anteriorly and medially** above the optic nerves and chiasm may produce symptoms and signs of a suprasellar mass. Krayenbühl (1941) described a case in which a large carotid bifurcation aneurysm produced a remarkably symmetric bitemporal field defect. Walsh (1964) described a 64-year-old woman who experienced progressive loss of vision in the right eye. Within 1 year, she had lost all vision in the eye and had begun to lose vision in the left eye. When first examined,

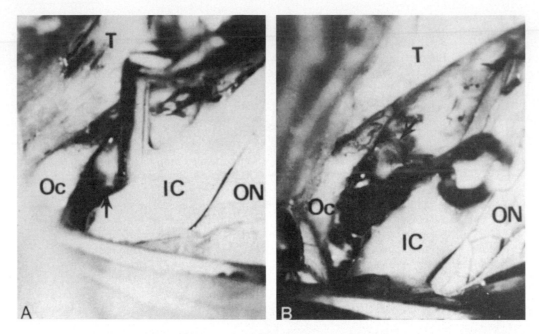

Figure 53.126. Oculomotor nerve paresis related to clipping of an internal carotid-anterior choroidal artery aneurysm. The paresis developed immediately after successful clipping of the aneurysm, and it did not improve substantially over the next 12 days. *A*, At reoperation, the aneurysm was found to be completely obliterated (*arrow*) by the Sugita clip, but the clip had slipped laterally and was compressing the edge of the tentorium (*T*). The tentorial edge was, in turn, compressing the ipsilateral oculomotor nerve (*Oc*). *B*, After replacement of the Sugita clip by a medium, curved Yaşargil clip, the aneurysm (*arrow*) remains occluded, the tentorium is no longer compressed, and it no longer compresses the oculomotor nerve. The patient's paresis resolved completely 2 months after this operation. *IC*, internal carotid artery; *ON*, optic nerve. (From Wakai S, Eguchi T, Asano T, et al. Oculomotor palsy caused by aneurysm clip: Report of two cases. Neurosurgery *9*:429–432, 1981.)

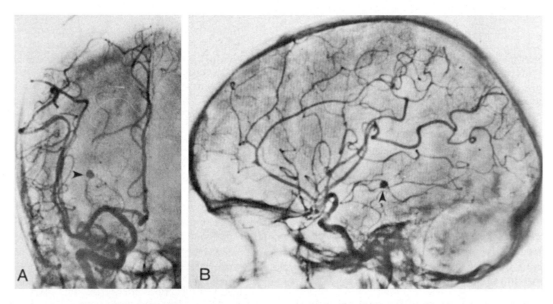

Figure 53.127. Aneurysm of the distal anterior choroidal artery. The patient had experienced an acute subarachnoid hemorrhage. *A*, Right carotid angiogram, anteroposterior view, shows an aneurysm (*arrowhead*) located in the region of the basal nuclei, possibly within the right lateral ventricle. *B*, Lateral view shows that the aneurysm arises from the distal, intraventricular portion of the right anterior choroidal artery (*arrowhead*). (From Papo I, Salvolini U, Caruselli G. Aneurysm of the anterior choroidal artery with intraventricular hematoma and hydrocephalus: Case report. J Neurosurg *39*: 255–260, 1973.)

fused treatment and apparently became completely blind several years later. Walsh (1964) stated that among 37 other patients with carotid bifurcation aneurysms, two had bitemporal field defects, but he did not provide any details of these cases.

Peiris and Ross Russell (1980) described four patients with carotid bifurcation aneurysms, three of whom had loss of central vision. Two of the patients had a distal optic nerve (anterior chiasmal) syndrome (Fig. 53.129). One of them, a 59-year-old woman, had vision of 20/40 in the right eye with marked constriction of the visual field, particularly nasally. Left eye vision was 20/30, and there was a relative superior temporal defect. She had a right-sided aneurysm that compressed the ipsilateral optic nerve and anterior chiasm. The other patient was a 52-year-old woman with vision of 20/40 OD and 20/200 OS. She had a slight temporal depression of the right visual field and a complete temporal hemianopia in the left visual field. This patient had a right-sided aneurysm that expanded superomedially to compress the contralateral optic nerve. The third patient had a right-sided carotid bifurcation aneurysm that compressed both optic nerves, the

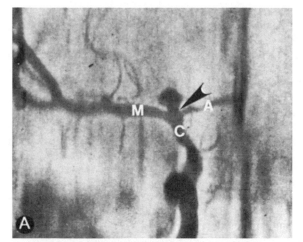

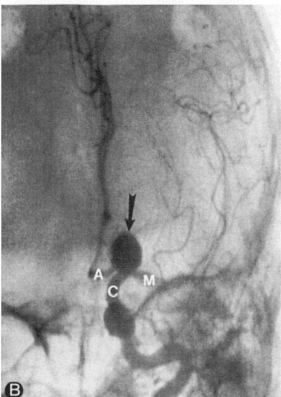

Figure 53.128. Aneurysms located at the terminal bifurcation of the internal carotid artery. *A*, Small aneurysm arises from the bifurcation of the internal carotid artery (*C*) into the anterior (*A*) and middle (*M*) cerebral arteries. The neck of the aneurysm can be identified (*arrowhead*), and the aneurysm was easily clipped. *B*, Large aneurysm (*arrow*) arises from the bifurcation of the internal carotid artery. The neck of the aneurysm is not visible in this projection.

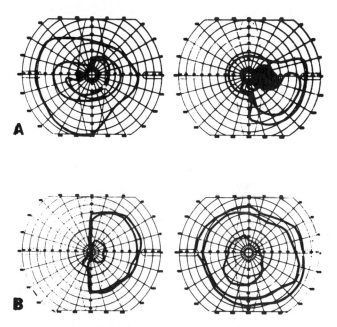

Figure 53.129. Syndrome of the distal optic nerve (anterior chiasmal syndrome) in two patients with aneurysms arising from the terminal bifurcation of the internal carotid artery. *A*, Syndrome of the distal right optic nerve. The right eye has visual acuity of 20/40 with a nasal hemianopic defect and superior field constriction. Visual acuity in the left eye is 20/30 and there is a relative superior temporal quadrantanopia. The aneurysm arose from the terminal bifurcation of the right internal carotid artery. *B*, Syndrome of the distal left optic nerve. The right eye has visual acuity of 20/40 with slight superior temporal depression of the visual field. Visual acuity in the left eye is 20/200, and there is a complete temporal hemianopia. The aneurysm arose from the terminal bifurcation of the *right* internal carotid but crossed the midline superior to the optic chiasm to compress the *left* optic nerve. (From Peiris JB, Ross Russell RW. Giant aneurysms of the carotid system presenting as visual field defect. J Neurol Neurosurg Psychiatry *43*:1053–1064, 1980.)

the patient could not perceive light with the right eye. Visual acuity in the left eye was 20/400, and the visual field of the left eye showed a central scotoma. The right optic disc was slightly pale, whereas the left optic disc appeared normal or slightly pale. The patient was found to have a large, globular aneurysm located above the optic chiasm. The patient re-

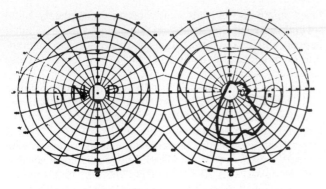

Figure 53.130. Bilateral optic neuropathy in a patient with an aneurysm arising from the terminal bifurcation of the right internal carotid artery. The aneurysm compressed both optic nerves, the optic chiasm, and the right optic tract. Visual acuity in the right eye was 20/70, and there was severe constriction of the visual field. The left eye was blind. (From Peiris JB, Ross Russell RW. Giant aneurysms of the carotid system presenting as visual field defect. J Neurol Neurosurg Psychiatry 43:1053–1064, 1980.)

optic chiasm, and the right optic tract. The patient had vision of 20/80 in the right eye with severe constriction of the visual field (Fig. 53.130). The left eye was blind.

Huber (1976) described a 56-year-old man who suddenly lost vision in the left eye and was found to have vision of 20/40 OD and hand motions OS. He was thought to have experienced an attack of either retrobulbar optic neuritis or ischemic optic neuropathy; however, visual field testing showed an asymmetric bitemporal hemianopia. The patient was found to have a partially thrombosed aneurysm originating from the bifurcation of the left ICA.

A carotid bifurcation aneurysm that expands **posteriorly and medially** can compress the posterior aspect of the optic chiasm, the ipsilateral optic tract, or both, producing a homonymous field defect that may be complete or incomplete (Figs. 53.131–53.134). When incomplete, the defect is invariably incongruous and often scotomatous (Kodama et al., 1978). When complete, there is always an RAPD in the eye contralateral to the damaged tract (ipsilateral to the hemianopia), and there may be hemianopic optic nerve and retinal nerve fiber layer atrophy (see Chapter 8). The hemianopia

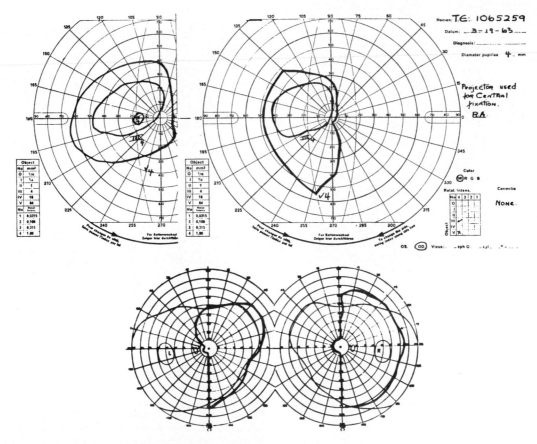

Figure 53.131. Homonymous hemianopias caused by aneurysms arising from the terminal bifurcation of the internal carotid artery. *Above,* Complete right homonymous hemianopia in a 73-year-old woman who also had markedly decreased vision in both eyes and left optic disc pallor. The patient was found to have a large aneurysm arising from the terminal bifurcation of the left internal carotid artery. It was thought that the patient's visual deficits resulted from compression of the left posterior chiasm and the left optic tract. *Below,* Incomplete left homonymous hemianopia with macular sparing in a 60-year-old man with an aneurysm originating at the bifurcation of the right internal carotid artery. The aneurysm compressed the right optic tract without compressing the optic chiasm. Visual acuity was 20/30 OD and 20/40 OS. (From Peiris JB, Ross Russell RW. Giant aneurysms of the carotid system presenting as visual field defect. J Neurol Neurosurg Psychiatry 43:1053–1064, 1980.)

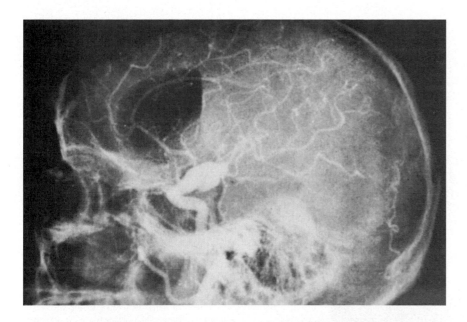

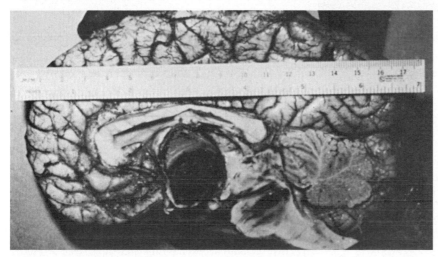

Figure 53.132. Angiographic and gross appearance of a large aneurysm that arose from the terminal bifurcation of the left internal carotid artery and produced a complete right homonymous hemianopia that initially was thought to have been caused by a stroke in the territory of the left posterior cerebral artery. The patient then developed progressive dementia, and an angiogram was performed. *Top,* A left internal carotid arteriogram demonstrates only a portion of the lumen of a giant bifurcation aneurysm. The patient subsequently died. *Bottom,* Sagittal section showing medial surface of the right hemisphere. A huge, partially thrombosed aneurysm has expanded into the 3rd ventricle, obstructing the ventricle, and producing hydrocephalus. The aneurysm apparently had compressed the left optic tract without damaging the optic chiasm or either of the optic nerves sufficiently to produce loss of visual acuity.

may be associated with ipsilateral, contralateral, or bilateral loss of visual acuity and color vision if there is also compression of one or both optic nerves. Walsh (1964) examined 37 patients with bifurcation aneurysm, three of whom had homonymous field defects (one of which was "questionable"). Walsh and Hoyt (1969i) described a 73-year-old woman who had experienced several accidents, while both driving and walking, involving objects on the right side. She was found to have a right homonymous hemianopia associated with decreased vision in the left eye. The decreased visual acuity in the left eye was thought to be caused by a cataract, and the patient was thought to have had a stroke. Four months later, however, she experienced acute loss of vision in the right eye. At this time, visual acuity was counting fingers at 3 feet in each eye, and there was a persistent right homonymous hemianopia (Fig. 53.131*A*). The right optic disc appeared normal, whereas the left disc was pale. The patient was found to have a thrombosed aneu-

rysm of the carotid bifurcation. The aneurysm was compressing both optic nerves and the left optic tract. After aneurysmorrhaphy, the patient had slight return of vision in the right eye. One of the four patients with a bifurcation aneurysm described by Peiris and Ross Russell (1980) was a 70-year-old man with a right-sided aneurysm and a complete optic tract syndrome. He had visual acuity of 20/30 OD and 20/40 OS with a complete, left, macular-sparing, homonymous hemianopia (Fig. 53.131*B*).

A carotid bifurcation aneurysm that expands **inferiorly** may compress the oculomotor nerve, producing an oculomotor nerve paresis (Cogan and Mount, 1963) (Fig. 53.135). It may also compress the pituitary gland, producing panhypopituitarism. Gallagher et al. (1957) described a 54-year-old woman who developed a frontal lobe syndrome characterized by disturbances of attention and memory, alternating elation and depression, memory lapses, confusion, and a tendency to repeat statements. The patient's right eye was blind,

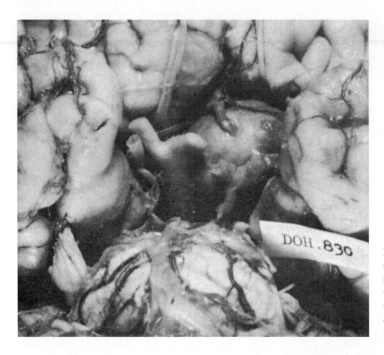

Figure 53.133. Basal view of an unruptured aneurysm arising from the terminal bifurcation of the left internal carotid artery. The aneurysm originates above and lateral to the optic chiasm and left optic tract, but it has expanded inferiorly and medially to such an extent that it compresses and displaces these structures to the right. The optic nerves and the anterior portion of the optic chiasm appear to be unaffected by the aneurysm. (Courtesy of Dr. Richard Lindenberg.)

the right pupil nonreactive to direct light stimulation, and the right optic disc was pale. The left eye was normal. Skull x-rays showed complete destruction of the dorsum sellae, erosion of the anterior and posterior clinoid processes, and absence of the floor of the sella turcica. Arteriography, performed under anesthesia, demonstrated a giant aneurysm arising from the right ICA near its terminal bifurcation (Fig. 53.136). The patient did not regain consciousness after arteriography. Her blood pressure dropped, and her respirations become shallow. Hypopituitarism was suspected, and she was treated with hydrocortisone, adrenocorticotropic hormone (ACTH), and thyroid extract with marked improvement. Subsequent endocrinologic evaluation revealed panhypopituitarism. A similar patient with hypopituitarism caused by a carotid bifurcation aneurysm was described by Shantharam and Clift (1974). The patient was a 55-year-old

woman with bifrontal headache, weight loss, alopecia, cold sensitivity, and increased sleep requirements. She had been hypertensive for many years but spontaneously had become normotensive in the previous 18 months. Her visual examination revealed a bitemporal hemianopia. The patient was treated medically with desiccated thyroid and hydrocortisone.

Dust et al. (1981) described a patient who developed a mild right ptosis, diplopia thought to be related to an oculomotor nerve paresis, and right hemicranial pain in the distribution of the first division of the trigeminal nerve. The patient was found to have a bifurcation aneurysm, the sac of which extended **superiorly**. It was thought by Dust et al. (1981) that the patient's symptoms and signs were produced by the aneurysm, but it is hard to understand how such an aneurysm produced them, because the aneurysm was well above the cavernous sinus and interpeduncular fossa. In fact, the patient may have had an inflammatory Tolosa-Hunt syndrome (see Chapter 36) and an asymptomatic unrelated aneurysm.

When aneurysms that arise from the region of the bifurcation of the ICA expand **posteriorly**, they may eventually attain sufficient size to produce obstructive hydrocephalus (Morota et al., 1988) (Fig. 53.132). They also may compress the ventral brainstem and produce symptoms and signs mimicking a posterior fossa neoplasm. Duff and Gossmann (1975) described a 13-year-old girl who developed progressively severe occipital headaches over a 2-year-period. She then began to have episodes of vomiting, lethargy, unsteadiness of gait, and difficulty with both speech and swallowing. She was found to have saccadic ocular pursuit movements, vestibular nystagmus, mild bilateral facial weakness, dysarthric speech, difficulty swallowing, and difficulty protruding the tongue. She also had an increased jaw jerk reflex,

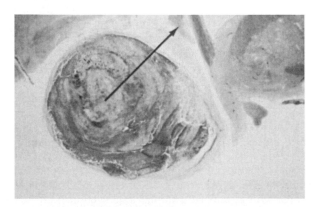

Figure 53.134. Histopathologic appearance of a laminated, thrombosed bifurcation aneurysm that is compressing the ipsilateral optic tract (*arrow*). (Courtesy of Dr. Richard Lindenberg.)

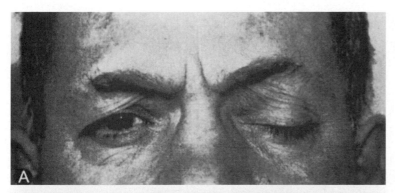

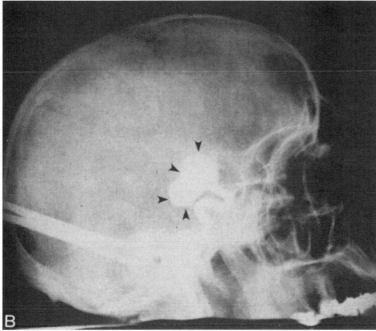

Figure 53.135. Oculomotor nerve paresis from an aneurysm arising from the terminal bifurcation of the ipsilateral internal carotid artery. *A,* The patient has a left oculomotor nerve paresis. The paresis developed after an episode of severe pain around the left eye. There was no evidence of trigeminal neuropathy. *B,* Left cerebral angiogram, lateral view, shows large aneurysm arising from the terminal bifurcation of the left internal carotid artery and projecting posterior and inferiorly (*arrowheads*), where it presumably compressed the left oculomotor nerve in the subarachnoid space. (From Cogan DG, Mount HTJ. Intracranial aneurysms causing ophthalmoplegia. Arch Ophthalmol *70:* 757–771, 1963.)

generalized weakness of the extremities with hyperactive reflexes, bilateral extensor plantar responses, and bilateral ankle clonus. The patient was thought to have a brainstem neoplasm, but cerebral arteriography disclosed a giant aneurysm measuring about 60 mm in diameter arising near the bifurcation of the right ICA. The aneurysm projected over the petrous ridge into the ventral midbrain and rostral pons (Fig. 53.137). The neck of the aneurysm was subsequently clipped, and the sac was opened and emptied of its contents. Postoperatively, the patient had a complete right oculomotor nerve paresis, but her preoperative neurologic deficits cleared rapidly.

Aneurysms Arising from the Anterior Cerebral Artery

Unlike aneurysms that arise at most other locations, aneurysms of the ACA are more common in men (Kongable et al., 1996). They may be associated with vascular anomalies, including an azygous origin in which both ACAs arise from a single trunk (Nardı et al., 1990; Sanders et al., 1993) and fenestrations in the artery (Friedlander and Oglivy, 1996).

Aneurysms that originate from the ACA may arise at any

location. Those that arise from the precommunicating (A-1) segment, proximal to the anterior communicating artery, account for 1–2% of all aneurysms (Locksley, 1969; Pia, 1979; Yaşargil and Smith, 1982; Kassell and Torner, 1983a; Wakabayashi et al., 1985; Weir, 1987; Takeuchi et al., 1991; Suzuki et al., 1992) (Fig. 53.138). These aneurysms usually produce symptoms when they rupture (Handa et al., 1984). In a cooperative study (Locksley, 1969), 35 of 41 (85%) A-1 aneurysms first produced symptoms when they ruptured. Unruptured A-1 aneurysms may, however, cause loss of vision from compression of the optic nerves, chiasm, tract, or a combination of these structures (Jefferson, 1937; Henderson, 1955; Versavel et al., 1988; Tajima et al., 1993). The loss of vision may occur shortly before rupture, presumably because of sudden enlargement of the aneurysm, or it may be unassociated with rupture. The symptoms and signs produced by A-1 aneurysms are identical with those produced by aneurysms arising from the proximal portion of the A-2 (postcommunicating) segment of the ACA and from the anterior communicating artery (see below). For this reason, many investigators consider them together as "anterior cere-

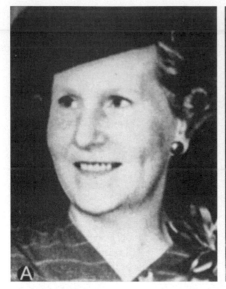
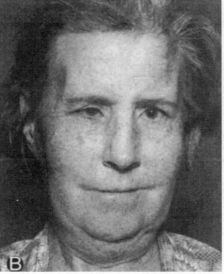
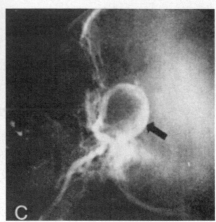

Figure 53.136. Panhypopituitarism from giant bifurcation aneurysm. The patient was a 54-year-old woman whose chief complaint was headache. Six weeks before admission, she became very weak, lost weight despite a good appetite, and spoke only in a mumble. *A*, Appearance of patient 10 years previously. *B*, Appearance of patient at time of admission. *C*, Right cerebral arteriogram shows a large, partially calcified aneurysm arising near the terminal bifurcation of the right internal carotid artery. The patient underwent ligation of the right common carotid artery in the neck, and her panhypopituitarism was treated medically. (From Gallagher PG, Dorsey JF, Stefanini M, et al. Large intracranial aneurysm producing panhypopituitarism and frontal lobe syndrome. Neurology *6*:830–837, 1957.)

bral-anterior communicating aneurysms'' (Höök and Norlén 1964b; Odom, 1964; Walsh, 1964).

The pattern of visual loss caused by an aneurysm arising from the A-1 or A-2 segment of the ACA depends on a number of factors, including the size and direction of growth of the aneurysm and the length of the intracranial portion of the optic nerves (e.g., if the optic chiasm is normal in position, prefixed, or postfixed). In addition, the presence of associated vascular and other anomalies in patients with these aneurysms (Henderson, 1955; Hoff et al., 1975; Senter and Miller, 1982; Kawakita et al., 1991; Maurer et al., 1991; S. Sugita et al., 1995) may affect the symptoms and signs produced by them.

An A-1 or proximal A-2 aneurysm may produce monocular loss of visual acuity and visual field from compression of the ipsilateral optic nerve (Fig. 53.139). The loss of vision is usually slowly progressive, but it may be sudden, rapidly progressive, and associated with ipsilateral orbital, frontal, or temple pain (Henderson, 1955). When loss of vision is slowly progressive, delay in diagnosis may result in subsequent visual loss in the opposite eye from compression of the contralateral optic nerve (Henderson, 1955). When loss of vision is rapidly progressive, the patient may be thought to have experienced an attack of retrobulbar optic neuritis or ischemic optic neuropathy (Huber, 1976; Norwood et al., 1986), even though the ipsilateral optic disc may be pale, thereby providing clear evidence of preexisting optic nerve damage. In these cases, any type of field defect may be present but there seems to be a preponderance of inferior field defects from compression of the superior portion of the nerve by the aneurysm (Norwood et al., 1986). Although

the aneurysm initially may compress the optic nerve, it eventually may extend or erode into the nerve and become almost surrounded by it (Milliser et al., 1968).

Some patients with A-1 aneurysms experience visual loss that fluctuates or spontaneously improves. Such patients may not seek medical attention, or if they do, they may be thought to have nonorganic visual loss. Miller (1991f) described a 32-year-old woman who complained of headache and intermittent visual loss that lasted several minutes at a time. Visual acuity was 20/40 OD and 20/30 OS, and visual fields showed irregular nasal constriction. Pupillary responses were normal, and both optic discs appeared normal. The patient was thought by the ophthalmologist who initially examined her to have nonorganic visual loss because of the fluctuating nature of the visual loss, the irregularly constricted fields, and the normal appearance of the fundi. However, a skull X-ray showed a partially calcified mass in the suprasellar region, and an arteriogram revealed a large, bilobed aneurysm originating from the A-1 segment of the right ICA and extending medially. At craniotomy, the aneurysm was compressing both optic nerves and the anterior portion of the chiasm.

Although most aneurysms that damage the optic nerves affect either the ipsilateral nerve or both nerves, an A-1 aneurysm may occasionally cross the midline and compress only the **contralateral** optic nerve without producing clinical evidence of damage to the ipsilateral optic nerve. In this setting, there is unilateral visual loss on the side opposite the aneurysm, and the origin of the aneurysm may not be clear unless a complete angiographic study with selective catheterization of all major vessels is performed.

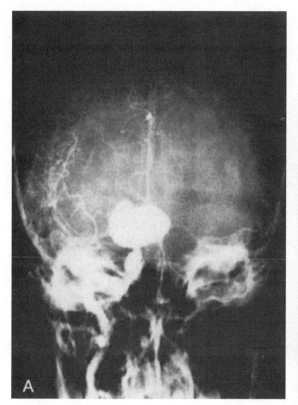

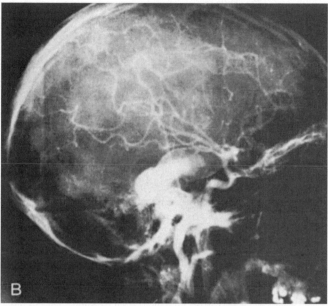

Figure 53.137.   Giant aneurysm arising from the terminal bifurcation of the internal carotid artery and producing symptoms suggesting a posterior fossa tumor. The patient was a 13-year-old girl with increasing headaches, vomiting, lethargy, unsteadiness of gait, and difficulty with articulation and swallowing. She had mild bilateral facial weakness, saccadic eye movements, and vestibular nystagmus that was both vertical and horizontal. Speech was dysarthric, and the patient had difficulty swallowing and in protruding the tongue. She had generalized extremity weakness, hyperactive muscle stretch reflexes, extensor plantar responses, and bilateral ankle clonus. A brain scan suggested a posterior fossa mass, and a cerebral angiogram was performed. The angiogram shows a giant aneurysm arising from the terminal bifurcation of the right internal carotid artery and projecting posteriorly over the petrous ridge into the ventral mesencephalon and rostral pons. *A*, Anteroposterior view; *B*, Lateral view. The neck of the aneurysm was clipped, and an aneurysmorrhaphy was performed. The patient subsequently made a complete recovery. (From Duff TA, Gossmann HH. Giant aneurysm of the internal carotid artery simulating posterior fossa tumour in a 13-year-old girl. Neurochirurgia *18*:190–193, 1975.)

An A-1 aneurysm may compress the optic chiasm, producing a bitemporal field defect. The field defect may be associated with unilateral or bilateral loss of visual acuity and color vision if one or both optic nerves are also damaged. Jefferson (1937) and Henderson (1955) emphasized the tendency for the bitemporal defects seen in patients with ACA aneurysm to be asymmetric. Jefferson (1937) also emphasized that the defects were usually **inferior** rather than superior, because the aneurysm is invariably located above the chiasm (Fig. 53.139). This is important in clinical diagnosis, because the most common suprasellar lesions, pituitary adenomas, are infrachiasmal and thus tend to produce superior field defects. Pieris and Ross Russell (1980) described a 62-year-old man with an aneurysm arising from the A-1 segment of the left ACA (Fig. 53.140). The aneurysm expanded downward and medially to compress the right optic nerve and chiasm, producing loss of vision in the right eye. There was loss of the superior visual field in the right eye, temporal more than nasal. The left eye had an inferotemporal quadrantanopic defect.

Versavel et al. (1988) described a 55-year-old woman with a 2-month history of blurred vision in the left homonymous hemifield who was found to have 20/20 visual acuity in both eyes associated with an incomplete, incongruous, left homonymous hemianopia (Fig. 53.141*A*). An evaluation revealed a giant aneurysm arising from the A-1 segment of the right ACA (Figs. 53.141*B* and 53.141*C*). The aneurysm was trapped by placing one aneurysm clip proximal to it and one distal to it on the ACA. Postoperatively, the patient had no new neurologic deficits, and over the next 6 months, the visual field defect completely resolved (Fig. 53.141*D*). The field defect in this patient was clearly caused by aneurysmal compression of the right optic tract.

Aneurysms originating from the **distal segments** of the ACA account for 2–5% of all intracranial aneurysms (Laitinen and Snellman, 1960; Locksley, 1969; Yaşargil and Carter, 1974; Wisoff and Flamm, 1987; Hernesniemi et al., 1992). These aneurysms are commonly called ''pericallosal artery aneurysms'' (Maiuri et al., 1990), but many of them actually arise at the origin of the callosomarginal artery. Thus, Yaşargil and Carter recommended that they be called **distal anterior cerebral artery aneurysms** (Fig. 53.142).

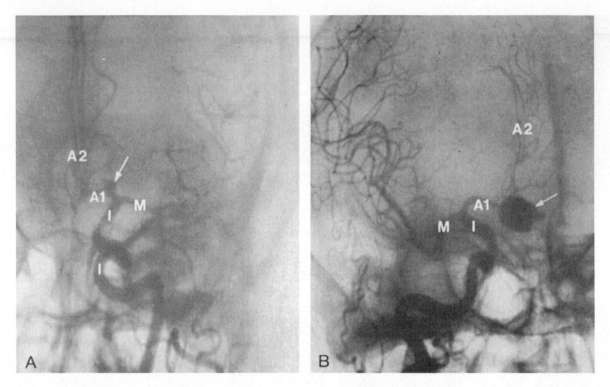

Figure 53.138.   Aneurysms arising from the A-1 segment of the anterior cerebral artery, proximal to its junction with the anterior communicating artery. *A*, A small aneurysm (*arrow*) arises from the anterior cerebral artery just distal to its origin from the terminal bifurcation of the internal carotid artery. *B*, A large aneurysm (*arrow*) arises just proximal to the junction of the anterior cerebral artery with the anterior communicating artery. *A1*, A-1 segment of anterior cerebral artery; *A2*, A-2 segment of anterior cerebral artery; *I*, internal carotid artery; *M*, middle cerebral artery. (From Karyenbühl HA, Yaşargil MG. Cerebral Angiography. Philadelphia, JB Lippincott, 1968.)

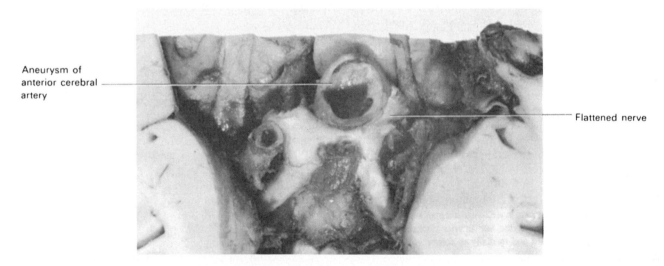

Figure 53.139.   Compression of the optic nerve by an aneurysm arising from the proximal portion of the ipsilateral anterior cerebral artery. Basal view of a pathologic specimen shows a large aneurysm arising from the proximal left anterior cerebral artery. The aneurysm has compressed and flattened the left optic nerve. The right optic nerve is normal as is the anterior portion of the optic chiasm. (From Lindenberg R, Walsh FB, Sacks JG. Neuropathology of Vision: An Atlas. Philadelphia, Lea & Febiger, 1973.)

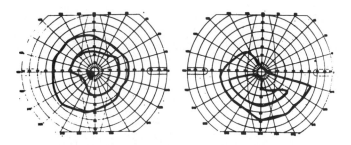

Figure 53.140. Visual field defects in a 62-year-old man with an aneurysm arising from the A-1 segment of the left anterior cerebral artery. The aneurysm expanded downward and medially to compress the right optic nerve and the optic chiasm. Visual acuity in the right eye was finger counting. The right visual field shows a severe superior loss, temporal more than nasal. Visual acuity in the left eye was 20/30, but there is an inferior temporal field defect in this eye. (From Peiris JB, Ross Russell RW. Giant aneurysms of the carotid system presenting as visual field defect. J Neurol Neurosurg Psychiatry *43*:1053–1064, 1980.)

Distal ACA aneurysms seem to be associated with a higher prevalence of multiple aneurysms, AVMs, and other vascular anomalies of the circle of Willis than are aneurysms in other locations (Becker and Newton, 1979; Preul et al., 1992). In a study by Wisoff and Flamm (1987), 14 of 20 patients (70%) with distal ACA aneurysm had anomalies of the circle of Willis, 11 patients (55%) had at least one intracranial aneurysm in another location, and three patients (15%) had an AVM arising from the ACA from which the aneurysm originated. These findings suggest that aneurysms that arise from the distal ACA occur during embryogenesis as part of a generalized disturbance in the development of cerebral vessels.

Distal ACA aneurysms usually first produce symptoms when they rupture (Ohno et al., 1990). They tend to be smaller in size at the time of rupture than most intracranial aneurysms (less than 5 mm in diameter in 20 of 30 cases reported by Ohno et al., 1990), leading to the conclusion that they have a propensity to bleed easily. In a cooperative study (Locksley, 1969), 66 of 69 such aneurysms (96%) presented with SAH, whereas 65 of 84 patients (77%) reported by Hernesniemi et al. (1992) bled. The remainder were diagnosed as incidental findings on angiography performed for other reasons, usually other vascular lesions. Unruptured distal ACA aneurysms almost never produce any focal neurologic or neuro-ophthalmologic symptoms or signs; however, Walsh and Hoyt (1969j) described a patient who developed a bitemporal hemianopia from a huge aneurysm that arose from the distal ACA near the origin of the pericallosal artery (Fig. 53.143). Wisoff and Flamm (1987) evaluated 20 patients with aneurysm of the distal ACA. Six of these patients had unruptured aneurysms, but the symptoms that led to diagnosis were not related to the aneurysm, except in the case of a 60-year-old woman who experienced a TIA in the territory supplied by the affected ACA. Of the other five patients with unruptured aneurysms, three had seizures caused by an AVM supplied by the same ACA from which the asymptomatic aneurysm arose, one patient had a calcified but probably asymptomatic aneurysm detected during CT scanning after minor head trauma, and one patient had an asymptomatic aneurysm of the distal ACA discovered during an evaluation for a right Horner's syndrome that was found to have been caused by an unruptured aneurysm arising from the petrous portion of the right ICA. Giant aneurysms of the distal anterior circulation are exceptionally rare (Maiuri et al., 1990). Such aneurysms may present with seizures (Obrien et al., 1997).

Aneurysms Arising from the Middle Cerebral Artery

Middle cerebral aneurysms are relatively common and occur as frequently as aneurysms that arise from the junction of the internal carotid and posterior communicating arteries (Locksley, 1969; Nishimoto et al., 1985). In a study from Finland, 561 of 1314 aneurysm patients (43%) had MCA aneurysms (Rinne et al., 1996). In addition, 39% of these patients had multiple aneurysms. This increased incidence of multiplicity with MCA aneurysms was also noted by Proust et al. (1994). MCA aneurysms seem to occur more frequently in families (Ronkainen et al., 1993; Bromberg et al., 1995b; Ronkainen et al., 1995b).

Middle cerebral aneurysms may arise at the bifurcation of the ICA (see above), from the M-1 segment of the MCA proximal to its main branchings (Nardi et al., 1996), from the origin of the M-2 segments of the artery in the insula deep within the Sylvian fissure, and, rarely, from vessels distal to the main branchings (M-3 and M-4 segments) (Figs. 53.41 and 53.144). Hosoda et al. (1995) estimated that M-1 segment aneurysms made up 3% of all intracranial aneurysms and 13% of all MCA aneurysms. Most aneurysms that originate from the MCA arise at the origin of the M-2 segments, usually between them (Fig. 53.144*B–E*). When an aneurysm arises at this location, its sac is formed in part by the walls of one or more of the segments. In a cooperative study (Locksley, 1969), 324 of 529 middle cerebral aneurysms (61%) arose from the origin of the M-2 segments. In the Finnish series, 81% of MCA aneurysms were located at the middle cerebral bifurcation (Rinne et al., 1996) (Fig. 53.41). Distal MCA aneurysms are somewhat more likely to be infectious (Corr et al., 1995) or neoplastic. MCA aneurysms are also more likely to be associated with polycystic kidney disease (Lozano and Leblanc, 1992).

Patients with MCA aneurysms have an increased incidence of other vascular anomalies. Takahashi et al. (1994) and Koyama et al. (1995) reported cases in which a ruptured aneurysm arose at the origin of a duplicated MCA, and several authors reported aneurysms at MCA fenestrations (Deruty et al., 1992a; Finlay and Canham, 1994; Nakamura et al., 1994). Kuwabara and Naitoh (1990) and Han et al. (1994) described patients with ruptured aneurysms at the origin of an accessory MCA. In the case reported by Han et al. (1994), the ipsilateral MCA was aplastic. Radiation to a parietal astrocytoma preceded the development of a MCA aneurysm in a patient reported by Casey et al. (1993).

MCA aneurysms usually first become symptomatic when they rupture. In a cooperative study (Locksley, 1969), 488 of 529 MCA aneurysms (92%) first produced symptoms when they ruptured. As noted above, rupture of an MCA aneurysm usually causes severe damage to the ipsilateral

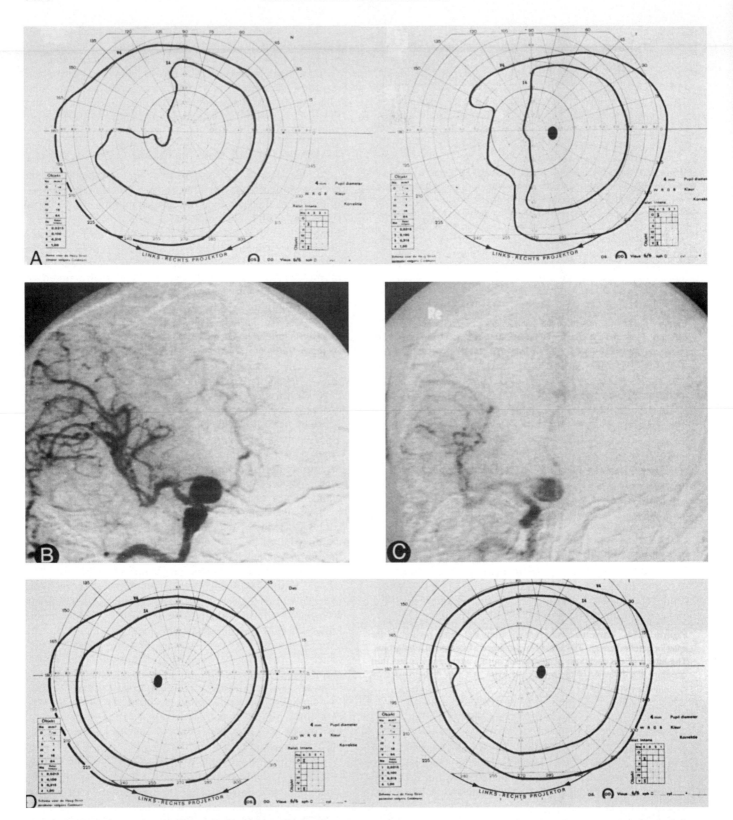

Figure 53.141. Homonymous hemianopia from damage to the optic tract caused by an aneurysm arising from the A-1 segment of the anterior cerebral artery. The patient was a 55-year-old woman with a 2-month history of blurred vision. Visual acuity was 20/20 in both eyes. *A,* Visual field shows an incomplete, incongruous, left homonymous hemianopia. *B* and *C,* Right carotid angiogram shows a large aneurysm arising from the proximal portion of the right anterior cerebral artery (*B,* Lateral view; *C,* Anteroposterior view). *D,* 6 months after trapping of the aneurysm, the visual field is normal in both eyes. (From Versavel M, Witmer JP, Matricali B. Giant aneurysm arising from the anterior cerebral artery and causing an isolated homonymous hemianopia. Neurosurgery 22:560–563, 1988.)

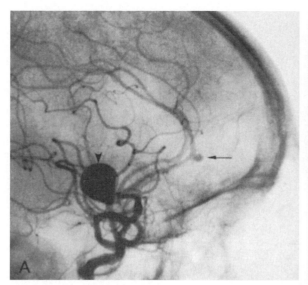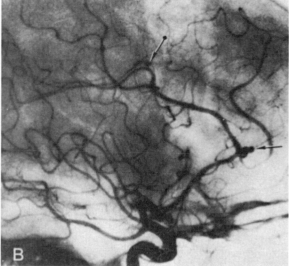

Figure 53.142. Aneurysms of the distal anterior cerebral artery. *A,* The patient has two aneurysms, a large aneurysm at the junction of the right anterior cerebral artery and the anterior communicating artery (*arrowhead*), and a smaller aneurysm that arises near the origin of the frontopolar artery (*arrow*). *B,* The patient has two aneurysms originating from the distal anterior cerebral artery (*arrows*). (From Huber P. Cerebral Angiography, 2nd ed. New York, Springer-Verlag, 1982.)

cerebral hemisphere (Fig. 53.145). Blood spreads into the subarachnoid space, producing the usual signs of SAH, and also dissects into the substance of the hemisphere, producing contralateral hemiplegia or hemiparesis, hemianesthesia, and, commonly, homonymous hemianopia (Henderson, 1955; Höök and Norlén, 1958). If the bleeding aneurysm is located on a posterior branch of the MCA, it may produce a sudden homonymous hemianopia that is the only focal clinical sign associated with the nonlocalizing signs of an ictus. The hemianopia usually is complete, but we have observed both superior and inferior quadrantic defects. The

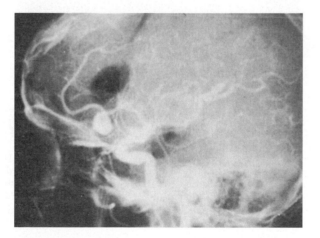

Figure 53.143. Large aneurysm arising from the distal portion of the anterior cerebral artery. The aneurysm produced a bitemporal hemianopia. The lumen of the aneurysm demonstrated in this arteriogram is less than one-third the diameter of the suprasellar mass that was demonstrated by pneumoencephalography.

visual field defects are often permanent, but they occasionally improve as cerebral edema subsides. Aphasia may occur in patients with rupture of an MCA aneurysm of the dominant hemisphere.

Unruptured aneurysms of the MCA usually cause no neurologic or ophthalmologic signs unless they give rise to emboli that cause TIAs or infarcts (Przelomski et al., 1986; Kobayashi et al., 1989; Raps et al., 1993), or they become large enough to act as a temporal lobe mass (Fig. 53.146). A giant MCA aneurysm may also be the nidus for thrombus leading to occlusion of the proximal and distal artery with potentially devastating consequences (Sugita et al., 1991).

An unruptured giant aneurysm of the MCA may compress the venous outflow of the cavernous sinus, thus producing a sphenocavernous syndrome characterized by unilateral ophthalmoplegia, ipsilateral proptosis, and even ipsilateral visual loss associated with evidence of an optic neuropathy (see Chapter 8). Miller (1991g) examined a patient who developed decreased vision in the right eye associated with binocular diplopia and right-sided proptosis (Figs. 53.147A–C). The patient was thought to have a right orbital mass, but a CT scan showed a large, well-circumscribed mass in the right temporal lobe (Figs. 53.147D and 53.147E). The mass had a rim of calcium surrounding it. An arteriogram demonstrated a giant, partially thrombosed aneurysm of the right MCA arising near the bifurcation of the M-1 segment (Fig. 53.147F).

The most common neuro-ophthalmologic manifestation of an unruptured MCA aneurysm is a contralateral homonymous visual field defect. The defect may be the only sign of the aneurysm, or it may be associated with other manifestations, including visual hallucinations in the affected homonymous field and weakness, numbness, or both on the side

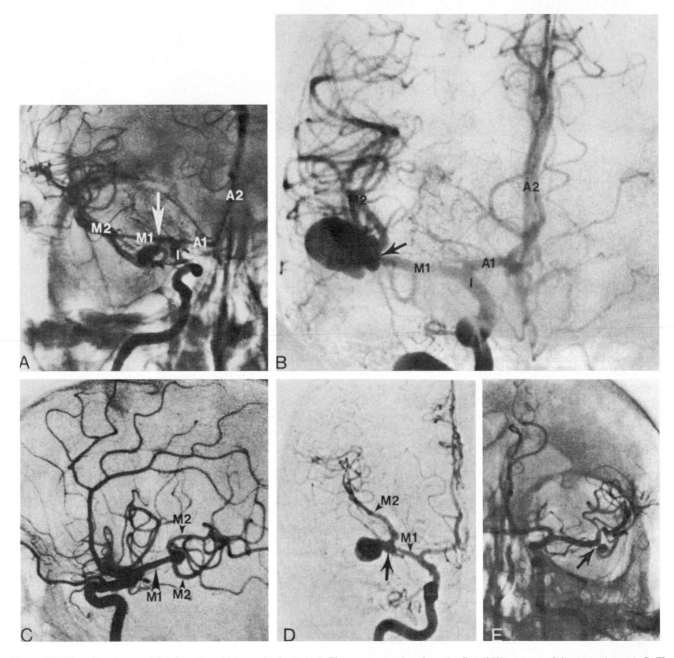

Figure 53.144. Aneurysms arising from the middle cerebral artery. *A,* The aneurysm arises from the first (*M1*) segment of the artery (*arrow*). *B,* The aneurysm arises from the bifurcation of the M-1 segment into the two M-2 segments (*arrow*). *I,* internal carotid artery; *A1,* A-1 segment of the anterior cerebral artery; *A2,* A-2 segment of the anterior cerebral artery; *M1,* M-1 segment of the middle cerebral artery; *M2,* M-2 segments of the middle cerebral artery. *C,* Oblique view showing the origin of the aneurysm from the bifurcation of the M-1 segment (*M1*) into two M-2 segments (*M2*). *D,* Cerebral angiogram, anteroposterior view, in another patient shows an aneurysm that originates from the M-1 bifurcation (*arrow*) and projects laterally. *E,* A small aneurysm originates from the M-1 bifurcation. Note that the neck of this aneurysm is clearly visible (*arrow*).

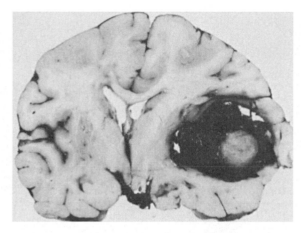

Figure 53.145. Intracerebral hemorrhage from a large middle cerebral artery aneurysm. (Courtesy of Dr. Richard Lindenberg).

age to the optic tract or the optic radiation in the temporal lobe. Walsh (1964) observed contralateral homonymous field defects in two of 12 patients with an MCA aneurysm and commented that such lesions usually damage the optic tract. We agree with this statement, having examined several such patients who had other evidence of damage to the optic tract; i.e., 20/20 visual acuity in both eyes, an RAPD in the eye contralateral to the aneurysm (e.g., ipsilateral to the hemianopia), and hemianopic optic nerve and retinal nerve fiber layer atrophy. Patients in whom an MCA aneurysm becomes sufficiently large to produce a visual field defect may also experience seizures. In other patients, seizures are the only sign of the unruptured aneurysm (Kamrin, 1966; Sengupta et al., 1978; Pasqualin et al., 1979; McCulloch and Bryan, 1982; Whittle et al. 1985; Pásztor et al., 1986; Przelomski et al. 1986; Miyagi et al., 1991). The seizures may be grand mal, focal, or psychomotor (Sengupta et al., 1978). Tanaka et al. (1994) described a 20-month-old infant who developed partial complex seizures as the sole manifestation of an aneurysm of the MCA which subsequently spontaneously thrombosed.

Gross (1987) described a 39-year-old man who developed right hemiparkinsonism with ipsilateral hemiparesis and was found to have a giant, thrombosed aneurysm of the left MCA. After removal of the aneurysm, the patient experienced complete resolution of the hemiparkinsonism, although he had a mild, persistent, right hemiparesis. This

of the field defect (contralateral to the aneurysm). When the aneurysm arises from the left MCA, it may cause aphasia and other disturbances of speech and language. Höök and Norlén (1958) examined 80 patients with an MCA aneurysm, eight of whom had an homonymous visual field defect. The defect was associated with intracerebral hemorrhage in six of these patients, but in two patients, an unruptured MCA aneurysm produced a homonymous hemianopia from dam-

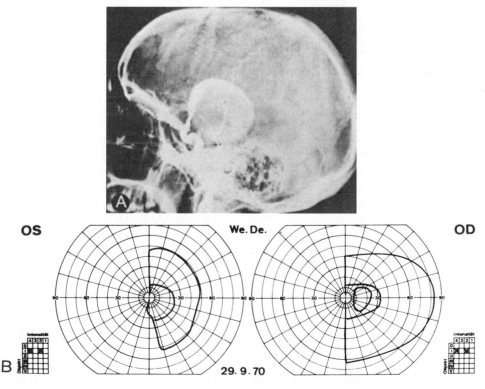

Figure 53.146. Homonymous hemianopia from giant unruptured aneurysm arising from the trifurcation of the right middle cerebral artery. *A*, Cerebral angiogram, lateral view, shows a giant aneurysm arising from the right middle cerebral artery. *B*, Visual fields show a complete left homonymous hemianopia from compression of the right optic tract by the aneurysm. (From Huber A. Eye signs of intracranial aneurysms. Neuro-ophthalmology 2:203–216, 1982.)

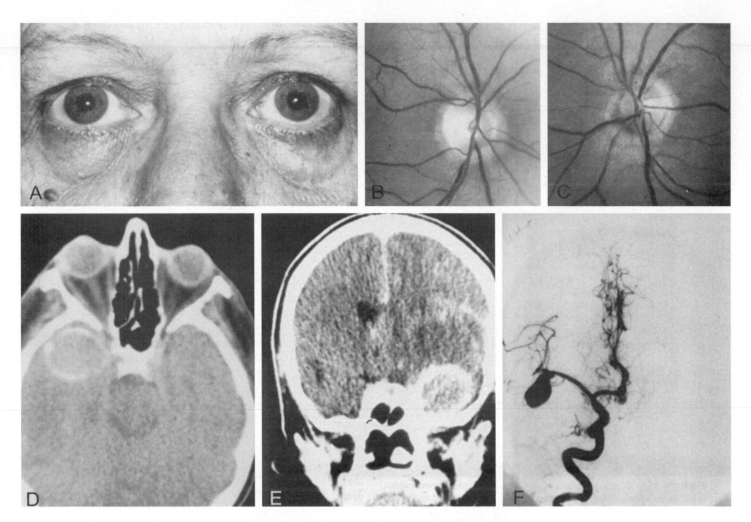

Figure 53.147. Pseudo-orbital apex syndrome from giant, calcified middle cerebral artery aneurysm. The patient was a 73-year-old woman with progressive visual loss in the right eye, right proptosis, and binocular diplopia. Movements of the right eye were limited in all directions. *A*, Appearance of the patient showing mild right proptosis and a right hypertropia (note relative position of the light reflexes in the two eyes). *B*, Right optic disc shows temporal pallor. *C*, Left optic disc is normal. *D*, CT scan, axial view, shows a giant egg-shaped mass in the right temporal lobe. The mass has a calcified rim. *E*, Coronal view of the mass shows its relationship to the base of the skull. *F*, Right lateral angiogram shows an aneurysm of the right middle cerebral artery near the bifurcation of the M-1 segment. The aneurysm projects downward and forward. Discrepancy between the size of the mass on CT scan and the angiographic appearance of the mass is caused by the substantial amount of clot within the aneurysm.

patient's symptoms and signs probably were caused by compression of the left internal capsule and basal ganglia by the aneurysm.

Kumabe et al. (1990) reported the case of a 39-year-old man who developed right-sided eye pain without any other neurologic deficit. A CT scan showed a huge irregular mass in the right temporal lobe, and cerebral arteriography revealed a giant thrombosed aneurysm of the right MCA. The patient subsequently developed papilledema, dysarthria, and mild left hemiparesis, and he became increasingly confused and disoriented. He refused treatment and eventually died.

Unruptured MCA aneurysms that produce neurologic symptoms and signs are not always large. Small aneurysms that leak or undergo a small rupture may produce temporal lobe seizures indistinguishable from those produced by giant aneurysms (Sengupta et al., 1978; Pásztor et al., 1986). Eller

(1986) described a 69-year-old woman who suffered a stroke characterized by a left hemiparesis and extinction of the left visual field. She was found to have a relatively small (18-mm) aneurysm of the right MCA. MR imaging showed a clot inside the aneurysm, and it was thought that the patient's stroke had resulted from an embolus originating from within the aneurysm. Antunes and Correll (1976) and Stewart et al. (1980) reported similar cases.

Aneurysms Arising from the Anterior Communicating Artery

Aneurysms that arise from the anterior communicating artery account for 25–30% of all intracranial aneurysms (Locksley, 1969; Hacker et al., 1983; Weir, 1987) (Fig. 53.148). Thus, this location is one of the most frequent sites of aneurysm formation (Nakagawa and Hashi, 1994). Like

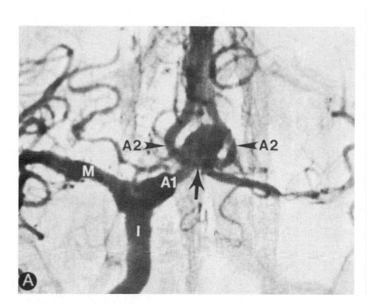
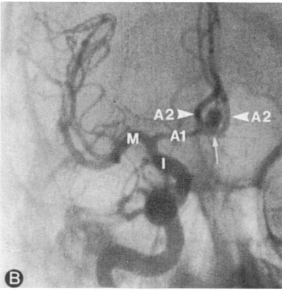

Figure 53.148. Aneurysms arising from the anterior communicating artery. *A* and *B*, Angiograms from two different patients with aneurysms arising from the anterior communicating artery (*arrows*). In all cases, the aneurysm is located between the A-2 segments of the anterior cerebral arteries (*A2*). *A1*, A-1 (proximal) segment of the anterior cerebral artery; *I*, internal carotid artery; *M*, middle cerebral artery.

distal ACA aneurysms, anterior communicating artery aneurysms are often associated with anomalies of local vessels (Inoue et al., 1992), including triplicate redundancy (Yamagami et al., 1992). This location may be under-represented in patients with familial aneurysms (Leblanc et al., 1995) and polycystic kidney disease (Schievink et al., 1992a), but increases in frequency in older patients (Noterman et al., 1995). Anterior communicating artery aneurysms usually become symptomatic when they rupture. In a cooperative study (Locksley, 1969), 711 of 747 such aneurysms (95%) initially presented with SAH. The rupture rate may increase with age (Inagawa et al., 1992). Anterior communicating artery aneurysms may also develop de novo following occlusion of one of the ICAs (Ladzinski et al., 1994; Maiuri et al., 1995; Timperman et al., 1995).

Unruptured anterior communicating aneurysms produce visual symptoms and signs that are indistinguishable from those produced by aneurysms arising from the A-1 and proximal A-2 segments of the ACA (Walsh, 1964; Huber, 1976,

1982; Tajima et al., 1993). Visual loss may be slowly progressive or sudden in onset and may be associated with headache or eye pain. Because the anterior communicating artery is a midline vessel, aneurysms that arise from it usually produce bilateral visual loss, but they also may cause unilateral loss of vision (Durston and Parsons-Smith, 1970; Caprioli et al., 1983; Takahashi et al., 1983; Chan et al., 1997). The optic nerves, optic chiasm, and even the optic tract (Date et al., 1997) may be affected by these aneurysms (Figs. 53.149–53.151).

Patients with bilateral visual loss commonly have a bitemporal hemianopia that may be asymmetric. Takahashi et al. (1983) described a 59-year-old man who experienced an SAH in 1956. He apparently was treated with conservative therapy at that time, although it is not clear whether the cause of the hemorrhage was identified. Twenty years later, the patient developed blurred vision. Visual acuity at this time was 20/70 OD and 20/20 OS, associated with an asymmetric bitemporal hemianopia. The right optic disc was pale; the

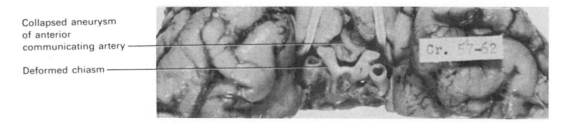

Figure 53.149. Pathologic appearance of an aneurysm that arose from the anterior communicating artery and compressed the anterior portion of the optic chiasm. The aneurysm has collapsed during processing, but the deformity of the optic chiasm is obvious, with widening and squaring of the normal anterior angle. The patient probably had a bitemporal visual field defect. (From Lindenberg R, Walsh FB, Sacks JG. Neuropathology of Vision: An Atlas. Philadelphia, Lea & Febiger, 1973.)

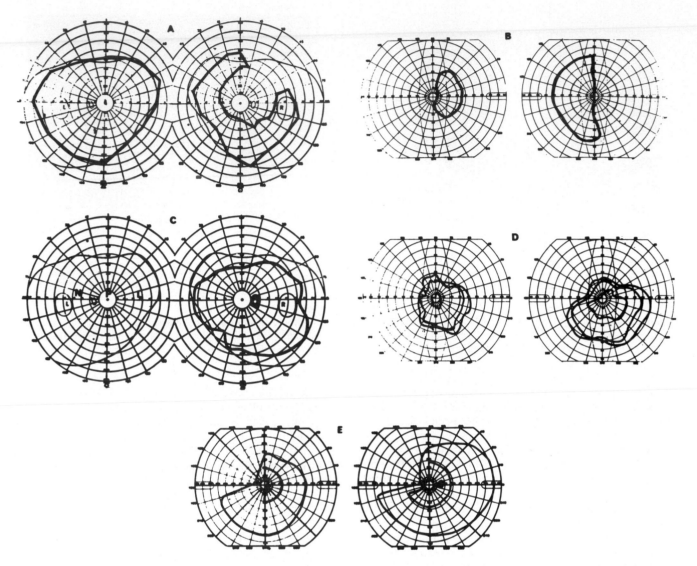

Figure 53.150. Visual field defects in five patients with aneurysms arising from the anterior communicating artery. *A*, Visual fields in a 62-year-old woman with vision of 20/60 OD and 20/20 OS. The visual field of the right eye shows a central scotoma that breaks out to the superior temporal periphery. The visual field of the left eye is normal. In this patient, only the right optic nerve was compressed by the aneurysm. *B*, Visual fields in a 61-year-old man with visual acuity of 20/30 OD and 20/200 OS. The visual field of the right eye shows a complete temporal hemianopia. The visual field of the left eye also shows a complete temporal hemianopia, and there also is constriction of the nasal field. In this case, the aneurysm compressed primarily the nasal portions of both optic nerves, but the left optic nerve was affected more than the right optic nerve. *C*, Visual fields in a 48-year-old man. The right eye has 20/15 visual acuity with a full visual field. The left eye is blind. Although both optic nerves were compressed by the aneurysm, there was clinical evidence of damage only to the left optic nerve. *D*, Visual fields in a 34-year-old man with visual acuity of 20/40 OD and 20/100 OS. Both visual fields show diffuse constriction, perhaps more superiorly than inferiorly. In this case, the aneurysm expanded medially and downward, compressing both the optic nerves. *E*, Visual fields in a 53-year-old man with visual acuity of 20/30 OD and 20/200 OS. There is an incomplete left homonymous hemianopia, denser above, associated with a central scotoma in the left eye. In this case, the right optic tract was damaged as was the left optic nerve. This is a most unusual pattern of visual acuity and field loss. (From Peiris JB, Ross Russell RW. Giant aneurysms of the carotid system presenting as visual field defect. J Neurol Neurosurg Psychiatry *43*:1053–1064, 1980.)

left disc was normal. Neuroimaging studies demonstrated a suprasellar, thrombosed aneurysm arising from the anterior communicating artery. At surgery, the aneurysm was found to be compressing the anterior portion of the optic chiasm, mainly on the right side. Similar cases were described by other investigators (Hojer-Pedersen and Haase, 1981; Aoki, 1988) (Fig. 53.151). More than a single pathologic process

may be present in such cases. Yuki et al. (1996) reported the case of a 60-year-old woman with bilateral optic neuropathies and a bitemporal visual field defect. CT scanning and MR imaging revealed a cystic intrasellar mass with suprasellar extension. The lesion proved to be a Rathke cleft cyst. In addition, however, the patient had an anterior communicating aneurysm embedded in the central portion of the optic

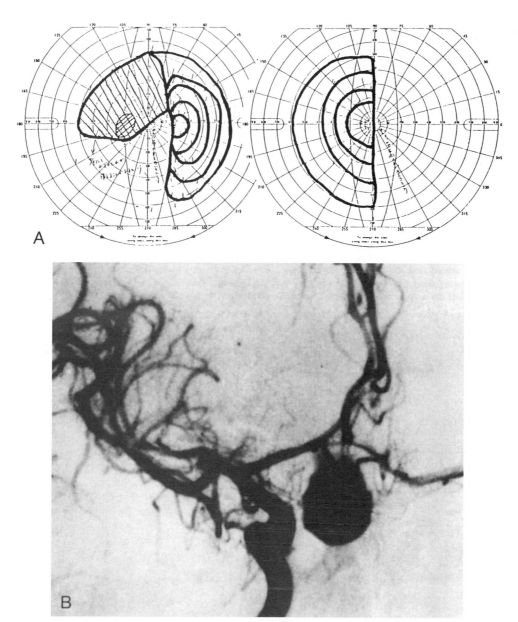

Figure 53.151. Optic chiasmal syndrome in a patient with a giant anterior communicating artery aneurysm. The patient was a 47-year-old man with decreased vision in both eyes. *A,* Visual field demonstrates an asymmetric bitemporal hemianopia. *B,* Right carotid angiogram shows a large aneurysm of the anterior communicating artery that projects downward onto the optic chiasm and into the sella turcica. The patient underwent clipping of the aneurysm followed by aneurysmorrhaphy; however, the bitemporal hemianopia did not improve. (From Aoki N. Partially thrombosed aneurysm presenting as the sudden onset of bitemporal hemianopsia. Neurosurgery 22:564–566, 1988.)

chiasm. Clipping of the aneurysm and drainage of the cyst resulted in improvement in visual function.

Peiris and Ross Russell (1980) described five patients with visual loss caused by an unruptured anterior communicating aneurysm. The patients, four of whom were men, ranged in age from 34 to 62 years. All five patients had asymmetric loss of visual function without a consistent pattern. Two patients had one eye that was normal with respect to both visual acuity and visual field. One of these patients had no light perception in the opposite eye (Fig. 53.150C). In the other patient, the affected eye had 20/60 acuity with a central scotoma that broke out to the temporal periphery (Fig. 53.150A). Both of these patients thus presented with unilateral optic neuropathy.

Of the other three patients described by Peiris and Ross Russell (1980), one patient had visual acuity of 20/40 OD and 20/100 OS with irregular constriction of both visual fields (Fig. 53.150D). This patient thus exhibited evidence of bilateral optic neuropathy. A second patient had visual acuity of 20/30 OD and 20/200 OS, a bitemporal hemianopia, and constriction of the remaining nasal field in the left eye (Fig. 53.150B). This patient had a left optic neuropathy combined with a chiasmal syndrome. The third patient described by Peiris and Ross Russell (1980) with bilateral visual loss from an anterior communicating aneurysm had visual acuity of 20/30 OD and 20/200 OS with an incomplete, incongruous left homonymous hemianopia (Fig. 53.150E). The visual findings in this patient were probably caused by damage to the left optic nerve and the right optic tract. Golding et al. (1980) described a patient with a giant, thrombosed, anterior communicating aneurysm who had a homonymous hemianopia from either compression or ischemia of the right optic tract.

Norwood et al. (1986) described two patients with anterior communicating aneurysms and loss of vision. One of the patients, a 40-year-old man, had a 6-month history of bilateral, progressive visual loss. His initial examination revealed vision of 20/200 OU with inconsistent central scotomas and pale optic discs. He was thought to be suffering from nutritional optic neuropathy until neuroimaging studies revealed the true cause of the bilateral optic neuropathy. A second patient described by Norwood et al. (1986) was a 49-year-old woman who experienced sudden left retrobulbar pain followed by blindness in the left eye. Visual acuity was 20/20 OD and light perception OS. The right visual field was full, and both optic discs were normal. The patient was thought to have experienced an attack of retrobulbar optic neuritis, but neuroimaging studies revealed an anterior communicating aneurysm.

Anterior communicating aneurysms that enlarge without rupture may attain sufficient size to produce symptoms and signs in addition to visual loss (Jefferson, 1937; Meadows, 1951). They may compress the undersurface of one or both frontal lobes, resulting in dementia and other symptoms and signs of frontal lobe dysfunction (Peiris and Ross Russell, 1980; Bokemeyer et al., 1990). These aneurysms also may expand into the sella turcica and compress the pituitary gland. If the anterior lobe of the gland is damaged, the patient may develop symptoms and signs of panhypopituitarism (Van 'T Hoff et al., 1961; White and Ballantine, 1961; Nukta and Taylor, 1987). If the posterior lobe is damaged, the patient may develop diabetes insipidus. Austin and Maceri (1993) described a patient who presented with pulsatile tinnitus and was found to have an anterior communicating artery aneurysm. It is difficult to understand how an aneurysm in this location could have produced this syndrome, but the tinnitus resolved after the aneurysm was clipped.

Aneurysms Arising from the Vertebrobasilar Arterial System

Only 5–15% of all clinically documented saccular aneurysms arise from the vertebral and basilar arteries or their branches (Duvoisin and Yahr, 1965; Locksley, 1969; Stehbens, 1972; Yoshimoto et al., 1978; Kassell and Torner, 1983a; Hacker et al., 1983; Nishimoto et al., 1985; Weir, 1987; Marks, 1996), although the results of an autopsy study performed by McDonald and Korb (1939) suggested that the true figure is closer to 25%. The discrepancy between clinical and autopsy figures probably is related to a previous tendency for physicians to obtain incomplete angiographic studies. For example, in a cooperative study (Sahs et al., 1969), only 27% of patients with over 2600 aneurysms underwent vertebral angiography.

Aneurysms that originate from the vertebrobasilar arterial system, like aneurysms that arise from the ICA and its branches, usually present with SAH (Locksley, 1969; Sutton, 1971; Nijensohn et al., 1974; Hudgins et al., 1983; Solomon and Stein, 1988). Nevertheless, unruptured saccular aneurysms originating from the vertebrobasilar arterial system may enlarge sufficiently to produce a variety of neurologic deficits, including: (a) progressive cranial nerve, brainstem, or cerebellar dysfunction; (b) TIAs or stroke; and (c) seizures. In fact, a substantial percentage of aneurysms larger than 2.5 cm in diameter (giant aneurysms) are located in the vertebrobasilar distribution (Tulleken, 1976; Drake, 1979; Hosobuchi, 1979; Sundt and Piepgras, 1979; Storrs et al., 1982).

Some posterior circulation aneurysms originate at the junction of the vertebral and basilar arteries and therefore cannot be said to arise specifically from one artery or the other (Figs. 53.152–53.154). Most vertebrobasilar system aneurysms, however, have a precise origin from the vertebral artery, the basilar artery, or one of their branches.

Aneurysms Arising from the Vertebral Artery and Its Branches

Aneurysms originating from the vertebral artery or one of its branches account for about 4–5% of all intracranial aneurysms (Stehbens, 1972; Yoshimoto et al., 1978; Kassell and Torner, 1983a; Hacker et al., 1983; Nishimoto et al., 1985; Weir, 1987). They occur with the same frequency in adults and children (Stehbens, 1972).

ANEURYSMS ARISING FROM THE VERTEBRAL ARTERY

Aneurysms that originate from the vertebral artery usually arise near the origin of the posterior inferior cerebellar artery

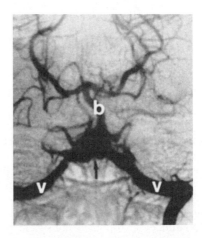

Figure 53.152. Cerebral angiogram, anteroposterior view, shows an aneurysm (*arrow*) arising from the junction of the vertebral (*v*) and basilar (*b*) arteries.

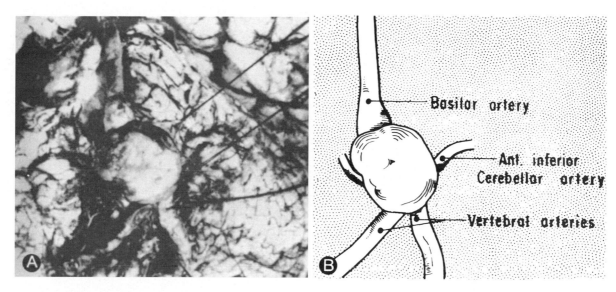

Figure 53.153. Vertebrobasilar junction aneurysm. The patient presented with dizzy spells and difficulty swallowing. He died 6 weeks after onset of symptoms of progressive infarction of the brainstem. Ocular signs consist of vertical nystagmus and bilateral paresis of upward gaze. *A*, Basal view of the brain shows a large aneurysm arising from the junction of the vertebral and basilar arteries. *B*, Artist's sketch of the photograph on the *left*. (From Cogan DG, Mount HTJ. Intracranial aneurysms causing ophthalmoplegia. Arch Ophthalmol *70*:757–771, 1963.)

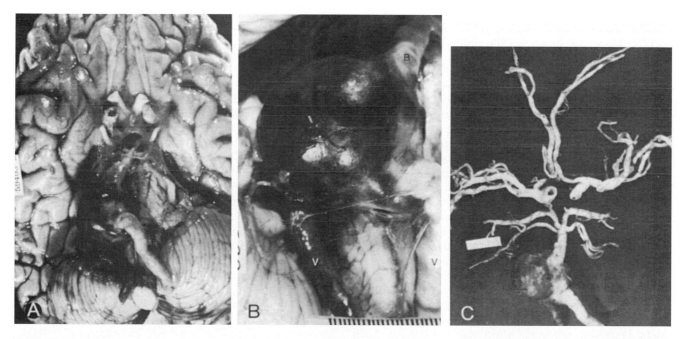

Figure 53.154. Giant intracranial aneurysm arising from the junction of the vertebral and basilar arteries. The patient initially developed a right abducens nerve paresis. He then began to have difficulty walking, and he subsequently became increasingly confused. In the midst of an evaluation, he suddenly deteriorated, became progressively obtunded, and died. An autopsy was performed. *A*, There is a giant saccular aneurysm at the junction of the vertebral and basilar arteries. *B*, Higher power view of *A*, shows the aneurysm located between the two vertebral arteries (*V*) and the basilar artery (*B*). The aneurysm is compressing the brainstem at the pontomedullary junction. *C*, The circle of Willis has been dissected out, and the location of the aneurysm at the vertebrobasilar junction is more easily appreciated. (From Cohen AR, Aleksic S, Budzilovich GN, et al. Giant intracranial aneurysm presenting as a posterior fossa mass. Surg Neurol *20*:160–164, 1983.)

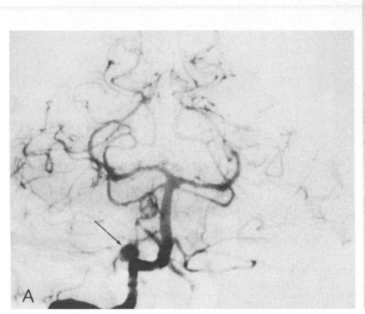

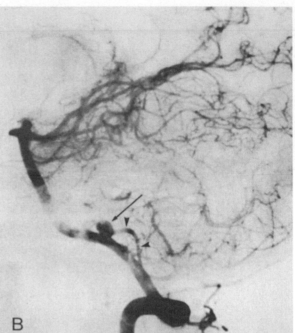

Figure 53.155.   Vertebral artery aneurysm arising near the origin of the posterior inferior cerebellar artery. *A*, Cerebral angiogram, anteroposterior view, shows the aneurysm (*arrow*) arising from the right vertebral artery. *B*, Lateral view shows the relationship of the aneurysm (*arrow*) to the origin and course of the right posterior inferior cerebellar artery (*arrowheads*). (From Fox JL. Intracranial Aneurysms, Vol I. New York, Springer-Verlag, 1983.)

(PICA) (Ferrante et al., 1992) (Fig. 53.155). Such aneurysms are often associated with a vascular anomaly of the vertebral artery, such as duplication (Antunes et al., 1991) or a fenestration (Arai et al., 1989; Okamura et al., 1995). They usually become symptomatic when they rupture (Yamaura, 1988; Andoh et al., 1992a). In a retrospective series reported by Andoh et al. (1992a), 33 of 38 vertebral aneurysms had ruptured at the time of diagnosis, including 18 of 20 (90%) saccular aneurysms. Some, however, progressively enlarge until they produce increased ICP from compression of the brainstem and cerebellum or from obstruction of the 4th ventricle (Yaskin and Alpers, 1944; Paulson et al., 1959; Bull, 1962; Tommasi-Davenas et al., 1989; Nagahiro et al., 1995) (Figs. 53.156–53.158). In such cases, nonlocalizing unilateral or bilateral abducens paresis may be present, although papilledema usually does not occur. In other cases, enlargement of the aneurysm may be associated with transient or permanent neurologic symptoms and signs that result from a variety of mechanisms (Höök et al., 1963; Steinberger et al., 1984; Maruyama et al., 1989; Kurokawa et al., 1990).

The aneurysm can compress the ventral surface of the caudal brainstem, producing direct neuronal damage. Such a mechanism was probably responsible for the horizontal gaze paresis that occurred in a 45-year-old woman with a large aneurysm arising from the origin of the PICA (Morgan and Honan, 1988). The patient also had dysesthesia of the left side of the body, left-sided incoordination, and an ataxic gait. An aneurysm at the origin of the PICA also may compress or stretch the lower cranial nerves as they emerge from the ventral surface of the brainstem, producing single or

multiple, unilateral or bilateral, cranial neuropathy (see Table in Tulleken, 1976; Amacher et al., 1981). An aneurysm can interrupt the blood supply to the brainstem, cerebellum, and spinal cord by compressing the arteries that supply these areas, thereby producing local or generalized neuronal ischemia (Paulson et al., 1959). Bilateral abducens nerve paresis is not uncommon in this setting (Höök et al., 1986), although unilateral abducens nerve paresis also may occur. The paresis initially may be isolated (Arseni et al., 1969), but it usually is associated with occipital or neck pain (Coppeto and Chan, 1982) or with other cranial neuropathies and brainstem signs (Arseni et al., 1969). Vestibular nystagmus often is present (Thron and Bockenheimer, 1979). Other symptoms and signs produced by aneurysms that arise from the vertebral artery near the origin of the PICA and that damage neural structures, interrupt their blood supply, or both, include decreased hearing, tinnitus, vertigo, dysarthria, dysphagia, respiratory difficulty, hemiparesis or paraparesis, unilateral or bilateral paresthesia and sensory deficits, and ataxia (Yaskin and Alpers, 1944; Paulson et al., 1959; Jannetta et al., 1966; see the Table in Tulleken, 1976; Miller and Newton, 1978; Thron and Bockenheimer, 1979; Massey et al., 1984; Hahn et al., 1986; Kurokawa et al., 1990).

An aneurysm of the vertebral artery may be the source of emboli that produce TIAs suggesting atherosclerotic disease of the vertebrobasilar arterial circulation (Maruyama et al., 1989) (Fig. 53.159). Tommasi-Davenas et al. (1989) described a 30-year-old man who experienced three episodes of transient right homonymous hemianopia before developing progressive hiccup, vomiting, orthostatic dizziness, and pos-

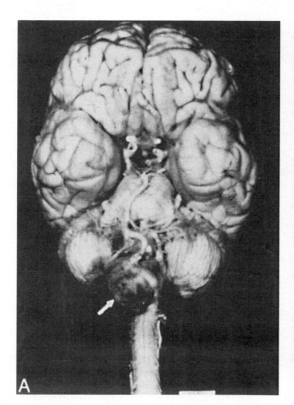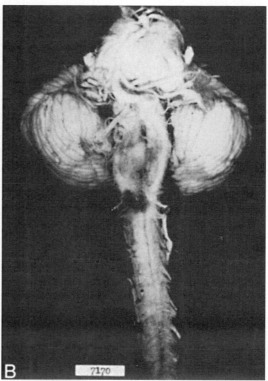

Figure 53.156. Aneurysm of the vertebral artery compressing the caudal brainstem and upper cervical spinal cord. *A,* Ventral view of the brain of a 62-year-old man who had experienced an episode of headache and loss of consciousness 6 years previously. An evaluation at that time revealed bloody cerebrospinal fluid. The patient subsequently complained of diplopia that resolved over 4 months. Over the next 5 years, he experienced intermittent occipital headaches. He then began to experience difficulty swallowing and numbness of the right arm and signs. These symptoms initially were transient, but they subsequently became constant. At the same time, the patient developed numbness of the 4th and 5th fingers of the left hand, diplopia, difficulty breathing, and headache that was so severe that he refused to move his head. A tumor of the upper cervical cord was suspected after a myelogram showed a partial obstruction between C4 and C7. The patient died shortly after a cervical laminectomy. *A,* Ventral view of the patient's brain and spinal cord shows a large aneurysm (*arrow*) arising from the vertebral artery. *B,* The aneurysm has been removed, revealing severe compression of the upper cervical spinal cord and the caudal medulla. The compression completely obliterated the 4th ventricle. (From Paulson G, Nashold BS Jr, Margolis G. Aneurysms of the vertebral artery: Report of 5 cases. Neurology 9:590–598, 1959.)

tural hypotension that led to an evaluation. The patient was found to have a giant, thrombosed aneurysm originating from the distal portion of the left vertebral artery and extending into the 4th ventricle. It is possible that the patient's initial episodes of transient hemianopia were caused by emboli from the partially thrombosed aneurysm.

An unruptured, saccular aneurysm arising at the origin of the PICA need not be large to produce neurologic dysfunction. Maroon et al. (1978) described a 54-year-old woman with left hemifacial spasm caused by a saccular aneurysm at the origin of the PICA from the vertebral artery (Fig. 53.160). The aneurysm measured about 3 mm in transverse diameter and 5 mm in length. The patient underwent craniotomy, at which time the dome of the aneurysm was found to be deforming, stretching, and angulating the facial nerve as well as indenting the brainstem at the root entry zone of the facial nerve. The neck of the aneurysm was clipped, and the dome was mobilized away from the facial nerve and the brainstem. A small piece of polyvinyl chloride nonabsorbable sponge was inserted between the dome of the aneurysm and the brainstem to maintain the new position of the aneu-

rysm. Postoperatively, the patient had complete resolution of hemifacial spasm. Additional cases of saccular aneurysms producing hemifacial spasm were reported by Nagata et al. (1992) and by Moriuchi et al. (1996).

The symptoms and signs produced by unruptured aneurysms of the vertebral artery and its branches are usually slowly progressive, but they may occur suddenly even in the absence of evidence of SAH. When neurologic dysfunction is caused by sudden enlargement of the aneurysm with compression of adjacent neural structures, the symptoms and signs are usually permanent. Walsh and Hoyt (1969k) described an 18-year-old girl who experienced choking spells, difficulty with speech, and neck stiffness caused by an unruptured aneurysm of the left vertebral artery that was compressing the medulla and upper cervical cord. The aneurysm subsequently ruptured, producing bilateral abducens nerve paresis, vestibular nystagmus, and mild right ptosis. The patient died after an operation that was complicated by severe bleeding from the aneurysm.

Acute neurologic dysfunction may also develop when the blood supply to parts of the brainstem is interrupted by an

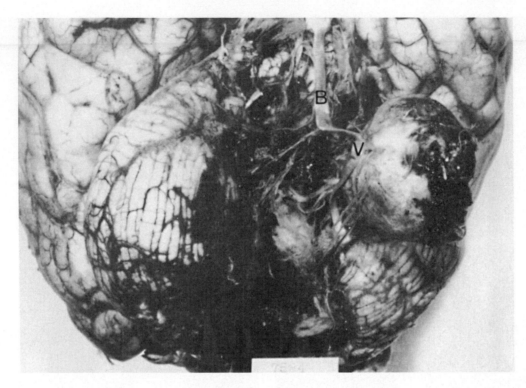

Figure 53.157. Giant aneurysm of the vertebral artery with brainstem compression. The patient was a 53-year-old man with occipital headaches of increasing severity, progressive weakness of the legs, a staggering gait, dizziness, vertigo, and tinnitus. He had vestibular nystagmus, a fine tremor of the outstretched hands, and he fell toward the left and backward when he attempted to stand still with his feet together and his eyes closed. A right vertebral angiogram showed an aneurysm of the right vertebral artery. A craniotomy was performed, the aneurysm was trapped, and clot was removed from within the lesion. The patient died 2 days after surgery. View of the ventral surface of the brain at autopsy with the aneurysm reflected to the left shows its origin from the vertebral artery (*V*). *B*, basilar artery. (From Paulson G, Nashold Jr BS, Margolis G. Aneurysms of the vertebral artery: Report of 5 cases. Neurology 9:590–598, 1959.)

unruptured aneurysm. The interruption may be caused by aneurysmal compression of adjacent arteries or thrombosis within the aneurysm (Uranishi et al., 1995). In such cases, the neurologic deficits may be permanent (Cohen et al., 1983) or transient (Steinberger et al., 1984). West and Todman (1991) reported a patient with a 12-year history of cluster headache who was found to have an aneurysm arising from the junction of the vertebral and posterior inferior cerebellar arteries. The patient's headaches resolved following clipping of the aneurysm.

Technically, vertebral artery aneurysms may be difficult to approach if they arise from the proximal artery just after dural penetration. Extradural control of vertebral artery blood flow may be required for adequate clipping (Aoki et al., 1993).

ANEURYSMS ARISING FROM THE POSTERIOR INFERIOR CEREBELLAR ARTERY

Most aneurysms that are said to arise from the PICA actually arise from the junction of that artery with the vertebral artery (Figs. 53.155 and 53.160). Such aneurysms account for only about 2% of all intracranial aneurysms and 9% of all aneurysms arising from the vertebrobasilar arterial system (Hacker et al., 1983; Lee et al., 1989; Blard et al., 1997).

Rarely, the origin of the PICA is extracranial (Chen and Chen, 1997). In this setting, a proximally located aneurysm may actually be extracranial (Tanaka et al., 1993), even within the spinal canal (Hakozaki et al., 1996). Even less commonly, the PICA arises from the ICA. Manabe et al. (1991) reported this anomaly in a patient with multiple aneurysms. In another patient with a PICA aneurysm, the PICA arose from a branch of the contralateral PICA and supplied both cerebellar hemispheres (Hlavin et al., 1991).

Saccular aneurysms that arise from the distal portion of the PICA are rare (see Table 2 in Yamamoto et al., 1984; Beyerl and Heros, 1986; Dernbach et al., 1988a; Madsen and Heros, 1988; Lee et al., 1989; Mintz and Cosgrove, 1990; Kashiwagi et al., 1992; Reynier et al., 1992; Salomao et al., 1992; Yoshida and Yamamoto, 1992; Price and Miller, 1994; Uranishi et al., 1994; Zingale et al., 1994; Bilge et al., 1995; Chen and Chen, 1997) (Figs. 53.161 and 53.162). Andoh et al. (1992b) described 15 cases. More than half of these aneurysms arose from the telovelotonsillar segment of the artery. One patient had two aneurysms arising from the same peripheral PICA. Another aneurysm was located at the internal auditory meatus. Even more rare are bilateral distal PICA aneurysms (Sano et al., 1993). When large, these aneurysms may be mistaken for vestibular schwannomas (Morris et al., 1995). Distal aneurysms of the PICA usually occur

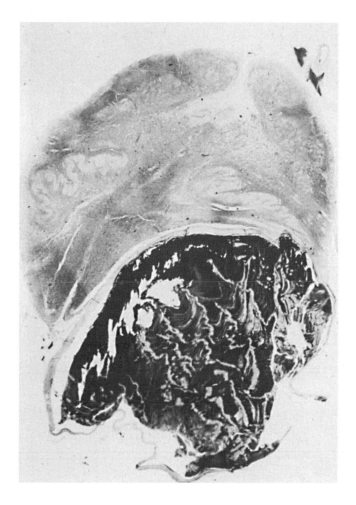

Figure 53.158. Severe compression of the ventral brainstem from a partially thrombosed aneurysm of the vertebral artery. The patient had progressive symptoms and signs of compression of the medulla, including vomiting, slurred speech, difficulty swallowing, and ataxia.

in adults, but they may become symptomatic in childhood, even in the neonatal period (Jane, 1961; Pickering et al., 1970).

Some distal PICA aneurysms are related to previous surgery or infection. Kojima et al. (1996) reported the case of de novo development of a distal PICA aneurysm in a 73-year-old woman who 6 years previously had undergone clipping of a vertebral-PICA aneurysm, and Kurino et al. (1994) found *Aspergillus* species in the vessel wall of a patient who experienced an SAH from a PICA aneurysm while being treated for meningitis.

Trauma may produce a pseudoaneurysm of the PICA. Teitelbaum et al. (1995a) reported a patient in whom a PICA pseudoaneurysm developed after a transoral biopsy of a tumor, and Morard and de Tribolet (1991) published the case of a PICA aneurysm associated with an occipital fracture. Pau et al. (1994) described three patients in whom an aneurysm of the PICA was associated with an AVM that was fed in part by the same vessel.

Both vertebral-PICA junction aneurysms and distal PICA aneurysms usually present with subarachnoid, intracerebellar, or intraventricular hemorrhage (Uranishi et al., 1994; Urbach et al., 1995; Blard et al., 1997). The manifestations in such cases are usually nonspecific; however, Miller (1997) described a unique case in which a woman with pseudotumor

cerebri and a mild Chiari malformation developed cortical blindness and simultagnosia after a lumboperitoneal shunt and was found to have a PICA aneurysm associated with SAH and angiographic evidence of vasospasm (Fig 53.163). It was postulated that the lumboperitoneal shunt caused an abrupt lowering of the patient's ICP, resulting in further downward displacement of the cerebellar tonsils and rupture of the previously asymptomatic aneurysm.

Unruptured vertebral-PICA and distal PICA aneurysms occasionally produce neurologic symptoms and signs related to mass effect. These include hydrocephalus with and without papilledema, vestibular nystagmus, abducens nerve paresis, trigeminal neuropathy, diminished or absent corneal reflex, decreased hearing, tinnitus, vertigo, dysarthria, dysphagia, respiratory difficulty, hemiparesis or paraparesis, unilateral or bilateral paresthesia and sensory deficits, and ataxia (Yaskin and Alpers, 1944; Paulson et al., 1959; Alexander et al., 1966; Miller and Newton, 1978; Yoshii et al., 1979) (Fig. 53.164). A large aneurysm arising from the PICA may present as a mass in the region of the foramen magnum (Judice and Connolly, 1978; Richmond and Schmidt, 1993). Downbeat nystagmus may be seen in such cases.

The use of noninvasive neuroimaging studies, particularly MR angiography and spiral CT angiography, permits the identification of asymptomatic PICA aneurysms (Price and

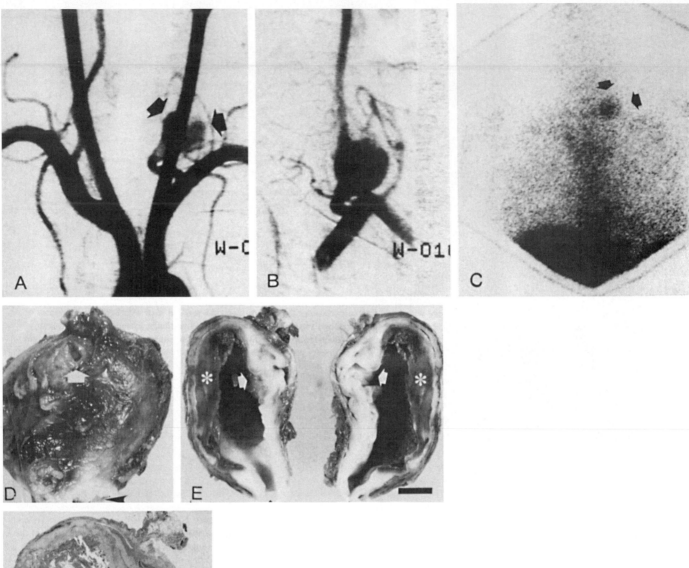

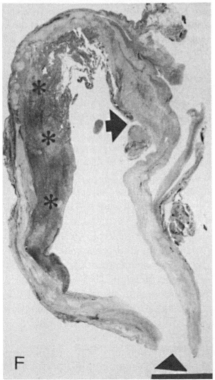

Figure 53.159. Aneurysm of the extracranial portion of the vertebral artery that caused transient ischemic attacks. The patient was a 40-year-old man with episodes of diplopia, sensory impairment, and weakness of either side of the extremities. All episodes occurred suddenly, and they resolved within 24 hours. The only permanent neurologic deficit was a left homonymous quadrantanopia. *A,* Digital subtraction aortogram shows a giant saccular aneurysm (*arrows*) arising from the left vertebral artery at the C7 level. *B,* The aneurysm is seen in its entirety on an oblique view of a left subclavian angiogram. *C,* An indium-111 platelet scintigram of the neck in this patient performed 50 hours after injection of labeled autologous platelets shows a well-defined focus of abnormal activity within the aneurysm (*arrows*). The patient was treated with aspirin, but the attacks continued. Accordingly, he underwent an aneuryectomy combined with an end-to-end anastomosis of the left vertebral artery using an artery graft from the left radial artery. *D,* Photograph of excised aneurysm of the left vertebral artery shows the proximal (*arrowhead*) and distal (*arrow*) portions of the excised vertebral artery. *E,* Photograph of bisected aneurysm shows mural thrombus (*asterisks*) in the aneurysmal sac. Bar = 5 mm. *F,* Histopathologic appearance of aneurysm shows entrance (*arrowhead*) and exit (*arrow*) of vertebral artery. The wall of the vessel is thickened and lined by an extensive mural thrombus (*asterisks*). Bar = 5 mm. (From Maruyama M, Asai T, Kuriyama Y, et al. Positive platelet scintigram of a vertebral aneurysm presenting thromboembolic transient ischemic attacks. Stroke *20*:687–690, 1989.)

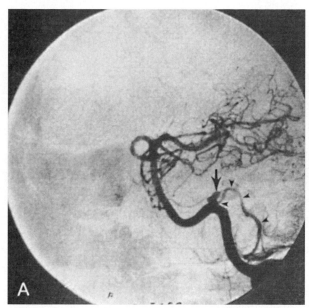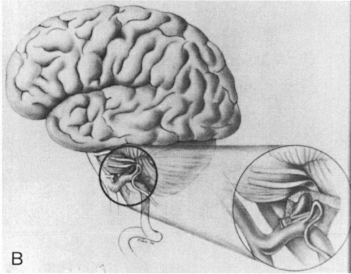

Figure 53.160. Hemifacial spasm caused by compression of the facial nerve by an artery arising at the junction of the vertebral and posterior inferior cerebellar arteries. The patient was a 54-year-old woman with a 6-year history of typical left hemifacial spasm. *A*, Cerebral angiography shows a small saccular aneurysm *(arrow)* arising from the left vertebral artery at the origin of the posterior inferior cerebellar artery *(arrowheads)*. The patient underwent posterior fossa craniectomy at which time the aneurysm was identified. The left facial nerve was "deformed, stretched, and angulated across the dome of the aneurysm." The neck of the aneurysm was clipped, and the dome was mobilized away from its adherent position to the facial nerve and brainstem. A piece of polyvinyl chloride nonabsorbable sponge then was inserted between the dome of the aneurysm and the brainstem to maintain the aneurysm in its new position. *B*, Schematic representation of aneurysmal compression of the facial nerve before and after clipping and mobilization of the aneurysm. (From Maroon JC, Lunsford LD, Deeb ZL. Hemifacial spasm due to aneurysmal compression of the facial nerve. Arch Neurol 35:545–546, 1978.)

Miller, 1994). It is likely that as more such studies are performed, the number of asymptomatic PICA aneurysms detected will increase significantly.

Aneurysms Arising from the Basilar Artery and Its Branches

About 3–9% of all intracranial aneurysms arise from the basilar artery or from one of its main branches: the anterior inferior cerebellar, superior cerebellar, and posterior cerebral arteries (Locksley, 1969; Stehbens, 1972; Yoshimoto et al., 1978; Hacker et al., 1983; Kassell and Torner, 1983a; Nishimoto et al., 1985; Weir, 1987). Most of these aneurysms do not produce symptoms until they rupture, at which time they cause SAH that is associated with a high morbidity and mortality (Nijensohn et al., 1974). Occasionally, these aneurysms enlarge sufficiently to produce progressive neurologic symptoms and signs from mass effect, obstruction of the ventricular system, thrombosis, or compression of the brainstem, cranial nerves, and adjacent arteries.

ANEURYSMS ARISING FROM THE BASILAR ARTERY

Aneurysms that originate from the basilar artery may arise: (*a*) near its origin from the two vertebral arteries, often in a fenestration of the artery (Andrews et al., 1986; Campos et al., 1987; Miyagi et al., 1990; Hoshimaru et al., 1992; Sanders et al., 1993; Picard et al., 1993; Crivelli et al., 1993; Graves et al., 1996); (*b*) along its course near the origin of the anterior inferior or superior cerebellar arteries; or (*c*) most often, at its terminal bifurcation into the posterior cerebral arteries (Höök et al., 1963; Duvoisin and Yahr, 1965; Sharr and Kelvin, 1973; Drake, 1979; Marchel et al., 1992) (Fig. 53.165). A fenestration of the basilar artery may be mistaken for an aneurysm if it thromboses (Kalia et al., 1992).

Basilar aneurysms usually rupture before they become large enough to produce focal or diffuse neurologic signs (Locksley, 1969; Nijensohn et al., 1974) (Fig. 53.166). In some cases, however, the rupture is localized and produces symptoms and signs suggesting a posterior fossa tumor or stroke (Höök et al., 1963), and, in others, unruptured aneurysms enlarge sufficiently to cause progressive neurologic symptoms and signs that are related to the size, location, and direction of projection of the aneurysm.

Basilar artery aneurysms are uncommonly associated with infection. Perry et al. (1992) reported the case of basilar aneurysm development and rupture in a patient with *Streptococcus milleri* meningitis, and Calopa et al. (1990) described a giant basilar aneurysm in a 42-year-old man with mitral valve regurgitation and *Streptococcus morbillorum* subacute bacterial endocarditis. Patients with bacterial aneurysms of the basilar artery associated with bacterial endocarditis often

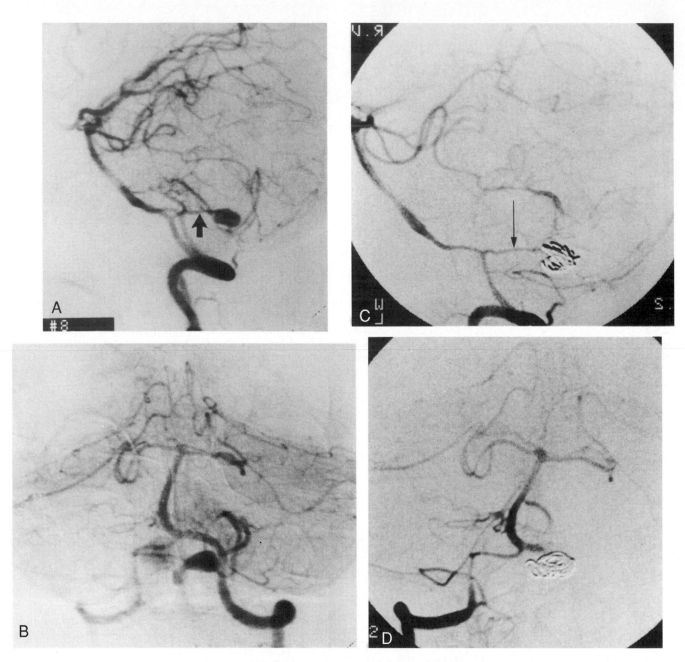

Figure 53.161.   Preoperative and postoperative appearance of an aneurysm of the distal posterior inferior cerebellar artery (PICA). The patient was a 63-year-old woman who suffered right-sided neck pain and headaches for 8 months. *A* and *B,* Left vertebral angiography prior to surgery demonstrates an irregular bilobed fusiform aneurysm arising from the posterior medullary segment of the right PICA. The patient underwent transarteriolar coil embolization of the aneurysm using 14 0.018-inch platinum coils interwoven with Dacron fibers to promote thrombosis. Coil length ranged from 20 to 21 mm in length and 3 to 7 mm in diameter. *C* and *D,* Postoperative angiography demonstrates complete occlusion of the aneurysm with no further filling. Flow to the proximal anterior and lateral medullary segments of the right PICA are preserved. The patient's headaches disappeared without further neurologic consequence. (From Dowd CF, Halbach VV, Higashida RT, et al. Endovascular coil embolization of unusual posterior inferior cerebellar artery aneurysms. Neurosurgery *27:* 954–961, 1990.)

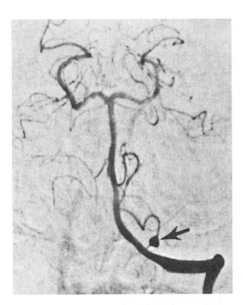

Figure 53.162. Aneurysm of the distal portion of the posterior inferior cerebellar artery (PICA) (*arrow*). The aneurysm was asymptomatic. It was discovered during a complete angiogram in a patient with a subarachnoid hemorrhage from another aneurysm arising from the internal carotid arterial system.

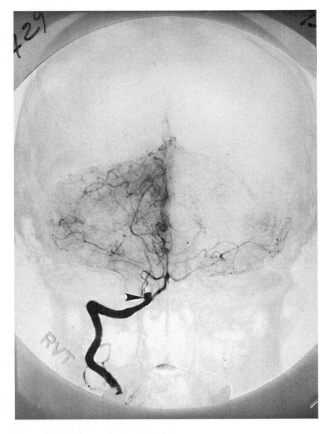

Figure 53.163. Angiographic appearance of ruptured vertebral-posterior inferior cerebellar artery aneurysm in a 42-year-old woman who experienced bilateral visual loss and simultagnosia shortly after undergoing an apparently uncomplicated lumboperitoneal shunt procedure for pseudotumor cerebri. Right vertebral angiogram, anteroposterior view, shows a saccular aneurysm at the junction of the vertebral and posterior inferior cerebellar arteries (*arrowhead*). Note diffuse vasospasm. (From Miller NR. Bilateral visual loss and simultagnosia after lumboperitoneal shunt for pseudotumor cerebri. J Neuroophthalmol *17*:36–38, 1997.)

have similar aneurysms arising from the intracranial branches of the ICA (Kuki et al., 1994).

Fungal mycotic aneurysms may also arise from the basilar artery. Radhakrishnan et al. (1994) reported four cases of mycotic aneurysms of the basilar artery and its branches, all of which were caused by *Aspergillus* species. Iihara et al. (1990) published a case of a 78-year-old who initially had an aspergillus granuloma of the cavernous sinus and subsequently succumbed to a ruptured mycotic aneurysm of the basilar artery. Chou et al. (1993) reported a middle aged adult male who died of a pontine stroke after rupture of a

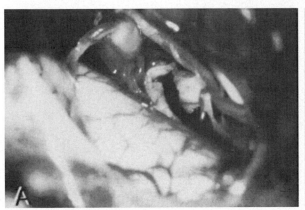

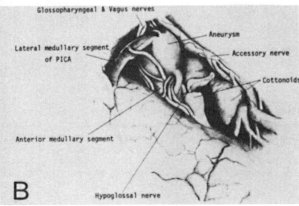

Figure 53.164. Aneurysm of the distal posterior inferior cerebellar artery (PICA) in a 39-year-old man who experienced sudden vertigo, nausea, and vomiting. He had mild truncal ataxia. He underwent an angiogram that showed an aneurysm of the distal portion of the right PICA. He subsequently underwent suboccipital craniectomy and wrapping of the aneurysm. *A*, Photograph of the aneurysm at the time of surgery. Note that the aneurysm arises from the lateral medullary segment of the PICA. *B*, Drawing of the aneurysm and the operative site. (From Yamamoto I, Tsugane R, Ohya M, et al. Peripheral aneurysms of the posterior inferior cerebellar artery. Neurosurgery *15*:839–845, 1984.)

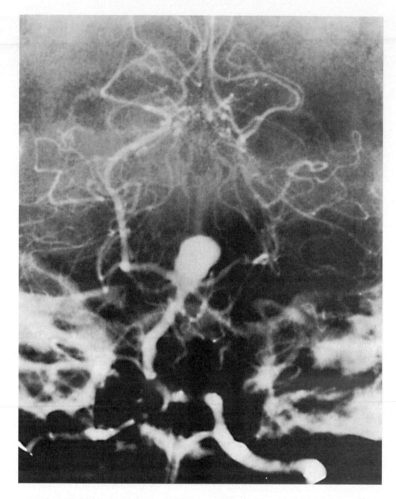

Figure 53.165. Aneurysm originating at the bifurcation of the basilar artery.

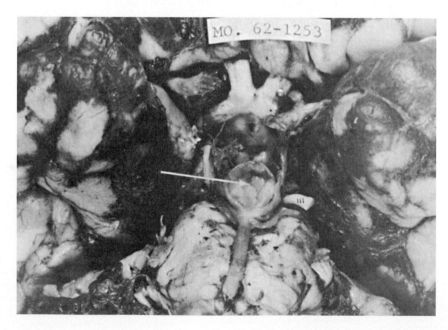

Figure 53.166. Ruptured aneurysm of the rostral basilar artery bifurcation (*arrow*). This lesion is located in the interpeduncular fossa. Note its relationship to the oculomotor nerve (*3rd*). (Courtesy of Dr. Richard Lindenberg.)

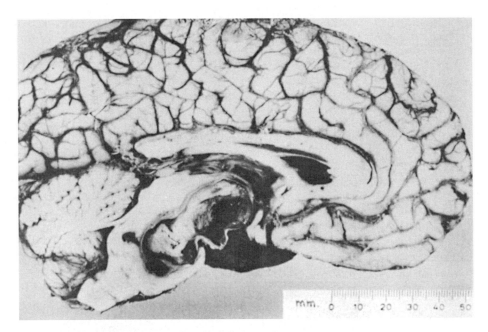

Figure 53.167. Gross appearance of a giant basilar artery aneurysm that caused hydrocephalus and brainstem signs. The patient was a 51-year-old woman who developed progressive confusion and difficulty walking. She had a moderately severe left hemiparesis. She initially was thought to have suffered a stroke, but over the next year, she developed a feeling of numbness on the right side of the face and of the inside of the mouth, and her gait became less steady. She complained of persistent headache and frequent vomiting. A CT scan showed a large mass projecting into the 3rd ventricle from behind. The patient underwent a ventriculoatrial shunt to relieve the obstructive hydrocephalus. A cerebral angiogram showed a large aneurysm of the basilar artery. The patient subsequently deteriorated, and she died shortly after undergoing an unsuccessful attempt to clip the aneurysm. The photograph shows a midsagittal section through the brain. A large aneurysm arising from the terminal bifurcation of the basilar artery extends forward into the left side of the pons and extends superiorly to elevate the floor of the 3rd ventricle. Most of the aneurysm is filled with laminated thrombus. (From Stark RJ. Supranuclear ophthalmoplegia with basilar artery aneurysms. Surg Neurol *12*:447–452, 1979.)

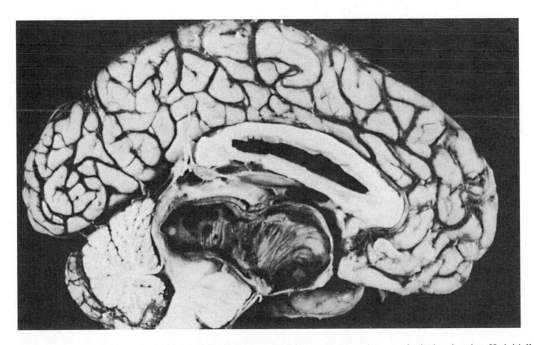

Figure 53.168. Midsagittal section through the brain of a 45-year-old man who developed progressive neurologic deterioration. He initially had symptoms and signs of hydrocephalus, but he gradually developed progressive evidence of brainstem dysfunction. Midsagittal section through the brain shows a large aneurysm arising from the terminal bifurcation of the basilar artery. The aneurysm contains laminated thrombus. Note the indentation of the upper pons, the midbrain, and the 3rd ventricle. The lateral ventricles are markedly dilated.

mycotic aneurysm in the setting of CNS aspergillosis. We saw a 74-year-old woman with a large-cell lymphoma of the clivus who developed a progressive brainstem syndrome related to a fungal mycotic aneurysm of the basilar artery. The aneurysm subsequently ruptured, with fatal results.

Patients with systemic vasculitis may develop basilar artery aneurysms. Asai et al. (1989) reported the case of a patient with SLE who was found to have multiple aneurysms, one of which was located at the terminal bifurcation of the basilar artery.

Severe headaches occur in most patients with both ruptured and unruptured basilar aneurysms (Höök et al., 1963; Trobe et al., 1978b). The headaches usually are suboccipital, but they may be nonspecific and even ocular or periorbital (Lightman et al., 1984). They are often aggravated by motion of the head (Rush et al., 1981).

Giant basilar aneurysms may compress the 3rd ventricle, 4th ventricle, or cerebral aqueduct to such an extent that hydrocephalus develops (Bull, 1962; Sutton, 1971; Drake, 1979; Stark, 1979; Naheedy et al., 1982; Bose et al., 1983; Piek et al., 1983; Musiek et al., 1987; Goetz et al., 1990) (Figs. 53.167 and 53.168). Affected patients may experience changes in personality, loss of recent memory, headache, and ataxia. Dementia may be the most prominent, and, occasionally, the only sign (Sutton, 1952; Bull, 1962). Other patients also have evidence of compression of the brainstem, cerebellum, or both. Signs of pontine compression include abducens nerve paresis, horizontal gaze paresis, facial weakness, hearing loss, and vestibular nystagmus (Bull, 1962; Naheedy et al., 1982). Mesencephalic compression may result in a dorsal midbrain syndrome (Stark, 1979).

Patients with hydrocephalus caused by a basilar aneurysm

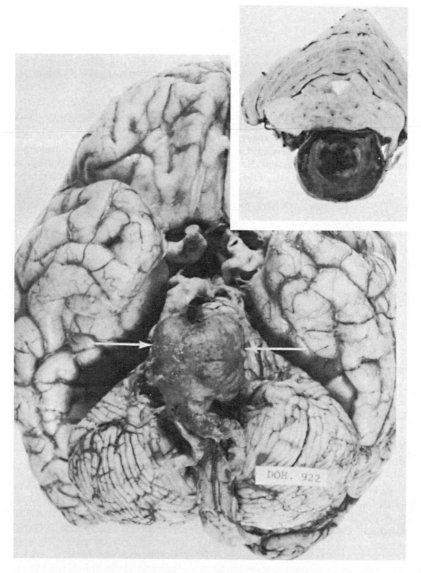

Figure 53.169. A huge aneurysm (*arrows*) arising from the basilar artery has mimicked a prepontine tumor. *Inset* shows marked compression of the pons, although the cerebral aqueduct and 4th ventricle are patent. (Courtesy of Dr. Richard Lindenberg.)

occasionally have papilledema (Stark, 1979). Walsh and Hoyt (19691) described a 27-year-old man who began to experience occipital headaches. About 1 year later, his speech became thick and slurred, he had difficulty swallowing, and he began to stagger while walking. An examination at this time revealed severe dysarthria, absence of the gag reflex, and severe bilateral papilledema. He also had slight ataxia and generalized hyperreflexia, especially on the left. The patient was thought to have a cerebellar tumor, but exploratory surgery failed to disclose such a lesion. He died shortly after surgery. A postmortem examination revealed a large aneurysm of the basilar artery that compressed and displaced the pons and also occluded the cerebral aqueduct.

Some patients with basilar aneurysms, particularly those that are larger than 2.5 cm, develop symptoms and signs of brainstem compression, cranial neuropathy, or both without evidence of hydrocephalus (Figs. 53.169 and 53.170). These patients initially may be thought to harbor a brainstem or cerebellopontine angle (CPA) neoplasm (Sutton, 1952; Höök et al., 1963; Bull, 1962; Duvoisin and Yahr, 1965;

Steckel, 1965; Jannetta et al., 1966; Sutton, 1971; Sharr and Kelvin, 1973; Michael, 1974; see Table in Tulleken, 1976; Drake, 1979; Amacher et al., 1981; Spincemaille et al., 1985). Such patients may develop vestibular nystagmus as well as various unilateral and bilateral cranial neuropathies. The trigeminal, abducens, facial, vestibulocochlear, and glossopharyngeal nerves are most commonly damaged, but even the oculomotor nerve may be affected by an aneurysm located near the terminal bifurcation of the artery (Case Records of the Massachusetts General Hospital, 1959). Horizontal gaze paresis may result from damage to the abducens nuclei or the pontine paramedian reticular formation, whereas vertical gaze paresis may result from damage to the mesencephalon, and an INO also may occur (Rad and Piscol, 1971; Tulleken, 1976; Steinberger et al., 1984; Spincemaille et al., 1985; Kumabe et al., 1990). Hemiparesis and hemisensory loss are common in such patients (Goto et al., 1993).

Not all patients with unruptured symptomatic basilar aneurysm have multiple neurologic deficits. **Dementia** is the only finding in some patients with aneurysms arising from

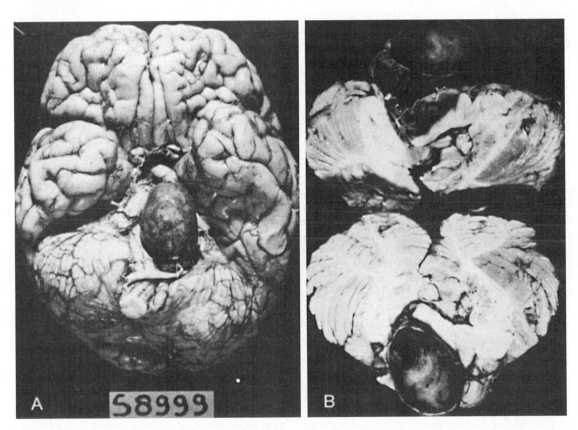

Figure 53.170. Brainstem compression by a giant saccular aneurysm arising from the basilar artery. The patient initially developed an unsteady gait, dysarthria, and intermittent vomiting. He subsequently developed a left abducens and facial nerve paresis, diminished corneal reflex, and progressive somnolence. His condition deteriorated over the next 6 months. He developed a complete left horizontal gaze palsy, marked dysarthria, and dysphagia. Sensation was diminished for all modalities on the right side of the body except for the face, and there was slight hyperreflexia of the right extremities. Neuroimaging studies suggested a posterior fossa tumor compressing the pons and medulla. The patient underwent a suboccipital craniectomy, at which time a giant, partially thrombosed aneurysm arising from the basilar artery was found. No treatment was possible, and the operation was terminated. The patient died 10 days later. *A*, View of the base of the brain shows a giant aneurysm that arises from the basilar artery. The lesion compresses the medulla and pons and displaces them to the right. *B*, Section through the aneurysm and adjacent brain shows almost total destruction of the brainstem. (From Tulleken CAF. Giant aneurysms of the posterior fossa presenting as space occupying lesions. Clin Neurol Neurosurg *79*:161–186, 1976.)

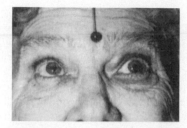
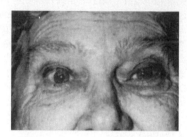
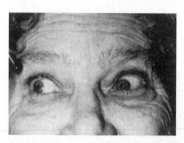
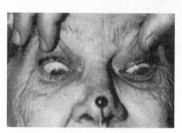

the origin of the basilar artery and projecting into the 3rd ventricle (Sutton, 1952; Bull, 1969; Sutton, 1971). Hydrocephalus from compression of the 3rd ventricle plays a role in the production of the dementia in some of these patients, but in others, hydrocephalus is absent or minimal, and the etiology of the dementia is unclear.

Michael (1974) described a patient with a basilar aneurysm who developed an **isolated abducens paresis** that persisted for 1 year before other symptoms and signs led to the correct diagnosis. The paresis resolved after treatment of the aneurysm. Hedera and Friedland (1993) reported a 36-year-old patient with Duane's retraction syndrome (see Chapter 28) who developed a giant aneurysm at the vertebrobasilar artery junction. The authors suggested a possible etiologic connection.

An **isolated oculomotor nerve palsy** may be caused by an unruptured basilar artery aneurysm, particularly one that arises near the origin of the superior cerebellar artery (SCA). Walsh and Hoyt (1969m) described a patient who experienced retrobulbar headache and then developed an ipsilateral dilated pupil without ptosis or ophthalmoparesis. The pupillary dilation was the only neurologic abnormality for 2 weeks. The patient then experienced recurrent headaches and developed other signs of an oculomotor nerve paresis. Angiography revealed an aneurysm at the junction of the basilar and superior cerebellar arteries. In other patients with saccular aneurysms of the basilar artery, an isolated complete or incomplete oculomotor nerve paresis is the first sign of the aneurysm (Trobe et al., 1978b; Guy et al., 1985; Boccardo et al., 1986; Guy and Day, 1989; Batjer and Purdy, 1990). The patients reported by Guy and co-workers (Guy et al., 1985; Guy and Day, 1989) had isolated involvement of the **superior division** of the oculomotor nerve (Figs. 53.171 and 53.172). With large basilar tip aneurysms, evidence of midbrain dysfunction may accompany ophthalmoplegia. An 82-year-old woman with a basilar tip aneurysm that had previously ruptured developed an oculomotor nerve palsy associated with contralateral weakness (Weber's syndrome) (Fukudome et al., 1994). Oculomotor nerve disturbances are common following surgery for basilar tip aneurysms. Such abnormalities result from damage to perforating vessels during surgery (dissection, clipping, or both) or from vasospasm (Goto et al., 1993). The oculomotor nerve dysfunction may be unilateral or bilateral. Recovery of oculomotor nerve function is variable in such cases. Some patients recover completely within several weeks; others experience neurologic recovery that may or may not be associated with aberrant regeneration of the oculomotor nerve (secondary oculomotor nerve synkinesis). Others show no recovery at all. Slavin and Einberg (1996) described a patient who developed a delayed-onset abduction defect associated with co-contraction of the ipsilateral medial and lateral rectus muscles on attempted abduction after surgery to clip a basilar tip aneurysm. The authors postulated that this unusual ocular movement disorder was caused by a secondary synkinesis between the oculomotor and abducens nerves.

Lustbader and Miller (1988) reported a patient in whom a painless, pupil-sparing but otherwise complete oculomotor nerve paresis was the only sign of an aneurysm arising from

Figure 53.171. Isolated superior division oculomotor nerve paresis in a patient with an aneurysm of the terminal bifurcation of the basilar artery. The patient was a 72-year-old woman with left temporal headaches and progressive vertical diplopia for over 2 years. The patient has a paresis of the superior division of the left oculomotor nerve. She has a mild left ptosis and limitation of upgaze of the left eye; however, she has normal adduction and depression of the left eye and her pupils are equal and normally reactive to light. (From Guy JR, Day AL. Intracranial aneurysms with superior division paresis of the oculomotor nerve. Ophthalmology 96:1071–1076, 1989.)

the basilar artery. The patient was a 65-year-old woman with hypertension who presented to the Wilmer Eye Institute of the Johns Hopkins Hospital with a 1-month history of complete ptosis of the right eye. She absolutely denied any headache, and she had no pain or discomfort in the right orbital region. When first examined, the patient had a complete right oculomotor nerve paresis, characterized by absent adduction, elevation, and depression of the right eye and a complete right ptosis (Fig. 53.173). The right eye abducted fully, and there was intorsion of the eye when the patient attempted to look down and to the right, indicating normal function of

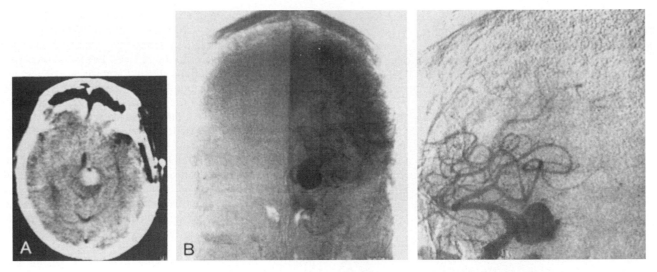

Figure 56.172. Neuroimaging studies obtained on the patient whose appearance is seen in Figure 53.171. *A*, CT scan shows an enhancing mass lesion in the region of the ventral mesencephalon. *B*, Left vertebral angiogram shows an aneurysm arising from the terminal bifurcation of the basilar artery in anteroposterior (*left*) and lateral (*right*) views. (From Guy J, Savino PJ, Schatz NJ, et al. Superior division paresis of the oculomotor nerve. Ophthalmology *96*:1071–1076, 1989.)

the ipsilateral abducens and trochlear nerves, respectively. Both pupils measured 3 mm in diameter in light and 5 mm in darkness, and both constricted briskly to light stimulation. The remainder of the ocular examination was normal. Edrophonium chloride (Tensilon) (10 mg) was injected intravenously without improvement in ptosis or extraocular muscle function. Topical 10% cocaine was placed in both eyes and produced equal dilation of both pupils. An erythrocyte sedimentation rate was normal, and a glucose tolerance test also gave normal results. A diagnosis of presumed vasculopathic oculomotor nerve paresis was made, and it was elected to observe the patient at regular intervals. One month later (2 months after the onset of ptosis), the examination findings were unchanged, and the patient continued to deny headache,

pain, or periorbital discomfort, but a CT scan that was performed because the condition had not improved revealed a bilobed mass in the region of the junction of the basilar and posterior cerebral arteries (Fig. 53.174). Cerebral angiography subsequently disclosed an aneurysm originating from the tip of the basilar artery and projecting toward the right side (Fig. 53.175).

One or both trochlear nerves may be damaged by a basilar tip aneurysm or its surgery. In most cases, trochlear nerve dysfunction is associated with unilateral or bilateral oculomotor nerve palsies, and the diagnosis of superior oblique weakness may be difficult unless the significance of absent torsion on attempted downgaze is appreciated. Trochlear nerve function may or may not eventually recover. If it does

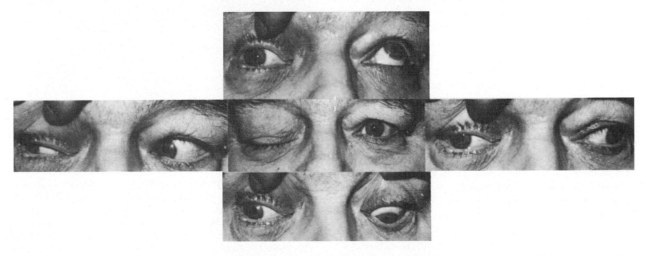

Figure 53.173. Complete, pupil-sparing oculomotor nerve paresis in a 65-year-old woman who denied ocular or orbital pain. (From Lustbader JM, Miller NR. Painless, pupil-sparing but otherwise complete oculomotor nerve paresis caused by basilar artery aneurysm. Arch Ophthalmol *106*:583–584, 1988.)

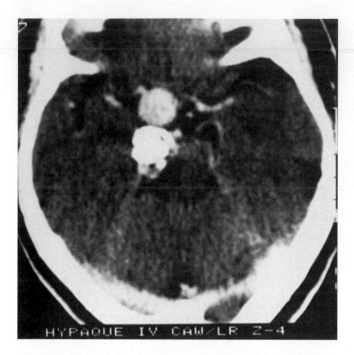

Figure 53.174. CT scan performed in the patient whose appearance is seen in Figure 53.173 shows a bilobed mass. One lobe of the mass enhances after contrast material is given intravenously. The other lobe has the characteristics of calcium. (From Lustbader JM, Miller NR. Painless, pupil-sparing but otherwise complete oculomotor nerve paresis caused by basilar artery aneurysm. Arch Ophthalmol *106*:583–584, 1988.)

rysm ''half the size of a pea'' on the left side of the basilar artery. No treatment was given. Sutton (1971) described a 53-year-old woman with systemic hypertension who experienced sudden deafness in the left ear, left facial weakness, and ataxia. These deficits did not improve over the next several months. Four months later, she developed acute diplopia and weakness of the left arm. The patient was subsequently found to have a large basilar aneurysm.

Acute neurologic deficits that occur in patients with giant aneurysms may result from emboli that arise within the aneurysm (Calopa et al., 1990), from an intracranial ''steal'' phenomenon, or from extension of an aneurysmal thrombus (Steinberger et al., 1984). Whether or not these symptoms and signs are permanent depends on their precise cause and the extent of collateral flow to the damaged area of the brain.

Visual loss occasionally may occur in patients with an unruptured basilar artery aneurysm, although it is much more common in patients with aneurysms arising from the internal carotid, anterior cerebral, and anterior communicating arteries (see above). Patients who develop hydrocephalus from obstruction of the 3rd ventricle by a basilar aneurysm may become blind from postpapilledema optic atrophy (Jefferson, 1953). In other patients, a basilar aneurysm, usually one arising from the terminal bifurcation, extends forward and upward beneath the floor of the 3rd ventricle to compress the optic chiasm and produce a chiasmal syndrome characterized by bitemporal field defects and variable loss of visual acuity and color perception

not do so, surgery, prism therapy, or both may be used to correct residual torsion or vertical misalignment.

Neurologic symptoms and signs caused by an unruptured basilar aneurysm may occasionally be acute and either transient or permanent. When the symptoms and signs are transient, they mimic typical TIAs that occur in patients with atherosclerotic cerebrovascular occlusive disease (see Chapter 55). Salde (1934) described a 42-year-old man who experienced three episodes of transient right hemiparesis. Each episode lasted about 10 minutes, and all three episodes occurred over a 1-month period. A complete neurologic examination was normal except for right hyperreflexia. A pneumoencephalogram was interpreted as showing a tumor of the pons, but cerebral arteriography revealed a giant saccular aneurysm arising from the mid-portion of the basilar artery. Two patients with similar transient neurologic deficits thought to have been caused by a saccular aneurysm located at the vertebrobasilar junction were described by Steinberger et al. (1984).

Patients with a basilar aneurysm may develop acute, permanent neurologic deficits. Höök et al. (1963) described a 37-year-old man who experienced attacks of right-sided head pain radiating toward the right eye. A neurologic examination showed only a right homonymous hemianopia. The patient was thought to have had a stroke, and no further evaluation was performed. About 9 months later, however, the patient experienced a transient confusional state that lasted 24 hours. An evaluation at that time disclosed an aneu-

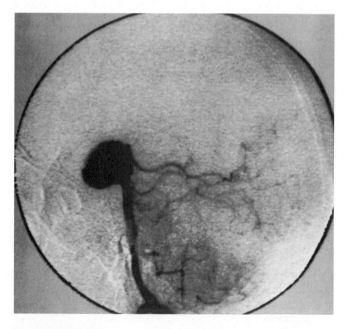

Figure 53.175. Vertebral angiogram, lateral view, in the patient whose appearance is seen in igure 53.173 and whose CT scan is shown in Figure 53.174. The angiogram shows a large aneurysm arising from the terminal bifurcation of the basilar artery. The aneurysm projects inferiorly and anteriorly, presumably compressing the right oculomotor nerve. (From Lustbader JM, Miller NR. Painless, pupil-sparing but otherwise complete oculomotor nerve paresis caused by basilar artery aneurysm. Arch Ophthalmol *106*: 583–584, 1988.)

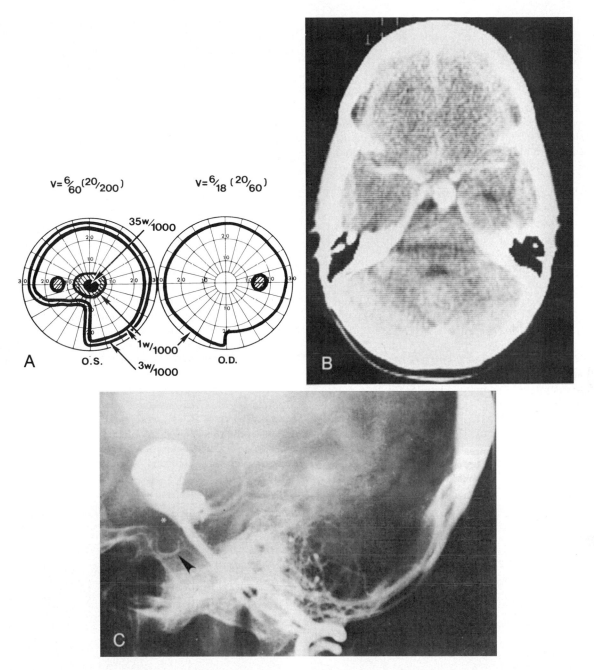

Figure 53.176. Optic chiasmal syndrome from a basilar aneurysm. The patient was a 10-year-old boy with a 4-month history of occipital headaches and blurred vision. Visual acuity was 20/60 OD and 20/200 OS. There was reduced color vision in both eyes. There was no relative afferent pupillary defect. Ophthalmoscopy was said to be normal. *A,* Visual fields show an inferior bitemporal defect combined with a dense central scotoma in the left eye. *B,* Axial computed tomographic scan after intravenous injection of iodinated contrast material shows a well-circumscribed, enhancing lesion in the posterior suprasellar region. The lesion measures about 2 cm in diameter. *C,* Vertebral angiogram, lateral view, shows a giant, bilobed aneurysm arising from the terminal bifurcation of the basilar artery. The aneurysm extends anterosuperiorly into the suprasellar region (*asterisk*). Note the location of the sella turcica (*arrowhead*). The patient's visual field defect improved after the aneurysm was clipped. (From Rush JA, Balis GA, Drake CG. Bitemporal hemianopsia in basilar artery aneurysm. J Clin Neuroophthalmol *1*:129–133, 1981.)

(Jefferson, 1937, 1953; Walsh, 1964; Sutton, 1971; Drake, 1979; Rush et al., 1981) (Fig. 53.176). Höök et al. (1963) described a patient in whom an unruptured aneurysm arose from the segment of the basilar artery between the origins of the superior cerebellar and posterior cerebral arteries.

The patient had pain around the right eye, a complete right homonymous hemianopia, and episodes of confusion with visuospatial disorientation (peduncular hallucinosis; see Chapter 9). The symptoms and signs in this patient probably resulted from interruption of the blood supply to the dominant posterior parietal cortex and compression of the cerebral peduncle by the aneurysm.

Basilar artery aneurysms occasionally compress the temporal lobe. Patients in whom this occurs may experience seizures (Amacher et al., 1981). When the lower brainstem is compressed, other symptoms may result from direct compression or associated ischemia. De Mattos et al. (1992) described a 70-year-old man with atherosclerosis who developed palatal myoclonus and was found to have a giant basilar artery aneurysm. The role of the aneurysm in the development of his symptoms remains unclear.

ANEURYSMS ARISING FROM THE ANTERIOR INFERIOR CEREBELLAR ARTERY

Aneurysms arising from the peripheral portion of the AICA are rare (Kline and Johnson, 1984; Fukuya et al., 1987; Kaech et al., 1987; Chen, 1990; Honda et al., 1994; Spallone et al., 1995; Yokoyama et al., 1995). In an unusual case, meningitis related to neurocysticercosis was accompanied by an aneurysm of the distal AICA (Soto-Hernandez et al., 1996). The surrounding inflammatory reaction suggested a possible etiologic role.

Nearly all aneurysms of the distal portion of the AICA arise from the arterial loops near the internal acoustic meatus. Patients with unruptured aneurysms at this site may therefore complain of symptoms similar to those caused by neoplasms in the CPA (e.g., vestibular schwannoma or meningioma) (see Chapters 40 and 44). Such patients may experience unilateral hearing loss (Rinehart et al., 1992), vertigo, tinnitus, and facial weakness that may be acute or slowly progressive (Fox, 1983; Nishimoto et al., 1983; Dailey et

al., 1986; Fukuya et al., 1987; Honda et al., 1994; Kamiya et al., 1994; Spallone et al., 1995) (Fig. 53.177). Abducens nerve paresis occasionally may occur. Lower cranial nerve dysfunction may also occur but is more commonly caused by trauma at the time of surgery (Yokoyama et al., 1995). Hearing loss is frequently permanent and facial weakness may worsen after clipping of the aneurysm (Chen, 1990).

ANEURYSMS ARISING FROM THE SUPERIOR CEREBELLAR ARTERY

Aneurysms that arise from the SCA are more common than those arising from the AICA but less common than those arising from the PICA. Most SCA aneurysms arise from the central portion of the artery (Kawaguti et al., 1995), but they may also arise more distally (Matricali and Seminara, 1986; Kubota et al., 1994; Milner et al., 1994; Nakahara et al., 1994); even from a vermian branch (Vassilakis et al., 1993). McDermott and Sellar (1994) reported three cases of SCA aneurysms associated with an AVM fed in part by the involved SCA. In one patient, the aneurysm spontaneously thrombosed following thrombosis of the malformation. A previous case was reported by Mabuchi et al. (1992). Other purportedly etiologic associations have been published. A 1.5-cm distal SCA aneurysm was found in a neonate who presented with seizures following birth trauma (Piatt and Clunie, 1992), Kawamata et al. (1991) found a SCA aneurysm in one of their three patients with SLE, and a mycotic aneurysm was seen in a patient with endocarditis (Hojer et al., 1993). Quattrocchi et al. (1990) reported the case of an adult with a traumatic SCA aneurysm.

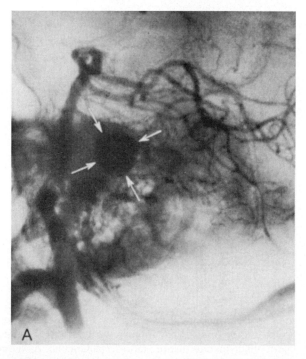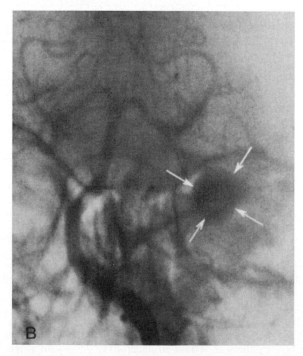

Figure 53.177. Aneurysm of the anterior inferior cerebellar artery (AICA). The patient was a 69-year-old man with progressive deafness, tinnitus, and right facial pain. A cerebral angiogram shows a large aneurysm of the right AICA at the internal auditory meatus (*arrows*). *A*, Lateral view; *B*, Anteroposterior view. (From Krayenbühl HA, Yaşargil MG. Cerebral Angiography. Philadelphia, JB Lippincott, 1968.)

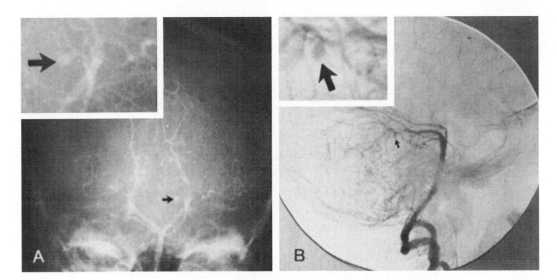

Figure 53.178. Aneurysm of the peripheral portion of the superior cerebellar artery (SCA). The patient was a 13-year-old girl who experienced an acute subarachnoid hemorrhage, following which she became comatose. She later developed ocular bobbing. Angiography disclosed an aneurysm of the left SCA. The patient underwent craniotomy at which time the aneurysm sac was adherent to the pons, and there was a small hematoma within the pons. The aneurysm was trapped, and the patient subsequently made a slow recovery. *A,* Vertebral angiogram, lateral view, shows a small saccular aneurysm of the peripheral portion of the left SCA (*arrow*). *B,* Lateral view of the aneurysm (*arrow*). *Insets* show magnified views of the area of the aneurysm. (From Sherman DG, Salmon JH. Ocular bobbing with superior cerebellar artery aneurysm: Case report. J Neurosurg *47:*596–598, 1977.)

Patients with an SCA aneurysm usually do not become symptomatic until the aneurysm ruptures, at which time they often develop signs of mesencephalic or pontine dysfunction in the setting of SAH (Lapresle and Said, 1977; Sherman and Salmon, 1977) (Figs. 53.178 and 53.179). Terson's syndrome occurs in some cases (Takeuchi et al., 1997). Harada et al. (1991) described peduncular hallucinosis, presumably caused by vasospasm, in a patient who experienced rupture of an SCA aneurysm. Unruptured aneurysms occasionally may produce oculomotor nerve paresis or other evidence of mesencephalic dysfunction (Vincent and Zimmerman, 1980; Guy and Day, 1989). Trochlear nerve palsies may occur in patients with SCA aneurysms (Agostinis et al., 1992; Collins et al. 1992). In the case reported by Collins et al. (1992), the trochlear nerve palsy resolved after clipping of an SCA aneurysm that was found at surgery to be adherent to and compressing the trochlear nerve.

ANEURYSMS ARISING FROM THE POSTERIOR CEREBRAL ARTERY

Aneurysms that arise from the PCA rather than from the terminal bifurcation of the basilar artery are rare (Drake and Amacher, 1969; Pia and Fontana, 1977; Chang et al., 1986; Simpson and Parker, 1986; Fukushima, 1988; Sevrain et al., 1990; Kumar et al., 1991; Putty et al., 1990–1991; Branley et al., 1992; Gerber and Neil-Dwyer, 1992; Scholten et al., 1992; Strobel et al., 1992; Yamashita et al., 1992; Sakata et al., 1993; Milner et al., 1994; Orita et al., 1994; Yacubian et al., 1994; Byrne et al., 1995b; Kawaguti et al., 1995; Kurihara et al., 1995; Pereira et al., 1995; Ferrante et al., 1996; Huang et al., 1996) (Figs. 53.180 and 53.181). Not a single example was found among 290 aneurysms reviewed by Krayenbühl and Yaşargil (1958). Even in the extensive

autopsy study performed by McDonald and Korb (1939), PCA aneurysms were seen in only 3% of cases. Gerber and Neil-Dwyer (1992) accumulated a surgical series of 15 cases, and Sakata et al. (1993) reported their experience with 11 cases. Two cases of traumatic pseudoaneurysms of the PCA were published in 1994. In one, a nail caused a direct injury to the PCA (Rezai et al., 1994); in the other, the pseudoaneurysm was ascribed to damage to the PCA from the edge of the tentorium cerebelli following blunt trauma (Casey and Moore, 1994). Mycotic aneurysms occasionally arise from the distal PCA (Barami and Ko, 1994), and Orita et al. (1992) reported a 73-year-old woman with SLE who experienced rupture of a PCA aneurysm.

As is the case with other saccular intracranial aneurysms, PCA aneurysms usually become symptomatic when they rupture (see Table 4 in Pia and Fontana, 1977). The resulting subarachnoid and intracranial hemorrhage is often catastrophic and may be associated with rapid neurologic deterioration and death (Pia and Fontana, 1977; Scott et al., 1988). PCA aneurysms may not be recognized until autopsy (Branley et al., 1992).

An unruptured PCA aneurysm may be asymptomatic and discovered by chance (Pia and Fontana, 1977), or it may produce a variety of different symptoms and signs depending on the size, location, and direction of projection of the aneurysm. Unruptured symptomatic PCA aneurysms tend to be larger, present earlier, and have a higher incidence of mass effect than aneurysms arising from other vessels (Ferrante et al. 1996). The only symptom in some patients is nonspecific headache (Amacher et al., 1981). Kaplan and Hahn (1984) described two children in whom persistent headaches were the only evidence of a PCA aneurysm. In one patient, the headaches were triggered by sudden movement of the head,

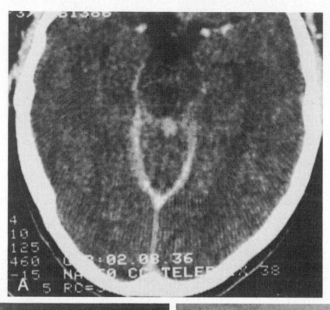

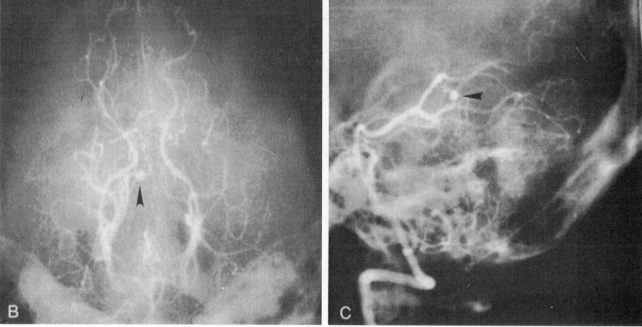

Figure 53.179. Aneurysm of the superior cerebellar artery (SCA). The patient was a 45-year-old woman with a history of headaches. Neurologic examination was normal except for a stiff neck. *A*, Axial computed tomographic scan after intravenous injection of iodinated contrast material shows a small enhancing lesion in the ambient cistern just to the right of the culmen of the cerebellum. *B*, Vertebral angiogram, anteroposterior view, shows an aneurysm (*arrowhead*) arising either from a branch of the right posterior cerebral artery (PCA) or from the right SCA. *C*, Vertebral angiogram, oblique view, shows that the aneurysm arises from the peripheral segment of the right SCA between the branches of the PCA (*arrowhead*). The aneurysm was clipped, and the patient recovered uneventfully. (From Matricali B, Seminara P. Aneurysm arising from the medial branch of the superior cerebellar artery. Neurosurgery *18*:350–352, 1986.)

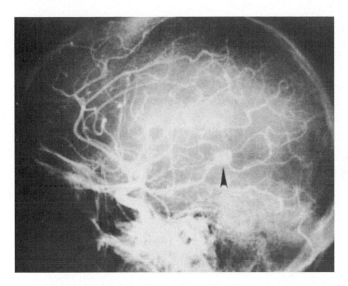

Figure 53.180. Aneurysm of the posterior cerebral artery (PCA). The patient was a 14-year-old girl who experienced an acute subarachnoid hemorrhage. The cerebral angiogram shows an aneurysm of the P-3 segment of the left PCA (*arrowhead*). Note that the PCA arises directly from the left internal carotid artery (fetal configuration). (From Simpson RK Jr, Parker WD. Distal posterior cerebral artery aneurysm: Case report. J Neurosurg 64:669–672, 1986.)

were located in the parieto-occipital region, and lasted less than 1 hour. The second patient had midfrontal headaches that seemed to be triggered by stress and excitement, were alleviated by resting, and had recently increased in frequency and duration.

Some PCA aneurysms become large enough to produce increased ICP (Fig. 53.182). In such patients, visual loss from bilateral optic neuropathy may result. Obrador et al. (1967) described a 20-year-old girl with a 2-year history of abnormal sensations of smell and a 1-year history of progressive, bilateral visual loss. The patient's neurologic examination was normal except for slight loss of tone in the left arm. Visual acuity was hand motions in each eye, and bilateral optic atrophy was present. The patient was found to have increased ICP caused by a giant aneurysm originating from the right PCA, which arose directly from the right ICA through a dilated posterior communicating artery. The aneurysm displaced the ventricular system to the left and produced a filling defect in the posterior portion of the 3rd ventricle. The aneurysm was completely removed without any major complications. The patient's only residual neurologic defect was astereognosis in the left hand, but her visual acuity did not improve after surgery.

Höök et al. (1963) found no visual field defects in five patients with unruptured PCA aneurysms, although Pool and Potts (1965) hypothesized that unruptured PCA aneurysms should occasionally cause contralateral homonymous field defects resulting from impaired circulation to the visual cortex. Although Pool and Potts (1965) were unaware of any instances in which an unruptured PCA aneurysm produced a homonymous hemianopia, it is clear that such a phenomenon does occur. Hanafee and Jannetta (1966) described one pa-

tient in whom an unruptured PCA aneurysm caused an acute homonymous hemianopia. The patient initially was thought to have had a stroke from the effects of atherosclerotic cerebrovascular disease. A similar patient was described by Mochimatsu et al. (1987). The patient was a 36-year-old woman who experienced the sudden onset of headache, nausea, and numbness of the left side of the body. She was slightly confused, and she had neck stiffness, left-sided hemiparesis, hemihypesthesia, and homonymous hemianopia. Neuroimaging studies revealed a large, partially thrombosed, unruptured aneurysm arising from the distal portion of the right PCA at the origin of the right posterior temporal artery. A right homonymous hemianopia also was present in a 69-year-old woman who developed severe aphasia from a giant saccular aneurysm arising from the basilar segment of the left PCA (Belec et al., 1988).

Because of the proximity of the initial segment of the PCA to the mesencephalon, the oculomotor nerve, and the trochlear nerve, unruptured PCA aneurysms may produce symptoms and signs caused by compressive or ischemic damage to these structures. Hyland and Barnett (1953) described a patient who developed left-sided headaches and a left oculomotor nerve paresis. Six weeks later, he became drowsy and developed a right hemiplegia. He then deteriorated rapidly and died. Postmortem examination revealed a large, recently thrombosed aneurysm arising from the left PCA. The aneurysm compressed the mesencephalon, left thalamus, and left oculomotor nerve. There had been no gross rupture of the aneurysm, but considerable blood had leaked into adjacent tissue. A somewhat similar case was reported by Hanafee and Jannetta (1966), who described a patient with an acute oculomotor nerve paresis associated with a contralateral hemiplegia (Weber's syndrome). The patient was thought to have had a hypertensive or atherosclerotic stroke until angiography revealed a large PCA aneurysm that compressed the ventral surface of the mesencephalon. Kerns et al. (1979) described a patient who developed an acute right oculomotor nerve paresis associated with a severe retrobulbar headache and who was found to have a mild left hemiparesis. The patient had a large aneurysm with a broad origin from the left PCA at its junction with the left posterior communicating artery. The aneurysm was found at craniotomy to be compressing the right cerebral peduncle and the right oculomotor nerve as it emerged from the brainstem. A similar patient was described by Huang et al. (1996). The patient was a 2-year-old child who presented with seizures and then developed an oculomotor nerve paresis and an **ipsilateral** hemiparesis caused by compression of the contralateral cerebral peduncle by a large PCA aneurysm.

Drake and Amacher (1969) described eight patients with PCA aneurysms. One of the patients was a 52-year-old woman who experienced left orbital and temple pain and simultaneous diplopia. She was found to have an incomplete, left oculomotor nerve paresis. Angiography revealed a saccular aneurysm arising from the left PCA near its junction with the posterior communicating artery. The patient refused operation, and she eventually experienced complete recovery of oculomotor nerve function. Over the next 6 years, she developed no new neurologic symptoms or signs.

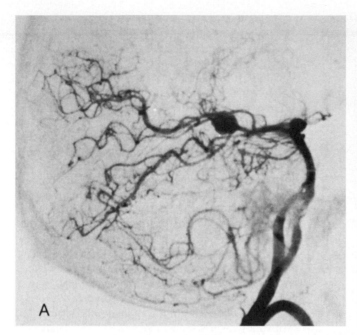
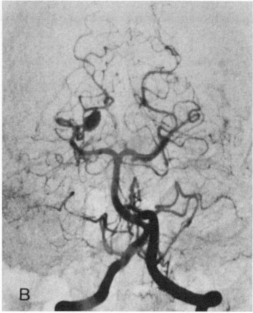

Figure 53.181.   Aneurysm of the posterior cerebral artery (PCA). The aneurysm arises from the perimesencephalic segment of the right PCA. *A,* Lateral view; *B,* Anteroposterior view. (From Huber P. Cerebral Angiography, 2nd ed. New York, Georg Thieme Verlag, 1982.)

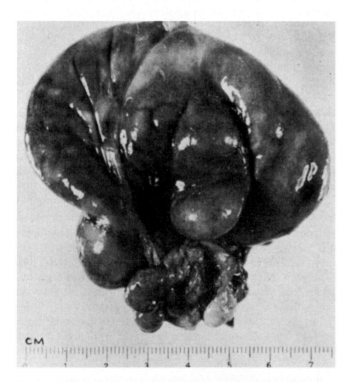

Figure 53.182.   Giant aneurysm of the posterior cerebral artery in a 20-year-old woman with progressive loss of vision in both eyes and bilateral optic atrophy. A cerebral angiogram demonstrated a giant aneurysm arising from the distal portion of the right posterior cerebral artery. The artery was occluded with an aneurysm clip, and the aneurysm was excised. (From Obrador S, Dierssen G, Hernandez JR. Giant aneurysm of the posterior cerebral artery: Case report. J Neurosurg *26:*413–416, 1967.)

Acute onset of ophthalmoplegia in a patient with a PCA aneurysm may indicate aneurysmal thrombosis. Griffiths et al. (1994) reported a patient who developed an acute painful oculomotor nerve palsy 2 days after angiography revealed a P-1 segment aneurysm. CT scan demonstrated a clot in the aneurysm and follow up angiography at 6 months revealed complete thrombosis of the aneurysm. It is possible, however, for a PCA aneurysm to thrombose without producing any symptoms (Kumar et al., 1991).

Neurologic dysfunction caused by a PCA aneurysm is not always related to damage to the brainstem or the proximal portions of the cranial nerves. Coppeto and Hoffman (1981) described a 75-year-old man who developed a cavernous sinus syndrome caused by an unruptured PCA aneurysm. The patient developed left retrobulbar and temple pain that was continuous for 1 month. It resolved spontaneously but recurred 1 month later, this time accompanied by diplopia and drooping of the left upper eyelid. Examination at this time revealed normal visual sensory function in both eyes. The right eye moved fully in all directions, and the right pupil had normal responses to light and near stimuli. The left eye could not elevate, adduct, or depress, and it showed no torsion on attempted down and left gaze. The left pupil was smaller than the right and was nonreactive. It showed evidence of sympathetic denervation by pharmacologic testing. There was partial left ptosis associated with mild swelling and a prominent venous pattern on the left upper eyelid. Left proptosis of 3.5 mm was measured. The patient was thought to have a left "Tolosa-Hunt syndrome," and he was treated with oral corticosteroids with prompt improvement in pain. Six months later, however, he began to experience unsteadiness of gait. He not only had ophthalmoparesis but also showed aberrant regeneration of the oculomotor nerve.

A vertebral angiogram revealed a large aneurysm arising from the left PCA. The aneurysm compressed the left side of the mesencephalon, shifted the brainstem toward the right, and extended forward to compress the posterior portion of the left cavernous sinus.

Seizures, which may be motor or sensory, occasionally occur in patients with a PCA aneurysm (Obrador et al., 1967; Amacher et al., 1981; Ley-Valle et al., 1983; Putty et al., 1990–1991; Yacubian et al., 1994). Even infants may be affected in this manner (Putty et al., 1990–1991). The patient described by Obrador et al. (1967) complained of episodes in which she would experience an abnormal sensation of smell. At surgery, there was marked compression of the right temporal lobe by a PCA aneurysm. A patient described by Ley-Valle et al. (1983) had a 2-year history of ''petit mal'' seizures and was found to have a giant, calcified, PCA aneurysm compressing the left temporal lobe. A 30-year-old man with an 18-year history of complex partial seizures was found to have a partially thrombosed giant aneurysm of the right PCA (Yacubian et al., 1994). Selective amygdalohippocampectomy and occlusion of the PCA abolished the seizures without inducing any neurologic or visual deficits.

SUMMARY OF NEURO-OPHTHALMOLOGIC SIGNS OF UNRUPTURED INTRACRANIAL SACCULAR ANEURYSMS

Neuro-ophthalmologic signs are among the most important focal neurologic manifestations of unruptured intracranial saccular aneurysms. It must be remembered, however, that aneurysms that become symptomatic because of direct interference with the function of adjacent neural and vascular structures are much less common than are aneurysms that become symptomatic when they rupture. About 90% of intracranial aneurysms become symptomatic when they bleed into the subarachnoid space or into the substance of the brain (Locksley, 1969; Fox, 1983; Weir, 1987). Because acute enlargement leading to mass effect may be associated with limited rupture, it is not always possible to separate aneurysms on this basis.

Local mass effect may compromise the afferent visual pathways—the optic nerves (Fig. 53.139), optic chiasm (Figs. 53.85, 53.87–53.89, 53.120, 53.149), optic tracts (Figs. 53.120 and 53.121), lateral geniculate bodies, retrogeniculate optic radiations, and occipital cortex—producing decreased vision, visual field defects, or both. In a retrospective series of 132 unruptured aneurysms by Raps et al. (1993), visual acuity loss (10 patients) was more common than oculomotor nerve palsies (two patients). In most series, however, aneurysms more often affect the ocular motor nerves, causing ocular misalignment and limitation of movement and producing diplopia. The majority of intracranial aneurysms that produce focal neuro-ophthalmologic signs arise from the junction of the internal carotid and posterior communicating arteries (Figs. 53.111–53.118). These are the aneurysms that most often compress or otherwise damage the oculomotor nerve in the subarachnoid space. It is a moot point to determine if these are truly unruptured aneurysms, as local expansion from limited rupture may precede the onset of symptoms.

Involvement of the trochlear and abducens nerves is most common in the cavernous sinus, where associated involvement of the trigeminal nerve may present as pain or numbness (Figs. 53.67–53.73 and 53.75). Isolated atypical facial pain unassociated with SAH is probably more frequently associated with a dolichoectatic basilar artery (Okada et al., 1994). Posterior fossa aneurysms can exceptionally produce isolated numbness (Zager, 1991). Less commonly there is involvement of the intra-axial brainstem structures responsible for organizing eye movements, leading to gaze palsies, nystagmus, or skew deviation.

Adnexal abnormalities can occur rarely from local orbital effects but occasionally related to other cranial nerve dysfunction, particularly the facial nerve. Less specific symptoms include headache, which almost universally accompanies rupture but which may also occur with unruptured aneurysms (Raps et al., 1993).

Oculomotor Nerve Paresis

Paresis of the oculomotor nerve is the hallmark of the internal carotid-posterior communicating artery aneurysm (Figs. 53.113–53.117), although it also may be caused by intracavernous (Figs. 53.74–53.76, 53.83, and 53.84), terminal carotid (Fig. 53.135), basilar (Figs. 53.171–53.175), superior cerebellar, and posterior cerebral artery aneurysms. The patient typically presents with: (a) severe, unilateral, frontal headache; (b) ptosis; (c) limited elevation, depression, and adduction of the eye; and (d) a dilated, nonreactive or poorly reactive pupil. Onset may take 2–3 days and may occur a week or more following SAH (Harris and Udvarhelyi, 1957). Absence of an affected pupil in the setting of a **complete** acute oculomotor nerve paresis almost always excludes a diagnosis of aneurysm (see, however, Lustbader and Miller, 1988). Truly isolated ptosis is only rarely caused by an aneurysm (Good, 1990) as is isolated pupillary paralysis. The absence of pain is unusual, but it does not exclude the diagnosis of aneurysm. Unfortunately, the frequency, character, and duration of the pain does not help separate microvascular from aneurysmal oculomotor nerve palsies (Capo et al., 1992; Renowden et al., 1993). Transient oculomotor nerve dysfunction related to an aneurysm is also possible (Greenspan and Reeves, 1990). As noted above, when an oculomotor nerve paresis occurs in the setting of minor head trauma, an evaluation for an underlying aneurysm or other intracranial lesion is mandatory (Walter et al., 1994).

The most difficult clinical situation relates to the patient with an acute incomplete oculomotor nerve palsy. If the pupil is involved, a thorough workup for a possible aneurysm is always appropriate, whether or not there is associated pain. If the pupil is not involved, however, the appropriate management is somewhat controversial. In our opinion, it depends on whether or not the oculomotor nerve paresis is otherwise complete or incomplete. If the oculomotor nerve paresis is incomplete, an aneurysm is possible, and a workup is appropriate; however, it is uncommon for a complete pupil-sparing oculomotor nerve palsy to be secondary to an aneu-

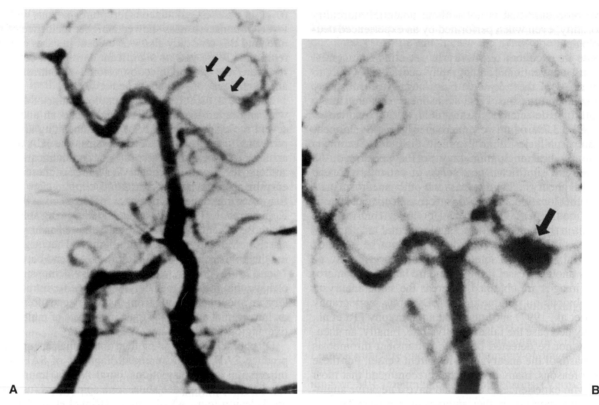

Figure 53.184.   Angiographic appearance of a ruptured intracranial aneurysm that initially could not be detected because of vasospasm after a subarachnoid hemorrhage. The patient was a 23-year-old right-handed man with a 2-week history of severe continuous left-sided throbbing headache. He had a mild right hemiparesis and dense right homonymous hemianopsia. A computed tomographic scan demonstrated a 1-cm high-density lesion in the left anterior perimesencephalic cistern and magnetic resonance imaging confirmed an acutely thrombosed 1-cm posterior cerebral artery aneurysm. *A,* Selective left vertebral angiogram obtained initially shows segmental vasospasm (*arrows*) but no opacification of the aneurysm. *B,* Left vertebral artery angiogram obtained 3 months later demonstrates a 1-cm fusiform aneurysm (*arrow*) with distal opacification of the left posterior cerebral artery. No neck was appreciated. Vasospasm acutely hid the aneurysm. With follow-up, however, the aneurysm was appreciated. (From Atkinson JL, Lane JI, Colbassani HJ, et al. Spontaneous thrombosis of posterior cerebral artery aneurysm with angiographic reappearance: Case report. J Neurosurg *79:*434–437, 1993.)

et al., 1991a), this complication usually occurs only when all of the perimesencephalic cisterns are filled with blood (Rinkel et al., 1992). A case of a basilar aneurysm simulating nonaneurysmal perimesencephalic SAH was reported by Friedman (1996).

MR imaging is a very sensitive way to identify a clot within the wall of a blood vessel. Therefore, for dissecting aneurysms as well as those containing clot, MR imaging may be a very sensitive tool. Artifact induced by iophendylate (Pantopaque) within the basal cisterns may be mistaken for clot within an aneurysm (Lidov et al., 1996). Moving blood creates a dark area on MR imaging—**the flow void**. Large aneurysms may thus be recognized on standard-sequence MR imaging scanning with accurate determination of size and luminal characteristics (Kurihara et al., 1995). Although standard-sequences MR imaging is relatively insensitive to acute hemorrhage and is limited in its maximum resolution, specialized MR sequences can be used to recognize acute hemorrhage. In 20 patients with proven acute SAH, fluid-attenuated inversion recovery (FLAIR) sequences demonstrated the SAH as well as CT scanning without any false-positive results in a matched control group (Noguchi et al., 1995).

Any ferromagnetic material results in significant image

distortion on MR imaging. Although aneurysm clips were once made of such material, most neurosurgeons use nonferromagnetic clips, especially titanium or silver clips, which produce the least MR distortion (Piepgras et al., 1995; Kato et al., 1996a; Ooker et al., 1996). Nevertheless, even clips said to be nonferromagnetic may contain some ferromagnetic material (Kanal et al., 1996), and a ferromagnetic clip placed in the field of an MR imaging machine may experience significant torque, resulting in potentially disasterous consequences. Klucznik et al. (1993), for example, reported a patient who developed a fatal intracerebral hemorrhage while undergoing MR imaging. Postmortem examination in this patient revealed that the hemorrhage resulted from a tear in the MCA adjacent to a torqued ferromagnetic clip. Embolization coils do not produce a significant MR artifact (Hartman et al., 1997).

Virtual reconstruction of the major intracranial vessels based on flowing blood is possible with dynamic MR sequences—MR angiography (Chong et al., 1994; Kaufman et al., 1995). These images are of two types that are generated in two different ways: phase-contrast (PC) and time-of-flight (TOF). Both techniques have advantages and disadvantages (Huston et al., 1991). The major weaknesses are the relatively poor resolution in PC MR angiograms and the lack

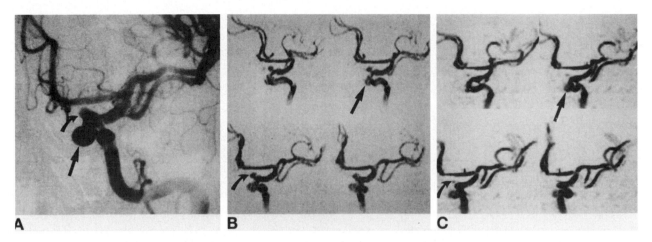

Figure 53.185. Comparison of conventional angiography with time-of-flight (TOF) and phase-contrast (PC) magnetic resonance (MR) angiography in detecting intracranial aneurysms. *A*, Conventional left internal carotid angiogram, oblique view, shows a 7-mm left carotid siphon aneurysm (*straight arrow*) and a 3-mm ophthalmic artery aneurysm (*curved arrow*). *B*, TOF MR angiogram; *C*, PC MR angiogram. The 7-mm carotid siphon aneurysm was detected with both TOF (*straight arrow in B*) and PC (*straight arrow in C*) angiography. The 3-mm ophthalmic aneurysm was not initially recognized on either TOF or PC angiography, although it can be identified in retrospect on both sequences (*curved arrows in B and C*). The small ophthalmic artery aneurysm was displayed better with the 512-TOF than with the PC technique (From Huston J 3rd, Nichols DA, Luetmer PH, et al. Blinded prospective evaluation of sensitivity of MR angiography to known intracranial aneurysms: Importance of aneurysm size. AJNR *15*:1607–1614, 1994.)

of recognition of slowly flowing blood in TOF studies (Fig. 53.185). Ikawa et al. (1994) compared PC and TOF MR angiography in detection of 27 intracerebral aneurysms confirmed by conventional angiography. Sensitivity was 70.4% with the PC method and 92.6% with the TOF method. Huston et al. (1994) also concluded that TOF MR angiography is more sensitive than PC angiography or standard MR imaging for detection of aneurysms. Araki et al. (1994) failed to identify with PC MR angiography three aneurysms that were seen using the TOF method (Fig. 53.186). The technique of

overlapping segments (MOTSA) further improves the sensitivity of TOF MR angiography (Blatter et al., 1992), as does increasing the magnetic field strength (Korogi et al., 1997).

Because of its noninvasive nature, MR angiography offers a major advantage in screening for aneurysms (Ross et al., 1990; Sevick et al., 1990; Gouliamos et al., 1992; Schuierer et al., 1992; Huston et al., 1993; Harrison et al., 1997; Tateiwa et al., 1997) and other vascular lesions (Awad et al., 1992; Yoshimoto et al., 1997). The sensitivity and specificity in the diagnosis of aneurysms, including internal carotid-pos-

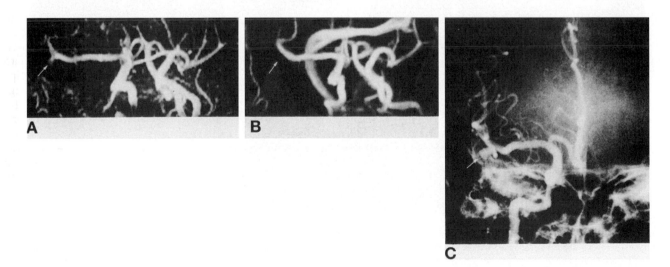

Figure 53.186. Comparison of ability of time-of-flight (TOF) and phase-contrast (PC) magnetic resonance (MR) angiographic techniques to detect intracranial aneurysms. *A*, Projection image of 3-D TOF MR angiogram from a 63-year-old woman admitted because of acute loss of consciousness demonstrates an unruptured aneurysm at the trifurcation of the right middle cerebral artery (*arrow*). *B*, Projection image of 3-D PC MR angiogram with velocity encoded value of 45 cm/sec viewed from the same direction as *A* does not show the aneurysm (*arrow*). *C*, Conventional cerebral angiogram shows the aneurysm at the trifurcation on the right middle cerebral artery (*arrow*) (From Araki Y, Kohmura E, Tsukaguchi I. A pitfall in detection of intracranial unruptured aneurysms on three-dimensional phase-contrast MR angiography. AJNR *15*:1618–1623, 1994.)

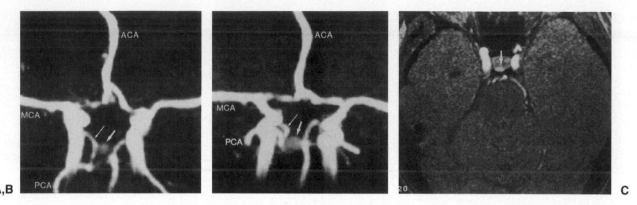

Figure 53.187. Pituitary gland causing artifact mimicking intracranial aneurysm on magnetic resonance (MR) angiography. *A* and *B*, On both of two 3-D time-of-flight MR angiographic images taken in slightly different planes, the circle of Willis shows a circular area of intermediate signal intensity (*large arrows*) which is intimately associated with the right posterior communicating artery (*small arrows*). The appearance of the signal suggests an aneurysm. *C*, Standard axial MR image, however, demonstrates that the apparent aneurysm is actually a partial signal arising from the pituitary gland. (From Uberoi R, Murphy P, Jones A. The "pituitary pseudoaneurysm" artefact with 3D TOF MRA of the circle of Willis. J Comput Assist Tomogr *19*:822–823, 1995.)

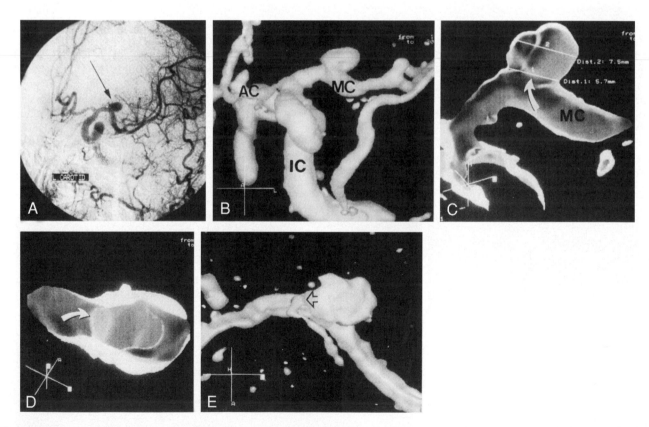

Figure 53.188. Three-dimensional reconstructions of an intracranial aneurysm from magnetic resonance imaging data. *A*, Left middle cerebral artery aneurysm (*arrow*) is depicted in an anterior/posterior digital subtraction angiogram. *B–D*, 3-D display phase-contrast MR angiograms depict the aneurysmal sac and its orifice (*arrow in C and D*), which are measured in anterior and posterior views in *B* and *C* and from beneath in *D*. *E*, A 3-D display, time-of-flight MR angiogram depicts a vascular branch (*arrow*) that originates from the aneurysmal sac. Many artifacts are related to background noise. *AC,* anterior cerebral artery; *IC,* internal carotid artery; *MC,* middle cerebral artery (From Bontozoglou NP, Spanos H, Lasjaunias P, et al. Intracranial aneurysms: Endovascular evaluation with three-dimensional-display MR angiography. Radiology *197*:876–879, 1995.)

terior communicating aneurysms that cause an oculomotor nerve paresis, is generally good compared with conventional angiography (Tomsak et al., 1991; Harrison et al., 1997). As noted above, Ikawa et al. (1994) reported a sensitivity of 92.4% using TOF MR angiography in 27 patients with intracranial aneurysms confirmed using conventional angiography. Wilcock et al. (1996) compared TOF MR angiography with conventional angiography in 39 patients with SAH. Ten patients had no aneurysm by either method. The remaining 29 patients had 37 aneurysms. Using conventional angiography as the gold standard, Wilcock et al. (1996) calculated the sensitivity of TOF MR angiography for the detection of aneurysms to be 81% and specificity to be 100% but cautioned that all available imaging data must be considered. In a similar study from Germany, Falk et al. (1996) detected 33 of 38 aneurysms with diameters ranging from 3 to 50mm in diameter in 30 patients. From Japan, Horikoshi et al. (1994) reported a sensitivity of 79% and a specificity of 92% using TOF angiography. The technique was less sensitive in the region of the carotid siphon, where only 60% of the aneurysms could be detected. Korogi et al. (1994) noted a much greater sensitivity of TOF MR angiography for aneurysms on the anterior or middle cerebral artery than for aneurysms arising from the proximal intradural segment of the ICA. In this area, the pituitary gland may produce a false-positive study (Uberoi et al., 1995) (Fig. 53.187). Bosmans et al. (1995) applied additional sequences to initially negative TOF studies and demonstrated aneurysms in 13 of 14 angiographically proven cases. Atlas et al. (1997) estimated that 95% of aneurysms greater than 3 mm in size can be detected by MR angiography. Although movement artifact can degrade the images (Sankhla et al., 1996), images can be improved by using band-limited interpolation (Du et al., 1994) and including the source images (Korogi et al., 1996). Three-dimensional reconstructions can be made from MR angiographic data, producing a virtual vascular endoscopic picture (Bontozoglou et al., 1995; Maeder et al., 1996) (Fig. 53.188).

Despite the high sensitivity and specificity of aneurysm detection using MR angiography, false-positive and false-negative results still are not uncommon (Fig. 53.189). False-

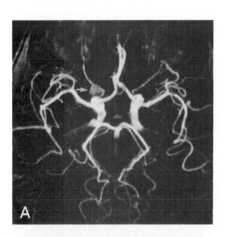
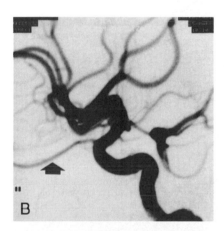
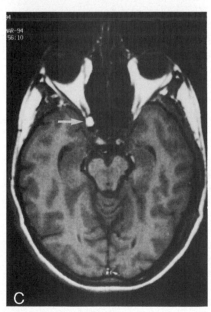
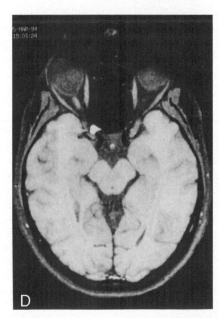

Figure 53.189. False-positivity of magnetic resonance (MR) angiography in detecting intracranial aneurysms. *A*, MR angiogram of a 33-year-old woman who presented with retrobulbar pain appears to demonstrate a 6-mm aneurysm arising from a right ophthalmic artery (*arrow*). *B*, Digital subtraction intra-arterial angiography demonstrates no lesion (*arrow indicates the ophthalmic artery*). *C*, Standard T1-weighted axial MR image demonstrates a lesion with high-signal intensity (*arrow*) within the right optic canal. *D*, Fat-suppressed T1-weighted spin-echo axial MR image confirms a lesion within the optic canal above the optic nerve. The lesion was thought to be a thrombosed varix. (From Wilcock DJ, Jaspan T, Worthington BS. Comparison of magnetic resonance angiography with conventional angiography in the detection of intracranial aneurysms in patients presenting with subarachnoid hemorrhage. Clin Radiol *50*: 526–532, 1995.)

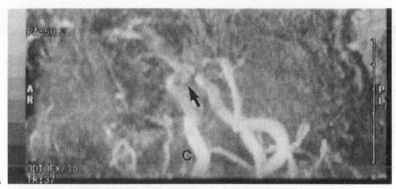

A

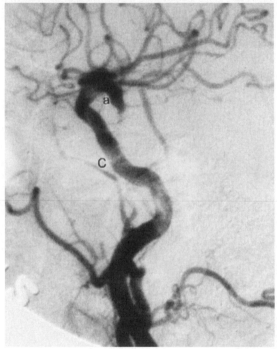

B

Figure 53.190. False-negativity of magnetic resonance (MR) angiography in a patient with a ruptured intracranial aneurysm. The patient was a 76-year-old woman who presented with progressive diplopia and retrobulbar pain. She had 2 mm of right ptosis and a right pupil that was larger than the left and sluggishly reactive. There was limitation in elevation, adduction and depression on the right side. An aneurysm was suspected, and the patient initially underwent MR angiography. *A*, 3-D time-of-flight MR angiogram shows no definite lesion. *Arrow* points to area of the approximate origin of the posterior communicating artery from the internal carotid artery (*C*). *B*, Subtraction angiogram demonstrates a 10-mm aneurysm (*a*) arising from origin of the right posterior communicating artery from the right internal carotid artery (*C*). (From Weinberg DA. Negative MRI versus real disease. Surv Ophthalmol *40*:312–319, 1996.)

positive results can be caused by subacute thrombus and high-signal structures, which may masquerade as vascular abnormalities. Nevertheless, the false-positive rate for MR angiography is sufficiently low that in rare settings, usually related to allergy to iodinated contrast material or severe renal disease, surgery is undertaken on the basis of the MR angiography alone (Parenti et al., 1995).

False-negative MR angiographic results constitute a more significant problem. In particular, small aneurysms may not be appreciated because of the limits of resolution of MR angiography. In one prospective study, aneurysms less than 5 mm could not reliably be detected with an acceptable sensitivity using TOF MR angiography (Huston et al., 1994). Although such aneurysms have a lower likelihood of hemorrhage, they are not immune to rupture (N. Yasui et al., 1996; Ortiz et al., 1997). Felber et al. (1995) reported that TOF MR angiography failed to detect three aneurysms that were 3 mm or less in diameter, one of which subsequently ruptured. Indeed, it is not unusual for MR angiography to give negative results prior to rupture of a small aneurysm (Keane and Ahmadi, 1991; Vanninen et al., 1996; Weinberg, 1996) (Fig. 53.190). In addition, interpretation of reconstructions can also

be difficult or impossible when there is a sizeable hematoma, local susceptibility artifacts from aneurysm clips or coils may also reduce the signal from vascular structures (Wilcock et al., 1995), and even large aneurysms may not be detected because of loss of signal from saturation effects or dephasing related to slow or complex flow. Turtz et al. (1995) reported an 11-mm pericallosal aneurysm that was not detected with TOF MR angiography (Fig. 53.191). Thus, one cannot cannot rely on MR angiography, regardless of the technique that is used, to exclude an intracranial aneurysm (Puskar and Ruggieri, 1995). In the appropriate setting, it may be necessary to perform conventional angiography in order to feel confident that an aneurysm has been eliminated from consideration. Once an aneurysm is identified, however, MR angiography can be used to follow it or to assess its status after treatment (Sevick et al., 1990; Harrison et al., 1997).

MR angiography can be used not only to detect and follow an intracranial aneurysm but also to determine the patency of the circle of Willis, an important consideration in determining the management of patients with intracranial aneurysms. In a study performed by Patrux et al. (1994), the sensitivity of MR angiography was 89.2% for the anterior

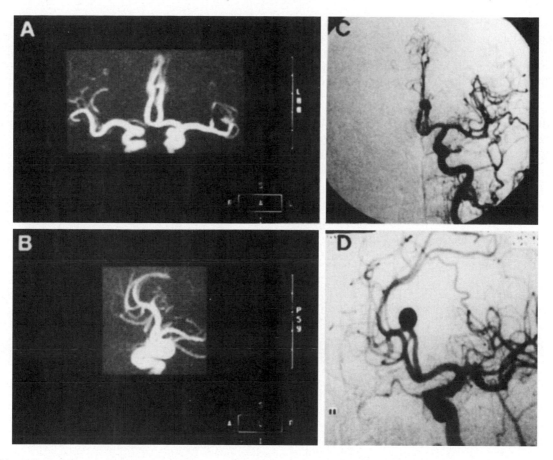

Figure 53.191. Failure of phase-contrast (PC) magnetic resonance (MR) angiography to demonstrate an intracranial aneurysm in an elderly woman with vertigo. *A* and *B*, Lateral 3-dimensional PC MR angiographic images show no evidence of the large pericallosal artery aneurysm seen in conventional angiographic images (*C* and *D*).(From Turtz A, Allen D, Koenigsberg R, et al. Nonvisualization of a large cerebral aneurysm despite high-resolution magnetic resonance angiography: Case report. J Neurosurg *82*:294–295, 1995.)

communicating artery, 81.3% for the posterior communicating arteries, and 100% for the anterior, middle, and posterior cerebral arteries.

As noted above, the sensitivity of CT scanning to acute hemorrhage makes it the most popular initial diagnostic procedure in identifying SAH. It also may be helpful in identifying which of several aneurysms on angiography is responsible for the bleed. Occasionally, however, adhesions and obliteration of the subarachnoid cisterns from a previous hemorrhage alters the direction of hemorrhage, resulting in a hematoma that is located at a distance from the ruptured aneurysm (Lee et al., 1996). In addition, when an aneurysm ruptures medially, a hematoma may occur on the side contralateral to the aneurysm, resulting in inaccurate lateralization of the causative aneurysm. This may have disasterous consequences in patients with multiple aneurysms or in patients in whom a limited angiogram is performed. It is also important to remember that conventional CT scanning cannot always distinguish giant aneurysms from vascular tumors. This is particularly important in the sellar region, where an aneurysm may masquerade as a pituitary tumor and vice versa (Kayath et al., 1991; Barontini et al., 1994).

Dynamic acquisition of CT data offers the potential for

reconstruction of the intracranial vascular pathways (Anderson et al., 1997; Blumke and Fishman, 1994; Hope et al., 1996; Hsiang et al., 1996; Kalender et al., 1994; Ogawa et al., 1996; Rieger et al., 1996; Wilms et al., 1996). Spiral (also called helical or dynamic) CT angiography offers the additional advantage of multiplanar presentation with three-dimensional capability (Dietrich et al., 1995) and simultaneous representation of the bony landmarks of the cranium and skull base (Aoki et al., 1992). Resolution of spiral CT angiography is at least equivalent to MR angiography and is probably even better, particularly when narrow collimation is used (Kallmes et al., 1996).

Alberico et al. (1995) reported that CT angiography showed 23 of 24 aneurysms and two of two AVMs (sensitivity, 96%; specificity, 100%). The size of the aneurysms ranged from 2 to 40 mm (mean, 7.9 mm). In a similar prospective study of 23 patients suspected of harboring an aneurysm, CT angiography diagnosed 15 of 17 aneurysms in 14 of 15 patients (Liang et al., 1995). Using conventional angiography as the reference standard, CT angiography gave one false-positive and two false-negative findings, resulting in a sensitivity of 88% (14 of 15 patients with aneurysms correctly diagnosed) for aneurysms as small as 2 mm and a specificity of 89% (eight of nine patients without an aneurysm correctly diagnosed). Tanabe et al. (1995) compared the ability of CT angiography and MR angiography to detect 67 aneurysms identified by conventional angiography in 11 patients with SAH and 30 patients without SAH (i.e., with unruptured aneurysms). CT angiography detected all 67 aneurysms, including several that were smaller than 2 mm in diameter. MR angiography did not have the same sensitivity, and Tanabe et al. (1995) thus concluded that CT angiography is superior to MR angiography in detecting intracranial aneu-

rysms. In another study, Tsuchiya et al. (1994) compared the sensitivity of CT angiography with that of MR angiography in patients with 17 intracranial aneurysms detected by conventional angiography. These investigators found that seven of the aneurysms were better delineated with CT angiography than with MR angiography (Fig. 53.192), both techniques demonstrated five aneurysms equally well, and MR angiography delineated three aneurysms better than CT angiography. Both techniques failed to detect two very small aneurysms.

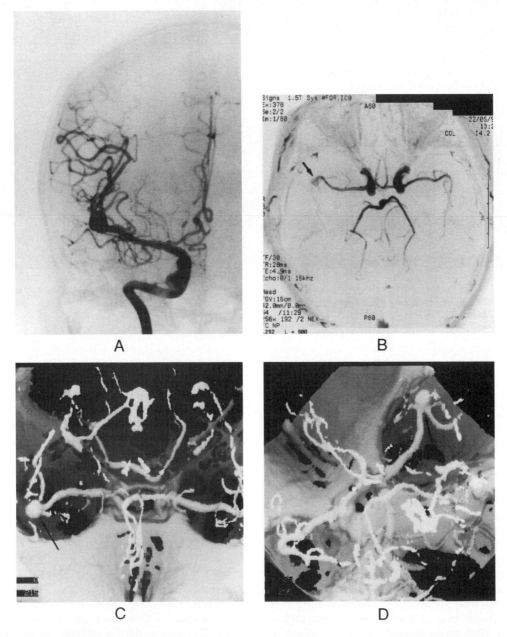

Figure 53.192. Comparison of ability of magnetic resonance (MR) angiography and spiral computed tomographic (CT) angiography to identify a right middle cerebral artery aneurysm in a 77-year-old woman. *A*, Right internal carotid artery angiogram demonstrates a middle cerebral artery aneurysm. *B*, Axial 3-D time-of-flight MR angiogram depicts the aneurysm (*arrow*); however, note signal loss from saturation effects in the aneurysm and the distal middle cerebral artery branches. *C*, Spiral CT angiogram, anterior-superior view clearly demonstrates the aneurysm (*arrow*), and *D*, spiral CT angiogram, left posterior-superior view, clearly shows its neck (*arrow*). (From Tsuchiya K, Makita K, Furui S. 3D-CT angiography of cerebral aneurysms with spiral scanning: Comparison with 3D time-of-flight MR angiography. Radiat Med *12*:161–166, 1994.)

Like MR angiography, spiral CT angiography has limitations of resolution. As noted above, Tsuchiya et al. (1994) reported that both spiral CT angiography and MR angiography failed to detect two small aneurysms (among 17 total aneurysms) that were detected by conventional angiography. Schwartz et al. (1994) found neither MR angiography nor spiral CT angiography to be sensitive to aneurysms smaller than 3 mm, and Tampieri et al. (1995) found that spiral CT angiography failed to detect 50% of aneurysms smaller than 3 mm that were detected with conventional angiography. On the other hand, spiral CT angiography was employed in a series of 32 patients with oculomotor nerve palsies (Teasdale et al., 1990). A total of 17 aneurysms were detected in 13 patients. All aneurysms detected with conventional angiography were also identified by spiral CT angiography, suggesting that spiral CT angiography is a sensitive method of screening patients with acute oculomotor nerve pareses in whom an aneurysm is considered a possible etiology. According to Dr. Robert McFadzean, one of the co-authors of the study by Teasdale et al. (1990), a subsequent long-term follow-up study of patients with acute oculomotor nerve pareses confirmed the sensitivity of spiral CT angiography in the detection of aneurysms that produce acute oculomotor nerve pareses. Dissecting aneurysms can also be detected using this technique (Soper et al., 1995).

There are no major disadvantages to performing spiral CT angiography except for the necessity of injecting iodinated contrast material, to which some patients are allergic. Acquisition times are less than standard CT scanning (Wilms et al., 1995). Thus, exposure to radiation is minimal, and the studies are relatively insensitive to movement artifact. Another advantage of spiral CT angiography is that it is less expensive than either MR angiography or digital subtraction angiography (Harbaugh et al., 1995; Harrison et al., 1997).

The mutiplanar capacity of spiral CT angiography as well as the bone definition that is possible with CT technology combine to make spiral CT angiography ideal for planning a surgical approach (Harbaugh et al., 1995; Kato et al., 1995; Tampieri et al., 1995). Thus, in selected cases, spiral CT angiography is sufficient for preoperative evaluation (Alberico et al., 1995), and surgery may be performed without conventional angiography (Rusyniak et al., 1992; Harrison et al., 1997). Le Roux et al. (1993) operated on 25 patients with aneurysmal SAH complicated by intracerebral hemorrhage on the basis of spiral CT angiography alone. In all patients, the preoperative Glasgow Coma Scale score was less than 5, and brainstem compression was evident. An intracerebral hematoma was present in the frontal or temporal lobe and was often associated with intraventricular hemorrhage (17 patients) and significant (>1 cm) midline shift (18 patients). Spiral CT angiography correctly identified the ruptured aneurysm in all patients. The aneurysm arose from the MCA in 18 patients, the posterior communicating artery in two patients, the terminal carotid bifurcation in three patients, and the anterior communicating artery in two patients. All patients underwent conventional angiography after surgery to confirm aneurysm obliteration, at which time 11 unruptured aneurysms were identified, nine of which (82%) had been detected with spiral CT angiography. Although this sensitivity is quite good, it is still possible that basing surgery on the results of spiral CT angiography alone may result in

the failure to detect other incidental aneurysms that might be amenable to clipping at the time of the initial craniotomy (Le Roux et al., 1993). An additional cautionary note was voiced by Nagasawa et al. (1995), who found that spiral CT angiography had difficulty in recognizing aneurysms in the paraclinoid region. There is also a learning curve in assessing the results of spiral CT angiography as there is in most studies that rely on interpretation of images. Significant interobserver differences were found in a study performed by Vieco et al. (1995) of 30 aneurysms in 22 patients. One observer had a sensitivity of 97% and a specificity of 100%, whereas the other observer had a sensitivity of 77% and a specificity of 87%.

Spiral CT angiography has potential uses other than those described above. For example, it can be used to localize lesions for stereotactic surgery (Elowiz et al., 1995). On the basis of our experience and despite the limitations described above, we agree with those authors who predict that this technique will eventually be the preferred method of following patients after aneurysm surgery (Ahmadi et al., 1993; Dorsch et al., 1995; Harrison et al., 1997) and the optimum method of screening patients at high risk for the development of de novo aneurysms (familial aneurysms, polycystic kidney disease, etc.) (Chapman et al., 1992; Schievink, 1997b) (Figs. 53.193–53.195).

A number of noninvasive techniques can be used to aid in the diagnosis of aneurysms, although none is as sensitive as either spiral CT angiography or MR angiography. For example, color Doppler flow imaging detected 30 of 33 aneurysms in 35 patients evaluated by Wardlaw and Cannon (1996). However, Klotzsch et al. (1996) were able to detect only 27–47% of aneurysms with color Doppler imaging. Thus, the future of this technique in identifying aneurysms is unclear, although it may be an effective way to monitor their status after treatment (Wardlow et al., 1996).

NATURAL HISTORY

In order to determine the appropriate treatment for a patient with an unruptured symptomatic or asymptomatic aneurysm, one must know the risk of rupture of the aneurysm as well as the morbidity and mortality of such an initial rupture. Similarly, treatment of a patient with a ruptured, intracranial, saccular aneurysm must be based on the risk and complications of a second hemorrhage from that aneurysm.

Natural History of Unruptured Saccular Aneurysms

Unruptured, intracranial, saccular aneurysms are usually discovered in one of two settings. First, an asymptomatic aneurysm may be found during an evaluation for an unrelated symptom (Zacks et al., 1980). Included in this group are unruptured aneurysms that are found when another aneurysm ruptures (about 15% of intracranial saccular aneurysms are multiple—see above). Second, an unruptured aneurysm may become symptomatic by virtue of its size, location, and effect on adjacent neural and vascular structures. Such an aneurysm may be discovered during an evaluation for focal neurologic symptoms and signs, seizures, or transient neurologic dysfunction. Unruptured aneurysms may do one of five things: (a) remain unchanged, (b) increase in size, (c) rupture, (d) thrombose, or (e) spontaneously disappear.

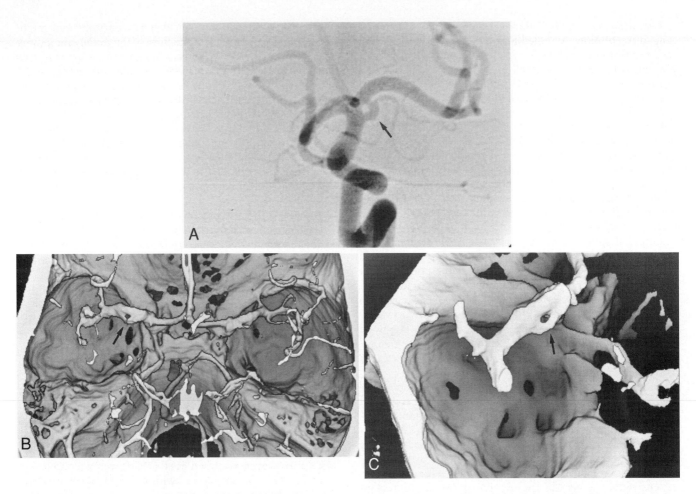

Figure 53.193.   Spiral computed tomographic (CT) angiography in a patient with a suspected intracranial aneurysm. The patient was a 51-year-old woman involved in a motor vehicle accident. MR imaging showed changes suggesting an intracranial aneurysm arising from the left middle cerebral artery (MCA). *A*, Conventional angiogram, anteroposterior view, shows a suspicious area (*arrow*) at the proximal M-1 segment of the left MCA. *B*, Spiral CT angiogram demonstrates that the abnormality (*arrow*) is actually a duplicated M-1 segment, rather than an aneurysm. *C*, An enlarged, rotated view of the spiral CT angiogram clearly shows the fenestrated M-1 segment that was initially mistaken for an aneurysm, even on conventional angiography. (Courtesy of Drs. C. Douglas Phillips and Jonas H. Goldstein.)

The risk of rupture of a previously unruptured intracranial saccular aneurysm is estimated to be 1–2% per year (McKissock et al., 1960; Heiskanen, 1981; Wiebers et al., 1981; Jane et al., 1985; Yasui et al., 1997). Wiebers et al. (1981) identified 65 patients with 81 unruptured, intracranial aneurysms; 71% of these aneurysms were asymptomatic. All patients were then followed for at least 5 years after aneurysm diagnosis or until death (mean follow-up of 98.5 months). During the follow-up period, eight of the 81 aneurysms (10%) ruptured. Wiebers et al. (1981) performed a multivariate discriminant analysis to assess the relation of several independent variables to aneurysm rupture and found that the only variable of unquestionable significance was aneurysm size. All eight ruptured aneurysms were 10 mm or more in diameter. Although this is an important statistic, it must be remembered that 60% of ruptured intracranial aneurysms are 3–10 mm in diameter, that almost 40% of ruptured aneurysms are less than 6 mm in diameter (Orz et al., 1997), and that 50% of all aneurysms that produce a

sudden fatal SAH are 6–9 mm in diameter (Weir, 1987; Inagawa and Hirano, 1990a). It is therefore inappropriate to assume that as long as an unruptured aneurysm remains less than 10 mm in diameter, it will never rupture (Solomon and Correll, 1988).

Juvela et al. (1993b) followed 142 patients with 181 unruptured aneurysms until death or SAH intervened or for at least 10 years after the unruptured aneurysm was diagnosed. The median follow-up time was 13.9 years (range 0.8–30.0 years). During 1944 patient-years of follow-up study, there were 27 first episodes of hemorrhage from a previously unruptured aneurysm, giving an average annual rupture incidence of 1.4%. Fourteen of these episodes were fatal. The cumulative rate of bleeding was 10% at 10 years, 26% at 20 years, and 32% at 30 years after the diagnosis. As in the study by Wiebers et al. (1981), the only predictor for rupture was the size of the aneurysm. Yasui et al. (1997) reported similar results.

Rupture rates are nevertheless significantly less for small

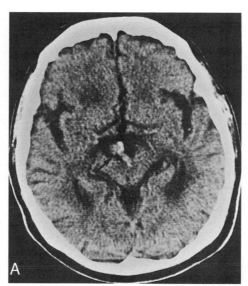

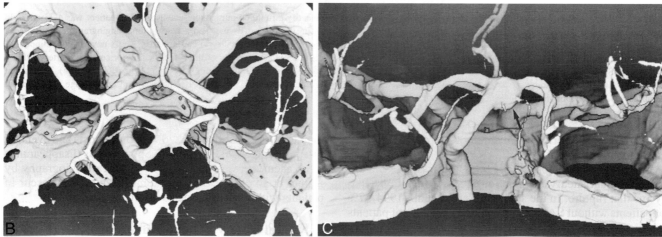

Figure 53.194. Spiral computed tomographic (CT) scanning in a 63-year-old hypertensive man with presyncope and dehydration. *A,* An axial CT scan shows an area of calcification in the region of the head of the basilar artery. The patient was considered to be a poor risk for conventional angiography; accordingly, spiral CT angiography was performed. *B* and *C,* Two different orientations on spiral CT scanning beautifully demonstrate an aneurysm at the head of the basilar artery (*arrows*). Note that the aneurysm incorporates both posterior cerebral arteries and has no neck. (Courtesy of Drs. C. Douglas Phillips and Jonas H. Goldstein.)

aneurysms than for large ones. Of 49 patients with unruptured aneurysms followed without surgical intervention, eight subsequently experienced an aneurysmal SAH (with a mortality of 88%) during a mean follow-up of 4.3 years (Mizoi et al., 1995). The mean size of the ruptured aneurysms was significantly larger than that of the unruptured aneurysms. Indeed, none of the 26 aneurysms smaller than 4 mm in diameter ruptured during the follow-up period. The incidence of rupture may also vary with location. In another study, 11 of 14 (78.6%) M-1 aneurysms greater than 5 mm in diameter ruptured, whereas only one of seven (14.3%) aneurysms whose diameter was 5 mm or less ruptured (Hosoda et al., 1995).

The increase in the incidence of rupture with increasing aneurysm size is explained by Laplace's law, which relates the circumferential tension to the systolic pressure and the radius of the aneurysm. Hademenos et al. (1994) modified Laplace's law to accommodate an expression for wall thickness and the elastic modulus for collagen. These investigators concluded that the critical size for aneurysm rupture is 4.8 mm.

It might be expected that the larger an aneurysm, the more likely it is to rupture. This is not the case. Once an aneurysm reaches a certain size, factors such as increasing thickness of the aneurysm wall as well as thrombosis and calcification within the aneurysm combine to reduce the risk of rupture. Thus, so-called "giant aneurysms" often do not rupture but rather create symptoms by local mass effect (Symon, 1992). Some giant aneurysms do bleed, however. Vargas et al. (1994) reported that of seven patients with giant aneurysms affecting the visual system who refused surgery, three eventually ruptured, one fatally. Similarly, Hamburger et al.

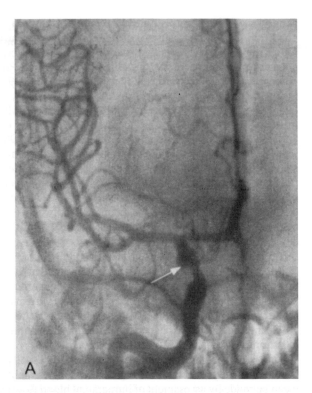 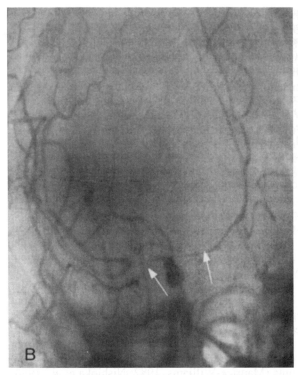

Figure 53.197. Cerebral vasospasm after subarachnoid hemorrhage from a ruptured intracranial aneurysm. *A*, Right internal carotid arteriogram, anteroposterior view, shows an unruptured aneurysm arising just proximal to the terminal bifurcation of the right internal carotid artery (*arrow*). The aneurysm subsequently ruptured. *B*, There is marked spasm of the anterior and middle cerebral arteries (*arrows*) and their branches associated with a large intracerebral hematoma.

Koike et al., 1981; Meyer et al., 1983; Mickey et al., 1984; Knuckey et al., 1985; Voldby et al., 1985a; Dernbach et al., 1988b). These changes almost certainly are caused by disturbed cerebral autoregulation at the microcirculatory level (Petruk et al., 1974; Jakubowski et al., 1982; Voldby et al., 1985a, 1985b; Dernbach et al., 1988b).

In view of the potential devastating effects of vasospasm and its frequency, attempts have been made to recognize patients at increased risk and to diagnosis it before the onset of irreversible neurologic complications. A rapid increase in flow velocities of 50 cm/s or more during a 24-hour period on transcranial Doppler seem to be a strong predictor of symptomatic vasospasm, as seven of 12 patients developed delayed ischemic deficits, five with permanent neurologic sequelae (Ekelund et al., 1996). Elevation of the flow is usually seen at the onset of vasospasm, although its presence is not necessarily diagnostic in and of itself. Meixensberg et al. (1996) identified a subgroup of patients that, despite elevation of flow velocities, did not develop neurologic deficits. He termed this phenomenon "hyperemia," and noted that the elevated flow velocities in such patients were invariably bilateral and symmetric. It should be emphasized that hypertensive patients with SAH have **low** flow velocities. Thus, even a mild elevation of velocity in these patients may indicate significant vasospasm (Ekelund et al., 1995).

The risks of developing vasospasm and subsequent fixed neurologic deficits increases with the amount of subarachnoid blood (Inagawa et al., 1995). In a study by Hirashima

et al. (1995), the total amount of subarachnoid blood on admission and on the day after operation, as determined by CT scanning, was more in the cerebral infarction group than in the noninfarction group. Patients with the greatest amount of SAH had the highest incidence of infarction. CT scanning can quantify the amount of hemorrhage (Hirashima et al., 1995), correlating with the potential for vasospasm.

Rabb et al. (1994) performed a univariate analysis of patients with aneurysmal SAH. These investigators concluded that age under 20 was a major factor associated with a higher risk of vasospasm, and that in patients with a poor outcome, the amount of SAH and the clinical grade also correlated with vasospasm.

A number of medical markers have been investigated to determine if they can be used to predict the development of vasospasm after SAH. For example, Schisano et al. (1994) found that fibrinogen degradation products in the CSF were significantly elevated in patients with severe neurologic deficits caused by delayed cerebral ischemia. Endothelin is a potent vasoconstrictor peptide thought to be related to vasospasm (Suzuki et al., 1992; Hamann et al., 1993). Shirakami et al. (1994) reported that the immunoreactivity of endothelin in both plasma and CSF rose after SAH and aneurysm clipping. It then declined but rose again in patients who developed symptomatic vasospasm. Using microdialysis techniques, Nilsson et al. (1996) and Säveland et al. (1996) detected a marked rise in extracellular levels of both glutamate and aspartate in seven patient after aneurysmal SAH.

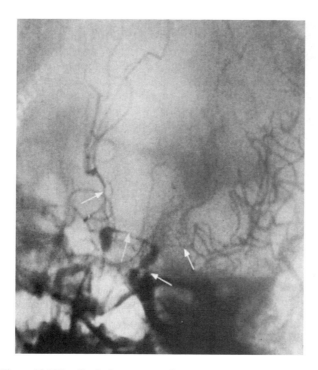

Figure 53.198. Cerebral vasospasm after aneurysmal subarachnoid hemorrhage. The patient had rupture of an anterior communicating artery aneurysm. Cerebral arteriogram, anteroposterior view, shows marked spasm of the distal portion of the internal carotid artery, the proximal portion of the middle cerebral artery, and the A-1 and A-2 portions of the anterior cerebral artery (*arrows*) associated with an intracerebral hematoma.

The levels of these amino acids correlated well with the subsequent neurologic course in all cases. The detection of free radicals in the serum, CSF, or both may also be related to the development of vasospasm (Mcdonald and Weir, 1994), but evidence for such an association is weak.

The manifestations of delayed cerebral ischemia may be focal, generalized, or both. Focal neurologic symptoms depend on the vessel involved. Hemiparesis, aphasia, and homonymous visual field defects can all occur. Three patients developed vivid visual hallucinations associated with abnormal sleep-waking rhythms, suggesting a diagnosis of peduncular hallucinosis following aneurysmal bleed (Yano et al., 1994). The hallucinations disappeared with administration of an increased dose of dobutamine, suggesting that they were a manifestation of delayed cerebral ischemia related to SAH. Generalized manifestations of delayed cerebral ischemia include seizures and alterations in mentation and consciousness.

TREATMENT AND RESULTS

The treatment of a patient with an intracranial saccular aneurysm depends on a number of factors, including the age and general condition of the patient, the size, shape, and location of the aneurysm, and whether or not the aneurysm has ruptured. A patient who has experienced SAH, intracerebral hemorrhage, or both from aneurysm rupture requires treatment different from that for a patient with an unruptured symptomatic or asymptomatic aneurysm.

Treatment of Unruptured Intracranial Saccular Aneurysms

As noted above, a patient with an unruptured intracranial saccular aneurysm has a risk of hemorrhage from that aneurysm of about 1–2% per year (McKissock et al., 1960; Weibers et al., 1981; Winn et al., 1983; Jane et al., 1985; Juvela et al., 1993b; Yasui et al., 1997). Because rupture of an aneurysm is ultimately associated with a potential 70–80% mortality and significant morbidity and because even small aneurysms have a significant risk of rupture (Orz et al., 1997), most investigators recommend definitive surgical therapy for almost all unruptured saccular aneurysms (Yasui et al., 1997). This, however, depends on the age, general health, and neurologic status of the patient and on the size and location of the aneurysm (Ausman et al., 1989; Rice et al., 1990; Linskey et al., 1991a; Leblanc and Worsely, 1995). The intraoperative and postoperative risks of surgery must thus be weighed against the cumulative risk of leaving the aneurysm untreated.

Direct Surgical Approach

Most saccular aneurysms are treated by applying a spring-action metal clip to the neck of the aneurysm using an operating microscope, microneurosurgical instruments, and anesthesia that is oriented toward the neurosurgical patient (Hollin and Decker, 1977; Drake, 1984; Weir, 1987) (Figs. 53.199–53.202) In some cases, particularly those involving giant intracranial aneurysms, complete circulatory arrest, hypothermia, and cerebral protection using barbiturates are useful adjuncts to surgery (Sundt et al., 1972; Spetzler et al., 1988; Pacult et al., 1993; Greene et al., 1994; Kato et al., 1996c). The specific surgical approach used depends on the size and location of the aneurysm and the preference of the neurosurgeon (Yaşargil and Fox, 1975; Rhoton and Perlmutter, 1980; Heros et al., 1982; Fox, 1983; MacFarlane et al., 1983; Yamada et al., 1984a, 1984b; Aoki, 1987; Archer et al., 1987; Sugita et al., 1987; Weir, 1987; Fox, 1988; Bojanowski et al., 1988; Giannotta and Maceri, 1988; Nutik, 1988a; Solomon and Stein, 1988; Vajda et al., 1988; Deruty et al., 1996).

The surgical approach to unruptured aneurysms of the basilar artery is a particular challenge (Marks, 1996; Kawase et al., 1996; Lawton et al., 1997). Several modifications of skull base approaches allow neurosurgeons to safely reach this area (Tulleken and Luiten, 1986; Sekhar et al., 1994; Day et al., 1997). These include the use of a pterional bone flap (Yamada et al., 1984a; Heros and Lee, 1993; Tanaka et al., 1995; Harland et al., 1996; Nagasawa et al., 1996), a partial petrous dissection (Harsh and Sekhar, 1992; Selfert et al., 1996), and an orbitozygomatic temporopolar en bloc section (Ikeda et al., 1991a; Day et al., 1994; Neil-Dwyer et al., 1997). An approach through the temporal horn decreases the chance of damaging the basal veins (Sakaki et al., 1995). A combined transcallosal, transventricular approach can give alternative access to the basilar apex (de los Reyes et al., 1992b). The basilar tip may also be accessed through the 3rd ventricle (Kodama et al., 1995). A transclival approach offers a direct view but has the potential for a major postoperative CSF leak (de los Reyes et al., 1992a; Ogilvy et al., 1996).

3158

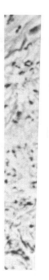

al., 1994). An aneurysm being treated with balloon occlusion can also rupture during placement of the balloon (Taki et al., 1992). Finally, aneurysms can continue to grow even when occluded with a balloon (Hirasawa et al., 1992). In an experimental study in rabbits with long-term follow-up, nine of 10 balloon-occluded aneurysms eventually recurred (Heilman et al., 1992). Vargas et al. (1994) reported neurologic complications in seven of 12 patients following endovascular balloon occlusion of giant aneurysms affecting the visual system (temporary in four patients and severe and permanent in three). Silicone balloons may have a worse record because of their low thrombogenicity (Miyachi et al., 1992b). Because of these and other complications, direct occlusion of intracranial aneurysms using detachable balloons is mainly of historical interest.

The many limitations and complications in the use of detachable balloons led to the development of **thrombogenic metallic wires or coils** that can be packed into an aneurysm cavity (Dowd et al., 1990; Guglielmi et al., 1992b; Knuckey et al., 1992; Houdart, 1996; Melisch et al., 1997; Vinuela et al., 1997) (Fig. 53.211). Some coils are simply packed into the aneurysm, gradually forming a mass within the sac. Others have a memorized shape so that although they are intro-

duced into the aneurysm as a linear wire, they immediately form pretzel, helical, or other complex shapes after they are detached into the aneurysm sac. The use of such detachable coils decreases the risk of inadvertent malposition both within the aneurysm and within the parent vessel (Graves et al., 1993). The thickness, length, and material of the coils determines the friction of the coil through the catheter and its stability once in place (Marks et al., 1996). Coil embolization can be used to treat both unruptured and ruptured aneurysms (Gurian et al., 1995b; Teitelbaum et al., 1995b; Raymond et al., 1997; Roy et al., 1997; Vinuela et al., 1997). Coils are less likely to be displaced from the aneurysm and to compromise the parent vessel when compared to balloons, but both complications are possible (Guglielmi et al., 1992b; Vázquez-Barquero et al., 1994; Spetzler et al., 1997). The use of balloons to hold the coils in place may reduce the risk of these complications (Levy et al., 1997). The ability to achieve complete occlusion of an aneurysm with detachable coils is critically dependent on the size of the aneurysm neck. Complete aneurysm thrombosis was observed in 85% of small-necked (Fig. 53.161) aneurysms but only 15% of wide-necked aneurysms (Fernandez Zubillaga et al., 1994).

Overall, the results of aneurysm occlusion with coils, par-

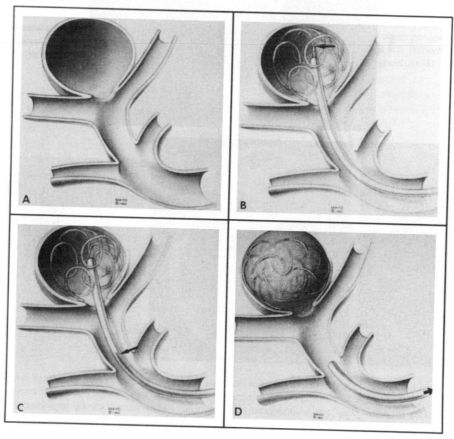

Figure 53.211. Occlusion of aneurysm with Guglielmi detachable coils. *A,* Diagram of basilar tip aneurysm before treatment. *B,* Microcatheter has been placed inside the aneurysm and first coil has been delivered inside the aneurysm but not yet detached. *Arrow* depicts junction between guide wire and coil. *C,* Coil has been detached and guide wire has been withdrawn approximately into the micro-catheter (*arrow*). *D,* Appearance of aneurysm after completion of treatment. Aneurysm is filled and excluded from intracranial circulation by combination of thrombosis and multiple coils. Microcatheter is being withdrawn from the basilar artery (*arrow*). (From Nichols DA, Meyer FB, Piepgras DG, et al. Endovascular treatment of intracranial aneurysms. Mayo Clin Proc 69:272–285, 1994.)

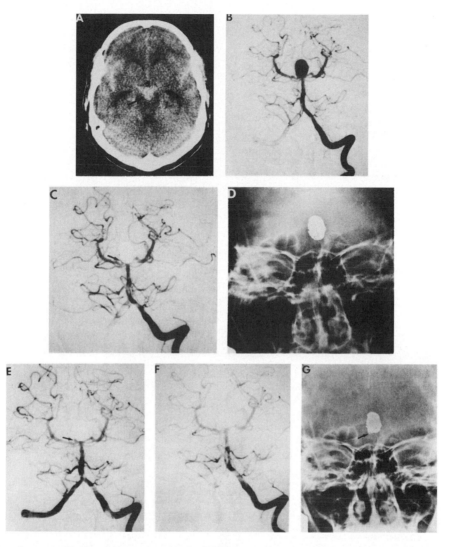

Figure 53.212. Occlusion of a ruptured basilar tip aneurysm using Guglielmi detachable coils in a 39-year-old man with sudden onset of severe headache and decreased level of consciousness. *A,* Axial computed tomographic scan demonstrates diffuse subarachnoid hemorrhage, most prominent in region of the interpeduncular cistern (*arrow*). *B,* Angiogram of the left vertebral artery, Towne view, demonstrates basilar tip aneurysm 16 mm in maximum diameter. *C,* Angiogram of left vertebral artery, Towne view, obtained immediately after treatment of aneurysm. Seven coils, a total of 180 cm in length, were detached within aneurysm. Note remaining patent portion of aneurysm (*arrow*). *D,* Plain skull radiograph, unsubtracted Towne view, demonstrates position and configuration of detached coils after initial treatment. *E,* Angiogram of left vertebral artery, Towne view, obtained 6 weeks after treatment demonstrates slight interval enlargement of aneurysmal remnants (*arrow*). *F,* Aneurysmal remnant was successfully treated by detaching a single additional coil 8 cm in length and 2 mm in diameter. *G,* Plain skull radiograph, unsubtracted Towne view, demonstrates position of additional detached coil (*arrow*). (From Nichols DA, Meyer FB, Piepgras DG, et al. Endovascular treatment of intracranial aneurysms. Mayo Clin Proc *69:*272–285, 1994.)

ticularly detachable coils, are encouraging (Vinuela et al., 1997) (Figs. 53.212 and 53.214). If the parent vessel is compromised, however, the artery may need to be occluded endovascularly (Fig. 53.214), and subsequent thrombosis and distal ischemia may produce new neurologic defects. For example, a patient reported by Guglielmi et al. (1992b) developed an homonymous hemianopia following coil embolization of a giant basilar tip aneurysm. Nevertheless, in a series of seven patients with giant unruptured aneurysms treated by placement of coils, only one patient developed a transient neurologic deficit, and none of the patients had a permanent neurologic or visual deficit (Vargas et al., 1994).

Early neuro-ophthalmologic results of endovascular surgery using detachable coils are also encouraging. Vargas et al. (1994) reported the New York University experience in 26 consecutive patients with giant aneurysms associated with visual loss. Of these patients, 21 had optic neuropathy (13 monocular and eight bilateral), and five had homonymous visual field defects caused by damage to one of the optic tracts. Embolization of the aneurysm was performed in 19 patients. Detachable balloons were used in 12 patients and Guglielmi detachable coils in seven (Figs. 53.97 and 53.215). Vision improved in seven patients, was unchanged in 11, and worsened in one patient. Of the seven patients

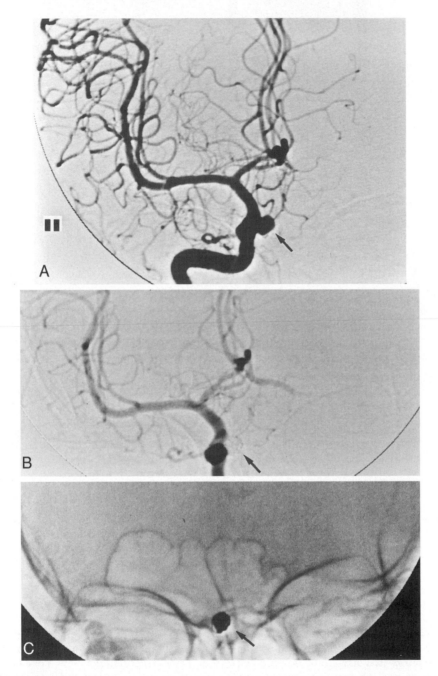

Figure 53.213. Occlusion of ruptured paraophthalmic artery aneurysm using Guglielmi detachable coils. The patient was a 66-year-old man with an acute subarachnoid hemorrhage. *A,* Right internal carotid angiogram shows medially pointing paraophthalimc artery aneurysm (*arrow*). *B,* Aneurysm has been obliterated with coils. Note patent right internal carotid artery with normal flow through both the anterior and middle cerebral arteries. *C,* Plan skull radiograph shows position of coils. (Courtesy of Dr. M. Lee Jensen.)

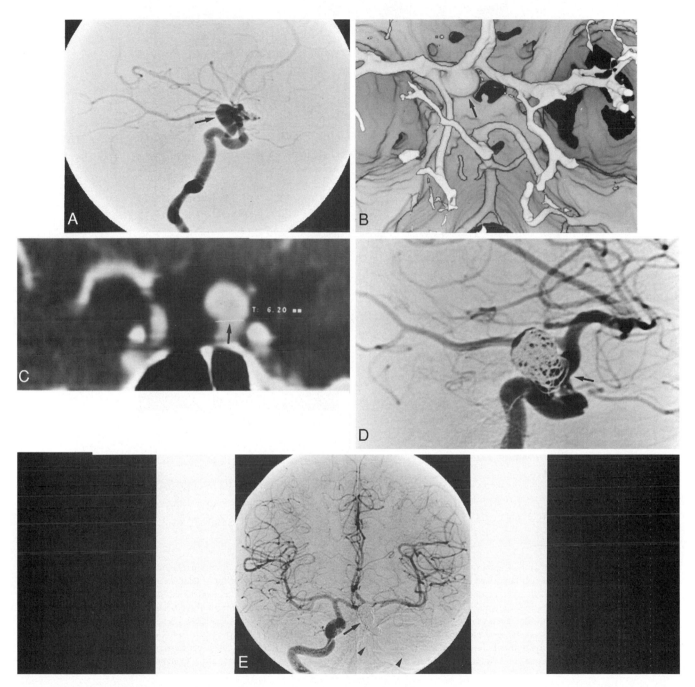

Figure 53.214. Occlusion of a distal paraophthalmic aneurysm using Guglielmi detachable coils complicated by protrusion of coils into the parent vessel. *A*, Left internal carotid angiogram shows large left paraophthalmic aneurysm. *B*, Three-dimensional spiral computed tomographic (CT) angiogram confirms position of aneurysm (*arrow*) and shows somewhat broad neck. *C*, Neck of aneurysm is measured directly using spiral CT angiographic imaging. *D*, Guglielmi detachable coils are placed into the aneurysm. Note, however, protrusion of coils into the lumen of the internal carotid artery. Because of the coil protrusion, it was elected to occlude the internal carotid artery using two proximal detachable balloons. *E*, Right internal carotid arteriogram, anteroposterior view, shows left internal carotid artery occluded by two proximal balloons (*arrowheads*). Aneurysm is completely obliterated by coils (*arrow*). Note excellent cross-filling, with right internal carotid artery filling both left anterior cerebral and middle cerebral arteries. (Courtesy of Drs. C. Douglas Phillips and Jonas H. Goldstein.)

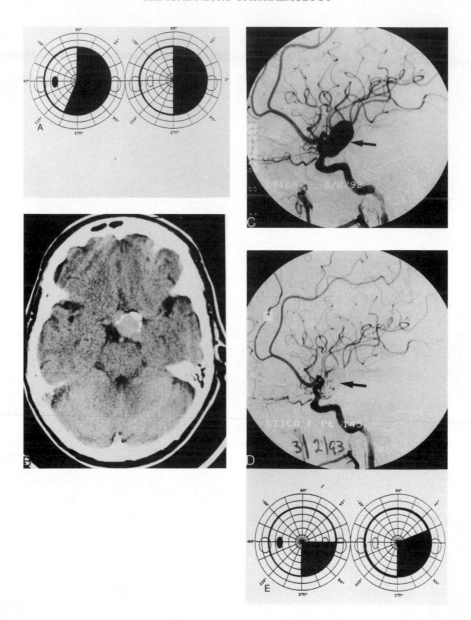

Figure 53.215. Results of coil embolization of a large internal carotid-posterior communicating artery lesion that had caused a right homonymous field defect. *A*, Perimetry using a tangent (Bjerrum) screen at 1 meter shows a dense complete right homonymous hemianopia with slight extension into the inferonasal field of the left eye. *B*, Axial non-contrast computed tomographic scan shows a mass with a calcified rim on the left side of the suprasellar cistern. *C*, Lateral digital subtraction angiogram demonstrates a large aneurysm (*arrow*) arising at the origin of the posterior communicating artery. The patient underwent embolization of the aneurysm with Guglielmi detachable coils on two separate occasions. *D*, 1 year after the initial embolization and 6 months after a second embolization, repeat angiography reveals that the aneurysm is obliterated by the coils (*arrow*). *E*, The visual field, performed 6 months after the first embolization, shows improvement in both eyes, now being primarily an inferior, incongruous quadrantic homonymous defect. (From Vargas ME, Kupersmith MJ, Setton A, et al. Endovascular treatment of giant aneurysms which cause visual loss. Ophthalmology *101*:1091–1098, 1994.)

who refused treatment, monocular blindness with dementia developed in two, a complete homonymous hemianopia and dementia developed in one, and one patient became bilaterally blind. In addition, three of seven aneurysms hemorrhaged, one fatally. An additional case of progressive visual loss despite coil embolization of a giant aneurysm was recorded by Litofsky et al. (1994) (Fig. 53.216).

Because endovascular techniques result in thrombosis of an aneurysm without reduction in its size there is concern about using these techniques to treat unruptured aneurysms that present with mass effect. A total of 26 patients with such aneurysms who underwent endovascular occlusion were followed for a mean of 60 months by Halbach et al. (1994). Of these, the symptoms and signs resolved in 13 patients (50%), improved in 11 (42.3%), and remained unchanged in two (7.7%). A comparison of the 13 patients whose symptoms and signs resolved with the 11 patients whose manifestations improved revealed that the former

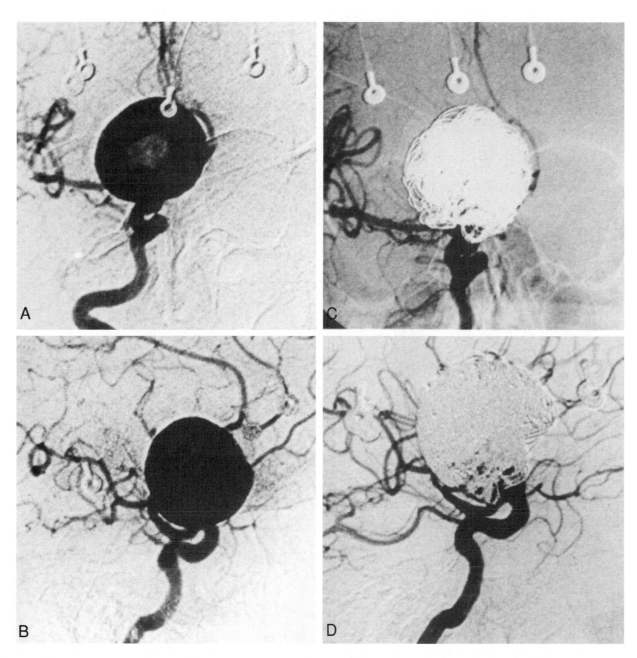

Figure 53.216. Progressive visual failure despite successful endovascular occlusion of a giant carotid-ophthalmic aneurysm with Guglielmi detachable coils. The patient was a 57-year-old woman who presented with a 1-year history of progressive right-sided visual loss. She was found to have visual acuity of 20/200 with a nasal field cut. Magnetic residence imaging demonstrated a 3.6 cm globoid lesion consistent with a giant aneurysm of the right internal carotid artery. Right internal carotid arteriogram, anteroposterior (*A*) and lateral (*B*) views, shows a giant carotid-ophthalmic aneurysm. The aneurysm was treated with coil embolization. Post-treatment angiogram, anteroposterior (C) and lateral (*D*) views, shows that the aneurysm is completely obliterated by the coils. Four days after the coiling procedure, the patient was readmitted with progressive visual loss with severe headache and disorientation. Visual acuity had declined to 20/800. The patient subsequently underwent surgical evacuation of the coils and clipping of the aneurysm. Postoperatively, visual acuity returned to 20/20. (From Litofsky NS, Vinuela F, Giannotta SL. Progressive visual loss after electrothrombosis treatment of a giant intracranial aneurysm: Case report. Neurosurgery *34*:548–550, 1994.)

group had less wall calcification (30% vs 60%) and a shorter duration of symptoms. In addition, patients with resolution of neurologic manifestations were more likely to have totally occluded aneurysms on late follow-up arteriograms than those who had improvement or were unchanged.

Modifications of and alternatives to coil embolization are undergoing investigation. In an effort to make the coils more thrombogenic and therefore less likely to leave the aneurysm only partly occluded, collagen-coated microcoils are being developed (Dawson et al., 1995), and surface modifications

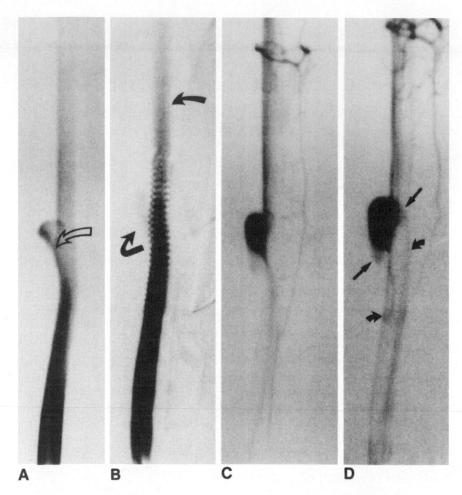

Figure 53.217.   Treatment of experimentally produced carotid aneurysm with a percutaneously placed stent. *A,* Early phase of angiogram demonstrates typical flow pattern demonstrating the aneurysm (*open arrow*). *B,* The aneurysm neck is bridged with a self-expanding experimental nitinol stent. The flow is seen to be directed towards the distal part of the parent vessel. The inflow zone is seen to be shifted toward the proximal portion of the ostium (*curved arrow*). The flow itself is seen to be directed centrally and more distally (*superior curved arrow*). *C,* Late-phase carotid angiogram demonstrates outflow of contrast material before placement of stent. *D,* After placement of the stent, the late phase demonstrates hang-up of contrast material (*straight arrows*). Note contrast material trapped within filaments of the proximal stent (*short curved arrows*) (From Wakhloo AK, Schellhammer F, de Vries J, et al. Self-expanding and balloon-expandable stents in the treatment of carotid aneurysms: An experimental study in a canine model. AJNR *15*:493–502, 1994.)

to existing coils have been described (Ahuja et al., 1993) including protein coating and ion implantation (Murayama et al., 1997). So far, however, these coils tend to be stiffer and nonretrievable. Coil or balloon migration might be impeded by the use of N-butyl-2-cyanoacrylate glue to keep the material in place (Teng et al., 1994). Liquid endovascular materials are being explored, including ethylenevinyl alcohol polymer (Nishi et al., 1996).

Percutaneously placed vascular stents may be used to treat unruptured intracranial aneurysms (Marin and Veith, 1996; Singer et al., 1997) (Fig. 53.217). Although this procedure is still largely experimental with respect to intracranial aneurysms (Geremia et al., 1994; Grotenhuis et al., 1994; Szikora et al., 1994; Turjman et al., 1994a; Wakhloo et al., 1994; Massoud et al., 1995; Link et al., 1996; Lieber et al. 1997) (Figs. 53.218 and 53.219), it is used to treat patients with ICA stenosis and to occlude aneurysms arising from the extracranial portion of the ICA (Mase et al., 1995; Nicholson et al.,

1995; Miyachi et al., 1997) (Fig. 53.220). It would seem to be particularly applicable to treatment of fusiform aneurysms or aneurysms with a very broad neck, and coils could be placed outside the stent selectively to protect vessels arising from the aneurysm. Work is continuing to improve the long-term patency of these stents (Link et al., 1996) while insuring complete obliteration of the aneurysm.

Also still largely at the experimental stage is the use of intravascular endoscopy. This may permit direct visualization of endovascular intervention (Miyachi et al., 1992a).

Endovascular surgical procedures may be used intraoperatively (Mizoi et al., 1993, 1994). This natural progression from intraoperative angiography may help guide surgical clipping (Barrow et al., 1992). In particular, suction decompression of a large aneurysm can make dissection and clipping substantially easier (Batjer and Samson, 1990; Albert et al., 1993; Sinson et al., 1996). Barnett et al. (1994) reported the use of intraoperative angiography together with

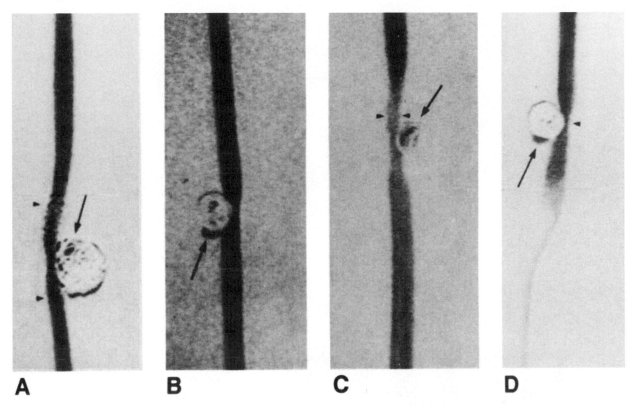

Figure 53.218. Results of subtotal aneurysm packing with Guglielmi detachable coils with and without previous stent implantation in experimentally produced aneurysm in dogs. *A*, Digital subtraction angiography immediately after subtotal aneurysm packing with coils through a stent (*arrowheads*) shows residual aneurysm filling within the inflow zone (*arrow*). *B*, Residual filling (*arrow*) within the dome of the contralateral aneurysm treated with coils alone. *C*, Digital subtraction angiography 4 weeks later demonstrates unchanged filling (*arrow*) within the stented and coiled aneurysm. The stented portion of the lumen of the carotid artery is narrowed by approximately 35% (*arrowheads*). *D*, Unchanged residual flow (*arrow*) within the non-stented aneurysm 4 weeks after treatment. Mild stenosis of the carotid artery adjacent to the aneurysm neck (*arrow head*) is related to surgery and postoperative scar tissue formation. Note the circular appearance of the stenosis (From Szikora I, Guterman LR, Wells KM, et al. Combined use of stents and coils to treat experimental wide-necked carotid aneurysms: Preliminary results. AJNR *15*:1091–1102, 1994.)

intraoperative balloon occlusion of the ICA and electroencephalography to optimize the timing of an extracranial-intracranial bypass before occlusion of the carotid artery and to provide intraoperative documentation of graft patency. This technique may permit changes in both the approach and the specific technique used to occlude an aneurysm at surgery. Indeed, Derdeyn et al. (1995) reported that the use of intraoperative endovascular techniques led to clinically significant changes in surgical therapy in five of 66 cases. The surgery of basilar artery aneurysms may particularly benefit from this type of approach (Bailes et al., 1992; Albert et al., 1993).

When endovascular therapy fails, surgery is occasionally necessary (Civit et al., 1996). In the UCLA experience, 21 of 196 patients who underwent endovascular surgery for aneurysms subsequently required craniotomy (Gurian et al., 1995a). This was a result of complications of embolization in six cases (four of whom improved following surgery; two died), failure of embolization in five, and partial occlusion in 10. Of the 15 patients in the latter two groups, 14 (93%) had an excellent or good outcome with complete aneurysm occlusion. Continued enlargement of a giant aneurysm following incomplete balloon occlusion is an indication for surgical intervention with revascularization (Kurokawa et al., 1992).

Results of Surgery on Unruptured Aneurysms

The results of surgery on unruptured intracranial saccular aneurysms are generally excellent, particularly when the aneurysm can be clipped. The surgical risks associated with operating on unruptured aneurysms are much less than those of surgery on ruptured ones (see below). The sac of the aneurysm is usually not adherent to adjacent brain tissue, and it can be dissected away fairly easily. In addition, delayed cerebral ischemia (vasospasm) rarely follows surgery on an unruptured aneurysm, compared with rates of occurrence both before and after surgery on ruptured aneurysms. Most series that describe the results of surgery on patients with unruptured aneurysms report mortality rates of 0–5% and morbidity rates under 10% (Moyes, 1971; Samson et al., 1977; Yoshimoto et al., 1979; Salazar, 1980; Wirth et al., 1983; Heiskanen, 1986; Freger et al., 1987; Heiskanen and Poranen, 1987; Jomin et al., 1987). King et al. (1994) published a meta-analysis of the results of surgery in unruptured aneurysms. These investigators reviewed 28 articles containing data on 733 patients and concluded that the expected mortality rate for surgery on unruptued aneurysms should be 1.0% or less, with a morbidity rate of 4.1%. In a subsequent series of 76 aneurysms in 69 patients, there was no

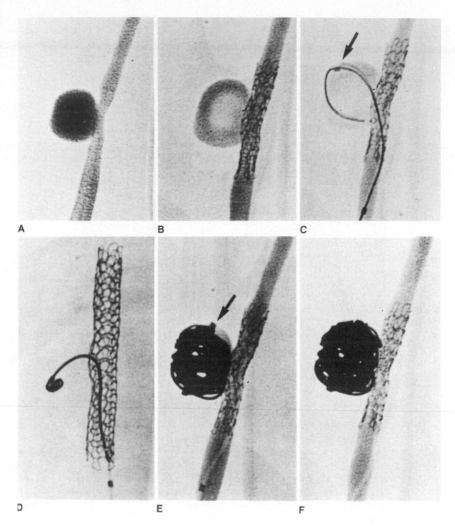

Figure 53.219. Treatment of experimental aneurysms with Guglielmi detachable coils combined with percutaneously placed stent in adult swine. *A*, Right carotid angiogram shows an 8-mm aneurysm created on the carotid artery. *B*, Following placement of a balloon-inflatable Strecker stent, the aneurysm is still seen to be seen patent. *C*, A micro-guidewire is introduced into the aneurysm through the stent mesh. The tip of the catheter appears as a black dot (*arrow*). *D*, The first coil is placed within the aneurysm. *E*, The aneurysm is almost completely occluded with coils. A small coil of 2 mm × 4 cm is visible in the inflow zone of the aneurysm (*arrow*). *F*, Post-treatment control angiogram shows complete occlusion of the aneurysm with 5 coils (total length 82 cm) (From Turjman F, Massoud TF, Ji C, et al. Combined stent implantation and endosaccular coil placement for treatment of experimental wide-necked aneurysms: A feasibility study in swine. AJNR *15*:1087–1090, 1994.)

mortality, although morbidity was 7.2% (Asari and Ohmoto, 1994b). Over a follow-up period averaging 50 months, 53 patients (76.8%) had a good or fair outcome, 11 (15.9%) had a poor outcome, and five (7.3%) died from causes unrelated to the aneurysms. In another series, 90 patients harboring 119 incidental aneurysms less than 25 mm in diameter underwent surgery without any surgical mortality or morbidity (Mizoi et al., 1995).

As a general rule, the larger the aneurysm, the greater the risk of the procedure. Mortality and morbidity are therefore highest for patients with giant aneurysms (Symon and Vajda, 1984). In these patients, multiple clips and even resection of portions of the aneurysmal wall may be necessary (Tanaka et al., 1994).

In an attempt to better classify the risks of operating on unruptured aneurysms Khanna et al. (1996) reviewed their experience on 172 patients. Major morbidity occurred in 12 patients (6.9%) and five patients (2.9%) died. These authors concluded that the main factors associated with an increased operative morbidity in patients with unruptured aneurysms are a posterior fossa location of the aneurysm, a large size of the aneurysm, and advanced age of the patient. Nevertheless, if one considers the risk of hemorrhage from a previously unruptured aneurysm (1% per year) and the morbidity and mortality of such a hemorrhage (70–80%), the risks of surgery for unruptured intracranial saccular aneurysms, both symptomatic and asymptomatic, seem so low that such surgery should be offered to most patients.

King et al. (1995) used mathematical modeling techniques to assess the cost-effectiveness of elective surgery for the

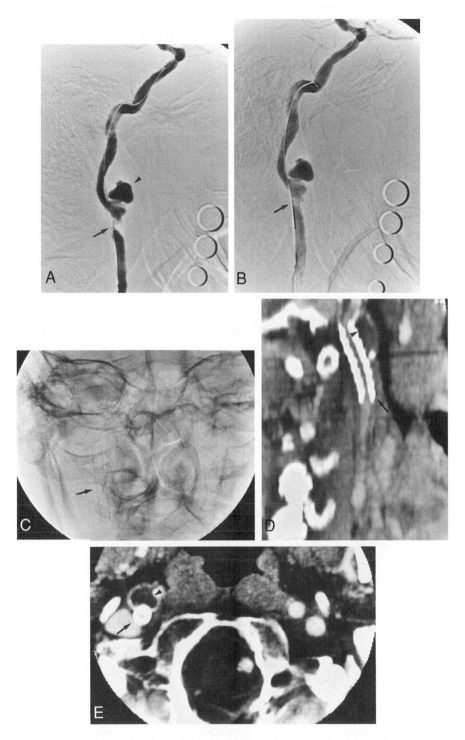

Figure 53.220. Use of percutaneously placed vascular stent to treat stenosis and pseudoaneurysm formation in the extracranial portion of the right internal carotid artery of a 57-year-old man who complained of episodes of transient visual loss in the right eye and numbness of the left upper extremity. *A*, Digital subtraction intra-arterial angiogram shows marked (80%) stenosis (*arrow*) associated with a distal pseudoaneurysm (*arrowhead*). *B*, After balloon angioplasty, repeat angiogram shows widening of the previously stenotic segment, but the pseudoaneurysm persists. Accordingly, a stent was placed. *C*, Plain skull x-ray shows location of stent (*arrow*). *D* and *E*, One year after treatment, spiral computed tomographic angiography shows intact stent (*arrow*) with normal flow. Pseudoaneurysm is completely thrombosed (*arrowhead*). (Courtesy of Drs. C. Douglas Phillips and Jonas H. Goldstein.)

treatment of asymptomatic, unruptured, intracranial aneurysms. Using baseline model assumptions for a 50-year-old patient, they estimated that elective aneurysm surgery provides an average of 0.88 additional quality-adjusted life years compared with nonsurgical treatment. Prompt elective surgery for asymptomatic, unruptured, intracranial aneurysms thus is a cost-effective use of medical resources provided that: (*a*) surgical morbidity and mortality remain at or below the low levels reported above; (*b*) the patient has a life expectancy of at least 13 additional years; and (*c*) the patient experiences a decrease in quality of life from knowingly living with an unruptured aneurysm.

The major exception to this dictum is the aneurysm located within the cavernous sinus (Kupersmith et al., 1992). Such an aneurysm usually is treated by occlusion of the ICA, often in association with an STA-MCA bypass. Not only does this treatment have a significant risk of cerebral ischemia, but intracavernous aneurysms have a much lower

morbidity and mortality from rupture than do intradural aneurysms. As noted in the section on intracavernous aneurysms above, rupture of such an aneurysm usually produces a carotid-cavernous sinus fistula, not a subarachnoid or intraparenchymal hemorrhage, and the fistula almost always can be treated successfully by occlusion with a detachable balloon or thrombogenic coils without occlusion of the ICA (see Chapter 54). Thus, decisions about treatment of aneurysms within the cavernous sinus should depend mainly on the symptoms they produce. In symptomatic patients, endovascular obliteration of the aneurysm is usually associated with a significantly lower morbidity than a direct surgical approach (Polin et al., 1996). The possibility of late distal embolization, however, remains. We saw two patients with late visual loss following endovascular occlusion of intracavernous aneurysms.

When obliteration of an unruptured aneurysm requires occlusion of the parent vessel, the risks of resultant neurologic

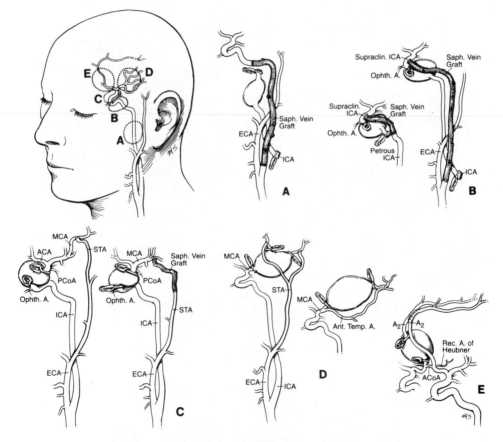

Figure 53.221.   Surgical approaches to revascularization of the anterior circulation. Overview shows the anterior circulation and common locations for aneurysms. *A*, Internal carotid artery (*ICA*) aneurysm at the cranial base is trapped and revascularized with a cervical to petrous carotid bypass with saphenous (*Saph.*) vein graft. *ECA*, external carotid artery. *B*, Cavernous ICA aneurysm is trapped and revascularized with a petrous to supraclinoid (C5 to C3) carotid bypass with a saphenous (*Saph.*) vein graft or, alternatively, with a cervical to supraclinoid carotid artery bypass. *Ophth. A.*, ophthalmic artery; *Supraclin.*, supraclinoid; *ECA*, external carotid artery. *C*, Supraclinoid ICA is trapped and revascularized with a superficial temporal artery (*STA*) to middle cerebral artery (*MCA*) bypass or, alternatively, with an STA-MCA bypass using a saphenous (*Saph.*) vein interposition graft. *PcoA*, posterior communicating artery; *ACA*, anterior cerebral artery; *Ophth. A.*, ophthalmic artery; *ECA*, external carotid artery. *D*, middle cerebral artery (*MCA*) aneurysm is trapped and revascularized with a double-barrel STA-MCA bypass or, alternatively, with an anterior temporal artery (*Ant. Temp. A.*) to MCA in situ bypass. *ECA*, external carotid artery. *E*, Anterior cerebral artery aneurysm is trapped and revascularized with an A-2 to A-2 in situ bypass. *Rec. A.*, recurrent artery; *ACoA*, anterior communicating artery. (From Lawton MT, Hamilton MG, Morcos JJ, et al. Revascularization and aneurysm surgery: Current techniques, indications, and outcome. Neurosurgery *38*:83–92, 1996.)

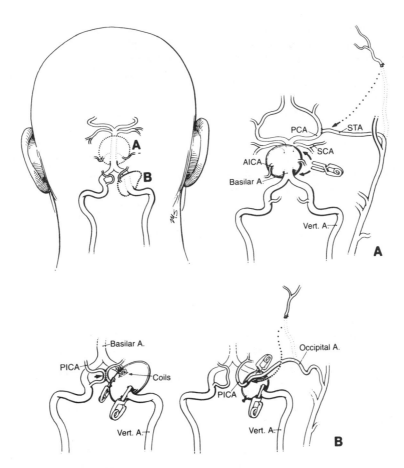

Figure 53.222. Surgical approaches to revascularization of the posterior circulation. Overview showing the posterior circulation and common locations for aneurysms. *A,* Midbasilar artery is occluded proximally or distally to the aneurysm and revascularized with a superficial temporal artery (*STA*) to posterior cerebral artery (*PCA*) bypass. *AICA,* anterior inferior cerebellar artery; *Vert.,* vertebral; *A,* artery; *SCA,* superior cerebellar artery. *B,* Vertebral artery aneurysm is trapped between a clip on the proximal vertebral artery and endovascular coils placed distally in the vertebral artery. Revascularization was accomplished with a posterior inferior cerebellar artery (*PICA*) to internal carotid artery (*ICA*) in situ bypass. The clip at the origin of the PICA prevents retrograde filling of the aneurysm. Alternatively, an occipital artery to PICA bypass is shown. *Vert A.,* vertebral artery. (From Lawton MT, Hamilton MG, Morcos JJ, et al. Revascularization and aneurysm surgery: Current techniques, indications, and outcome. Neurosurgery *38*:83–92, 1996.)

dysfunction depend on the vessel location and possible collateral flow. When collateral flow is inadequate, the distal area should be revascularized, usually with distal branches of the external carotid artery (Figs. 53.221 and 53.222). The superficial temporal and occipital arteries are the most commonly employed branches of the external carotid either used alone or with saphenous vein extenders (Spetzler et al., 1990; Fitzpatrick et al., 1993; Lawton et al., 1996). A radial artery graft can be used to revascularize the PCA (Wakui et al., 1992). Late patency of these procedures is excellent, approaching 90% even when vein grafts are required (Regli et al., 1995). Most graft failures (76%) occur during the first year after surgery, with 42% of all graft failures being identified during the first 24 hours after operation. When grafts fail late, only 20% of patients develop new neurologic symptoms as opposed to 72% when the occlusion is early (Regli et al., 1995).

Microvascular surgery can be adapted to individual situations. An A-3 to A-3 side-to-side anastomosis was used to revascularize the territory of the pericallosal artery following surgery for an aneurysm of the anterior communicating artery (Mabuchi et al., 1995), and manipulation of MCA aneurysms may be made significantly safer with an STA-MCA or a similar type of bypass (Bederson and Spetzler, 1992; Suzuki et al., 1992; Kimura et al., 1993).

Failure to control hypertension can result in an intracerebral hemorrhage from saphenous bypass failure (Nagasawa et al., 1994). In addition, revascularization may not prevent recurrent TIAs caused by collateral embolization (Takeuchi et al., 1995) or distal infarction (Cahill, 1992).

Treatment of Ruptured Intracranial Saccular Aneurysms

Treatment of an unruptured, intracranial saccular aneurysm consists of an attempt to occlude or obliterate the aneurysm without rupturing it or reducing blood flow to critical areas of the brain in the process. When an aneurysm has already ruptured, treatment is much more complicated (Ausman et al., 1985, 1989; Batjer and Samson, 1989). A patient who survives an SAH caused by rupture of an intracranial aneurysm has the potential to return to a productive life, but only if the effects of SAH as well as its cause are treated effectively (Yoshimoto et al., 1979; Drake, 1984; Laine, 1986; Marsh et al., 1987; Solomon and Fink, 1987; Biller et al., 1988; Guy et al., 1995).

All patients with aneurysmal SAH should be admitted to a hospital for emergency evaluation and treatment. The optimum care of these patients is provided by a team composed of neurologists, neurosurgeons, neuroradiologists, neuroanesthesiologists, and intensive care specialists in a stroke or neurologic intensive care unit (Biller et al., 1988; Guy et al., 1995).

Treatment of Delayed Cerebral Ischemia

Because subarachnoid blood may play an etiologic role in inducing vasospasm, the treatment of a ruptured aneurysm includes an attempt to reduce the amount of blood products in the subarachnoid space. In general, early surgery of ruptured aneurysms permits additional intervention designed to reduce the incidence of clinical vasospasm (Kassell et al., 1982a). Intracisternal (Stolke and Seifert, 1992) or intrathecal (Ohman et al., 1991b) application of tissue plasminogen activator (TPA) results in radical resolution of residual clot. Preliminary series using this substance reported encouraging results in the rate of clearance of subarachnoid blood and also in preventing or ameliorating vasospasm (Findlay et al., 1991; Zabramski et al., 1991). In one series, a single intracistern application of recombinant TPA was administered to 51 patients at the time of surgery to clip a ruptured aneurysm (Findlay et al., 1995). The results were compared with those from a control group of 49 patients whose ruptured aneurysms were clipped but who were not given TPA. The incidence of angiographically documented vasospasm measured between the 7th and 11th days following SAH was similar between the two groups, with arterial narrowing detected in 74.4% of control subjects and 64.6% of patients treated with TPA, although there was a trend toward less severe vasospasm in the treated group. In another study, TPA resulted in a 56% reduction in severe vasospasm in patients with thick subarachnoid clots (Sasaki et al., 1992, 1994). In addition, when TPA was administered intrathecally 24 hours after surgery, no vasospasm occurred even when a low dose of TPA was used. In this study, there was no dose-dependent risk of bleeding, which occurred in 7.5% of 53 patients. Aggressive treatment with TPA after emergent occlusion of aneurysms in 12 patients with Hunt and Hess neurologic Grades III–V led to complete clearing of cisternal hemorrhage within 72 hours in 10 surviving patients and angiographic evidence of mild vasospasm in only one patient (Kinugasa et al., 1995). Vasospasm may, however, occur despite the use of intrathecal TPA. Steinberg et al. (1994a) reported four of eight patients with aneurysmal SAH who developed angiographic and clinical vasospasm with delayed neurologic deterioration, despite treatment with intracisternal TPA after early aneurysm clipping. One patient did not clear a massive SAH with TPA; one patient had extremely poor collateral flow with occlusion of one cervical

ICA and 80% stenosis of the other cervical ICA; and the other two patients had an SAH 7–12 days after a sentinel hemorrhage.

Some authors advocate a combination of cisternal drainage (Inagawa et al., 1991) and intrathecal injection of urokinase to prevent vasospasm following SAH. In a series of 60 patients, the incidence of permanent neurologic deficits caused by vasospasm was 31% (five of 16 patients) without cisternal drainage, 15% (five of 34 patients) with drainage alone, and 10% (one of 10 patients) with drainage combined with urokinase injection (Moriyama et al., 1995c). CSF drainage significantly reduced the incidence of permanent neurologic deficits caused by vasospasm but significantly increased the incidence of hydrocephalus requiring shunt procedures.

In a retrospective review, 111 patients with aneurysmal SAH treated with early surgery and intrathecal thrombolytic therapy (60 treated with urokinase for 7 days, 22 treated with TPA every 6–8 hours for 5 days, and 29 treated with neither) were assessed for evidence of vasospasm and outcome (Usui et al., 1994). The severity of angiographic vasospasm and the incidence of infarction in patients treated with either thrombolytic agent were less than in patients without treatment, despite a larger amount of initial subarachnoid blood clot in both thrombolytic groups. Only TPA therapy reduced the incidence of symptomatic vasospasm. There were no significant differences among the three groups in overall outcome at 3 months possibly related to the size of the series.

Of 55 patients following aneurysmal hemorrhage who had intracranial irrigation with pH 8.0 Hartmann solution containing 1 mg/ml of methylprednisolone after early (before day 3) clipping, only six (11%) developed evidence of vasospasm (Suzuki et al., 1994).

Treatment of vasospasm (Warnell, 1996) is one of the most important means of reducing morbidity in patients with SAH. Patients with severe vasospasm and delayed cerebral ischemia have lost the capability of autoregulation of cerebral blood flow (Jakubowski et al., 1982; Voldby et al., 1985b). The affected cerebral arteries have narrowed lumens and a fixed, high resistance. The arteriolar and capillary beds in affected areas of the brain become maximally dilated in an effort to augment collateralization (Grubb et al., 1977). Cerebral blood flow therefore responds in a passive fashion to changes of systemic blood pressure and cardiac output. Under these conditions, intravascular volume expansion and consequent augmentation of systemic cardiovascular parameters might be expected to significantly increase cerebral blood flow in ischemic areas (Denny-Brown, 1951; Kosnik and Hunt, 1976). Red blood cell aggregability increases after SAH (Mori et al., 1995) but this may be reversed by volume expansion (Mori et al., 1996). The hemodilution induced by volume expansion should reduce whole blood viscosity, thereby improving blood flow in the microcirculation (Wood et al., 1982).

Volume expansion is the most widely used and successful treatment of delayed cerebral ischemia after SAH (Kosnik and Hunt, 1976; Giannotta et al., 1977; Pritz et al., 1978; Kudo et al., 1981; Montgomery et al., 1981; Kassell et al.,

1982b; Heros et al., 1983; Rosenwasser et al., 1983; Milhorat and Krautheim, 1986; Solomon and Fink, 1987; Biller et al., 1988; Creissard et al., 1988; Ausman et al., 1989; Archer et al., 1996). Volume expansion may be achieved through the use of hydroxyethyl starch (Hadeishi et al., 1990). At least 70% of ischemic deficits that develop after SAH can be reversed by a combination of increased cardiac output and increased arterial pressure if treatment is initiated before infarction occurs (Kassell et al., 1982b), but this treatment may cause recurrent rupture of an untreated aneurysm. Volume expansion therapy therefore is reserved in most cases for postoperative patients. Some authors recommend giving calcium-channel blocking drugs to patients undergoing volume expansion in the belief that these agents further improve the results (Medlock et al., 1992), whereas others believe that these drugs add little or nothing to volume expansion (Origitano et al., 1992; Mercier et al., 1993).

Patients with a ruptured aneurysm may harbor additional unruptured aneurysms, and this may affect the decision to raise a patient's blood pressure after SAH, unless all of the unruptured aneurysms can be treated at the time of the initial surgery. In a series of 199 patients with aneurysmal SAH who underwent early surgery, 31 had one or more unprotected aneurysms postoperatively (Swift and Solomon, 1992). All patients were treated with prophylactic volume expansion with mean central venous pressure during treatment of 10.3 cm H_2O and mean arterial blood pressure 141/76 mm Hg (volume expansion was continued for 7 to 10 days). No patient suffered rupture of an unprotected aneurysm during hypervolemic treatment. We agree with Archer et al. (1996) that systolic blood pressure be maintained between 120 and 150 mm Hg until surgery, at which time it should be increased to between 160 and 200 mm Hg with a cardiac index of >3.5 L/min. Hypervolemic therapy may also contribute to the increasing frequency of medical complications, especially cardiac decompensation and pulmonary edema, particularly in the elderly (Yoshimoto and Kwak, 1995). To avoid this, careful monitoring of cardiac parameters, especially pulmonary wedge pressure, is critical (Levy and Giannotta, 1991; Shimoda et al., 1991).

The results of laboratory and clinical studies suggest that calcium channel-blocking agents can improve the outcome in patients after SAH. Initial laboratory studies suggested that the calcium channel-blocker **nimodipine** blocked muscular contraction and prevented vasospasm (Allen and Bahr, 1979); however, both laboratory and clinical studies subsequently demonstrated that nimodipine neither reverses nor prevents angiographic arterial narrowing after SAH (Allen et al., 1983; Krueger et al., 1985; Nosko et al., 1985; Mee et al., 1988). Instead, nimodipine seems to dilate the intraparenchymal arterioles of the brain and to promote leptomeningeal collateral circulation (Auer, 1981). In animal models of cerebral ischemia, nimodipine improves the outcome after ischemic insults to the brain (Harris et al., 1982; Nosko et al., 1986), and in controlled clinical trials, nimodipine significantly reduces the morbidity and mortality associated with delayed cerebral ischemia, particularly in sicker patients and in patients with angiographic evidence of vasospasm (Allen et al., 1983; Auer, 1984; Ljunggren et al., 1984; Frerebeau et al., 1988; Jan et al., 1988; Petruk et al., 1988; Seiler et

al., 1988; Öhman and Heiskanen, 1989; Pickard et al., 1989; Gilsbach et al., 1990; Ohman et al., 1991a; Langlois et al., 1992). The nimodipine effect seems to be dose related, with worsening of flow parameters documented by transcranial Doppler when the administration rate is lowered (Zygmunt and Delgado-Zygmunt, 1995). Nimodipine is generally used routinely in the management of patients with aneurysmal SAH (Findlay, 1997).

Frazee et al. (1988) reported that another calcium channel-blocking agent, **diltiazem**, prevents or reduces vasospasm after experimental SAH in nonhuman primates. Kawano et al. (1995) reported the efects of high-dose diltiazem (5 mg/kg/min) injection combined with dextran and hydrocortisone administered continuously via a central line in 48 patients. Symptomatic vasospasm occurred in five patients (10.4%), four of whom recovered, although one had severe neurologic deficits. A low-density area on CT scanning was observed in two patients. A total of 30 patients (62.5%) had good recovery, 10 patients (20.8%) had moderate disability, three (6.3%) had severe disability, and three (6.3%) had vegetative survival. Two patients died of the initial brain damage. There were no severely hypotensive side effects. However, three patients showed atrioventricular blockage on electrocardiogram possibly associated with the calcium-channel blocker. There is also experimental evidence that calcium-channel blocking agents improve the blood flow in patients after SAH by improving red blood cell deformability and by inhibiting platelet aggregation (Dale et al., 1983). A number of other calcium-channel blockers may also be effective in lowering the incidence and severity of vasospasm (Shibuya et al., 1992). Regardless of their mechanism of action, calcium channel-blocking substances should play a major role in the treatment of patients with SAH, especially after rupture of an intracranial aneurysm.

Calcium-channel blockers may drop blood pressure to less than ideal levels. To avoid this complication, low doses of the drugs are often used. In the Cooperative Aneurysm Study, 365 patients at 21 neurosurgical centers were entered into a randomized double-blind trial comparing high-dose (0.15 mg/kg/hr) nicardipine with a 50% lower dose (0.075 mg/kg/hr) administered by continuous intravenous infusion for up to 14 days following SAH (Haley et al., 1994). The incidence of symptomatic vasospasm was 31% in both groups, and the overall 3-month outcomes were nearly identical. These data suggest that, from a clinical standpoint, the results of high-dose and low-dose nicardipine treatment are nearly equivalent, but administration of low-dose nicardipine is associated with fewer side effects. In a previous report, high-dose nicardipine was associated with a reduced incidence of symptomatic vasospasm in patients with recent aneurysmal SAH but not with an improvement in overall outcome at 3 months when compared with standard management in North America (Haley et al., 1993).

In order to avoid the potential systemic cardiovascular effects of calcium channel blockers, these agents are often administered intrathecally (Shibuya et al., 1994). Intrathecal administration of nicardipine decreased the incidence of symptomatic vasospasm by 26% and angiographic vasospasm by 20% and increased good clinical outcome at 1 month after the hemorrhage by 15%. Of 50 patients, nine complained of headache, probably secondary to nicardipine-induced vasodilation. Two patients developed meningitis.

Tirilazad mesylate, a nonglucocorticoid 21-aminosteroid, reduces vasospasm following SAH and reduces infarct size from focal cerebral ischemia in experimental models. A total of 1023 patients were enrolled in a prospective randomized, double-blind, vehicle-controlled trial at 41 neurosurgical centers in Europe, Australia, and New Zealand (Kassell et al., 1996). All patients were also treated with intravenously administered nimodipine. Patients receiving 6 mg/kg per day of tirilazad had a reduced mortality, a greater reduction in vasospasm, and a greater frequency of good recovery on the Glasgow Outcome Scale 3 months after SAH than patients who did not receive this drug, although the difference in incidence of vasospasm reduction between the two groups was not statistically significant. Subsequent studies did not confirm this beneficial effect (Haley et al., 1997). Preliminary studies also suggest that the serine protease inhibitor **FUT-175** can reduce the incidence of symptomatic vasospasm when administered at the time of admission (Yanamoto et al., 1992). Paradoxically, administration of thromboxane A_2 synthetase inhibitor, initially believed to protect against vasospasm (Tokiyoshi et al., 1991), is associated with an **increase** in the incidence of vasospasm (Yano et al., 1993).

Papaverine has a direct effect on smooth muscle, leading to muscle relaxation. This substance can be infused directly into vessels in spasm. Results are generally good when papaverine is directly infused into an artery with vasospasm (Kaku et al., 1992; Kassell et al., 1992). Of 21 patients, 16 (76%) experienced good angiographic results, and 11 (52%) obtained objective clinical improvement within 48 hours in one study (McAuliffe et al., 1995). In another study, angiographic improvement occurred in 18 of 19 treatment sessions (95%). Results were excellent in three sessions, moderately better in eight, and mildly better in seven (Clouston et al., 1995). The best angiographic results often were obtained with superselective infusion. Seven of the 14 (50%) treated patients showed dramatic acute clinical improvement within 24 hours of papaverine therapy, and there was no clinical evidence of recurrent vasospasm in these patients. Recurrence of angiographic vasoconstriction was demonstrated in three patients, and one showed marked clinical improvement after a second treatment. Intra-arterial papaverine may be supplemented with intravenous high-dose **nicardipine** (Yoshimura et al., 1995) in treating vasospasm. **Nitroglycerine** administered intravenously by infusion may also act directly on the smooth vascular muscle of intracranial arteries to reduce the incidence and severity of vasospasm (Sasanuma et al., 1991).

A number of potential complications may result from papaverine infusion. Significant elevations in ICP, blood pressure, and pulse rate can occur during papaverine infusion, although cerebral perfusion pressure does not statistically change. Infusion in the common carotid artery resulted in transient severe brainstem depression in one patient reported by Barr et al. (1994) and in profound bradycardia and hypotension with a subsequent significant increase in ICP and a marked decrease in cerebral perfusion pressure in an elderly patient reported by McAuliffe et al. (1995). Clyde et al. (1996) reported a 48-year-old man in whom infusion of papaverine to control vasospasm 10 days after rupture of an anterior communicating aneurysm resulted in a paradoxic worsening of vasospasm and a subsequent stroke. Monocular blindness developed in one patient after infusion of papaverine near the ophthalmic artery (Clouston et al., 1995). Three patients experienced transient neurologic events associated with intra-arterial infusion of papavarine in the vertebrobasilar system (Mathis et al., 1994). Two of these patients developed severe respiratory depression. A 63-year-old woman had a transient respiratory arrest followed by rapid progressive loss of brainstem function 25 minutes after infusions of papaverine into her left vertebral and left internal carotid arteries. Miller et al. (1995) described a patient who experienced two episodes of severe immune-related thrombocytopenia following intra-arterial administration of papaverine. Pritz (1994a) described pupillary dilation after intracisternal administration of papaverine.

Balloon angioplasty can be used to expand focal areas of vasospasm (Barnwell et al., 1989; Bracard et al., 1990; Pistoia et al., 1991, Higashida et al., 1992) (Fig. 53.223). The effect of this procedure on vasospasm may be monitored using dynamic digital subtraction angiography (DSA) to measure local transit time (Touho, 1995). Fujii et al. (1995b) described four patients who were Hunt and Hess grade IV following aneurysmal SAH complicated by symptomatic vasospasm. All four patients were treated with early clipping of the ruptured aneurysm and balloon angioplasty. Two patients recovered sufficiently to return to their previous occupations, whereas one patient remained bedridden, and one died. Among 19 cases of high-grade symptomatic vasospasm treated with balloon angioplasty in another study, vasospastic arteries were significantly dilated (diameter of more than 75% of diameter on admission) in 83% (Fujii et al., 1995c). There was no recurrence of vasospasm or chronic atherosclerotic changes on repeat angiography. Clinical improvement within 24 hours after angioplasty was observed in 63% of cases (seven of 17 cases with consciousness disturbance, five of 16 cases with motor weakness, and one of seven cases with aphasia). Outcomes at the time of discharge were excellent in 10 cases, good in three, and fair in four. Two patients died. SPECT scanning before and after angioplasty confirmed improvement of cerebral blood flow in three of five cases investigated. In another series, Finlik et al. (1997) reported improvement in 13 of 14 patients following angioplasty. The main complication of balloon angioplasty is vessel rupture (Linskey et al., 1991b). Higashida et al. (1992) reported arterial rupture in two of 28 cases. Experimental studies demonstrate the potential for damage to the vessel wall and disruption of collagen and myocytes (Fujiwara et al., 1990; Konishi et al., 1992; Yamamoto et al., 1992; Kobayashi et al., 1993; Fujiwara et al., 1994; Ohkawa et al., 1996).

Timing of Aneurysm Surgery and Its Relationship to Neurologic Status

In 1968, Hunt and Hess proposed a grading system for the clinical condition of patients after SAH to better assess the value of various methods of surgical treatment. This grading system, or a variant of it, is used by almost all neurosurgeons in assessing the results of surgery (Table 53.2)

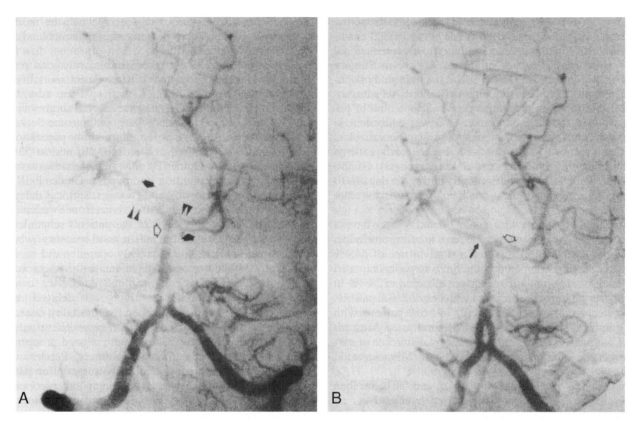

Figure 53.223. Balloon angioplasty for treatment of vasospasm. *A,* Left vertebral artery angiogram in a 41-year-old gentleman with recurrent skull base myxoid chondrosarcoma obtained 12 days after original surgery demonstrates vasospasm within the distal basilar artery (*open arrow*), both proximal posterior cerebral arteries (*double arrowheads*), and both proximal superior cerebellar arteries (*closed arrows*). *B,* Repeat left vertebral angiogram after angioplasty of proximal portions of both posterior cerebral arteries shows dilation of both proximal posterior cerebral arteries. A focal area of narrowing persists at the origin of the right posterior cerebral artery (*closed arrow*) and the proximal left posterior cerebral artery (*open arrow*). (From Pistoia F, Horton JA, Sekhar L, et al. Imaging of blood flow changes following angioplasty for treatment of vasospasm. AJNR *12*:446–448, 1991.)

although other grading systems based on the Glasgow Coma Scale can also be used (Goton et al., 1996; Oshira et al., 1997b).

Rebleeding and cerebral ischemia occur most often during the first 14 days after SAH from a ruptured aneurysm (Kassell and Torner, 1983b) and often within the first few hours (Yasui et al., 1994). Rates of rebleed steadily climb during the first 2 weeks of hospitalization in unoperated patients (Steiger et al., 1994), reaching cumulative rates of 23% within 2 weeks and 42% within 4 weeks. Indeed, the most important predictive factors for prognosis in patients with surgically treated, ruptured aneurysms are preoperative neurologic status, postoperative cerebral ischemia (vasospasm), preoperative systemic hypertension, and age (Arteriola i Fortuny and Prieto-Valiente, 1981b; Chyatte et al., 1988; Inagawa et al., 1988). The pattern and distribution of complications after surgery performed within 4 days of SAH do not differ substantially from those in patients who undergo surgery later in the course of their illness (Sonesson et al., 1987; Chyatte et al., 1988). Therefore, early surgery might offer the best prognosis to the majority of patients.

Hunt and Miller (1977) were among the first investigators to report the results of aneurysm surgery performed within 1 week of SAH. In their series, 75 of 104 patients (72%) survived surgery. Since that time, excellent results of early

surgery for ruptured intracranial aneurysm have been reported in numerous series. Mizukami et al. (1982) described 64 patients who underwent aneurysm surgery within 4 days of SAH. Of grade I and II patients, 87% had an excellent result after surgery, and 85% of grade III patients also had an excellent outcome. Only one of 13 grade IV or V patients had even a good outcome, however. Ljunggren and his colleagues (Ljunggren et al., 1981, 1984, 1985; Säveland et al., 1986a, 1986b) performed a careful analysis of a population of patients who had experienced SAH from a ruptured intracranial aneurysm and who underwent surgery within 4 days of SAH. Of 105 patients, 79 (75.2%) had a good recovery with minimal or no neurologic deficit. In addition, 11 of 21 (52.4%) grade III or IV patients had a fair to good outcome when evaluated 1 year after surgery. Auer et al. (1986) reported the results of a 6-month follow-up on patients who underwent surgery within 1 week of aneurysm rupture. In this series, 85% of patients grade IV or better had an excellent or good outcome (96% of grade I and II patients, 90% of grade III patients, and 50% of grade IV patients). Other investigators described similar results in both adults and children (Maurice-Williams and Marsh, 1985; Nishimoto et al., 1985; Medhkour et al., 1986; Milhorat and Krautheim, 1986; Thierry et al., 1987; Adams et al., 1988; Ferrante et al., 1988;

postoperative hypertension may increase the risk of seizure activity following aneurysm treatment (Ohman, 1990). Although some physicians advocate treating patients with prophylactic antiseizure medications for 1 year or more (Rabinowicz et al., 1991), prophylaxis is usually advised only during the immediate postoperative period (Baker et al., 1995b).

Medical therapy may eventually play a role in prevention and therapy of aneurysms. Futami et al. (1995a) demonstrated that exogenous basic fibroblast growth factor induces a proliferative response of smooth muscle cells in aneurysmal lesions in rats, leading to a strengthening of the wall. Treatment of at-risk patients or patients with known asymptomatic aneurysms with such a substance might prevent subsequent aneurysm development or rupture.

Results of Surgery on Ruptured Aneurysms

The majority of aneurysms are treated after they rupture. The prognosis for patients following surgery for a ruptured intracranial aneurysm is largely dependent on the effects of the SAH itself, the complications at surgery, and any associated episodes of vasospasm (Säveland and Brandt, 1994). Multiple series emphasize a good long-term prognosis for patients who survive the acute event, but a problem in comparing such series is that few use published guidelines to describe the clinical status of treated patients. For example, van Gijn et al. (1994) found that of 161 articles reporting the initial clinical status of patients with a ruptured intracranial aneurysm, only 30 (19%) used an unequivocal grading system (World Federation of Neurological Surgeons Scale or Glasgow Coma Scale). Nevertheless, as mentioned above, the best predictor of outcome is the clinical grade of the patient at the time of admission (Proust et al., 1995). In the series reported by Säveland and Brandt (1994), only two of 51 Hunt and Hess grade V patients made a good recovery after aneurysm surgery.

The most devastating complication of aneurysm surgery is intraoperative rupture of the aneurysm. Not only does this increase immediate mortality, but it also increases the risk of vasospasm in those who survive (Mustaki et al., 1996). Intraoperative rupture depends on a number of factors, including the amount of dissection required to clip the aneurysm, the blood pressure before and during surgery, and the amount of clot. Shigeta et al. (1992) reported intraoperative rupture of five of 20 dorsal ICA aneurysms. Attempts at deliberately lowering blood pressure during surgery but before clipping failed to lower the rate of rupture during surgery (Inomata et al., 1992). Intraoperative rupture may be reduced by the use of temporary clipping of the parent vessel (Ogilvy et al., 1996), but this technique is associated with its own risk of stroke (see above), especially if the clip is maintained for more than 20 minutes or the aneurysm ruptures despite attempts at prevention.

The specifics of fatal vascular complications of aneurysm surgery were investigated by postmortem angiography in a consecutive prospective series of 63 patients in Helsinki (Karhunen, 1991). Operative vascular complications occurred in 28 (44%) of the cases, with massive intraoperative bleeding resulting from rupture of the aneurysm or adjacent major artery during dissection or clip application in 16 (25%). Clip-induced obstruction of cerebral arteries was detected in seven cases (11%), and in six of the patients, an adjacent cerebral vessel was inadvertently clipped. In one case, kinking of the clip caused obstruction of the right ACA, resulting in a frontal infarct. In another case, intraoperative rupture of the ICA and inadvertent ligation of the left PICA occurred during attempted clipping of a ruptured basilar aneurysm. Other types of complications occurred in four cases (6%) and included slippage of the aneurysm clip with subsequent rebleeding, clipping of an unruptured aneurysm instead of the ruptured one, and displacement of the clip beneath the ruptured aneurysm. Operations on ruptured basilar artery aneurysms were significantly more prone to complications than operations on aneurysms in other locations.

Aneurysm size is not necessarily a poor prognostic factor in patients with aneurysmal SAH. In a series of 35 patients with a giant aneurysm of the anterior circulation treated surgically, complete obliteration of the aneurysm was achieved in 34 cases (97%) and patency of all parent arteries in 30 cases (86%) without revascularization (Gewirtz and Awad, 1996). Overall mortality was 6% in the surgical cohort, with good or excellent clinical outcome in 71%. Mortality and poor outcome occurred exclusively in the setting of recent hemorrhage.

As with other highly technical procedures, such as coronary artery bypass surgery outcomes of aneurysm surgery might be expected to vary with the volume of surgery. Indeed, in a study from New York, there was a 43% reduction in mortality rate in hospitals performing more than 30 craniotomies per year for cerebral aneurysm compared with hospitals performing less surgery (8.8% versus 15.5%) (Solomon et al., 1996).

In the sections above, we commented on several changes in the management of patients with ruptured aneurysms, including a switch to earlier surgery and a more aggressive treatment of vasospasm. That such factors lead to an improvement in outcome can be shown by the results over time at several individual institutions. For example, Moriyama et al. (1995a) reported a retrospective analysis of 571 patients with aneurysmal SAH evaluated by means of Glasgow Outcome Scale 6 months after the ictus. Over a 30-year period, patients in good clinical condition at follow-up increased from 8.7% to 60.7%, and mortality decreased from 28.7% to 10.7%. Elderly (over 70 years old) patients were evaluated separately (Moriyama et al., 1995b), and although the results were not as dramatic, these patients also had an improvement in prognosis over time, particularly with respect to the poorest grades. Similarly, Maurice-Williams and Kitchen (1994) noted that over four successive 100-patient cohorts, 1-year overall management mortality decreased steadily from 38% to 24%, and 1-year surgical mortality decreased from 19% to 3%. Simultaneously, the percentage of patients with excellent outcome (Glasgow Outcome Score 5 at 1 year) rose from 73% to 90%. Because neither the population nor the surgical timing changed during this period, the authors attributed the improved results to increased surgical experience.

An improvement in results over several years in Seattle, Washington, was attributed to improvements in critical-care techniques and the improved management of vasospasm by Le Roux et al. (1995). These authors observed a significant increase in the number of favorable outcomes: 74.5% of patients treated during the first management period (1983–1987), 87% of patients treated during the second period (1987–1990), and 93.5% of patients treated during the third management period (1990–1993) experienced favorable outcomes.

Several groups analyzed their results by location of the aneurysm. Of particular interest to neuro-ophthalmologists is that patients with paraclinoid aneurysms tend to have a good prognosis. Of 87 patients with such aneurysms reviewed by Batjer et al. (1994), surgery resulted in a good outcome in 77 (86.5%), fair in eight (9%), and poor in three (3%). Only one patient died. Surgical clipping of an aneurysm in contact with the optic nerve can lead to recovery of vision even if the patient was completely without light perception preoperatively (Tajima et al., 1993).

As general rule, patients with posterior fossa aneurysms have a worse prognosis than patients with aneurysms arising from the ICA and its branches. Nevertheless, in a series of 49 cases from Sweden, good overall management outcomes at 6 months were achieved in 30 cases (61%), with a mortality of 27%, even though 69% of patients were grade III–V on admission and one-third were over 60 years old (Hillman et al., 1996).

Several authors have focused on the postoperative results in patients with poor preoperative neurologic function (Hunt and Hess grades IV and V). In a retrospective study of 159 patients, favorable outcome (assessed by the Glasgow Outcome Scale) occurred in 53.9% of Hunt and Hess Grade IV, and in 24.1% of Grade V patients (Le Roux et al., 1996). Outcome was largely determined by the initial hemorrhage and subsequent development of intractable intracranial hypertension or cerebral infraction. It was emphasized that in spite of the morbidity, a significant percentage of patients did well, arguing against withholding therapy even in the poorest grade patients. Similar results were reported by Spetzger and Gilsbach (1994), who found that overall outcome was favorable in 41 of 76 (54%) poor-grade patients, with a mortality of 28%.

The age of a patient may affect the outcome of surgery for a ruptured aneurysm. According to Stachniak et al. (1996), mortality increases with age, although the duration of hospitalization, numbers of procedures and complications in the surgical intensive care unit (SICU), number of days in the SICU and the hospital, costs for SICU and ward care, total cost (SICU plus ward costs), the Acute Physiology and Chronic Health Evaluation (APACHE) II score at admission and discharge, the Hunt-Hess grade at admission and immediately preoperatively, and the quality of life score do not. The authors of this study concluded that treatment for aneurysmal SAH should not be withheld because of age, and this was also the opinion of Fridriksson et al. (1995), who found that two-thirds of 76 patients aged 70–74 years returned to independent living in good mental condition after clipping of a ruptured aneurysm. Among matched patients who were refused surgery because of age, 75% suffered morbidity and mortality, with more than half of the patients dying within

the first 3 months. In another series of patients over 60, 81 patients with good a neurologic grade underwent surgery for a ruptured aneurysm, and six patients underwent surgery for a symptomatic unruptured aneurysm (O'Sullivan et al., 1994a). The surgical mortality was 1.1%, and a favorable outcome at discharge was achieved in 83.9% of patients. These results contrasted with those of 21 unoperated patients who had a mortality of 47.6% and a favorable outcome at discharge in only 38.1%. Mortality was even higher (68.6%) in 51 patients who did not undergo angiography, although this was a retrospective study, and it is likely the patients who did not undergo angiography were deemed too ill to do so. Nevertheless, it seems clear from available data that elderly patients with a ruptured intracranial aneurysm may achieve a good neurologic outcome, even when their preoperative neurologic status is poor.

Surgery for a ruptured aneurysm should not be withheld because a patient has evidence of infection by the human immunodeficiency virus (HIV) or has AIDS. Five of six HIV-positive patients with aneurysmal SAH did well with at least 1 year follow-up after clipping (Maniker and Hunt, 1996). These patients had no higher incidence of postoperative infections or other complications than did patients without HIV infection operated by the same group of surgeons.

Late complications of otherwise successfully treated aneurysms includes a low frequency of rerupture. This almost always occurs in patients who are incompletely treated because of a slipped clip, incomplete clipping leaving a residual neck, or wrapping or other reinforcement procedures. The frequency of late rebleed in patients incompletely treated is the same as in untreated patients (Kamitani et al., 1995). Although wrapping, coating, and incomplete clipping procedures provide some protection against rebleeding in the first 6 months, they provide little or no protection in the period extending beyond 5 years after surgery.

Even when the results of aneurysm surgery are "good," patients are often left with significant morbidity. This morbidity may be difficult to quantify. For example, neuropsychiatric disturbances and disturbances in mentation are present in many patients following an aneurysmal SAH, even when the patients otherwise seem to be doing well. In a sample of 20 patients who had intracranial aneurysm surgery, 13 had a "good recovery," but 18 had evidence of some neuropsychiatric impairment (Beristain et al., 1996). Thus, the Karnofsky Scale and Glasgow Outcome Scale may not be sufficiently sensitive to detect residual cognitive or psychologic impairment. Irle et al. (1992) reported disturbances of memory in 25% of patients after repair of a ruptured anterior communicating artery aneurysm, and Hutter et al. (1995) found cognitive deficits in visual short-term memory (46%) and in the three parameters of a reaction-time task ranging from 31 to 65% in patients after surgery to treat a ruptured aneurysm. Hutter et al. (1995) also found deficits in verbal long-term memory (28%), concentration (5–13%), and language (11%). The quality of life was reduced in the SAH patients according to a self-rating scale in motivation (50%), interests (47%), mental capacity (47%), free-time activities (52%), social relationships (39%), concentration (70%), fine motor co-ordination

(25%), and sleep (47%). Frequent headaches were reported by 77% of the patients, and depression was found in 30% of the patients. Life satisfaction was significantly reduced in 37% of the patients, whereas 48% suffered from increased emotional lability, and in 41%, motivation was significantly reduced. Negative job consequences, such as loss of a job or demotion, were reported by 16% of the patients investigated, and an additional 15% had retired. Tidswell et al. (1995) also found impairment in executive functions and some aspects of memory in comparison with normative data in a series of 37 patients following aneurysmal clipping. Overall, 65% of the patients were impaired in at least one cognitive domain, with 19% showing executive impairments alone, 14% showing memory impairments alone, and 32% showing deficits in both domains. In another prospective study of memory, however, the grade at discharge proved to be the best predictor of impairment of cognition and memory at follow-up assessments (Ogden et al., 1993). Older subjects did not recover to the same extent as younger subjects by the 12-month assessment. Aneurysm site was not shown to be associated with performance on any test at any time, and the other complications of SAH had only minimal predictive value. Despite excellent clinical results, Deruty et al. (1994) found that only 67% of patients had resumed their previous activity at the same level. Some of the difference in outcome may be related to the size of the ruptured aneurysm. Rosenorn and Eskeson (1994) found that after 2 years, more patients with small- and medium-sized ruptured aneurysms had resumed their previous occupation (49% versus 34%), regained a normal daily functional capacity (55% vs 44%), and had a normal mental status (29% and 32%, respectively, versus 23%) than patients with large aneurysms that were treated following rupture.

On rare occasions, rerupture occurs from a previously clipped aneurysm. In most cases, this is related to a malpositioned or slipped clip (Giannotta and Litofsky, 1995). Reoperation on patients in whom this complication occurs generally produces good results. In a series of 20 patients in whom rerupture of an aneurysm occurred despite clipping of the responsible aneurysm, only two patients had moderate disability and one severe disability after a second operation (Giannotta and Litofsky, 1995).

Endovascular Surgical Results

Initially utilized only in patients considered inoperable (van Rooij et al., 1996) or in patients with giant (Casasco et al., 1992) or incompletely clipped aneurysms (Fraser et al., 1994), endovascular surgical approaches are being widely employed (Fig. 53.224). Several centers utilize endovascular surgery routinely in all aneurysms of the posterior circulation; others in selected cases. In comparing the results of series among institutions, it is important to recognize the preoperative status of the patient (including the clinical grade following hemorrhage), the location of the aneurysm, and the presence of vasospasm. As a rule, patients in endovascular series tend to be admitted with delay, severe vasospasm, a poor Hunt and Hess grading, and involvement of the vertebrobasilar arterial network (Marchal et al., 1996).

Endovascular techniques can be used to treat acutely bleeding aneurysms. Although the initial applications involved balloons to occlude parent vessels or trap the aneurysm, coils are most often used to occlude and thrombose a ruptured aneurysm (Teitelbaum et al., 1995b; Raymond et al., 1997; Vinuela et al., 1997). Such treatment can produce excellent results. Casasco et al. (1993) reported that of 71 intracranial aneurysms treated by placement of minicoils inside the aneurysmal sac, outcome was good in 84.5% at 1 year, with morbidity and mortality rates of 4.2% and 11.3%, respectively. In this series, 29 aneurysms were in the anterior circulation, and 42 were in the posterior circulation. Vinuela et al. (1997) treated 403 patients with ruptured intracranial aneurysms within 15 days of acute SAH using Guglielmi detachable coils. Fifty-seven percent of the aneurysms were in the posterior circulation, and 43% were in the anterior circulation. Complete occlusion of the aneurysm was achieved in 71% of aneurysms with a small neck, 35% of large aneurysms, and 50% of giant aneurysms. A small neck remnant was observed in 21% of small aneurysms with a small neck, 57% of large aneurysms, and 50% of giant aneurysms. There was an 8.9% immediate morbidity rate related to the technique. Technical complications included aneurysm perforation in 2.7% of cases, unintentional parent artery occlusion in 3%, and untoward cerebral embolization in 2.5%. Seven deaths (1.7%) were related to technical complications.

Because of the high morbidity associated with a direct surgical approach to aneurysms at the tip of the basilar artery, it is not surprising that some of the first endovascular series addressed basilar tip aneurysms (Fig. 53.212). In a series from University of California San Francisco, treatment with electrolytically detachable coils resulted in complete aneurysm occlusion in seven of 33 patients (21.2%) (McDougall et al., 1996). In 17 of the patients (51.5%), greater than 90% but less than 100% aneurysm occlusion was achieved. Angiographically, four of 19 (21%) aneurysms were 100% occluded, and 12 of 19 (63.2%) were more than 90% but less than 100% occluded. One patient experienced major permanent morbidity from thrombosis of the basilar tip region a few hours after coil placement, and one treated patient experienced further hemorrhage 6 months later. Raymond et al. (1997) treated 31 patients with ruptured and unruptured aneurysms of the basilar bifurcation. Technical complications occurred in seven patients. Most were asymptomatic, but one patient died after aneurysm rupture during treatment, and one had residual diplopia at 4 months. Six months after treatment, repeat angiography revealed complete obliteration of the aneurysm in only 42% of cases.

There is a similarly low morbidity and mortality from embolization with aneurysms in other locations but also a similar high rate of incomplete occlusion. In a series of 50 patients, complete embolization of the aneurysms was thought to have been achieved in 100% of small, 95% of large, and 85% of giant aneurysms, but follow-up angiography of 42 aneurysms demonstrated some degree of refilling in 17% of small, 19% of large, and 50% of giant aneurysms (Byrne et al., 1995a). As noted above, among 403 patients with ruptured aneurysms treated by coil embolization by

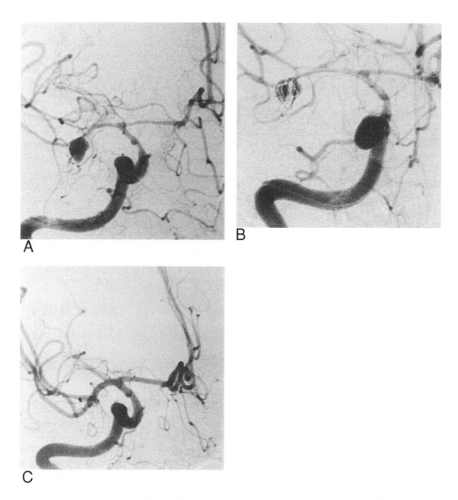

Figure 53.224. Treatment of ruptured aneurysm complicated by vasospasm using thrombogeneic coils. *A*, Digital subtraction angiogram demonstrates an aneurysm arising from the right middle cerebral artery with vasospasm affecting the supraclinoid segment of the right internal carotid and the proximal segments of the right anterior and middle cerebral arteries. *B*, Digital subtraction angiogram during placement of thrombogenic coils. *C*, Follow-up angiogram 8 months after treatment demonstrating complete recovery of vascular lumenal diameter with resolution of vasospasm and a complete occlusion of the previously noted middle cerebral artery aneurysm. (From Byrne JV, Molyneux AJ, Brennan RP, et al. Endosaccular treatment of inoperable intracranial aneurysms with platinum coils. J Neurol Neurosurg Psychiatry *59*:616–620, 1995.)

Vinuela et al. (1997), complete occlusion of the aneurysm was achieved in 71% of aneurysms with a small neck, 35% of large aneurysms, and 50% of giant aneurysms. A small neck remnant was observed in 21% of small aneurysms with a small neck, 57% of large aneurysms, and 50% of giant aneurysms.

Incomplete occlusions using detachable balloons or coils are worrisome, because histopathologic studies demonstrate that without total occlusion and thrombosis, endothelialization does not take place (Molyneux et al., 1995). In addition, in a study in pigs, three of four incompletely occluded aneurysms ruptured during the follow-up period (Byrne et al., 1994). Experimentally, Guglielmi detachable coils induce a cellular response within several hours of aneurysm occlusion (Tenjin et al., 1995). By 2 weeks after coil placement, endothelialization can be demonstrated, and by 3 months remodeling of the aneurysm has progressed to produce a media-like structure in the former aneurysm, associated with a minimal inflammatory reaction (Mawad et al., 1995).

Even with incomplete occlusion of ruptured aneurysms using endovascular techniques results in a significant reduction in the rate of rebleeding. Graves et al. (1995) reported no rebleeding in 13 patients following coil occlusion, three of whom had incomplete occlusion, over a mean follow-up period of 16 months (range, 6–36 month). This is lower than expected for untreated patients. Patient outcome, as measured by the Glasgow Outcome Scale, was good in nine of 13 patients (69%) and poor in only one of 13 patients (8%), with death in three of 13 (23%) patients. Meisel et al. (1995) reported subsequent aneurysmal growth in only one of eight patients occluded with Guglielmi detachable coils. This is interesting because the rebleed rates in patients with incomplete surgical occlusion seem to be the same as if they were untreated (Kamitani et al., 1995).

A number of complications can occur with endovascular surgery for ruptured (as well as unruptured) intracranial aneurysms. Besides inability to occlude the aneurysm, these include intraoperative aneurysm rerupture, distal coil or balloon migration or embolization, and parent-artery occlusion or progressive thrombosis. Balloon occlusion seems to have a significantly higher rate of complications than the use of detachable coils. Following balloon occlusion, thrombosis may extend beyond the desired confines. If recognized early, this can be treated with thrombolytics. In a case of basilar artery thrombosis after endovascular occlusion of a recently ruptured wide-necked basilar apex aneurysm with a nondetachable silicone balloon, prompt thrombolytic therapy prevented a potentially disastrous outcome (Kwan et al., 1995).

Coils are not completely free of risk. In one patient with a basilar artery aneurysm, the aneurysmal wall was perforated during coil packing (angiographically demonstrated contrast-medium extravasation), but this remained "clinically asymptomatic" (Reul et al., 1995). Wantanabe et al. (1995) reported retrieving a migrated detachable coil using a snare type endovascular retrieving device, and Standard et al. (1994) retrieved a fractured Guglielmi detachable coil using a dual guidewire technique.

Cellulose acetate polymer has been developed for use as a thrombotic material (Mandai et al., 1992a) and is advocated as an emergency means of treating acutely bleeding aneurysms (Kinugasa et al., 1992, 1994b). In experimental animals, injection of the polymer was capable of completely thrombosing an aneurysm with subsequent endothelialization of the former aneurysmal orifice (Sugiu et al., 1995). Overfilling of the aneurysm, however, caused parent artery occlusion in three of 24 experimental aneurysms. There was incomplete occlusion of five aneurysms possibly associated with persistent risk of rupture (although this did not occur). Kinugasa et al. (1994b) utilized cellulose acetate polymer to acutely thrombose aneurysms in 12 patients with Hunt and Hess neurologic Grades III–V. Subsequent aggressive therapy with TPA allowed clipping of seven partially thrombosed aneurysms and five multiple aneurysms during delayed surgery. Eight patients improved clinically and had a good recovery, two had severe disability, and two died.

FUSIFORM ANEURYSMS (ARTERIAL ECTASIA, DOLICHOECTASIA)

GENERAL CONSIDERATIONS

Large arteries of the carotid and vertebrobasilar systems may occasionally become enlarged and tortuous (Fig. 53.225). This process is called by a variety of names, the most common of which are **dolichoectasia** (from the Greek words *dolichos,* meaning "elongation," and *ectasia,* meaning "distension"), **ectasia**, and **fusiform aneurysm** (Smoker et al., 1986). Some authors simply describe such arteries as "tortuous" (Kerber et al., 1972; Rao and Woodlief, 1979).

The intracranial arteries most commonly affected by fusiform aneurysms or dolichoectasia are the three largest: the internal carotid, the vertebral, and the basilar. Other large arteries that originate from these vessels, particularly the anterior cerebral, middle cerebral, posterior cerebral, and anterior communicating arteries, may also be affected in rare patients (Hopkins and Poser, 1973; Scotti, 1974; Eldevik and Gabrielsen, 1975; Coppeto and Hoffman, 1981; Goldstein and Tibbs, 1981; Little et al., 1981; Massey et al.,

1984; Nakasu et al., 1984; Blumenkopf and Huggins, 1985; Tamura et al., 1985; Shigemori et al., 1988; Atkinson et al., 1993).

Many investigators believe that dolichoectasia results from atherosclerosis (Svien and Peserico, 1959; Hayes et al., 1967; Waberzinek et al., 1971; Schindler and Hase, 1973; Nijensohn et al., 1974; Moseley and Holland, 1979; Yu et al., 1982); however, in some cases, there is no evidence of atherosclerosis, even on histopathologic investigation (Ley, 1950; Greitz and Löfstedt, 1954; Hultén-Gyllensten et al., 1959; Bergaust, 1963; Shokunbi et al., 1988). In addition, arterial ectasia occasionally is found in children who have no evidence of atherosclerosis (Sacks and Lindenberg, 1969; Ferry et al., 1974; Johnson et al., 1977; Little et al., 1981, 1986) and in patients with other disorders characterized by mesodermal dysgenesis, such as von Recklinghausen's neurofibromatosis (NF-1) (Frank et al., 1989; Muhonen et al., 1991; Benatar, 1994) and FMD (Belen et al., 1996). Malig-

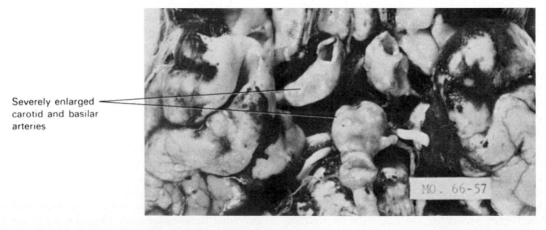

Severely enlarged carotid and basilar arteries

Figure 53.225. View of the base of the brain in a patient with diffuse ectasia (*dolichoectasia*) of the supraclinoid portion of both internal carotid arteries and the basilar artery. (From Lindenberg R, Walsh FB, Sacks JG. Neuropathology of Vision: An Atlas. Philadelphia, Lea & Febiger, 1973.)

nant cells weakening the vessel wall can also produce fusiform dilatation (Mori et al., 1990; Iihara et al., 1991; Hung et al., 1992; Friedman and Rapoport, 1996; Komeichi et al., 1996). Moriyama et al. (1992) published the case of a 51-year-old woman who developed multiple fusiform aneurysms within the ports of 50 Gy irradiation delivered after resection of a pituitary adenoma. Infectious causes may also lead to fusiform dilation. Masago et al. (1992) and Takeshita et al. (1992) reported fusiform aneurysms in the setting of aspergillosis. There is a single case report of multiple giant fusiform aneurysms in a patient with lymphomatoid granulomatosis (Capone et al., 1994), and Lang et al. (1992) reported an HIV-positive 8-year-old with multiple fusiform aneurysms. Sutton (1994) reported fusiform dilation of one or both ICAs in 11 patients previously operated for craniopharyngioma. Presumably the walls of the affected arteries were weakened by previous surgery. None of these patients developed symptoms, and all were followed without intervention. Because of these findings, some investigators believe that atherosclerosis plays little (Hassler, 1961; Waberzinek et al., 1971) or no (Ley, 1950; Boeri and Passerini, 1964) role in the pathogenesis of arterial ectasia.

The studies of Hegedüs (1985) seem to support this latter view. This investigator performed histopathologic examinations of ectatic arteries and arteries from patients with advanced atherosclerosis, including 40 arteries from which a saccular aneurysm arose. She found that defects in the elastic lamina and deficiency of reticular fibers in the muscular layer were common pathologic features in ectatic basilar arteries and in arteries with saccular aneurysm, but that such abnormalities were more conspicuous in ectatic arteries. In other atherosclerotic arteries sampled from patients with neither saccular aneurysm nor ectasia, the density of reticular fibers in the media was preserved. Hegedüs (1985) therefore concluded that atherosclerosis may not play a basic role in the pathogenesis of arterial ectasia, but that a severe deficiency of reticular fibers in the media associated with extensive defects in the elastic lamina is the cause of this condition (Fig. 53.226). The cause of the deficiency of reticular fibers is unknown, but it does not seem to be caused by either aging or atherosclerosis. The process has been ascribed, therefore, to an inborn error of collagen metabolism.

Rigamonti et al. (1994) reported the results of an experimental study in which he and his colleagues produced fusiform arterial dilation in white rabbits injected with porcine elastase. They postulated the importance of the elastic lamellae for the maintenance of tubular shape and length of the carotid artery and its possible pathophysiologic role in dolichoectasia.

Whatever the cause of arterial ectasia, the result is that an affected vessel undergoes thinning of its walls with replacement of normal elastic and reticular fibers by fibrous tissue. The vessel increases in length and becomes tortuous. Its lumen may dilate from thinning of the wall, or it may become narrowed by subsequent intimal proliferation. Blood pressure may play a contributory role. Of 15 patients reported by Okada et al. (1994) with megadolichobasilar anomalies, 12 had severe hypertension.

Ectatic and dolichoectatic arteries behave quite differently

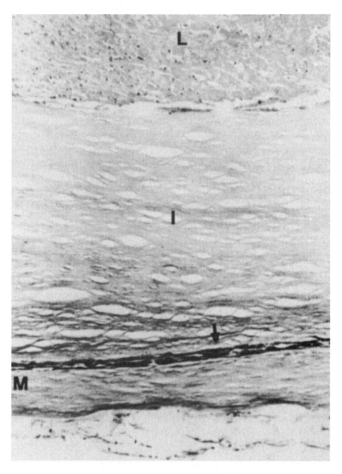

Figure 53.226. Histopathology of an ectatic intracranial artery. Reticular fibers are absent in the muscular layer (*M*), and they have a tendency to change into collagen fibers in the thickened intima (*I*). *Arrow* indicates the elastic lamina. *L*, lumen of vessel. (From Hededüs K. Ectasia of the basilar artery with special reference to possible pathogenesis. Surg Neurol 24: 463–469, 1985.)

from saccular aneurysms. They do not arise from arterial bifurcations, almost always become symptomatic in middle-aged or elderly patients, are frequently calcified, and tend to be quite large. Most importantly, about 90% of saccular aneurysms first become symptomatic when they rupture, whereas fusiform aneurysms rarely cause SAH. Instead, they produce neurologic symptoms and signs by direct pressure on adjacent neural tissue (particularly cranial nerves), by impairment of circulation in adjacent neural tissue from direct compression of smaller feeding arteries and arterioles, by obliteration of nutrient vessels derived from the diseased artery, and by giving rise to emboli. In a series of 120 posterior fossa fusiform aneurysms reported by Drake and Peerless (1997), 50% presented with mass effect, 20% with hemorrhage, and 6% with TIAs.

Rupture of fusiform aneurysms may occur, however. This is particularly true of aneurysms involving the vertebral arteries. Andoh et al. (1992a) reviewed their experience with 38 aneurysms of the vertebral artery, of which 10 (38%) were fusiform. All 10 of the fusiform aneurysms eventually ruptured, producing SAH.

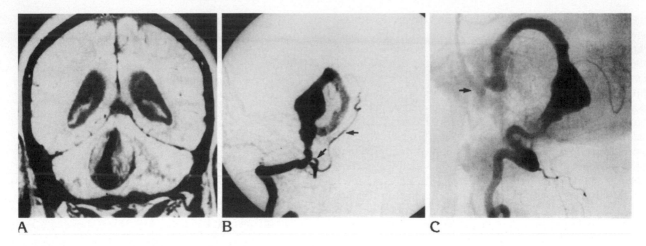

Figure 53.227. Giant serpentine (fusiform) aneurysm creating mass effect. *A*, T1-weighted coronal magnetic resonance image demonstrates a large midline posterior fossa mass of heterogeneous signal intensity representing thrombus of various age. *B*, Digital subtraction angiogram, anteroposterior view, demonstrates ectatic vascular channel involving the vertebral artery distal to the posterior inferior cerebellar artery (PICA) (*arrows*). *C*, Digital subtraction angiogram, lateral view, demonstrates the same ectatic fusiform aneurysm involving the intracranial vertebral artery originating just distal to the PICA and ending at its junction to form the basilar artery (From Aletich VA, Debrun GM, Monsein LH, et al. Giant serpentine aneurysms: A review and presentation of five cases. AJNR *16*:1061–1072, 1995.)

The specific symptoms and signs produced by ectatic arteries are related to their location, size, and extent (see Appendix 2). Thrombus may form within the lumen of a fusiform aneurysm leading to distal embolization and associated transient or permanent neurologic sequelae. When thrombosed, they may mimic intracranial tumors. This is particularly true of a subset of fusiform aneurysms called **giant serpentine aneurysms** (Aletich et al., 1995; Mawad and Klucznik, 1995) (Fig. 53.227).

The treatment of fusiform aneurysms is also different from that of saccular aneurysms (Little et al., 1981). Because fusiform aneurysms have no neck, they cannot be clipped. Surgical treatment, when appropriate, nevertheless is directed toward isolating the aneurysm from the intracranial circulation. In some cases, the ectatic region may be excised without permanent neurologic deficit (Segal and McLaurin, 1977). This is particularly true when the process affects a branch of the MCA. In many cases, however, excision or trapping of the aneurysm produces severe permanent neurologic deficits. In other cases, the affected artery is ligated proximal to the lesion (Bhushan et al., 1978; Little et al., 1981), or the vessel is occluded using an inflatable balloon (Weir, 1987; Higashida et al., 1989; Makita et al., 1993). Detachable thrombogenic coils can also be utilized to occlude a dolichoectatic vessel. Their advantage over a detachable balloon includes occlusion of a shorter segment of normal artery, no traction on the parent vessel, and possibly safer and easier catheterization techniques (Gobin et al. 1996). With feeding artery occlusion, a bypass procedure may be used to provide blood flow to the territory normally supplied by the occluded vessel. A distal clip combined with an STA-MCA bypass procedure may permit the obliteration of the aneurysm by retrograde clot progression (Horowitz et al., 1994); however, in some cases, the collateral flow provided by the revascularization procedure allows the aneurysm to continue to enlarge (Isla et al., 1994).

In patients who cannot tolerate loss of distal flow in the parent vessel of a fusiform aneurysm, the involved arterial segment may be reconstructed. Sometimes this is possible with an end-to-end anastomosis. Ikeda et al. (1991b) were able to reconstruct a PICA after excising the aneurysmal segment. In other cases, a venous interpositional graft may be used. Lee and Sekhar (1996) described removal of a fusiform MCA aneurysm and reconstructing the wall with a saphenous vein. In still other cases, the aneurysm can be wrapped or mobilized to decompress adjacent neural tissue. Fujitsu et al. (1994) described the use of a dacron mesh silastic sheet to reinforce a fusiform aneurysm that they reconstructed using aneurysm clips. The sheet may be tailored to avoid impinging on the surrounding cranial nerves or perforating vessels.

Dealing with dolichoectatic aneurysms of the basilar is a major challenge. However, proximal endovascular balloon occlusion may produce long-term satisfactory results (Aymard et al., 1992).

Anson et al. (1996) reviewed the experience of the Barrow Neurological Institute in treating a series of 40 patients with 41 fusiform or dolichoectatic aneurysms. Surgical procedures included direct clipping, trapping with bypass, proximal occlusion, resection with reanastomosis, transposition, aneurysmorrhaphy with thrombectomy, and wrapping. There was no surgical mortality, and the outcome at late follow-up was good (Glasgow Outcome Scale scores 1–2) in 78% of patients, although the patients with posterior circulation aneurysms did not do as well as those with anterior circulation aneurysms. Cardiopulmonary bypass, hypothermic circulatory arrest, and barbiturate cerebral protection are often utilized during resection of large fusiform aneurysms (Greene et al., 1994).

Medical therapy using antiplatelet drugs or anticoagulants may prevent permanent neurologic damage from emboli in selected patients with fusiform aneurysms (Nishizaki et al., 1986; Echiverri et al., 1989). Other patients with specific neurologic symptoms may benefit from medical therapy. Martins and Ferro (1989), for example, described a patient with severe atypical facial pain thought to be caused by a dolichoectatic basilar artery in whom baclofen produced complete pain relief.

An exciting potential treatment of fusiform aneurysms is the endovascular placement of support. Wakhloo et al. (1994) published their experience in placement of balloon-expandable tantalum and self-expanding nitinol stents in 14 dogs after creation of experimentally constructed aneurysms. Compromise of the lumen of the parent vessel occurred in some animals, with subtotal and complete thrombosis in two. Massoud et al. (1995) reported the UCLA experience with arterial stents and detachable coils in treating experimentally created fusiform aneurysms in swine. Recognizing the importance of maintaining intact perforators originating from the aneurysm, they attempted to locally pack uninvolved segments of the aneurysm with thrombus inducing coils. Technical difficulties remain.

CLINICAL MANIFESTATIONS, TREATMENT, AND PROGNOSIS ACCORDING TO SITE

Fusiform Aneurysms of the Internal Carotid Artery and Its Branches

Dolichoectasia of the intracranial portions of the ICAs and their branches may be asymptomatic, or it may cause a variety of symptoms and signs that are related to the location and extent of the condition (Blumenkopf and Huggins, 1985; Braunsdorf, 1987; Unsöld, 1989a, 1989b). Thus, dolichoectasia of the petrous portion of the ICA may produce lower cranial neuropathies, whereas dolichoectasia of the intracavernous portion of the artery can enlarge the sella turcica and simulate a pituitary tumor (Anderson, 1976), causing diplopia that often is painful (Fig. 53.228). Little et al. (1981) described two patients with unilateral abducens paresis caused by a fusiform aneurysm of the intracavernous portion of the ICA. A 43-year-old woman with a 3-year history of progressive diplopia was noted to have weakness of abduction of the right eye that was associated with an esotropia of 35 prism diopters (Miller, 1991h). Before her examination in the Neuro-ophthalmology Unit at the Johns Hopkins Hospital, she had undergone several CT scans, several lumbar punctures, numerous serologic studies, and MR imaging. These studies were all unremarkable except that MR imaging, which was of poor quality, suggested a lesion in the cavernous sinus. An isolated right abducens nerve paresis was diagnosed and repeat MR imaging was obtained, which showed a tortuous, enlarged intracavernous portion of the right ICA. An arteriogram confirmed this finding. The patient subsequently underwent strabismus surgery that eliminated her diplopia. Pritz (1994b) reported the rare case of a nontraumatic fusiform aneurysm of the cavernous portion of the ICA that presented with epistaxis from a small rupture.

As early as the 19th century, investigators observed that ectasia affecting the supraclinoid portion of the ICA had potentially severe effects on the adjacent optic nerves and

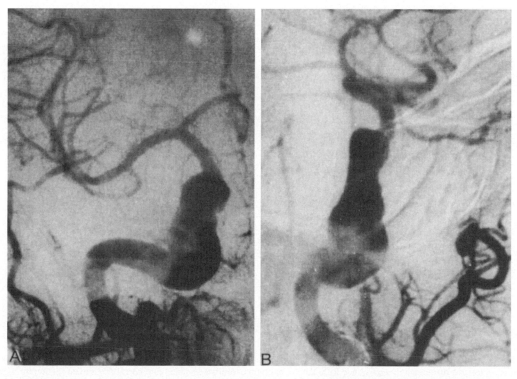

Figure 53.228. Dolichoectasia of the petrous and cavernous segments of the internal carotid artery in a patient who developed a painful oculmotor nerve paresis. The internal carotid artery was ligated, after which the patient's pain and paresis resolved.

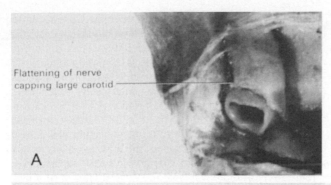

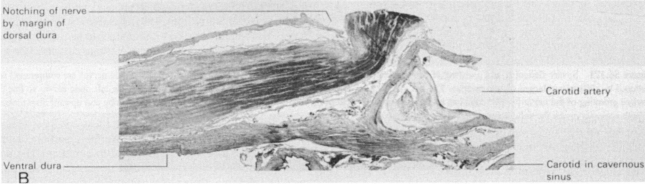

Flattening of nerve capping large carotid

Notching of nerve by margin of dorsal dura

Carotid artery

Ventral dura

Carotid in cavernous sinus

Figure 53.229.   Dolichoectasia of the supraclinoid portion of the left internal carotid artery causing flattening and upward displacement of the left optic nerve against the dural fold overlying the optic canal. *A*, Gross view shows flattening and upward displacement of the nerve by the enlarged carotid artery. *B*, Longitudinal section through the right optic nerve shows its upward displacement by the enlarged artery. Note notching and atrophy of the nerve by the superior dural fold that normally overhangs the intracranial end of the optic canal. (From Lindenberg R, Walsh FB, Sacks JG. Neuropathology of Vision: An Atlas. Philadelphia, Lea & Febiger, 1973.)

chiasm (Liebrecht, 1901). The ipsilateral optic nerve frequently was flattened by the diffusely enlarged sclerotic artery that often compressed the nerve against the dural fold overlying the superior portion of the intracranial end of the optic canal (Figs. 53.229–53.232). Histologic examination

of affected nerves showed patchy loss of myelin and reduction of axons. These original studies were purely anatomic; however, Knapp (1932, 1940) subsequently reported several patients who had nasal and altitudinal field defects associated with optic disc cupping and who were found to have

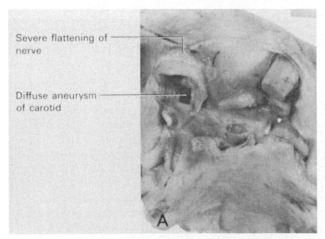

Severe flattening of nerve

Diffuse aneurysm of carotid

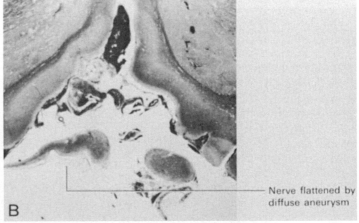

Nerve flattened by diffuse aneurysm

Figure 53.230.   Flattening of the left optic nerve by a dolichoectatic carotid artery. *A*, The nerve has been reduced to a thin sheet of tissue by the diffusely enlarged carotid artery. Note the difference in appearance from the normal right carotid artery and optic nerve. *B*, Coronal section through the intracranial portions of both optic nerves in the same case shows that the left optic nerve is flat and atrophic, whereas the right optic nerve has a normal shape and consistency. (From Lindenberg R, Walsh FB, Sacks JG. Neuropathology of Vision: An Atlas. Philadelphia, Lea & Febiger, 1973.)

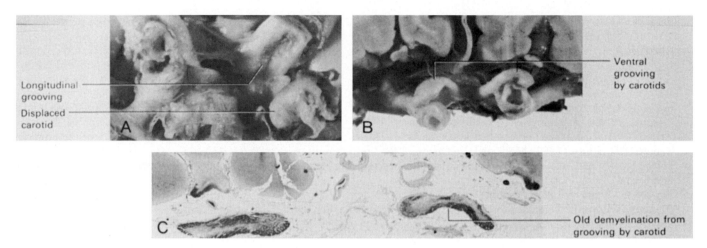

Figure 53.231. Severe flattening and grooving of both optic nerves by dolichoectatic internal carotid arteries. *A,* Both optic nerves are compressed and flattened by diffusely enlarged carotid arteries. The left carotid artery has been displaced away from the undersurface of the left optic nerve, so that the marked grooving of the nerve by the vessel can be seen. *B,* Coronal view of the nerves in the same case shows marked thinning and upward displacement of both optic nerves by the enlarged, ectatic vessels. Note ventral grooving of the nerves. *C,* Histopathologic transverse sections through both optic nerves shows thinning and demyelination caused by chronic compression by dolichoectatic carotid arteries. (From Lindenberg R, Walsh FB, Sacks JG. Neuropathology of Vision: An Atlas. Philadelphia, Lea & Febiger, 1973.)

dolichoectatic ICAs. Knapp (1932, 1940) suggested that the visual symptoms and signs in these patients with "soft" or "low-tension" glaucoma might be caused either from direct compression of the intracranial portion of the optic nerve by an ectatic, sclerotic ICA or by obliteration of the small nutrient vessels supplying the optic nerves and chiasm and originating from the affected portion of the ICA.

McLean and Ray (1947) reported the case of a 61-year-old man who was told in 1935 that he had glaucoma, although his intraocular pressures were consistently less than 20 mm IIg. In 1939, he underwent an iridectomy because of an increasing field defect. At that time, visual acuity was 20/20 OD and 1/200 OS. After the iridectomy, the patient continued to lose visual acuity and visual field in both eyes, although at no time did he experience pain or redness of either eye. By December 1945, 10 years after the diagnosis of glaucoma was first made, the patient's visual acuity was 20/70 OD and 3/200 OS. Both visual fields showed substan-

tial superior loss. Intraocular pressure was 22 mm Hg in the right eye and 18 mm Hg in the left eye. Both optic discs were pale, but neither was significantly cupped. The patient underwent craniotomy by Dr. Ray, who observed that both optic nerves appeared atrophic. The nerves were flattened where they crossed the ICAs. Each ICA contained a calcified plaque in its wall directly under the nerve. The plaques could be seen hammering against the optic nerves with each heartbeat. This observation suggested that pulsating pressure of a sclerotic, calcified plaque adjacent to the optic nerve could explain some cases of optic atrophy and might also be responsible for the development of the "soft glaucoma" described by Knapp (1932, 1940).

Schloffer (1934) described a 65-year-old woman who complained of loss of vision in the right eye of 5 years' duration, a recent defect in the field of vision in the left eye, headaches, dizziness, and diplopia. Examination revealed that vision was grossly defective in both eyes. The right

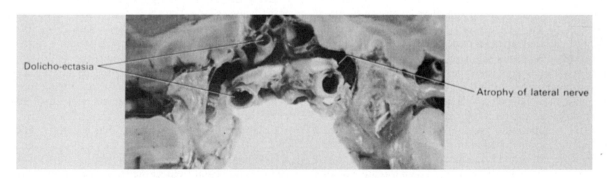

Figure 53.232. Dolichoectasia of the supraclinoid portion of both internal carotid arteries causing flattening and atrophy of both optic nerves. Note that both anterior cerebral arteries are also enlarged. (From Lindenberg R, Walsh FB, Sacks JG. Neuropathology of Vision: An Atlas. Philadelphia, Lea & Febiger, 1973.)

optic disc was pale, and the left was swollen. The patient was thought to have the Foster Kennedy syndrome (see Chapters 8, 10, and 38); however, when a craniotomy was performed, no tumor was found. The patient died, and at necropsy, the intracranial portions of both ICAs adjacent to the optic nerves were enlarged and firm. They were compressing and distorting both optic nerves.

Subsequently, a number of investigators (Glees, 1938; Adson, 1941; Yaskin and Schlezinger, 1942; Tassman, 1944; Taptas, 1948; Ley, 1950; Mitts and McQueen, 1965) reported elderly patients who underwent intracranial exploration because of optic atrophy in one eye and optic disc swelling in the other. In all cases, the features of the Foster Kennedy syndrome were said to be present, but there was always decreased visual acuity in the eye with disc swelling. In no case, was the expected tumor found. Instead, each patient had a fusiform dilation of the intracranial portion of the ICA and sometimes of the ophthalmic artery. Unsöld (1989b) described a 66-year-old woman with a 1-week history of blurred vision, a 2-day history of darkness in front of the left eye, and frontal headaches. Visual acuity was 20/25 OD and 20/100 OS. The visual field of the right eye showed a relative inferior nasal defect (Fig. 53.233A). The visual field of the left eye showed a dense inferior altitudinal defect (Fig. 53.233B). There was a left RAPD. The right optic disc was slightly pale, and the left optic disc was swollen (Fig. 53.233C). Thin-section CT scanning showed dolichoectasia of the left ICA. The patient underwent a craniotomy, at which time the left optic nerve was found to be flattened and pressed up against the dural fold overlying the superior portion of the intracranial end of the optic canal (Fig. 53.233D). The nerve was decompressed. Postoperatively, visual acuity improved to 20/50 OS, the visual field showed minimal improvement (Fig. 53.233E), and the disc swelling resolved (Fig. 53.233F). Unsöld (1989b) did not explain the cause of optic disc pallor in the right eye.

The possible association between dolichoectatic carotid arteries and low-tension glaucoma is intriguing. Stroman et al. (1995) performed a prospective study in which they used high-resolution MR imaging to assess 20 patients with low-tension glaucoma and 20 age-matched control subjects. These investigators found no difference between the two groups in the diameter or length of the intracranial portion of the optic nerves, the cross-sectional area of the supraclinoid portion of the ICAs, or the distance from the intracranial optic nerves to the supraclinoid portion of the ipsilateral ICA. There was, however, a relative decrease in the cross section of the intracranial segment of the optic nerve and an increase in changes consistent with small-vessel ischemia. In a subsequent study, Golnik et al. (1996) found that 20 patients with unexplained optic neuropathy had a statistically closer relationship of the intracranial segment of the optic nerve to the supraclinoid portion of the ipsilateral carotid artery than did age-matched control subjects. These vessels, however, were not dilated. Jacobson et al. (1997) reviewed MR imaging findings in 100 visually asymptomatic patients and determined that there was contact between the intracranial portions of one or both optic nerves and the supraclinoid portion of the ipsilateral ICA in 70% of cases. There ap-

peared to be true compression of one optic nerve by the ipsilateral ICA in five patients and bilateral compression in 12 patients. The estimated odds of compression were significantly increased as the diameter of the supraclinoid portion of the ICA increased. These investigators concluded that supraclinoid ICA contact with the intracranial portion of the optic nerve occurs frequently compared with anatomic compression and that the risk of compression of the optic nerve is directly proportional to the diameter of the supraclinoid portion of the ICA.

Patients with dolichoectasia of the ICAs may lose vision suddenly or in a slow, progressive fashion. Walsh and Hoyt (1969n) described a 58-year-old man who experienced sudden painless loss of vision in the inferior portion of the field of the right eye. One week later, the patient was found to have visual acuity of 20/15 OD and 20/20 OS, associated with complete loss of the lower half of the visual field of the right eye. The visual field of the left eye showed a relative superotemporal defect. The right optic disc was swollen, but the left disc appeared normal. The patient underwent a craniotomy, at which time the right ICA was found to be markedly dilated (Fig. 53.234). The artery elevated the right optic nerve, flattening it and pushing it against the A-1 segment of the right ACA. The left ICA and the left optic nerve appeared normal. The right optic canal was unroofed, but the patient had no return of visual function in either eye. In this case, it is likely that the visual field defect in the right eye was caused not by pressure on the inferior optic nerve from the ectatic ICA, but by pressure on the **superior** portion of the nerve from either the ACA or the dural shelf of the optic canal. The visual field defect in the left eye probably was caused by damage to Wilbrand's knee in the distal portion of the right optic nerve, adjacent to the optic chiasm or to the chiasm itself (see Chapter 4).

Sakaguchi and Hirayama (1985) described a case similar to that reported by Walsh and Hoyt (1969n), except that their patient had no optic disc swelling in either eye. The patient was a 56-year-old woman who had lost almost all vision in the left eye over several days. Six months earlier she had lost visual acuity and superior visual field in the right eye. When she was first examined, the right eye had visual acuity of 20/100 with complete loss of the superior field. The left eye had only bare hand motions vision in a small inferior paracentral island. The right optic disc was normal; the left optic disc was pale. Neuroimaging studies demonstrated ectasia of the intracranial portions of both ICAs. Because of further deterioration of vision in the patient's right eye, craniotomy was performed, at which time both optic nerves were found to be compressed by the ectatic portions of the ICAs. Both optic canals were unroofed. Visual function initially improved in the right eye, but worsened suddenly 3 weeks after surgery.

Colapinto et al. (1996) described a patient who experienced painless loss of vision in the right eye over 2 weeks. An evaluation revealed visual acuity of 20/40 OD and 20/20 OS. The visual field of the right eye was constricted; the visual field of the left eye was normal. The optic discs were normal in appearance. Neuroimaging revealed dolichoectasia of the supraclinoid portion of the right internal carotid

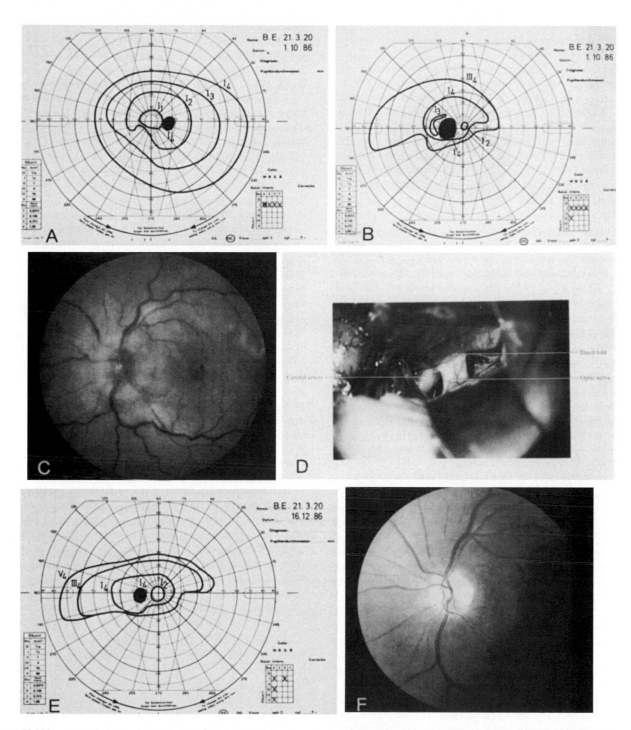

Figure 53.233. Dolichoectasia of the left internal carotid artery causing progressive visual loss and optic disc swelling. The patient was a 66-year-old woman with decreased vision in the left eye and frontal headache. Visual acuity in the right eye was 20/25; visual acuity in the left eye was 20/100. *A*, Right visual field shows a relative inferior nasal defect. *B*, Visual field in the left eye shows a dense inferior altitudinal defect. *C*, The left optic disc is swollen. *D*, View of the left optic nerve at craniotomy shows it to be flattened and displaced upward against the dural fold overlying the superior portion of the intracranial end of the optic canal. *E*, Postoperative visual field is relatively unchanged, although visual acuity in this eye improved to 20/50. *F*, The optic disc has become pale. (From Unsöld R. In Compressive Optic Nerve Lesions at the Optic Canal. Editors, Unsöld R, Seeger W. Berlin, Springer-Verlag, 1989.)

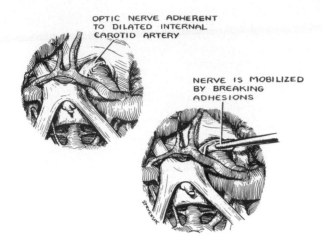

OPTIC NERVE ADHERENT
TO DILATED INTERNAL
CAROTID ARTERY

NERVE IS MOBILIZED
BY BREAKING
ADHESIONS

Figure 53.234. Illustration of operative findings in a 58-year-old man with sudden loss of the inferior portion of the visual field of the right eye. The patient had 20/15 vision in this eye, but the right optic disc was swollen. At craniotomy, the right optic nerve was found to be compressed by a dolichoectatic carotid artery. The nerve was decompressed, but the patient had no improvement in visual field.

artery. The patient underwent a right pterional craniotomy. At surgery, the supraclinoid portion of the right ICA elevated and compressed the intracranial portion of the right optic nerve. The dural sheath was therefore opened, and the optic canal was unroofed. The patient subsequently experienced marked improvement in visual function in the right eye.

Bilateral dolichoectasia of the intracranial portions of the ICAs may produce extremely asymmetric visual dysfunction. Hinshaw et al. (1985) described a 19-year-old girl with a 4-year history of episodic, transient left-sided weakness and bilateral blindness. After one episode of weakness, there was no recovery of strength. At that time, an examination revealed mild left hemiparesis. Visual acuity was finger counting at 10 cm OD and 20/25 OS. There was a right RAPD and right optic atrophy. The left ocular fundus was said to be normal. There was no reproducible response in the right eye to pattern or flash stimulation. In addition, the latency to pattern stimulation in the left eye was significantly prolonged. A CT scan showed evidence of infarction in the right hemisphere in the distribution of the right ACA. Cerebral angiography revealed severe dolichoectasia of the intracranial portions of both ICAs, the A-1 segments of both ACAs, and the proximal portions of both MCA. The right ACA was occluded. CT cisternography showed that the abnormal vessels were compressing and distorting the intracranial optic nerves and the optic chiasm. No surgery was attempted, and the patient had no change in visual symptoms over the next 18 months.

Visual loss in patients with dolichoectatic ICAs is not always acute. Miller (1991i) described two patients in whom dolichoectatic intracranial ICAs seemed to be responsible for bilateral, symmetric, slowly progressive optic neuropathy. The first patient was a 63-year-old man whose medical history was unremarkable except for alcohol abuse many years previously. The patient complained of progressive

blurred vision in both eyes of 2 months' duration. He had previously been examined by a retinal specialist who found mild age-related macular degeneration that did not seem to be consistent with the degree of visual loss. The patient was subsequently referred to the Neuro-Ophthalmology Unit of the Johns Hopkins Hospital. When the patient was first examined, visual acuity was 20/80 in both eyes. He had decreased color vision in both eyes, bilateral central scotomas, and mild bilateral optic atrophy with no significant cupping. The patient underwent a CT scan, serologic studies including serum vitamin B_{12} and red blood cell folate assay, and a lumbar puncture. All of these studies yielded normal results. He was placed on 60 mg of prednisone per day for 4 weeks, but he continued to lose vision in both eyes. When visual acuity became reduced to 20/300 OU, it was recommended to the patient that he undergo craniotomy and exploration of the optic nerves. He initially refused, but his visual acuity continued to drop until it reached 2/200 OD and 4/200 OS. The central scotomas now were quite large, and the peripheral visual fields were constricted. The patient had severe, bilateral optic atrophy. He now agreed to undergo craniotomy. At surgery, the patient was found to have diffusely enlarged, firm, internal carotid and ophthalmic arteries that were flattening the optic nerves and pushing them upward against the dural shelves at the intracranial end of the optic canals. Both optic canals were unroofed using a high-speed drill under microscopic control. Postoperatively, the patient was blind in the left eye; however, within 24 hours, he began to regain his sight. Eventually, visual acuity improved to 20/400 OD and 20/300 OS, with enlargement of the peripheral visual fields and shrinkage of the central scotomas in both eyes. It remained at this level during the next 7 years.

The second patient was a 65-year-old man being treated for chronic open-angle glaucoma. The patient did indeed have intraocular pressures in the high 20s and low 30s, with almost 100% cupping of both optic discs; however, he also had visual acuity of 20/40 in each eye with bilateral central scotomas and marked pallor of both optic discs, even in areas where there was a residual neural rim. Accordingly, it was decided to evaluate the patient further. He underwent a CT scan that suggested dolichoectatic ICAs, and an arteriogram confirmed this impression. Because of the mild visual loss, intracranial surgery was not recommended; however, over the next 3 months, the patient's visual acuity dropped to 20/100 OD and 20/60 OS. Craniotomy therefore was recommended to the patient. The patient agreed, and, at operation, both intracranial portions of the ICAs were observed to be diffusely enlarged, firm, and yellow-white. Both optic nerves were elevated by the ectatic arteries such that there was grooving superiorly where they passed beneath the dural shelves of the optic canals. The dura was excised, and both optic canals were unroofed using a high-speed drill under microscopic control. The procedure seemed to relieve the pressure on the optic nerves, and although the patient did not experience visual improvement after surgery, he did not experience further loss of visual acuity or visual field over the subsequent 5 years.

The optic neuropathy caused by dolichoectasia of the internal carotid and anterior cerebral arteries occurs equally in men and women. Most patients experience visual symptoms after 40 years of age. Visual loss is usually bilateral, but one eye may be affected weeks, months, or years before the other. The visual loss may be insidious in onset and slowly progressive, suggesting a compressive lesion, or it may be acute and nonprogressive, suggesting optic neuritis or ischemic optic neuropathy. Visual field defects are often altitudinal, but all types of field defects may occur, even central and cecocentral scotomas (Miller, 1991i). Nonspecific visual field constriction is not uncommon (Colapinto et al., 1996). Many patients have normal or pale optic discs when they are first examined, but some patients have swelling of one optic disc, usually in the eye with the more recent visual symptoms. When the opposite disc is pale in such patients, the diagnosis of Foster Kennedy syndrome may be considered, even though the patient has loss of vision in the eye with disc swelling.

The disc swelling that occurs in these patients probably is caused by ectasia-related thrombotic or embolic compro-mise of the short posterior ciliary arteries that arise from the ophthalmic artery and supply the retrolaminar and laminar portions of the optic disc, thus producing a true anterior ischemic optic neuropathy.

Patients with dolichoectatic ICAs and visual loss who are found to have optic atrophy in one or both eyes when first examined may have had a previous attack of anterior ischemic optic neuropathy with disc swelling that progressed to optic atrophy, or the process may, in fact, have been a posterior (retrobulbar) ischemic optic neuropathy in which the optic disc was initially normal and eventually became pale. Patients in whom acute visual loss with evidence of optic neuropathy is associated with a normal-appearing optic disc almost certainly have experienced an attack of posterior ischemic optic neuropathy (Sakaguchi and Hirayama, 1985). However, slowly progressive unilateral or bilateral visual loss associated with progressive optic atrophy in patients with dolichoectatic ICAs may be caused by the direct effects of optic nerve compression, ischemia, or both.

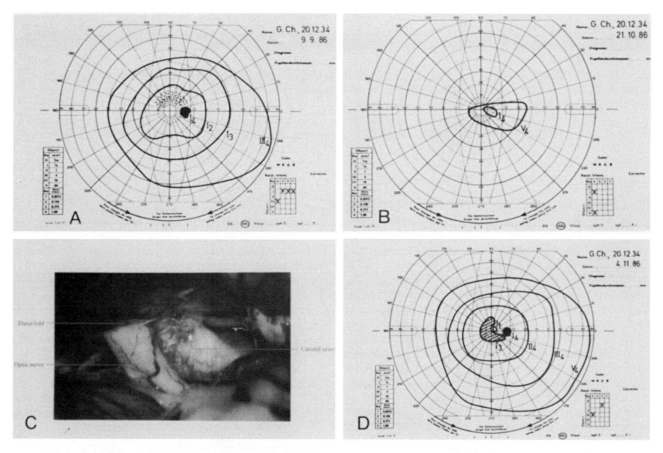

Figure 53.235. Improvement in visual function after surgical decompression of an optic nerve being compressed by a dolichoectatic internal carotid artery. The patient was a 52-year-old woman with progressive visual loss in the right eye. When she first was evaluated, visual acuity in the right eye was 20/100. *A,* Visual field in the right eye at the time of initial examination shows a superior arcuate defect. Visual acuity in the right eye progressively worsened to 20/500, and the visual field in this progressively constricted *(B).* A craniotomy was performed. *C,* View of the right optic nerve at surgery shows compression of the right optic nerve by a whitish, dolichoectatic internal carotid artery. The nerve is displaced upward and medially against the dural fold lining the superior portion of the optic canal. The nerve was decompressed by opening the dura and unroofing the optic canal. *D,* Two weeks after surgery, visual acuity in the right eye has returned to about 20/30, and the right visual field shows marked improvement. (From Unsöld R. In Compressive Optic Nerve Lesions at the Optic Canal. Editors, Unsöld R, Seeger W. Berlin, Springer-Verlag, 1989.)

The ischemic nature of the optic neuropathy caused by dolichoectatic ICAs may explain the lack of significant visual improvement in most patients after surgical decompression of the affected optic nerves (Mitts and McQueen, 1965). Nevertheless, visual improvement may occur after surgery for this condition. Sanford et al. (1935) described a patient in whom surgical exploration revealed tortuous ophthalmic arteries compressing the optic nerves against the superior portion of the optic canals and their dural shelves. The shelves were opened, and the canals were unroofed. The patient subsequently experienced improvement in vision in both eyes. Unsöld (1989b) described two patients who experienced progressive unilateral visual loss from dolichoectasia of the ipsilateral ICA and who improved after decompression of the optic nerves. One patient was a 52-year-old woman who had progressive loss of vision in the right eye associated with increasing optic atrophy. When the patient was first examined, the visual acuity in the right eye

was 20/100, and there was a superior arcuate visual field defect in that eye (Fig. 53.235A). Visual acuity in the eye eventually decreased to 20/500 and was associated with marked constriction of the visual field (Fig. 53.235B). A craniotomy revealed an ectatic ICA compressing the right optic nerve upward against the dural fold overlying the intracranial end of the optic canal (Fig. 53.235C). The nerve was decompressed, and within a week of surgery, visual acuity in the right eye had improved to about 20/30, and the visual field in that eye had enlarged substantially (Fig. 53.235D). The second patient described by Unsöld (1989b) was a 41-year-old hypertensive man who noted progressive visual loss in the right eye. The patient initially was thought to have optic neuritis, but vision eventually dropped to about 20/70 in the eye, and an evaluation revealed evidence of a compressive lesion. At craniotomy, the optic nerve was found to be compressed by a dolichoectatic ICA, and it was decompressed by unroofing the optic canal. Postoperatively, visual

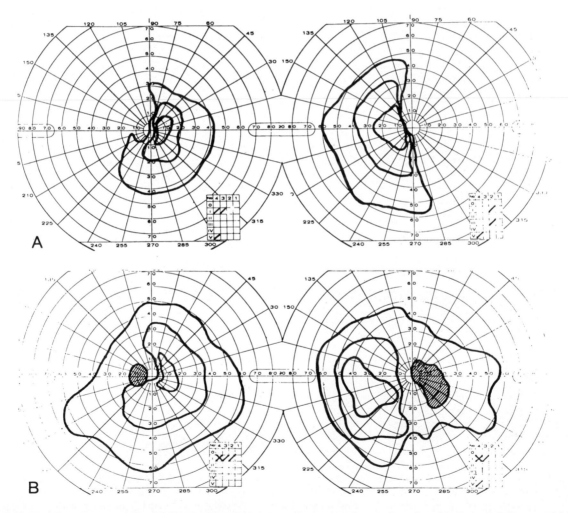

Figure 53.236. Bitemporal hemianopia from dolichoectatic carotid arteries with improvement after opening of both dural shelves over lying the optic canals and unroofing of both optic canals. The patient was a 68-year-old woman with a 6-month history of progressive visual loss. Visual acuity was 20/200 OD and 20/600 OS. *A,* Visual fields at time of initial examination show bitemporal hemianopia with central scotomas. *B,* Visual fields performed after surgery show substantial improvement, although patient's visual acuity did not improve. (From Matsuo K, Kobayashi S, Sugita K. Bitemporal hemianopsia associated with sclerosis of the intracranial internal carotid arteries. J Neurosurg *53*:566–569, 1980.)

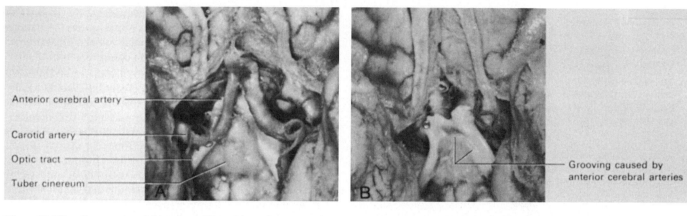

Anterior cerebral artery —

Carotid artery —

Optic tract —

Tuber cinereum —

Grooving caused by anterior cerebral arteries

Figure 53.237. Compression of the **undersurface** of the optic nerves and optic chiasm by dolichoectatic anterior cerebral arteries. *A,* The arteries compress the optic nerves and chiasm from below rather than from above. *B,* After removal of the vessels, the marked compression and grooving of the nerves and chiasm can be seen. (From Lindenberg R, Walsh FB, Sacks JG. Neuropathology of Vision: An Atlas. Philadelphia, Lea & Febiger, 1973.)

acuity in the right eye improved to 20/40, and the visual field defect improved. As noted above, the 63-year-old patient with bilateral dolichoectatic ICAs treated with bilateral optic canal decompressions had definite improvement in visual acuity and visual field in both eyes after surgery. von Wild and Busse (1990) and Colapinto et al. (1996) reported similar results. It therefore is reasonable to conclude that at least some patients with optic neuropathy in the setting of dolichoectasia of the internal carotid, anterior cerebral, or ophthalmic arteries, perhaps those without optic disc swelling, have the potential for visual improvement after decompression of the optic nerves, either by optic canal decompression using a high-speed microsurgical drill under microscopic control or by otherwise separating the optic nerves from the vessels compressing them.

Only rarely do bitemporal field defects occur in patients with ectasia of the supraclinoid portion of the ICA (Matsuo et al., 1980; von Wild and Busse, 1990) (Fig. 53.236). Such defects indicate damage to the nasal crossing fibers in the center of the chiasm and therefore cannot be ascribed to direct pressure by a laterally situated artery. Either the dilated vessels must act as a mass beneath the chiasm as described by Bergaust (1963) (Fig. 53.237), or the process must specifically compromise the vascular supply to the center of the chiasm (Walsh and Gass, 1960; Mitts and McQueen, 1965). Hilton and Hoyt (1966) described an elderly patient with bitemporal hemianopia and bilateral optic atrophy who underwent angiography that showed evidence of marked atherosclerosis and ectasia of both ACAs and the intracranial portions of both ICAs (Figs. 53.238 and 53.239). Lee and Schatz (1975) described similar cases.

In some patients, ectasia of the A-1 or proximal A-2 segments of the ACAs cause them to compress one or both optic nerves from above (Fig. 53.240), thus producing progressive visual loss. Post et al. (1981) described a 51-year-old woman who experienced decreased vision in the right eye after a massive gastrointestinal hemorrhage and then began to lose vision in the left eye about 1 year later. When she was first examined, her visual acuity was 20/200 OD and 20/40 OS.

Color vision was markedly impaired in both eyes, both visual fields were constricted (Fig. 53.241*A*), and there was a right RAPD. The right optic disc was pale; the left disc appeared normal. Angiography demonstrated dolichoectatic ACAs (Figs. 53.241*B* and 53.241*C*). The patient eventually underwent craniotomy at which time both ACAs were found to be elongated and tortuous. Both vessels were compressing the left optic nerve (Fig. 53.241*D*). Adhesions between these vessels and the nerve were lysed, and the vessels were separated from the nerve by a piece of muscle that was placed between the nerve and the arteries. Eight months after surgery, visual acuity had improved to 20/60 OD and 20/25 OS. Color vision was normal in the left eye, and the left visual field was less constricted (Fig. 53.241*E*).

Ectasia of the proximal portions of the ACAs may cause

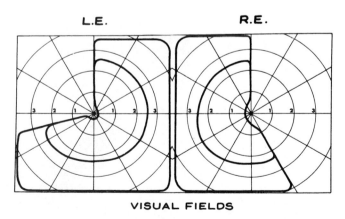

L.E.   **R.E.**

VISUAL FIELDS

ISOPTERS : 5W/1000 AND 25W/1000

Figure 53.238. The atherosclerotic optic chiasmal syndrome. There is a bitemporal hemianopia with reduction in central vision in both eyes. (From Hilton GF, Hoyt WF. An arteriosclerotic chiasmal syndrome: Bitemporal hemianopia associated with fusiform dilatation of the anterior cerebral arteries. JAMA *196*:1018–1020, 1966.)

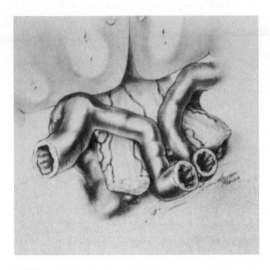

Figure 53.239. Artist's drawing of findings at surgery in the patient whose visual fields are depicted in Figure 53.238. The intracranial portions of both internal carotid arteries are diffusely enlarged, as are the A-1 and A-2 segments of both anterior cerebral arteries. Note that the distal portions of the A-1 segments and the proximal portions of the A-2 segments are extended between and slightly below both optic nerves. (From Hilton GF, Hoyt WF. An arteriosclerotic chiasmal syndrome: Bitemporal hemianopia associated with fusiform dilatation of the anterior cerebral arteries. JAMA *196*:1018–1020, 1966.)

them to prolapse downward between the optic nerves such that they compress the nasal fibers of both nerves, the anterior portion of the optic chiasm, or both (Schatz and Schlezinger, 1976; von Wild and Busse, 1990) (Fig. 53.242). We believe, however, that compression from such lesions is not as important in the production of bitemporal field defects as is associated obliteration of small arterioles of the superior and inferior chiasmal plexus (Hilton and Hoyt, 1966).

An homonymous visual field defect is an extremely rare finding in patients with a dolichoectasia of the ICA. Little et al. (1981) reported one such example among 11 patients with dolichoectasia of the intracranial vessels. The homonymous defect may result either from compression of the ipsilateral optic tract by the ectatic vessel (Fig. 53.243) or from emboli that originate within this portion of the artery and obstruct vessels supplying the postchiasmal visual sensory pathway.

Fusiform aneurysms of the distal anterior circulation (anterior and middle cerebral arteries) usually do not present with neuro-ophthalmologic symptoms. These patients may have a long history of headaches usually diagnosed as migraine. Rare rupture or thrombosis of the aneurysm may bring it to clinical attention, usually with a change in mental status and increased headache (Hara et al., 1993). Borzone et al. (1993) reported two cases of giant fusiform aneurysms of the MCA (Fig. 53.244). Fusiform aneurysms may be difficult to recognize without superselective angiography (Nakahara et al., 1995).

In about 20% of normal patients, the PCA arises from the ICA (Von Mitterwallner, 1955) (see Chapter 52). In such cases, the PCA is located laterally and inferiorly to the posterior communicating artery, in the same general region as the subarachnoid portion of the oculomotor nerve. A dolichoectatic PCA that arises from the ICA thus may produce an acute oculomotor nerve paresis, either from compression of the nerve or from interruption of its blood supply. Hopkins and Poser (1973) described a patient in whom ectasia of a PCA that originated from the ICA was thought to be responsible for a recurrent, painful, oculomotor nerve paresis. The patient, an 81-year-old woman, had complete left ptosis, moderate difficulty depressing the left eye, and inability to adduct that eye. The left eye intorted on attempted downgaze, indicating an intact trochlear nerve, and abduction and elevation of the left eye were normal. The left pupil was dilated and nonreactive to both direct and consensual illumi-

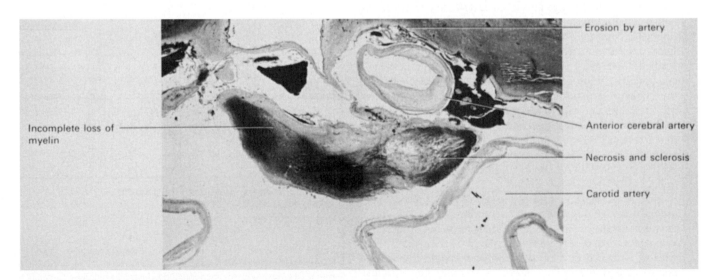

Figure 53.240. Compression of the left portion of the optic chiasm from below by a dolichoectatic internal carotid artery and from above by a dolichoectatic anterior cerebral artery. (From Lindenberg R, Walsh FB, Sacks JG. Neuropathology of Vision: An Atlas. Philadelphia, Lea & Febiger, 1973.)

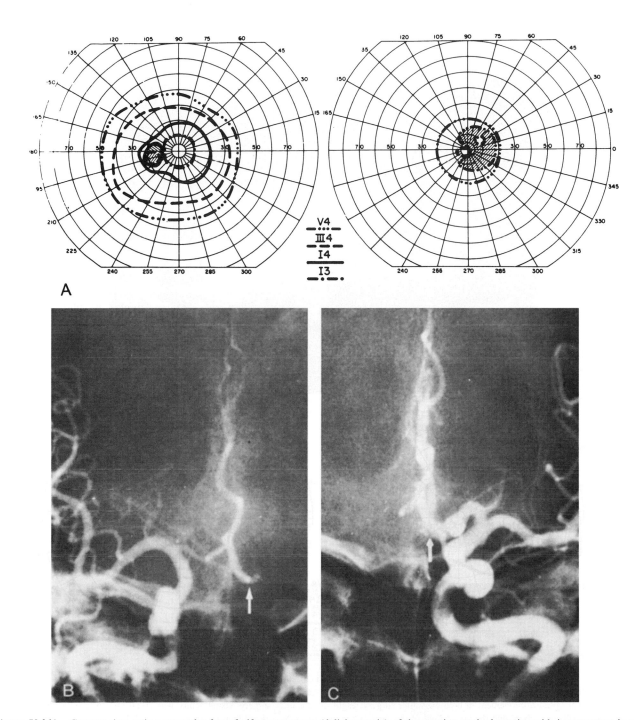

Figure 53.241. Compressive optic neuropathy from fusiform aneurysm (dolichoectasia) of the anterior cerebral arteries with improvement in visual function after decompression. The patient was a 51-year-old woman with progressive loss of vision in both eyes. Visual acuity was 20/200 OD and 20/40 OS. *A*, The right visual field is markedly constricted; the left visual field shows mild constriction. *B*, Right internal carotid angiogram, anteroposterior view, shows looping of A-1 segment of the right anterior cerebral artery *(arrow)*. *C*, Left internal carotid angiogram, anteroposterior view, shows enlargement and looping of left anterior cerebral artery *(arrow)*. The patient underwent craniotomy and exploration of the suprasellar region. At the time of surgery, loops of the right and left anterior cerebral arteries were seen to compress the optic nerves.

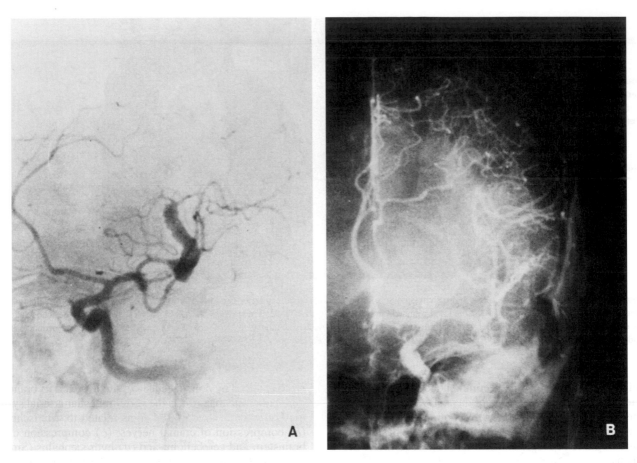

Figure 53.244.   Giant fusiform aneurysm of the middle cerebral artery. *A*, Anterior-posterior digital subtraction angiogram demonstrating a giant fusiform aneurysm of the prefrontal branch of the middle cerebral artery in a 53-year-old man admitted because of the onset of focal seizures. *B*, Following clipping of the proximal aneurysm with spontaneous collapse, the posterior angiography demonstrates complete exclusion of the aneurysm (From Borzone M, Altomonte M, Baldini M, et al. Giant fusiform aneurysm in middle cerebral artery branches: A report of two cases and a review of the literature. Acta Neurochir *125*:184–187, 1993.)

reported only two cases of dolichoectasia of the vertebral artery compared with 11 examples of basilar artery dolichoectasia. Fusiform aneurysms of the vertebral artery also are less common than saccular aneurysms affecting that vessel. Yamaura (1988) found only 12 cases of vertebral artery dolichoectasia among 94 cases of vertebral artery aneurysm. No patient with such a lesion had experienced subarachnoid or intracranial hemorrhage. Six fusiform aneurysms were asymptomatic but were associated with a symptomatic intracranial aneurysm in another location, one was an incidental finding in a patient being evaluated for an unrelated problem, and five fusiform aneurysms were symptomatic by virtue of mass effect although no clinical details were provided. A contrary view was expressed by Andoh et al. (1992a), who reported a series of 38 aneurysms of the vertebral artery seen over a 10-year interval, 10 of which were fusiform. All of the fusiform aneurysms in this series presented with evidence of SAH. Dolichoectasia of one or both vertebral arteries most often is associated with dolichoectasia of the basilar artery.

Dolichoectatic dilation of the vertebral artery may be related to dissection. Mizutani and Aruga (1992) reported five

cases of vertebral dissection with widely dilated tortuous arteries. MR imaging revealed the true nature of these dissecting aneurysms by demonstrating intimal flaps, a double lumen, or subacute clot in the false lumen. The findings of Mizutani and Aruga (1992) suggest that some cases of dolichoectasia of the vertebral arteries reported in the literature may actually have been caused by dissections.

In most series, the complaints of patients with vertebral artery dolichoectasia are related to dysfunction of the cerebellum and caudal brainstem. Yamada et al. (1984b) described three patients with dolichoectatic vertebral arteries. All three patients had nonspecific complaints including headache, dizziness, and unsteady gait. Sugita et al. (1988) also described three patients with dolichoectatic vertebral arteries. All three patients complained of headache, and all three had truncal ataxia and hemiparesis. Two of the patients also had dysarthria and dysphagia, and one patient had nystagmus, the nature of which was not described. Although none of the patients reported by Yamada et al. (1984b) or Sugita et al. (1988) had significant visual complaints, Slavin and LoPinto (1987) described a 66-year-old woman who

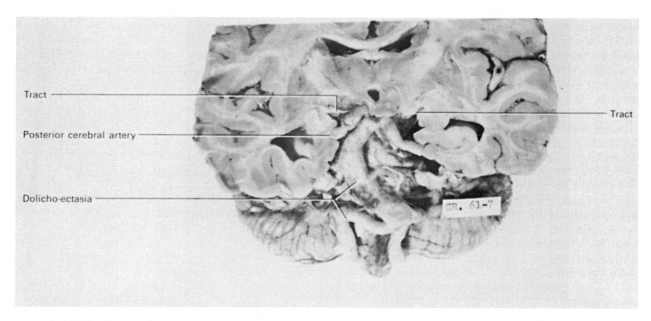

Tract

Tract

Posterior cerebral artery

Dolicho-ectasia

Figure 53.245. Diffuse dolichoectasia of the major arteries of the vertebrobasilar arterial system. The brain has been sectioned coronally, and the view is from in front and slightly below. Note dolichoectasia of the right vertebral artery, the basilar artery, and both posterior cerebral arteries. Also note that the right optic tract is compressed by the dolichoectatic right posterior cerebral artery which also erodes the adjacent internal capsule and mammillary body. The ectatic left posterior cerebral artery *(arrowhead)* compresses the left oculomotor nerve *(asterisk)*. The patient had a left homonymous hemianopia. (From Lindenberg R, Walsh FB, Sacks JG. Neuropathology of Vision: An Atlas. Philadelphia, Lea & Febiger, 1973.)

experienced sudden monocular and binocular tilting of images of distant objects. She denied other neurologic symptoms, including diplopia, oscillopsia, vertigo, weakness, paresthesias, and difficulty walking. An evaluation revealed compression of the lateral medulla by a dolichoectatic left vertebral artery. This patient's visual symptom was thought to be similar to the type of environmental tilting seen by some patients with the syndrome of lateral medullary infarction (Wallenberg's syndrome) (see Chapters 29 and 55). A

patient with dolichoectatic vertebral arteries described by Echiverri et al. (1989) complained of intermittent vertical diplopia and an unsteady gait. The patient had bilateral limb and gait ataxia and a left hemiparesis. The cause of his diplopia was not discussed, however.

Rare patients have dolichoectasia of one of the branches of the vertebral artery. Massey et al. (1984) described a 60-year-old woman who began to experience difficulty swallowing, dizziness, and left-sided weakness. Although she

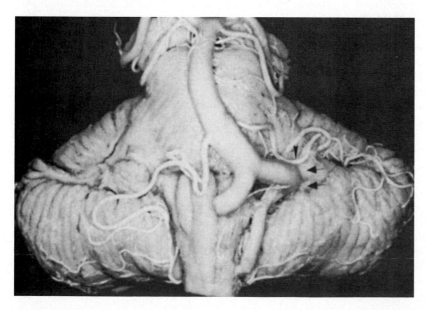

Figure 53.246. Dolichoectasia of the right vertebral artery. The artery is displaced laterally and superiorly into the region of the right cerebellopontine angle *(arrows)*. Note superior displacement of the right posterior inferior cerebellar artery *(arrowhead)*. (From Kerber CW, Margolis MT, Newton TH. Tortuous vertebrobasilar system: A cause of cranial nerve signs. Neuroradiology *4*:74–77, 1972.)

had normal pupillary responses and eye movements, she had horizontal, gaze-evoked nystagmus, an absent gag reflex, bilateral paresis of the palate, and a mild left hemiparesis. An evaluation revealed dolichoectasia of the right PICA beginning at its origin from the right vertebral artery. Ligation of the right vertebral artery resulted in improvement of the patient's dysphagia and resolution of the other neurologic deficits. Dernbach et al. (1988a) described a man who experienced sudden nausea, vomiting, gait ataxia, and dysarthria at age 33. He was treated for a presumed inner ear infection, and his symptoms and signs resolved. Eight years later, he awakened with a severe occipital headache, sonophobia, and photophobia that resolved over 5 days. At age 47 (14 years after his "inner ear infection" and 6 years after his headache), he experienced sudden loss of his right peripheral visual field. The patient was found to have an incongruous, incomplete, right homonymous hemianopia and left-beating, gaze-evoked nystagmus. Neuroimaging studies showed a mass in the 4th ventricle, and angiography demonstrated a giant, fusiform aneurysm arising from a small branch of the right PICA. A smaller aneurysm was present slightly proximal to the larger one. The patient was treated by obliterating both aneurysms with clips. According to Dernbach et al. (1988a), the patient "did well" postoperatively. Ligation of fusiform aneurysms of the PICA may be carried out without inducing new neurologic symptoms if the origin is distal to the tonsillomedullary segment (Yamaguchi et al., 1996).

Fusiform Aneurysms of the Basilar Artery and Its Branches

As is the case with ICA dolichoectasia, patients with dolichoectasia of the basilar artery and its branches may be asymptomatic, with the abnormality being found during a screening examination for unrelated symptoms or during a routine autopsy (Nijensohn et al., 1974; Yu et al., 1982) (Fig. 53.247). Most patients who become symptomatic from this condition are 50 years of age or older and have atherosclerotic or hypertensive vascular disease. Men are affected more often than women (Nijensohn et al., 1974; Nishizaki et al., 1986; Smoker et al., 1986; Echiverri et al., 1989).

Dolichoectasia of the basilar artery may cause a variety of neurologic difficulties. Smoker et al. (1986) reviewed 288 cases of basilar artery dolichoectasia and added 20 cases of their own. Nishizaki et al. (1986) added another 23 cases. Neurologic deficits among these 331 cases included isolated cranial neuropathy, multiple cranial neuropathies, mixed ischemic and compressive deficits, and evidence of hydrocephalus. Symptoms and signs of SAH were extremely uncommon. In a series of 30 patients with a megadolichobasilar artery reported by D'Andrea et al. (1992), nine had TIAs or an ischemic stroke, seven had subarachnoid or intracerebral hemorrhage, and seven had single or multiple cranial nerve deficits. In the other seven cases, the condition was asymptomatic. Of 15 patients reported by Okada et al. (1994), 11 presented with strokes or TIAs, two had unilateral facial pain consistent with trigeminal neuralgia, and the remaining two patients had severe headaches.

Dysfunction of a single cranial nerve may be the only

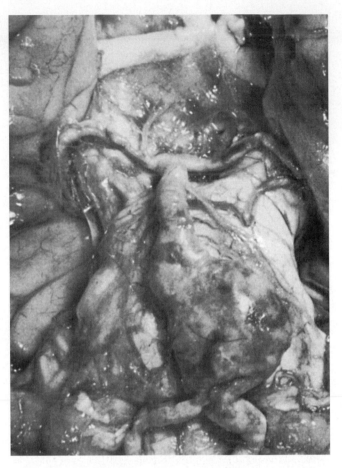

Figure 53.247. Dolichoectasia of the proximal portion of the basilar artery. The patient had died after a myocardial infarction and was not known to have experienced any neurologic dysfunction. Note some ectasia of the left vertebral artery.

sign of a dolichoectatic basilar artery. The most common cranial nerves affected are the facial and the trigeminal nerves (Smoker et al., 1986). Damage to the facial nerve most often causes hemifacial spasm (Dettori et al., 1966; Tridon et al., 1971; Kerber et al., 1972; Kramer and Eckman, 1972; Nappi et al., 1977; Nishizaki et al., 1986; Smoker et al., 1986; Digre et al., 1988), but isolated facial paresis occasionally occurs. Trigeminal nerve damage may be manifest as typical trigeminal neuralgia, atypical facial pain, or trigeminal neuropathy with decreased corneal sensation and facial hypesthesia and dysesthesia (Dandy, 1944; Dehaene et al., 1975; Waga et al., 1979; Miner et al., 1980; Lye, 1986; Smoker et al., 1986; Martins and Ferro, 1989) (Figs. 53.248 and 53.249). Other individual cranial nerves, including the vestibulocochlear (Buttner et al., 1995), glossopharyngeal, vagus, and hypoglossal, may become compromised. Even the ocular motor nerves may become damaged. At least five cases of isolated oculomotor nerve paresis, with and without pupillary involvement, are documented in the literature (Boeri and Passerini, 1964; Trobe et al., 1978b; Weisberg, 1981; Smoker et al., 1986; Scuccimarra et al., 1988) (Fig. 53.250). Isolated trochlear and abducens nerve paresis also

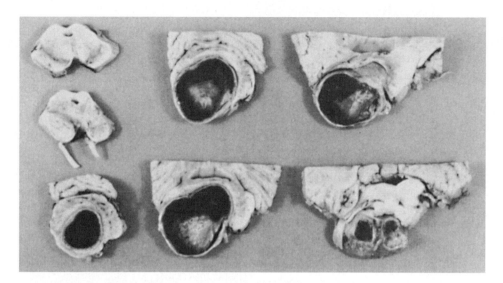

Figure 53.248. Massive dolichoectasia of the basilar artery that caused trigeminal neuralgia. The patient was a 78-year-old man who initially developed trigeminal neuralgia. Signs of brainstem failure eventually occurred, and these led to the patient's death. Serial sections through the brainstem show a massive, "fusiform" aneurysm that has invaginated into the pons. Note that the vertebral arteries are also enlarged and atherosclerotic. There is extensive premortem thrombosis within the affected arteries. (From Weir B. Aneurysms Affecting the Nervous System. Baltimore, Williams & Wilkins, 1987.)

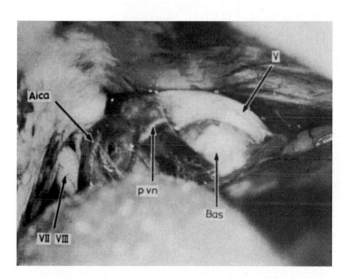

Figure 53.249. Basilar artery ectasia causing trigeminal neuralgia. The patient was a 71-year-old man with an 8-year history of left trigeminal neuralgia affecting the first and second divisions of the trigeminal nerve. The patient initially responded to carbamazepine, but he was unable to tolerate the drug on a long-term basis. An angiogram showed evidence of ectasia of the basilar artery, and it was decided to perform a posterior fossa microvascular decompression of the trigeminal nerve. *A,* Surgical view shows that the left trigeminal nerve *(V)* is compressed and elevated by the dilated, tortuous basilar artery *(Bas). Aica,* anterior inferior cerebellar artery; *VII VIII,* facial and vestibuloacoustic nerves; *p vn,* petrosal vein. (From Lye RH. Basilar artery ectasia: An unusual cause of trigeminal neuralgia. J Neurol Neurosurg Psychiatry *49:*22–28, 1986.)

occur in patients with dolichoectasia of the basilar artery but with much less frequency (Smoker et al., 1986).

Multiple unilateral and bilateral cranial neuropathies occur more commonly than isolated cranial neuropathy in patients with dolichoectasia of the basilar artery and its branches. Any of the cranial nerves (except for the olfactory and optic nerves) may be affected. Oculomotor nerve paresis may occur bilaterally (Moschner et al., 1997) or in combination with other cranial neuropathies (Boeri and Passerini, 1964; Jamieson, 1964; Sacks and Lindenberg, 1969; Carella et al., 1973; Azar-Kia et al., 1976; Trobe et al., 1978b; Weisberg, 1981; Resta et al., 1984; Durand and Samples, 1989) (Fig. 53.251), as may trochlear nerve paresis (Echiverri et al., 1989), but the nerves most often affected are those that course through the cerebellopontine angle (i.e., the trigeminal, abducens, facial, and vestibulocochlear nerves) (Wells, 1922; Scott and Stauffer, 1964; Wallace and Jaffe, 1967; Pribram et al., 1969; Tridon et al., 1971; Kerber et al., 1972; Neagoy and Dohn, 1974; Frasson et al., 1977; Peterson et al., 1977; Rao and Woodlief, 1979; Thron and Bockenheimer, 1979; Smoker et al., 1986; Echiverri et al., 1989). The symptoms and signs in such patients thus mimic those produced by CPA neoplasms, such as vestibular schwannomas and meningiomas (Le Beau and Daum, 1960; Bull, 1969; see Chapters 38, 40, and 44). Some patients develop both hemifacial spasm **and** ipsilateral trigeminal neuralgia, whereas others develop progressive trigeminal, abducens, and facial paresis (Echiverri et al., 1989). Progressive paresis of the lower cranial nerves may develop, mimicking the symptoms and signs produced by tumors in the region of the clivus and foramen magnum (e.g., chordoma, nasopharyngeal carcinoma, meningioma) (Thron and Bockenheimer, 1979; Nishizaki et al., 1986). In some cases, both upper and lower cranial nerves are affected, a consequence of the extensive nature and erratic

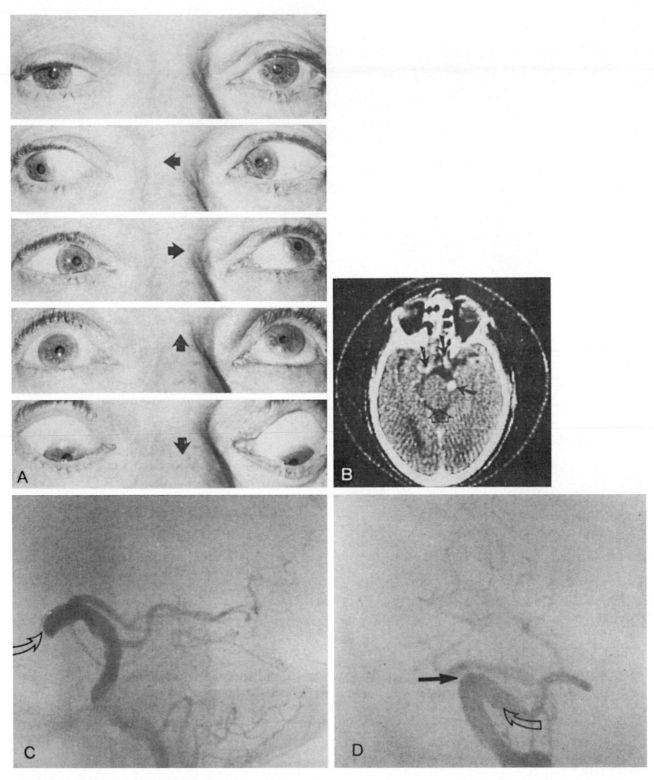

Figure 53.250. Isolated oculomotor nerve paresis caused by a fusiform aneurysm (*dolichoectasia*) of the basilar artery. The patient was a 61-year-old hypertensive man with a 3-year history of diplopia. *A*, Appearance of the patient shows a moderate right ptosis associated with marked limitation of elevation and mild limitation of depression and adduction of the right eye. The right pupil is the same size as the left. It reacted normally to light and near stimulation. *B*, A CT scan shows small areas of opacification consistent with enlargement of the basilar artery in the perimesencephalic, parasellar, and suprasellar cisterns *(solid arrows)*. The brainstem is displaced to the left *(open arrow)*. *C* and *D*, Vertebral angiogram, lateral and anteroposterior views, respectively, shows marked dolichoectasia of the basilar artery. At its most distal portion *(solid arrow)*, it is causing a mass effect on the right posterior cerebral artery which also is somewhat ectatic and dilated. The anterior portion of the basilar artery extends into the left suprasellar cistern *(open arrows)*. (From Trobe JD, Glaser JS, Quencer RC. Isolated oculomotor paralysis: The product of saccular and fusiform aneurysms of the basilar artery. Arch Ophthalmol *96*:1236–1240, 1978.)

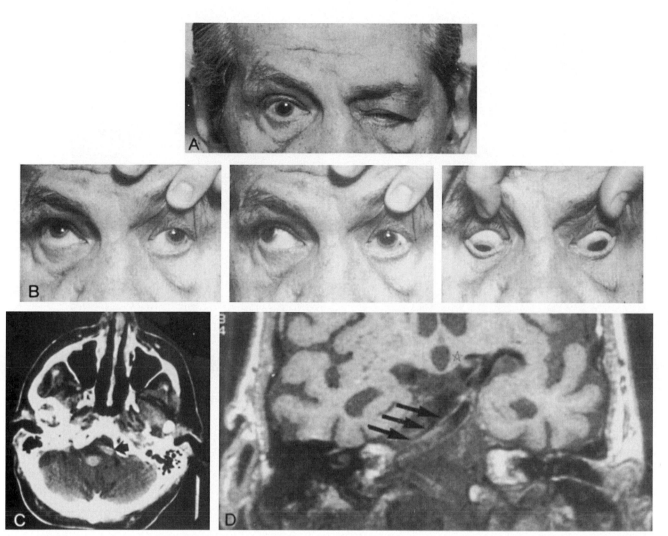

Figure 53.251. Multiple cranial nerve pareses caused by a dolichoectatic basilar artery. The patient was a 74-year-old man with diplopia. *A,* The patient has a left ptosis. In addition, however, the left face is weak. Note mild ectropion of the left lower eyelid and sagging of the skin below the left eyelid. *B,* The patient has limitation of elevation, adduction, and depression of the left eye consistent with a left oculomotor nerve paresis. The patient also had reduced corneal sensation on the left. Because of apparent left oculomotor, trigeminal, and facial neuropathies, the patient underwent neuroimaging studies. *C,* CT scan, axial view, shows two regions of enhancement, one of which seems to be an elongated structure *(arrow). D,* Coronal MR image shows marked tortuosity and enlargement of the left vertebral and the basilar arteries *(arrows)* with compression of the hypothalamus by the top of the basilar artery *(star).* No treatment was recommended. The patient improved spontaneously about 6 weeks later. (From Durand JR, Samples JR. Dolichoectasia and cranial nerve palsies: A case report. J Clin Neuroophthalmol 9:249–253, 1989.)

course of the ectatic artery. The patient reported by Durand and Samples (1989) had a left oculomotor nerve paresis combined with a left trigeminal sensory neuropathy and a left facial nerve paresis (Fig. 53.251). Most patients with multiple cranial neuropathies from basilar artery dolichoectasia have unilateral symptoms and signs, but evidence of bilateral dysfunction develops in some patients.

A variety of **acute brainstem and cerebellar** symptoms and signs may develop in patients with dolichoectasia of the basilar artery and its branches. In some cases, the symptoms and signs develop acutely and resolve within about 24 hours. Patients in whom this occurs may be thought to have suffered a TIA from atherosclerotic verte-

brobasilar insufficiency (Alajouanine et al., 1948; Nijensohn et al., 1974; Nishizaki et al., 1986; Echiverri et al., 1989) (Fig. 53.252). In other cases, neurologic symptoms and signs develop suddenly, do not resolve, and may even progress. Patients may develop vestibular nystagmus, conjugate horizontal and vertical gaze paresis, vertigo, dysarthria, ataxia, and hemiparesis (Case Records of the Massachusetts General Hospital, 1953; Boeri and Passerini, 1964; Dettori et al., 1966; Deeb et al., 1979; Stark, 1979; Thron and Bockenheimer, 1979; Weisberg, 1981; Yu et al., 1982; Resta et al., 1984; Hegedüs, 1985; Nishizaki et al., 1986; Smoker et al., 1986; Echiverri et al., 1989; Pessin et al., 1989a). Patients in whom these abnormalities

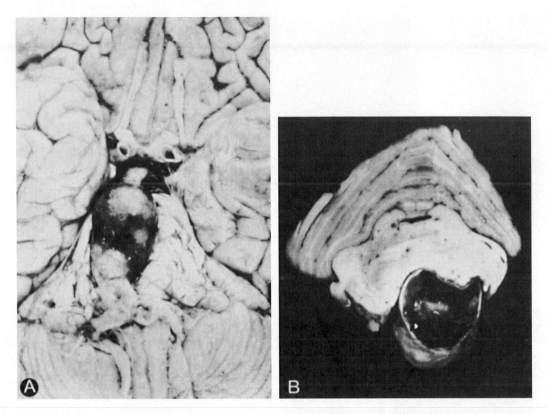

Figure 53.252. Fusiform aneurysm of the basilar artery (dolichoectasia) causing transient ischemic attacks. The patient was a 50-year-old man with hyperlipidemia and angina pectoris who experienced episodes of binocular diplopia that lasted 1-3 minutes. During one of these episodes he also experienced transient left hemiparesis, paresthesias, nausea, and vomiting. The patient was thought to have vertebrobasilar atherosclerotic disease, and he was treated with anticoagulation. He died 4 months later from rupture of the thoracic aorta. *A*, View of the base of the brain in this patient shows a large fusiform aneurysm (*dolichoectasia*) of the midportion of the basilar artery. *B*, Cross-section of the pons shows marked compression by the aneurysm. Note that the "aneurysm" is filled with premortem thrombus and atheroma. (From Nijensohn DE, Saez RJ, Reagan TJ. Clinical significance of basilar artery aneurysms. Neurology *24*:301–305, 1974.)

occur may be thought to have experienced an atherosclerotic or hypertensive pontine stroke unless basilar artery ectasia is detected by neuroimaging studies. In fact, these disturbances are caused by a combination of factors, including direct compression of the ventral brainstem and cerebellum by the dolichoectatic artery, ischemia and infarction secondary to the mass effect, and hemodynamic changes resulting from vascular stasis and thrombosis within the aneurysm (Case Records of the Massachusetts General Hospital, 1953; Shirakuni et al., 1985; Nishizaki et al., 1986; Smoker et al., 1986; Pessin et al., 1989a; Watanabe et al., 1994; Ildan et al., 1995). These patients often have a rapidly progressive, downhill course ending in death (Case Records of the Massachusetts General Hospital, 1953; Marchau et al., 1988); however, some eventually stabilize and even improve (Thron and Bockenheimer, 1979; Pessin et al., 1989a).

Hydrocephalus develops in some patients with basilar artery dolichoectasia (Greitz and Löfstedt, 1954; Breig et al., 1967; Ekbom et al., 1969; Greitz et al., 1969; Sutton, 1971; Tonali et al., 1973; Rozario et al., 1978; Scotti et al., 1978; Moseley and Holland, 1979; Healy et al., 1981; Nishizaki et al., 1986; Smoker et al., 1986; Echiverri et

al., 1989). In most cases, increased ICP is caused by obstruction of the 3rd or 4th ventricle, the floor of which is compressed and elevated by the ectatic portion of the artery (Fig. 53.248). In other patients, an ectatic basilar artery extends into the floor of the 3rd ventricle and exerts a water-hammer pulse that is transmitted toward the foramina of Monro, thus impairing outflow from the lateral ventricles (Breig et al., 1967).

Coppeto (1988) described three women with long-standing, recurrent, classic migraine. All three patients had expanding hemianopic scintillating scotomas with characteristic "build-up" (see Chapter 56). Each patient was eventually found to have severe basilar or vertebrobasilar dolichoectasia. One patient underwent partial occlusion of the dolichoectatic basilar artery segment, after which she had no further visual disturbances during an 8-year follow-up period. Coppeto (1988) suggested that the ectasia and the migraine in these patients may have been independent phenomena, or that some patients may be at risk for accelerated degeneration and subsequent ectasia of cephalic arteries after years of severe migraine.

Dolichoectasia of the PCA and other branches of the basilar artery may cause neurologic dysfunction in the absence

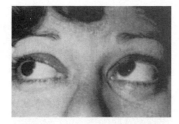
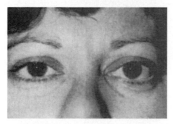
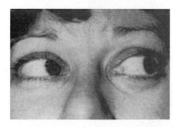
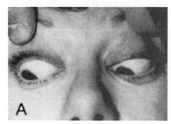
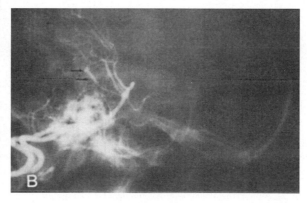

Figure 53.253. Superior division oculomotor nerve paresis caused by infarction of the mesencephalon associated with hemorrhage from a dolichoectatic superior cerebellar artery. The patient was a 35-year-old woman who developed left hemibody numbness, headache, difficulty with balance, and diplopia. *A,* The patient has a right, superior division, oculomotor nerve paresis. *B,* Vertebral angiography, lateral view, shows a fusiform aneurysm (dolichoectasia) of the right superior cerebellar artery. The patient underwent a craniotomy at which time it was observed that the artery was *not* compressing the right oculomotor nerve. It was postulated that the patient had experienced a brainstem infarct that affected, in part, the fascicular fibers of the superior division of the oculomotor nerve. (From Guy J, Day AL. Intracranial aneurysms with superior division paresis of the oculomotor nerve. Ophthalmology *96:* 1071–1076, 1989.)

of basilar artery ectasia itself. Boeri and Passerini (1958) described two patients in whom an oculomotor nerve paresis was thought to have been caused by compression of the oculomotor nerve by a tortuous, ectatic PCA that originated from the basilar artery. Guy and Day (1989) described a 35-year-old woman who developed left hemibody numbness, diplopia, headache, and difficulty with balance. She was found to have a right superior division oculomotor nerve paresis (Fig. 53.253*A*), right-beating nystagmus on right lateral gaze, dysmetria of the right upper extremity, decreased sensation to pin prick over the left face and body, and truncal ataxia. An evaluation revealed dolichoectasia of the right SCA (Fig. 53.253*B*). Because the right oculomotor nerve was not compressed by the dolichoectatic vessel, the patient was thought to have had an infarction of the brainstem affecting, in part, the fasciculi of the superior division of the oculomotor nerve. Zager (1991) reported isolated trigeminal sensory loss related to a fusiform partially thrombosed aneurysm of the AICA. The aneurysm indented the pons at the trigeminal root entry zone.

DISSECTING ANEURYSMS

GENERAL CONSIDERATIONS

A dissecting aneurysm represents blood within the wall of an artery. This presumably results from a breach in the endothelium and subjacent layers of an artery that permits circulating blood to dissect into the arterial wall, separating the layers and collapsing the intima upon itself (Figs. 53.254 and 53.255). Alternatively, hemorrhage beginning within the vasa vasorum of a large artery may rupture into the lumen (Foster et al., 1991). Because there is no vasa vasorum intracranially, it is less likely that this plays a major role in intra-

cranial dissection. Dissecting aneurysms that affect the aorta and other extracranial arteries produce a plane of cleavage within the tunica media, whereas intracranial arterial dissections usually separate the internal elastic lamina from the medial layer (Stehbens, 1972; O'Connell et al., 1985). This has a tendency to emphasize luminal narrowing over external diameter expansion. In either setting, a false lumen that dissects the vessel wall for a varying distance along the artery is created. The blood within the false lumen may return to

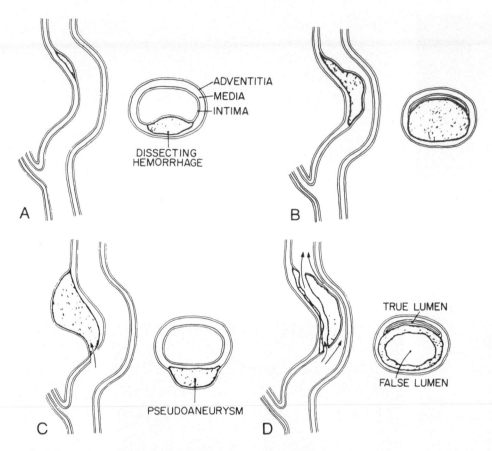

Figure 53.254. Schematic illustration of types of dissecting aneurysms. *A*, Lateral (*left*) and cross-sectional (*right*) views of the internal carotid artery demonstrate the initial phase of intramedial and subintimal dissecting aneurysm. The three basic arterial layers (adventitia, media, and intima) are delineated. *B*, Comparable views of an intramedial hemorrhage. The hemorrhage has reduced substantially the lumen of the artery. *C*, Comparable views of an intramedial hemorrhage that dissects into the subadventitial, rather than the subintimal plane as in *A* and *B*. In this case, the lumen of the artery is not compromised, and a pseudoaneurysm develops. *D*, A dissecting hemorrhage has ruptured through the intima, establishing a communication with the true lumen of the artery. In this case, recanalization may occur, enlarging the lumen of the artery, the lumen of the aneurysm, or both. (From Friedman WA, Day AL, Quisling RG Jr, et al. Cervical carotid dissecting aneurysms. Neurosurgery 7:207–214, 1980.)

the true lumen of the artery distal to the original site of damage, thus reestablishing flow within the vessel. It also may completely occlude the vessel, or it may rupture through the entire wall, producing severe hemorrhage (Figs. 53.254 and 53.255). The false lumen often undergoes resolution but occasionally the second lumen may stabilize (Mizutani, 1996).

The diagnosis of dissection, originally made by postmortem examination, can be suspected clinically and confirmed using a variety of neuroimaging techniques, including MR imaging, MR angiography, spiral CT angiography, and conventional angiography (Nohjoh et al., 1995; Mascalchi et al., 1997). Dissecting aneurysms have a variable angiographic appearance that reflects different anatomic possibilities: a tapering column ("string sign"), a blunt occlusion, a thin residual lumen, a series of dilations resembling a "string of pearls," delayed emptying from an apparently dilated segment of artery, and a double lumen (Engeset et al., 1967; Ojemann et al., 1972; Ehrenfeld and Wylie, 1976; Yonas et al., 1977; Fisher et al., 1978; Houser et al., 1984; Goldberg et al., 1986; Herman and Spetzler, 1990)

(Fig. 53.256). Besides creating a double lumen, arterial narrowing, and focal areas of dilation, dissection may also produce intramural pseudoaneurysms (Boström and Liliequist, 1967; Ehrenfeld and Wylie, 1976; Mokri et al., 1977; Fisher et al., 1978; Friedman et al., 1980; Hodge and Lee, 1982). These are particularly common in dissections of the ICA. Petro et al. (1987) observed pseudoaneurysms in five of nine dissections in eight patients. These areas can undergo subsequent enlargement (Boström and Liliequist, 1967; Petro et al., 1987), although most involute with time. In a series of 13 patients with pseudoaneurysms of the ICA, four were unchanged, six were smaller, and three resolved (Houser et al., 1984). Petro et al. (1987) estimated that pseudoaneurysm formation occurs in up to 5% of patients with dissections of the ICA. Dissection often evolves angiographically. One patient with repeat studies progressed from a double lumen appearance to a "string of pearls" and then to complete resolution (Amagasa et al., 1988). Indeed, in our experience, spontaneous resolution is not uncommon (Adams et al., 1982, Houser et al., 1984).

Standard MR imaging as well as MR angiography can be

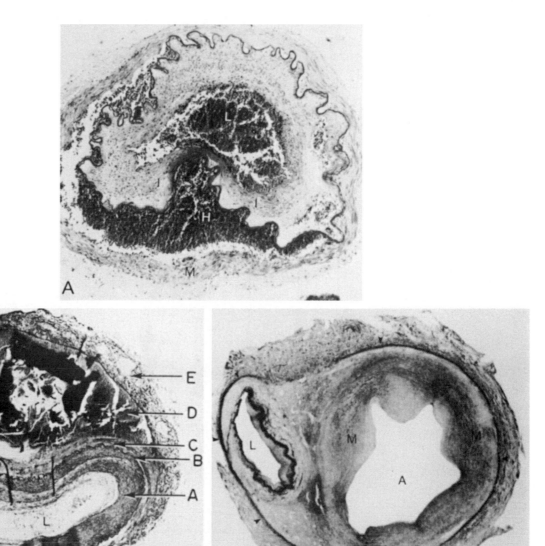

Figure 53.255. The effects of dissecting aneurysms on the parent artery. *A,* Acute dissection of the internal carotid artery with extension into the anterior cerebral artery. The media (*M*) of the artery is separated from the thickened intima (*I*) by acute hemorrhage (*H*). The lumen of the artery (*L*) is occluded by the hemorrhage. (From Yamashita M, Tanaka K, Matsuo T, et al. Cerebral dissecting aneurysms in patients with moyamoya disease: Report of two cases. J Neurosurg *58*:120–125, 1983.) *B,* Dissecting aneurysm of the vertebral artery. A hematoma (*D*) separates the adventitia (*E*) from the media (*C*). The elastic lamina (*B*) and the endothelium (*A*) are intact, and the lumen of the artery (*L*) is open. (From Yonas H, Agamanolis D, Takaoka Y, et al. Dissecting intracranial aneurysms. Surg Neurol *8*:407–415, 1977.) *C,* Cross-section of an internal carotid artery at the level of a dissecting aneurysm. The arterial lumen (*L*) is compressed but open. The larger lumen of the aneurysm (*A*) is also open. The sac of the aneurysm has formed within the media of the artery (*M*), and both of the lumens are surrounded by the external elastic lamina (*arrowheads*). (From Mokri B, Piepgras DG, Houser OW. Traumatic dissections of the extracranial internal carotid artery. J Neurosurg *68*:189–197, 1988.)

used to diagnose and follow dissections (Goldberg et al., 1986; Edelman et al., 1988; Lieschke et al., 1988; Waespe et al., 1988; Rae-Grant et al., 1989; Rothrock et al., 1989; Herman and Spetzler, 1990; Kucharczyk, 1990; Panisset and Eidelman, 1990; Quint and Spickler, 1990; Pacini et al., 1991; Leys et al., 1997; Mascalchi et al., 1997). Routine spin-echo images show thickening of the arterial wall with abnormal increased signal intensity. The earliest sign of basi-

lar thrombosis may be loss of the normal flow void (Biller et al., 1988). Flow-sensitive sequences can confirm the degree of luminal stenosis. The lesion within the wall is hyperintense on both T1- and T2-weighted sequences during the subacute phase (Goldberg et al., 1986; Lieschke et al., 1988; Rae-Grant et al., 1989; Quint and Spickler, 1990; Pacini et al., 1991; Matsuyama et al., 1993). MR imaging is usually positive when CT is negative (Rae-Grant et al., 1989; Her-

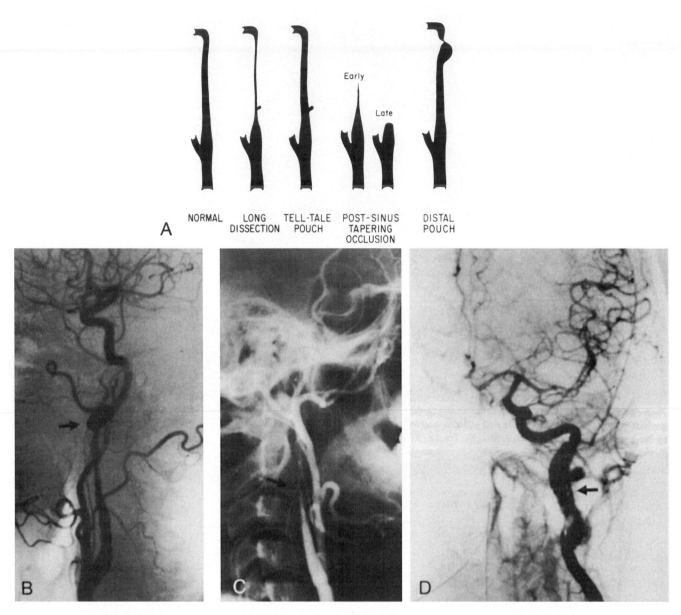

Figure 53.256.   Angiographic appearance of dissecting aneurysms. *A*, Schematic illustration of the various radiographic changes that may be seen in an artery affected by a dissection. (From Fisher CM, Ojemann RG, Roberson GH. Spontaneous dissection of cervico-cerebral arteries. Can J Neurol Sci *5*: 9–19, 1978.) *B–D*, Arteriographic appearance of dissections affecting the cervical portion of the internal carotid artery. *B*, Pseudoaneurysm (*arrow*) of the distal cervical carotid artery associated with proximal narrowing of the lumen. *C*, Tapered occlusion (*arrow*) that begins just distal to the carotid sinus. *D*, Double lumen (*arrow*) with irregularity of the entire lumen.

man and Spetzler, 1990; Panisset and Eidelman, 1990; Quint and Spickler, 1990; Pacini et al., 1991) and may even be positive when conventional angiography is negative (Panisset and Eidelman, 1990; Foster et al., 1991).

MR imaging is sensitive to ischemic complications from dissections, although not always acutely. Evidence of pontine infarction is not present on unenhanced MR imaging for at least 12 hours (Biller et al., 1988), but after this, such infarcts are well delineated by MR imaging (Baker and Carr, 1987; Povlsen et al., 1987; Biller et al., 1988; Rae-Grant et al., 1989). MR imaging is also extremely useful in monitor-

ing patients with dissections. In one of the cases reported by Goldberg et al. (1986), MR imaging demonstrated resolution of a mural thrombus. Rothrock et al. (1989) also used MR to demonstrate partial improvement at 7 weeks, with complete resolution at 3 1/2 months. Waespe et al. (1988) used MR imaging to show resolution of an ICA dissection at 9 months, and Panisset and Eidelman (1990) described "essentially complete" resolution of the wall hematoma using MR imaging in one patient at 6 months and in another patient at 2 months. Because dissections often involve the proximal portion of the ICA, it is important to make certain that the images extend far enough down in the neck to image the entire lesion (Foster et al., 1991).

A mural thrombus in an artery with a dissection may be confused with surrounding interstitial fat at the skull base using MR imaging (Goldberg et al., 1986). Sequences designed to minimize chemical shift and motion artifact and to suppress fat signal may improve the resolution and diagnosis of dissection in such cases (Edelman et al., 1988; Pacini et al., 1991). We agree with Panisset and Eidelman (1990) that MR imaging is the diagnostic procedure of choice for screening patients with suspected ICA dissection. However, angiography is still necessary to demonstrate patency of the vessel and status of the distal circulation, which are important in planning therapeutic strategies, with particular respect to the institution of anticoagulation. This view is supported others (Sturzenegger, 1994). The role of spiral CT angiography in the diagnosis and management of dissections is unclear, but based on our experience and that of others (Soper et al., 1995; Vieco et al., 1997), we suspect that it has a sensitivity and specificity at least that of MR angiography.

Ultrasound may play an adjunctive role in the diagnosis and follow-up of patients with arterial dissections. In a study of several ultrasonographic techniques performed by de Bray et al. (1994), continuous-wave Doppler imaging revealed signs of severe obstruction (i.e., occlusion, extensive submandibular tight stenoses, significant slowdowns in the carotid and ophthalmic vessels, retrograde ophthalmic blood flow) of the affected ICAs in 40 of 42 cases (96%) of ICA dissection, Color Doppler flow imaging suggested a dissection in 34 of the 42 cases (82%) of the cases, and standard duplex scanning suggested dissection (i.e., tapering stenoses or occlusion, segmental ectasia, tubular vessel, peripheral residual channel, or rare irregular "membrane") in 30 of the 42 cases (72%). Bakke et al. (1996) reported false-negative results using pulsed-Doppler ultrasonography in three of 14 patients with ICA dissection.

Dissecting aneurysms may originate in any artery at any location. They may develop in any of the major extracranial vessels, including the aorta, the innominate artery, the subclavian artery, and the common carotid artery (Graham et al., 1988); however, they most often affect the extracranial portion of the internal carotid and vertebral arteries. As trauma plays an important role, those locations where the major arteries are in contact with bony prominences are particularly vulnerable. These include the transverse processes of C2 and C3 (Stringer and Kelly, 1980; Zelenock et al., 1982) or the styloid process (Sundt et al., 1986), which may come in contact with the carotid in the neck or at the skull base. Dissecting aneurysms also may develop in the major intracranial arteries and in the intracranial portions of the internal carotid and vertebral arteries (Stehbens, 1972; Manz et al., 1979; Mizutani et al., 1982; Manz and Luessenhop, 1983).

The true incidence of dissection is difficult to ascertain. Biller et al. (1986) reported cervicocephalic dissection in 19 of 4531 patients (0.4%) undergoing angiography for acute cerebrovascular symptoms. In patients with a completed stroke, however, the incidence of dissection is significantly higher. Bogouslavsky et al. (1987) quoted a figure of 2.5%

based on a review of 1200 cases, and in a series of 41 patients younger than 30 years of age with ischemic strokes, dissections were the cause in 22% (nine patients) (Bogousslavsky and Regli, 1987). The frequency of dissection-related stroke is even higher in young patients with vertebrobasilar symptoms, ranging from 28 to 35% (Greselle et al., 1987; Yamaura, 1988).

Most patients have a single dissecting aneurysm, but some patients have more. Fourteen of 42 patients (33%) with spontaneous carotid dissections seen at the Mayo Clinic had at least one other vessel affected by a dissection (Houser et al., 1984). Many, but not all, of these patients have a systemic disorder characterized by abnormalities of connective tissue (see above). The aneurysms may affect both internal carotid arteries, both vertebral arteries, or the internal carotid and vertebral arteries on one or both sides (Boström and Liliequist, 1967; Lloyd and Bahnson, 1971; Pilz and Hartjes, 1976; Ringel et al., 1977; Mas et al., 1985; Yoshii et al., 1986; Leys et al., 1987). Some patients harbor both a dissecting aneurysm and a saccular aneurysm (Davies, 1987).

Dissecting aneurysms occur more frequently in men than in women in most series, perhaps men are somewhat more likely than women to experience head and neck trauma. In the series reported by Houser et al. (1984), however, women outnumbered men by a small margin.

Dissections can occur in patients of all ages. The peak age for spontaneous carotid system dissections is about 50 (O'Connell et al., 1985), and the average age of patients with spontaneous vertebral dissections is similar (Yamaura et al., 1990). This is almost a decade younger than congenital saccular (average 56.7 years) or fusiform atherosclerotic (average 58.9 years) aneurysms (Yamaura, 1988). Most dissections that occur in children affect the intracranial carotid system, particularly the middle and anterior cerebral arteries and the intracranial portion of the ICA, but extracranial carotid dissections can occur in this age group (Patel et al., 1995) as can traumatic dissections involving the vertebral artery (Horowitz and Niparko, 1994). Young and middle-aged adults usually develop dissecting aneurysms involving the cervical portions of the internal carotid and vertebral arteries and the vessels that comprise the intracranial portion of the vertebrobasilar arterial system. A familial risk of dissection has been reported (Schievink et al., 1991b, 1995c, 1996a). In these patients, there is a significantly increased risk of recurrent dissection.

Dissecting carotid and vertebrobasilar aneurysms may develop after blunt or penetrating injury to the head or neck, or they may arise spontaneously. Traumatic dissecting aneurysms usually arise in the extracranial portions of the carotid and vertebral arteries, the intracranial segments of the ICA, and the MCA (O'Connell et al., 1985). The basilar artery and its branches are almost never affected unless iatrogenically (Toyota and Ferguson, 1994).

Patients with spontaneous dissecting aneurysms sometimes have a predisposing disorder, especially connective tissue disease. Spontaneous dissecting aneurysm may occur in patients with alpha-1-antitrypsin deficiency (Schievink et al., 1994b, 1996b), lentiginosis (Schievink et al., 1995d), FMD (Pilz and Hartjes, 1976; Ringel et al., 1977; Hugenholz et al., 1982; Sato and Hata, 1982; Garcia-Merino et al., 1983; Sellier et al., 1983; Houser et al., 1984; Chiras et al., 1985; Mas et al., 1985; O'Connell et al., 1985; Bogousslavsky et al., 1987; Francis et al., 1987; Benrabah et al., 1988; Vles et al., 1990; Chin et al., 1996; Arunodaya et al., 1997; Manninen et al., 1997), moyamoya disease (Yamashita et al., 1983), cystic medial necrosis (Ramsay and Mosquera, 1948; Wolman, 1959; Thapedi et al., 1970; Lloyd and Bahnson, 1971; Chang et al., 1991), Marfan's syndrome (Austin and Schaefer, 1957; Croisile et al., 1988; Youl et al., 1990), Ehlers-Danlos syndrome (Rubinstein and Cohen, 1964; Graf, 1965; Schoolman and Kepes, 1967; Schievink et al., 1990; Youl et al., 1990; Schievink et al., 1991a; Pollack et al., 1997), polycystic kidney disease (Kulla et al., 1982; Larranaga et al., 1995), syphilis (Turnbull, 1915; Sato et al., 1971; Sato and Hata, 1982), mixed connective tissue disease (Ohki et al., 1994), atherosclerosis (Yonas et al., 1977; Adams et al., 1982), and congenital anomalies of the arterial walls (Johnson et al., 1977; Steiner et al., 1986). Patients with dissection also have a higher incidence of saccular aneurysms. In a retrospective study of 164 patients with dissecting aneurysms Schievink et al. (1992c) found saccular aneurysms in nine patients (5.5%). Spontaneous dissecting aneurysms also occur with increased frequency in patients with migraine (Sinclair, 1953; Spudis et al., 1962; Alexander et al., 1979; Mokri et al., 1988a; D'Anglejan-Chatillon et al., 1989; Hinse et al., 1991), with redundancy of the carotid artery (Ben Hamouda-M'Rad et al., 1995), and in patients with various vasculitides, including giant cell arteritis (Chang et al., 1975; Hatanaka et al., 1986; Lomeo et al., 1989; Youl et al., 1990; Takahashi et al., 1992).

In many patients, no specific cause for a dissection is found (Sato et al., 1971; Grosman et al., 1980; Pessin et al., 1989b). In others, what seems to be a spontaneous dissection is actually the result of relatively minor neck trauma (Rae-Grant et al., 1989; see Table 1 in Trosch et al., 1989; Mourad et al., 1997).

Hypertension may play a contributory role in both carotid and vertebral artery dissections. Sellier et al. (1983) reported that 22 of 46 patients (48%) with spontaneous carotid dissections had a history of hypertension, and Mokri et al. (1986) reported hypertension in 14 of 36 patients (39%) with spontaneous carotid dissection at the Mayo Clinic. Hypertension was also present in a total of 29 of 54 patients (54%) with vertebral artery dissections reported in three separate series (Friedman and Drake, 1984; Chiras et al., 1985; Mokri et al., 1988a).

The symptoms and signs that result from a dissecting aneurysm depend on a number of factors, including the site of the aneurysm, whether it is traumatic or spontaneous in origin, whether or not blood flow is maintained in the affected vessel, and whether or not the aneurysm ruptures into the extravascular space (see above).

Of nonlocalizing or incompletely localizing symptoms associated with dissections, headache, facial pain, and neck pain are the most common. Indeed, some type of head or neck pain may be the only manifestation of a dissection (Biousse et al., 1992; Silbert et al., 1997). In the Mayo Clinic series, 92% of patients with spontaneous carotid dissection had headache (Mokri et al., 1986). Scott et al. (1960) also

reported a high frequency of headache with carotid dissection, as did Biousse et al. (1994). The frequency is slightly lower in patients with posterior fossa dissection; 72% in the series reported by Berger and Wilson (1984). Yamaura et al. (1990) reported headache in all but one case of intracranial vertebral dissection. Silbert et al. (1995, 1997) reviewed the characteristics of headache and facial pain in 161 patients with dissection seen at the Mayo Clinic. In patients with dissections of the ICA, headaches were limited to the anterior head in 60% of patients. They were steady in 73% and pulsating in 25%. In contrast, patients with vertebral dissections had headaches that were distributed posteriorly in 83% of patients. These headaches were steady in 56% and pulsating in 44%. Neck pain was present in 26% of patients with carotid dissections and in 46% of patients with vertebral dissections. Ten percent of patients with carotid dissection had eye, facial, or ear pain without headache.

The natural history of arterial dissections is variable. The most important factor is location, both in terms of the vessel involved, but also the location within the wall. If the dissection is subintimal, the lumen is most likely stenotic, and there is a high risk of thrombosis. When the dissection is more subadventitial, the artery usually appears dilated, and there is a higher risk of rupture. Spontaneous resolution is common (Yoshimoto et al., 1997), but dissections may also progress. Narrowing can progress to complete occlusion. Of 42 patients seen at the Mayo clinic with craniocervical dissection, 15% progressed (Houser et al., 1984). Although most authors report that patients with dissections have a good prognosis regardless of treatment (Hart and Easton, 1983; Biller et al., 1986; Mokri et al. 1986), others emphasize that most patients who die from a spontaneous or traumatic dissection do so immediately and thus are never evaluated at the tertiary centers from which large series of patients are most often reported (Bogousslavsky et al., 1987). Thus, the prognosis for patients with a dissection may only be good if the patient does not die at the time the dissection occurs. It is also clear that the prognosis is significantly worse if an extracranial dissection extends intracranially (de Bray et al., 1997). In such cases, a fatal outcome is not uncommon (Anderson and Schechter, 1959; Brice and Crompton, 1964; Boström and Liliequist, 1967; Thapedi et al., 1970; Ojemann et al., 1972; Brown and Armitage, 1973; Nomose and New, 1973; Grosman et al., 1980; Bradac et al., 1981; Nass et al., 1982; Berkovic et al., 1983; Kalyan-Raman et al., 1983; Farrell et al., 1985; Linden et al., 1987). Most of these fatalities are related to increased ICP secondary to massive infarction, followed by subsequent herniation (Steiner et al., 1986). Individual case reports document survival even with intracranial extension, however (Pacini et al., 1991).

In contrast to saccular aneurysms, intracranial involvement with dissection has a better prognosis in the posterior fossa than in the anterior circulation, although as might be expected, a basilar artery dissection has a worse prognosis than a dissection limited to one vertebral artery.

Of patients who survive an acute dissection, most with carotid dissection tend to do well (Ehrenfeld and Wylie, 1976; Fisher et al., 1978; Shuster et al., 1985; Eljamel et al., 1989). Mokri et al. (1986) reported excellent or complete recovery in 36 patients with spontaneous carotid dissection. Even traumatic dissections with late onset seem to have a generally good prognosis (Lai et al., 1960; Pozzati et al., 1982, 1989). Despite the generally appreciated lower mortality and overall improved prognosis, there are significant neurologic sequelae in a substantial number of patients. Of 46 cases of spontaneous carotid dissection reported by Sellier et al. (1983), the clinical course was "favorable" in 25, but 21 patients (46%) had a residual neurologic deficit. Similarly, of 23 survivors of spontaneous carotid dissection, 11 were left with significant residual dysfunction (Bogousslavsky et al., 1987). The prognosis associated with traumatic ICA dissection is complicated by the additional potential of associated cranial damage. Of 24 cases reported by Watridge et al. (1989), two died from progressive thrombosis, one died from sepsis, and two died from concomitant brain injuries. Three patients recovered completely, whereas six had minimal neurologic sequelae, nine had moderate deficits, and one patient remained in a persistent vegetative state. Patients recovering from vertebral dissection may have a better prognosis. Of 15 patients with spontaneous vertebral dissection reported by Chiras et al. (1985), 13 returned to normal, and there were "slight neurologic sequelae" in two. Kitanaka et al. (1994b) followed five patients with vertebral artery dissection with serial angiograms. No further progression of dissection or associated SAH occurred in any of the cases, and all patients returned to their previous lifestyles. In the serial angiograms in five patients, the findings continued to change during the first few months after onset. Four cases ultimately showed "angiographic cure," whereas fusiform aneurysmal dilation of the affected vessel persisted in one case.

Traumatic carotid dissections improve less than corresponding spontaneous dissections. Mokri et al. (1986, 1988b) reported that although 87% of patients with spontaneous ICA dissections improved, only 55% of patients with traumatic ICA dissections showed evidence of improvement, and only two-thirds of these patients (or about 37% of the total) improved to normal. The prognosis for recovery of a complete arterial occlusion related to a dissection may be even worse, although even a completely occluded carotid may recanalize (Geeraert and Al-Saigh, 1987). Whereas stenosis tends to improve in the majority, pseudoaneurysm seems to resolve slightly less well (Sellier et al., 1983). Of thirteen patients restudied by Houser et al. (1984), four showed resolution, six decreased in size, and three remained unchanged; none enlarged. Vertebral dissections also tend to undergo change, improving spontaneously in the majority of cases (Adams et al., 1982; Berger and Wilson, 1984; Friedman and Drake, 1984). In a series of 19 patients, Mas et al. (1987) noted normalization in 12 (63%) and marked improvement in five (26%). Progression to occlusion was uncommon, occurring in only two cases (11%). Basilar artery occlusion following vertebral dissection can occur. In most cases this has devastating consequences, but collateral blood flow will sometimes limit manifestations to minimal symptoms (Okumura et al., 1995).

Because the most common cause of delayed onset symptoms in patients with dissection is progressive thrombosis or distal embolization (Sellier et al., 1983; Houser et al., 1984; Bogousslavsky et al., 1987), most medical treatment is aimed at preventing further clotting. Biousse et al. (1995a) studied 80 patients with cervical carotid dissection for the timing of completed infarcts following the onset of symptoms. A total of 42 patients developed completed infarcts (cerebral or retinal); nine initially and 33 after a delay. Whereas time to onset was as much as 31 days, 82% of events occurred within 1 week. To prevent these complications, Biousse et al. (1995a) recommended immediate anticoagulation in all patients with a spontaneous dissection of the cervical portion of the ICA.

Standard anticoagulation, initially with heparin and later with oral coumadin, is the mainstay of nonsurgical treatment. The risk of embolization is increased in patients with complete occlusion of the affected vessel (Aarabi and McQueen, 1978), and evidence of such embolization may be seen on angiography (Katirji et al., 1985). This phenomenon was documented in 15% of patients in one series of 42 patients with spontaneous carotid dissection (Houser et al., 1984) and in 24% of 46 patients in another (Sellier et al., 1983). If there is angiographic evidence of a thrombus, the frequency of distal embolization may be even higher; 37% of patients had evidence of emboli in a series of patients with carotid dissection and stroke reported by Bogousslavsky et al. (1987).

Anticoagulation can cause significant complications in patients with dissections, particularly those in whom the dissection extends intracranially (Caplan et al., 1985, 1988; Youl et al., 1990). The risk of anticoagulation in such patients is related to the chance of full-thickness compromise of the vascular wall, resulting in SAH. Mokri et al. (1988a) estimated an incidence of 10% in patients with vertebral artery dissection, and Berger and Wilson (1984) reported SAH in seven of 27 patients with posterior fossa dissections. Recurrent hemorrhage is associated with a significant increase in mortality (Shimoji et al., 1984). Although this complication is well described (Manz and Luessenhop, 1983; Shimoji et al., 1984; Caplan et al., 1988; Yamaura, 1988; Kawamata et al., 1994), some authors consider it a rare phenomenon. None of the patients reported by Mas et al. (1987) experienced rebleeding. Yamaura (1988), however, reported recurrent hemorrhage in five of 21 patients with vertebral dissection (24%), and two patients reported in a later series by Yamaura et al. (1990) and who rebled (at 5 and 15 days, respectively) died. Takai et al. (1993) and Kawamata et al. (1994) reported rebleeding in patients in whom the length of the vertebral dissection precluded more than a proximal clip. Mizutani et al. (1995) reported on 42 patients with vertebral dissections; 30 rebled, 14 of whom died (12 directly related), for a mortality of 46.7%. Only one patient who did not rebleed died (mortality of 8.3%). Of the 30 hemorrhages, 17 (56.7%) occurred within 24 hours after the first SAH, and 24 (80%) occurred within the first week. Surgery did not prevent rebleeds if it did not completely isolate the involved segment.

Despite the risk of stroke and SAH in patients with dissections, most patients have a good prognosis regardless of treatment. Frumkin and Baloh (1990) reviewed the results of treatment in patients with Wallenberg's syndrome following dissection induced by neck manipulation. Five patients treated with anticoagulation did well but so did 12 untreated patients. Patients may have recurrent distal ischemia even if anticoagulated. Extension of dissection despite anticoagulation also occurs (Duman and Stephens, 1963). Pacini et al. (1991) reported a patient who developed a Horner's syndrome related to extension of a carotid dissection despite anticoagulation with heparin. A 57-year-old man who developed a vertebral dissection after carrying a heavy weight on his shoulder developed recurrent episodes of occipital ischemia despite anticoagulation (Katirji et al., 1985). Of seven patients anticoagulated for cervicocephalic dissection, three developed hemorrhagic complications: an intracerebellar bleed requiring shunting in one and extracerebral gastrointestinal hemorrhage in two (Biller et al., 1986). Watridge et al., (1989) described a case of subdural hematoma in one of 17 patients undergoing anticoagulation for traumatic carotid dissection. Intracerebral hematomas also occur in this setting (Kunze and Schiefer, 1971; Hochberg et al., 1975). Rupture of a dissecting aneurysm (Adams et al., 1982; Hochberg et al., 1975), the most feared complication of anticoagulation, is fortunately very uncommon and may not be increased by anticoagulation.

There is little data on the efficacy of antiplatelet agents in patients with arterial dissections. Some authors recommend them (Biller et al., 1986), but three of four patients reported by Eljamel et al. (1990) continued to have TIAs despite such treatment. Some authors advocate the combined use of anticoagulation and antiplatelet agents (Ishikawa et al., 1994).

The surgical approach to dissecting aneurysms is dependent on the location and extent of the dissection as well as on potential collateral flow (Burklund, 1970). Because there is no neck to clip, surgical therapy may consist of ligation (Yonas et al., 1977), trapping (Sekino et al., 1982), wrapping (Yamaura et al., 1990), resection (Schievink et al., 1994c), or reconstruction (Yokoh et al., 1986) of the affected area with or without revascularization (Lee and Sekhar, 1996). In the anterior circulation, lack of adequate collaterals may be managed with an STA-MCA bypass (Adams et al., 1982). In addition, endovascular occlusion of an affected vessel may be achieved with a detachable balloon, or coils may be placed to induce thrombosis (Halbach et al., 1993).

CLINICAL MANIFESTATIONS, TREATMENT, AND PROGNOSIS ACCORDING TO SITE

Dissecting Aneurysms of the Internal Carotid Artery and Its Branches

Dissecting aneurysms may develop in the ICA or any of its major branches, particularly the MCA (O'Connell et al., 1985). Aneurysms can arise in the extracranial segment of the ICA and remain extracranial or extend intracranially. Dissecting aneurysms may also originate in the intracranial portions of the ICA. These aneurysms may remain confined to the ICA or may extend along its major branches. Rarely, dissecting aneurysms occur along the external carotid or its branches (Fujii et al., 1995).

Dissecting Aneurysms of the Extracranial Portion of the Internal Carotid Artery

Traumatic dissections of the cervical segment of the ICA usually occur after blunt head or neck injury of marked or moderate severity. Motor vehicle accidents commonly cause such aneurysms, as do fist fights, falls, blows to the neck or head with various objects, compression of the ICA, hanging by the neck, local surgery, and manipulative neck therapy (Yamada et al., 1967; Robertson, 1981; Chandler, 1982; Chiras et al., 1982; Hart and Easton, 1983; Cellerier and Georget, 1984; Mokri et al., 1986; Dunne et al., 1987; Watridge et al., 1989; Leys et al., 1997).

In some cases, a dissection of the extracranial portion of the ICA occurs after relatively minor neck trauma. Trosch et al. (1989) reported the case of a young woman who participated in a drinking game, swallowing several shots of whiskey in rapid succession and throwing her head back in a whiplike fashion. The next morning, she experienced a bitemporal headache. Over the next 5 days, she developed a right hemiparesis, expressive aphasia, and tinnitus. Angiography revealed a dissection of the extracranial portion of the left ICA. Mourad et al. (1997) described a young woman who developed sudden right-sided neck pain immediately after a telephone conversation that lasted 32 minutes. During the entire conversation, she held the handset between her right ear and shoulder by flexing her head to the side, thereby allowing her to continue ironing. Dissection can also occur following other types of apparently trivial trauma (Table 53.3). Many of these episodes are associated with athletic activity (Table 53.4). Others occur after "unusual exertion" (Adelman et al., 1974). The minimal severity of trauma capable of producing dissection makes it difficult to distinguish traumatic from spontaneous dissection. Further complicating the issue is that there may be a considerable delay from the time of trauma to the onset of symptoms of dissection (Northcroft and Morgan, 1944–1945; Boyd and Watson, 1956; Lai et al., 1960; Crissey and Bernstein, 1974; Pozzati et al., 1982; Reverdin et al., 1986; Mokri et al., 1988b; Pozzati et al., 1989; Rae-Grant et al., 1989). Thus, the distinction between traumatic and spontaneous dissections is not always clear.

Intraoral trauma may cause a dissecting aneurysm of the cervical portion of the carotid artery. This occurs most often in children who fall on a foreign object (such as a pencil) that they are carrying in the mouth, sustaining trauma to the peritonsillar region (Bickerstaff, 1964; Pitner, 1966). Carotid artery dissection during or following angiography may result from direct needle puncture (Fig. 53.257) or, less commonly, from arterial catheterization (Tangchai and Pisitbutr, 1971; Vitek, 1973; Huckman et al., 1979).

Trauma to the head and neck can produce a dissecting aneurysm by several mechanisms. Direct neck or intraoral trauma may contuse and tear the wall of the ICA. Abrupt, severe rotation of the head may cause a dissecting aneurysm when the ICA is damaged by a prominent styloid process (Sundt et al., 1986). Hyperextension and rotation of the neck may stretch the artery against the transverse processes of the C2 and C3 vertebrae, causing intimal tears and arterial

Table 53.3
Dissection Association with Trivial Trauma

Brushing teeth	Hart and Easton, 1983
Eating	Fisher, 1978
Laughing	Hart and Easton, 1983
Nose blowing	Hart and Easton, 1983; Katirji et al., 1985 (case 3); Roome and Aberfeld, 1977
Shaving	Fisher et al., 1978
Coughing	Fisher et al., 1978; Hart and Easton, 1983; Britton and Guiloff, 1988; Sellier et al., 1983
Violent sneezing	Sellier et al., 1983; Gutowski et al., 1992
Childbirth	Périer et al., 1964; Chiras et al., 1985; Wiebers and Mokri, 1985; Brass, 1970
Extension while painting the ceiling	Okawara and Nibbelink, 1975; Saeed et al., 1990
Turning head while leading a parade	Hart and Easton, 1983
Turning head while backing up car	Hilton-Jones and Warlow, 1985
Old whiplash injury	Hart and Easton, 1983
Car sliding on ice	O'Connell et al., 1985
Neck flexing with child scolding	Waespe et al., 1988
Straightening up after bending	Fisher et al., 1978
Head banging during punk rock dancing	Jackson et al., 1983
Tree falling on back	Waespe et al., 1988
Drinking game	Trosch et al., 1989
MVA without apparent injury	Newman et al., 1989
Peritonsillar trauma	Bickerstaff, 1964; Woodhurst et al., 1980
Riding a roller coaster	Biousse et al., 1995b
Seizure	Young et al., 1991
Telephone call	Mourad et al., 1997

dissection (Stringer and Kelly, 1980; Zelenock et al., 1982). Abrupt, severe neck flexion may directly compress the ICA between the angle of the mandible and the upper cervical column, causing arterial contusion and dissection (Zelenock et al., 1982).

Many patients who experience trauma sufficient to produce a dissecting aneurysm of the cervical portion of the ICA have no signs of direct injury to the neck (Yamada et al., 1967). The only indication of the trauma may be mild bruises or abrasions of the skin; however, fractures of the mandible, cervical spine, or base of the skull may be present in such patients.

The most common cause of direct damage to the ICA is percutaneous puncture of the artery for angiography. This was first reported by Idbohrn (1951) in a 40-year-old man who suddenly lost consciousness following an intramural injection of iodinated contrast material. Multiple other cases were subsequently reported (Rowbotham et al., 1953; de Grood, 1954; Serois et al., 1954; Boyd-Wilson, 1962). Small dissecting aneurysms were found in nine of 75 patients autopsied within 8 months of death (Crawford, 1956). Simi-

larly Rimpau (1957) found evidence of blood in the wall of 11 of 92 autopsied cases following percutaneous angiography. In a subsequent study, a puncture site was found in the opposite wall in nearly all cases, indicating that the artery was transfixed during puncture (Rimpau and Seils, 1957). Fleming and Park (1959) identified nine cases of clinical dissection in a series of 900 direct percutaneous injections. Less commonly, dissection is associated with retrograde catheterization to reach the cervical arteries (Tangchai and Pisitbutr, 1971; Vitek, 1973; Huckman et al., 1979). Angioplasty also has the potential to induce dissection.

The clinical picture of patients who develop traumatic dissections of the extracranial ICA varies considerably. When a patient sustains severe injuries to multiple organs or is comatose, the dissection may go unrecognized. The patient may subsequently recover and have no neurologic deficit, or residual deficits may be incorrectly attributed to "head injury" (Mokri et al., 1988b).

Many patients who develop a traumatic dissecting aneurysm of the extracranial ICA experience delayed, focal cerebral ischemic symptoms and signs (Watridge et al., 1989). These disturbances may develop weeks, months, or even years after the injury (Crissey and Bernstein, 1974; Batzdorf et al., 1979; Perry et al., 1980; Sundt et al., 1986; Pozzati et al., 1989). A 24-year-old man developed acute left hemiparesis, blindness in the right eye, and a right Horner's syndrome 3 weeks after he was involved in a motorcycle accident (Miller, 1991j). The patient was found to have a dissection of the extracranial portion of the right ICA. The

Table 53.4
Athletics and Dissection

Gymnastics	Nagler, 1973
Swimming	Tramo et al., 1985; Greselle et al., 1987
Badminton	Saeed et al., 1990; Chang et al., 1991
Diving into water	Fisher et al., 1978
Heavy lifting	Lieschke et al., 1988
Basketball	O'Connell et al., 1985
Tennis	Hart and Easton, 1983; Manz and Luessenhop, 1983; Roualdes et al., 1985; Hilton-Jones and Warlow, 1985
Skiing	Ringel et al., 1977; Hart and Easton, 1983
Volleyball	Hart and Easton, 1983
Polo	O'Connell et al., 1985
Hockey	Fisher et al., 1978; Reverdin et al., 1986
Football	Hart, 1978; Mokri et al., 1988b
Bowling	Hart, 1978
Trampoline exercises	Hart, 1985
Waterskiing	Mokri et al., 1988b
Skydiving	Mokri et al., 1988b; Reverdin et al., 1986
Bicycling	Bogousslavsky et al., 1987 (2); Pikula et al., 1973
Jogging	Bogousslavsky et al., 1987; Kline et al., 1987
Weight lifting	Kline et al., 1987
Yoga	Hilton-Jones and Warlow, 1985 (Case 3); Hanus et al., 1977; Nagler, 1973
Archery	Sorensen, 1978
Squash	Fisher, 1981

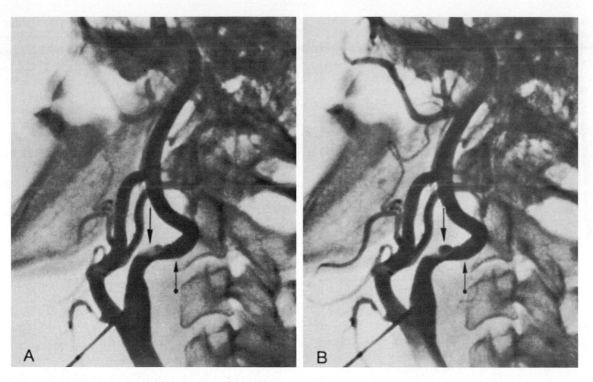

Figure 53.257. Iatrogenic dissecting aneurysm of the extracranial portion of the internal carotid artery. The aneurysm developed after failed angiography. *A*, The *arrow* shows early opacification of the aneurysm. The *ball-tipped arrow* points to a minute lesion of the intima. *B*, A later phase of the angiogram shows progressive filling of the aneurysm. (From Huber P. Cerebral Angiography, 2nd ed. Stuttgart, Georg Thieme Verlag, 1982.)

blindness was caused by a combined central retinal artery occlusion and ischemic optic neuropathy.

Although narrowing of the true lumen of the affected artery may be responsible for the development of delayed neurologic deficits (Pozzati et al., 1989), occlusion of the vessel or thromboembolism from the aneurysm site are more common causes (Fig. 53.258). Most patients make a good recovery (Chiras et al., 1982; Pozzati et al., 1989), but some are left with severe neurologic deficits, and a few die from massive cerebral infarction and edema (Mokri et al., 1988b).

Patients with a traumatic dissecting aneurysm affecting the cervical portion of the ICA occasionally experience an acute, focal, unilateral headache associated with Horner's syndrome. The headache is often distinctive (West et al., 1976; Mokri et al., 1979; Fisher, 1981). It typically affects the ipsilateral forehead just above the orbit, the portions of the face just lateral or below the orbit, or the orbit itself and is associated with neck pain that extends from just above the clavicle to the area behind the ear (Fisher, 1981). In such patients, a bruit may be heard, and a pulsating mass may be felt in the neck. Pulsatile tinnitus may occur with a petrous dissection (Saeed et al., 1990) or extension of the dissection to the base of the skull (Waespe et al., 1988). A subjective bruit occurs in up to 39% of patients with a spontaneous carotid dissection (Fisher, 1981; Mokri et al., 1986). Less frequently, an objective bruit is present (Sellier et al., 1983; Mokri et al., 1986).

When a dissection of the ICA extends to the base of the brain, it may produce single or multiple cranial neuropathies.

A patient reported by Vighetto et al. (1990) developed a left hypoglossal neuropathy associated with an ipsilateral Horner's syndrome from a traumatic dissection of the extracranial portion of the left ICA.

Spontaneous dissecting aneurysms that affect the extracranial portion of the ICA are not uncommon (Gautier and Pertuiset, 1983; Bogousslavsky et al., 1984; Gauthier et al., 1985; Mokri et al., 1986; Bogousslavsky et al., 1987; Leys et al., 1997) (Fig. 53.259). Some present as a pulsating neck mass (Itoh et al., 1987), but most produce no external signs. External rupture of the aneurysm rarely, if ever, occurs (Mokri et al., 1986).

Spontaneous extracranial ICA aneurysms produce neurologic symptoms and signs similar to those produced by traumatic dissecting aneurysms. Some cause acute, unilateral headache. The headache, which may be spontaneous or induced by coughing or straining (Britton and Guiloff, 1988), is often associated with ipsilateral oculosympathetic paresis (Mokri et al., 1986; Bogousslavsky et al., 1987; Itoh et al., 1987; Benrabah et al., 1988; Gautier and Loron, 1989; Assaf et al., 1993; Brown et al., 1995). As noted above, the headache that occurs in such patients is often typical. It is centered in and around the orbit and is associated with pain that radiates from just above the clavicle to just behind the ear (Fisher, 1981). An oculosympathetic paresis that accompanies the headache consists of a Horner's syndrome that is almost always postganglionic (see Chapters 24 and 36). Biousse et al. (1994) found a painful Horner's syndrome in 31% of 65 patients with dissections of the cervical portion of the ICA; it

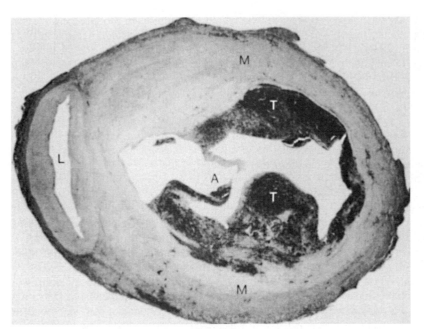

Figure 53.258. Thromboembolism from dissecting aneurysm. The patient was a 23-year-old man who suffered an injury to the neck while playing football. He was found to have a dissecting aneurysm of the right internal carotid artery. Cross-section of the artery through the aneurysm shows that the lumen of the artery (*L*) is compressed but open. The aneurysm is located within the media (*M*) of the artery, and its lumen (*A*) is filled with organized thrombus (*T*). (From Mokri B, Piepgras DG, Houser OW. Traumatic dissections of the extracranial internal carotid artery. J Neurosurg *68*:189–197, 1988.)

was the only manifestation in 16%. In most patients, the headache resolves within several months, although the Horner's syndrome may be permanent (Mokri et al., 1979).

Patients with a spontaneous dissecting aneurysm of the extracranial portion of the ICA often experience TIAs or permanent, focal neurologic deficits from thromboembolism related to the aneurysm (Hart and Easton, 1983; Gauthier et al., 1985; Mokri et al., 1986; Biousse et al., 1995a) or from

occlusion of the artery (Pozzati et al., 1990). The TIAs are nonspecific and cannot be differentiated from those that result from cerebrovascular or cardiovascular atherosclerotic disease. Some are characterized by transient monocular visual loss (Ehrenfeld and Wylie, 1976; Fisher et al., 1978; Bashour et al., 1985; Marchal et al., 1985; Verreault and Cote, 1986; Bogousslavsky et al., 1987; Kline et al., 1987; Mas et al., 1987; Duker and Belmont, 1988; Saeed et al.,

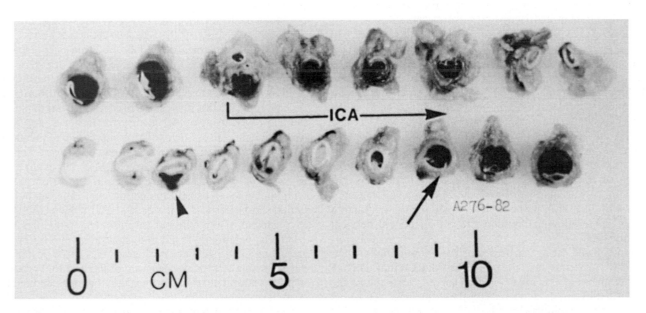

Figure 53.259. Spontaneous dissection of the left common and internal carotid arteries in a patient with Ehlers-Danlos syndrome. The patient died after repeated cardiac arrests. Serial cross-sections through the affected arteries show a continuous dissection of the common carotid artery (*lower row*) and internal carotid artery (*ICA, upper row*). The *arrow* points to the origin of the dissection in the common carotid artery. A small intramural hematoma is seen at the site of previous angiography (*arrowhead*). (From Lach B, Nair SG, Russell NA, et al. Spontaneous carotid-cavernous fistula and multiple arterial dissections in Type IV Ehlers-Danlos syndrome: Case report. J Neurosurg *66*:462–467, 1987.)

1990; Pacini et al., 1991). About 30–50% of patients experience an acute stroke. In about 20% of these patients, the stroke is preceded by a TIA (Bogousslavsky et al., 1987). In the remainder, the stroke is the first sign of the aneurysm. Bogousslavsky et al. (1987) found that 30 of 1200 (2.5%) consecutive patients with a first stroke had a spontaneous dissection with occlusion of the cervical ICA. Six of these patients (20%) experienced monocular blindness as an initial symptom of the disorder. In one of the patients, monocular blindness was the only symptom. Four patients initially experienced hemicranial headache, ipsilateral neck pain, and ipsilateral blindness. A sixth patient experienced monocular blindness associated with ipsilateral tinnitus.

Visual loss in patients with spontaneous dissecting ICA aneurysms may be caused by embolic occlusion of the ophthalmic artery, the central retinal artery, one or more of the retinal branch arteries (including the cilioretinal artery), or one or more of the short posterior ciliary arteries (Camuzet et al., 1984; Newman et al., 1989; Rivkin et al., 1990). Hyland (1933) reported a 58-year-old man with intracranial extension of a thrombus in the ICA that produced loss of vision associated with pallid swelling of the optic disc, consistent with anterior ischemic optic neuropathy. In another case, a 31-year-old woman with sudden onset of headache, facial pain and decreased vision was found to have a dissecting aneurysm of the ipsilateral ICA (Jentzer, 1954). In a review of aortic dissection by Hirst et al. (1958), five of nine patients with complaints of decreased vision were found to have extension of the dissection into the common carotid or innominate arteries. O'Dwyer et al. (1980) described central retinal artery occlusion from dissection. Visual loss may also result from occlusion of the ICA by the dissection itself, either by extension of the dissection into the ophthalmic artery or by generalized reduction in blood flow to the eye (Newman et al., 1989). Duker and Belmont (1988) described a 64-year-old man who experienced transient loss of vision in the right eye. The right eye had visual acuity of 20/50, mild flare in the anterior chamber, neovascularization of the iris, generalized narrowing of retinal arteries, and blot hemorrhages in the midperipheral retina. The left eye was normal. Intraocular pressures were 22 mm Hg in both eyes. A diagnosis of the ocular ischemic syndrome was made (see Chapter 55), and the patient underwent cerebral angiography that disclosed a spontaneous dissection of the right ICA. The patient was treated with panretinal photocoagulation and maintained 20/60 vision in the right eye, associated with disappearance of both iris neovascularization and retinal hemorrhages. Ramadan et al. (1991) described three patients with scintillating scotomata resembling migraine aura associated with cervical ICA dissections.

When a dissecting aneurysm of the extracranial portion of the ICA extends up to the base of the skull, it may damage one or more of the lower cranial nerves, particularly the vagus and hypoglossal nerves (Bradac et al., 1981; Havelius et al., 1982; Goldberg et al., 1986; Mokri et al., 1987; Waespe et al., 1988; Panisset and Eidelman, 1990). Hommel et al. (1984) described a patient in whom a dissecting aneurysm of the ICA produced unilateral glossopharyngeal, vagal, and hypoglossal neuropathy. Davies (1987) reported a patient in whom a similar aneurysm produced a unilateral paresis of the vagus nerve. Panisset and Eidelman (1990) described two cases with multiple lower cranial neuropathies. One patient developed glossopharyngeal, vagal, and hypoglossal neuropathies; the other patient developed unilateral trigeminal, facial, glossopharyngeal, vagal, and hypoglossal neuropathies. Delayed hemilingual paresis was described by Pica et al. (1996), and Zipp et al. (1993) reported isolated unilateral hypoglossal nerve paralysis as the only manifestation in a 41-year-old patient with an cervical ICA dissection that extended to the base of the skull. Bilbao et al. (1997) described a 43-year-old woman in whom an acute postganglionic Horner's syndrome associated with mild periocular discomfort was the only sign of a spontaneous dissection of the petrous segment of the ipsilateral ICA.

Spontaneous dissecting aneurysms of the cervical portion of the ICA may extend intracranially, producing neurologic symptoms and signs related to the intracranial extension. Maitland et al. (1983) described a 37-year-old woman who awoke with severe, bilateral, retrobulbar headache. Later that day, the pain extended into the left side of the face, the teeth, and the neck. The headache progressively worsened over the next 12 days, and the patient began to experience a bitter, unpleasant taste, like "tooth decay." She then developed sudden, horizontal diplopia, worse to the left. Complete neurologic and general physical examinations were normal except for a left abducens nerve paresis that became complete within 48 hours. Arteriography demonstrated a dissecting aneurysm of the left ICA beginning in the high cervical region and extending into the inferior cavernous sinus. The patient was treated with analgesics. Her headaches continued for 2 weeks and then disappeared. The abducens nerve paresis resolved completely within 2 months. The paresis was probably caused by expansion of the wall of the cavernous portion of the ICA with either direct compression or interruption of blood supply of the adjacent abducens nerve.

Cranial neuropathies other than abducens nerve paresis may also be caused by intracranial extension of a dissecting ICA aneurysm. Paralysis of the tongue from compression of the hypoglossal nerve at the base of the skull may occur (Fisher et al., 1978). Dysgeusia may result from damage to the chorda tympani by the aneurysm (Fisher et al., 1978), although it may also be caused by compression of the glossopharyngeal nerve in the neck as it passes forward between the ICA and the internal jugular vein (Maitland et al., 1983). Mokri et al. (1986) found dysgeusia in one of 36 patients with spontaneous carotid dissection, and other authors reported similar cases (Francis et al., 1987; Kline et al., 1987). Involvement of the external carotid artery (Devoize et al., 1985) can potentially result in dysgeusia by interrupting the ascending pharyngeal artery. Lane et al. (1980) described a patient with a dissecting aneurysm of the ICA that produced hypoglossal and glossopharyngeal neuropathies without perversion of taste.

Ocular motor disturbances are uncommon in patients with an intracranial extension of a cervical ICA dissection. Schievink et al. (1993) reported transient ocular motor disorders in four of 155 patients with spontaneous carotid dissection seen at the Mayo Clinic. The oculomotor nerve was involved in two patients, the trochear nerve in one, and the abducens nerve in one. Three patients had ipsilateral headache or facial pain, one had bilateral headaches, and three had oculosympathetic palsy. None had any associated cerebral or retinal ischemic symptoms.

Newman et al. (1989) reported a 42-year-old man who lost vision in the right eye over 24 hours and then developed right-sided jaw and neck pain as well as an abnormal taste in the mouth. He was found to have a central retinal artery occlusion in the right eye, a partial right abducens nerve paresis, and slightly decreased sensation in the region supplied by the ophthalmic division of the right trigeminal nerve. A cerebral angiogram revealed complete occlusion of the right ICA beginning at its origin in the neck. The right ophthalmic artery could not be visualized. Newman et al. (1989) postulated that the central retinal artery occlusion that occurred in this patient resulted from extension of the dissection or its attendant thrombus across or into the origin of the right ophthalmic artery, although they could not ignore the possibility that the occlusion was caused by emboli originating from the occluded artery.

Intracranial extension of an extracranial ICA dissection may also cause interruption of the postchiasmal afferent visual pathways. Two patients reported by Fisher et al. (1978) had transient homonymous visual field defects. One had intracranial extension of a dissection of the ICA on the side contralateral to the field defect; the other had a contralateral MCA dissection. This may not be a rare phenomenon. Two of 14 patients with spontaneous ICA dissections reported by Bogousslavsky et al. (1984) developed contralateral homonymous visual field defects. We believe that the incidence of homonymous visual field defects in patients with spontaneous ICA dissections is significantly higher than reported in the literature because such patients often have a hemiplegia and the field defect in such cases is likely to be ignored.

Neuro-ophthalmologic manifestations other than those described above occasionally occur in patients with spontaneous ICA dissections. For example, Newman et al. (1989) attributed the ipsilateral mydriasis that occurred in one patient to ciliary body ischemia related to occlusion of the ophthalmic artery.

The prognosis of patients with spontaneous dissecting aneurysms of the cervical portion of the ICA is variable (Hart and Easton, 1983; Bogousslavsky et al., 1984; Gauthier et al., 1985; Mokri et al., 1986; Bogousslavsky et al., 1987; Kushner, 1988; Pozzati et al., 1990). Some patients develop severe, permanent neurologic deficits or die from thromboembolism associated with the lesion (Anderson and Schechter, 1959; Brice and Crompton, 1964; Boström and Liliequist, 1967; Thapedi et al., 1970; Ojemann et al., 1972; Brown and Armitage, 1973; Nomose and New, 1973; Bradac et al., 1981; Bogousslavsky et al., 1984; Farrell et al., 1985), whereas others have a much more benign course with no lasting neurologic disturbance (Shuster et al., 1985; Mokri et al., 1986; Eljamel et al., 1989, 1990). Clearly, occlusion of the affected ICA is associated with a significant mortality and morbidity (Pozzati et al., 1990), but the percentage of patients in whom this occurs varies depending on the series

(Bogousslavsky et al., 1984; Mokri et al., 1986; Kushner, 1988).

There is no general agreement regarding the treatment of patients with either traumatic or spontaneous dissections of the extracranial portion of the ICA (Mokri et al., 1986; Bogousslavsky et al., 1987; Dunne et al., 1987). During the acute phase of the disease, anticoagulant therapy may prevent the intraluminal clotting that is associated with a poor prognosis, but recanalization of the artery can occur both with and without anticoagulant therapy (Mokri et al., 1986; Bogousslavsky et al., 1987; Eljamel et al., 1989, 1990). Anticoagulation may be appropriate for patients with symptoms or signs of focal, but not profound, cerebral ischemia (Stringer and Kelly, 1980; Ajir and Tibbetts, 1981; Dragon et al., 1981; Mas et al., 1985; Mokri et al., 1986; Eljamel et al., 1989, 1990). Such therapy is probably also contraindicated in patients with severe visceral injuries. In patients without any symptoms or signs of cerebral ischemia, many investigators do not recommend anticoagulation because of possible side effects. In such patients, antiplatelet therapy (e.g., aspirin) may be helpful, although there is no proof that this is the case (Andersen et al., 1980; Monfort et al., 1981; Garcia-Merino et al., 1983; Mas et al., 1985; Mokri et al., 1986).

Emergency surgery may be indicated in some patients with ICA dissections. If the dissection is confined to the proximal portion of the ICA, it may be possible to excise the aneurysm and repair the affected segment at the same time (Schievink et al., 1994c). More commonly, the dissection extends to the base of the skull. Direct repair of the affected segment usually is not possible in such cases, but a bypass procedure such as an STA-MCA anastomosis may be beneficial. In some cases, both a bypass procedure and excision of the aneurysm are performed (Garcia-Merino et al., 1983).

Measurement of retinal artery pressure may be valuable in the management of patients with dissecting aneurysms of the ICA. Several investigators (Gee et al., 1980; Mokri et al., 1986) described a reproducible relationship between an increase in retinal artery pressure and a decrease in, or resolution of, the luminal stenosis that accompanies dissection. Eljamel et al. (1989, 1990) recommended Doppler blood flow and duplex ultrasonographic studies both to diagnose and to follow patients with strokes or TIAs related to dissecting aneurysms of the extracranial ICA. Color doppler flow imaging may also be helpful in such patients (de Bray et al., 1994; Bartels, 1996).

Dissecting Aneurysms of the Intracranial Portion of the Internal Carotid Artery

Most dissecting aneurysms that affect the intracranial portion of the ICA arise extracranially and extend intracranially. Both traumatic and spontaneous dissecting aneurysms arising in the intracranial portion of the ICA are exceptionally rare. Nevertheless, they can produce transient or permanent cerebral ischemia from thrombosis or embolism related to the site of the aneurysm (Pessin et al., 1989b). In exceptional cases, the dissection may separate the medial and adventitial layers of the vessel wall and result in SAH, intraparenchymal hemorrhage, or both (Kunze and Schiefer, 1971; Adams et al., 1982).

Because of the small number of patients encountered, the optimum treatment of intracranial ICA dissections is unclear. The potential of these lesions to rupture and produce intracranial hemorrhage is significant, and the use of anticoagulants or vasopressors may promote such hemorrhage (Hochberg et al., 1975). Anticoagulation is therefore probably contraindicated in such patients. A direct surgical approach to these lesions is usually not possible because they cannot be clipped, and trapping procedures are often associated with significant mortality and morbidity. Some patients seem to benefit from a combination of ligation of the ICA combined with extracranial-intracranial bypass (Adams et al., 1982).

Dissecting Aneurysms of the Branches of the Internal Carotid Artery

Many dissecting aneurysms that affect the major branches of the ICA actually arise within the ICA itself and extend into its branches (Kunze and Schiefer, 1971; Kitani et al., 1987) (Fig. 53.255A). Dissecting aneurysms nevertheless may arise within the major branches of the ICA. The MCA is affected in over 90% of the cases (Ramsay and Mosquera, 1948; Sinclair, 1953; see Table 1 in Sato et al., 1971; Grosman et al., 1980; Mizutani et al., 1982; Steiner et al., 1986; Graber et al., 1992; Adams and Trevenen, 1996). The ACA is less commonly affected (Guridi et al., 1993; Kidooka et al., 1993; Yano et al., 1995; Araki et al., 1996).

Most patients with dissecting aneurysms of the intracranial branches of the ICA have experienced significant head trauma or have a congenital or acquired defect of connective tissue. Two patients were reported in whom dissecting aneurysms of the MCA developed after intracranial surgery. In one case, a dissecting aneurysm occurred after resection of a saccular aneurysm (Bigelow, 1955). In the other case, a dissecting aneurysm developed after removal of a large sphenoid wing meningioma (Heye et al., 1989). Patients with dissecting aneurysms affecting the intracranial branches of the ICA often experience massive infarction, and most die within 1 week of onset of symptoms (Steiner et al., 1986).

Intracranial hemorrhage may occur in patients with an intracranial dissecting aneurysm (Ramsay and Mosquera, 1948; Guridi et al., 1993; Yano et al., 1995). In some cases, early STA-MCA bypass results in neurologic stabilization and improvement (Kitani et al., 1987), although hemorrhage is usually a poor prognostic sign.

Occasionally, an intracranial dissecting aneurysm develops after apparently insignificant head trauma. Amagasa et al. (1988) described a 44-year-old man who sustained a blow to the occiput when he was involved in a rear-end collision while driving a car. He lost consciousness for a moment but then recovered completely and drove home. About 30 minutes after the accident, he developed weakness of his right arm and leg and difficulty with speech. He was hospitalized and found to have a right hemiparesis and mild motor aphasia. An evaluation revealed an apparent dissecting aneu-

rysm of the left ACA. The patient was briefly treated with an osmotic agent. No other therapy was given. Adams and Trevenen (1996) described a 12-year-old girl who hit her head on a coffee table, causing an abrasion but no loss of consciousness. The following day, she had a seizure and then developed right-sided weakness. A CT scan revealed changes consistent with an ischemic infarct in the territory of the left MCA. The child died despite supportive therapy. Postmortem examination revealed left MCA dissection with an intact ICA and no evidence of vasculitis. Sharif et al. (1995) also reported a case in which minor trauma was associated with a fatal intracranial dissection. Occasionally, dissection of the MCA is associated with the development of a saccular aneurysm (Graber et al., 1992; Piepgras et al., 1994).

Dissecting Aneurysms of the Vertebral and Basilar Arteries and Their Branches

About 40% of dissecting intracranial aneurysms affect the vertebral and basilar arteries and their branches (Manz and Luessenhop, 1983; see Table 1 in Berger and Wilson, 1984). Most of the cases that affect the extracranial portion of the vertebral artery are caused by neck trauma from automobile accidents, fights, sports activities, and, occasionally, chiropractic manipulation of the neck (Cellerier and Georget, 1984; Dunne et al., 1987; Mas et al., 1989; Rae-Grant et al., 1989; Frumkin and Baloh, 1990; Leys et al., 1997; Scazzeri et al., 1997) (Fig. 53.260 and Table 53.1) or are associated with systemic disorders of connective tissue (Youl et al., 1990; Ohki et al., 1994). Rarely, pseudoaneurysms develop (Davidson et al., 1975). Kaplan et al. (1993) reported a vertebral pseudoaneurysm that developed in a 41-year-old woman 1 month after an uncomplicated pregnancy and delivery. The onset was heralded by neck stiffness followed by intense neck and head pain and paresthesias that extended into the left arm, thumb, and forefinger. Evidence of SAH was found on lumbar puncture. Another case of vertebral dissection following neck manipulation occurred in a 50-year-old man with myelopathy secondary to basilar impression who was treated with 8 pounds of cervical traction (Dickinson et al., 1995).

Most of the cases that originate in the intracranial portion of the vertebral artery, the basilar artery, and their branches are spontaneous and occur in young, hypertensive patients (Manz and Luessenhop, 1983; Berger and Wilson, 1984; Caplan et al., 1988; Hart, 1988; Mokri et al., 1988a) (Fig. 53.261). In some cases, a spontaneous dissection produces the neck pain and stiffness that cause the patient to seek relief by cervical manipulation. The manipulation then induces hemorrhage within the dissecting aneurysm, resulting in a stroke (Mas et al., 1989).

Dissecting aneurysms of the vertebral artery may affect the extracranial portion, intracranial portion, or both (de Bray et al. 1997) (Figs. 53.260 and 53.261). Patients with dissecting aneurysms of the extracranial portion of the vertebral artery usually complain of neck pain and headache, and they usually develop focal ischemic symptoms and signs of brainstem and cerebellar dysfunction (Yonas et al., 1977; Miyazaki et al., 1984; Chiras et al., 1985; Hart, 1988; Mokri et al., 1988a; Rae-Grant et al., 1989; Yamaura et al., 1990;

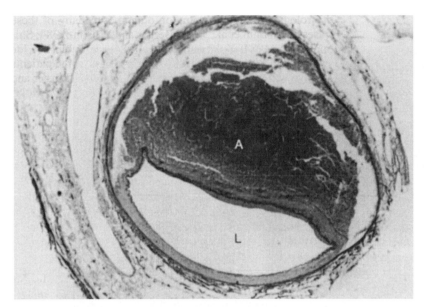

Figure 53.260. Dissecting aneurysm of the extracranial vertebral artery after cervical manipulation. The patient was a 43-year-old truck driver who experienced intermittent headaches and discomfort in the neck after driving long distances. He was treated by a chiropractor with local manipulation of the neck. Immediately after a therapeutic twist of the neck by the chiropractor, he developed acute vertigo and transient loss of consciousness. When he regained consciousness, he complained of persistent vertigo and oscillopsia. He was found to have conjugate gaze deviation to the left, a right horizontal gaze paresis, and horizontal jerk nystagmus on left lateral gaze. Vertebral angiography showed a dissecting aneurysm of the right vertebral artery. The patient experienced a respiratory arrest 42 hours after neck manipulation and died shortly thereafter. Cross-section through the right vertebral artery shows a dissecting aneurysm located between the adventitia and the media of the vessel. The lumen of the artery (*L*) is open, and there is thrombus within the lumen of the aneurysm (*A*). (From Dunne JW, Conacher GN, Khangure M, et al. Dissecting aneurysms of the vertebral arteries following cervical manipulation: A case report. J Neurol Neurosurg Psychiatry *50*:349–353, 1987.)

Youl et al., 1990). There is a high incidence of bilaterality with extracranial vertebral dissection (Massoud and Molyneux, 1994), estimated at 40 to 61% (Mas et al., 1987; Mokri et al., 1988a).

Pulsatile tinnitus may occur in patients with extracranial vertebral artery dissections (Mas et al., 1987). Involvement of the basilar artery may produce "hissing" in the ear (Greselle et al., 1987).

Lower cranial neuropathies, ataxia, vestibular nystagmus, and hemiparesis are common, as are respiratory arrest and coma. Evidence of glossopharyngeal dysfunction often occurs (Scholefield, 1924; Senter and Miller, 1982; Mas et al., 1987; Caplan et al., 1988; Yamaura et al., 1990). The vagus nerve may also be affected. Lower cranial nerve palsies may occur after surgery for a vertebral artery dissection. For example, Yamaura et al. (1990) described the development of an accessory nerve palsy following clipping of a vertebral artery dissecting aneurysm. Hypoglossal dysfunction seems to be an uncommon complication of vertebral artery dissections, although tongue atrophy associated with bilateral vertebral dissections was reported by Caplan et al. (1985). Surgery in the posterior fossa for a dissecting vertebral aneurysm can also cause damage to the hypoglossal nerve (Yamaura et al., 1990). Kitanaka et al. (1994a) reviewed their experience with 24 vertebral dissections. Nineteen patients underwent 20 procedures, some of which consisted of trapping and others, proximal clipping. Most patients developed postoperative lower cranial nerve palsies (trapping more so than clipping). In one-half of these cases, the major disability was attributable to a lower cranial nerve palsy (dysphagia or hoarseness) and respiratory dysfunction.

Facial palsy may rarely occur. Matsumoto et al. (1991) reported hemifacial spasm in a 58-year-old woman with a vertebral artery dissection. The spasm was relieved by microvascular decompression of the root exit zone of the facial nerve and wrapping of the aneurysm.

The portion of the lateral medulla supplied by the PICA is particularly vulnerable to ischemia, and Wallenberg's syndrome is a common complication of both traumatic and spontaneous vertebral artery dissections (Contamin et al., 1982; Shimoji et al., 1984; Caplan et al., 1985; Chiras et al., 1985; Dunne et al., 1987; Mas et al., 1987; Hart, 1988; Mokri et al., 1989; Frumkin and Baloh, 1990; Yamaura et al., 1990; Nater et al., 1991; Kawaguchi et al., 1993; Matsuyama et al., 1993; Nagahiro et al., 1993; Hosoya et al., 1994; Mizushima et al., 1994; Sturzenegger, 1994) (Fig. 53.262). These patients often complain of ocular tilt (Charles et al., 1992) and have an associated nystagmus with a torsional component that may cause oscillopsia (Braun et al., 1983; Caplan et al., 1985; Roualdes et al., 1985; Dunne et al., 1987; Mokri et al., 1988a; Frumkin and Baloh, 1990) and a skew deviation that produces vertical diplopia. The descending sympathetics in the central tegmental tract are also affected, and these patients thus have a central Horner's syndrome. In a study of 22 patients with Wallenberg's syndrome, Okuchi et al. (1990) found evidence of aneurysmal dilation and luminal stenosis diagnostic of dissection in seven of 15 patients with vertebral stenosis or occlusion. In a similar study of 16 patients with Wallenberg's syndrome, Hosoya et al. (1994) diagnosed definite dissection in seven, probable dissection in three, and possible dissection in three. Seven of 14 patients with spontaneous vertebral dissection showed evidence of Wallenberg's syndrome in a series reported by Sturzenegger (1994).

When a dissection in the PICA is distal to the perforating branches to the medulla the patient may be asymptomatic. Trapping of the aneurysm may then be accomplished without inducing neurologic symptoms (Kopera et al., 1992). When the dissection is located more proximally, a bypass procedure utilizing the occipital artery may protect the distal circulation (Kawaguchi et al., 1993; Nagahiro et al., 1993).

A locked-in syndrome occurs in some patients with extracranial dissection of the vertebral artery (Périer et al., 1966; Redondo-Marco and Walb, 1967; Escourolle et al., 1973;

Table 53.5
Subarachnoid Hemorrhage Associated with Dissecting Aneurysms

Turnbull, 1915	MCA related to syphilis found at autopsy
Ramset and Mosquera, 1948	47yo M occipital HA, hemiplegia, LOC 2wks, cystic medial degeneration of the MCA
Jentzer, 1954	autopsy 2nd carotoid 8½ years after transient episode HA & monocular blindness
Crompton, 1965	autopsy case distal vertebral
Gherardi and Lee, 1967	26yo hypertensive F w/PAN: HA, coma, ACA on autopsy
Kunze and Schiefer, 1971	34yo M HA, hemiparesis, LOC, MCA
Hirsh and Roessmann, 1975	11yo F pain in neck after calisthenics then LOC, basilar w/fibromuscular dysplasia
Karasawa et al., 1976	
Yonas et al., 1977	42yo F occipital HA, distal vertebral
Waga et al., 1978	53yo M 3d HA, distal vertebral treated with ligation proximal to dissection
Alexander et al., 1979	69yo M, vertebrobasilar junction w/evidence prior hemorrhage
Takita et al., 1979	33yo M vertebrovasilar
Yamaura, 1981	
Sugita, 1982	
Senter and Miller, 1982	45yo HA, neck pain, vertebral treated with ligation
Adams et al., 1982	39yo F HA followed by pontine syndrome, basilar on post
Adams et al., 1982	75yo F HA, vomiting, intracranial ICA, treated with ICA ligation
Pilz, 1982	43yo F vertebral
Manz and Luessenhop, 1983	57yo M basilar/PICA died after massive rebleed
Berger and Wilson, 1984	46yo M vertebral clipping aneurysm
Berger and Wilson, 1984	39yo M vertebral clipping aneurysm
Berger and Wilson, 1984	21yo F PCA clipping aneurysm
Berger and Wilson, 1984	57yo M basilar aneurysm wrapping
Friedman and Drake, 1984	14 cases SAH (11 vertebral, 2 basilar, 1 PICA)
Shimoji et al., 1984	7 cases SAH (vertebral artery)
Yamada et al., 1984b	3 cases SAH (cases 4, 5, 6, vertebral)
Farrell et al., 1985	63yo M vertebral
Yoshii et al., 1986	47yo M vertebral died 9d
Yoshii et al., 1986	53yo M vertebral died 7d
Biller et al., 1986	basilar
Ide et al., 1986	37yo M vertebral
Caplan et al., 1988	case 4
Mokri et al., 1988a	incidence of 10% in vertebral dissection
Yamaura, 1988	rebleed rate of 5/21 presenting with SAH secondary to vertebral dissection
Yamaura et al., 1990	21/24 with SAH; only 2 died 19 operated
Youl et al., 1990	44yo F vertebral SLE
Sasaki et al., 1991	5 cases vertebral
Takahashi et al., 1992	22yo F PICA aneurysm with angiitis
Kaplan et al., 1993	41yo F post partum presumed traumatic vertebral pseudoaneurysm
Takai et al., 1993	38yo M vertebral aneurysm post prox clip
Guridi et al., 1993	72yo F anterior cerebral artery
Halbach et al., 1993	9/16 patients vertebral
Endo et al., 1993	3 vertebrobasilar
Guridi et al., 1993	72yo F anterior cerebral
Kawamata et al., 1994	post proximal clip
Fransen and de Tribolet, 1994	
Ohki et al., 1994	41yo F mixed connective tissue disease posterior cerebral artery
Kitanaka et al., 1994b	16/24 vertebral dissection
Kawaguchi et al., 1994	14/36 vertebral dissection
Tsukahara et al., 1995	5 vertebral artery
Yano et al., 1995	27yo M anterior cerebral
Nohjoh et al., 1995	59yo F vertebral dissection
Mizuntani et al., 1995	30/42 vertebral dissections subsequent rupture

et al., 1988a). The reasons for this higher incidence of SAH was investigated by Endo et al. (1993), who examined the affected arterial walls in three autopsied cases of vertebral dissection and rupture. These investigators found that in all three cases, the dissection was between the media and adventitia, and the rupture site was in the thin adventitia. This is more superficial than the usual subintimal dissection plane that occurs in most anterior circulation intracranial dissections.

Caplan et al. (1988) described four overlapping clinical syndromes caused by intracranial dissections of the vertebral artery: (*a*) brainstem infarction caused by subintimal dissection extending into the basilar artery, usually affecting young adults and commonly resulting in death; (*b*) SAH caused by subadventitial or transmural dissection; (*c*) aneurysmal dilation producing a mass effect on the brainstem and lower cranial nerves; and (*d*) chronic dissection caused by connective tissue defects, resulting in extensive bilateral aneurysm formation and repeated TIAs, small strokes, and SAH (see also Hart, 1988).

Because SAH is more common with dissections of the vertebrobasilar circulation (Table 53.5), most cases of Terson's syndrome associated with dissecting aneurysms are associated with posterior fossa dissection (Waga et al., 1978; Shimoji et al., 1984; Farrell et al., 1985; Yoshii et al., 1986). Of 14 cases of dissection resulting in SAH, vitreous blood was present in three (Friedman and Drake, 1984). In 21 patients with SAH following vertebral dissection, Yamaura et al. (1990) found Terson's syndrome in five.

Transient phenomena occurring in patients with intracranial vertebral artery dissections include episodes of bilateral visual loss or hemifield loss. Mas et al. (1985) described two patients with bilateral transient visual blurring related to bilateral ICA and vertebral artery dissections, and Greselle et al. (1987) described transient cortical blindness in a patient with a unilateral vertebral artery dissection. In many reports, the exact form of visual disturbance is not clear. Of 15 patients with vertebral dissections reported by Chiras et al. (1985), two were said to have experienced a transient "visual disorder." In a series of 25 cases of spontaneous vertebral dissections reported by Mokri et al., 1988a), occipital lobe infarction with homonymous visual loss occurred in two. The infarction in such cases may be related to either extension of thrombosis or distal embolization from a proximal vertebral dissection (Bladin, 1974; Quint and Spickler, 1990). A filling defect in the PCA distal to a vertebral occlusion in a 57-year-old laborer supports the concept of distal embolization (Katirji et al., 1985).

Dissecting aneurysms that arise in the basilar artery are more common than those that arise in the vertebral artery. These aneurysms often extend into one or more of the major branches of the basilar artery, particularly the superior cerebellar and PCA arteries (Friedman and Drake, 1984), and they almost always produce catastrophic neurologic dysfunction from mass effect, thromboembolism, intracranial hemorrhage, or a combination of these (Adams et al., 1982; Bugiani et al., 1983; Gautier and Pertuiset, 1983; Manz and Luessenhop, 1983; see Table 1 in Berger and Wilson, 1984) (Fig. 53.264). Affected patients initially develop headache followed by evidence of progressive brainstem and cerebellar dysfunction. Tetraplegia and coma are common, and most patients die or have permanent, severe, neurologic deficits (Manz and Luessenhop, 1983; Berger and Wilson, 1984). When the proximal perforators are affected, there may be pontine dysfunction. Nakaso et al. (1995) reported a 47-year-old man who had the abrupt onset of dysarthria and weakness in his left upper and lower extremities during his work. He had hypesthesia of the left face, absent gag reflex, dysarthria, and left hemiparesis with ataxia. On the 2nd hospital day, he developed paralysis of conjugate eye movement to the

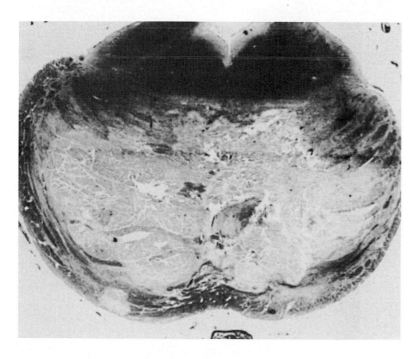

Figure 53.264. Infarction of the base of the pons in a patient with a dissecting aneurysm of the basilar artery. The patient was a 31-year-old woman who was a heavy smoker and who was using oral contraceptives. She developed acute headache, dizziness, unsteady gait, dysphagia and vomiting. She had diffuse brainstem signs and gradually developed a locked-in syndrome. She died 16 days after the onset of neurologic symptoms and signs. Postmortem examination revealed a dissecting aneurysm of the midportion of the basilar artery. Cross-section through the pons shows a massive infarction sparing only the tegmentum. (From Bugiani O, Piola P, Tabaton M. Nontraumatic dissecting aneurysm of the basilar artery. Eur Neurol 22:256–260, 1983.)

right, left central facial palsy, and left hemiplegia, and hyperhidrosis of the left side of the body; i.e., Foville's syndrome (see Chapter 28).

Most basilar artery dissections are spontaneous but Toyota and Ferguson (1994) reported a case of iatrogenic fatal basilar dissection following clipping of a basilar tip aneurysm. Abducens nerve paresis is common in patients with dissections of the basilar artery, and oculomotor nerve paresis may result when the aneurysm extends into the superior cerebellar or posterior cerebral arteries (Périer et al., 1964; Campiche et al., 1969; Manz and Luessenhop, 1983). Berger and Wilson (1984) described a 43-year-old man with a dissecting aneurysm of the tip of the basilar artery that extended into both proximal segments of the PCAs and the SCA on the right side. The patient's initial symptoms were diplopia on lateral gaze and difficulty with balance, followed by difficulty adducting the right eye. He was found to have a right INO, a right abducens nerve paresis, and vestibular nystagmus.

Other motility disorders that occur in patients with basilar artery dissections include vertical gaze impairment (Dunne et al., 1987) and horizontal gaze palsy (Katirji et al., 1985). Oculomotor nerve palsy is uncommon but may occur when the dissection affects the distal portion of the artery (Périer et al., 1964; Campiche et al., 1969; Manz and Luessenhop, 1983).

Some patients develop dissecting aneurysms limited to one of the branches of the basilar artery, particularly the posterior cerebral and superior cerebellar arteries (Fisher et al., 1978; Kalyan-Raman et al., 1983; Berger and Wilson, 1984; Ohki et al., 1994). These aneurysms may produce symptoms by mass effect, rupture, or ischemic effect on the brainstem (Fig. 53.265). Sasaki et al. (1992) reported a dissecting aneurysm of the P-3 segment of the right PCA after mild head injury. The patient was treated with surgical occlusion after he experienced repeated intramural hemorrhages associated with neuroimaging evidence of enlarge-

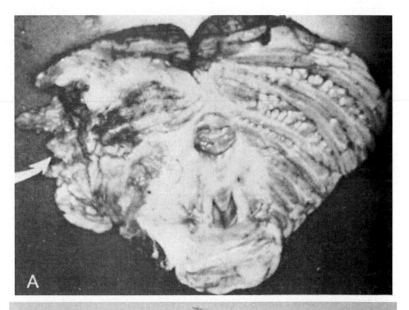

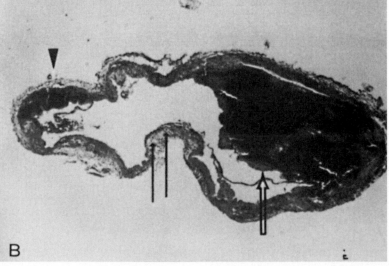

Figure 53.265. Dissecting aneurysm of the superior cerebellar artery in a patient with fibromuscular dysplasia. The patient was a 38-year-old man who developed bifrontal headache followed by severe vertigo, diplopia, and projectile vomiting. The patient suffered a cardiac arrest and died 3 days later. *A,* There is a large infarction affecting the lateral half of the right cerebellar hemisphere. *B,* Cross-section through the right superior cerebellar artery shows a dissection within its wall (*arrowhead*). Blood is present in the lumen of the artery (*open arrow*), and some portions of the wall of the artery are ectatic (*double arrows*). (From Kalyan-Raman UP, Kowalski RV, Lee RH, et al. Dissecting aneurysm of superior cerebellar artery: Its association with fibromuscular dysplasia. Arch Neurol *40*:120–122, 1983.)

ment of the aneurysm. Proximal ligation produced thrombosis of the aneurysm without resulting in infarction in the territory of the affected PCA.

There is no ideal treatment for dissecting aneurysms of the vertebrobasilar arterial system (Berger and Wilson, 1984; Mokri et al., 1988a). The affected artery may be ligated or clipped proximally (Drake, 1975), but such surgery may lead to fatal SAH or severe thromboembolic neurologic deficit (Friedman and Drake, 1984). Yamada et al. (1984b) reported two patients with dissecting aneurysms of the vertebral artery in whom the aneurysm originated distal to the PICA. The vertebral artery was therefore clipped distal to the PICA, resulting in good neurologic recovery. An alternative treatment for such aneurysms is midcervical occlusion of the vertebral artery using a detachable balloon or a surgical clip (Weinstein, 1984; Tsukahara et al., 1995). This procedure preserves extracranial collateral flow through suboccipital

muscular branches of the vertebral artery. Good results may be achieved with both surgical and nonsurgical approaches. In a series of 36 patients with posterior circulation dissections, 84% of the surgically managed patients and 71% of the nonsurgical cases had a favorable outcome (good recovery or moderate disability) (Kawaguchi et al., 1994).

When the aneurysm arises in the basilar artery or one of its major branches, it is doubtful that any therapy is of benefit, although microvascular bypass procedures are sometimes employed (Nagahiro et al., 1993). Proximal ligation may not always prevent subsequent neurologic problems including rupture (Takai et al., 1993; Kawamata et al., 1994; Mizutani et al., 1995). The prognosis may be better if the segment can be trapped safely. Endovascular approaches may permit occlusion of the parent artery or occlusion of the secondary pseudoaneurysm with preservation of the parent artery. In the study of Halbach et al., 1993, 15 of 16 patients with vertebral dissections so treated were cured.

CONCLUSIONS

Intracranial aneurysms occur with high frequency and have a significant impact on public health. Most aneurysms present with subarachnoid hemorrhage, but 10% cause symptoms by mass effect, distal embolization, or thrombosis. Early clinical recognition and the use of improved and improving diagnostic techniques permit accelerated intervention, which itself continues to improve, with resultant

decrease in overall mortality and morbidity and improvement in long-term prognosis. Aggressive treatment to prevent or reverse delayed secondary ischemia and endovascular techniques for both ruptured and unruptured aneurysms promise to have a continuing impact on the outlook for patients with intracranial aneurysms.

REFERENCES

Aarabi B. Traumatic aneurysms of brain due to high velocity missile head wounds. Neurosurgery 22:1056–1063, 1988.

Aarabi B. Management of traumatic aneurysms caused by high-velocity missile head wounds. Neurosurg Clin North Am 6:775–797, 1995.

Aarabi B, McQueen JD. Traumatic internal carotid occlusion at the base of the skull. Surg Neurol 10:233–236, 1978.

Abad JM, Alvarez F, Blazquez MG. An unrecognized neurological syndrome: Sixth-nerve palsy and Horner's syndrome due to traumatic intracavernous carotid aneurysm. Surg Neurol 16:140–144, 1981.

Abdel-Khalek MN, Richardson J. Retinal macroaneurysm: Natural history and guide lines for treatment. Br J Ophthalmol 70:2–11, 1986.

Abe K, Fujino Y, Demizu A, et al. The effect of prostaglandin E1 on local cerebral blood flow during cerebral-aneurysm clip ligation. Eur J Anaesthesiol 8:359–363, 1991.

Abe K, Iwanaga H, Inada E. Effect of nicardipine and diltiazem on internal carotid artery blood flow velocity and local cerebral blood flow during cerebral aneurysm surgery for subarachnoid hemorrhage. J Clin Anesth 6:99–105, 1994.

Abe T, Matsumoto K, Aruga T. Primitive trigeminal artery variant associated with intracranial ruptured aneurysm and cerebral arteriovenous malformation: Case report. Neurol Med Chir 34:104–107, 1994.

Abe T, Nemoto S, Iwata T, et al. Rupture of a cerebral aneurysm during embolization for a cerebral arteriovenous malformation. AJNR 16:1818–1820, 1995.

Abiko S, Orita T. A case of "true" posterior communicating artery aneurysm. No Shinkei Geka 9:1181–1185, 1981.

Acqui M, Ferrante L, Fraioli B, et al. Association between intracranial aneurysms and pituitary adenomas. Neurochirurgia 30:177–181, 1987.

Adachi K, Kudo M, Chen MN, et al. Cerebral aneurysm associated with multiple endocrine neoplasia, type 1: Case report. Neurol Med Chir 33:309–311, 1993.

Adams C, Trevenen C. Middle cerebral artery dissection. Neuropediatrics 27:331–332, 1996.

Adams HP Jr, Nibbelink DW, Torner JC, et al. Antifibrinolytc therapy in patients with aneurysmal subarachnoid hemorrhage: A report of the cooperative aneurysm study. Arch Neurol 38:25–29, 1981.

Adams HP Jr, Aschenbrener CA, Kassell NF, et al. Intracranial hemorrhage produced by spontaneous dissecting intracranial aneurysm. Arch Neurol 39:773–775, 1982.

Adams HP Jr, Kassell NF, Kongable GA, et al. Intracranial operation within seven days of aneurysmal subarachnoid hemorrhage: Results in 150 patients. Arch Neurol 45:1065–1069, 1988.

Adamson J, Humphries SE, Ostergaard JR, et al. Are cerebral aneurysms atherosclerotic? Stroke 25:963–966, 1994.

Adelman LS, Doe FD, Sarnat HB. Bilateral dissecting aneurysms of the internal carotid arteries. Acta Neuropathol 29:93–97, 1974.

Adeloye A, Ngu VA, Odeku EL. Traumatic aneurysm of the first portion of the vertebral artery. Br J Surg 75:312, 1970.

Adson AW. Surgical treatment of vascular diseases altering the function of the eyes. Trans Am Acad Ophthalmol Otolaryngol 46:95–111, 1941.

Af Björkesten G, Troupp H. Changes in the size of intracranial arterial aneurysms. J Neurosurg 19:583–588, 1962.

Agostinis C, Caverni L, Moschini L, et al. Paralysis of fourth cranial nerve due to superior-cerebellar artery aneurysm. Neurology 42:457–458, 1992.

Ahmad I, Tominaga T, Suzuki M, et al. Primitive trigeminal artery associated with cavernous aneurysm: Case report. Surg Neurol 41:75–79, 1994.

Ahmadi J, Keane JR, McCormick GS, et al. Ischemic chiasmal syndrome and hypopituitarism associated with progressive cerebro-vascular occlusive disease. AJNR 5:367–372, 1984.

Ahmadi J, Tung H, Giannotta SL, et al. Monitoring of infectious intracranial aneurysms by sequential computed tomographic/magnetic resonance imaging studies. Neurosurgery 32:45–49; discussion 49–50, 1993.

Ahuja AA, Hergenrother RW, Strother CM, et al. Platinum coil coatings to increase thrombogenicity: A preliminary study in rabbits. AJNR 14:794–798, 1993.

Ajir F, Tibbetts JC. Post-traumatic occlusion of the supraclinoid internal carotid artery. Neurosurgery 9:173–176, 1981.

Alajouanine TH, Le Beau J, Houdart R. La symptomatologie tumorale des volumineux anévrysmes des artères vertébrales et basilaires. Rev Neurol 80:321–337, 1948.

Alberico RA, Patel M, Casey S, et al. Evaluation of the circle of Willis with three-dimensional CT angiography in patients with suspected intracranial aneurysms. AJNR 16:1571–1578; discussion 1579–1580, 1995.

Albert FK, Forsting M, Aschoff A, et al. Clipping of proximal paraclinoid aneurysms with support of the balloon-catheter "trapping-evacuation" technique. Technical note. Acta Neurochir 125:138–141, 1993.

Alberts MJ, Quinones A, Graffagnino C, et al. Risk of intracranial aneurysms in families with subarachnoid hemorrhage. Can J Neurol Sci 22:121–125, 1995.

Aletich VA, Debrun GM, Monsein LH, et al. Giant serpentine aneurysms: A review and presentation of five cases. AJNR 16:1061–1072, 1995.

Alexander CB, Burger PC, Gorgee JA. Dissecting aneurysms of the basilar artery in two patients. Stroke 10:294–299, 1979.

Alexander E Jr, Davis CH Jr, Pikula L. Aneurysm of the posterior inferior cerebellar artery filling the fourth ventricle: Case report. J Neurosurg 24:99–101, 1966.

Alexander TD, Macdonald RL, Weir B, et al. Intraoperative angiography in cerebral aneurysm surgery: A prospective study of 100 craniotomies. Neurosurgery 39:10–17, 1996.

Allen GS, Bahr AL. Cerebral arterial spasm: X. Reversal of acute and chronic spasm in dogs with orally administered nifedipine. Neurosurgery 4:43–47, 1979.

Allen GS, Ahn HS, Preziosi TJ, et al. Cerebral arterial spasm: A controlled trial of nimodipine in patients with subarachnoid hemorrhage. N Engl J Med 308:619–624, 1983.

Alleyne CH Jr, Krisht A, Yoo FK, et al. Bilateral persistent trigeminal arteries associated with cerebral aneurysms and aortic arch vessel anomaly. South Med J 90:434–438, 1997.

Almeida GM, Pindaro J, Plese P, et al. Intracranial arterial aneurysms in infancy and childhood. Childs Brain 3:193–199, 1977.

Alpers BJ. Aneurysms of the circle of Willis. Morphological and clinical considerations. In Intracranial Aneurysms and Subarachnoid Hemorrhage. Editors, Fields WS, Sahs AL, pp 5–21. Springfield, IL, Charles C Thomas, 1965.

Alpers BJ, Schlezinger NS, Tassman IM. Bilateral internal carotid aneurysm involving cavernous sinus. Arch Ophthalmol 46:403–407, 1951.

al-Rodhan NR, Piepgras DG, Sundt TM Jr. Transitional cavernous aneurysms of the internal carotid artery. Neurosurgery 33:993–996; discussion 997–998, 1993.

Amacher AL, Drake CG, Ferguson GG. Posterior circulation aneurysms in young people. Neurosurgery 8:315–320, 1981.

Amagasa M, Sato S, Otabe K. Posttraumatic dissecting aneurysm of the anterior cerebral artery: Case report. Neurosurgery 23:221–225, 1988.

Amalric P, Dauban F, Courtois M, et al. Signes cliniques et angiographiques des macro-anevrysmes arteriels retiniens. Bull Soc Ophtalmol Fr 79:109–111, 1979.

Ambler Z, Ulc M, Ledinsky Q. Aneurysma der A. carotis int. im extra-kraniellen Verlauf. Neurochirurgia 10:169–175, 1967.

Amirjamshidi A, Rahmat H, Abbassioun K. Traumatic aneurysms and arteriovenous fistulas of intracranial vessels associated with penetrating head injuries occurring during war: Principles and pitfalls in diagnosis and management. A survey of 31 cases and review of the literature. J Neurosurg 84:769–780, 1996.

Amtoft-Nielsen A. Cerebrovaskulaere insulter forarsaget af manipulation af columna cervicalis. Ugeskr Laeger 146:3267–3270, 1984.

Anand VK, Raila FA, McAuley JR, et al. Giant pseudoaneurysm of the extracranial vertical artery. Otolaryngol Head Neck Surg 109:1057–1060, 1993.

Andersen CA, Collins GJ, Rich NM, et al. Spontaneous dissection of the internal carotid artery associated with fibromuscular dysplasia. Am Surg 46:263–266, 1980.

Anderson DR. Ultrastructure of the optic nerve head. Arch Ophthalmol 83:63–73, 1970.

Anderson GB, Findlay JM, Steinke DE, et al. Experience with computed tomographic angiography for the detection of intracranial aneurysms in the setting of acute subarachnoid hemorrhage. Neurosurgery 41:522–528, 1997.

Anderson J. Intracranial aneurysm of internal carotid. Br Med J 2:872, 1885.

Anderson RD. Tortuosity of the cavernous carotid arteries causing sellar expansion simulating pituitary adenoma. AJR 126:1203–1210, 1976.

Anderson RD, Leibeskind A, Schechter MM, et al. Aneurysms of the internal carotid artery in the carotid canal of the petrous temporal bone. Radiology 102:639–642, 1972.

Anderson RM, Schechter MM. A case of spontaneous dissecting aneurysm of the internal carotid artery. J Neurol Neurosurg Psychiatry 22:195–201, 1959.

Andoh T, Shirakami S, Nakashima T, et al. Clinical analysis of a series of vertebral aneurysm cases. Neurosurgery 31:987–993, 1992a.

Andoh T, Itoh T, Yoshimura S, et al. Peripheral aneurysms of the posterior inferior cerebellar artery; analysis of 15 cases. No Shinkei Geka 20:683–690, 1992b.

Andrews BT, Brant-Zawadzki M, Wilson CB. Variant aneurysms of the fenestrated basilar artery. Neurosurgery 18:204–207, 1986.

Anguita M, Romo E, Vinals M, et al. Curacion con tratamiento medico de un aneurisma micotico intracraneal en un paciente con endocarditis infecciosa con hemocultivos negativos y miocardiopatia hipertrofica. Rev Esp Cardiol 44:556–559, 1991.

Anson JA, Lawton MT, Spetzler RF. Characteristics and surgical treatment of dolichoectatic and fusiform aneurysms. J Neurosurg 84:185–193, 1996.

Antunes JL, Correll JW. Cerebral emboli from intracranial aneurysms. Surg Neurol 6:7–10, 1976.

Antunes JL, Valenca A, Ferro JM, et al. Ruptured saccular aneurysm associated with duplication of the vertebral artery. Surg Neurol 36:207–209, 1991.

Aoki N. Interhemispheric approach for carotid-ophthalmic artery aneurysm clipping: Case report. J Neurosurg 67:293–295, 1987.

Aoki N. Partially thrombosed aneurysm presenting as the sudden onset of bitemporal hemianopsia. Neurosurgery 22:564–566, 1988.

Aoki N, Sakai T, Kaneko M. Traumatic aneurysm of the middle meningeal artery presenting as delayed onset of acute subdural hematoma. Surg Neurol 37:59–62, 1992.

Aoki N, Sakai T, Oikawa A. Vertebral artery aneurysm at the level of the cervicomedullary junction: Case report. Neurol Med Chir 33:100–102, 1993.

Aoki S, Sasaki Y, Machida T, et al. Cerebral aneurysms: Detection and delineation using 3-D-CT angiography. AJNR 13:1115–1120, 1992.

Aoyagi N, Hayakawa I. Study on early re-rupture of intracranial aneurysms. Acta Neurochir 138:12–18, 1996.

Arai K, Endo S, Hirashima Y, et al. Posterior inferior cerebellar artery aneurysm associated with fenestration of the vertebral artery: Case report. Neurol Med Chir 29:29–31, 1989.

Araki C, Handa H, Handa J, et al. Traumatic aneurysm of the intracranial extradural portion of the internal carotid artery: Report of a case. J Neurosurg 23:64–67, 1965.

Araki T, Ouchi M, Ikeda Y. A case of anterior cerebral artery dissecting aneurysm. No Shinkei Geka 24:87–91, 1996.

Araki Y, Kohmura E, Tsukaguchi I. A pitfall in detection of intracranial unruptured aneurysms on three-dimensional phase-contrast MR angiography. AJNR 15:1618–1623, 1994.

Archer DJ, Young S, Uttley D. Basilar aneurysms: A new transclival approach via maxillotomy. J Neurosurg 67:54–58, 1987.

Archer DP, Bissonnette B, Ravussin P. Augmentation de la performance cardiaque pour la prevention et le traitement de l'ischemie cerebrale retardee par vasospasme. Ann Fr Anesth Reanim 15:359–365, 1996.

Arruga J, De Rivas P, Espinet HL, et al. Chronic isolated trochlear nerve palsy produced by intracavernous internal carotid artery aneurysm. Report of a case. J Clin Neuroophthalmol 11:104–108, 1991.

Arseni C, Ghitescu N, Cristescu A, et al. The pseudotumoral form of aneurysms of the posterior cranial fossa. Neurochirurgia 12:123–127, 1969.

Arseni C, Ghitescu N, Critescu A, et al. Intrasellar aneurysms simulating hypophyseal tumors. Eur Neurol 3:321–329, 1970.

Artiola i Fortuny L, Prieto-Valiente L. Long-term prognosis in surgically treated intracranial aneurysms. Part 1: Mortality. J Neurosurg 54:26–34, 1981a.

Artiola i Fortuny L, Prieto-Valiente L. Long-term prognosis in surgically trated intracranial aneurysms. Part 2: Morbidity. J Neurosurg 54:35–43, 1981b.

Arunodaya GR, Vani S, Shankar SK, et al. Fibromuscular dysplasia with dissection of basilar artery presenting as "locked-in-syndrome." Neurology 48:1605–1608, 1997.

Asai A, Matsutani M, Kohno T, et al. Multiple saccular cerebral aneurysms associated with systemic lupus erythematosus: Case report. Neurol Med Chir 29:245–247, 1989.

Asano T, Takakura K, Sano K, et al. Effects of a hydroxyl radical scavenger on delayed ischemic neurological deficits following aneurysmal subarachnoid hemorrhage: Results of a multicenter, placebo-controlled double-blind trial. J Neurosurg 84:792–803, 1996.

Asari S, Ohmoto T. Growth and rupture of unruptured cerebral aneurysms based on the intraoperative appearance. Acta Med Okayama 48:257–262, 1994a.

Asari S, Ohmoto T. Long-term outcome of surgically treated unruptured cerebral aneurysms. Clin Neurol Neurosurg 96:230–235, 1994b.

Asari S, Nakamura S, Yamada O, et al. Traumatic aneurysm of peripheral cerebral arteries: Report of two cases. J Neurosurg 46:795–803, 1977.

Asdourian GK, Goldberg MF, Jampol L, et al. Retinal macroaneurysms. Arch Ophthalmol 95:624–628, 1977.

Assaf M, Sweeney PJ, Kosmorsky G, et al. Horner's syndrome secondary to angiogram negative, subadventitial carotid artery dissection. Can J Neurol Sci 20:62–64, 1993.

Atkinson JL, Sundt TM Jr, Houser OW, et al. Angiographic frequency of anterior circulation intracranial aneurysms. J Neurosurg 70:551–555, 1989.

Atkinson JL, Lane JI, Colbassani HJ, et al. Spontaneous thrombosis of posterior cerebral artery aneurysm with angiographic reappearance. Case report. J Neurosurg 79:434–437, 1993.

Atlas SW, Sheppard L, Goldberg HI, et al. Intracranial aneurysms: detection and characterization with MR angiography with use of an advanced postprocessing technique in a blinded-reader study. Radiology 203:807–814, 1997.

Attali P, Sterkers M, Coscas G. Les macroanévrysmes artériels rétiniens. J Fr Ophtalmol 7:697–710, 1984.

Atzor KR, Stolz H, Kauczor HU, et al. 3D-high resolution imaging of tumors and aneurysms at the cranial base-comparison of CT and MR. Comput Biol Med 25:277–291, 1995.

Auer AI, Nunnelee JD. Internal carotid artery aneurysm. A case report. J Cardiovasc Surg 37:21–23, 1996.

Auer LM. Pial arterial vasodilatation by intravenous nimodipine in cats. Drug Res 31:1423–1425, 1981.

Auer LM. Acute operation and preventive nimodipine improve outcome in patients with ruptured cerebral aneurysms. Neurosurgery 15:57–66, 1984.

Auer LM, Schneider GH, Auer T. Computerized tomography and prognosis in early aneurysm surgery. J Neurosurg 65:217–221, 1986.

Ausman JI, Diaz FG, Sadasivan B, et al. Giant intracranial aneurysm surgery: The role of micro-vascular reconstruction. Surg Neurol 34:8–15, 1990.

Ausman JL, Diaz FG, Malik GM, et al. Current management of cerebral aneurysms: Is it based on facts or myths? Surg Neurol 24:625–635, 1985.

Ausman JL, Diaz FG, Malik GM, et al. Management of cerebral aneurysms: Further facts and additional myths. Surg Neurol 32:21–35, 1989.

Austin G, Fisher S, Dickson D, et al. The significance of the extracellular matrix in intracranial aneurysms. Ann Clin Lab Sci 23:97–105, 1993.

Austin JR, Maceri DR. Anterior communicating artery aneurysm presenting as pulsatile tinnitus. J Otorhinolaryngol Relat Spec 55:54–57, 1993.

Austin MG, Schaefer RF. Marfan's syndrome with unusual blood vessel manifestations. Arch Pathol Lab Med 64:205–209, 1957.

Avins LR, Krummenacher TK. Valsalva maculopathy due to a retinal arterial macroaneurysm. Ann Ophthalmol 15:421–423, 1983.

Awad I, Sawhny B, Little JR. Traumatic postsurgical aneurysm of the intracavernous carotid artery: A delayed presentation. Surg Neurol 18:54–57, 1982.

Awad IA, Mckenzie R, Magdinec M, et al. Application of magnetic resonance angiography to neurosurgical practice: A critical review of 150 cases. Neurol Res 14: 360–368, 1992.

Aymard A, Hodes JE, Rufenacht D, et al. Endovascular treatment of a giant fusiform aneurysm of the entire basilar artery. AJNR 13:1143–1146, 1992.

Azar-Kia B, Palacios E, Spak M. The megadolichobasilar artery anomaly and expansion of the internal auditory meatus. Neuroradiology 11:109–111, 1976.

Babu RP, Sekhar LN, Wright DC. Extreme lateral transcondylar approach: Technical improvements and lessons learned. J Neurosurg 81:49–59, 1994.

Bailes JE, Deeb ZL, Wilson JA, et al. Intraoperative angiography and temporary balloon occlusion of the basilar artery as an adjunct to surgical clipping: Technical note. Neurosurgery 30:949–953, 1992.

Baker CJ, Fiore A, Connolly ES Jr, et al. Serum elastase and alpha-1-antitrypsin levels in patients with ruptured and unruptured cerebral aneurysms. Neurosurgery 37: 56–61; discussion 61–62, 1995a.

Baker CJ, Prestigiacomo CJ, Solomon RA. Superior perioperative anticonvulsant prophylaxis for the surgical treatment of low-risk patients with intracranial aneurysms. Neurosurgery 37:863–870; discussion 870–871, 1995b.

Baker RS, Carr WA. Pontine infarction: Angiography and magnetic resonance imaging. Surv Ophthalmol 32:141–143, 1987.

Bakke SJ, Smith HJ, Kerty E, et al. Cervicocranial artery dissection. Detection by Doppler ultrasound and MR angiography. Acta Radiol 37:529–534, 1996.

Ball MJ. Pathogenesis of the ''sentinel headache'' preceding berry aneurysm rupture. Can Med Assoc J 112:78–79, 1975.

Ballantyne AJ. The ocular manifestations of spontaneous subarachnoid hemorrhage. Br J Ophthalmol 27:383–414, 1943.

Banach MJ, Flamm ES. Supraclinoid internal carotid artery fenestration with an associated aneurysm. Case report. J Neurosurg 79:438–441, 1993.

Bandoh K, Sugimura J, Hosaka Y, et al. Ruptured intracranial mycotic aneurysm associated with acute subdural hematoma: Case report. Neurol Med Chir 27: 56–59, 1987.

Banfield GK, Brasher PF, Deans JA, et al. Intrapetrous carotid artery aneurysm presenting as epistaxis and otalgia. J Laryngol Otol 109:865–867, 1995.

Banna M, Lasjaunias P. Intracavernous carotid aneurysm associated with proptosis in a 13-month-old girl. AJNR 12:969–970, 1991.

Bannerman RM, Ingall GB, Graf CJ. The familial occurrence of intracranial aneurysms. Neurology 20:283–292, 1969.

Barami K, Ko K. Ruptured mycotic aneurysm presenting as an intraparenchymal hemorrhage and nonadjacent acute subdural hematoma: Case report and review of the literature. Surg Neurol 41:290–293, 1994.

Barnett DW, Barrow DL, Joseph GJ. Combined extracranial-intracranial bypass and intraoperative balloon occlusion for the treatment of intracavernous and proximal carotid artery aneurysms. Neurosurgery 35:92–97; discussion 97–98, 1994.

Barnwell SL, Higashida RT, Halbach VV, et al. Transluminal angioplasty of intracerebral vessels for cerebral arterial spasm: Reversal of neurological deficits after delayed treatment. Neurosurgery 25:424–429, 1989.

Barontini F, Ammannati F, Gagliardi R, et al. A further case of giant intrasellar carotid aneurysm mimicking a pituitary adenoma: The relevance of a multivariate approach in differential diagnosis. Ital J Neurol Sci 15:369–372, 1994.

Barr HWK, Blackwood W, Meadows SP. Intracavernous carotid aneurysms: A clinical-pathological report. Brain 94:607–622, 1971.

Barr JD, Mathis JM, Horton JA. Transient severe brain stem depression during intraarterial papaverine infusion for cerebral vasospasm. AJNR 15:719–723, 1994.

Barrett JH, Lawrence VL. Aneurysms of the internal carotid artery as a complication of mastoidectomy. Arch Otolaryngol 72:366–368, 1960.

Barrow DL, Prats AR. Infectious intracranial aneurysms: Comparison of groups with and without endocarditis. Neurosurgery 27:562–572; discussion 572–573, 1990.

Barrow DL, Reisner A. Natural history of intracranial aneurysms and vascular malformations. Clin Neurosurg 40:3–39, 1993.

Barrow DL, Boyer KL, Joseph GJ. Intraoperative angiography in the management of neurovascular disorders. Neurosurgery 30:153–159, 1992.

Bartels E. Dissektion der extrakraniellen Vertebralarterie. Farbduplexsonographische Befunde und Verlaufsbeobachtung bei 20 Patienten. Ultraschall Med 17:55–63, 1996.

Barth A, de Tribolet N. Growth of small saccular aneurysms to giant aneurysms: Presentation of three cases. Surg Neurol 41:277–280, 1994.

Barth A, Nabavi A, Stein H, et al. Die perimesenzephale Subarachnoidalblutung—Ein eigenstandiges Krankheitsbild einer nichtaneurysmatischen Subarachnoidalblutung mit gutartigem Verlauf. Zentralbl Neurochir 57:108–112, 1996.

Bartleson JD, Trautmann JC, Sundt TM Jr. Minimal oculomotor nerve paresis secondary to unruptured intracranial aneurysm. Arch Neurol 43:1015–1020, 1986.

Bashour TT, Crew JP, Dean M, et al. Ultrasonic imaging of common carotid artery dissection. J Clin Ultrasound 13:210–211, 1985.

Bassett CR, Lemmen LF. Subdural hematoma associated with bleeding intracranial aneurysm. J Neurosurg 9:443–450, 1950.

Batjer HH, Purdy PD. Enlarging thrombosed aneurysm of the distal basilar artery. Neurosurgery 26:695–700, 1990.

Batjer HH, Samson DS. Causes of morbidity and mortality from surgery of aneurysms of the distal basilar artery. Neurosurgery 25:904–915, 1989.

Batjer HH, Samson DS. Retrograde suction decompression of giant paraclinoidal aneurysms. Technical note. J Neurosurg 73:305–306, 1990.

Batjer HH, Suss RA, Samson D. Intracranial arteriovenous malformations associated with aneurysms. Neurosurgery 18:29–35, 1986.

Batjer HH, Frankfurt AI, Purdy PD, et al. Use of etomidate, temporary arterial occlusion, and intraoperative angiography in surgical treatment of large and giant cerebral aneurysms. J Neurosurg 68:234–240, 1988.

Batjer HH, Kopitnik TA, Giller CA, Samson DS. Surgery for paraclinoidal carotid artery aneurysms. J Neurosurg 80:650–658, 1994.

Batzdorf U, Bentson JR, Machleder HI. Blunt trauma to the high cervical carotid artery. Neurosurgery 5:195–201, 1979.

Baudrillard JC, Rousseaux P, Lerais JM, et al. Anévrysmes mycotiques fongiques et abcès cérébraux multiples à Scedosporium Apiospermum: Apropos d'une observation avec revue de la littérature. J Radiol 66:321–326, 1985.

Beadles CF. Aneurisms of the larger cerebral arteries. Brain 30:285–336, 1907.

Beatty RA. Dissecting hematoma of the internal carotid artery following chiropractic cervical manipulation. J Trauma 17:248–249, 1977.

Beatty RA. Splitting of the optic nerve by a carotid-ophthalmic artery aneurysm: Case report. J Neurosurg 65:560–562, 1986.

Becker DH, Newton TH. Distal anterior cerebral artery aneurysm. Neurosurgery 4: 495–503, 1979.

Becker DH, Silverberg GD, Nelson DH, et al. Saccular aneurysm of infancy and early childhood. Neurosurgery 2:1–7, 1978.

Bederson JB, Spetzler RF. Anastomosis of the anterior temporal artery to a secondary trunk of the middle cerebral artery for treatment of a giant M1 segment aneurysm: Case report. J Neurosurg 76:863–866, 1992.

Beiran I, Dori D, Pikkel J, et al. Recurrent retinal artery obstruction as a presenting symptom of ophthalmic artery aneurysm: A case report. Graefes Arch Clin Exp Ophthalmol 233:444–447, 1995.

Belec L, Cesaro P, Brugieres P, et al. Tumor-simulating giant serpentine aneurysm of the posterior cerebral artery. Surg Neurol 29:210–215, 1988.

Belen D, Bolay H, Firat M, et al. Unusual appearance of intracranial fibromuscular dysplasia: A case report. Angiology 476:627–632, 1996.

Ben Hamouda-M'Rad I, Biousse V, Bousser MG, et al. Internal carotid artery redundancy is significantly associated with dissection. Stroke 26:1962, 1995.

Benatar MG. Intracranial fusiform aneurysms in von Recklinghausen's disease: Case report and literature review. J Neurol Neurosurg Psychiatry 57:1279–1280, 1994.

Benoit BG, Wortzman G. Traumatic cerebral aneurysms: Clinical features and natural history. J Neurol Neurosurg Psychiatry 36:127–138, 1973.

Benrabah R, Bousser MG, Cabanis EA, et al. Syndrome de Claude Bernard-Horner douloureux revalateur d'une dissection spontanée de l'artère carotide interne interet du cilan ultrasonique cervical: A propos de 2 observations. Bull Soc Ophtalmol Fr 88:763–770, 1988.

Berenstein A, Ransohoff J, Kupersmith M, et al. Transvascular treatment of giant aneurysms of the cavernous carotid and vertebral arteries: Functional investigation and embolization. Surg Neurol 21:3–12, 1984.

Bergaust B. Unusual course of internal carotid artery accompanied by bitemporal hemianopsia. Acta Ophthalmol 41:270–278, 1963.

Berger MS, Wilson CB. Intracranial dissecting aneurysms of the posterior circulation: Report of six cases and review of the literature. J Neurosurg 61:882–894, 1984.

Bergsneider M, Frazee JG, DeSalles AA. Thalamostriate artery aneurysm within the third ventricle. Case report. J Neurosurg 81:463–465, 1994.

Beristain X, Gaviria M, Dujovny M, et al. Evaluation of outcome after intracranial aneurysm surgery: The neuropsychiatric approach. Surg Neurol 45:422–428; discussion 428–429, 1996.

Berkovic SF, Spokes RL, Anderson RM, et al. Basilar artery dissection. J Neurol Neurosurg Psychiatry 46:126–129, 1983.

Bersani D, Lanchier C, Lippa A, et al. Pseudo-anevrysme de la carotide interne. J Radiol 73:115–119, 1992.

Berson EL, Freeman MI, Gay AJ. Visual field defects in giant suprasellar aneurysms of the internal carotid artery: Report of three cases. Arch Ophthalmol 76:52–58, 1966.

Bevan H, Sharma K, Bradley W. Stroke in young adults. Stroke 21:382–386, 1990.

Beyerl BD, Heros RC. Multiple peripheral aneurysms of the posterior inferior cerebellar artery. Neurosurgery 19:285–289, 1986.

Bhatoe HS, Suryanarayana KV, Gill HS. Recurrent massive epistaxis due to traumatic intracavernous internal carotid artery aneurysm. J Laryngol Otol 109:650–652, 1995.

Bhushan C, Hodges FJ, Posey J. Successful surgical treatment of giant aneurysm of the basilar artery: Case report. J Neurosurg 49:124–128, 1978.

Bickerstaff ER. Etiology of acute hemiplegia in childhood. Br Med J 2:82–87, 1964.

Bidzinski J, Marchel A, Sherif A. Risk of epilepsy after aneurysm operations. Acta Neurochir 119:49–52, 1992.

Bidzinski J, Marchel A. W sprawie profilaktyki padaczki po operacjach tetniakow wewnatrzczaszkowych. Neurol Neurochir Pol 29:213–220, 1995.

Bigar F, Witmer R. Progrediente aneurysmatische retinale Arteriopathie. Fortschr Ophthalmol 79:488–491, 1983.

Bigelow NH. The association of polycystic kidneys with intracranial aneurysms and other related disorders. Am J Med Sci 225:485–494, 1953.

Bigelow NH. Intracranial dissecting aneurysms. Arch Pathol 60:271–275, 1955.

Bilbao R, Amoros S, Murube J. Horner syndrome as an isolated manifestation of an intrapetrous internal carotid artery dissection. Am J Ophthalmol 123:562–564, 1997.

Bilge T, Barut S, Sahin Y, et al. Distal posterior inferior cerebellar artery aneurysm association with multiple aneurysms. Acta Neurol Belg 95:37–41, 1995.

Biller J, Hingtgen WL, Adams HP, et al. Cervicocephalic arterial dissections. A ten-year experience. Arch Neurol 43:1234–1238, 1986.

Biller J, Godersky JC, Adams HP Jr. Management of aneurysmal subarachnoid hemorrhage. Stroke 19:1300–1305, 1988.

Bingham WF. Treatment of mycotic intracranial aneurysms. J Neurosurg 46:428–437, 1977.

Biousse V, Woimant F, Amarenco P, et al. Pain as the only manifestation of internal carotid artery dissection. Cephalalgia 12:314–317, 1992.

Biousse V, D'Anglejan-Chatillon J, Massiou H, et al. Head pain in non-traumatic carotid artery dissection: A series of 65 patients Cephalalgia 14:33–36, 1994.

Biousse V, D'Anglejan-Chatillon J, Touboul PJ, et al. Time course of symptoms in extracranial carotid artery dissections. A series of 80 patients. Stroke 26:235–239, 1995a.

Biousse V, Chabriat H, Amarenco P, et al. Roller-coaster-induced vertebral artery dissection. Lancet 346(8977):767, 1995b.

Bird AC, Nolan B, Gargano FP, et al. Unruptured aneurysm of the supraclinoid carotid artery: A treatable cause of blindness. Neurology 20:445–454, 1970.

Bisland T, Topilow A. Subhyaloid hemorrhage and exophthalmos due to ruptured intraventricular aneurysm: A case occurring in toxemia of pregnancy. Arch Ophthalmol 47:470–476, 1952.

Biumi F. Observations Anatomicae, Scholiis ilustratae. Observatio V. In Thesaurus Dissertationum. Editor, Sandifort E, Vol 3. Milan, S & J Luchtmans, 1765.

Black BK, Hicks SP. The relation of hypertension to arterial aneurysms of the brain. US Armed Forces Med J 3:1813–1818, 1952.

Black WC. Intracranial aneurysm in adult polycystic kidney disease: Is screening with MR angiography indicated? Radiology 191:18–20, 1994.

Blackall J. Observations on the Nature and Cure of Dropsies. 2nd ed, pp 132–135, London, Longman, Hurst, Rees, Orme and Brown, 1814.

Bladin PF. Dissecting aneurysm of carotid and vertebral arteries. A clinical and angiographic study of early diagnosis, natural history, and pathophysiology of cerebral lesions. A study of four cases. Vasc Surg 8:203–223, 1974.

Bladin PF, Merory J. Mechanisms in cerebral lesions in trauma to the high cervical portion of the vertebral artery—Rotation injury. Proc Austr Assoc Neurol 12:35–41, 1975.

Blard JM, Finiels PJ, Combalbert A, et al. Anévrysmes symptomatiques de l'artère cérébelleuse postéro-inférieure: Étude rétrospective multicentrique de 29 cas. Rev Neurol 153:41–50, 1997.

Blatter DD, Parker DL, Ahn SS, et al. Cerebral MR angiography with multiple overlapping thin slab acquisition: Part II. Early clinical experience. Radiology 183:379–389, 1992.

Bleckmann H. Pulsierendes Makroaneurysma einer retinalen Arterie. Klin Monatsbl Augenheilkd 182:91–93, 1983.

Blumenkopf B, Huggins MJ. Tuberous sclerosis and multiple intracranial aneurysms: Case report. Neurosurgery 17:797–800, 1985.

Blumenthal EZ, Gomori JM, Dotan S. Recurrent abducens nerve palsy caused by dolichoectasia of the cavernous internal carotid artery. Am J Ophthalmol 124:255–257, 1997.

Blumke DA, Fishman EK. Spiral CT. Initial experience with vascular applications. Clin Imaging 18:107–112, 1994.

Boccardo M, Ruelle A, Banchero MA. Isolated oculomotor palsy caused by aneurysm of the basilar artery bifurcation. J Neurol 233:61–62, 1986.

Boecher-Schwarz HG, Ungersboeck K, Ulrich P, et al. Transcranial Doppler diagnosis of cerebral vasospasm following subarachnoid hemorrhage: Correlation and analysis of results in relation to the age of patients. Acta Neurochir 127:32–36, 1994.

Boecher-Schwarz HG, Ungersboeck K, Ulrich P, et al. Pre- and intraoperative methods of controlling cerebral circulation in giant aneurysm surgery. Neurosurg Rev 18:85–93, 1995.

Boeri R, Passerini A. La megadolicobasilaire. Nunt Radiol 24:580–591, 1958.

Boeri R, Passerini A. The megadolichobasilar anomaly. J Neurol Sci 1:475–484, 1964.

Boghen D. Pupil sparing oculomotor palsy. Ann Neurol 14:698, 1983.

Bogousslavsky J, Regli F. Ischemic stroke in adults younger than 30 years of age. Cause and prognosis. Arch Neurol 44:479–482, 1987.

Bogousslavsky J, Regli F, Despland P-A. Anévrysmes disséquants spontanés de l'artère carotide interne: Évaluation prospective du pronostic et de la reperméabilisation artérielle dans 14 cas. Rev Neurol 140:625–636, 1984.

Bogousslavsky J, Despland P-A, Regli F. Spontaneous carotid dissection with acute stroke. Arch Neurol 44:137–140, 1987.

Bohmfalk GL, Story JL, Wissinger JP, et al. Bacterial intracranial aneurysm. J Neurosurg 48:369–382, 1978.

Bojanowski WM, Spetzler RF, Carter LP. Reconstruction of the MCA bifurcation after excision of a giant aneurysm: Technical note. J Neurosurg 68:974–977, 1988.

Bokemeyer C, Frank B, Brandis A, et al. Giant aneurysm causing frontal lobe syndrome. J Neurol 237:47–50, 1990.

Bonita R, Thomson S. Subarachnoid hemorrhage: Epidemiology, diagnosis, management, and outcome. Stroke 16:591–594, 1985.

Bontozoglou NP, Spanos H, Lasjaunias P, et al. Intracranial aneurysms: Endovascular evaluation with three-dimensional-display MR angiography. Radiology 197:876–879, 1995.

Borzone M, Altomonte M, Baldini M, et al. Giant fusiform aneurysm in middle cerebral artery branches: A report of two cases and a review of the literature. Acta Neurochir 125:184–187, 1993.

Bose B, Northrup B, Osterholm J. Giant basilar artery aneurysm presenting as a third ventricular tumor. Neurosurgery 13:699–702, 1983.

Bosmans H, Wilms G, Marchal G, et al. Characterisation of intracranial aneurysms with MR angiography. Neuroradiology 37:262–266, 1995.

Boström K, Liliequist B. Primary dissecting aneurysm of the extracranial part of the internal carotid and vertebral arteries: A report of three cases. Neurology 17:179–186, 1967.

Botterell EH, Lloyd LA, Hoffman HJ. Oculomotor palsy due to supraclinoid internal carotid artery berry aneurysm: A long-term study of the results of surgical treatments on the recovery of third-nerve function. Am J Ophthalmol 54:609–616, 1962.

Bour P, Taghavi I, Bracard S, et al. Aneurysms of the extracranial internal carotid artery due to fibromuscular dysplasia: Results of surgical management. Ann Vasc Surg 6:205–208, 1992.

Bousquet Ch, Lejeune JP, Christiaens JL. Traumatic aneurysm of the supraclinoid internal carotid artery: Case report. Surg Neurol 31:319–322, 1989.

Boyd JF, Watson AJ. Dissecting aneurysm due to trauma. Scott Med J 1:326–329, 1956.

Boyd-Wilson JS. Iatrogenic carotid occlusion medial dissection complicating arteriography. World Neurol 3:507–511, 1962.

Bracard S, Picard L, Marchal JC, et al. Role of angioplasty in the treatment of symptomatic vascular spasm occurring in the post-operative course of intracranial ruptured aneurysms. J Neuroradiol 17:6–19, 1990.

Brackett CE Jr, Morantz RA. Special problems associated with subarachnoid hemorrhage. In Neurological Surgery. Editor, Youmans R, Vol 3, pp 1807–1820. Philadelphia, WB Saunders, 1982.

Bradac GB, Kaernbach A, Bolk-Weischedel D, et al. Spontaneous dissecting aneurysm of cervical cerebral arteries: Report of six cases and review of the literature. Neuroradiology 21:149–154, 1981.

Bramwell B. Two enormous intracranial aneurysms. Edinburgh Med J 32:911–922, 1886–1887.

Brandt L, Sonesson B, Ljunggren B, et al. Ruptured middle cerebral artery aneurysm with intracerebral hemorrhage in younger patients appearing moribund: Emergency operation? Neurosurgery 20:925–929, 1987.

Branley MG, Wright KW, Borchert MS. Third nerve palsy due to cerebral artery aneurysm in a child. Aust NZ J Ophthalmol 20:137–140, 1992.

Brass K. Bilaterale Hirnerweichung bei bilateralen dissezierenden Aneurysmen der Carotides internae intra partum. Vichows Arch A Path Anat 349:163–169, 1970.

Braun IF, Pinto RS, DeFilipp GJ, et al. Brain stem infarction due to chiropractic manipulation of the cervical spine. South Med J 76:1507–1510, 1983.

Braun J, Gdal-On M, Goldsher D, et al. Traumatic carotid aneurysm secondary to cavernous sinus penetration by wood: CT features. J Comput Assist Tomogr 11:525–528, 1987.

Braunsdorf WE. Fusiform aneurysm of basilar artery and ectatic internal carotid arteries associated with glycogenosis Type 2 (Pompe's disease). Neurosurgery 21:748–749, 1987.

Brega KE, Seltzer WK, Munro LG, et al. Genotypic variations of type III collagen in patients with cerebral aneurysms. Surg Neurol 46:253–256, 1996.

Breig A, Ekbom K, Greitz T, et al. Hydrocephalus due to elongated basilar artery: A new clinicoradiological syndrome. Lancet 1:874–875, 1967.

Brennan RW, Bergland RM. Acute cerebellar hemorrhage: Analysis of clinical findings and outcome in 12 cases. Neurology 27:527–532, 1977.

Brenner H, Pendl G. Hirngefässaneurysmen mit ausschliesslich ophthalmologischen Symptomen. Bericht Dtsch Ophthalmol Ges 72:85–91, 1974.

Brent BD, Goncc M, Diamond JG. Pars plana vitrectomy for complications of retinal arterial macroaneurysms: A case series. Ophthalmic Surg 24:534–536, 1993.

Brice JG, Crompton MR. Spontaneous dissecting aneurysm of the cervical internal carotid artery. Br Med J 2:790–792, 1964.

Brick JF, Roberts T. Cerebral arteriovenous malformation coexistent with intracranial aneurysm and persistent trigeminal artery. South Med J 80:398–400, 1987.

Brihaye J, Mouawad E, Jeanmart L. L'anévrysme de la bifurcation carotidienne intracranienne. Acta Neurol. Belge 76:129–141, 1976.

Brill CB, Peyster RG, Hoover ED, et al. Giant intracranial aneurysm in a child with tuberous sclerosis: CT demonstration. J Comput Assist Tomogr 9:377–380, 1985.

Brint SU, Yoon WB, Hier DB, et al. Normalization of transcranial Doppler middle cerebral artery velocities after aneurysm clipping. Surg Neurol 47:541–546, 1997.

Britton TC, Guiloff RJ. Carotid artery disease presenting as cough headache. Lancet 2:1406, 1988.

Brodribb AJM. Vertebral aneurysm in a case of Ehlers-Danlos syndrome. Br J Surg 57:148–151, 1970.

Bromberg JE, Rinkel GJ, Algra A, et al. Outcome in familial subarachnoid hemorrhage. Stroke 26:961–963, 1995a.

Bromberg JE, Rinkel GJ, Algra A, et al. Familial subarachnoid hemorrhage: Distinctive features and patterns of inheritance. Ann Neurol 38:929–934, 1995b.

Brott T, Mandybur TI. Case-control study of clinical outcome after aneurysmal subarachnoid hemorrhage. Neurosurgery 19:891–895, 1986.

Brown DM, Sobol WM, Folk JC, et al. Retinal arteriolar macroaneurysms: Long-term visual outcome. Br J Ophthalmol 78:534–538, 1994.

Brown GC, Weinstock F. Arterial macroaneurysm on the optic disk presenting as a mass lesion. Ann Ophthalmol 17:519–520, 1985.

Brown J Jr, Danielson R, Donahue S, et al. Horner's syndrome in subadventitial carotid artery dissection and the role of magnetic resonance angiography. Am J Ophthalmol 119:811–813, 1995.

Brown OL, Armitage JL. Spontaneous dissecting aneurysms of the cervical internal carotid artery: Two case reports and a survey of the literature. AJR 118:648–653, 1973.

Brown RAP. Cystic disease of the kidneys and intracranial aneurysms: The etiology and interrelationship of these conditions: Review of current literature and report of seven cases in which both conditions coexisted. Glasgow Med J 32:333–347, 1951.

Brownlee RD, Tranmer BI, Sevick RJ, et al. Spontaneous thrombosis of an unruptured anterior communicating artery aneurysm. An unusual cause of ischemic stroke. Stroke 26:1945–1949, 1995.

Brunberg JA, Frey KA, Horton JA, et al. [15O]H2O positron emission tomography determination of cerebral blood flow during balloon test occlusion of the internal carotid artery. AJNR 15:725–732, 1994.

Brust JCM, Dickinson PCT, Hughes JEO, et al. The diagnosis and treatment of cerebral mycotic aneurysms. Ann Neurol 27:238–246, 1990.

Bucciero A, Carangelo B, Vizioli L. Giant basilar artery aneurysm associated with moya-moya disease. Case report and review of the literature. Acta Neurol 16:121–128, 1994.

Buckingham MJ, Crone KR, Ball WS, et al. Traumatic intracranial aneurysms in childhood: Two cases and a review of the literature. Neurosurgery 22:398–408, 1988.

Bugiani O, Piola P, Tabaton M. Nontraumatic dissecting aneurysm of the basilar artery. Eur Neurol 22:256–260, 1983.

Bull J. Massive aneurysms at the base of the brain. Brain 92:535–570, 1969.

Bull JWD. Contribution of radiology to the study of intracranial aneurysms. Br Med J 2:1701–1708, 1962.

Bullock R, van Dellen JR, van den Heever CM. Intracranial mycotic aneurysm. S Afr Med J 60:970–973, 1981.

Burklund CW. Spontaneous dissecting aneurysm of cervical carotid artery. A report of surgical treatment in two patients. Johns Hopkins Med J 126:154–159, 1970.

Burleson AC, Strother CM, Turitto VT. Computer modeling of intracranial saccular and lateral aneurysms for the study of their hemodynamics. Neurosurgery 37:774–782; discussion 782–784, 1995.

Burton C, Velasco F, Dorman J. Traumatic aneurysm of a peripheral cerebral artery: Review and case report. J Neurosurg 28:468–474, 1968.

Busby DR, Slemmons DH, Miller TF Jr. Fatal epistaxis via carotid aneurysm and eustachian tube. Arch Otolaryngol 87:295–298, 1968.

Butler AB, Partain RA, Netsky MC. Primary intraventricular hemorrhage: A mild and remediable form. Neurology 22:675–687, 1972.

Buttner U, Ott M, Helmchen C, et al. Bilateral loss of eighth nerve function as the only clinical sign of vertebrobasilar dolichoectasia. J Vestib Res 5:47–51, 1995.

Byers PH, Holbrook KA. Molecular basis of clinical heterogeneity in the Ehlers-Danlos syndrome. Ann NY Acad Sci 460:298–310, 1985.

Byrne JV, Hubbard N, Morris JH. Endovascular coil occlusion of experimental aneurysms: Partial treatment does not prevent subsequent rupture. Neurol Res 16:425–427, 1994.

Byrne JV, Adams CB, Kerr RS, et al. Endosaccular treatment of inoperable intracranial aneurysms with platinum coils. Br J Neurosurg 9:585–592, 1995a.

Byrne JV, Molyneux AJ, Brennan RP, et al. Embolisation of recently ruptured intracranial aneurysms. J Neurol Neurosurg Psychiatry 59:616–620, 1995b.

Cabezudo JM, Carrillo R, Vaquero J, et al. Intracavernous aneurysm of the carotid artery following transsphenoidal surgery: Case report. J Neurosurg 54:118–121, 1981.

Cahill DW. Supergiant anterior circulation aneurysms. Neurol Res 14(2 Suppl):204–207, 1992.

Calopa M, Rubio F, Aguilar M, et al. Giant basilar aneurysm in the course of subacute bacterial endocarditis. Stroke 21:1625–1627, 1990.

Campiche R, Anzil AP, Zander E. Dissecting aneurysm of the basilar artery. Arch Suisses Neurol Neurochir Psychiatr 104:209–223, 1969.

Campos J, Fox AJ, Venuela F, et al. Saccular aneurysms in basilar artery fenestration. AJNR 8:233–236, 1987.

Camuzet F, Mathis A, Grandperret A, et al. Anévrysme disséquant de la carotide interne avec manifestations ophtalmologiques. Rev Otoneuroophtalmol 56:27–29, 1984.

Canhao P, Pinto AN, Ferro H, et al. Smoking and aneurysmal subarachnoid hemorrhage: A case-control study. J Cardiovasc Risk 1:155–158, 1994.

Canhao P, Ferro JM, Pinto AN, et al. Perimesencephalic and nonperimesencephalic subarachnoid hemorrhages with negative angiograms. Acta Neurochir 132:14–19, 1995.

Cantu RC, LeMay M, Wilkinson HA. The importance of repeated angiography in the treatment of mycotic-embolic intracranial aneurysms. J Neurosurg 25:189–193, 1966.

Capanna AH. Traumatic intracranial aneurysm and Gradenigo's syndrome secondary to gunshot wound. Surg Neurol 22:263–266, 1984.

Caplan L. Intracerebral hemorrhage revisited. Neurology 38:624–627, 1988.

Caplan LR, Zarins CK, Hemmati M. Spontaneous dissection of the extracranial vertebral arteries. Stroke 16:1030–1038, 1985.

Caplan LR, Baquis GD, Pessin MS, et al. Dissection of the intracranial vertebral artery. Neurology 38:868–877, 1988.

Capo H, Warren F, Kupersmith MJ. Evolution of oculomotor nerve palsies. J Clin Neuroophthalmol 12:21–25, 1992.

Capone PM, Mechtler LL, Bates VE, et al. Multiple giant intracranial aneurysms associated with lymphomatoid granulomatosis. A magnetic resonance imaging and angiographic study. J Neuroimaging 4:109–111, 1994.

Caprioli J, Fagadau W, Lesser R. Acute monocular visual loss secondary to anterior communicating artery aneurysm in a patient with sickle cell disease. Ann Ophthalmol 15:873–876, 1983.

Caram PC, Sharkey PC, Alvord EC. Thalamic angioma and aneurysm of the choroidal artery with intraventricular hematoma. J Neurosurg 17:347–352, 1960.

Carella A, Caruso G, Lambert P. Hemifacial spasm due to elongation and ectasia of the distal segment of the vertebral artery: Report of two cases. Neuroradiology 6:233–236, 1973.

Carls FR, Engelke W, Locher MC, et al. Complications following arthroscopy of the temporomandibular joint: Analysis covering a 10-year period (451 arthroscopies). J Craniomaxillofac Surg 24:12–15, 1996.

Carmichael R. The pathogenesis of non-inflammatory cerebral aneurysms. J Pathol Bacteriol 62:1–19, 1950.

Carruthers J, Blach RK. Vitrectomy in subarachnoid hemorrhage. Br Med J 2:404, 1976.

Carter JE, Montgomery RJ. The impossible aneurysm: Canalicular and orbital apex aneurysms of the ophthalmic artery. Neuro-ophthalmology 9:103–110, 1989.

Casasco A, Arnaud O, Gobin P, et al. Anevrysmes geants intracraniens. Traitement endovasculaire electif par des spires metalliques. Neurochirurgie 38:18–26, 1992.

Casasco AE, Aymard A, Gobin YP, et al. Selective endovascular treatment of 71 intracranial aneurysms with platinum coils. J Neurosurg 79:3–10, 1993.

Case records of the Massachusetts General Hospital. Case 39451. N Engl J Med 249:776–779, 1953.

Case records of the Massachusetts General Hospital. N Engl J Med 261:89 92, 1959.

Case records of the Massachusetts General Hospital. Case 10-1993.

N Engl J Med 328:717–725, 1993.

Casey AT, Moore AJ. A traumatic giant posterior cerebral artery aneurysm mimicking a tentorial edge meningioma. Br J Neurosurg 8:97–99, 1994.

Casey AT, Marsh HT, Uttley D. Intracranial aneurysm formation following radiotherapy. Br J Neurosurg 7:575–579, 1993.

Castier P, Francois P, Constantinides G, et al. Macroanevrysmes arteriels retiniens. Bull Soc Ophtalmol Fr 84:485–489, 1984.

Castrén JA. Pathogenesis and treatment of Terson-syndrome. Acta Ophthalmol 41:430–434, 1963.

Cellerier P, Georget AM. Dissection des artères vertébrales après manipulation du rachis cervical: A propos d'un cas. J Radiol 65:191–196, 1984.

Chace R, Hedges TR III. Retinal artery occlusion due to moyamoya disease. J Clin Neuroophthalmol 4:31–34, 1984.

Chadan N, Thierry A, Sautreaux JL, et al. Rupture anevrysmale et toxicomanie a la cocaine. Neurochirurgie 37:403–405, 1991.

Chambers EF, Rosenbaum AE, Norman D, et al. Traumatic aneurysms of cavernous internal carotid artery with secondary epistaxis. AJNR 2:405–409, 1981.

Chambi I, Tasker RR, Gentili F, et al. Gauze-induced granuloma (''gauzoma''): An uncommon complication of gauze reinforcement of berry aneurysms. J Neurosurg 72:163–170, 1990.

Chan JW, Hoyt WF, Ellis WG, Gress D: Pathogenesis of acute monocular blindness from leaking anterior communicating artery aneurysm: Report of six cases. Neurology 48:680–683, 1997.

Chandler WF. Carotid Artery Injuries. Mt Kisco, NY. Futura, 1982.

Chandra B. Treatment of subarachnoid hemorrhage from ruptured intracranial aneurysm with tranexamic acid: A double-blind clinical trial. Ann Neurol 3:502–504, 1978.

Chang CM, Ng HK, Leung SY, et al. Fatal bilateral vertebral artery dissection in a patient with cystic medial necrosis. Clin Neurol Neurosurg 93:309–311, 1991.

Chang GY, Ahn PC. Postcoital vertebral artery dissection. Am Fam Phys 54:2195–2196, 1996.

Chang HS, Fukushima T, Takakura K, et al. Aneurysms of the posterior cerebral artery: Report of ten cases. Neurosurgery 19:1006–1011, 1986.

Chang V, Rewcastle NB, Harwood-Nash DCF, et al. Bilateral dissecting aneurysms of the intracranial internal carotid arteries in an 8-year-old boy. Neurology 25:573–579, 1975.

Chapman AB, Rubinstein D, Hughes R, et al. Intracranial aneurysms in autosomal dominant polycystic kidney disease. N Engl J Med 327:916–920, 1992.

Chapman AB, Johnson AM, Gabow PA. Intracranial aneurysms in patients with autosomal dominant polycystic kidney disease: How to diagnose and who to screen. Am J Kidney Dis 22:526–531, 1993.

Charamis J, Tsamparlakis J, Scouras J, et al. Les manifestations ophtalmologiques des anévrysmes artériels intracraniens. Bull Mem Soc Fr Ophtalmol 87:213–218, 1976.

Charles N, Froment C, Rode G, et al. Vertigo and upside down vision due to an infarct in the territory of the medial branch of the posterior inferior cerebellar artery caused by dissection of a vertebral artery. J Neurol Neurosurg Psychiatry 55:188–189, 1992.

Chason JL, Hindman WM. Berry aneurysm of the circle of Willis: Results of a planned autopsy study. Neurology 8:41–44, 1958.

Chaudhary MY, Puljic S, Clauss RH. Bilateral false aneurysms after carotid endarterectomy. Neuroradiology 18:215–216, 1979.

Chauveau D, Pirson Y, Verellen-Dumoulin C, et al. Intracranial aneurysms in autosomal dominant polycystic kidney disease. Kidney Int 45:1140–1146, 1994.

Chen CJ, Chen ST. Extracranial distal aneurysm of posterior inferior cerebellar artery. Neuroradiology 39:344–347, 1997.

Chen HJ, Liou CW, Chen L. Metastatic atrial myxoma presenting as intracranial aneurysms with hemorrhage: Case report. Surg Neurol 40:61–64, 1993.

Chen ST, Liu YH. Moyamoya disease associated with bilateral persistent primitive trigeminal arteries: Report of a case. J Formos Med Assoc 92:385–387, 1993.

Chen ZP. Anterior inferior cerebellar artery aneurysm: Report of 2 cases. Chung Hua Wai Ko Tsa Chih 28:490–491, 511, 1990.

Chester AC, Harris JP, Schreiner GE. Polycystic kidney disease. Am Family Physician 16:94–101, 1977.

Chew EY, Murphy RP. Acquired retinal macroaneurysms. In Retina. Editors, Schachat AP, Murphy RP, 2nd ed, Vol 2, pp 1499–1502, 1994.

Cheynet F, Gere E, Chossegros C, et al. Faux anevrysmes traumatiques associes aux fractures fermees de la mandibule. A propos de 3 cas. Rev Stomatol Chir Maxillofac 93:6–12, 1992.

Chiras J, Bories J, Fredy D, et al. Traumatismes fermés de la carotide extra-cranienne. J Radiol 63:329–336, 1982.

Chiras J, Marciano S, Vega Molina J, et al. Spontaneous dissecting aneurysm of the extracranial vertebral artery (20 cases). Neuroradiology 27:327–333, 1985.

Chiu NC, DeLong GR, Heinz ER. Intracranial fibromuscular dysplasia in a 5-year-old child. Pediatr Neurol 14:262–264, 1996.

Chong BW, Kerber CW, Boxton RB, et al. Blood flow dynamics in the vertebrobasilar System: Correlation of a transparent elastic model and MR angiography. AJNR 15:733–745, 1994.

Chou SM, Chong YY, Kinkel R. A proposed pathogenetic process in the formation of Aspergillus mycotic aneurysm in the central nervous system. Ann Acad Med Singapore 22:518–525, 1993.

Chyatte D, Lewis I. Gelatinase activity and the occurrence of cerebral aneurysms. Stroke 28:799–804, 1997.

Chyatte D, Fode NC, Sundt TM Jr. Early versus late intracranial aneurysm surgery in subarachnoid hemorrhage. J Neurosurg 69:326–331, 1988.

Chyatte D, Reilly J, Tilson MD. Morphometric analysis of reticular and elastin fibers in the cerebral arteries of patients with intracranial aneurysms. Neurosurgery 26:939–943, 1990.

Chyatte D, Chen TL, Bronstein K, et al. Seasonal fluctuation in the incidence of intracranial aneurysm rupture and its relationship to changing climatic conditions. J Neurosurg 81:525–530, 1994.

Civit T, Auque J, Marchal JC, et al. Aneurysm clipping after endovascular treatment with coils: Report of eight patients. Neurosurgery 38:955–960, 1996.

Clare CE, Barrow DL. Infectious intracranial aneurysms. Neurosurg Clin N Am 3:551–566, 1992.

Clarke E, Walton JN. Subdural haematoma complicating intracranial aneurysm and angioma. Brain 76:378–404, 1953.

Clarke P, Whittaker M. Traumatic aneurysm of the internal carotid artery and rupture of the duodenum following seat belt injury. Injury 12:158–160, 1980.

Clarkson JG, Flynn HW Jr, Daily MJ. Vitrectomy in Terson's syndrome. Am J Ophthalmol 90:549–552, 1980.

Cleary PE, Kohner EM, Hamilton AM, et al. Retinal macroaneurysms. Br J Ophthalmol 59:355–361, 1975.

Clouston JE, Numaguchi Y, Zoarski GH, et al. Intraarterial papaverine infusion for cerebral vasospasm after subarachnoid hemorrhage. AJNR 16:27–38, 1995.

Clyde BL, Firlik AD, Kaufmann AM, et al. Paradoxical aggravation of vasospasm with papaverine infusion following aneurysmal subarachnoid hemorrhage. Case report. J Neurosurg 84:690–695, 1996a.

Clyde BL, Resnick DK, Yonas H, et al. The relationship of blood velocity as measured by transcranial doppler ultrasonography to cerebral blood flow as determined by stable xenon computed tomographic studies after aneurysmal subarachnoid hemorrhage. Neurosurgery 38:896–904, 1996b.

Cogan DG. Ophthalmic manifestations of bilateral non-occipital cerebral lesions. Br J Ophthalmol 49:281–297, 1965.

Cogan DG, Mount HTJ. Intracranial aneurysms causing ophthalmoplegia. Arch Ophthalmol 70:757–771, 1963.

Cohen AR, Aleksic S, Budzilovich GN, et al. Giant intracranial aneurysm presenting as a posterior fossa mass. Surg Neurol 20:160–164, 1983.

Collier J. Observations on cerebral hemorrhage due to causes other than arteriosclerosis. Br Med J 2:519–521, 1931.

Collins TE, Mehalic TF, White TK, et al. Trochlear nerve palsy as the sole initial sign of an aneurysm of the superior cerebellar artery. Neurosurgery 30:258–261, 1992.

Colopinto EV, Cabeen MA, Johnson LN. Optic nerve compression by a dolichoectatic internal carotid artery: Case report. Neurosurgery 39:604–606, 1996.

Connolly ES Jr, Fiore AJ, Winfree CJ, et al. Elastin degradation in the superficial temporal arteries of patients with intracranial aneurysms reflects changes in plasma elastase. Neurosurgery 40:903–908, 1997.

Constantinides G, Hochart G. Macroanevrysme arteriel retinien: A propos d'un cas. Bull Soc Ophtalmol Fr 81:579–581, 1981.

Contamin F, Hauw JJ, Singer B, et al. Syndrome de Wallenberg par hémodissection (anévrysme disséquant) de l'artère vertébrale. Rev Neurol 138:337–343, 1982.

Coppeto JR. Vertebrobasilar degeneration and chronic visual migraine. Neuroophthalmology 8:1–7, 1988.

Coppeto JR, Chan YS. Abducens nerve paresis caused by unruptured vertebral artery aneurysm. Surg Neurol 18:385–387, 1982.

Coppeto JR, Hoffman H. Tolosa-Hunt syndrome with proptosis mimicked by giant aneurysm of posterior cerebral artery. Arch Neurol 38:54–55, 1981.

Coppeto JR, Lessell S. Dorsal midbrain syndrome from giant aneurysm of the posterior fossa: Report of two cases. Neurology 33:732–736, 1983.

Corr P, Wright M, Handler LC. Endocarditis-related cerebral aneurysms: Radiologic changes with treatment. AJNR 16:745–748, 1995.

Cosgrove GR, Villemure JG, Melancon D. Traumatic intracranial aneurysm due to arterial injury at surgery: Case report. J Neurosurg 58:291–294, 1983.

Cossu M, Pau A, Turtas S, et al. Subsequent bleeding from ruptured intracranial aneurysms treated by wrapping or coating: A review of the long-term results in 47 cases. Neurosurgery 32:344–346; discussion 347, 1993.

Cox TA, Wurster JB, Godfrey WA. Primary aberrant oculomotor regeneration due to intracranial aneurysm. Arch Neurol 36:570–571, 1979.

Coyne TJ, Wallace MC. Bilateral third cranial nerve palsies in association with a ruptured anterior communicating artery aneurysm. Surg Neurol 42:52–56, 1994.

Crawford MD, Sarner M. Ruptured intracranial aneurysms: Community study. Lancet 21:1254–1257, 1965.

Crawford T. The pathological effects of cerebral arteriography. J Neurol Neurosurg Psychiatry 19:217–221, 1956.

Crawford T. Some observations on the pathogenesis and natural history of intracranial aneurysms. J Neurol Neurosurg Psychiatry 22:259–266, 1959.

Creissard P, Sevrain L, Freger P, et al. Le vasospasme et l'ischémie dans une série de 60 anévrismes opérés tot. Neurochirurgie 34:157–160, 1988.

Crissey MM, Bernstein EF. Delayed presentation of carotid intimal tear following blunt craniocervical trauma. Surgery 75:543–549, 1974.

Crivelli G, Bianchi M, Dario A, et al. Saccular aneurysm associated with proximal basilar artery fenestration. Case report. J Neurosurg Sci 37:29–34, 1993.

Croisile B, Deruty R, Pialat J, et al. Anévrysme de la carotide supra-clinoï dienne et méga-dolicho-artères cervicales dans un syndrome de Marfan. Neurochirurgie 34:342–347, 1988.

Crompton JL, Moore CE. Painful third nerve palsy: How not to miss an intracranial aneurysm. Aust J Ophthalmol 9:113–115, 1981.

Crompton MR. Subtentorial changes following the rupture of cerebral aneurysms. Brain 88:75–84, 1965.

Cucco G. Manifestazioni oculari nella sindrome da emorragia subaracnoidea. Ann Ottal 77:454–462, 1951.

Cullen JF, Haining WM, Crombie AL. Cerebral aneurysms presenting with visual field defects. Br J Ophthalmol 50:251–256, 1966.

Cullom ME, Savino PJ, Sergott RC, et al. Relative pupillary sparing third nerve palsies. To arteriogram or not? J Neuroophthalmol 15:136–140; discussion 140–141, 1995.

Cunha e Sa MJ, Stein BM, Solomon RA, et al. The treatment of associated intracranial aneurysms and arteriovenous malformations. J Neurosurg 77:853–859, 1992.

Cunningham RD, Sewell JJ. Aneurysm of the ophthalmic artery with drusen of the optic nerve head. Am J Ophthalmol 72:743–745, 1971.

Curnes JT, Shogry ME, Clark DC, et al. MR angiographic demonstration of an intracranial aneurysm not seen on conventional angiography. AJNR 14:971–973, 1993.

D'Andrea F, Maiuri F, Gangemi M, et al. Megadolichobasilar anomaly. Clinical and diagnostic considerations on 30 cases. Acta Neurol 14:611–619, 1992.

D'Angelo V, Fiumara E, Gorgoglione L, et al. Surgical treatment of a cerebral mycotic aneurysm using the stereo-angiographic localizer. Surg Neurol 44:263–264, 1995.

D'Anglejan-Chatillon J, Ribeiro V, Mas JL, et al. Migraine: A risk factor for dissection of cervical arteries. Headache 29:560–561, 1989.

Dailey EJ, Holloway JA, Murto RE, et al. Evaluation of ocular signs and symptoms in cerebral aneurysms. Arch Ophthalmol 71:463–474, 1964.

Dailey RA, Wilson DJ, Putnam D. Superficial temporal-artery aneurysm. Ophthalmic Surg 25:328–329, 1994.

Dailey RW, Robertson WD, Nugent RA, et al. Computed tomography of anterior inferior cerebellar artery aneurysm mimicking an acoustic neuroma. J Comput Assist Tomogr 10:881–884, 1986.

Dale J, Landmark KH, Myhre E. The effects of nifedipine, a calcium antagonist, on platelet function. Am Heart J 105:103–105, 1983.

Damasio H, Seabra-Gomes R, da Silva JP, et al. Multiple cerebral aneurysms and cardiac myxoma. Arch Neurol 32:269–270, 1975.

Dandy WE. Intracranial aneurysm of the internal carotid artery. Ann Surg 107:654–659, 1938.

Dandy WE. Treatment of internal carotid aneurysm within the cavernous sinus and cranial chamber. Ann Surg 109:689–711, 1939.

Dandy WE. Intracranial Arterial Aneurysms. Ithaca, NY, Comstock Publishing Associates, Cornell University Press, 1944.

Daneshmend TK, Hewer RL, Bradshaw JR. Acute brain stem stroke during neck manipulation. Br Med J 288:189, 1984.

Date I, Akioka T, Ohmoto T. Penetration of the optic chiasm by a ruptured anterior communicating artery aneurysm: Case report. J Neurosurg 87:324–326, 1997.

Daus W, Kasmann B, Alexandridis E. Terson-Syndrom. Komplizierte klinische Verlaufe. Ophthalmologe 89:77–81, 1992.

Davidson KC, Weiford EC, Dixon GD. Traumatic vertebral artery pseudoaneurysm following chiropractic manipulation. Radiology 115:651–652, 1975.

Davies L. A case of vagal palsy due to dissecting aneurysm of the carotid artery. Med J Aust 147:352–353, 1987.

Davis GG, Swalwell CI. Acute aortic dissections and ruptured berry aneurysms associated with methamphetamine abuse. J Forensic Sci 39:1481–1485, 1994.

Davis GG, Swalwell CI. The incidence of acute cocaine or methamphetamine intoxication in deaths due to ruptured cerebral (berry) aneurysms. J Forensic Sci 41:626–628, 1996.

Davis RH, Daroff RB, Hoyt WF. Hemicrania, oculosympathetic paresis, and subcranial carotid aneurysm: Raeder's paratrigeminal syndrome (Group 2): Case report. J Neurosurg 29:94–96, 1968.

Dawson RC, Krisht AF, Barrow DL, et al. Treatment of experimental aneurysms using collagen-coated microcoils. Neurosurgery 36:133–139; discussion 139–140, 1995.

Day AL. Visual loss with ophthalmic segment aneurysms. J Neurosurg 72:342A, 1990a.

Day AL. Aneurysms of the ophthalmic segment. A clinical and anatomical analysis. J Neurosurg 72:677–691, 1990b.

Day JD, Giannotta SL, Fukushima T. Extradural temporopolar approach to lesions of the upper basilar artery and infrachiasmatic region. J Neurosurg 81:230–235, 1994.

Day JD, Fukushima T, Giannotta, SL. Cranial base approaches to posterior circulation aneurysms. J Neurosurg 87:544–554, 1997.

de Bray JM, Lhoste P, Dubas F, et al. Ultrasonic features of extracranial carotid dissections: 47 cases studied by angiography. J Ultrasound Med 13:659–664, 1994.

de Bray JM, Penisson-Besnier I, Dubas F, et al. Extracranial and intracranial vertebrobasilar dissections: diagnosis and prognosis. J Neurol Neurosurg Psychiatry 63:46–51, 1997.

de Grood MPAM. Anévrysme disséquant carotidien comme complication de l'angiographie carotidienne. Rev Neurol 90:661, 1954.

De Jesús O. The clinoidal space: Anatomical review and surgical implications. Acta Neurochir 139:361–365, 1997.

de los Reyes RA, Kantrowitz AB, Detwiler PW, et al. Transoral-transclival clipping of a giant lower basilar artery aneurysm. Surg Neurol 38:379–382, 1992a.

de los Reyes RA, Kantrowitz AB, Boehm FH, et al. Transcallosal, transventricular approach to a basilar apex aneurysm. Neurosurgery 31:597–601; discussion 601–602, 1992b.

de Oliveira E, Tedeschi H, Siqueira MG, et al. Anatomical and technical aspects of the contralateral approach for multiple aneurysms. Acta Neurochir 138:1–11; discussion 11, 1996.

de Paepe A, van Landegem W, de Keyser F, et al. Association of multiple intracranial aneurysms and collagen type III deficiency. Clin Neurol Neurosurg 90:53–56, 1988.

de Wazieres B, Coppere B, Durieu I, et al. Manifestations vasculaires et/ou cardiaques du syndrome d'Ehlers-Danlos de type IV. 9 observations. Presse Med 24:1381–1385, 1995.

De Caro R, Serafini MT, Galli S, et al. Anatomy of segmental duplication in the human basilar artery. Possible site of aneurysm formation. Clin Neuropathol 14:303–309, 1995.

De Marinis P, Punzo A, Colangelo M, et al. Giant aneurysm of the calloso-marginal artery. Childs Nerv Syst 7:353–355, 1991.

De Mattos JP, De Rosso AL, Zayen E, et al. Segmental myoclonus and basilar artery. Giant aneurysm. Case report. Arq Neuropsiquiatr 50:528–530, 1992.

Debrun G, Fox A, Drake CG, et al. Giant unclippable aneurysms: Treatment with detachable balloons. Am J Neuroradiol 2:167–173, 1981.

Debrun GM, Aletich VA, Miller NR, et al. Three cases of spontaneous direct carotid cavernous fistulas associated with Ehlers-Danlos syndrome type IV. Surg Neurol 46:247–252, 1996.

Deeb ZL, Jannetta PJ, Rosenbaum AE, et al. Tortuous vertebrobasilar arteries causing cranial nerve syndromes: Screening by computed tomography. J Comput Assist Tomogr 3:774–778, 1979.

Dehaene I, Pattyn G, Calliauw L. Megadolichobasilar anomaly, basilar impression and occipito-vertebral anastomosis. Clin Neurol Neurosurg 78:131–138, 1975.

Delfini R, Domenicucci M, Ferrari M. Association of intracranial meningiomas and aneurysms. Report of three cases and review of the literature. J Neurosurg Sci 34:51–56, 1990.

Dell S. Asymptomatic cerebral aneurysm: Assessment of its risk of rupture. Neurosurgery 10:162–166, 1982.

Dellen JRV. Intracavernous traumatic aneurysms. Surg Neurol 13:203–207, 1980.

DeLuca J. Cognitive dysfunction after aneurysm of the anterior communicating artery. J Clin Exp Neuropsychol 14:924–934, 1992.

DeLuca J, Cicerone KD. Confabulation following aneurysm of the anterior communicating artery. Cortex 27:417–423, 1991.

DeLuca J, Diamond BJ. Aneurysm of the anterior communicating artery: A review of neuroanatomical and neuropsychological sequelae. J Clin Exp Neuropsychol 17:100–121, 1995.

Demierre B, Safran AB. Paralysies due III nerf cranien d'origines ischémique et anévrysmale: La signification de la douleur dans le diagnostic différentiel. J Fr Ophtalmol 4:133–141, 1981.

Denny-Brown D. The treatment of recurrent cerebrovascular symptoms and the question of "vasospasm." Med Clin North Am 35:1457–1474, 1951.

Derdeyn CP, Moran CJ, Cross DT, et al. Intraoperative digital subtraction angiography: A review of 112 consecutive examinations. AJNR 16:307–318, 1995.

Dernbach PD, Sila CA, Little JR. Giant and multiple aneurysms of the distal posterior inferior cerebellar artery. Neurosurgery 22:309–312, 1988a.

Dernbach PD, Little JR, Jones SC, Ebrahim ZY. Altered cerebral autoregulation and C02 reactivity after aneurysmal subarachnoid hemorrhage. Neurosurgery 22:822–826, 1988b.

Deruty R, Mottolese C, Lapras C, et al. Résultats à long-terme du traitement de l'anévrysme intra-cranien rompu: Etude d'une série de 328 patients hospitalisés de 1972 à 1984. Neurochirurgie 34:1–7, 1988.

Deruty R, Mottolese C, Soustiel JF, et al. Association of cerebral arteriovenous malformation and cerebral aneurysm. Diagnosis and management. Acta Neurochir 107:133–139, 1990.

Deruty R, Pelissou-Guyotat I, Mottolese C, et al. Fenestration of the middle cerebral artery and aneurysm at the site of the fenestration. Neurol Res 14:421–424, 1992a.

Deruty R, Pelissou-Guyotat I, Mottolese C, et al. Ruptured occult arteriovenous malformation associated with an unruptured intracranial aneurysm: Report of three cases. Neurosurgery 30:603–606; discussion 606–607, 1992b.

Deruty R, Pelissou-Guyotat I, Mottolese C, et al. Long-term outcome after treatment of the ruptured intracranial aneurysm: 73 cases admitted from day 0 to day 3 after subarachnoid hemorrhage. Neurol Res 16:83–88, 1994.

Deruty R, Pelissou-Guyotat I, Mottolese C, et al. Management of unruptured cerebral aneurysms. Neurol Res 18:39–44, 1996.

DeSouza TG, Berlad L, Shapiro K, et al. Pheochromocytoma and multiple intracerebral aneurysms. J Pediatr 108:947–949, 1986.

Destian S, Tung H, Gray R, et al. Giant infectious intracavernous carotid artery aneurysm presenting as intractable epistaxis. Surg Neurol 41:472–476, 1994.

Dettori P, Cristi G, Dalbuono S. Anomalia megadolichobasilaire. Radiol Med 52:1259–1272, 1966.

Devoize JL, Rouanet J, Cellerier P, et al. Paralysie bénigne des quatre derniers nerfs crâniens. Arguments en faveur d'un mécanisme ischémique. Presse Med 14:1328–1330, 1985.

Dewachter A, De Laey JJ. Acquired retinal macroaneurysm. Bull Soc Ophtalmol Belge 201:105–111, 1982.

Diaz FG, Ohaegbulam S, Dujovny M, et al. Surgical alternatives in the treatment of cavernous sinus aneurysms. J Neurosurg 71:846–853, 1989.

Dickinson LD, Tuite GF, Colon GP, et al. Vertebral artery dissection related to basilar impression: Case report. Neurosurgery 36:835–838, 1995.

Dierssen G, Montiaga F, Vazquez A, et al. Three cases of ruptured intracranial aneurysm in a family. Neurochirurgia 33:85–87, 1990.

Dietl S, Schuhmacher M, Menninger H, et al. Subarachnoid hemorrhage associated with bilateral internal carotid artery aneurysms as a Manifestation of Behçet's Disease. J Rheumatol 21:4:775–776, 1994.

Dietrich J, Gunther L, Fried H. Dreidimensionale Computertomographie in der Diagnostik und Operationsplanung von intrakraniellen Aneurysmen. Zentralbl Neurochir 56:34–39, 1995.

Diggs LW, Brookoff D. Multiple cerebral aneurysms in patients with sickle cell disease. South Med J 86:377–379, 1993.

Digre KB, Corbett JJ, Smoker WRK, et al. CT and hemifacial spasm. Neurology 38:1111–1113, 1988.

Ding MX. Traumatic aneurysm of the intracavernous part of the internal carotid artery presenting with epistaxis: Case report. Surg Neurol 30:65–67, 1988.

Diraz A, Kobayashi S, Okudera H, et al. Suprachiasmal carotid-ophthalmic artery aneurysm: Report of two cases. Neurol Med Chir 32:952–956, 1992.

Diraz A, Kobayashi S, Toriyama T, et al. Surgical approaches to the anterior communicating artery aneurysm and their results. Neurol Res 15:273–280, 1993.

Dixon JM. Angioid streaks and pseudoxanthoma elasticum. Am J Ophthalmol 34:1322–1323, 1951.

Dobrin PB. Mechanical properties of arteries. Physiol Rev 58:397–460, 1978.

Dobrin PB, Baker WH, Gley WC. Elastolytic and collagenolytic studies of arteries: Implications for the mechanical properties of aneurysms. Arch Surg 119:405–409, 1984.

Doherty WB, Trubek M. Significant hemorrhagic retinal lesions in bacterial endocarditis (Roth's spots). JAMA 97:308–313, 1931.

Dolenc VV. A combined epi- and subdural direct approach to carotid-ophthalmic artery aneurysms. J Neurosurg 62:667–672, 1985.

Donauers E, Reif J, al-Khalaf B, et al. Intraventricular hemorrhage caused by aneurysms and angiomas. Acta Neurochir 122:23–31, 1993.

Dorsch NW, Young N, Kingston RJ, et al. Early experience with spiral CT in the diagnosis of intracranial aneurysms. Neurosurgery *36*:230–236; discussion 236–238, 1995.

Dott NM. Intracranial aneurysms: Cerebral arterio-radiography: Surgical treatment. Edinburgh Med J *40*:219–234, 1933.

Doubler FH, Marlow SB. A case of hemorrhage into the optic-nerve sheaths as a direct extension from a diffuse intra-meningeal hemorrhage caused by rupture of aneurysm of a cerebral artery. Arch Ophthalmol *46*:533–536, 1917.

Dowd CF, Halbach VV, Higashida RT, et al. Endovascular coil embolization of unusual posterior inferior cerebellar artery aneurysms. Neurosurgery *27*:954–961, 1990.

Dragon R, Saranchak H, Lakin P, et al. Blunt injuries to the carotid and vertebral arteries. Am J Surg *141*:497–500, 1981.

Drake CG. Ligation of the vertebral (unilateral or bilateral) or basilar artery in the treatment of large intracranial aneurysms. J Neurosurg *43*:255–274, 1975.

Drake CG. Giant intracranial aneurysms: Experience with surgical treatment in 174 patients. Clin Neurosurg *26*:12–95, 1979.

Drake CG. Evolution of intracranial aneurysm surgery. Can J Surg *27*:549 555, 1984.

Drake CG, Amacher AL. Aneurysms of the posterior cerebral artery. J Neurosurg *30*: 468–474, 1969.

Drake CG, Peerless SJ: Giant fusiform intracranial aneurysms: review of 120 patients treated surgically from 1965 to 1992. J Neurosurg *87*:141–162, 1997.

Drake CG, Vanderlinden RG, Amacher AL. Carotid-ophthalmic aneurysms. J Neurosurg *29*:24–31, 1968a.

Drake CG, Vanderlinden RG, Amacher AL. Carotid-choroidal aneurysms. J Neurosurg *29*:32–36, 1968b.

Drake CG, Peerless SJ, Ferguson GG. Hunterian proximal arterial occlusion for giant aneurysms of the carotid circulation. J Neurosurg *81*:656–665, 1994.

Drapkin AJ, Rose WS. Serial development of 'de novo' aneurysms after carotid ligation: Case report. Surg Neurol *38*:302–308, 1992.

Du YP, Parker DL, Davis WL, et al. Reduction of partial-volume artifacts with zero-filled interpolation in three-dimensional MR angiography. J Magn Reson Imaging *4*:733–741, 1994.

Duff TA, Gossmann HH. Giant aneurysm of the internal carotid artery simulating posterior fossa tumour in a 13-year-old girl. Neurochirurgia *18*:190–193, 1975.

Duffy GP. The "warning leak" in spontaneous subarachnoid hemorrhage. Med J Aust *1*:514–516, 1983.

Duke-Elder S. Textbook of Ophthalmology. Vol 5, p 5405. London, Henry Kimpton, 1952.

Duker JS, Belmont JB. Ocular ischemic syndrome secondary to carotid artery occlusion. Am J Ophthalmol *106*:750–752, 1988.

Dumas R, Guard O. Les accidents vasculaires du tronc cerebral survenant a la suite de manipulations cervicales. Ann Med Phys *22*:62–70, 1979.

Dumas S, Shults WT. Abducens paresis: A rare presenting sign of posterior-inferior cerebellar artery aneurysm. J Clin Neuro-Ophthalmol *2*:55–60, 1982.

Duman S, Stephens JW. Post-traumatic middle cerebral artery occlusion. Neurology *13*:613–616, 1963.

Dunne JW, Conacher GN, Khangure M, et al. Dissecting aneurysms of the vertebral arteries following cervical manipulation: A case report. J Neurol Neurosurg Psychiatry *50*:349–353, 1987.

Duong H, Melancon D, Tampieri D, et al. The negative angiogram in subarachnoid hemorrhage. Neuroradiology *38*:15–19, 1996.

Durand JR, Samples JR. Dolichoectasia and cranial nerve palsies: A case report. J Clin Neuroophthalmol *9*:249–253, 1989.

Durston JHJ, Parsons-Smith BG. Blindness due to aneurysm of anterior communicating artery: With recovery after carotid ligation. Br J Ophthalmol *54*:170–176, 1970.

Dust G, Reineck M, Behrens-Baumann W, et al. Schmerzhafte Ophthalmoplegie ohne Mydriasis: Oculomotoriusparese und Läsion sympathischer Fasern (Raeder-Syndrom) durch Druck Aneurysmas der A. carotis interna. Nervenarzt *52*:85–89, 1981.

Duvoisin RC, Yahr MD. Posterior fossa aneurysms. Neurology *15*:231–241, 1965.

Easton JD, Sherman DG. Cervical manipulation and stroke. Stroke *8*:594–597, 1977.

Ebina K, Iwabuchi T. Preliminary experimental study on a newly-developed coating material (liquid cellulose) for cerebral aneurysms. Acta Neurochir *125*:161–168, 1993.

Ebner R. Angiography for 3rd nerve palsy in children. J Clin Neuro-Ophthalmol *10*: 154–155, 1990.

Echiverri HC, Rubino FA, Gupta SR, et al. Fusiform aneurysm of the vertebrobasilar arterial system. Stroke *20*:1741–1747, 1989.

Ecker AD, Riemenschneider PA. Arteriographic demonstration of spasm of the intracranial arteries: with special reference to saccular aneurisms. J Neurosurg *8*: 660–667, 1951.

Edelman RR, Atkinson DJ, Silver MS, et al. FRODO pulse sequences: A new means of eliminating motion, flow, and wraparound artifacts. Radiology *166*:231–236, 1988.

Editorial: Intracerebral haematoma from aneurysm rupture: Operation in moribund patients? Lancet *2*:1186–1187, 1987.

Egnor MR, Page LK, David C. Vertebral artery aneurysm—A unique hazard of head banging by heavy metal rockers. Case report. Pediatr Neurosurg *17*:135–138, 1991–1992.

Ehrenfeld WK, Wylie EJ. Spontaneous dissection of the internal carotid artery. Arch Surg *111*:1294–1301, 1976.

Eichler A, Story JL, Bennett DE, et al. Traumatic aneurysm of a cerebral artery: Case report. J Neurosurg *31*:72–76, 1969.

Ekbom K, Greitz T, Kugelberg E. Hydrocephalus due to ectasia of the basilar artery. J Neurol Sci *8*:465–477, 1969.

Ekelund A, Säveland H, Romner B, et al. Transcranial Doppler ultrasound in hypertensive versus normotensive patients after aneurysmal subarachnoid hemorrhage. Stroke *26*:2071–2074, 1995.

Ekelund A, Säveland H, Romner B, et al. Is transcranial Doppler sonography useful in detecting late cerebral ischaemia after aneurysmal subarachnoid hemorrhage? Br J Neurosurg *10*:19–25, 1996.

El Khamlichi A, Amrani F, El Azzusi M, et al. Hypoplasie bilatérale des carotides internes associée a un anévrysme de la communicante postérieure droite: A propos d'une observation. Neurochirurgie *35*:23–30, 1989.

Eldevik OP, Gabrielsen TO. Fusiform aneurysmal dilatation of pericallosal artery: A sign of lipoma of corpus callosum. Acta Radiol *347(Suppl)*:71–76, 1975.

Eljamel MSM, Humphrey PRD, Shaw MDM. Spontaneous dissection of the cervical carotid artery: The role of Doppler studies and conservative management. J Neurol Neurosurg Psychiatry *52*:1461–1462, 1989.

Eljamel MSM, Humphrey PRD, Shaw MDM. Dissection of the cervical internal carotid artery. The role of Doppler/Duplex studies and conservative management. J Neurol Neurosurg Psychiatry *53*:379–383, 1990.

Eller TW. MRI demonstration of clot in a small unruptured aneurysm causing stroke. J Neurosurg *65*:411–412, 1986.

Elowiz EH, Johnson WD, Milhorat TH. Computerized tomography (CT) localized stereotactic craniotomy for excision of a bacterial intracranial aneurysm. Surg Neurol *44*:265–269, 1995.

Endo S, Nishijima M, Nomura H, et al. A pathological study of intracranial posterior circulation dissecting aneurysms with subarachnoid hemorrhage: Report of three autopsied cases and review of the literature. Neurosurgery *33*:732–738, 1993.

Engel U. Hirnbasisaneurysma und tuberose Hirnsklerose. Zentralbl Pathol *138*:67–70, 1992.

Engeset A, Nelson JW, Munthe-Kaas AW. Acute cerebral vascular insufficiaency in young patients. Acta Neurol Scand *(Suppl 31)*:122, 1967.

Epelbaum S, Laurent C, Morin G, et al. Endocardite a Neisseria mucosa compliquee d'anevrysmes intracerebraux. Arch Fr Pediatr *50*:231–233, 1993.

Eppinger H. Pathogenesis (Histogenesis und Aetiologie) der Aneurysmen einschlieslich des Aneurysma equi verminosum. Pathologisch-anatomisch studien. Arch Klin Chir *35(Suppl 1)*:1–563, 1887.

Epstein F, Ransohoff J, Budzilovich GN. The clinical significance of junctional dilation of the posterior communicating artery. J Neurosurg *33*:529–531, 1970.

Escourolle R, Gautier JC, Rosa A, et al. Anévrysme disséquant vertébro-basilaire. Rev Neurol *128*:95–104, 1973.

Espinasse-Berrod MA, David T, Parent de Curzon H, et al. Le syndrome de Terson: A propos de 7 cas. J Fr Ophtalmol *11*:43–51, 1988.

Faggioli GL, Freyrie A, Stella A, et al. Extracranial internal carotid artery aneurysms: Results of a surgical series with long-term follow-up. J Vasc Surg *23*:587–594; discussion 594–595, 1996.

Fahmy JA. Symptoms and signs of intracranial aneurysms: With particular reference to retinal hemorrhage. Acta Ophthalmol *50*:129–136, 1972a.

Fahmy JA. Vitreous hemorrhage in subarachnoid hemorrhage: Terson's syndrome. Report of a case with macular degeneration. Acta Ophthalmol *50*:137–143, 1972b.

Fahmy JA. Papilloedema associated with ruptured intracranial aneurysms. Acta Ophthalmol *50*:793–802, 1972c.

Fahmy JA. Fundal hemorrhages in ruptured intracranial aneurysms: I. Material, frequency and morphology. Acta Ophthalmol. *51*:289–298, 1973a.

Fahmy JA. Fundal hemorrhages in ruptured intracranial aneurysms: II. Correlation with clinical course. Acta Ophthalmol *51*:299–304, 1973b.

Fahmy JA, Knudsen V, Anderson SR. Intraocular hemorrhage following subarachnoid hemorrhage. Acta Ophthalmol *47*:550–559, 1969.

Falk A, Schmieder K, Hentsch A, et al. 3-D-MT-TONE-Magnetresonanzangiographie zum Nachweis intrakranieller Aneurysmen im Vergleich zur digitalen Subtraktionsangiographie: Eine prospektive Studie. Rofo Fortschr Geb Rontgenstr Neuen Bildgeb Verfahr *164*:31–37, 1996.

Faria MA Jr, Fleischer AS, Spector RH. Bilateral giant intracavernous aneurysms treated by bilateral carotid ligation. Surg Neurol *14*:207–210, 1980.

Farley MK, Clark RD, Fallor MK, et al. Spontaneous carotid-cavernous fistula and the Ehlers-Danlos syndromes. Ophthalmology *90*:1337–1342, 1983.

Farrell MA, Gilbert JJ, Kaufmann JCE. Fatal intracranial arterial dissection: Clinical pathological correlation. J Neurol Neurosurg *48*:111–121, 1985.

Farris BK, Smith JL, David NJ. The nasal junction scotoma in giant aneurysms. Ophthalmology *93*:895–905, 1986.

Feder R, Camp WA. Superior branch palsy of oculomotor nerve and pupillary constriction caused by intracranial carotid artery aneurysm. Ann Neurol *5*:493–495, 1979.

Feely M, Kapoor S. Third nerve palsy due to posterior communicating artery aneurysm: The importance of early surgery. J Neurol Neurosurg Psychiatry *50*: 1051–1052, 1987.

Fehlings MG, Gentili F. The association between polycystic kidney disease and cerebral aneurysms. Can J Neurol Sci *18*:505–509, 1991.

Feindel W, Penfield W, McNaughton F. The tentorial nerves and localization of intracranial pain in man. Neurology *10*:555–563, 1960.

Felber S, Bosch S, Henkes H, et al. Magnetresonanzangiographie intrakranieller Aneurysmen nach Subarachnoidalblutungen. Radiologe *35*:822–829, 1995.

Felsberg GJ, Tien RD, Haplea S, et al. Muslin-induced optic arachnoiditis (''gauzoma''): Findings on CT and MR. J Comput Assist Tomogr *17*:485–487, 1993.

Feman SS. The natural history of the first clinically visible features of diabetic retinopathy. Trans Am Ophthalmol Soc *92*:745–773, 1994.

Ferguson GG, Drake CG. Carotid-ophthalmic aneurysms: Visual abnormalities in 32 patients and the results of treatment. Surg Neurol *16*:1–8, 1981.

Fernandez-Real JM, Fernandez-Castaner M, Villabona C, et al. Giant intrasellar aneurysm presenting with panhypopituitarism and subarachnoid hemorrhage: Case report and literature review. Clin Investig *72*:302–306, 1994.

Fernandez Zubillaga A, Guglielmi G, Vinuela F, et al. Endovascular occlusion of intracranial aneurysms with electrically detachable coils: correlation of aneurysm neck size and treatment results. AJNR *15*:815–820, 1994.

Ferrante L, Fortuna A, Celli P, et al. Intracranial arterial aneurysms in early childhood. Surg Neurol *29*:39–56, 1988.

Ferrante L, Acqui M, Mastronardi L, et al. Posterior inferior cerebellar artery (PICA) aneurysm presenting with SAH and contralateral crural monoparesis: A case report. Surg Neurol *38*:43–45, 1992.

Ferrante L, Acqui M, Trillo G, et al. Aneurysms of the posterior cerebral artery—do they present specific characteristics. Acta Neurochir *138*:840–852, 1996.

Ferry PC, Keiber C, Peterson D, et al. Arteriectasis, subarachnoid hemorrhage in a three-month-old infant. Neurology *24*:494–500, 1974.

Fessler RD, Esshaki CM, Stankewitz RC, et al. The neurovascular complications of cocaine. Surg Neurol *47*:339–345, 1997.

Fichte C, Streeten BW, Friedman AH. A histopathologic study of retinal arterial aneurysms. Am J Ophthalmol *85*:509–518, 1978.

Findlay JM. Current management of aneurysmal subarachnoid hemorrhage guidelines from the Canadian Neurosurgical Society. Can J Neurol Sci *24*:161–170, 1997.

Findlay JM, Weir BK, Kassell NF, et al. Intracisternal recombinant tissue plasminogen activator after aneurysmal subarachnoid hemorrhage. J Neurosurg *75*:181–188, 1991.

Findlay JM, Kassell NF, Weir BK, et al. A randomized trial of intraoperative, intracisternal tissue plasminogen activator for the prevention of vasospasm. Neurosurgery *37*:168–176; discussion 177–178, 1995.

Finkemeyer H. Ein säckchenförmiges Aneurysma der A. cerebri media als postoperative Komplikation. Zentralbl Neurochir *15*:302–315, 1955.

Finlay HM, Canham PB. The layered fabric of cerebral artery fenestrations. Stroke *25*:1799–1806, 1994.

Finney HL, Roberts TS, Anderson RE. Giant intracranial aneurysm associated with Marfan's syndrome: Case report. J Neurosurg *45*:342–347, 1976.

Firlik AD, Kaufmann AM, Jungreis CA, et al. Effect of transluminal angioplasty on cerebral blood flow in the management of symptomatic vasospasm following aneurysmal subarachnoid hemorrhage. J Neurosurg *86*:830–839, 1997.

Fischer J, Mustafa H. Endoscopic-guided clipping of cerebral aneurysms. Br J Neurosurg *8*:559–565, 1994.

Fisher A, Som PM, Mosesson RE, et al. Giant intracranial aneurysms with skull base erosion and extracranial masses: CT and MR findings. J Comput Assist Tomogr *18*:939–942, 1994.

Fisher CM. The pathologic and clinical aspects of thalamic hemorrhage. Trans Am Neurol Assoc *84*:56–59, 1959.

Fisher CM. Ocular bobbing. Arch Neurol *30*:383–392, 1964.

Fisher CM. Some neuro-ophthalmologic observations. J Neurol Neurosurg Psychiatry *30*:383–392, 1967.

Fisher CM. Clinical syndromes in cerebral thrombosis, hypertensive hemorrhage, and ruptured saccular aneurysm. Clin Neurosurg *22*:117–147, 1975.

Fisher CM. The headache and pain of spontaneous carotid dissection. Headache *22*:60–65, 1981.

Fisher CM, Picard EH, Polak A, et al. Acute hypertensive cerebellar hemorrhage: I. Diagnosis and surgical treatment. J Nerv Ment Dis *140*:38–57, 1965.

Fisher CM, Ojemann RG, Roberson GH. Spontaneous dissection of cervico-cerebral arteries. Can J Neurol Sci *5*:9–19, 1978.

Fitzpatrick BC, Spetzler RF, Ballard JL, et al. Cervical-to-petrous internal carotid artery bypass procedure. Technical note. J Neurosurg *79*:138–141, 1993.

Fleischer AS, Guthkelch AN. Management of high cervical-intracranial internal carotid artery traumatic aneurysms. J Trauma *27*:330–332, 1987.

Fleischer AS, Patton JM, Tindall GT. Cerebral aneurysms of traumatic origin. Surg Neurol *4*:233–239, 1975.

Fleming JFR, Park AM. Dissecting aneurysms of the carotid artery following arteriography. Neurology *9*:1–6, 1959.

Florin RE. Bilateral symmetrical aneurysms of the internal carotid arteries with spontaneous carotid cavernous fistula. Calif Med *89*:352–355, 1958.

Fodstad H, Forsell A, Lilliequist B, et al. Antifibrinolysis with tranexamic acid in aneurysmal subarachnoid hemorrhage: A consecutive controlled clinical trial. Neurosurgery *8*:158–165, 1981.

Fogelholm R. Subarachnoid hemorrhage in middle Finland: Incidence, early prognosis and indications for neurosurgical treatment. Stroke *12*:296–301, 1981.

Forbus WD. On the origin of miliary aneurysms of the superficial cerebral arteries. Johns Hopkins Med Bull *47*:239–284, 1930.

Ford FR, Clark D. Thrombosis of the basilar artery with softenings in the cerebellum and brain stem due to manipulation of the neck. A report of two cases with one post-mortem examination; reasons are given to prove that damage to the vertebral arteries is responsible. Bull Johns Hopkins Hosp *98*:37–42, 1956.

Foster RE, Kosmorsky GS, Sweeney PJ, et al. Horner's syndrome secondary to spontaneous carotid dissection with normal angiographic findings. Arch Ophthalmol *109*:1499–1500, 1991.

Fox AJ. Angiography for third nerve palsy in children. J Clin Neuro-Ophthalmol *9*:37–38, 1989.

Fox AJ, Vinuela F, Pelz DM, et al. Use of detachable balloons for proximal artery occlusion in the treatment of unclippable cerebral aneurysms. J Neurosurg *66*:40–46, 1987.

Fox JL. Intracranial Aneurysms. Vol 1. New York, Springer-Verlag, 1983.

Fox JL. Microsurgical treatment of ventral (paraclinoid) internal carotid artery aneurysms. Neurosurgery *22*:32–39, 1988.

Fox R, Pope FM, Narcisi P, et al. Spontaneous carotid cavernous fistula in Ehlers Danlos syndrome. J Neurol Neurosurg Psychiatry *51*:984–986, 1988.

Francis KR, Williams DP, Troost BT. Facial numbness and dysesthesia. New features of carotid artery dissection. Arch Neurol *44*:345–346, 1987.

François J. Acquired macroaneurysms of the retinal arteries. Int Ophthalmol *1*:153–161, 1979.

François P, Hochart G, Ribiere M. Les macro-anevrysmes arteriels attitude du photocoagulateur. Bull Soc Ophtalmol Fr *87*:385–387, 1987.

Frank E, Brown BM, Wilson DF. Asymptomatic fusiform aneurysm of the petrous carotid artery in a patient with von Recklinghausen's neurofibromatosis. Surg Neurol *32*:75–78, 1989.

Franks AJ. Prognostic factors in ruptured aneurysms of the circle of Willis: The significance of systemic hypertension. Neuropathol Appl Neurobiol *4*:61–70, 1978.

Fransen P, de Tribolet N. Dissecting aneurysm of the posterior inferior cerebellar artery. Br J Neurosurg *8*:381–386, 1994.

Fraser KW, Halbach VV, Teitelbaum GP, et al. Endovascular platinum coil embolization of incompletely surgically clipped cerebral aneurysms. Surg Neurol *41*:4–8, 1994.

Frasson F, Ferrari G, Fugazzola C, et al. Megadolichobasilar anomaly causing brainstem syndrome: A case report. Neuroradiology *13*:279–281, 1977.

Frazee JG, Cahan LD, Winter J. Bacterial intracranial aneurysms. J Neurosurg *53*:633–641, 1980.

Frazee JG, Bevan JA, Bevan RD, et al. Early treatment with diltiazem reduces delayed cerebral vascular narrowing after subarachnoid hemorrhage. Neurosurgery *23*:611–615, 1988.

Freger P, Meneses de Sousa M, Sevrain L, et al. Faut-il opérer les anévrysmes asymptomatiques? A propos de 114 anévrysmes asymptomatiques opérés. Neurochirurgie *33*:462–468, 1987.

Frerebeau Ph, Janny P, Taquoi G, et al. Traitement curatif du vasospasme des hémorragies méningées d'origine anévrysmale par la nimodipine intraveineuse: Etude coopératif multicentrique. Neurochirurgie *34*:383–388, 1988.

Fridriksson SM, Hillman J, Säveland H, et al. Intracranial aneurysm surgery in the 8th and 9th decades of life: Impact on population-based management outcome. Neurosurgery *37*:627–31; discussion 631–632, 1995.

Friedlander RM, Oglivy CS. Aneurysmal subarachnoid hemorrhage in a patient with bilateral A1 fenestrations associated with an azygos anterior cerebral artery. Case report and literature review. J Neurosurg *84*:681–684, 1996.

Friedman AH, Drake CG. Subarachnoid hemorrhage from intracranial dissecting aneurysm. J Neurosurg *60*:325–334, 1984.

Friedman DP. Ruptured aneurysm of the basilar artery simulating nonaneurysmal perimesencephalic subarachnoid hemorrhage. AJR *167*:283–284, 1996.

Friedman DP, Rapoport RJ. Giant fusiform oncotic aneurysm: MR and angiographic findings. AJR *167*:538–539, 1996.

Friedman WA, Day AL, Quisling RG, et al. Cervical carotid dissecting aneurysms. Neurosurgery *7*:207–213, 1980.

Friedman WA, Chadwick GM, Verhoeven FJ, et al. Monitoring of somatosensory evoked potentials during surgery for middle cerebral artery aneurysms. Neurosurgery *29*:83–88, 1991.

Fries G, Perneczky A, van Lindert E, et al. Contralateral and ipsilateral microsurgical approaches to carotid-ophthalmic aneurysms. Neurosurgery *41*:333–343, 1997.

Fritz VU, Maloon A, Tuch P. Neck manipulation as a cause of stroke. S Afr Med J *66*:844–846, 1984.

Frizzell RT, Vitek JJ, Hill DL, et al. Treatment of a bacterial (mycotic) intracranial aneurysm using an endovascular approach. Neurosurgery *32*:852–854, 1993.

Frizzell RT, Kuhn F, Morris R, et al. Screening for ocular hemorrhages in patients with ruptured cerebral aneurysms: A prospective study of 99 patients. Neurosurgery *41*:529–534, 1997.

Frumkin LR, Baloh RB. Wallenberg's syndrome following neck manipulation. Neurology *40*:611–615, 1990.

Fujii S, Kajikawa H, Yamamura K, et al. Spontaneous dissecting aneurysm of the superficial temporal artery: A case report. No Shinkei Geka *23*:797–800, 1995.

Fujii Y, Tanaka R, Takeuchi S, et al. Serial changes in hemostasis after intracranial surgery. Neurosurgery *35*:26–33, 1994.

Fujii Y, Takeuchi S, Sasaki O, et al. Hemostasis in spontaneous subarachnoid hemorrhage. Neurosurgery 37:226–234, 1995a.

Fujii Y, Takahashi A, Ezura M, et al. Balloon angioplasty immediately after surgical clipping for symptomatic vasospasm on admission. Report of four cases. Neurosurg Rev 18:79–84, 1995b.

Fujii Y, Takahashi A, Yoshimoto T. Effect of balloon angioplasty on high grade symptomatic vasospasm after subarachnoid hemorrhage. Neurosurg Rev 18:7–13, 1995c.

Fujii Y, Takeuchi S, Sasaki O, et al. Ultra-early rebleeding in spontaneous subarachnoid hemorrhage. J Neurosurg 84:35–42, 1996.

Fujimura M, Sugawara T, Higuchi H, et al. A ruptured aneurysm at the distal end of the basilar artery fenestration associated with multiple fenestrations of the vertebrobasilar system: Case report. Surg Neurol 47:469–472, 1997.

Fujitsu K, Ishiwata Y, Gondo G, et al. Wrap-clipping with a Dacron mesh silastic sheet. Technical note. J Neurosurg 80:336–337, 1994.

Fujiwara N, Ohkawa M, Tanabe M, et al. The effect of PTA on cerebral vessels in experimental vasospasm: A histopathological study. Nippon Igaku Hoshasen Gakkai Zasshi 54:378–388, 1994.

Fujiwara S, Fujii K, Nishio S, et al. Long-term results of wrapping of intracranial ruptured aneurysms. Acta Neurochir 103:27–29, 1990.

Fujiwara T, Mino S, Nagao S, et al. Metastatic choriocarcinoma with neoplastic aneurysms cured by aneurysm resection and chemotherapy. Case report. J Neurosurg 76:148–151, 1992.

Fukazawa S, Imai S, Saito A, et al. Fibromuscular dysplasia of the cervical arteries associated with a distal vertebral trunk aneurysm. Case report. Neurol Med Chir 30:899–903, 1990.

Fukudome Y, Okada Y, Utsunomiya H, et al. A case of Weber's syndrome due to gradual expansion of a basilar bifurcation aneurysm. Rinsho Shinkeigaku 34:183–185, 1994.

Fukushima T. Comments on Scott BA, Weinstein Z, Pulliam MW: Computed tomographic diagnosis of ruptured giant posterior cerebral artery aneurysms. Neurosurgery 22:557–558, 1988.

Fukuya T, Kishikawa T, Ikeda J, et al. Aneurysms of the peripheral portion of the anterior inferior cerebellar artery: Report of two cases. Neuroradiology 29:493–496, 1987.

Furuya K, Sasaki T, Yoshimoto Y, et al. Histologically verified cerebral aneurysm formation secondary to embolism from cardiac myxoma. Case report. J Neurosurg 83:170–173, 1995.

Futami K, Yamashita J, Tachibana O, et al. Basic fibroblast growth factor may repair experimental cerebral aneurysms in rats. Stroke 26:1649–1654, 1995a.

Futami K, Yamashita J, Tachibana O, et al. Immunohistochemical alterations of fibronectin during the formation and proliferative repair of experimental cerebral aneurysms in rats. Stroke 26:1659–1664, 1995b.

Gabianelli EB, Klingele TG, Burde RM. Acute oculomotor nerve palsy in childhood. Is arteriography necessary? J Clin Neuro-Ophthalmol 9:33–36, 1989.

Gale AN, Crockard HA. Transient unilateral mydriasis with basilar aneurysm. J Neurol Neurosurg Psychiatry 45:565–566, 1982.

Gallagher PG, Dorsey JF, Stefanini M, et al. Large intracranial aneurysm producing panhypopituitarism and frontal lobe syndrome. Neurology 6:829–837, 1957.

Gallina E, Gallo O, Boccuzzi S, et al. Aneurisma post-traumatico intracranico della carotide interna come causa di epistassi: Considerazioni su due casi. Acta Otorhinolaryngol Ital 10:607–613, 1990.

Gallo P, Fabiao Neto OM, Raupp SF, et al. Cerebral metastasis from choriocarcinoma and oncotic aneurysms. Case report. Arq Neuropsiquiatr 51:275–280, 1993.

Garcia-Merino JA, Gutierrez JA, Lopez-Lozano JJ, et al. Double lumen dissecting aneurysms of the internal carotid artery in fibromuscular dysplasia: Case report. Stroke 14:815–818, 1983.

Gauthier G, Rohr J, Wildi E, et al. L'hématome disséquant spontané de l'artère carotide interne: Revu générale de 205 cas publiés dont 10 personnels. Arch Suisses Neurol Psychiatr 136:53–74, 1985.

Gautier JC, Pertuiset BF. Les anévrysmes disséquants spontanés des artères cérébrales. Ann Med Interne 134:458–464, 1983.

Gautier JC, Loron Ph. Anévrysmes disséquants de l'artère carotide interne et syndrome de Claude Bernard-Horner isolé. Rev Neurol 145:328–329, 1989.

Gautier JC, Awada A, Majdalani A. Ophthalmoplegia with contralateral hemiplegia: Occlusion of the internal carotid artery due to thrombosis of an intracavernous aneurysm. Stroke 17:1321–1322, 1986.

Gay S, Miller EJ. Collagen in the Physiology and Pathology of Connective Tissue, pp 46–62. Stuttgart, Gustav Fischer Verlag, 1978.

Gee W, Kaupp HA, McDonald KM, et al. Spontaneous dissection of internal carotid arteries: Spontaneous resolution documented by serial ocular pneumoplethysmography and angiography. Arch Surg 115:944–949, 1980.

Geeraert AJ, Al-Saigh AH. Spontaneous dissection of the carotid artery: An unusual cause of stroke in younger patients. Can Med Assoc J 136:51–53, 1987.

George B, Mourier KL, Gelbert F, et al. Vascular abnormalities in the neck associated with intracranial aneurysms. Neurosurgery 24:499–508, 1989.

Gerber CJ, Neil-Dwyer G. A review of the management of 15 cases of aneurysms of the posterior cerebral artery. Br J Neurosurg 6:521–527, 1992.

Gerber S, Dormont D, Sahel M, et al. Complete spontaneous thrombosis of a giant intracranial aneurysm. Neuroradiology 36:316–317, 1994.

Geremia G, Haklin M, Brennecke L. Embolization of experimentally created aneurysms with intravascular stent devices. AJNR 15:1223–1231, 1994.

Gewirtz RJ, Awad IA. Giant aneurysms of the anterior circle of Willis: Management outcome of open microsurgical treatment. Surg Neurol 45:409–420; discussion 420–421, 1996.

Gherardi GJ, Lee HY. Localized dissecting hemorrhage and arteritis. JAMA 199:219–220, 1967.

Gianetti AV, Perpetuo FO. Granuloma formation and arterial thrombosis following cotton wrapping of an intracranial aneurysm. A case report. Arq Neuropsiquiatr 50:534–538, 1992.

Giannakopoulos G, Nair S, Snider C, et al. Implications for the pathogenesis of aneurysm formation: Metastatic choriocarcinoma with spontaneous splenic rupture. Case report and a review. Surg Neurol 38:236–240, 1992.

Giannotta SL, Litofsky NS. Reoperative management of intracranial aneurysms. J Neurosurg 83:387–393, 1995.

Giannotta SL, Maceri DR. Retrolabyrinthine transsigmoid approach to basilar trunk and vertebrobasilar artery junction aneurysms: Technical note. J Neurosurg 69:461–466, 1988.

Giannotta SL, McGillicuddy JE, Kindt GW. Diagnosis and treatment of postoperative cerebral vasospasm. Surg Neurol 8:286–290, 1977.

Gibbs JR, O'Gorman P. Fibrinolysis in subarachnoid hemorrhage. Postgrad Med 42:779–784, 1967.

Gibo H, Lenkey C, Rhoton AL Jr. Microsurgical anatomy of the supraclinoid portion of the internal carotid artery. J Neurosurg 55:560–574, 1981.

Giller CA, Mathews D, Walker B, et al. Prediction of tolerance to carotid artery occlusion using transcranial Doppler ultrasound. J Neurosurg 81:15–19, 1994.

Gillingham FJ. The management of ruptured intracranial aneurysm. Ann R Coll Surg Engl 23:89–117, 1958.

Gillingham FJ. The management of ruptured intracranial aneurysms. Scott Med J 12:377–383, 1967.

Gilsbach JM, Reulen HJ, Ljunggren B, et al. Early aneurysm surgery and preventive therapy with intravenously administered nimodipine: A multicenter, double-blind, dose-comparison study. Neurosurgery 26:458–464, 1990.

Giombini S, Ferraresi S, Pluchino F. Reversal of oculomotor disorders after intracranial aneurysm surgery. Acta Neurochir 112:19–24, 1991.

Gire C, Lamoureux S, Ghodbane D, et al. Rupture d'anvrisme cérébrale associée à une coarctation aortique. Rev Neurol 153:357–358, 1997.

Giuffrè G, Montalto FP, Amodei G. Development of an isolated retinal macroaneurysm of the cilioretinal artery. Br J Ophthalmol 71:445–448, 1987.

Glassock ME, Smith PG, Bond AG, et al. Management of aneurysms of the petrous portion of the internal carotid by resection and primary anastomosis. Laryngoscope 93:1445–1452, 1983.

Gledhill JA, Moore DF, Bell D, et al. Subarachnoid hemorrhage associated with MDMA abuse. J Neurol Neurosurg Psychiatry 56:1036–1037, 1993.

Glees M. Dem Foster Kennedyschen Syndrom ähnliche Veränderungen der Sehnerven durch Arteriosklerose. Klin Monatsbl Augenheilkd 100:865–873, 1938.

Gobin YP, Counord JL, Flaud P, et al. In vitro study of haemodynamics in a giant saccular aneurysm model: Influence of flow dynamics in the parent vessel and effects of coil embolisation. Neuroradiology 36:530–536, 1994.

Gobin YP, Vinuela F, Gurian JH, et al. Treatment of large and giant fusiform intracranial aneurysms with Guglielmi detachable coils. J Neurosurg 84:55–62, 1996.

Godel V, Blumenthal M, Regenbogen L. Arterial macroaneurysm of the retina. Ophthalmologica 175:125–129, 1977.

Goetz C, Seifert V, Haubitz B. Foramen Monroi—Blockade durch ein Riesenaneurysma der Arteria basilaris. Fallbeschreibung und Literaturubersicht. Neurochirurgia 33:122–126, 1990.

Gold DH, La Piana FG, Zimmerman LE. Isolated retinal arterial aneurysms. Am J Ophthalmol 82:848–857, 1976.

Goldberg HI, Grossman RI, Gomori JM, et al. Cervical internal carotid artery dissecting hemorrhage: Diagnosis using MR. Radiology 158:157–161, 1986.

Goldin RR, Silver ML. Ophthalmic artery aneurysm. Radiology 68:727–729, 1957.

Golding R, Peatfield RC, Shawdon HH, et al. Computer tomographic features of giant intracranial aneurysms. Clin Radiol 31:41–48, 1980.

Goldstein SJ, Tibbs PA. Recurrent subarachnoid hemorrhage complicating cerebral arterial ectasia. J Neurol Neurosurg Psychiatry 55:139–142, 1981.

Golnik KC, Hund PW 3rd, Stroman GA, et al. Magnetic resonance imaging in patients with unexplained optic neuropathy. Ophthalmology 103:515–520, 1996.

Gomori JM, Weinberger G, Shachar E, et al. Multiple intracranial aneurysms and neurofibromatosis: A case report. Australas Radiol 35:271–273, 1991.

Good EF. Ptosis as the sole manifestation of compression of the oculomotor nerve by an aneurysm of the posterior communicating artery. J Clin Neuro-Ophthalmol 10:59–61, 1990.

Goto K, Imai H, Nakazato O, et al. Inferior branch palsy of the oculomotor nerve following clipping of basilar apex aneurysm. Rinsho Shinkeigaku 33:203–206, 1993.

Gotoh O, Tamura A, Yasui N, et al. Glasgow Coma Scale in the prediction of outcome after early aneurysm surgery. Neurosurgery 39:19–24, 1996.

Gouliamos A, Gotsis E, Vlahos L, et al. Magnetic resonance angiography compared to intra-arterial digital subtraction angiography in patients with subarachnoid hemorrhage. Neuroradiology 35:46–49, 1992.

Graber D, Flurin-Chollet V, Chaix Y, et al. Dissection de l'artere sylvienne avec anevrysme sequellaire chez une enfant de 6 ans. Arch Fr Pediatr *49*:445–448, 1992.

Graf CJ. Spontaneous carotid-cavernous fistula: Ehlers-Danlos syndrome and related conditions. Arch Neurol *13*:662–672, 1965.

Graham JM, Miller T, Stinnett DM. Spontaneous dissection of the common carotid artery: Case report and review of the literature. J Vasc Surg *7*:811–813, 1988.

Graves VB, Strother CM, Rappe AH. Treatment of experimental canine carotid aneurysms with platinum coils. AJNR *14*:787–793, 1993.

Graves VB, Strother CM, Duff TA, et al. Early treatment of ruptured aneurysms with Guglielmi detachable coils: Effect on subsequent bleeding. Neurosurgery *37*:640–647; discussion 647–648, 1995.

Graves VB, Strother CM, Weir B, et al. Vertebrobasilar junction aneurysms associated with fenestration: Treatment with Guglielmi detachable coils. AJNR *17*:35–40, 1996.

Grayson MC, Soni SR, Spooner VA. Analysis of the recovery of third nerve function after direct surgical intervention for posterior communicating aneurysms. Br J Ophthalmol *58*:118–125, 1974.

Green D, Joynt RJ. Vascular accidents to the brain stem associated with neck manipulation. JAMA *170*:522–524, 1959.

Green WR. Retina. In Ophthalmic Pathology: An Atlas and Textbook. Editor, Spencer, WH, pp 667–1331. Philadelphia, WB Saunders, 1996.

Green WR, Hackett ER, Schlezinger NS. Neuroophthalmologic evaluation of oculomotor nerve paralysis. Arch Ophthalmol *72*:154–167, 1964.

Greene KA, Marciano FF, Hamilton MG, et al. Cardiopulmonary bypass, hypothermic circulatory arrest and barbiturate cerebral protection for the treatment of giant vertebrobasilar aneurysms in children. Pediatr Neurosurg *21*:124–133, 1994.

Greene KA, Marciano FF, Dickman CA, et al. Anterior communicating artery aneurysm paraparesis syndrome: Clinical manifestations and pathologic correlates. Neurology *45*:45–50, 1995.

Greenspan BN, Reeves AG. Transient partial oculomotor nerve paresis with posterior communicating artery aneurysm. A case report. J Clin Neuro-Ophthalmol *10*:56–58, 1990.

Greitz T, Löfstedt S. The relationship between the third ventricle and the basilar artery. Acta Radiol *42*:85–100, 1954.

Greitz T, Ekbom K, Kugelberg E. Occult hydrocephalus due to ectasia of the basilar artery. Acta Radiol *9*:310–316, 1969.

Greselle JF, Zenteno M, Kien P, et al. Spontaneous dissection of the vertebro-basilar system. J Neuroradiol *14*:115–123, 1987.

Griffith JQ Jr, Jeffers WA, Fry WE. Papilledema associated with subarachnoid hemorrhage: Experimental and clinical study. Arch Intern Med *61*:880–889, 1938.

Griffiths PD, Gholkar A, Sengupta RP. Oculomotor nerve palsy due to thrombosis of a posterior communicating artery aneurysm following diagnostic angiography. Neuroradiology *36*:614–615, 1994.

Griffiths PD, Worthy S, Gholkar A. Incidental intracranial vascular pathology in patients investigated for carotid stenosis. Neuroradiol *38*:25–30, 1996.

Grimson BS, Thompson HS. Raeder's syndrome: A clinical review. Surv Ophthalmol *24*:199–210, 1980.

Gros C, Vlahovitch B, Labauge R, et al. Les anévrysmes extra-craniens de la carotide interne. Neurochirurgie *16*:367–382, 1970.

Grosman H, Fornasier VL, Bonder D, et al. Dissecting aneurysm of the cerebral arteries: Case report. J Neurosurg *53*:693–697, 1980.

Gross M. Giant middle cerebral aneurysm presenting as hemiparkinsonism. J Neurol Neurosurg Psychiatry *50*:1075–1084, 1987.

Grossi RJ, Onofrey D, Tvetenstrand C, et al. Mycotic carotid aneurysm. J Vasc Surg *6*:81–83, 1987.

Grotenhuis JA, de Vries J, Tacl S. Angioscopy-guided placement of balloon-expandable stents in the treatment of experimental carotid aneurysms. Minim Invasive Neurosurg *37*:56–60, 1994.

Grubb RL, Raichle ME, Eichling JO, et al. Effects of subarachnoid hemorrhage on cerebral blood volume, blood flow, and oxygen utilization in humans. J Neurosurg *46*:446–453, 1977.

Guest PG, Schnetler J. Traumatic cavernous carotid aneurysm resulting in blindness. Br J Oral Maxillofac Surg *30*:395–397, 1992.

Guglielmi G, Vinuela F, Dion J, et al. Persistent primitive trigeminal artery-cavernous sinus fistulas: Report of two cases. Neurosurgery *27*:805–808; discussion 808–809, 1990.

Guglielmi G, Vinuela F, Dion J, et al. Electrothrombosis of saccular aneurysms via endovascular approach. Part 2: Preliminary clinical experience. J Neurosurg *75*:8–14, 1991.

Guglielmi G, Vinuela F, Briganti F, et al. Carotid-cavernous fistula caused by a ruptured intracavernous aneurysm: Endovascular treatment by electrothrombosis with detachable coils. Neurosurgery *31*:591–596; discussion 596–597, 1992a.

Guglielmi G, Vinuela F, Duckwiler G, et al. Endovascular treatment of posterior circulation aneurysms by electrothrombosis using electrically detachable coils. J Neurosurg *77*:515–524, 1992b.

Guidetti B, La Torre E. Carotid-ophthalmic aneurysms: A series of 16 cases treated by direct approach. Acta Neurochir *22*:289–304, 1970.

Guidetti B, La Torre E. Management of carotid-ophthalmic aneurysms. J Neurosurg *42*:438–442, 1975.

Guijarro Castro C, Fernandez Carril JM, Guerrero A, et al. Agenesia de la carotida interna y multiples dilataciones aneurismaticas de la arteria comunicante posterior. Neurologia *9*:199–201, 1994.

Guiolet M, Jouhaud F, Malbrel C, et al. Maladie d'Ehlers-Danlos—fistule artério-veineuse. Bull Soc Ophtalmol Fr *84*:267–268, 1984.

Guirguis S, Tadros FW. An internal carotid aneurysm in the petrous temporal bone. J Neurol Neurosurg Psychiatry *24*:84–85, 1961.

Gumprecht H, Winkler R, Gerstner W, et al. Therapeutic management of grade IV aneurysm patients. Surg Neurol *47*:54–58, 1997.

Gupta RK, Mehta VS, Misra NK. Unilateral proptosis secondary to partially thrombosed giant carotid ophthalmic artery aneurysm. J Neurol Neurosurg Psychiatry *53*:925, 1990.

Gupta SK, Gupta OP, Singh MM, et al. Giant aneurysm of the internal carotid artery in the carotid canal. J Laryngol Otol *93*:299–305, 1979.

Gurian JH, Martin NA, King WA, et al. Neurosurgical management of cerebral aneurysms following unsuccessful or incomplete endovascular embolization. J Neurosurg *83*:843–853, 1995a.

Gurian JH, Vinuela F, Gobin YP, et al. Aneurysm rupture after parent vessel sacrifice: Treatment with Guglielmi detachable coil embolization via retrograde catheterization: Case report. Neurosurgery *37*:1216–1220; discussion 1220–1221, 1995b.

Guridi J, Gallego J, Monzon F, et al. Intracerebral hemorrhage caused by transmural dissection of the anterior cerebral artery. Stroke *24*:1400–1402, 1993.

Gutman I, Levartovski S, Goldhammer Y, et al. Sixth nerve palsy and unilateral Horner's syndrome. Ophthalmology *93*:913–916, 1986.

Gutowski NJ, Murphy RP, Beale DJ. Unilateral upper cervical posterior spinal artery syndrome following sneezing. J Neurol Neurosurg Psychiatry *55*:841–843, 1992.

Guy J, Day AL. Intracranial aneurysms with superior division paresis of the oculomotor nerve. Ophthalmology *96*:1071–1076, 1989.

Guy J, Savino PJ, Schatz NJ, et al. Superior division paresis of the oculomotor nerve. Ophthalmology *92*:777–784, 1985.

Guy J, McGrath BJ, Borel CO, et al. Perioperative management of aneurysmal subarachnoid hemorrhage: Part 1. Operative management. Anesth Analg *81*:1060–1072, 1995.

Haberback-Modesto MA, Edner G, Greitz T. Bilateral aneurysms of the juxtasellar segment of the internal carotid artery. Acta Neurochir *57*:235–245, 1981.

Hacker RJ, Krall JM, Fox JL. Data I. In Intracranial Aneurysms. Editor, Fox JL, pp 19–62. New York, Springer-Verlag, 1983.

Haddad FS, Haddad GF, Taha J. Traumatic intracranial aneurysms caused by missiles: Their presentation and management. Neurosurgery *28*:1–7, 1991.

Hadeishi H, Mizuno M, Suzuki A, et al. Hyperdynamic therapy for cerebral vasospasm. Neurol Med Chir *30*:317–323, 1990.

Hademenos GJ, Massoud T, Valentino DJ, et al. A nonlinear mathematical model for the development and rupture of intracranial saccular aneurysms. Neurol Res *16*:376–384, 1994.

Hadley MN, Martin NA, Spetzler RF, et al. Multiple intracranial aneurysms due to *Coccidioides immitis* infection: Case report. J Neurosurg *66*:453–456, 1987.

Hadley MN, Septzler RF, Martin NA, et al. Middle cerebral artery aneurysm due to *Nocardia asteroides*: Case report of aneurysm excision and extracranial-intracranial bypass. Neurosurgery *22*:923–928, 1988.

Hahn FJ, Ong E, McComb R, et al. Peripheral signal void ring in giant vertebral aneurysm: MR and pathology findings. J Comput Assist Tomogr *10*:1036–1038, 1986.

Hahn YS, McLone DG. Traumatic bilateral ophthalmic artery aneurysms: A case report. Neurosurgery *21*:86–89, 1987.

Hahn YS, Welling B, Reichman OH, et al. Traumatic intracavernous aneurysm in children: Massive epistaxis without ophthalmic signs. Childs Nerv Syst *6*:360–364, 1990.

Hainsworth PJ, Mendelow AD. Giant intracranial aneurysm associated with Marfan's syndrome: A case report. J Neurol Neurosurg Psychiatry *54*:471–472, 1991.

Haisa T, Matsumiya K, Yoshimasu N, et al. Foreign-body granuloma as a complication of wrapping and coating an intracranial aneurysm. Case report. J Neurosurg *72*:292–294, 1990.

Hakozaki S, Suzuki M, Kidoguchi J, et al. Posterior inferior cerebellar artery aneurysm located in the spinal canal: Case report. Neurol Med Chir *36*:314–316, 1996.

Halbach VV, Higashida RT, Dowd CF, et al. Treatment of carotid-cavernous fistulas associated with Ehlers-Danlos syndrome. Neurosurgery *26*:1021–1027, 1990a.

Halbach VV, Higashida RT, Hieshima GB, et al. Aneurysms of the petrous portion of the internal carotid artery: Results of treatment with endovascular or surgical occlusion. AJNR *11*:253–257, 1990b.

Halbach VV, Higashida RT, Dowd CF, et al. Endovascular treatment of vertebral artery dissections and pseudoaneurysms. J Neurosurg *79*:183–191, 1993.

Halbach VV, Higashida RT, Dowd CF, et al. The efficacy of endosaccular aneurysm occlusion in alleviating neurological deficits produced by mass effect. J Neurosurg *80*:659–666, 1994.

Haley EC Jr, Kassell NF, Torner JC. The International Cooperative Study on the Timing of Aneurysm Surgery. The North American experience. Stroke *23*:205–214, 1992.

Haley EC Jr, Kassell NF, Torner JC. A randomized controlled trial of high-dose intravenous nicardipine in aneurysmal subarachnoid hemorrhage. A report of the Cooperative Aneurysm Study. J Neurosurg *78*:537–547, 1993.

Haley EC Jr, Kassell NF, Torner JC, et al. A randomized trial of two doses of nicardipine in aneurysmal subarachnoid hemorrhage. A report of the Cooperative Aneurysm Study. J Neurosurg 80:788–796, 1994.

Haley EC Jr, Kassell NF, Apperson-Hansen C, et al. A randomized, double-blind, vehicle-controlled trial of tirilazad mesylate in patients with aneurysmal subarachnoid hemorrhage: A cooperative study in North America. J Neurosurg 86:467–474, 1997.

Hall DP, Young SA. Frontal lobe cerebral aneurysm rupture presenting as psychosis. J Neurol Neurosurg Psychiatry 55:1207–1208, 1992.

Halloul Z, Lippert H, Meyer F. Monstroses extrakranielles Aneurysma der Arteria carotis. Zentralbl Chir 120:245–248, 1995.

Hamada H, Endo S, Fukuda O, et al. Giant aneurysm in the cavernous sinus causing subarachnoid hemorrhage 13 years after detection: A case report. Surg Neurol 45:143–146, 1996.

Hamada J, Kitamura I, Kurino M, et al. Abnormal origin of bilateral ophthalmic arteries. Case report. J Neurosurg 74:287–289, 1991.

Hamada J, Hashimoto N, Tsukahara T. Moyamoya disease with repeated intraventricular hemorrhage due to aneurysm rupture. Report of two cases. J Neurosurg 80:328–331, 1994.

Hamada T, Inoue T, Hitotsumatsu T, et al. Symptomatic bilateral extracranial internal carotid artery aneurysms—Successfully treated by unilateral aneurysmectomy and saphenous vein graft. Fukuoka Igaku Zasshi 85:128–132, 1994.

Hamann G, Isenberg E, Strittmatter M, et al. Absence of elevation of big endothelin in subarachnoid hemorrhage. Stroke 24:383–386, 1993.

Hamburger C, Schonberger J, Lange M. Management and prognosis of intracranial giant aneurysms. A report on 58 cases. Neurosurg Rev 15:97–103, 1992.

Hamby WB. Intracranial Aneurysms. Springfield, IL, Charles C Thomas, 1952.

Hamer J. Die okulomotorius parese bei nicht rupturierten zerebralen aneurysmen. Acta Neurol 8:73, 1981a.

Hamer J. Incidence and prognosis of oculomotor palsy after subarachnoid hemorrhage due to ruptured aneurysms of the posterior communicating artery. In The Cranial Nerves. Editors, Sammii M, Jannetta PJ, pp 237–240. Berlin, Springer-Verlag, 1981b.

Hamer J. Prognosis of oculomotor palsy in patients with aneurysms of the posterior communicating artery. Acta Neurochir 66:173–185, 1982.

Hamilton MG, Dold ON. Spontaneous disappearance of an intracranial aneurysm after subarachnoid hemorrhage. Can J Neurol Sci 19:389–391, 1992.

Hamm KD, Pothe H, Steube D, et al. Zur Problematik traumatischer infraklinoidaler Aneurysmen. Neurochirurgie 31:88–92, 1988.

Han DH, Gwak HS, Chung CK. Aneurysm at the origin of accessory middle cerebral artery associated with middle cerebral artery aplasia: Case report. Surg Neurol 42:388–391, 1994.

Hanafee W, Jannetta PJ. Aneurysm as a cause of stroke. AJR 98:647–652, 1966.

Hancock DO. A case of complete bilateral ophthalmoplegia due to an intrasellar aneurysm. J Neurol Neurosurg Psychiatry 26:81–82, 1963.

Handa J, Handa H. Severe epistaxis caused by traumatic aneurysm of cavernous carotid artery. Surg Neurol 5:241–243, 1976.

Handa J, Kikuchi H, Iwayama K, et al. Traumatic aneurysm of the internal carotid artery. Acta Neurochir 17:161–177, 1967.

Handa J, Shimizu Y, Matsuda M, et al. Traumatic aneurysm of the middle cerebral artery. AJR 109:127–129, 1970.

Handa J, Matsuda I, Handa H. Association of brain tumor and intracranial aneurysms. Surg Neurol 6:25–29, 1976.

Handa J, Nakasu Y, Matsuda M, et al. Aneurysms of the proximal anterior cerebral artery. Surg Neurol 22:486–490, 1984.

Hanley JR, Pearson NA, Young AW. Impaired memory for new visual forms. Brain 113:1131–1148, 1990.

Hannachi N, Beard T, Ben Ismail M. Les complications neurologiques des endocardites infectieuses. Arch Mal Coeur Vaiss 84:81–86, 1991.

Hanus SH, Homer TD, Harter DH. Vertebral artery occlusion complicating yoga exercises. Arch Neurol 34:574–575, 1977.

Hara K, Shirouzu T, Watanabe T, et al. Completely thrombosed giant fusiform aneurysm in a young patient: Case report. Neurol Med Chir 33:103–107, 1993.

Harada Y, Ishimitsu H, Miyata I, et al. Peduncular hallucinosis associated with ruptured basilar-superior cerebellar artery aneurysm: Case report. Neurol Med Chir 31:526–528, 1991.

Harbaugh RE, Schlusselberg DS, Jeffery R, et al. Three-dimensional computed tomographic angiography in the preoperative evaluation of cerebrovascular lesions. Neurosurgery 36:320–326; discussion 326–327, 1995.

Hardin CA. Surgical treatment of extracranial carotid aneurysms with excision and arterial restoration. Vasc Surg 7:247–252, 1973.

Hardy RE, Obianyo I, Shu HS, et al. Unilateral moyamoya disease, intracranial aneurysm, and a pituitary adenoma: A case report. J Natl Med Assoc 83:827–830, 1991.

Harino S, Motokura M, Nishikawa N, et al. Chronic ocular ischemia associated with the Eisenmenger's syndrome. Am J Ophthalmol 117:302–307, 1994.

Harr DL, Quencer RM. Acute cavernous sinus syndrome. J Clin Neuro-Ophthalmol 1:291–294, 1981.

Harris P, Udvarhelyi GB. Aneurysms arising at the internal carotid-posterior communicating artery junction. J Neurosurg 14:180–191, 1957.

Harris RJ, Branston NM, Symon L, et al. The effects of a calcium antagonist, nimodi-

pine, upon physiologic responses of the cerebral vasculature and its possible influence upon focal cerebral ischaemia. Stroke 13:759–766, 1982.

Harrison MJ, Johnson BA, Gardner GM, et al. Preliminary results on the management of unruptured aneurysms with magnetic resonance angiography and computed tomographic angiography. Neurosurgery 40:947–957, 1997.

Harrison TH, Odom GL, Kunkle EC. Internal carotid aneurysm arising in carotid canal. Arch Neurol 8:328–331, 1963.

Harsh GR 4th, Sekhar LN. The subtemporal, transcavernous, anterior transpetrosal approach to the upper brain stem and clivus. J Neurosurg 77:709–717, 1992.

Hart RG. Vertebral artery dissection. Neurology 38:987–989, 1988.

Hart RG, Easton JD. Dissections of cervical and cerebral arteries. Neurol Clin 1:155–182, 1983.

Hart RG, Kagan-Hallet K, Joerns SE. Mechanisms of intracranial hemorrhage in infective endocarditis. Stroke 18:1048–1056, 1987.

Hartland SP, Hussein A, Gullan RW. Modification of the standard pterional approach for aneurysms of the anterior circle of Wills. Br J Neurosurg 10:149–153, 1996.

Hartman J, Nguyen T, Larsen D, et al. MR artifacts, heat production, and ferromagnetism of Guglielmi detachable coils. AJNR 18:497–501, 1997.

Hassler O. Morphological studies on the large cerebral arteries: With reference to the etiology of subarachnoid hemorrhage. Acta Psychiatr Neurol Scand 36(Suppl 154):60–67, 1961.

Hassler O. On the etiology of intracranial aneurysms. In Intracranial Aneurysms and Subarachnoid Hemorrhage. Editors, Fields WS, Sahs AL, pp 25–39. Springfield, IL, Charles C Thomas, 1965.

Hassler O, Saltzman GF. Histologic changes in infundibular widening of the posterior communicating artery: A preliminary report. Acta Pathol 46:305–312, 1959.

Hassler O, Saltzman GF. Angiographic and histologic changes in infundibular widening of the posterior communicating artery. Acta Radiol 1:321–327, 1963.

Hatam A, Greitz T. Ectasia of cerebral arteries in acromegaly. Acta Radiol 12:410–418, 1972.

Hatanaka K, Yutani C, Fujieda T, et al. Polymyositis associated with dissecting aneurysm of arteries and intracerebral hemorrhage. Acta Pathol Jpn 36:1217–1223, 1986.

Hatashita S, Nitta T, Koga N, et al. Traumatic aneurysm of the intracavernous carotid artery. Neurol Med Chir 23:885–890, 1983.

Hatayama T, Shima T, Okada Y, et al. Ruptured distal anterior cerebral artery aneurysms presenting with acute subdural hematoma: report of two cases. No Shinkei Geka 22:577–582, 1994.

Hattori T, Kobayashi H. Fenestration of the supraclinoid internal carotid artery associated with carotid bifurcation aneurysm. Surg Neurol 37:284–288, 1992.

Hauerberg J, Andersen BB, Eskesen V, et al. Importance of the recognition of a warning leak as a sign of a ruptured intracranial aneurysm. Acta Neurol Scand 83:61–64, 1991.

Havelius U, Hindfelt B, Brismar J, et al. Carotid fibromuscular dysplasia and paresis of lower cranial nerves (Collet-Sicard syndrome). J Neurosurg 56:850–853, 1982.

Hayashi M, Taira T, Terasaka N, et al. Intracavernous internal carotid artery aneurysm associated with persistent trigeminal artery variant: Case report. No Shinkei Geka 22:67–70, 1994.

Hayashi S, Arimoto T, Itakura T, et al. The association of intracranial aneurysms and arteriovenous malformation of the brain: Case report. J Neurosurg 55:971–975, 1981.

Hayashi S, Takahashi H, Shimura T, et al. A case of multiple cerebral aneurysm which showed rapid growth caused by left atrial myxoma. No Shinkei Geka 23:977–980, 1995.

Hayes W, Bernhardt H, Young J. Fusiform arteriosclerotic aneurysm of the basilar artery. Vasc Surg 1:171–178, 1967.

Haykowsky MJ, Findlay JM, Ignaszewski AP. Aneurysmal subarachnoid hemorrhage associated with weight training: Three case reports. Clin J Sport Med 6:52–55, 1996.

Hayreh SS. An experimental study of the central retinal vein occlusion. Trans Ophthalmol Soc UK 84:586–598, 1964.

Hazarika P, Sahota JS, Nayak DR, et al. Congenital internal carotid artery aneurysm. Int J Pediatr Otorhinolaryngol 28:63–68, 1993.

Healy JF, Wells MV, Rosenkrantz H. Computed tomographic demonstration of enlarged ectatic basilar artery associated with obstruction of the anterior third ventricle. Comput Radiol 5:239–245, 1981.

Heck AF. Manifestations of spontaneous subarachnoid hemorrhage in the orbit and bulbus oculi: Report of previously undescribed hemorrhagic phenomena in the conjunctivae. Neurology 11:701–708, 1961.

Hedera P, Friedland RP. Duane's syndrome with giant aneurysm of the vertebral basilar arterial junction. J Clin Neuroophthalmol 13:271–274, 1993.

Hegedüs K. Ectasia of the basilar artery with special reference to possible pathogenesis. Surg Neurol 24:463–469, 1985.

Heilman CB, Kwan ES, Wu JK. Aneurysm recurrence following endovascular balloon occlusion. J Neurosurg 77:260–264, 1992.

Heiskanen O. Risk of bleeding from unruptured aneurysms in cases with multiple intracranial aneurysms. J Neurosurg 55:424–426, 1981.

Heiskanen O. Risks of surgery for unruptured intracranial aneurysms. J Neurosurg 65:451–453, 1986.

Heiskanen O, Poranen A. Surgery of incidental intracranial aneurysms. Surg Neurol 28:432–436, 1987.

Helmchen C, Nahser HC, Yousry T, et al. Therapie zerebraler Aneurysmen und arteriovenoser Gefassmalformationen bei der hereditaren hamorrhagischen Teleangiektasie (Morbus Rendu-Osler-Weber). Nervenarzt 66:124–128, 1995.

Helmer FA. Oncotic aneurysm: Case report. J Neurosurg 45:98–100, 1976.

Henderson JW. Intracranial arterial aneurysms: A study of 119 cases, with special reference to the ocular findings. Trans Am Ophthalmol Soc 53:349–462, 1955.

Henderson WG, Torner JC, Nibbelink DW. Intracranial aneurysms and subarachnoid hemorrhage: Report on a randomized treatment study. IV-B. Regulated bedrest—statistical evaluation. Stroke 8:579–589, 1977.

Hepler RS, Cantu RC. Aneurysms and third nerve palsies: Ocular status of survivors. Arch Ophthalmol 77:604–608, 1967.

Herb E, Kehler U. Macro-aneurysm in the basal ganglia region. Clin Neurol Neurosurg 94:319–322, 1992.

Herman JM, Spetzler RF. MR imaging in carotid artery dissection. J Neurosurg 72:987–988, 1990.

Herman JM, Rekate HL, Spetzler RF. Pediatric intracranial aneurysms: Simple and complex cases. Pediatr Neurosurg 17:66–72; discussion 73, 1991–1992.

Hernesniemi J, Tapaninaho A, Vapalahti M, et al. Saccular aneurysms of the distal anterior cerebral artery and its branches. Neurosurgery 31:994–998; discussion 998–999, 1992.

Heros RC, Lee SH. The combined pterional/anterior temporal approach for aneurysms of the upper basilar complex: Technical report. Neurosurgery 33:244–250; discussion 250–251, 1993.

Heros RC, Ojemann RG, Crowell RM. Superior temporal gyrus approach to middle cerebral artery aneurysms: Technique and results. Neurosurgery 10:308–313, 1982.

Heros RC, Zervas NT, Varsos V. Cerebral vasospasm after subarachnoid hemorrhage: An update. Ann Neurol 14:599–608, 1983.

Heye N, Iglesias JR, Henkes H, et al. Dissecting aneurysm of middle cerebral artery following resection of meningioma. J Neurol Neurosurg Psychiatry 52:683, 1989.

Hieshima GB, Higashida RT, Wapenski J, et al. Balloon embolization of a large distal basilar artery aneurysm: Case report. J Neurosurg 65:413–416, 1986a.

Hieshima GB, Higashida RT, Halbach VV, et al. Intravascular balloon embolization of a carotid-ophthalmic artery aneurysm with preservation of the parent vessel. AJNR 7:916–918, 1986b.

Higashi K, Hatano M, Yamashita T, et al. Coexistence of posterior inferior cerebellar artery aneurysm and arteriovenous malformation fed by the same artery. Surg Neurol 12:405–408, 1979.

Higashida RT, Halbach VV, Hieshima GB, et al. Cavernous carotid artery aneurysm associated with Marfan's syndrome: Treatment by balloon embolization therapy. Neurosurgery 22:297–300, 1988a.

Higashida RT, Halbach VV, Hieshima GB, et al. Treatment of a giant carotid ophthalmic artery aneurysm by intravascular balloon embolization therapy. Surg Neurol 30:382–386, 1988b.

Higashida RT, Halbach VV, Cahan LD, et al. Detachable balloon embolization therapy of posterior circulation intracranial aneurysms. J Neurosurg 71:512–519, 1989.

Higashida RT, Halbach VV, Dowd C, et al. Endovascular detachable balloon embolization therapy of cavernous carotid artery aneurysms: Results in 87 cases. J Neurosurg 72:857–863, 1990.

Higashida RT, Halbach VV, Dowd CF, et al. Intracranial aneurysms: Interventional neurovascular treatment with detachable balloons—Results in 215 cases. Radiology 178:663–670, 1991.

Higashida RT, Halbach VV, Dowd CF, et al. Intravascular balloon dilatation therapy for intracranial arterial vasospasm: Patient selection, technique, and clinical results. Neurosurg Rev 15:89–95, 1992.

Hijdra A, van Gijn J. Early death from rupture of an intracranial aneurysm. J Neurosurg 57:765–768, 1982.

Hijdra A, Vermeulen M, van Gijn J, et al. Rerupture of intracranial aneurysms: A clinicoanatomic study. J Neurosurg 67:29–33, 1987.

Hillman J, Säveland H, Jakobsson KE, et al. Overall management outcome of ruptured posterior fossa aneurysms. J Neurosurg 85:33–38, 1996.

Hilton GF, Hoyt WF. An arteriosclerotic chiasmal syndrome: Bitemporal hemianopia associated with fusiform dilatation of the anterior cerebral arteries. JAMA 196:1018–1020, 1966.

Hilton-Jones D, Warlow CP. Non-penetrating arterial trauma and cerebral infarction in the young. Lancet 1:1435–1438, 1985.

Hinse P, Thie A, Lachenmayer L. Dissection of the extracranial vertebral artery: Report of four cases and review of the literature. J Neurol Neurosurg Psychiatry 54:863–869, 1991.

Hinshaw DB Jr, Jordan KR, Hasso AN, et al. CT cisternography of dolichoectatic arterial compression of the optic chiasm. AJNR 6:837–839, 1985.

Hiranandani LH, Chandra O, Malpani NK, et al. An internal carotid aneurysm in the petrous temporal bone. J Laryngol Otol 76:703–706, 1962.

Hirano A, Imaizumi T, Kato T, et al. A case of growing up aneurysms with occlusion of basilar artery. No Shinkei Geka 23:693–698, 1995.

Hirasawa T, Tsubokawa T, Katayama Y, et al. Growth of a giant aneurysm following complete thrombosis by detachable balloon occlusion. Surg Neurol 38:283–286, 1992.

Hirashima Y, Endo S, Horie Y. An anterior communicating artery aneurysm complicated by chronic subdural haematoma. Neurol Surg 9:1041–1045, 1981.

Hirashima Y, Kurimoto M, Takaba M, et al. The use of computed tomography in the prediction of delayed cerebral infarction following acute aneurysm surgery for subarachnoid hemorrhage. Acta Neurochir 132:9–13, 1995.

Hirose S, Shimada S, Yamaguchi N, et al. Ruptured aneurysm associated with arachnoid cyst: Intracystic hematoma without subarachnoid hemorrhage. Surg Neurol 43:353–356, 1995.

Hirsh CS, Roessmann U. Arterial dysplasia with ruptured basilar artery aneurysm: Report of a case. Human Pathol 6:749–758, 1975.

Hirst AE Jr, Johns VJ Jr, Kime SW Jr. Dissecting aneurysms of the aorta: A review of 505 cases. Medicine 37:217–279, 1958.

Hlavin ML, Takaoka Y, Smith AS. A "PICA communicating artery" aneurysm: Case report. Neurosurgery 29:926–929, 1991.

Ho KL. Neoplastic aneurysm and intracranial hemorrhage. Cancer 50:2935–2940, 1982.

Hochberg FH, Bean CS, Fisher CM, et al. Stroke in a 15-year-old girl secondary to terminal carotid dissection. Neurology 25:725–729, 1975.

Hodes JE, Fletcher WA, Goodman DF, et al. Rupture of cavernous carotid artery aneurysm causing subdural hematoma and death: Case report. J Neurosurg 69:617–619, 1988.

Hodge CJ Jr, Lee SH. Spontaneous dissecting cervical carotid artery aneurysm. Neurosurgery 10:93–95, 1982.

Hoff J, Winestock D, Hoyt WF. Giant suprasellar aneurysm associated with optic stalk agenesis and unilateral anophthalmos: Case report. J Neurosurg 43:495–498, 1975.

Hoh H, Palmowski A. Central subretinal hemorrhage from a retinal arterial macroaneurysm—Two-step treatment with laser and vitreoretinal surgery. Ger J Ophthalmol 1:335–337, 1992.

Hojer C, Bewermeyer H, Hildebrandt G, et al. Ruptur und erfolgreiche Operation eines mykotischen Aneurysmas der A. cerebelli superior. Nervenarzt 64:404–406, 1993.

Hojer-Pedersen E, Haase J. Giant anterior communicating artery aneurysm with bitemporal hemianopsia: Case report. Neurosurgery 8:703–706, 1981.

Holemans JA, Cox TC. CT and MRI of intracavernous carotid artery aneurysm with occlusion of the cervical internal carotid artery. J Comput Assist Tomogr 19:1006–1007, 1995.

Holland PM. Evolution of a retinal arterial macroaneurysm. Ann Ophthalmol 16:1167–1170, 1984.

Hollin SA, Decker RE. Microsurgical treatment of internal carotid artery aneurysms. J Neurosurg 47:142–149, 1977.

Holt JM, Gordon-Smith EC. Retinal abnormalities in diseases of the blood. Br J Ophthalmol 53:145–160, 1969.

Holtzman RNN, Taylor Dickinson PC, Hughes JEO, et al. Cerebral mycotic aneurysms: Presentation and outcome. Ann Neurol 24:129, 1988.

Hommel M, Pollak P, Gaio JM, et al. Paralysies du nerf grand hypoglosse par deux anévrismes et un anévrisme disséquant de l'artère carotide interne. Rev Neurol 140:415–421, 1984.

Honda Y, Tanaka R, Kameyama S. Ruptured distal anterior inferior cerebellar artery aneurysm: Case report. Neurol Med Chir 34:763–767, 1994.

Höök O, Norlén G. Aneurysms of the middle cerebral artery: A report of 80 cases. Acta Chir Scand 235(Suppl):5–39, 1958.

Höök O, Norlén G. Aneurysms of the internal carotid artery. Acta Neurol Scand 40:200–212, 1964a.

Höök O, Norlén G. Aneurysms of the anterior communicating artery. Acta Neurol Scand 40:219–240, 1964b.

Höök O, Norlén G, Guzman J. Saccular aneurysms of the vertebral-basilar arterial system. Acta Neurol Scand 39:271–304, 1963.

Hope JK, Wilson JL, Thomson FJ. Three-dimensional CT angiography in the detection and characterization of intracranial berry aneurysms. AJNR 17:437–445, 1996.

Hopkins EW, Poser CM. Posterior cerebral artery ectasia: An unusual cause of ophthalmoplegia. Arch Neurol 29:279–280, 1973.

Horikoshi T, Fukamachi A, Nishi H, et al. Detection of intracranial aneurysms by three-dimensional time-of-flight magnetic resonance angiography. Neuroradiology 36:203–207, 1994.

Horikoshi T, Nukui H, Mitsuka S, et al. Partial resection of the gyrus rectus in pterional approach to anterior communicating artery aneurysms. Neurol Med Chir 32:136–139, 1992.

Horiuchi T, Kyoshima K, Oya F, et al. Fenestrated oculomotor nerve caused by internal carotid-posterior communicating artery aneurysm: Case report. Neurosurgery 40:397–399, 1997.

Horn SW. The "locked-in" syndrome following chiropractic manipulation of the cervical spine. Ann Emerg Med 12:648–650, 1983.

Hornibrook J, Rhode JC. Fatal epistaxis from an aneurysm of the intracranial internal carotid artery. Aust NZ J Surg 51:206–208, 1981.

Horowitz IN, Niparko NA. Vertebral artery dissection with bilateral hemiparesis. Pediatr Neurol 11:252–254, 1994.

Horowitz MB, Yonas H, Jungreis C, et al. Management of a giant middle cerebral artery fusiform serpentine aneurysm with distal clip application and retrograde thrombosis: Case report and review of the literature. Surg Neurol 41:221–225, 1994.

Hoshimaru M, Hashimoto N, Kikuchi H, et al. Aneurysm of the fenestrated basilar artery: Report of two cases. Surg Neurol 37:406–409, 1992.

Hosobuchi Y. Direct surgical treatment of giant intracranial aneurysms. J Neurosurg *51*:743–756, 1979.

Hosoda K, Fujita S, Kawaguchi T, et al. Saccular aneurysms of the proximal (M1) segment of the middle cerebral artery Neurosurgery *36*:441–446, 1995.

Hosoya T, Watanabe N, Yamaguchi K, et al. Intracranial vertebral artery dissection in Wallenberg syndrome. AJNR *15*:1161–1165, 1994.

Houdart E: Traitement par spires (coils) a detachement controle electrique de 315 anevrysmes intracraniens. Bull Acad Nat Med *180*:1173–1186, 1996.

Housepian EM, Pool JL. A systematic analysis of intracranial aneurysms from the autopsy file of the Presbyterian Hospital, 1914 to 1956. J Neuropathol Exp Neurol *17*:409–423, 1958.

Houser OW, Mokri B, Sundt TM Jr, et al. Spontaneous cervical cephalic arterial dissection and its residuum: Angiographic spectrum. AJNR *5*:27–34, 1984.

Hove B, Andersen BB, Christiansen TM. Intracranial oncotic aneurysms from chorio-carcinoma. Case report and review of the literature. Neuroradiology *32*:526–528, 1990.

Hsiang JN, Liang EY, Lam JM, et al. The role of computed tomographic angiography in the diagnosis of intracranial aneurysms and emergent aneurysm clipping. Neurosurgery *38*:481–487, 1996.

Huang LT, Shih TY, Lui CC. Posterior cerebral artery aneurysm in a two-year-old girl. J Formos Med Assoc *95*:170–172, 1996.

Huber A. Eye Signs and Symptoms in Brain Tumors. Editor and Translator, Blodi FC, 3rd ed, pp 317–337. St Louis, CV Mosby, 1976.

Huber A. Ocular symptomatology of sellar aneurysms. In Neuroophthalmology Update. Editor, Smith JL, pp 261–270. New York, Masson, 1977.

Huber A. Eye signs and symptoms of intracranial aneurysm. Neuroophthalmology *2*: 203–216, 1982.

Huber A, Klöti R, Landolt E. Terson's syndrome. Neuroophthalmology *8*:223–233, 1988.

Hubert P. Hematome sous-dural aigu pur de la convexite par rupture d'un anevrisme de l'artere communicante anterieure. A propos d'un cas chez une femme enceinte. Neurochirurgie *40*:363–368, 1994.

Huckman MS, Shenk GI, Neems RL, et al. Transfemoral cerebral arteriography versus direct percutaneous carotid and brachial arteriography: A comparison of complication rates. Radiology *132*:93–97, 1979.

Hudgins RJ, Day AL, Quisling RG, et al. Aneurysms of the posterior inferior cerebellar artery: A clinical and anatomical analysis. J Neurosurg *58*:381–387, 1983.

Hudomel J, Imre G. Photocoagulation treatment of solitary aneurysm near the macula lutea. Acta Ophthalmol *51*:633–638, 1973.

Hugenholz H, Pokrupa R, Montpetit VJA, et al. Spontaneous dissecting aneurysm of the extracranial vertebral artery. Neurosurgery *10*:96–100, 1982.

Huige WMM, Van Vliet AGM, Bastiaensen LAK. Early symptoms of subarachnoid hemorrhage due to aneurysms of the posterior communicating artery. Doc Ophthalmol *70*:251–256, 1988.

Hultén-Gyllensten JL, Löfstedt S, von Reis G. Observations on generalized arteriectasis. Acta Med Scand *163*:125–130, 1959.

Hung KS, Lee TC, Lui CC. Aneurysm of superior branch of anterior choroidal artery mimicking carotid bifurcation aneurysm: Case report. Acta Neurochir *138*: 1464–1467, 1996.

Hung PC, Wang HS, Chou ML, et al. Multiple cerebral aneurysms in a child with cardiac myxoma. J Formos Med Assoc *91*:818–821, 1992.

Hunt WE, Hess RM. Surgical risk as related to time of intervention in the repair of intracranial aneurysms. J Neurosurg *28*:14–20, 1968.

Hunt WE, Miller CA. The results of early operation for aneurysm. Clin Neurosurg *24*:208–215, 1977.

Huppman JL, Gahton V, Bowers VD, et al. Neurofibromatosis and arterial aneurysms. Am Surg *62*:311–314, 1996.

Huston J III, Rufenacht DA, Ehman RL, et al. Intracranial aneurysms and vascular malformations: Comparison of time-of-flight and phase-contrast MR angiography. Radiology *181*:721–730, 1991.

Huston J III, Torres VE, Sulivan PP, et al. Value of magnetic resonance angiography for the detection of intracranial aneurysms in autosomal dominant polycystic kidney disease. J Am Soc Nephrol *3*:1871–1877, 1993.

Huston J III, Nichols DA, Luetmer PH, et al. Blinded prospective evaluation of sensitivity of MR angiography to known intracranial aneurysms: Importance of aneurysm size. AJNR *15*:1607–1614, 1994.

Huston J 3rd, Torres VE, Wiebers DO, et al. Follow-up of intracranial aneurysms in autosomal dominant polycystic kidney disease by magnetic resonance angiography. J Am Soc Nephrol *7*:2135–2141, 1996.

Hutchinson J. Aneurysm of the internal carotid within the skull diagnosed eleven years before the patient's death. Spontaneous cure. Trans Clin Soc *8*:127, 1875.

Hutter BO, Gilsbach JM, Kreitschmann I. Is there a difference in cognitive deficits after aneurysmal subarachnoid hemorrhage and subarachnoid hemorrhage of unknown origin? Acta Neurochir *127*:129–135, 1994.

Hutter BO, Gilsbach JM, Kreitschmann I. Quality of life and cognitive deficits after subarachnoid hemorrhage. Br J Neurosurg *9*:465–475, 1995.

Hyland HH. Thrombosis of intracranial arteries. Report of three cases involving, respectively, the anterior cerebral, basilar and internal carotid arteries. Arch Neurol Psychiatr *30*:342–356, 1933.

Hyland HH, Barnett HJM. The pathogenesis of cranial nerve palsies associated with intracranial aneurysms. Proc R Soc Med *47*:141–146, 1953.

Hylton PD, Reichman OH. Endaneurysmal microendarterectomy in the treatment of giant cerebral aneurysms: Technical note. Neurosurgery *23*:674–679, 1988.

Idbohrn H. A complication of percutaneous carotid angiography. Acta Radiol *36*: 155–161, 1951.

Ide Y, Fukushima T, Yamamoto M, et al. Vertebral dissecting aneurysm associated with medial mucoid degeneration. Neurol Med Chir *26*:888–894, 1986.

Iihara K, Makita Y, Nabeshima S, et al. Aspergillosis of the central nervous system causing subarachnoid hemorrhage from mycotic aneurysm of the basilar artery: Case report. Neurol Med Chir *30*:618–623, 1990.

Iihara K, Kikuchi H, Nagata I. Left atrial myxoma with cerebral oncotic aneurysms with special reference to the importance of serial angiography. No Shinkei Geka *19*:857–860, 1991.

Ikawa F, Sumida M, Uozumi T, et al. Comparison of three-dimensional phase-contrast magnetic resonance angiography with three-dimensional time-of-flight magnetic resonance angiography in cerebral aneurysms. Surg Neurol *42*:287–292, 1994.

Ikawa F, Kiya K, Kitaoka T, et al. Indication of early surgery in elderly patients with ruptured intracranial aneurysms—The comparison between surgical and conservative therapy. No To Shinkei *48*:59–63, 1996.

Ikeda K, Yamashita J, Hashimoto M, et al. Orbitozygomatic temporopolar approach for a high basilar tip aneurysm associated with a short intracranial internal carotid artery: A new surgical approach. Neurosurgery *28*:105–110, 1991a.

Ikeda A, Yamaguchi T, Yamamoto I, et al. Excision and end-to-end anastomosis of a fusiform aneurysm of the distal posterior inferior cerebellar artery associated with ischemia: Case report. Neurol Med Chir *31*:351–355, 1991b.

Ikui H, Mimatsu T. The pathogenesis of optic nerve sheath hemorrhage: Report I. Optic nerve sheath hemorrhage in hypertension. Jpn J Ophthalmol *5*:154–167, 1961.

Ikui H, Inomata H, Hayashi J. The pathogenesis of optic nerve sheath hemorrhage. Jpn J Ophthalmol *11*:67–78, 1967.

Ildan F, Uzuneyupoglu Z, Boyar B, et al. Traumatic giant aneurysm of the intracavernous internal carotid artery causing fatal epistaxis: Case report. J Trauma *36*: 565–567, 1994.

Ildan F, Cetinalp E, Bagdatoglu H, et al. Giant fusiform aneurysm of the vertebrobasilar artery presenting with stroke. Neurosurg Rev *18*:135–138, 1995.

Ildan F, Gocer AI, Bagdatoglu H, et al. Intracranial arterial aneurysm complicating Behçet's disease. Neurosurg Rev *19*:53–56, 1996.

Inagawa T. Effect of early operation on cerebral vasospasm. Surg Neurol *33*:239–246, 1990.

Inagawa T. Cerebral vasospasm in elderly patients treated by early operation for ruptured intracranial aneurysms. Acta Neurochir *115*:79–85, 1992.

Inagawa T, Hirano A. Ruptured intracranial aneurysms: An autopsy study of 133 patients. Surg Neurol *33*:117–123, 1990a.

Inagawa T, Hirano A. Autopsy study of unruptured incidental intracranial aneurysms. Surg Neurol *34*:361–365, 1990b.

Inagawa T, Kamiya K, Ogasawara H, et al. Rebleeding of ruptured intracranial aneurysms in the acute stage. Surg Neurol *28*:93–99, 1987.

Inagawa T, Yamamoto M, Kamiya K, et al. Management of elderly patients with aneurysmal subarachnoid hemorrhage. J Neurosurg *69*:332–339, 1988.

Inagawa T, Matsuda Y, Kamiya K, et al. Saccular aneurysm of the distal anterior choroidal artery: Case report. Neurol Med Chir *30*:498–502, 1990.

Inagawa T, Kamiya K, Matsuda Y. Effect of continuous cisternal drainage on cerebral vasospasm. Acta Neurochir *112*:28–36, 1991.

Inagawa T, Hada H, Katoh Y. Unruptured intracranial aneurysms in elderly patients. Surg Neurol *38*:364–370, 1992.

Inagawa T, Ohbayahi N, Hada H. Rapid spontaneous diminution of cisternal blood on computed tomography in patients with subarachnoid hemorrhage. Surg Neurol *44*:356–363, 1995.

Inomata S, Mizuyama K, Sato S, et al. The effect of deliberate hypotensive anesthesia on the prognosis of patients who underwent early surgeries for ruptured cerebral aneurysm. Masui *41*:207–213, 1992.

Inoue R, Katayama S, Kasai N, et al. Middle cerebral artery occlusion with unilateral moyamoya like vessels and with ruptured anterior cerebral artery aneurysm—Its relation to the antiphospholipid antibody syndrome. No To Shinkei *46*:995–998, 1994.

Inoue T, Matsushima T, Fujii K, et al. Microsurgical and angiographic analysis of anterior communicating artery aneurysms with associated anomalies. Fukuoka Igaku Zasshi *83*:397–402, 1992.

Irikura T, Sakai H, Nakahara S, et al. Isolated intraventricular hemorrhage due to a ruptured vertebral artery aneurysm. No Shinkei Geka *18*:469–473, 1990.

Irle E, Wowra B, Kunert HJ, et al. Memory disturbances following anterior communicating artery rupture. Ann Neurol *31*:473–480, 1992.

Ishiguro M, Nakagawa T, Yamamura A, et al. De novo aneurysm associated with a persistent primitive trigeminal artery: Case report. No Shinkei Geka *23*: 1017–1020, 1995.

Ishii R. Regional cerebral blood flow in patients with ruptured intracranial aneurysms. J Neurosurg *50*:587–594, 1979.

Ishikawa S, Sasaki U, Shima T, et al. Extracranial aneurysm of the internal carotid artery at the base of the skull. Neurol Surg *3*:337–342, 1975.

Ishikawa A, Kanazawa Y, Hikasa T, et al. Dissection of the extracranial vertebral artery: A case report. No Shinkei Geka *22*:1077–1080, 1994.

Isla A, Alvarez F, Roda JM, et al. Serpentine aneurysm: Regrowth after a superficial temporal artery-middle cerebral artery bypass and internal carotid artery ligation: Case report. Neurosurgery 34:1072–1074, 1994.

Islak C, Ogut G, Numan F, et al. Persistent nonmigrated ventral primitive ophthalmic artery. Report on one case. J Neuroradiol 21:46–49, 1994.

Isoda H, Mohazab HR, Ramsey RG. Spontaneous disappearance of a ruptured anterior communicating artery aneurysm. AJR 167:536–537, 1996.

Itoh Y, Itoyama Y, Fukumura A, et al. Dissecting aneurysm of the cervical internal carotid artery: Cervical CT scan findings and treatment. Neurol Med Chir 27: 564–568, 1987.

Iwata H, Hata Y, Matsuda T, et al. Solidifying liquid with novel initiation system for detachable balloon catheters. Biomaterials 13:891–896, 1992.

Jackson MA, Hughes RC, Ward SP, et al. "Headbanging" and carotid dissection. Br Med J 287:1262, 1983.

Jacobson DM, Warner JJ, Broste SK. Optic nerve contact and compression by the carotid artery in asymptomatic patients. Am J Ophthalmol 123:677–683, 1997.

Jafar JJ, Weiner HL. Surgery for angiographically occult cerebral aneurysms. J Neurosurg 79:674–679, 1993.

Jain DC, Ahuja GK, Goulatia RK. Intracranial internal carotid artery aneurysm as a cause of Raeder's paratrigeminal syndrome. Surg Neurol 16:357–359, 1981.

Jain KK. Saccular aneurysm of the ophthalmic artery. Am J Ophthalmol 69:997–998, 1970.

Jakobsson KE, Carlsson C, Elfverson J, et al. Traumatic aneurysms of cerebral arteries: A study of five cases. Acta Neurochir 71:91–98, 1984.

Jakobsson KE, Saveland H, Hillman J, et al. Warning leak and management outcome in aneurysmal subarachnoid hemorrhage. J Neurosurg 85:995–999, 1996.

Jaksche H, Donauer E, Kivelitz R, et al. Aneurysmen als seltene Ursache chronisch subduraler Hämatome. Neurochirurgia 31:93–95, 1988.

Jakubowski J, Kendall B. Coincidental aneurysms with tumours of pituitary origin. J Neurol Neurosurg Psychiatry 41:972–979, 1978.

Jakubowski J, Bell BA, Symon L, et al. A primate model of subarachnoid hemorrhage: Change in regional cerebral metabolism in patients with ruptured intracranial aneurysms. J Neurosurg 13:601–611, 1982.

James IM. Changes in cerebral blood flow and in systemic arterial pressure following spontaneous subarachnoid hemorrhage. Clin Sci 35:11–22, 1968.

Jamieson KG. Aneurysms of the vertebrobasilar system. J Neurosurg 21:781–797, 1964.

Jan M, Buchheit F, Tremoulet M. Therapeutic trial of intravenous nimodipine in patients with established cerebral vasospasm after rupture of intracranial aneurysms. Neurosurgery 23:154–157, 1988.

Jane JA. A large aneurysm of the posterior inferior cerebellar artery in a 1-year-old child. J Neurosurg 18:245–247, 1961.

Jane JA, Winn HR, Richardson AE. The natural history of intracranial aneurysms: Rebleeding rates during the acute and long-term period and implications for surgical management. Clin Neurosurg 24:176–184, 1977.

Jane JA, Kassell NF, Torner JC, et al. The natural history of aneurysms and arteriovenous malformations. J Neurosurg 62:321–323, 1985.

Jannetta PJ, Hanafee W, Weidner W, et al. Pneumoencephalographic findings suggesting aneurysm of the vertebral-basilar junction: Differentiation of cases simulating mass lesions. J Neurosurg 24:530–535, 1966.

Jefferson G. Compression of the chiasma, optic nerves, and optic tracts by intracranial aneurysms. Brain 60:444–497, 1937.

Jefferson G. On the saccular aneurysms of the internal carotid artery in the cavernous sinus. Br J Surg 26:267–302, 1938.

Jefferson G. Isolated oculomotor palsy caused by intracranial aneurysm. Proc R Soc Med 40:419–432, 1947.

Jefferson G. Concerning injuries, aneurysms, and tumours involving the cavernous sinus. Trans Ophthalmol Soc UKK 73:117–152, 1953.

Jensen FK, Wagner A. Intracranial aneurysm following radiation therapy for medulloblastoma: A case report and review of the literature. Acta Radiol 38:37–42, 1997.

Jentzer A. Dissecting aneurysm of the left internal carotid artery. Angiology 5: 232–234, 1954.

Jho HD, Ko Y. Glabellar approach: Simplified midline anterior skull base approach. Minim Invasive Neurosurg 40:62–67, 1997.

Jimenez JP, Goree JA, Parker JC Jr. An unusual association of multiple meningiomas, intracranial aneurysms, and cerebrovascular atherosclerosis in two young women. AJR 112:281–288, 1971.

John DG, Porter MJ, van Hasselt CA. Beware bleeding from the ear. J Laryngol Otol 107:137–139, 1993.

Johnsen S, Okamoto G, Kooiker J. Fusiform basilar aneurysm in a child. Neurology 27:334–336, 1977.

Johnson AC, Graves VB, Pfaff JP Jr. Dissecting aneurysm of intracranial arteries. Surg Neurol 7:49–52, 1977.

Johnston I. Direct surgical treatment of bilateral intracavernous internal carotid artery aneurysms: Case report. J Neurosurg 51:98–102, 1979.

Johnston JA, Parkinson D. Intracranial sympathetic pathways associated with the sixth cranial nerve. J Neurosurg 39:236–243, 1974.

Jomin M, Lesoin F, Lozes G, et al. Surgical prognosis of unruptured intracranial arterial aneurysms: Report of 50 cases. Acta Neurochir 84:85–88, 1987.

Jones BH, Mendelson M. Oculomotor nerve compression. Ann Emergency Med 15: 1255–1256, 1986.

Jones HR Jr, Siekert RG. Neurological manifestations of infective endocarditis. Review of clinical and therapeutic challenges. Brain 112:1295–1315, 1989.

Jones HR Jr, Siekert RG, Geraci JE. Neurologic manifestations of bacterial endocarditis. Ann Intern Med 71:21–28, 1969.

Joondeph BC, Joondeph HC, Blair NP. Retinal macroaneurysms treated with the yellow dye laser. Retina 9:187–192, 1989.

Judice D, Connolly ES. Foramen magnum syndrome caused by a giant aneurysm of the posterior inferior cerebral artery: Case report. J Neurosurg 48:639–641, 1978.

Julien I, De Boucaud D. Fistule carotido-caverneuse spontanée et maladie d'Ehlers-Danlos. Presse Med 79:1241–1242, 1971.

Juvela S. Rebleeding from ruptured intracranial aneurysms. Surg Neurol 32:323–326, 1989.

Juvela S. Minor leak before rupture of an intracranial aneurysm and subarachnoid hemorrhage of unknown etiology. Neurosurgery 30:7–11, 1992a.

Juvela S. Alcohol consumption as a risk factor for poor outcome after aneurysmal subarachnoid hemorrhage. Br Med J 304:1663–1667, 1992b.

Juvela S. Aspirin and delayed cerebral ischemia after aneurysmal subarachnoid hemorrhage. J Neurosurg 82:945–952, 1995.

Juvela S. Prevalence of risk factors in spontaneous intracerebral hemorrhage and aneurysmal subarachnoid hemorrhage. Arch Neurol 53:734–740, 1996.

Juvela S, Hillbom M, Numminen H, et al. Cigarette smoking and alcohol consumption as risk factors for aneurysmal subarachnoid hemorrhage. Stroke 24:639–646, 1993a.

Juvela S, Porras M, Heiskanen O. Natural history of unruptured intracranial aneurysms: a long-term follow-up study. J Neurosurg 79:174–182, 1993b.

Kaech D, de Tribolet N, Lasjaunias P. Anterior inferior cerebellar artery aneurysm, carotid bifurcation aneurysm, and dural arteriovenous malformation of the tentorium in the same patient. Neurosurgery 21:575–582, 1987.

Kageji T, Murayama Y, Matsumoto K. Spontaneous middle cerebral artery occlusion with moyamoya-like vessels associated with contralateral middle cerebral artery aneurysm: A case report. No Shinkei Geka 20:177–181, 1992.

Kagstrom E, Palma L. Influence of antifibrinolytic treatment on the morbidity in patients with subarachnoid hemorrhage. Acta Neurol Scand 48:257, 1972.

Kahana L, Lebovitz H, Lusk W, et al. Endocrine manifestations of intracranial extrasellar lesions. J Clin Endocrinol Metab 22:304–324, 1962.

Kahn SG, Frenkel M. Intravitreal hemorrhage associated with rapidly increasing intracranial pressure (Terson's syndrome). Am J Ophthalmol 80:37–43, 1975.

Kaim A, Mader I, Kirsch E, et al. Die perimesenzephale Subarachnoidalblutung: Klinische und computertomographische Aspekte. Rofo Fortschr Geb Rontgenstr Neuen Bildgeb Verfahr 162:274–281, 1995.

Kak VK, Gleadhill CA, Bailey IC. The familial incidence of intracranial aneurysms. J Neurol Neurosurg Psychiatry 33:29–33, 1970.

Kaku Y, Yonekawa Y, Tsukahara T, et al. Superselective intra-arterial infusion of papaverine for the treatment of cerebral vasospasm after subarachnoid hemorrhage. J Neurosurg 77:842–847, 1992.

Kalender WA, Wedding K, Polacin A, et al. Grundlagen der Gefassdarstellung mit spiral-CT. Aktuelle Radiol 4:287–297, 1994.

Kalia KK, Ross DA, Gutin PH. Multiple arterial fenestrations, multiple aneurysms, and an arteriovenous malformation in a patient with subarachnoid hemorrhage. Surg Neurol 35:45–48, 1991.

Kalia KK, Pollack IF, Yonas H. A partially thrombosed, fenestrated basilar artery mimicking an aneurysm of the vertebrobasilar junction: Case report. Neurosurgery 30:276–278, 1992.

Kallmes DF, Evans AJ, Woodcock RJ, et al. Optimization of parameters for the detection of cerebral aneurysms: CT angiography of a model. Radiology 200: 403–405, 1996.

Kalyan-Raman UP, Kowalski RV, Lee RH, et al. Dissecting aneurysm of superior cerebellar artery: Its association with fibromuscular dysplasia. Arch Neurol 40: 120–122, 1983.

Kamitani H, Masuzawa H, Kanazawa I, et al. A long-term follow-up study in direct cerebral aneurysm surgery. Acta Neurochir 133:134–140, 1995.

Kamiya K, Inagawa T, Yamamoto M, et al. Subdural hematoma due to ruptured intracranial aneurysm. Neurol Med Chir 31:82–86, 1991.

Kamiya K, Nagai H, Koide K, et al. Peripheral anterior inferior cerebellar artery aneurysms. Surg Neurol 42:46–51, 1994.

Kamiyama K, Sakurai Y, Suzuki J. Case report: Aneurysm of the posterior communicating artery itself: Report of a successfully treated case. Neurol Med Chir 20: 80–84, 1980.

Kamrin R. Temporal lobe epilepsy caused by unruptured middle cerebral artery aneurysm. Arch Neurol 14:421–427, 1966.

Kanai H, Nagai H, Wakabayashi S, et al. A large aneurysm of the persistent primitive hypoglossal artery. Neurosurgery 30:794–797, 1992.

Kanal E, Shellock FG, Lewin JS. Aneurysm clip testing for ferromagnetic properties: Clip variability issues. Radiology 200:576–578, 1996.

Kanaya N, Sato K, Komeichi T, et al. Rupture of asymptomatic mycotic aneurysm after valve replacement in infective endocarditis. Masui 42:1359–1362, 1993.

Kang S, Yang T, Kim T, et al. Sudden unilateral blindness after intracranial aneurysm surgery. Acta Neurochir 139:221–226, 1997.

Kanshepolsky J, Danielson H, Flynn RE. Vertebral artery insufficiency and cerebellar infarct due to manipulation of the neck. Bull Los Angeles Neurol Soc 37:62–66, 1972.

Kanter MC, Hart RG. Cerebral mycotic aneurysms are rare in infective endocarditis. Ann Neurol 28:590–591, 1990.

Kaplan PA, Hahn FJ. Aneurysms of the posterior cerebral artery in children. AJNR 5:771–774, 1984.

Kaplan SS, Ogilvy CS, Gonzalez R, et al. Extracranial vertebral artery pseudoaneurysm presenting as subarachnoid hemorrhage. Stroke 24:1397–1399, 1993.

Karasawa H, Matsumoto H, Naito H, et al. Angiographically unrecognized microaneurysms: Intraoperative observation and operative technique. Acta Neurochir 139:416–419, 1997.

Karasawa J, Kikuchi H, Furuse S, et al. Surgery of vertebral aneurysms at the origin of PICA. No Shinkei Geka 4:1157–1163, 1976.

Karhunen PJ. Neurosurgical vascular complications associated with aneurysm clips evaluated by postmortem angiography. Forensic Sci Int 51:13–22, 1991.

Kashihara K, Ito H, Yamamoto S, et al. Raeder's syndrome associated with intracranial internal carotid artery aneurysm. Neurosurgery 20:49–51, 1987.

Kashiwagi S, Tew JM Jr, van Loveren HR, et al. Trapping of giant basilar trunk aneurysms: Report of two cases. J Neurosurg 69:442–445, 1988.

Kashiwagi S, Tsuchida E, Shiroyama Y, et al. Paraplegia due to a ruptured aneurysm of the distal posterior inferior cerebellar artery. J Neurol Neurosurg Psychiatry 55:836–837, 1992.

Kashiwagi S, Tsuchida E, Goto K, et al. Balloon occlusion of a spontaneous carotid-cavernous fistula in Ehlers-Danlos syndrome Type IV. Surg Neurol 39:187–190, 1993.

Kasoff I, Kelly DL Jr. Pupillary sparing in oculomotor palsy from internal carotid aneurysm: Case report. J Neurosurg 42:713–717, 1975.

Kassell NF, Drake CG. Timing of aneurysm surgery. Neurosurgery 10:514–519, 1982.

Kassell NF, Torner JC. Size of intracranial aneurysms. Neurosurgery 12:291–297, 1983a.

Kassell NF, Torner JC. Aneurysmal rebleeding: A preliminary report from the cooperative aneurysm study. Neurosurgery 13:479–481, 1983b.

Kassell NF, Torner JC. The International Cooperative Study on Timing of Aneurysm Surgery: An update. Stroke 15:566–570, 1984.

Kassell NF, Adams HP, Torner JC, et al. Effect of early operation for ruptured aneurysms on prevention of delayed ischemic symptoms. J Neurosurg 57:622–628, 1982a.

Kassell NF, Peerless SJ, Durward QJ, et al. Treatment of ischemic deficits from vasospasm with intravascular volume expansion and induced arterial hypertension. Neurosurgery 11:337–343, 1982b.

Kassell NF, Torner JC, Adams HP. Antifibrinolytic therapy in the acute period following aneurysmal subarachnoid hemorrhage: Preliminary observations from the cooperative aneurysm study. J Neurosurg 61:225–230, 1984.

Kassell NF, Torner JC, Haley EC Jr, et al. The International Cooperative Study on the Timing of Aneurysm Surgery. Part 1: Overall management results. J Neurosurg 73:18–36, 1990a.

Kassell NF, Torner JC, Jane JA, et al. The International Cooperative Study on the Timing of Aneurysm Surgery. Part 2: Surgical results. J Neurosurg 73:37–47, 1990b.

Kassell NF, Helm G, Simmons N, et al. Treatment of cerebral vasospasm with intra-arterial papaverine. J Neurosurg 77:848–852, 1992.

Kassell NF, Haley EC Jr, Apperson-Hansen C, et al. Randomized, double-blind, vehicle-controlled trial of tirilazad mesylate in patients with aneurysmal subarachnoid hemorrhage: A cooperative study in Europe, Australia, and New Zealand. J Neurosurg 84:221–228, 1996.

Kaste M, Ramsay M. Tranexamic acid in subarachnoid hemorrhage: A double-blind study. Stroke 10:519–522, 1979.

Katano H, Nagai H, Mase M, et al. Measurement of regional cerebral blood flow with H2(15)O positron emission tomography during Matas test: Report of three cases. Acta Neurochir 135:70–77, 1995.

Katirji MB, Reinmuth OM, Latchaw RE. Stroke due to vertebral artery injury. Arch Neurol 42:242–248, 1985.

Kato Y, Sano H, Katada K, et al. Usefulness of simulation of surgical approaches to cerebral aneurysms by helical scanning CT (HES-CT). Minim Invasive Neurosurg 38:99–104, 1995.

Kato Y, Sano H, Katada K, et al. Effects of new titanium cerebral aneurysm clips on MRI and CT images. Minim Invasive Neurosurg 39:82–85, 1996.

Kaufman DI, Siebert JE, Pernicone JR. Magnetic resonance angiography relevant to Neuroophthalmology. In Neuroophthalmological Disorder. Diagnostic Work-Up and Management. Editors, Tusa RJ, Newman SA, pp 367–404. New York, Marcel Dekker, Inc, 1995.

Kaufmann AM, Reddy KK, West M, et al. Alkaptonuric ochronosis and multiple intracranial aneurysms. Surg Neurol 33:213–216, 1990.

Kawaguchi S, Sakaki T, Kamada K, et al. Dissecting aneurysm of the posterior inferior cerebellar artery: Case report. Neurol Med Chir 33:634–637, 1993.

Kawaguchi S, Sakaki T, Tsunoda S, et al. Management of dissecting aneurysms of the posterior circulation. Acta Neurochir 131:26–31, 1994.

Kawaguchi S, Sakaki T, Morimoto T, et al. Characteristics of intracranial aneurysms associated with moyamoya disease: A review of 111 cases. Acta Neurochir 138:1287–1294, 1996.

Kawaguti T, Yokoyama H, Tsutsumi K, et al. Surgical treatment of aneurysms at basilar artery and posterior cerebral artery associated with moyamoya disease: A case report. No Shinkei Geka 23:807–811, 1995.

Kawakami K, Kayama T, Kondo R, et al. A case of mycotic ICA petrous portion aneurysm treated with endovascular surgery. No Shinkei Geka 24:253–257, 1996.

Kawakita S, Yasuda M, Kuroiwa T, et al. A ruptured aneurysm in the hypoplastic proximal anterior cerebral artery (A1 portion): Case report. No Shinkei Geka 19:773–776, 1991.

Kawamata T, Kagawa M, Kubo O, et al. Clinicopathological studies of three cases of cerebral aneurysms associated with systemic lupus erythematosus. No Shinkei Geka 19:633–639, 1991.

Kawamata T, Tanikawa T, Takeshita M, et al. Rebleeding of intracranial dissecting aneurysm in the vertebral artery following proximal clipping. Neurol Res 16:141–144, 1994.

Kawano T, Kazekawa K, Nakashima S, et al. Combined drug therapy with diltiazem, dextran, and hydrocortisone (DDH therapy) for late cerebral vasospasm after aneurysmal subarachnoid hemorrhage: Assessment of efficacy and safety in an open clinical study. Int J Clin Pharmacol Ther 33:513–517, 1995.

Kawase T, Bertalanffy H, Otani M, et al. Surgical approaches for vertebro-basilar trunk aneurysms located in the midline. Acta Neurochir 138:402–410, 1996.

Kayath MJ, Lengyel AM, Nogueira R, et al. Giant aneurysms of the sellar region simulating pituitary adenomas: A diagnosis to be considered. J Endocrinol Invest 14:975–979, 1991.

Kayazawa F. Bilateral retinal arterial macroaneurysms. Ann Ophthalmol 12:1218–1222, 1980.

Keane JR. Contralateral gaze deviation with supratentorial hemorrhage: Three pathologically verified cases. Arch Neurol 32:119–122, 1975.

Keane JR. Aneurysms and third nerve palsies. Ann Neurol 14:696–697, 1983.

Keane JR. The pretectal syndrome: 206 patients. Neurology 40:684–690, 1990.

Keane JR, Ahmadi J. Third-nerve palsies and angiography. Arch Neurol 48:470, 1991.

Keane JR, Talalla A. Posttraumatic intracavernous aneurysm: Epistaxis with monocular blindness preceded by chromatopsia. Arch Ophthalmol 87:701–705, 1972.

Keller E, Ries F, Grunwald F, et al. Multimodaler Karotisokklusionstest zur Bestimmung des Infarktrisikos vor therapeutischem Karotis-interna-Verschluss. Laryngorhinootologie 74:307–311, 1995.

Keller E, Ries F, Urbach H, et al. Endovaskularer Ballonokklusionstest der A. carotis interna mit erweitertem hamodynamischen Monitoring zur Bestimmung der Durchblutungsreserve vor geplantem Karotisverschluss. Rofo Fortschr Geb Rontgenstr Neuen Bildgeb Verfahr 164:324–330, 1996.

Kennedy JE, Wise GN. Clinicopathological correlation of retinal lesions. Arch Ophthalmol 74:658–662, 1965.

Kennerdell JS, Maroon JC. Intracanalicular meningioma with chronic optic disc edema. Ann Ophthalmol 7:507–512, 1975.

Keogh AJ, Sharma RR, Vanner GK. The anterior interhemispheric trephine approach to anterior midline aneurysms: Results of treatment in 72 consecutive patients. Br J Neurosurg 7:5–12, 1993.

Kerber CW, Margolis MT, Newton TH. Tortuous vertebrobasilar system: A cause of cranial nerve signs. Neuroradiology 4:74–77, 1972.

Kerns JM, Smith DR, Jannotta FS, et al. Oculomotor nerve regeneration after aneurysm surgery. Am J Ophthalmol 87:225–233, 1979.

Kerr FWL, Hollowell OW. Location of pupillomotor and accommodation fibers in the oculomotor nerve: Experimental observations on paralytic mydriasis. J Neurol Neurosurg Psychiatry 27:473–481, 1964.

Khalil M, Lorenzetti DWC. Acquired retinal macroaneurysms. Can J Ophthalmol 14:163–168, 1979.

Khanna RK, Malik GM, Qureshi N. Predicting outcome following surgical treatment of unruptured intracranial aneurysms: A proposed grading system. J Neurosurg 84:49–54, 1996.

Khayata MH, Aymard A, Casasco A, et al. Selective endovascular techniques in the treatment of cerebral mycotic aneurysms: Report of three cases. J Neurosurg 78:661–665, 1993.

Khayata MH, Spetzler RF, Mooy JJ, et al. Combined surgical and endovascular treatment of a giant vertebral artery aneurysm in a child. Case report. J Neurosurg 81:304–307, 1994.

Khurana RK, Genut AA, Yannakakis GD. Locked-in syndrome with recovery. Ann Neurol 8:439–441, 1980.

Kidooka M, Okada T, Sonobe M, et al. Dissecting aneurysm of the anterior cerebral artery: Report of two cases. Surg Neurol 39:53–57, 1993.

Kieck CF, de Villiers JC. Vascular lesions due to transcranial stab wounds. J Neurosurg 60:42–46, 1984.

Kikuchi K, Kowada M. Case report: Saccular aneurysm of the intraorbital ophthalmic artery. Br J Radiol 67:1134–1135, 1994.

Kikuchi K, Watanabe K, Sugawara A, et al. Multiple fungal aneurysms: Report of a rare case implicating steroid as predisposing factor. Surg Neurol 24:253–259, 1985.

Kim C, Kikuchi H, Hashimoto N, et al. Histopathological study of induced cerebral aneurysms in primates. Surg Neurol 32:45–50, 1989.

Kimura M, Tanaka A, Matsuno H, et al. Use of STA-MCA anastomosis for clipping of giant middle cerebral artery aneurysm: Case report. Neurol Med Chir 33:774–778, 1993.

Kindl R, Nigbur H, Horsch S. Das extrakranielle Aneurysma der Arteria carotis interna. Eine Vasa 22:256–259, 1993.

King AB. Successful surgical treatment of an intracranial mycotic aneurysm complicated by a subdural hematoma. J Neurosurg 17:788–791, 1960.

King JT Jr, Berlin JA, Flamm ES. Morbidity and mortality from elective surgery for asymptomatic, unruptured, intracranial aneurysms: A meta-analysis. J Neurosurg 81:837–842, 1994.

King JT Jr, Glick HA, Mason TJ, et al. Elective surgery for asymptomatic, unruptured, intracranial aneurysms: A cost-effectiveness analysis. J Neurosurg 83:403–412, 1995.

King RB, Saba MI. Forewarnings of major subarachnoid hemorrhage due to congenital berry aneurysm. NY State J Med 74:638–639, 1974.

Kinugasa K, Mandai S, Terai Y, et al. Direct thrombosis of aneurysms with cellulose acetate polymer. Part II: Preliminary clinical experience. J Neurosurg 77:501–507, 1992.

Kinugasa K, Mandai S, Tsuchida S, et al. Direct thrombosis of a pseudoaneurysm after obliteration of a carotid-cavernous fistula with cellulose acetate polymer: Technical case report. Neurosurgery 35:755–759; discussion 759–760, 1994a.

Kinugasa K, Mandai S, Tsuchida S, et al. Cellulose acetate polymer thrombosis for the emergency treatment of aneurysms: Angiographic findings, clinical experience, and histopathological study. Neurosurgery 34:694–701; discussion 700–701, 1994b.

Kinugasa K, Kamata I, Hirotsune N, et al. Early treatment of subarachnoid hemorrhage after preventing rerupture of an aneurysm. J Neurosurg 83:34–41, 1995.

Kirchhof K, Vogt-Schaden M, Forsting M. Fusiformes Basilarisaneurysma bei M. Rechlinghausen. Rofo Fortschr Geb Rontgenstr Neuen Bildgeb Verfahr 165:412–414, 1996.

Kirollos RW, Tyagi AK, Marks PV, et al. Muslin induced granuloma following wrapping of intracranial aneurysms—the role of infection as an additional precipitating factor: Report of two cases and review of the literature. Acta Neurochir 139:411–415, 1997.

Kissel JT, Burde RM, Klingele TG, et al. Pupil-sparing oculomotor palsies with internal carotid-posterior communicating artery aneurysms. Ann Neurol 13:149–154, 1983.

Kitanaka C, Sasaki T, Eguchi T, et al. Intracranial vertebral artery dissections: Clinical, radiological features, and surgical considerations. Neurosurgery 34:620–626; discussion 626–627, 1994a.

Kitanaka C, Tanaka J, Kuwahara M, et al. Nonsurgical treatment of unruptured intracranial vertebral artery dissection with serial follow-up angiography. J Neurosurg 80:667–674, 1994b.

Kitani R, Itouji T, Noda Y, et al. Dissecting aneurysms of the anterior circle of Willis arteries: Report of two cases. J Neurosurg 67:296–300, 1987.

Klein R, Meuer SM, Moss SE, et al. Retinal microaneurysm counts and 10-year progression of diabetic retinopathy. Arch Ophthalmol 113:1386–1391, 1995.

Kleinpeter G, Schatzer R, Bock F. Is blood pressure really a trigger for the circadian rhythm of subarachnoid hemorrhage? Stroke 26:1805–1810, 1995.

Kline DG, Johnson JH. Anterior inferior cerebellar artery aneurysms. J Neurosurg 60:1115, 1984.

Kline LB, Vitek JJ, Raymon BC. Painful Horner's syndrome due to spontaneous carotid artery dissection. Ophthalmology 94:226–230, 1987.

Klingler M. Compression des nerfs et du chiasma optique par des anévrysmes. Confin Neurol 11:261–270, 1951.

Klotzsch C, Nahser HC, Fisher B, et al. Visualization of intracranial aneurysms by transcranial duplex sonography. Neuroradiology 38:555–559, 1996.

Klucznik RP, Carrier DA, Pyka R, et al. Placement of a ferromagnetic intracerebral aneurysm clip in a magnetic field with a fatal outcome. Radiology 187:855–856, 1993.

Knapp A. Association of sclerosis of the cerebral basal vessels with optic atrophy and cupping. Arch Ophthalmol 8:637–648, 1932.

Knapp A. Course in certain cases of atrohy of the optic nerve with cupping and low tension. Arch Ophthalmol 23:41–47, 1940.

Knosp E, Müller G, Perneczky A. The paraclinoid carotid artery: Anatomical aspects of a microneurosurgical approach. Neurosurgery 22:896–901, 1988.

Knuckey NW, Fox RA, Surveyor I, et al. Early cerebral blood flow and computerized tomography in predicting ischemia after cerebral aneurysm rupture. J Neurosurg 62:850–855, 1985.

Knuckey NW, Epstein MH, Haas R, et al. Distal anterior choroidal artery aneurysm: Intraoperative localization and treatment. Neurosurgery 22:1084–1087, 1988.

Knuckey NW, Haas R, Jenkins R, et al. Thrombosis of difficult intracranial aneurysms by the endovascular placement of platinum-Dacron microcoils. J Neurosurg 77:43–50, 1992.

Kobayashi H, Hayashi M, Kawano H, et al. Magnetic resonance imaging of emoblism from intracranial aneurysms. Surg Neurol 32:225–230, 1989.

Kobayashi H, Ide H, Aradachi H, et al. Histological studies of intracranial vessels in primates following transluminal angioplasty for vasospasm. J Neurosurg 78:481–486, 1993.

Kobayashi S, Kyoshima K, Gibo H, et al. Carotid cave aneurysms of the internal carotid artery. J Neurosurg 70:216–221, 1989.

Kochi N, Tani E, Yokota M, et al. Neoplastic cerebral aneurysm from lung cancer: Case report. J Neurosurg 60:640–643, 1984.

Kodama N, Sato T, Suzuki J. Homonymous hemianopsia caused by chiasmal compression due to intracranial aneurysm. Neurol Med Chir 18:91–100, 1978.

Kodama N, Sasaki T, Sakurai Y. Transthird ventricular approach for a high basilar bifurcation aneurysm: Report of three cases. J Neurosurg 82:664–668, 1995.

Kodama S, Asakura T, Kadota K, et al. A case of systemic lupus erythematosus with subarachnoid hemorrhage due to ruptured aneurysm. No Shinkei Geka 18:571–575, 1990.

Kodama N, Sato M, Sasaki T. Treatment of ruptured cerebral aneurysm in moyamoya disease. Surg Neurol 46:62–66, 1996.

Koeleveld RF, Heilman CB, Klucznik RP, et al. De novo development of an aneurysm: Case report. Neurosurgery 29:756–759, 1991.

Koenigsberg AD, Solomon GD, Kosmorsky G. Psuedoaneurysm within the cavernous sinus presenting as cluster headache. Headache 34:111–113, 1994.

Koga N. Ruptured cerebral aneurism associated with chronic subdural haematoma and unusual extravasation of contrast medium during angiography. J Clin Radiol 30:905–908, 1985.

Kohno K, Ueda T, Kadota O, et al. Subdural hemorrhage caused by de novo aneurysm complicating extracranial-intracranial bypass surgery: case report. Neurosurgery 38:1051–1055, 1996.

Kohshi K, Yokota A, Konda N, et al. Hyperbaric oxygen therapy adjunctive to mild hypertensive hypervolemia for symptomatic vasospasm. Neurol Med Chir 33:92–99, 1993.

Koike T, Ishii R, Ihara I. Cerebral circulation and metabolism in patients with ruptured aneurysms—With special reference to vasospasm and infarction. J Cereb Blood Flow Metab 1:S522–S523, 1981.

Kojima A, Nakamura T, Takayama H, et al. A case of de novo aneurysm of the distal posterior inferior cerebellar artery with intraventricular hemorrhage. No Shinkei Geka 24:469–473, 1996.

Kojima Y, Saito A, Kim I. The role of serial angiography in the management of bacterial and fungal intracranial aneurysms—Report of two cases and review of the literature. Neurol Med Chir 29:202–216, 1989.

Komatsu Y, Narushima K, Kobayashi E, et al. Aspergillus mycotic aneurysm: Case report. Neurol Med Chir 31:346–350, 1991.

Komatsu Y, Yasuda S, Shibata T, et al. Management for subarachnoid hemorrhage with negative initial angiography. No Shinkei Geka 22:43–49, 1994.

Komeichi T, Igarashi K, Takigami M, et al. A case of metastatic choriocarcinoma associated with cerebral thrombosis and aneurysmal formation. No Shinkei Geka 24:463–467, 1996.

Komiyama M, Khosla VK, Tamura K, et al. A provocative internal carotid artery balloon occlusion test with 99mTc-HM-PAO CBF mapping: Report of three cases. Neurol Med Chir 32:747–752, 1992.

Komiyama M, Tamura K, Nagata Y, et al. Aneurysmal rupture during angiography. Neurosurgery 33:798–803, 1993.

Komiyama M, Yasui T, Tamura K, et al. "Kissing aneurysms" of the internal carotid artery. Neurol Med Chir 34:360–364, 1994.

Kondo S, Hashimoto N, Kikuchi H, et al. Cerebral aneurysms arising at nonbranching sites: An experimental study. Stroke 28:398–403, 1997.

Kondziolka D, Bernstein M, ter Brugge K, et al. Acute subdural hematoma from ruptured posterior communicating artery aneurysm. Neurosurgery 22:151–154, 1988.

Kong KH, Chan KF. Ruptured intracranial mycotic aneurysm: A rare cause of intracranial hemorrhage. Arch Phys Med Rehabil 76:287–289, 1995.

Kongable GL, Lanzino G, Germanson TP, et al. Gender-related differences in aneurysmal subarachnoid hemorrhage. J Neurosurg 84:43–48, 1996.

Konishi Y, Kadowaki C, Hara M, et al. Aneurysms associated with moyamoya disease. Neurosurgery 16:484–491, 1985.

Konishi Y, Maemura E, Shiota M, et al. Treatment of vasospasm by balloon angioplasty: Experimental studies and clinical experiences. Neurol Res 14:273–281, 1992.

Kopczynski S, Drewniak K. Tetniak tetnicy mozgowej domniemanego pochodzenia kilowego. Pol Tyg Lek 25:1465–1466, 1970.

Kopera M, Majchrzak H, Ladzinski P, et al. Tetniak rozwarstwiajacy tetnicy mozdzkowej tylnej dolnej. Neurol Neurochir Pol 26:897–901, 1992.

Korogi Y, Takahashi M, Mabuchi N, et al. Intracranial aneurysms: Diagnostic accuracy of three-dimensional, Fourier transform, time-of-flight MR angiography. Radiology 193:181–186, 1994.

Korogi Y, Takahashi M, Mabuchi N, et al. Intracranial aneurysms: Diagnostic accuracy of MR angiography with evaluation of maximum intensity projection and source images. Radiology 199:199–207, 1996.

Korogi Y, Takahashi M, Mabuchi N, et al. MR angiography of intracranial aneurysms: A comparison of 0.5 T and 1.5 T. Comput Med Imaging Graph 21:111–116, 1997.

Korovessis P, Michalopoulos B, Vassilakos P. Delayed recognition of a vascular complication, carotid artery aneurysm, 60 years after operation for muscular torticollis: A case report. Clin Orthop 275:258–262, 1992.

Kosierkiewicz TA, Factor SM, Dickson DW. Immunocytochemical studies of atherosclerotic lesions of cerebral berry aneurysms. J Neuropathol Exp Neurol 53:399–406, 1994.

Kosnik EJ, Hunt WE. Postoperative hypertension in the management of patients with intracranial arterial aneurysms. J Neurosurg 45:148–154, 1976.

Kothandaram P, Dawson BH, Kruyt RC. Carotid-ophthalmic aneurysms: A study of 19 patients. J Neurosurg 34:544–548, 1971.

Kotwica Z. Middle cerebral artery aneurysm developing apparently de novo. Neurochirurgia 36:70–72, 1993.

Koyama S, Kotani A, Sasaki J, et al. Ruptured aneurysm at the origin of duplication of the middle cerebral artery: Case report. Neurol Med Chir 35:671–673, 1995.

Kramer RA, Eckman PB. Hemifacial spasm associated with redundancy of the vertebral artery. AJR 115:133–136, 1972.

Kraus E, Koschorek F, Scheil F, et al. Timing and factors influencing operative outcome in intracranial aneurysms. Neurochirurgia 29:215–218, 1986.

Kraus GE, Herman JM, Marciano F, et al. Ruptured giant aneurysm of an occluded middle cerebral artery in a severe-grade patient: Case report. Neurosurgery 36: 169–171; discussion 171–172, 1995.

Krauss HR, Slamovits TL, Sibony PA, et al. Carotid artery aneurysm simulating pituitary adenoma. J Clin Neuro-Ophthalmol 2:169–174, 1982.

Krayenbühl H. Das Hernaneurysma. Schweiz Arch Neurol Psychiatr 47:155–236, 1941.

Krayenbühl H, Yaşargil MG. Das Hirnaneurysma. Basel JR. Gcigy, 1958.

Krieger D, Adams HP, Albert F, et al. Pure motor hemiparesis with stable somatosensory evoked potential monitoring during aneurysm surgery: Case report. Neurosurgery 31:145–150, 1992.

Kriplani A, Relan S, Misra NK, et al. Ruptured intracranial aneurysm complicating pregnancy. Int J Gynaecol Obstet 48:201–206, 1995.

Krivosic-Horber R, Leclerc X, Doumith S, et al. Anesthesie-reanimation pour occlusion endovasculaire des anevrismes intracraniens rompus par des spires electriquement detachables. Ann Fr Anesth Reanim 15:354–358, 1996.

Krueger BR, Okazaki H. Vertebral-basilar distribution infarction following chiropractic cervical manipulation. Mayo Clin Proc 55:322–332, 1980.

Krueger C, Weir B, Nosko M, et al. Nimodipine and chronic vasospasm in monkeys: II. Pharmacologic studies of vessels in spasm. Neurosurgery 16:137–140, 1985.

Krupp W, Heienbrok W, Muke R. Management results attained by predominantly late surgery for intracranial aneurysms. Neurosurgery 34:227–233; discussion 233–234, 1994.

Krysl J, Noel de Tilly L, Armstrong D. Pseudoaneurysm of the internal carotid artery: Complication of deep neck space infection. AJNR 14:696–698, 1993.

Kubo S, Nakagawa H, Imaoka S. Systemic multiple aneurysms of the extracranial internal carotid artery, intracranial vertebral artery, and visceral arteries: Case report. Neurosurgery 30:600–602, 1992.

Kubota S, Tatara N, Miyoshi A, et al. An evaluation of temporary clipping during aneurysmal surgery: A retrospective study. No Shinkei Geka 20:1247–1254, 1992.

Kubota S, Ohmori S, Tatara N, et al. A ruptured peripheral, superior cerebellar artery aneurysm: A case report and a review of the literature as to surgical approaches. No Shinkei Geka 22:279–283, 1994.

Kucharczyk W. High resolution magnetic resonance imaging of vascular lesions at the skull base: A review. Can Assoc Rad J 41:14–18, 1990.

Kudo T. Postoperative oculomotor palsy due to vasospasm in a patient with a ruptured internal carotid artery aneurysm: A case report. Neurosurgery 19:274–277, 1986.

Kudo T. An operative complication in a patient with a true posterior communicating artery aneurysm: Case report and review of the literature. Neurosurgery 27: 650–653, 1990.

Kudo T, Suzuki S, Iwabuchi T. Importance of monitoring the circulating blood volume in patients with cerebral vasospasm after subarachnoid hemorrhage. Neurosurgery 9:514–520, 1981.

Kuether TA, Nesbit GM, Clark WM, et al. Rotational vertebral artery occlusion: A mechanism of vertebrobasilar insufficiency. Neurosurgery 41:427–433, 1997.

Kuki S, Yoshida K, Suzuki K, et al. Successful surgical management for multiple cerebral mycotic aneurysms involving both carotid and vertebrobasilar systems in active infective endocarditis. Eur J Cardiothorac Surg 8:508–510, 1994.

Kulla L, Deymeer F, Smith TW, et al. Intracranial dissecting and saccular aneurysms in polycystic kidney disease: Report of a case. Arch Neurol 39:776–778, 1982.

Kumabe T, Kaneko U, Ishibashi T, et al. Two cases of giant serpentine aneurysm. Neurosurgery 26:1027–1033, 1990.

Kumar S, Rao VR, Mandalam KR, et al. Disappearance of a cerebral aneurysm—An unusual angiographic event. Clin Neurol Neurosurg 93:151–153, 1991.

Kunkle EC, Muller JC, Odom GL. Traumatic brain-stem thrombosis: Report of a case and analysis of the mechanism of injury. Ann Intern Med 36:1329–1335, 1952.

Kunze S, Schiefer W. Angiographic demonstration of a dissecting aneurysm of the middle cerebral artery. Neuroradiology 2:201–206, 1971.

Kupersmith MJ, Krohn D. Cupping of the optic disc with compressive lesions of the anterior visual pathway. Ann Ophthalmol 16:948–953, 1984.

Kupersmith MJ, Berenstein A, Choi IS, et al. Percutaneous transvascular treatment of giant carotid aneurysms: Neuro-ophthalmologic findings. Neurology 34: 328–335, 1984.

Kupersmith MJ, Hurst R, Berenstein A, et al. The benign course of cavernous carotid artery aneurysms. J Neurosurg 77:690–693, 1992.

Kurihara N, Takahashi S, Higano S, et al. Evaluation of large intracranial aneurysm with three-dimensional MRI. J Comput Assist Tomogr 19:707–712, 1995.

Kurino M, Kuratsu J, Yamaguchi T, et al. Mycotic aneurysm accompanied by aspergillotic granuloma: A case report. Surg Neurol 42:160–164, 1994.

Kurita H, Shiokawa Y, Segawa H, et al. Delayed parent artery narrowing occurring months after aneurysm surgery: A complication after aneurysm surgery—Technical case report. Neurosurgery 36:1225–1229, 1995.

Kuroiwa T, Tanabe H, Takatsuka H, et al. Bilateral distal anterior cerebral artery aneurysms associated with polycystic kidney and liver disease: A case report. No Shinkei Geka 20:905–908, 1992.

Kuroiwa T, Morita H, Tanabe H, et al. Significance of ST segment elevation in electrocardiograms in patients with ruptured cerebral aneurysms. Acta Neurochir 133:141–146, 1995.

Kurokawa Y, Okamura T, Watanabe K. Transcerebellar thrombectomy for the successful clipping of thrombosed giant vertebral-posterior inferior cerebellar artery aneurysm: Case report. Surg Neurol 33:217–220, 1990.

Kurokawa Y, Abiko S, Okamura T, et al. Direct surgery for giant aneurysm exhibiting progressive enlargement after intraaneurysmal balloon embolization. Surg Neurol 38:19–25, 1992.

Kushner M. Spontaneous dissection of the internal carotid artery. Arch Neurol 45: 138, 1988.

Kuwabara S, Naitoh H. Ruptured aneurysm at the origin of the accessory middle cerebral artery: Case report. Neurosurgery 26:320–322, 1990.

Kuzniecky R, Melmed C, Schipper H. Carotid-ophthalmic aneurysm: An uncommon cause of acute monocular blindness. Can Med Assoc J 136:727–728, 1987.

Kwak R, Ito S, Yamamoto N, et al. Significance of intracranial aneurysms associated with moyamoya disease: I. Differences between intracranial aneurysms associated with moyamoya disease and usual saccular aneurysms—Review of the literature. Neurol Med Chir 24:97–103, 1984a.

Kwak R, Emori T, Nakamura T, et al. Significance of intracranial aneurysms associated with moyamoya disease: II. Cause and site of hemorrhage—Review of the literature. Neurol Med Chir 24:104–109, 1984b.

Kwan E, Hieshima GB, Higashida RT, et al. Interventional neuroradiology in neuroophthalmology. J Clin Neuro-Ophthalmol 9:83–97, 1989.

Kwan ES, Kwon OJ, Borden JA. Successful thrombolysis in the vertebrobasilar artery after endovascular occlusion of a recently ruptured large basilar tip aneurysm. AJNR 16(4 Suppl):847–851, 1995.

Lach B, Nair SG, Russell NA, et al. Spontaneous carotid-cavernous fistula and multiple arterial dissections in Type IV Ehlers-Danlos syndrome: Case report. J Neurosurg 66:462–467, 1987.

Ladzinski P, Majchrzak H, Machowski J, et al. Tetniak tetnicy laczacej przedniej jako mozliwe pozne powiklanie podwiazania tetnicy szyjnej wewntrznej. Neurol Neurochir Pol 28:933–938, 1994.

Lai MD, Hoffman HB, Adamkiewicz JJ. Dissecting aneurysms of internal carotid artery after non-penetrating neck injury. Case report. Acta Radiol 5:290–295, 1960.

Laine E. Rappel historique de la chirurgie des anévrysmes intracraniens. Neurochirurie 32:459–470, 1986.

Laitinen L, Snellman A. Aneurysms of the pericallosal artery: A study of 14 cases verified angiographically and treated mainly by direct surgical attack. J Neurosurg 17:447–458, 1960.

Lakhanpal SK, Glasier CM, James CA, et al. MR and CT diagnosis of carotid pseudoaneurysm in children following surgical resection of craniopharyngioma. Ped Radiol 25:249–251, 1995.

Lam CH, Montes J, Farmer JP, et al. Traumatic aneurysm from shaken baby syndrome: Case report. Neurosurgery 39:1252–1255, 1996.

Lan MY, Liu JS, Chang YY, et al. Fibromuscular dysplasia associated with intracranial giant aneurysm: Report of a case. J Formos Med Assoc 94:692–694, 1995.

Landau K, Horton JC, Hoyt WF, et al. Aneurysm mimicking intracranial growth of optic nerve sheath meningioma. J Clin Neuroophthalmol 10:185–187, 1990.

Landolt AM, Millikan CH. Pathogenesis of cerebral infarction secondary to mechanical carotid artery occlusion. Stroke 1:52–62, 1970.

Lane RJ, Weisman RA, Savino PJ, et al. Aneurysm of the internal carotid artery at the base of the skull: An unusual cause of cranial neuropathies. Otolaryngol Head Neck Surg 88:230–232, 1980.

Lanfermann H, Gross-Fengels W, Steinbrich W. Intrakranielle Aneurysmen. Vergleich zwischen magnetischer Resonanztomographie und Arteriographie. Rofo Fortschr Geb Rontgenstr Neuen Bildgeb Verfahr 157:118–123, 1992.

Lang C, Jacobi G, Kreuz W, et al. Rapid development of giant aneurysm at the base of the brain in an 8-year-old boy with perinatal HIV infection. Acta Histochem Suppl 42:83–90, 1992.

Lange-Cosack H. In Handbuch der Neurochirurgie. Editors, Olivecrona H, Tönnis H, Vol 4, Pt 2, p 100. Berlin, Springer-Verlag, 1966.

Langlois O, Proust F, Rabehenoina C, et al. Vasospasme, chirurgie precoce et nimodipine. Une serie de 120 cas consecutifs d'anevrismes rompus operes. Neurochirurgie 38:160–164, 1992.

Lanzino G, Andreoli A, Tognetti F, et al. Orbital pain and unruptured carotid-posterior communicating artery aneurysms: The role of sensory fibers of the third cranial nerve. Acta Neurochir 120:7–11, 1993a.

Lanzino G, Kassell NF, Germanson T, et al. Plasma glucose levels and outcome after aneurysmal subarachnoid hemorrhage. J Neurosurg 79:885–891, 1993b.

Lanzino G, Kassell NF, Germanson TP, et al. Age and outcome after aneurysmal subarachnoid hemorrhage: Why do older patients fare worse? J Neurosurg 85: 410–418, 1996.

Lapresle J, Said G. Déviation forcée des yeux vers le bas et on dedans et mouvements oculaires périodiques au cours d'une hémorragie anévrysmale de la calotte mésencéphalique. Rev Neurol 133:497–503, 1977.

Larranaga J, Rutecki GW, Whittier FC. Spontaneous vertebral artery dissection as a complication of autosomal dominant polycystic kidney disease. Am J Kidney Dis 25:70–74, 1995.

Larson JJ, Tew JM Jr, Tomsick TA, et al. Treatment of aneurysms of the internal carotid artery by intravascular balloon occlusion: long-term follow-up of 58 patients. Neurosurgery 36:23–30; discussion 30, 1995.

Lassman LP, Ramani PS, Sengupta RP. Aneurysms of peripheral cerebral arteries due to surgical trauma. Vasc Surg 8:1–5, 1974.

Laszlo FA, Varga C, Doczi T. Cerebral oedema after subarachnoid hemorrhage. Pathogenetic significance of vasopressin. Acta Neurochir 133:122–133, 1995.

Latka D, Szydlik W, Kozub D, et al. Nowopowstale wewnatrzczaszkowe tetniaki workowate ujawnione w okresie kilku lat od operacji tetniaka o innej lokalizacji—Opis 2 przypadkow. Neurol Neurochir Pol 29:613–621, 1995.

Law WR, Nelson ER. Internal carotid aneurysm as a cause of Raeder's paratrigeminal syndrome. Neurology 18:43–46, 1968.

Lawton MT, Hamilton MG, Morcos JJ, et al. Revascularization and aneurysm surgery: Current techniques, indications, and outcome. Neurosurgery 38:83–92; discussion 92–94, 1996.

Lawton MT, Daspit CP, Spetzler RF. Technical aspects and recent trends in the management of large and giant midbasilar artery aneurysms. Neurosurgery 41:513–521, 1997.

Lazorthes Y, Sonilhac F, Lagarrigue J, et al. La surveillance des potentiels evoques somesthesiques dans la chirurgie des anevrysmes sylviens. Neurochirurgie 38:333–346, 1992.

Le Beau J, Daum S. Pseudo-tumeurs vasculaires de l'angle pontocérébelleux. Sem Hop Paris 36:1839–1842, 1960.

Le Cam B, Guivarch G, Boles JM, et al. Neurologic complications in a group of 86 patients with bacterial endocarditis. Eur Heart J 5(Suppl C):97–100, 1984.

Le Roux PD, Dailey AT, Newell DW, et al. Emergent aneurysm clipping without angiography in the moribund patient with intracerebral hemorrhage: the use of infusion computed tomography scans. Neurosurgery 33:189–197; discussion 197, 1993.

Le Roux PD, Elliott JP, Downey L, et al. Improved outcome after rupture of anterior circulation aneurysms: A retrospective 10-year review of 224 good-grade patients. J Neurosurg 83:394–402, 1995.

Le Roux PD, Elliott JP, Newell DW, et al. Predicting outcome in poor-grade patients with subarachnoid hemorrhage: A retrospective review of 159 aggressively managed cases. J Neurosurg 85:39–49, 1996.

Leblanc R. Familial cerebral aneurysms. A bias for women. Stroke 27:1050–1054, 1996.

Leblanc R, Lozano AM, van der Rest M, et al. Absence of collagen deficiency in familial cerebral aneurysms. J Neurosurg 70:837–840, 1989a.

Leblanc R, Lozano A, van der Rest M. Collagen deficiency in cerebral aneurysms. Stroke 20:561, 1989b.

Leblanc R, Lozano A, van der Rest M. Type III collagen mutations and cerebral aneurysms. Stroke 20:1432–1433, 1989c.

Leblanc R, Lozano AM, van der Rest M. Familial cerebral aneurysm and type III collagen deficiency. J Neurosurg 72:157–158, 1990.

Leblanc R, Worsley KJ, Melanson D, et al. Angiographic screening and elective surgery of familial cerebral aneurysms: A decision analysis. Neurosurgery 35:9–18; discussion 18–19, 1994.

Leblanc R, Melanson D, Tampieri D, et al. Familial cerebral aneurysms: A study of 13 families. Neurosurgery 37:633–638, 1995.

Leblanc R, Worsley KJ. Surgery of unruptured, asymptomatic aneurysms: A decision analysis. Can J Neurol Sci 22:30–35, 1995.

Ledic S, Vujicic M, Citic R, et al. Zatvorene traumatske intrakranijalne ekstraduralne lezije unutrasnje karotidne arterije. Vojnosanitetski Pregled 49:317–324, 1992.

Lee AG, Mawad ME, Baskin DS. Fatal subarachnoid hemorrhage from the rupture of a totally intracavernous carotid artery aneurysm. Neurosurgery 38:596–598, 1996.

Lee JP, Wang AD. Epistaxis due to traumatic intracavernous aneurysm: Case report. J Trauma 30:619–622, 1990.

Lee KC, Joo JY, Lee KS. False localization of rupture by computed tomography in bilateral internal carotid artery aneurysms. Surg Neurol 45:435–440; discussion 440–441, 1996.

Lee KF, Schatz NJ. Ischemic chiasmal syndrome. Acta Radiol Suppl 347:131–148, 1975.

Lee KS, Gower DJ, Branch CL Jr, et al. Surgical repair of aneurysms of the posterior inferior cerebellar artery—A clinical series. Surg Neurol 31:85–91, 1989.

Lee KS, Liu SS, Spetzler RF, et al. Intracranial mycotic aneurysm in an infant: Report of a case. Neurosurgery 26:129–133, 1990.

Lee SY, Sekhar LN. Treatment of aneurysms by excision or trapping with arterial reimplantation or interpositional grafting. Report of three cases. J Neurosurg 85:178–185, 1996.

Leipzig MJ, Brown FD. Treatment of mycotic aneurysms. Surg Neurol 23:403–407, 1985.

Leipzig TJ, Redelman K, Horner TG. Reducing the risk of rebleeding before early aneurysm surgery: A possible role for antifibrinolytic therapy. J Neurosurg 86:220–225, 1997.

Leishman R. The eye in general vascular disease, hypertension, and arteriosclerosis. Br J Ophthalmol 41:641–701, 1957.

Leivo S, Hernesniemi J, Luukkonen M, et al. Early surgery improves the cure of aneurysm-induced oculomotor palsy. Surg Neurol 45:430–434, 1996.

Leng SZ, Lu XQ, Pang SQ. Etiological analysis of 246 cases of oculomotor palsy. Chung Hua Yen Ko Tsa Chih 30:31–33, 1994.

Lepoire J, Montaut J, Renard M, et al. Anévrysme sacculaire de la carotide cervicale: Complication d'une angiographie carotidienne percutanée. Neurochirurgie 10:275–281, 1964.

Lepore FE, Glaser JS. Misdirection revisited: A critical appraisal of acquired oculomotor nerve synkinesis. Arch Ophthalmol 98:2206–2209, 1980.

Lerner DN. Nasal septal perforation and carotid cavernous aneurysm: Unusual manifestations of systemic lupus erythematosus. Otolaryngol Head Neck Surg 115:163–166, 1996.

Lesoin F, Rousseaux M, Autricque A, et al. Anévrysmes intracaverneux post-traumatiques: Deux observations. Neurochirurgie 34:50–54, 1988.

Lesser RL. A most atypical exotropia. Presented at the 29th Annual Frank B. Walsh Meeting, Baltimore, MD, April 5–6, 1997.

Levin HS, Goldstein FC, Ghostine SH, et al. Hemispheric disconnection syndrome persisting after anterior cerebral artery aneurysm rupture. Neurosurgery 21:831–838, 1987.

Levin P, Gross SW. Meningioma and aneurysm in the same patient. Arch Neurol 15:629–632, 1966.

Levy DI, Ku A. Balloon-assisted coil placement in wide-necked aneurysms: Technical note. J Neurosurg 86:724–727, 1997.

Levy ML, Giannotta SL. Cardiac performance indices during hypervolemic therapy for cerebral vasospasm. J Neurosurg 75:27–31, 1991.

Lewis AI, Tomsick TA, Tew JM Jr. Management of tentorial dural arteriovenous malformations: Transarterial embolization combined with stereotactic radiation or surgery. J Neurosurg 81:851–859, 1994.

Lewis R, Lampe H. An aneurysm of the external carotid artery presenting as a parotid mass: A case report. J Otolaryngol 22:413–414, 1993.

Lewis RA, Norton EWD, Gass JDM. Acquired arterial macroaneurysms of the retina. Br J Ophthalmol 60:21–30, 1976.

Ley A. Compression of the optic nerve by fusiform aneurysm of the carotid artery. J Neurol Neurosurg Psychiatry 13:75–86, 1950.

Leys D, Lesoin F, Pruvo JP, et al. Bilateral spontaneous dissection of extracranial vertebral arteries. J Neurol 234:237–240, 1987.

Leys D, Lucas C, Gobert M, et al. Cervical artery dissections. Eur Neurol 37:3–12, 1997.

Ley-Valle A, Vilalta J, Sahuquillo J, et al. Giant calcified aneurysm on the posterior cerebral artery in a nine-year-old child. Surg Neurol 20:396–398, 1983.

Liang EY, Chan M, Hsiang JH, et al. Detection and assessment of intracranial aneurysms: Value of CT angiography with shaded-surface display. AJR 165:1497–1502, 1995.

Liapis CD, Gugulakis A, Misiakos E, et al. Surgical treatment of extracranial carotid aneurysms. Int Angiol 13:290–295, 1994.

Lidov MW, Silvers AR, Mosesson RE, et al. Pantopaque simulating thrombosed intracranial aneurysms on MRI. J Comput Assist Tomogr 20:225–227, 1996.

Lie JT, Kim HS. Fibromuscular dysplasia of the superior mesenteric artery and coexisting cerebral berry aneurysms. Angiology 28:256–260, 1977.

Lieber BB, Stancampiano AP, Wakhloo AK. Alteration of hemodynamics in aneurysm models by stenting: Influence of stent porosity. Ann Biomed Eng 25:460–469, 1997.

Liebrecht K. Sehnerv und Arteriosclerose. Arch Augenheilkd 44:193–225, 1901.

Lieschke GJ, Davis S, Tress BM, et al. Spontaneous internal carotid artery dissection presenting as hypoglossal nerve palsy. Stroke 19:1151–1155, 1988.

Lieske JC, Toback FG. Autosomal dominant polycystic kidney disease. J Am Soc Nephrol 3:1442–1450, 1993.

Lightman S, Tyers A, Leaver P. Basilar aneurysm: An unusual cause of pain in a blind eye. Neuroophthalmology 4:39–41, 1984.

Lin BH, Vieco PT. Intracranial mycotic aneurysm in a patient with endocarditis caused by Cardiobacterium hominis. Can Assoc Radiol J 46:40–42, 1995.

Lin TK. Delayed intracerebral hematoma caused by traumatic intracavernous aneurysm: Case report. Neurosurgery 36:407–410, 1995.

Linden MD, Chou SM, Furlan AJ, et al. Cerebral arterial dissection. A case report with histopathologic and ultrastructural findings. Cleve Clin J Med 54:105–114, 1987.

Link J, Feyerabend B, Grabener M, et al. Dacron-covered stent-grafts for the percutaneous treatment of carotid aneurysms: Effectiveness and biocompatibility—Experimental study in swine. Radiology 200:397–401, 1996.

Linn FH, Wijdicks EF, van der Graaf Y, et al. Prospective study of sentinel headache in aneurysmal subarachnoid hemorrhage. Lancet 344:590–593, 1994.

Linskey ME, Sekhar LN, Hirsch W Jr, et al. Aneurysms of the intracavernous carotid artery: Clinical presentation, radiographic features, and pathogenesis. Neurosurgery 26:71–79, 1990a.

Linskey ME, Sekhar LN, Hirsch W Jr, et al. Aneurysms of the intracavernous carotid artery: Natural history and indications for treatment. Neurosurgery 26:933–938, 1990b.

Linskey ME, Sekhar LN, Horton JA, et al. Aneurysms of the intracavernous carotid artery: A multidisciplinary approach to treatment. J Neurosurg 75:525–534, 1991a.

Linskey ME, Horton JA, Rao GR, et al. Fatal rupture of the intracranial carotid artery during transluminal angioplasty for vasospasm induced by subarachnoid hemorrhage. Case report. J Neurosurg 74:985–990, 1991b.

Linskey ME, Jungreis CA, Yonas H, et al. Stroke risk after abrupt internal carotid artery sacrifice: Accuracy of preoperative assessment with balloon test occlusion and stable xenon-enhanced CT AJNR 15:829–843, 1994.

Litofsky NS, Vinuela F, Giannotta SL. Progressive visual loss after electrothrombosis treatment of a giant intracranial aneurysm: Case report. Neurosurgery 34: 548–550; discussion 551, 1994.

Litt AW. MR angiography of intracranial aneurysms: Proceed but with caution. AJNR 15:1615–1616, 1994.

Litten M. Ueber septische Erkrankungen. Z Klin Med 2:378, 1880.

Little JR, St Louis P, Weinstein M, et al. Giant fusiform aneurysm of the cerebral arteries. Stroke 12:183–188, 1981.

Little JR, Larkins MV, Lüders H, et al. Fusiform basilar artery aneurysm in a 33-month-old child. Neurosurgery 19:631–634, 1986.

Little JR, Rosenfeld JV, Awad IA. Internal carotid artery occlusion for cavernous segment aneurysm. Neurosurgery 25:398–404, 1989.

Liu MY, Shih CJ, Wang YC, et al. Traumatic intracavernous carotid aneurysm with massive epistaxis. Neurosurgery 17:569–573, 1985.

Ljunggren B, Brandt L, Kagstrom E, et al. Results of early operations for ruptured aneurysms. J Neurosurg 54:473–479, 1981.

Ljunggren B, Säveland H, Brandt L, et al. Early operation and overall outcome in aneurysmal subarachnoid hemorrhage. J Neurosurg 62:547–551, 1985.

Ljunggren B, Brandt L, Sundbarg G, et al. Early management of aneurysmal subarachnoid hemorrhage. Neurosurgery 11:412–418, 1982.

Ljunggren B, Brantit L, Säveland H, et al. Outcome in 60 consecutive patients treated with early aneurysm operation and intravenous nimodipine. J Neurosurg 61: 864–873, 1984.

Lloret MD, Escudero JR, Hospedales J, et al. Mycotic aneurysm of the carotid artery due to Salmonella enteritidis associated with multiple brain abscesses. Eur J Vasc Endovasc Surg 12:250–252, 1996.

Lloyd J, Bahnson HT. Bilateral dissecting aneurysms of the internal carotid arteries. Am J Surg 122:549–551, 1971.

Locksley HB. Report on the cooperative study of intracranial aneurysms and subarachnoid hemorrhage: V. Natural history of subarachnoid hemorrhage, intracranial aneurysms and arteriovenous malformations. Based on 6368 cases in the cooperative study. J Neurosurg 25:321–368, 1966.

Locksley HB. Natural history of subarachnoid hemorrhage, intracranial aneurysms and arteriovenous malformations. Based on 6,368 cases in the cooperative study. In Intracranial Aneurysms and Subarachnoid Hemorrhage: A Cooperative Study. Editors, Sahs AL, Perret GE, Locksley HB, et al., pp 37–108. Philadelphia, LB Lippincott, 1969.

Lomeo RM, Silver RM, Brothers M. Spontaneous dissection of the internal carotid artery in a patient with polyarteritis nodosa. Arth Rheum 32:1625–1626, 1989.

Longstreth WT, Nelson LM, Koepsell TD, et al. Subarachnoid hemorrhage and hormonal factors in women. A population-based case-control study. Ann Intern Med 121:168–173, 1994.

Lougheed WM, Marshall BM. The diploscope in intracranial aneurysms surgery: Results in 40 patients. Can J Surg 12:75–82, 1969.

Low M, Perktold K, Raunig R. Hemodynamics in rigid and distensible saccular aneurysms: A numerical study of pulsatile flow characteristics. Biorheology 30: 287–298, 1993.

Lozano AM, Leblanc R. Cerebral aneurysms and polycystic kidney disease: A critical review. Can J Neurol Sci 19:222–227, 1992.

Lozano AM, Leblanc R. Familial intracranial aneurysms. J Neurosurg 66:522–528, 1987.

Lustbader JM, Miller NR. Painless, pupil-sparing but otherwise complete oculomotor nerve paresis caused by basilar artery aneurysm. Arch Ophthalmol 106:583–584, 1988.

Lutcavage GJ. Traumatic facial artery aneurysm and arteriovenous fistula. Case report. J Oral Maxillofac Surg 50:402–405, 1992.

Lye RH. Basilar artery ectasia: An unusual cause of trigeminal neuralgia. J Neurol Neurosurg Psychiatry 49:22–28, 1986.

Lynch JC, Andrade R. Unilateral pterional approach to bilateral cerebral aneurysms. Surg Neurol 39:120–127, 1993.

Lyness SS, Wagman AD. Neurologic deficit following cervical manipulation. Surg Neurol 2:121–124, 1974.

Maass U. Die syphilis als häufigste Ursache der Aneurysmen an der Gehirnbasis. Beitr Pathol Anat 98:307–322, 1937.

Mabuchi S, Kamiyama H, Abe H. Distal aneurysms of the superior cerebellar artery and posterior inferior cerebellar artery feeding an associated arteriovenous malformation: Case report. Neurosurgery 30:284–287, 1992.

Mabuchi S, Kamiyama H, Kobayashi N, et al. A3-A3 side-to-side anastomosis in the anterior communicating artery aneurysm surgery: Report of four cases. Surg Neurol 44:122–127, 1995.

Macdonald RL, Weir BK. Cerebral vasospasm and free radicals. Free Radic Biol Med 16:633–643, 1994.

Macdonald RL, Wallace MC, Coyne TJ. The effect of surgery on the severity of vasospasm J Neurosurg 80:433–439, 1994.

MacDonald JD, Gyorke A, Jacobs JM, et al. Acute phase vascular endothelial injury: A comparison of temporary arterial occlusion using an endovascular occlusive balloon catheter versus a temporary aneurysm clip in a pig model. Neurosurgery 34:876–881; discussion 881, 1994.

MacFarlane MR, McAllister VL, Whitby DJ, et al. Posterior circulation aneurysms: Results of direct operations. Surg Neurol 20:399–413, 1983.

Madsen JR, Heros RC. Giant peripheral aneurysm of the posterior inferior cerebellar artery treated with excision and end-to-end anastomosis. Surg Neurol 30: 140–143, 1988.

Maeder PP, Meuli RA, de Tribolet N. Three-dimensional volume rendering for magnetic resonance angiography in the screening and preoperative workup of intracranial aneurysms. J Neurosurg 85:1050–1055, 1996.

Magnan PE, Branchereau A, Cannoni M. Traumatic aneurysms of the internal carotid artery at the base of the skull. Two cases treated surgically. J Cardiovasc Surg 33:372–379, 1992.

Mahaley MS Jr, Spock A. An unusual case of intracranial aneurysm. In Neuro-ophthalmology Symposium of the University of Miami and the Bascom Palmer Eye Institute. Editor, Smith JL, pp 158–166. St Louis, CV Mosby, 1968.

Mahmoud NA. Traumatic aneurysm of the internal carotid artery and epistaxis (review of literature and report of a case). J Laryngol Otol 93:629–656, 1979.

Maitland CG, Black JL, Smith WA. Abducens nerve palsy due to spontaneous dissection of the internal carotid artery. Arch Neurol 40:448–449, 1983.

Maiuri F, Gangemi M, Corriero G, et al. Anterior communicating artery aneurysm presenting with sudden paraplegia. Surg Neurol 25:397–398, 1986.

Maiuri F, Corriero G, D'Amico L, et al. Giant aneurysm of the pericallosal artery. Neurosurgery 26:703–706, 1990.

Maiuri F, Iaconetta G, Gallicchio B, et al. Olfactory groove meningioma and multiple aneurysms. Case report. Acta Neurol 14:1–5, 1992.

Maiuri F, Spaziante R, Iaconetta G, et al. 'De novo' aneurysm formation: Report of two cases. Clin Neurol Neurosurg 97:233–238, 1995.

Majamaa K, Savolainen ER, Myllyla VV. Synthesis of structurally unstable type III procollagen in patients with cerebral artery aneurysm. Biochim Biophys Acta 1138:191–196, 1992.

Makabe R. Netzhautblutung bei Makroaneurysma der Netzhautarterien. Klin Monatsbl Augenheilkd 178:471–472, 1981.

Maki Y, Nakada Y, Watanabe O, et al. Bilateral saccular aneurysms of the internal carotid artery in the cavernous sinus. Brain Nerve 22:379–385, 1970.

Makita K, Tsuchiya K, Furui S, et al. Nondissecting vertebral fusiform aneurysm: Embolization using wire-directed detachable balloons. AJNR 14:340–342, 1993.

Malecha MJ, Rubin R. Aneurysms of the carotid arteries associated with von Recklinghausen's neurofibromatosis. Pathol Res Pract 188:145–147, 1992.

Malik JM, Kamiryo T, Goble E, et al. Stereotactic laser-guided approach to distal middle cerebral artery aneurysms. Acta Neurochir 132:138–144, 1995.

Malisch TW, Guglielmi G, Vinuela F, et al. Intracranial aneurysms treated with the Guglielmi detachable coil: Midterm clinical results in a consecutive series of 100 patients. J Neurosurg 87:176–183, 1997.

Manabe H, Oda N, Ishii M, et al. The posterior inferior cerebellar artery originating from the internal carotid artery, associated with multiple aneurysms. Neuroradiology 33:513–515, 1991.

Mandai S, Kinugasa K, Ohmoto T. Direct thrombosis of aneurysms with cellulose acetate polymer. Part I: Results of thrombosis in experimental aneurysms. J Neurosurg 77:497–500, 1992a.

Mandai S, Nishino S, Itoh T, et al. A case of fibromuscular dysplasia associated with intra- and extracranial multiple aneurysms. No Shinkei Geka 20:611–615, 1992b.

Maniker AH, Hunt CD. Cerebral aneurysm in the HIV patient: A report of six cases. Surg Neurol 46:49–54, 1996.

Mann W, Gilsbach J, Amedee R, et al. Diseases of the intrapetrous carotid artery. Arch Otorhinolaryngol 245:69–73, 1988.

Manninen HI, Kolvisto T, Saari T, et al. Dissecting aneurysms of all four cervicocranial arteries in fibromuscular dysplasia: treatment with self-expanding endovascular stents, coil embolization, and surgical ligation. AJNR 18:1216–1220, 1997.

Manninen PH, Patterson S, Lam AM, et al. Evoked potential monitoring during posterior fossa aneurysm surgery: A comparison of two modalities. Can J Anaesth 41:92–97, 1994.

Manschot WA. The fundus oculi in subarachnoid hemorrhage. Acta Ophthalmol 22: 281–299, 1944.

Manschot WA. Subarachnoid hemorrhage: Intraocular symptoms and their pathogenesis. Am J Ophthalmol 38:501–505, 1954.

Manschot WA, Hampe JF. The origin of ocular symptoms in spontaneous subarachnoid hemorrhages. Acta XVI Concilium Ophthalmologicum, pp 356–357. London, British Medical Association, 1950.

Manz HJ, Luessenhop AJ. Dissecting aneurysm of intracranial vertebral artery: Case report and review of literature. J Neurol 230:25–35, 1983.

Manz HJ, Vester J, Lavenstein B. Dissecting aneurysm of cerebral arteries in childhood and adolescence: Case report and literature review of 20 cases. Virchows Arch. 384:325–335, 1979.

Marchal JC, Vespignani H, Bracard S, et al. Les dissections spontanees de la carotide interne extra-cranienne. A propos de trois observations. Utilite de l'occlusion-anastomose preventive. Neurochirurgie 31:199–205, 1985.

Marchal JC, Lescure JP, Bracard S, et al. Hemorragies sous-arachnoidiennes par rupture anevrismale. Chirurgie ou embolisation? Ann Fr Anesth Reanim 15: 342–347, 1996.

Marchau MMB, Vallaeys J, Vanhoonen G. Thrombosis of a giant aneurysm of the basilar artery. Neurosurgery 22:612–613, 1988.

Marchel A, Bidzinski J, Bojarski P. Formation of new aneurysms. Report of five cases. Acta Neurochir 112:96–99, 1991.

Marchel A, Bidzinski J, Bojarski P. Analiza kliniczna i wyniki leczenia operacyjnego chorych z tetniakami ukladu kregowo-podstawnego. Neurol Neurochir Pol 26: 192–200, 1992.

Margolis MT, Stein RL, Newton TH. Extracranial aneurysms of the internal carotid artery. Neuroradiology 4:78–89, 1972.

Marin ML, Veith FJ. Endovascular stents and stented grafts for the treatment of aneurysms and other arterial lesions. Adv Surg 29:93–109, 1996.

Marks MP, Lane B, Steinberg GK, et al. Intranidal aneurysms in cerebral arteriovenous malformations: Evaluation and endovascular treatment. Radiology 183:355–360, 1992.

Marks MP, Tsai C, Chee H. In vitro evaluation of coils for endovascular therapy. AJNR 17:29–34, 1996.

Marks P. Posterior circulation aneurysms. Br J Neurosurg 10:337–341, 1996.

Markwalder TM, Meienberg O. Acute painful cavernous sinus syndrome in unruptured intracavernous aneurysms of the internal carotid artery: Possible pathogenetic mechanisms. J Clin Neuroophthalmol 3:31–35, 1983.

Marmor M, Wertenbaker C, Berstein L. Delayed ophthalmoplegia following head trauma. Surv Ophthalmol 27:126–132, 1982.

Maroon JC, Lunsford LD, Deeb ZL. Hemifacial spasm due to aneurysmal compression of the facial nerve. Arch Neurol 35:545–546, 1978.

Maroun FB, Murray GP, Jacob JC, et al. Familial intracranial aneurysms: Report of three families. Surg Neurol 25:85–88, 1986.

Marsh H, Maurice-Williams RS, Lindsay KW. Differences in the management of ruptured intracranial aneurysms: A survey of practice amongst British neurosurgeons. J Neurol Neurosurg Psychiatry 50:965–970, 1987.

Martinez AJ, Sotelo-Avila C, Alcala H, et al. Granulomatous encephalitis, intracranial arteritis, and mycotic aneurysm due to a free-living ameba. Acta Neuropathol 49:7–12, 1980.

Martini E. Intracranial dissecting aneurysm: Report of a case. Arch Psychiatr Nervenkrankh 227:17–21, 1979.

Martins IP, Ferro JM. Atypical facial pain, ectasia of the basilar artery, and baclofen: A case report. Headache 29:581–583, 1989.

Maruki C, Suzukawa K, Koike J, et al. Cardiac malignant fibrous histiocytoma metastasizing to the brain: Development of multiple neoplastic cerebral aneurysms. Surg Neurol 41:40–44, 1994.

Maruyama M, Asai T, Kuriyama Y, et al. Positive platelet scintigram of a vertebral aneurysm presenting thromboembolic transient ischemic attacks. Stroke 20: 687–690, 1989.

Mas JL, Goeau C, Bousser MG, et al. Spontaneous dissecting aneurysms of the internal carotid and vertebral arteries: Two case reports. Stroke 16:125–129, 1985.

Mas JL, Bousser MG, Corone P, et al. Anévrysme disséquant des artères vertébrales extracraniennes et grossesse. Rev Neurol 143:761–764, 1987.

Mas JL, Henin D, Bousser MG, et al. Dissecting aneurysm of the vertebral artery and cervical manipulation: A case report with autopsy. Neurology 39:512–515, 1989.

Masago A, Fukuoka H, Yoshida T, et al. Intracranial mycotic aneurysm caused by Aspergillus—Case report. Neurol Med Chir 32:904–907, 1992.

Mascalchi M, Bianchi MC, Mangiafico S, et al. MRI and MR angiography of vertebral artery dissection. Neuroradiology 39:329–340, 1997.

Mase M, Banno T, Yamada K, et al. Endovascular stent placement for multiple aneurysms of the extracranial internal carotid artery: Technical case report. Neurosurgery 37:832–835, 1995.

Massey CE, El Gammal T, Brooks BS. Giant posterior inferior cerebellar artery aneurysm with dysphagia. Surg Neurol 22:467–471, 1984.

Masson RL Jr, Day AL. Aneurysmal intracerebral hemorrhage. Neurosurg Clin North Am 3:539–550, 1992.

Massoud TF, Molyneux AJ. Spontaneous dissection of both intracranial vertebral arteries. Neuroradiology 36:224–225, 1994.

Massoud TF, Guglielmi G, Vinuela F, et al. Saccular aneurysms in moyamoya disease: Endovascular treatment using electrically detachable coils. Surg Neurol 41: 462–467, 1994.

Massoud TF, Turjman F, Ji C, et al. Endovascular treatment of fusiform aneurysms with stents and coils: Technical feasibility in a swine model. AJNR 16: 1953–1963, 1995.

Masuda J, Yutani C, Waki R, et al. Histopathological analysis of the mechanisms of intracranial hemorrhage complicating infective endocarditis. Stroke 23:843–850, 1992.

Masuzawa T, Shimabukuro H, Furuse M, et al. Pulseless disease associated with a ruptured intracranial aneurysm. Neurol Med Chir 24:490–494, 1984.

Mathiesen T, Edner G, Ulfarsson E, et al. Cerebrospinal fluid interleukin-1 receptor antagonist and tumor necrosis factor-α following subarachnoid hemorrhage. J Neurosurg 87:215–220, 1997.

Mathis JM, DeNardo A, Jensen ME, et al. Transient neurologic events associated with intraarterial papaverine infusion for subarachnoid hemorrhage-induced vasospasm. AJNR 15:1671–1674, 1994.

Matricali B, Seminara P. Aneurysm arising from the medial branch of the superior cerebellar artery. Neurosurgery 18:350–352, 1986.

Matson DD. Intracranial arterial aneurysms in childhood. J Neurosurg 23:578–583, 1965.

Matsuda M, Matsuda I, Handa H, et al. Intracavernous giant aneurysm associated with Marfan's syndrome. Surg Neurol 12:119–121, 1979.

Matsuda M, Shiino A, Handa J. Sequential changes of cerebral blood flow after aneurysmal subarachnoid hemorrhage. Acta Neurochir 105:98–106, 1990.

Matsuda M, Kidooka M, Nakazawa T, et al. Intraoperative monitoring of somatosensory evoked potentials in patients with cerebral aneurysm—Correlation between central conduction time and postoperative neurological status. Neurol Med Chir 31:13–17, 1991.

Matsumara M, Wada H, Ohwada A, et al. Unruptured intracranial aneurysms and polycystic kidney disease. Acta Neurochir 79:94–99, 1986.

Matsumoto K, Kato A, Fujii K, et al. Bilateral giant intracavernous carotid artery aneurysms mimicking a cavernous sinus neoplasm: Case report. Neurol Med Chir 36:583–585, 1996.

Matsumoto K, Saijo T, Kuyama H, et al. Hemifacial spasm caused by a spontaneous dissecting aneurysm of the vertebral artery. Case report. J Neurosurg 74:650–652, 1991.

Matsumoto T, Yamaura I, Morimura T, et al. A case of aneurysm of the peripheral middle cerebral artery presenting putaminal hemorrhage—Pitfall in diagnosis. No To Shinkei 44:1133–1136, 1992.

Matsumura H, Iwai F, Ichikizaki K. Ischemic myocardial disorder in acute phase subarachnoid hemorrhage: Clinical study of 52 patients. No Shinkei Geka 19: 349–357, 1991.

Matsuo K, Kobayashi S, Sugita K. Bitemporal hemianopsia associated with sclerosis of the intracranial internal carotid artery. J Neurosurg 53:566–569, 1980.

Matsuyama T, Hoshida T, Sakaki T. A characteristic magnetic resonance image of a dissecting aneurysm in the vertebrobasilar system. No Shinkei Geka 21:819–821, 1993.

Maurer J, Maurer E, Perneczky A. Surgically verified variations in the A1 segment of the anterior cerebral artery. Report of two cases. J Neurosurg 75:950–953, 1991.

Maurer JJ, Mills M, German WJ. Triad of unilateral blindness, orbital fractures and massive epistaxis after head injury. J Neurosurg 18:837–840, 1961.

Maurice-Williams RS. Ruptured intracranial aneurysms: Has the incidence of early rebleeding been over-estimated? J Neurol Neurosurg Psychiatry 45:774–779, 1982.

Maurice-Williams RS, Harvey PK. Isolated palsy of the fourth cranial nerve caused by an intracranial aneurysm. J Neurol Neurosurg Psychiatry 52:679, 1989.

Maurice-Williams RS, Kitchen ND. Ruptured intracranial aneurysms—Learning from experience. Br J Neurosurg 8:519–527, 1994.

Maurice-Williams RS, Marsh H. Ruptured intracranial aneurysms: The overall effect of treatment and the influence of patient selection and data presentation on the reported outcome. J Neurol Neurosurg Psychiatry 48:1208–1212, 1985.

Mawad ME, Klucznik RP. Giant serpentine aneurysms: Radiographic features and endovascular treatment. AJNR 16:1053–1060, 1995.

Mawad ME, Mawad JK, Cartwright J Jr, et al. Long-term histopathologic changes in canine aneurysms embolized with Guglielmi detachable coils. AJNR 16:7–13, 1995.

Mayer PL, Awad I. Subarachnoid hemorrhage and choir singing. J Neurosurg 81: 159–160, 1994.

Mayer PL, Awad IA, Todor R, et al. Misdiagnosis of symptomatic cerebral aneurysm: Prevalence and correlation with outcome at four institutions. Stroke 27: 1558–1563, 1996.

McAuliffe W, Townsend M, Eskridge JM, et al. Intracranial pressure changes induced during papaverine infusion for treatment of vasospasm. J Neurosurg 83:430–434, 1995.

McCollum CH, Wheeler WG, Noon GP, et al. Aneurysms of the extracranial carotid artery: Twenty-one years' experience. Am J Surg 137:196–200, 1979.

McConachie NS, Jacobson I. Bilateral aneurysms of the cavernous internal carotid arteries following yttrium-90 implantation. Neuroradiology 36:611–613, 1994.

McCormick WF, Schmalstieg EJ. The relationship of arterial hypertension to intracranial aneurysms. Arch Neurol 34:285–288, 1977.

McCormick WF, Nofzinger JD. Saccular intracranial aneurysms: An autopsy study. J Neurosurg 22:155–159, 1965.

McCulloch D, Bryan A. Cerebral aneurysm presenting with epilepsy. Postgrad Med 58:94–97, 1982.

McDermott VG, Sellar RJ. Superior cerebellar artery aneurysms associated with infratentorial arteriovenous malformations. Clin Imaging 18:209–212, 1994.

McDonald CA, Korb M. Intracranial aneurysms. Arch Neurol Psychiatr 42:298–328, 1939.

McDougall CG, Halbach VV, Dowd CF, et al. Endovascular treatment of basilar tip aneurysms using electrolytically detachable coils. J Neurosurg 84:393–399, 1996.

McFadzean RM, Hadley DM, McIlwaine GG. Optochiasmal arachnoiditis following muslin wrapping of ruptured anterior communicating artery aneurysm. J Neurosurg 75:393–396, 1991.

McIvor NP, Willinsky RA, TerBrugge KG, et al. Validity of test occlusion studies prior to internal carotid artery sacrifice. Head Neck 16:11–16, 1994.

McKinna AJ. Eye signs in 611 cases of posterior fossa aneurysms: Their diagnostic and prognostic value. Can J Ophthalmol 18:3–6, 1983.

McKissock W, Richardson AE, Walsh L. Posterior communicating aneurysms: A controlled trial of the conservative and surgical treatment of ruptured aneurysms of the internal carotid artery at or near the point of origin of the posterior communicating artery. Lancet *1*:1203–1206, 1960.

McLaughlin MR, Jho HD, Kwon Y. Acute subdural hematoma caused by a ruptured giant intracavernous aneurysm: Case report. Neurosurgery 38:388–392, 1996.

McLean JM, Ray BS. Soft glaucoma and calcification of the internal carotid arteries. Arch Ophthalmol 38:154–158, 1947.

McLellan NJ, Prasad R, Punt J. Spontaneous subhyaloid and retinal hemorrhages in an infant. Arch Dis Child *61*:1130–1132, 1986.

Meadows SP. Symptoms and signs of anterior communicating artery aneurysms. In Modern Trends in Neurology. Editor, Feiling A, p 39. London, Butterworth, 1951.

Meadows SP. Intracavernous aneurysms of the internal carotid artery: Their clinical features and natural history. Arch Ophthalmol 62:566–574, 1959.

Medhkour A, Leblanc G, Francoeur J, et al. Chirurgie précoce des anévrysmes intra-craniens. Neurochirurgie 32:418–422, 1986.

Medlock MD, Dulebohn SC, Elwood PW. Prophylactic hypervolemia without calcium channel blockers in early aneurysm surgery. Neurosurgery 30:12–16, 1992.

Mee E, Dorrance D, Lowe D, et al. Controlled study of nimodipine in aneurysm patients treated early after subarachnoid hemorrhage. Neurosurgery 22:484–491, 1988.

Meguro K, Rowed DW. Traumatic aneurysm of the posterior inferior cerebellar artery caused by fracture of the clivus. Neurosurgery 16:666–668, 1985.

Mehalic T, Farhat SM. Vertebral artery injury from chiropractic manipulation of the neck. Surg Neurol 2:125–129, 1974.

Mehler MF. The clinical spectrum of ocular bobbing and ocular dipping. J Neurol Neurosurg Psychiatry *51*:725–727, 1988.

Mehta V, Holness RO, Connolly K, et al. Acute hydrocephalus following aneurysmal subarachnoid hemorrhage. Can J Neurol Sci 23:40–45, 1996.

Meier P, Wiedermann P. Glaskörper- und Fundusveränderungen beim Terson-syndrom: Drei Falldarstellungen. Klin Monatsbl Augenheilkd 209:244–248, 1996.

Meisel HJ, Rodesch G, Alvarez H, et al. Der Einsatz von GDC coils zur Behandlung inoperabler Aneurysmen: Erster Erfahrungsbericht. Zentralbl Neurochir 56:27–33, 1995.

Meixensberger J, Hamelbeck B, Dings J, et al. Critical increase of blood flow velocities after subarachnoid hemorrhage: Vasospasm versus hyperaemia. Zentralbl Neurochir 57:70–75, 1996.

Mercier P, Alhayek G, Rizk T, et al. Les anticalciques sont-ils reellement utiles en chirurgie anevrysmale cerebrale? Neurochirurgie 39:149–156, 1993.

Merkus JW, Nieuwenhuijzen GA, Jacobs PP, et al. Traumatic pseudoaneurysm of the superficial temporal artery. Injury 25:468–471, 1994.

Merva W, Jamshidi S, Kurtzke JF. Posterior communicating artery giant aneurysm as a cause of seizures. Neurology 35:620–622, 1985.

Merwarth HR, Feiring E. Modifications of induced nystagmus by acute cerebral lesions. Brooklyn Hosp J *1*:99–106, 1939.

Mettinger KL. Fibromuscular dysplasia and the brain: II. Current concept of the disease. Stroke *13*:53–58, 1982.

Mettinger KL, Ericson K. Fibromuscular dysplasia and the brain: I. Observations on angiogramic, clinical and genetic characteristics. Stroke *13*:46–52, 1982.

Meyer CHA, Lowe D, Meyer M, et al. Progressive change in cerebral blood flow during the first three weeks of subarachnoid hemorrhage. Neurosurgery *12*:58–76, 1983.

Meyer FB, Sundt TM Jr, Fode NC, et al. Cerebral aneurysms in childhood and adolescence. J Neurosurg 70:420–425, 1989.

Meyer FB, Morita A, Puumala MR, et al. Medical and surgical management of intracranial aneurysms Mayo Clin Proc 70:153–172, 1995.

Meyer YJ, Batjer HH. Resolution of a recurrentresidual bacterial aneurysm during antibiotic therapy. Neurosurgery 26:537–539, 1990.

Meyerson L, Lazar SJ. Intraorbital aneurysm of the ophthalmic artery. Br J Ophthalmol 55:199–204, 1971.

Michael WF. Posterior fossa aneurysms simulating tumours. J Neurol Neurosurg Psychiatry 37:218–223, 1974.

Micheli F, Schteinschnaider A, Plaghos LL, et al. Bacterial cavernous sinus aneurysm treated by detachable balloon technique. Stroke 20:1751–1754, 1989.

Mickey B, Vorstrup S, Voldby B, et al. Serial measurement of regional cerebral blood flow in patients with SAH using 133Xe inhalation and emission computerized tomography. J Neurosurg 60:916–922, 1984.

Milenkovic Z, Duric S, Stefanovic I, et al. Multiple intrakranijalne aneurizme i asimetricni Willisov prsten. Med Pregl 48:32–35, 1995.

Milhorat TH. Acute hydrocephalus after aneurysmal subarachnoid hemorrhage. Neurosurgery 20:15–20, 1987.

Milhorat TH, Krautheim M. Results of early and delayed operations for ruptured intracranial aneurysms in two series of 100 consecutive patients. Surg Neurol 26:123–128, 1986.

Miller AJ, Cuttino JT. On the mechanism of production of massive preretinal hemorrhage following rupture of a congenital medial-defect intracranial aneurysm. Am J Ophthalmol *31*:15–24, 1948.

Miller CA, Hill SA, Hunt WE. "De novo" aneurysms: A clinical review. Surg Neurol 24:173–180, 1985.

Miller EM, Newton TH. Extra-axial posterior fossa lesions simulating intraaxial lesions on computed tomography. Radiology *127*:675–679, 1978.

Miller JA, Cross DT, Moran CJ, et al. Severe thrombocytopenia following intraarterial papaverine administration for treatment of vasospasm. J Neurosurg 83:435–437, 1995.

Miller NR. Walsh and Hoyt's Clinical Neuroophthalmology. 4th ed, Vol 4, pp 2079–2080. Baltimore, Williams & Wilkins, 1991a.

Miller NR. Walsh and Hoyt's Clinical Neuroophthalmology. 4th ed, Vol 4, pp 2086–2087. Baltimore, Williams & Wilkins, 1991b.

Miller NR. Walsh and Hoyt's Clinical Neuroophthalmology. 4th ed, Vol 4, p 2092. Baltimore, Williams & Wilkins, 1991c.

Miller NR. Walsh and Hoyt's Clinical Neuroophthalmology. 4th ed, Vol 4, p 1999. Baltimore, Williams & Wilkins, 1991d.

Miller NR. Walsh and Hoyt's Clinical Neuroophthalmology. 4th ed, Vol 4, p 2010. Baltimore, Williams & Wilkins, 1991e.

Miller NR. Walsh and Hoyt's Clinical Neuroophthalmology. 4th ed, Vol 4, p 2042. Baltimore, Williams & Wilkins, 1991f.

Miller NR. Walsh and Hoyt's Clinical Neuroophthalmology. 4th ed, Vol 4, p 2050. Baltimore, Williams & Wilkins, 1991g.

Miller NR. Walsh and Hoyt's Clinical Neuroophthalmology. 4th ed, Vol 4, p 2102. Baltimore, Williams & Wilkins, 1991h.

Miller NR. Walsh and Hoyt's Clinical Neuroophthalmology. 4th ed, Vol 4, pp 2105–2106. Baltimore, Williams & Wilkins, 1991i.

Miller NR. Walsh and Hoyt's Clinical Neuroophthalmology. 4th ed, Vol 4, p 2138. Baltimore, Williams & Wilkins, 1991j.

Miller NR. Bilateral visual loss and simultagnosia after lumboperitoneal shunt for pseudotumor cerebri. J Neuroophthalmol *17*:36–38, 1997.

Miller NR, Savino PJ, Schneider T. Rapid growth of an intracranial aneurysm causing apparent retrobulbar optic neuritis. J Neuroophthalmol *15*:212–218, 1995.

Miller RG, Burton R. Stroke following chiropractic manipulation of the spine. JAMA 229:189–190, 1974.

Milliser RV, Greenberg SR, Neiman BH. Congenital or berry aneurysm in the optic nerve. J Clin Pathol *21*:335–338, 1968.

Milner JW Jr, Hardjasudarma M, Megison RP. Aneurysms of the posterior cerebral and superior cerebellar arteries in a child. Can Assoc Radiol J *45*:130–133, 1994.

Mimata C, Kitaoka M, Nagahiro S, et al. Differential distribution and expressions of collagens in the cerebral aneurysmal wall. Acta Neuropathol 94:197–206, 1997.

Minakawa T, Kolke T, Fujii Y, et al. Long-term results of ruptured aneurysms treated by coating. Neurosurgery *21*:660–663, 1987.

Miner ME, Rea GL, Handel S, et al. Trigeminal neuralgia due to dolichoectasia: Angiographic and CT findings in a patient with the EEC syndrome. Neuroradiology 20:163–166, 1980.

Minion DJ, Lynch TG, Baxter BT, et al. Pseudoaneurysm of the external carotid artery following radical neck dissection and irradiation: A case report and review of the literature. Cardiovasc Surg 2:607–611, 1994.

Minola E, Maculotti L. Lesioni vascolari multiple in paziente con sindrome di Ehlers-Danlos di tipo IV. Pathologica 86:61–65, 1994.

Mintz A, Cosgrove GR. Multiple peripheral aneurysms of the posterior inferior cerebellar artery associated with a cerebellar arteriovenous malformation: Case report. Neurosurgery 26:533–537, 1990.

Mishima H, Kim YK, Shiomi K, et al. Ruptured anterior communicating artery aneurysm associated with inter-optic course of anterior cerebral artery: Report of a case and review of the literature. No Shinkei Geka 22:495–498, 1994.

Misra BK, Whittle IR, Steers AJW, et al. De novo saccular aneurysms. Neurosurgery 23:10–15, 1988.

Misra M, Mohanty AB, Rath S. Giant aneurysm of internal carotid artery presenting features of retrobulbar neuritis. Indian J Ophthalmol 39:28–29, 1991.

Mitchell N, Angrist A. Intracranial aneurysms—A report of thirty-six cases. Ann Intern Med *19*:909–921, 1943.

Mitchell SW. Aneurysm of an anomalous artery causing anteroposterior division of the chiasm and optic nerves and producing bitemporal hemianopsia. J Nerv Ment Dis *14*:44–62, 1889.

Mitts MG, McQueen JD. Visual loss associated with fusiform enlargement of the intracranial portion of the internal carotid artery. J Neurosurg 23:33–37, 1965.

Miyachi S, Negoro M, Handa T, et al. Vascular endoscopy for intravascular surgery—An experimental study. Neurol Med Chir 32:323–327, 1992a.

Miyachi S, Negoro M, Handa T, et al. Histopathological study of balloon embolization: Silicone versus latex. Neurosurgery 30:483–489, 1992b.

Miyachi S, Ishiguchi T, Taniguichi K, et al. Endovascular stenting of a traumatic dissecting aneurysm of the extracranial internal carotid artery: Case report. Neurol Med Chir 37:270–274, 1997.

Miyagi J, Shigemori M, Hirohata M, et al. Fenestrated basilar artery with ruptured cerebral aneurysms: Case report. No Shinkei Geka *18*:1129–1133, 1990.

Miyagi J, Shigemori M, Sugita Y, et al. Giant aneurysm of the middle cerebral artery presenting with complex partial seizure: Case report. Neurol Med Chir *31*:953–956, 1991.

Miyahara S, Cheng CL, Kitamura K. Intracranial aneurysm due to arterial injury at surgery. Neurol Surg 5:991–994, 1977.

Miyamoto S, Kikuchi H, Karasawa J, et al. Study of the posterior circulation in moyamoya disease. J Neurosurg 65:454–460, 1986.

Miyaoka M, Sato K, Ishii S. A clinical study of the relationship of timing to outcome of surgery for ruptured cerebral aneurysms. A retrospective analysis of 1622 cases. J Neurosurg 79:373–378, 1993.

Miyatake S, Kikuchi H, Kondoh S, et al. Treatment of a giant aneurysm of the cavernous internal carotid artery associated with a persistent primitive trigeminal artery: Case report. Neurosurgery 26:315–319, 1990.

Miyauchi M, Shionoya S. Aneurysm of the extracranial internal carotid artery caused by fibromuscular dysplasia. Eur J Vasc Surg 5:587–591, 1991.

Miyazaki S, Yamaura A, Kamata K, et al. A dissecting aneurysm of the vertebral artery. Surg Neurol 21:171–174, 1984.

Miyazawa T, Watanabe M, Hasegawa T, et al. A case of posterior communicating artery aneurysm associated with vascular anomaly of circle of Willis. Neurol Surg 11:541–546, 1983.

Mizoi K, Takahashi A, Yoshimoto T, et al. Combined endovascular and neurosurgical approach for paraclinoid internal carotid artery aneurysms. Neurosurgery 33:986–992, 1993.

Mizoi K, Yoshimoto T, Takahashi A, et al. Direct clipping of basilar trunk aneurysms using temporary balloon occlusion. J Neurosurg 80:230–236, 1994.

Mizoi K, Yoshimoto T, Nagamine Y, et al. How to treat incidental cerebral aneurysms: A review of 139 consecutive cases. Surg Neurol 44:114–120; discussion 120–121, 1995.

Mizukami M, Kawase T, Usami T, et al. Prevention of vasospasm by early operation with removal of subarachnoid blood. Neurosurgery 10:301–307, 1982.

Mizuno M, Nakajima S, Sampei T, et al. Serial transcranial Doppler flow velocity and cerebral blood flow measurements for evaluation of cerebral vasospasm after subarachnoid hemorrhage. Neurol Med Chir 34:164–171, 1994.

Mizushima H, Sasaki K, Kunii N, et al. Dissecting aneurysm in the proximal region of the posterior inferior cerebellar artery presenting as Wallenberg's syndrome—Case report. Neurol Med Chir 34: 307–310, 1994.

Mizutani T. Middle cerebral artery dissecting aneurysm with persistent patent pseudolumen. Case report. J Neurosurg 84:267–268, 1996.

Mizutani T, Aruga T. ''Dolichoectatic'' intracranial vertebrobasilar dissecting aneurysm. Neurosurgery 31:765–773; discussion 773, 1992.

Mizutani T, Goldberg HI, Parr J, et al. Cerebral dissecting aneurysm and intimal fibroelastic thickening of cerebral arteries. J Neurosurg 56:571–576, 1982.

Mizutani T, Aruga T, Kirino T, et al. Recurrent subarachnoid hemorrhage from untreated ruptured vertebrobasilar dissecting aneurysms. Neurosurgery 36:905–911; discussion 912–913, 1995.

Mochimatsu Y, Fujitsu K, Hayashi A, et al. Giant aneurysm of the distal posterior cerebral artery: Case report. Neurol Med Chir 27:214–217, 1987.

Mohr JP, Rubinstein LV, Kase CS, et al. Gaze palsy in hemispheral stroke: The NINCDS stroke data bank. Neurology 34(Suppl 1):199, 1984.

Mokri B, Piepgras DG. Cervical internal carotid artery aneurysm with calcific embolism to the retina. Neurology 31:211–214, 1981.

Mokri B, Houser OW, Sundt TM Jr. Idiopathic regressing arteriopathy. Ann Neurol 2:466–472, 1977.

Mokri B, Sundt TM Jr, Houser OW. Spontaneous internal carotid dissection, hemicrania, and Horner's syndrome. Arch Neurol 36:677–680, 1979.

Mokri B, Piepgras DG, Sundt TM Jr, et al. Extracranial internal carotid artery aneurysms. Mayo Clin Proc 57:310–321, 1982.

Mokri B, Sundt TM Jr, Houser OW, et al. Spontaneous dissection of the cervical internal carotid artery. Ann Neurol 19:126–138, 1986.

Mokri B, Piepgras DG, Wiebers DO, et al. Familial occurence of spontaneous dissection of the internal carotid artery. Stroke 18:246–251, 1987.

Mokri B, Houser OW, Sandok BA, et al. Spontaneous dissections of the vertebral arteries. Neurol 38:880–885, 1988a.

Mokri B, Piepgras DG, Houser OW. Traumatic dissections of the extracranial internal carotid artery. J Neurosurg 68:189–197, 1988b.

Molinari GF, Smith L, Goldstein MN, et al. Pathogenesis of cerebral mycotic aneurysms. Neurology 23:325–332, 1973.

Molyneux AJ, Ellison DW, Morris J, et al. Histological findings in giant aneurysms treated with Guglielmi detachable coils. Report of two cases with autopsy correlation. J Neurosurg 83:129–132, 1995.

Monfort JC, Degos JD, Eizenbaum JF, et al. Aspect artériographique de dysplasie fibro-musculaire révélé par une dissection de la carotide. Ann Med Interne 132:333–336, 1981.

Moniz E. L'encephalographie arterielle, son importance dans la localisation des tumeurs cerebrales. Rev Neurol 2:72–90, 1927.

Moniz E. Aneurysme intra-cranien de la carotide interne droite rendu visible par l'arteriographie cerebrale. Rev d'Oto-Neurol Ophthal 11:746–748, 1933.

Montgomery EB, Grubb RL, Raichle ME. Cerebral hemodynamics and metabolism in postoperative cerebral vasospasm and treatment with hypertensive therapy. Ann Neurol 9:502–506, 1981.

Moore D, Budde RB, Hunter CR, et al. Massive epistaxis from aneurysm of the carotid artery. Surg Neurol 11:115–117, 1979.

Morard M, de Tribolet N. Traumatic aneurysm of the posterior inferior cerebellar artery: Case report. Neurosurgery 29:438–441, 1991.

Morawetz RB, Karp RB. Evolution and resolution of intracranial bacterial (mycotic) aneurysms. Neurosurgery 15:43–49, 1984.

Moreau P, Albat B, Thevenet A. Surgical treatment of extracranial internal carotid artery aneurysm. Ann Vas Surg 8:409–416, 1994.

Moret J, Morax M, Sachs M, et al. Traitement endovasculaire des anevrysmes carot-

idiens geants a manifestations ophtalmologiques. Bull Soc Ophtalmol Fr 87:29–332, 1987.

Morgagni JB. De Sedibus et Causis Morborum per Anatomen Indagatis, Book 1, letters 3 & 4, Venetis, Remodiniana, 1769.

Morgan DW, Honan W. Lateral gaze palsy due to giant aneurysm of the posterior fossa. J Neurol Neurosurg Psychiatry 52:883–886, 1988.

Morgenstern LB, Hankins LL, Grotta JC. Anterior choroidal artery aneurysm and stroke. Neurology 47:1090–1092, 1996.

Mori K, Arai H, Nakajima K, et al. Hemorheological and hemodynamic analysis of hypervolemic hemodilution therapy for cerebral vasospasm after aneurysmal subarachnoid hemorrhage. Stroke 26:1620–1626, 1995.

Mori K, Mishina H, Shimoji T, et al. Rupture of intracranial aneurysm due to intravascular metastasis of choriocarcinoma. Case report. Neurol Med Chir 30:858–862, 1990.

Mori K, Cho K, Suda K, et al. Changes in red blood cell aggregation rate after aneurysmal subarachnoid hemorrhage. No Shinkei Geka 24:541–548, 1996.

Mori T, Fujimoto M, Sakae K, et al. A case of subarachnoid hemorrhage with acute subdural hematoma due to head injury: A case report. No Shinkei Geka 23:249–252, 1995.

Morimatsu M, Hirai S, Yamauchi H, et al. A case of ''moyamoya'' disease presenting as Balint's syndrome. Neurol Med 6:416–422, 1977.

Morioka M, Marubayashi T, Masumitsu T, et al. Wrapping of intracranial aneurysms with gauze sponge. Neurol Med Chir 31:135–140, 1991.

Moriuchi S, Nakagawa H, Yamada M, et al. Hemifacial spasm due to compression of the facial nerve by vertebral artery-posterior inferior cerebellar artery aneurysm and elongated vertebral artery: Case report. Neurol Med Chir 36:884–887, 1996.

Moriyama E, Matsumoto Y, Meguro T, et al. Progress in the management of patients with aneurysmal subarachnoid hemorrhage: A single hospital review for 20 years. Part I: Younger patients. Surg Neurol 44:522–527, 1995a.

Moriyama E, Matsumoto Y, Meguro T, et al. Progress in the management of patients with aneurysmal subarachnoid hemorrhage: A single hospital review for 20 years. Part II: Aged patients. Surg Neurol 44:528–533, 1995b.

Moriyama E, Matsumoto Y, Meguro T, et al. Combined cisternal drainage and intrathecal urokinase injection therapy for prevention of vasospasm in patients with aneurysmal subarachnoid hemorrhage. Neurol Med Chir 35:732–736, 1995c.

Moriyama T, Shigemori M, Hirohata Y, et al. Multiple intracranial aneurysms following radiation therapy for pituitary adenoma: A case report. No Shinkei Geka 20:487–492, 1992.

Morota N, Ohtsuka A, Kameyama S, et al. Obstructive hydrocephalus due to a giant aneurysm of the internal carotid bifurcation. Surg Neurol 29:227–231, 1988.

Morris DP, Ballagh RH, Hong A, et al. Thrombosed posterior-inferior cerebellar artery aneurysm: A rare cerebellopontine angle tumour. J Laryngol Otol 109:429–430, 1995.

Morris KM, Shaw MD, Foy PM. Smoking and subarachnoid hemorrhage: A case control study. Br J Neurosurg 6:429–432, 1992.

Morriss FH Jr, Spock A. Intracranial aneurysm secondary to mycotic orbital and sinus infection: Report of a case implicating Penicillium as an opportunistic fungus. Am J Dis Child 119:357–362, 1970.

Moschner C, Moser A, Kömpf D. Bilateral oculomotor nerve palsy due to dolichoectasia of the basilar artery. Neuroophthalmology 17:39–43, 1997.

Moseley I, Holland J. Ectasia of the basilar artery: The breadth of the clinical spectrum and the diagnostic value of computed tomography. Neuroradiology 18:83–91, 1979.

Moskowitz MA, Rosenbaum AE, Tyler HR. Angiographically monitored resolution of cerebral mycotic aneurysms. Neurology 24:1103–1108, 1974.

Motuo Fotso MJ, Brunon J, Outhel R, et al. Anevrysmes familiaux, anevrysmes multiples et anevrysmes ''de novo.'' A propos de deux observations. Neurochirurgie 39:225–230, 1993.

Mount LA, Antunes JL. Results of treatment of treatment of intracranial aneurysms by wrapping and coating. J Neurosurg 42:189–193, 1975.

Mourad J-J, Girerd X, Safar M. Carotid-artery dissection after a prolonged telephone call. N Engl J Med 337:516–517, 1995.

Moyer DJ, Flamm ES. Anomalous arrangement of the origins of the anterior choroidal and posterior communicating arteries. Case report. J Neurosurg 76:1017–1018, 1992.

Moyes PD. Surgical treatment of multiple aneurysms and incidentally-discovered unruptured aneurysms. J Neurosurg 35:291–295, 1971.

Mueller S, Sahs AL. Brain stem dysfunction related to cervical manipulation. Report of three cases. Neurology 26:547–550, 1976.

Muhonen MG, Godersky JC, VanGilder JC. Cerebral aneurysms associated with neurofibromatosis. Surg Neurol 36:470–475, 1991.

Muller PJ, Deck HJN. Intraocular and optic nerve sheath hemorrhage in cases of sudden intracranial hypertension. J Neurosurg 41:160–166, 1974.

Murata J, Sawamura Y, Takahashi A, et al. Intracerebral hemorrhage caused by a neoplastic aneurysm from small-cell lung carcinoma: Case report. Neurosurgery 32:124–126, 1993.

Murayama Y, Viñuela F, Suzuki Y, et al. ION implantation and protein coating of detachable coils for endovascular treatment of cerebral aneurysms: Concepts and preliminary results in swine models. Neurosurgery 40:1233–1243, 1997.

Murthy JMK, Naidu KV. Aneurysm of the cervical internal carotid artery following chiropractic manipulation. J Neurol Neurosurg Psychiatry 51:1237–1238, 1988.

Musiek FE, Geurkink NA, Spiegel P. Audiologic and other clinical findings in a case of basilar artery aneurysm. Arch Otolaryngol Head Neck Surg 113:772–776, 1987.

Mustaki JP, Bissonnette B, Archer D, et al. Risques peroperatoires lors de chirurgie cerebraleanevrismale. Ann Fr Anes Rean 15:328–337, 1996.

Nabawi P, Tan WS, Spigos DG. Carotid-ophthalmic artery aneurysm: A report of two cases. Radiologie 23:137–138, 1983.

Nadeau SE, Trobe JD. Pupil sparing in oculomotor palsy: A brief review. Ann Neurol 13:143–148, 1983.

Nadel AJ, Gupta KK. Macroaneurysms of the retinal arteries. Arch Ophthalmol 94:1092–1096, 1976.

Nagahiro S, Goto S, Yoshioka S, et al. Dissecting aneurysm of the posterior inferior cerebellar artery: Case report. Neurosurgery 33:739–741; discussion 741–742, 1993.

Nagahiro S, Takada A, Goto S, et al. Thrombosed growing giant aneurysms of the vertebral artery: Growth mechanism and management. J Neurosurg 82:796–801, 1995.

Nagahiro S, Hamada J-I, Sakamoto Y, et al. Follow-up evaluation of dissecting aneurysms of the vertebrobasilar circulation by using gadolinium-enhanced magnetic resonance imaging. J Neurosurg 87:385–390, 1997.

Nagamine Y, Takahashi S, Sonobe M. Multiple intracranial aneurysms associated with moyamoya disease: Case report. J Neurosurg 54:673–676, 1981.

Nagasawa S, Ohta T, Kajimoto Y, et al. Giant thrombosed vertebral artery aneurysm treated by extracranial-intracranial bypass and aneurysmectomy: Case report. Neurol Med Chir 34:311–314, 1994.

Nagasawa S, Deguchi J, Arai M, et al. Usefulness of thin axial images of computerized tomography angiography for surgery on paraclinoidal carotid artery aneurysms. No Shinkei Geka 23:677–684, 1995.

Nagata S, Matsushima T, Fujii K, et al. Hemifacial spasm due to tumor, aneurysm, or arteriovenous malformation. Surg Neurol 38:204–209, 1992.

Nagayama Y, Okamoto S, Konishi T, et al. Cerebral berry aneurysms and systemic lupus erythematosus. Neuroradiology 33:466, 1991.

Nagler W. Vertebral artery obstruction by hyperextension of the neck: Report of three cases. Arch Phys Med Rehabil 54:237–240, 1973.

Naheedy MH, Tyler HR, Wolf MA, et al. Diagnosis of thrombotic giant basilar artery aneurysm on computed tomographic scan. Arch Neurol 39:64–65, 1982.

Nakagawa F, Kobayashi S, Takemae T, et al. Aneurysms protruding from the dorsal wall of the internal carotid artery. J Neurosurg 65:303–308, 1986.

Nakagawa T, Hashi K. The incidence and treatment of asymptomatic, unruptured cerebral aneurysms. J Neurosurg 80:217–223, 1994.

Nakahara I, Pile-Spellman J, Hacein-Bey L, et al. Usefulness of non-detachable balloons in endovascular treatment for cerebral aneurysms. Neurol Med Chir 34:353–359, 1994.

Nakahara I, Taki W, Tanaka M, et al. Dolichoectasia of the middle cerebral artery: Case report. Neurol Med Chir 35:822–824, 1995.

Nakahara K, Nakayama K, Takahashi Y, et al. Two cases of distal superior cerebellar artery aneurysm. No To Shinkei 46:1075–1079, 1994.

Nakahara T, Nonaka N, Kinoshita K, et al. Subarachnoid hemorrhage and aneurysmal change of cerebral arteries due to metastases of chorioepithelioma. Neurol Surg 3:777–782, 1975.

Nakai H, Kawata Y, Aizawa S, et al. Unilateral agenesis of the internal carotid artery in a patient with ruptured aneurysm of the anterior communicating artery: A case report. No Shinkei Geka 20:893–898, 1992.

Nakajima S, Atsumi H, Bhalerao AH, et al. Computer-assisted surgical planning for cerebrovascular neurosurgery. Neurosurgery 41:403–410, 1997.

Nakamura H, Takada A, Hide T, et al. Fenestration of the middle cerebral artery associated with an aneurysm: Case report. Neurol Med Chir 34:555–557, 1994.

Nakaso K, Nakayasu H, Isoe K, et al. A case of dissecting aneurysm of the basilar artery presented as superior pons type of Foville's syndrome. Rinsho Shinkeigaku 35:1040–1043, 1995.

Nakasu Y, Saito A, Handa J. Fusiform aneurysm of the anterior communicating artery. Surg Neurol 21:183–188, 1984.

Nakayama M, Niiro M, Hirahara K, et al. A case of ruptured aneurysm associated with persistent primitive trigeminal artery and metopism. No Shinkei Geka 22:651–655, 1994.

Nakazima H, Tanabe Y, Ishikawa H, et al. Analysis of 7 cases with intracavernous aneurysm. Nippon Ganka Gakkai Zasshi 95:1268–1274, 1991.

Nakstad P, Nornes H, Hauge HN. Traumatic aneurysms of the pericallosal arteries. Neuroradiology 28:335–338, 1986.

Nappi G, Moglia A, Poloni M, et al. Hemifacial spasm associated with dolichomegavertebrobasilar anomaly. Eur Neurol 15:94–101, 1977.

Nardi PV, Esposito S, Greco R, et al. Aneurysms of azygous anterior cerebral artery. Report of two cases treated by surgery. J Neurosurg Sci 34:17–20, 1990.

Nardi PV, Gigli R, Brunori A, et al. Aneurysms of the sphenoid segment of the middle cerebral artery. J Neurosurg Sci 40:93–97, 1996.

Nass R, Hays A, Chutorian A. Intracranial dissecting aneurysms in childhood. Stroke 13:204–207, 1982.

Nater B, Regli F, Bogousslavsky J. Syndrome de Wallenberg sur dissection de l'artere vertebrale. Rev Med Suisse Romande 111:39–41, 1991.

Nathal E. Foreign-body "gauzomas." J Neurosurg 74:529–530, 1991.

Nathal E, Yasui N, Suzuki A, et al. Ruptured anterior communicating artery aneurysm causing bilateral abducens nerve paralyses: Case report. Neurol Med Chir 32:17–20, 1992.

Neagoy DR, Dohn DF. Hemifacial spasm secondary to vascular compression of the facial nerve. Cleve Clin Q 41:205–214, 1974.

Negoro M, Kageyama N, Ishiguchi T. Cerebrovascular occlusion by catheterization and embolization: Clinical experience. AJNR 4:362–365, 1983.

Nehls DG, Flom RA, Carter LP, et al. Multiple intracranial aneurysms: Determining the site of rupture. J Neurosurg 63:342–348, 1985.

Neil-Dwyer G, Bartlett JR, Nicholls AC, et al. Collagen deficiency and ruptured cerebral aneurysms: A clinical and biochemical study. J Neurosurg 59:16–20, 1983.

Neil-Dwyer G, Lang DA, Evans BT. The effect of orbitozygomatic access for ruptured basilar and related aneurysms on management outcome. Surg Neurol 47:354–358, 1997.

New PFJ, Price DL, Carter B. Cerebral angiography in cardiac myxoma: Correlation of angiographic and histopathological findings. Radiology 96:335–345, 1970.

Newcombe AL, Munns GF. Rupture of aneurysm of circle of Willis in the newborn. Pediatrics 3:769–772, 1949.

Newman NJ, Kline LB, Leifer D, et al. Ocular stroke and carotid artery dissection. Neurology 39:1462–1464, 1989.

Newton TH, Potts DG. Radiology of the skull and brain. In Aneurysms. Editor, Allcock JM, p 2451. St Louis, CV Mosby, 1974.

Nibbelink DW, Torner JC, Henderson WC. Intracranial aneurysms and subarachnoid hemorrhage: A cooperative study: Antifibrinolytic therapy in recent onset subarachnoid hemorrhage. Stroke 6:622–629, 1975.

Nichols DA, Meyer FB, Piepgras DG, et al. Endovascular treatment of intracranial aneurysms. Mayo Clin Proc 69:272–285, 1994.

Nichols DA, Brown RD Jr, Thielen KR, et al. Endovascular treatment of ruptured posterior circulation aneurysms using electrolytically detachable coils. J Neurosurg 87:374–380, 1997.

Nicholson A, Cook AM, Dyet JF, et al. Case report: Treatment of a carotid artery pseudoaneurism with a polyester covered nitinol stent. Clin Radiol 50:872–873, 1995.

Nijensohn DE, Saez RJ, Reagan TJ. Clinical significance of basilar artery aneurysms. Neurology 24:301–305, 1974.

Nilsson IM, Anderson L, Bjorkman SE. Epsilon-aminocaproic acid (E-ACA) as a therapeutic agent: Based on five years' clinical experience. Acta Med Scand 180(Suppl 448):5–46, 1966.

Nilsson OG, Säveland H, Boris-Moller F, et al. Increased levels of glutamate in patients with subarachnoid hemorrhage as measured by intracerebral microdialysis. Acta Neurochir (Suppl) 67:45–47, 1996.

Nishi S, Taki W, Nakahara I, et al. Embolization of cerebral aneurysms with a liquid embolus, EVAL mixture: Report of three cases. Acta Neurochir 138:294–300, 1996.

Nishihara J, Kumon Y, Matsuo Y, et al. A case of distal anterior choroidal artery aneurysm: Case report and review of the literature. Neurosurgery 32:834–837; discussion 837, 1993.

Nishimoto A, Takeuchi S. Abnormal cerebrovascular network related to the internal carotid arteries. J Neurosurg 29:255–260, 1968.

Nishimoto A, Fujimoto S, Tsuchimoto S, et al. Anterior inferior cerebellar artery aneurysm: Report of three cases. J Neurosurg 59:697–702, 1983.

Nishimoto A, Ueta K, Onbe H, et al. Nationwide co-operative study of intracranial aneurysm surgery in Japan. Stroke 16:48–52, 1985.

Nishimura S, Suzuki M, Mizoi K, et al. Multiple cerebral aneurysms associated with aortitis syndrome: Case report. Neurol Med Chir 34:821–824, 1994.

Nishioka H, Torner JC, Graf CJ, et al. Cooperative study of intracranial aneurysms and subarachnoid hemorrhage: A long-term prognostic study: II. Ruptured intracranial aneurysms managed conservatively. Arch Neurol 41:1142–1146, 1984.

Nishioka T, Kondo A, Aoyama I, et al. Subarachnoid hemorrhage possibly caused by a saccular carotid artery aneurysm within the cavernous sinus. Case report. J Neurosurg 73:301–304, 1990.

Nishiyama K, Fuse S, Shimizu J, et al. A case of fibromuscular dysplasia presenting with Wallenberg syndrome, and developing a giant aneurysm of the internal carotid artery in the cavernous sinus. Rinsho Shinkeigaku—Clinical Neurology 32:1117–1120, 1992.

Nishizaki T, Tamaki N, Takeda N, et al. Dolichoectatic basilar artery: A review of 23 cases. Stroke 17:1277–1281, 1986.

Noble KG. Retinal macroaneurysms. Ophthalmology 91:108–109, 1984.

Noda S, Hayasaka S, Setogawa T, et al. Ocular symptoms of moyamoya disease. Am J Ophthalmol 103:812–816, 1987.

Noguchi K, Ogawa T, Inugami A, et al. Acute subarachnoid hemorrhage: MR imaging with fluid-attenuated inversion recovery pulse sequences. Radiology 196:773–777, 1995.

Nohjoh T, Houkin K, Takahashi A, et al. Ruptured dissecting vertebral artery aneurysm detected by repeated angiography: Case report. Neurosurgery 36:180–182; discussion 182–183, 1995.

Nomose KJ, New PFJ. Non-atheromatous stenosis and occlusion of the internal carotid artery and its main branches. AJR 118:550–566, 1973.

Norrgard O, Ängquist KA, Fodstad H, et al. Intracranial aneurysms and heredity. Neurosurgery 20:236–239, 1987.

Northcroft GB, Morgan AD. A fatal case of traumatic thrombosis of the internal carotid artery. Br J Surg 32:105–107, 1944–1945.

Norwood EG, Kline LB, Chandra-Sekar B, et al. Aneurysmal compression of the anterior visual pathways. Neurology 36:1035–1041, 1986.

Nosko M, Weir B, Krueger C, et al. Nimodipine and chronic vasospasm in monkeys: I. Clinical and radiological findings. Neurosurgery 16:129–136, 1985.

Nosko M, Norris SL, Weir B, et al. Nimodipine and chronic vasospasm in monkeys: III. Cardiopulmonary effects. Neurosurgery 18:261–265, 1986.

Noterman J, Georges P, Brotchi J. Arteriovenous malformation associated with multiple aneurysms in the posterior fossa: A case report with a review of the literature. Neurosurgery 21:387–391, 1987.

Noterman J, Dewitte O, Baleriaux D, et al. Les hemorragies sous-arachnoidiennes (HSA) au-dela de 65 ans. Etude retrospective d'une serie de 72 patients dont 65 cas d'origine anevrismale. Neurochirurgie 41:51–57, 1995.

Nouhuys FV, Deutman AF. Argon laser treatment of retinal macroaneurysms. Int Ophthalmol 1:45–53, 1980.

Nukta EM, Taylor HC. Panhypopituitarism secondary to an aneurysm of the anterior communicating artery. Can Med Assoc J 137:413–415, 1987.

Nukui H, Imai S, Fukamachi A, et al. Bilaterally symmetrical giant aneurysms of the internal carotid artery within the cavernous sinus, associated with an aneurysm of the basilar artery. Neurol Surg 5:479–484, 1977.

Nusynowitz RN, Stricof DD. Pseudoaneurysm of the cervical internal carotid artery with associated hypoglossal nerve paralysis. Demonstration by CT and angiography. Neuroradiology 32:229–231, 1990.

Nutik S. Carotid paraclinoid aneurysms with intradural origin and intracavernous location. J Neurosurg 48:526–533, 1978.

Nutik SL. Ventral paraclinoid aneurysms. J Neurosurg 69:340–344, 1988a.

Nutik SL. Removal of the anterior clinoid process for exposure of the proximal intracranial carotid artery. J Neurosurg 69:529–534, 1988b.

Nyberg-Hansen R, Loken AD, Tenstad O. Brainstem lesion with coma for five years following manipulation of the cervical spine. J Neurol 218:97–105, 1978.

O'Boynick P, Green KD, Batnitzky S, et al. Aneurysm of the left middle cerebral artery caused by myxoid degeneration of the vessel wall. 25:2283–2286, 1994.

O'Connell BK, Towfighi J, Brennan RW, et al. Dissecting aneurysms of head and neck. Neurology 35:993–997, 1985.

O'Connor PS, Tredici TJ, Green RP. Pupil-sparing third nerve palsies caused by aneurysm. Am J Ophthalmol 95:395–400, 1983.

O'Dwyer JA, Moscow N, Trevor R, et al. Spontaneous dissection of the carotid artery. Radiology 137:379–385, 1980.

O'Laoire SA. Epilepsy following neurosurgical intervention. Acta Neurochir Suppl 50:52–54, 1990.

O'Neill OR, Barnwell SL, Silver DJ. Middle meningeal artery aneurysm associated with meningioma: Case report. Neurosurgery 36:396–398, 1995.

O'Sullivan MG, Dorward N, Whittle IR, et al. Management and long-term outcome following subarachnoid hemorrhage and intracranial aneurysm surgery in elderly patients: An audit of 199 consecutive cases. Br J Neurosurg 8:23–30, 1994a.

O'Sullivan MG, Whyman M, Steers JW, et al. Acute subdural haematoma secondary to ruptured intracranial aneurysm: Diagnosis and management. Br J Neurosurg 8:439–445, 1994b.

Oba M, Niizuma H, Kodama N, et al. Villaret's syndrome due to extra-cranial internal carotid aneurysm: A case report. Neurol Surg 11:751–754, 1983.

Obrador S, Dierssen G, Hernandez JR. Giant aneurysm of the posterior cerebral artery: Case report. J Neurosurg 26:413–416, 1967.

Obrien D, Odell MW, Eversol A. Delayed traumatic cerebral aneurysm after brain injury. Arch Phys Med Rehab 78:883–885, 1997.

Obuchowski NA, Modic MT, Magdinec M. Current implications for the efficacy of noninvasive screening for occult intracranial aneurysms in patients with a family history of aneurysms. J Neurosurg 83:42–49, 1995.

Oda M, Niizuma H, Kodama N, et al. Villaret's syndrome due to extra-cranial internal carotid aneurysm: A case report. Neurol Surg 11:751–754, 1983.

Odom GL. Ophthalmic involvement in neurological vascular lesions. In Neuro-Ophthalmology Symposium. Editor, Smith JL, pp 213–216. Springfield, IL, Charles C Thomas, 1964.

Ogasawara K, Numagami Y, Kitahara M. A case of ruptured true posterior communicating artery aneurysm thirteen years after surgical occlusion of the ipsilateral cervical internal carotid artery. No Shinkei Geka 23:359–363, 1995.

Ogawa A, Tominaga T, Yoshimoto T, et al. Intraorbital ophthalmic artery aneurysm: Case report. Neurosurgery 31:1102–1104; discussion 1104, 1992.

Ogawa R. Okudera T, Noguchi K, et al. Cerebral aneurysms: Evaluation with three-dimensional CT angiography. AJNR 17:447–454, 1996.

Ogden JA, Mee EW, Henning M. A prospective study of impairment of cognition and memory and recovery after subarachnoid hemorrhage. Neurosurgery 33:572–586; discussion 586–587, 1993.

Ogden JA, Utley T, Mee EW. Neurological and psychosocial outcome 4 to 7 years after subarachnoid hemorrhage. Neurosurgery 41:25–34, 1997.

Ogilvy CS, Crowell RM, Heros RC. Surgical management of middle cerebral artery aneurysms: Experience with transsylvian and superior temporal gyrus approaches. Surg Neurol 43:15–22; discussion 22–24, 1995.

Ogilvy CS, Carter BS, Kaplan S, et al. Temporary vessel occlusion for aneurysm surgery: Risk factors for stroke in patients protected by induced hypothermia and

hypertension and intravenous mannitol administration. J Neurosurg 84:785–791, 1996a.

Ogilvy CS, Barker FG 2nd, Joseph MP, et al. Transfacial transclival approach for midline posterior circulation aneurysms. Neurosurgery 39:736–741, 1996b.

Ohkata N, Ikota T, Tashiro T, et al. A case of multiple extracranial vertebral artery aneurysms associated with neurofibromatosis. No Shinkei Geka 22:637–641, 1994.

Ohkawa M, Fujiwara N, Tanabe M, et al. Cerebral vasospastic vessels: Histologic changes after percutaneous transluminal angioplasty. Radiology 198:179–184, 1996.

Ohki M, Nakajima M, Sato K, et al. A case of dissecting aneurysm associated with mixed connective tissue disease. No To Shinkei 46:855–858, 1994.

Ohkubo T, Hirakata A, Miki D, et al. Vitrectomy for Terson's syndrome. Folia Ophthalmol Jpn 47:1515–1519, 1996.

Ohman J. Hypertension as a risk factor for epilepsy after aneurysmal subarachnoid hemorrhage and surgery. Neurosurgery 27:578–581, 1990.

Öhman J, Heiskanen O. Timing of operation for ruptured supratentorial aneurysms: A prospective randomized study. J Neurosurg 70:55–60, 1989.

Ohman J, Servo A, Heiskanen O. Long-term effects of nimodipine on cerebral infarcts and outcome after aneurysmal subarachnoid hemorrhage and surgery. J Neurosurg 74:8–13, 1991a.

Ohman J, Servo A, Heiskanen O. Effect of intrathecal fibrinolytic therapy on clot lysis and vasospasm in patients with aneurysmal subarachnoid hemorrhage. J Neurosurg 75:197–201, 1991b.

Ohno K, Monma S, Suzuki R, et al. Saccular aneurysms of the distal anterior cerebral artery. Neurosurgery 27:907–912; discussion 912–913, 1990.

Ohyama T, Ohara S, Momma F. Aneurysm of the cervical internal carotid artery associated with Marfan's syndrome: Case report. Neurologia Medico-Chirurgica 32:965–968, 1992.

Ojemann RG, Fisher CM, Rich JC. Spontaneous dissecting aneurysm of the internal carotid artery. Stroke 3:434–440, 1972.

Oka K, Maehara F, Tomonaga M. Aneurysm of the lenticulostriate artery—Report of four cases. Neurol Med Chir 31:582–585, 1991.

Okada Y, Shima T, Nishida M, et al. Clinicopathoradiological studies in 15 cases of megadolichobasilar anomaly. No To Shinkei 46:257–262, 1994.

Okamura T, Yamamoto M, Ohta K, et al. A case of ruptured cerebral aneurysm associated with fenestrated vertebral artery in osteogenesis imperfecta. No Shinkei Geka 23:451–455, 1995.

Okawara S, Nibbelink D. Vertebral artery occlusion following hyperextension and rotation of the head. Stroke 5:640–642, 1974.

Okawara SH. Warning signs prior to rupture of an intracranial aneurysm. J Neurosurg 38:575–580, 1973.

Okuchi K, Watabe Y, Hiramatsu K, et al. Dissecting aneurysm of the vertebral artery as a cause of Wallenberg's syndrome. No Shinkei Geka 18:721–727, 1990.

Okudaira Y, Arai H, Sato K. Cerebral blood flow alteration by acetazolamide during carotid balloon occlusion: Parameters reflecting cerebral perfusion pressure in the acetazolamide test. Stroke 27:617–621, 1996.

Okumura Y, Nikaido Y, Yokoyama K, et al. A case of basilar artery occlusion caused by vertebrobasilar artery dissection presenting with mild clinical symptoms. No Shinkei Geka 23:463–467, 1995.

Olmsted WW, McGee TP. The pathogenesis of peripheral aneurysms of the central nervous system: A subject review from the AFIP. Radiology 123:661–666, 1977.

Onishi H, Ito H, Kuroda E, et al. Intracranial mycotic aneurysm associated with transsphenoidal surgery for the pituitary adenoma. Surg Neurol 31:149–154, 1989.

Onishi H, Yamashita J, Enkaku F, et al. Anomalous origin of the anterior cerebral artery and congenital skull dysplasia: Case report. Neurol Med Chir 32:296–299, 1992.

Onoue H, Abe T, Tashibu K, et al. Two undesirable results of wrapping of an intracranial aneurysm. Neurosurg Rev 15:307–309, 1992.

Ooka K, Shibuya M, Suzuki Y. Motion and image artifacts of various intracranial aneurysm clips in a magnetic field. Acta Neurochir 138:1241–1245, 1996.

Orgul S, Flammer J. Perilimbal aneurysms of conjunctival vessels in glaucoma patients. Ger J Ophthalmol 4:94–96, 1995.

Origitano TC, Reichman OH, Anderson DE. Prophylactic hypervolemia without calcium channel blockers in early aneurysm surgery. Neurosurgery 31:804–806, 1992.

Orita T, Kajiwara K, Izumihara A. Ruptured aneurysm at the peripheral branch of the posterior cerebral artery with systemic lupus erythematosus. No To Shinkei 44:733–737, 1992.

Orita T, Tsurutani T, Izumihara A, et al. Distal posterior cerebral artery aneurysms—Three case reports. Neurol Med Chir 34:692–696, 1994.

Ortiz JR, Newman NJ, Barrow DL. CREST-associated multiple intracranial aneurysms and bilateral optic neuropathies. J Clin Neuroophthalmol 11:233–240, 1991.

Ortiz O, Voelker J, Eneorji F. Transient enlargement of an intracranial aneurysm during pregnancy: case report. Surg Neurol 47:527–531, 1997.

Orz Y, Kobayashi S, Osawa M, et al. Aneurysm size: A prognostic factor for rupture. Br J Neurosurg 11:144–149, 1997.

Osenbach RK, Blumenkopf B, McComb B, et al. Ocular bobbing with ruptured giant distal posterior inferior cerebellar artery aneurysm. Surg Neurol 25:149–152, 1986.

Oshiro EM, Rini DA, Tamargo RJ. Contralateral approaches to bilateral cerebral aneurysms: A microsurgical anatomic study. J Neurosurg 86:163–169, 1997a.

Oshiro EM, Walter KA, Piantadosi S, et al. A new subarachnoid hemorrhage grading system based on the glasgow coma scale: A comparison with the hunt and hess and world federation of neurological surgeons scales in a clinical series. Neurosurgery 41:140–147, 1997b.

Osler W. Malignant endocarditis. Br Med J 1:467–470, 1885a.

Osler W. Malignant endocarditis. Lancet 1:415–418, 1885b.

Ostergaard JR. Association of intracranial aneurysm and arteriovenous malformation in childhood. Neurosurgery 14:358–362, 1984.

Ostergaard JR, Hog E. Incidence of multiple intracranial aneurysms: Influence of arterial hypertension and gender. J Neurosurg 63:49–55, 1985.

Ostergaard JR, Oxlund H. Collagen type III deficiency in patients with rupture of intracranial saccular aneurysms. J Neurosurg 67:690–696, 1987.

Ostergaard JR, Reske-Nielsen E, Oxlund H. Histological and morphometric observations on the reticular fibers in the arterial beds of patients with ruptured saccular aneurysms. Neurosurgery 20:554–558, 1987.

Ott KH, Kase CS, Ojemann RG, et al. Cerebellar hemorrhage: Diagnosis and treatment. Arch Neurol 31:160–167, 1974.

Overton MC III, Calverton TH Jr. Iatrogenic cerebral cortical aneurysm: Case report. J Neurosurg 24:672–675, 1966.

Oxlund H, Andreassen TT. The roles of hyaluronic acid, collagen, and elastin in the mechanical properties of connective tissue. J Anat 131:611–620, 1980.

Oyakawa RT, Michels RG, Blase WP. Vitrectomy for nondiabetic vitreous hemorrhage. Am J Ophthalmol 96:517–525, 1983.

Oyama H, Ueda M, Kida Y, et al. Subarachnoid hemorrhage of unknown origin associated with Weber-Christian disease: Case report. Neurol Med Chir 35:454–457, 1995.

Oyesiku NM, Barrow DL, Eckman JR, et al. Intracranial aneurysms in sickle-cell anemia: Clinical features and pathogenesis. J Neurosurg 75:356–363, 1991.

Oyesiku NM, Colohan AR, Barrow DL, et al. Cocaine-induced aneurysmal rupture: An emergent factor in the natural history of intracranial aneurysms? Neurosurgery 32:518–525; discussion 525–526, 1993.

Pacini R, Simon J, Ketonen L, et al. Chemical-shift imaging of a spontaneous internal carotid artery dissection: Case report. AJNR 12:360–362, 1991.

Pacult A, Gratzick G, Voegele D, et al. Surgical clipping of difficult intracranial aneurysms using deep hypothermia and total circulatory arrest. South Med J 86:898–902, 1993.

Pakarinen S. Incidence, etiology, and prognosis of primary subarachnoid hemorrhage: A study based on 589 cases diagnosed in a defined urban population during a defined period. Acta Neurol Scand 43(Suppl 29):1–128, 1967.

Palestine AG, Robertson DM, Goldstein BG. Macroaneurysms of the retinal arteries. Am J Ophthalmol 93:164–171, 1982.

Panisset M, Eidelman BH. Multiple cranial neuropathy as a feature of internal carotid artery dissection. Stroke 21:141–147, 1990.

Pankey GA. Acute bacterial endocarditis at the University of Minnesota Hospitals, 1939–1959. Am Heart J 64:583–591, 1962.

Pant B, Arita K, Kurisu K, et al. Incidence of intracranial aneurysm associated with pituitary adenoma. Neurosurg Rev 20:13–17, 1997.

Papo I, Salvolini U, Caruselli G. Aneurysm of the anterior choroidal artery with intraventricular hematoma and hydrocephalus: Case report. J Neurosurg 39:255–260, 1973.

Pare L, Delfino R, Leblanc R. The relationship of ventricular drainage to aneurysmal rebleeding. J Neurosurg 76:422–427, 1992.

Parekh HC, Prabhu SS, Keogh AJ. De novo development of saccular aneurysms: Report of two cases. Br J Neurosurg 9:695–698, 1995.

Parenti G, Fiori L, Gasparotti R. Ruptured cerebral aneurysms operated on with only MRA. Reports of two cases. J Neurosurg Sci 39:21–25, 1995.

Parinaud H. Clinique nerveuse: Paralysie des mouvements associés des yeux. Arch Neurol (Paris) 5:145–172, 1883.

Park CC, Shin ML, Simard JM. The complement membrane attack complex and the bystander effect in cerebral vasospasm. J Neurosurg 87:294–300, 1997.

Parkin PJ, Wallis WE, Wilson JL. Vertebral artery occlusion following manipulation of the neck. NZ Med J 88:441–443, 1978.

Parkinson D. Bernard, Mitchell, Horner syndrome and others? Surg Neurol 11:221–223, 1979.

Parkinson D, West M. Traumatic intracranial aneurysms. J Neurosurg 52:11–20, 1980.

Parkinson D, Jain KK, Johnston JB. Saccular aneurysm of the ophthalmic artery: Report of an unusual case. Can J Surg 4:229–232, 1961.

Parkinson D, Johnston I, Chaudhuri A. Sympathetic connections of the fifth and sixth cranial nerves. Anat Rec 191:221–226, 1978.

Pasqualin A, DaPian R, Colamaria V, et al. Giant unruptured aneurysm of the middle cerebral artery manifesting as epilepsy. J Neurosurg Sci 23:303–310, 1979.

Pasqualin A, Massa C, Cavazzani P, et al. Intracranial aneurysms and subarachnoid hemorrhage in children and adolescents. Childs Nerv Syst 2:185–190, 1986.

Pasquier B, Courderc P, Pasquier D, et al. Hémodissection pariétale oblitérante ou anévrisme disséquant vertébrale-basilaire. Sem Hop Paris 52:1519–1527, 1976.

Pásztor E, Vajda J, Juhász J, et al. The surgery of middle cerebral artery aneurysms. Acta Neurochir 82:92–101, 1986.

Patel AN, Richardson AE. Ruptured intracranial aneurysms in the first two decades of life: A study of 58 patients. J Neurosurg 35:571–576, 1971.

Patel H, Smith RR, Garg BP. Spontaneous extracranial carotid artery dissection in children. Pediatr Neurol 13:55–60, 1995.

Patel RL, Richards P, Chambers DJ, et al. Infective endocarditis complicated by ruptured cerebral mycotic aneurysm. J R Soc Med 84:746–747, 1991.

Paterson JH, McKissock WA. A clinical survey of intracranial angiomas with special reference to their mode of progression and surgical treatment: A report of 110 cases. Brain 79:233–266, 1956.

Pathirana N, Refsum SE, McKinstry CS, et al. The value of repeat cerebral angiography in subarachnoid hemorrhage. Br J Neurosurg 8:141–146, 1994.

Paton L. Ocular symptoms in subarachnoid hemorrhage. Trans Ophthalmol Soc UK 44:110–126, 1924.

Patrick JT. Magnetic resonance imaging of petrous carotid aneurysms. J Neuroimaging 6:177–179, 1996.

Patrux B, Laissy JP, Jouini S, et al. Magnetic resonance angiography (MRA) of the circle of Willis: A prospective comparison with conventional angiography in 54 subjects. Neuroradiology 36:193–197, 1994.

Pau A, Cossu M, Turtas S. Association of aneurysm and arteriovenous malformation on the posterior inferior cerebellar artery. Report of three further cases and review of the literature. Acta Neurol 16:52–57, 1994.

Paullus WS Jr, Norwood CW, Morgan HW. False aneurysm of the cavernous carotid artery and progressive external ophthalmoplegia after transsphenoidal hypophysectomy. J Neurosurg 51:707–709, 1979.

Paulson G, Nashold BS Jr, Margolis G. Aneurysms of the vertebral artery: Report of 5 cases. Neurology 9:590–598, 1959.

Payne JW, Adamkiewicz J Jr. Unilateral internal ophthalmoplegia with intracranial aneurysm: Report of a case. Am J Ophthalmol 68:349–352, 1969.

Pecker J, Hoel J, Javalet A, et al. Paralysie du moteur oculaire externe par anévrysme intra-petreux traumatique de la carotide interne. Presse Med 68:1023–1024, 1960.

Peerless SJ, Drake CG, Fox AJ. In discussion of Swearington B, Heros RC. Common carotid occlusion for unclippable carotid aneurysms: An old but still effective operation. Neurosurgery 21:295, 1987.

Peerless SJ, Hernesniemi JA, Gutman FB, et al. Early surgery for ruptured vertebrobasilar aneurysms. J Neurosurg 80:643–649, 1994.

Peiris JB, Ross Russell RW. Giant aneurysms of the carotid system presenting as visual field defect. J Neurol Neurosurg Psychiatry 43:1053–1064, 1980.

Pelissou I, Sindou M, Pierluca P, et al. Anévrysmes "de novo": Apropos d'un cas opéré. Neurochirurgie 33:399–404, 1987.

Pelissou-Guyotat I, Deruty R, Mottolese C, et al. The use of Teflon as wrapping material in aneurysm surgery. Neurol Res 16:224–227, 1994.

Peltones S, Jevela S, Kaste M, et al. Hemostasis and gibrinolysis activation after subarachoid hemorrhage. J Neurosurg 87:207–214, 1997.

Perata HJ, Tomsick TA, Tew JM Jr. Feeding artery pedicle aneurysms: association with parenchymal hemorrhage and arteriovenous malformation in the brain. J Neurosurg 80:631–634, 1994.

Pereira R, Ramalho M, Pereira A, et al. Aneurisma gigante da arteria cerebral posterior (segmento P3): Relato de caso. Arq Neuropsiquiatr 53:481–484, 1995.

Périer O, Cauchie C, Demanet JC. Hématome intramural par dissection pariétale ("anévrysme disséquant") du tronc basilaire. Acta Neurol Belge 64:1064–1074, 1964.

Périer O, Brihaye J, Dhaene R. Hémodissection pariétale oblitérante (anévrisme disséquant) du tronc basilaire. Acta Neurol Psychiatr Beige 66:123–141, 1966.

Perneczky A, Czech T. Prognosis of oculomotor palsy following subarachnoid hemorrhage due to aneurysms of the posterior communicating artery. Zentralbl Neurochir 45:189–195, 1984.

Perret G, Nishioka H. Arteriovenous malformations: An analysis of 545 cases of cranio-cerebral arteriovenous malformations and fistulae reported to the Cooperative Study. J Neurosurg 25:467–490, 1966.

Perret G, Nishioka H. Arteriovenous malformations: An analysis of 545 cases of cranio-cerebral arteriovenous malformations and fistulae reported to the Cooperative Study. In Intracranial Aneurysms and Subarachnoid Hemorrhage: A Cooperative Study. Editors, Sahs AL, Perret GE, Locksley HB, et al., pp 200–222. Philadelphia, JB Lippincott, 1969.

Perria L, Viale GL, Rivano C. Anévrysmes de la jonction carotide internechoroï dienne antérieure. Acta Neurochir 21:153–166, 1969.

Perria L, Viale GL, Rivano C. Further remarks on the surgical treatment of carotid-choroidal aneurysms. Acta Neurochir 24:253–262, 1971.

Perry HD, Zimmerman LE, Benson WE. Hemorrhage from isolated aneurysm of a retinal artery: Report of two cases simulating malignant melanoma. Arch Ophthalmol 95:281–283, 1977.

Perry JR, Bilbao JM, Gray T. Fatal basilar vasculopathy complicating bacterial meningitis. Stroke 23:1175–1178, 1992.

Perry MO, Snyder WH, Thai ER. Carotid artery injuries caused by blunt trauma. Ann Surg 192:74–77, 1980.

Pertuiset B, Sichez JP, Arthuis F. Traitement chirurgical des anévrysmes artériels sacculaires supra-clinoï diens admis dans les trois semaines suivant la rupture. Neurochirurgie 33(Suppl 1):1–106, 1987.

Pessin MS, Chimowitz MI, Levine SR, et al. Stroke in patients with fusiform vertebrobasilar aneurysms. Neurology 39:16–21, 1989a.

Pessin MS, Adelman LS, Barbas N. Spontaneous intracranial carotid artery dissection. Stroke 20:1100–1103, 1989b.

Peterson NT, Duchesneau PM, Westbrook EL, et al. Basilar artery ectasia demonstrated by computed tomography. Radiology 122:713–715, 1977.

Petro GR, Witwer GA, Cacayorin ED, et al. Spontaneous dissection of the cervical carotid artery: Correlation of arteriography, CT, and pathology. AJR 148: 393–398, 1987.

Petruk KC, Weir BK, Overton TR, et al. The effect of graded hypocapnia and hypercapnia on regional cerebral blood flow and cerebral vessel caliber in the rhesus monkey: Study of cerebral hemodynamics following subarachnoid hemorrhage and traumatic internal carotid spasm. Stroke 5:230–246, 1974.

Petruk KC, West M, Mohr G, et al. Nimodipine treatment in poor-grade aneurysm patients: Results of a multicenter double-blind placebo-controlled trial. J Neurosurg 68:505–517, 1988.

Petty JM. Epistaxis from aneurysm of the internal carotid artery due to a gunshot wound: Case report. J Neurosurg 30:741–743, 1969.

Pfausler B, Belcl R, Metzler R, et al. Tersons syndrome in spontaneous subarachnoid hemorrhage—A prospective study in 60 consecutive patients. J Neurosurg 85: 392–394, 1996.

Phelps CD. The association of pale-centered retinal hemorrhages with intracranial bleeding in infancy. Am J Ophthalmol 72:348–350, 1971.

Phillips LH, Whisnant JP, O'Fallon WM, et al. The unchanging pattern of subarachnoid hemorrhage in a community. Neurology 30:1034–1040, 1980.

Pia HW. Classification of aneurysms of the internal carotid artery system. Acta Neurochir 40:5–31, 1978.

Pia HW. Aneurysm of the anterior cerebral artery. In Cerebral Aneurysms: Advances in Diagnosis and Therapy. Editors, Pia HW, Langmaid C, Zierski J, pp 109–115. Berlin, Springer-Verlag, 1979.

Pia HW, Fontana H. Aneurysms of the posterior cerebral artery: Locations and clinical pictures. Acta Neurochir 38:13–35, 1977.

Pia HW, Obrador S, Martin JG. Association of brain tumours and arterial intracranial aneurysms. Acta Neurochir 27:189–204, 1972.

Piatt JH Jr, Clunie DA. Intracranial arterial aneurysm due to birth trauma. Case report. J Neurosurg 77:799–803, 1992.

Pica RA Jr, Rockwell BH, Raji MR, et al. Traumatic internal carotid artery dissection presenting as delayed hemilingual paresis. AJNR 17:86–88, 1996.

Picard L, Roy D, Bracard S, et al. Aneurysm associated with a fenestrated basilar artery: Report of two cases treated by endovascular detachable balloon embolization. AJNR 14:591–594, 1993.

Picard L, Bracard S, Anxionnat R, et al. Traitement endovasculaire des anevrismes intracraniens. Ann Fr Anesth Reanim 15:348–353, 1996.

Pickard JD, Murray GD, Illingworth R, et al. Effect of oral nimodipine on the incidence of cerebral infarction and outcome at three months following subarachnoid hemorrhage: The British aneurysm nimodipine trial (BRANT). J Neurol Neurosurg Psychiatry 52:140, 1989.

Pickering LK, Hogan GR, Gilbert EF. Aneurysm of the posterior inferior cerebellar artery: Rupture in a newborn. Am J Dis Child 119:155–158, 1970.

Piek J, Lim DP, Bock WJ. Obstructive hydrocephalus caused by a growing, giant aneurysm on the upper basilar artery. Surg Neurol 20:288–290, 1983.

Piepgras A, Guckel F, Weik T, et al. Titananeurysmaclips und ihre Vorteile in der bildgebenden Diagnostik. Radiologe 35:830–833, 1995.

Piepgras DG, McGrail KM, Tazelaar HD. Intracranial dissection of the distal middle cerebral artery as an uncommon cause of distal cerebral artery aneurysm. Case report. J Neurosurg 80:909–913, 1994.

Pikula B, Plamenac P, Ferkovic M. Anévrisme disséquant (hématome disséquant) d'une artère cérébrale après un effort physique intense. Rev Neurol 128:125–130, 1973.

Piller P, Herman D, Kennel P, et al. Les anevrysmes post-traumatiques de la carotide interne. Rev Stomatol Chir Maxillofac 93:1–5, 1992.

Pilz P, Hartjes HJ. Fibromuscular dysplasia and multiple dissecting aneurysms of intracranial arteries: A further cause of moyamoya syndrome. Stroke 7:393–398, 1976.

Pinto AN, Ferro JM, Canhao P, et al. How often is a perimesencephalic subarachnoid hemorrhage CT pattern caused by ruptured aneurysms? Acta Neurochir 124: 79–81, 1993.

Piotrowski WP, Pilz P, Chuang IH. Subarachnoid hemorrhage caused by a fungal aneurysm of the vertebral artery as a complication of intracranial aneurysm clipping. Case report. J Neurosurg 73:962–964, 1990.

Pistoia F, Horton JA, Sekhar L, et al. Imaging of blood flow changes following angioplasty for treatment of vasospasm. AJNR 12:446–448, 1991.

Pitner SE. Carotid thrombosis due to intraoral trauma: An unusual complication of a common childhood accident. N Engl J Med 274:764–767, 1966.

Pluta R, Boock RJ, Afshar JK, et al. Source and cause of endothelin-1 release into cerebrospinal fluid after subarachnoid hemorrhage. J Neurosurg 87:287–293, 1997.

Poli P, Peillon C, Ladha E, et al. Anevrysmes intracraniens multiples en rapport avec une maladie de Recklinghausen. A propos d'un cas. J Mal Vasc 19:253–255, 1994.

Polin RS, Shaffrey ME, Jensen ME, et al. Medical management in the endovascular treatment of carotid-cavernous aneurysms. J Neurosurg 84:755–761, 1996.

Pollack JS, Custer PL, Hart WM, et al. Ocular complications in Ehlers-Danlos syndrome type IV. Arch Ophthalmol 115:416–419, 1997.

Pollard ZF. Aneurysm causing third nerve palsy in a 15-year-old boy. Arch Ophthalmol 106:1647–1648, 1988.

Pool JL. Cerebral vasospasm. N Engl J Med 259:1259–1264, 1958.

Pool JL. Early treatment of ruptured intracranial aneurysms of the circle of Willis with special clip technique. Bull NY Acad Med 35:357–369, 1959.

Pool JL, Potts DG. Aneurysms and Arteriovenous Anomalies of the Brain: Diagnosis and Treatment. New York, Hoeber Medical Division, Harper and Row, 1965.

Pool JL, Wood EH, Maki Y. On the cases with abnormal vascular networks in the cerebral basal region in the United States. In A Disease with Abnormal Intracranial Vascular Networks—Spontaneous Occlusion of the Circle of Willis. Editor, Kudo T, pp 63–68. Tokyo, Igaku-Shoin, 1967.

Pope FM. Type III collagen mutations and cerebral aneurysms. Stroke 20:1432, 1989.

Pope FM, Nicholls AC, Narcisi P, et al. Some patients with cerebral aneurysms are deficient in type III collagen. Lancet 1:973–975, 1981.

Pope FM, Limburg M, Schievink WI. Familial cerebral aneurysms and type III collagen deficiency. J Neurosurg 72:156–158, 1990.

Pope FM, Kendall BE, Slapak GI, et al. Type III collagen mutations cause fragile cerebral arteries. Br J Neurosurg 6:551–574, 1991.

Portney GL, Roth AM. Optic cupping caused by an intracranial aneurysm. Am J Ophthalmol 84:98–103, 1977.

Pospiech J, Kalff R, Reinhardt V, et al. Brain abscess and infections aneurysm of extravascular origin. Zentralbl Neurochir 51:219–222, 1990.

Post KD, Flamm ES, Goodgold A, et al. Ruptured intracranial aneurysms: Case morbidity and mortality. J Neurosurg 46:290–295, 1977.

Post KD, Gittinger JW Jr, Stein BM. Visual improvement after surgical manipulation of dolichoectatic anterior cerebral arteries. Surg Neurol 15:321–324, 1981.

Povlsen UJ, Kjaer L, Arlien-Soborg P. Locked-in syndrome following cervical manipulation. Acta Neurol Scand 76:486–488, 1987.

Pozzati E, Gaist G, Poppi M. Resolution of occlusion in spontaneously dissected carotid arteries. Report of two cases. J Neurosurg 56:857–860, 1982.

Pozzati E, Giuliani G, Poppi M, et al. Blunt traumatic carotid dissection with delayed symptoms. Stroke 20:412–416, 1989.

Pozzati E, Giuliani G, Acciarri N, et al. Long-term follow-up of occlusive cervical carotid dissection. Stroke 21:528–531, 1990.

Prabhu SS, Keogh AJ, Parekh HC, et al. Optochiasmal arachnoiditis induced by muslin wrapping of intracranial aneurysms. A report of two cases and a review of the literature. Br J Neurosurg 8:471–476, 1994.

Pratt-Thomas HR, Berger KE. Cerebellar and spinal injuries after chiropractic manipulation. JAMA 133:600–603, 1947.

Prêtre R, Reverdin A, Kalonji T, et al. Blunt carotid artery injury: Difficult therapeutic approaches for an underrecognized entity. Surgery 115:375–381, 1994.

Prêtre R, Kürsteiner K, Reverdin A, et al. Blunt carotid artery injury: Devastating consequences of undetected pseudoaneurysms. J Trauma 39:1012–1014, 1995.

Preul M, Tampieri D, Leblanc R. Giant aneurysm of the distal anterior cerebral artery: Associated with an anterior communicating artery aneurysm and a dural arteriovenous fistula. Surg Neurol 38:347–352, 1992.

Pribek RA. Brain stem vascular accident following neck manipulation. Wis Med J 62:141–143, 1963.

Pribram HFW, Hudson JD, Joynt RJ. Posterior fossa aneurysms presenting as mass lesions. AJR 105:334–340, 1969.

Price DB, Miller LJ. MR angiography of peripheral posterior inferior cerebellar artery aneurysms. J Comput Assist Tomogr 18:539–541, 1994.

Pritz MB, Giannotta SL, Kindt GW, et al. Treatment of patients with neurological deficits associated with cerebral vasospasm by intravascular volume expansion. Neurosurgery 3:364–368, 1978.

Pritz MB. Pupillary changes after intracisternal injection of papaverine. Surg Neurol 41:281–282; discussion 283, 1994a.

Pritz MB. Ruptured nontraumatic fusiform aneurysm of the cavernous carotid presenting with multiple episodes of epistaxis. Surg Neurol 42:293–296, 1994b.

Proust F, Langlois O, Rabehenoina C, et al. Les anevrysmes multiples decouverts a l'occasion d'une hemorragie meningee. A propos de 60 cas. Neurochirurgie 40: 10–17, 1994.

Proust F, Hannequin D, Langlois O, et al. Causes of morbidity and mortality after ruptured aneurysm surgery in a series of 230 patients. The importance of control angiography. Stroke 26:1553–1557, 1995.

Provenzale JM, Gorecki JP, Koen JL. Cerebral aneurysms associated with seizures but without clinical signs of rupture: seemingly distinctive MR imaging findings in two patients. AJR 167:230–232, 1996.

Pruitt AA, Rubin RH, Karchmer AW, et al. Neurologic complications of bacterial endocarditis. Medicine 57:329–343, 1978.

Przelomski MM, Fisher M, Davidson RI, et al. Unruptured intracranial aneurysm and transient focal cerebral ischemia: A follow-up study. Neurology 36:584–587, 1986.

Psinakis A, Kokolakis S, Theodossiadis PG, et al. Macroanévrysme artériel rétien pulsatile: Traitement par photocoagulation au laser argon. J Fr Ophtalmol 12: 673–676, 1989.

Puchner MJ, Lohmann F, Valdueza JM, et al. Monozygotic twins not identical with respect to the existence of intracranial aneurysms: A case report. Surg Neurol 41:284–289, 1994.

Punt J. Some observations on aneurysms of the proximal internal carotid artery. J Neurosurg 51:151–154, 1979.

Puskar G, Ruggieri PM. Intracranial aneurysms. MRI Clin North Am 3:467–483, 1995.

Putty TK, Luerssen TG, Campbell RL, et al. Magnetic resonance imaging diagnosis of a cerebral aneurysm in an infant. Case report and review of the literature. Pediatr Neurosurg 16:48–51, 1990–1991.

Quattrocchi KB, Nielsen SL, Poirier V, et al. Traumatic aneurysm of the superior cerebellar artery: Case report and review of the literature. Neurosurgery 27:476–479, 1990.

Quint DJ, Spickler EM. Magnetic resonance demonstration of vertebral artery dissection. Report of two cases. J Neurosurg 72:964–967, 1990.

Rabb CH, Tang G, Chin LS, et al. A statistical analysis of factors related to symptomatic cerebral vasospasm. Acta Neurochir 127:27–31, 1994.

Rabinowicz AL, Ginsburg DL, DeGiorgio CM, et al. Unruptured intracranial aneurysms: Seizures and antiepileptic drug treatment following surgery. J Neurosurg 75:371–373, 1991.

Rabow L, Algers G, Elfversson J, et al. Does a routine operation for intracranial aneurysm incur brain damage? Acta Neurochir 133:13–16, 1995.

Rácz P, Bobest M, Szilvássy I. Significance of fundal hemorrhage in predicting the state of the patient with ruptured intracranial aneurysm. Ophthalmologica 175:61–66, 1977.

Rad M, Piscol K. Parinaudisches Syndrom und internucleäre Ophthalmoplegie bei raumforderndem Basilarisaneurysma. Z Neurol 199:319–331, 1971.

Radhakrishnan VV, Saraswathy A, Rout D, et al. Mycotic aneurysms of the intracranial vessels. Indian J Med Res 100:228–231, 1994.

Rae-Grant AD, Lin F, Yaeger BA, et al. Post traumatic extracranial vertebral artery dissection with locked-in syndrome: A case with MRI documentation and unusually favourable outcome. J Neurol Neurosurg Psychiatry 52:1191–1193, 1989.

Raeder JG. Paratrigeminal paralysis of oculo-pupillary sympathetic. Brain 47:149–158, 1924.

Ragland RL, Gelber ND, Wilkinson HA, et al. Anterior communicating artery aneurysm rupture: An unusual cause of acute subdural hemorrhage. Surg Neurol 40:400–402, 1993.

Rahmat H, Abbassioun K, Amirjamshidi A. Pulsating unilateral exophthalmos due to traumatic aneurysm of the intraorbital ophthalmic artery: Case report. J Neurosurg 60:630–632, 1984.

Raitta C. Ophthalmic artery aneurysm: Causing optic atrophy and enlargement of the optic foramen. Br J Ophthalmol 52:707–709, 1968.

Raja IA. Aneurysm-induced third nerve palsy. J Neurosurg 36:548–551, 1972.

Rajshekhar V, Harbaugh RE. Results of routine ventriculostomy with external ventricular drainage for acute hydrocephalus following subarachnoid hemorrhage. Acta Neurochir 115:8–14, 1992.

Ramadan NM, Tietjen GE, Levine SR, et al. Scintillating scotomata associated with internal carotid artery dissection: Report of three cases. Neurology 41:1084–1087, 1991.

Ramirez-Lassepas M. Antifibrinolytic therapy in subarachnoid hemorrhage caused by ruptured intracranial aneurysm. Neurology 31:316–322, 1981.

Ramsay TL, Mosquera VT. Dissecting aneurysm of the middle cerebral artery. Ohio State Med J 44:168–170, 1948.

Ranganadham P, Dinakar I, Mohandas S, et al. A rare presentation of posterior communicating artery aneurysm. Clin Neurol Neurosurg 94:225–227, 1992.

Ranjan A, Joseph T. Giant aneurysm of anterior ethmoidal artery presenting with intracranial hemorrhage. Case report. J Neurosurg 81:934–936, 1994.

Rao KG, Woodlief RM. CT simulation of cerebellopontine tumor by tortuous vertebrobasilar artery. AJR 132:672–673, 1979.

Rapport R, Murtagh FR. Ophthalmoplegia due to spontaneous thrombosis in a patient with bilateral cavernous carotid aneurysms. J Clin Neuro-Ophthalmol 1:225–229, 1981.

Raps EC, Rogers JD, Galetta SL, et al. The clinical spectrum of unruptured intracranial aneurysms. Arch Neurol 50:265–268, 1993.

Raskind R. An intracranial arterial aneurysm associated with a recurrent meningioma: Report of a case. J Neurosurg 23:622–625, 1965.

Ratcheson RA, Wirth FP. Ruptured Cerebral Aneurysms: Perioperative Management. Baltimore, Williams & Wilkins, 1994.

Ray BS, Wolff HG. Experimental studies on headache: Pain-sensitive structures in the head and their significance in headache. Arch Surg 41:813–856, 1940.

Raymond J, Roy D, Bojanowski M, et al. Endovascular treatment of acutely ruptured and unruptured aneurysms of the basilar bifurcation. J Neurosurg 86:211–219, 1997.

Raymond LA, Tew J. Large suprasellar aneurysms imitating pituitary tumour. J Neurol Neurosurg Psychiatry 41:83–87, 1978.

Reader AL III, Massey EW. Fibromuscular dysplasia of the carotid artery: A cause of congenital Homer's syndrome? Ann Ophthalmol 10:326–330, 1980.

Reddy K, Lesiuk H, West M, et al. False aneurysm of the cavernous carotid artery: A complication of transsphenoidal surgery. Surg Neurol 33:142–145, 1990.

Redondo-Marco JA, Walb D. Zur Frage des Aneurysma dissecans am intrakraniellen Gefässsystem. Acta Neurochir 16:278–290, 1967.

Regli L, Piepgras DG, Hansen KK. Late patency of long saphenous vein bypass grafts to the anterior and posterior cerebral circulation. J Neurosurg 83:806–811, 1995.

Regli L, Nater B, Regli F, et al. Cephalée sentinelle: Symptome premonitoire trop souvent meconnu d'une rupture d'anevrisme intracranien. Schweiz Med Wochenschr 127:668–674, 1997.

Reiber ME, Burkey BB. Intracavernous carotid pseudoaneurysm after blunt trauma: Case report and discussion. Head Neck 16:253–258, 1994.

Reichenthal E, Savitz MH, Rothman AS, et al. Ruptured intracranial aneurysms as a cause of subdural haematoma: Potential diagnostic pitfalls and the surgical management of the acute patient. Neurochirurgia 29:219–224, 1986.

Reina A, Seal RB. False cerebral aneurysm associated with metastatic carcinoma of the brain: Case report. J Neurosurg 41:380–382, 1974.

Remy P, Massin H, Blampain JP. Bacterial aneurysm of the internal carotid: A rare condition. Eur J Vasc Surg 8:524–526, 1994.

Rengachary SS. Comments on Aarabi B. Traumatic aneurysms of brain due to high velocity missile head wounds. Neurosurgery 22:1062, 1988.

Renowden SA, Harris KM, Hourihan MD. Isolated atraumatic third nerve palsy: Clinical features and imaging techniques. Br J Radiol 66:1111–1117, 1993.

Renowden SA, Molyneux AJ, Anslow P, et al. The value of MRI in angiogram-negative intracranial hemorrhage. Neuroradiology 36:422–425, 1994.

Repka MX, Miller NR, Penix JO, et al. Optic neuropathy from the use of intracranial muslin. J Clin Neuro-Ophthalmol 4:147–150, 1984.

Repka MX, Miller NR, Penix JO, et al. Optic neuropathy from the use of intracranial muslin. In Neuro-ophthalmology Now! Editor, Smith JL, pp 29–32. New York, Field, Rich and Associates, 1986.

Resende LADL, Asseis EA, Costa LDS, et al. Sindrome de Marfan aneurismas intracranianos gigantes. Arg Neuro-Psiquiatr (Sao Paulo) 42:294–297, 1984.

Resta M, Gentile MA, DiCuonzo F, et al. Clinical-angiographic correlations in 132 patients with megadolichovertebrobasilar anomaly. Neuroradiology 26:213–216, 1984.

Reul J, Spetzger U, Fricke C, et al. Endovaskulare Behandlung zerebraler arterieller Aneurysmen mit selektiv ablosbaren Platinspiralen. Dtsch Med Wochenschr 120:669–675, 1995.

Reverdin A, Ramadan A, Berney J, et al. Complications tardives de traumatismes fermés de la carotide extracrânienne: A propos de deux cas. Neurochirurgie 32:216–220, 1986.

Reynier Y, Lena G, Vincentelli F, et al. Anévrysmes de la bifurcation de la carotide interne. Réflexions techniques à propos d'une série de 10 cas. Neurochirurgie 35:242–245, 1989.

Reynier Y, Alliez B, Diaz A. Anevrysme distal de l'artere cerebelleuse postero-inferieure. Considerations anatomiques et chirurgicales. Neurochirurgie 38:358–361, 1992.

Rezai AR, Lee M, Kite C, et al. Traumatic posterior cerebral artery aneurysm secondary to an intracranial nail: Case report. Surg Neurol 42:312–315, 1994.

Rhonheimer C. Zur Symptomatologie der sellären Aneurysmen: Ein Beitrag zur Differentialdiagnose der Chiasmasyndrome. Klin Monatsbl Augenheilkd 134:1–34, 1959.

Rhoton AL Jr, Perlmutter D. Microsurgical anatomy of anterior communicating artery aneurysms. Neurol Res 2:217–251, 1980.

Rice BJ, Peerless SJ, Drake CG. Surgical treatment of unruptured aneurysms of the posterior circulation. J Neurosurg 73:165–173, 1990.

Richardson AE, Jane JA, Yashon D. Prognostic factors in the untreated course of posterior communicating aneurysms. Arch Neurol 14:172–176, 1966.

Richardson JC, Hyland HH. Intracranial aneurysms. Medicine 20:1–83, 1941.

Richardson JTE. Arterial spasm and recovery from subarachnoid hemorrhage. J Neurol Neurosurg Psychiatry 39:1134–1136, 1976.

Richmond BK, Schmidt JH 3rd. Giant posterior inferior cerebellar artery aneurysm associated with foramen magnum syndrome. W V Med J 89:494–495, 1993.

Riddoch G, Goulden C. On the relationship between subarachnoid and intraocular hemorrhage. Br J Ophthalmol 9:209–233, 1925.

Rieger J, Hosten N, Neumann K, et al. Initial clinical experience with spiral CT and 3D arterial reconstruction in intracranial aneurysms and arteriovenous malformations. Neuroradiology 38:245–251, 1996.

Rigamonti D, Saleh J, Liu AM, et al. Dolichoectatic aneurysm of common carotid artery: An animal model with histological correlation. Pathobiology 62:8–13, 1994.

Riise R. Ocular symptoms in saccular aneurysms of the internal carotid artery (A survey of 100 cases). Acta Ophthalmol 47:1012–1020, 1969.

Rimpau A. Zur Morphologie der Carotispunktion. Virchows Arch 330:156–171, 1957.

Rimpau A, Seils H. Pathologisch-anatomische Befunde an der Punktionsstelle bei der Hirnarteriographie und Betrachtungen zur Punktionstechnik. Fortsch Roentgenstrahl 87:191, 1957.

Rinehart R, Harre RG, Roski RA, et al. Aneurysm of the anterior inferior cerebellar artery producing hearing loss. Ann Otol Rhinol Laryngol 101:705–706, 1992.

Ringel SP, Brick JF. Carotid-ophthalmic artery aneurysm masquerading as optic neuritis. J Neurol Neurosurg Psychiatry 49:460, 1986.

Ringel SP, Harrison SH, Norenberg MD, et al. Fibromuscular dysplasia: Multiple "spontaneous" dissecting aneurysms of the major cervical arteries. Ann Neurol 1:301–304, 1977.

Rinkel GJ, Wijdicks EF, Vermeulen M, et al. The clinical course of perimesencephalic nonaneurysmal subarachnoid hemorrhage. Ann Neurol 29:463–468, 1991a.

Rinkel GJ, Wijdicks EF, Vermeulen M, et al. Nonaneurysmal perimesencephalic subarachnoid hemorrhage: CT and MR patterns that differ from aneurysmal rupture. AJNR 12:829–834, 1991b.

Rinkel GJ, Wijdicks EF, Hasan D, et al. Outcome in patients with subarachnoid hemorrhage and negative angiography according to pattern of hemorrhage on computed tomography. Lancet *338*:964–968, 1991c.

Rinkel GJ, Wijdicks EF, Vermeulen M, et al. Acute hydrocephalus in nonaneurysmal perimesencephalic hemorrhage: Evidence of CSF block at the tentorial hiatus. Neurology *42*:1805–1807, 1992.

Rinkel GJ, van Gijn J, Wijdicks EF. Subarachnoid hemorrhage without detectable aneurysm. A review of the causes. Stroke *24*:1403–1409, 1993.

Rinne JK, Hernesniemi JA. De novo aneurysms: Special multiple intracranial aneurysms. Neurosurgery *33*:981–985, 1993.

Rinne J, Hernesniemi J, Puranen M, et al. Multiple intracranial aneurysms in a defined population: Prospective angiographic and clinical study. Neurosurgery *35*: 803–808, 1994.

Rinne J, Hernesniemi J, Niskanen M, et al. Management outcome for multiple intracranial aneurysms. Neurosurgery *36*:31–37; discussion 37–38, 1995.

Rinne J, Hernesniemi J, Niskanen M, et al. Analysis of 561 patients with 690 middle cerebral artery aneurysms: Anatomic and clinical features as correlated to management outcome. Neurosurgery *38*:2–11, 1996.

Rivera M, Gonzalo A, Urdanibia JF, et al. Magnetic resonance angiography and intracranial aneurysms in polycystic kidney disease. A preliminary study. Contrib Nephrol *115*:167–170, 1995.

Rivierez M, Landau-Ferey J, Grob R, et al. Value of electroencephalogram in prediction and diagnosis of vasospasm after intracranial aneurysm rupture. Acta Neurochir *110*:17–23, 1991.

Rivkin MJ, Hedges TR III, Logigian EL. Carotid dissection presenting as posterior ischemic optic neuropathy. Neurology *40*:1469, 1990.

Rizzo JF 3rd. Visual loss after neurosurgical repair of paraclinoid aneurysms. Ophthalmology *102*:905–910, 1995.

Roach MR, Drake CG. Ruptured cerebral aneurysms caused by microorganisms. N Engl J Med *273*:240–244, 1965.

Robertson DM. Macroaneurysms of the retinal arteries. Trans Am Acad Ophthalmol Otolaryngol *77*:55–67, 1973.

Robertson EG. Intracranial aneurysm. Med J Aust *2*:381–390, 1936.

Robertson EG. Cerebral lesions due to intracranial aneurysms. Brain *72*:150–185, 1949.

Robertson JT. Neck manipulation as a cause of stroke. Stroke *12*:1, 1981.

Roche JL, Choux M, Czorny A, et al. L'anévrisme artériel intra-cranien chez l'enfant: Etude coopérative. A propos de 43 observations. Neurochirurgie *34*:243–251, 1988.

Rodesch G, Noterman J, Thys JP, et al. Treatment of intracranial mycotic aneurysm: Surgery or not: A case report. Acta Neurochir *85*:63–68, 1987.

Roeltgen DP, Weimer GR, Patterson LF. Delayed neurologic complications of left atrial myxoma. Neurology *31*:8–13, 1981.

Román-Campos G, Edwards KR. Painful ophthalmoplegia: Oculomotor nerve palsy without mydriasis due to compression by aneurysm. Headache *19*:43–46, 1979.

Romaniuk CS, Bartlett RJ, Kavanagh G, et al. Case report: An unusual cause of epistaxis: Non-traumatic intracavernous carotid aneurysm. A case report with 12 year follow-up and review of the literature. Br J Radiol *66*:942–945, 1993.

Romodanov AP, Shcheglov VI. Intravascular occlusion of saccular aneurysms of the cerebral arteries by means of a detachable balloon catheter. In Advances and Technical Standards in Neurosurgery. Editor, Krayenbühl H, Vol 9, pp 25–49 New York, Springer-Verlag, 1982.

Ronkainen A, Hernesniemi J. Subarachnoid hemorrhage of unknown etiology. Acta Neurochir *119*:29–34, 1992.

Ronkainen A, Hernesniemi J, Ryynanen M. Familial subarachnoid hemorrhage in east Finland, 1977–1990. Neurosurgery *33*:787–796; discussion 796–797, 1993.

Ronkainen A, Hernesniemi J, Ryynanen M, et al. A ten percent prevalence of asymptomatic familial intracranial aneurysms: Preliminary report on 110 magnetic resonance angiography studies in members of 21 Finnish familial intracranial aneurysm families. Neurosurgery *35*:208–212; discussion 212–213, 1994.

Ronkainen A, Puranen MI, Hernesniemi JA, et al. Intracranial aneurysms: MR angiographic screening in 400 asymptomatic individuals with increased familial risk. Radiology *195*:35–40, 1995a.

Ronkainen A, Hernesniemi J, Tromp G. Special features of familial intracranial aneurysms: Report of 215 familial aneurysms. Neurosurgery *37*:43–46; discussion 46–47, 1995b.

Ronkainen A, Hernesniemi J, Puranen M, et al. Familial intracranial aneurysms. Lancet *349*:380–384, 1997.

Roome NS, Aberfeld DC. Spontaneous dissecting aneurysm of the internal carotid artery. Arch Neurol *34*:251–252, 1977.

Rosa A, Masmoudi K, Mizon JP. Typical and atypical ocular bobbing: Pathology through five case reports. Neuro-ophthalmology *7*:285–290, 1987.

Rosenberg ML. Spontaneous vertical eye movements in coma. Ann Neurol *20*: 635–637, 1986.

Rosenberg SI, Flamm ES, Hoffer ME, et al. The retrolabyrinthine transsigmoid approach to midbasilar artery aneurysms. Laryngoscope *102*:100–104, 1992.

Rosenorn J, Eskesen V. Patients with ruptured intracranial saccular aneurysms: Clinical features and outcome according to the size Br J Neurosurg *8*:73–78, 1994.

Rosenrn J, Eskesen V, Schmidt K, et al. The risk of rebleeding from ruptured intracranial aneurysms. J Neurosurg *67*:329–332, 1987a.

Rosenrn J, Eskesen V, Schmidt K, et al. Clinical features and outcome in 1076 patients with ruptured intracranial saccular aneurysms: A prospective consecutive study. Ugeskr Laeger *49*:2908–2911, 1987b.

Rosenwasser RH, Delgado TE, Bucheit WA, et al. Control of hypertension and proxphylaxis against vasospasm in cases of subarachnoid hemorrhage: A preliminary report. Neurosurgery *12*:658–661, 1983.

Rosenwasser RH, Jallo JI, Getch CC, et al. Complications of Swan-Ganz catheterization for hemodynamic monitoring in patients with subarachnoid hemorrhage. Neurosurgery *37*:872–875; discussion 875–876, 1995.

Ross JS, Masaryk TJ, Modic MT, et al. Intracranial aneurysms: Evaluation by MR angiography. AJNR *11*:449–455, 1990.

Rosset E, Roche PH, Magnan PE, et al. Surgical management of extracranial internal carotid artery aneurysms. Cardiovasc Surg *2*:567–572, 1994.

Rossitti S, Lofgren J. Optimality principles and flow orderliness at the branching points of cerebral arteries. Stroke *24*:1029–1032, 1993.

Rothrock JF, Lim V, Press G, et al. Serial magnetic resonance and carotid duplex examinations in the management of carotid dissection. Neurology *39*:686–692, 1989.

Röttgen P. Intrakranielle Aneurysmen mit Chiasmasyndromen. Zbl Neurochir *29*: 285–292, 1968.

Roualdes G, Lartigue C, Boudigue MD, et al. Dissection de l'artere vertebrale dans sa portion extra-cranienne apres un match de tennis. Presse Med *14*:2108, 1985.

Roux FX, Panthier JN, Tanghe YM, et al. Syndrome de Terson et complications intra-oculaires dans les hemorragies meningees (26 cas). Neurochirurgie *37*:106–110, 1991.

Rowbotham GF, Hay RK, Kirby AR, et al. Technique and the dangers of cerebral angiography. J Neurosurg *10*:602–607, 1953.

Rowe JG, Hosni AA. A common carotid artery aneurysm causing severe dysphagia. J Laryngol Otology *108*:67–68, 1994

Rowed DW, Walters BC. Iatrogenic false aneurysm following repair of intracranial aneurysm. Can J Neurol Sci *21*:346–349, 1994.

Roy C, Noseda G, Arzimanoglou A, et al. Maladie de Rendu-Osler revelee par la rupture d'un anevrysme arteriel cerebral chez un nourrisson. Arch Fr Pediatr *47*: 741–742, 1990.

Roy D, Raymond J, Bouthillier A, et al. Endovascular treatment of ophthalmic segment aneurysms with Guglielmi detachable coils. AJNR *18*:1207–1215, 1997.

Rozario RA, Levine HL, Scott RM. Obstructive hydrocephalus secondary to an ectatic basilar artery. Surg Neurol *9*:31–34, 1978.

Ruben S, Afshar F. Visual failure following subarachnoid hemorrhage from rupture of an anterior communicating artery aneurysm. J Neurol Neurosurg Psychiatry *54*:1017–1018, 1991.

Rubinstein MK, Cohen NH. Ehlers-Danlos syndrome associated with multiple intracranial aneurysms. Neurology *14*:125–132, 1964.

Rubinstein MK, Wilson G, Levin DC. Intraorbital aneurysms of the ophthalmic artery: Report of a unique case and review of the literature. Arch Ophthalmol *80*:42–44, 1968.

Rucker CW. Paralysis of the third, fourth, and sixth cranial nerves. Am J Ophthalmol *46*:787–794, 1958.

Rucker CW. The causes of paralysis of the third, fourth, and sixth cranial nerves. Am J Ophthalmol *61*:1293–1298, 1966.

Ruggieri PM, Poulos N, Masaryk TJ, et al. Occult intracranial aneurysms in polycystic kidney disease: Screening with MR angiography. Radiology *191*:33–39, 1994.

Rush JA, Younge BR. Paralysis of cranial nerves III, IV, and VI: Cause and prognosis in 1,000 cases. Arch Ophthalmol *99*:76–79, 1981.

Rush JA, Balis GA, Drake CG. Bitemporal hemianopsia in basilar artery aneurysm. J Clin Neuro-Ophthalmol *1*:129–133, 1981.

Russegger L, Grunert V. A thrombosed giant MCA aneurysm in a ten-week-old infant. Neurochirurgia *30*:186–189, 1987.

Russell EJ, Goldberg K, Oskin J, et al. Ocular ischemic syndrome during carotid balloon occlusion testing. AJNR *15*:258–262, 1994.

Rusyniak WG, Peterson PC, Okawara SH, et al. Acute subdural hematoma after aneurysmal rupture; evacuation with aneurysmal clipping after emergent infusion computed tomography: Case report. Neurosurgery *31*:129–131; discussion 131–132, 1992.

Ryba M, Pastuszko M, Iwanska K, et al. Cyclosporine A prevents neurological deterioration of patients with SAH—A preliminary report. Acta Neurochir *112*:25–27, 1991.

Ryba M, Grieb P, Pastuszko M, et al. Successful prevention of neurological deficit in SAH patients with 2-chlorodeoxyadenosine. Acta Neurochir *124*:61–65, 1993.

Ryu SJ. Intracranial hemorrhage in patients with polycystic kidney disease. Stroke *21*:291–294, 1990.

Sachdev VP, Drapkin AJ, Hollin SA, et al. Subarachnoid hemorrhage following intranasal procedures. Surg Neurol *8*:122–125, 1977.

Sacks JG, Lindenberg R. Dolicho-ectatic intracranial arteries: Symptomatology and pathogenesis of arterial elongation and distension. Johns Hopkins Med J *125*: 95–105, 1969.

Sadar ES, Jane JA, Lewis LW, et al. Traumatic aneurysms of the intracranial circulation. Surg Gynecol Obstet *137*:59–67, 1973.

Sadasivan B, Ma S, Dujovny M, et al. Use of experimental aneurysms to evaluate wrapping materials. Surg Neurol *34*:3–7, 1990.

Saeed SR, Hinton AE, Ramsden RT, et al. Spontaneous dissection of the intrapetrous internal carotid artery. J Laryngol Otol *104*:491–493, 1990.

Sahlman A, Salo J, Kostiainen S, et al. Extracranial carotid artery aneurysms. Vasa 20:369–373, 1991.

Sahrakar K, Boggan JE, Salamat MS. Traumatic aneurysm: A complication of stereotactic brain biopsy: Case report. Neurosurgery 36:842–846, 1995.

Sahs AL, Meyers R. The coexistence of intracranial aneurysms and polycystic kidney disease. Trans Am Neurol Assoc 76:147–150, 1951.

Sahs AL, Perret GE, Locksley HB, et al. Intracranial Aneurysms and Subarachnoid Hemorrhage: A Cooperative Study. Philadelphia, JB Lippincott, 1969.

Saifuddin A, Dathan JRE. Adult polycystic kidney disease and intracranial aneurysms. Br Med J 295:596, 1987.

Saito I, Shigeno T, Aritake K, et al. Vasospasm assessed by angiography and computerized tomography. J Neurosurg 51:466–475, 1979.

Saito K, Baskaya MK, Shibuya M, et al. False traumatic aneurysm of the dorsal wall of the supraclinoid internal carotid artery: Case report. Neurol Med Chir 35:886–891, 1995.

Saito R, Yazaki T, Kawase T, et al. Traumatic intracranial aneurysms after removal of tuberculum sellae meningioma: Case report. No Shinkei Geka 20:973–977, 1992.

Saitoh H, Hayakawa K, Nishimura K, et al. Rerupture of cerebral aneurysms during angiography. AJNR 16:539–542, 1995.

Sakaguchi S, Hirayama A. A case of optic nerve compression by sclerotic internal carotid arteries. Folia Ophthalmol Jpn 36:406–411, 1985.

Sakaki T, Morimoto T, Utsumi S. Cerebral transmural angiitis and ruptured cerebral aneurysms in patients with systemic lupus erythematosus. Neurochirurgia 33:132–135, 1990.

Sakaki T, Takeshima T, Tominaga M, et al. Recurrence of ICA-PCoA aneurysms after neck clipping. J Neurosurg 80:58–63, 1994.

Sakaki T, Matsuyama T, Yabuno T, et al. Approach through the temporal horn of the lateral ventricle for clipping of large dorsal type basilar bifurcation aneurysms. Acta Neurochir 133:17–21, 1995.

Sakata S, Fujii K, Matsushima T, et al. Aneurysm of the posterior cerebral artery: report of eleven cases—Surgical approaches and procedures. Neurosurgery 32:163–167; discussion 167–168, 1993.

Sako K, Nakai H, Takizawa K, et al. Aneurysm surgery using temporary occlusion under SEP monitoring. No Shinkei Geka 23:35–41, 1995.

Salar G, Mingrino S. Traumatic intracranial internal carotid aneurysm due to gunshot wound: Case report. J Neurosurg 49:100–102, 1978.

Salazar JL. Surgical treatment of asymptomatic and incidental intracranial aneurysms. J Neurosurg 53:20–21, 1980.

Salde WR. Massive basilar artery aneurysm. Vase Surg 8:74–81, 1934.

Salgado AV, Furlan AJ, Keys TF. Mycotic aneurysm, subarachnoid hemorrhage, and indications for cerebral angiography in infective endocarditis. Stroke 18:1057–1060, 1987.

Salmon JH, Blatt ES. Aneurysm of the internal carotid artery due to closed trauma. J Thorac Cardiovasc Surg 56:28–32, 1968.

Salomao JF, Leibinger RD, Lima YM, et al. Aneurisma da porcao distal da arteria cerebelar posterior e inferior em crianca. Arq Neuropsiquiatr 50:229–233, 1992.

Samson D, Batjer HH, Bowman G, et al. A clinical study of the parameters and effects of temporary arterial occlusion in the management of intracranial aneurysms. Neurosurgery 34:22–28; discussion 28–29, 1994.

Samson DS, Hodosh RM, Clark WK. Surgical management of unruptured asymptomatic aneurysms. J Neurosurg 46:731–734, 1977.

San-Galli F, Leman C, Kien P, et al. Cerebral arterial fenestrations associated with intracranial saccular aneurysms. Neurosurgery 30:279–283, 1992.

Sanchez R, Alfaro A, Perla C, et al. Hemorragia subdural de origen aneurismatico. Neurologia 9:65–68, 1994.

Sanders WP, Sorek PA, Mehta BA. Fenestration of intracranial arteries with special attention to associated aneurysms and other anomalies. AJNR 14:675–680, 1993.

Sandok BA. Fibromuscular dysplasia of the internal carotid artery. In Neurologic Clinics. Editor, Barnett HJM, Vol 1, pp 17–26. Philadelphia, WB Saunders, 1983.

Sanford HS, Craig WM, Wagener WP. An unusual chiasmal lesion and its operative treatment. Mayo Clin Proc 10:721–725, 1935.

Sankhla SK, Gunawardena WJ, Coutinho CM, et al. Magnetic resonance angiography in the management of aneurysmal subarachnoid haemorrhage: A study of 51 cases. Neuroradiology 38:724–729, 1996.

Sano H, Jain VK, Kato Y, et al. Bilateral giant intracavernous aneurysms: Technique of unilateral operation. Surg Neurol 29:35–38, 1988.

Sano K. Grading and timing of surgery for aneurysmal subarachnoid hemorrhage. Neurol Res 16:23–26, 1994.

Sano K, Hayano M, Ibuchi Y. A case of distal aneurysms of bilateral posterior inferior cerebellar arteries. No Shinkei Geka 21:645–648, 1993.

Sarner M, Rose FC. Clinical presentation of ruptured intracranial aneurysm. J Neurol Neurosurg Psychiatry 30:67–70, 1967.

Sarwar M. Abducens nerve paralysis due to giant aneurysm in the medial carotid canal: Case report. J Neurosurg 46:121–123, 1977.

Sarwar M, Banitzky S, Schechter MM. Tumorous aneurysms. Neuroradiology 12:79–97, 1976.

Sasaki J, Miura S, Ohishi H, et al. Neurofibromatosis associated with multiple intracranial vascular lesions: Stenosis of the internal carotid artery and peripheral aneurysm of the Heubner's artery; report of a case. No Shinkei Geka 23:813–817, 1995.

Sasaki O, Ogawa H, Koike T, et al. A clinicopathological study of aneurysms of the intracranial vertebral artery. J Neurosurg 75:874–882, 1991.

Sasaki O, Koizumi T, Ito Y, et al. Dissecting aneurysm of the posterior cerebral artery treated with proximal ligation. Surg Neurol 37:394–401, 1992.

Sasaki S, Asada K, Kodama T, et al. Surgical treatment of infective endocarditis. Kyobu Geka 47:209–214, 1994.

Sasaki T, Ohta T, Kikuchi H, et al. Preliminary clinical trial of intrathecal rt-PA (TD-2061) for the prevention of cerebral vasospasm in patients with aneurysmal subarachnoid hemorrhage. No To Shinkei 44:1001–1008, 1992.

Sasaki T, Ohta T, Kikuchi H, et al. A phase II clinical trial of recombinant human tissue-type plasminogen activator against cerebral vasospasm after aneurysmal subarachnoid hemorrhage. Neurosurgery 35:597–604; discussion 604–605, 1994.

Sasanuma J, Goto T, Ogayama H, et al. Clinical effect of nitroglycerin (GTN) on prevention of cerebral vasospasm. No Shinkei Geka 19:227–232, 1991.

Sato K, Fujiwara S, Kameyama M, et al. Follow-up study on ruptured aneurysms treated by wrapping. Neurol Med Chir 30:734–737, 1990.

Sato M, Yamaguchi K, Tadaki T, et al. Traumatic carotid-cavernous aneurysm after removal of cancer of the upper jaw: A case report. No Shinkei Geka 23:515–519, 1995.

Sato O, Bascom JF, Logothetis J. Intracranial dissecting aneurysm: Case report. J Neurosurg 35:483–487, 1971.

Sato O, Kobayashi M, Kamitani H, et al. Intracranial aneurysms in geriatric patients: Angiographic features and angioautotomographic analyses. Neuroradiology 16:147–149, 1978.

Sato S, Hata J. Fibromuscular dysplasia: Its occurrence with a dissecting aneurysm of the internal carotid artery. Arch Pathol Lab Med 106:332–335, 1982.

Säveland H, Brandt L. Which are the major determinants for outcome in aneurysmal subarachnoid hemorrhage? A prospective total management study from a strictly unselected series. Acta Neurol Scand 90:245–250, 1994.

Säveland H, Ljunggren B, Brandt L, et al. Delayed ischemic deterioration in patients with early aneurysm operation and intravenous nimodipine. Neurosurgery 18:146–150, 1986a.

Säveland H, Sonesson B, Ljunggren B, et al. Outcome evaluation following subarachnoid hemorrhage. J Neurosurg 64:191–196, 1986b.

Säveland H, Nilsson OG, Boris-Moller F, et al. Intracerebral microdialysis of glutamate and aspartate in two vascular territories after aneurysmal subarachnoid hemorrhage. Neurosurgery 38:12–19; discussion 19–20, 1996.

Scazzeri F, Mascalchi M, Calabrese R, et al. Case report: MRI and MR angiography of basilar artery dissection in a child. Neuroradiology 39:654–657, 1997.

Scharfetter F, Födisch HJ, Menardi G, et al. Falsches Aneurysma der Arteria gyri angularis durch Gefassverletzung bei einer Ventrikelpunktion. Acta Neurochir 33:123–132, 1976.

Schatz NJ, Schlezinger NS. Noncompressive causes of chiasmal disease. In Symposium on Neuro-ophthalmology: Transactions of the New Orleans Academy of Ophthalmology, pp 90–97. St Louis, CV Mosby, 1976.

Schechter DC. Cervical carotid aneurysms. NY State J Med 1:892–901, 1979a.

Schechter DC. Cervical carotid aneurysms. NY State J Med 2:1042–1048, 1979b.

Scheie HG, Hogan TF Jr. Angioid streaks and generalized arterial disease. Arch Ophthalmol 57:855–868, 1957.

Schellhas KP, Latchaw RE, Wendling LR, et al. Vertebrobasilar injuries following cervical manipulation. JAMA 244:1450–1453, 1980.

Schenk VWD, Solleveld H. Multiple aneurysms in a case of acromegaly. Psychiatr Neurol Neurochir 71:309–317, 1968.

Schievink WI. Intracranial aneurysms. N Engl J Med 336:28–40, 1997a.

Schievink WI. Genetics of intracranial aneurysms. Neurosurgery 40:651–663, 1997b.

Schievink WI, van der Werf DJM, Hageman LM, et al. Referral pattern of patients with aneurysmal subarachnoid hemorrhage. Surg Neurol 29:367–371, 1988.

Schievink WI, Karemaker JM, Hageman LM, et al. Circumstances surrounding aneurysmal subarachnoid hemorrhage. Surg Neurol 32:266–272, 1989.

Schievink WI, Limburg M, Oorthuys JWE, et al. Cerebrovascular disease in Ehlers-Danlos syndrome Type IV. Stroke 21:626–632, 1990.

Schievink WI, Piepgras DG, Earnest F IV, et al. Spontaneous carotid-cavernous fistulae in Ehlers-Danlos syndrome Type IV. J Neurosurg 74:991–998, 1991a.

Schievink WI, Mokri B, Michels VV, et al. Familial association of intracranial aneurysms and cervical artery dissections. Stroke 22:1426–1430, 1991b.

Schievink WI, Torres VE, Piepgras DG, et al. Saccular intracranial aneurysms in autosomal dominant polycystic kidney disease. J Am Soc Nephrol 3:88–95, 1992a.

Schievink WI, Piepgras DG, Wirth FP. Rupture of previously documented small asymptomatic saccular intracranial aneurysms. Report of three cases. J Neurosurg 76:1019–1024, 1992b.

Schievink WI, Mokri B, Piepgras DG. Angiographic frequency of saccular intracranial aneurysms in patients with spontaneous cervical artery dissection. J Neurosurg 76:62–66, 1992c.

Schievink WI, Mokri B, Garrity JA, et al. Ocular motor nerve palsies in spontaneous dissections of the cervical internal carotid artery. Neurology 43:1938–1941, 1993.

Schievink WI, Schaid DJ, Rogers HM, et al. On the inheritance of intracranial aneurysms. Stroke 25:2028–2037, 1994a.

Schievink WI, Prakash UB, Piepgras DG, et al. Alpha 1-antitrypsin deficiency in intracranial aneurysms and cervical artery dissection. Lancet 343:452–453, 1994b.

Schievink WI, Piepgras DG, McCaffrey TV, et al. Surgical treatment of extracranial internal carotid artery dissecting aneurysms. Neurosurgery 35:809–815, 1994c.

Schievink WI, Schaid DJ, Michels VV, et al. Familial aneurysmal subarachnoid hemorrhage: A community-based study. J Neurosurg 83:426–429, 1995a.

Schievink WI, Wijdicks EF, Parisi JE, et al. Sudden death from aneurysmal subarachnoid hemorrhage. Neurology 45:871–874, 1995b.

Schievink WI, Wijdicks EF, Piepgras DG, et al. The poor prognosis of ruptured intracranial aneurysms of the posterior circulation. J Neurosurg 82:791–795, 1995c.

Schievink WI, Michels VV, Mokri B, et al. Brief report: A familial syndrome of arterial dissections with lentiginosis. N Engl J Med 332:576–579, 1995d.

Schievink WI, Mokri B, Piepgras DG, et al. Recurrent spontaneous arterial dissections: Risk in familial versus nonfamilial disease. Stroke 27:622–624, 1996a.

Schievink WI, Katzmann JA, Piepgras DG, et al. Alpha-1-antitrypsin phenotypes among patients with intracranial aneurysms. J Neurosurg 84:781–784, 1996b.

Schievink WI, Parisi JE, Piepgras DG, et al. Intracranial aneurysms in Marfan's syndrome: An autopsy study. Neurosurgery 41:866–871, 1997.

Schindler E, Hase U. Die Megadolichobasilaris als Ursache eines Hirnstamm-Syndroms. Z Neurol 205:221–228, 1973.

Schisano G, Franco A, Nina P, et al. Monitoring of fibrin and fibrinogen degradation products (FDP) in the cerebrospinal fluid of patients with subarachnoid hemorrhage due to ruptured aneurysm. Report of 55 cases. J Neurosurg Sci 38:77–86, 1994.

Schloffer H. Erwägnungen über die operative Entlastung des intrakraniellen Optikusabschnittes. Zugleich ein Beitrag zum Foster Kennedyschen Syndrom. Med Klin 30:421–425, 1934.

Schmitt HP. Rupturen und thrombosen der arteria vertebralis nach gedeckten mechanischen insulten. Schweiz Arch Neurol Neurochir Psychiatr 119:363–379, 1976.

Scholefield BG. A case dissecting aneurysm of basilar artery. Guys Hosp Rep 74:485–487, 1924.

Scholten FG, ter Berg HW, Hofstee N, et al. Giant aneurysm of the posterior cerebral artery in a one-year-old child. Eur J Radiol 15:56–58, 1992.

Schoolman A, Kepes JJ. Bilateral spontaneous carotid-cavernous fistulae in Ehlers-Danlos syndrome. J Neurosurg 26:82–86, 1967.

Schramm J, Zentner J, Pechstein U. Intraoperative SEP monitoring in aneurysm surgery. Neurol Res 16:20–22, 1994.

Schramm J, Koht A, Schmidt G, et al. Surgical and electrophysiological observations during clipping of 134 aneurysms with evoked potential monitoring. Neurosurgery 26:61–70, 1990.

Schuierer G, Huk WJ, Laub G. Magnetic resonance angiography of intracranial aneurysms: Comparison with intra-arterial digital subtraction angiography. Neuroradiology 35:50–54, 1992.

Schutz H, Fleming JFR, Humphreys RP, et al. Normal pressure hydrocephalus—High pressure normocephalus. Can J Neurosci 7:211–219, 1980.

Schwartz RB, Tice HM, Hooten SM, et al. Evaluation of cerebral aneurysms with helical CT: Correlation with conventional angiography and MR angiography. Radiology 192:717–722, 1994.

Schwarz GA, Geiger JK, Spano AV. Posterior inferior cerebellar artery syndrome of Wallenberg after chiropractic manipulation. Arch Intern Med 97:352–354, 1956.

Scodary DJ, Tew JM Jr, Thomas GM, et al. Radiation-induced cerebral aneurysms. Acta Neurochir 102:141–144, 1990.

Scott BA, Weinstein Z, Pulliam MW. Computed tomographic diagnosis of ruptured giant posterior cerebral artery aneurysms. Neurosurgery 22:557–558, 1988.

Scott GE, Neuberger KT, Denst J. Dissecting aneurysms of intracranial arteries. Neurology 10:22–27, 1960.

Scott M, Stauffer HM. A case of aneurysmal malformation of the vertebral and basilar arteries causing cranial nerve involvement. AJR 92:836–837, 1964.

Scotti G. Internal carotid origin of a tortuous posterior cerebral artery. Arch Neurol 31:273–275, 1974.

Scotti G, DeGrandi C, Colombo A. Ectasia of the intracranial arteries diagnosed by computed tomography: Megadolichobasilar artery: CT diagnosis. Neuroradiology 15:183–184, 1978.

Scuccimarra A, Russo A, Cafarelli F. Paralysie du III par mégadolicho-artère basilaire. Neurochirurgie 34:137–138, 1988.

Secher-Hansen E. Subarachnoid hemorrhage and sudden unexpected death. Acta Neurol Scand 40:115–130, 1964.

Seftel DM, Kolson H, Gordon BS. Ruptured intracranial carotid artery aneurysm with fatal epistaxis. Arch Otolaryngol 70:52–60, 1959.

Segal HD, McLaurin RL. Giant serpentine aneurysm: Report of two cases. J Neurosurg 46:115–120, 1977.

Seifert V, Stolke D. Posterior transpetrosal approach to aneurysms of the basilar trunk and vertebrobasilar junction. J Neurosurg 85:373–379, 1996.

Seiler RW, Reulen HJ, Huber P, et al. Outcome of aneurysmal subarachnoid hemorrhage in a hospital population: A prospective study including early operation, intravenous nimodipine, and transcranial Doppler ultrasound. Neurosurgery 23:598–604, 1988.

Sekhar LN, Heros RC. Origin, growth, and rupture of saccular aneurysms: A review. Neurosurgery 8:248–260, 1981.

Sekhar LN, Patel SJ. Permanent occlusion of the internal carotid artery during skull-base and vascular surgery: Is it really safe? Am J Otol 14:421–422, 1993.

Sekhar LN, Kalia KK, Yonas H, et al. Cranial base approaches to intracranial aneurysms in the subarachnoid space. Neurosurgery 35:472–481; discussion 481–483, 1994.

Sekino H, Nakamura N, Katoh Y, et al. Dissecting aneurysms of the vertebro-basilar system: Clinical and angiographic observations. No Shinkei Geka 9:125–133, 1982.

Sekino H, Katoh Y, Kanki T, et al. Iatrogenic traumatic intracranial aneurysm: Case report. Neurol Med Chir 25:945–951, 1985.

Sellier N, Chiras J, Benhamou M, et al. Spontaneous dissection of the internal carotid artery. J Neuroradiology 10:243–259, 1983.

Seltzer J, Hurteau EF. Bilateral symmetrical aneurysms of internal carotid artery within the cavernous sinus. J Neurosurg 14:448–451, 1957.

Sengupta RP, Gryspeerdt GL, Hankinson J. Carotid-ophthalmic aneurysms. J Neurol Neurosurg Psychiatr 39:837–853, 1976.

Sengupta RP, Saunders M, Clark RP. Unruptured intracranial aneurysms: An unusual source of epilepsy. Acta Neurochir 40:45–53, 1978.

Senter HJ, Miller DJ. Interoptic course of the anterior cerebral artery associated with anterior cerebral artery aneurysm: Case report. J Neurosurg 56:302–304, 1982.

Serbinenko FA. Balloon catheterization and occlusion of major cerebral vessels. J Neurosurg 41:125–145, 1974.

Serbinenko FA, Filatov JM, Spallone A, et al. Management of giant intracranial ICA aneurysms with combined extracranial-intracranial anastomosis and endovascular occlusion. J Neurosurg 73:57–63, 1990.

Serdaru M, Schaison M, Lhermitte F. Pupil sparing in oculomotor palsy and Claude Bernard Homer syndrome. Ann Neurol 14:697–698, 1983.

Setoyama M, Shimada T, Kanzaki T, et al. Cutaneous arterial fibromuscular dysplasia: A case report and electron-microscopic study. J Dermatol 21:205–210, 1994.

Setton A, Davis AJ, Bose A, et al. Angiography of cerebral aneurysms. Neuroimaging Clin North Am 6:705–738, 1996.

Sevick RJ, Tsuruda JS, Schmalbrock P. Three-dimensional time-of-flight MR angiography in the evaluation of cerebral aneurysms. J Comput Assist Tomogr 14:874–881, 1990.

Sevrain L, Rabehenoina C, Hattab N, et al. Les anevrismes a expression clinique grave d'emblee (grades IV et V de Hunt et Hess). Une serie de 66 cas. Neurochirurgie 36:287–296, 1990.

Shantharam VV, Clift GV. Suprasellar aneurysm: An unusual cause of hypopituitarism. JAMA 229:1473, 1974.

Shapiro SA, Campbell RL, Scully T. Hemorrhagic dilation of the fourth ventricle: An ominous predictor. J Neurosurg 80:805–809, 1994.

Sharif AA, Remley KB, Clark HB. Middle cerebral artery dissection: A clinicopathologic study. Neurology 45:1929–1931, 1995.

Sharr MM, Kelvin FM. Vertebrobasilar aneurysms: Experience with 27 cases. Eur Neurol 10:129–143, 1973.

Shaw HE Jr, Landers MB III. Vitreous hemorrhage after intracranial hemorrhage. Am J Ophthalmol 80:207–213, 1975.

Shaw HE Jr, Landers MB III, Sydnor CF. The significance of intraocular hemorrhage due to subarachnoid hemorrhage. Ann Ophthalmol 9:1403–1405, 1977.

Sherman DG, Salmon JH. Ocular bobbing with superior cerebellar artery aneurysm: Case report. J Neurosurg 47:596–598, 1977.

Sherman DG, Hart RG, Easton JD. Abrupt change in head position and cerebral infarction. Stroke 12:2–6, 1981.

Sherman MR, Smialek JE, Zane WE. Pathogenesis of vertebral artery occlusion following cervical spine manipulation. Arch Pathol Lab Med 111:851–853, 1987.

Shibuya M, Suzuki Y, Sugita K, et al. Effect of AT877 on cerebral vasospasm after aneurysmal subarachnoid hemorrhage. Results of a prospective placebo-controlled double-blind trial. J Neurosurg 76:571–577, 1992.

Shibuya M, Suzuki Y, Enomoto H, et al. Effects of prophylactic intrathecal administrations of nicardipine on vasospasm in patients with severe aneurysmal subarachnoid hemorrhage. Acta Neurochir 131:19–25, 1994.

Shibuya S, Igarashi S, Amo T, et al. Mycotic aneurysms of the internal carotid artery: Case report. J Neurosurg 44:105–108, 1976.

Shigemori M, Shirahama M, Hara K, et al. Traumatic aneurysms of intracranial internal carotid arteries: Case reports. Neurol Med Chir 22:241–247, 1982.

Shigemori M, Kawaba T, Yoshitake Y, et al. Fusiform aneurysm of the proximal anterior cerebral artery. J Neurol Neurosurg Psychiatry 51:451, 1988.

Shigemori M, Tokunaga T, Miyagi J, et al. Multiple brain tumors of different cell types with an unruptured cerebral aneurysm: Case report. Neurol Med Chir 31:96–99, 1991.

Shigeta H, Kyoshima K, Nakagawa F, et al. Dorsal internal carotid artery aneurysms with special reference to angiographic presentation and surgical management. Acta Neurochir 119:42–48, 1992.

Shih TY. Delayed oculomotor palsy from focal subarachnoid hematoma. J Clin Neuro-ophthalmol 13:218–219, 1993.

Shike T, Hoshino H, Takagi K, et al. Bacterial intracavernous carotid aneurysm presented as massive epistaxis. Rinsho Shinkeigaku 35:531–536, 1995.

Shimizu T, Suzuki N, Ottomo M. A fungal aneurysm in a patient with presumed Tolosa-Hunt syndrome. No Shinkei Geka 19:477–483, 1991.

Suzuki M, Onuma T, Sakurai Y, et al. Aneurysms arising from the proximal (A1) segment of the anterior cerebral artery. A study of 38 cases. J Neurosurg 76: 455–458, 1992.

Suzuki R, Masaoka H, Hirata Y, et al. The role of endothelin-1 in the origin of cerebral vasospasm in patients with aneurysmal subarachnoid hemorrhage. J Neurosurg 77:96–100, 1992.

Suzuki S, Takahashi T, Ohkuma H, et al. Management of giant serpentine aneurysms of the middle cerebral artery—Review of literature and report of a case successfully treated by STA-MCA anastomosis only. Acta Neurochir 117:23–29, 1992.

Suzuki S, Ogane K, Souma M, et al. Efficacy of steroid hormone in solution for intracranial irrigation during aneurysmal surgery for prevention of the vasospasm syndrome. Acta Neurochir 131:184–188, 1994.

Suzuki S, Ohkuma H, Sekiya T, et al. A flexible aneurysm clip applier. Technical note. Acta Neurochir 135:201–202, 1995.

Suzuki T, Nagai R, Yamazaki T, et al. Rapid growth of intracranial aneurysms secondary to cardiac myxoma. Neurology 44:570–571, 1994.

Sved PD, Morgan MK, Weber NC. Delayed referral of patients with aneurysmal subarachnoid hemorrhage. Med J Aust 162:310–311, 1995.

Svien HJ, Peserico L. Occlusion of the third ventricle by tortuous, bulbous, calcified basilar artery. Neurology 9:836–838, 1959.

Swearingen B, Heros RC. Common carotid occlusion for unclippable carotid aneurysms: An old but still effective operation. Neurosurgery 21:288–295, 1987.

Swift DM, Solomon RA. Unruptured aneurysms and postoperative volume expansion. J Neurosurg 77:908–910, 1992.

Symon L. Surgical experiences with giant intracranial aneurysms. Acta Neurochir 118:53–58, 1992.

Symon L, Vajda J. Surgical experiences with giant intracranial aneurysms. J Neurosurg 61:1009–1028, 1984.

Symonds CP. Contributions to the clinical study of intracranial aneurysms. Guy's Hosp Rep 72:139–158, 1923.

Szikora I, Guterman LR, Wells KM, et al. Combined use of stents and coils to treat experimental wide-necked carotid aneurysms: Preliminary results. AJNR 15: 1091–1102, 1994.

Taira T, Tamura Y, Kawamura H. Intracranial aneurysm in a child with Klippel-Trenaunay-Weber syndrome: Case report. Surg Neurol 36:303–306, 1991.

Tajima A, Ito M, Ishii M. Complete recovery from monocular blindness caused by aneurysmal compression to optic nerve: Report of two cases. Neurol Med Chir 33:19–23, 1993.

Takahashi I, Takamura H, Gotoh S, et al. Dissecting aneurysm of the posterior inferior cerebellar artery: A case report. No Shinkei Geka 20:277–281, 1992.

Takahashi K, Nagao K, Momokawa T, et al. Two treated cases of infectious endocarditis with subsequent rupture of cerebral aneurysm. Nippon Kyobu Geka Gakkai Zasshi 38:2426–2430, 1990.

Takahashi T, Kanatani I, Isayama Y, et al. Visual disturbance due to internal carotid aneurysm. Ann Ophthalmol 13:1014–1024, 1983.

Takahashi T, Suzuki S, Ohkuma H, et al. Aneurysm at a duplication of the middle cerebral artery. AJNR 15:1166–1168, 1994.

Takahashi Y, Shigemori M, Tokunaga T, et al. A case of bacterial aneurysm following Hardy's operation. No Shinkei Geka 19:665–669, 1991.

Takai N, Ezuka I, Sorimachi T, et al. Vertebral artery dissecting aneurysm rebleeding after proximal occlusion: Case report. Neurol Med Chir 33:765–768, 1993.

Takeshita M, Kagawa M, Kubo O, et al. Clinicopathological study of bacterial intracranial aneurysms. Neurol Med Chir 31:508–513, 1991a.

Takeshita M, Kubo O, Onda H, et al. A case showing the infraoptic course of the anterior cerebral artery associated with anterior cerebral artery aneurysm. No Shinkei Geka 19:871–876, 1991b.

Takeshita M, Izawa M, Kubo O, et al. Aspergillotic aneurysm formation of cerebral artery following neurosurgical operation. Surg Neurol 38:146–151, 1992.

Takeuchi K. Occlusive disease of the carotid artery. Recent Adv Res Nerv Sys 5: 511–543, 1961.

Takeuchi K, Shimizu K. Hypoplasia of the bilateral internal carotid arteries. No To Shinkei 9:37–43, 1957.

Takeuchi S, Tanaka R, Koike T, et al. Frequent TIA in the territory fed by the anastomosed STA after combined therapeutic ICA occlusion and extracranial-intracranial bypass: Case report. Acta Neurochir 133:206–210, 1995.

Takeuchi T, Ogawa H, Kimura S. Aneurysm in the horizontal segment of the anterior cerebral artery confirmed by cerebral vasospasm: Case report. Neurol Med Chir 31:272–276, 1991.

Takeuchi T, Kasahara E, Iwasaki M, et al. Necessity of cerebral angiography in thunderclap headache patients who show no evidence of subarachnoid hemorrhage: Investigation of 350 cases. No Shinkei Geka 22:925–931, 1994.

Takeuchi T, Kasahara E, Iwasaki M, et al. Necessity for searching for cerebral aneurysm in thunderclap headache patients who show no evidence of subarachnoid hemorrhage: Investigation of 8 minor leak cases on operation. No Shinkei Geka 24:437–441, 1996.

Takeuchi T, Kasahara E, Iwasaki M, et al. Terson's syndrome which arose from ruptured right superior cerebellar artery aneurysm: A case report and 32 series investigations. No Shinkei Geka 25:259–264, 1997.

Taki W, Handa H, Yamagata S, et al. Balloon embolization of a giant aneurysm using a newly developed catheter. Surg Neurol 12:363–365, 1979.

Taki W, Nishi S, Yamashita K, et al. Selection and combination of various endovascular techniques in the treatment of giant aneurysms. J Neurosurg 77:37–42, 1992.

Taki W, Nakahara I, Nishi Sh, et al. Pathogenetic and therapeutic considerations of carotid-cavernous sinus fistulas. Acta Neurochir 127:6–14, 1994.

Takita K, Shirato H, Akasaka T, et al. Dissecting aneurysm of the vertebro-basilar artery: A case report and review of previous cases. No To Shinkei 31:1211–1218, 1979.

Tamaki M, Ohno K, Matsushima Y, et al. Coexistence of cerebral aneurysm and angiographically occult AVM in the occipital lobe: A case report. No Shinkei Geka 20:267–271, 1992.

Tamatani S, Toyama M, Kawaguchi T, et al. Evaluation of the surgical results of the interhemispheric approach in comparison with the pterional approach for anterior communicating artery aneurysms. No Shinkei Geka 20:657–661, 1992.

Tampieri D, Leblanc R, Oleszek J, et al. Three-dimensional computed tomographic angiography of cerebral aneurysms. Neurosurgery 36:749–754; discussion 754–755, 1995.

Tampieri D, Melancon D, Ethier R. The role of computed tomographic angiography in the assessment of intracranial vascular disease. Neuroimaging Clin North Am 6:759–767, 1996.

Tamura M, Tsukahara Y, Yodonawa M. Fusiform aneurysm of the anterior cerebral artery (A1 segment). No Shinkei Geka 13:1337–1340, 1985.

Tanabe M, Inoue Y, Hori T. Spontaneous thrombosis of an aneurysm of the middle cerebral artery with subarachnoid hemorrhage in a 6-year-old child: Case report. Neurol Res 13:202–204, 1991.

Tanabe S, Ohtaki M, Uede T, et al. Diagnosis of ruptured and unruptured cerebral aneurysms with three-dimensional CT angiography (3D-CTA). No Shinkei Geka 23:787–795, 1995.

Tanaka A, Kimura M, Yoshinaga S, et al. Extracranial aneurysm of the posterior inferior cerebellar artery: Case report. Neurosurgery 33:742–744; discussion 744–745, 1993.

Tanaka F, Nishizawa S, Yonekura Y, et al. Changes in cerebral blood flow induced by balloon test occlusion of the internal carotid artery under hypotension. Eur J Nucl Med 22:1268–1273, 1995.

Tanaka K, Hirayama K, Hattori H, et al. A case of cerebral aneurysm associated with complex partial seizures. Brain Dev 16:233–237, 1994.

Tanaka S, Kimura Y, Furukawa M. Pseudoaneurysm of the carotid artery with hemorrhage into the hypopharynx. J Laryngol Otol 109:889–891, 1995.

Tanaka Y, Takeuchi K, Akai K. Intracranial ruptured aneurysm accompanying moya moya phenomenon. Acta Neurochir 52:35–43, 1980.

Tanaka Y, Kobayashi S, Kyoshima K, et al. Multiple clipping technique for large and giant internal carotid artery aneurysms and complications: Angiographic analysis. J Neurosurg 80:635–642, 1994.

Tanaka Y, Kobayashi S, Sugita K, et al. Characteristics of pterional routes to basilar bifurcation aneurysm. Neurosurgery 36:533–538; discussion 538–540, 1995.

Tangchai P, Pisitbutr M. Angiographic dissecting aneurysm of internal carotid artery: An autopsy case report. J Med Assoc Thai 54:598–601, 1971.

Taptas JN. Les dilatations et allongements de l'artère carotide interne. Rev Neurol 80:338, 1948.

Tarel V, Pellat J, Naegele B, et al. Troubles mnesiques apres rupture d'anevrysme de l'artere communicante anterieure. 22 cas. Rev Neurol 146:746–751, 1990.

Tashima-Kurita S, Matsushima T, Kato M, et al. Moyamoya disease: Posterior cerebral artery occlusion and pattern-reversal visual-evoked potential. Arch Neurol 46: 550–553, 1989.

Tashima T, Takaki T, Hikita T, et al. Bacterial intracranial aneurysm associated with infective endocarditis: A case showing enlargement of aneurysm size. No Shinkei Geka 23:985–989, 1995.

Tasker AD, Byrne JV. Basilar artery fenestration in association with aneurysms of the posterior cerebral circulation. Neuroradiology 39:185–189, 1997.

Tassman IS. Foster Kennedy syndrome with fusiform aneurysm of internal carotid arteries. Arch Ophthalmol 32:125–127, 1944.

Tateiwa Y, Hoya T, Yoshimura N. Compression of the optic nerve by bilateral internal carotid aneurysms identified by magnetic resonance angiography. Folia Ophthalmol Jpn 48:400–403, 1997.

Tatter SB, Crowell RM, Ogilvy CS. Aneurysmal and microaneurysmal "angiogram-negative" subarachnoid hemorrhage. Neurosurgery 37:48–55, 1995.

Taylor CL, Yuan Z, Selman WR, et al. Cerebral arterial aneurysm formation and rupture in 20,767 elderly patients: Hypertension and other risk factors. J Neurosurg 83:812–819, 1995.

Taylor CL, Selman WR, Kiefer SP, et al. Temporary vessel occlusion during intracranial aneurysm repair. Neurosurgery 39:893–905, 1996.

Taylor PE. Delayed postoperative hemorrhage from intracranial aneurysm after craniotomy for tumor. Neurology 11:225–231, 1961.

Teal JS, Bergeron RT, Rumbaugh CL, et al. Aneurysms of the petrous or cavernous portions of the internal carotid artery associated with non-penetrating head trauma. J Neurosurg 38:568–574, 1973.

Teasdale E, Macpherson P, Statham P. Non-invasive investigation for oculomotor palsy due to aneurysm. J Neurol Neurosurg Psychiatry 52:929, 1989.

Teasdale E, Statham P, Straiton J, et al. Non-invasive radiological investigation for oculomotor palsy. J Neurol Neurosurg Psychiatry 53:549–553, 1990.

Teitelbaum GP, Halbach VV, Larsen DW, et al. Treatment of massive posterior epistaxis by detachable coil embolization of a cavernous internal carotid artery aneurysm. Neuroradiology *37*:334–336, 1995a.

Teitelbaum GP, Dowd CF, Larsen DW, et al. Endovascular management of biopsy-related posterior inferior cerebellar artery pseudoaneurysm. Surg Neurol *43*: 357–359, 1995b.

Tekkok IH, Ventureyra EC. Spontaneous intracranial hemorrhage of structural origin during the first year of life. Childs Nerv Syst *13*:154–165, 1997.

Teng MM, Chen CC, Lirng JF, et al. N-butyl-2-cyanoacrylate for embolisation of carotid aneurysm. Neuroradiology *36*:144–147, 1994.

Tenjin H, Fushiki S, Nakahara Y, et al. Effect of Guglielmi detachable coils on experimental carotid artery aneurysms in primates. Stroke *26*:2075–2080, 1995.

ter Berg JWM, Van Meel GJ, Blom WAM, et al. Ophthalmological abnormalities in (relatives of) patients with familial intracranial aneurysms. A collagen deficiency? Neuro-ophthalmology *9*:213–218, 1989.

ter Berg HWM, Bijlsma JB, Veiga Pires JA, et al. Familial association of intracranial aneurysms and multiple congenital anomalies. Arch Neurol *43*:30–33, 1986.

ter Berg HW, Dippel DW, Limburg M, et al. Familial intracranial aneurysms: A review. Stroke *23*:1024–1030, 1992.

Terada T, Tsuura M, Kinoshita Y, et al. Stenotic kinking of the cavernous internal carotid artery with a giant intra-cavernous aneurysm: Case report. Neuroradiology *36*:608–610, 1994.

Terada Y, Kikawa I, Wanibuchi Y. Late rupture of a mycotic cerebral aneurysm after mitral valve replacement for bacterial endocarditis in the inactive stage. Med J Aust *159*:567, 1993.

Terai Y, Sugiu K, Mandai S, et al. Unbranched-site aneurysm of intracranial internal carotid artery. No Shinkei Geka *20*:741–748, 1992.

Terry JE, Stout T. A pupil-sparing oculomotor palsy from a contralateral giant intra-cavernous carotid aneurysm. J Am Optom Assoc *61*:640–645, 1990.

Terson A. De l'hémorrhagie dans le corps vitré au cours de l'hémorrhagie cérébrale. Clin Ophtalmol *6*:309–312, 1900.

Terson A. Le syndrome de l'hématome du corps vitré et de l'hémorrhagie intracranienne spontanés. Ann Oculist *163*:666–673, 1926.

Tertel KJ 2nd, Beydoun NM, Thompson WC 3rd. Extracranial carotid artery aneurysm. Ann Otol Rhinol Laryngol *102*:961–963, 1993.

Teuscher AU, Meienberg O. Ischaemic oculomotor nerve palsy: Clinical features and vascular risk factors in 23 patients. J Neurol *232*:144–149, 1985.

Tezel TH, Gunalp I, Tezel G. Morphometrical analysis of retinal arterial macroaneurysms. Doc Ophthalmol *88*:113–125, 1994a.

Tezel TH, Gunalp I, Tezel G. Morphometric analysis of exudative retinal arterial macroaneurysms: A geometrical approach to exudate curves. Ophthal Res *26*: 332–339, 1994b.

Thapedi IM, Ashenhurst EM, Rozdilsky B. Spontaneous dissecting aneurysms of the internal carotid artery in the neck. Arch Neurol *23*:549–554, 1970.

Thielen KR, Nichols DA, Fulgham JR, et al. Endovascular treatment of cerebral aneurysms following incomplete clipping. J Neurosurg *87*:184–189, 1997.

Thierry A, Sautreaux JL, Lopin-Pelikan MC, et al. Les complications observées dans la chirurgie des anévyrsmes du polygone de Willis dans une optique d'intervention précoce. Neurochirurgie *33*:469–473, 1987.

Thompson JR, Harwood-Nash DC, Fitz CR. Cerebral aneurysms in children. AJR *118*:163–175, 1975.

Thomson AT. A case of aneurisms within the skull, terminating in apoplexy and paralysis, with clinical remarks. Lond Edinburgh Monthly J Med Sci 2:557–563, 1842.

Thron A, Bockenheimer S. Giant aneurysms of the posterior fossa suspected as neoplasms on computed tomography. Neuroradiology *18*:93–97, 1979.

Thun F, Lanfermann H. Intrakranielle Riesenaneurysmen verursacht durch Strahleneinwirkung. Radiology *31*:244–246, 1991.

Tidswell P, Dias PS, Sagar HJ, et al. Cognitive outcome after aneurysm rupture: Relationship to aneurysm site and perioperative complications. Neurology *45*: 875–882, 1995.

Timberlake WH, Kubik CS. Follow-up report with clinical and anatomical notes on 280 patients with subarachnoid hemorrhage. Trans Am Neurol Assoc *77*:26–30, 1952.

Timperman PE, Tomsick TA, Tew JM Jr, et al. Aneurysm formation after carotid occlusion. AJNR *16*:329–331, 1995.

Titer EM, Laureno R. Inverse/reverse ocular bobbing. Ann Neurol *23*:103–104, 1988.

Todd NV, Tocher JL, Jones PA, et al. Outcome following aneurysm wrapping: A 10-year follow-up review of clipped and wrapped aneurysms. J Neurosurg *70*: 841–846, 1989a.

Todd NV, Tocher J, Jones PA, et al. Recurrent subarachnoid hemorrhage in patients with wrapped aneurysms. J Neurol Neurosurg Psychiatry *52*:926, 1989b.

Todd NV, Howie JE, Miller JD. Norman Dott's contribution to aneurysm surgery. J Neurol Neurosurg Psychiatry *53*:455–458, 1990.

Tokimura H, Atsuchi M, Tokimura Y, et al. Direct surgical management of aneurysms in the cavernous sinus: A report of 5 cases. No Shinkei Geka *19*:15–20, 1991.

Tokimura H, Todoroki K, Asakura T, et al. Coexistence of extracranial internal carotid artery aneurysm and multiple intracranial aneurysms: Case report. Neurol Med Chir *32*:292–295, 1992.

Tokiyoshi K, Ohnishi T, Nii Y. Efficacy and toxicity of thromboxane synthetase inhibitor for cerebral vasospasm after subarachnoid hemorrhage. Surg Neurol *36*:112–118, 1991.

Tokuda T, Ono Y, Nishiya H, et al. An autopsy case of fungal (Mucor) cerebral aneurysm. Kansenshogaku Zasshi *69*:438–443, 1995.

Tokuda Y, Inagawa T, Katoh Y, et al. Intracerebral hematoma in patients with ruptured cerebral aneurysms. Surg Neurol *43*:272–277, 1995.

Tokuno T, Ban S, Shingu T, et al. Traumatic anterior cerebral artery aneurysm difficult to distinguish from congenital cerebral aneurysm: Case report. No Shinkei Geka *22*:1073–1076, 1994.

Tommasi-Davenas C, Demiaux B, Kzaiz M, et al. Anévrysme gént thrombosé de l'artère vertébrale gauche développé dans le quatriéme ventricule. Rev Neurol *145*:799–801, 1989.

Tomsak RL. Muslin optic neuropathy. J Clin Neuro-Ophthalmol *5*:71–72, 1985.

Tomsak RL, Costin JA, Hanson M. Carotid-ophthalmic artery aneurysm presenting as unilateral disc edema with choroidal folds. In Neuro-ophthalmology Focus 1980. Editor, Smith JL, pp 181–187. New York, Masson, 1979.

Tomsak RL, Masaryk TJ, Bates JH. Magnetic resonance angiography (MRA) of isolated aneurysmal third nerve palsy. J Clin Neuroophthalmol *11*:16–18, 1991.

Tonali P, Laudisio A, Belloni G, et al. Functional obstructive hydrocephalus. Neuroradiology *5*:220–222, 1973.

Tönnis W, Walter W. Die Behandlung der sackförmigen intrakraniellen Aneurysmen. In Klinik und Behandlung der Raumbeengenden Intrakraniellen Prozesse. Editors, Olivecrona H, Tönnis W, Vol 4, Pt 2, pp 212–363. Berlin, Springer-Verlag, 1966.

Toosi SH, Malton M. Terson's syndrome: Significance of ocular findings. Ann Ophthalmol *19*:7–12, 1987.

Torner JC, Nibbelink DW, Burmeister LF. Statistical comparisons of end results of a randomized study. In Aneurysmal Subarachnoid Hemorrhage: Report of the Cooperative Study. Editors, Sahs AL, Nibbelink DW, Torner JC, pp 249–276. Baltimore, Urban & Schwarzenberg, 1981.

Touho H. Hemodynamic evaluation with dynamic DSA during the treatment of cerebral vasospasm: A retrospective study. Surg Neurol *44*:63–73; discussion 73–74, 1995.

Touho H, Karasawa J, Shishido H, et al. Continuous alprenolol infusion for control of hypertension in the acute stage of ruptured intracranial aneurysms. Neurol Med Chir *31*:396–400, 1991.

Touho H, Karasawa J, Ohnishi H, et al. Assessment of delayed cerebral vasospasm using intracisternal echography—technical note. Surg Neurol *44*:319–325, 1995.

Toyota BD, Ferguson GG. Basilar artery dissection: An early postoperative complication of aneurysm clipping. Case report. J Neurosurg *81*:139–142, 1994.

Tramo MJ, Hainline B, Petito F, et al. Vertebral artery injury and cerebellar stroke while swimming: Case report. Stroke *16*:1039–1042, 1985.

Tridon P, Masingue M, Picard L, et al. Hémispasme faciale et mégadolichobasilaire à symptomatologie pseudo-tumorale. Rev Otoneuroophtalmol *43*:279–286, 1971.

Trippel OH, Haid SP, Kornmesser TW, et al. Extracranial carotid aneurysms. In Aneurysms: Diagnosis and Treatment. Editors, Bergan JJ, Yao JST, pp 493–504. New York, Grune & Stratton, 1982.

Trobe JD, Glaser JS, Post JD. Meningiomas and aneurysms of the cavernous sinus. Arch Ophthalmol *96*:457–467, 1978a.

Trobe JD, Glaser JS, Quencer RC. Isolated oculomotor paralysis: The product of saccular and fusiform aneurysms of the basilar artery. Arch Ophthalmol *96*: 1236–1240, 1978b.

Trobe JD, Glaser JS, Cassady JC, et al. Non glaucomatous excavation of the optic disc. Arch Ophthalmol *98*:1046–1050, 1980.

Trosch RM, Hasbani M, Brass LM. "Bottoms up" dissection. N Engl J Med *320*: 1564–1565, 1989.

Tsuchiya K, Makita K, Furui S. 3D CT angiography of cerebral aneurysms with spiral scanning: Comparison with 3D-time-of-flight MR angiography. Radiat Med *12*: 161–166, 1994.

Tsugu A, Matsumae M, Ikeda A, et al. A case report: Persistent primitive hypoglossal artery aneurysm. No Shinkei Geka *18*:95–100, 1990.

Tsuji T, Abe M, Tabuchi K. Aneurysm of a persistent primitive olfactory artery. Case report. J Neurosurg *83*:138–140, 1995.

Tsukahara T, Wada H, Satake K, et al. Proximal balloon occlusion for dissecting vertebral aneurysms accompanied by subarachnoid hemorrhage. Neurosurgery *36*:914–919; discussion 919–920, 1995.

Tsuruta K, Kasai N, Katayama S. A case of polycystic kidney associated with new growth of cerebral aneurysm after aneurysmal operation. No Shinkei Geka *22*: 877–880, 1994.

Tu RK, Cohen WA, Maravilla KR, et al. Digital subtraction rotational angiography for aneurysms of the intracranial anterior circulation: Injection method and optimization. AJNR *17*:1127–1136, 1996.

Tulleken CA. Giant aneurysms of the posterior fossa presenting as space occupying lesions. Clin Neurosurg *79*:161–186, 1976.

Tulleken CAF, Luiten MLFB. The basilar artery bifurcation *in situ* approached via the Sylvian route (50 ×): An anatomical study in human cadavers. Acta Neurochir *80*:109–115, 1986.

Tureen L. Lesions of the fundus associated with brain hemorrhage. Arch Neurol Psychiatr *42*:664–678, 1939.

Turjman F, Massoud TF, Ji C, et al. Combined stent implantation and endosaccular coil placement for treatment of experimental wide-necked aneurysms: A feasibility study in swine. AJNR *15*:1087–1090, 1994.

Turjman F, Massoud TF, Ji C, et al. Combined stent implantation and endosaccular coil placement for treatment of experimental wide-necked aneurysms: A feasibility study in swine. AJNR 15:1087–1090, 1994a.

Turjman F, Massoud TF, Vinuela F, et al. Aneurysms related to cerebral arteriovenous malformations: superselective angiographic assessment in 58 patients. AJNR 15: 1601–1605, 1994b.

Turnbull HM. Alterations in arterial structure and their relation to syphilis. Q J Med 8:201–253, 1915.

Turss R. Vitrektomie bei Terson-syndrom. Fortschr Ophthalmol 81:257–259, 1984.

Turtz A, Allen D, Koenigsberg R, et al. Nonvisualization of a large cerebral aneurysm despite high-resolution magnetic resonance angiography: Case report. J Neurosurg 82:294–295, 1995.

Turut P, Pfaelzer I, Regnaut B, et al. La vitrectomie dans le syndrome de Terson. Bull Soc Ophtalmol Fr 84:1129–1132, 1984.

Tytle TL, Loeffler CL, Steinberg TA. Fistula between a posterior communicating artery aneurysm and the cavernous sinus. AJNR 16:1808–1810, 1995.

Uberoi R, Murphy P, Jones A. The "pituitary pseudoaneurysm" artefact with 3D TOF MRA of the circle of Willis. J Comput Assist Tomogr 19:822–823, 1995.

Uhthoff W. Ophthalmic experiences and considerations on the surgery of cerebral tumors and tower skull. The Bowman Lecture. Trans Ophthalmol Soc UK 34: 47–123, 1914.

Ukkola V, Heikkinen ER. Epilepsy after operative treatment of ruptured cerebral aneurysms. Acta Neurochir 106:115–118, 1990.

Umezu H, Seki Y, Aiba T, et al. Aneurysm arising from the petrous portion of the internal carotid artery: Case report. Radiat Med 11:251–255, 1993.

Unal OF, Hepgul KT, Turantan MI, et al. Extracranial carotid artery aneurysm in a child misdiagnosed as a parapharyngeal abscess: A case report. J Otolaryngol 21:108–111, 1992.

Ungerman AH, Loubeer L. Spontaneous subarachnoid hemorrhage, diagnosis, management, and prognosis: Presentation of two cases resembling Dietl's crisis and six fatal cases of ruptured intracranial aneurysm (two luetic). J Oklahoma Med Assoc 40:445–450, 1947.

Unsöld R. The concept of optic nerve compression by dolichoectatic arteries revisited. The literature and why it became forgotten. In Compressive Optic Nerve Lesions at the Optic Canal. Editors, Unsöld R, Seeger W, pp 35–37. Berlin, Springer-Verlag, 1989a.

Unsöld R. Selected case reports. In Compressive Optic Nerve Lesions at the Optic Canal. Editors, Unsöld R, Seeger W, pp 87–128. Berlin, Springer-Verlag, 1989b.

Uranishi R, Ochiai C, Tejima T, et al. A distal posterior inferior cerebellar artery aneurysm in the fourth ventricle: A case report. No Shinkei Geka 22:1035–1038, 1994.

Uranishi R, Ochiai C, Okuno S, et al. Cerebral aneurysms associated with von Recklinghausen neurofibromatosis: Report of two cases. No Shinkei Geka 23: 237–242, 1995.

Urbach H, Meyer B, Cedzich C, et al. Posterior inferior cerebellar artery aneurysm in the fourth ventricle. Neuroradiology 37:267–269, 1995.

Ushikoshi S, Houkin K, Itoh F, et al. Ruptured aneurysm of the middle meningeal artery associated with occlusion of the posterior cerebral artery. Case report. J Neurosurg 84:269–271, 1996.

Usui M, Saito N, Hoya K, et al. Vasospasm prevention with postoperative intrathecal thrombolytic therapy: A retrospective comparison of urokinase, tissue plasminogen activator, and cisternal drainage alone. Neurosurgery 34:235–244; discussion 244–245, 1994.

Utoh J, Miyauchi Y, Goto H, et al. Endovascular approach for an intracranial mycotic aneurysm associated with infective endocarditis. J Thorac Cardiovasc Surg 110: 557–559, 1995.

Vajda J, Juhász J, Pásztor E, et al. Contralateral approach to bilateral and ophthalmic aneurysms. Neurosurgery 22:662–668, 1988.

van Alphen HA, Gao YZ. Multiple cerebral de novo aneurysms. Clin Neurol Neurosurg 93:13–18, 1991.

van den Berg JS, Limburg M, Hennekam RC. Is Marfan syndrome associated with symptomatic intracranial aneurysms? Stroke 27:10–12, 1996.

van der Meulen JH, Weststrate W, van Gijn J, et al. Is cerebral angiography indicated in infective endocarditis? Stroke 23:1662–1667, 1992.

van Dijk MA, Chang PC, Peters DJ, et al. Intracranial aneurysms in polycystic kidney disease linked to chromosome 4. J Am Soc Nephrol 6:1670–1673, 1995.

van Gijn J, Hijdra A, Wijdicks EFM, et al. Acute hydrocephalus after aneurysmal subarachnoid hemorrhage. J Neurosurg 63:355–362, 1985.

van Gijn J, Bromberg JE, Lindsay KW, et al. Definition of initial grading, specific events, and overall outcome in patients with aneurysmal subarachnoid hemorrhage. A survey. Stroke 25:1623–1627, 1994.

van Rens GH, Bos PJM, van Dalen JTW. Vitrectomy in two cases of bilateral Terson syndrome. Doc Ophthalmol 56:155–159, 1983.

van Rooij WJ, Sluzewski M, Wijnalda D, et al. Endovasculaire behandeling van inoperabele cerebrale aneurysma's met Guglielmi-spiraaltjes; eerste ervaringen in Nederland. Ned Tijdschr Geneeskd 140:491–495, 1996.

van Rossum J, Wintzen AR, Endtz JL, et al. Effect of tranexamic acid on rebleeding after subarachnoid hemorrhage: A double-blind controlled clinical trial. Ann Neurol 2:238–242, 1977.

Van 'T Hoff W, Hornabrook RW, Marks V. Hypopituitarism associated with intracranial aneurysms. Br Med J 2:1190–1194, 1961.

Van der Linden M, Bruyer R. Troubles de la memoire et signes de dysfonctionnement

frontal chez vingt-neuf patients operes d'un anevrysme de l'artere communicante anterieure. Acta Neurol Belg 92:255–277, 1992.

Van Uitert RL, Solomon GE. White-centered retinal hemorrhages: A sign of intracranial hemorrhage. Neurology 29:236–239, 1979.

Vanderlinden RG, Chisholm LD. Vitreous hemorrhage and sudden increased intracranial pressure. J Neurosurg 41:167–176, 1974.

Vangelista S, Pirrone R, Agrillo U, et al. Aneurismi micotici intracranici: Considerazioni a proposito di due casi clinici. Riv Neurol 54:309–314, 1984.

Vanhoorne M, De Rouck A, Bacquer D. Epidemiological study of the systemic ophthalmological effects of carbon disulfide. Arch Environ Health 51:181–188, 1996.

Vanninen RL, Hernesniemi JA, Puranen MI, et al. Magnetic resonance angiographic screening for asymptomatic intracranial aneurysms: The problem of false negatives: Technical case report. Neurosurgery 38:838–840; discussion 840–841, 1996.

Vargas ME, Kupersmith MJ, Setton A, et al. Endovascular treatment of giant aneurysms which cause visual loss. Ophthalmology 101.1091–1098, 1994.

Varma R, Miller NR. Primary oculomotor nerve synkinesis caused by an extracavernous intradural aneurysm. Am J Ophthalmol 118:83–87, 1994.

Vassilakis D, Sirmos C, Selviaridis P. Aneurysm of the vermian branch of the superior cerebellar artery. J Neurosurg Sci 37:243–245, 1993.

Vassiliou GA, Dielas E, Doris MS. Acquired cranial nerve lesions affecting the ocular system. In International Congress of Ophthalmology. Editors, Henkind P, Shimizu K, Blodi FC, et al, Vol 2, pp 945–947. Philadelphia, JB Lippincott, 1982.

Vazquez Anon V, Aymard A, Gobin YP, et al. Balloon occlusion of the internal carotid artery in 40 cases of giant intracavernous aneurysm: Technical aspects, cerebral monitoring, and results. Neuroradiology 34:245–251, 1992.

Vázquez-Barquero A, Quintana F, Austin O, et al. Emergency embolectomy of middle cerebral artery occlusion due to microcoil migration: Case report. Surg Neurol 42:135–137, 1994.

Velikay M, Datlinger P, Stolbam U, Wedrichm A, et al. Retinal detachment with severe proliferative vitreoretinopathy in Terson syndrome. Ophthalmology 101: 35–37, 1994.

Ventureyra EC, Higgins MJ. Traumatic intracranial aneurysms in childhood and adolescence. Case reports and review of the literature. Childs Nerv Syst 10:361–379, 1994.

Ventureyra ECG, Choo SH, Benoit BG. Super giant globoid intracranial aneurysm in an infant: Case report. J Neurosurg 53:411–416, 1980.

Verbalis JG, Nelson PB, Robinson AG. Reversible panhypopituitarism caused by a suprasellar aneurysm: The contribution of mass effect to pituitary dysfunction. Neurosurgery 10:604–611, 1982.

Vermeer SE, Rinkel GJ, Algra A. Circadian fluctuations in onset of subarachnoid hemorrhage. New data on aneurysmal and perimesencephalic hemorrhage and a systematic review. Stroke 28:805–808, 1997.

Vermeij FH, Hasan D, Vermeulen M, et al. Predictive factors for deterioration from hydrocephalus after subarachnoid hemorrhage. Neurology 44:1851–1855, 1994.

Vermeulen M, van Gijn J. The diagnosis of subarachnoid hemorrhage. J Neurol Neurosurg Psychiatry 53:365–372, 1990.

Vermeulen M, van Gijn J, Hijdra A, et al. Causes of acute deterioration in patients with a ruptured intracranial aneurysm: A prospective study with serial CT scanning. J Neurosurg 60:935–939, 1984a.

Vermeulen M, Lindsay KW, Murray GD, et al. Antifibrinolytic treatment in subarachnoid hemorrhage. N Engl J Med 311:432–437, 1984b.

Verreault J, Cote C. Flip-flop phenomenon and dissection of extracranial carotid artery. Clin Nucl Med 11:251–253, 1986.

Versavel M, Witmer JP, Matricali B. Giant aneurysm arising from the anterior cerebral artery and causing an isolated homonymous hemianopia. Neurosurgery 22: 560–563, 1988.

Viale GL, Pau A. Carotid-ophthalmic aneurysms: Remarks on surgical treatment and outcome. Surg Neurol 11:141–145, 1979.

Vieco PT, Shuman WP, Alsofrom GF, et al. Detection of circle of Willis aneurysms in patients with acute subarachnoid hemorrhage: A comparison of CT angiography and digital subtraction angiography. AJR 165:425–430, 1995.

Vieco PT, Maurin EE 3rd, Gross CE. Vertebrobasilar dolichoectasia: Evaluation with CT angiography. AJNR 18:1385–1388, 1997.

Vighetto A, Lisovoski F, Revol A, et al. Internal carotid artery dissection and ipsilateral hypoglossal nerve palsy. J Neurol Neurosurg Psychiatry 53:530–531, 1990.

Vincent FM, Zimmerman JE. Superior cerebellar artery aneurysm presenting as an oculomotor nerve palsy in a child. Neurosurgery 6:661–664, 1980.

Vinduska V, Hejnal J, Karel W, et al. Aneurysm of the common carotid artery as a sequel of puncture angiography. Australas Radiol 37:115–118, 1993.

Vinuela F, Duckwiler G, Mawad M. Guglielmi detachable coil embolization of acute intracranial aneurysm: Perioperative anatomical and clinical outcome in 403 patients. J Neurosurg 86:475–482, 1997.

Vitek JJ. Femoro-cerebral angiography: Analysis of 2000 consecutive examinations: Special emphasis on carotid arteries catheterization in older patients. AJR 118: 633–647, 1973.

Vles JS, Hendriks JJ, Lodder J, et al. Multiple vertebro-basilar infarctions from fibromuscular dysplasia related dissecting aneurysm of the vertebral artery in a child. Neuropediatrics 21:104–105, 1990.

Voldby B, Enevoldsen EM, Jensen FT. Regional CBF, intraventricular pressure, and cerebral metabolism in patients with ruptured intracranial aneurysms. J Neurosurg 62:48–58, 1985a.

Voldby B, Enevoldsen EM, Jensen FT. Cerebrovascular reactivity in patients with ruptured intracranial aneurysms. J Neurosurg 62:59–67, 1985b.

von Wild K, Busse H. Neurovaskuläre Kompression des N. opticus als Ursache fortschreitender Sehfunktionsstörungen und ihre Dekompressionsbehandlung. Klin Monatsbl Augenheilkd 196:460–465, 1990.

Von Mitterwallner F. Variationsstatische Untersuchungen an den basalen Hirngefässen. Acta Anat 24:51–88, 1955.

Voris HC, Basile JXR. Recurrent epistaxis from aneurysm of the internal carotid artery: Case report with cure by operation. J Neurosurg 18:841–842, 1961.

Vukov JG. Intracavernous aneurysm with isolated 6th nerve palsy. Ann Ophthalmol 5:1071–1074, 1975.

Waberzinek G, Urbanek K, Klaus E. Beitrag zum klinishcen Bild der sogenannten Megadolichobasilaris. Nervenarzt 42:208–211, 1971.

Waespe W, Niesper J, Imhof HG, et al. Lower cranial nerve palsies due to internal carotid dissection. Stroke 19:1561–1564, 1988.

Waga S, Morikawa A. Aneurysm developing on the infundibular widening of the posterior communicating artery. Surg Neurol 11:125–127, 1979.

Waga S, Tochio H. Intracranial aneurysm associated with moyamoya disease in childhood. Surg Neurol 23:237–243, 1985.

Waga S, Ohtsubo K, Handa H. Warning signs in intracranial aneurysms. Surg Neurol 3:15–20, 1975.

Waga S, Fujimoto K, Morooka Y. Dissecting aneurysm of the vertebral artery. Surg Neurol 10:237–239, 1978.

Waga S, Morikawa A, Kojima T. Trigeminal neuralgia: Compression of the trigeminal nerve by an elongated and dilated basilar artery. Surg Neurol 11:13–16, 1979.

Waga S, Kojima T, Tochio H, et al. Aneurysm of the posterior communicating artery itself. Neurol Med Chir 24:495–498, 1984.

Waga S, Itoh H, Kojima T. Posterior inferior cerebellar artery aneurysm associated with arteriovenous malformation fed by the same artery. Surg Neurol 23:617–620, 1985.

Wakabayashi T, Fujita S, Ohbora Y, et al. Polycystic kidney disease and intracranial aneurysms: Early angiographic diagnosis and early operation for the unruptured aneurysm. J Neurosurg 58:488–491, 1983.

Wakabayashi T, Tamaki N, Yamashita H, et al. Angiographic classification of aneurysms of the horizontal segment of the anterior cerebral artery. Surg Neurol 24:31–34, 1985.

Wakai S, Fukushima T, Furihata T, et al. Association of cerebral aneurysm with pituitary adenoma. Surg Neurol 12:503–507, 1979.

Wakai S, Yoshimasu N, Eguchi T, et al. Traumatic intracavernous aneurysm of the internal carotid artery following surgery for chronic sinusitis. Surg Neurol 13:391–394, 1980.

Wakai S, Eguchi T, Asano T, et al. Oculomotor palsy caused by aneurysm clip: Report of two cases. Neurosurgery 9:429–432, 1981.

Wakhloo AK, Schellhammer F, de Vries J, et al. Self-expanding and balloon-expandable stents in the treatment of carotid aneurysms: An experimental study in a canine model. AJNR 15:493–502, 1994.

Wakui K, Kobayashi S, Takemae T, et al. Giant thrombosed vertebral artery aneurysm managed with extracranial intracranial bypass surgery and aneurysmectomy. Case report. J Neurosurg 77:624–627, 1992.

Walker AE, Allegre GW. The pathology and pathogenesis of cerebral aneurysms. J Neuropathol Exp Neurol 13:248–254, 1954.

Wallace S, Jaffe ME. Cerebral arterial ectasia with saccular aneurysms. Radiology 88:90–93, 1967.

Walsh FB. Clinical Neuro-Ophthalmology. 2nd ed, pp 820–821. Baltimore, Williams & Wilkins, 1957.

Walsh FB. Visual field defects due to aneurysms at the circle of Willis. Arch Ophthalmol 71:15–27, 1964.

Walsh FB, Gass JD. Concerning the optic chiasm: Selected pathologic involvement and clinical problems. Am J Ophthalmol 50:1031–1047, 1960.

Walsh FB, Hedges TR. Optic nerve sheath hemorrhage: The Jackson Memorial Lecture. Am J Ophthalmol 34:509–527, 1951.

Walsh FB, Hoyt WF. Clinical Neuro-Ophthalmology. 3rd ed, Vol 2, p 1741. Baltimore, Williams & Wilkins, 1969a.

Walsh FB, Hoyt WF. Clinical Neuro-Ophthalmology. 3rd ed, Vol 2, pp 1767–1768. Baltimore, Williams & Wilkins, 1969b.

Walsh FB, Hoyt WF. Clinical Neuro-Ophthalmology. 3rd ed, Vol 2, p 1743. Baltimore, Williams & Wilkins, 1969c.

Walsh FB, Hoyt WF. Clinical Neuro-Ophthalmology. 3rd ed, Vol 2, p 1746. Baltimore, Williams & Wilkins, 1969d.

Walsh FB, Hoyt WF. Clinical Neuro-Ophthalmology. 3rd ed, Vol 2, p 1754. Baltimore, Williams & Wilkins, 1969e.

Walsh FB, Hoyt WF. Clinical Neuro-Ophthalmology. 3rd ed, Vol 2, p 1755. Baltimore, Williams & Wilkins, 1969f.

Walsh FB, Hoyt WF. Clinical Neuro-Ophthalmology. 3rd ed, Vol 2, p 1766. Baltimore, Williams & Wilkins, 1969g.

Walsh FB, Hoyt WF. Clinical Neuro-Ophthalmology. 3rd ed, Vol 2, p 1765. Baltimore, Williams & Wilkins, 1969h.

Walsh FB, Hoyt WF. Clinical Neuro-Ophthalmology. 3rd ed, Vol 2, pp 1757–1758. Baltimore, Williams & Wilkins, 1969i.

Walsh FB, Hoyt WF. Clinical Neuro-Ophthalmology. 3rd ed, Vol 2, p 1760. Baltimore, Williams & Wilkins, 1969j.

Walsh FB, Hoyt WF. Clinical Neuro-Ophthalmology. 3rd ed, Vol 2, p 1770. Baltimore, Williams & Wilkins, 1969k.

Walsh FB, Hoyt WF. Clinical Neuro-Ophthalmology. 3rd ed, Vol 2, p 1770. Baltimore, Williams & Wilkins, 1969l.

Walsh FB, Hoyt WF. Clinical Neuro-Ophthalmology. 3rd ed, Vol 2, pp 1767 1768. Baltimore, Williams & Wilkins, 1969m.

Walsh FB, Hoyt WF. Clinical Neuro-Ophthalmology. 3rd ed, Vol 2, pp 1777–1778. Baltimore, Williams & Wilkins, 1969n.

Walsh FB, King AB. Ocular signs of intracranial saccular aneurysms: Experimental work on collateral circulation through the ophthalmic artery. Arch Ophthalmol 27:1–33, 1942.

Walshe TM, Davis KR, Fisher CM. Thalamic hemorrhage: A computed tomographic-clinical correlation. Neurology 5:638–647, 1977.

Walter KA, Newman NJ, Lessell S. Oculomotor palsy from minor head trauma: Initial sign of intracranial aneurysm. Neurology 44:148–150, 1994.

Wang AN, Winfield JA, Gücer G. Traumatic internal carotid artery aneurysm with rupture in the sphenoid sinus. Surg Neurol 25:77–81, 1986.

Wapenski JA, Hieshima GB, Halbach VV. Therapeutic intravascular balloon embolization of intracranial aneurysms. Neurology 37(Suppl):97, 1987.

Wardlaw JM, Cannon JC. Color transcranial "power" Doppler ultrasound of intracranial aneurysms. J Neurosurg 84:459–461, 1996.

Wardlaw JM, Cannon JC, Sellar RJ. Use of color power transcranial Doppler sonography to monitor aneurysmal coiling. AJNR 17:864–867, 1996b.

Warnell P. Advanced concepts in the management of cerebral vasospasm associated with aneurysmal subarachnoid hemorrhage. Axone 17:86–92, 1996.

Watanabe A, Hirano K, Mizukawa K, et al. Retrieval of a migrated detachable coil: Case report. Neurol Med Chir 35:249–250, 1995.

Watanabe K, Wakai S, Okuhata S, et al. Ruptured distal anterior cerebral artery aneurysms presenting as acute subdural hematoma: Report of three cases. Neurol Med Chir 31:514–517, 1991.

Watanabe T, Satz K, Yoshimoto T. Basilar artery occlusion caused by thrombosis of atherosclerotic fusiform aneurysm of the basilar artery. Stroke 25:1068–1070, 1994.

Watridge CB, Muhlbauer MS, Lowery RD. Traumatic carotid artery dissection: Diagnosis and treatment. J Neurosurg 71:854–857, 1989.

Weaver DF, Gates EM, Nielsen AE. Traumatic intracranial vascular lesions producing late massive nasal hemorrhage. Trans Am Acad Ophthalmol Otolaryngol 65:759–774, 1961.

Weil SM, van Loveren HR, Tomsick TA, et al. Management of inoperable cerebral aneurysms by the navigational balloon technique. Neurosurgery 21:296–302, 1987.

Weinberg DA, Kaufman OI, Siebert JD, et al. Negative MRI versus real disease. Surv Ophthalmol 40:312–319, 1996.

Weingeist TA, Goldman EJ, Folk JC, et al. Terson's syndrome: Clinicopathologic correlations. Ophthalmology 93:1435–1442, 1986.

Weinstein JM, Rufenacht DA, Partington CR, et al. Delayed visual loss due to trauma of the internal carotid artery. Arch Neurol 48:490–497, 1991.

Weinstein L, Schlesinger JJ. Pathoanatomic, pathophysiologic and clinical correlation in endocarditis. N Engl J Med 291:832–837, 1122–1126, 1974.

Weinstein PR. In discussion of Yamada K, Hayakawa T, Ushio Y, et al. Therapeutic occlusion of the vertebral artery for unclippable vertebral aneurysm: Relationship between site of occlusion and clinical outcome. Neurosurgery 15:838, 1984.

Weintraub MI, Sananman ML. Giant intracavernous aneurysm and sixth nerve palsy. Can J Ophthalmol 6:223–226, 1971.

Weir B. Aneurysms Affecting the Nervous System. Baltimore, Williams & Wilkins, 1987.

Weir BK. Vasospasme cerebral. Etude experimentale. Neurochirurgie 38:129–133, 1992.

Weisberg L. Atherosclerotic deformation of the basilar artery as visualized by computerized tomography. Comput Radiol 5:247–254, 1981.

Weissman JL, Johnson JT, Snyderman CH, et al. Thrombosed aneurysm of the cervical carotid artery: Avoiding a retrospective diagnosis. Radiology 190:869–871, 1994.

Welling DB, Glasscock ME III, Tarasidis N. Management of carotid artery hemorrhage in middle ear surgery. Otolaryngology—Head & Neck Surgery 109:996–999, 1993.

Wells HG. Intracranial aneurysms of the vertebral artery. Arch Neurol Psychiatr 1:311–322, 1922.

Wemple JB, Smith GW. Extracranial carotid aneurysm: Report of four cases. J Neurosurg 24:667–671, 1966.

Werner SC, Blakemore AH, King BG. Aneurysm of the internal carotid artery within the skull: Wiring and electrothermic coagulation. JAMA 116:578–582, 1941.

Werry H, Brewitt H. Pars-plana Vitrektomie beim Terson-Syndrom. Fortschr Ophthalmol 79:424–427, 1983.

West P, Todman D. Chronic cluster headache associated with a vertebral artery aneurysm. Headache 31:210–212, 1991.

West TET, Davies RJ, Kelly RE. Horner's syndrome and headache due to carotid artery disease. Br Med J 1:818–820, 1976.

CHAPTER 54

Carotid-Cavernous Sinus Fistulas

Neil R. Miller

A carotid-cavernous sinus fistula is an abnormal communication between the cavernous sinus and the carotid arterial system. Carotid-cavernous sinus fistulas can be classified by etiology (traumatic vs. spontaneous), velocity of blood flow (high vs. low), and anatomy (direct vs. dural; internal carotid vs. external carotid vs. both) (Parkinson, 1964, 1965, 1973; Barrow et al., 1985; Keltner et al., 1987; Debrun et al., 1988; Kwan et al., 1989; Taki et al., 1994; Debrun, 1995).

Some fistulas are characterized by a direct connection between the cavernous segment of the internal carotid artery and the cavernous sinus (Type I of Parkinson, 1965; Type A of Barrow et al., 1985) (Fig. 54.1). These fistulas usually are of the high flow type. Most often caused by a single traumatic tear in the arterial wall, they are called **direct** carotid-cavernous sinus fistulas (Kwan et al., 1989; Monsein and Rigamonti, 1996).

Other carotid-cavernous sinus fistulas are **dural** (Type 2 of Parkinson, 1964, 1965, 1973; Types B, C, and D or Barrow et al., 1985). Many of these lesions are actually congenital arteriovenous malformations that develop spontaneously or in the setting of atherosclerosis, systemic hypertension, or connective tissue disease and during or after childbirth. Dural carotid-cavernous sinus fistulas consist of a communication between the cavernous sinus and one or more meningeal branches of the internal carotid artery (Type B of Barrow et al., 1985) (Fig. 54.2), the external carotid artery (Type C of Barrow et al., 1985) (Fig. 54.3), or both (Type D of Barrow et al., 1985) (Fig. 54.4). These fistulas usually have low rates of arterial blood flow, and they almost always produce symptoms and signs spontaneously; i.e., without any antecedent trauma or manipulation. Because many dural carotid-cavernous sinus fistulas seem to be true congenital arteriovenous malformations, they are also discussed in Chapter 43 of this text in the section on "arteriovenous malformations."

In this chapter, we discuss both direct and dural carotid-cavernous sinus fistulas, allowing us to compare and contrast their pathology, causes, clinical manifestations, diagnosis, treatment, and prognosis.

DIRECT CAROTID-CAVERNOUS SINUS FISTULAS

Direct carotid-cavernous sinus fistulas represent from 70–90% of all carotid-cavernous sinus fistulas in most series (Keltner et al., 1987; Debrun et al., 1988). They occur in both men and women of all ages.

ANATOMY

A direct carotid-cavernous sinus fistula results from a single tear in the wall of the cavernous segment of the internal carotid artery. This produces a direct connection between the artery and one or more of the venous channels within the cavernous sinus. The arteriovenous connection is usually short, tangential, and endothelialized (Dandy and Follis, 1941; Parkinson, 1973; Daxecker and Hattinger, 1982) (Fig. 54.5). It thus is identical, in anatomy and hemodynamics, to traumatic arteriovenous fistulas elsewhere in the body.

A direct carotid-cavernous sinus fistula usually is located along the course of the cavernous segment of the internal

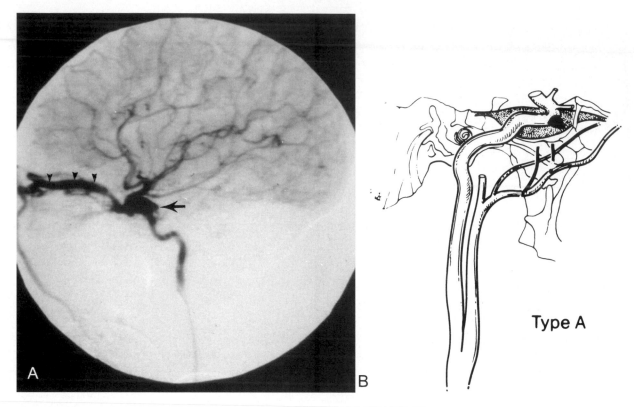

Figure 54.1. Appearance of a direct carotid-cavernous sinus fistula. *A,* Angiographic appearance after a selective injection of the left internal carotid artery shows a collection of contrast material in the cavernous sinus (*arrow*). Note that the fistula drains anteriorly into the superior ophthalmic vein (*arrowheads*). There was no contribution from the ipsilateral external carotid artery, nor was there any contribution from the contralateral internal or external carotid arteries. The patient was a 26-year-old woman who suffered a head injury in a motor vehicle accident and developed a red left eye associated with proptosis of the eye and binocular diplopia. *B,* Artist's drawing of a direct carotid-cavernous sinus fistula. Note that there is a single tear in the wall of the internal carotid artery. There is no contribution from either the extradural branches of the internal carotid artery of the extradural branches of the ipsilateral external carotid artery. (From Barrow DL, Spector RH, Braun IF, et al. J Neurosurg *62:*248–256, 1985.)

carotid artery (Debrun et al., 1981). It may project anteriorly, posteriorly, superiorly, or inferiorly. Helmke et al. (1994) studied 42 patients with direct carotid-cavernous sinus fistulas and found that 27 of the fistulas (64.3%) originated from the most proximal portion of the internal carotid artery within the cavernous sinus that runs superiorly and slightly anteriorly (called the C4 segment by Teufel, 1964), whereas 13 fistulas (31%) originated from the segment that runs anteriorly in the cavernous sinus (called the C2 segment by Teufel, 1964–see Chapter 52) (Fig. 52.7).

On rare occasions, a fistula may develop between the supraclinoid portion of the internal carotid artery or one of its branches and the cavernous sinus (Pelz et al., 1988). An unusual case of this latter type was reported by Kinugasa et al. (1995) who described a 24-year-old man who developed progressive left conjunctival hyperemia, chemosis, pulsating left proptosis, and a retroocular bruit one week after a head injury. An evaluation revealed a fistula between the left posterior communicating artery and the ipsilateral cavernous sinus. A similar case was reported by Tytle et al. (1995), who described a 46-year-old woman who developed a fistula between a posterior communicating artery aneurysm and the ipsilateral cavernous sinus several years after severe head trauma.

Rarely, a direct carotid-cavernous sinus fistula occurs spontaneously or after trauma in the setting of a persistent primitive trigeminal artery originating from the internal carotid artery within the cavernous sinus. Enomoto et al. (1977) reported the case of a 42-year-old woman in whom a carotid-cavernous sinus fistula resulted from the spontaneous rupture of an aneurysm originating at the junction of the right internal carotid artery and a persistent primitive trigeminal artery within the cavernous sinus. McKenzie et al. (1996) reported a patient who developed left-sided proptosis and conjunctival chemosis, a left abducens nerve paresis, and an audible orbitocranial bruit 6 months after a motor vehicle accident. Cerebral angiography demonstrated a traumatic fistula between a persistent trigeminal artery originating from the distal portion of the cavernous segment of the internal carotid artery and the caverous sinus.

PATHOGENESIS

Direct carotid-cavernous sinus fistulas most often result from head trauma (Fleishman et al., 1986; Taki et al., 1994; Monsein and Rigamonti, 1996). The most frequent settings are motor vehicle accidents, fights, and falls (McKinna, 1985; Kupersmith et al., 1986; Brosnahan et al., 1992;

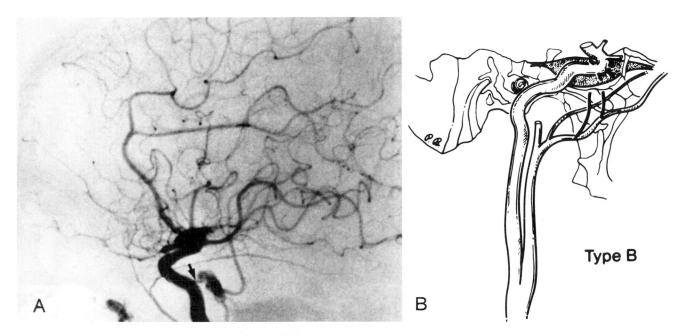

Figure 54.2. Appearance of dural carotid-cavernous sinus fistula in which the only contribution is from extradural branches of the internal carotid artery. *A,* A selective left internal carotid arteriogram shows a fistula at the posterior portion of the intracavernous carotid artery (*arrow*). The left external carotid arteriogram was normal. *B,* Artist's drawing shows that this type of fistula is fed only by extradural branches of the internal carotid artery with no contribution from the extradural branches of the ipsilateral external carotid artery (type B of Barrow et al.). (From Barrow DL, Spector RH, Braun IF, et al. J Neurosurg *62:*248–256, 1985.)

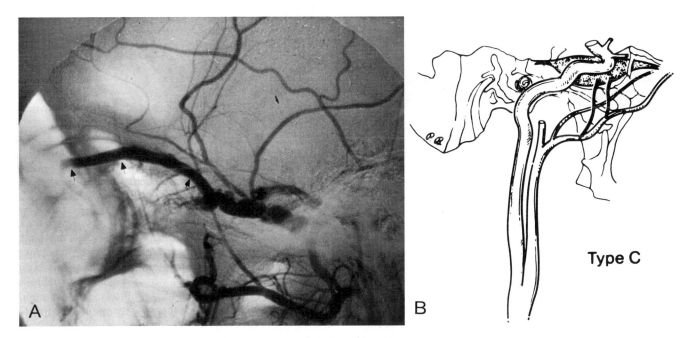

Figure 54.3. Appearance of dural carotid-cavernous sinus in which the only contribution is from extradural branches of the external carotid artery. *A,* A high-flow fistula is fed by extradural branches of the left external carotid artery, particularly the internal maxillary artery. The fistula drains anteriorly into the ipsilateral superior ophthalmic vein (*arrows*). There was no contribution from the ipsilateral internal carotid artery or from the contralateral internal or external carotid arteries. The patient was a 65-year-old woman with the gradual onset of redness and swelling of the left eye. *B,* Artist's drawing of the appearance of this type of fistula. Note that the only contribution is from the extradural branches of the external carotid artery (type C of Barrow et al.). (From Barrow DL, Spector RH, Braun IF, et al. J Neurosurg *62:*248–256, 1985.)

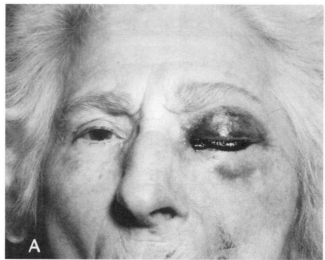

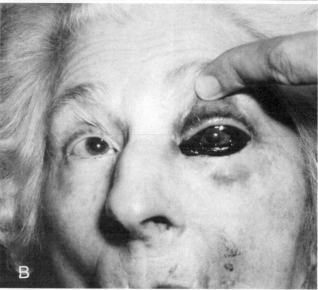

Figure 54.6. Appearance of a patient who developed a spontaneous *direct* carotid-cavernous sinus fistula after rupture of a previously asymptomatic intracavernous aneurysm. *A,* The patient has marked proptosis of the left eye, swelling and ecchymosis of the left upper and lower eyelids, and hemorrhagic conjunctival chemosis. *B,* There is diffuse hemorrhagic chemosis of the conjunctiva. Note that the patient is attempting to look upward to the left, but the left eye is almost completely immobile.

teriosclerosis (Rwiza et al., 1988), or an underlying connective tissue disorder such as fibromuscular dysplasia or Ehlers-Danlos syndrome (Hieshima et al., 1986a; Halbach et al., 1990; Taki et al., 1994; Debrun et al., 1996; Forlodou et al., 1996); however, Gossman et al. (1993) reported the occurrence of a spontaneous direct carotid-cavernous sinus fistula in an otherwise healthy 5-year-old boy with no history of head trauma and no evidence of a connective tissue disorder.

CLINICAL MANIFESTATIONS

The most common clinical manifestations of a direct carotid-cavernous sinus fistula are ocular in nature; however,

in some cases, the first manifestations of the fistula are neurologic or rhinologic.

Nonocular Manifestations

Although direct carotid-cavernous sinus fistulas are not usually thought to be life-threatening, there are, in fact, numerous reports of patients who have experienced significant epistaxis or intracranial hemorrhage from rupture of the fistula. de Schweinitz and Holloway (1908) first reported a patient with a traumatic carotid-cavernous sinus fistula who died after suddenly developing an intracerebral hematoma. At autopsy, the right cavernous sinus was found to have ruptured at the extreme posterior region adjacent to the apex of the petrous portion of the temporal bone. Sattler (1920) also described a case of intracerebral hematoma secondary to rupture of the cavernous sinus in a patient with a traumatic carotid-cavernous sinus fistula. In a review of the literature, he found 5 fatal cases of epistaxis and 3 intracerebral hematomas among 322 cases of carotid-cavernous sinus fistula. Numerous investigators subsequently described severe epistaxis or intracerebral hemorrhage, often fatal, in patients with traumatic carotid-cavernous sinus fistula (Hamby, 1964; Wilson and Markesbery, 1966; Lee et al., 1975; Turner et al., 1983; Dohrmann et al., 1985; Gaston et al., 1986; Hieshima et al., 1986b; Isamat et al., 1986; Kupersmith et al., 1986; O'Reilly et al., 1986; d'Angelo et al., 1988; Shimizu et al., 1988; Lin et al., 1992; Millman and Giddings, 1994). In most cases, the hemorrhage occurs shortly after the trauma. In other cases, however, the hemorrhage occurs months or even years later.

Subarachnoid hemorrhage has been described as a complication of traumatic carotid-cavernous sinus fistula (Sedzimir and Occleshaw, 1967; Mullan, 1979). Unlike epistaxis, it usually occurs months or years after the injury.

Based on Sattler's (1920) review of the literature, a 3% incidence of spontaneous intracerebral hemorrhage caused by carotid-cavernous sinus fistula has been quoted by some investigators (Walker and Allegré, 1956; Hamby, 1964). d'Angelo et al. (1988) defined a group of carotid-cavernous sinus fistulas that they considered most likely to produce intracerebral hemorrhage. The most important angiographic characteristic of these "high-risk" fistulas is a pattern of dilated and tortuous cerebral veins. We have examined an 18-year-old girl who developed a right-sided traumatic carotid-cavernous sinus fistula after she was involved in a motor vehicle accident. She was referred for treatment of the fistula, at which time cerebral angiography revealed prominent, dilated cerebral vessels. Dr. Gerard Debrun, head of the Interventional Radiology Division at The Johns Hopkins Hospital, agreed that this radiographic picture constituted a potentially life-threatening condition that required immediate intervention. Because the right internal carotid artery was occluded, and because the fistula was fed by the right vertebral artery and the left carotid circulation, the patient underwent trapping and intraoperative embolization of the fistula without complication. At the time of craniotomy, the veins in the Sylvian fissure were noted to be dilated and "arterialized," and it was easy to understand how such vessels could rupture and produce subarachnoid hemorrhage, intracerebral hematoma, or both. The patient recovered completely after surgery, and postoperative angiography showed normal venous flow in the previously arterialized cortical veins.

Rare direct carotid-cavernous sinus fistulas may cause a steal phenomenon in cerebral vessels, the result of which may be a debilitating or even fatal stroke. Iida et al. (1995) described such a case.

Ocular Manifestations

The direction of blood flow through a direct carotid-cavernous sinus fistula may be posterior, into the superior and inferior petrosal sinuses, or anterior, into the orbital veins. Although posteriorly draining fistulas may occasionally cause isolated ocular motor nerve pareses, the most severe ocular manifestations occur in patients with anterior redirection of arterial blood through normal orbital venous channels. These manifestations are caused by a combination of diminished arterial flow to the cranial nerves within the cavernous sinus, stasis of both venous and arterial circulation within the eye and orbit, and an increase in episcleral and orbital venous pressure.

The ocular manifestations of a direct carotid-cavernous sinus fistula usually are ipsilateral to the side of the fistula, but they may be bilateral (Fig. 54.7), or even contralateral (54.8) (Ramos and Mount, 1953; Kunc and Dulik, 1954; White et al., 1958; Jamieson et al., 1960; David et al., 1964; Graham, 1966; Bickerstaff, 1970; Madsen, 1970; Hawkins, 1986; Kupersmith et al., 1986). The lateralization of ocular manifestations depends on the venous drainage of the cavernous sinuses, especially the connections between the two sinuses through the intercavernous sinuses and the basilar sinus (see Chapter 52), and the presence or absence of thrombosis within a sinus or a superior ophthalmic vein on one side. In rare cases, usually after trauma, bilateral carotid-cavernous sinus fistulas may occur (West, 1980).

Proptosis

Proptosis is one of the most common signs observed in patients with a direct carotid-cavernous sinus fistula, occurring in almost all patients if the fistula is left untreated (Madsen, 1970; McKinna, 1985; Jorgensen and Guthoff, 1986; Kupersmith et al., 1986; Nowe et al., 1989; Brosnahan et al., 1992) (Fig. 54.9). In most cases, proptosis develops rapidly on the side of the fistula, becoming pronounced within a few days. Some cases have been described in which proptosis has developed months or even years after head trauma. Most likely in such cases, the internal carotid artery was injured at the time of trauma, but a fistula did not develop until shortly before proptosis appeared.

In some patients, proptosis develops not only on the side of the fistula but also on the opposite side. Of 32 patients with unilateral, direct carotid-cavernous sinus fistulas examined by Kupersmith et al. (1986), 2 had bilateral proptosis. In about one-third of cases with bilateral proptosis, proptosis develops simultaneously on both sides (Sattler, 1920). In the

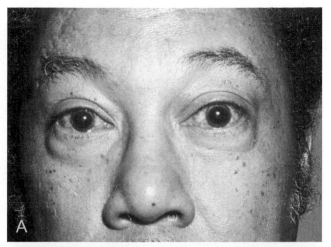

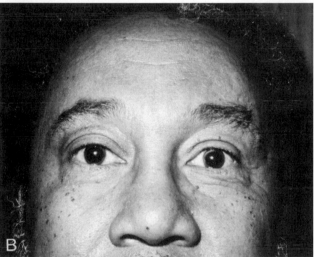

Figure 54.7. Bilateral ocular manifestations in a patient with a unilateral direct carotid-cavernous sinus fistula. The patient was a 56-year-old man who experienced apparently mild, blunt head trauma in a motor vehicle accident. Three weeks after the injury the left eye became somewhat red and swollen. The right eye became red and slightly swollen about 2 weeks later. The patient was assumed to have a chronic conjunctivitis until he developed binocular diplopia. Angiography confirmed a direct (traumatic) carotid-cavernous sinus fistula originating from the left internal carotid artery. *A,* The conjunctival vessels of **both** eyes are dilated. Although the left eye clearly is slightly proptotic, the right eye also is slightly prominent. The left eye is slightly exotropic. *B,* After balloon occlusion of the fistula, both eyes appear normal.

remainder, the second eye becomes affected days to weeks after the first eye.

Once proptosis begins, it increases slowly for several weeks until it finally stabilizes. The eye usually is pushed directly forward, but it may be deviated when ocular motor paresis is present (see below). The severity of proptosis varies considerably. Some patients have only a few millimeters of proptosis; most have 10 mm or less. Among 27 patients examined by Kupersmith et al. (1986), proptosis ipsilateral to the fistula ranged from 3 to 10 mm. On the other hand,

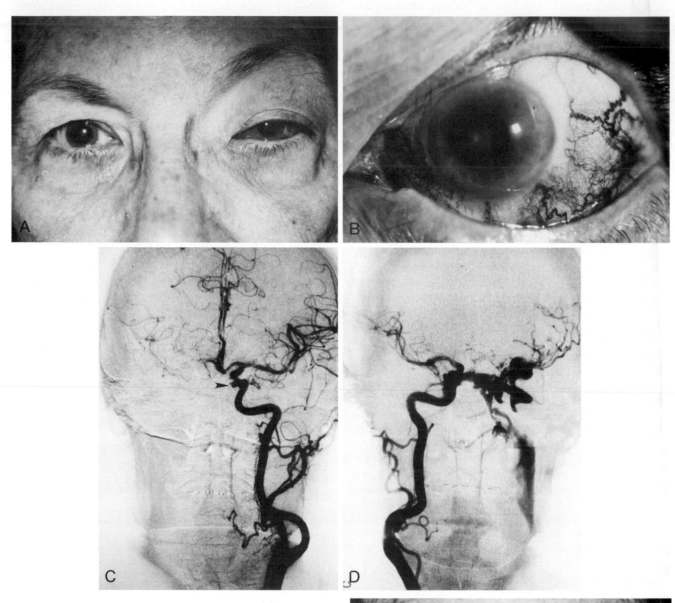

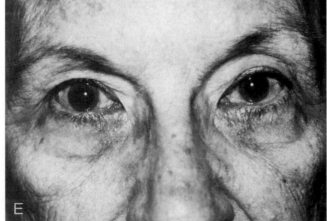

Figure 54.8.   Contralateral ocular manifestations from a direct carotid-cavernous sinus fistula. The patient was a 65-year-old woman who developed swelling, redness, and protrusion of the left eye. *A,* External appearance of the patient at presentation reveals swelling of the left upper eyelid and redness of the left eye. The right eye appears normal. *B,* Close-up of left eye, showing typical dilated, arterialized conjunctival vessels, with minimal conjunctival chemosis. *C,* Selective left common carotid arteriogram, anteroposterior view, shows no evidence of a fistula, although there is a small aneurysm within the cavernous sinus (*arrowhead*). *D,* Selective right common carotid artery, anteroposterior view, reveals a direct carotid-cavernous sinus fistula with immediate crossover to the left side via the intercavernous sinus and subsequent drainage through the left superior ophthalmic vein and superficial cerebral veins. *E,* 2 months after occlusion of the *right-sided* fistula via a transarterial endovascular approach, the appearance of the left eye has returned to normal.

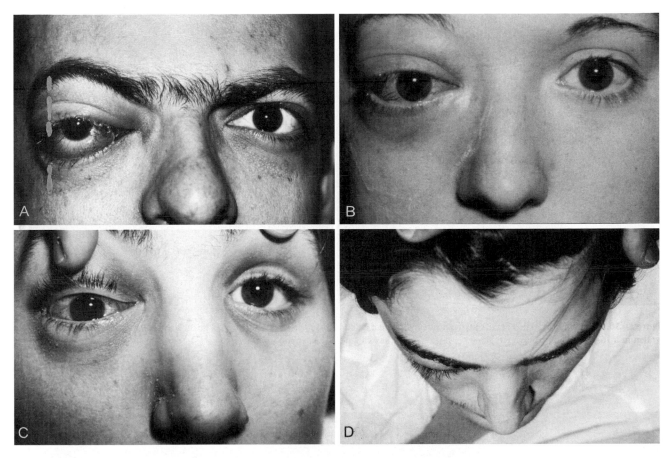

Figure 54.9. Proptosis from direct carotid-cavernous sinus fistula. Note that in all cases, the proptotic eye also has dilated conjunctival and episcleral vessels. *A,* Marked right proptosis associated with dilated conjunctival vessels and diffuse chemosis of the inferior conjunctiva in a 28-year-old man who was injured in a motor vehicle accident. The patient had a right-sided direct carotid-cavernous sinus fistula. *B,* Moderate proptosis and dilated conjunctival vessels in a 21-year-old woman who was injured in a motor vehicle accident. *C,* Moderate right proptosis in a 16-year-old boy who was injured in a skiing accident. *D,* Same patient seen in *C* viewed from above. Note ease with which right proptosis can be seen.

Birch-Herschfeld (1930) described a patient with 16 mm of proptosis, and we have seen similar patients.

Most patients who have significant proptosis caused by a direct carotid-cavernous sinus fistula also are aware of a cranial bruit or have evidence of ocular pulsation, although this is not invariably the case (Hamby, 1966). Burton and Goldberg (1970) described a 54-year-old woman who developed a spontaneous, direct carotid-cavernous sinus fistula from rupture of an intracavernous carotid aneurysm. The patient had severe proptosis and conjunctival chemosis but neither a subjective nor an objective bruit.

Eyelid and Facial Changes

In the early stages of a direct carotid-cavernous sinus fistula, the eyelids may become moderately or even severely swollen (Brosnahan et al., 1992) (Fig. 54.10). With time, the persistent swelling can become associated with progressive and even grotesque changes in the eyelid and its vasculature (Fig. 54.11). Ultimately, racemose undulating dilation of periorbital vessels may produce chronic dermal cyanosis and thickening that resembles the changes seen in patients with congenital facial arteriovenous malformations (Fig. 54.12). When the superior ophthalmic vein is enlarged, the medial portion of the upper eyelid may be considerably stretched and swollen.

Chemosis of Conjunctiva

Conjunctival chemosis occurs in most patients with a direct carotid-cavernous sinus fistula (Madsen, 1970; Nowe et al., 1989; Brosnahan et al., 1992). This swelling of the conjunctiva may develop before proptosis becomes apparent, and it may become quite marked (Figs. 54.6, 54.13, and 54.14). Because the tarsus of the upper eyelid is thicker and firmer than the tarsus of the lower eyelid, the superior bulbar and palpebral conjunctiva usually remains nonchemotic, and the chemosis is invariably limited to the interpalpebral bulbar conjunctiva and the inferior palpebral conjunctiva, regardless of the rate of blood flow through the fistula. In severe cases, the inferior palpebral conjunctiva may actually prolapse through the interpalpebral fissure (Figs. 54.13 and 54.14). Prolapsed conjunctiva that is not kept well-lubricated may become necrotic and infected.

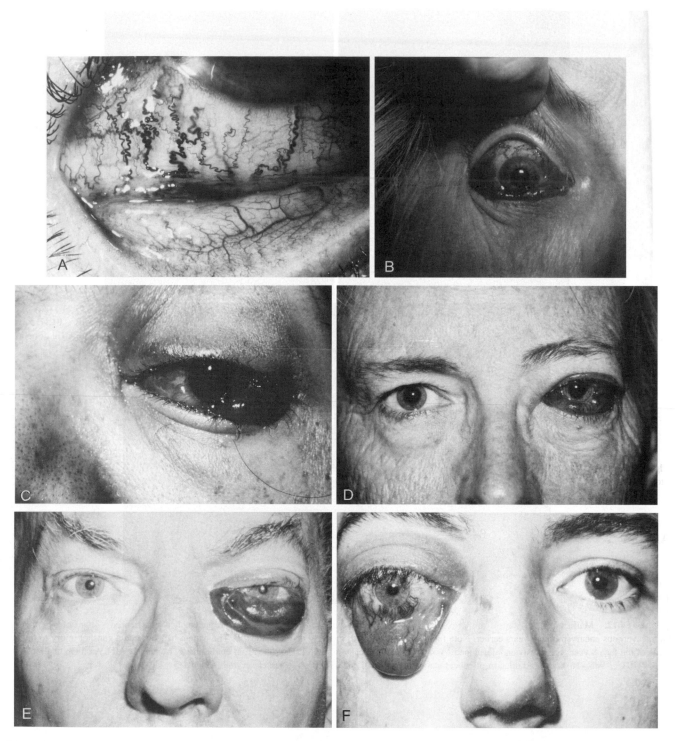

Figure 54.13. Conjunctival chemosis in patients with direct carotid-cavernous sinus fistulas. *A*, Mild chemosis primarily limited to the conjunctiva in the right inferior fornix. In this patient, the dilated tortuous conjunctival and episcleral veins overshadow the chemosis. *B*, Moderate inferior chemosis of the conjunctiva. *C*, Conjunctival chemosis that is mild nasally and severe temporally. *D*, Moderate chemosis of the left interpalpebral conjunctiva. Note inferior displacement of the left lower eyelid. *E*, Severe conjunctival chemosis. *F*, Severe chemosis, expansion, and prolapse of the inferior palpebral conjunctiva.

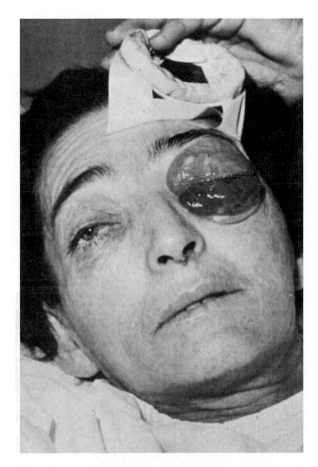

Figure 54.14. Severe unilateral conjunctival chemosis and bilateral proptosis from a direct carotid-cavernous sinus fistula.

Arterialization of the Conjunctiva and Episcleral Veins

As arterial blood is forced anteriorly into the orbital veins, the conjunctival and episcleral veins become dilated, tortuous, and filled with arterial blood (Fig. 54.15). This **arterialization** of conjunctival vessels is a hallmark of a carotid-cavernous sinus fistula. Although it initially may be mistaken for conjunctivitis or episcleritis, the peculiar dilation and tortuousity of the affected vessels usually is quite distinctive.

The extent of arterialization of the conjunctival and episcleral veins is variable. It may be generalized or limited to only two or three vessels. Active arterial bleeding from such arterialized vessels rarely may occur. Walsh and Hoyt (1969) described a patient who experienced episodes in which a small stream of blood was projected from a mass of conjunctival vessels.

Ocular Pulsation

Ocular pulsation is caused by transmission of the pulse wave from the internal carotid or ophthalmic artery to the dilated ophthalmic veins. Birch-Hirschfeld (1930) stated that increased ocular pulsation is present in 95% of patients with direct carotid-cavernous sinus fistula. He thought that patients without such pulsation had experienced retrobulbar hemorrhage; however, it is more likely that patients in whom ocular pulsation is not increased despite evidence of a direct carotid-cavernous sinus fistula have experienced thrombosis of the superior ophthalmic vein. Brosnahan et al. (1992) reported ocular pulsations in 5 of 11 patients with direct carotid-cavernous sinus fistulas that they examined.

Abnormal ocular pulsation may be visible and palpable or only palpable. Visible ocular pulsation usually is more readily detected from the side than from the front, but it is possible to overlook a pulsation that can be easily palpated. Palpable ocular pulsation is detected as a sensation of thrusts of blood passing in the vessels being felt or as a heaving sensation of the eye against fingers that have been placed on the closed eyelid overlying the affected eye. In fact, the increased pulse does not affect just the eye, but also the vessels of the eyelids, the orbit, and frequently the temporal fossa.

As a rule, patients are not conscious of increased ocular pulsation, even when it is as much as 6 mm. They are much more aware of other disturbances, especially swelling of the eyelid, redness of the eye, and buzzing or swishing sounds that can be heard (bruit; see below).

Increased ocular pulsation probably develops as soon as a newly formed carotid-cavernous sinus fistula begins to drain anteriorly. It may be detected within hours after trauma by observation, palpation, or other means. Tonometry is an effective method of detecting increased ocular pulsation, even when such pulsation is not visible. A tonometer can detect not only increased intraocular pressure (usually on the side of the lesion; see below) but also increased ocular pulsation. If a Schiötz tonometer is used, the indicator hand will have an abnormally wide swing on one side compared with the other (Boyes and Ralph, 1954). Similarly, the meirs of an applanation tonometer will have an exaggerated to-and-fro movement on one side, and a pneumotonometer can be used to measure directly the abnormal ocular pulse, which may be 2 to 5 times that of the normal eye (Golnik and Miller, 1992) (Figs. 54.16 and 54.17). These instruments also can be used to determine if a fistula has been successfully closed after treatment (see below).

Pulsating Exophthalmos

When a direct, high-flow, carotid-cavernous sinus fistula drains anteriorly to the orbit, it may produce both visible ocular pulsation and proptosis: **pulsating exophthalmos** (de Schweinitz and Holloway, 1908; Martin and Mabon, 1943; Madsen, 1970). In this setting, the exophthalmos almost always is associated with conjunctival chemosis, arterialization of conjunctival vessels, and a bruit that is audible to both the patient and the examiner (see below). When a patient with previous head trauma develops pulsating exophthalmos associated with these other signs, the diagnosis of direct carotid-cavernous sinus fistula is usually obvious.

Pulsating exophthalmos can be caused by conditions other than a direct carotid-cavernous sinus fistula, however. Both

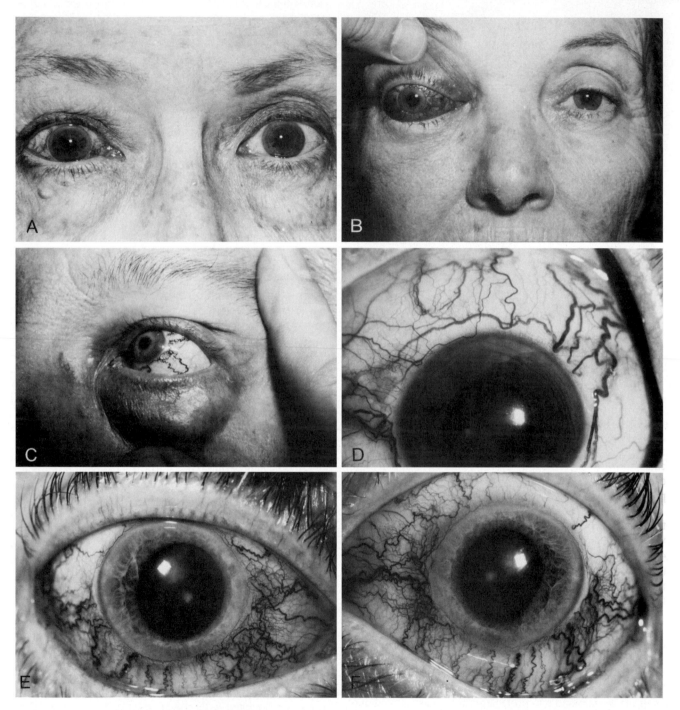

Figure 54.15. Dilated, tortuous, and arterialized conjunctival vessels in six patients with direct carotid-cavernous sinus fistulas. These vessels are typically bright red. Also note associated chemosis of the interpalpebral conjunctiva in several of the eyes.

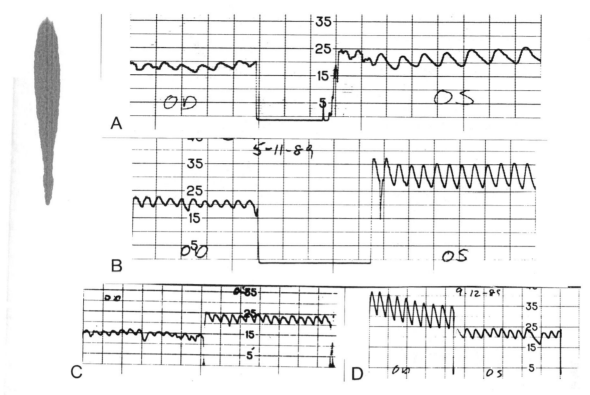

Figure 54.16. Asymmetric ocular pulse amplitudes in four different patients with unilateral carotid-cavernous sinus fistula. All amplitudes were recorded with a pneumotonometer. Note that in all cases, the intraocular pressure is higher in the eye with the larger pulse amplitude.

spontaneous, high-flow, carotid-cavernous sinus fistulas (see below) and orbital arteriovenous fistulas occasionally produce pulsating exophthalmos indistinguishable from that caused by direct carotid-cavernous sinus fistulas. In such cases, the correct diagnosis usually is not made until appropriate neuroimaging studies are performed.

Other causes of pulsating exophthalmos include congenital absence of the sphenoid bone, as seen in patients with von Recklinghausen's neurofibromatosis (NF-1; see Chapter 49), and acquired dehiscence of the frontal or sphenoid bones (e.g., after trauma). In these conditions, the cranial pulse is transmitted to the eye, which is also pushed forward by the frontal or temporal lobe (LeWald, 1933; Verbiest, 1953). There is no associated bruit.

An arteriovenous fistula between the internal carotid artery and the jugular vein produced pulsating exophthalmos in a patient described by Terry and Mysel (1934). The fistula was in the upper part of the neck. At operation, the vein was dissected free from the artery. When both the vein and the common carotid artery were ligated, the ocular pulsation and an accompanying bruit disappeared. A traumatic middle meningeal arteriovenous fistula may also arterialize orbital veins and produce pulsating exophthalmos (Gerlach et al., 1962) (Figs. 54.18 and 54.19).

Tumors in the orbit rarely produce pulsating exophthalmos. The tumors usually are vascular and slow growing (Rottgen, 1950). In such cases, ocular pulsation and bruit appear late, and the condition usually is not confused with a direct carotid-cavernous sinus fistula.

Corneal Damage

Exposure keratopathy is the most frequent corneal sign encountered in patients with a direct carotid-cavernous sinus fistula. It usually is related to the severity of proptosis, unless a traumatic facial nerve paresis also is present. The keratopathy may be aggravated by trigeminal neuropathy caused by the injury or by the effect of the fistula on the trigeminal nerve within the cavernous sinus (Dandy and Follis, 1941). In rare cases, **filamentary keratitis** may develop in the setting of trigeminal sensory neuropathy, even though proptosis is not severe (Fig. 54.20).

Although exposure keratopathy is the most common corneal sign in patients with direct carotid-cavernous sinus fistula, it is not the only sign. The cornea also may become turbid and hazy in patients with secondary glaucoma or anterior segment ischemia (see below).

Bruit

In many patients with a direct carotid-cavernous sinus fistula, the initial symptom is a buzzing, swishing, or roaring sound that is synchronous with the heartbeat. This **bruit** (from the French word for noise) is principally systolic in timing, and it usually increases when the heart

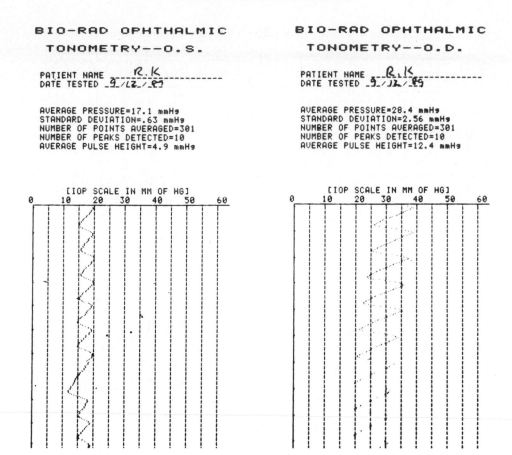

Figure 54.17. Quantitative analysis of ocular pulse amplitudes in a patient with a right-sided direct carotid-cavernous sinus fistula. Note that this particular machine calculates not only the average intraocular pressure but also the average height of the ocular pulse.

is beating actively; e.g., during exercise. The bruit usually decreases in amplitude when the patient is at rest or when the affected internal carotid artery is compressed, although failure of carotid compression to eliminate a bruit heard over the eye does not exclude the possibility of a carotid-cavernous sinus fistula. Ramos and Mount (1953) described a patient with a direct carotid-cavernous sinus fistula in whom the associated bruit was not eliminated by compression of either or both internal carotid arteries. Arteriography showed that the bruit persisted because of a large, right, posterior communicating artery that carried blood anteriorly from the basilar artery when the carotid arteries were compressed.

A bruit present in a patient with a direct carotid-cavernous sinus fistula may be heard only by the patient or by both the patient and the examiner. It is extremely unusual for a patient to be unaware of a bruit that can be heard by the examiner. Indeed, the bruit that results from a direct carotid-cavernous sinus fistula is often a great source of annoyance (Madsen, 1970), preventing the patient from working, relaxing, and even sleeping. Some patients are so distressed from the constant sound that they may threaten to commit suicide if something is not done to eliminate it. A bruit that is produced by a direct carotid-

cavernous sinus fistula is heard best when a stethoscope is placed over the affected eye, but it can often be heard over much of the head.

Several authors have reported an objective bruit in every one of their patients with traumatic carotid-cavernous sinus fistulas (Kupersmith et al., 1986; Brosnahan et al., 1992); however, other authors have emphasized that not all patients with a direct carotid-cavernous sinus fistula have a bruit, even if they have significant ocular symptoms and signs (Martin and Mabon, 1943; Burton and Goldberg, 1970). It also must be emphasized that a bruit is not pathognomonic of a carotid-cavernous sinus fistula. Bruits are common in otherwise healthy infants and young children (Hamburger, 1931), and they also may be heard in children with anemia or rickets. They occasionally may be heard over the skull in some patients with increased intracranial pressure. A bruit may represent the transmitted sound of a cardiac murmur, or it may be caused by a vascular anomaly in the orbit. We even have heard a bruit in several patients with meningiomas of the sphenoid ridge.

Diplopia

Diplopia occurs in about 60–70% of patients with a direct carotid-cavernous sinus fistula. The diplopia may be caused the fistula, ischemia from alterations in the blood flow in the vasa nervorum of the ocular motor nerves, or both. In this setting, diplopia and ophthalmoparesis may not develop until several days to weeks after other symptoms and signs of the fistula.

Of the three ocular motor nerves, the abducens nerve is most often affected by a direct carotid-cavernous sinus

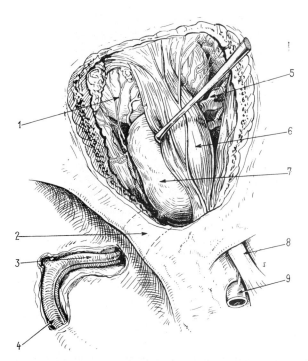

Figure 54.18. Middle meningeal-sphenoparietal arteriovenous fistula that produced pulsating exophthalmos. The fistula developed as a complication of a skull fracture. The patient underwent exploratory surgery at which time the roof of the orbit was removed, the contents examined, and the connection between the orbit and the middle meningeal artery was identified. Artist's drawing of the surgical findings shows the globe (*1*), the area of bone removed at surgery to expose the arteriovenous communication (*2*), the middle meningeal artery with the sphenoparietal vein beneath it (*3 and 4*), enlarged orbital veins (*5*), the levator palpebrae superioris and superior rectus muscles (*6*), the dilated aneurysmal sac (*7*), the optic nerve (*8*), and the internal carotid artery showing the origin of the ophthalmic artery (*9*). (From Gerlach J, Spuler H, Vichweger G. Klin Monatsbl Augenheilkd *140*:344–356, 1962.)

by dysfunction of one or more of the ocular motor nerves, the extraocular muscles, or both, and the degree of limitation of eye movement varies from mild limitation in only one direction to complete ophthalmoplegia.

When a direct carotid-cavernous sinus fistula is caused by trauma, the ocular motor nerves may be damaged at the time of initial injury, especially when the injury is severe enough to cause a basal skull fracture. Ophthalmoparesis usually is present immediately after injury in such patients, but it may not be appreciated if the patient is comatose or has substantial facial and orbital damage.

When a direct carotid-cavernous sinus fistula results from rupture of an intracavernous aneurysm, ocular motor nerve paresis actually may occur before rupture from compression of one or more nerves, with the abducens nerve most often damaged. A careful history invariably indicates that diplopia began weeks to hours before the aneurysm ruptured.

Ophthalmoparesis also may be caused by damage to one or more of the ocular motor nerves by the fistula itself. This damage may be caused by compression of the nerve(s) by

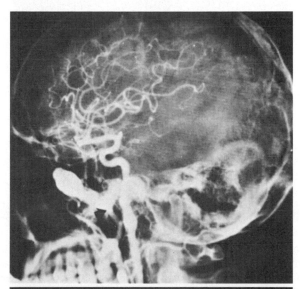

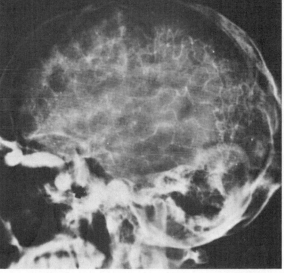

Figure 54.19. Fistula between the middle meningeal artery and the inferior petrosal vein. The patient was a 32-year-old man who developed pulsating exophthalmos 12 years after fracture of the skull, zygoma, and left lateral orbital wall. The patient was thought to have a carotid-cavernous sinus fistula. *Top,* Carotid arteriogram, lateral view, shows an enlarged middle meningeal artery (*arrow*) and early opacification of the enlarged inferior petrosal sinus and its tributaries. *Bottom,* Carotid arteriogram, lateral view, in a late arterial phase shows opacification of the cavernous sinus (*arrow*) and an enlarged superior ophthalmic vein. (From Pool JL, Potts DG. Aneurysms and Arteriovenous Anomalies of the Brain: Diagnosis and Treatment. New York, Hoeber Medical Division, Harper & Row, 1965.)

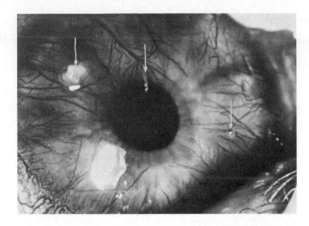

Figure 54.20. Neovascularization of the cornea and filamentary keratitis (*arrows*) in a patient with a carotid-cavernous sinus fistula.

fistula (Sattler, 1920; Henderson and Schneider, 1959; Madsen, 1970; Kupersmith et al., 1986; Brosnahan et al., 1992). The abducens nerve may be the only one of the ocular motor nerves affected (McIlwaine et al., 1991) (Fig. 54.21), or it may be damaged along with the oculomotor nerve, trochlear nerve, or both (Fig. 54.22). The particular vulnerability of the abducens nerve to damage from a carotid-cavernous sinus fistula is related to its location within the cavernous sinus. Whereas the oculomotor and trochlear nerves are located in the deep layer of the lateral wall of the cavernous sinus, the abducens nerve is located within the body of the sinus, between the lateral wall of the cavernous segment of the internal carotid artery and the lateral wall of the sinus. The abducens nerve thus is more likely to be damaged by the hemodynamic and mechanical changes that occur when the fistula develops. Among 33 patients with 34 traumatic direct carotid-cavernous sinus fistulas, Kupersmith et al. (1986) described abducens nerve paresis in 28 (85%).

Even though abducens nerve paresis is the most common ocular motor nerve paresis that occurs in patients with a direct carotid-cavernous fistula, either oculomotor and trochlear nerve paresis may develop in such patients, not only from the initial trauma but also as a direct result of the fistula itself. In an autopsy case, Dandy and Follis (1941) found one oculomotor nerve compressed by a projecting pouch of the dilated cavernous sinus. Elliot (1954) described two patients with traumatic carotid-cavernous sinus fistula who developed isolated oculomotor nerve paresis. Kupersmith et al. (1986) reported oculomotor nerve paresis in 22 of 33 patients (67%) and trochlear nerve paresis in 17 of 33 patients (49%) with traumatic carotid-cavernous sinus fistula, but it is not clear in what percentage of these cases only one nerve was affected.

We have examined a 31-year-old man who developed vertical diplopia 1 week after he was injured in a motorcycle accident. The patient was thought by the referring physician to have an isolated, traumatic trochlear nerve paresis, but upon evaluation in the Neuro-Ophthalmology Unit of The Johns Hopkins Hospital, he complained of a subjective cranial bruit that had begun about 24 hours after the accident. His examination revealed normal visual sensory function, a right hypertropia that increased on left lateral gaze and head tilt to the right and decreased on right lateral gaze and head tilt to the left, 2 mm of right proptosis, and mild chemosis of the conjunctiva of the right eye. Neuroimaging studies confirmed a right-sided, direct carotid-cavernous sinus fistula that was successfully occluded with a detachable balloon (see below). Within 48 hours after occlusion of the fistula, the patient's hypertropia began to improve. Two weeks after treatment, the patient's eye movements were normal, and he had no diplopia.

Mechanical restriction of the extraocular muscles, instead of, or in addition to, ocular motor nerve paresis, may cause diplopia in patients with a direct carotid-cavernous fistula.

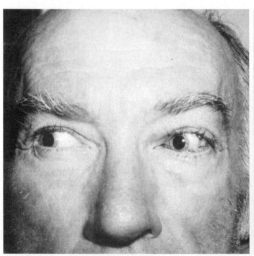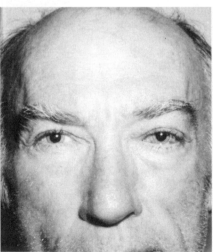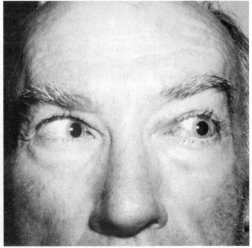

Figure 54.21. Isolated abducens nerve paresis in a patient with a traumatic carotid-cavernous sinus fistula. The patient has mild abduction weakness of the left eye, but the rest of the eye movements are normal. The patient's pupils were dilated with mydriatics before these photographs were taken.

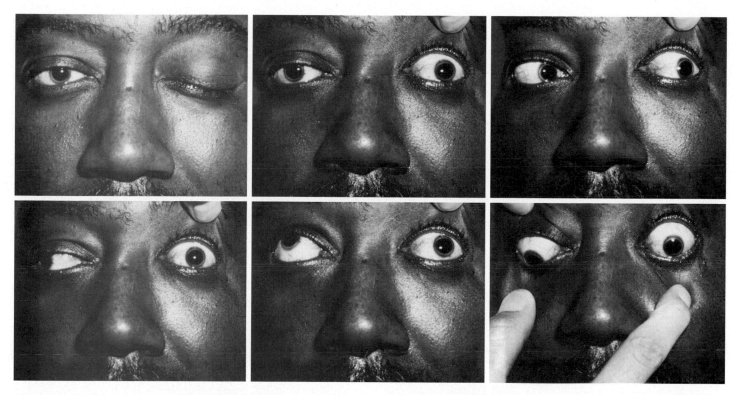

Figure 54.22. Abducens, oculomotor, and trochlear nerve pareses in a patient with a direct carotid-cavernous sinus fistula. The patient had been injured in a motor vehicle accident. Note that the patient has weakness of abduction of the left eye (*top right*), consistent with a left abducens nerve paresis, but he also has a complete left ptosis (*top left*), a left exotropia (*top center*), and limitation of adduction, elevation, and depression of the left eye consistent with an oculomotor nerve paresis. The left eye did not intort on attempted downgaze.

The restriction is the result of venous stasis and orbital edema, often with enlargement of the extraocular muscles themselves (Dandy and Follis, 1941). In this setting, ophthalmoparesis and diplopia occur at the same time as, or shortly after, signs of orbital congestion.

Patients with a direct carotid-cavernous sinus fistula, ophthalmoparesis, and diplopia who do not have significant proptosis, chemosis, and orbital edema almost always have neuropathic limitation of eye movement. When signs of orbital congestion are prominent, it may be impossible to determine whether ophthalmoparesis is neuropathic, myopathic, or both unless there is evidence of damage to the parasympathetic or sympathetic pupillomotor fibers. Even in this setting, limitation of eye movement may be **both** neuropathic and myopathic (Fig. 54.23).

Visual Loss

Visual loss associated with a direct carotid-cavernous sinus fistula may be immediate or delayed. Immediate visual loss is usually caused by ocular or optic nerve damage that occurs at the time of head injury (Walker and Allegré, 1956; Kupersmith et al., 1986; Brosnahan et al., 1992). When visual loss is associated with a lacerated or ruptured globe, extensive arterial bleeding may complicate attempted repair or enucleation (Purcell, 1979). Delayed visual loss is usually caused by retinal dysfunction, but it may be related to vitre-

ous hemorrhage, anterior ischemic optic neuropathy, or even corneal ulceration (Henderson and Schneider, 1959; Sanders and Hoyt, 1969; Spencer et al., 1973). Dandy and Follis (1941) suggested that the optic nerve could be damaged in patients with long-standing fistulas from compression of the nerve by a distended cavernous sinus or from retrobulbar ischemia, and Hedges et al. (1985) described a patient in whom one of these two mechanisms was thought to be responsible for an optic neuropathy that occurred 7 weeks after development of a traumatic carotid-cavernous sinus fistula. The optic neuropathy resolved after the fistula was successfully occluded.

Visual loss is the rule rather than the exception in patients with a direct carotid-cavernous sinus fistula. In 1908, de Schweinitz and Holloway found that only 11.1% of patients with direct carotid-cavernous sinus fistulas had normal vision. In Sattler's (1920) series of direct carotid-cavernous sinus fistulas, 73% had impaired vision, with almost 50% being blind or nearly so. Kupersmith et al. (1986) described visual loss in 16 of 33 patients.

The pathophysiology of visual loss from retinal or choroidal dysfunction in patients with direct carotid-cavernous sinus fistula is complex. Retinal and choroidal blood flow are reduced by (*a*) a drop in effective ophthalmic artery perfusion pressure secondary to the hemodynamic alterations caused by the fistula, (*b*) an increase in venous pressure caused by arterialization of the orbital venous bed, and (*c*)

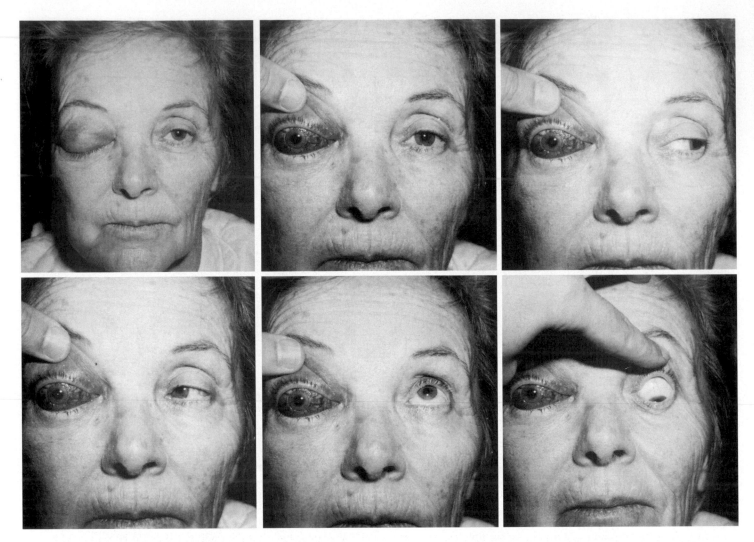

Figure 54.23. Combined mechanical and neuropathic limitation of eye movement in a patient with a traumatic right-sided direct carotid-cavernous sinus fistula. The right eye is immobile. There is a complete right ptosis and anisocoria with the right pupil larger than the left, indicating damage to the right oculomotor nerve; however, the right eye also is substantially proptotic, and forced duction testing indicated some degree of mechanical limitation of eye movement.

obstruction or thrombosis of the ophthalmic venous system (Grove, 1984; Kupersmith, 1993; Kupersmith et al., 1996). The result is chronic hypoxia leading to choroidal effusion or detachment on the one hand, or stasis retinopathy, central retinal vein occlusion, or nonrhegmatogenous retinal detachment on the other.

Many patients with a direct carotid-cavernous sinus fistula initially complain of vague dimming of vision and an inability of the affected eye to adapt quickly to changes in brightness. In some patients, the peripheral visual field becomes constricted, although central vision is usually normal unless macular edema or choroidal detachment occurs.

Ophthalmoscopic Abnormalities

Dilation of retinal veins is usually present in patients with a direct carotid-cavernous sinus fistula (Fig. 54.24). When the degree of dilation is mild, it may not be appreciated during direct ophthalmoscopy, although it usually is obvious when indirect ophthalmoscopy is performed and the appearance of one ocular fundus is compared with the appearance of the other. In severe cases, **optic disc swelling** and **intraretinal hemorrhage** may occur in patients with a direct carotid-cavernous sinus fistula (Brosnahan et al., 1992). All of these manifestations are caused by venous stasis and impaired retinal blood flow, with secondary ischemia or hypoxia. Disc swelling is usually mild, but may occasionally be severe. Retinal hemorrhages are both flame-shaped (located in the nerve fiber layer) and punctate (located in the outer retinal layers) (Fig. 54.25). In extremely rare cases, subhyaloid (preretinal) or vitreous hemorrhage may be present (Madsen, 1970). Thus, the ophthalmoscopic appearance ranges from one of mild **stasis retinopathy** to one of frank **central retinal vein occlusion** (Kupersmith et al., 1996) (Fig. 54.26).

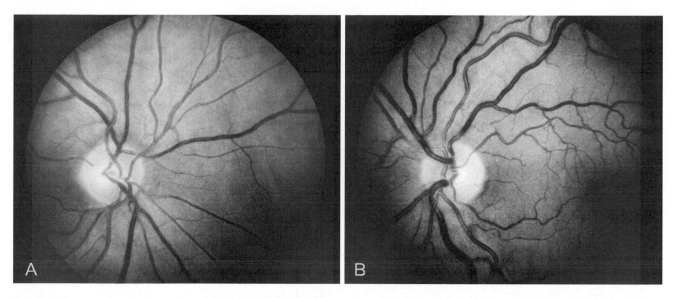

Figure 54.24. Unilateral dilation of retinal veins on the side of a direct carotid-cavernous sinus fistula. The patient was a 25-year-old woman with a traumatic left-sided carotid-cavernous sinus fistula. *A,* The ophthalmoscopic appearance of the right posterior pole is normal. The retinal vessels are of normal caliber. *B,* Ophthalmoscopic view of the left posterior pole shows moderate dilation of retinal veins unassociated with retinal hemorrhage.

In extremely rare instances, nonrhegmatogenous **retinal detachment** (Cogan, 1960) or **choroidal effusion or detachment** (Woillez et al., 1967; Kupersmith et al., 1996; Berk et al., 1997) can develop. In such patients, successful treatment of the fistula is associated with spontaneous resolution of the retinal or choroidal process; however, we agree with Kupersmith et al. (1996) that improvement in visual

function is more likely to occur in patients with choroidal effusion or detachment than in patients with stasis retinopathy, central retinal vein occlusion, or retinal detachment.

Trigeminal Nerve Dysfunction

Ocular and orbital pain are rarely present in patients with a direct carotid-cavernous sinus fistula unless there is signifi-

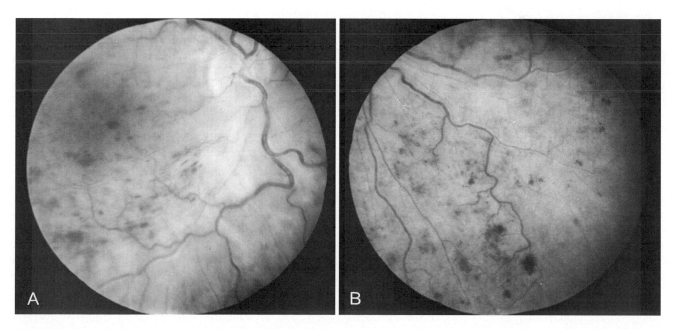

Figure 54.25. Retinal hemorrhages and mild optic disc swelling in patients with direct carotid-cavernous sinus fistula. *A,* In one patient with a right-sided fistula, the right optic disc is mildly swollen and hyperemic. The posterior pole shows numerous flame-shaped (superficial) and punctate (deep) intraretinal hemorrhages. *B,* In another patient with a direct carotid-cavernous sinus fistula, the eye on the side of the lesion shows numerous intraretinal hemorrhages, most of which are punctate.

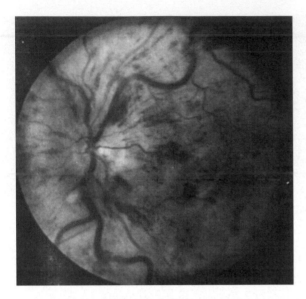

Figure 54.26. Central retinal vein occlusion in a patient with a direct carotid-cavernous sinus fistula.

cant corneal exposure or ulceration. Nevertheless, occasional patients complain of facial pain in the distribution of the 1st, and rarely the 2nd, division of the trigeminal nerve. Similarly, rare patients experience a decrease in corneal sensation, facial sensation, or both on the side of the fistula (Madsen, 1970). Presumably, both pain and hypesthesia are related to ischemia or compression of the ophthalmic and maxillary divisions of the trigeminal nerve within the cavernous sinus.

Glaucoma

Glaucoma is a potential complication of untreated direct carotid-cavernous sinus fistula (Sugar and Meyer, 1940; Madsen, 1970). It develops in 30–50% of patients (Elliot, 1954; Henderson and Schneider, 1959; Brosnahan et al., 1992).

At least four types of glaucoma can occur in patients with direct carotid-cavernous sinus fistula. The most common type is caused by increased episcleral venous pressure (Fig. 54.27). Intraocular pressure in such cases is usually mildly elevated, but we have encountered patients with intraocular pressures as high as 50–60 mm Hg, and other investigators have described similar patients (Kupersmith et al., 1986). According to Weekers and Delmarcelle (1952), intraocular pressure rises millimeter for millimeter with a corresponding increase in episcleral venous pressure in this type of glaucoma. Excessively high intraocular pressure may be associated with the development of central retinal artery occlusion.

In some patients with severe proptosis and chemosis, glaucoma is caused by orbital congestion. Intraocular pressure usually is quite high in such cases, and the elevated pressure may be difficult, if not impossible, to control.

Neovascular glaucoma occurs in some patients with a direct carotid-cavernous sinus fistula (Fig. 54.28). It is always associated with evidence of chronic retinal hypoxia and reti-

nal neovascularization, and it is particularly common after central retinal vein occlusion (Swan and Raaf, 1951; Weiss et al., 1963; Duke, 1967; Spencer et al., 1973).

Rare patients with direct carotid-cavernous sinus fistula develop angle closure glaucoma without rubeosis iridis or neovascularization of the anterior chamber angle. In such patients, arterialization of orbital venous drainage channels causes elevated pressure in the vortex veins, central retinal vein, and episcleral vessels. Engorgement of the choroidal bed increases the volume of the posterior compartment, producing a forward shift in the iris-lens diaphragm. Hyperemia of the ciliary body and iris may contribute further to shallowing of the anterior chamber (Harris and Rice, 1979).

DIAGNOSIS

A direct carotid-cavernous sinus fistula should be suspected in any patient who suddenly develops chemosis, proptosis, and a red eye. When this occurs after a head injury, the diagnosis should be obvious. Even when there is no history of trauma, one should consider the possibility of a ruptured intracavernous aneurysm, particularly if there is a history of preexisting diplopia.

A patient suspected of having a direct carotid-cavernous sinus fistula should be questioned about a subjective bruit, and careful auscultation of the eye and orbital region should be performed using the bell of the stethoscope. In addition, the intraocular pressure and ocular pulse should be measured. We have found the pneumotonometer to be an ideal instrument for performing such measurements (Golnik and Miller, 1992) (Figs. 54.16 and 54.17), because it provides a permanent quantitative record of the findings. However, any tonometer can be used.

When a careful history and clinical examination support the diagnosis of a direct carotid-cavernous sinus fistula, appropriate confirmation should be obtained. Computed tomographic (CT) scanning, magnetic resonance (MR) imaging, and orbital ultrasonography can be used to confirm the diagnosis, showing enlargement of extraocular muscles, dilation of one or both superior ophthalmic veins, and enlargement of the affected cavernous sinus (Keltner et al., 1987; Atta et al., 1996) (Fig. 54.29). Duplex carotid ultrasonography can be used to detect the fistula and to determine its flow rate (H.-J. Lin et al., 1994), and transorbital or transcranial color doppler imaging can also be used to show one or both enlarged superior ophthalmic vein within which the blood flow is toward, rather than away from, the eye (Kotval et al., 1990; Flaharty et al., 1991; S.-K. Lin et al., 1994; Zhao et al., 1995). The ultimate diagnostic test, however, is cerebral arteriography (Figs. 54.1–54.4, and 54.8). The angiographic technique should include selective catheterization of the ipsilateral common carotid artery, the ipsilateral internal and external carotid arteries, the contralateral internal carotid artery with compression of the ipsilateral internal carotid artery, and the dominant vertebral artery also with compression of the ipsilateral internal carotid artery. This techique permits the neurointerventionalist to determine the exact location and morphology of the fistula, the rate and direction of blood flow through the fistula, the anatomy of the venous

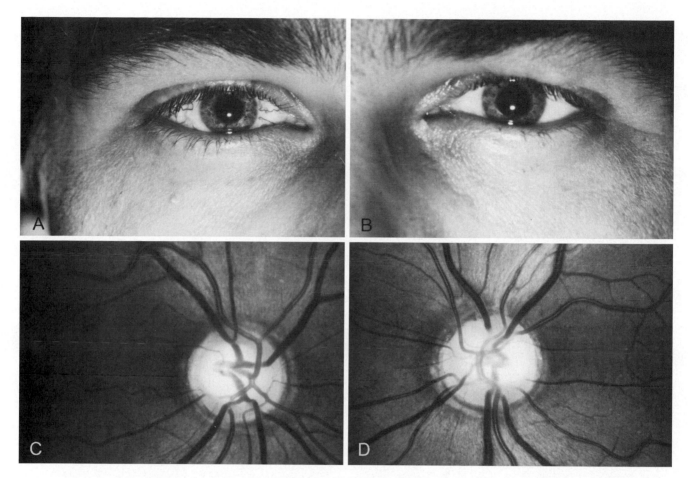

Figure 54.27. Chronic glaucoma from raised episcleral venous pressure in a patient with a right-sided traumatic carotid-cavernous sinus fistula. The patient had refused treatment of the fistula, and he was noncompliant with regard to antiglaucoma medication. Intraocular pressure in the right eye consistently measured between 30 and 35 mm Hg. *A,* External appearance of patient's right eye shows minimal proptosis and several dilated, tortuous conjunctival veins. *B,* The left eye appears normal. *C,* Ophthalmoscopic view of the right optic disc shows moderate glaucomatous cupping. The cup to disc ratio is about 0.6. *D,* Ophthalmoscopic view of the left optic disc shows a normal optic disc with no significant cupping.

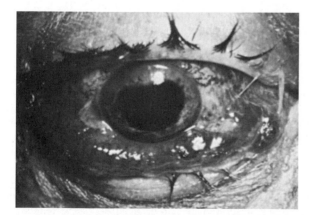

Figure 54.28. Neovascular glaucoma in a patient with a direct carotid-cavernous sinus fistula. The patient had proptosis, chemosis of the conjunctiva, arterialized conjunctival and episcleral veins, elevated intraocular pressure, corneal edema, and iridoplegia.

drainage of the fistula, the presence of absence of a vascular steal phenomenon, the patency of the circle of Willis, and the anatomy of the carotid bifurcation on the side of the fistula (Debrun et al., 1989; Wilms et al., 1989; Debrun, 1995). Only in this way can the optimum treatment of the fistula and the potential risks of such treatment be determined.

NATURAL HISTORY

Almost all patients have progressive ocular difficulties if a direct carotid-cavernous sinus fistula is left untreated. Over months to years, there is increasing proptosis, chemosis, and visual loss. de Schweinitz and Holloway (1908) emphasized that only 11% of patients with untreated fistulas retained normal central vision. The most severe complications are central retinal vein occlusion and secondary glaucoma.

As noted above, rhinologic and neurologic complications can occur in patients with direct carotid-cavernous sinus fistulas. Such complications may occur at the time of the development of the fistula, shortly thereafter, or months to years

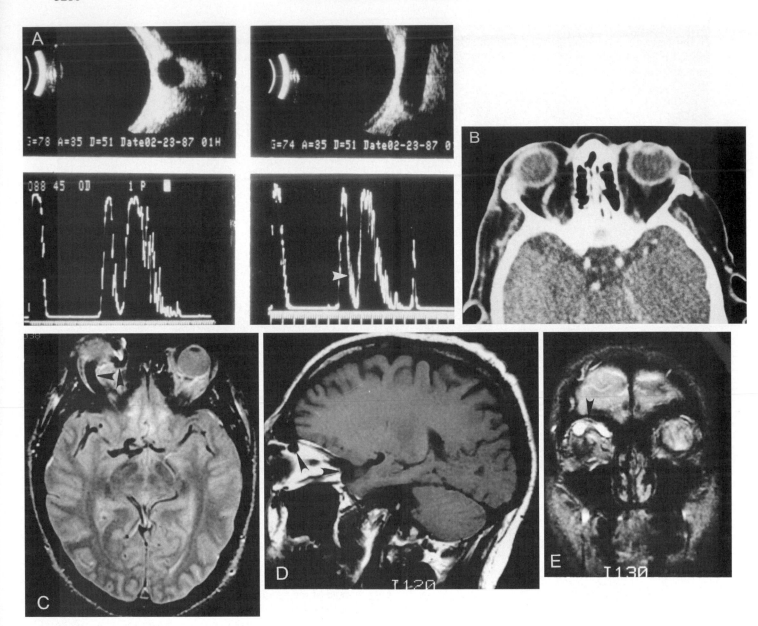

Figure 54.29. Diagnostic tests in patients with clinical evidence of a direct carotid-cavernous sinus fistula. *A,* Orbital ultrasonography (A and B modes) shows enlargement of one of the veins in the orbit that connects the superior and inferior ophthalmic veins. The lower right A-scan shows blurring of the spikes within the vein (*arrowhead*). This appearance is caused by rapid blood flow within the vessel. *B,* Computed tomogram, axial view, shows an enlarged superior ophthalmic vein in a patient with a direct carotid-cavernous sinus fistula on that side. *C–E,* Magnetic resonance images in a patient with a carotid-cavernous sinus fistula. *C,* T2-weighted axial image, shows an enlarged superior ophthalmic vein on the side of the fistula. The vein appears as a black curvilinear structure beginning at the apex of the orbit and continuing forward in the superolateral orbit as a curvilinear tubular structure (*arrowhead*). A small portion of the nasal component of the vein is also seen (*arrowhead*). *D,* T2-weighted sagittal image shows the most posterior and anterior components of the enlarged vein (*arrowheads*). *E,* Short TR and TE image, coronal view, shows the enlarged superior ophthalmic vein as a white curvilinear structure that curves from lateral to medial in the anterosuperior orbit (*arrowhead*).

later. The most significant of these complications are epistaxis, subarachnoid hemorrhage, intracerebral hemorrhage, and cerebral infarction (Hamby, 1964; Wilson and Markesbery, 1966; Sedzimir and Occleshaw, 1967; Lee et al., 1975; Mullan, 1979; Turner et al., 1983; Dohrmann et al., 1985; Gaston et al., 1986; Hieshima et al., 1986b; Isamat et al., 1986; Kupersmith et al., 1986; O'Reilly et al., 1986;

d'Angelo et al., 1988; Shimizu et al., 1988; Lin et al., 1992; Millman and Giddings, 1994; Iida et al., 1995). For example, the patient described by Lin et al. (1992) experienced two intracerebral hemorrhages during pregnancy and one during the puerperium 5½ years after the trauma that initially produced the fistula.

We have examined a 34-year-old man who suffered head

trauma with basal skull fracture when the car that he was driving was struck by another vehicle. He subsequently developed bilateral red eyes, right more than left, proptosis of the right eye, and conjunctival chemosis. Visual acuity was 20/20 OU, with normal color vision and normal visual fields. Intraocular pressures were 28 mm Hg OD and 22 mm Hg OS. Both fundi showed dilated retinal veins with scattered intraretinal hemorrhages. He had a subjective bruit, and an objective bruit was best heard over the right eye, although it could be heard over the entire skull. Arteriography showed a right-sided direct carotid-cavernous sinus fistula. Treatment was recommended but was refused by the patient. Over the next 5 years, he experienced increasing redness of both eyes associated with a mild increase in stasis retinopathy and a slight decrease in visual acuity to 20/30 OU. Five years after injury, he experienced a sudden, severe headache and abruptly lost consciousness. He was brought to the emergency room of The Johns Hopkins Hospital, where he was found to have a dense left hemiparesis, a stiff neck, and papilledema. An echoencephalogram demonstrated a shift from right to left, and an arteriogram demonstrated an avas-

cular mass in the right frontotemporal region compatible with an intraparenchymal hemorrhage. The patient was treated with supportive therapy. He died 25 days after admission to the hospital. At autopsy, he was found to have a right-sided direct carotid-cavernous fistula that had ruptured into the frontotemporal region, producing both a subarachnoid hemorrhage and an intracerebral hematoma.

TREATMENT

The optimum treatment of a direct carotid-cavernous sinus fistula is closure of the abnormal arteriovenous communication with preservation of internal carotid artery patency. A variety of procedures can be used to close the fistula, but many (e.g., ligation of the internal carotid artery, occlusion of the fistula using the nondetachable balloon tip of a Fogarty catheter, occlusion of the fistula by occlusion of the artery both proximal and distal to the fistula) also occlude the internal carotid artery (Walker and Allegré, 1956; Hamby and Dohn, 1964; Hamby, 1966; Stern et al., 1967; Prolo and Hanbery, 1971; Chowdhary, 1978). When the artery is oc-

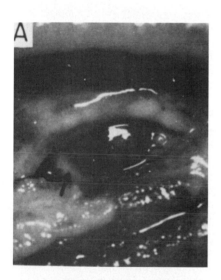
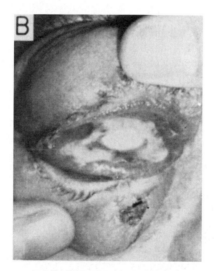
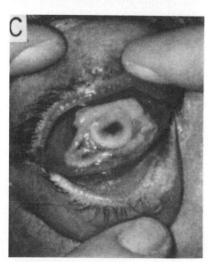
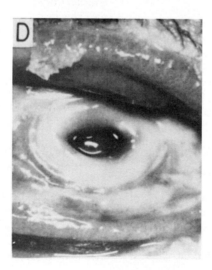

Figure 54.30. Ischemic ocular necrosis before and after attempted treatment of a direct carotid-cavernous sinus fistula. The patient was a 39-year-old man who had suffered multiple fractures, including a basal skull fracture, when he was struck by an automobile. Shortly thereafter, he developed marked proptosis of the right eye associated with swelling of the eyelids and chemosis of the conjunctiva. Arteriography showed a right-sided direct carotid-cavernous sinus fistula. *A,* Preoperative appearance of the patient shows patchy necrosis of the eyelids, conjunctiva, and cornea (*arrow*). About 3 weeks after injury, the patient underwent attempted treatment of the fistula. The right internal carotid artery was clipped above the fistula, muscle emboli were introduced into the intracavernous segment of the vessel, and both the right internal and right external carotid arteries were ligated in the neck. *B,* After surgery, the lid edema and erythema are reduced, but the cornea is completely opacified and the conjunctiva is sloughing. *C* and *D,* Progressive necrosis, perforation, and sloughing of the cornea 7 and 9 days after operation. (From Spencer WH, Thompson HS, Hoyt WF. Br J Ophthalmol *57*:145–152, 1973.)

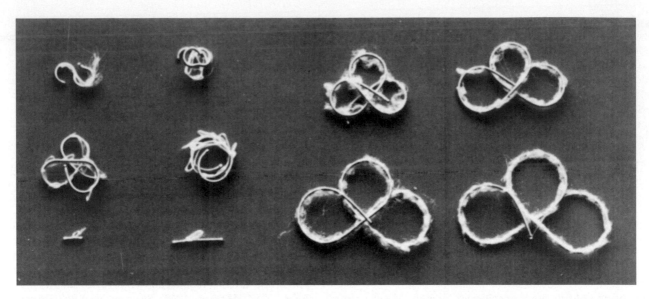

Figure 54.31. Flower coils. These complex helical platinum coils coated with dacron fibers promote thrombogenicity when used in the treatment of intracranial malformations. (From Higashida RT, Halbach VV, Dowd CF, et al. Neurosurg Clin North Am *5(3)*:413–425, 1994.)

cluded, the patient may suffer extensive neurologic deficits from hypoxic damage to the ipsilateral cerebral hemisphere. In addition, occlusion of the internal carotid artery may so reduce arterial blood flow to the eye that the patient develops hypotony, proliferative retinopathy, neovascular glaucoma, blindness, and even devastating ischemic necrosis of the eyelids and orbital contents (Renpenning and Wacaser, 1963; Hashi et al., 1969; Sanders and Hoyt, 1969; Ohta et al., 1971; Spencer et al., 1973; Kalina and Kelly, 1978; Palestine et al., 1981) (Fig. 54.30).

Several techniques permit successful closure of a direct carotid-cavernous fistula without occlusion of the internal carotid artery (Debrun et al., 1989; Kwan et al., 1989; Taki et al., 1994). Direct obliteration of the fistula can be performed by surgical repair of the damaged portion of the intracavernous internal carotid artery (Parkinson, 1967, 1973; Isamat et al., 1986; LeRoux et al., 1990; Lewis et al., 1995). This procedure can be difficult to perform, requires a craniotomy, and has significant potential morbidity. Nevertheless, it may be successful in closing the fistula without sacrificing the internal carotid artery, particularly when combined with intraoperative angiography and temporary balloon occlusion of the internal carotid artery (LeRoux et al., 1990). This technique is usually used when endovascular coil or balloon embolization of the fistula (see below) cannot be performed for technical reasons (LeRoux et al., 1990; Lewis et al., 1995).

Endovascular closure of a direct carotid-cavernous sinus fistula can be performed by many techniques. For instance, a copper or bronze wire or thrombogenic needles can be inserted into the fistula and a direct current can be applied to the metal until a thrombus develops (Hosobuchi, 1975; Conley et al., 1975; Wilson et al., 1976; Mullan, 1979). In this procedure, the material is introduced either through the superior ophthalmic vein or directly into the sinus, which is reached by craniotomy or through the paranasal sinuses.

Again, however, the procedure is associated with a definite morbidity and mortality.

Endovascular closure of direct carotid-cavernous sinus fistulas is most often accomplished by embolization using a variety of agents, primarily platinum coils and detachable balloons (Barker et al., 1994; Khayata et al., 1994; Taki et al., 1994; Guglielmi et al., 1995; Monsein and Rigamonti, 1996). These materials are usually introduced into the cavernous sinus through the internal carotid artery, but in selected cases, they may be introduced either transvenously through the inferior petrosal sinus or the superior ophthalmic vein, or directly into the cavernous sinus using via a craniotomy, transethmoidal transsphenoidal approach, or even a direct puncture through the superior orbital fissure (Barker et al., 1994; Teng et al., 1995).

The most common coils used for closure of a direct carotid-cavernous sinus fistula are platinum "flower" coils and electrolytically detachable coils. Flower coils have complex shapes (Fig. 54.31), but they can be straightened so that they can be delivered via a microcatheter that is advanced up the internal carotid artery, through the hole in its wall, and into the cavernous sinus or is placed in the superior ophthalmic vein and advanced directly into the cavernous sinus. Once the flower coils are released, they revert to their original shape (Fig. 54.32), thus promoting thrombosis in the area of the fistula. Electrolytically detachable coils are normally circular in shape (Fig. 54.33), but they can be straightened so that they can be introduced into the cavernous sinus via a guidewire within a microcatheter that, as noted above, can be advanced up the internal carotid artery and through the hole in the wall of the artery into the cavernous sinus or can be placed in the superior ophthalmic vein and advanced directly into the cavernous sinus. Once the catheter is in place, the coil is pushed out of the catheter by means of a stainless steel coil pusher (Fig. 54.34). As the

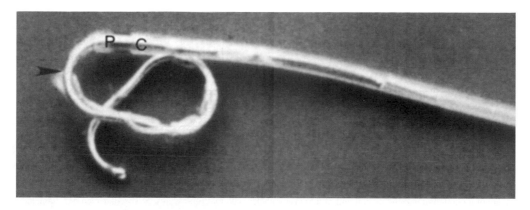

Figure 54.32.   Platinum flower coil going through a microcatheter (*C*) with the help of a coil pusher (*P*). Note that the coil is straight within the catheter, but once it exits the catheter (*arrowhead*), it begins to regain its original coiled shape. (From Khayata MH, Dean BL, Spetzler RF. Neurosurg Clin North Am *5(3)*:475–484, 1994.)

coil exits the catheter, it resumes its normal circular shape (Fig. 54.35). Once the coil is in place within the cavernous sinus, it is detached by applying a small electrical current to the connection between it and the guidewire (Figs. 54.34 and 54.36).

Detachable, flow-guided balloons are used to close most direct carotid-cavernous sinus fistulas (Fig. 54.37). The balloon initially is attached to the end of a catheter that is introduced into the cavernous sinus by an endovascular arterial route and out through the tear in the internal carotid artery (Serbinenko, 1974; Debrun et al., 1978; Serbinenko, 1979; Debrun et al., 1981; Laroche et al., 1984; Debrun et al., 1988; Wilms et al., 1989; Barnwell and O'Neill, 1994; Taki et al., 1994; Lewis et al., 1995), by a venous route through

the inferior petrosal sinus or superior ophthalmic vein directly into the cavernous sinus (Mullan, 1974; Manelfe and Berenstein, 1980; Shimizu et al., 1988; Debrun et al., 1989; Hanneken et al., 1989; Debrun, 1994; Barnwell and O'Neill, 1994; Spinelli et al., 1994; Miller et al., 1995), or, rarely, by a direct opening in the cavernous sinus when endovascular techniques fail or are not possible (Kobayashi et al., 1991). Once the balloon enters the cavernous sinus, it is inflated and detached, occluding the fistula but leaving the internal carotid artery patent (Figs. 54.35, 54.36, and 54.38). Some fistulas are so large that two or more balloons must be used to occlude them. Bömer and Kommerell (1994) reported a case in which four balloons were needed to close the fistula, and we have seen similar cases. Although there are some

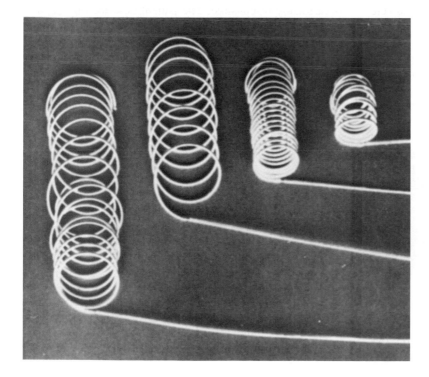

Figure 54.33.   Guglielmi electrolytic detachable coil system. The coils are available in a variety of diameters, coil sizes, and lengths. The coil is made from platinum and is connected to a stainless steel introducer and pusher wire by a solder junction. The solder junction separates by connecting the proximal end of the stainless steel guidewire to a small electric current. (From Higashida RT, Halbach VV, Dowd CF, et al. Neurosurg Clin North Am *5(3)*:413–425, 1994.)

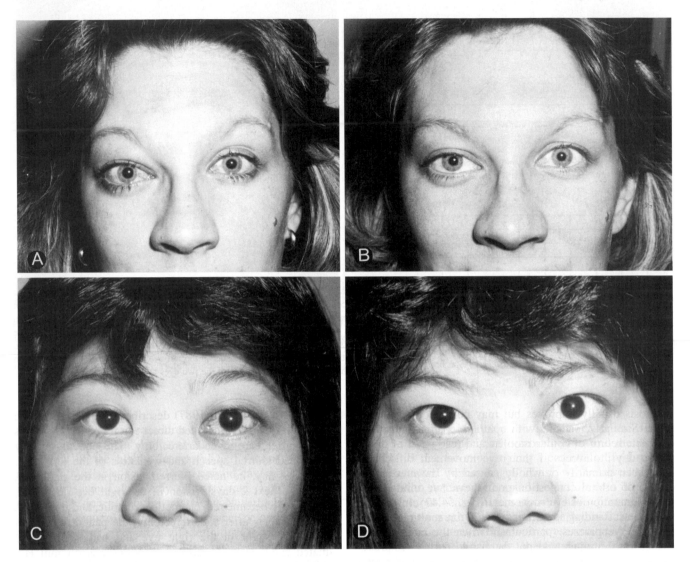

Figure 54.40. Immediate and long-term improvement in ocular manifestations after successful balloon occlusion of direct carotid-cavernous sinus fistulas. *A,* Preoperative appearance of a 32-year-old woman who developed a traumatic right-sided carotid-cavernous sinus fistula. The patient has mild right proptosis and dilated conjunctival vessels on the right. *B,* 48 hours after successful occlusion of the fistula with preservation of the right internal carotid artery, the patient's redness is improved. She still has mild, although reduced, proptosis. *C,* Preoperative appearance of a 21-year-old Asian woman who developed a left-sided direct carotid-cavernous sinus fistula after an automobile accident. The patient has moderate proptosis and redness of the left eye. She also had intermittent horizontal diplopia. *D,* 2 weeks after successful balloon occlusion of the fistula via the superior ophthalmic vein, the left eye appears normal. Both the redness and proptosis have completely resolved. The patient no longer has diplopia. *E,* Preoperative appearance of the eyes of a 56-year-old man who developed a left-sided direct carotid-cavernous sinus fistula after a motor vehicle accident. Note that both eyes are slightly red and proptotic. The patient also had generalized limitation of left eye movement. *F,* 4 weeks after successful balloon occlusion of the fistula via an endoarterial route, the patient has a normal appearance. *G,* Preoperative appearance of a 27-year-old woman with a traumatic right-sided carotid-cavernous fistula. The patient has moderate right proptosis and redness of the right eye. She also had generalized limitation of eye movement. *H,* 3 months after successful balloon occlusion of the fistula, the right eye appears normal. There is no longer any redness or proptosis, and the eye moves normally in all directions. *I,* Preoperative appearance of a 16-year-old boy who developed a left-sided carotid-cavernous sinus fistula after a motor vehicle accident. The left eye is proptotic and red, there is moderate left ptosis, and there is limitation of eye movement in all directions. *J,* 24 hours after successful balloon occlusion of the fistula, the patient's eye is already less red and proptotic, the left upper eyelid is less ptotic, and eye movement is improved.

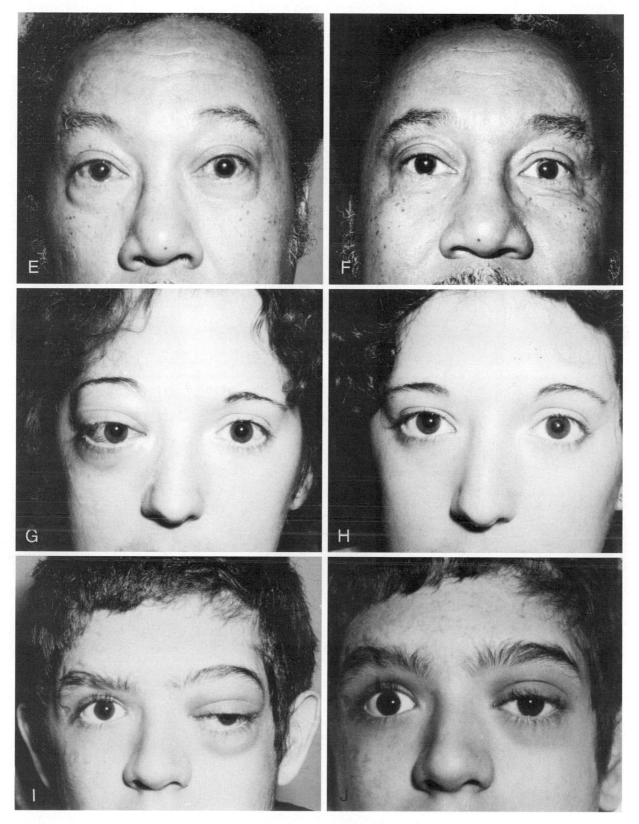

Figure 54.40. *(continued)*

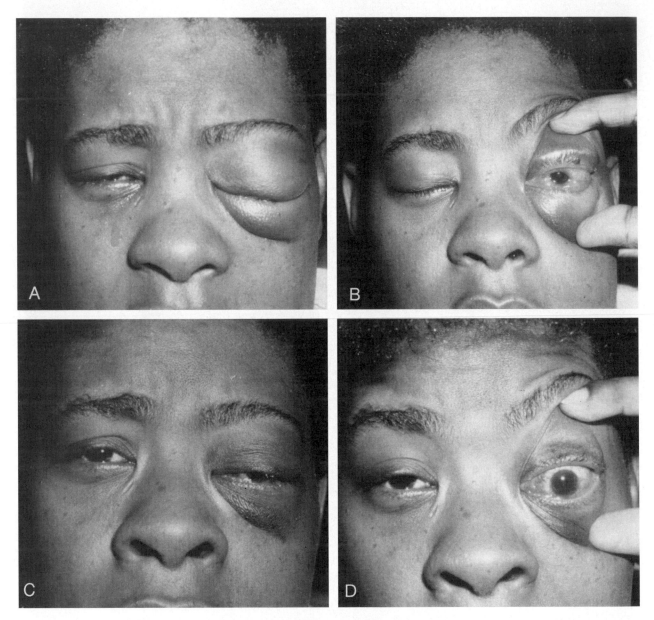

Figure 54.41. Rapid improvement in ocular manifestations of a direct carotid-cavernous sinus fistula after successful closure of the fistula with preservation of the ipsilateral internal carotid artery. *A* and *B,* Preoperative appearance of a 44-year-old woman with a left-sided carotid-cavernous sinus fistula that was initially mistaken for a cavernous sinus thrombosis. The patient has severe left upper and lower eyelid swelling, redness and proptosis of the left eye, and almost complete ophthalmoparesis. *C* and *D,* 5 days after successful balloon occlusion of the fistula, there is marked improvement in the appearance of the eyelids, reduction in proptosis and conjunctival chemosis, and improvement in movement of the left eye.

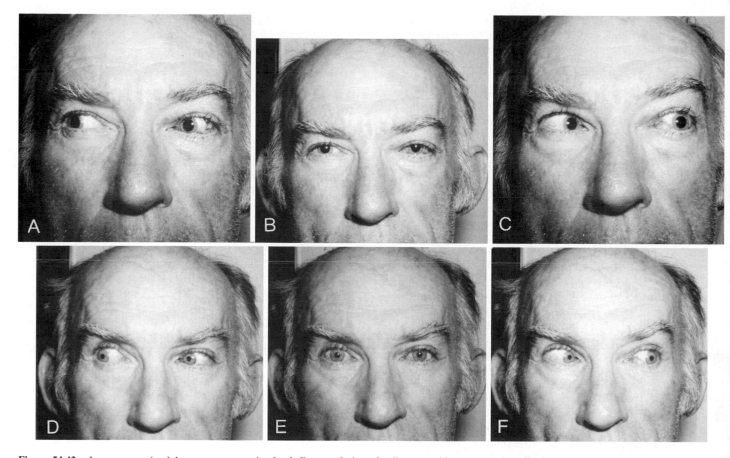

Figure 54.42. Improvement in abducens nerve paresis after balloon occlusion of a direct carotid-cavernous sinus fistula. The patient is a 65-year-old man who developed a left-sided direct carotid-cavernous sinus fistula after an automobile accident. *A–C,* The patient has mild proptosis and redness of the left eye as well as mild left abducens nerve paresis. *D-F,* 72 hours after successful balloon occlusion of the fistula, the patient's appearance has improved, and the abducens nerve paresis has resolved.

DURAL CAROTID-CAVERNOUS SINUS FISTULAS
(DURAL ARTERIOVENOUS MALFORMATIONS)

Because at least some dural carotid-cavernous sinus fistulas are thought to be congenital arteriovenous fistulas that spontaneously become symptomatic later in life (from atherosclerosis, hypertension, or other vascular disorders), they are discussed in Chapter 43 of this text. We have chosen to review the nature, manifestations, and treatment of these lesions in this chapter also to allow the reader to compare and contrast them with direct carotid-cavernous sinus fistulas.

ANATOMY

The internal and external carotid arteries (along with the vertebral artery) supply meningeal branches to the dura mater of the cranial cavity. Dural carotid-cavernous sinus fistulas arise from some of these branches.

Meningeal Branches of the Internal Carotid Artery

Meningeal branches of the internal carotid artery originate from its cavernous segment and supply the dura of the cavernous sinus, the dura of the clivus, and portions of the tentorium cerebelli (Pribram et al., 1966) (Figs. 52.8–52.11, and 52.12). Two of these branches, the meningohypophyseal trunk and the artery of the inferior cavernous sinus, provide the afferent supply of most dural carotid-cavernous sinus fistulas (Barrow et al., 1985).

As noted in Chapter 52, the meningohypophyseal trunk originates from the apex of the initial proximal curve of the cavernous segment of the internal carotid artery and usually gives off three branches: the tentorial artery (artery of Bernasconi-Cassonari), the inferior hypophyseal artery, and the dorsal meningeal artery (Figs. 52.6 and 52.7). Of these branches, any of which may arise separately from the internal carotid artery, the dorsal meningeal artery supplying the dura of the clivus most often participates in dural carotid-cavernous sinus fistulas. This vessel may anastomose within the dura of the clivus with collateral branches of the ascending pharyngeal artery, a branch of the external carotid artery (see below).

The artery of the inferior cavernous sinus arises from the lateral aspect of the cavernous segment of the internal carotid artery and curves over the abducens nerve, after which it usually divides into three main branches that supply the dura and cranial nerves within the cavernous sinus (Lasjaunias et al., 1977) (Figs. 52.9 and 52.10). A superior (tentorial) ramus supplies the roof of the cavernous sinus and the oculomotor and trochlear nerves as they enter the sinus. This branch may occasionally give rise to the tentorial artery. An anterior ramus usually divides into a medial and a lateral branch. The medial branch supplies the dura of the superior orbital fissure and the oculomotor, trochlear, and abducens nerves as they enter the orbit. This branch may anastomose with the ophthalmic artery. The lateral branch courses to the foramen rotundum, supplies the dura in this region of the temporal fossa, and terminates as the artery of the foramen rotundum. It may anastomose with middle meningeal branches of the internal maxillary artery and thus provide collateral pathways between the internal and external carotid arteries (Parkinson, 1964, 1965; Pribram et al., 1966; Wallace et al., 1967; Margolis and Newton, 1969). The posterior ramus of the artery of the inferior cavernous sinus also divides into a medial and a lateral branch. The medial branch courses to the region of the foramen ovale and supplies the abducens nerve, the gasserian ganglion, and the motor root of the trigeminal nerve. It may anastomose with the accessory meningeal artery of the proximal internal maxillary artery. The lateral branch supplies the gasserian ganglion and adjacent dura. It may anastomose with the cavernous branch of the middle meningeal artery as that artery emerges from the foramen spinosum. Branches of the artery of the inferior cavernous sinus are the most common contributors to dural carotid-cavernous sinus fistulas.

Meningeal Branches of the External Carotid Artery

The meningeal supply from the external carotid artery originates from the internal maxillary, ascending pharyngeal, and occipital arteries (Fig. 52.97). The internal maxillary artery is the source of the middle meningeal and the accessory meningeal arteries, branches of which supply the dura in the region of the foramen spinosum and foramen ovale, respectively. As noted above, these branches may anastomose with branches of the artery of the inferior cavernous sinus from the internal carotid artery. The ascending pharyngeal artery gives rise to a neuromeningeal trunk that supplies the dura of the clivus and that may anastomose with the dorsal meningeal artery.

Anatomic Types of Dural Carotid-Cavernous Sinus Fistulas

Since the blood supply to the region of the cavernous sinus is provided by interconnecting branches of the internal and external carotid arteries, it is not surprising that dural carotid-cavernous sinus fistulas may be separated anatomically into three types: (a) shunts between meningeal branches of the internal carotid artery and the cavernous sinus, (b) shunts between meningeal branches of the external carotid artery and the cavernous sinus, and (c) shunts between meningeal branches of both the internal and external carotid arteries and the cavernous sinus (Peeters and Kröger,

1979; Barrow et al., 1985) (Figs. 54.2–54.4). Of these types, the third is by far the most common (Debrun et al., 1988).

PATHOGENESIS

Dural carotid-cavernous sinus fistulas usually become symptomatic spontaneously. The pathogenesis of these fistulas is controversial (Fleishman et al., 1986; Debrun et al., 1988; Berlit et al., 1993). Lie (1968) suggested that at least some of these fistulas are congenital. Newton and Hoyt (1970) speculated that spontaneous dural carotid-cavernous sinus fistulas form after rupture of one or more of the thin-walled dural arteries that normally traverse the cavernous sinus. After rupture, extensive preformed dural arterial anastomoses not directly involved in the fistula may dilate and contribute collateral blood supply, resulting in an angiographic appearance indistinguishable from a congenital vascular malformation (Aminoff, 1973). Indeed, sequential arteriography demonstrates that the feeder vessels of dural carotid-cavernous sinus fistulas change with time as the vessels spontaneously open and close (Takahashi and Nakano, 1980). Although the theory of Newton and Hoyt (1970) is favored by some investigators (Barrow et al., 1985), it fails to explain why spontaneous dural carotid-cavernous sinus fistulas are more common in elderly women than in men. Brismar and Brismar (1976) and Seeger et al. (1980) noted a high incidence of venous thrombosis in patients with dural carotid-cavernous sinus fistula. They thought the venous occlusion was the result of the fistula; however, Houser et al. (1979) suggested that most dural carotid-cavernous sinus fistulas develop because of venous thrombosis in the cavernous sinus. In this setting, the meningeal network in the cavernous sinus occurs as a collateral response to the thrombosis. This theory is favored by most investigators since it also explains the pathogenesis of arteriovenous fistulas that develop in the sigmoid and other dural sinuses (Chaudhary et al., 1982; Sundt and Piepgras, 1983; Grove, 1984; Shults, 1984; Viñuela et al., 1984; Graeb and Dolman, 1986; Parkinson, 1986; Debrun et al., 1988).

Certain factors may predispose to the development of symptomatic dural carotid-cavernous sinus fistulas. These include pregnancy, systemic hypertension, atherosclerotic vascular disease, connective tissue disease (e.g., Ehlers-Danlos syndrome), and minor trauma (Francois et al., 1955; Walker and Allegré, 1956; Parkinson, 1964; Graf, 1965; Hamby, 1966; Newton and Hoyt, 1970; Julien and De Boucaud, 1971; Taniguchi et al., 1971; Slusher et al., 1979; Toya et al., 1981; Farley et al., 1983; Guiolet et al., 1984; Lach et al., 1987; Fox et al., 1988; Schievink et al., 1991; Taki et al., 1994) (Fig. 54.43). Mironov (1995) reported the case of a 30-year-old man who suffered head trauma with a bilateral basal skull fracture. A few weeks later, he experienced progressive proptosis and developed an audible bruit. An evaluation revealed that he had a dural carotid-cavernous sinus fistula caused by rupture of a primitive intracavernous anastomosis between an accessory meningeal artery and a redundant deep recurrent ophthalmic artery.

CLINICAL MANIFESTATIONS

Dural carotid-cavernous sinus fistulas usually occur in middle-aged or elderly women, but they may produce symp-

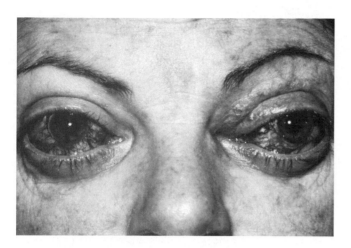

Figure 54.43. External appearance of a 39-year-old woman with Ehlers-Danlos syndrome who developed spontaneous bilateral dural carotid cavernous sinus fistulas. The fistulas were successfully closed using an endovascular approach, but the patient died several months later from unrelated vascular complications of the underlying disease.

toms at any age, even in infancy (Biglan et al., 1981; Konishi et al., 1990; Yamamoto et al., 1995). The symptoms and signs produced by these lesions are influenced by a number of factors, including the size of the fistula, location within the cavernous sinus, rate of flow, and especially whether drainage is posterior, anterior, or both (Lasjaunias et al., 1986). The route of drainage of the fistula is probably related to its basic anatomic configuration, although Grove (1984) postulated that many, if not all, fistulas initially drain posteriorly into the inferior petrosal sinus, basilar venous plexus, or both. He believed that when this normal pathway for drainage becomes thrombosed, the fistula begins to drain anteriorly, producing visual symptoms and signs. Hawke et al. (1989) described a patient in whom this process seemed to have occurred. The patient developed a painful oculomotor nerve paresis that was thought to be caused by an intracranial aneurysm. An arteriogram showed a dural carotid-cavernous sinus fistula that was draining posteriorly (Fig. 54.44). Several weeks after arteriography, the patient developed ipsilateral redness, conjunctival chemosis, and proptosis. A repeat arteriogram now showed that the inferior petrosal sinus had become occluded and that the fistula was draining anteriorly through the superior and inferior ophthalmic veins (Fig. 54.45).

Posteriorly Draining Fistulas

When dural carotid-cavernous sinus fistulas drain posteriorly into the superior and inferior petrosal sinuses, they usually are asymptomatic. In some cases, however, such fistulas produce a cranial neuropathy. Rizzo et al. (1982) described a 38-year-old woman who spontaneously developed a left trigeminal sensory neuropathy characterized by facial numbness and paresthesia. She also had long-standing tinnitus in the left ear that had recently become pulsatile. An examination revealed dulled sensation to touch and pinprick

along the distribution of the left maxillary and mandibular divisions of the trigeminal nerve. Corneal sensation was normal bilaterally, and the muscles of mastication had normal strength. A bruit was heard over the left temporal and mastoid areas. There were no signs of orbital disease. The patient was found to have a dural carotid-cavernous sinus fistula fed by terminal branches of the left middle meningeal artery. After trapping of the fistula, the bruit and pulsatile tinnitus disappeared immediately. Over the next 2 months, the facial numbness and paresthesia improved. Rizzo et al. (1982) speculated that the trigeminal neuropathy was caused by vascular compromise of the gasserian ganglion.

Numerous authors have reported patients in whom a posteriorly draining spontaneous dural carotid-cavernous sinus fistula produced an isolated ocular motor nerve paresis unassociated with clinical evidence of orbital congestion (see Table in Acierno et al., 1995; Lee, 1996) (Figs. 54.44–54.46). In most cases, the onset of the paresis is sudden and only one of the ocular motor nerves is affected. The oculomotor nerve is most often affected and usually is associated with ipsilateral orbital or ocular pain, a presentation that initially suggests an intracranial aneurysm (Hawke et al., 1989; Pérez Sempere et al., 1991; Kurata et al., 1993; Lee, 1996). Miyachi et al. (1993) reported five such patients. The paresis was complete and associated with an unreactive ipsilateral pupil in two patients. The paresis was incomplete in the other three patients, with one patient having a sluggish pupil on the side of the paresis and the other two patients having a normally reactive ipsilateral pupil. All patients were older women in whom angiography showed a low flow fistula causing early filling of the

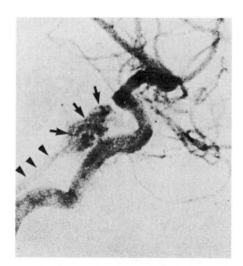

Figure 54.44. Posteriorly draining dural carotid-cavernous sinus fistula (shunt) causing an acute, painful oculomotor nerve paresis. The patient was a 58-year-old woman who developed an acute right-sided fronto-orbital headache. Four weeks later she developed diplopia, and 7 days after this, she developed right ptosis and a dilated right pupil. She was thought to have an intracranial aneurysm, and an arteriogram was performed. Selective right carotid arteriogram, lateral view, shows a dural arteriovenous fistula of the cavernous sinus (*arrows*) that drains posteriorly into the inferior petrosal sinus (*arrowheads*). (From Hawke SHB, Mullie MA, Hoyt WF, et al. Arch Neurol *46*:1252–1255, 1989.)

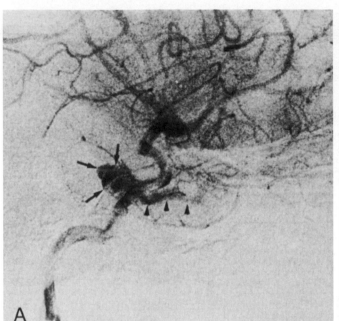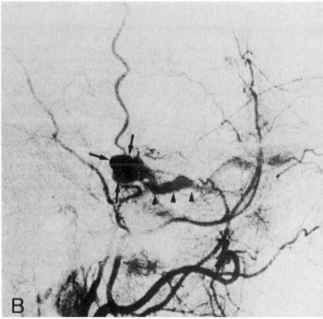

Figure 54.45. Cerebral angiography in the patient described in *Figure 54.44* several weeks later, after the patient developed redness, conjunctival chemosis, and proptosis of the right eye. *A,* Repeat selective right internal carotid arteriogram, lateral view, shows that the dural carotid-cavernous sinus fistula (*arrows*) now drains anteriorly (*arrowheads*) rather than posteriorly. *B,* Selective right external carotid arteriogram shows that the fistula (*arrows*) also fills from extradural branches of the external carotid artery. The anterior drainage of the fistula into the right superior ophthalmic vein is clearly seen (*arrowheads*). (From Hawke SHB, Mullie MA, Hoyt WF, et al. Arch Neurol *46*:1252–1255, 1989.)

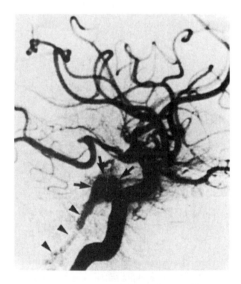

Figure 54.46. Selective right internal carotid arteriogram, lateral view, in a 57-year-old woman who had developed acute, right-sided temporal and orbital pain that was followed within 2 hours by the development of a complete right oculomotor nerve paresis. The patient had no signs or symptoms of orbital disease. The angiogram shows a large dural carotid-cavernous sinus fistula (*arrows*) that drains posteriorly into the inferior petrosal sinus (*arrowheads*) rather than anteriorly into the orbit. (From Hawke SHB, Mullie MA, Hoyt WF, et al. Arch Neurol *46*:1252–1255, 1989.)

superoposterior cavernous sinus and drainage posteriorly into the inferior petrosal sinus. Two of the patients experienced spontaneous resolution of the oculomotor nerve paresis 6 weeks to 3 months after onset of symptoms. Two other patients experienced resolution of the palsy after treatment with hemostatic agents and embolization, and one patient resolved after medical treatment alone.

Kosmorsky et al. (1988) described two patients with dural carotid-cavernous sinus fistulas who developed acute, painful ophthalmoplegia without conjunctival chemosis, dilation of conjunctival vessels, or proptosis. One patient had a right trochlear nerve paresis. The other patient had mild bilateral abducens nerve paresis and a partial left oculomotor nerve paresis. Posterior drainage of the fistula into the inferior petrosal sinus was thought to be responsible for the ocular motor nerve pareses in both cases. Other authors have reported similar cases involving either the trochlear nerve or the abducens nerve (Newton and Hoyt, 1970; Nukui et al., 1978; Phelps et al., 1982; Kataoka et al., 1985; Kurata et al., 1993; Selky and Purvin, 1994; Sogg, 1996). We have seen several cases of unilateral abducens nerve paresis but no cases of trochlear nerve paresis in this setting.

Posterior drainage of a spontaneous, dural carotid-cavernous sinus fistula also was thought to be responsible for the development of a left facial nerve paresis in two patients, one described by Kapur et al. (1982) and the other by Moster et al. (1988). In both patients, the paresis may have been caused by compression of the facial nerve by increased venous pressure or redirection of the arterial supply of the nerve by the fistula. The patient described by Moster et al. (1988) also had ocular symptoms and signs caused by simultaneous anterior drainage of the fistula (see below).

The cranial neuropathies that are caused by a posteriorly draining dural carotid-cavernous sinus fistula are usually the initial sign of the fistula. In many of these cases, failure to diagnose and treat the fistula leads eventually to a change in the direction of the flow of blood in the fistula. The flow becomes anterior, and the patient develops evidence of orbital congestion. In other cases, the blood flow in the fistula initially is anterior, producing orbital manifestations. With time, however, the anterior drainage ceases, and posterior flow is associated with the development of the cranial neuropathy.

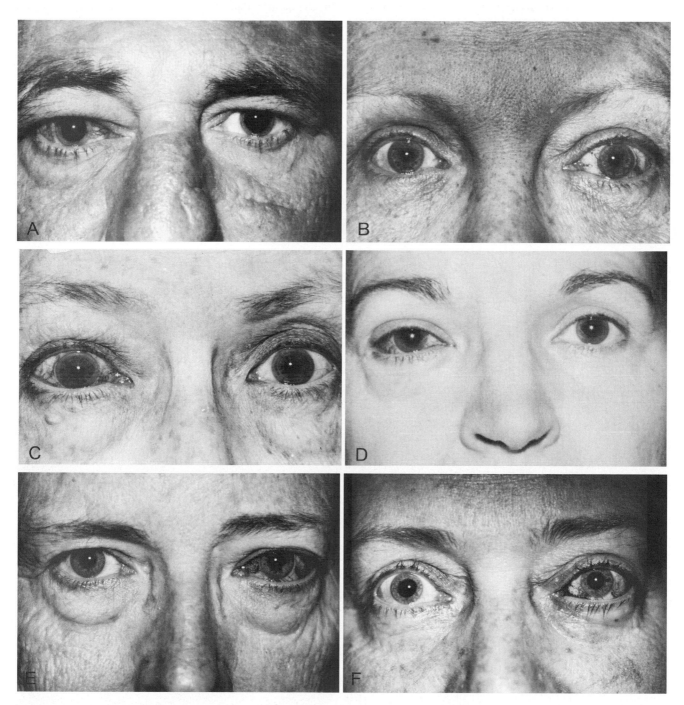

Figure 54.47. Appearance of six different patients with spontaneous dural carotid-cavernous sinus fistulas (shunts). *A–F,* Note that all patients have monocular redness of the eyes with minimal if any proptosis, chemosis of the conjunctiva, or eyelid swelling. This appearance often is mistaken for that of chronic conjunctivitis, episcleritis, or dysthyroid orbitopathy.

Anteriorly Draining Fistulas

Like their direct counterparts, dural carotid-cavernous sinus fistulas usually produce visual symptoms and signs when they drain anteriorly into the superior and inferior ophthalmic veins. The clinical manifestations of patients with dural carotid-cavernous fistulas that drain anteriorly are therefore similar to but usually much less severe than those of patients with direct fistulas, since most dural fistulas contain blood flowing at a low rate. Indeed, dural fistulas usually produce an important and rather characteristic syndrome that nevertheless is often misdiagnosed (Newton and Hoyt, 1968, 1970; Taniguchi et al., 1971; Brismar and Brismar, 1976; Costin et al., 1978; de Keizer, 1979; Slusher et al., 1979; de Keizer, 1981; Phelps et al., 1982; Grove, 1984; Viñuela et al., 1984; Jorgensen and Guthoff, 1986; Keltner et al., 1986, 1987; Jorgensen and Guthoff, 1988; Kupersmith et al., 1988; Shiga et al., 1994). Unlike direct fistulas, there often is no objective or subjective bruit. Even when a subjective bruit is present, the patient may not mention it, either because it is mild or because the patient does not associate the sound with his or her ocular symptoms and signs. In the mildest cases, there is redness of one or occasionally both eyes caused by dilation and arterialization of both conjunctival and episcleral veins (Fig. 54.47). The appearance may suggest conjunctivitis, episcleritis, or thyroid eye disease; however, careful examination of the dilated vessels demonstrates a typical tortuous corkscrew appearance that is virtually pathognemonic of a dural carotid-cavernous sinus fistula (Fig. 54.48). There also may be minimal eyelid swelling, conjunctival chemosis, proptosis, or a combination of these findings (Nowe et al., 1989). Diplopia from abducens nerve paresis may be present (Fig. 54.49). Ophthalmoscopy may be normal, or there may be mild dilation of retinal veins.

In more advanced cases, particularly those with a high flow rate, the symptoms and signs are identical with those in patients with a direct carotid-cavernous sinus fistula (Levasseur et al., 1992). Proptosis, chemosis, and dilation of conjunctival vessels are obvious (Fig. 54.50). Diplopia may result from ophthalmoparesis caused by ocular motor nerve paresis, orbital congestion, or both, and it may be painful, initially suggesting an orbital inflammatory process or even the so-called Tolosa-Hunt syndrome of painful ophthalmoplegia (Brazis et al., 1994; Procope et al., 1994; see below). Raised episcleral venous pressure may produce increased intraocular pressure which occasionally can be quite

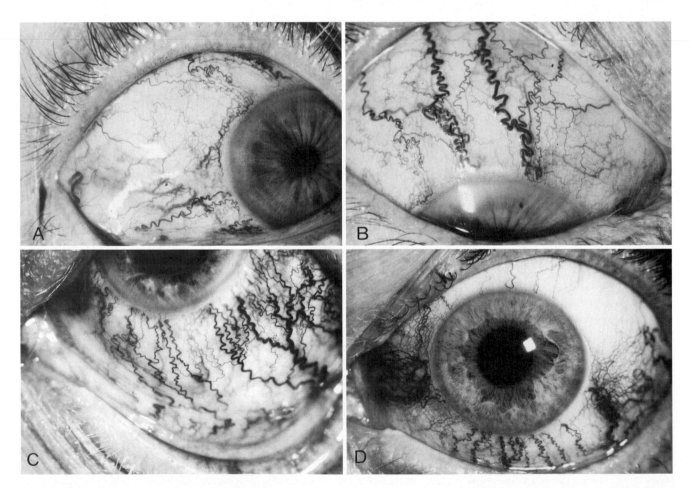

Figure 54.48. Appearance of conjunctival and episcleral vessels in four patients with spontaneous, dural carotid-cavernous sinus fistulas. *A–D*, note dilation, tortuosity, and corkscrew appearance of the veins.

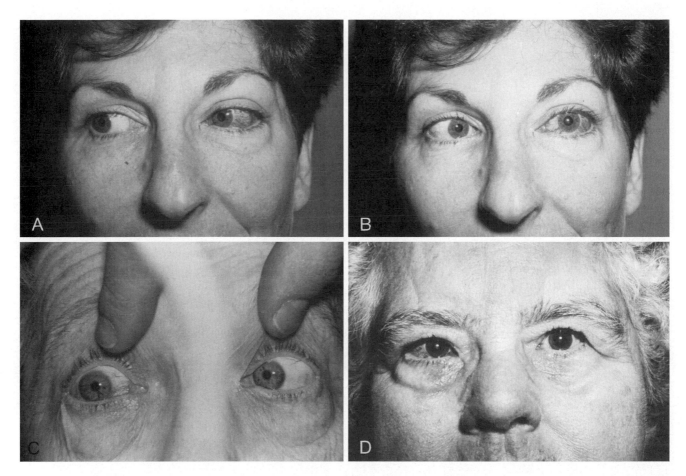

Figure 54.49. Abducens nerve pareses in patients with dural carotid-cavernous sinus fistula. *A* and *B*, In a 34-year-old woman with a left-sided fistula, the left eye adducts fully on attempted right lateral gaze; however, when the patient attempts to look to the left, the left eye abducts only to just beyond the midline. Note the mild left proptosis and the dilated conjunctival veins of the left eye. *C*, A 75-year-old woman with a right-sided, spontaneous, dural carotid-cavernous sinus fistula shows moderate weakness of abduction of the right eye on attempted right lateral gaze. Note prominent conjunctival vessels of the right eye compared with the normal left eye. *D*, An 80-year-old woman with a right-sided dural carotid-cavernous sinus fistula. Note the obvious right esotropia of about 40 prism diopters when the patient fixates with the left eye. Also note the prominent conjunctival vessels in the right eye. The patient has no proptosis or conjunctival chemosis.

high (Phelps et al., 1982; Keltner et al., 1986). Angle closure glaucoma may develop in rare cases from elevated orbital venous pressure, congestion of the iris and choroid, and forward displacement of the iris-lens diaphragm (Harris and Rice, 1979; Buus et al., 1989; Fiore et al., 1990). Ophthalmoscopic abnormalities include venous stasis retinopathy with intraretinal hemorrhages, central retinal vein occlusion, proliferative retinopathy, retinal detachment, vitreous hemorrhage, choroidal folds, choroidal effusion, choroidal detachment, optic disc swelling, and neovascular or angle closure glaucoma (Harbison et al., 1978; Harris et al., 1980; Hines and Guy, 1986; Pollock and Miller, 1986; Brunette and Boghen, 1987; Fiore et al., 1990; Komiyama et al., 1990a; Gonshor and Kline, 1991; Kojima et al., 1991; Yamada et al., 1991; Kupersmith et al., 1996) (Fig. 54.51).

Visual loss, although less frequent than in patients with direct carotid-cavernous fistula, occurs in 20–30% of patients with dural carotid-cavernous sinus fistulas (Newton and Hoyt, 1970; de Keizer, 1979; Grove, 1984). It may be caused by ischemic optic neuropathy, chorioretinal dysfunction, or uncontrolled glaucoma (Kupersmith et al., 1988, 1996).

The ocular manifestations of dural carotid-cavernous sinus fistulas almost always are ipsilateral to the fistula or bilateral (Fig. 54.52), but they may be purely contralateral (Graeleau and Namin, 1954; Bynke and Efsing, 1970; Kurokawa et al., 1995; Martin et al., 1995). We have seen a patient with bilateral dural carotid-cavernous sinus fistulas that caused only left-sided ocular manifestations. The left-sided fistula drained anteriorly into the left orbit via the left superior ophthalmic vein. The right-sided fistula drained across the intercavernous sinus and then anteriorly into the left orbit.

Although most dural fistulas are unilateral, spontaneous bilateral dural fistulas may occur (Schoolman and Kepes, 1967; West, 1980; Rwiza et al., 1988; Haugen et al., 1990) (Figs. 54.43 and 54.50*D*). Patients with bilateral dural carotid-cavernous sinus fistulas often have severe systemic hy-

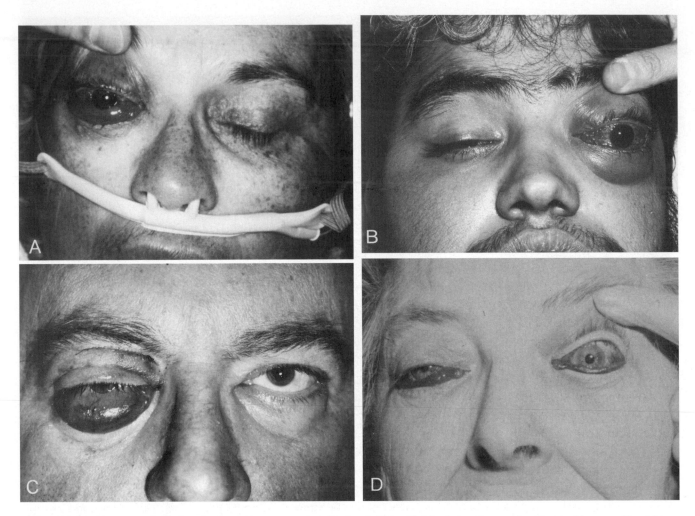

Figure 54.50. Appearance of high-flow dural carotid-cavernous sinus fistulas. *A,* Right-sided fistula in a hypertensive 63-year-old woman. The right eye is moderately proptotic, and there is significant chemosis of the conjunctiva. *B,* Left-sided spontaneous fistula in a 34-year-old man with factor VIII deficiency. Note marked proptosis, redness, and conjunctival chemosis of the left eye. The eye could not move well in any direction. *C,* Right-sided fistula in a 50-year-old man with severe diabetes mellitus and renal failure. Note marked right proptosis, lid swelling, and severe conjunctival chemosis. *D,* Bilateral dural fistulas in a 77-year-old woman. Note bilateral ptosis, proptosis, redness, and conjunctival chemosis. The appearance of these four patients is indistinguishable from the appearance of patients with high-flow direct carotid-cavernous sinus fistulas.

pertension, atherosclerosis, or some type of systemic connective tissue disease, particularly Ehlers-Danlos syndrome (Fig. 54.43).

In extremely rare instances, anteriorly-draining, dural carotid-cavernous sinus fistulas produce cranial neuropathies other than ocular motor nerve paresis. Moster et al. (1988) described a 73-year-old woman with an otherwise typical presentation of a spontaneous, dural carotid-cavernous sinus fistula (redness and prominence of the right eye, right proptosis, right ophthalmoparesis, increased intraocular pressure in the right eye) who also developed right facial weakness within 24 hours after ocular signs began. Cerebral angiography revealed that the fistula drained not only anteriorly into the superior ophthalmic vein but also posteriorly into the inferior petrosal sinus. It was postulated by Moster et al. (1988) that the facial nerve paresis resulted from compression of the facial nerve by increased venous pressure

and from redirection of the arterial supply by the fistula (i.e., a steal syndrome).

Intracranial hemorrhage is an unusual complication of a dural carotid-cavernous sinus fistula. Harding et al. (1984) described two patients with unilateral periorbital pain, proptosis, chemosis of the conjunctiva, and ophthalmoparesis who were found to have dural carotid-cavernous sinus fistulas. Both patients experienced a spontaneous intracerebral hemorrhage within 18 months after the onset of signs and symptoms of the fistula. The clinical manifestations of the hemorrhage were focal seizures and signs of unilateral hemisphere dysfunction. The hematomas in both patients occurred in the region drained by the superficial middle cerebral vein ipsilateral to the shunt, and it was postulated that the hemorrhage occurred from locally increased venous pressure.

Because the symptoms and signs of a dural carotid-cav-

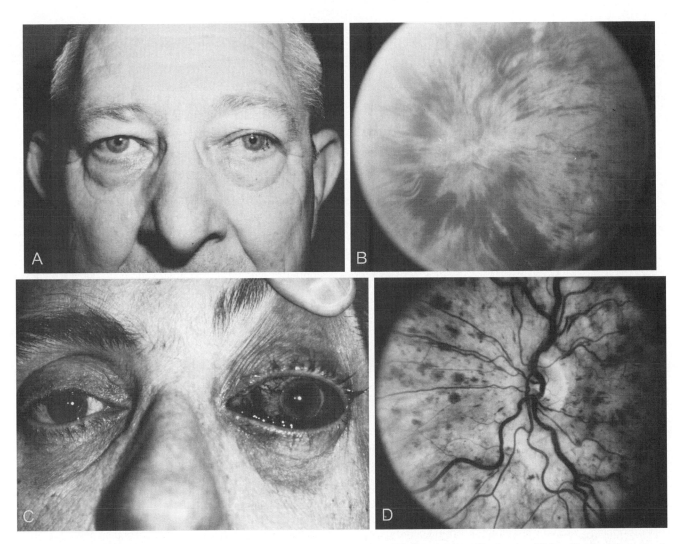

Figure 54.51. Central retinal vein occlusion in two patients with spontaneous, dural carotid-cavernous sinus fistulas. *A* and *B*, In a 67 year old hypertensive man with a left-sided fistula. *A*, External appearance of the patient shows mild proptosis of the left eye and dilation of conjunctival and episcleral veins of that eye. *B*, Appearance of the left ocular fundus shows changes consistent with a central retinal vein occlusion. Note marked swelling of the left optic disc, dilation of retinal veins, and typical "blood and thunder" appearance of the retina with diffuse intraretinal hemorrhages and exudates. The visual acuity in this eye was 20/300 and did not improve as the hemorrhages cleared. *C* and *D*, In a 62-year-old otherwise healthy woman. *C*, External appearance shows moderate proptosis of left eye, associated with conjunctival chemosis and arterialization of conjunctival and episcleral vessels. The patient noted progressive visual loss in the left eye over several days. *D*, Ophthalmoscopic appearance of left ocular fundus shows changes consistent with a mild central retinal vein occlusion. Left optic disc is normal, but retinal veins are dilated, and there are numerous intraretinal "dot and blot" hemorrhages. The visual acuity in this eye was 20/80, but it improved to 20/20 as the hemorrhages cleared spontaneously.

ernous sinus fistula often are mild, usually developing spontaneously and rather slowly, patients with this lesion often are misdiagnosed initially. When the patient simply has a chronic red eye, perhaps with minimal eyelid swelling (Fig. 54.53), he or she may be thought to have a chronic conjunctivitis or blepharoconjunctivitis that is refractory to topical therapy. In patients who develop diplopia from abducens nerve paresis, the significance of a slightly red eye may be missed. We have seen such a patient, a 65-year-old woman who was referred to the Neuro-Ophthalmology Unit of the Johns Hopkins Hospital for evaluation of horizontal diplopia. The patient, who had long-standing systemic hypertension, stated that the diplopia had developed rather suddenly

about 2 months earlier. It was initially intermittent and present only in right lateral gaze; however, it had become constant within the last several weeks, and it was now present in primary position. The examination revealed an apparently isolated right abduction weakness associated with an esotropia in primary position. The esotropia increased in attempted right lateral gaze and decreased on gaze to the left. It was thought that the patient had a vasculopathic abducens nerve paresis, and she was told to return for follow-up evaluation in 4 weeks. When she returned, her diplopia and abduction weakness were about the same. This time, however, it was observed that the right eye was slightly injected with dilation of conjunctival and episcleral vessels (Fig. 54.54). The pa-

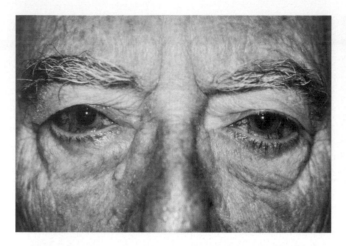

Figure 54.52. Bilateral ocular manifestations in a patient with a right-sided spontaneous dural carotid-cavernous sinus fistula. The patient has bilateral red eyes, with dilated, tortuous conjunctival and episcleral veins.

tient was asked if she heard any abnormal sounds in her head. She answered that she heard a constant swishing noise that seemed to originate from behind the right eye. In retrospect, the sound had begun about the time the patient had first noted diplopia. When asked why she had not reported this problem during her first visit, she explained that she hadn't been asked and did not think it was related to her double vision. A bilateral, selective internal and external carotid arteriogram demonstrated a right-sided carotid-cavernous sinus fistula fed by dural branches from both the internal and the external carotid arteries.

In patients with evidence of orbital congestion, red eye, conjunctival chemosis, etc., diagnoses other than a spontaneous dural carotid-cavernous sinus fistula, such as dysthyroid orbitopathy, orbital pseudotumor, orbital cellulitis, episcleritis, spheno-orbital meningioma, or even Tolosa-Hunt syndrome, may be considered (Newton and Hoyt, 1970; Tan-

iguchi et al., 1971; Brismar and Brismar, 1976; Costin et al., 1978; Klepach et al., 1978; de Keizer, 1979; Slusher et al., 1979; Merlis et al., 1982; Phelps et al., 1982; Grove, 1984; Fleishman et al., 1986; Jorgensen and Guthoff, 1986, 1988; Brazis et al., 1994; Procope et al., 1994; Shiga et al., 1994; Oestreicher and Frueh, 1995) (Fig. 54.55). The correct diagnosis in such cases may then not be made until symptoms and signs worsen, new symptoms and signs develop, or appropriate diagnostic studies are performed.

Conversely, since the disorders mentioned above often produce clinical manifestations similar to those produced by a carotid-cavernous sinus fistula, they may be the cause of symptoms and signs initially attributed to a carotid-cavernous sinus fistula. In addition, trauma to the posterior orbit in the region of the superior orbital fissure may produce such manifestations (Llorente Pendás and Albertos Castro, 1995), and we and others have seen patients with congenital or acquired anomalous intracranial venous drainage who developed clinical manifestations suggesting a carotid-cavernous sinus fistula (Tech et al., 1995). The correct diagnosis in virtually all cases is made by appropriate neuroimaging studies, particularly cerebral angiography (see below).

DIAGNOSIS

The diagnosis of dural carotid-cavernous sinus fistula should be considered in any patient who spontaneously develops a red eye, chemosis of the conjunctiva, abducens nerve paresis, or mild orbital congestion with proptosis. Auscultation of the orbit occasionally may disclose a bruit, but this is relatively uncommon. Tonometry, however, usually shows asymmetry of the ocular pulse with a greater pulse amplitude on the side of the lesion. The asymmetry in the amplitude of the ocular pulse can be appreciated using any tonometer, although we prefer to use a pneumotonometer which provides a direct measurement and an objective record of the pulse (Golnik and Miller, 1992) (Fig. 54.56). This instrument or a similar one also can be used to determine if

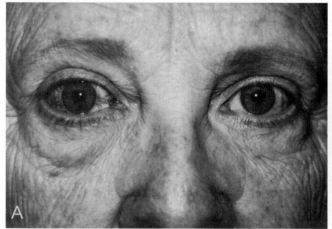
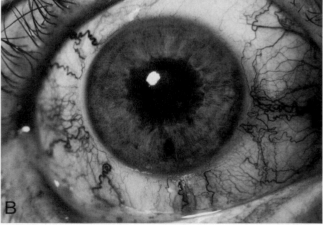

Figure 54.53. Spontaneous dural carotid-cavernous sinus fistula mistaken for chronic conjunctivitis. *A,* Redness and minimal swelling of the right eye of a 66-year-old woman who was thought to have chronic conjunctivitis but who, in fact, had an ipsilateral spontaneous dural carotid-cavernous sinus fistula. *B,* Magnified view of right eye shows dilated, corkscrew conjunctival and episcleral veins typical for a dural carotid-cavernous sinus fistula.

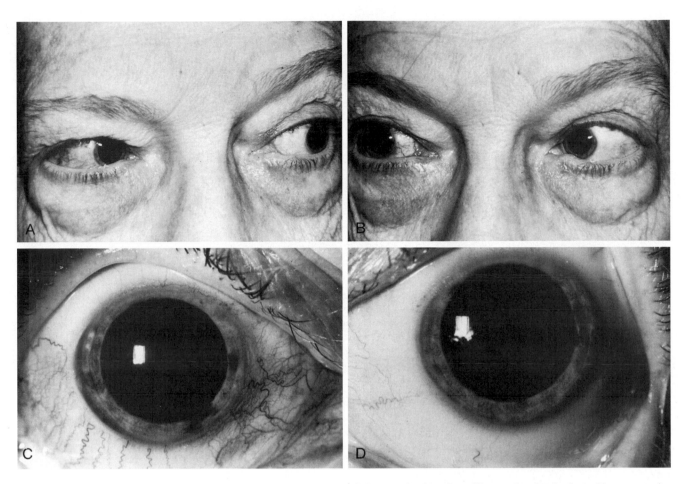

Figure 54.54. Abducens nerve paresis thought to have been caused by systemic hypertension in patient with a spontaneous dural carotid-cavernous sinus fistula. The patient was a 65-year-old woman with known systemic hypertension who developed acute horizontal diplopia. *A* and *B,* The patient has mild weakness of abduction of the right eye. She was initially thought to have a vasculopathic right abducens nerve paresis. In retrospect, however, the conjunctival and episcleral veins of the right eye are dilated and tortuous compared with those of the left eye. Higher magnification of photographs of the right eye (*C*) shows obvious dilation and tortuosity of conjunctival and episcleral veins compared with the appearance of the same vessels of the left eye (*D*). The correct diagnosis was made when the abnormal vessels were noted during a follow-up examination.

an untreated fistula is resolving or if a treated fistula has been successfully closed (see below).

When a dural carotid-cavernous sinus fistula is suspected, CT scanning, MR imaging, orbital ultrasonography, duplex carotid sonography, transorbital and transcranial color doppler imaging, or a combination of these tests may be of benefit in confirming the diagnosis (Merrick et al., 1980; Zilkha and Daiz, 1980; Phelps et al., 1982; de Keizer, 1983; Moster and Kennerdell, 1983; Grove, 1984; Gomori et al., 1986; Jorgensen and Guthoff, 1986; Keltner et al., 1987; Jorgensen and Guthoff, 1988; Kotval et al., 1990; Flaharty et al., 1991; Spector, 1991; Muttaquin et al., 1992; Soulier-Sotto et al., 1992; H.-J. Lin et al., 1994; S.K. Lin et al., 1994; Zhao et al., 1995; Atta et al., 1996). The gold-standard diagnostic test, however, is, as in the case of the direct carotid-cavernous sinus fistula, an arteriogram (Debrun et al., 1981; Grove, 1984; Fleishman et al., 1986; Debrun et al., 1988; Debrun, 1995). Some investigators have advocated performing intravenous digital subtraction angiography to diagnose dural ca-

rotid-cavernous sinus fistulas (Modic et al., 1982), but we and others believe that intra-arterial subtraction angiography gives much better resolution and is therefore the preferred technique (Viñuela et al., 1983; Debrun et al., 1988; Kosmorsky et al., 1988). Since most dural carotid-cavernous sinus fistulas are fed either by meningeal branches of the external carotid artery or by meningeal branches of both the internal and external carotid arteries, whereas others are fed by arteries from both sides or are fed by unilateral arteries but produce bilateral symptoms and signs, selective angiography of **both** internal and external carotid arteries on **both** sides should always be performed (Rosenbaum and Schechter, 1969; Bickerstaff, 1970; Bynke and Efsing, 1970; de Keizer, 1981; Grove, 1984; Viñuela et al., 1984; Barrow et al., 1985; Grossman et al., 1985; Fleishman et al., 1986; Debrun et al., 1988; Kosmorsky et al., 1988; Debrun, 1995). Such angiography has a relatively low morbidity and mortality that is less than 1% in most centers, except in patients with connective tissue disorders such as Ehlers-Danlos syndrome, in

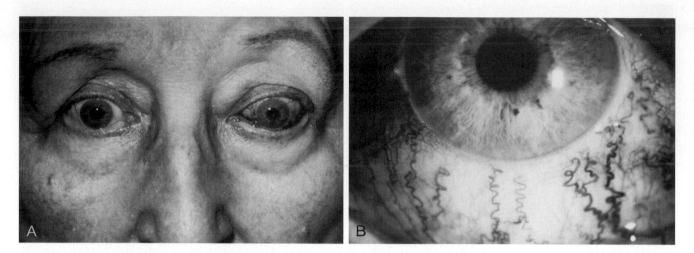

Figure 54.55. Spontaneous dural carotid-cavernous sinus fistula mistaken for dysthyroid orbitopathy. The patient was a 78-year-old woman with redness of the left eye and mild vertical binocular diplopia. *A,* On attempted downgaze, the patient has bilateral upper eyelid retraction. The left eye is also red and swollen. *B,* Magnified view of the left eye shows typical dilated, tortuous, and corkscrew shaped conjunctival and episcleral veins. An evaluation revealed no clinical or laboratory evidence of thyroid disease; however, echography showed a dilated left superior ophthalmic vein, and cerebral angiography revealed a left-sided dural carotid-cavernous sinus fistula fed by branches of the left external and left internal carotid arteries.

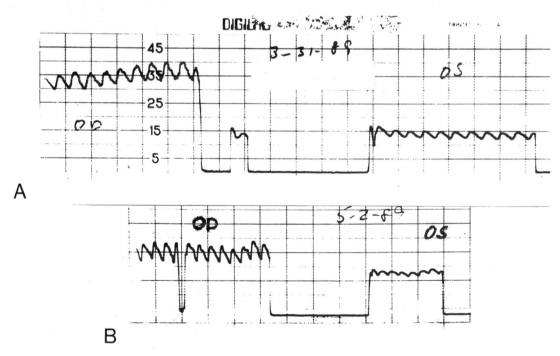

Figure 54.56. Measurements of intraocular pressure and ocular pulse amplitudes in two patients with spontaneous, dural carotid-cavernous sinus fistulas. Both patients had developed progressive redness and mild swelling of the right eye. *A,* In a 71-year-old woman who had been treated for several weeks for a "chronic conjunctivitis," the intraocular pressure in the right eye is elevated to 35 mm Hg compared with 15 mm Hg in the left eye, and the amplitude of the ocular pulse in the right eye is about 3 times that in the left eye. Cerebral angiography revealed a dural carotid-cavernous sinus fistula fed by branches from the right internal and external carotid arteries. *B,* In a 65-year-old man who was thought to have dysthyroid orbitopathy, the intraocular pressure is slightly elevated to 25 mm Hg compared with 17 mm Hg in the left eye, and the ocular pulse amplitude in the right eye is about 3 times that in the left eye. Cerebral angiography revealed a right-sided dural carotid-cavernous sinus fistula.

whom the risks are much greater because of excessive fragility of the extracranial and intracranial vessels. Indeed, Schievink et al. (1991) reported a morbidity rate of 36% and a mortality rate of 12% for diagnostic angiography in 17 patients with a dural carotid-cavernous sinus fistula in the setting of Ehlers-Danlos syndrome.

NATURAL HISTORY

The majority of patients with a dural carotid-cavernous sinus fistula have no difference in mortality from that of the normal population, since the lesion usually affects only the eyes. Spontaneous intracranial hemorrhage is exceptionally rare (Harding et al., 1984). Thus, when one considers the natural history of a dural carotid-cavernous sinus fistula, one is really considering the ocular morbidity.

Between 20 and 50% of dural carotid-cavernous sinus fistulas, regardless of whether they drain anteriorly or posteriorly, close spontaneously, after angiography, or after air flight travel (Bickerstaff, 1970; Newton and Hoyt, 1970; Taniguchi et al., 1971; Voigt et al., 1971; Bennett et al., 1973; Klepach et al., 1978; Palestine et al., 1981; Ishikawa et al., 1982; Merlis et al., 1982; Phelps et al., 1982; Grove, 1984; Nishijima et al., 1984; Nukui et al., 1984; Viñuela et al., 1984; Debrun et al., 1988; Kupersmith et al., 1988; Haugen et al., 1990; Miyachi et al., 1993; Shiga et al., 1994; Yamamoto et al., 1995) (Figs. 54.57 and 54.58). In some cases, the symptoms and signs begin to resolve within days to weeks after angiography. In others, they do not resolve until months to years after the fistula has become symptomatic.

We believe it is appropriate to follow clinically patients who have mild ocular manifestations to see if the fistula will close spontaneously. During the waiting period, we and others advise patients not to alter their lifestyle. Sacks and Gerson (1990) found that even vigorous exercise does not increase intraocular pressure in such patients and thus would appear to pose no risk to visual loss from glaucoma, even in patients with somewhat increased intraocular pressure. Patients being followed should be examined at regular intervals so that their visual function, intraocular pressure, and ophthalmoscopic appearance can be monitored.

Patients whose fistulas do not close spontaneously occasionally lose vision from central retinal vein occlusion (Hines and Guy, 1986; Pollock and Miller, 1986; Brunette and Boghen, 1987; Komiyama et al., 1990a; Kojima et al., 1991) (Fig. 54.51). Although such patients often have long-standing increased intraocular pressure, they rarely develop loss of either visual acuity or visual field from glaucomatous optic nerve damage. Persistent proptosis, chemosis, and redness of the eye may be associated with significant irritation and epiphora from exposure keratopathy. Limitation of eye movement from ocular motor nerve paresis, orbital congestion, or both may produce persistent, bothersome diplopia necessitating prism therapy or occlusion of one eye.

Patients with a dural carotid-cavernous sinus fistula may experience acute worsening of ocular manifestations. Although this clinical deterioration has been attributed to an increase in blood flow through the malformation, we and others have shown that in many cases, the deterioration actually results from spontaneous *thrombosis* of the superior ophthalmic vein (Sergott et al., 1987; Golnik and Miller, 1992). Within several weeks after this abrupt change, most patients begin to improve spontaneously, and most achieve complete resolution of symptoms and signs (Fig. 54.59). Systemic corticosteroids given when deterioration occurs may lessen the severity of symptoms and signs and perhaps reduce the length of time until recovery occurs.

Patients in whom a dural carotid-cavernous sinus fistula persists or in whom such a fistula is not recognized may experience major hemorrhagic and other complications when they undergo intraocular or orbital surgery performed for other reasons, such as cataract or strabismus. Nevertheless, Slochower and Dowhan (1991) reported the successful cataract extraction and insertion of an intraocular lens in a 76-year-old man with an ipsilateral low-flow dural fistula that was diagnosed by ultrasonography and CT scanning, but who never underwent diagnostic angiography. Unfortunately, the patient subsequently experienced a central retinal vein occlusion in that eye, followed by neovascular glaucoma. We believe that this patient would have been better served by diagnostic angiography and attempted closure of the fistula via a transvenous approach through the inferior petrosal sinus or superior ophthalmic vein.

TREATMENT

Although some investigators have advocated direct surgery (Wilson et al., 1976; Nishijima et al., 1984), conventional radiation therapy (Bitoh et al., 1982; Yasunaga et al., 1987; Yen et al., 1996), stereotactic radiosurgery (Kubota et al., 1993; Barcia-Salorio et al., 1994), or intermittent self-compression of the affected internal carotid artery (Higashida et al., 1986; Halbach et al., 1987; Kwan et al., 1989) for treatment of dural carotid-cavernous sinus fistula, we and others believe that endovascular embolization is the optimum treatment for those lesions producing progressive or unacceptable symptoms and signs including visual loss, diplopia, intolerable bruit, and severe proptosis (Ishimori et al., 1967; Tress et al., 1983; Viñuela et al., 1984; Barrow et al., 1985; Grossman et al., 1985; Hieshima et al., 1986b; Courtheoux et al., 1987; Debrun et al., 1988; Kupersmith et al., 1988; Debrun et al., 1989; Barnwell and O'Neill, 1994; Taki et al., 1994). A number of synthetic and natural materials have been used for embolization, including absorbable gelatin (Gelfoam), silastic, platinum coils, low-viscosity silicone rubber, autogenous clot, muscle or dura, tetradecyl sulfate (a sclerosing agent), polyvinyl alcohol particles (Ivalon), oxidized cellulose (Oxycel), and isobutyl-2-cyanoacrylate glue (Bucrylate). The most successful of these materials are polyvinyl alcohol particles, isobutyl-2 cyanoacrylate glue, and platinum flower coils or electrolytically detachable platinum coils (Viñuela et al., 1984; Barrow et al., 1985; Halbach et al., 1987; Debrun et al., 1988; Kupersmith et al., 1988; Guglielmi et al., 1992; Barnwell and O'Neill, 1994; Khayata et al., 1994; Kinugasa et al., 1994; Touho et al., 1995).

In patients with a fistula fed only by meningeal branches of the external carotid artery or by meningeal branches from

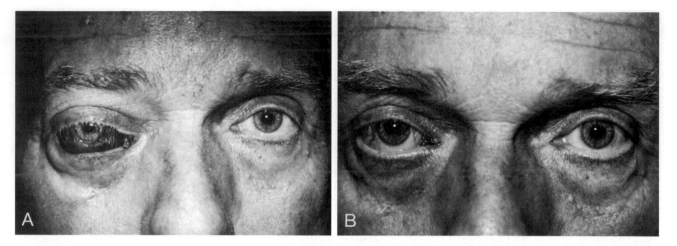

Figure 54.58. Spontaneous closure of a dural carotid-cavernous sinus fistula after cerebral angiography. The patient was a 59-year-old man who developed progressive redness and swelling of the right eye. *A,* The patient's right eye is swollen and red. There is significant conjunctival chemosis. Ocular pulse amplitudes were asymmetric, with the higher pulse on the right side. Cerebral angiography confirmed a right-sided dural carotid-cavernous sinus fistula fed by branches of the right internal and external carotid arteries. It was elected to follow the patient without intervention. Within 1 week after the angiogram, the patient began to experience reduction in swelling and redness of the right eye. *B,* 1 month after the angiogram, the patient has minimal swelling and redness of the right eye. Intraocular pressure and ocular pulse amplitudes are normal and symmetric.

of the significant risk of neurologic and visual sequelae (De-brun et al., 1981; Kupersmith et al., 1988).

Successful closure of dural carotid-cavernous sinus fistulas by standard particulate or glue embolization is possible in 70–95% of cases (Viñuela et al., 1984; Berenstein et al., 1986; Hieshima et al., 1986b; Kupersmith et al., 1988). When transvenous balloon or coil occlusion of the fistula is used, the rate of successful closure approaches 100% (Miller et al., 1995). The complication rates of both procedures are extremely low but include hemorrhage at the catheter site or in the orbit, local infection, sepsis, and both transient and permanent neurologic deficits, particularly ocular motor nerve pareses (Kupersmith et al., 1988). Complications are particularly common in patients with connective tissue disor-

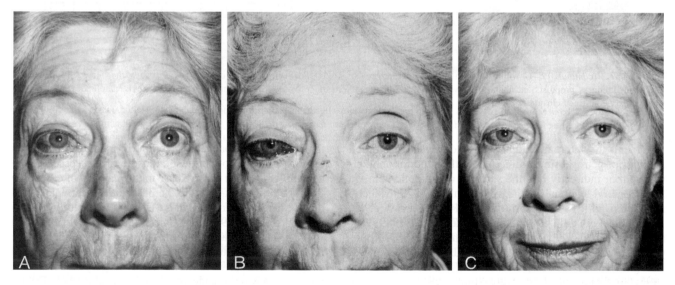

Figure 54.59. Worsening of ocular appearance in the setting of spontaneous closure of a dural carotid-cavernous sinus fistula. The patient was a 73-year-old woman who developed a red right eye. *A,* Appearance of the patient when she was first examined. Note mild redness of the right eye, associated with swelling of the right eyelid and mild proptosis. An evaluation revealed a right-sided dural carotid-cavernous sinus fistula fed by branches of the right internal and external carotid arteries. It was elected to follow the patient without intervention. Two months later, she experienced an abrupt increase in the swelling and redness of the right eye. *B,* Appearance of the right eye now shows increased redness, swelling, conjunctival chemosis, and proptosis. Color doppler imaging showed that the right superior ophthalmic vein was occluded, and a cerebral arteriogram confirmed that the fistula was in the process of spontaneously occluding. *C,* 1 month after the onset of worsening and 3 months after the onset of visual manifestations, the right eye shows only minimal redness and swelling. The patient had a normal appearance 3 months later.

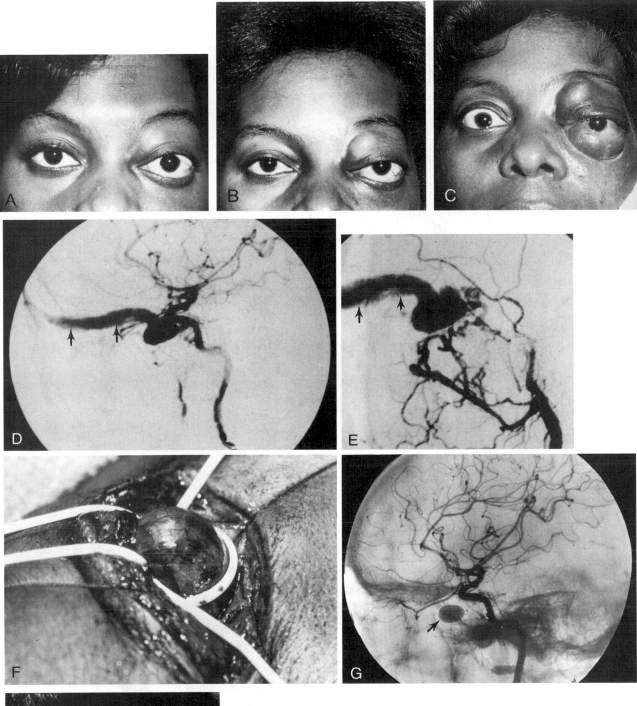

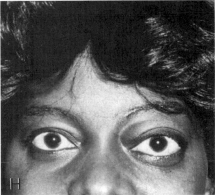

Figure 54.60. Occlusion of a dural carotid-cavernous sinus fistula using a detachable balloon introduced through the superior ophthalmic vein. The patient was a 35-year-old woman with a long-standing dural carotid-cavernous sinus fistula. *A–C,* Progressive left proptosis, chemosis, and eyelid distortion over a 5-year period. Note superior nasal bulge in the left upper eyelid caused by an enlarging superior ophthalmic vein. *D,* Selective left internal carotid angiogram, lateral view, shows contribution to the fistula by extradural branches of the left internal carotid artery. *E,* Selective left external carotid angiogram shows contribution to the fistula by extradural branches of the left external carotid artery. *F,* Appearance of the left superior ophthalmic vein at the time of treatment. Note marked enlargement with thickened wall. *G,* After placement of the balloon in the cavernous sinus (*arrow*), a selective internal carotid angiogram shows no evidence of the fistula. A selective left external angiogram gave similar results. *H,* Appearance of the patient 3 months after the procedure. Note marked reduction in proptosis, chemosis, and redness of the left eye.

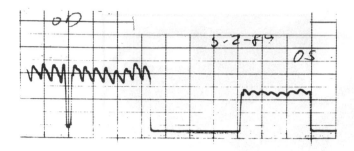

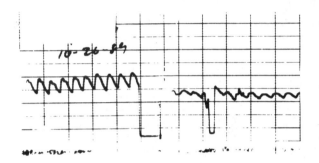

Figure 54.62. Ocular pulse amplitudes in a patient with a right-sided spontaneous dural carotid-cavernous sinus fistula that was fed by branches from both the right internal and external carotid arteries. The fistula initially was treated by particulate embolization of the right external carotid artery. *Top,* The preoperative intraocular pressure in the right eye is elevated to 25 mm Hg compared with a pressure of 17 mm Hg in the left eye, and the ocular pulse amplitude in the right eye is about 3–4 times that in the left eye. *Bottom,* Almost 6 months after embolization of the fistula, there is almost no change in the asymmetry of either the intraocular pressures or the ocular pulse amplitudes, indicating persistence of the fistula.

ocular pulse amplitude using a pneumotonometer or similar instrument before and after this type of treatment (Golnik and Miller, 1992). We are less concerned about incomplete closure or recurrence if we have closed the fistula using one or more detachable balloons or platinum coils. Nevertheless, if a preexisting pulse asymmetry remains after treatment, the fistula probably is still open (Fig. 54.62), and repeat embolization or transvenous balloon occlusion of the fistula may then be necessary. Even if the ocular pulse pressures are normal, we also perform postoperative angiography to make certain that the fistula is not still open and draining posteriorly.

As with direct carotid-cavernous sinus fistulas, symptoms and signs usually begin to improve within hours to days after successful, permanent closure of a dural carotid-cavernous sinus fistula (Palestine et al., 1981; Kupersmith et al., 1988). Any preexisting bruit immediately disappears, and intraocular pressure immediately returns to normal. Proptosis, conjunctival chemosis, redness of the eye, and ophthalmoparesis (whether caused by orbital congestion or ocular motor nerve paresis) usually resolve completely within weeks to months (Fig. 54.63), and most patients have a normal or near-normal

external appearance within 6 months. Choroidal and retinal pathology also resolve over the same period of time. As is the case with patients who have direct carotid-cavernous sinus fistulas, patients with visual loss caused by choroidal effusion or detachment usually experience substantial if not complete recovery of visual function, whereas patients with visual loss caused by retinal dysfunction (e.g., central retinal vein occlusion, retinal detachment) usually have persistently poor visual function (Kupersmith et al., 1996).

Not all patients with dural carotid-cavernous sinus fistulas experience immediate improvement in their signs and symptoms, particularly when techniques other than endovascular closure of the fistula are used to treat the fistula. For instance, stereotactic radiosurgery was advocated as a treatment for low-flow dural fistulas by Barcia-Salorio et al. (1994). These investigators treated 22 patients with such fistulas with radiosurgery between 1977 and 1992. During a follow-up period that ranged from 15 months to 14 years (mean: 49.76 months), 20 of the 22 fistulas (91%) closed in a mean period of 7.5 months (range: 2–20 months). There were no recurrences and no complications. Kubota et al. (1993), however, described a 38-year-old man who developed severe proptosis, conjunctival chemosis, loss of vision, and secondary glaucoma **after** treatment of a dural fistula with stereotactic radiosurgery. The intraocular pressure became normal within 1 week, and the other manifestations resolved after 6 weeks. It is likely that in this case the radiosurgery caused thrombosis of the ipsilateral superior ophthalmic vein, resulting in worsening of orbital congestion of the type normally seen in patients in whom the fistula undergoes spontaneous closure (Sergott et al., 1987; Golnik and Miller, 1992).

Patients who undergo successful balloon or coil embolization of a dural carotid-cavernous sinus fistula may experience both transient and permanent complications. The most common transient complications are ocular motor nerve pareses and facial or orbital pain. Taniguchi et al. (1994) reported the occurrence of an ophthalmic artery occlusion that occurred 1 day after embolization of a dural carotid-cavernous sinus fistula via the ipsilateral middle meningeal artery using polyvinyl alcohol particles. It was postulated by the authors that emboli reached the ophthalmic artery via the lacrimal artery, which generally anastomoses between and middle meningeal artery and the ophthalmic artery or via the fistula itself.

Occasionally, treatment of a dural carotid-cavernous sinus fistula will produce a dural fistula in another location. Nakagawa et al. (1992) reported the case of a 43-year-old woman who developed signs of orbital congestion associated with a left abducens palsy and was found to have a left-sided dural carotid-cavernous sinus fistula fed mainly by the meningeal branches of both internal maxillary arteries, the left ascending pharyngeal artery, and the meningohypophyseal and inferolateral trunks of both internal carotid arteries. The patient underwent transarterial embolization of the left sided feeding arteries using gelfoam introduced via the internal maxillary artery. Transvenous embolization of the left cavernous sinus was then performed using spring coils introduced through the left superior ophthalmic vein. The patient's ocular signs improved slightly but then recurred, and repeat angiography

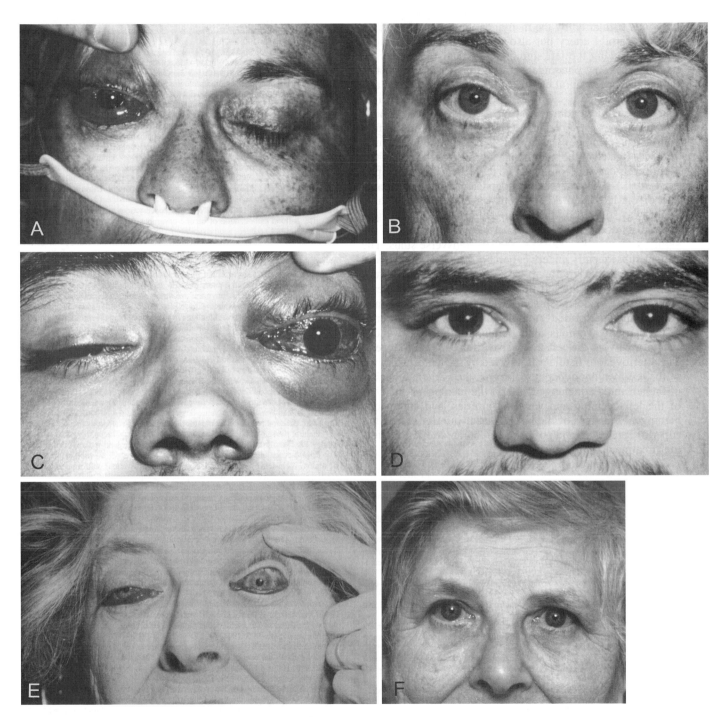

Figure 54.63. Improvement in ocular signs and symptoms after transvenous occlusion of a dural carotid-cavernous sinus fistula using a detachable balloon technique. *A,* Preoperative appearance of a 65-year-old woman with a right-sided, spontaneous, dural carotid-cavernous sinus fistula. Note marked eyelid swelling, proptosis, redness, and conjunctival chemosis. *B,* 2 months after transvenous occlusion of the fistula through the inferior petrosal sinus, the right eye is normal except for about 2 mm of proptosis and slight dilation of conjunctival veins. *C,* Preoperative appearance of a 34-year-old man with a left-sided dural carotid-cavernous fistula. Note marked left-sided eyelid swelling and erythema, proptosis, conjunctival chemosis, and dilation of conjunctival vessels. The left eye had markedly limited movement. *D,* 3 months after balloon occlusion through the left superior ophthalmic vein, the patient has a normal appearance. Eye movements also were normal. *E,* Bilateral proptosis, ptosis, redness, and chemosis of the conjunctiva in a patient with bilateral dural carotid-cavernous sinus fistulas. Both eyes were almost entirely immobile. *F,* 3 months after transvenous balloon occlusion of the fistulas, the patient has a normal appearance.

Takahashi A, Yoshimoto T, Kawakami K, et al. Transvenous copper wire insertion for dural arteriovenous malformations of cavernous sinus. J Neurosurg 70:751–754, 1989.

Takahashi M, Nakano Y. Magnification angiography of dural carotid-cavernous fistulae, with emphasis on clinical and angiographic evolution. Neuro-radiology 19:249–256, 1980.

Takahashi M, Killeffer F, Wilson G. Iatrogenic carotid cavernous fistula: Case report. J Neurosurg 30:498–500, 1969.

Taki W, Nakahara I, Nishi Sh, et al. Pathogenetic and therapeutic considerations of carotid-cavernous sinus fistulas. Acta Neurochir 127:6–14, 1994.

Taniguchi I, Kazuo K, Miyazaki D, et al. Ophthalmic artery occlusion after neuroradiological embolization to treat spontaneous carotid-cavernous sinus fistula. Folia Ophthalmol Jpn 45:668–671, 1994.

Taniguchi RM, Goree JA, Odom GL. Spontaneous carotid-cavernous shunts presenting diagnostic problems. J Neurosurg 35:384–391, 1971.

Tech KE, Becker CJ, Lazo A, et al. Anomalous intracranial venous drainage mimicking orbital or cavernous arteriovenous fistula. AJNR 16:171–174, 1995.

Teng MMH, Lirng J-F, Chang T, et al. Embolization of carotid cavernous fistula by means of direct puncture through the superior orbital fissure. Radiology 194:705–711, 1995.

Terry TL, Mysel P. Pulsating exophthalmos due to internal jugular aneurysm: Use of thorium dioxide solution in localization. JAMA 103:1036–1041, 1934.

Teufel J. Einbau der Arteria carotis interna in den Canalis caroticus unter Berücksichtigung des transbasalen Venenabflusses. Morph Jb 106:188–274, 1964.

Touho H, Furuoka N, Ohnishi H, et al. Traumatic arteriovenous fistula treated by superselective embolisation with microcoils: Case report. Neuroradiology 37:65–67, 1995.

Toya S, Shiobara R, Izumi J, et al. Spontaneous carotid-cavernous fistula during pregnancy or in the postpartum stage: Report of two cases. J Neurosurg 54:252–256, 1981.

Tress BM, Thomson KR, Klug GL, et al. Management of carotid-cavernous fistulas by surgery combined with interventional radiology. J Neurosurg 59:1076–1081, 1983.

Turner DM, Vangilder JC, Mojtahedi S, et al. Spontaneous intracerebral hematoma in carotid-cavernous fistula: Report of three cases. J Neurosurg 59:680–686, 1983.

Tytle TL, Loeffler CL, Steinberg TA. Fistula between a posterior communicating artery aneurysm and the cavernous sinus. AJNR 16:1808–1810, 1995.

Uflacker R, Lima S, Ribas G, et al. Carotid-cavernous fistulas: Embolization through the superior ophthalmic vein approach. Radiology 159:175–179, 1986.

Verbiest H. Post-traumatic pulsating exophthalmos caused by perforation of an eroded orbital roof by a hydrocephalic brain. J Neurosurg 10:264–271, 1953.

Viñuela F, Debrun GM, Fox AJ, et al. Detachable calibrated-leak balloon for superse-

lective angiography and embolization of dural arteriovenous malformations. J Neurosurg 58:817–823, 1983.

Viñuela F, Fox A, Debrun G, et al. Spontaneous carotid-cavernous fistulas: Clinical, radiological, and therapeutic consideration. J Neurosurg 60:976–984, 1984.

Voigt K, Sauer M, Dichgans J. Spontaneous occlusion of a bilateral caroticocavernous fistula studied by serial angiography. Neuroradiology 2:207–211, 1971.

Walker AE, Allegré GE. Carotid-cavernous fistulas. Surgery 39:411–422, 1956.

Wallace S, Goldberg HI, Leeds NE, et al. Cavernous branches of the internal carotid artery. AJR 101:34–46, 1967.

Walsh FB, Hoyt WF. Clinical Neuro-Ophthalmology. 3rd ed, p 1719. Baltimore, Williams & Wilkins, 1969.

Weekers R, Delmarcelle Y. Pathogenesis of intraocular hypertension in cases of arteriovenous aneurysm. Arch Ophthalmol 48:338–343, 1952.

Weiss DI, Shaffer RN, Nehrenberg TR. Neovascular glaucoma complicating carotid-cavernous fistula. Arch Ophthalmol 69:304–307, 1963.

Wepsic JG, Pruett RC, Tarlov E. Carotid-cavernous fistula due to extradural subtemporal retrogasserian rhizotomy. J Neurosurg 37:498–500, 1972.

West CGH. Bilateral carotid-cavernous fistulae: A review. Surg Neurol 13:85–90, 1980.

White JC, Love JG, Goldstein NP. Carotid-cavernous fistula on the left side with ocular symptoms on right side: Report of case. Mayo Clin Proc 33:441–445, 1958.

Wilms G, Peene P, Nowe G, et al. Angiographic diagnosis and treatment of posttraumatic carotid-cavernous sinus fistulas. Bull Soc Belge Ophtalmol 231:83–89, 1989.

Wilson CB, Markesbery W. Traumatic carotid-cavernous fistula with fatal epistaxis: Report of a case. J Neurosurg 24:111–113, 1966.

Wilson WB, Bringewald PR, Hosobuchi Y, et al. Transient third nerve palsy after electrometallic thrombosis of carotid cavernous fistulae. J Neurol Neurosurg Psychiatry 39:854–860, 1976.

Woillez M, Blervacque A, Dufour D. Décollement annulaire antérieur de la choriorétine après fistule carotido-caverneuse. Bull Soc Ophtalmol Fr 67:819–822, 1967.

Yamada M, Ikeda N, Mimura O, et al. Choroidal detachment associated with spontaneous carotid cavernous fistula. Acta Soc Ophthalmol Jpn 95:704–709, 1991.

Yamamoto T, Asai K, Lin YW, et al. Spontaneous resolution of symptoms in an infant with a congenital dural caroticocavernous fistula. Neuroradiology 37:247–249, 1995.

Yasunaga T, Takada C, Uozumi H, et al. Radiotherapy of spontaneous carotid-cavernous sinus fistulas. Int J Radiat Onc Biol Phys 13:1909–1913, 1987.

Yen M-Y, Yen S-H, Teng MM-H, et al. Radiotherapy of dural carotid-cavernous sinus fistulas. Neuro-ophthalmology 16:133–142, 1996.

Zhao Y, Duan Y, Cao T. Application of transcranial color doppler flow imaging in the carotid cavernous sinus fistulae. Chung Hua I Hsueh Tsa Chih 75:141–143, 1995.

Zilkha A, Daiz AS. Computed tomography in carotid cavernous fistula. Surg Neurol 14:325–329, 1980.

CHAPTER 55

Cerebrovascular Disease

Nancy J. Newman

ISCHEMIC CEREBROVASCULAR DISEASE	HEMORRHAGIC CEREBROVASCULAR DISEASE
Definitions	Pathophysiology
Pathology	General Symptoms and Signs
Pathophysiology	Causes
Collateral Circulation to the Brain and Orbit	Signs and Symptoms by Location
Symptoms and Signs	Diagnosis
Diagnosis	Treatment
Prognosis	Prognosis
Management	

Cerebrovascular disease is the most common devastating condition that affects the central nervous system (CNS). The mortality from cerebrovascular disease in the United States and most developed countries is exceeded only by the direct effects of heart disease and cancer (Gorelick, 1995; American Heart Association, 1996). The short- and long-term disability suffered by the approximately 3 million stroke survivors in the United States and the economic costs to society are staggering. Patients with strokes may have not only significant neurologic deficits but also substantial visual difficulties (Lansche, 1968; Isaeff et al., 1974).

Cerebrovascular disease results from two major causes: (*a*) ischemia and (*b*) hemorrhage. Ischemic disease is a far more common cause of stroke than is hemorrhage, accounting for about 80% of strokes compared with 20% from hemorrhage (Bogousslavsky et al., 1988a; see Table 3.1 in Caplan, 1993). In this chapter, we discuss the mechanisms for both ischemic and hemorrhagic cerebrovascular disease, the syndromes of neuro-ophthalmologic importance that they produce, and the prevention and treatment of stroke. The reader interested in pursuing these subjects in more detail should read the World Health Organization's special report: "Stroke—1989: Recommendations on stroke prevention, diagnosis, and therapy" (WHO/MNH Task Force on Stroke and Other Cerebrovascular Disorders, 1989) and the special report from the National Institute of Neurological Disorders and Stroke entitled "Classification of Cerebrovascular Diseases III" (Whisnant et al., 1990a). Comprehensive textbooks on cerebrovascular disease are also available, including those by Barnett et al. (1986, 1992), Caplan and Stein (1986), Millikan et al. (1987), Warlow et al. (1987), and Caplan (1993).

ISCHEMIC CEREBROVASCULAR DISEASE

Ischemic cerebrovascular disease is a major cause of morbidity and mortality both in older patients (Kurtzke, 1969; Kuller et al., 1970) and in young adults (Humphrey and Newton, 1960; Louis and McDowell, 1967; Fogelholm and Aho, 1973; Hindfelt and Nilsson, 1977; Grindal et al., 1978; Chopra and Prabhakar, 1979; Dalal, 1979; Marshall, 1982; Hart and Miller, 1983; Klein and Seland, 1984; Bogousslavsky et al., 1988a; Chancellor et al., 1989; Stern et al., 1991a, 1991b; Adams et al., 1995; Barinagarrementeria et al., 1996; Rohr et al., 1996). Even children may have an ischemic stroke (Awerbuch et al., 1989; Higgins et al., 1989; Biller, 1994).

The causes of ischemic stroke are numerous, and the treatment for many of these conditions is controversial. This overview of ischemic cerebrovascular disease includes definitions and discussions of pathology, pathophysiology, aspects of collateral circulation that relate to cerebrovascular ischemia, clinical features, diagnosis, and treatment.

DEFINITIONS

Hypoxia is a reduction in the normal concentration of tissue oxygen. In **anoxia,** which rarely occurs, no oxygen is present in the tissue.

Traditionally, hypoxia is divided into four types:

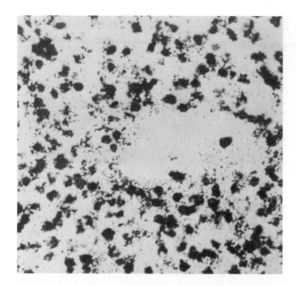

Figure 55.10. Perivascular accumulation of phagocytes in the white matter of a 42-year-old man who died from the effects of severe hypotension. (From Brierley JB, Graham DI. Hypoxia and vascular disorders of the central nervous system. In Greenfield's Neuropathology. Editors, Adams JH, Corsellis JAN, Duchen LW, 4th ed, pp 125–207. New York, John Wiley & Sons, 1984.)

Within 4–5 days after infarction, **phagocytic** activity is seen in the affected region (Brierley and Brown, 1982) (Fig. 55.10). The phagocytes are derived from circulating monocytes and adventitial fibroblasts in the walls of intact blood vessels. The activity of phagocytic, adventitial fibroblasts causes thickening of the walls of remaining blood vessels and the laying down of reticulin and collagen (Brierley and Brown, 1982). At the same time, there is both hypertrophy and proliferation of fiber-forming and gemistocytic astrocytes, some of which are binucleated, at the periphery of the infarct. The result is gliomesodermal cyst formation with increasing thickening of cyst walls.

After several months, large and small cysts appear that are either empty or contain varying numbers of lipid-filled phagocytes. The outer wall of a cyst or slit in the cerebral cortex may consist of the pia and the heavily gliotic first layer of the cortex, or it may be formed entirely from thickened pia mater from which a small number of delicate collagen fibrils pass toward surviving blood vessels adjacent to the cyst.

PATHOPHYSIOLOGY

Ischemic cerebrovascular disease can be produced by three different mechanisms: (*a*) thrombosis, (*b*) embolism, and (*c*) decreased systemic perfusion (Pessin et al., 1979; Kistler et al., 1984a; Caplan and Stein, 1986; Bogousslavsky et al., 1988a; Caplan, 1993; Mohr et al., 1997). In some patients, the particular mechanism responsible is obvious, whereas in others, more than one mechanism may be responsible, and, in still others, the cause of cerebral ischemia is unclear (Sacco et al., 1989a).

The factors that contribute to an ischemic stroke are both environmental and genetic (WHO/MNH Task Force on Stroke and Other Cerebrovascular Disorders, 1989; Bronner et al., 1995; Gorelick, 1995; Sacco, 1995). Recognition of specific environmental factors that predispose to stroke in a particular patient may significantly affect that patient's prognosis both before and after a stroke has occurred. Such factors include diet, cigarette use, alcohol consumption, weight, and physical fitness.

Many genetic disorders also are associated with an increased risk of stroke (Natowicz and Kelley, 1987; Berciano, 1988; WHO/MNH Task Force on Stroke and Other Cerebrovascular Disorders, 1989; Stern et al., 1991a, 1991b). Some are transmitted as simple mendelian disorders (i.e., single gene defects); whereas others are caused by chromosomal disorders, have a multifactorial genetic basis, or probably are inherited in some fashion as yet undiscovered. The recognition of a genetic disorder as the cause of a stroke has important implications:

1. Specific remedies or palliative measures may be instituted in some patients;
2. Problems in other organ systems may be anticipated;
3. The natural history and prognosis for the disorder can be specified; and
4. Appropriate diagnosis and counseling of the proband's parents, siblings, or children can be offered, often leading to prevention of disease in other family members.

In the discussion that follows, we emphasize both the environmental and the genetic factors that influence the risk of stroke.

Thrombosis

General Considerations

Thrombosis (from the Greek word meaning curdling) is an obstruction to blood flow caused by a localized process within one or more blood vessels. It results from narrowing or occlusion of the lumen of an affected vessel by an alteration of the vessel wall, clot formation, or both.

The frequency with which in-situ thrombosis causes ischemic cerebrovascular disease is unclear, partly because of biases within studies designed to study this subject and partly because more than one mechanism may be responsible (i.e., embolism from a thrombosed artery). Nevertheless, about 60–70% of all ischemic cerebrovascular disease is caused by thrombosis (Barnett et al., 1992; Caplan, 1993).

Thrombosis may affect large extracranial arteries, large intracranial arteries, or small intracranial arteries. In some patients, both large extracranial and small intracranial arteries are affected.

Causes

The most common cause of thrombosis is damage to the arterial wall through atherosclerosis, which chiefly affects the larger extracranial and intracranial vessels (Mohr and Pessin, 1986). Torvik et al. (1989) studied the histologic appearance of specimens from 11 patients with thrombi at the bifurcation of the common carotid artery to determine local factors in the vessel wall that precipitated the thrombi. Severe atherosclerotic stenosis was frequent, but it was not a prerequisite for thrombus formation. Other factors thought to be important for thrombogenesis in these specimens included ulcerations in the wall, intraplaque hemorrhage, and massive plaque rupture. Ulceration in plaques may allow the luminal contents to be in contact with the inside of the plaque which, in turn, triggers the release of various tissue factors and promotes clot formation. Patients who appear to be at higher risk for thrombogenesis and subsequent stroke are those who have heterogeneous plaques or plaques with hemorrhage within them, especially if the plaque narrows the lumen of the affected vessel by more than 70–75% (Bornstein et al., 1990; Dempsey et al., 1990; Gomez, 1990). However, plaque ulceration by itself may not be a reliable predictor of stroke risk. In addition, smaller intracranial vessel walls more often are damaged from the effects of systemic hypertension than from plaques (Chester et al., 1978).

Other diseases that affect arterial walls and are capable of producing thrombosis-induced neurologic symptoms and signs include migraine, infectious and noninfectious arteritis, spontaneous and traumatic dissection, fibromuscular dysplasia, sickle cell disease, radiation angiopathy, amyloid angiopathy, and neoplastic angiopathy. Arterial walls may be mechanically constricted or compressed against external structures, such as bony prominences or dural folds in patients with cervical spondylosis, increased intracranial pressure (ICP), and extrinsic head and neck masses (e.g., hematoma or tumor). Compression of arterial walls against external structures sufficient to cause thrombosis and neurologic deficit may also result from chiropractic manipulation and other forms of blunt and penetrating trauma (Frisoni and Anzola, 1990; Donzis and Factor, 1997). Occasionally, a clot forms within the lumen of a normal artery because of a primary hematologic problem, such as erythrocytosis, thrombocytosis, leukemia, and hemoglobinopathy, or because of a hypercoagulability state that reflects an inherited clotting abnormality or that has developed in association with some other disorder, such as systemic vasculitis, inflammatory bowel disease, or cancer, or in association with oral contraceptive use. Finally, drug abuse is an important cause of ischemic and hemorrhagic stroke in adolescents and young adults. Heroin, amphetamines, cocaine, and intravenously injected drugs synthesized for oral use are most often responsible.

It should be emphasized that multiple factors often combine to increase the risk of stroke (Bronner et al., 1995; Gorelick, 1995; Sacco, 1995). Especially in the young patient, no overt cause for stroke may be found, or many possible causes may be elucidated (Stern et al., 1991a, 1991b; Adams et al., 1995). Even in the young patient, atherosclerosis is one of the leading contributors to ischemic stroke.

ATHEROSCLEROSIS

Atherosclerosis (from the Greek words *athērē,* gruel, and *sklērōsis,* hardness) is a descriptive term for thickened, hardened, lipid-rich lesions of medium and large muscular and elastic arteries. It is the most common form of **arteriosclero-**sis, the generic term used to described thickened arteries of all sizes.

Factors Predisposing to Atherosclerosis. A number of factors are associated with an increased prevalence of atherosclerosis and thus heart disease and stroke (Kannel et al., 1971; Wolf et al., 1977a, 1977b; Whisnant et al., 1978; Wolf et al., 1983a; Kistler et al., 1984a; Dyken et al., 1984; Davis et al., 1986, 1987; Medical Research Council Working Party, 1988; WHO/MNH Task Force on Stroke and Other Cerebrovascular Disorders, 1989; Yatsu and Fisher, 1989; Folsom et al., 1990; Shaper et al., 1991; Lai et al., 1994; Bronner et al., 1995; Gorelick, 1995; Sacco, 1995; Whisnant et al., 1996; Sacco et al., 1997). These include hyperlipidemia, cigarette smoking, hypertension, diabetes mellitus, and obesity. These factors are particularly prevalent in younger patients with atherosclerosis (Klein and Seland, 1984), although they are important in patients of all ages.

There is a definite association between chronic **hyperlipidemia**—primarily the elevation of plasma cholesterol concentration, triglyceride concentration, or both—and an increased incidence of atherosclerotic disease (Duncan et al., 1977; Takeya et al., 1984; Tell et al., 1988; Iso et al., 1989). Patients with homozygous familial hypercholesterolemia, for example, may have plasma cholesterol concentrations of 500–1000 mg/dL or higher (normal is about 220 mg/dL). Such patients often develop advanced atherosclerosis, usually at a very young age. The precise role of lipids and lipoproteins in the etiology of atherosclerosis is not completely clear, but lipoproteins are thought to enter arterial walls through intact or damaged vascular endothelium and cause or complicate atherosclerotic plaques (St. Clair et al., 1986). Serum lipids or specific lipid subfractions may act differently on intracranial and extracranial arteries and on small and large intracranial vessels. Interestingly, a meta-analysis of randomized, controlled trials of cholesterol reduction and the risk of stroke in middle-aged men did not show a clear reduction in stroke mortality or morbidity (Atkins et al., 1993). However, hypercholesterolemia and other elevations of serum lipids are clearly associated with carotid atherosclerosis which, in turn, is associated with an increased risk of stroke. Furthermore, in a case-control study, Hachinski et al. (1996) demonstrated that elevated low-density lipoprotein cholesterol and triglyceride levels were significant independent risk factors in patients with stroke or transient ischemic attack. Indeed, the newest class of cholesterol-lowering agents (statin drugs) provide large reductions in cholesterol, reduce the risk of stroke, and lower overall stroke mortality (Herbert et al., 1997).

Cigarette smoking is one of the most important risk factors associated with an increased incidence of atherosclerosis. Stroke, myocardial infarction, and intermittent claudication are all more prevalent in smokers than in nonsmokers (Abbott et al., 1986; Wolf, 1986; Colditz et al., 1988; Donnan et al., 1989; Gill et al., 1989; Gorelick et al., 1989; Love et al., 1990; Ingall et al., 1991; Robbins et al., 1994; Calori et al., 1996). Indeed, the duration of smoking is thought to be the strongest predictor of severe atherosclerosis affecting the extracranial portion of the carotid artery (Whisnant et al., 1990b). The mechanism by which cigarette smoking affects atherosclerosis is unclear, but 1 year from the cessation of

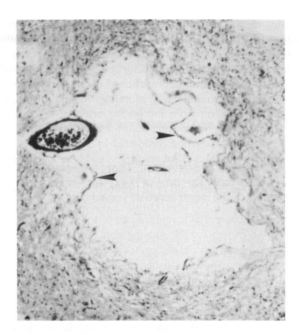

Figure 55.15. Histopathologic appearance of a lacune. Note that the lesion is a tiny cavity that contains very few cells and is lined by a narrow border of fibrillary gliosis (*arrowheads*). (From Brierley JB, Graham DI. Hypoxia and vascular disorders of the central nervous system. In Greenfield's Neuropathology. Editors, Adams JH, Corsellis JAN, Duchen LW, 4th ed, pp 125–207. New York, John Wiley & Sons, 1984.)

rand, 1902; Fisher, 1965a, 1969; Bamford and Warlow, 1988; Weisberg, 1988; see, however, Landau, 1989).

Lacunes are small, discrete, often irregular lesions that range in size from 1 to 20 mm (Fig. 55.15), although only 17% of lacunes are larger than 10 mm (Fisher, 1965a). Histologically, they are tiny cavities within which are fine strands of connective tissue resembling cobwebs. They contain very few cells and are limited by a narrow border of fibrillary gliosis.

The most common locations of lacunar infarcts are the putamen and globus pallidum, followed by the pons, thalamus, caudate nucleus, internal capsule, and corona radiata (Caplan, 1993). Lacunes are rare in the cerebral peduncles, pyramids, and cerebral white matter, and they do not occur in the cerebral or cerebellar cortex.

Patients with systemic hypertension may develop a severe **encephalopathy** rather than focal ischemic infarction (Oppenheimer and Fishberg, 1928; Pickering, 1948). Hypertensive encephalopathy is characterized by an altered state of consciousness and severe headache. Nausea, vomiting, and visual disturbances may develop, but seizures and focal signs are rare (Chester et al., 1978). The neuropathologic changes observed in patients with hypertensive encephalopathy are similar to those that occur in patients with focal ischemic damage. Vascular alterations include fibrinoid necrosis of arterioles and thrombosis of arterioles and capillaries (Fig. 55.16). These changes produce parenchymal lesions consisting of microinfarcts and petechial hemorrhages (Chester et al., 1978). These lesions may occur in any part of the CNS, but they are most common in the brainstem. Similar lesions

also affect the eyes, kidneys, and other organs (Figs. 55.17–55.19).

MIGRAINE AND VASOSPASM

Well-documented examples of ischemic stroke in patients with classic or common migraine are infrequent compared with the frequency of migraine in the general population (Guest and Woolf, 1964; Fisher, 1971a; Dorfman et al., 1979; Kupersmith et al., 1979; Featherstone, 1986; Broderick and Swanson, 1987; Bogousslavsky et al., 1988b; Moen et al., 1988; Mohr, 1988; Rothrock et al., 1988a; Chancellor et al., 1989; Caplan, 1991c; Buring et al., 1995; Tzourio et al., 1995). In young and otherwise healthy adults, however, migraine is a relatively common cause of stroke (Fig. 55.20). Bogousslavsky and Regli (1987) evaluated 41 patients under 30 years of age who suffered ischemic stroke and concluded that migraine was the cause of the stroke in six of the patients (15%). Broderick and Swanson (1987) concluded that migraine was the cause of stroke in 25% of patients 50 years of age or younger in Rochester, Minnesota, evaluated from 1976 to 1979. In a review of 72 women younger than 45 years of age with ischemic stroke, Tzourio et al. (1995) found a strong association with migraine, especially if the women were contraceptive users or smokers. A similar association was noted in a larger epidemiologic study performed by Merikangas et al. (1997). Migrainous stroke is more common in migraineurs with aura than in migraineurs without aura, but this association is of little value in distinguishing patients with migraine destined for stroke from the general migraine population (Rothrock et al., 1993; Carolei et al., 1996).

The mechanism for stroke is uncertain, but it is possible that prolonged vasoconstriction causes prolonged distal ischemia and even clot formation within the constricted vessel.

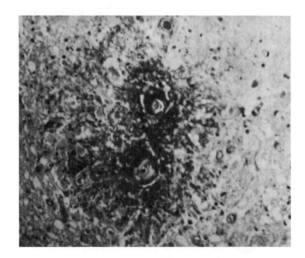

Figure 55.16. Histopathologic appearance of intracranial vessels in a patient with hypertensive encephalopathy. Two branches of a small intracerebral artery show necrosis of their walls and fibrinous exudate. The surrounding brain shows early rarefaction and dissolution. (From Brierley JB, Graham DI. Hypoxia and vascular disorders of the central nervous system. In Greenfield's Neuropathology. Editors, Adams JH, Corsellis JAN, Duchen LW, 4th ed, pp 125–207. New York, John Wiley & Sons, 1984.)

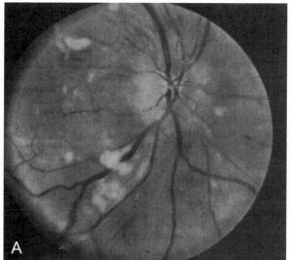

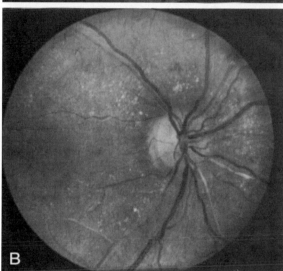

Figure 55.17. Ophthalmoscopic appearance of changes in the ocular fundus in patients with acute and chronic hypertension. *A*, Acute hypertensive retinopathy. Note swelling of optic disc, narrowing of retinal arteries, and numerous cotton wool patches (soft exudates). *B*, Chronic hypertensive retinopathy. Note severe narrowing and occlusion of retinal arteries and arterioles and hard exudates. (From Hoyt WF, Beeston D. The Ocular Fundus in Neurologic Disease. St Louis, CV Mosby, 1966.)

Platelets are activated during migraine, and the endothelium of the vessel wall may release factors that promote local thrombosis in the constricted segment (Caplan, 1993). Local atherosclerosis may also promote the vasoconstrictive effect (Hayreh et al., 1997). In addition, some young patients with apparent migraine-related stroke also have mitral valve prolapse (MVP) (Procacci et al., 1975, 1976; Herman, 1987, 1989), and others have circulating polyclonal immunoglobulins that bind negatively charged or neutral phospholipids—antiphospholipid antibodies—in their serum, which also may predispose to infarction (Frohman et al., 1989; Briley et al., 1989; Digre et al., 1989; Levine and Welch, 1989a; Shuaib and Barcley, 1989; Brey et al., 1990; Kushner,

1990; Levine et al., 1990a; Valesini et al., 1990). Migraine is discussed further in Chapter 56 of this text.

Migrainous accompaniments occur in older patients with or without associated headache (Fisher, 1968b; Fisher, 1980) and may represent temporary local vasoconstriction. Women are affected more frequently than men (Caplan, 1993). Sensory modalities are preferentially involved. The first symptoms tend to be "positive" (i.e., shimmering of vision). There is a build-up of symptoms over several minutes, with attacks usually lasting 15–30 minutes. Different attacks may involve different vascular territories and may alternate sides; headache, if present, usually follows the neurologic symptoms. Spells may occur over years. Transient global amnesia may represent a migraine accompaniment (Caplan et al., 1981). However, local atherosclerosis may also predispose vessels to superimposed vasoconstriction (Hayreh et al., 1997).

Vasospasm can cause transient monocular or binocular visual loss (Harbison et al., 1988; Burger et al., 1991; Winterkorn and Teman, 1991; Winterkorn et al., 1993). For ex-

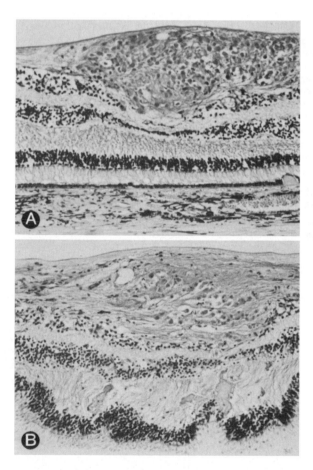

Figure 55.18. Histopathologic appearance of hypertensive retinopathy. *A*, Typical cytoid body located in the nerve fiber layer of the retina. Note numerous dilated axons. *B*, Edema surrounds the cytoid bodies and extends into the outer plexiform layer. This edema is responsible for the fluffy white appearance like that of a cotton-wool spot. These lesions result from focal ischemia and infarction of the nerve fiber layer. (Courtesy of Dr. William Spencer.)

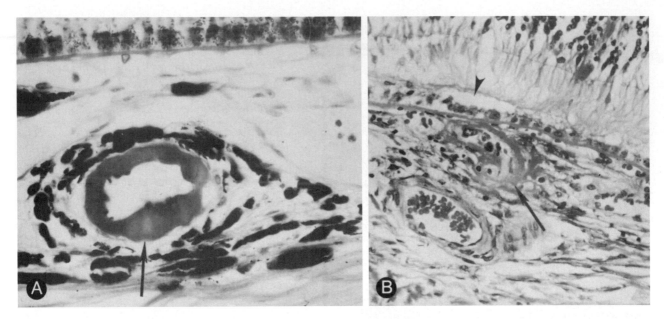

Figure 55.19. Histopathologic changes in the walls of choroidal arteries in a patient with hypertensive encephalopathy. *A,* Wall of artery is thickened by a homogeneous material (*arrow*). The endothelium of the vessel is intact. *B,* Thrombosed choroidal artery with fibrinoid necrosis (*arrow*). Adjacent retinal pigment epithelium is disrupted (*arrowhead*). (From Green WR. Retina. In Ophthalmic Pathology. An Atlas and Textbook. Editor, Spencer WH, 3rd ed, Vol 2, pp 589–1292. Philadelphia, WB Saunders, 1985.)

ample, Winterkorn et al. (1993) described nine patients with frequent attacks of presumed vasospastic amaurosis fugax, several of whom had evidence of systemic coagulopathies or vasculitides. All patients experienced dramatic cessation of the visual episodes after treatment with calcium-channel blocking drugs, especially nifedipine, although one must be cautious in assuming an underlying pathophysiology of vasospasm on the basis of a positive drug effect (Fig. 55.21).

Disorders other than migraine that are associated with vasospasm are rare. Call et al. (1988b) described a syndrome

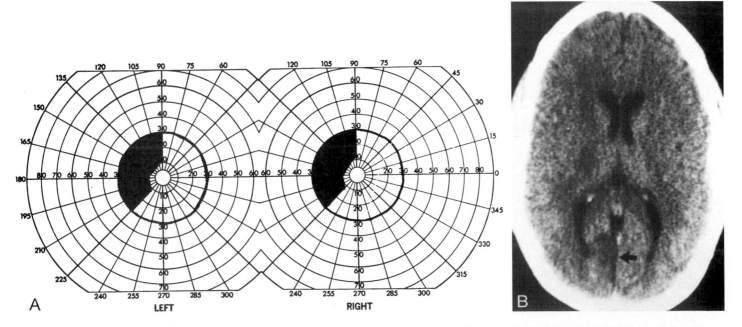

Figure 55.20. Occipital lobe infarct caused by migraine. *A,* The patient has a left homonymous hemianopic scotoma that is exquisitely congruous. *B,* CT scan shows a right occipital lobe infarction (*arrow*). (From Kupersmith MJ, Warren FA, Hass WK. The non-benign aspects of migraine. Neuro-ophthalmology *7:*1–10, 1987.)

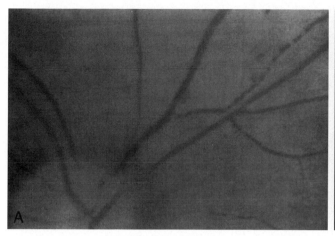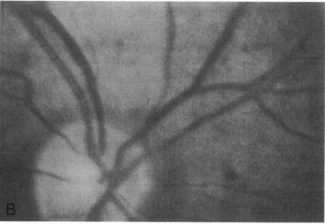

Figure 55.21. Presumed vasospasm causing transient monocular visual loss in a 62-year-old man with up to seven episodes per week lasting 5 to 120 minutes. *A*, Retinal view during an attack of visual loss showing disc pallor, constriction of retinal arterioles, and rouleaux formation in venules, indicating sluggish blood flow. *B*, Retinal view of same eye after 18 months of treatment with a calcium-channel blocker, showing perfusion of arterioles and veins with normal blood flow. (From Winterkorn MS, Kupersmith MJ, Wirtschafter JD, et al. Brief report: Treatment of vasospastic amaurosis fugax with calcium-channel blockers. N Engl J Med *329:*396–398, 1996.)

of reversible cerebral segmental vasoconstriction of all sized arteries in young women, especially during the puerperium. Clinically, fluctuating multifocal neurologic signs are accompanied by headache, seizures, and altered consciousness. Many of these patients have a previous history of migraine. Savino et al. (1990) reported four patients who experienced visual loss after an intranasal injection of anesthetic in preparation for nasal surgery. In all cases, the anesthetic was mixed with epinephrine. One patient had a branch retinal artery occlusion, one had a central retinal artery occlusion (CRAO), one had anterior ischemic optic neuropathy (AION), and one of the patients had a posterior ischemic optic neuropathy (PION). In no instance was there any ophthalmoscopic evidence of embolism. Savino et al. (1990) postulated that the visual loss resulted from vasospasm induced by the anesthetic/sympathomimetic solution. Vasospasm is also one of the mechanisms by which cocaine and other recreational drugs induce thrombosis (see below).

ARTERITIS

Both infectious and noninfectious inflammation can damage an arterial wall sufficiently to predispose to thrombosis. Infectious causes include acute bacterial meningitis and chronic basal meningitis as well as the focal arteritis associated with herpes zoster infection. Noninfectious causes are more common and include a large group of disorders often classified as the **rheumatic diseases** (Sigal, 1987; Jabs, 1989). These disorders include systemic and CNS vasculitides, such as temporal (giant cell) arteritis, Takayasu's arteritis (pulseless disease), isolated (granulomatous) angiitis of the CNS, Churg-Strauss syndrome, microangiopathy of brain and retina (Susac's syndrome), and polyarteritis nodosa as well as the connective tissue diseases (systemic lupus erythematosus [SLE], scleroderma, Sjögren's syndrome), and Behçet's disease. These disorders are discussed in more detail in Chapter 57 of this text.

Infectious Arteritis. In patients with **acute bacterial** meningitis, the pial arteries also are inflamed. They may become occluded and produce a stroke (Figs. 55.22 and 55.23). *Listeria monocytogenes* produces such a condition, which has a predilection for the lower brainstem.

In patients with **syphilis**, the spirochete probably invades cerebral arteries at the time of the meningitis of secondary syphilis. The resulting meningovascular syphilis is characterized by apoplectic attacks of hemiplegia, headache, seizures, cerebrospinal fluid (CSF) pleocytosis, and positive serology. Cerebral angiography shows variable findings in patients with stroke in the setting of neurosyphilis. Some patients show evidence of cerebral arteritis, some show both atherosclerotic changes and arteritis, and some show no abnormal findings (Landi et al., 1990). **Lyme disease** may rarely cause strokes, presumably from meningovascular inflammation (Uldry et al., 1987; Halperin et al., 1989; Pachner et al., 1989; Rahn and Malawista, 1991).

Chronic basal meningitis, usually caused by the tubercle bacillus, by fungi such as *Cryptococcus neoformans, Histoplasma capsulatum,* or *Coccidioides imitis,* or by parasites such as *Cysticercus,* can cause an obliterative arteritis that damages intracranial vessels and results in an acute stroke (Sole-Llenas and Pons-Tortella, 1978; Rodriguez-Carbajal et al., 1989; Fesenmeier et al., 1990). The proximal middle cerebral artery and the arteries in the posterior perforated substance are most often affected, although Veenendaal-Hilbers et al. (1988) reported two cases of basilar artery occlusion in patients with chronic basal meningovasculitis caused by *Borrelia burgdorferi* (Lyme disease). Regardless of the causative organism, most cases of arterial occlusion associated with a chronic basal meningitis have a typical histopathologic picture. An exudate surrounds the arteries, producing thickening and inflammation of the walls. Eventually, occlusion of the affected vessels occurs, and an infarct, usually in the basal ganglia or mesencephalon, results (Fig.

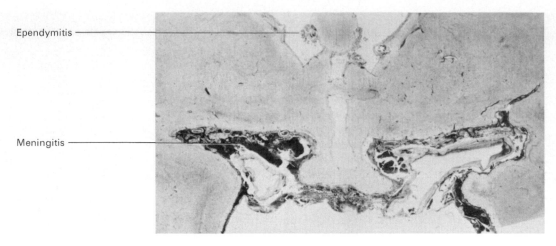

Ependymitis

Meningitis

Figure 55.22. Acute bacterial meningitis producing an ischemic stroke. The patient was a 27-year-old woman with eclampsia who developed respiratory difficulties and circulatory collapse. She died a few hours after admission to the hospital. Autopsy showed a swollen brain with a purulent meningitis over its surface. The meningitis was caused by a staphylococcal middle ear infection. Cross-section through the optic chiasm shows pus filling the basal cistern. Note that the basal arteries are completely surrounded by the inflammatory material. Such arteries may become occluded and produce a stroke. (From Lindenberg R, Walsh FB, Sacks JG. Neuropathology of Vision: An Atlas. Philadelphia, Lea & Febiger, 1973.)

55.24). Other fungi, particularly *Mucor* and *Aspergillus,* can cause a necrotizing arteritis that may occlude both large and small intracranial and intraorbital arteries, causing cerebral infarction, blindness, or both (Bank et al., 1962; Bentwich et al., 1968; Ferry and Abedi, 1983; Qingli et al., 1989; Galetta et al., 1990).

Herpes zoster can produce a necrotizing intracranial arteritis that primarily affects the anterior and middle cerebral arteries (Walker et al., 1973; MacKenzie et al., 1981) and, rarely, the posterior cerebral artery (Powers, 1986), (Fig. 55.25). The condition may occur after an attack of herpes zoster ophthalmicus, resulting in a delayed ischemic cerebral

infarction on the side of the affected eye (Pratesi et al., 1977; Doyle et al., 1983; Fryer et al., 1984; Pfeifer et al., 1989) (Fig. 55.26). In such cases, the classic neurologic sign is a hemiparesis or hemiplegia that is contralateral to the affected eye. Cerebral infarction may also occur after an attack of herpes zoster oticus (Joy et al., 1989), and brainstem infarction can occur in patients with cervical herpes zoster (Snow and Simcock, 1988; Ross et al., 1991).

Patients infected with the human immunodeficiency virus (HIV-1) have up to 40 times the risk of stroke compared with age-matched controls (Mizusawa et al., 1988; Engstrom et al., 1989; Berger et al., 1990; Park et al., 1990; Kieburtz et al., 1993; but also see Pinto, 1996). This likely reflects the increased prevalence of opportunistic infections like those noted above, but it may also be related to primary HIV-1 infection or immune-mediated vascular damage. Chronic infections and weight loss can also cause an increase in acute plasma reactants, thus promoting thrombosis.

Recognition of those rare instances in which arteritis is caused by a specific microbial infection is critical for effective treatment. Infectious agents and their neuro-ophthalmologic effects are discussed in Chapters 60–69 of this text.

Noninfectious Arteritis. Most cases of arteritis that produce stroke with and without neuro-ophthalmologic symptoms and signs are noninfectious. The most common and important is **temporal (giant cell) arteritis** (see Chapter 57 for a more extensive discussion). Although the branches of the external carotid artery, especially the superficial temporal and occipital arteries, are most frequently affected, the internal carotid, vertebral, subclavian, coronary, femoral, and even intracranial arteries can be affected, especially the ophthalmic arteries (Klein et al., 1975; Cull, 1979) (Fig. 55.27). The lesions that most frequently cause stroke are located in the distal extracranial portion of the internal carotid artery just as it enters the carotid siphon and in the

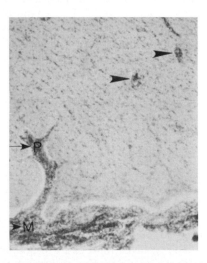

Figure 55.23. Perivascular inflammation and occlusion of intracranial vessels by bacterial meningitis. The basal surface of the brain is covered by a purulent leptomeningitis (*M*). Note that the inflammation extends into the brain parenchyma and occludes several small arterioles (*P* and *arrowheads*), producing microinfarction.

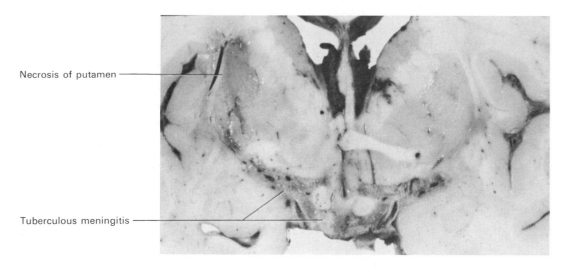

Necrosis of putamen ——————

Tuberculous meningitis ——————

Figure 55.24. Chronic tuberculous meningitis producing a stroke. The patient was a 22-year-old man who died 1 month after suffering a mild head injury in a motorcycle accident. Cross-section through the brain at the level of the optic chiasm shows extensive tuberculous meningitis filling the basal cistern and encasing the optic chiasm and the arteries at the base of the brain. The left putamen is discolored and separated from the claustrum because of an infarction caused by endarteritis. (From Lindenberg R, Walsh FB, Sacks JG. Neuropathology of Vision: An Atlas. Philadelphia, Lea & Febiger, 1973.)

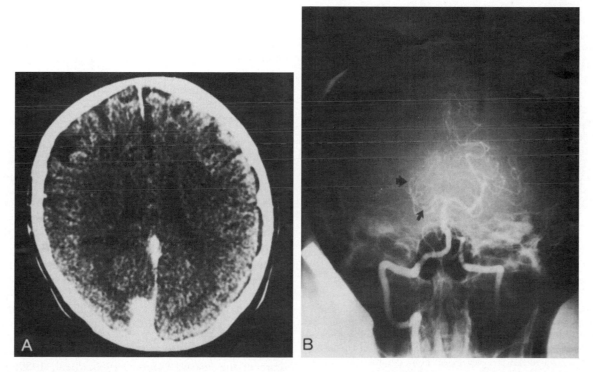

Figure 55.25. Occipital infarction in a patient with herpes zoster. The patient was a 68-year-old man who had previously experienced an attack of herpes zoster maxillaris. About 3 months later, he experienced transient episodes of left face and arm numbness, and he then noted blurred vision to the left. Neurologic examination revealed only a congruous homonymous hemianopic paracentral scotoma sparing the macula. *A,* A CT scan obtained after intravenous injection of contrast material shows an enhancing infarction in the medial right occipital lobe. *B,* Selective right vertebral arteriogram, anteroposterior view, shows bead-like segmental narrowing of the proximal right posterior cerebral artery (*small arrow*) with complete occlusion of the distal portion of the artery (*large arrow*). (From Powers JM. Herpes zoster maxillaris with delayed cerebral infarction. J Clin Neuroophthalmol *6:*113–115, 1986.)

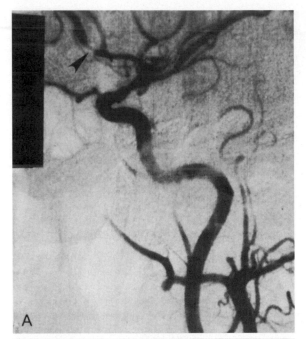

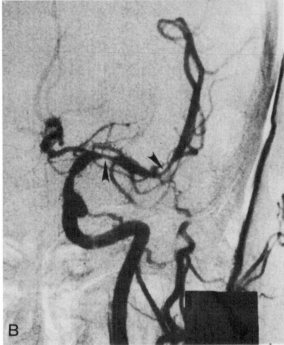

Figure 55.26. Ischemic infarction in a patient with herpes zoster ophthalmicus. The patient was a 60-year-old man with chronic lymphatic leukemia who developed herpes zoster ophthalmicus on the left side. Eight weeks later he complained of right hand numbness, and he subsequently became increasingly confused. He then developed severe dysphasia and a right hemiparesis. *A,* Left common carotid arteriogram, lateral view, shows high-grade segmental stenosis of the proximal A-2 portion of the left anterior cerebral artery (*arrowhead*). *B,* Left common carotid arteriogram, antero-posterior view, shows segmental narrowing of the proximal portion and the region of the trifurcation of the left middle cerebral artery (*arrowheads*). (From MacKenzie RA, Forbes GS, Karnes WE. Angiographic findings in herpes zoster arteritis. Ann Neurol *10:*458–464, 1981.)

distal extracranial vertebral arteries (Sindermann et al., 1970; Wilkinson and Ross Russell, 1972; Caselli et al., 1988).

Often called pulseless disease, **Takayasu's arteritis** was originally described in young Japanese females (Takayasu, 1908; Shimizu and Sano, 1951). Most cases are characterized by severe occlusive disease of the aortic arch and its branches, resulting in absent neck and limb pulses and occasionally in generalized stroke or focal neurologic deficits (Lupi-Herrera et al., 1977; Ishikawa, 1978; Fraga and LaValle, 1980; Hall et al., 1985; Shelhamer et al., 1985; Wolfe, 1989; Lewis et al., 1993) (Fig. 55.28). Headache, dizziness, syncope, and blurred vision are common in such patients. Neuro-ophthalmologic manifestations include ischemia of the orbit, retina, choroid, or anterior segment (Lewis et al., 1993).

Isolated angiitis of the CNS is an idiopathic, recurrent vasculitis confined to the vessels of the brain and spinal cord (Cupps et al., 1983; Moore and Cupps, 1983; Sigal, 1987; Moore, 1989; Hankey, 1991; Vollmer et al., 1993). It usually occurs in young adults, but it occasionally occurs in children (Levin et al., 1989). The condition, which primarily affects small and, sometimes, medium-sized blood vessels, is also called ''granulomatous angiitis'' because the affected vessels are surrounded by an infiltrate composed of lymphocytes, macrophages, and giant cells (Kolodny et al., 1968; Vanderzant et al., 1988; Moore, 1989) (Fig. 55.29). These vessels can thrombose, causing microinfarction. The disease usually begins with diffuse cerebral dysfunction characterized by headache, seizures, lethargy, and confusion, but some patients present with focal symptoms and signs of an acute stroke (Burger et al., 1977), and others present with the clinical picture of multiple infarcts (Koo and Massey, 1988). As the disorder progresses, focal deficits become increasingly prominent. Eventually, about 75% of patients develop multiple, localized lesions of the cerebrum, cerebellum, or brainstem (Moore, 1989). Cranial nerve paresis may occur late in the course of the disease. The nerves most commonly affected are the ocular motor, trigeminal, and facial nerves.

Isolated granulomatous angiitis of the CNS should be suspected when angiography shows multiple localized areas in which vessels are segmentally narrowed or occluded (Fig. 55.30); however, about half of all angiograms appear normal. Biopsy of the leptomeninges, brain parenchyma, or both confirms the diagnosis. Without treatment, most patients with isolated granulomatous angiitis of the CNS experience recurrent strokes and usually die within 1–3 years of the onset of symptoms. Treatment with aggressive immunosuppressive therapy, primarily systemic corticosteroids combined with cyclophosphamide, can result in remission or cure of the disease (Moore, 1989; Sigal, 1989; Hankey, 1991).

Other systemic vasculitides rarely associated with stroke include polyarteritis nodosa, Wegener's granulomatosis, the hypersensitivity vasculitides, and allergic angiitis and granulomatosis, often called the **Churg-Strauss syndrome** (Churg and Strauss, 1950; Chumbley et al., 1977; Oonishi and Ishiko, 1980). This condition forms part of the spectrum

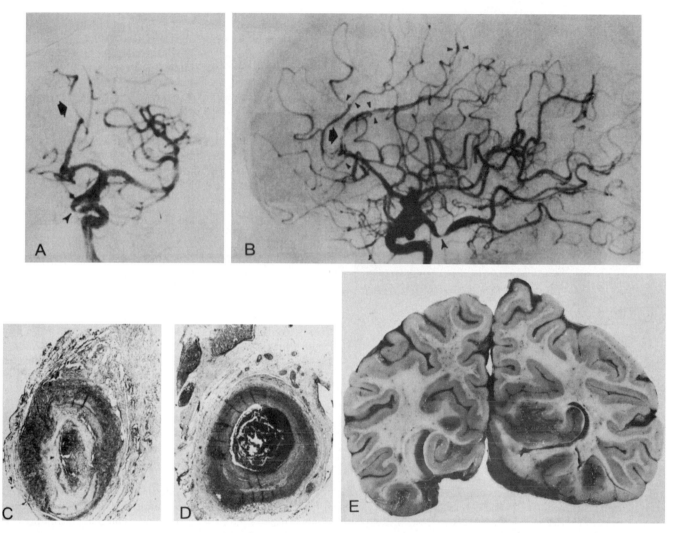

Figure 55.27. Giant cell arteritis producing stroke. *A* and *B*, Right internal carotid arteriogram, anteroposterior and lateral views, in a patient with a left hemiparesis, left homonymous hemianopia, fever, headaches, an elevated erythrocyte sedimentation rate, and a positive temporal artery biopsy. The arteriogram shows marked irregular narrowing of the genu of the left anterior cerebral artery (*large arrows*). There are scattered areas of dilation and narrowing of the pericallosal and callosmarginal arteries and their branches (*small arrowheads*), and there is stenosis and fusiform dilation of the proximal left posterior cerebral artery (*large arrowheads*). Also note an incidental small aneurysm of the supraclinoid portion of the internal carotid artery. (From Enzmann D, Scott WR. Intracranial involvement of giant cell arteritis. Neurology *27:*794–797, 1977.) *C* and *D*, Cross-sections of vertebral arteries from 2 patients with biopsy proven giant cell arteritis, both of who developed neurologic symptoms and signs consistent with disease in the territory of the vertebrobasilar arterial system. Both vessels are occluded by granulomatous inflammation consistent with giant cell arteritis. (From Wilkinson IMS, Russell RWR. Arteries of the head and neck in giant cell arteritis. Arch Neurol *27:*378–391, 1972.) *E*, Bilateral nonsimultaneous infarcts in a 79-year-old man with cortical blindness, an elevated erythrocyte sedimentation rate, a flat visual evoked response, and a positive temporal artery biopsy. There is an old infarct in the right optic radiation and a more extensive, recent infarct in the region of the left calcarine fissure. (From Chisholm IH. Cortical blindness in cranial arteritis. Br J Ophthalmol *59:*332–333, 1975.)

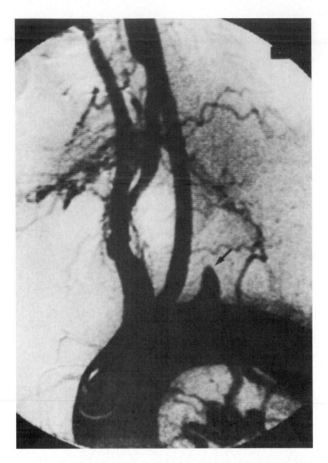

Figure 55.28. Takayasu's disease. Angiogram of aortic arch demonstrates tapered occlusion of the left subclavian artery (*arrow*) and no filling of the right subclavian artery. Multiple dilated collateral channels are seen at the base of the neck and in the upper thoracic region. (From Goldberg HI. Cerebral angiography. In Stroke. Pathophysiology, Diagnosis, and Management. Editors, Barnett HJM, Mohr JP, Stein BM, et al., Vol 1, pp 221–244. New York, Churchill Livingstone, 1986.)

of disseminated systemic necrotizing vasculitis, of which classic polyarteritis nodosa is the best recognized entity. Cerebral ischemia is rare in polyarteritis nodosa but may be caused by cerebral arteritis, hypertension, or renal disease (Ford and Siekert, 1965; Akova et al., 1993). Churg-Strauss syndrome shares with polyarteritis nodosa the pathologic features of fibrinoid necrosis of small- and medium-sized muscular arteries, causing damage to multiple organs, but there is, in addition, a substantial degree of inflammatory damage to small vessels such as capillaries and venules, which does not occur in polyarteritis nodosa. Churg-Strauss syndrome is characterized clinically by an allergic diathesis, adult-onset asthma, fever, transient pulmonary infiltrations, eosinophilia, and tissue infiltration by eosinophils and granulomas, none of which are common in polyarteritis nodosa.

Neuro-ophthalmologic complications in Churg-Strauss syndrome include ocular motor neuropathies (Rackemann and Green, 1939; Weinstein et al., 1983) and visual loss (Ibanez Bermudez et al., 1983; Weinstein et al., 1983; Dagi and Currie, 1985; Acheson et al., 1993). Interestingly, these

complications may result not from the direct effects of vasculitis, but from a hypercoagulable state that predisposes to thromboembolism. This phenomenon is best exemplified by the case reported by Dagi and Currie (1985). These investigators described a 46-year-old Asian woman with Churg-Strauss syndrome who experienced sudden visual loss in the right eye and was found to have widespread retinal branch artery occlusions. Affected vessels contained white material, some located at bifurcations and some located along the course of the vessels. There were no vitreous cells, nor was there any vascular sheathing. Fluorescein angiography performed 36 hours after visual loss showed focal arterial occlusions without flow and a single area of focal leakage of dye from the first inferior temporal bifurcation; however, there was no evidence of more widespread leakage from arteries, veins, or the optic disc that usually occurs in patients with retinal vasculitis (Karel et al., 1974). The patient was treated with low molecular weight dextran, heparin, and prednisone. Within 24 hours, her vision had improved from 20/200 to 20/50 in the affected eye, and the white material had disappeared.

An unusual but apparently distinct form of vasculitis that affects the brain and retina was initially described in two patients by Pfaffenbach and Hollenhorst (1973) who ascribed the process to CNS lupus despite inconclusive laboratory tests. Susac et al. (1979) subsequently recognized the unique features of the disease and called it **microangiopathy of brain and retina**. The condition is similar to granulomatous angiitis; however, it specifically causes obliteration of the large retinal arteries in both eyes in addition to the arteries of the brain and meninges (Fig. 55.31). The condition occurs almost exclusively in women from 18 to 40 years of age (Coppeto et al., 1984a; Monteiro et al., 1985; Swanson et al., 1985; McFadyen et al., 1987; Heiskala et al., 1988; Mass et al., 1988; Bogousslavsky et al., 1989; Susac, 1994; Notis et al., 1995; Vila et al., 1995; Wildemann et al., 1996). The clinical features include multiple branch retinal arterial occlusions and encephalopathy characterized by early disturbances in behavior and memory. Hearing loss is so common that the condition is sometimes called a "retinocochleocerebral" arteriolopathy (Bogousslavsky et al., 1989). There are no consistent laboratory or radiographic abnormalities except for minimal CSF pleocytosis and an increased concentration of protein in the spinal fluid. The disease may occasionally respond to treatment with calcium-antagonist therapy, systemic corticosteroids, other immunosuppressive agents, intravenous immunoglobulins, or even hyperbaric oxygen, but there is no invariably successful treatment (Li et al., 1996; Wildemann et al., 1996). Coppeto et al. (1984a) postulated that this syndrome is a viral-induced immune-mediated disease, but there is no firm evidence to support this hypothesis.

Johnson et al. (1994) reviewed the course of 16 patients with idiopathic recurrent branch retinal arterial occlusions and confirmed that the long-term visual, neurologic, and systemic prognosis of this syndrome appears to be favorable. Eight of these patients had associated vestibuloauditory symptoms, transient sensorimotor symptoms, or both, but there were no serious permanent neurologic deficits or recur-

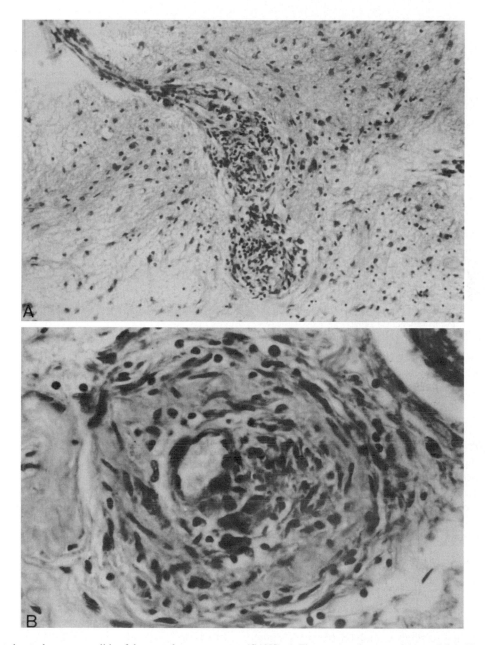

Figure 55.29. Isolated granulomatous angiitis of the central nervous system (GANS). *A*, The segmental nature of the angiitis is illustrated by the nodular aggregates of inflammatory cells along a small leptomeningeal artery as it penetrates the rarefied and gliotic cerebellar cortex. *B*, Cross-section of an affected leptomeningeal vessel shows proliferation of mononuclear and epithelioid cells surrounded by a rim of lymphocytes and fibroblasts in the periphery. (From Koo EH, Massey EW. Granulomatous angiitis of the central nervous system: Protean manifestations and response to treatment. J Neurol Neurosurg Psychiatry *51:*1126–1133, 1988.)

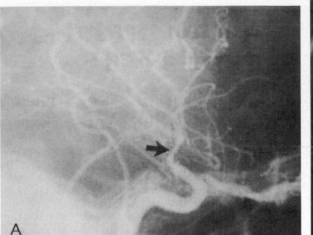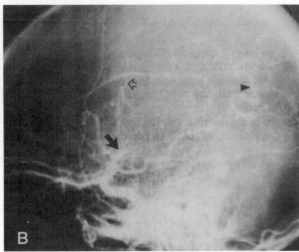

Figure 55.30.   Cerebral angiography in two patients with isolated granulomatous angiitis of the central nervous system (GANS). *A,* In a 35-year-old man with right-sided headaches, left hemiparesis, and moderate weakness of the right arm, a common carotid arteriogram, lateral view, shows a long segment of stenosis of the supraclinoid portion of the internal carotid artery. Biopsy of the middle cerebral artery revealed changes consistent with GANS. *B,* In a 40-year-old woman with left hemiplegia, mild aphasia, and mild right hemiparesis, a selective left common carotid arteriogram, lateral view, shows occlusion of the supraclinoid segment of the left internal carotid artery associated with neovascularization (*closed arrow*). There are extensive collaterals from the external circulation (*open arrow*) and the posterior circulation (*arrowhead*). Biopsy of the leptomeninges confirmed the diagnosis of GANS. (From Moore PM. Diagnosis and management of isolated angiitis of the central nervous system. Neurology *39:*167–173, 1989.)

rent systemic thromboembolic events. Most patients had one or more vaso-occlusive risk factors, but no particular factor was common to all patients, suggesting that the etiology of this syndrome is likely heterogeneous and perhaps multifactorial. Many of these patients may have a mild or partial form of Susac's syndrome.

All of the **connective tissue diseases** can be complicated by stroke, but true cerebral infarction is seldom caused directly by vasculitis (Caplan and Stein, 1986; Futrell and Millikan, 1989). Patients with SLE, for example, may experience transient neurologic or visual symptoms similar to those experienced by patients with migraine and probably caused by vasospasm (Brandt et al., 1975a; Brandt and Lessell, 1978; Shaw et al., 1979). Patients with SLE usually develop permanent visual or neurologic deficits because large and medium-sized vessels become occluded or obliterated by thrombosis caused by an associated coagulopathy, especially thrombotic thrombocytopenic purpura (TTP) (Trevor et al., 1972; Hart et al., 1984; Devinsky et al., 1988; Futrell and Millikan, 1989), because associated hypertension from renal disease results in occlusion of small vessels (Feinglass et al., 1976), or because they develop embolism from associated cardiac valvular disease (Galve et al., 1988; Futrell and Millikan, 1989; Roldan et al., 1996). Most patients with visual or neurologic deficits in the setting of SLE have scant evidence of inflammation of intracranial arteries (Johnson and Richardson, 1968), but intracranial vasculitis does occur occasionally (Graham et al., 1985; Bryant et al., 1986; Sakaki et al., 1990; Yigit et al., 1996). In scleroderma, most strokes are caused by hypertension, whereas CNS ischemia in rheumatoid arthritis is usually caused by a hypercoagulable state or marantic endocarditis (Caplan et al., 1984).

Sarcoidosis may cause a cerebral vasculitis. TIAs, strokes, and evidence of meningeal, hypothalamic, and pituitary dysfunction are the clinical features of angiitic neurosarcoidosis (Brown et al., 1989), a disorder that can also affect the spinal cord, peripheral nervous system, and muscle. In rare cases, an intracranial sarcoid granuloma compresses an adjacent vessel, and produces TIAs or a stroke (Corse and Stern, 1990). The visual sensory and ocular motor systems are frequently affected in such cases (Caplan et al., 1983). Ocular sarcoid may also cause retinal vascular occlusions. Sarcoidosis is discussed in Chapter 70 of this text.

Behçet's disease may be characterized by cerebral arteritis. Patients with this disorder have symptoms and signs of ocular and meningeal inflammation. Strokes are uncommon, however (Kawakita et al., 1967; Chajek and Fainaru, 1975; Herskovitz et al., 1988; Masai et al., 1996).

Malignant atrophic papulosis, also called **Degos' disease**, is a cutaneovisceral disorder characterized by a typical skin rash and gastrointestinal perforation. The condition, which is frequently fatal and for which there is no treatment, is caused by a vasculopathy that may affect intracranial and extracranial vessels, causing an ischemic or hemorrhagic stroke (Degos, 1979). There is pathologic evidence to suggest that the nervous system vasculopathy in this disease is not associated with a true vasculitis (Subbiah et al., 1996).

Romano et al. (1989) described a previously healthy, developmentally normal 34-month-old boy who was stung repeatedly on the inner upper lip by a wasp that was removed from the boy's mouth. The child received no stings in the posterior pharynx. There was immediate swelling around the area of the sting, and the boy was treated with diphenhydramine. Five days later, the child developed progressive neuro-

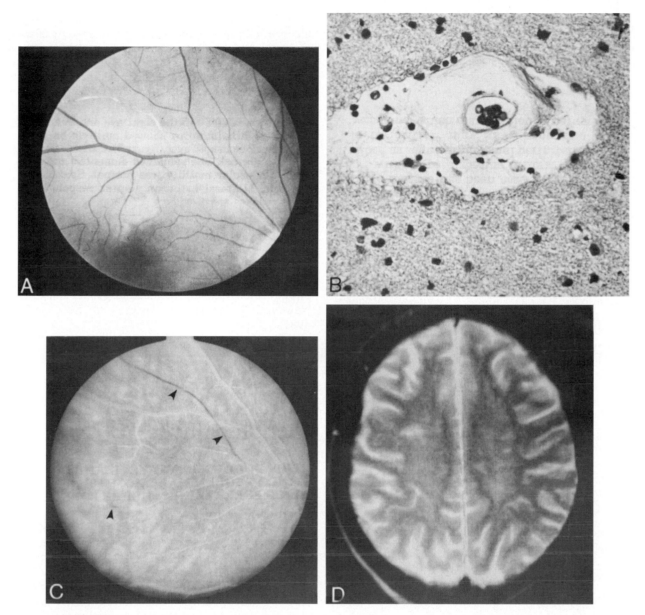

Figure 55.31. Microangiography of brain and retina. *A,* Ophthalmoscopic appearance of the right ocular fundus in a 40-year-old woman with headache, confusion, inappropriate behavior, generalized hyperactive muscle stretch reflexes, ankle clonus, and bilateral extensor plantar reflexes. Note narrowed superior temporal retinal artery and subtle nerve fiber layer infarcts. The distal portion of the artery has a "silver streak" appearance. *B,* Brain biopsy from right frontal cortex in the same patient shows sclerosis of media and adventitia of a small cortical vessel. Similar changes also were seen in small pial vessels. (From Susac JO, Hardman JM, Selhorst JB. Microangiopathy of the brain and retina. Neurology *29:*313–316, 1979.) *C,* Fluorescein angiogram of the right ocular fundus in a 19-year-old woman with headaches, confusion, an unsteady gait, hearing loss, and loss of visual acuity in the right eye. The patient was ataxic, incontinent, and had bilateral extensor plantar responses. Visual acuity was 20/50 OD and 20/20 OS. The fluorescein angiogram shows marked distal arteriolar sheathing and occlusions (*arrowheads*). *D,* MR image, axial view, in the same patient shows areas of increased signal (T-2 weighted image). (From Bogousslavsky J, Gaio JM, Caplan LR, et al. Encephalopathy, deafness and blindness in young women: A distinct retinocochleocerebral arteriolopathy? J Neurol Neurosurg Psychiatry *52:*43–46, 1989.)

logic symptoms and signs and was found to have a mild right spastic hemiparesis and a nonfluent aphasia. He also had a vesicular rash around the mouth. Evaluation revealed occlusion of the left internal carotid artery at its supraclinoid portion. All other intracranial and neck vessels were normal. Romano et al. (1989) postulated that the carotid occlusion was caused by an immune response that produced an arteritis with thrombus formation in the internal carotid artery. Although this may be the case, it is difficult to explain why only one artery was affected in this patient. The wasp sting and the signs of carotid occlusion may have been temporally related, but it is unclear if they were causally related.

Patients with allergic, hypersensitivity, and systemic vasculitis may respond to treatment with corticosteroids or other immunosuppressive agents. Vasculitis and its neuro-ophthalmologic sequelae are discussed in Chapter 57 of this text.

SPONTANEOUS AND TRAUMATIC DISSECTION

The development of thrombosis in patients with both traumatic and nontraumatic **dissections** of the extracranial and intracranial portions of the carotid, vertebral, and basilar arteries and their branches is discussed in Chapter 53 of this text. It suffices here simply to state that such patients may experience both acute strokes and chronic, progressive neurologic dysfunction related to dissection (Gauthier et al., 1985; Bogousslavsky and Regli, 1987; Bogousslavsky et al., 1987a; Pozzati et al., 1990; Hicks et al., 1994) (Fig. 55.32).

FIBROMUSCULAR DYSPLASIA

Fibromuscular dysplasia is a disorder of medium-diameter systemic arteries. It is characterized by segmental, nonatheromatous, stenosing lesions that can affect any or all three layers of the vessel wall. The most common form of fibromuscular dysplasia affects the media. Constricting bands are composed of fibrous dysplastic tissue and proliferating

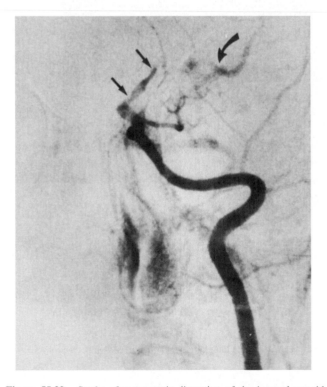

Figure 55.32. Stroke after traumatic dissection of the internal carotid artery. The patient was an 8-year-old boy who experienced minor head trauma. Cerebral angiogram, frontal projection, demonstrates nonuniform, severe stenosis of the supraclinoid segment of the internal carotid artery. The stenotic region has a flattened, twisted contour (*straight arrows*). The stenosis tapers to a complete occlusion, but the middle cerebral artery is reconstituted about 2 cm lateral to its origin through lenticulostriate artery collateral circulation (*curved arrow*).

smooth muscle cells in the media. These constricting rings alternate with areas of luminal dilation caused by thinning of the media and disruption of the elastic membrane (Sandok, 1983). The arteries most often affected are the renal, vertebral, and the common, external, and internal carotid arteries.

Fibromuscular dysplasia occurs five times more often in women than in men. The average age of an affected patient is 49 years, and more than 80% of patients are over 50 years of age (Reader and Massey, 1980).

Although most patients with fibromuscular dysplasia are asymptomatic, this disorder may produce neurologic symptoms and signs in a variety of ways: (*a*) by association with the development of one or more intracranial aneurysms, although whether or not this association is fortuitous is unclear (see Chapter 53); (*b*) by predisposing to both intracranial and extracranial arterial dissection (see Chapter 53); and (*c*) by producing TIAs or strokes from thrombosis of affected arteries (Fig. 55.33). In the last setting, narrowing and irregularity of the lumen of affected vessels predisposes to thrombus formation (Connett and Lansche, 1965; Palubinskas and Newton, 1965; Reader and Massey, 1980; Ketz and Gaspar, 1981).

MOYAMOYA

Moyamoya disease is a disorder characterized by: (*a*) a network of fine vessels with a cloud-like, mesh appearance (*moyamoya* is the Japanese word for puff of smoke) located at the base of the brain, (*b*) congenital atresia or acquired stenosis (or occlusion) of one or both internal carotid arteries, and (*c*) prominent ethmoid and meningeal anastomotic channels (Takeuchi and Shimizu, 1957; Takeuchi, 1961; Nishimoto and Takeuchi, 1968; Suzuki and Takaku, 1969; Galligioni et al., 1971; Suzuki, 1983; Bruno et al., 1988) (Fig. 55.34). The pathologic changes consist of a variety of abnormalities, including thinning of the vessel wall, intimal thickening, medial necrosis, discontinuity of the internal elastic membrane of some vessels, and dilation of arterioles, but with a characteristic absence of inflammation. The syndrome can be idiopathic or related to a number of diseases, such as sickle-cell disease, neurofibromatosis, fibromuscular dysplasia, and radiation-induced cerebral vasculopathy (see below).

Acute subarachnoid hemorrhage is the most common initial clinical manifestation of moyamoya disease in patients over 21 years old (Fox, 1983). Patients who are under 21 years of age usually present with focal neurologic symptoms and signs that are often transient. Ischemic cerebral infarction also may occur in both younger and older patients (Miyamoto et al., 1986; Yoshida et al., 1986; Bruno et al., 1988). In some patients, a variety of visual deficits caused by occlusion of the internal carotid arteries, posterior cerebral arteries, basilar artery, or a combination of these vessels are the initial or at least a prominent sign of disease. Deficits associated with carotid circulation ischemia include the ocular ischemic syndrome, neovascular glaucoma, CRAO, central retinal vein occlusion (CRVO), ION, and the optic chiasmal syndrome. Visual deficits associated with posterior circulation (posterior cerebral-basilar artery) ischemia include

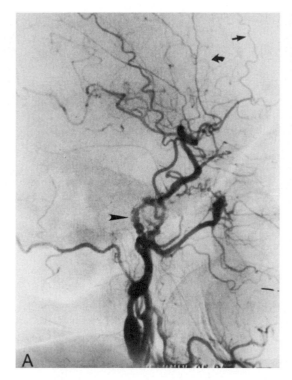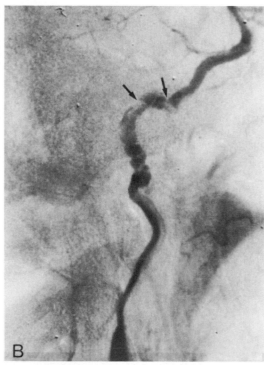

Figure 53.33. Hemodynamically significant fibromuscular dysplasia in the distal cervical and petrous segments of the internal carotid artery. *A,* Common carotid arteriogram, lateral view, shows typical "string of beads" configuration of fibromuscular dysplasia in the distal cervical and proximal petrous portion of the internal carotid artery (*arrowhead*). Circulation in distal branches of the superficial temporal artery (*straight arrow*) leads circulation in the branches of the ipsilateral middle cerebral artery (*curved arrow*), thus indicating the hemodynamic effect of the fibromuscular dysplasia. *B,* Internal carotid arteriogram, lateral view, shows several band-like regions of constriction (*arrows*) between dilated regions of the affected artery. (From Goldberg HI. Cerebral angiography. In Stroke. Pathophysiology, Diagnosis, and Management. Editors, Barnett HJM, Mohr JP, Stein BM, et al., Vol 1, pp 221–244. New York, Churchill Livingstone, 1986.)

homonymous hemianopia, generalized visual field constriction, Bálint's syndrome, and cortical blindness (Hoare and Keogh, 1974; Arita et al., 1977; Morimatsu et al., 1977; Schoenberg et al., 1977; Schrager et al., 1977; Karasawa et al., 1978; Coakham et al., 1979; Slamovits et al., 1981; Valvo et al., 1982; Suzuki, 1983; Ahmadi et al., 1984; Chace and Hedges, 1984; Miyamoto et al., 1986; Yoshida et al., 1986; Noda et al., 1987; Tashima-Kurita et al., 1989).

It is thought that the primary event in the development of moyamoya disease is early occlusion of one or both internal carotid arteries, although the process may also affect the posterior cerebral and basilar arteries. Collateral vessels then develop as a secondary phenomenon, presumably to compensate for reduced arterial blood flow through the compromised major vessels.

Saccular aneurysms may develop in patients with moyamoya disease. These may arise from network vessels, collateral vessels, or from normal vessels of the vertebrobasilar or, less frequently, the carotid circulation. They usually become symptomatic when they rupture, but they may also produce ischemic or compressive symptoms and signs (Kwak et al., 1984a, 1984b) (see Chapter 53).

SICKLE CELL DISEASE

Homozygous **sickle cell anemia** (hemoglobin SS disease) and **sickle hemoglobin C disease** (hemoglobin SC disease)

predispose to stroke (Greer and Schotland, 1962; Portnoy and Herion, 1972; Wood, 1977; Fabian and Peters, 1984; Prohovnik et al., 1989; Moser et al., 1996) (Fig. 55.35). Patients with sickle cell anemia are much more likely to develop neurologic symptoms and signs than are patients with hemoglobin SC disease (Powars et al., 1978), and patients with sickle trait (hemoglobin SA disease) only rarely suffer stroke (Diggs and Jones, 1952; Pensler and Radke, 1980; Handler and Perkins, 1982; Greenberg and Massey, 1985; Reyes, 1989). Ischemic cerebral infarction is more common in young patients, whereas hemorrhagic infarction is more common in adults. In patients with ischemic infarction, small lenticulostriate arteries become blocked, resulting in white matter infarcts (Reyes, 1989). PION occurs in some patients (Perlman et al., 1994). Large intracranial and extracranial arteries may also become obliterated.

The cause of ischemic stroke in patients with sickle cell disease and sickle trait was originally thought to be blockage of capillaries by deformed red blood cells. Although this does occur in some patients, it is not the primary cause of stroke. Within blocked arteries, fibrous tissue and smooth muscle proliferate, forming a heaped-up mass of fibromuscular tissue that compromises the lumen (Stockman et al., 1972; Boros et al., 1976) (Fig. 55.36). Sludging of sickled red blood cells apparently irritates the arteries to produce

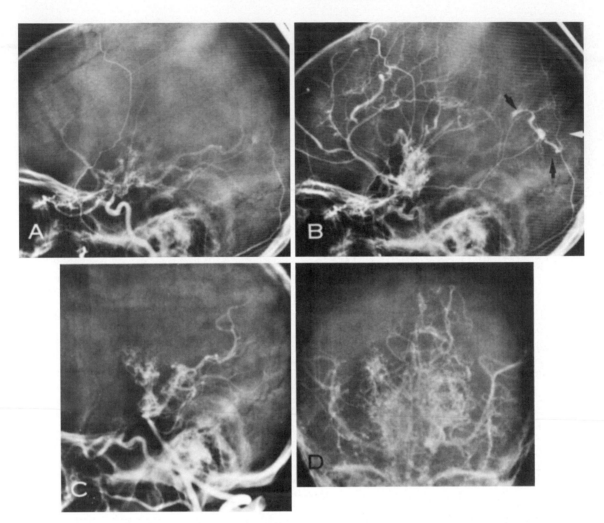

Figure 55.34. Moyamoya disease. The patient was a 3-year-old child with multiple, progressive, arterial occlusions. *A*, Left carotid arteriogram, lateral view, shows occlusion of the left internal carotid artery. There is a fine network of vessels at the base of the brain consisting of dilated perforating branches of the internal carotid and posterior communicating arteries. These vessels supply most of the cerebral circulation. The ophthalmic artery is enlarged, and there is extensive enlargement and proliferation of the branches of this artery, some of which anastomose with meningeal branches that, in turn, anastomose with cortical arteries across the subdural space. *B*, Left carotid arteriogram, lateral view, later phase than *A*, shows the basal network of vessels more clearly. Prominent transdural anastomoses are filling (*arrows*). *C*, Right brachial arteriogram, lateral view, shows preservation of the basilar arterial system. This system not only contributes to the basal network of moyamoya vessels but also supplies the middle cerebral arteries on both sides. *D*, Right brachial arteriogram, anteroposterior view, later phase than *C*, shows filling of most middle cerebral branches on both sides. (From Taveras JM, Wood EH. Diagnostic Neuroradiology. Vol 2. Baltimore, Williams & Wilkins, 1976.)

this intimal hypertrophy, because similar lesions are found in experimental animals when vascular endothelium is mechanically denuded (Ross and Glomset, 1976) or when the endothelium is exposed to platelet aggregates (Fujimoto et al., 1985). It is possible that aggregation of sickled erythrocytes is sufficient in itself to occlude small vessels, whereas hemoglobin-platelet-fibrin aggregates together injure the endothelium of larger arteries to produce large vessel occlusion (Caplan, 1993).

RADIATION ANGIOPATHY

Radiation therapy may produce fibrinoid or hyaline changes with endothelial proliferation and perivascular fibrosis in the walls of affected arteries (Murros and Toole,

1989) (see Chapter 48). These changes predispose to accelerated atherosclerosis and to thrombosis (Fig. 55.37). In humans, morphologic changes first appear about 3 months after irradiation. At this time, light microscopy reveals degeneration of vascular endothelium, vacuolization and thickening of the intima, and changes in elastic fibers (Gassmann, 1899). At the same time, electron microscopy demonstrates swelling and detachment of endothelial cells, splitting of basement membranes, and subintimal foam cells (Ackerman, 1972). Silverberg et al. (1978) described nine patients with radiation-induced damage to the carotid arteries. Four of the patients presented with transient monocular loss of vision (see below), four experienced a stroke, and one patient developed headaches and was found to have bilateral carotid

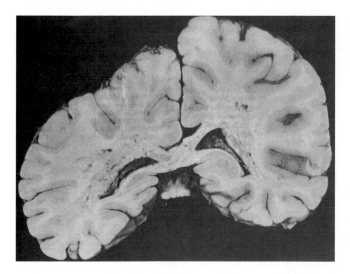

Figure 55.35. Stroke in sickle cell trait. The patient was a 32-year-old woman who developed an acute right hemiparesis, slurred speech, and cortical blindness. Neuroimaging studies showed evidence of bilateral parieto-occipital infarction. The patient subsequently died of recurrent staphylococcal septicemia. Coronal section through the brain shows bilateral infarctions in parieto-occipital white matter, in the optic radiations, and in the splenium of the corpus callosum. (From Reyes MG. Subcortical cerebral infarctions in sickle cell trait. J Neurol Neurosurg Psychiatry *52:*516–518, 1989.)

bruits. Similar patients were described by other investigators (see Table 2 in Murros and Toole, 1989). Radiation treatment of optic glioma or craniopharyngioma can cause a postradiation vasculopathy resembling moyamoya disease (Kestle et al., 1993; Bitzer and Topka, 1995). Even moderate radiation doses, such as those used in the treatment of Graves' ophthalmopathy can cause CRAO (Noble, 1994).

AMYLOID ANGIOPATHY

Cerebral amyloid angiopathy is characterized by infiltration of intracranial vessels, most often in the frontal, parietal, and occipital lobes, with amyloid material (Fig. 55.38). This disorder is discussed in more detail later in this chapter in the section on ''Hemorrhagic Cerebrovascular Disease,'' because the most prominent clinical and pathologic feature of the disorder is intracerebral hemorrhage. Nevertheless, small, scattered, nonhemorrhagic infarcts may occasionally develop in patients with this condition (Scheinberg and Cathcart, 1978; Okazaki et al., 1979; Cosgrove et al., 1985).

NEOPLASTIC ANGIOPATHY

A condition called **neoplastic angioendotheliosis** was described by Beal and Fisher (1982) in two patients. The disorder was characterized by a malignant proliferation of blood vessel endothelial cells. Small vessels were packed with tumor cells, and the occluded vessels were surrounded by microinfarcts. Progressive neurologic deterioration occurred in both patients. **Meningeal carcinomatosis** can also cause vascular occlusive disease, presumably by compressing or invading blood vessels (Schaible and Golnik, 1993).

MISCELLANEOUS SYSTEMIC DISORDERS AFFECTING THE ARTERIAL WALL

A variety of systemic disorders other than those described above may be associated with thrombosis-induced neuro-

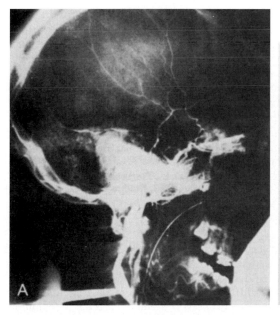
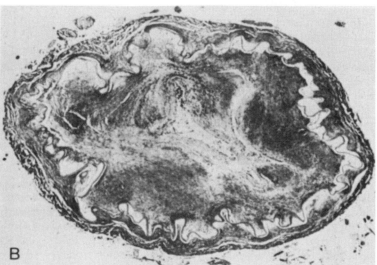

Figure 55.36. Pathogenesis of stroke in sickle cell disease and sickle cell trait. *A,* Left carotid arteriogram, lateral view, shows complete occlusion of the internal carotid artery distal to the origin of the ophthalmic artery. *B,* Cross-section of the left internal carotid artery obtained after the death of the patient shows a marked endarteritic process nearly occluding the vessel lumen. (From Boros L, Thomas C, Weiner WJ. Large cerebral vessel disease in sickle cell anemia. J Neurol Neurosurg Psychiatry *39:*1236–1239, 1976.)

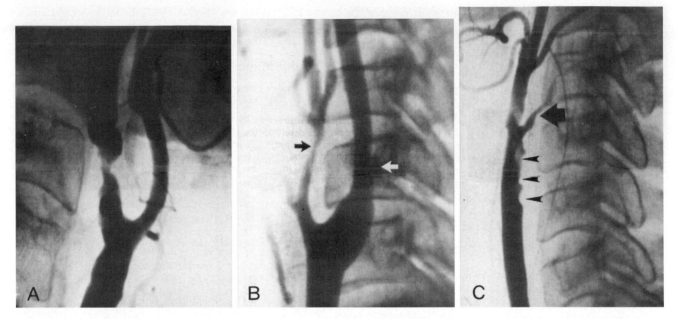

Figure 55.37. Radiation angiopathy affecting the carotid arterial system in 3 patients. All 3 patients had received radiation therapy for lymphoproliferative malignancy. *A,* Ulcerated plaque of the internal carotid artery with maximum stenosis several centimeters distal to the bifurcation after radiation therapy for Hodgkin's disease. *B,* Ulcerated, stenotic plaque of the internal carotid artery (*white arrow*) and severe, extensive stenosis of the external carotid artery (*black arrow*) distal to a normal-appearing bifurcation after radiation for Hodgkin's disease. *C,* An unusual occlusion of the internal carotid artery distal to the bifurcation (*arrow*) but with involvement beginning proximal to the bifurcation (*arrowheads*) after radiation therapy for large cell lymphoma. (From Silverberg GD, Britt RH, Goffinet DR. Radiation-induced carotid artery disease. Cancer *41:*130–137, 1978.)

logic dysfunction. Vascular occlusive disease and stroke occur in young children with **Menkes' kinky hair syndrome**. Inherited diseases that affect connective tissue, such as **homocystinuria**, the **Ehlers-Danlos syndromes**, **pseudoxanthoma elasticum**, and even **neurofibromatosis** may predispose to stroke (Natowicz and Kelley, 1987; Rizzo and Lessell, 1994; North et al., 1995), but documented cases are few, and neuropathology is scanty.

Homocystinuria is an autosomal-recessive disease in which accumulated homocysteine causes injury to the vascular endothelium, promoting thrombosis. Homozygous patients can suffer arterial and venous occlusions at a relatively young age (Harker et al., 1974; Boers et al., 1985). Heterozygotes may also be susceptible to accelerated cerebrovascular disease, including the development of retinal arterial and vein occlusions (Brattstrom et al., 1984; Wenzler et al., 1993; Biousse et al., 1997). Dietary folate supplementation may reduce the rate of development of atherosclerosis and the risk for related cardiovascular and cerebrovascular events by decreasing circulating homocysteine levels, even in patients without known abnormalities in the gene linked to homocystinuria (Boushey et al., 1995; Stampfer and Malinow, 1995).

Fabry's disease is an inborn error of glycosphingolipid metabolism that results from the defective activity of the lysosomal enzyme, α-galactosidase A (Desnick and Sweeley, 1983). The enzymatic defect is transmitted by an X-linked gene and results in progressive deposition of the glycosphingolipid, trihexosyl ceramide (ceramide trihexoside), in various tissues, particularly in the vascular endothelium (Natowicz and Kelley, 1987; de Veber et al., 1990). In affected males, clinical onset of the disease typically occurs in childhood or adolescence and is characterized by episodic crises of pain in the extremities and by cutaneous vascular lesions. With time, cardiovascular and renal manifestations develop, and death often occurs in the 3rd to 5th decades from the effects of vascular disease of the heart or kidneys. Because Fabry's disease is associated with an abnormality of blood vessels, stroke is common in patients with this disorder (Bethune et al., 1961; Wise et al., 1962; Wallace and Cooper, 1965; Lou and Reske-Nielson, 1971; Tagliavini et al., 1982; de Veber et al., 1990; Mitsias and Levine, 1996) and in female carriers (heterozygotes) (Bird and Lagunoff, 1978). Elongated, ectatic, tortuous vertebral and basilar arteries are the most frequent cause of recurrent cerebrovascular symptoms, including hemiparesis, vertigo, diplopia, dysarthria, nystagmus, headache, and ataxia (Mitsias and Levine, 1996). Although the most common ocular manifestation of Fabry's disease is a whorl-like corneal opacification that is present in over 90% of patients (Spaeth and Frost, 1965), many patients also have tortuosity of conjunctival vessels, retinal vessels, or both (Franceschetti, 1976). Calmettes et al. (1959) described a central vein occlusion in a 40-year-old man with Fabry's disease, and Sher et al. (1978) described a 16-year-old boy with Fabry's disease who developed a CRAO. Meckler (1990) reported the case of a 24-year-old man who developed diplopia and was found to have a left oculomotor nerve paresis that spared the pupil. The patient also had mild hyperreflexia of the lower extremities. The cause of the oculomotor nerve paresis could not be determined. The paresis eventually resolved, but over the next 18 months, it

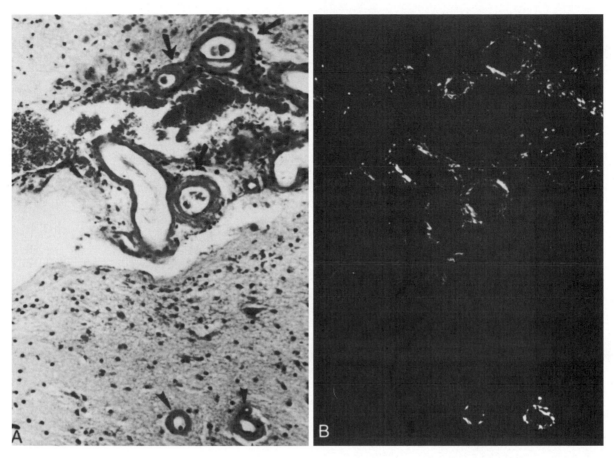

Figure 55.38. Cerebral amyloid angiopathy. *A*, The arteries in the leptomeninges (*arrows*) and in the superficial cortex (*arrowheads*) contain amyloid within the vessel wall. *B*, Same field as in *A* photographed using polarized light. Note birefringence of amyloid deposits in the vessel walls. (From Kase CS, Mohr JP. General features of intracerebral hemorrhage. In Stroke. Pathophysiology, Diagnosis, and Management. Editors, Barnett HJM, Mohr JP, Stein BM, et al., Vol 1, pp 497–523. New York, Churchill Livingstone, 1986.)

recurred intermittently in association with left facial paresis, mild unsteadiness of gait, and dementia. The patient eventually developed a left hemiparesis and hemisensory deficit, right hemiataxia, episodic vomiting, hypothermia, recurrent fevers, and arthralgias. Neuroimaging studies, initially normal, eventually showed multiple intracranial lesions. Ophthalmologic examination eventually revealed corneal opacities consistent with Fabry's disease, and the condition was confirmed by demonstration of a reduced concentration of α-galactosidase A in the serum. Fabry's disease is also discussed in Chapter 51 of this text.

Rizzo and Lessell (1994) reviewed the cerebrovascular complications of **neurofibromatosis type 1**. They emphasized that patients with this disorder may develop stenosis and occlusion of large and small vessels, both systemically and intracranially, aneurysms that may occasionally present as arterial dissections, arteriovenous fistulae, moyamoya disease, spontaneous vascular rupture, and arterial adventitial infiltration by neurofibroma or ganglioneuroma. Retinal vascular occlusive disease also occurs in such patients (Moadel et al., 1994). Neurofibromatosis and other phacomatoses are discussed in Chapter 49 of this text.

The disorder known as **delayed cerebral ischemia** occurs after subarachnoid hemorrhage, at least in part from the effects of vasospasm (Solomon and Fink, 1987). This condition is discussed in Chapter 53 of this text.

ARTERIAL WALL CONSTRICTION AND COMPRESSION

The arteries of the head and neck may be constricted in such a way as to predispose to thrombosis. The two vertebral arteries ascend from the base of the neck through the foramina in the transverse processes of the upper six vertebrae and wind behind the upper articular processes of the atlas to enter the cranial cavity through the foramen magnum (see Chapter 52). Disorders such as **cervical spondylosis**, a degenerative disease of the spine that affects the lower cervical vertebrae, may cause thickening of the bone and ligamentous structures, resulting in constriction of the vertebral arteries as they pass through this region (Tatlow and Bammer, 1957; Hardin et al., 1960; Sheehan et al., 1960; Brain, 1963; Hardin, 1963; Gorvai, 1964; Bakay and Leslie, 1965; Bala and Langford, 1967; Bauer, 1984; Chin, 1993; Rosengart et al., 1993). The constriction may be constant, or it may occur

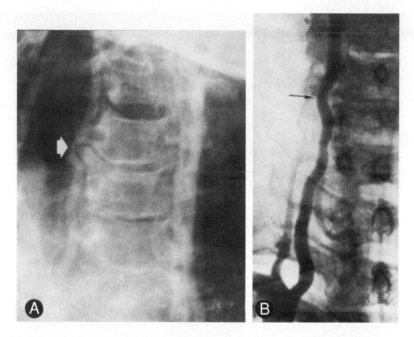

Figure 55.39. Constriction of the vertebral artery by cervical spine disease. *A*, The vertebral artery is significantly narrowed by a large osteophyte (*arrow*) in a patient with severe cervical spondylosis. *B*, The vertebral artery is displaced but not narrowed by a cervical osteophyte. In this patient, turning the head or chiropractic manipulation could cause occlusion of the artery. (From Huber P. Cerebral Angiography. 2nd ed. New York, Georg Thieme Verlag, 1982.)

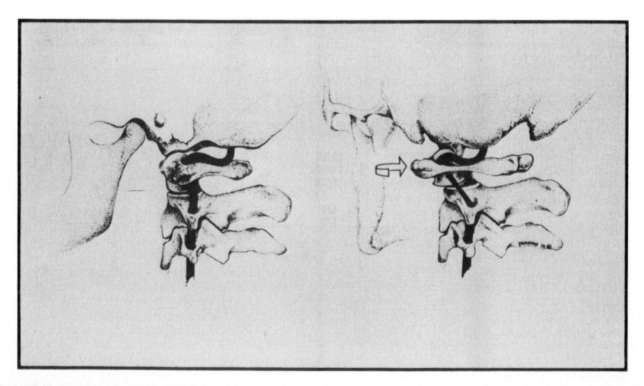

Figure 55.40. Schematic drawing of vertebral artery injury with abrupt cervical rotation. The vertebral artery is subject to stretch and mechanical trauma between C-1 and C-2 when the neck is vigorously rotated and extended. (From Barnett HJM. Progress towards stroke prevention. Neurology *30:*1212–1225, 1980.)

only when the patient's head is rotated in a certain manner (Fig. 55.39). Similar problems may occur in patients with other acquired and congenital abnormalities of the bones and ligaments through which the carotid and vertebral arteries pass in their respective courses (Coria et al., 1982; Bauer, 1984). Sell et al. (1994) reported a 44-year-old woman with episodes of transient blindness on turning her head, caused by extrinsic compression of a vertebral artery by a tight anterior scalene muscle. Chiropractic and other **manipulation** of the cervical region may also produce injury to the vertebral or carotid arterial wall, predisposing to thrombosis or embolism and to dissection, with subsequent thrombosis or embolism (see Chapter 53) (Blaine, 1925; Pratt-Thomas and Berger, 1947; Schwartz et al., 1956; Green and Joynt, 1959; Smith and Estridge, 1962; Pribek, 1963; Mehalic and Farhat, 1974; Sullivan et al., 1975; Frizoni and Anzola, 1990; Frumkin and Baloh, 1990; Lee et al., 1995; Peters et al., 1995; Jumper and Horton, 1996; Donzis and Factor, 1997) (Fig. 55.40).

Occlusion of the internal carotid artery, vertebral artery, or their branches occasionally may be used to treat aneurysms, fistulas, or other vascular abnormalities that are thought to pose a threat to the neurologic status of the patient and that cannot be treated in any other fashion (see Chapter 53). Occlusion of these vessels also may occur inadvertently during attempted treatment of vascular and other lesions. Whether inadvertent or premeditated, **iatrogenic** occlusion of any artery that is part of the carotid or vertebrobasilar system has a definite risk of producing stroke, death, or both (Landolt and Millikan, 1970) (Fig. 55.41).

Trauma may produce a hematoma that can constrict the common or internal carotid artery in the neck, and traumatic intracranial hematomas may rarely occlude adjacent intracranial vessels, thus adding to an already significant neurologic deficit. **Tumors** that arise in the neck and at the base of the brain may occlude or constrict arteries in these regions, producing thrombosis and stroke (Molsen, 1980; Spallone, 1981; Oppido et al., 1989) (Fig. 55.42). In particular, paragangliomas commonly compress the internal carotid artery in the neck or at its entrance into the skull (see Chapter 46), and patients who experience an acute stroke are found to have occlusion of the intracavernous portion of the internal carotid artery by an intracavernous meningioma or by a pituitary adenoma that has extended into the adjacent cavernous sinus (Salomez et al., 1981; Oppido et al., 1989; Schnur and Clar, 1989). Unruptured **aneurysms** occasionally com-

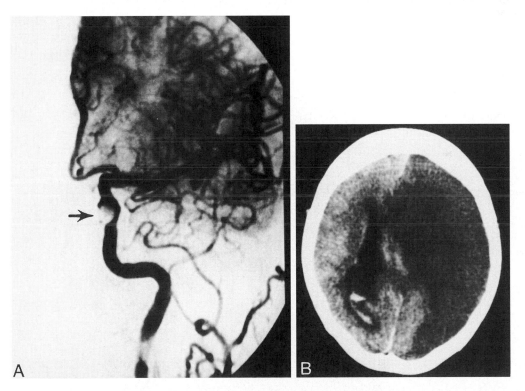

Figure 55.41. Iatrogenic occlusion of the internal carotid artery. The patient was a 56-year-old woman with a left-sided, direct carotid-cavernous sinus fistula that resulted from rupture of an intracavernous carotid aneurysm. Although the fistula was closed successfully with a detachable balloon, the balloon protruded into the left internal carotid artery. About 6 hours after the conclusion of the procedure, the patient developed a massive left hemisphere stroke consistent with occlusion of the left internal carotid artery. She died 3 days after the procedure. *A,* Left common carotid arteriogram, anteroposterior view, shows detachable balloon protruding into the lumen of the intracavernous portion of the left internal carotid artery (*arrow*). Although the artery is not occluded, there is substantial reduction in the size of the lumen. *B,* Unenhanced CT scan, axial view, performed after the patient developed clinical evidence of a stroke, shows massive hypointensity throughout most of the left cerebral hemisphere with a marked mass effect, consistent with a massive infarction in the territories of the left anterior and middle cerebral arteries. Note relative preservation of the medial left occipital lobe, indicating preservation of the territory of the posterior cerebral artery.

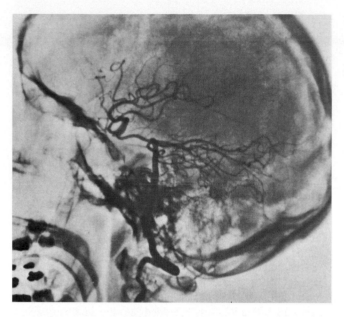

Figure 55.42. Occlusion of the internal carotid artery by a large cranio-pharyngioma. Brachial arteriogram shows complete occlusion of the internal carotid artery. The basilar artery is patent but is displaced posteriorly by the tumor. (From Huber P. Cerebral Angiography. 2nd ed. New York, Georg Thieme Verlag, 1982.)

press an adjacent normal vessel, producing thrombosis and subsequent neurologic dysfunction (Sato et al., 1990; see Chapter 53).

Local mechanical factors may also be responsible for retinal stroke, including preretinal arterial loops, meningeal carcinomatosis, and optic neuritis/perineuritis (Schaible and Golnik, 1993; Reichel et al., 1994; Winterkorn et al., 1994).

Increased intracranial pressure occasionally forces intracranial arteries against bony prominences or dural folds (Lindenberg, 1955) (Figs. 55.43 and 55.44). Compression of arteries may be particularly severe if ICP rises acutely and is accompanied by a dysfunction of the systemic cerebral circulation. Lindenberg (1955) performed an extensive pathologic study of 250 cases that macroscopically demonstrated alterations caused by vascular compression. He concluded that the individual arteries prone to be compressed and the locations at which compression occurred were:

1. The stem of the anterior cerebral artery where it turns around the caudal portion of the gyrus rectus and its branches where they pass the edge of the falx;
2. The stem of the middle cerebral artery where it turns around the insula and its branches where they pass through the caudal portion of the sylvian fissure;
3. The stem and cortical branches of the posterior cerebral artery where they run across the tentorial edge and its brainstem branches where they pass through the interpeduncular fossa (this probably is responsible for the devel-

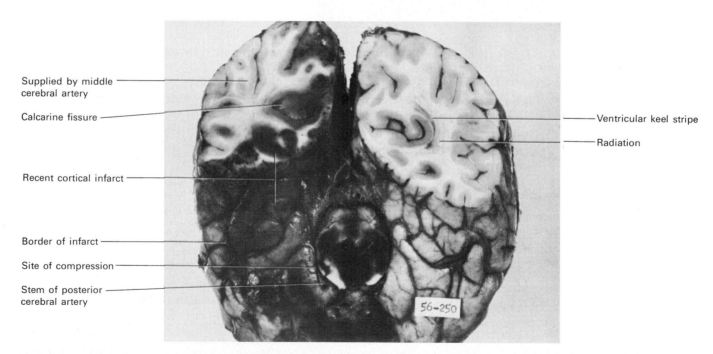

Figure 55.43. Infarction of the left posterior cerebral hemisphere and the brainstem from vascular compression caused by increased intracranial pressure. The patient was a woman who developed a subdural hematoma after trauma. Although the hematoma was removed, she died shortly thereafter. The lesions shown are secondary and are caused by vascular compression. The left uncus is markedly herniated, and it has compressed the stem of the adjacent posterior cerebral artery against the edge of the tentorium cerebelli, resulting in occlusion of the artery and hemorrhagic necrosis of the cortex throughout the region normally supplied by the artery. (From Lindenberg R, Walsh FB, Sacks JG. Neuropathology of Vision: An Atlas. Philadelphia, Lea & Febiger, 1973.)

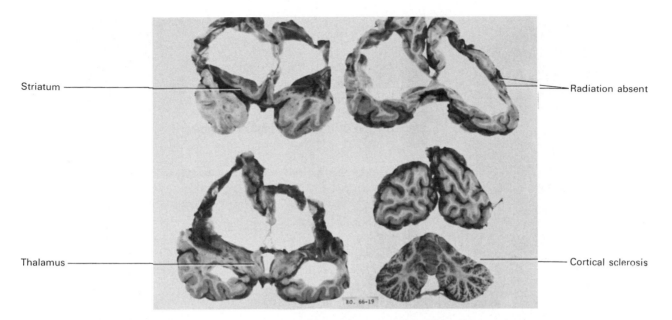

Striatum

Thalamus

Radiation absent

Cortical sclerosis

Figure 55.44. Cerebral atrophy from increased intracranial pressure after meningitis. The patient was a 9-year-old girl who developed marked increased intracranial pressure after meningitis caused by *Haemophilus influenzae*. The patient was cortically blind. She died during a seizure. The photographs show that both optic radiations have been destroyed as part of the severe loss of cortex and white matter in the supply territories of the anterior and middle cerebral arteries at the convexity of the brain. The tissues supplied by the posterior cerebral arteries and those bordering them are relatively well preserved. The basal ganglia and thalami are sclerotic. Bilateral atrophy of the cerebellar cortex also is the result of vascular compression. (From Lindenberg R, Walsh FB, Sacks JG. Neuropathology of Vision: An Atlas. Philadelphia, Lea & Febiger, 1973.)

opment of transient and permanent cortical blindness and homonymous hemianopia that occur in association with hydrocephalus, particularly after acute shunt malfunction—see Hoyt, 1960; Kojima et al., 1984; Tycheson and Hoyt, 1984);

4. The anterior choroidal artery and its branches where they are closest to the tentorial edge;
5. The intracranial portion of the internal carotid artery where it enters the cranium;
6. The superior cerebellar artery and its branches where they cross the lower aspect of the tentorial edge;
7. The posterior inferior cerebellar artery and its branches where they are closest to the posterior rim of the foramen magnum;
8. The paramedian branches that supply the middle pons where they branch off the basilar artery; and
9. The terminal branches of all cerebral and cerebellar arteries where they run through the sulci to supply the inner portions of the cortex.

HYPERCOAGULABILITY

A variety of **hematologic disorders** that are associated with a hypercoagulable state may predispose to thrombus formation (Hart and Kanter, 1990). Platelet, red blood cell, white blood cell, and serologic disorders all have the potential to cause thrombosis, although they do so by quite different mechanisms. In **leukemia**, patients with high white blood cell counts, usually greater than 100,000/mL, develop stasis and thrombosis in small arterioles and capillaries, resulting in microinfarcts. Patients with **absolute erythrocytosis** (e.g., polycythemia vera, erythroleukemia) and **essential thrombocythemia** (essential thrombocytosis) may develop visual and neurologic symptoms from the thrombotic effects of increased blood viscosity.

Ischemic stroke as a presenting manifestation of **essential thrombocythemia** is probably underrecognized (Jabaily et al., 1983; Benassi et al., 1989; Muller et al., 1990; Michiels et al., 1993; Arboix et al., 1995). Mundall et al. (1972a, 1972b) described a patient with essential thrombocythemia whose major symptom was recurrent, transient, monocular visual loss. The patient had a platelet count that ranged from 400,000 to over 1 million. Of the 17 patients with primary thrombocythemia described by Michiels and colleagues (1993), four patients complained of scintillating scotomas, and two patients had sudden episodes of transient monocular visual loss. Other patients have abnormal platelet aggregability that may predispose to thrombosis, even when the absolute platelet count is normal.

Polycythemia can cause stroke in both neonates (Clancy et al., 1985; Golden, 1985) and adults (Chievitz and Thiede, 1962; Silverstein et al., 1962; Kremer et al., 1972; Hoyt, 1978) (Fig. 55.45). Most cases of polycythemia are idiopathic or are caused by nongenetic abnormalities of oxygen delivery, but some cases seem to be transmitted in an autosomal-dominant or autosomal-recessive fashion (Natowicz and Kelley, 1987).

It has already been emphasized that patients with **hemoglobinopathies**, such as sickle cell disease, may experience ischemic (and hemorrhagic) stroke. Although it is clear that

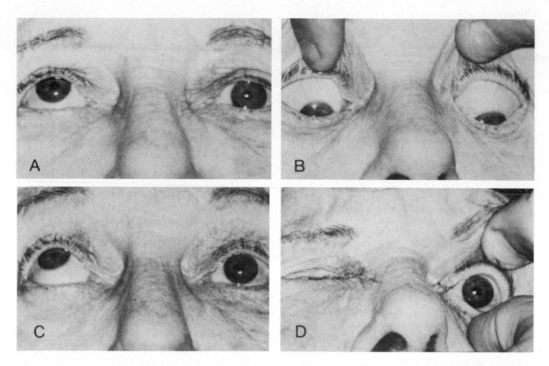

Figure 55.45. Double elevator palsy from mesencephalic stroke in a patient with polycythemia vera. *A,* When patient fixes with the paretic left eye, there is a 30 prism diopter right hypertropia. *B,* In downgaze, there is no significant paresis or ocular misalignment. *C,* On attempted upgaze, there is marked limitation of the left eye. *D,* The left eye shows no Bell's phenomenon. (From Hoyt CS. Acquired ''double elevator'' palsy and polycythemia vera. J Pediatr Ophthalmol Strabismus *15:*362–365, 1978.)

the mechanism for thrombosis in such patients is primarily an alteration in the wall of affected vessels, at least some patients develop neurologic symptoms and signs from simple thrombosis of small vessels because of sickled erythrocytes.

Some patients have congenital or acquired deficits in one or more of the plasma proteins or other substances that regulate coagulation, such as protein S, protein C, and antithrombin III, natural inhibitors of coagulation (Stenflo, 1976; Coller et al., 1987; Smith and Ens, 1987; Nelson et al., 1989; Sacco et al., 1989b; Ernerudh et al., 1990; Golub et al., 1990; Hart and Kanter, 1990; Kohler et al., 1990; Camerlingo et al., 1991; Barinagarrementeria et al., 1994; Schafer, 1994; Rees et al., 1995; Simioni et al., 1995; Vignes et al., 1996). The deficiencies may be quantitative or qualitative, making diagnostic assay occasionally problematic. These disorders most frequently cause venous clotting, such as deep vein thrombosis, but arterial occlusions may also occur. Abnormalities of the hemostatic system probably account for 15–28% of unexplained systemic vascular thrombosis in young patients, and this may manifest as retinal arterial occlusion (Golub et al., 1990; Greven et al., 1991; Vine and Samama, 1993; Vignes et al., 1996). In one study of 50 patients with stroke younger than 45 years of age, three patients had inherited protein C deficiency (Camerlingo, 1991). In another study of 36 patients under the age of 40 with cerebral infarction of undetermined cause, nine patients (25%) had a deficiency of one natural anticoagulant, most frequently protein S (six cases) (Barinagarrementeria et al.,

1994). Deficiencies of protein C, antithrombin III, and plasminogen were noted in one patient each. Combined deficiencies of coagulant inhibitors in the same patient may increase the risk for cerebral ischemia (Koller et al., 1994). Resistance to activated protein C is the most frequently found laboratory abnormality in patients with idiopathic deep vein thrombosis. It appears to be caused by an inherited mutation in the gene coding for coagulation factor V (so-called Factor V Leiden). Although heterozygosity for this factor is quite common, it is not usually considered a factor in cerebral ischemia (Greengard et al., 1994; Forsyth and Dolan, 1995; Rees et al., 1995; Ridker et al., 1995; Larsson et al., 1996; Press et al., 1996; but also see Halbmayer et al., 1994). However, a propensity for venous thrombosis combined with a patent foramen ovale (PFO) might increase the risk of right-to-left shunting and cerebral embolism (see below). Whether or not additional vascular risk factors, such as cigarette use or oral contraceptives in combination with coagulant inhibitor deficiencies, also predispose to increased stroke risk is unknown.

Elevated levels of factor VIII may contribute to hypercoagulability and brain ischemia (Kosik and Furie, 1980). Indeed, increased factor VIII activity likely contributes to the ischemic neurologic deficits associated with **inflammatory bowel disease**, particularly ulcerative colitis and regional enteritis (Hogan et al., 1957; Kehoe and Newcomber, 1964; Silverstein and Present, 1971; Mayeux and Fahn, 1978; Schneiderman et al., 1979; Heuer et al., 1982; Duker et al., 1987; Johns, 1991; Keyser and Hass, 1994; Lossos et al.,

1995). Affected patients may develop CRAO, recurrent retinal branch artery occlusion, ION, cerebral thromboembolism, cerebral venous thrombosis, transient brainstem ischemia, massive cerebral and brainstem infarction, or a combination of these phenomena. The cause of the cerebral and retinal vascular complications of inflammatory bowel disease is thought to be a hypercoagulable state characterized by thrombocytosis, short partial thromboplastin time, and elevated serum fibrinogen and factor VIII concentrations. Platelet counts and coagulation factors become normal in some patients when the intestinal inflammation is successfully treated (Schneiderman et al., 1979).

Patients with systemic **cancer** may develop a hypercoagulable syndrome, resulting in systemic and cerebral infarctions. In most cases, the syndrome is caused by disseminated intravascular coagulation (DIC) characterized by thrombocytopenia, a reduction in fibrinogen, and a decrease in the prothrombin time. The proportion of patients with malignancy-related DIC who develop neurologic complications is about 15% (Schwartzman and Hill, 1982) (Figs. 55.46 and 55.47). Lymphomas, leukemias (particularly acute promyelocytic leukemia), and adenocarcinomas are the neoplasms most often described in these patients (Collins et al., 1975; Schwartzman and Hill, 1982; Morimatsu et al., 1985). Paraneoplastic marantic endocarditis may produce stroke in patients with mucin-secreting adenocarcinomas and lymphomas (Biller et al., 1982) (Figs. 55.48 and 55.49). Mucin-secreting adenocarcinomas also may produce a clinical picture of stroke or encephalopathy, characterized pathologically by occlusion of large, medium-sized, and microscopic arteries with resultant cerebral infarction (Amico et al., 1989). In such cases, widespread intravascular mucin pre-

sumably produces a hypercoagulable state. Patients with one of the **paraproteinemias** (e.g., multiple myeloma; Waldenström's macroglobulinemia) may experience ischemic or hemorrhagic strokes from the effects of increased blood viscosity from increased serum proteins (see Chapter 45). Paraneoplastic thromboembolic disorders are discussed in Chapter 47 of this text.

The use of **oral contraceptive agents** is associated with an increased risk of thrombotic cerebrovascular and ocular disease (Walsh et al., 1965; Shafey and Scheinberg, 1966; Anderson and Martin, 1969; Nicholson and Walsh, 1969; Sartwell et al., 1969; Vessey and Doll, 1969; Davidson, 1971; Collaborative Group for the Study of Stroke in Young Women, 1973, 1975; Gombos et al., 1975; Trux et al., 1976; Varga, 1976; Jick et al., 1978; Stowe et al., 1978; Royal College of General Practitioners' Oral Contraceptive Study, 1981; Vessey et al., 1984; Xuereb and Pullicino, 1988; Norris, 1989; Pullicino and Xuereb, 1989; Hannaford et al., 1994; Spitzer et al., 1996) (Fig. 55.50). The most common vessels affected are the internal carotid artery at its siphon, the origin of the middle cerebral artery, and the distal extracranial portion of the vertebral artery (Bickerstaff, 1975) (Fig. 55.51). Among women with stroke or transient monocular visual loss, independent risk factors include smoking, social class, hypertension, and oral contraceptive use, with the detrimental effect of oral contraceptives persisting in former users who continue to smoke (Hannaford et al., 1994). A population-based, case-control study in the United States looked specifically at the risk of stroke in women using low-estrogen oral contraceptives (Petitti et al., 1996). Stroke was rare, and the authors concluded that oral contraceptives that contain low amounts of estrogen are generally

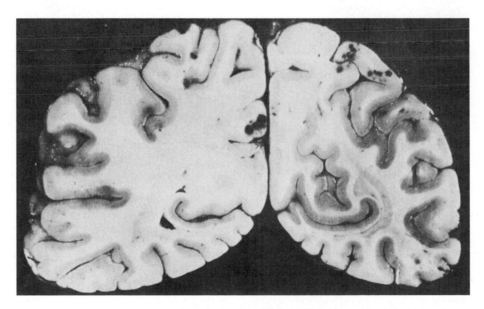

Figure 55.46. Neurologic complications of paraneoplastic disseminated intravascular coagulopathy (DIC). The patient was a 54-year-old woman with carcinoma of the breast who developed seizures and delirium before death. Coronal section through the occipital lobes shows scattered small hemorrhages in the cortex and white matter. Similar lesions were present throughout the cerebral and cerebellar hemispheres. (From Collins RC, Al-Mondhiry H, Chernik NL, et al. Neurologic manifestations of intravascular coagulation in patients with cancer: A clinicopathologic analysis of 12 cases. Neurology 25:795–806, 1975.)

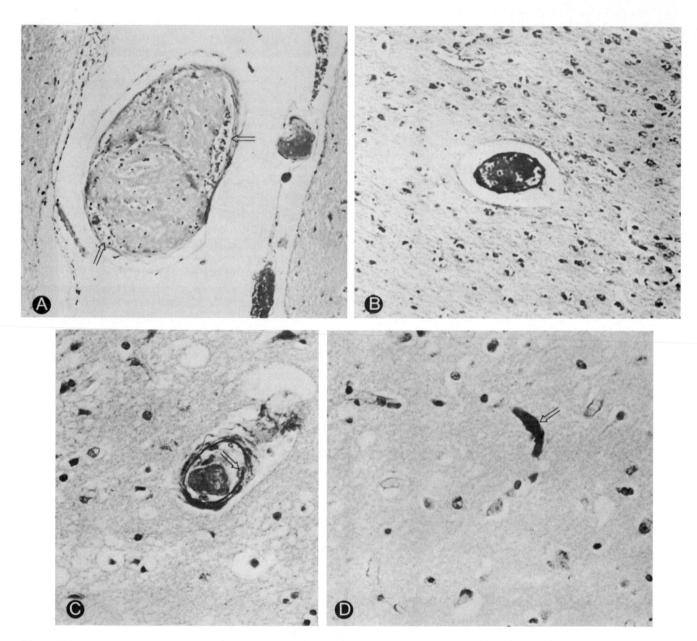

Figure 55.47. Histopathologic appearance of intracranial vessels in patients with paraneoplastic disseminated intravascular coagulopathy (DIC). *A*, A thrombosed meningeal vein shows peripheral recanalization (*arrows*). *B*, Thrombosis of a medium-sized penetrating vein with fragmentation and rarefaction of adjacent tissue. *C*, A small penetrating artery contains thrombotic material filling only the central portion of the lumen. There is moderate endothelial swelling (*arrow*). Surrounding tissue shows vacuolization and fragmentation. *D*, Distended, thrombosed capillary (*arrow*) is seen in longitudinal section. (From Collins RC, Al-Mondhiry H, Chernik NL, et al. Neurologic manifestations of intravascular coagulation in patients with cancer: A clinicopathologic analysis of 12 cases. Neurology *25:*795–806, 1975.)

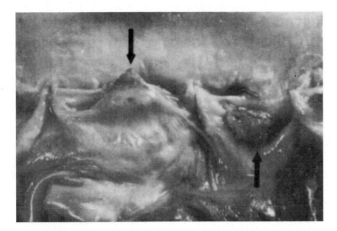

Figure 55.48. Paraneoplastic nonbacterial thrombotic (marantic) endocarditis. Aortic valve shows large, friable, polypoid vegetations (*arrows*). These vegetations are large and more friable than rheumatic vegetations, and they are not confined to the contact edges of the leaflets of the valve. (From Biller J, Challa VR, Toole JF, et al. Nonbacterial thrombotic endocarditis: A neurologic perspective of clinicopathologic correlations of 99 patients. Arch Neurol *39:*95–98, 1982.)

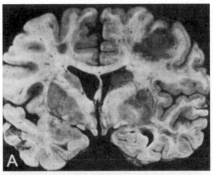
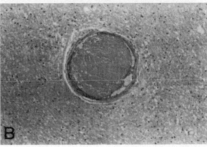

Figure 55.49. Paraneoplastic nonbacterial thrombotic (marantic) endocarditis. *A,* Coronal section through the brain of a patient who died of neurologic complications from the disease shows recent infarction in the left insular cortex, left central white matter, and right parietal lobe. *B,* Small arteriole in affected white matter is occluded and distended by embolic material. The surrounding white matter is edematous. (From Biller J, Challa VR, Toole JF, et al. Nonbacterial thrombotic endocarditis: A neurologic perspective of clinicopathologic correlations of 99 patients. Arch Neurol *39:*95–98, 1982.)

safe with respect to the risk of stroke. It should be noted, however, that other risk factors for stroke, especially smoking, increased the risk of stroke in these women. Similar results were reported in an international, multicenter, case-control study of the risk of ischemic stroke in women using combined oral contraceptives (WHO Collaborative Study of

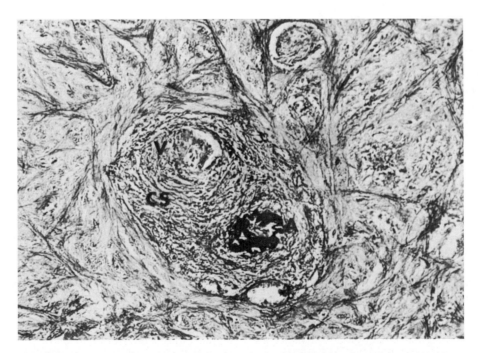

Figure 55.50. Central retinal artery and vein occlusion in a 40-year-old woman who was taking oral contraceptives at the time of loss of vision. The patient had no other risk factors for vascular occlusive disease, and a systemic evaluation disclosed no other explanation for the process. *A,* Central retinal artery; *V,* central retinal vein; *CS,* common sheath enclosing the artery and vein. (From Stowe GC III, Zakov ZN, Albert DM. Central retinal vascular occlusion associated with oral contraceptives. Am J Ophthalmol *86:*798–801, 1978.)

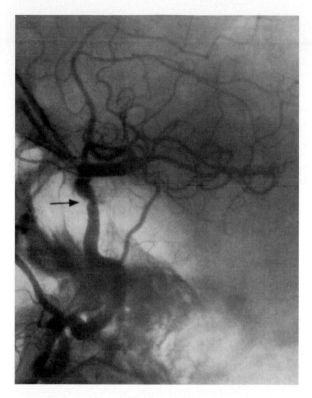

Figure 55.51. Severe stenosis of the internal carotid artery at the sinus (*arrow*) in a young woman who developed transient ischemic attacks consisting of monocular visual loss and contralateral hemiparesis. The patient had no risk factors for cerebrovascular occlusive disease except that she had been taking oral contraceptives for 10 years.

Cardiovascular Disease and Steroid Hormone Contraception, 1996a). The overall odds ratio of ischemic stroke was 2.99 in Europe, with the risk being lower in persons under age 35 years, in nonsmokers, in patients without hypertension, and in women using oral contraceptive preparations containing low doses of estrogen. Although the exact mechanism by which oral contraceptives predispose to thrombotic stroke is unclear, it may be related to hypercoagulability (Caplan, 1993).

Hypercoagulability may also be responsible for thrombotic strokes that occur during **pregnancy** (Chancellor et al., 1989; Wiebers, 1985). It is claimed that pregancy increases the risk of focal ischemic cerebrovascular events about 13 times the expected rate for age (Wiebers, 1985); however, this high frequency may result from a selection bias and the lack of precise diagnosis (Grosset et al., 1995; Sharshar et al., 1995). Initial investigations suggested that most of these strokes were the result of arterial occlusions that occurred primarily during the 2nd and 3rd trimesters of pregnancy and the 1st week after delivery (Wiebers, 1985); however, a subsequent population-based study concluded that the risks of both cerebral infarction and intracerebral hemorrhage are increased in the 6 weeks after delivery, but not during pregnancy itself (Kittner et al., 1996).

Persons who abuse **anabolic steroids** or who undergo **estrogen therapy** for infertility or gender identity disorders

may be at risk for cerebrovascular thrombosis. The mechanism may be hypercoagulability (Akhter et al., 1994; Biller and Saver, 1995; Pálfi et al., 1997).

Abnormalities of the body's normal fibrinolytic system may predispose to thrombosis (Hart, 1990; Caplan, 1993). Abnormalities of tissue plasminogen activator or its inhibitors, plasminogen deficiencies, and dysfibrinogenemias can all increase the tendency for thrombus formation.

In an earlier section of this chapter, we emphasized that patients with various types of vasculitis, particularly the connective tissue diseases and the Churg-Strauss syndrome, may develop cerebral and ocular ischemia that is caused in most cases not by the direct effects of the vasculitis but by thromboembolic phenomena related to a hypercoagulable state (Trevor et al., 1972; Hart et al., 1984; Dagi and Currie, 1985).

MISCELLANEOUS VASCULOPATHIES

Patients with an increased concentration of **antiphospholipid antibodies** in the serum have an increased risk of thrombotic and embolic neurologic, visual, and systemic events (Frohman et al., 1989; Shuaib and Barcley, 1989; Brey et al., 1990; Coull and Goodnight, 1990; Gerber and Cantor, 1990; Kushner, 1990; Levine et al., 1990a; The Antiphospholipid Antibodies in Stroke Study Group, 1990; Valesini et al., 1990; DeWitt and Caplan, 1991; Montalban et al., 1991; Pope et al., 1991; Canoso, 1993; The Antiphospholipid Antibodies in Stroke Study (APASS) Group, 1993; Hartnett et al., 1994; Feldmann and Levine, 1995; Levine et al., 1995; The Antiphospholipid Antibodies in Stroke Study Group, 1997; Weichens et al., 1997). These circulating antibodies include the lupus anticoagulant and anticardiolipin antibodies. Clinical manifestations include thrombophlebitis, pulmonary embolism, migraine, miscarriages, venous thrombosis, and arterial occlusions. The mechanism of increased coagulability and thrombosis is unclear but is probably related in part to immune-mediated damage to endothelium. Patients may also have cardiac valvular vegetations similar to Libman-Sachs endocarditis (Young et al., 1989). Some of these patients have other findings diagnostic of SLE, but the majority have the primary antiphospholipid antibody syndrome, without other evidence of systemic disease. The higher the immunoglobulin (Ig) G anticardiolipin titers, the greater the risk of recurrent thrombo-occlusive events (Levine et al., 1995; The Antiphospholipid Antibodies in Stroke Study Group, 1997). The presence of antiphospholipid antibodies is the most frequently identified abnormal hematologic factor in patients with retinal vascular occlusion (Castanon et al., 1995). All patients younger than 45 years of age with a history of thromboembolic events should be hematologically screened, especially if they have other manifestations of the syndrome, including migraines, miscarriages, or splinter hemorrhages of the nail beds (Digre et al., 1989). Anticardiolipin antibodies may be an independent risk factor for ischemic stroke even in older patients, especially when present in high titers (The APASS Group, 1993). However, in a prospective controlled study of 262 unselected patients with acute stroke, Muir et al. (1994)

found no evidence to support the hypothesis that anticardio-lipin antibodies are an independent risk factor for stroke in young patients. Interestingly, they did find that a higher titer of IgG anticardiolipin antibodies among older patients with stroke correlated with the number of vascular risk factors, suggesting that in some patients, anticardiolipin antibodies is a nonspecific marker of vascular disease. Empiric treatment of the antiphospholipid antibody syndrome includes antiplatelet agents, anticoagulants, and immunosuppressants (Feldmann and Levine, 1995). In a study of 147 patients with the antiphospholipid antibody syndrome, Khamashta et al. (1995) determined that treatment with high-intensity warfarin (normalized ratio of 3) with or without low-dose aspirin (75 mg per day) was significantly more effective than treatment with low-intensity warfarin with or without low-dose aspirin or treatment with aspirin alone in preventing further thrombotic events.

Sneddon's syndrome is a progressive, noninflammatory, occlusive arteriopathy of medium-sized vessels that is characterized by idiopathic livedo reticularis and stroke (Sneddon, 1965; Bruyn et al., 1987; Geschwind et al., 1995; Sitzer et al., 1995; Tourbah et al., 1997). The disorder occasionally is familial and may be transmitted in an autosomal-dominant fashion (Rebollo et al., 1983; Ascott and Boyle, 1986). Geschwind et al. (1995) reported the pathologic findings from a brain biopsy and concluded that Sneddon's syndrome is not a vasculitis but an autoimmune vasculopathy like the antiphospholipid antibody syndrome, with an immune-mediated prothrombotic state that facilitates the formation of arterial thrombi, causing in situ thrombosis of cerebral vessels, cerebral embolism, or both (Sitzer et al., 1995). Kalashnikova et al. (1990) detected a high concentration of anticardiolipin antibodies in six of 17 patients with Sneddon's syndrome. They suggested that the similarity of clinical symptoms and immunologic disturbances between Sneddon's syndrome and the antiphospholipid syndrome may indicate a common pathogenesis in at least some cases (Martinez-Menendez et al., 1990). Tourbah et al. (1997) found antiphospholipid antibodies in 11 of 26 patients with Sneddon's syndrome, but there was no difference in disease severity among patients with and without these antibodies. After evaluating the location and severity of infarction with magnetic resonance (MR) imaging, these investigators concluded that the vascular territories that are first affected in Sneddon's syndrome seem to be the end-perfusion territories of the cortical arteries, suggesting a hypercoagulable state.

Cerebral autosomal-dominant arteriopathy with subcortical infarcts and leukoencephalopathy (**CADASIL**) is an inherited disease of the small arteries of the brain occurring in mid-adulthood (Tournier-Lasserve et al., 1991; Chabriat et al., 1995, 1996; Ducros et al., 1996). CADASIL is characterized by recurrent subcortical ischemic events in patients in the 5th decade of life, leading to dementia and, in a third of patients, death, about 20 years after the first symptoms. Subcortical dementia is associated with frontal symptoms, a pseudobulbar syndrome, gait difficulties, and incontinence. Other frequent symptoms include early attacks of migraine with aura in 22% of patients and severe mood disorders with depressive or manic episodes after the onset of cerebral

ischemia in 20% of cases. Most patients have no vascular risk factors. All symptomatic patients have prominent signal abnormalities on MR imaging, with hyperintense lesions on T2-weighted images, typical of small deep infarctions in the white matter and basal ganglia. These signal abnormalities are sometimes noted in asymptomatic persons with an affected parent and probably antedate the clinical symptoms by about 15 years. Pathologically, there is a widespread vasculopathy affecting the leptomeningeal and perforating arteries of the brain, distinct from atherosclerotic and amyloid angiopathies. The arterial media is thickened by an eosinophilic granular and electron-dense material of unknown origin (Baudrimont et al., 1993). Similar abnormalities are present within the vessels of muscle and skin biopsies of patients with CADASIL (Ruchoux et al., 1995). CADASIL is transmitted with an autosomal-dominant pattern of inheritance, with penetrance usually complete between 30 and 40 years of age (Chabriat et al., 1995). The CADASIL gene, which has been characterized (Joutel et al., 1996), is located on the short arm of chromosome 19 (Tournier-Lasserve et al., 1993). There are at least 50 families with CADASIL, but the exact frequency of the disease is unknown. Sporadic cases of CADASIL also occur. The disease thus should be suspected in patients with recurrent subcortical infarctions leading to dementia, and in patients with TIAs, migraine with aura, or severe mood disorders in whom MR imaging discloses widespread signal abnormalities in the subcortical white matter and basal ganglia.

DRUG ABUSE

Thrombotic ischemic stroke can occur in drug abusers (Kaku and Lowenstein, 1990). In **heroin** addicts, strokes are invariably ischemic and frequently follow the reintroduction of intravenous heroin after a period of abstention (Woods and Strewler, 1972; Brust and Richter, 1976; Caplan et al., 1982a; Caplan, 1993). In such patients, symptoms and signs of cerebral ischemia may develop immediately after injection but more often occur about 6–24 hours later. Heroin addicts also have a number of serologic and systemic abnormalities, including eosinophilia, elevated immune and gamma globulins, false-positive syphilis serology, Coombs-positive hemolysis, and lymph node hypertrophy (Caplan et al., 1982a). In addition, heroin often is adulterated with various fillers and foreign substances. It seems most likely that the cerebral ischemia that occurs in abusers of heroin results from immune complex deposition or other hyperimmune mechanisms triggered by chronic or periodically introduced unusual antigens.

Necrotizing angiitis may develop in patients who chronically abuse **amphetamines**. The lesions of this disorder resemble those of polyarteritis nodosa (see Chapter 57). Angiography shows segmental changes in intracerebral vessels with prominent beading (Rumbaugh et al., 1971a) (Fig. 55.52). Most patients in whom amphetamine-induced necrotizing angiitis occurs experience intracerebral hemorrhage (Yu et al., 1983), but they also may develop cerebral ischemia (Rothrock et al., 1988b).

Cocaine may produce ischemic stroke (see Table 2 in

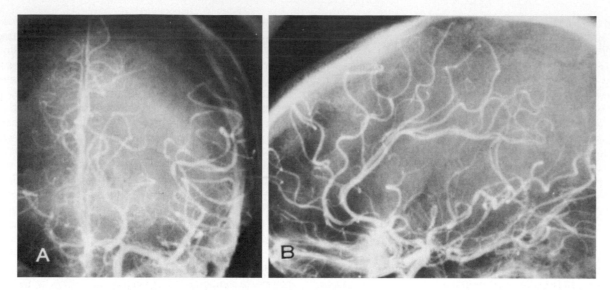

Figure 55.52. Segmental spasm and beading of intracranial arteries in a 20-year-old abuser of amphetamines who developed acute right hemiparesis and aphasia. She then became obtunded. *A* and *B*, Left internal carotid arteriogram shows marked segmental spasm of many branches of the intracranial arteries, particularly those of the middle cerebral artery. The patient improved after withdrawal of drugs. (From Taveras JM, Wood EH. Diagnostic Neuroradiology. Vol 2. Baltimore, Williams & Wilkins, 1976.)

Klonoff et al., 1989; Krendel et al., 1990; Levine et al., 1990b; Daras et al., 1991; Levine et al., 1991; Fessler et al., 1997), although its use is more often associated with hemorrhagic stroke (Klonoff et al., 1989; Green et al., 1990; Nolte et al., 1996; Fessler et al., 1997). Libman et al. (1993) reported a 40-year-old woman with habitual intranasal cocaine abuse, who experienced multiple episodes of transient monocular visual loss. During a witnessed episode, she developed a relative afferent pupillary defect (RAPD) and had diffuse severe narrowing of the retinal arterioles, leading the authors to postulate a vasospastic mechanism. Cocaine-induced stroke may occur after any route of administration, including inhalation, intranasal, intravenous, and intramuscular routes (Fessler et al., 1997). Smoking crack cocaine is associated with the highest frequency of brain infarction. Strokes associated with cocaine use may be caused by cerebral vasculitis (Kaye and Fainstat, 1987; Krendel et al., 1990), by hypertension resulting from vasoconstriction with a secondary increase in blood pressure and cardiac output, by local cerebrovascular vasoconstriction, or by increased endovascular synthesis of thromboxane with platelet aggregation (Klonoff et al., 1989; Levine et al., 1990b; Konzen et al., 1995; Martinez et al., 1996; Fessler et al., 1997).

Patients who intravenously inject substances synthesized for oral use may develop an obliterative arteritis from the effects of the **fillers** added to the drugs to maintain them in pill form. Common fillers include talc and microcrystalline cellulose. When a pill such as methylphenidate (Ritalin) or Talwin with pyribenzamine is ground into powder, dissolved in water, and injected intravenously or intra-arterially, particles may be trapped by lung arterioles and other small arteries, producing an obliterative arteritis (Szwed, 1970; Caplan et al., 1982b). Pulmonary arteriovenous shunts develop and are probably the pathway by which particles reach the intra-

cranial and intraocular arteries, producing blindness, visual field loss, seizures, and stroke (Atlee, 1972; Caplan et al., 1982b).

In addition to the mechanisms described above, patients who abuse drugs may develop a variety of infectious and inflammatory systemic disorders, including hepatitis, bacterial and fungal infections, and acquired immunodeficiency syndrome (AIDS), many of which can produce thrombotic ischemic cerebrovascular disease.

Embolism

General Considerations

An **embolus** (from the Greek, *embolos,* a wedge or stopper) is a piece of material that lodges in a blood vessel and blocks the flow of blood. In contrast to a thrombus, an embolus is not caused by a localized process originating within the vessel but rather has formed elsewhere. Emboli arise proximal to the vessel in which they lodge.

Embolism is responsible for 15–30% of ischemic strokes (Mohr et al., 1978; Kunitz et al., 1984; Cerebral Embolism Task Force, 1986a, 1986b, 1989; Brickner, 1996). Embolism is particularly important as an underlying cause of stroke in young adults (Lisovoski and Rousseaux, 1991). The most common sources of cerebral and ocular emboli are the heart, the major arteries, and the veins (Caplan et al., 1983; Caplan, 1993) (Table 55.1). Caplan (1993) cogently argued that the treatment of brain embolism should depend on the nature of the embolic material, if discoverable or predictable, and not on the particular source (i.e., a cardiac or intra-arterial origin). Hence, the appearance of emboli may not only provide important information as to the origin of the embolic material but may also guide therapy.

Emboli may be composed of clotted blood, fibrin, plate-

Table 55.1
Causes of Cerebral Embolism

I. Cardiac origin
  A. Arrhythmia
  B. Myocardial infarction with mural thrombus
  C. Infective endocarditis (acute and subacute)
  D. Noninfective thrombotic (marantic) endocardial vegetations
  E. Cardiomyopathy
  F. Cardiac valvular disease
    1. Stenosis
    2. Regurgitation
    3. Mitral valve prolapse (Barlow's syndrome)
    4. Prosthetic valves
  G. Congenital heart abnormalities (venous thrombosis with paradoxical embolus)
  H. Iatrogenic
    1. Cardiac catheterization
    2. Cardiac surgery
II. Noncardiac origin
  A. Arteriosclerosis
    1. Monckeberg's focal calcific arteriosclerosis
    2. Atherosclerosis
      a. Aorta
      b. Extracranial carotid arteries
      c. Extracranial vertebral arteries
      d. Intracranial arteries
  B. Arterial Dissection
    1. Extracranial carotid or vertebral arteries
    2. Intracranial arteries
  C. Pulmonary vein thrombosis
  D. Miscellaneous
    1. Fat
    2. Tumor
    3. Air
    4. Aneurysm with secondary thrombus formation
    5. Iatrogenic (neck and thoracic surgery)
    6. Undetermined

lets, atheromatous tissue, cholesterol crystals, calcium, organisms (e.g., bacteria, fungi), air, fat, tumor cells, or foreign material. They usually lodge at the bifurcation of a vessel, but they may stop at any location.

Appearance of Emboli

Emboli not infrequently travel to and lodge within retinal vessels. Because the retinal vessels can be seen with an ophthalmoscope, emboli within them, many of which have a distinctive appearance, can be detected (Hoyt, 1972; Arruga and Sanders, 1982; Ellenberger and Epstein, 1986; Miller, 1996; Mitchell et al., 1997). The most common emboli that travel to the retinal arterial circulation are cholesterol emboli, platelet-fibrin emboli, and emboli composed of calcium. Less common varieties of retinal emboli include tumor emboli from cardiac myxoma and metastatic neoplasms, fat emboli from fractures of long bones, septic emboli, talc emboli, and miscellaneous emboli of depotdrugs, silicone, or air that occur after injections in the region of the face or scalp (Hollenhorst, 1976).

CHOLESTEROL EMBOLI (HOLLENHORST PLAQUES)

Witmer and Schmid (1958) described what they thought were **cholesterol** emboli in retinal arterioles, but Hollenhorst (1961) first recognized and stressed the significance of these plaques in retinal arterioles of patients with atherosclerotic disease. Unlike the white appearance of platelet-fibrin emboli, the particles described by Hollenhorst (1961) had a bright, glistening, yellow or orange appearance, particularly when the light of the ophthalmoscope was shined slightly away from them (Fig. 55.53). Also, unlike platelet-fibrin emboli, these particles did not seem to block the flow of blood within affected vessels. Hollenhorst (1961) observed these bright plaques in patients with thrombosis of the carotid arterial system, both before and after endarterectomy. In some patients, they changed position and moved peripherally through the retinal vessels. In others, they seemed stationary, but pressure on the eye caused them to move within the vessel, to change color, and, occasionally, to fragment, move distally, and disappear. Hollenhorst (1961) concluded that these plaques were cholesterol crystals that arose from ulcerating atheromatous plaques in the aorta or carotid arteries. He removed the material from such a lesion at autopsy, stirred it with blood, and found that flakes of cholesterol floated to the top of the fluid. When this material was injected into the common carotid artery of a dog, it appeared in the retinal arterioles, and its appearance in these vessels was similar to that of the glistening plaques in humans.

Both Hollenhorst (1961) and Ross Russell (1961) described patients with transient loss of vision in one eye associated with the appearance of cholesterol emboli in retinal vessels. David et al. (1963) examined the eyes from a 67-year-old man who died after a stroke that followed surgery for carotid thrombosis. Before death, at least six "shiny copper-yellow" plaques were seen at bifurcations of the retinal arteries in the left eye (Fig. 55.54). The "brilliant reflection" of these plaques was "particularly apparent when the eye moved slightly or was being compressed." Microchemical analysis proved that the retinal emboli were composed of cholesterol, neutral fat, phospholipid, glycolipid, and calcium. An embolus in the middle cerebral artery was composed of similar material. The source of these emboli was thought to be an atheromatous plaque located at the bifurcation of the ipsilateral common carotid artery.

Irefin and Selhorst (1988) described two patients in whom diagnostic manual manipulation of an atheromatous internal carotid artery was followed by loss of vision in the ipsilateral eye and the appearance of previously unobserved "bright yellow" emboli in several of the retinal arterioles. One of the patients subsequently underwent surgery during which the common carotid artery was ligated and a segment of the diseased wall removed. Microscopic analysis of the excised segment demonstrated a large atheromatous plaque.

From these and other reports, it is clear that cholesterol emboli have a distinctive ophthalmoscopic appearance. They are yellow, orange, or copper-colored refractile structures that are globular or rectangular in shape (Arruga and Sanders, 1982; Younge, 1989; Miller, 1996), with the appearance changing somewhat, depending on the direction of the oph-

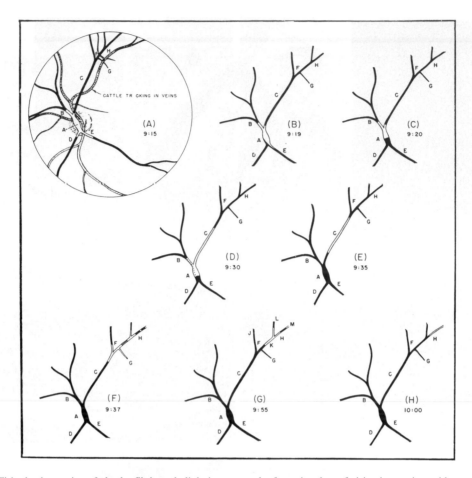

Figure 55.58. CM Fisher's observation of platelet-fibrin emboli during an attack of transient loss of vision in a patient with carotid stenosis. The attack began at 8:55 AM. *A,* Observation of the fundus began at 9:15 AM when the patient had no vision in the eye except for a superior temporal quadrant. A white segment occupied the main stem of the artery. The upper retinal veins contained interrupted segments of blood. *B,* At 9:19 AM, the inferior arterioles had cleared. *C,* One minute later, the patient reported return of vision in the upper half of the visual field. *D,* At 9:30 AM, the white segment moved upward in the retinal branches, and trickles of blood passed through the segment AB. *E,* At 9:35 AM, the patient could see in the inferior temporal visual field of the eye. *F–H,* Over the next 23 minutes, the embolus gradually moved more distally in the superior temporal arteriole, and vision gradually returned to normal. *A–M,* Specific segments of the retinal arterioles. (From Fisher CM. Observations of the fundus oculi in transient monocular blindness. Neurology *9:*333–347, 1959.)

partial or total blindness of the left eye that usually occurred once or twice a day. A left carotid arteriogram showed marked stenosis at the bifurcation of the left common carotid artery. During each of two attacks observed by Fisher (1959a), a long white mass slowly passed through the retinal arteries, became temporarily impacted at bifurcations, and then passed on, gradually fragmenting (Fig. 55.58). Adjacent veins showed "cattle tracking" when the blood column was arrested.

Ross Russell (1961) observed particles similar to those observed by Fisher (1959a) in one eye of a patient with thrombosis of the ipsilateral internal carotid artery. The artery was explored, and a thrombus, composed of fibrin and platelets and extending to the origin of the ophthalmic artery, was removed.

Ashby et al. (1963) successfully photographed white emboli in a patient who was experiencing recurrent, unilateral visual loss in the setting of thrombosis of the ipsilateral inter-

nal carotid artery. The initial photographs showed a white plug occluding the initial bifurcation of the central retinal artery at the optic disc (Fig. 55.59). The embolus remained in this location for 3–4 minutes, then suddenly began to move through the retinal arteries toward the periphery. At this time, the retinal arteries and veins, which had previously seemed narrow, dilated. Ashby et al. (1963) suggested that the embolus initially blocked flow in the retinal arterial system, resulting in hypoxic changes in the retinal arterial walls. The changes caused vascular dilation, allowing the embolus to move distally, which eliminated the vascular occlusion.

McBrien et al. (1963) examined the retina of a 37-year-old man with ipsilateral internal carotid artery stenosis in whom white intravascular particles identical with those described by Fisher (1959a) and Ross Russell (1961) had been observed. The patient died after endarterectomy. Flat preparations of the retina showed positive fat staining with oil red O, confined to the opaque material within the arteries (Fig.

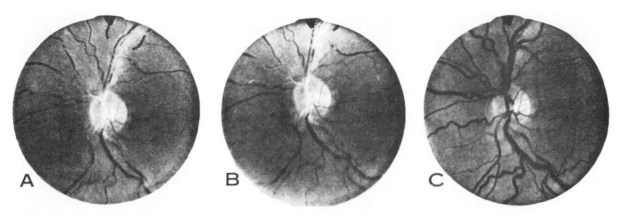

Figure 55.59. Photographic appearance of platelet-fibrin emboli during an attack of transient monocular loss of vision in the left eye. *A*, At 3 1/2 minutes after the onset of the attack, white embolic material is advancing into the superior nasal and temporal arteries. A white zone on either side of the artery is deprived of blood and thus is pale compared with the surrounding retina. *B*, At 4 minutes after the onset, the embolus is mainly in the upper temporal artery. Small superior venules running directly to the optic disc are almost empty. *C*, Almost 5 minutes after the onset of the attack, the embolus has vanished, the fundus is hyperemic, and the retinal veins are distended. Vision is returning at this time, and vision is normal 30 seconds later. (From Ashby M, Oakley N, Lorentz I, et al. Recurrent transient monocular blindness. Br Med J 2:894–897, 1963.)

55.60). This material also stained positively with periodic acid-Schiff (PAS) stain. The specimen was then digested with trypsin and re-examined. The opacities were observed to be within arterial lumina, birefringent in polarized light, and histologically compatible with aggregates of platelets (Fig. 55.60).

From the descriptions of Fisher (1959a), Ross Russell (1961) and McBrien et al. (1963), it is clear that platelet-fibrin emboli appear as dull, gray-white plugs (Fig. 55.61). Usually mobile, they adopt a long, smooth shape before breaking up in the retinal arterioles (Miller, 1996). These emboli usually arise either from the walls of atherosclerotic arteries or from the heart, particularly from its valves. Platelet-fibrin emboli can form in patients with coagulopathies, and Magargal et al. (1985) reported a patient who developed a branch retinal artery occlusion with a visible platelet-fibrin embolus after excessive use of oxymethazolone hydrochloride 0.5% nasal spray. The embolus was thought to be caused by sympathomimetic drug-induced platelet aggregation.

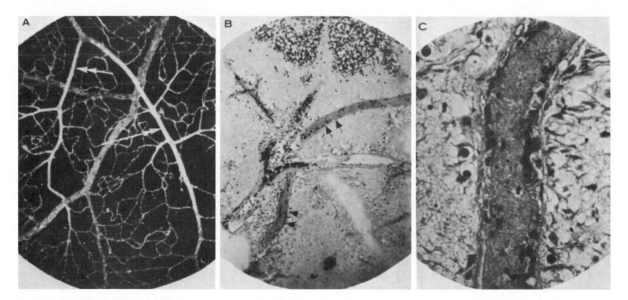

Figure 55.60. Pathology of platelet emboli. The patient was a 37-year-old man who had emboli to the retinal vessels from ipsilateral carotid artery stenosis. He died after attempted thromboendarterectomy. *A*, Trypsin digest preparation of the inferior nasal vessels showing long, thin emboli in two branches of the artery just beyond its bifurcation (*arrows*). *B*, Flat preparation of a superior temporal arteriole shows impacted microemboli (*arrows*). *C*, Higher power of the same region as *B* shows the granular nature of the material, which is PAS-positive and stains negatively for fibrin. (From McBrien DJ, Bradley RD, Ashton N. The nature of retinal emboli in stenosis of the internal carotid artery. Lancet 1:697–699, 1963.)

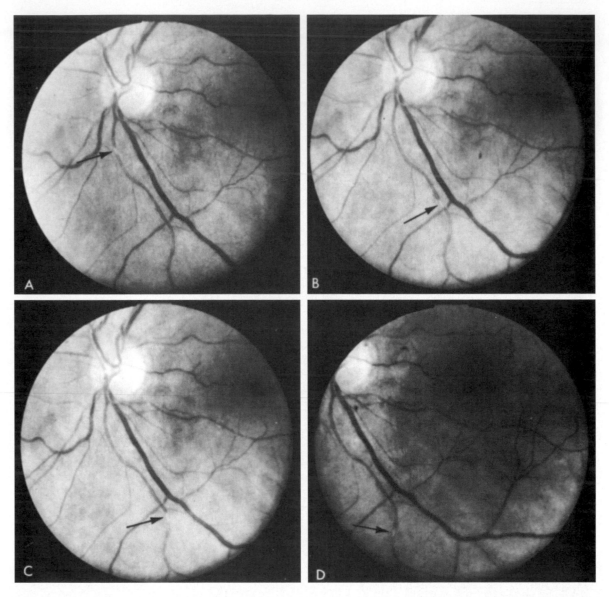

Figure 55.61. Gradual movement of platelet-fibrin embolus through a retinal arteriole. *A*, The embolus appears as a gray-white plug that is located just beyond the first bifurcation of the inferior temporal retinal artery (*arrow*). Note dilation of the inferior temporal retinal vein. *B–D*, Over several minutes, the embolus moves distally within the artery. (From Green WR. Retina. In Ophthalmic Pathology. An Atlas and Textbook. Editor, Spencer WH, 3rd ed, Vol 2, pp 589–1292. Philadelphia, WB Saunders, 1985.)

CALCIUM EMBOLI

Emboli composed of **calcium** may lodge in the retinal and cerebral arteries of patients with rheumatic heart disease, calcific aortic stenosis, calcification of the mitral valve annulus, and other disorders of the heart and great vessels that predispose to formation of calcium (Holley et al., 1963a; Penner and Font, 1969; Patrinely et al., 1982; Younge, 1989; Shanmugam et al., 1997) (Figs. 55.62 and 55.63).

Baghdassarian et al. (1970) described a 41-year-old man with rheumatic heart disease characterized by mitral stenosis and insufficiency, atrial fibrillation, pulmonary hypertension, and congestive heart failure who died 11 days after mitral valve replacement. The patient had a history of a pre-

vious stroke characterized by a right hemiparesis and an incongruous right homonymous hemianopia. About 4 weeks before surgery, the patient experienced a 25-minute episode of visual loss in the right eye followed by complete recovery of vision. Two hours after the episode, an ophthalmoscopic examination showed a "chalk white" embolus in the superior nasal artery of the right eye just beyond the first bifurcation and a similar particle in the superior temporal artery of the left eye at the disc margin. At the time of admission for surgery, the embolus in the right eye had moved distally to the second bifurcation of the superior nasal artery, whereas the plaque in the left eye was still located in the superior temporal artery at the disc margin. Ten days after surgery,

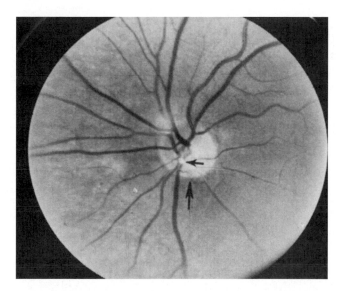

Figure 55.62. Calcific embolus in the inferior temporal retinal artery of a patient with aortic stenosis (*small arrow*). A collateral vessel (*large arrow*) supplies the obstructed artery distal to the embolus. Calcific emboli usually are large, round or ovoid, chalky, and nonrefractile (see also Fig. 55.65).

the patient had loss of vision in the left eye. At this time, the ophthalmoscopic appearance of the right fundus was unchanged, but the left fundus now showed three new white emboli lodged in branches of the inferior temporal artery in addition to the previously seen embolus in the superior temporal artery. The day after these observations were made, the patient had a cardiac arrest and could not be resuscitated. Postmortem examination of the left eye showed large calcific granules obstructing the inferior nasal retinal artery, the central retinal artery, and one of the short posterior ciliary arter-

ies (Fig. 55.64). All of these emboli stained positively with alizarin red and Von Kossa stains, confirming the presence of calcium.

Brockmeier et al. (1981) described four patients with retinal artery occlusion, loss of vision, and aortic valvular disease, two of whom were noted to have emboli in occluded retinal vessels. In both patients with visible emboli, there was a single, large, round, white particle in the obstructed vessel. Two of the four patients (the two in whom no emboli were observed) subsequently underwent open heart surgery, at which time they were found to have bicuspid aortic valves with substantial calcification. The other heart valves were normal. Both patients had replacement of the aortic valve, after which they had no further episodes of visual loss.

Mokri and Piepgras (1981) described a 72-year-old woman who had sudden loss of vision in the nasal half of the field of vision of the left eye and was found to have a large, white embolus lodged in the inferior temporal artery of the left retina (Fig. 55.65A). The embolus was thought to be composed of calcium. An evaluation disclosed a partially calcified aneurysm about 4 cm in diameter arising from the cervical portion of the left internal carotid artery just above its origin from the common carotid artery (Fig. 55.65B). The aneurysm was later resected, and histologic examination revealed atherosclerotic changes associated with significant deposition of lipid and calcium (Fig. 55.65C).

Stefánsson et al. (1985) observed retinal emboli in a patient with calcific aortic stenosis who underwent cardiac catheterization. During the procedure, the patient complained of blurred vision and was found to have two retinal emboli in the left eye. The authors did not describe the exact appearance of these emboli, but a photograph of the patient's left retina shows that both were located at third arterial bifurcations (Fig. 55.66). One embolus was quite small, whereas

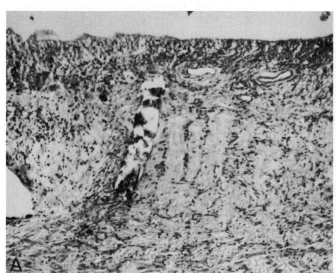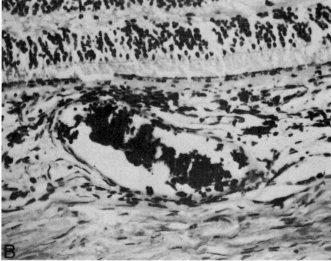

Figure 55.63. Histopathologic appearance of calcific retinal and choroidal emboli. *A*, Embolus in central retinal artery. *B*, Similar embolus in a choroidal artery. (From Green WR. Retina. In Ophthalmic Pathology. An Atlas and Textbook. Editor, Spencer WH. 3rd ed, Vol 2, pp 589–1292. Philadelphia, WB Saunders, 1985.)

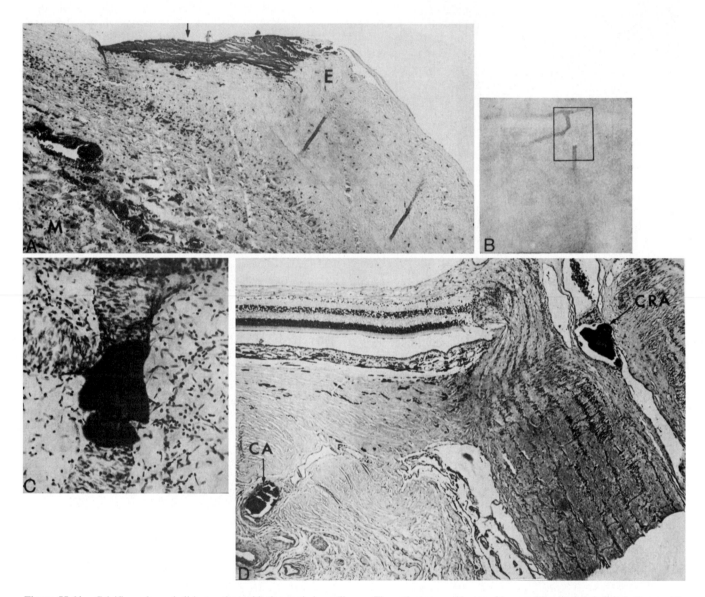

Figure 55.64. Calcific ocular emboli in a patient with rheumatic heart disease. The patient was a 41-year-old man with retinal emboli in both eyes. He died shortly after undergoing mitral valve replacement. *A*, Section from the wall of the left atrium shows calcification (*arrow*). *E*, Endocardium; *M*, myocardium. *B*, Gross appearance of the left inferior nasal retinal artery shows a chalk white embolus. *C*, Flat preparation of the area outlined in *B* shows that the embolus consists of calcium. *D*, Posterior segment of the left eye shows a calcified embolus (*arrow*) in the central retinal artery (*CRA*) and a similar embolus in a short posterior ciliary artery (*CA*). (From Baghdassarian SA, Crawford JB, Rathbun JE. Calcific emboli of the retinal and ciliary arteries. Am J Ophthalmol *69*:372–375, 1970.)

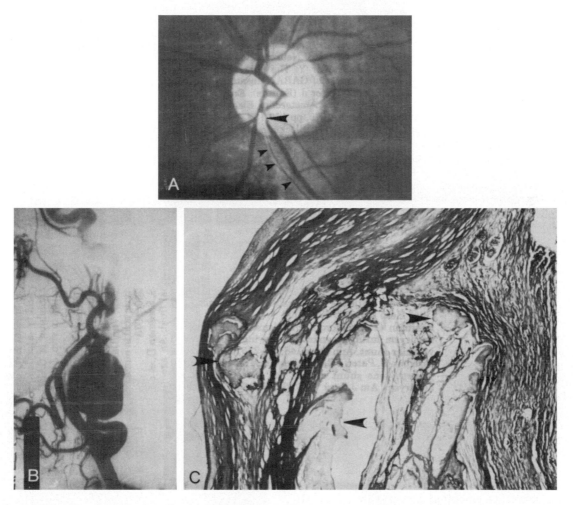

Figure 55.65. Calcific retinal embolus originating from a partially calcified aneurysm of the ipsilateral internal carotid artery. The patient was a 72-year-old woman who experienced sudden visual loss in the left eye. *A,* A large, round, chalk white embolus is lodged in the inferior temporal artery (*large arrowhead*). Note occlusion and narrowing of the vessel distal to the embolus (*small arrowheads*). *B,* Common carotid arteriogram, lateral view, shows a large saccular aneurysm in the midsection of the cervical portion of the left internal carotid artery. The aneurysm was resected without complication. *C,* Histopathologic appearance of part of the wall of the aneurysm shows atherosclerotic changes with large deposits of calcium (*arrowheads*). (From Mokri B, Piepgras DG. Cervical internal carotid artery aneurysm with calcific embolism to the retina. Neurology *31:*211–214, 1981.)

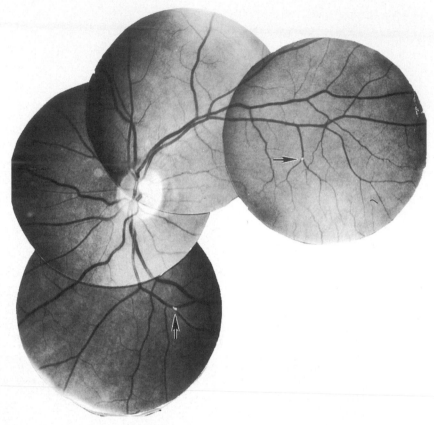

Figure 55.66. Probable calcific emboli in the left eye of a patient with calcific aortic stenosis who developed blurred vision during cardiac catheterization. The composite photograph of the left ocular fundus shows two emboli (*arrows*). One is lodged at the third bifurcation of the superior temporal retinal artery, and the other is lodged at the third bifurcation of the inferior temporal retinal artery. Neither embolus is refractile or long and narrow. (From Stefénsson E, Coin JT, Lewis WR III, et al. Central retinal artery occlusion during cardiac catheterization. Am J Ophthalmol *99:*586–589, 1985.)

the other was somewhat larger and appeared white. These emboli probably were composed of calcium.

Like platelet-fibrin and cholesterol emboli, emboli composed of calcium have a unique appearance (Miller, 1996). They are usually large, round or ovoid, ''chalk'' white, and nonrefractile (Fig. 55.67). They most often lodge in the first or second arterial bifurcation and may overlie the optic disc (Younge, 1989). Unlike cholesterol emboli and platelet-thrombin emboli, which tend to pass through the retinal circulation or resolve over time, calcific emboli tend to lodge permanently in retinal vessels, occasionally resulting in the development of collateral vessels forming shunts around the embolic blockage (Winterkorn and Ptachewich, 1995) (Fig. 55.68). Because calcium emboli usually arise from the heart or great vessels, it is not surprising that patients with such emboli are at significant risk for stroke, heart attack, and death (Howard and Ross Russell, 1987).

TUMOR EMBOLI

A variety of tumors can undergo hematogenous dissemination. Carcinoma, sarcoma, lymphoproliferative tumors, and atrial myxoma are all capable of spreading via the circulation (Fig. 55.69). The appearance of tumor emboli in retinal vessels is nonspecific. Anderson and Lubow (1973) described a 13-year-old boy with an atrial myxoma who had a ''shiny, smooth, cream-cheese-like material'' obstructing the central retinal artery and several of its retinal branches. Five months later, the material had disappeared from the

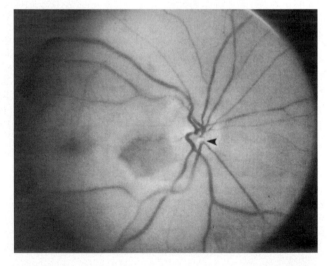

Figure 55.67. Central retinal artery occlusion caused by a calcific embolus lodged at the initial bifurcation of the central retinal artery. The embolus (*arrowhead*) is difficult to see because of the surrounding retinal edema. Note sparing of a portion of the peripapillary temporal retina supplied by a small cilioretinal artery. (From Younge BR. The significance of retinal emboli. J Clin Neuroophthalmol *9:*190–194, 1989.)

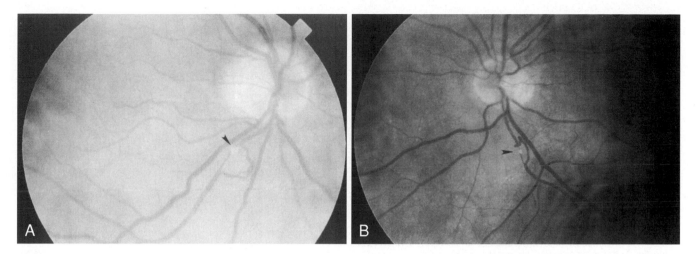

Figure 55.68. Collateral shunting around calcific retinal emboli. A woman with rheumatic heart disease experienced inferior retinal infarctions from cardiac emboli prior to valve replacement in her 20s. At age 53, funduscopic examination revealed calcific emboli in the inferior branch arterioles of the right (*A*) and left (*B*) eyes with collateral vessels bypassing the segment of vascular occlusion (*arrows*). (From Winterkorn JMS, Ptachewich Y. Calcific retinal emboli and collateral shunting in a woman with rheumatic heart disease. Arch Ophthalmol *113:*1464–1465, 1995.)

retinal vasculature. In another patient with an atrial myxoma, Campbell (1974) described a "large, grey, nonrefractile embolus" occluding the central retinal artery at the optic disc. Cogan and Wray (1975) described "white material" in the retinal arteries of a patient with a cardiac myxoma. The material disappeared 20 months after it was first seen.

FAT EMBOLI

Systemic intravascular dissemination of neutral fat globules is most often a complication of trauma to the long bones (Grossling and Pelligrini, 1982). The underlying pathology of this process is incompletely understood, but evidence suggests that fat emboli result from release of fat from damaged long bones and from coalescence of fat globules in the circulation after disruption of blood lipid stability (Oh and Mital, 1978). Loss of lipid stability seems to be caused by a neurohumoral stress response that also produces an increase in the blood concentration of free fatty acids. Endothelial cell damage results from the toxic effects of free fatty acids and from capillary obstruction by fat globules, with associated platelet aggregation, release of vasoactive substances, and production of a coagulopathy (Hagley, 1983a). Loss of capillary integrity is the likely cause of the widespread microinfarction and hemorrhage seen in various tissues including the brain (Hagley, 1983b) (see below).

Nontraumatic fat embolism occurs in clinical settings other than severe trauma. These include diabetes mellitus, acute pancreatitis, alcoholic fatty liver disease, prolonged steroid therapy, contusion of fatty viscera during surgery, intravascular lipid infusion, and autologous fat injection (Evarts, 1970; Goulon et al., 1974; Inkeles and Walsh, 1975; McCarthy and Norenberg, 1988; Dreizen and Framm, 1989). Respiratory insufficiency is the most common clinical manifestation of the fat embolism syndrome, but neurologic manifestations occur in up to 80% of cases (Jacobson et al., 1986).

Variable impairment of consciousness is present in all patients with neurologic complications of fat embolism, and seizures and focal signs occur frequently (McCarthy and Norenberg, 1988). The typical neuropathologic picture is widespread distribution of embolic fat droplets in both gray and white matter with diffuse, petechial hemorrhagic infarcts and occasional focal pale infarcts in white matter (Kamenar and Burger, 1980).

Fat emboli were first described clinically in retinal vessels and confirmed histologically by Cogan et al. (1964). These investigators described a 59-year-old man who suffered a left hemisphere stroke characterized by aphasia. The patient underwent a percutaneous left carotid arteriogram that was complicated by mild systemic hypotension lasting about 2 minutes. Shortly after arteriography, the patient became comatose, and his eyes deviated to the left. Over the next several hours, he regained consciousness, at which time an examination revealed a right hemiparesis, a temporal hemianopia in the right eye, and blindness in the left eye with the retinal vessels of that eye containing about a dozen white emboli (Fig. 55.70). Many of the emboli were quite long and located at various points along the vessels, not just at bifurcations. A left carotid endarterectomy revealed that the lumen of the vessel was filled with a soft, friable thrombus, which was completely removed. The patient failed to improve after surgery, and he died of septicemia about 1 month later. At postmortem examination, the retinal emboli were globules that showed bright fluorescence under ultraviolet light and vivid staining with Sudan IV stain for fat (Fig. 55.71).

Dreizen and Framm (1989) reported the case of a 44-year-old woman who developed severe right hemicranial pain and total loss of vision in the right eye following an injection of autologous fat into the glabellar region to remove facial wrinkles. The patient could not perceive light in the right eye. The right optic disc was pale and swollen, and many

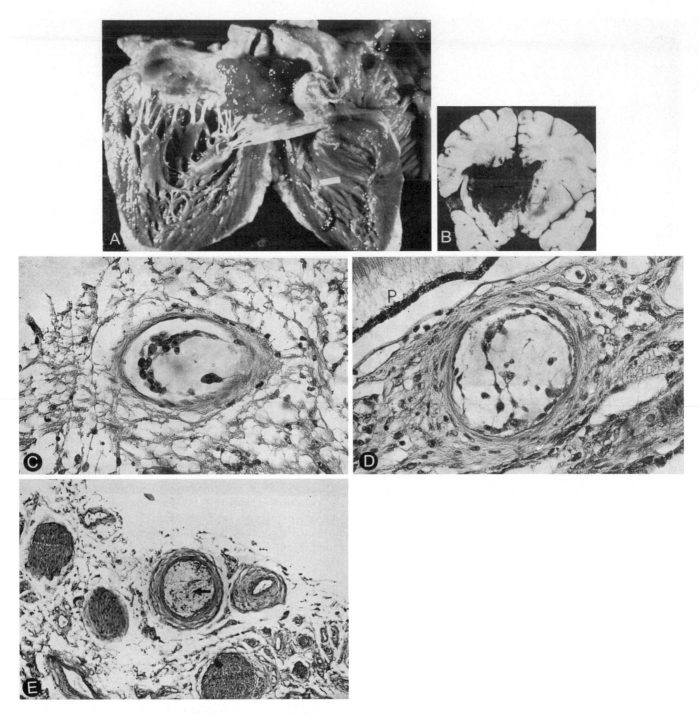

Figure 55.69. Atrial myxoma with metastases to the brain, orbit, and eye. The patient was a 37-year-old woman who developed joint pain and intermittent fever and then suddenly collapsed. The patient died shortly thereafter. *A,* A large, gelatinous atrial myxoma is present in the left atrium of the heart. *B,* Coronal section through the brain shows a hemorrhagic infarct in the region of the left internal capsule and basal ganglia. *C,* A retinal arteriole contains metastatic cells from the myxoma. *D,* Another embolus from the myxoma occludes a choroidal artery. *P,* Retinal pigment epithelium. *E,* A posterior ciliary artery is occluded by an embolus from the myxoma (*arrow*). (From Jampol LM, Wong AS, Albert DM. Atrial myxoma and central retinal artery occlusion. Am J Ophthalmol *75:*242–249, 1973.)

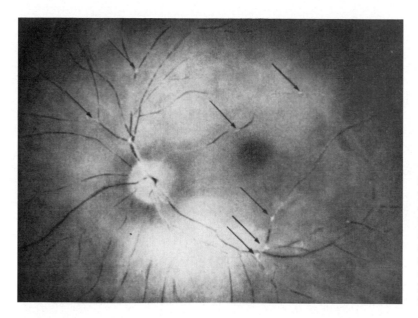

Figure 55.70. Fat emboli in the retina. The patient was a 59-year-old man who developed neurologic and visual difficulties after a percutaneous carotid arteriogram. The patient was noted to have numerous white emboli in the retinal vessels of the left eye. The patient died of septicemia 1 month later. The appearance of the left ocular fundus at autopsy shows numerous emboli in the retinal arterioles (*arrows*). These emboli were visible during life. (From Cogan DG, Kuwabara T, Moser H. Fat emboli in the retina following angiography. Arch Ophthalmol *71:*308–313, 1964.)

of the retinal arterioles were segmentally occluded with **opaque, yellow** material (Fig. 55.72). Two-and-a-half months after visual loss, the patient still had no vision in the right eye. The right optic disc was now pale, the retinal arterioles still contained some emboli, there was mottling of the retinal pigment epithelium in the posterior pole, and the peripheral fundus demonstrated several areas of segmental retinal epithelial mottling, each of which had a wedge-shaped configuration. Dreizen and Framm (1989) postulated that autologous fat was inadvertently injected into a distal forehead branch of the ophthalmic artery. Under pressure exerted by the syringe, the fat was forced retrograde into the main trunk of the ophthalmic artery. Once the pressure from the syringe ceased, the fat travelled in an orthograde fashion into the ocular branches of the ophthalmic artery, producing infarction of the choroid, retina, and optic nerve.

ORGANISM EMBOLI (SEPTIC EMBOLI)

Septic emboli occur most often in patients with subacute and acute bacterial endocarditis (Reese and Shafer, 1978), but they may develop in other settings. For example, Kilmartin and Barry (1996) reported septic retinal emboli in a 36-year-old man after dental surgery in which a periapical abscess was drained (see also King et al., 1993).

Septic emboli usually consist of white blood cells, some of which contain organisms (Friedenwald and Rones, 1930, 1931) (Fig. 55.73). Rarely are free organisms identified in retinal or choroidal vessels. In rare cases, septic emboli appear as gray-white plugs in one or more retinal arteries (Manor and Sachs, 1973). In other cases, they are surrounded by a localized intraretinal hemorrhage. The appearance is thus that of a "Roth spot"—a focal hemorrhage with a white or gray center (Roth, 1872a, 1872b; Litten, 1878; Dellmann, 1919; Dienst and Gartner, 1944; Kennedy and Wise, 1965; Duane et al., 1980; Green, 1996) (Fig. 55.74). Such lesions develop when septic emboli cause disruption of the vessel

wall, resulting in hemorrhage with a central area of organisms and white blood cells. The lesions may heal without spreading to other areas, or they may extend into the vitreous to produce a suppurative endophthalmitis (Green, 1996). Thus, by the time an ophthalmologist examines the patient, there is more likely to be a diffuse infiltrative retinitis, choroiditis, or endophthalmitis than individual retinal emboli.

AIR EMBOLI

Air embolism occasionally occurs when air is injected into an organ or tissue of the body, after chest injuries, and during pulmonary, cardiac, or neurologic surgery (Schlaepfer, 1922; Walker, 1933; Weyrauch, 1940). In some of these cases, the emboli reach the retinal vessels and produce severe visual loss that usually recovers over several hours to days (Walsh and Goldberg, 1940).

The appearance of air in the retinal vessels was described by Wong (1941) in a patient suffering from tuberculosis. During aspiration of an effusion in the chest, the patient suddenly lost consciousness and died within a few minutes. When Wong (1941) examined the patient before death, both retinas were pale. The retinal arteries were of normal size and contour, and they were of even caliber. At irregular intervals between columns of blood in the retinal arteries, there were pale, silvery sections that varied from 1–4 vessel diameters in length. These sections appeared successively at the bifurcation of the central retinal artery, moved distally, and disappeared rapidly from view in the retinal periphery. Wong (1941) subsequently injected air into the carotid artery of dogs and observed in the retina an appearance identical with what he had seen in his patient (see also Wever, 1914). Walsh and Goldberg (1940) also injected air into the carotid artery of an anesthetized dog and immediately noted "glistening rods" within the retinal arterioles identical with those observed by Wong (1941). The emboli were most clearly

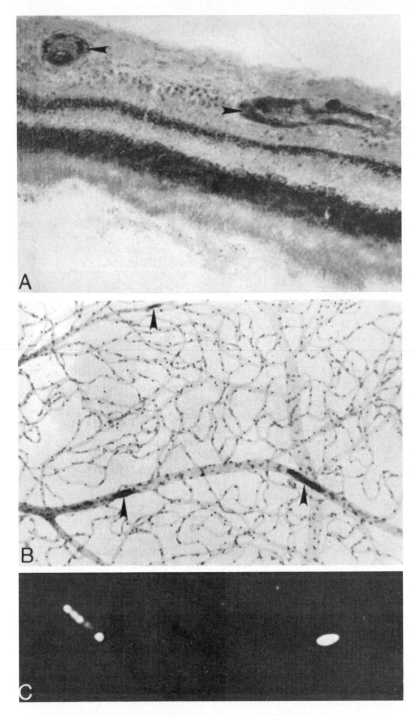

Figure 55.71. Pathologic appearance of fat emboli in the retina. Same patient as described in Figure 55.69. *A,* Cross-section of retina in posterior portion of globe, stained with hematoxylin and Sudan. The dark appearance of the vessel walls (*arrowheads*) is positive reaction for fat. *B,* Flat mount of retinal vessels stained with hematoxylin and Sudan. Three emboli stain positively for fat (*arrowheads*). *C,* The emboli show bright fluorescence when photographed using ultraviolet light. (From Cogan DG, Kuwabara T, Moser H. Fat emboli in the retina following angiography. Arch Ophthalmol *71:*308–313, 1964.)

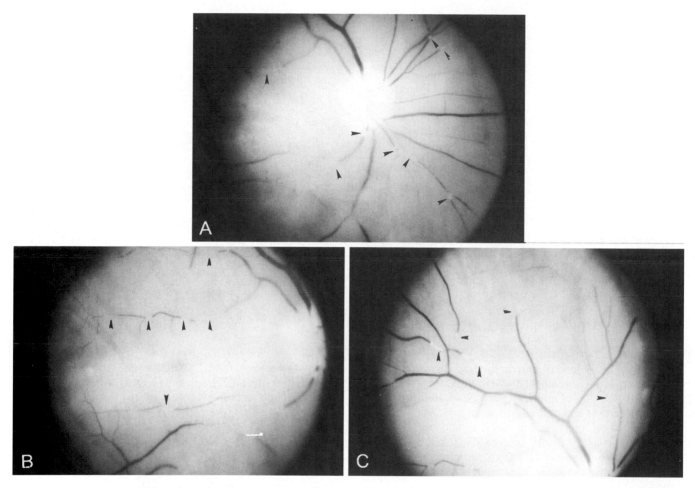

Figure 55.72. Clinical appearance of fat emboli in retinal arteries. The patient was a 44-year-old woman who developed loss of vision in the right eye after an injection of autologous fat into the glabellar region to remove wrinkles. *A*, The right optic disc is swollen, the retina is edematous, and the retinal arteries are segmentally occluded with opaque, yellow material (*arrowheads*). *B*, The retinal arteries above and below the macula show segmental occlusion by fat emboli (*arrowheads*). *C*, Segmental occlusion by emboli of branches of the superior temporal artery (*arrowheads*). (From Dreizen NG, Framm L. Sudden unilateral visual loss after autologous fat injection into the glabellar area. Am J Ophthalmol *107*:85–87, 1989.)

visible at vascular bifurcations and disappeared within about 1 minute, leaving the retinas pale and edematous. Sachsenweger (1958) noted that an air embolus in a retinal arteriole has a convex meniscus at either end, whereas a platelet embolus has a concave meniscus at both ends (Fig. 55.75). Air emboli can also be seen in conjunctival vessels.

FOREIGN BODY EMBOLI

Any foreign material that is allowed access to the arterial (and occasionally the venous) circulation has the potential to cause embolic stroke, visual loss, or both. The foreign material usually is introduced into the systemic circulation by the patient or iatrogenically. The most common settings for emboli of foreign material are: (*a*) retrobulbar, intranasal, peritonsillar, and scalp injections of drugs, usually corticosteroids; (*b*) intravascular injection of drugs designed for oral use; (*c*) vascular diagnostic studies including cardiac catheterization and angiography of the neck vessels; (*d*) endoarterial embolization procedures; and (*e*) placement of a

prosthetic heart valve (McGrew et al., 1978a). Rarely, trauma causes fragments of cartilagenous material from the vertebral disc space to enter the spinal vascular system and, occasionally, the vertebral arteries.

Retrobulbar and, more commonly, sub-Tenon injections of systemic corticosteroids are performed for a variety of ophthalmic conditions. Corticosteroid suspensions also are injected in the conchae nasalis to treat allergic rhinitis, in the peritonsillar fossae to decrease postoperative pain, and in the scalp to treat alopecia areata, psoriatic plaques, discoid lupus erythematosus, and lichen planopiliaris (Evans et al., 1980). All of these routes of injection have the potential to cause visual loss.

Although intranasal or retrobulbar injections of anesthetics may cause visual loss by inducing vasospasm, especially when the solution contains epinephrine (Savino et al., 1990), most cases of visual loss that follow injections of corticosteroids and other substances to the head and neck are probably caused by high-pressure injection of material

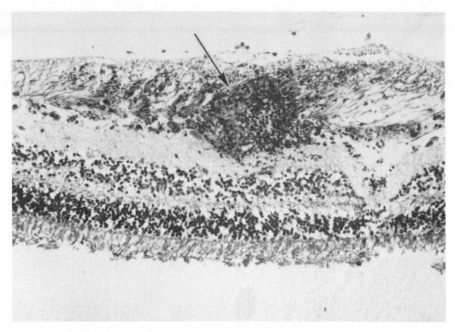

Figure 55.73. Retinal embolus (*arrow*) consisting of white blood cells, some of which contain bacteria, in a patient with subacute bacterial endocarditis. (From Green WR. Retina. In Ophthalmic Pathology. An Atlas and Textbook. Editor, Spencer WH. 3rd ed, Vol 2, pp 589–1292. Philadelphia, WB Saunders, 1985.)

with embolic potential into highly vascular tissue (Selmanowitz and Osentreich, 1974; McGrew et al., 1978b; Mabry, 1979, 1981; Lemagne et al., 1990). Retrograde arterial flow permits emboli to lodge in vascular beds far distant from the site of injection. For this reason, injections to such diverse areas as the scalp, peritonsillar fossa, and conchae nasalis can cause visual loss from embolic retinal disease. Ophthalmoscopic examinations in such patients support this theory.

Francois and Van Langenhone (1970) reported a case of blindness that resulted after a retrobulbar injection of aqueous methylprednisolone. Whitish, flocculent material was

seen in numerous retinal arteries of the affected eye. Ellis (1978) described a 38-year-old woman with presumed retrobulbar optic neuritis who was treated with retrobulbar injection of 1.5 cc of a solution of 1% xylocaine mixed with a combination of betamethasone acetate and betamethasone disodium phosphate (Celestone Soluspan). About 15–20

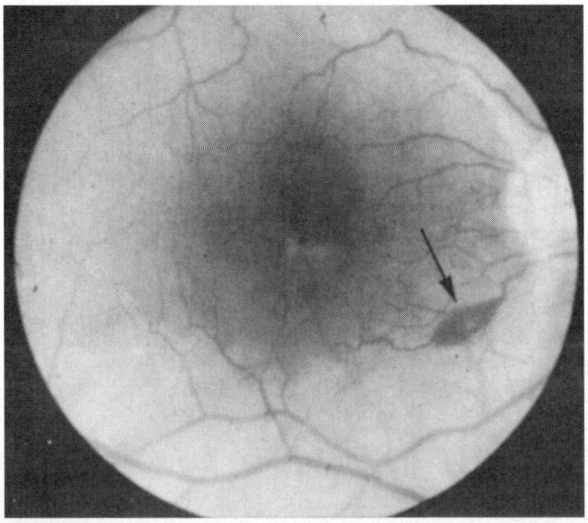

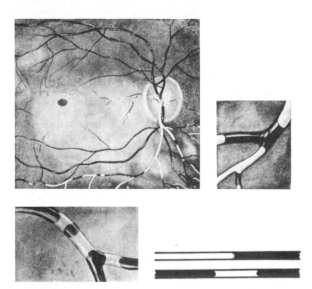

Figure 58.75. Air emboli in retinal arteries. *Top left,* Air emboli in the fundus of a 27-year-old man 2 days after embolization. *Top right,* magnified drawing shows that the air emboli have a convex meniscus at each end. *Bottom left,* Drawing of platelet-fibrin emboli shows that they have a concave meniscus at each end. *Bottom right,* A comparison of air embolus with a convex meniscus at one end (*above*) and a platelet-fibrin embolus (*below*) with a concave meniscus at both ends. (From Sachsenweger R. Zur Differentialdiagnose der Luftembolie des Netzhautkreislaufes. Klin Monatsbl Augenheilkd *133:*788–797, 1958.)

Figure 55.74. Clinical appearance of a Roth spot in a patient with subacute bacterial endocarditis. The lesion consists of an intraretinal-white spot surrounded by hemorrhage.

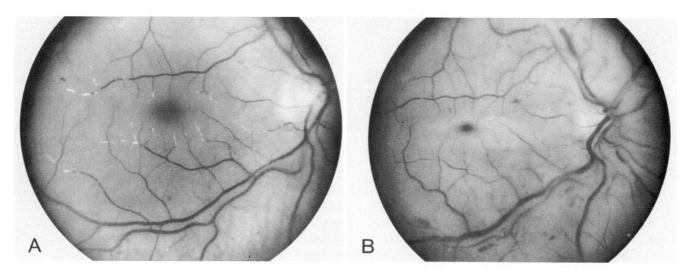

Figure 55.76. Retinal emboli after retrobulbar injection of corticosteroids. The patient was a 38-year-old woman with presumed retrobulbar optic neuritis in the right eye. She was given a retrobulbar injection of a solution of 1% lidocaine, betamethasone acetate, and betamethasone disodium phosphate. Within 15–20 seconds after injection, the patient complained of loss of vision in the eye. *A*, Ophthalmoscopic view of the right posterior pole shows clumps of white, flocculent material in several small arterioles and capillaries. The patient was treated with inhalation of a mixture of 10% CO_2 and 90% O_2 and with intravenous injection of hydrocortisone sodium succinate and mannitol without improvement. *B*, The retinal emboli have disappeared 48 hours after loss of vision. There is now diffuse retinal edema, a cherry-red spot in the macula, attenuation of retinal arterioles, and scattered intraretinal hemorrhages. The patient never regained vision in this eye. (From Ellis PP. Occlusion of the central retinal artery after retrobulbar corticosteroid injection. Am J Ophthalmol 85:352–356, 1978.)

seconds after injection, the patient experienced complete loss of vision in the eye. Ophthalmoscopic examination revealed mild retinal edema in the affected eye. Clumps of white flocculent material were seen within several of the small retinal arterioles and capillaries (Fig. 55.76*A*). Within 48 hours, all of the foreign material had disappeared. The patient now had diffuse retinal edema, a cherry-red spot in the macula, attenuation of retinal arterioles, and several small intraretinal hemorrhages (Fig. 55.76*B*). The patient never regained vision in the eye.

Egbert et al. (1996) reported the case of a 4-month-old infant who suffered an ophthalmic artery occlusion after an intralesional injection of corticosteroids into an ipsilateral upper eyelid capillary hemangioma. The event was witnessed during simultaneous indirect ophthalmoscopy, allowing immediate discontinuation of the procedure and treatment with paracentesis. Although fluorescein angiography 20 minutes later showed delayed retinal and choroidal filling and large areas of retinal and choroidal ischemia, follow-up fluorescein angiography and clinical examination revealed complete resolution of the abnormalities.

Blindness caused by retinal emboli can develop in patients after inadvertent intra-arterial injection of corticosteroid preparations into the turbinates for various otorhinolaryngologic disorders (Byers, 1979; Whiteman et al., 1980; Garland et al., 1989; Wilkinson et al., 1989). In such cases, numerous emboli composed of white, flocculent material are seen in both retinal and choroidal vessels (Fig. 55.77). The emboli usually disappear within several days. Visual acuity at the time of the embolic event is usually reduced to the level of hand motions or counting fingers, but acuities ranging from

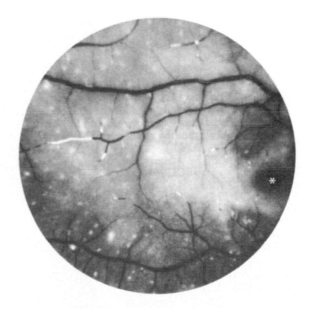

Figure 55.77. Retinal emboli after intranasal injection of corticosteroids. The patient was a 34-year-old woman who received an intranasal injection of methylprednisolone acetate after an endonasal procedure that was performed for allergic rhinitis and nasal polyps. On awakening from anesthesia, she complained of lack of vision in the right eye. Photograph of the right ocular fundus obtained 24 hours after the injection shows embolic material in terminal retinal arterioles and in the choroidal vessels. Retinal edema is present, and there is a cherry-red spot in the macula (*asterisk*). (From Whiteman DW, Rosen DA, Pinkerton RMH. Retinal and choroidal microvascular embolism after intranasal corticosteroid injection. Am J Ophthalmol 89:851–853, 1980.)

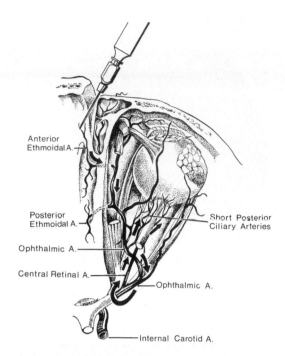

Anterior
Ethmoidal A.

Posterior
Ethmoidal A.

Ophthalmic A.

Central Retinal A.

Short Posterior
Ciliary Arteries

Ophthalmic A.

Internal Carotid A.

Figure 55.78. Pathway by which embolic material is thought to reach retinal and choroidal vessels after intranasal injection. The material is inadvertently injected into the anterior ethmoidal artery from which it passes in retrograde fashion into the ophthalmic artery and then forward into the ocular circulation. (From Whiteman DW, Rosen DA, Pinkerton RMH. Retinal and choroidal microvascular embolism after intranasal corticosteroid injection. Am J Ophthalmol *89*:851–853, 1980.)

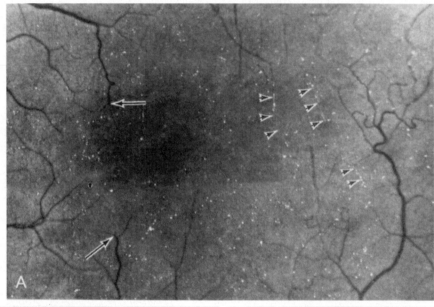

A

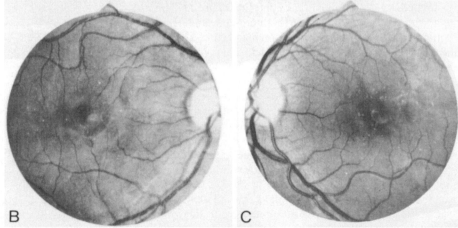

B   C

Figure 55.79. Ophthalmoscopic appearance of talc emboli in patients who are intravenous drug abusers. *A*, Monochromatic photograph at 570 nm demonstrates talc particles in ghost vessels (*arrowheads*) and focal attenuation of small terminal venules (*arrows*). (From Friberg TR, Gragoudas ES, Regan CDJ. Talc emboli and macular ischemia in intravenous drug abuse. Arch Ophthalmol *97*:1089–1091, 1979.) *B* and *C*, Photographs of right and left eyes, respectively, in another patient who had intravenously injected methylphenidate tablets each day for at least 1 year. The right fundus photograph shows small, yellow-white dots throughout the macular region. The left fundus photograph shows a similar picture. (From Schatz H, Drake M. Self-injected retinal emboli. Ophthalmology *86*:468–483, 1979.)

no perception of light to 20/20 have been recorded. The eventual visual outcome is similarly variable. Most patients have a persistent visual deficit (Garland et al., 1989), although some patients recover completely (Wilkinson et al., 1989). The embolic material, after being injected intranasally, is thought to reach the ocular circulation via the anterior ethmoidal artery. The material presumably passes in retrograde fashion through this artery to the ophthalmic artery and then to the retinal and choroidal vessels (Fig. 55.78).

Drug abusers who inject substances synthesized for oral use or certain illegal drugs into their veins or arteries may develop retinal and choroidal emboli associated with permanent or transient loss of vision (Atlee, 1972; Lee and Sapira, 1973; Murphy et al., 1978; Brucker, 1979; Friberg et al., 1979; Kresca et al., 1979; Schatz and Drake, 1979; Tse and Ober, 1980; Keane, 1981; Siepser et al., 1981). In some cases, the emboli occur from purposeful or inadvertent injection of the substance into an artery (Lindell et al., 1972; Begg et al., 1980; Keane, 1981). In other cases, intravenous injection, by a patient with a known or unknown cardiac septal defect or with pulmonary arteriovenous shunts acquired from the consequences of chronic intravenous drug abuse, results in arterial emboli (Schatz and Drake, 1979). Most of the emboli are composed of talc, cornstarch, or microcrystalline cellulose, the fillers and binders used in medications such as methylphenidate chloride (Ritalin) tablets (Hahn et al., 1969) and in illegal drugs such as cocaine and heroin (Siepser et al., 1981). They appear as numerous tiny, yellow-white, glistening, refractile particles that usually lodge at the distal aspect of the smallest retinal arterioles but that may be located at large vessel bifurcations (Figs. 55.79–55.81).

Emboli consisting of a variety of foreign materials, including plastic, talc, cotton, and particulate contaminants of contrast material may be produced during angiography of the heart and great vessels (Silberman et al., 1960; Levine and Henry, 1963; Genee and Honegger, 1969; Kay and Wilkins, 1969; Duquesnel et al., 1973; Brekkan et al., 1975; Nehen et al., 1978; Moulene et al., 1981; Hartel et al., 1982; Soong et al., 1982; Hallermann and Singh, 1984; Singh, 1990) (Fig. 55.82). Such emboli may also be produced during open-heart surgery (Aguilar et al., 1971).

Congenital anastomoses involving small branches of the internal and external carotid arteries exist in most patients, providing a potential pathway for embolization to the eye, brain, or both through the latter vessel. This explains how cholesterol or platelet-fibrin emboli that originate in the external carotid artery can spontaneously reach the retinal vessels (Burnbaum et al., 1977), and how foreign body emboli can reach the retina during attempted particulate embolization of the external carotid artery system for treatment of epistaxis, arteriovenous malformations (AVMs), or dural carotid-cavernous sinus fistulas (Mames et al., 1991).

Most emboli that occur in patients with artificial heart valves are composed of blood products, such as fibrin and platelets, or infected material that has formed on the valve

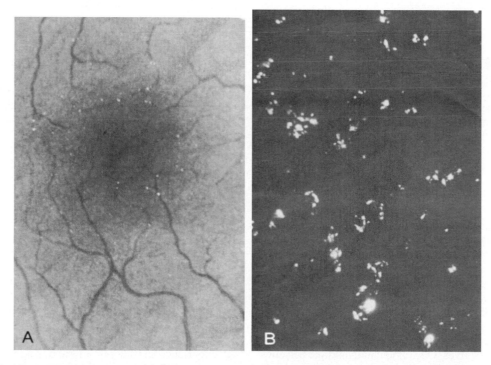

Figure 55.80. Refractile appearance of talc emboli. *A*, Magnified view of emboli in the retina show the small, yellow-white particles in terminal arterioles in the macula. *B*, Photograph of crushed talc particles obtained using polarized light shows refractile nature of the talc crystals. Note variable size and shape of the particles. (From Schatz H, Drake M. Self-injected retinal emboli. Ophthalmology *86:*468–483, 1979.)

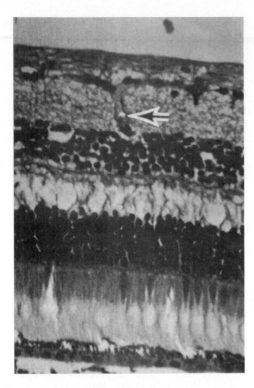

Figure 55.81. Histopathologic appearance of talc embolus in a retinal arteriole. Note bright "crystalline" appearance (*arrow*). (From Schatz H, Drake M. Self-injected retinal emboli. Ophthalmology *86:*468–483, 1979.)

and then become dislodged. In rare instances, however, the valve itself is defective or deteriorates in such a way that it produces emboli composed of valve material (Crawford et al., 1973; Pluth and Danielson, 1974; Moggio et al., 1978; Shah et al., 1978). Ide et al. (1971) described a 26-year-old man who underwent placement of a prosthetic aortic valve made of silicone rubber. Seven years later, he began to experience episodes during which he would see showers of small floaters in one or both eyes. The episodes would last 10–15 minutes and then resolve. Visual acuity was 20/20 in each eye, but numerous white specks were seen in the retinal and choroidal vessels of both eyes (Fig. 55.83). The particles, irregular and variable in size, were thought to be emboli originating from the prosthetic valve, which therefore was replaced. The replaced silicone ball showed yellowish discoloration and marked surface irregularities. Although the retinal particles may have been composed of blood products, Ide et al. (1971) emphasized that their ragged appearance and silver-gray tinged white color seemed characteristic of small slivers of silicone.

Rush et al. (1980) reported two patients who developed permanent visual loss caused by retinal emboli that were thought to be composed of foreign material from cloth-covered artificial heart valves. One patient had multiple episodes of transient loss of vision in both eyes (as well as an episode of dysphasia and agraphia that lasted 1 week) that began about 10 months after placement of a cloth-covered mitral

ball valve prosthesis for treatment of recurrent mitral stenosis and congestive heart failure related to old rheumatic heart disease. Both eyes showed retinal emboli at various times over the next 6 years. When the prosthetic valve was finally replaced 7 years after its placement, the valve showed fragmentation and shredding of the cloth covering with many areas of cloth loss. After replacement of the valve by a different type of prosthesis without a cloth cover, the patient had no further episodes of visual or neurologic dysfunction over the next 2 years. The second patient described by Rush et al. (1980) was a 52-year-old man with a cloth-covered mitral valve prosthesis for treatment of mitral regurgitation, pulmonary hypertension, and congestive heart failure. Six years later, the patient noted acute blurred vision and was found to have multiple retinal emboli, most of which were large, dull, and "fluffy" or "fuzzy" in appearance, simulating exudates (Fig. 55.84). Rush et al. (1980) suspected that these emboli were composed of foreign material from the prosthetic valves rather than of blood products, like fibrin, platelets, or cholesterol.

Causes of Embolism

CARDIAC DISEASE

Embolic cerebrovascular disease is most often caused by **cardiac disease** (Cerebral Embolism Task Force, 1986a, 1989; Kittner et al., 1990). Arrhythmias, valvular disease, endocarditis, ischemic lesions, cardiomyopathies, and tumors are all potential sources of emboli that originate in the heart (Furlan, 1987; Kittner et al., 1990; Sirna et al., 1990; Bogousslavsky et al., 1991; Yamanouchi et al., 1997). Emboli also may be produced iatrogenically during cardiac manipulation. Although cardiac emboli lodge more frequently in the anterior circulation, transcranial Doppler studies show that embolism to the posterior intracranial circulation is more common than previously believed (Caplan, 1993; Venketasubramanian, 1993).

Arrhythmias. Arrhythmias are the most common cause of cardiac-related, embolic cerebrovascular disease, and they may be the most common cause of all emboli to the brain (Norris et al., 1978; Cerebral Embolism Task Force, 1986a, 1989). Abnormal heart rhythms most likely to produce emboli are chronic atrial fibrillation (AF), paroxysmal AF, and the abnormal rhythms that develop in patients with disturbances of cardiac conduction.

Chronic AF is the most common arrhythmia that produces cerebral embolism (Starkey and Warlow, 1986; Petersen, 1990; The Stroke Prevention in Atrial Fibrillation Investigators, 1990a, 1990b; Wolf et al., 1991). From 6 to 24% of all ischemic strokes occur in patients with AF (Norris et al., 1978; Wolf et al., 1978a, 1978b; Greenland et al., 1981; Nishide et al., 1983; Harrison and Marshall, 1984; Kelley et al., 1984; Kuramoto et al., 1984; Olsen et al., 1985; Norrving and Nilsson, 1986; Foulkes et al., 1988; Bogousslavsky et al., 1990), and from 35 to 65% of patients with chronic AF experience an ischemic stroke during their lifetime (Hinton et al., 1977; Sherman et al., 1984; see Table 1 in Halperin and Hart, 1988; D'Olhaberriague et al., 1989; Yamanouchi et al., 1997). In most of these cases, the stroke is embolic

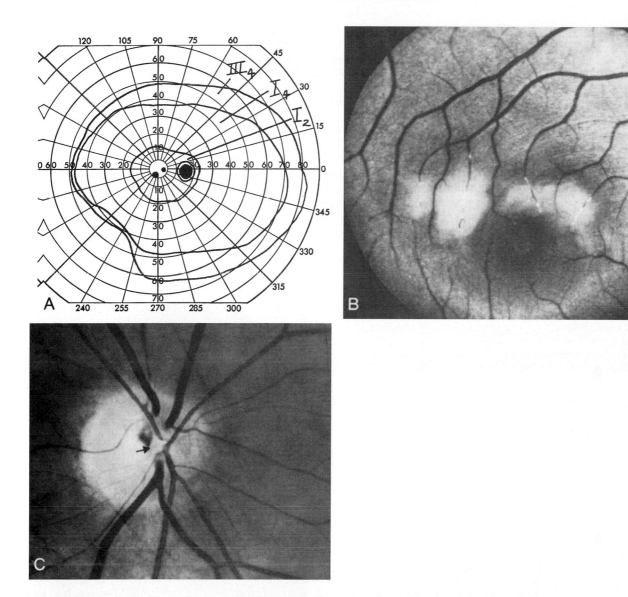

Figure 55.82. Foreign body emboli to the retina after vascular diagnostic studies. *A,* Visual field defect in the right eye of a patient who underwent percutaneous femoral cerebral angiography as part of an evaluation for severe headache and nuchal rigidity. The results of the angiogram were normal. At the conclusion of the procedure, however, the patient complained of blurred vision in the right eye. Visual field shows two small paracentral scotomas. *B,* Appearance of right ocular fundus shows multiple retinal emboli and parifoveal edema. The emboli were thought to be foreign contaminants rather than endogenous particles of platelets, fibrin, or cholesterol. (From Hartel WC, Spoor TC, Hammer ME. Retinal embolism following percutaneous femoral cerebral angiography. J Clin Neuroophthalmol *2:*49–54, 1982.) *C,* Appearance of the right optic disc in a 57-year-old man who lost vision in the right eye during cardiac catheterization that was performed after the patient had experienced a myocardial infarction. A green, crystalline foreign body is seen within the central retinal artery on the optic disc (*arrow*). The retinal arteries are constricted, and the retinal veins are dilated. The foreign body was thought to be a fragment from the catheter. (From Hallermann D, Singh G. Iatrogenic central retinal embolization: A complication of cardiac catheterization. Ann Ophthalmol *16:*1025–1027, 1984.)

and caused by the AF (Jorgensen and Torvik, 1966; Mohr et al., 1978; Wolf et al., 1978a, 1978b; Bogousslavsky et al., 1990); however, in up to 30% of cases, the stroke is unrelated to the AF, and both are separate consequences of atherosclerosis (van Merwijk et al., 1990).

Embolic infarction related to AF is an important cause of fatal massive cerebral infarction in the elderly. Yamanouchi

et al. (1989) studied 3408 consecutive autopsied elderly patients and found that 86 of the 132 massive infarctions (65%) were cardioembolic. Many of these patients were known to have AF. In the Framingham Study, AF was a powerful independent risk factor for stroke, especially in the elderly (Wolf et al., 1991). D'Olhaberriague et al. (1989) performed a prospective evaluation of 72 patients with chronic AF and

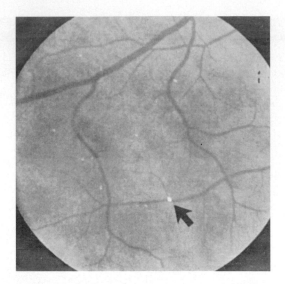

Figure 55.83. Foreign body emboli from artificial heart valve. The patient was a 26-year-old man who had undergone placement of a prosthetic aortic valve made of silicone rubber. Seven years later, he began to experience episodes during which he would see showers of small floaters. The right fundus shows numerous white specks in retinal vessels and in the choroidal circulation. The particles have an irregular shape and a variable size. A particularly large particle is lodged at the bifurcation of a retinal arteriole. The silicone valve was replaced. The old valve showed yellowish discoloration and numerous surface irregularities. The ocular emboli were thought to have originated from the valve. The patient had no further episodes of visual loss over the next 9 months, and the appearance of the ocular fundi did not change over this period. (From Ide CH, Almond CH, Hart WM, et al. Hematogenous dissemination of microemboli: Eye findings in a patient with Starr-Edwards aortic prosthesis. Arch Ophthalmol 85:614–617, 1971.)

ischemic stroke. These investigators concluded that several variables were significantly associated with cardioembolic stroke, including onset during activity, peak deficit at onset, history of a TIA in a different territory, one or more previous infarcts in different territories, and a TIA lasting more than 1 hour. Chronic AF is usually caused by atherosclerotic or rheumatic heart disease, with the source of the cerebral embolus being a mural thrombus within the atrium (Hinton et al., 1977). Patients with chronic arteriosclerotic AF are five to seven times more likely to experience a stroke than are patients of identical age and sex with normal cardiac rhythm (Flegel et al., 1987; Flegel and Hanley, 1989), and patients with rheumatic AF are 17 times more likely to experience a stroke than are age-matched controls (Wolf et al., 1983b).

Paroxysmal AF also predisposes to embolic cerebrovascular disease (Petersen, 1990). Thrombi are thought to form in the heart and to break off as emboli during episodes of fibrillation (Wolf et al., 1983b). In some patients, cerebral embolism develops after cardioversion of AF (Caplan, 1993).

Several groups of investigators attempted to determine the risk factors for stroke in patients with chronic AF (Petersen, 1990). Halperin and Hart (1988) concluded that patients with AF at highest risk for stroke (over 6% per year) are those who also have mitral stenosis, a prosthetic mitral valve, or

congestive failure, and those who have had a previous stroke. Patients with AF at lower risk (less than 3% per year) are those under 60 years of age with either isolated or paroxysmal AF. Aronow et al. (1989) followed 110 elderly patients with chronic AF for 3 years for occurrence of stroke. These investigators found a strong association between hypertension and stroke. Other significant risk factors in this group of patients were left ventricular hypertrophy, left atrial enlargement, and previous myocardial infarction. Flegel and Hanley (1989) concluded that advanced age (over 75 years) and systolic hypertension (>160 mm Hg) were the most significant risk factors in the occurrence of a first stroke in patients with nonrheumatic AF. These investigators also found that patients who had one or more previous strokes were about twice as likely to have a subsequent stroke as patients who had no strokes, and, overall, they were **13.5** times more likely to experience a stroke than were normal

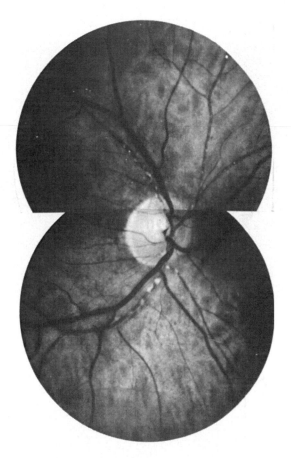

Figure 55.84. Foreign body emboli to the retina in a patient with a prosthetic heart valve. The patient was a 52-year-old man who had undergone placement of a cloth-covered, prosthetic mitral valve because of mitral regurgitation, pulmonary hypertension, and congestive heart failure. Six years later, he experienced blurred vision in the right eye. The fundus photograph of the right eye shows multiple retinal emboli, most of which are large, dull, and "fluffy." The largest emboli are in the superior and inferior temporal retinal arteries. Smaller emboli are seen in the superior and inferior nasal retinal arteries. (From Rush JA, Kearns TP, Danielson GK. Cloth-particle retinal emboli from artificial cardiac valves. Am J Ophthalmol 89:845–850, 1980.)

persons of the same age and sex. Other risk factors for embolic stroke in patients with AF include rheumatic heart disease, onset of AF within the preceding 3 months, an enlarged left atrium, and left ventricular dysfunction (Stroke Prevention in Atrial Fibrillation Investigators, 1992; Caplan, 1993). In patients with AF who have already experienced an initial episode of cerebral ischemia, the independent risk factors for subsequent stroke are history of previous thromboembolism, ischemic heart disease, enlarged heart, hypertension, AF for more than 1 year, and an ischemic lesion on computed tomographic (CT) scanning (van Latum et al., 1995; EAFT Study Group, 1996).

Cerebral embolism may occur in patients with both hereditary and acquired abnormalities of cardiac conduction, such as the **sick sinus syndrome** and other types of sinoatrial heart block (Rubenstein et al., 1972; Fairfax and Lambert, 1976; Fairfax et al., 1976; Lambert and Fairfax, 1976; Guntheroth and Motulsky, 1983; D.E. Ward et al., 1984; Onat, 1986; Natowicz and Kelley, 1987). Such patients have disturbances of the normal sinoatrial pacemaker, resulting in periods of sinus bradycardia, sinoatrial arrest, atrial tachycardia, AF, atrial flutter, or a combination of these abnormalities. All of these arrhythmias, associated with mechanical inactivity of the atria, predispose to formation of cardiac thrombi and subsequent embolization. Patients with sinoatrial disease who have periods of bradycardia alternating with tachycardia are at the greatest risk for embolization (Bathen et al., 1978).

Noninfective Valvular Disease. Abnormalities of the heart valves without associated infection may cause cerebral embolism. Some of the abnormalities of natural heart valves that predispose to embolism are calcification or stenosis of the valve, calcification of the annulus of the mitral valve, and mitral valve prolapse. Otherwise normal heart valves may develop noninfectious vegetations in certain settings. Debilitating diseases, particularly cancer, and an increased concentration of circulating antiphospholipid antibodies may predispose to the development of vegetations on otherwise normal cardiac valves. Finally, prosthetic heart valves may develop noninfectious vegetations.

Calcified or Stenotic Valves. Noninfected calcified and stenotic valves, particularly the mitral and aortic valves, can provide a template for deposition of platelet and fibrin clots that may eventually embolize. In addition, particles of cal-

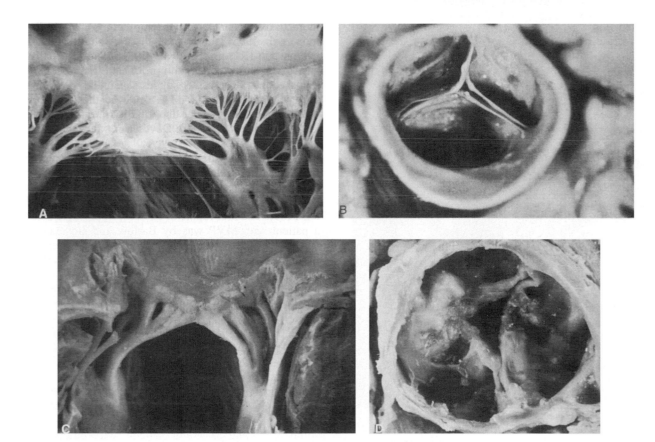

Figure 55.85. Normal vs. calcified, stenotic heart valves. *A*, Normal mitral valve. Note thin appearance of valve and chordae tendinae. *B*, Normal aortic valve. Note thin appearance of three sets of leaflets, and the normal apposition of the valves. *C*, Calcified, stenotic mitral valve. Note thickened chordae tendinae. *D*, Calcified aortic valve. Note abnormal displacement and poor apposition of leaflets caused by thickening and calcification. Calcified, stenotic heart valves may be a source of platelet, fibrin, and calcific emboli to the brain and eye. (From Younge BR. The significance of retinal emboli. J Clin Neuroophthalmol *9*:190–194, 1989.)

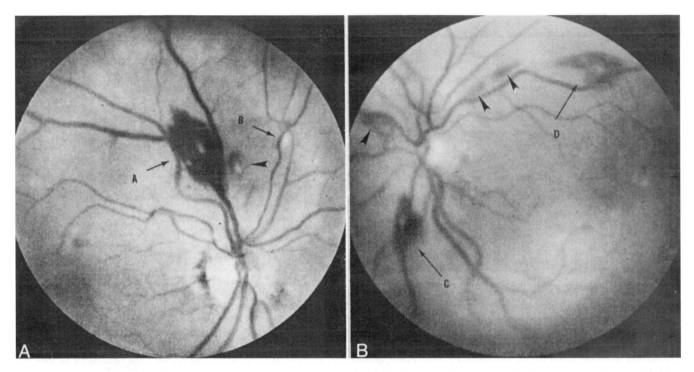

Figure 55.94. Ophthalmoscopic appearance of Roth spots in subacute bacterial endocarditis. The patient was a 57-year-old woman with subacute bacterial endocarditis who failed to respond to antibiotic therapy and died after a brief hospitalization. The day before death, the ocular fundi were examined ophthalmoscopically and photographs were obtained. *A*, The right ocular fundus contains one large, intraretinal white-centered hemorrhage (*A*), a smaller hemorrhage with a white edge (*arrowhead*), and a soft exudate (*B*). *B*, The left fundus contains two white-centered intraretinal hemorrhages (*C* and *D*) and several flame-shaped hemorrhages (*arrowheads*). (From Kennedy JE, Wise GN. Clinicopathologic correlation of retinal lesions: Subacute bacterial endocarditis. Arch Ophthalmol *74:*658–662, 1965.)

such patients may be severely damaged, producing akinetic segments or ventricular aneurysms. These abnormal regions serve as nidi for mural thrombi that eventually may embolize (Editorial, 1990) (Fig. 55.96 and 55.97). Such emboli occur most frequently in the first 3 months after myocardial infarction (Bean, 1958; Wolf et al., 1978b), but they may occur later if there is a persistent mural clot or an aneurysm (Cerebral Embolism Task Force, 1986a, 1989). The clots may be so small that they are undetectable on echocardiography or cardiac angiography.

Zimmerman (1965) described a 59-year-old man who experienced sudden loss of vision in the left eye 10 days after experiencing an acute myocardial infarction. Examination revealed a CRAO in the left eye. The patient died 62 hours after the onset of visual symptoms. At autopsy, the lumen of the central retinal artery was completely obstructed by a partially organized clot, composed of fibrin with enmeshed red and white blood cells (Fig. 55.98). The wall of the artery showed no evidence of atherosclerosis. Small emboli were seen in the vessels of the ciliary body and choriocapillaris.

Cardiomyopathies. Nonischemic diseases of the myocardium may be complicated by cerebral embolism (Easton and Sherman, 1980; Cerebral Embolism Task Force, 1986a, 1989). Fibrin-platelet or thrombin can deposit on the endocardial surface and subsequently embolize (Fig. 55.99). Stasis within the heart cavities caused by poor myocardial function, congestive heart failure, and arrhythmias that occur

in patients with cardiomyopathies may also predispose to formation of thrombi. Mural thrombi are particularly common in patients with inherited, idiopathic, and alcoholic cardiomyopathies (Vost et al., 1964; McDonald et al., 1972; Demakis et al., 1974; Taylor, 1983; Natowicz and Kelley, 1987; Gaffney et al., 1989), and in elderly patients with cardiac amyloidosis. In Case Records of the Massachusetts General Hospital (1975), a patient with sarcoid cardiomyopathy was described who developed severe personality and behavioral disturbances. Neurologic examination revealed defects in naming objects, poor recent memory, lability of mood, slight dysarthria, and mild left pyramidal signs. The patient subsequently died, and a postmortem examination revealed multiple old infarcts consistent with emboli from a mural thrombus in the left ventricle of the heart. Even idiopathic hypertrophic subaortic stenosis, a focal disorder of the muscle of the ventricular septum, can be complicated by cerebral embolism, particularly if there is associated AF, hypertension, mitral anulus calcification, or atrioventricular delay (Glancy et al., 1970; Russell et al., 1991). Cocaine can also cause a cardiomyopathy with subsequent brain embolism and stroke (Isner et al., 1986; Petty et al., 1990; Sauer, 1991).

Tumors. Cardiac **tumors,** although rare, are important and potentially treatable causes of cerebral embolism. The most common cardiac tumor is the **myxoma,** which occurs in both sexes with equal frequency and may become symp-

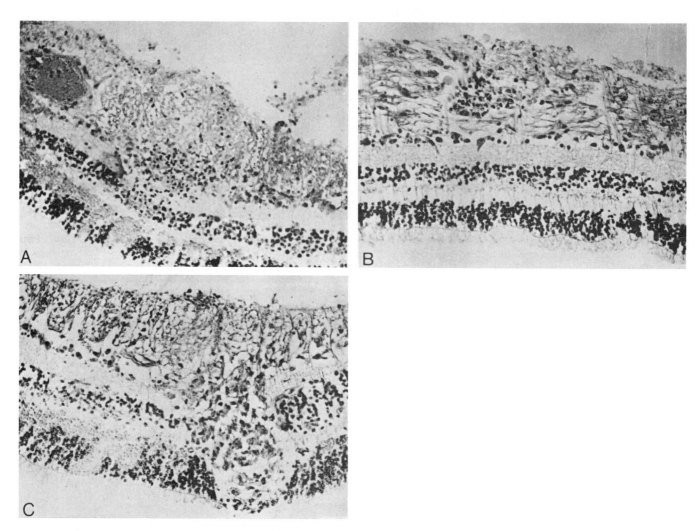

Figure 55.95. Pathology of Roth spots in subacute bacterial endocarditis. The patient's ocular fundi are shown in Figure 55.94. *A*, Histopathologic appearance of white-centered hemorrhage in the retina of the right eye marked *A* in Figure 55.94. Note edema and hemorrhage in the nerve fiber layer and outer plexiform layer with a central accumulation of polymorphonuclear leukocytes. *B*, Histopathologic appearance of white-centered retinal hemorrhage marked *C* in the left eye in Figure 55.94. Note central accumulation of polymorphonuclear leukocytes in the retinal nerve fiber layer. *C*, Histopathologic appearance of white-centered retinal hemorrhage in the retina of the left eye marked *D* in Figure 55.94. Note hemorrhage in the outer plexiform and nerve fiber layers with a central collection of mononuclear cells and polymorphonuclear leukocytes. (From Kennedy JE, Wise GN. Clinicopathologic correlation of retinal lesions: Subacute bacterial endocarditis. Arch Ophthalmol *74*:658–662, 1965.)

occurred in rapid succession. Ophthalmoscopic examination revealed dull yellow-white emboli in several retinal arteries. The emboli, first seen at the optic disc, travelled peripherally and then disappeared. Whenever an embolus travelled near the macula, the patient complained of blurred vision. As the embolus moved further peripherally, the patient's vision cleared. The episodes continued for 30 minutes and then resolved, leaving her with normal vision.

Transluminal angioplasty of a cephalic artery may result in distal embolization of debris released from a ruptured atherosclerotic plaque (Bockenheimer and Mathias, 1983; Smith et al., 1983). DeMonte et al. (1989) performed a transluminal angioplasty on a 57-year-old woman with symptomatic atherosclerotic stenosis at the origin of the left common carotid artery. The angioplasty was performed retrogradely through a distal arteriotomy after endarterectomy, and the postangioplasty effluent was collected and analyzed. The effluent contained cholesterol crystals and amorphous plaque debris, indicating a potential source for distal embolization (Fig. 55.103).

A particularly severe form of artery-to-artery embolization occurs in the syndrome called **diffuse disseminated atheroembolism** (DDA). DDA is a multisystem disorder in which showers of cholesterol-rich atheromatous emboli lodge in small and medium-sized arteries in numbers sufficient to infarct multiple organs (Goulet and Mackay, 1963). Patients with this syndrome may have abdominal pain, anemia, hematuria, an elevated erythrocyte sedimentation rate, and neurologic and visual dysfunction consistent with multiple infarctions. Such patients are thus often misdiagnosed as having a systemic infection, giant cell arteritis, other vasculitides, or disseminated neoplasm (Case Records of the Massachusetts General Hospital, 1973). DDA seems to be a clinical and pathologic entity separate from, but closely related to, atherosclerosis (Case Records of the Massachusetts General Hospital, 1967a). The frequency and severity of embolization in patients with DDA are far greater than they are in patients with atherosclerosis (Goulet and Mackay, 1963; Mauriz et al., 1968; Sieniewicz et al., 1969; Ramirez et al., 1978; Jacobson, 1991), and the plaques in DDA are unusually friable, so much so that seemingly minimal manipulation of vessels during arteriography or surgery may cause severe embolization (Mauriz et al., 1968; Case Records of the Massachusetts General Hospital, 1973; Ramirez et al., 1978; Rieben et al., 1979; Starr et al., 1979; Beal et al., 1981a).

Many cases of DDA are only diagnosed after death; however, Coppeto et al. (1984b) described three patients with DDA and neuro-ophthalmologic symptoms and signs, two of whom were diagnosed correctly before death. One patient was a 74-year-old man with dementia, multiple systemic and cerebral infarctions, an elevated sedimentation rate, a left homonymous paracentral scotoma, and transient monocular blindness and teichopsias. A diagnosis of DDA was made on pathologic review of a specimen of infarcted bowel. A second patient was a 68-year-old man with multiple systemic and cerebral embolic infarctions, syncope, microscopic hematuria, elevated sedimentation rate, and complaints that

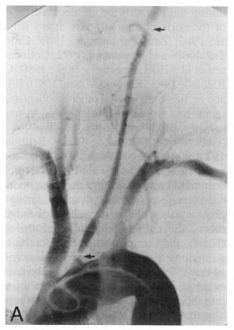 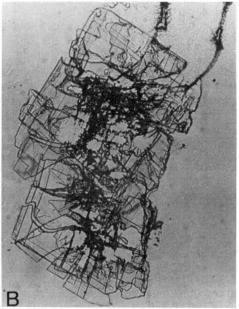

Figure 55.103. Gross appearance of cholesterol crystals collected by filtration of postangioplasty effluent in a 52-year-old woman who underwent transluminal angioplasty of an atherosclerotic stenosis at the origin of the common carotid artery. *A,* Preoperative aortic arch angiogram shows tandem stenosis of the left common carotid artery (*arrows*), occlusion of the left vertebral artery, and mild stenosis of the right common carotid, innominate, and both subclavian arteries. *B,* Cholesterol crystals in effluent. (From DeMonte F, Peerless SJ, Rankin RN. Carotid transluminal angioplasty with evidence of distal embolization: Case report. J Neurosurg *70:*138–141, 1989.)

objects seemed to jump to the side each time he closed and opened his eyes and that he was seeing ''comet-like'' phosphenes that traveled in an arc through the upper visual field of the right eye. The patient was found to have lateropulsion of saccades to the right. Review of previous surgical specimens demonstrated atheromatous emboli in sections from the kidney and big toe, confirming the diagnosis of DDA. Carotid endarterectomy was complicated by blindness in both eyes with extensive hemorrhages and cholesterol emboli. The third patient was a 70-year-old man with elevated erythrocyte sedimentation rate, microscopic hematuria, dementia, syncope, cerebral infarction, and a large, refractile particle at the first bifurcation of the inferior division of the central retinal artery. Autopsy revealed numerous, friable, ulcerated plaques throughout the aorta and both carotid arteries and microscopic examination of the pancreas, kidney, brain, and skin showed extensive atheroembolism. Jacobson (1991) reported two patients with clinical features consistent with giant cell arteritis who were found to have DDA. The diagnosis was established by muscle biopsy in one patient and kidney biopsy in the other.

Venous (Paradoxical) Emboli. Paradoxic embolism can result when an abnormal communication exists between the right and left sides of the heart, or when both cardiac ventricles communicate with the aorta (Jones et al., 1983; Biller et al., 1986; Harvey et al., 1986; Biller et al., 1987; Lechat et al., 1988; Webster et al., 1988; Sardesai et al., 1989). It is a major cause of otherwise unexplained stroke in young adults (Lechat et al., 1988; Mohr, 1988; Webster et al., 1988; Cabanes et al., 1993; Wisotsky and Engel, 1993; Hanna et al., 1994; Klotzsch et al., 1994; Nighoghossian et al., 1996).

Paradoxic emboli usually originate from venous thrombi that form in the veins of the lower extremities or the pelvis, but they may arise from any veins in the body. These emboli pass through an abnormal communication in the heart (usually an atrial septal defect, ventricular septal defect, or PFO), bypass the pulmonary circulation, and enter the systemic arterial circulation (Thompson and Evans, 1930) (Figs. 55.104 and 55.105).

Noninvasive methods of imaging the heart, such as spiral CT scanning and transesophageal echocardiography, reveal that the prevalence of a PFO is much higher than previously acknowledged (Fig. 55.106). A PFO is present in 18–35% of the normal population, and the frequency is even higher in patients with stroke of unknown etiology, especially young patients in whom it often is the only identifiable risk factor (Hanna et al., 1994; Klotzsch et al., 1994; Nighoghossian et al., 1996; Rauh et al., 1996; Petty et al., 1997). In one study, patients with cryptogenic stroke had a significantly higher prevalence of a PFO than did patients with an identifiable cause of stroke, in both younger and older patient groups (Di Tullio et al., 1992). Among stroke patients under the age of 50 years, the prevalence of a PFO was 48% in those with stroke of unknown origin, compared with 4% in those with stroke of determined cause. Another study suggested that a PFO may not be a risk factor for cerebral ischemia in patients over the age of 50 years (Jones et al., 1994). The degree of shunting across a PFO may be directly related to

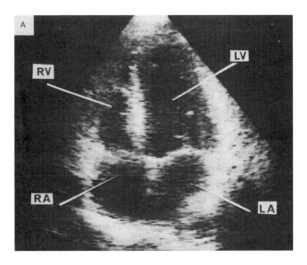

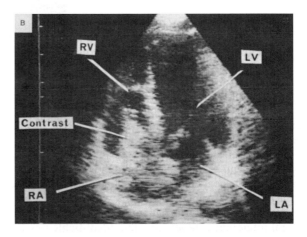

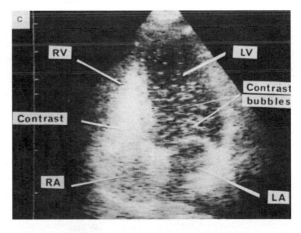

Figure 55.104. Patent foramen ovale diagnosed using two-dimensional contrast echocardiography. *A,* View of the heart before contrast injection shows the four chambers separated by an apparently intact septum. *B,* Immediately after injection of contrast material into a peripheral vein, the material appears in the right cavities. *C,* Contrast material completely fills the right cavities and appears in the left cavities through the patent foramen ovale. *LA,* left atrium; *LV,* left ventricle; *RA,* right atrium; *RV,* right ventricle. (From Lechat Ph, Mas JL, Lascault G, et al. Prevalence of patent foramen ovale in patients with stroke. N Engl J Med *318:*1148–1152, 1988.)

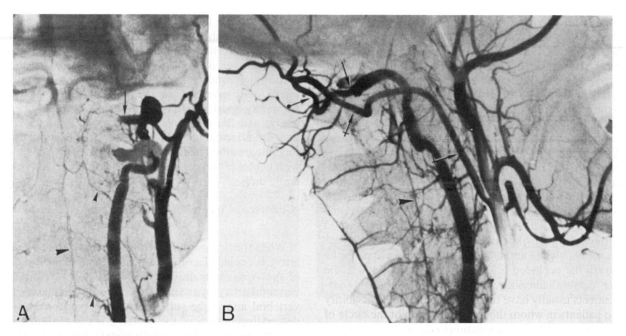

Figure 55.119. Collateral circulation after occlusion of the vertebral artery. The left vertebral artery is occluded between the atlas and the basilar artery (*arrow*). *A*, Cerebral angiogram, anteroposterior view, shows filling of anterior spinal artery (*large arrowhead*) via dilated radicular arteries (*small arrowheads*). *B*, Cerebral angiogram, lateral view, shows filling of a dilated, muscular branch of the vertebral artery (*dotted arrow*) proximal to the occlusion. This muscular branch anastomoses with the occipital artery (*crossed arrow*), a branch of the external carotid artery. *Large arrowhead*, anterior spinal artery. (From Huber P. Cerebral Angiography. 2nd ed. New York, Georg Thieme Verlag, 1982.)

tions of both the vertebral and basilar arteries are occluded, collateral flow to the brainstem and cerebellum may be achieved through the anterior spinal arteries, the posterior inferior cerebellar arteries, and from the internal carotid artery circulation via the posterior communicating arteries to the posterior cerebral arteries.

SYMPTOMS AND SIGNS

General Considerations

Topical diagnosis of sites of occlusion or stenosis of extracranial or intracranial arteries has many pitfalls. In most cases, occlusive atheromatous disease is a diffuse process that is compensated by development of an intricate system of collateral vascular circuits. The time-honored inductive type of reasoning employed in medicine, which is based on the analysis of a variety of clinical signs and symptoms and a stylized conception of the cerebrovascular tree, thus is often inadequate. Sudden appearance of focal neurologic signs may indicate dysfunction of a particular portion of the brain, but diagnosis of the vascular disorder that has produced these signs requires knowledge of the anatomic, pathologic, and physiologic factors involved. Generally speaking, a distinction between the clinical manifestations of **carotid** and **vertebrobasilar** insufficiency is both valid and useful. Nevertheless, this broad subdivision of cerebrovascular disease ignores important and sometimes clinically indistinguishable problems resulting from occlusions of main trunks of the aortic arch.

Transient disturbances of neurologic function—TIAs—are of major significance among the polysymptomatic manifestations of cerebrovascular disease. These episodes are caused by reversible dynamic events in a diseased vascular system (Rolak et al., 1990). Because TIAs may be caused by any disorder that transiently reduces blood flow to the brain, eye, or both, their prognostic significance varies with the age, sex, and—most importantly—with the cause of the TIA (Brust, 1977; Caplan, 1988a). Nevertheless, they frequently provide the initial clinical indication of potentially lethal atheromatous or other disease in extracranial or intracranial arteries (Horenstein et al., 1972; Janeway and Toole, 1972; Ramirez-Lassepas et al., 1973; Heyman et al., 1974; Toole et al., 1975; Pessin et al., 1977; Heyman et al., 1984a; Rolak et al., 1990). Indeed, perhaps as many as 75% of stroke victims experience a TIA days to months before a disabling or fatal stroke, especially those patients with extracranial carotid artery occlusive disease (see Table 1 in Brust, 1977; Caplan, 1977; Whisnant et al., 1977; Heyman et al., 1984a).

As noted in an earlier section of this chapter, a TIA is an abrupt, focal loss of neurologic function caused by ischemia. TIAs are characterized by a brief duration, a spontaneous resolution without residual neurologic deficit, and a tendency to recur (Heyman et al., 1974). The maximum duration for a TIA is somewhat controversial (see Table 1 in Brust, 1977; Pessin et al., 1977). Marshall (1964) and others (Ziegler and Hassanein, 1973; Ad Hoc Committee, 1975; Millikan et al., 1975) defined the maximum duration of a TIA as 24 hours; however, most TIAs resolve in a much shorter period of time, usually 1–4 hours, and vascular neurologic events that last longer than 4 hours often result in permanent neurologic sequelae (Acheson and Hutchinson, 1964; Levy, 1988; Werdelin and Juhler, 1988). Unfortunately, most studies concerned with the duration of TIAs have not separated patients according to the specific lesion producing the neurologic event (e.g., cardiac disease, extracranial arterial stenosis or occlusion, intracranial vascular disease, vasospasm), and they thus have limited usefulness (Caplan, 1988a). Furthermore, the age of the patient is an important distinction, because TIAs in young patients have many clinical and etiologic differences from those in older patients, with important diagnostic and therapeutic implications. In younger patients, TIAs are less likely to occur in the vertebrobasilar circulation and are more commonly associated with vasospasm, valvular heart disease, MVP, atrial septal defects, fibromuscular dysplasia, and oral contraceptive use (Carolei et al., 1993; Giovannoni and Fritz, 1993). However, even in young patients, a TIA or stroke is a strong marker for athcromatous ccrcbrovascular disease—especially if other risk factors are present.

The temporal pattern of recurrent TIAs is highly variable. Some patients have one or two attacks and then, within a matter of days, experience a stroke. Other patients experience several attacks per day or per week over several years without any permanent sequelae. Still others experience a flurry of attacks over a period of a few weeks and then remain free of symptoms for a year or more. Some TIAs affect the same area repeatedly, whereas others affect different parts of the nervous system at various times. Many TIAs are unaffected by activity, occurring at rest as often as during activity; others are precipitated by activity, changes in head position, or changes in posture.

Symptoms and Signs of Carotid Arterial System Ischemia

Historical Review

In a review of the ophthalmologic signs of occlusion of the internal carotid artery, Hager (1962) credited Virchow with the first autopsy description of this phenomenon in 1856. The patient reported by Virchow had lost all vision on the side of the thrombosed vessel; however, at autopsy, the lumina of the ophthalmic and central retinal arteries were patent. Subsequently, it was claimed that the clinical picture of a CRAO could be produced by thrombosis of the internal carotid artery, ophthalmic artery, or both. Gowers (1875) described a case of monocular blindness and contralateral hemiplegia. Postmortem examination in this patient revealed mitral stenosis, clots in the atria, an embolus in the left middle cerebral artery, and several small emboli in the central retinal artery.

In 1893, Elschnig, aware of the frequent autopsy finding of asymptomatic occlusion of the internal carotid artery, performed injection studies on cadavers and successfully demonstrated the rich collateral supply of the ophthalmic artery. He concluded that slowly progressive occlusions of the internal carotid or ophthalmic artery would not necessarily produce clinical symptoms or signs. Elschnig (1893) also stated that sudden occlusion of the internal carotid artery could

cause a momentary disturbance in ocular circulation, but that such a disturbance would not necessarily produce a permanent anatomic lesion. He did not, however, exclude the possibility of ocular changes with carotid thrombosis, because he recognized that permanent change might develop if collateral circulation were ineffective. His work was considered so authoritative that it almost completely eliminated interest in ophthalmologic problems associated with thrombosis of the internal carotid artery for the next 50 years.

In 1905, Chiari published a classic monograph on atheromatous occlusion of the internal carotid artery. He had found that soft thrombi in major intracranial branches of the internal carotid artery often arose from mural thrombosis on an atheromatous plaque located at the carotid bifurcation. He emphasized that atheromatous disease in the internal carotid artery was a common source of emboli in elderly patients. Following this work, Hunt (1914) described two patients who had neck wounds that produced thrombosis of the internal carotid artery, contralateral hemiplegia, and ipsilateral optic atrophy. Both patients had experienced episodes of transient visual dysfunction on the side of the thrombosis and transient neurologic dysfunction on the contralateral side. Hunt (1914) was the first to recognize the importance of these transient episodes, and he correctly ascribed them to ischemia.

Despite the work of both Chiari (1905) and Hunt (1914), many physicians throughout the first half of the 20th century thought that most strokes that occurred in the territory of the major branches of the internal carotid artery (e.g., the middle cerebral artery) were caused by primary occlusive disease in that vessel. In 1951, however, C. Miller Fisher (1951a, 1951b) reawakened interest in the ophthalmologic and neurologic manifestations of internal carotid artery disease when he emphasized that patients with thrombosis of the internal carotid artery could experience fleeting episodes of monocular blindness and then, months later, develop a catastrophic hemiplegia on the opposite side of the body. These and other observations made by Fisher played a prominent role in the understanding of carotid artery disease for the next 40 years (Estol, 1996).

It is now clear that both thrombosis and occlusion of the internal carotid artery are responsible for a majority of strokes that occur in the territory of that vessel and its major branches. In most cases, the site of disease is in the cervical segment of the artery (Sindermann et al., 1970).

Transient Ischemic Attacks From Intermittent Insufficiency in the Internal Carotid Artery

SYMPTOMS OF CAROTID ARTERIAL SYSTEM TIAS

TIAs that result from transient ischemia in the distribution of branches of the internal carotid artery have two distinctive clinical expressions: contralateral cerebral and ipsilateral (monocular) visual symptoms.

Neurologic Symptoms. Cerebral symptoms of a carotid circulation TIA include transient weakness of the arm or leg on one side of the body or of both extremities, weakness of one side of the tongue or face, temporary sensory disturbances on one side of the body, difficulty speaking, and episodes of mental confusion (Mules et al., 1971; see Table 1 in Heyman et al., 1984a). Dizziness is infrequent. Seizures may occasionally occur as part of a TIA (Patrick and Whitty, 1965), as may headaches (Medina et al., 1975).

Marshall (1964) studied the natural history of TIAs in a group of patients with cerebrovascular disease. He found that 16 of 34 (48%) patients with TIAs in the distribution of the internal carotid artery experienced a major stroke within 1 month of the first TIA. Marshall (1964) could not predict which patients with TIAs would later have a major stroke, but among those who did, 75% had one or two TIAs before the stroke.

Rothrock et al. (1988c) examined clinically and angiographically 47 consecutive patients with repetitive symptoms indicative of carotid circulation ischemia ("crescendo TIAs"). Twenty-six patients (55%) had anatomically significant lesions of the internal carotid artery and, among 20 patients with signs or symptoms suggesting cortical ischemia (e.g., dysphasia, hemiparesis) or transient monocular visual loss, 17 (85%) had abnormal angiograms consistent with symptom-producing carotid artery disease.

Ocular Symptoms. A variety of transient visual symptoms and signs may develop in patients with disease in the carotid arterial system. The hallmark of most of these disturbances is their **monocular nature**. Although homonymous and bitemporal visual field defects and bilateral simultaneous visual loss may result from diseased carotid arteries and their branches, particularly when the disease is bilateral (Lee and Schatz, 1975; Fisher and Yellin, 1985), over 90% of visual symptoms that occur in patients with carotid arterial disease affect only one eye, even when there is bilateral disease.

Transient Monocular Visual Loss (Amaurosis Fugax). The most common and perhaps most important ophthalmologic symptom of disease of the internal carotid arterial system is **transient monocular visual loss** (Heyman et al., 1984a; The Amaurosis Fugax Study Group, 1990). This condition also is called **amaurosis fugax** (from the Greek, *amauros,* meaning "dark," and *fugax,* meaning "fleeting") (Bernstein, 1988), but we and others (Fisher, 1989a) believe that this term has a less precise connotation and should be abandoned.

Patients with this symptom complain of acute, **monocular** loss of vision that may be partial or complete. Patients in whom partial visual loss occurs may describe the entire field of vision as being "blurred," or they may be aware that they cannot see in one part of the field, whereas the rest of the field seems normal. In particular, loss of vision may be restricted to the upper or lower half of the field (Bruno et al., 1990). Venables et al. (1984) reviewed the hospital records of 152 patients with recurrent episodes of transient monocular visual loss and concluded that 53% of patients always had complete monocular loss of vision, 32% always had partial visual loss, and 14% of patients had experienced episodes of both partial and complete visual loss. Ehrenfeld et al. (1966) described 44 patients with transient monocular blindness associated with ipsilateral carotid artery disease. Most of these patients described their episodes of blindness as if a window shade were being drawn over all or part of

the field of vision, producing partial or complete blindness that lasted until the "window shade" was released. When blindness was incomplete, many patients were aware of sharp borders between seeing and non-seeing areas. O'Sullivan et al. (1992) reported monocular visual loss in nine young adults and noted that the visual loss in five patients progressed in a "lacunar" pattern unlike the "curtain" pattern noted above. In their analysis of patients entered into the North American Symptomatic Carotid Endarterectomy Trial (NASCET) with transient monocular visual loss, Chan et al. (1996) reported sudden, painless, and generalized loss of vision in 53.4% of 556 patients and altitudinal visual loss with a descending or ascending shade in 28.8% of patients.

Some episodes of transient monocular visual loss are accompanied by a sensation of color, such as yellow or green. Others are accompanied by photopsias consisting of showers of stationary flecks of light that disappear quickly (Fisher, 1951a, 1951b, 1952; Wagener, 1957; Ashby et al., 1963; Pessin et al., 1977; Goodwin et al., 1984, 1987). Such "positive" visual phenomena are rare, but they nevertheless occur with sufficient frequency that, based on clinical symptoms alone, transient monocular visual loss caused by carotid artery disease cannot always be differentiated from that caused by retinal migraine; i.e., vasospasm (Cohen et al., 1984).

Most episodes of transient monocular visual loss last 2–30 minutes and then resolve spontaneously, usually over seconds to minutes. Marshall and Meadows (1968) found that 51 of 67 patients (75%) experienced episodes of monocular visual loss lasting 30 minutes or less, with 29 patients (43%) experiencing attacks lasting 5 minutes or less. Pessin et al. (1977) evaluated 33 patients with transient monocular visual loss. In all but three patients, the attacks lasted less than 15 minutes, and in 14 patients (42%), the episodes lasted 5 minutes or less. Among 35 patients with transient monocular visual loss evaluated by Goodwin et al. (1987), 22 patients (63%) had attacks lasting 5 minutes or less, eight (23%) had episodes of visual loss lasting 6–15 minutes, and only six patients (14%) had visual loss lasting more than 15 minutes. Rare patients experience transient monocular visual loss lasting several hours (Longfellow et al., 1962; Fujino et al., 1983). In the NASCET, the duration of the episodes of transient monocular visual loss ranged from 15 seconds to 23 hours, with a median duration of 4 minutes and only 8% lasting more than 1 hour (Chan et al., 1996).

Some patients experience only one episode of transient visual loss, but most have more than one. Episodes may occur at extremely variable intervals. Marshall and Meadows (1968) found that some patients experienced recurrent attacks during a single day, whereas other patients had intervals from several days to **10 years** between attacks.

In some patients, transient monocular visual loss results when the patient is exposed to bright light. Furlan et al. (1979a) described five such patients, all of whom were found to have severe, ipsilateral carotid occlusive disease. Other investigators subsequently reported similar patients (Donnan et al., 1982a; Ross Russell and Page, 1983). We saw such a patient, a 78-year-old physician who began to experience episodes of visual loss in the right eye that seemed to be associated with looking outside into the sunlight. Cerebral

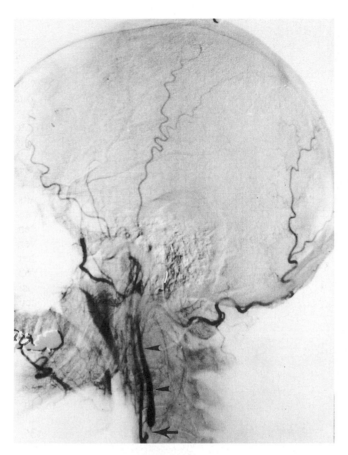

Figure 55.120. Cerebral angiogram in a patient with light-induced transient visual loss in the left eye. The patient was a 76-year-old man who began to experience visual loss in the left eye whenever he would look at a bright light. Left common carotid arteriogram, lateral view, shows a 99% stenosis of the left internal carotid artery just above its origin (*arrow*). Note that the artery is not completely occluded. There is slow filling distal to the stenosis (*arrowheads*). For this reason, the patient underwent an emergency endarterectomy (see Figure 55.121).

arteriography confirmed the presence of almost complete occlusion of the right internal carotid artery (Fig. 55.120), and an emergency endarterectomy was performed at which time a large thrombus was found and removed (Fig. 55.121). Postoperatively, the patient had normal visual function in the right eye and experienced no further episodes of visual loss in the eye. Wiebers et al. (1989) reported four patients with the extremely rare phenomenon of **bilateral, simultaneous, light-induced transient visual loss**. All four patients had bilateral severe stenosis or occlusion of the internal carotid arteries (Fig. 55.122).

Light-induced transient visual loss is caused by the inability of borderline ocular circulation to sustain the increased retinal metabolic activity associated with exposure to bright light (Brindley, 1959; Furlan et al., 1979a; Donnan et al., 1982a; Wiebers et al., 1989). Delay in the regeneration of visual pigments in the photoreceptor layer of the retina following exposure to bright light results in consequent blurred or absent vision that persists until regeneration of pigments

is achieved. Most cases of light-induced transient visual loss occur in patients with severe carotid artery disease that compromises flow to the orbital and ocular vessels; however, Safran and Boschi (1997) described a patient in whom painful visual loss occurred when the patient was exposed to bright light for 5–10 minutes. The patient had no evidence of carotid artery disease, but she had a long history of mi-

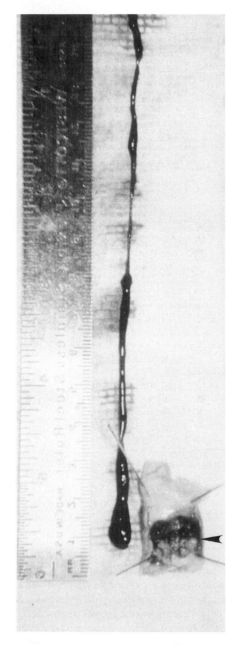

Figure 55.121. Operative findings in the patient whose angiogram results are shown in Figure 55.120. The patient underwent emergency carotid endarterectomy at which time an ulcerated plaque was found just above the carotid bifurcation. The plaque almost totally occluded the lumen of the internal carotid artery (*arrowhead*). A long thrombus extended from the plaque distally into the carotid siphon. The plaque was excised, and the thrombus was removed from the vessel.

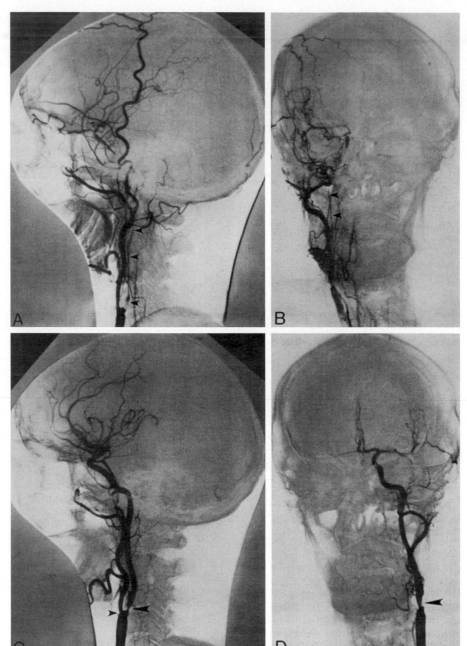

Figure 55.122. Cerebral angiography in a 68-year-old man with light-induced, *bilateral* transient loss of vision. *A* and *B*, Lateral and anteroposterior views, respectively, of right carotid arterial system show 99% stenosis of the right internal carotid artery with only a "string" of contrast extending from the origin of the right internal carotid artery to its cavernous segment (*arrowheads*). *C* and *D*, Lateral and anteroposterior views, respectively, of left carotid arterial system show 99% stenosis at origin of the left internal carotid artery (*large arrowheads*) and mild stenosis at the origin of the left external carotid artery (*small arrowheads*). (From Wiebers DO, Swanson JW, Cascino TL, et al. Bilateral loss of vision in bright light. Stroke *20:*554–558, 1989.)

graine and Raynaud's phenomenon. The visual loss in this patient seemed to result from light-induced vasospasm.

A phenomenon possibly related to light-induced transient visual loss is **postprandial transient visual loss**. Levin and Mootha (1997) described two women who developed transient visual loss lasting up to more than 1 hour after eating a meal. In one patient, the left eye was always affected. The other patient experienced bilateral simultaneous visual loss. Neuroimaging revealed 90% stenosis of the left internal carotid artery in the first patient and occlusion of the right internal carotid artery associated with 40–70% stenosis of the left internal carotid artery in the second patient. The

episodes of visual loss resolved in the first patient after carotid endarterectomy. The second patient had metastatic breast cancer and did not undergo treatment. Levin and Mootha (1997) postulated that the postprandial transient visual loss in these patients was related to a temporary retinal and choroidal hypoperfusion that occurred when blood flow that was already compromised by significant carotid artery disease was diverted to the gut following a meal—a mesenteric steal phenomenon.

Patients examined in the midst of an attack of transient, monocular visual loss may have an ipsilateral RAPD. They also may have ipsilateral pupillary dilation and paralysis, indicating ischemia of the ciliary and iris circulations. In some patients, the ophthalmoscopic appearance is that of spasmodic closure of the entire central retinal arterial tree (Wagenmann, 1897; Harbridge, 1906; Lundie, 1906; Ormond, 1918; Duane, 1954; Humphrey, 1979; Ellenberger and Epstein, 1986). The collapse of the arteries may be gradual, affecting one branch at a time, or it may be sudden and complete. In other cases, stationary or mobile emboli may be seen in the retinal arteries of the affected eye. The emboli usually are composed of platelet-fibrin particles, cholesterol, or calcium, but as has already been mentioned, they may be composed of a wide variety of material (see above). Bruno et al. (1990) prospectively evaluated 100 patients with transient monocular visual loss and found that an altitudinal or lateralized pattern of visual loss was more likely to be caused by embolic cerebrovascular disease than was complete or diffuse visual loss. Interestingly, Ormond (1918) described **mydriasis** of the pupil in the affected eye, indicating reduction of blood flow not only to the retina, choroid, and optic nerve, but also to the ciliary ganglion, the short ciliary nerves, or both.

Raymond et al. (1980) described a patient who experienced five episodes of inferior visual field loss in the left eye when he turned his head to the left. He then experienced an episode of decreased visual acuity and pain in the left eye after vigorous exercise. Later that day, he was found to have 20/20 vision in the left eye, but color vision in that eye was poor, and there was a left RAPD. Five days later, visual acuity was still normal in the left eye, and the left visual field was full when tested with kinetic perimetry; however, there was a persistent left RAPD. Ophthalmoscopy seemed normal, but fluorescein angiography showed delayed filling of the choroidal circulation with patchy choroidal filling defects. The patient was subsequently found to have a total occlusion of the left internal carotid artery.

Transient monocular loss of vision usually occurs as an isolated phenomenon, unassociated with other neurologic symptoms or signs. In particular, neither headache nor eye pain are common during an attack (Goodwin et al., 1987). Nevertheless, some patients, particularly young adults, experience headache at the time of visual loss (Tippin et al., 1989; O'Sullivan et al., 1992), and others experience transient monocular visual loss associated with contralateral hemiparesis, aphasia, or other features of hemisphere ischemia. Ropper (1985) described transient facial paresthesias associated with transient visual loss in the ipsilateral eye in five of 65 patients (8%) with transient monocular visual loss. Other patients may have had previous transient or permanent neurologic deficits before experiencing an attack of transient monocular visual loss. Among 44 patients with transient monocular visual loss examined by Sorensen (1983), six (14%) had experienced previous cerebral ischemic events, and two (5%) experienced a transient contralateral hemiparesis at the time of monocular visual loss. Among 152 patients with transient monocular visual loss whose hospital records were reviewed by Venables et al. (1984), 18% had previous or coincident TIAs affecting the ipsilateral cerebral hemisphere. Of 42 patients who experienced transient monocular visual loss and were randomized to the medical arm of a controlled trial of aspirin (Lemak et al., 1986), 15 (36%) had separate or concurrent hemisphere TIAs. In the NASCET, 26.1% of patients with transient monocular visual loss had a history of ipsilateral hemispheric TIAs or stroke (Chan et al., 1996).

Several authors separate transient monocular visual loss into several types based on the presumed underlying pathophysiology of the attacks (Wray, 1988; Burde, 1989). This approach is impractical because of the overlap in clinical features among the groups (see Table 1 in Burde, 1989). In our opinion, one should simply be mindful of the age of the patient and the numerous pathophysiologic mechanisms that can cause transient monocular visual loss. In most patients, a careful history, complete physical and ophthalmologic examinations, and appropriate diagnostic studies are sufficient to determine the source of the visual loss.

The most common identifiable cause of transient monocular visual loss, responsible for 25–90% of cases in various series, is atheromatous disease affecting the internal carotid or ophthalmic arteries (Behrman, 1951; Fisher, 1951b, 1952; Marshall and Meadows, 1968; Morax et al., 1970; Sandok et al., 1974; Mungas and Baker, 1977; Wilson and Ross Russell, 1977; Weinberger et al., 1980; De Bono and Warlow, 1981; Parkin et al., 1982; Pryse-Phillips, 1982; Adams et al., 1983; Goodwin et al., 1984; Fawcett et al., 1985; Lemak et al., 1986; Langsfeld and Lusby, 1988; Bruno et al., 1990; The Amaurosis Fugax Study Group, 1990; Carter, 1992; Perez-Burkhardt et al., 1994; Smit et al., 1994). Perez-Burkhardt et al. (1994) prospectively studied 81 patients with transient monocular visual loss with carotid duplex scanning and found greater than 70% ipsilateral stenosis in 55 patients. All 55 patients subsequently underwent carotid endarterectomy, and 42 of them (76%) had ulcerated carotid plaques. In such cases of transient monocular visual loss and ipsilateral carotid disease, atheromatous disease, either sufficient or insufficient to narrow these vessels, may predispose to the formation of emboli that transiently occlude the ophthalmic artery or one or more of its ocular branches. Alternatively, the internal carotid or ophthalmic artery is sufficiently narrow to reduce blood flow. This permits increased red blood cell aggregation and decreased red cell deformity that leads to increased blood viscosity and intermittent thrombosis. The result is transient visual loss from secondary reduction of blood flow to the ipsilateral eye (Slepyan et al., 1975; Ross and Morrow, 1984).

Transient visual loss caused by atheromatous disease of the common or internal carotid artery usually occurs in the eye on the side of the affected vessel. Occasionally, however, transient monocular visual loss occurs on the side **opposite** a stenotic or occluded artery (Aranibar et al., 1973). In such cases, the transient visual loss is probably not related directly to the carotid artery disease, but rather to associated vascular occlusive disease or systemic hypotension that, along with the diseased contralateral carotid artery, episodically compromises the flow to the eye.

Most patients with transient monocular visual loss caused by atheromatous disease of the internal or common carotid artery are over 50 years of age and have other evidence of disease, including ipsilateral or contralateral carotid bruits, systemic hypertension, claudication, and a history of other TIAs (Marshall and Meadows, 1968; Mungas and Baker, 1977; Wilson and Ross Russell, 1977; Perez-Burkhardt et al., 1994). Some patients, however, have no other symptoms or signs suggesting such disease. Feldon et al. (1977) described a 32-year-old obese, but otherwise healthy, woman who experienced recurrent attacks of monocular visual loss in the right eye. The episodes of visual loss lasted several minutes and were occasionally followed by vague, brief discomfort over the eye. The patient smoked 1 1/2 packs of cigarettes per day. The patient's ocular examination was normal; however, during an attack of visual loss, ophthalmoscopy revealed a white, nonrefractile embolus in the inferotemporal retinal artery of the right eye. Angiography revealed severe stenosis of the right internal carotid artery just distal to its origin. The patient underwent an endarterectomy after which she had no further episodes of visual loss. A similar patient was reported by Slavin et al. (1997). Harrison and Marshall (1977) emphasized that patients with transient monocular visual loss who have no history of cerebral ischemia nor any neurologic deficit on clinical examination may nevertheless have evidence of silent cerebral embolism from carotid artery disease when completely evaluated. Even in young patients, the most commonly identified single risk factor for cerebral ischemia is atherosclerotic disease (Lisovoski and Rousseaux, 1991). For these reasons, we agree with Slavin et al. (1997) that the possibility of atheromatous disease should be considered in **all** patients with transient monocular visual loss, even those who are young, healthy, and have no apparent risk factors for such disease.

From 10 to 40% of cases of transient monocular visual loss are caused by disorders other than primary atheromatous disease of the internal or common carotid artery (Bruno et al., 1990; The Amaurosis Fugax Study Group, 1990). In a prospective study of 41 patients with transient monocular visual loss or retinal artery occlusion, Smit et al. (1994) found ipsilateral carotid disease in only 27% of patients, a cardiac source in one patient, and no specific source of retinal emboli in 66% of cases (using conventional transthoracic echocardiography, 24-hour Holter monitoring, electrocardiography, and carotid duplex scanning). Although the heart can certainly be a source of emboli resulting in ocular stroke, it is unclear how commonly embolic material from the heart causes **transient** visual loss. Atheromatous (and nonatheromatous) **emboli** may reach the ocular vessels from the heart, aorta, innominate artery, and even the external carotid artery (Ehrenfeld and Lord, 1969; Barnett and Aldis, 1975; Barnett et al., 1977; Burnbaum et al., 1977; Burde, 1989). Weinberg et al. (1981) described a 48-year-old woman who experienced three episodes of transient visual loss in the left eye over a 4-month period. Each attack lasted a few minutes and resolved spontaneously. A complete examination disclosed a bruit at the level of the bifurcation of the left common carotid artery. Cerebral angiography demonstrated that the left ophthalmic artery originated not from the internal carotid artery but from the middle meningeal artery. In addition, the left external carotid artery had marked stenosis at its origin. The patient underwent uncomplicated left external carotid endarterectomy, after which she had no further episodes of visual loss over a 3-year follow-up period.

Patients with **giant cell (temporal) arteritis** may experience attacks of transient monocular visual loss indistinguishable from those produced by atheromatous disease (Hollenhorst et al., 1960). These episodes presumably result from intermittent inflammatory occlusion of the ophthalmic, posterior ciliary, or central retinal arteries (see Chapter 57).

Vasospasm, particularly that associated with **migraine,** may produce transient monocular visual loss without any of the positive visual phenomena that typically occur during an attack of migraine with visual aura. This mechanism may account for a large proportion of transient monocular visual loss of unknown etiology in young patients (Fisher, 1951b, 1952; Cogan, 1961; Marshall and Meadows, 1968; Burde, 1984; Cohen et al., 1984; Poole et al., 1987; Harbison et al., 1988; Booy, 1990; Burger et al., 1991; Winterkorn and Teman, 1991; O'Sullivan et al., 1992; Winterkorn et al., 1993—see Chapter 56). Imes and Hoyt (1989) described six patients with a variety of **exercise-induced** transient visual events (see also above), one of whom described typical transient monocular visual loss. Imes and Hoyt postulated that these episodes were a form of migraine aura without headache, and we agree. Disorders other than migraine that are associated with vasospasm (e.g., malignant hypertension and subarachnoid hemorrhage) may also produce transient monocular visual loss.

Intermittent **angle closure glaucoma** may cause brief episodes of monocular visual loss that are usually, but not invariably, associated with ipsilateral ocular pain (Chandler and Trotter, 1954; Ravits and Seybold, 1984). Such patients may experience simultaneous dilation of the pupil (Sarkies et al., 1985). These patients initially may be thought to have migraine until they are examined during an attack. We saw three such patients. Two of the patients were referred by neurologists to whom the patients had initially been referred by an ophthalmologist. One patient had already undergone a complete neurologic examination and cerebral arteriography by the time she was referred to us. The second patient had undergone a neurologic examination and was scheduled for a cerebrovascular evaluation when we made the correct diagnosis. In only one patient, a 63-year-old woman, was the diagnosis of intermittent angle closure glaucoma suspected by the ophthalmologist who initially saw the patient.

Patients with **increased intracranial pressure** may experience episodes of transient visual loss, although they are usually bilateral, last for only a few seconds to a minute, are often related to changes in position, and may occur dozens of times a day (see Chapter 10). These episodes of visual loss are thought to be related to the effects of increased ICP on the blood flow to the eye, perhaps where the central retinal artery penetrates the optic nerve sheath to enter the substance of the nerve or perhaps related to the increased crowding at the optic nerve head caused by papilledema.

Patients with **optic nerve sheath meningioma** may experience episodes of monocular, transient visual loss (Sibony et al., 1984). The episodes of visual loss in such patients are much more like those of patients with increased ICP than of patients with thromboembolic atheromatous disease. The duration of visual loss is brief, usually only a few seconds. The pathophysiology of the transient visual loss that occurs in these patients is unclear, but it may be caused by the effect of the meningioma on the central retinal artery where it enters the optic nerve or by swelling and crowding of the optic disc.

Hilton-Jones et al. (1982) described a patient who experienced frequent, stereotyped episodes of visual loss, associated with orbital and neck pain, who was found to have a large **frontal lobe tumor**. Each episode of visual loss lasted 5–30 minutes and occurred in both eyes simultaneously and symmetrically. These attacks thus differed from typical attacks of transient visual loss in that they were binocular and associated with pain, and they differed from the transient obscurations of vision that occur in association with papilledema in that they lasted about 20 minutes rather than a few seconds.

Transient, monocular visual loss is occasionally **gaze-evoked**, occurring only when the eye is turned in a certain direction and clearing as soon as the eye returns from that position of gaze. Patients with gaze-evoked visual loss usually have an **orbital mass** that interferes with the blood supply to the retina, optic nerve, or both when the eye is turned in a particular direction (Knapp et al., 1992) (see Chapter 38). Pascual et al. (1988) described a patient with pseudotumor cerebri (see Chapter 10) who experienced transient loss of vision in the left eye whenever she looked eccentrically. Each episode was characterized by disappearance of vision from the periphery to the center of the visual field. When the eye returned to primary gaze, vision cleared immediately. The left optic disc was swollen with splinter hemorrhages at the margin. The ophthalmoscopic appearance did not change during the episodes of visual loss. The pathogenesis of gaze-evoked visual loss in this patient is unclear, but it may have been caused by kinking of a swollen nerve sheath with secondary compression of the vascular supply to the optic nerve during eccentric gaze.

Reduced blood flow through nonoccluded and nonspastic vessels may be responsible for transient visual loss in some patients. Systemic hypotension from cardiac and noncardiac sources can produce it, as can orthostatic hypotension. Coppeto (1985) described a 78-year-old man with mild hypertension who began to experience episodes of transient monocular visual loss and other TIAs shortly after he was placed on a topical solution of 0.5% timolol maleate for glaucoma. He was taking the medication twice a day in the right eye only. The patient was found to be experiencing episodes of cardiac arrhythmia that corresponded to his episodes of neurologic and visual disturbance. The timolol maleate was discontinued, and the episodes of cardiac arrhythmia as well as the transient visual and neurologic deficits ceased and did not return over a follow-up period of over 4 years. Teman et al. (1995) postulated relative retinal hypoperfusion secondary to shunting of blood to the perineum as the underlying mechanism of transient monocular blindness during sexual intercourse.

Transient monocular visual loss occasionally can result from a reduction or diversion of blood flow in the ophthalmic artery caused by an AVM; i.e., a **steal phenomenon** (Kosary et al., 1973, Bogousslavsky et al., 1985a; Fritz et al., 1989; Xiong et al., 1993). The patient reported by Bogousslavsky

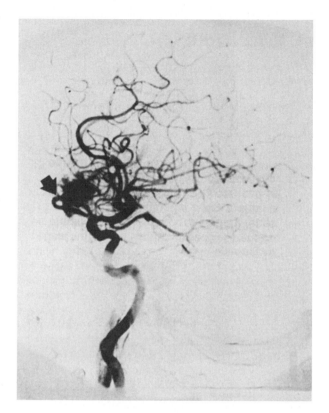

Figure 55.123. Arteriovenous malformation causing amaurosis fugax. The patient was a 46-year-old woman with a left-sided bruit and a 1-year history of episodes of transient monocular loss of vision in the left eye. Left internal carotid arteriogram, lateral view, shows a dural arteriovenous malformation in the left anterior cranial fossa. The anterior portion of the malformation is fed by a recurrent meningeal branch of the left ophthalmic artery (*arrow*). (From Bogousslavsky J, Vinuela F, Barnett HJM, et al. Amaurosis fugax as the presenting manifestation of dural arteriovenous malformation. Stroke 16:891–893, 1985.)

et al. (1985a) was a 46-year-old woman who was evaluated after she experienced three episodes of transient visual loss in the left eye. She was found to have a left anterior-middle fossa dural AVM with pial venous drainage. The malformation received its main supply from the left middle meningeal artery, but its anterior part was fed by the recurrent branch of the left ophthalmic artery (Fig. 55.123). The authors suggested that transient, episodic lowering of retinal artery pressure, caused by shunting of blood from the ophthalmic artery to the malformation, was the most likely explanation for the transient monocular visual loss in their patient.

Fritz et al. (1989) described a 57-year-old man who had three attacks of transient visual loss in the right eye over a 2-year period. He then developed a superior visual field defect in that eye. An evaluation revealed an AVM of the right anterior ethmoidal artery (Fig. 55.124). Because Doppler ultrasonography demonstrated a retrograde flow in the distal branches of the right ophthalmic artery, it was postulated that the malformation caused blood to be shunted from the ophthalmic artery to the anterior ethmoidal artery and away from the orbit. The AVM was completely excised. Postoper-

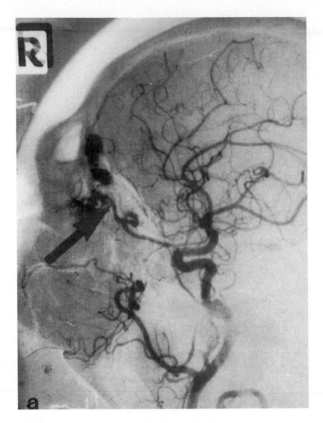

Figure 55.124. Arteriovenous malformation causing transient monocular loss of vision. The patient was a 57-year-old man who complained of episodes of transient loss of vision in the right eye. Right common carotid arteriogram, lateral view, shows a right frontopolar, dural arteriovenous malformation fed by the right anterior ethmoidal artery (*arrow*). It was postulated that the malformation was causing blood to be shunted away from the ophthalmic artery. The patient's symptoms resolved after the malformation was excised. (From Fritz W, Klein HJ, Schmidt K. Arteriovenous malformation of the posterior ethmoidal artery as an unusual cause of amaurosis fugax: The ophthalmic steal syndrome. J Clin Neuroophthalmol *9:* 165–168, 1989.)

atively, the pattern of flow in the right ophthalmic artery was normal, and the patient had no further episodes of visual loss.

Patients with **hyperviscosity** or **hypercoagulability** syndromes may have reduced blood flow through nonoccluded vessels resulting in transient visual loss. Mundall et al. (1972a, 1972b) described a 63-year-old woman who developed mild right-sided weakness and then began to experience episodes of transient blindness in the left eye. She was found to have a mild right hemiparesis and an incomplete right homonymous hemianopia that was denser inferiorly. Laboratory studies revealed a platelet count that ranged from 400,000 to 1,065,000 and averaged 740,000.

Not all cases of transient monocular visual loss are caused by reduced blood flow to the eye or orbit. Kosmorsky et al. (1985) reported transient monocular visual loss associated with erythropsia and color desaturation in a 73-year-old man. The patient was initially suspected of having atheromatous disease of the ipsilateral carotid artery; however, an exami-

nation during an episode of visual loss revealed a spontaneous **anterior chamber hemorrhage** (hyphema). Such hemorrhages are not uncommon in patients after cataract extraction (Swan, 1973; Watzke, 1980) and are particularly apt to occur after placement of an iris-fixated intraocular lens implant (Lieppman, 1982; Nicholson, 1982; Magargal et al., 1983). We examined a patient in whom a posterior-chamber intraocular lens was responsible for intermittent hyphemas that produced episodes of visual blurring that initially were thought to be caused by atherosclerotic carotid artery disease. Only when the patient was seen during one of these episodes and found to have a hyphema associated with elevated intraocular pressure in the eye was the actual cause of the visual episodes recognized.

In some patients with transient monocular visual loss, no definite cause is found despite exhaustive evaluations (Fisher, 1951b, 1952; Eadie, 1968; Eadie et al., 1968; Marshall and Meadows, 1968; Sorensen, 1983; Poole et al., 1987; Tippin et al., 1989; The Amaurosis Fugax Study Group, 1990; O'Sullivan et al., 1992). Most of these patients are young women who never develop permanent visual loss or neurologic deficits regardless of the number of episodes they experience. We suspect that in most such cases, the visual loss is caused by vasospasm; however, Digre et al. (1989) described six young adults under 45 years of age who experienced transient monocular visual loss and who were found to have elevated levels of antiphospholipid antibodies. Similar patients were described by Frohman et al. (1989). In these patients and in patients with otherwise unexplained transient (as well as permanent) neurologic deficits, antiphospholipid antibodies may somehow predispose to thrombosis (Briley et al., 1989; Digre et al., 1989; Levine and Welch, 1989a; Shuaib and Barcley, 1989; Kushner, 1990; Levine et al., 1990a; Castanon et al., 1995; Feldmann and Levine, 1995; Levine et al., 1995) (see above).

Miscellaneous Transient Ocular Symptoms. Ocular symptoms other than transient monocular visual loss that occur in patients with carotid artery disease are transient burning or watering of the ipsilateral eye (Hager, 1962) and transient homonymous visual field defects. The latter symptom may result from emboli to the middle cerebral artery, or it may result when the posterior cerebral artery originates from or communicates directly with the affected internal carotid artery rather than the basilar artery (Figs. 55.116 and 55.117). Transient homonymous hemianopia may also occur in patients with carotid artery disease in whom there is a persistent fetal channel between the internal carotid and vertebral or basilar artery. Such patients may also experience episodes of transient, **bilateral, simultaneous visual loss.** Such episodes occurred in a 67-year-old woman with severe obstructive atherosclerotic disease affecting both internal carotid arteries (Fisher and Yellin, 1985). The severity of visual loss was not the same in both eyes, however. In one eye, all vision was lost, whereas in the other eye, there was just cloudy vision. This asymmetry of simultaneous visual loss is usually not expected when the loss of vision is caused by vertebrobasilar arterial system disease.

PATHOPHYSIOLOGY OF CAROTID ARTERIAL SYSTEM TIAS

TIAs are caused by intermittent reduction of blood flow in arteries supplying clinically important neural or ocular structures. This reduction of blood flow may, in turn, be caused by any of the mechanisms described in earlier sections of this chapter: (*a*) thrombosis, (*b*) embolism, or (*c*) hypoperfusion (Mohr and Pessin, 1986). Pessin et al. (1977) evaluated 95 consecutive patients with TIAs and concluded that they formed three groups with respect to probable cause as determined by angiography. One group of patients had intracranial branch-artery occlusions above a normal carotid bifurcation or a carotid artery that was minimally atherosclerotic. In these and similar patients, **emboli**, probably originating in the heart, were most likely responsible for the TIAs (Millikan, 1965; Zatz et al., 1965; Ring, 1966; Moore and Hall, 1968; Davis et al., 1969; Moore and Hall, 1970; Yarnell et al., 1975; Duncan et al., 1976). Such findings do not eliminate the possibility of stagnation thrombus formation in distal branches of the symptomatic carotid artery territory; however, branch occlusions are more frequent in patients with otherwise normal carotid arteries, a fact that argues against a stagnation mechanism.

A second mechanism proposed by Pessin et al. (1977) to explain the pathogenesis of carotid system TIAs is **lacunar disease**. Patients in whom this mechanism is said to occur have no angiographic evidence of atherosclerotic disease affecting the extracranial portion, intracranial portion, or branches of the internal carotid artery in whose territory the TIA has occurred. Rapid lysis of embolic material, with a subsequent normal angiographic vessel, might account for some overlap with patients who have embolism. We examined two patients who experienced multiple attacks of transient monocular visual loss in the setting of normal cardiac studies and normal angiographic studies of the ipsilateral and contralateral internal and external carotid arteries. Both subsequently underwent exploratory carotid endarterectomy, and in both patients, significant atheromatous disease, with associated platelet-fibrin clot, was found. After endarterectomy, the episodes of transient visual loss stopped in both patients. Nevertheless, TIAs may precede pathologically documented lacunar infarctions (Fisher and Curry, 1965).

The final mechanism thought by Pessin et al. (1977) to be responsible for the majority of TIAs that occur in the territory of a carotid artery is severe **stenosis** or **occlusion** of the artery itself. Although TIAs may be caused by emboli arising from an atheromatous carotid lesion, transient intermittent obstruction of the carotid artery can clearly produce TIAs and stroke (Fisher, 1962; Moore and Hall, 1970; Duncan et al., 1976).

In order to determine which of these and other pathophysiologic processes (e.g., vasospasm) is responsible for TIAs in a specific patient, a thorough history, complete examination, and appropriate diagnostic evaluation are required (Toole and Yuson, 1977). The prognosis, and thus the appropriate treatment, of a patient with one or more TIAs cannot be determined unless the underlying cause is known.

Signs of Occlusive Disease of the Common Carotid Artery

Symptomatic extracranial cerebrovascular disease arises primarily from disease of the internal carotid artery. The incidence of occlusion of the **common carotid artery** in patients with signs of cerebral ischemia is only about 1–5% (Hass et al., 1968; Podore et al., 1981; Collice et al., 1983; Toole, 1984). Dyken et al. (1974) reviewed 279 consecutive angiograms and found only five that showed common carotid artery occlusion compared with 38 that showed occlusion of the internal carotid artery.

The most common lesion causing occlusion of the common carotid artery is an advanced atherosclerotic plaque located at the carotid bifurcation, causing retrograde thrombosis of the vessel, or at the origin of the common carotid artery, causing anterograde thrombosis (Keller et al., 1984; Toole, 1984; Mohr and Pessin, 1986) (Fig. 55.125). Like the internal carotid artery, the common carotid artery also can be occluded by vasculitis, fibromuscular dysplasia, emboli from the heart, radiation, and trauma (Levine and Welch, 1989b).

Predominant symptoms and signs in patients with occlusion of the common carotid artery are the same as those in patients with internal carotid artery occlusion. Levine and Welch (1989b) described visual symptoms and signs in 15 of 17 patients (88%) whom they evaluated. In some patients,

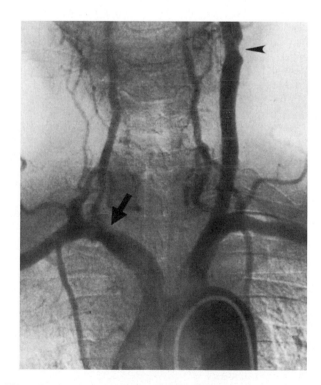

Figure 55.125. Occlusion of the common carotid artery. Aortic arch angiogram, anteroposterior view, shows occlusion of the right common carotid artery at its origin from the aortic arch (*arrow*). The patient also has an ulcerated plaque at the bifurcation of the left common carotid artery (*arrowhead*). (From Huber P. Cerebral Angiography. 2nd ed. New York, Georg Thieme Verlag, 1982.)

the visual disturbances were monocular and ipsilateral to the side of the occlusion. In others, they were bilateral and consisted of hemianopic field defects on the side contralateral to the occluded vessel. Levine and Welch (1989b) also found that motor weakness was common in patients with symptomatic occlusion of the common carotid artery, occurring in 88% of patients. Other symptoms and signs included sensory disturbances, dizziness or lightheadedness, and syncope. Symptoms were positional in two-thirds of patients.

Patients with occlusion of the common carotid artery are at high risk for myocardial ischemia, probably because they usually have several of the risk factors for the development of atherosclerosis. In the series reported by Levine and Welch (1989b), all 17 patients had at least one risk factor for stroke, with 14 of the 17 patients (82%) having two or more risk factors. The most common risk factor in this group of patients was cigarette smoking (see also Podore et al., 1981), with systemic hypertension a close second. Other risk factors in this group of patients included hyperglycemia and hyperlipidemia. These are the same risk factors that are commonly associated with atherosclerotic stenosis and occlusion of the internal carotid artery (Bogousslavsky et al., 1985b).

Signs of Occlusive Disease in the Internal Carotid Arterial System

The variability of symptoms and signs in patients with internal carotid artery stenosis or occlusion is simply an expression of the many effects that atheromatous and other disease can produce in the supply area of a major arterial trunk. Carotid occlusion or severe stenosis may be asymptomatic, produce transient neurologic episodes without permanent signs of neurologic or ophthalmologic abnormality, or produce an acute or slowly progressive stroke with physical signs indicating brain dysfunction in a portion of one cerebral hemisphere or in the supply area of a single arterial branch of the internal carotid artery (Vitek et al., 1972; Dyken et al., 1974; Cote et al., 1983; Fritz et al., 1985; Bogousslavsky et al., 1986a; Hennerici et al., 1987; Gorelick et al., 1988; Harrison and Marshall, 1988).

Persistent symptoms and signs that suggest occlusive disease of the carotid vascular system are of three types: (a) extracranial, (b) neurologic, and (c) ocular. In most patients, a careful history and examination, supplemented by appropriate diagnostic tests, are sufficient to arrive at the correct diagnosis; however, there may be considerable interobserver variation in the assessment of the neurologic history and, to a lesser extent, the neurologic examination in stroke patients (Sisk et al., 1970; Tomasello et al., 1982; Shinar et al., 1985). This variability has prompted a search for an optimum method of quantifying the results of neurologic testing (Asplund, 1987; Brott et al., 1989; Goldstein et al., 1989).

EXTRACRANIAL SIGNS

Stenosis of the **extracranial** portion of the internal carotid artery (or, for that matter, of the common carotid artery) frequently produces a sharply localized, systolic **bruit** that can be heard by auscultation over the carotid bifurcation (Matthews, 1961; Gilroy and Meyer, 1962; Ziegler et al.,

1971; David et al., 1973; Chambers and Norris, 1985). Bruits in the neck that are soft and high-pitched usually reflect significant stenosis with a low flow of blood (Patterson, 1988). Such bruits may be associated with ocular bruits heard by placing the bell of the stethoscope over one or both eyes (Cohen and Miller, 1956; Allen and Mustian, 1962; Fisher, 1957; Bousser et al., 1981; Chambers and Norris, 1985; Hu et al., 1988). Neck bruits that are loud and low-pitched usually suggest a large volume of blood flow without much obstruction (Patterson, 1988). As part of the NASCET, Sauve et al. (1994) concluded that cervical bruits alone were not sufficiently predictive of high-grade symptomatic carotid stenosis to be useful in selecting patients for angiography, because bruits were absent in over one-third of patients with high-grade stenosis.

Stenosis of the **intracranial** portion of the internal carotid artery may produce a **murmur** that is heard best over the eye on the side of the affected vessel. Occlusion of the internal carotid artery usually is not associated with a bruit or murmur; however, if the ipsilateral external carotid artery is stenotic, a bruit or murmur may be present (David et al., 1973; Sandok et al., 1974). In addition, a systolic murmur may be heard in the carotid or orbital region on the side **opposite** an occluded common or internal carotid artery (Bousser et al., 1981). This murmur results from the increased blood flow that occurs in a patent internal carotid artery contralateral to one that is occluded (Crevasse and Logue, 1958; Allen and Mustian, 1962). This murmur disappears when the patent vessel is compressed, but it is not influenced by compression of the occluded vessel.

Palpation of the internal carotid artery in the neck may be difficult or impossible to perform in some patients, but poor pulsation of the vessel, particularly when compared with the opposite side, may indicate occlusive disease in that vessel, and normal pulsation does not eliminate the possibility of significant disease in the vessel. In addition, although many investigators advocate manual compression of the internal carotid artery as a way to determine if that artery is stenotic or if the contralateral artery is occluded, we do not advocate compression of a potentially diseased vessel, because this maneuver may produce neurologic or visual defects from embolization.

NEUROLOGIC SIGNS

Occlusion of the Internal Carotid Artery. Spontaneous occlusion of the internal carotid artery may result from a variety of mechanisms (Fig. 55.126). Castaigne et al. (1970) performed a pathologic evaluation of 61 specimens of internal carotid artery occlusion from 50 patients. Thirty-seven specimens (61%) from 31 patients were occluded by primary atherosclerotic disease. In all of these specimens, the occlusion resulted from a thrombosis in or near a pre-existing atherosclerotic stenosis. Thirteen specimens (21%) from 12 patients were occluded by emboli. The remaining 11 specimens (18%) were occluded from miscellaneous or undetermined causes.

The clinical manifestations of occlusion of the internal carotid artery are the most variable of any cerebrovascular

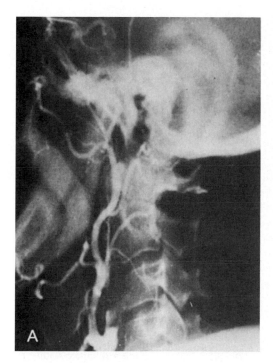
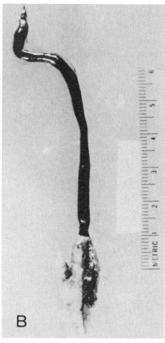

Figure 55.126. Complete occlusion of the internal carotid artery in a patient who had been experiencing ipsilateral monocular episodes of loss of vision. *A*, Common carotid arteriogram, lateral view, shows complete occlusion of the internal carotid artery. The patient underwent endarterectomy. *B*, Specimen removed at the time of surgery. At the bottom of the specimen is the cast of the carotid bulb. Attached to it is the thrombus that had propagated upward to the level of the cavernous sinus. (From Ehrenfeld WK, Hoyt WH, Wylie EJ. Embolization and transient blindness from carotid atheroma. Arch Surg *93:* 787–794, 1966.)

syndrome (Hultquist, 1942; Ford, 1952; Castaigne et al., 1970; Zülch and Gessaga, 1972). Some patients remain asymptomatic (Hennerici et al., 1987). Others develop focal or massive neurologic deficits. Still others experience seizures (Kilpatrick et al., 1990; Sung and Chu, 1990).

Occlusion, which occurs most frequently in the extracranial segment of the vessel just distal to the bifurcation of the common carotid artery, is not infrequently asymptomatic because of the adequacy of the intracranial collateral circulation provided by the circle of Willis. Such collateral flow, however, eventually may not be sufficient to protect the patient from subsequent stroke (Harrison and Marshall, 1988).

Hennerici et al. (1987) identified 284 patients with asymptomatic disease of the extracranial portion of the internal carotid artery. Forty-nine of these patients (17%) had occlusion of the vessel, 36 patients (13%) had severe stenosis, and the remaining 199 patients (70%) had mild to moderate stenosis. Over a follow-up period of 28–32 months, the mean annual mortality rate of these patients varied from 6.2% in patients with mild to moderate stenosis to 10.5% in patients with carotid occlusion. The percentage of patients experiencing a TIA during the follow-up period was about 8–10%, whereas the percentage of patients suffering a stroke varied from 2% in patients with mild to moderate stenosis to 12% in patients with carotid occlusion.

Bornstein and Norris (1989) followed 40 patients with unilateral carotid occlusion by serial clinical and Doppler examinations for over 6 years. These investigators divided the patients into two groups. The first group consisted of 19 patients who already had an occluded artery when they entered the study. The second group consisted of 21 patients who had asymptomatic stenosis when they entered the study, but in whom occlusion developed during the course of the

study. No strokes occurred in the first group during followup; the annual stroke rate in the second group was 3.8% for the territory of the occluded artery and 5.7% overall. The death rate was 6.6% annually for both groups, mainly from complications related to cardiac dysfunction.

In some patients, occlusion of the internal carotid artery produces only transient neurologic symptoms and signs. Cote et al. (1983) identified 47 patients with occlusion of the internal carotid artery, 27 of whom (57%) presented with TIAs. The remaining 20 patients had only minor neurologic deficits. These transient events were probably caused by intermittent relative hypotension. An infrequent but characteristic sign of carotid occlusive disease is the so-called "limb-shaking TIA," in which the patient experiences involuntary shaking and oscillation of the arm, hand, and, occasionally, leg contralateral to the occluded internal carotid artery (Baquis et al., 1985; Yanigahara et al., 1985). These episodes are caused by intermittent hypoperfusion with brain ischemia rather than seizure activity.

Some of the TIAs that occur in the distribution of an occluded internal carotid artery result from atherosclerotic disease located some distance distal to the occlusion (e.g., in the carotid siphon), whereas others result from emboli that originate from a thrombus that forms at the stump (distal end) of the occluded vessel (the stump embolization syndrome—Barnett et al., 1977, 1978; Ryan and Day, 1987). There also is some evidence that in the presence of an occluded internal carotid artery, an atherosclerotic **external carotid artery** may produce intracranial and ocular emboli (Ehrenfeld and Lord, 1969; Burnbaum et al., 1977) (Fig. 55.127). Of course, patients with an occluded internal carotid artery also may experience TIAs from disease located in other stenotic or ulcerated, but nonoccluded, vessels.

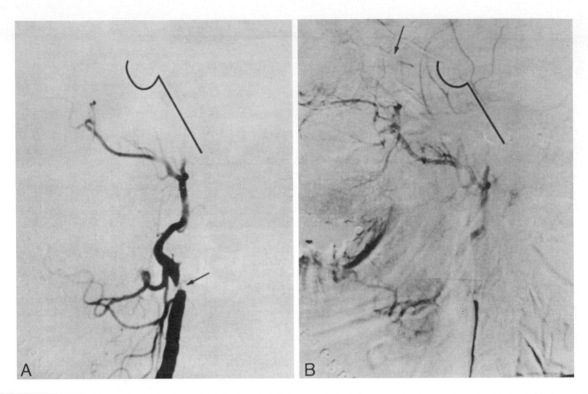

Figure 55.127. Amaurosis fugax from atherosclerotic disease of the external carotid artery. The patient was a 52-year-old man with recurrent episodes of transient loss of vision in the left eye. *A*, Left common carotid arteriogram shows complete occlusion of the left internal carotid artery and severe stenosis at the origin of the left external carotid artery (*arrow*). *B*, Later phase of the same arteriogram shows retrograde filling of the ophthalmic artery (*arrow*). Outline of the sella turcica and clivus is superimposed on each photograph. (From Burnbaum MD, Selhorst JB, Harbison JW, et al. Amaurosis fugax from disease of the external carotid artery. Arch Neurol *34:*532–535, 1977.)

When neurologic deficits result from occlusion of the internal carotid artery, they usually occur dramatically at the time of the occlusion. In some instances, occlusion of the internal carotid artery causes a massive infarction affecting the anterior two-thirds or all of the cerebral hemisphere including the basal ganglia. In this setting, death may result within hours to days. Most often the infarct affects all or some part of the territory supplied by the middle cerebral artery; however, when the anterior communicating artery is small or absent, the territory normally supplied by the ipsilateral anterior cerebral artery also is affected (Castaigne et al., 1970). If both anterior cerebral arteries arise from a common stem on one side, infarction may occur in the territories of both vessels. Not infrequently, the territory of the anterior choroidal artery also is affected in patients with occlusion of the internal carotid artery, and the territory supplied by the posterior cerebral artery is included in the infarction when this vessel originates from the internal carotid artery rather than from the distal portion of the basilar artery. Patients with unilateral carotid artery disease and a persistent anastomotic channel between the internal carotid artery and the basilar artery (e.g., a persistent trigeminal artery; see Chapter 52) may experience the unilateral or bilateral neurologic and visual symptoms usually associated with vertebrobasilar artery disease.

Heeney and Koo (1980) described a 65-year-old woman who developed acute cortical blindness and was found to have a left internal carotid artery bruit. Angiography revealed an ulcerated, atherosclerotic plaque in the left internal carotid artery and a persistent trigeminal artery. The patient was thought to have experienced embolism to the posterior cerebral arteries from the internal carotid artery via the persistent trigeminal artery. Pessin et al. (1989) reported the case of a 70-year-old man with no previous neurologic symptoms who experienced an acute, complete, left homonymous hemianopia. A neurologic examination was normal; however, he had a right cervical bruit, and a cholesterol embolus was observed in a branch retinal artery in the right eye. CT scanning demonstrated a right occipital infarct, and angiography showed that the right internal carotid artery communicated directly with the vertebrobasilar circulation through a fetal right posterior communicating artery. The patient was thought to have suffered an embolic occipital lobe stroke directly related to atheromatous disease in the right internal carotid artery. A similar patient was reported by Cohen (1989). The patient was a 63-year-old man who awoke from a nap with a severe headache and a left homonymous hemianopia. The neurologic examination was normal except for the visual field defect. A CT scan showed a lucency in the right occipital lobe consistent with an ischemic infarction. Cerebral angiography showed that the right posterior cerebral artery filled from a severely stenotic right internal carotid artery. Balcer et al. (1996) reported a patient with a carotid dissection who had infarctions in both the ipsilateral middle cerebral and posterior cerebral artery territories, the latter presumably resulting from an embolus that passed through the ipsilateral posterior communicating artery.

If one internal carotid artery has previously been silently occluded, occlusion or severe stenosis of the remaining artery may cause symptoms and signs of bilateral infarction. In some cases, the areas of infarction are massive and correspond to the territory of the major branches of one or both internal carotid arteries, whereas in others, lacunar infarctions result from hemodynamic cerebral ischemia (Waterston et al., 1990). Patients who experience massive infarction may become comatose, with quadriplegia and abnormal spontaneous to-and-fro conjugate eye movements (see Chapter 29). Patients with lacunar infarction may have one of several lacunar syndromes, such as ataxic hemiparesis or sensorimotor stroke.

Bilateral occlusion of the internal carotid arteries is rare. Fisher (1954) described 11 cases, all associated with severe neurologic deficits during life that caused or were primarily responsible for the patient's death. Clarke and Harrison (1956) also emphasized the progressive decline in cognitive function, evolving neurologic deficits, and poor outcome in patients with bilateral occlusion of the internal carotid arteries. In rare patients, a reversible dementia occurs from poor cerebral perfusion (Tatemichi et al., 1995). Nevertheless, some patients with bilateral carotid artery occlusion have no or only minor neurologic deficits (Hardy et al., 1962; Waltimo and Fogelholm, 1975). Wade et al. (1987) described the presenting characteristics and prognosis in 74 patients with bilateral occlusion of the internal carotid arteries in whom the initial deficits were not severe. Patients who presented with ischemic events affecting the territory of both carotid arteries were significantly more prone to subsequent cerebral infarction than those in whom symptoms were confined to the territory of only one artery.

Symptomatic occlusion of the internal carotid artery usually produces clinical manifestations resembling those of occlusion of the middle cerebral artery: contralateral hemiplegia, contralateral hemianesthesia, homonymous hemianopia, and aphasia when the lesion is left-sided (see below). In some cases, however, the ipsilateral eye has experienced a CRAO or ION. In such cases, the eye on the side of the lesion is blind or nearly so, and the contralateral eye has a temporal hemianopic field defect. This would not be expected with a middle cerebral artery stroke. Patients with this syndrome are often stuporous or semicomatose because of the sheer mass of swollen, necrotic brain. The eyes may be conjugately deviated toward the side of the infarction, although this deviation usually is of short duration and resolves soon after the onset of the stroke (Daroff and Hoyt, 1971; De Renzi et al., 1982; Mohr et al., 1984) unless there was damage to the contralateral frontal region (Steiner and Melamed, 1984). Headache, usually located above the ipsilateral eyebrow, may occur as the artery becomes occluded (Fisher, 1968a; Mohr et al., 1978; Edmeads, 1986; Gorelick et al., 1986; Britton and Guiloff, 1988; Wilson et al., 1989).

A surprising number of cases of total occlusion of the internal or common carotid artery present as acute hemiplegia without any premonitory signs (O'Day et al., 1970; Aleksic and George, 1973; Chokroverty and Rubino, 1975). Pa-

tients with this presentation initially may be thought to have suffered a small lacunar stroke. Other patients develop acute hemiparesis associated with contralateral orbital, temple, or hemicranial pain and blindness from CRAO or ischemic optic neuropathy. Some of these patients also have paresis of one or more ocular motor nerves on the side of the occlusion. Wilson et al. (1989) described two such patients. One of the patients had paresis of all three ocular motor nerves; the other had paresis of the oculomotor and abducens nerves with sparing of the trochlear nerve. In both patients, angiography showed a thrombus extending from the origin of the internal carotid artery to its intracranial bifurcation as well as occlusion of the proximal one-half to two-thirds of the ophthalmic artery.

Not all patients with occlusion of the internal carotid artery have severe hemispheric signs. One of the patients described by Wilson et al. (1989) developed severe left orbital and temple pain associated with acute loss of vision in the left eye, drooping of the left upper eyelid, and dilation of the left pupil. Examination revealed that the patient was blind in the left eye with the ocular fundus showing a picture consistent with CRAO. In addition, the patient had a left abducens nerve paresis and a complete left oculomotor nerve paresis with involvement of the pupil. He had no sensory or motor disturbances except for absent deep-tendon reflexes in the ankles. Four-vessel cerebral angiography showed complete occlusion of the left internal carotid artery at the bifurcation of the common carotid artery and retrograde filling of the terminal portion of the ophthalmic artery via the external carotid circulation. The proximal 20–25 mm of the ophthalmic artery was not visualized.

Some patients with occlusion of the internal carotid artery initially develop neurologic deficits caused by infarction at the borderzones with the middle cerebral artery territory (Wodarz, 1980). These "watershed" infarctions are thought to be caused by leptomeningeal emboli (Torvik, 1984), and they produce three stereotyped neurologic patterns (Bogousslavsky and Regli, 1986).

Anterior watershed infarctions produce hemiparesis predominating in the leg and sparing of the face. About 50% of patients also have a decrease in superficial and deep sensation in the same distribution. Patients with left-sided infarction show initial mutism, followed by a decrease in speech output with word-finding difficulty but with preservation of comprehension and repetition.

Posterior watershed infarctions produce an homonymous hemianopia that usually is incomplete, denser below, and associated with macular sparing (Sadun et al., 1983). Brachiofacial cortical hypesthesia often occurs in patients with this type of infarction, but motor weakness is both rare and mild. Patients with left-sided infarctions usually have a fluent aphasia characterized by semantic paraphasias and poor comprehension. Patients with right-sided infarctions show contralateral hemispatial neglect and anosognosia (Bisiach et al., 1990; Celesia et al., 1997; Coslett, 1997). Such patients often have a supranuclear horizontal gaze paresis with reduced or no spontaneous eye movements toward the side of the lesion (De Renzi et al., 1982; Goodwin and Kansu, 1986; Kelley and Kovacs, 1986; Kömpf and Gmeiner, 1989).

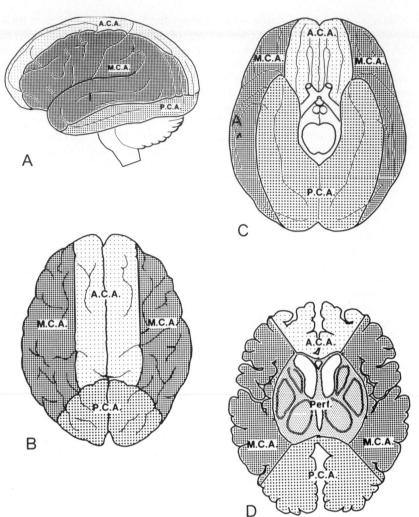

Figure 55.128. Cortical and subcortical supply of the cerebral hemispheres by the anterior (*A.C.A.*), middle (*M.C.A.*), and posterior (*P.C.A.*) cerebral arteries and their perforating branches (*perf.*). *A,* Lateral surface; *B,* Basal surface; *C,* Superior surface; *D,* Axial section through basal ganglia. (From Day AL. Arterial distributions and variants. In Cerebral Blood Flow. Editor, Wood JH, p 22. New York, McGraw-Hill, 1987.)

Subcortical watershed infarctions distal to an occluded internal carotid artery produce braciofacial hemiparesis with an accompanying hemisensory deficit. Patients with left-sided infarctions have expressive speech disturbances with good comprehension and repetition. These cases often are clinically indistinguishable from those traditionally labeled as middle cerebral or anterior cerebral artery thrombosis. The correct diagnosis in such cases is made after appropriate neuroimaging studies, particularly arteriography, are performed. In other cases, specific signs suggest selective ischemia in the territory supplied by a particular branch of the internal carotid artery. It must be remembered, however, that obstruction of the major branches of the internal carotid artery may result not from primary atheromatous disease in that vessel, but from an embolus that originated in the heart, internal carotid artery, or some other vessel (Gacs et al., 1983) or occasionally from compression by an extrinsic mass such as a tumor or aneurysm.

Occlusion of the Ophthalmic Artery and its Branches. There are never any neurologic signs of isolated occlusion of the ophthalmic artery or its branches, because the ophthalmic artery supplies only visual structures.

Occlusion of the Anterior Cerebral Artery. Through its cortical branches, this artery supplies the anterior three-quarters of the cerebral hemisphere, including the medial-orbital surface of the frontal lobe, the frontal pole, a strip of the lateral surface of the cerebral hemisphere along the superior border, and the anterior four-fifths of the corpus callosum (Fig. 55.128). The penetrating branches of the artery that arise near the circle of Willis run mainly to the anterior limb of the internal capsule and to the inferior part of the head of the caudate nucleus.

The clinical manifestations of occlusion of the anterior cerebral artery depend on the location and size of the infarct, which, in turn, relates to the site of the occlusion, the pattern of the circle of Willis, and other factors described above (Bogousslavsky and Regli, 1990). Occlusion of the anterior cerebral artery proximal to its junction with the anterior communicating artery may be asymptomatic because the collateral circulation from the contralateral side supplies the rest of the territory of the vessel (Fig. 55.129). Rare patients, however, develop an optic chiasmal syndrome from reduction or loss of blood supply from branches of the anterior cerebral and anterior communicating arteries (Lee and

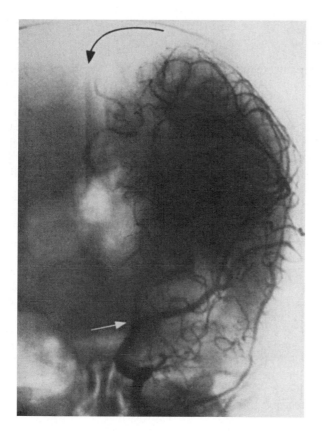

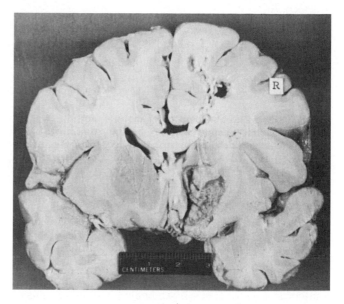

Figure 55.129. Occlusion of the anterior cerebral artery at its origin (*straight arrow*). Note that branches from the ipsilateral middle cerebral artery provide retrograde filling of some of the peripheral branches of the occluded artery (*curved arrow*). (From Krayenbühl HA, Yasargil MG. Cerebral Angiography. Philadelphia, JB Lippincott, 1968.)

Figure 55.130. Anterior cerebral artery occlusion. Coronal section through the brain in the plane of the anterior frontal and temporal lobes. There is infarction in the territories of both the proximal and the distal right anterior cerebral artery. Affected areas include the caudate, putamen, internal capsule, cingulate gyrus, and supplementary motor area. (From Brust JCM. Anterior cerebral artery. In Stroke. Pathophysiology, Diagnosis, and Management. Editors, Barnett HJM, Mohr JP, Stein BM, et al, Vol 1, pp 351–376. New York, Churchill Livingstone, 1986.)

Schatz, 1975). In addition, if there is no anterior communicating artery or if the anterior cerebral artery is occluded distal to its junction with the anterior communicating artery, several important neurologic syndromes can occur (Foix and Hillemand, 1925; Critchley, 1930; Chan and Ross, 1988; Bogousslavsky and Regli, 1990).

When the entire territory supplied by the anterior cerebral artery is infarcted, the neurologic signs are severe (Bogousslavsky and Regli, 1990). Severe contralateral **hemiplegia** consists of two elements. There is paralysis of the face, arm, and tongue from softening of the anterior limb of the internal capsule, and there is paralysis of the leg from softening of the paracentral lobule (Fig. 55.130). Cortical **anesthesia** over the leg results from softening of the mesial part of the posterior central convolution. **Apraxia affecting the left arm** is almost always present and results from damage to the corpus callosum, disconnecting the nondominant hemisphere from centers concerned with the organization of speech and skilled motor activity in the dominant hemisphere (Liepman and Maas, 1907; Geschwind and Kaplan, 1962; Geschwind, 1965) (Fig. 55.131). When the lesion is left-sided, the apraxia is obvious; however, when the lesion is on the right side, the apraxia is masked by the severe hemiplegia.

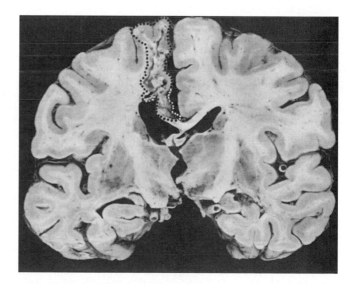

Figure 55.131. Infarct in the territory of the anterior cerebral artery. The region of the infarct is outlined by *dots*. Note that the infarct has damaged a portion of the corpus callosum, thus disconnecting the two hemispheres in this region. (From Zülch KJ. The Cerebral Infarct. Berlin, Springer-Verlag, 1985.)

Occlusion of the anterior cerebral artery just distal to the anterior communicating artery may produce several abnormal motor phenomena in addition to contralateral hemiparesis or hemiplegia and apraxia of the left upper extremity. A number of simple, reflex compulsive movements of the hand, particularly forced grasping and groping, may be present on the side opposite the lesion when the degree of hemiparesis is minimal (Walton, 1977). Abnormal motor behavior of a more complex and semipurposeful nature that occurs in the contralateral upper limb is called the "alien hand sign" (Brion and Jedynak, 1972; Bogen, 1985). In extreme cases, one hand acts at cross-purposes to the other. The term "intermanual conflict" is used to describe this behavior. McNabb et al. (1988) described three patients in whom occlusion of the dominant anterior cerebral artery was associated with a severe disturbance of upper extremity control that included impaired bimanual coordination, the alien hand sign, and intermanual conflict. All three patients had contralateral hemiparesis with the leg much worse than the arm, transcortical motor aphasia (see below), and other signs of hemispheric disconnection including ipsilateral apraxia and agraphia. This syndrome results from damage to the medial frontal region of the left frontal lobe that includes the supplementary motor cortex (Goldberg et al., 1981; McNabb et al., 1988) (Fig. 55.130).

Chan and Ross (1988) described a patient who developed pathologic left-handed mirror writing and demonstrated mirror movements of the left upper extremity during bimanual coordination tasks after infarction in the territory of the nondominant anterior cerebral artery. Because this patient had no neurologic or neuroimaging evidence of damage to the corpus callosum, Chan and Ross (1988) postulated that the syndrome resulted from damage to the right supplementary motor cortex.

Transcortical **motor aphasia** occurs when the left anterior cerebral artery is occluded (Bogousslavsky and Regli, 1990). The aphasia is characterized by reduced, nonfluent spontaneous speech despite normal reading, repetition, and auditory comprehension (Rubens, 1975; Racy et al., 1979; Alexander and Schmidt, 1980; Ross, 1980; McNabb et al., 1988). The aphasia results from softening in the centrum semiovale.

Severe disturbances of behavior occur after proximal anterior cerebral artery occlusion. Patients may have variable loss of intellect, marked emotional lability, and may be easily distracted. **Abulia**, a slowness and lack of spontaneity in all reactions, may be present, and the patient may tend to speak in a whisper. Dementia and even coma may occur. These disturbances result from injury to the ipsilateral frontal lobe.

Incontinence characterized by inability to control micturition with preservation of the urge to urinate results from infarction of the paracentral lobule in patients with anterior cerebral artery occlusion. The incontinence usually is transient in patients with unilateral lesions, but it may be permanent or protracted when the lesions are bilateral (Bogousslavsky and Regli, 1990).

When the anterior cerebral artery is occluded distal to the origin of its penetrating branches, the neurologic signs are somewhat less severe, but they are still quite extensive (Ford, 1952). Paralysis of the contralateral leg is often associated with mild transient weakness of the arm. This distribution of weakness—more severe in the lower extremity than the upper extremity—is a hallmark of anterior cerebral artery infarction. Cortical anesthesia over the contralateral paretic leg is often impressive. The patient may have difficulty touching a spot on the lower extremity touched by the examiner, be unable to identify numbers written on the foot with a pencil or finger, and extinguish bilateral tactile stimuli on the paralyzed foot or leg. Left-sided apraxia of the arm is present regardless of the side of the lesion, and forced grasping and groping are often present (see above).

Some patients with distal occlusion of the anterior cerebral artery develop localized infarction in the caudate nucleus. Such patients develop a syndrome characterized by a slight, transient hemiparesis, dysarthria, and behavioral and cognitive disturbances, including abulia, agitation, contralateral neglect, and difficulties with language (Caplan et al., 1990a). Similar findings may occur in patients with infarction of the caudate nucleus caused by occlusion of penetrating branches of the middle cerebral artery (see below).

About 60% of patients with infarction in the territory of the anterior cerebral artery evaluated by Bogousslavsky and Regli (1990) were caused by emboli from the heart or from the ipsilateral carotid artery. Causes in the remaining cases included primary occlusion of the anterior cerebral artery, internal carotid artery dissection with occlusion of the distal internal carotid artery, and vasospasm.

Occlusion of the Anterior Choroidal Artery. The syndrome of the anterior choroidal artery was initially described by Foix and colleagues (Foix and Hillemand, 1925; Foix et al., 1925) and was subsequently documented with anatomic or neuroimaging confirmation by others (Poppi, 1928a, 1928b; Ley, 1932; Abbie, 1933a, 1933b; Buge et al., 1979; Masson et al., 1983; T. Ward et al., 1984; Decroix et al., 1986; Helgason et al., 1986; Bruno et al., 1989; Fisher et al., 1989; Hupperts et al., 1994). The most common clinical sign is **hemiparesis**. The weakness affects the face, arm, and leg contralateral to the side of the occlusion. Contralateral **hemisensory loss** is often present. It may be severe at onset, but it usually is transient. A **homonymous visual field defect** occurs in many but not all patients with occlusion of an anterior choroidal artery. The defect may be quadrantic, hemianopic, or sectoral (see below). Most patients have no evidence of neglect, aphasia, or other abnormalities of higher cortical function; however, Cambier et al. (1983) described three patients in whom occlusion of the right anterior choroidal artery produced an infarction of the right internal capsule and caused visual neglect in the contralateral hemifield, constructional apraxia, alexia from visuospatial disturbance, and motor impersistence.

Decroix et al. (1986) described the findings in 16 patients with occlusion of the anterior choroidal artery, emphasizing that incomplete forms of the anterior choroidal artery syndrome were more frequent than complete forms. These investigators also found that left-sided spatial neglect often accompanied right-sided lesions, whereas slight disorders of speech occasionally accompanied left-sided lesions.

The visual field defect produced by occlusion of the anterior choroidal artery is caused by damage to the ipsilateral optic tract, lateral geniculate body, optic radiation, or a combination of these. Damage to the optic tract produces a homonymous hemianopia that may be complete or incomplete or a homonymous quadrantanopia. A complete or nearly complete homonymous hemianopia is invariably associated with other signs of an optic tract syndrome: normal visual acuity and color vision in both eyes, an RAPD on the side of the hemianopia (contralateral to the side of the lesion), and (eventually) bilateral retinal nerve fiber layer and optic nerve atrophy consistent with hemianopic field loss (Newman and Miller, 1983; see Chapters 8 and 38). Incomplete homonymous field defects caused by optic tract ischemia usually are extremely incongruous and may be scotomatous.

The lateral geniculate body has a dual blood supply (Frisén et al., 1978). The anterior hilum and the anterior and lateral aspects of the nucleus usually are supplied by branches of the anterior choroidal artery, whereas the remainder of the nucleus is supplied by the lateral posterior choroidal artery, a branch of the posterior cerebral artery (Abbie, 1933b; Francois et al., 1956; Galloway and Greitz, 1960; Fujino, 1962; Fujii et al., 1980). There usually are anastomoses between these arteries (Carpenter et al., 1954). When only the portion of the lateral geniculate body supplied by the anterior choroidal artery is ischemic, the resultant field defect is a homonymous, quadruple sectoranopia (Frisén, 1979; Shacklett et al., 1984; Helgason et al., 1986) (Figs. 55.132 and 55.133). More extensive damage to the lateral geniculate body can produce a complete homonymous hemianopia, an incomplete homonymous hemianopia that is extremely incongruous, or a homonymous horizontal sectoranopia (Gunderson and Hoyt, 1971; Frisén et al., 1979; Shacklett et al., 1984) (Fig. 55.134). When only the distal branches of the anterior choroidal artery are occluded, the

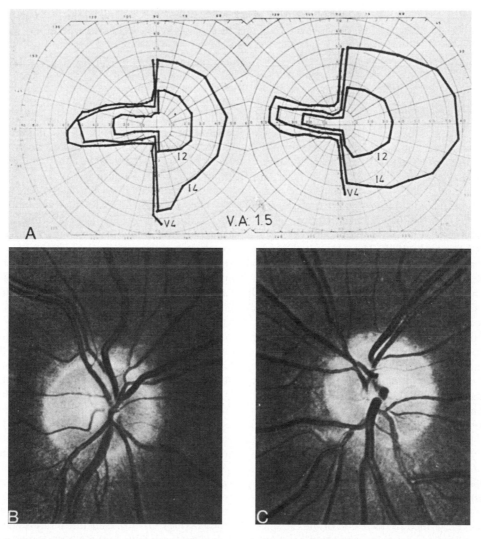

Figure 55.132. Quadruple sectoranopia and sectorial optic atrophy from occlusion of the distal anterior choroidal artery. Occlusion in this territory is thought to damage a portion of the lateral geniculate body. *A*, Visual fields show a relatively congruous quadruple sectoranopia. *B* and *C*, Fundus photographs show severe atrophy of retinal nerve fibers in broad regions above the optic disc with less atrophy below. (From Frisén L. Quadruple sectoranopia and sectorial optic atrophy: A syndrome of the distal anterior choroidal artery. J Neurol Neurosurg Psychiatry *42:*590–594, 1979.)

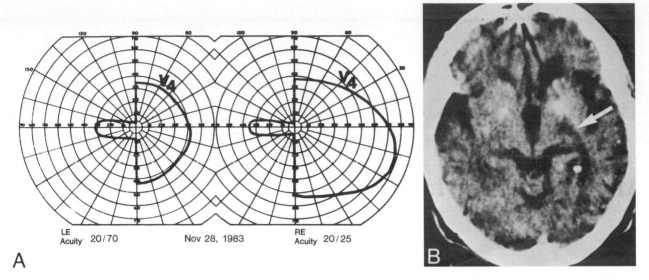

Figure 55.133. Quadruple sectoranopia from occlusion of the distal anterior choroidal artery. *A*, Visual field defect shows quadruple sectoranopia (see also Figure 55.132). *B*, Unenhanced CT scan shows infarct in the region of the right lateral geniculate body (*arrow*). (From Helgason C, Caplan LR, Goodwin J, et al. Anterior choroidal-artery territory infarction: Report of cases and review. Arch Neurol 43:681–686, 1986.)

field defect that is produced may be caused by an infarct in the optic radiation, and it may be unassociated with other neurologic symptoms or signs (Shacklett et al., 1984) (Fig. 55.135).

Occlusion of the anterior choroidal artery does not necessarily produce a visual field defect. Ligation of the artery was once used to treat Parkinson's disease under the assumption that deprivation of some of the blood supply to the basal ganglia might reduce or eliminate the extrapyramidal manifestations of the disease. Morello and Cooper (1955) examined five patients who underwent this operation. Four of the patients had no field defect. The fifth patient had a complete, superior, homonymous quadrantanopia with sparing of the macula. Walsh and Hoyt (1969b) performed kinetic perimetry on two patients in whom this procedure had been performed. One patient had no field defect. The other patient had a small, superior homonymous defect.

Abnormalities of eye movements may occasionally occur in patients with occlusion of the anterior choroidal artery. One of the patients described by Helgason et al. (1986) was drowsy, dysarthric, and had a complete right homonymous hemianopia and a right hemiplegia without sensory findings. The patient also had persistent head and conjugate eye deviation to the left (toward the side of the lesion and away from the hemianopia). Other patients have abnormal eye movements, particularly paresis of vertical gaze, caused by mesencephalic ischemia (Poppi, 1928a, 1928b; Buge et al., 1979; Viader et al., 1984). These abnormal eye movements may be associated with other evidence of oculomotor nerve dysfunction such as ptosis, pupillary dilation with poor reactivity, or both. They are ascribed to occlusion of the mesencephalic perforating branches of the anterior choroidal artery; however, they could also result from embolic occlusion of mesencephalic branches from other vessels occurring at the time of occlusion of the anterior choroidal artery.

The most common mechanism producing anterior choroidal artery occlusion is small-vessel occlusive disease (Bruno et al., 1989), although atherosclerotic and other disease of the extracranial portion of the common and internal carotid arteries may occasionally produce emboli that lodge in the anterior choroidal artery (Fisher et al., 1989). The most common risk factors identified in patients with infarction in the territory of the anterior choroidal artery are systemic hypertension, smoking, diabetes mellitus, and hypercholesterolemia. Emboli from the heart also may occlude the vessel. Massive infarcts in the territory of the anterior choroidal artery can also result from cardioembolic occlusion of the ipsilateral internal carotid artery (Levy et al., 1995). Temporal lobectomy for seizure control can iatrogenically cause anterior choroidal artery occlusion, presumably secondary to vasospasm from surgical manipulation (Anderson et al., 1989).

Occlusion of the Middle Cerebral Artery. The middle cerebral artery supplies the lateral part of the cerebral hemisphere through its **cortical branches** (Fig. 55.128). Its territory includes: (*a*) the cortex and white matter of the lateral and inferior aspects of the frontal lobe including motor areas 4 and 6 of Brodmann (Brodmann, 1909, 1918) and the motor speech area of Broca in the dominant hemisphere (area 44); (*b*) cortex and white matter of the parietal lobe including the sensory cortex and the angular and supramarginal gyri; and (*c*) superior parts of the temporal lobe and insula. Its **penetrating branches** supply the putamen, part of the head and body of the caudate nucleus, the outer globus pallidus, the posterior limb of the internal capsule, and the corona radiata (Fig. 55.136). Ischemic infarction in the territory supplied by the middle cerebral artery may be associated with focal neurologic deficits, seizures, or both (Kilpatrick et al., 1990; Sung and Chu, 1990).

The middle cerebral artery may be occluded at its origin,

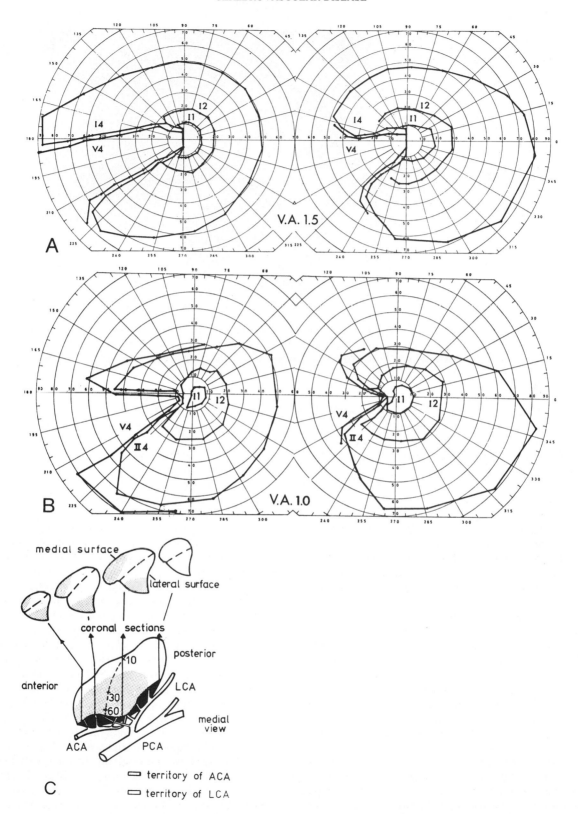

Figure 55.134. Homonymous horizontal sectoranopia from damage to the lateral geniculate body in the territory of the lateral choroidal artery. *A*, In a patient with a small arteriovenous malformation fed by branches of the distal anterior and lateral choroidal arteries. *B*, In a patient with presumed thrombosis of the lateral choroidal artery. *C*, Schematic representation of the blood supply of the lateral geniculate body from the anterior choroidal (*ACA*) and lateral choroidal (*LCA*) arteries. *PCA*, posterior cerebral artery. (From Frisén L, Holmegaard L, Rosencrantz M. Sectorial optic atrophy and homonymous, horizontal sectoranopia: A lateral choroidal artery syndrome? J Neurol Neurosurg Psychiatry *41*:374–380, 1978.)

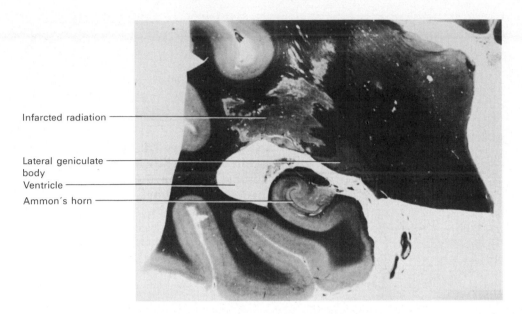

Infarcted radiation

Lateral geniculate body

Ventricle

Ammon's horn

Figure 55.135. Occlusion of the distal anterior choroidal artery producing an infarct of the optic radiation as it leaves the lateral geniculate body. Coronal section through the brain at the level of the lateral geniculate body shows an infarct of the left optic radiation with sparing of the lateral geniculate body. This infarct almost certainly produced a complete right homonymous hemianopia. (From Lindenberg R, Walsh FB, Sacks JG. Neuropathology of Vision. An Atlas. Philadelphia, Lea & Febiger, 1973.)

thus blocking flow in deep penetrating as well as superficial cortical branches, or its major branches may be individually occluded. Most occlusions of the middle cerebral artery or its branches are embolic, with the emboli originating from the heart or the extracranial portion of the internal carotid artery (Lhermitte et al., 1970; Fisher, 1975) (Fig. 55.137). The emboli usually pass beyond the origin of the vessel and lodge in the superficial cortical branches. Less than one in 20 emboli enter penetrating basal branches. Occasionally, the distal territory of the middle cerebral artery is rendered ischemic by failure of the systemic circulation (systemic hypoperfusion), especially if the internal carotid artery is severely stenotic. This may simulate embolic branch occlusion.

Occlusion of the origin of the middle cerebral artery by a thrombus is relatively infrequent. Lhermitte et al. (1970) found only two such examples among 47 cases of pathologically confirmed middle cerebral artery occlusion. However, other studies show that African-American and Asian patients have a higher prevalence of intracranial occlusive disease involving the carotid artery and its branches, including the middle cerebral artery, than Caucasian patients (Gorelick et al., 1984; Caplan et al., 1985; Caplan et al., 1986b; Feldmann et al., 1990).

Because many patients with occlusion or severe stenosis of the internal carotid artery have strokes in the distribution of the middle cerebral artery, Caplan et al. (1985) attempted to determine if the clinical picture of primary middle cerebral artery disease is different from that of middle cerebral artery disease that results from internal carotid artery occlusion. These investigators compared 20 patients with severe occlusive disease of the middle cerebral artery or its major division branches with 25 patients who had atheromatous disease

of the internal carotid artery. Patients with focal middle cerebral artery occlusion or severe stenosis were more often African-American, female, young, and had fewer TIAs than the patients with internal carotid artery disease. Neurologic signs in patients with middle cerebral artery disease evolved progressively during days to weeks, whereas patients with occlusive disease of the internal carotid artery more often had an acute onset of nonprogressive deficits.

Total occlusion of the middle cerebral artery produces: (*a*) contralateral hemiplegia, (*b*) contralateral hemianesthesia, (*c*) homonymous hemianopia, and (*d*) global aphasia if the lesion is on the left, sometimes with left-sided apraxia (Fig. 55.138). Such patients may show interesting syndromes caused by sparing of certain language or artistic abilities. For example, Basso and Capitani (1985) described an orchestra conductor who suffered a stroke caused by complete occlusion of the left middle cerebral artery. The stroke was characterized by a mild right hemiparesis, right homonymous hemianopia, global aphasia, and severe ideomotor apraxia. Although the aphasia and apraxia remained unchanged during the next 6 years, the patient's musical capacities were largely spared, and he was still able to understand and conduct music. Thus, music function abilities were primarily located in the nondominant (right) hemisphere in this patient.

Occlusion of the penetrating branches of the middle cerebral artery may produce: (*a*) contralateral hemiparesis, (*b*) contralateral hemihypesthesia, (*c*) homonymous hemianopia that may be complete or incomplete and congruous or incongruous, and (*d*) dysarthria that is more severe if the lesion is on the left side. When the penetrating branches of **both** middle cerebral arteries are occluded, the syndrome includes: (*a*) bilateral hemiparesis, (*b*) pseudobulbar symptoms including mask facies, dysarthria, dysphagia, and loss

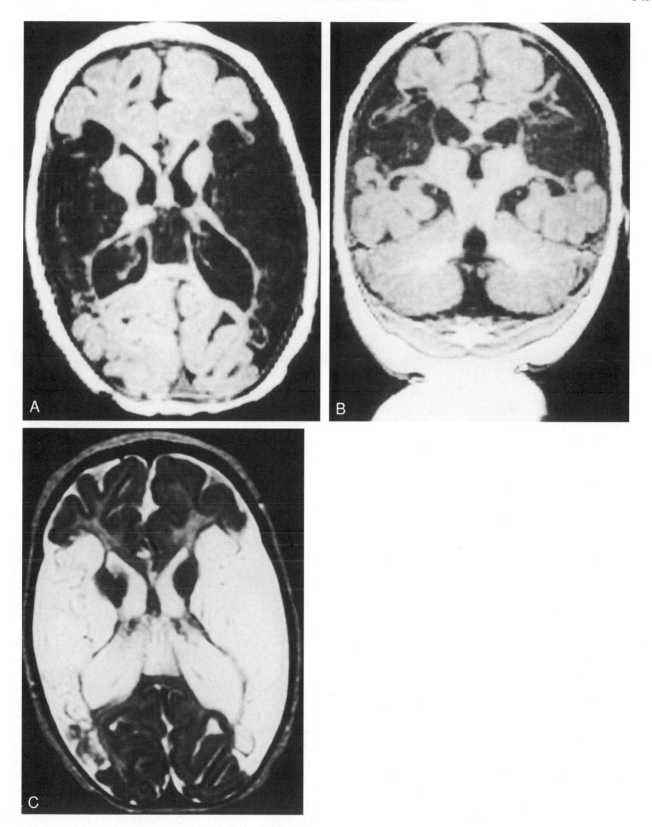

Figure 55.136. Bilateral intrauterine strokes in the territory of the middle cerebral arteries. This 6-month-old girl came to medical attention because of poor visual behavior and delayed development. There was no visual response and visual-evoked responses were not elicitable. Magnetic resonance imaging shows tissue loss suggesting occlusion of the middle cerebral arteries at their origins. *A*, T1-weighted axial image. *B*, T1-weighted coronal image. *C*, T2-weighted axial image.

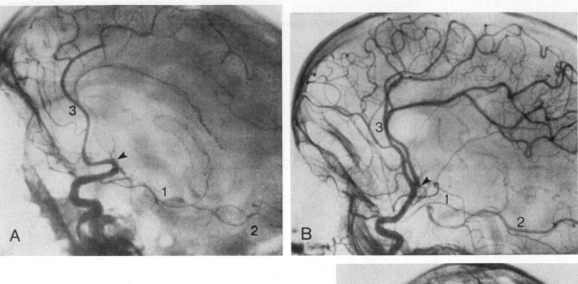

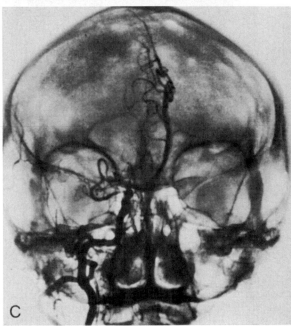

Figure 55.137.　Occlusion of the middle cerebral artery. *A*, Internal carotid arteriogram, lateral view, shows complete occlusion of the left middle cerebral artery at its origin (*arrowhead*). The anterior choroidal artery (*1*), posterior cerebral artery (*2*), and anterior cerebral artery (*3*) are visible. *B*, Complete occlusion of the middle cerebral artery at its origin (*arrowhead*). Again the anterior choroidal (*1*), posterior cerebral (*2*), and anterior cerebral (*3*) arteries are easily identified. *C*, Acute occlusion of the right middle cerebral artery at its origin. Note presence of cerebral edema that has shifted the A-2 segments of the right and left anterior cerebral arteries to the left. (From Huber P. Cerebral Angiography. 2nd ed. New York, Georg Thieme Verlag, 1982.)

of control of emotional reactions, (*c*) disturbances of gait out of proportion to the severity of hemiparesis, and (*d*) loss of bowel and bladder sphincter control.

When **penetrating deep branches** of the middle cerebral artery are blocked, an infarct of the internal capsule may result (Fisher, 1979). Patients with this condition develop a pure motor hemiplegia or hemiparesis affecting the face, arm, or leg. They have no sensory deficit, homonymous field defect, receptive aphasia, or apractagnosia.

Occlusion of the cortical branches of the middle cerebral artery results in: (*a*) hemiplegia with brachial predominance or monoplegia; (*b*) hemianesthesia, most marked in the arm; (*c*) homonymous hemianopia; and, when the lesion is on the left side, (*d*) global aphasia; and (*e*) ideomotor apraxia (Fig. 55.139).

When only certain branches of the middle cerebral artery are occluded, specific syndromes also occur. **Occlusion of**

the pre-Rolandic artery produces weakness of the mouth and tongue. When the left artery is occluded, dysarthria or motor aphasia are also present. When the condition is bilateral, the face, tongue, and jaw are completely paralyzed. **Occlusion of the Rolandic artery** produces branchial monoplegia with little or no aphasia and no sensory loss. **Occlusion of the anterior parietal artery** causes cortical anesthesia that is largely confined to the arm with loss of muscle tone, incoordination, and occasionally a mild hemiparesis. When the lesion is on the left side, sensory (fluent) aphasia and bilateral apraxia may result if the artery has an unusually large distribution. **Occlusion of the posterior branches** of the middle cerebral artery, including the posterior parietal, posterotemporal, and occipitoparietal, produces an isolated homonymous hemianopia when the lesion is on the right side. When the lesion is left-sided, the field defect is associated with an aphasia characterized by word deafness, an-

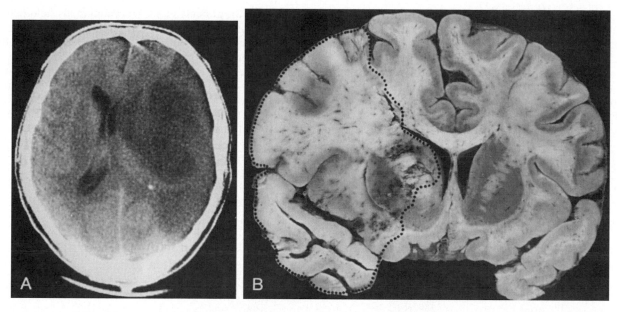

Figure 55.138. Infarction in the territory of the middle cerebral artery. *A*, CT scan, axial view, shows lucency in the entire territory supplied by the middle cerebral artery, including branches to the basal ganglia. Note marked edema with compression of the ipsilateral lateral ventricle and midline shift toward the contralateral side. *B*, Coronal section through pathologic specimen shows damage caused by complete infarct of the middle cerebral artery. Almost the entire hemisphere has been affected by the infarct (*dots*). (From Zülch KZ. The Cerebral Infarct. Berlin, Springer-Verlag, 1985.)

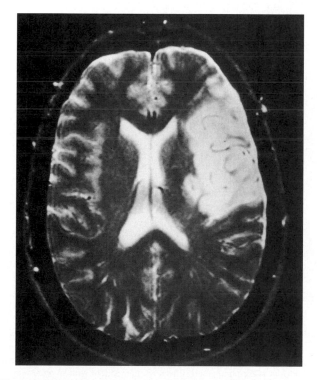

Figure 55.139. T2-weighted axial magnetic resonance image of an embolic infarction involving the cortical branches of the left middle cerebral artery. Note well-demarcated area of hyperintensity corresponding to area of infarction.

omia, paraphasia, alexia, and bilateral ideomotor apraxia. Regardless of the side of the lesion, the homonymous field defect is often associated with loss of low spatial frequency contrast sensitivity (Bulens et al., 1989), suggesting not only that visual processes are mediated by frequency selective channels but also that orientation selectivity is not confined to primary visual cortex neurons but also exists in the retrogeniculate visual pathway before the striate cortex (see Chapter 9).

Occlusion of the **angular branch** of the right middle cerebral artery, which supplies the inferior frontal gyrus and the inferior parietal lobule, can produce an acute confusional state (Mesulam et al., 1976). Affected patients show impairments of mental status that include agitation, inattentiveness, incoherent thought, and cognitive deficits. They also have impairments of higher cortical functions, such as anomia, dysgraphia, and dyscalculia. Some of these patients have visual hemineglect, a supranuclear horizontal gaze paresis with reduced or no spontaneous eye movements toward the side opposite the lesion, or both (De Renzi et al., 1982; Goodwin and Kansu, 1986; Kelley and Kovacs, 1986; Kömpf and Gmeiner, 1989). Other patients may demonstrate denial of eye closure acutely, not necessarily in association with other signs of neglect (Ellis and Small, 1994).

Patients who have occlusion of **distal pial branches** of the middle cerebral artery may develop a pattern of internal watershed infarction (Angeloni et al., 1990). This condition usually does not arise from occlusion of the main stem of the middle cerebral artery proximal to the origin of the lenticulostriate arteries, but rather it arises from occlusion of the main trunk of the middle cerebral artery just distal to the origin of the lenticulostriate arteries and proximal to the origin of the temporal pial branches, from occlusion distal to the origin of the temporal pial branches, and from occlusion of only peripheral pial branches.

The major neuro-ophthalmologic sign of middle cerebral artery occlusion is a contralateral homonymous hemianopia that may be complete or incomplete. It is most often caused by damage to the optic radiations, although the posterior pole of the striate cortex may also be affected (Figs.

55.140–142). In many cases, a homonymous field defect is the only neuro-ophthalmologic sign of a middle cerebral artery occlusion. As noted above, however, patients with damage to the right inferior parietal lobe may also have visual hemineglect in the field contralateral to the infarct, a supranuclear horizontal gaze paresis with reduced or no eye movements toward the side opposite the infarct, or both (De Renzi et al., 1982; Goodwin and Kansu, 1986; Kelley and Kovacs, 1986; Kömpf and Gmeiner, 1989).

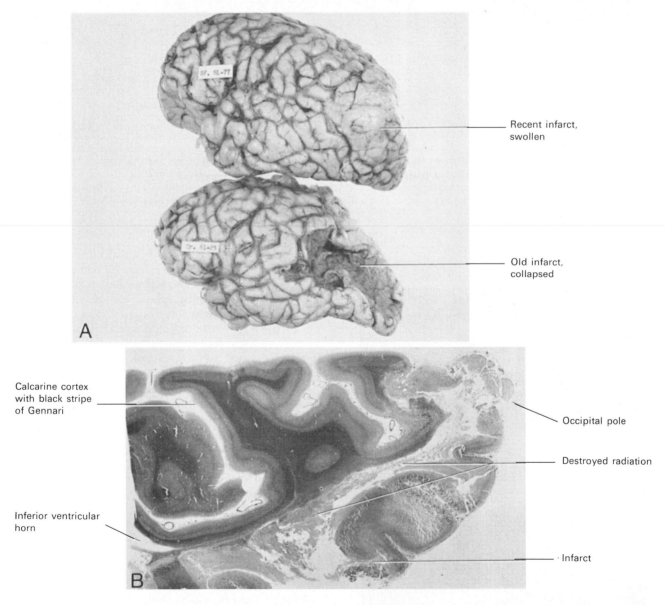

Figure 55.140. Destruction of the posterior visual sensory pathway from occlusion of the angular branch of the middle cerebral artery. The patient was an 85-year-old woman who experienced a myocardial infarction followed by a stroke. She died 6 weeks after the stroke. *A,* The hemisphere in the *upper portion* of the photograph is from this patient and shows an acute infarct that begins at the end of the sylvian fissure and extends into the posterior parietal and temporal regions toward the occipital pole. The hemisphere shown in the *lower portion* of the photograph is from another patient with an older infarct. The infarcts destroyed the entire optic radiation in both patients. *B,* Axial myelin section through the posterior half of the left hemisphere shows that the infarct has destroyed cortex and white matter up to the wall of the posterior horn of the lateral ventricle. The optic radiation has been totally destroyed. The infarct also has destroyed the calcarine cortex at the occipital pole. (From Lindenberg R, Walsh FB, Sacks JG. Neuropathology of Vision. An Atlas. Philadelphia, Lea & Febiger, 1973.)

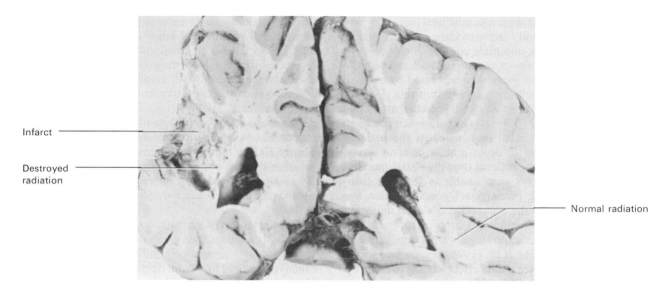

Figure 55.141. Destruction of the posterior visual sensory pathway from occlusion of the angular branch of the middle cerebral artery. The patient was a 30-year-old man with cardiac disease who had previously suffered a stroke. He suddenly collapsed at home and was dead on arrival to the hospital. Coronal section through the brain shows an infarct that extends from the surface of the brain to the wall of the lateral ventricle. The infarct has destroyed the cortex and white matter of the left lower parietal lobe, of the first and second posterior temporal convolutions, and the optic radiation. (From Lindenberg R, Walsh FB, Sacks JG. Neuropathology of Vision. An Atlas. Philadelphia, Lea & Febiger, 1973.)

Ohtsuka et al. (1988) described a patient with sudden onset of aphasia and a disturbance of consciousness who was found to have an occlusion of the M1 portion of the left middle cerebral artery. The patient underwent anastomosis of the left middle cerebral artery and the left superficial temporal artery. After recovery of consciousness, he had a mild right hemiparesis, mild aphasia, and Gerstmann's syndrome. He also complained of blurred and double vision during attempted near viewing. The patient's visual acuity and visual fields were normal, and eye movements were full, but hori-

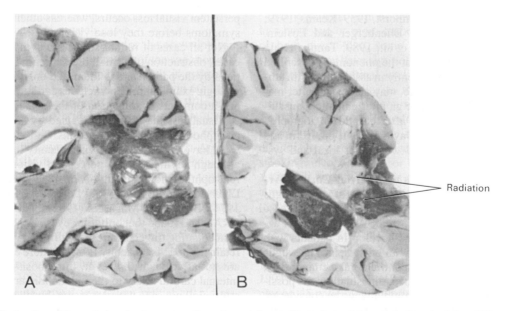

Figure 55.142. Destruction of the posterior visual sensory pathway by an infarct in the territory of the angular branch of the middle cerebral artery. The patient was a 65-year-old woman with systemic hypertension who experienced a stroke that caused left hemiplegia and an incomplete left homonymous hemianopia. She died 2 years later. *A,* Coronal section through the temporoparietal region on the right side shows that the infarct destroyed cortex and white matter bordering the right sylvian fissure and part of the first temporal convolution. The infarct disrupts the internal capsule by a dorsomedial extension that reaches the lateral angle of the lateral ventricle. *B,* A more posterior coronal section shows that the infarct interrupts only the middle third of the right optic radiation. (From Lindenberg R, Walsh FB, Sacks JG. Neuropathology of Vision. An Atlas. Philadelphia, Lea & Febiger, 1973.)

with carotid occlusive disease associated with CRAO, branch artery occlusion, or both varies from 11% to 85% (see Table 3 in Merchut et al., 1988). Patients with morphologically heterogeneous plaques of the extracranial carotid system as detected on noninvasive duplex ultrasound examination have a greater risk of retinal stroke and hemispheric infarction (Muller et al., 1993; O'Farrell and Fitzgerald, 1993; Iannuzzi et al., 1995). In patients with embolic retinal stroke who have no evidence of disease in the carotid arterial system, the heart is the most likely source of emboli (Kobayashi et al., 1997). In most cases, the emboli are of the platelet-fibrin or calcific type; in others, they are tumor emboli, usually from cardiac myxoma.

When patients with retinal stroke have ophthalmoscopically visible emboli in the retinal arterioles, a carotid or cardiac source is almost certain, and when the emboli have the typical appearance of cholesterol plaques, carotid artery disease is almost always responsible although the aorta is likely also a potential source of these emboli. Patients in whom such emboli are seen are at substantially higher risk for stroke and have a lower survival rate, usually from concurrent cardiac disease, than patients without emboli, whether or not such patients have suffered a retinal stroke (Pfaffenbach and Hollenhorst, 1973; Savino et al., 1977; Eckardt et al., 1983; Bruno et al., 1995).

Patients in whom CRAO is associated with ipsilateral carotid occlusive disease may experience neurologic symptoms before, simultaneously with, or after the CRAO. Wilson et al. (1989) described three patients in whom an acute CRAO occurred simultaneously with ipsilateral temple, orbit, or hemicranial pain and ipsilateral paresis of the ocular motor nerves. Two of the patients also experienced acute contralateral hemiparesis at the time of visual loss. All three patients were found to have occlusion of the internal carotid artery on the side of the blind, paretic eye.

The cause of CRAO in a patient with occlusion of the internal carotid artery may be embolic (Coats, 1905; Wolter, 1972; Wolter and Ryan, 1972) or thrombotic (Karjalainen, 1971; Merchut et al., 1988). Most occlusions of the central retinal artery occur in the region of the lamina cribrosa, regardless of the cause (Hayreh, 1971) (Fig. 55.98). In a young patient, retinal arterial occlusions are less likely to be caused by ipsilateral carotid stenosis and more likely to be related to cardiac embolism, a hypercoagulable state, or vasospasm (Greven et al., 1995).

There is no definitive treatment of a CRAO. Both medical and surgical approaches are disappointing (Henkes, 1954; Watson, 1969; Wise et al., 1971; Küchle, 1977; Magargal and Goldberg, 1977; Weidaw et al., 1978; Younge and Rosenbaum, 1978; Brown and Shields, 1979; Augsburger and Magargal, 1980; Kuritzky, 1990; Hausmann and Richard, 1991; Schmidt et al., 1992; Brown, 1994a; Mames et al., 1995; and see Table 1 in Mangat, 1995; Atebara et al., 1995). Conventional therapy for a CRAO includes ocular massage, anterior chamber paracentesis, topical medications to lower the intraocular pressure, intravenous or oral acetazolamide, and inhalation of a mixture of 95% oxygen and 5% carbon dioxide (carbogen), but the efficacy of these treatments is not proven (Atebara et al., 1995). Other agents proposed by investigators include sublingual nitroglycerin, oral warfarin, calcium-channel blocking agents, vasodilators, antiplatelet agents, intravenously injected heparin, urokinase, or tissue plasminogen activator (TPA), and intra-arterial urokinase or TPA. Anecdotal success must be weighed against the risk for major side effects. Werner et al. (1994), for example, reported a 66-year-old man with a remitting and relapsing CRAO that progressed despite aspirin and calcium-channel blocker therapy. Ophthalmic artery urokinase infusion improved the patient's visual acuity and visual field, but the procedure was complicated by a cerebral infarction.

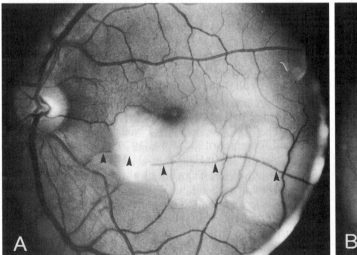 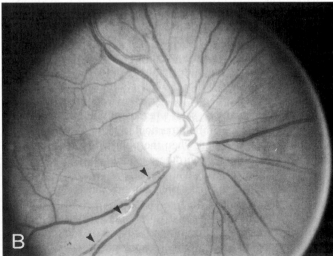

Figure 55.144. Branch artery occlusion in patients with carotid artery disease. *A*, Acute branch artery occlusion. Note area of retinal edema surrounding an obstructed inferotemporal branch artery (*arrowheads*). *B*, Old branch artery occlusion. Note irregular caliber of obstructed inferotemporal branch artery (*arrowheads*) associated with loss of nerve fiber layer in the area.

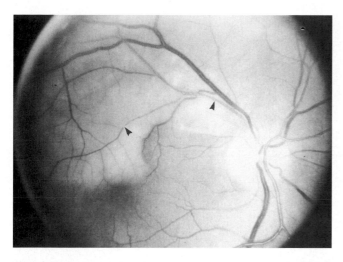

Figure 55.145. Acute branch artery occlusion associated with multiple emboli. Entire superotemporal region of retina is edematous. Note multiple emboli in the superior temporal branch artery and its tributaries (*arrowheads*).

Branch retinal artery occlusion may develop in patients with carotid artery disease (Hedges et al., 1985; Shah et al., 1985; Chawluk et al., 1988; Merchut et al., 1988; Brown, 1994a) (Fig. 55.144). The occlusion in such cases usually is caused by an embolus from the diseased vessel. Indeed, an embolus actually obstructs the vessel in some cases (Kollarits et al., 1972; Savino et al., 1977; Oshinskie, 1987) (Figs. 55.145–55.147). Obstruction of either the upper or lower branch of the central retinal artery results in typical visual field defects and ophthalmoscopic signs. When either all the upper or the lower branches are obstructed, the visual field defect has a border that runs horizontally through the point of fixation. In such cases, visual acuity may not be reduced.

The treatment of an acute branch retinal artery occlusion is usually similar to that for an acute CRAO. Anterior chamber paracentesis or ocular massage to lower intraocular pressure are the most commonly performed maneuvers. We have observed the fragmentation and disappearance of an embolus that produced an acute branch artery occlusion during and after such procedures. In such cases, visual acuity and visual field may improve dramatically. Dutton and Craig (1989) used long-duration, low-intensity argon laser photocoagulation to melt and dislodge a presumed cholesterol embolus that produced an acute branch artery occlusion in a 52-year-old woman after initial treatment consisting of ocular massage, rebreathing, and intravenous acetazolamide failed to dislodge the embolus. Unfortunately, although the embolus was successfully dislodged by this treatment, the patient's visual function did not improve afterward.

Ischemic Optic Neuropathy. Both AION and PION may occur in patients with carotid artery disease (Bettelheim, 1965; Eagling et al., 1974; Waybright et al., 1982; Sawle and Sarkies, 1987; Portnoy et al., 1989; Schönherr et al., 1990) and may even be the initial manifestation of internal carotid artery occlusion (Mori et al., 1983). In many cases, the optic neuropathy is not specifically related to the internal carotid artery disease but rather is a sign of widespread atherosclerosis affecting both large and small vessels. Alternatively, it may reflect shared risk factors, such as hypertension, diabetes mellitus, or cigarette smoking (Ellenberger and Epstein, 1986; Hayreh et al., 1994; Talks et al., 1995). Indeed, Arnold et al. (1995) reported that patients with nonarteritic AION had an increased prevalence of CNS white-

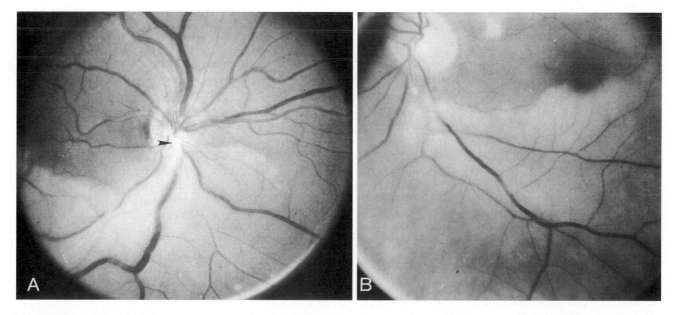

Figure 55.146. Embolic branch artery occlusion in patients with carotid artery disease. *A,* An embolus (*arrowhead*) has occluded the inferior temporal branch artery. Note marked inferotemporal retinal edema. The occluded artery is obscured by the edema. *B,* In another patient with an inferotemporal branch artery occlusion, an embolus occludes the artery just distal to its origin. Note marked inferotemporal retinal edema.

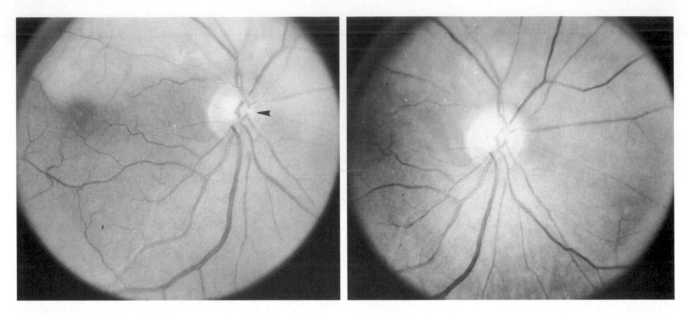

Figure 55.147. Embolic branch artery occlusion in a patient with carotid artery disease. *A*, At the time of acute loss of vision, there is an embolus at the bifurcation of the central retinal artery on the optic disc (*arrowhead*). There is retinal edema superiorly. *B*, Three months after visual loss, retinal edema has resolved, the superior retinal arteries are markedly narrowed, and the nerve fiber layer is no longer visible superiorly.

matter lesions consistent with small-vessel cerebrovascular disease on MR imaging (Awad et al., 1986), although others reported no such association (Jay and Williamson, 1987). Chung et al. (1994) reported a younger average age of onset of AION in smokers than in nonsmokers, a finding supported by baseline data from The Ischemic Optic Neuropathy Decompression Trial Study Group (1996). In a review of 406 cases of nonarteritic AION in patients aged 11–91, Hayreh et al. (1994) reported a multitude of accompanying systemic diseases and compared their prevalence with standard age-matched population survey prevalence rates. Patients with AION had significantly higher prevalence rates of arterial hypertension, diabetes mellitus, and gastrointestinal ulcer. When stratified by age, patients 45 years or older with AION also showed higher prevalence of ischemic heart disease and thyroid disease, and those between ages 45 and 65 years showed higher rates of chronic obstructive pulmonary disease and cerebrovascular disease. After onset of ION, patients with both hypertension and diabetes had a higher incidence of subsequent cerebrovascular disease. Guyer et al. (1985) found that patients who experienced an attack of nonarteritic AION had a higher prevalence of ischemic cerebrovascular events (stroke, TIA) than did an age- and sex-matched control population, a finding supported by the studies of Sawle et al. (1990) and Hayreh et al. (1994) who also reported a significantly increased mortality in such patients. However, Fry et al. (1993) prospectively evaluated patients with nonarteritic AION and found no increased prevalence of ipsilateral carotid artery disease. We believe that nonarteritic AION is a disease of small vessels and not directly related to carotid disease in the majority of cases.

The onset of ION is usually acute. It is characterized by painless loss of visual acuity, a visual field defect that is classically altitudinal or arcuate but which may be central (Fig. 55.148) (see Chapter 11), and an RAPD. The optic disc may show pallid or hyperemic swelling with peripapillary hemorrhages (i.e., AION) (Miller and Smith, 1966; Eagling et al., 1974; Hayreh, 1974a, 1974b; Boghen and Glaser, 1975; Hayreh, 1975, 1981a, 1981b) (Fig. 55.149), or it may be entirely normal (i.e., PION) (Hayreh, 1981c; Cullen and Duvall, 1983; Isayama et al., 1983; Shimo-Oku and Miyazaki, 1984; Sawle and Sarkies, 1987) (Figs. 55.150 and 55.151). Visual function usually stabilizes within several days to weeks, although it may improve or worsen in a stuttering fashion. The affected optic disc usually becomes pale beginning about 4 weeks after loss of vision (Fig. 55.152).

In some cases, ION caused by carotid artery disease is an isolated finding (Mori et al., 1983), whereas in other cases, it is associated with other evidence of ocular ischemia, such as choroidal infarction, retinal emboli, or iris and anterior chamber angle neovascularization (Brown, 1986a; Portnoy et al., 1989; Schönherr et al., 1990). We saw two patients who experienced acute AION and were found to have rubeosis iridis. Although neither patient had any history of neurologic difficulties, in each patient a complete evaluation revealed a severely stenotic ipsilateral internal carotid artery. We agree with Brown (1986a) that the finding of iris neovascularization in conjunction with AION (or PION), in the absence of diabetic retinopathy, a CRVO, or evidence of giant cell arteritis, strongly suggests concomitant (and causative) carotid occlusive disease.

Although monocular blindness combined with contralateral hemisphere symptoms and signs (e.g., hemiparesis) is a well-recognized entity in patients with carotid artery disease (Kussmaul, 1872; Hunt, 1914; Fisher, 1951b, 1952), it is generally assumed that the blindness is caused by retinal

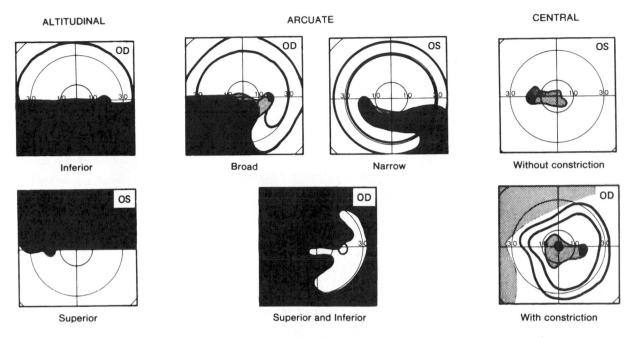

Figure 55.148. Typical visual field defects in anterior ischemic optic neuropathy. Altitudinal and arcuate defects are seen in the majority of cases, but central scotomas and peripheral constriction are not uncommon. (Redrawn from Boghen DR, Glaser JS. Ischaemic optic neuropathy. Brain *98*:689–708, 1975.)

ischemia. This concept is supported by the finding of emboli in retinal arterioles of many patients who experience transient monocular visual loss (see above). It is less well recognized that some patients with carotid artery disease experience the **simultaneous** occurrence of cerebral infarction and ipsilateral ION. This phenomenon is called the optico-pyramidal syndrome by some authors (Radovici and Lasco, 1948; Vergez, 1959; Castaigne et al., 1962; Boudouresques

et al., 1970), although Bogousslavsky et al. (1987b) recommended the term **optico-cerebral syndrome**, because signs other than motor weakness may be present.

Although all three patients described by Bogousslavsky et al. (1987b) had an AION, we have seen several patients with occlusion or severe stenosis of the internal carotid artery who presented with an acute hemisphere stroke and simultaneous monocular blindness caused by a PION in the ipsi-

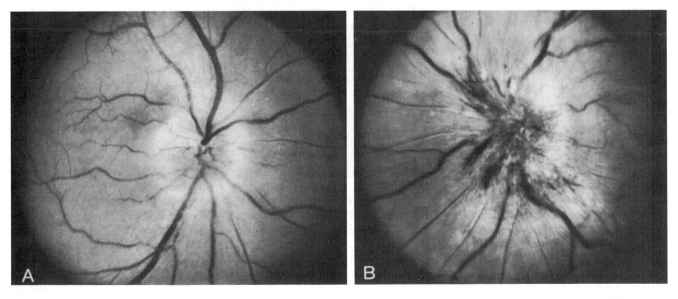

Figure 55.149. Ophthalmoscopic appearance of anterior ischemic optic neuropathy. *A*, Pallid swelling of the optic disc with a few small flame-shaped hemorrhages at the disc margin. *B*, Hyperemic swelling of the optic disc with numerous hemorrhages and a few soft exudates.

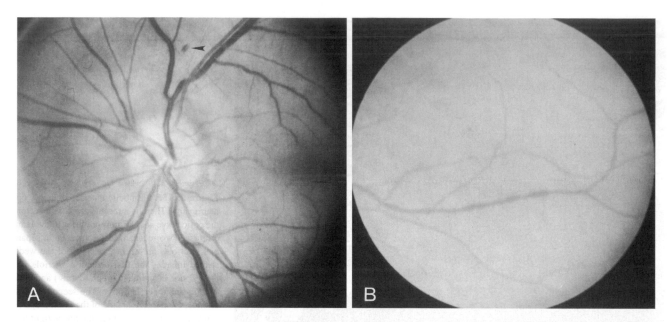

Figure 55.155. Mild venous stasis retinopathy. The patient was a 64-year-old man with vague symptoms of blurred vision in the left eye. *A*, The retinal veins are dilated. There is a single hemorrhage about one disc diameter above the optic disc (*arrowhead*). *B*, In the retinal periphery one of the veins has an irregular caliber.

was characterized by insidious onset, diminution or absence of venous pulsations, dilated and tortuous retinal veins, peripheral microaneurysms, and blossom-shaped hemorrhages in the midperipheral retina. Patients with this condition complained primarily of generalized blurred vision in the affected eye. Kearns and Hollenhorst (1963) subsequently called this condition **venous stasis retinopathy**, and this is the most common term used, although some authors call it "hypotensive retinopathy" (Green, 1983; Kahn et al., 1986a).

Venous stasis retinopathy is **not** the same entity as the nonischemic form of CRVO described by Hayreh (Hayreh, 1965, 1980, 1983; Ellenberger and Epstein, 1986; Kahn et al., 1986a). Kearns (1983) emphasized that patients with venous stasis retinopathy have a low retinal artery pressure, engorged retinal veins that are irregular in caliber, and hemorrhages, microaneurysms, and capillary dilations that are more often peripheral than in the posterior pole (see also McCrary, 1989) (Figs. 55.155 and 55.156). Such patients do not have swelling of the optic disc or optociliary (retinochoroidal) veins. Patients with the nonischemic form of CRVO have engorged retinal veins that are regular in caliber. Hemorrhages, microaneurysms, and capillary dilations are diffuse rather than peripheral. Disc swelling is common in such cases (Fig. 55.157). In addition, patients with venous stasis retinopathy often have other symptoms of carotid insufficiency, such as transient monocular loss of vision, decreased vision after exposure to bright light (see above), and, especially, orbital pain (Brown and Magargal, 1988). Patients with CRVO do not have such symptoms unless they have, in addition to the vein occlusion, unrelated carotid occlusive disease (see below).

The histopathologic features of venous stasis retinopathy

were beautifully described by Kahn et al. (1986a). In three eyes studied by these investigators, the retinal arterioles showed a normal 1:1 ratio between pericytes and endothelial cells in the posterior pole (Fig. 55.158*A*). At the midperiphery, however, there was a relatively greater loss of pericytes than endothelial cells, and at the equator and far periphery, there was marked loss of pericytes as well as microaneurysm formation (Fig. 55.158*B*).

Venous stasis retinopathy may occur as part of the ocular ischemic syndrome (see below), or it may occur in isolation (Kearns and Hollenhorst, 1963; Carter, 1984; Kahn et al., 1986a; McCrary, 1989). It is estimated that up to 20% of patients with carotid occlusive disease develop venous stasis retinopathy (Ross Russell and Page, 1983). Conversely, venous stasis retinopathy probably results most often from obstruction of the internal carotid artery near its bifurcation (Kearns, 1979; Magargal et al., 1982), although it can be caused by an occlusive process anywhere between the heart and the optic disc, not just within the internal carotid artery. Magargal et al. (1982) described a 58-year-old man who developed venous stasis retinopathy associated with an atheromatous plaque at the bifurcation of the central retinal artery on the optic disc of the left eye and an ulcerative plaque located at the origin of the ipsilateral internal carotid artery. Both systolic and diastolic ophthalmodynamometry measurements were significantly reduced on the left side. The patient underwent an uncomplicated left carotid endarterectomy at which time the lumen of the internal carotid artery was found to be 40–50% obstructed. The appearance of the retina did not change immediately after surgery, and ophthalmodynamometry readings also were unchanged. One year after surgery, however, visual acuity in the left eye was normal. Ophthalmoscopic examination at this time showed

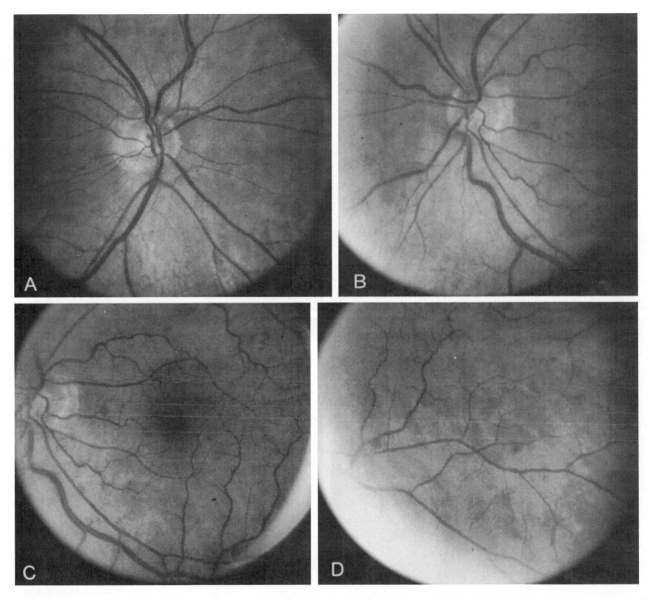

Figure 55.156. Moderate venous stasis retinopathy. The patient had blurred vision in the left eye. *A*, The right fundus is normal. Note normal caliber of retinal vessels and relationship of size of arteries to size of veins. *B*, The left optic disc is normal, but the retinal veins are dilated. There are a few hemorrhages in the posterior pole. *C*, The macular region shows a few small retinal hemorrhages and dilation of the capillaries. *D*, Multiple blot hemorrhages in the midperipheral retina.

on exposure to bright light (Jacobs and Ridgway, 1985). The early findings in chronic ocular ischemia suggest intraocular inflammation. The affected eye is often red, with a diffuse episcleral vascular injection, rather than a ciliary flush as would be expected in inflammatory disease (Countee et al., 1978; Kerty and Eide, 1989; Mills, 1989) (Fig. 55.159). Visual acuity is often poorer than would be expected from the inflammatory signs. The intraocular pressure is low or normal because of poor ocular perfusion, and there may be a few cells and minimal flare in the anterior chamber.

This "ischemic uveitis" is typically unresponsive to treatment with topical corticosteroids (Mills, 1989). The ocular fundus shows mild to severe retinopathy characterized by dilated and tortuous veins, narrowed retinal arteries, microaneurysms in close proximity to the retinal veins, small blossom-shaped hemorrhages that are most often located in the midperiphery, and, in some cases, sludging of blood within the veins (Hedges, 1962, 1963; Kearns and Hollenhorst, 1963; Knox, 1965; Brown and Magargal, 1988; Brown, 1994b; Mizener et al., 1997) (Fig. 55.160). Retinal arteriovenous communications may develop proximal to extensive areas of complete vascular closure (Bolling and Beuttner, 1990). Macular edema is common in some cases, although it may not be identified without fluorescein angiography (Brown, 1994b), and there may be one or more soft retinal exudates (cotton-wool spots) caused by infarction of the nerve fiber layer (Rosenberg et al., 1984; Brown and Magargal, 1988). The appearance thus may mimic diabetic retinopathy, except that the condition is unilateral and the microvascular changes are predominantly peripheral (Brown et al., 1982; Sturrock and Mueller, 1984). In some cases, there is spontaneous pulsation of the central retinal artery despite normal or low intraocular pressure, indicating that diastolic blood pressure is lower than intraocular pressure.

Some patients with the ocular ischemic syndrome have severe ocular discomfort or frank pain, even though intraocular pressure is low (Kearns and Hollenhorst, 1963). The pain is usually localized to the orbit and upper face, and it

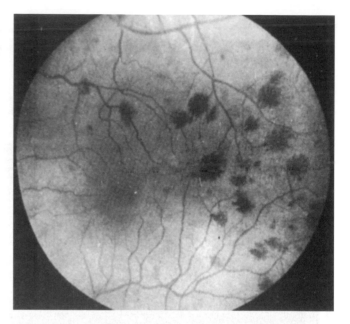

Figure 55.160. Venous stasis retinopathy in the ocular ischemic syndrome. There are blot hemorrhages above and temporal to the fovea. (From Sturrock GD, Mueller HR. Chronic ocular ischaemia. Br J Ophthalmol 68: 716–723, 1984.)

often decreases when the patient lies down. This sensation, which some investigators believe is pathognomonic of carotid occlusive disease (Kearns, 1979, 1983; Higgins, 1984; Brown and Magargal, 1988), probably results from ischemic damage to ocular and orbital branches of the trigeminal nerve (Knox, 1965; Kearns and Hollenhorst, 1963; Brown et al., 1982; Jacobs and Ridgway, 1985).

In eyes with persistent hypoperfusion, further evidence of panocular ischemia becomes evident, including neovascularization of the iris (rubeosis iridis), retina, optic disc, and anterior chamber angle (Brown et al., 1982; Jacobs and Ridgway, 1985; Mills, 1989; Mizener et al., 1997) (Fig. 55.161). Other signs of ocular ischemia include corneal edema, uveitis, cataract formation, and a mid-dilated and poorly reactive pupil (Michelson et al., 1971; Brown et al., 1982; Carter, 1985; Asai et al., 1988; Kerty and Eide, 1989; Mills, 1989; Mizener et al., 1997) (Fig. 55.161 and 55.162). Some patients develop vitreous hemorrhage from neovascularization of the optic disc, retina, or both (Knox, 1965; Hayreh and Podhajsky, 1982), whereas others develop hyphema from neovascularization of the iris and anterior chamber angle (Huckman and Haas, 1972; Fleck and Cullen, 1985) (Fig. 55.161B). These patients initially may present to the ophthalmologist when they develop blurred vision from the vitreous or anterior chamber blood (Fleck and Cullen, 1985).

Choroidal hypoxia also occurs with persistent hypoperfusion and may be associated with choroidal detachment and low intraocular pressure; however, severe glaucoma eventually may result from obstruction of outflow of aqueous humor by neovascularization of the anterior chamber angle (neovascular glaucoma) (Smith, 1962a; Hoefnagels, 1964; Young and Appen, 1981; Abedin and Simmons, 1982;

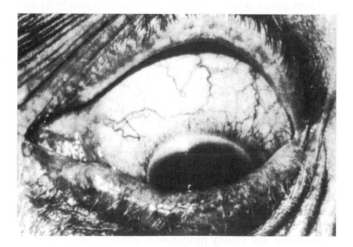

Figure 55.159. Dilated episcleral vessels in a patient with the ocular ischemic syndrome. (From Sturrock GD, Mueller HR. Chronic ocular ischaemia. Br J Ophthalmol 68:716–723, 1984.)

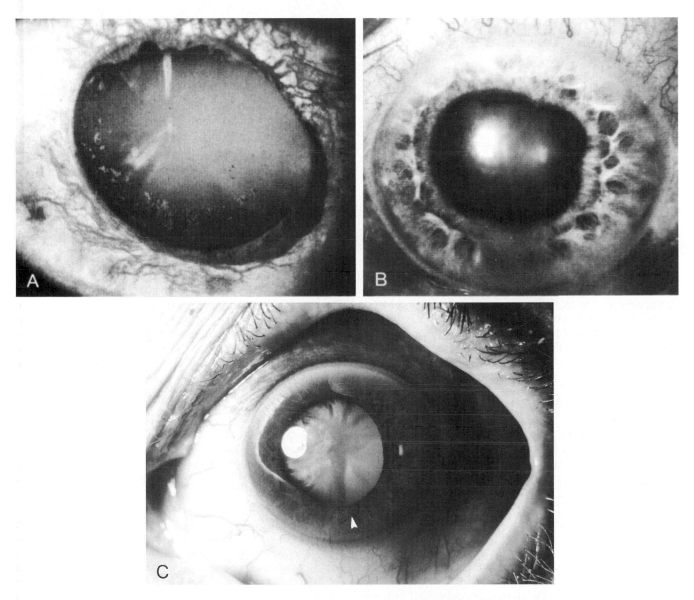

Figure 55.161. Anterior segment disturbances in patients with the ocular ischemic syndrome. *A*, Anterior segment ischemia with rubeosis iridis, ectropion uveae, and posterior synechiae. *B*, Anterior segment ischemia with dilated episcleral vessels, posterior synechiae, and small hyphema. (From Sturrock GD, Mueller HR. Chronic ocular ischaemia. Br J Ophthalmol *68:*716–723, 1984.) *C*, Anterior segment ischemia with rubeosis iridis (*arrowhead*) and dense cataract. (Courtesy of Dr. David Knox.)

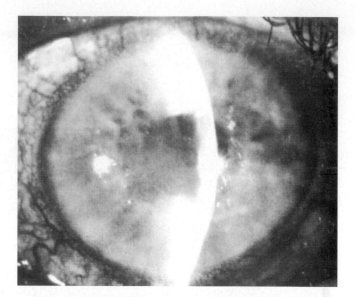

Figure 55.162. Severe corneal edema with bullous keratopathy from the effects of chronic ocular ischemia. (From Sturrock GD, Mueller HR. Chronic ocular ischaemia. Br J Ophthalmol *68:*716–723, 1984.)

Brown et al., 1984a; Higgins, 1984; Rosenberg et al., 1984; Pelosse et al., 1987; Fukuchi et al., 1988; Brown, 1994b; Mizener et al., 1997). Patients with neovascular glaucoma who previously were free of pain, develop severe pain with constant aching over the orbit, upper face, and temple on the affected side. The pain worsens when the patient shifts from the lying to the upright position (Cohen and McNamara, 1980; Carter, 1984). If intraocular pressure cannot be lowered to a normal level, the affected eye eventually becomes completely blind. Blindness may develop acutely from a CRAO caused by the combination of elevated intraocular pressure and low ocular perfusion pressure (Sanborn et al., 1980; Brown et al., 1982; Fukuchi et al., 1988), or it may develop slowly and insidiously from persistent panocular ischemia (Kahn et al., 1986a).

Most patients with the ocular ischemic syndrome have severe occlusion of both common or internal carotid arteries, although unilateral carotid or ophthalmic artery occlusion also may produce the syndrome (Young and Appen, 1981; Brown and Magargal, 1988; Dhooge and De Laey, 1989; Mizener et al., 1997). Some patients have unilateral occlusion of both the internal **and** external carotid arteries (Hoefnagels, 1964; Knox, 1965; Carter, 1985; Heros, 1986). The pathogenesis of the occlusion is usually atherosclerosis; however, other causes, such as trauma and dissection, can also be associated with carotid occlusion and the development of an ocular ischemic syndrome (Duker and Belmont, 1988). Other diseases that can cause the ocular ischemic syndrome include giant cell arteritis (Borruat et al., 1993) and vasospasm (Winterkorn and Beckman, 1995).

The mechanism by which reduction in orbital and ocular blood flow causes progressive ocular ischemia, tissue hypoxia, and neovascularization is somewhat controversial. Smith (1961) suggested that when arterial pressure within the eye falls because of carotid occlusion, tissue perfusion becomes insufficient to satisfy the metabolic needs of the retina. Ross and Morrow (1984) showed, however, that decreased flow in the ophthalmic artery results in increased

blood viscosity and in aggregation and deformation of erythrocytes, thus producing tissue ischemia. Galle et al. (1983) reported five patients with the ocular ischemic syndrome who had angiographic evidence of internal carotid artery occlusion combined with retrograde collateral flow to the brain via the ipsilateral external carotid and ophthalmic arteries. A similar patient was described by Kahn et al. (1986a).

These findings suggest that the panocular ischemia that occurs in patients with carotid occlusive disease may not be the result of internal carotid artery occlusion per se but may be the result of an ocular steal mechanism in which the collateral circulation shunts blood away from the eye to the brain (Kerty and Horven, 1995; Kerty et al., 1995). This mechanism may also contribute to retinal and optic disc neovascularization in patients with venous stasis retinopathy (Huckman and Haas, 1972; Kearns et al., 1979).

The prognosis for vision in eyes affected by untreated chronic ischemia is extremely poor because of the progressive nature of the disease. Although early retinopathy may resolve spontaneously with the development of collateral circulation (Hedges, 1962, 1963), significant loss of vision is almost always irreversible once tissue infarction occurs (Brown et al., 1981; Sturrock and Mueller, 1984; Dhooge and De Laey, 1989; Mizener et al., 1997).

As might be expected, patients with the ocular ischemic syndrome have poor cerebral perfusion (Yamaguchi et al., 1987). Such patients have a significant risk of stroke and heart attack (Sturrock and Mueller, 1984; L.N. Johnson et al., 1985). Early diagnosis of the syndrome is thus crucial in permitting reversal of visual loss and preventing associated neurologic and cardiac sequelae (Mizener et al., 1997).

The treatment of the ocular ischemic syndrome is aimed at preservation and improvement in visual function and treatment of the underlying process. The first requires a relative decrease in the oxygen requirements of the eye, thus reducing the drive for neovascularization. This is usually accomplished by ablation of retinal tissue by laser panretinal photocoagulation (Eggleston et al., 1980; Carter, 1984), peripheral

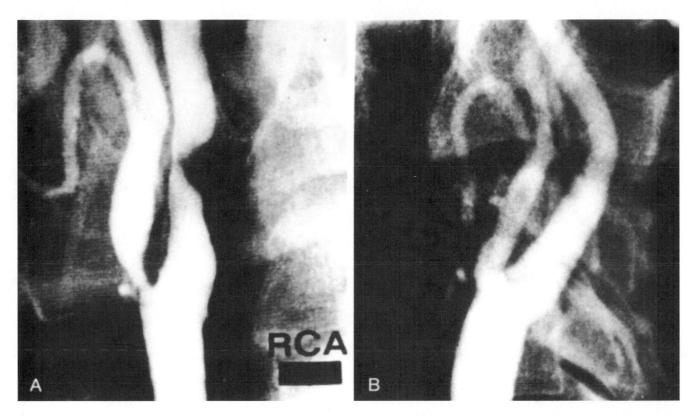

Figure 55.163. Results of endarterectomy performed to re-establish flow in a patient with severe ocular ischemia. *A,* Preoperative right common carotid arteriogram shows a large plaque producing severe stenosis of the right internal carotid artery about 3 cm above its origin. The external carotid artery also is severely stenotic. A combined internal and external carotid endarterectomy was performed. *B,* Postoperative angiogram shows a normal lumen in both the right internal and the right external carotid arteries. (From Ojemann RG, Crowell RM, Roberson GH, et al. Surgical treatment of extracranial carotid occlusive disease. *Clin Neurosurg 22:*214–263, 1975.)

retinal cryotherapy (Kiser et al., 1983), or both (Ros et al., 1987; Johnston et al., 1988). When severe carotid artery stenosis is the underlying condition, endarterectomy may be used to reestablish flow (Neupert et al., 1976; Rosenberg et al., 1984) (Fig. 55.163). When, as is usually the case, the artery is occluded, a superficial temporal artery to middle cerebral artery bypass procedure may be beneficial if the external carotid artery is patent (Kearns et al., 1979, 1980; Edwards et al., 1980; Young and Appen, 1981; Sundt et al., 1985; Mehdorn et al., 1986; Johnston et al., 1988) (Figs. 55.164 and 55.165). When the internal and external carotid artery are occluded, some form of revascularization of the external carotid artery may be of some benefit (Heros, 1986). Although certain drugs, such as pentoxyfylline (Trental) that reduce blood viscosity, reduce platelet aggregation, decrease clot formation, and increase clot lysis might be useful in improving blood flow to an eye with the ocular ischemic syndrome (Schröer, 1985), there are no data to support their use (Appen, 1987). If vasospasm is a contributing factor, calcium-channel blocking agents such as verapamil might be effective (Winterkorn and Beckman, 1995).

Unfortunately, no therapy is clearly effective in reversing the ocular ischemic syndrome. With early treatment, impressive visual return associated with resolution of the ocular condition may be expected (Neupert et al., 1976; Edwards

et al., 1980; Kearns et al., 1980; Shaw et al., 1981; Kiser et al., 1983; Ros et al., 1987; Johnston et al., 1988) (Fig. 55.166); however, patients with marked visual loss and pronounced ocular changes seldom improve even with therapy (Hayreh and Podhajsky, 1982; Carter, 1985; Mizener et al., 1997). Ros et al. (1987) evaluated 15 eyes from 14 patients with ocular ischemia from carotid artery obstruction. Only two of the 15 eyes were seen early enough in the course of the disease to achieve long-term improvement in visual function. On the other hand, Johnston et al. (1988) treated 13 affected eyes of 12 patients with panretinal photocoagulation and cerebrovascular surgery and achieved stabilization of visual acuity in 11 patients with visual acuity of 20/60 or better in nine patients.

Reestablishment of flow in a previously occluded or stenotic internal carotid artery may actually produce further visual difficulties. Several investigators showed experimentally and clinically that decreased perfusion of the ciliary body from obstruction of the internal (or common) carotid artery results in significantly decreased production of aqueous humor (Young and Appen, 1981; Rosenberg et al., 1984). Eyes with decreased aqueous humor production may have normal or low intraocular pressure, even when the anterior chamber angle is occluded by extensive neovascularization (Swan and Raaf, 1951; Huckman and Haas, 1972).

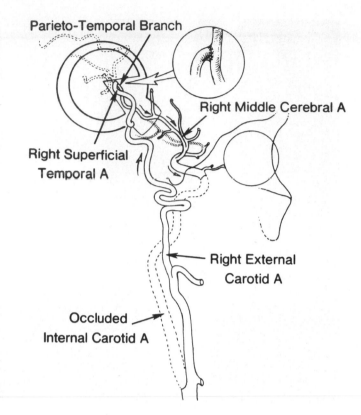

Figure 55.164. Schematic diagram shows the superficial temporal artery to middle cerebral artery bypass and the presumed direction of postoperative blood flow. (From Kearns TP, Siekert RG, Sundt TM Jr. The ocular aspects of bypass surgery of the carotid artery. Mayo Clin Proc *54:*3–11, 1979.)

When blood flow is restored in the carotid arterial system, perfusion to the ciliary body may improve, and production of aqueous humor returns to pre-ischemic levels, resulting in a dramatic increase in intraocular pressure (Hart and Haworth, 1971; Bullock et al., 1972; Huckman and Haas, 1972; Rosenberg et al., 1984; Coppeto et al., 1985; Heros, 1986). Such eyes may require aggressive ablation of the ciliary body to reduce intraocular pressure and preserve visual function. Eyes with neovascular glaucoma that become blind and remain painful despite therapy to lower intraocular pressure, may require treatment by either a retrobulbar injection of alcohol or enucleation (Knox, 1965; Hayreh and Podhajsky, 1982). Histopathologic examination of eyes with the ocular ischemic syndrome demonstrate extensive destruction of tissue, including iris atrophy, rubeosis iridis, peripheral anterior synechiae, ciliary body necrosis, extensive inner and outer retinal ischemic atrophy, and acellularity of retinal vessels (Michelson et al., 1971; Kahn et al., 1986a).

Optic Disc Neovascularization. It was mentioned above that neovascularization of the optic disc may occur in patients with carotid artery disease as part of the full ocular ischemic syndrome. Willerson and Aaberg (1978) also described optic disc neovascularization in a patient with complete occlusion of the left internal carotid artery and stenosis of the right internal carotid artery who had recently undergone a left carotid endarterectomy from which he awakened with severe loss of vision in the left eye. The examination showed evidence of a CRAO. Although there was no iris atrophy, iris neovascularization, or uveitis, and both lenses were clear, there was a neovascular frond covering most of

the left optic disc and extending into the vitreous. The retinal arteries contained multiple refractile emboli. Willerson and Aaberg (1978) postulated that the optic disc neovascularization in this patient was the result of chronic ocular ischemia, superimposed by an acute CRAO that was caused by emboli dislodged from the left internal carotid artery during endarterectomy.

Duker and Brown (1989) described neovascularization of the optic disc in three patients with a CRAO. Although one of the patients had an ulcerated, atherosclerotic plaque with 40% angiographic stenosis of the ipsilateral internal carotid artery, and a second patient had an ulcerated plaque with 70% stenosis of the ipsilateral internal carotid artery (and 50% stenosis of the contralateral internal carotid artery), there was no clinical evidence implicating carotid artery disease as the direct cause of the disc neovascularization.

Macular Edema. Patients with the ocular ischemic syndrome often have macular edema as part of the retinopathy that develops in this condition (Brown, 1986b; Brown and Magargal, 1988; Brown, 1994b). Odashima et al. (1986) described a 55-year-old man who experienced acute loss of central vision in the left eye and was found to have a "peculiar choroiditis-like mottled" edema of the macula in that eye. Fluorescein angiography revealed that arm-to-retina circulation time and submacular choroidal circulation time were delayed, and both systolic and diastolic ophthalmodynamometry readings were markedly reduced on the left compared with the right. Because cerebral angiography revealed 50% stenosis of the left internal carotid artery just above the carotid bifurcation, the maculopathy was thought to be

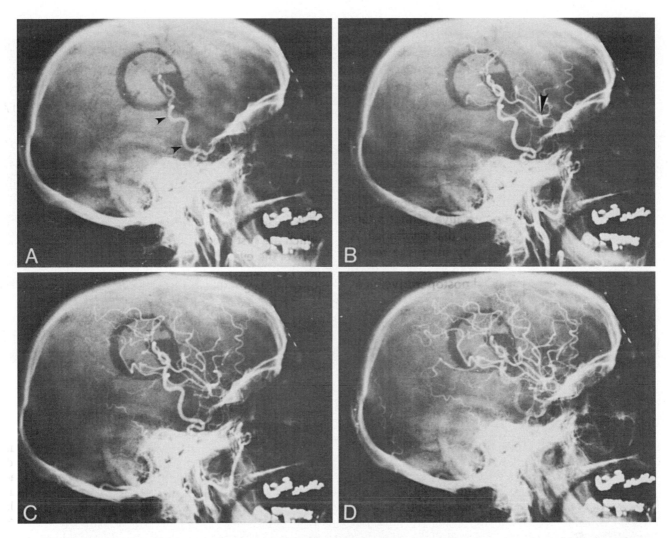

Figure 55.165. Patency of superficial temporal artery to middle cerebral artery bypass procedure shown by angiography. *A*, Initial phase of common carotid arteriogram (lateral view) shows filling of a dilated superficial temporal artery (*arrowheads*). *B*, Later phase shows beginning filling of branches of the middle cerebral artery with retrograde flow toward the origin of the middle cerebral artery (*arrowhead*). *C* and *D*, Progressive filling of middle cerebral artery system. (From Kearns TP, Siekert RG, Sundt TM Jr. The ocular aspects of bypass surgery of the carotid artery. Mayo Clin Proc *54:3*–11, 1979.)

induced by low perfusion of choroidal and retinal circulation. Although we agree that the maculopathy may have been caused by poor ocular perfusion, it is hard to understand why such poor perfusion would be caused by such a relatively minor stenosis. It seems more likely that small vessel changes caused by thrombosis or perhaps embolism from the site of stenosis were the cause of the poor ocular perfusion.

Choroidal Ischemia. Raymond et al. (1980) described a patient who had five episodes of inferior visual field loss in the left eye when he turned his head to the left. He then experienced an episode of decreased visual acuity and pain in the left eye after vigorous exercise. Later that day, he was found to have 20/20 vision in the left eye, although color vision in that eye was poor, and there was a left RAPD. Five days later, visual acuity and color vision were normal in the left eye, and the left visual field was full when tested with kinetic perimetry; however, there was a persistent left RAPD. Ophthalmoscopy seemed normal, but fluorescein angiography showed delayed filling of the choroidal circulation, patchy choroidal filling defects, and inadequate perfusion of the temporal aspect of the optic disc (Fig. 55.167). The patient was found to have a total occlusion of the left internal carotid artery. The ophthalmic artery filled in retrograde fashion from branches of the external carotid artery. It was thought that the patient's symptoms and signs were caused by compromise of the short posterior ciliary artery circulation. Perfusion problems should be considered in patients with monocular visual loss even if the cause of the problem is not detected on funduscopic examination. Appropriately timed and oriented fluorescein angiography may reveal occult vascular disease of either the choroid or retina in such patients (Rizzo, 1993).

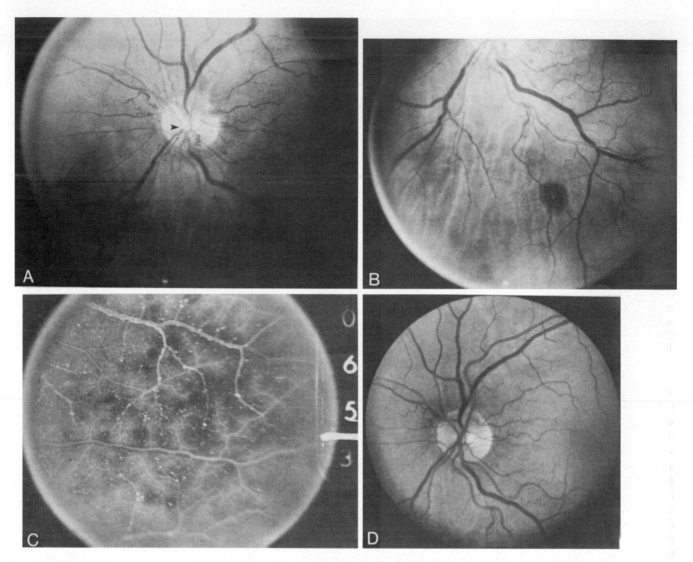

Figure 55.166. Improvement in venous stasis retinopathy and the ocular ischemia syndrome after endarterectomy. The patient was a 58-year-old man with blurred vision in the left eye. Visual acuity was 20/20 OD and 20/30 OS. *A,* The left ocular fundus shows a small atheromatous plaque at the bifurcation of the central retinal artery (*arrowhead*) with some sheathing of the superior nasal artery. The retinal veins are dilated, and there are multiple collateral vessels on the surface of the optic disc and in the peripapillary region. *B,* Ophthalmoscopic appearance of midperipheral retina shows several blot hemorrhages and irregularly dilated veins. *C,* Fluorescein angiogram of midperipheral retina shows numerous microaneurysms. Cerebral angiography showed severe stenosis of the extracranial portion of the left internal carotid artery, and the patient underwent uncomplicated endarterectomy. *D,* One year after onset of visual symptoms, visual acuity in the left eye was improved to 20/20, embolus is no longer visible, retinal veins are no longer dilated, and all hemorrhages and collateral vessels have disappeared. (From Magargal LE, Sanborn GE, Zimmerman A. Venous stasis retinopathy associated with embolic obstruction of the central retinal artery. J Clin Neuroophthalmol 2:113–118, 1982.)

Central Retinal Vein Occlusion. There is a strong association between atherosclerotic and arteriosclerotic disease of the central retinal artery and the development of a **CRVO** (Cassady, 1953; Morgan, 1955; Paton et al., 1964; Hayreh, 1965; Fujino et al., 1969; Clarkson, 1994). Atherosclerosis and arteriosclerosis of the central retinal artery within the optic nerve, where it is adjacent to and shares a common sheath with the central retinal vein, is believed to cause compression and irritative endothelial proliferation of the central retinal vein (Hayreh, 1980) (Fig. 55.54C). Several investigators (Brown et al., 1984b; Lazzaro, 1986) suggested

that patients with the ischemic form of CRVO also have a higher prevalence of obstructive carotid artery disease than would be expected for age and sex, although others have not found this to be the case (Zegarra et al., 1983). Indeed, the paper of Brown et al. (1984b) is seriously flawed, not only by the choice of digital subtraction **intravenous** angiography as the test by which these investigators determined the presence or absence of atherosclerotic disease affecting the carotid artery, but also by several assumptions made by the authors (Hayreh, 1984). Also, the article by Lazzaro (1986) does not explain why his patients with CRVO under-

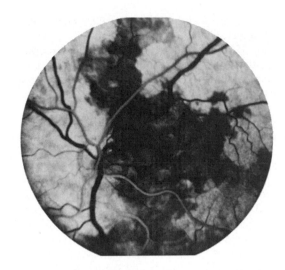

Figure 55.167. Choroidal ischemia producing exercise-related monocular visual loss in a patient with complete occlusion of the ipsilateral internal carotid artery. Fluorescein angiogram shows filling defects in the choroid and temporal portion of the optic disc. (From Raymond LA, Sacks JG, Choromokos E, et al. Short posterior ciliary artery insufficiency with hyperthermia (Uhthoff's symptom). Am J Ophthalmol 90:619–623, 1980.)

went cerebral angiography, although five of the 15 patients (33%) initially presented not with retinal vein occlusion but with transient monocular loss of vision associated with retinal emboli. In addition, we suspect that some of the confusion surrounding the proposed relationship between CRVO and carotid occlusive disease is related to errors in distinguishing the venous stasis retinopathy of Kearns and Hollenhorst (1963) from a CRVO (Kearns, 1983). We agree with Hayreh (1984) that atherosclerotic and arteriosclerotic disease of the **central retinal artery** plays a major role in the pathogenesis of a CRVO, but that there is no evidence that occlusive disease of the carotid artery has any direct relevance to the pathogenesis of CRVO. Patients with a CRVO certainly should undergo careful questioning regarding symptoms of carotid occlusive disease, but if these are absent, we see no reason to pursue further investigation.

Horner's Syndrome. Not all monocular signs of carotid artery disease affect visual acuity. Horner's syndrome may occur in patients with atherosclerotic carotid artery disease (Fig. 55.168). Most such patients have complete occlusion of the internal carotid artery, and the Horner's syndrome is associated with other symptoms and signs of carotid artery disease, such as contralateral hemiparesis and, when the lesion is on the left side, aphasia (Siegert, 1938; Milleti, 1950; Johnson and Walker, 1951; Walsh, 1957; O'Doherty and Green, 1958). Horner's syndrome that occurs in patients with occlusion of the internal carotid artery is almost always postganglionic. A preganglionic Horner's syndrome, characterized by ptosis, miosis, and ipsilateral facial anhidrosis, is usually associated with disease of the common or external carotid artery (O'Doherty and Green, 1958).

Patients with traumatic and spontaneous dissecting aneurysms that occlude or significantly obstruct the cervical portion of the internal carotid artery may develop an acute, ipsilateral Horner's syndrome that is usually associated with a focal, unilateral headache (Mokri et al., 1979; Bogousslavsky et al., 1987a; Itoh et al., 1987—see also Chapter 53). The Horner's syndrome is nearly always postganglionic in such patients (see Chapter 24), and the headache is often distinctive (West et al., 1976; Mokri et al., 1979; Fisher, 1981). It typically affects the ipsilateral forehead just above the orbit, the portions of the face just lateral or below the orbit, or the orbit itself. It is associated with neck pain that extends from just above the clavicle to the area behind the ear (Fisher, 1981). In such patients, a bruit may be heard, and a pulsating mass may be felt in the neck. In most patients, the headache resolves within several months, although the Horner's syndrome may be permanent (Mokri et al., 1979).

Corneal Arcus. Arcus of the cornea is an annular infiltration of lipid in the midperipheral cornea that is usually a natural consequence of aging. The condition usually is bilateral. It is present in about 60% of patients from 40–60 years of age and almost always present in patients 80 years of age and older (Duke-Elder, 1971). Smith and Susac (1973) described an 85-year-old man with open angle glaucoma who began to experience episodes of transient visual loss in the left eye. The patient had **unilateral** arcus of the right cornea in addition to findings consistent with bilateral glaucoma (Fig. 55.169A). A harsh, high-pitched, systolic bruit was heard in the region of the bifurcation of the left common carotid artery. The patient died after a myocardial infarction 2 years later. Autopsy revealed severe stenosis of the left internal carotid artery by an atherosclerotic plaque (Fig. 55.169B). The right internal carotid artery was patent. Smith and Susac (1973) postulated that a reduction in blood flow to the left eye from the atherosclerotic lesion somehow "protected" the patient from developing arcus in that cornea.

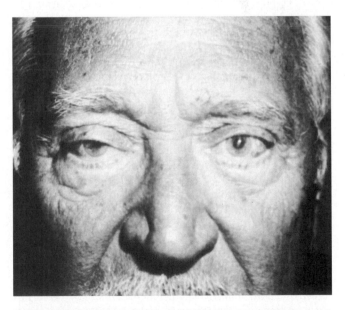

Figure 55.168. Right Horner's syndrome in an 82-year-old man with complete occlusion of the right internal carotid artery. The onset of ptosis was accompanied by the development of a mild left hemiparesis.

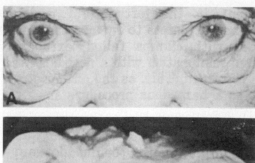

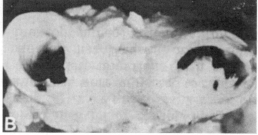

Figure 55.169. Unilateral corneal arcus associated with contralateral carotid artery occlusive disease. The patient was an 85-year-old man with glaucoma. *A,* External appearance of the patient shows right corneal arcus. The patient had a bruit in the region of the bifurcation of the left common carotid artery. The patient died 2 years later after a myocardial infarction. *B,* The right internal carotid artery is patent. The left internal carotid artery is almost occluded by a large atherosclerotic plaque. Occlusive disease of one carotid artery may somehow "protect" an eye from developing cornea arcus. (From Smith JL, Susac JO. Unilateral arcus senilis: Sign of occlusive disease of the carotid artery. JAMA *226:*676, 1973.)

These authors suggested that unilateral corneal arcus might be an important sign of contralateral carotid artery disease.

Iris Abnormalities. Abnormal iris transluminance and an increased prevalence of pseudoexfoliation may be markers of extracranial carotid artery disease (Repo et al., 1993, 1995). Hypoperfusion of the iris may contribute to the development of both stromal atrophy, which accounts for the transillumination defects in the iris, and pseudoexfoliation.

Ocular Motor Nerve Pareses. As noted above, patients with acute occlusion or severe stenosis of the internal carotid artery may experience paresis of one or more of the ocular motor nerves on the side of the occlusion. In some cases, only the oculomotor nerve becomes paretic (Balcer et al., 1997). In these cases, ischemia of the nerve probably results from reduction of blood flow through mesencephalic branches of the anterior choroidal artery. In other cases, unilateral paresis of more than one ocular motor nerve is associated with severe ipsilateral orbital and temple pain and ipsilateral visual loss from CRAO (Wilson et al., 1989). In these cases, small intracavernous branches from the internal carotid artery to the ocular motor nerves and the trigeminal nerve probably have become occluded. Unrecognized carotid artery dissection with propagation of the dissection or thrombosis should be considered as a possible underlying etiology in these cases.

Ptosis Unassociated with Either Oculomotor Nerve Paresis or Horner's Syndrome (Cerebral Ptosis). Ptosis not caused by either oculomotor nerve paresis or Horner's syndrome occasionally occurs in patients with stenosis or occlu-

sion of the internal carotid artery or its branches. Cerebral ptosis may be unilateral or bilateral.

Caplan (1974) described 13 patients with cerebral ptosis. Eight of these patients had unilateral ptosis. In six of the eight, the ptosis was on the side opposite the lesion (Fig. 55.170). Three of these six patients had acute hemiparesis, hemisensory loss, hemianopia, and either aphasia or apractagnosia on the side of the ptosis. All three of these patients were thought to have had a middle cerebral artery embolic stroke. Two of the six patients with contralateral ptosis had pure motor hemiparesis and were thought to have had a lacunar infarction, whereas one of the six patients had a slight right hemiparesis and aphasia associated with severe stenosis of the left internal carotid artery. Two of eight patients with unilateral ptosis had ptosis on the side of the infarct. Both patients were thought to have had an embolic ischemic stroke in the territory of the middle cerebral artery. Because both of these patients had contralateral hemiplegia that included the face, it is possible that they actually had bilateral cortical ptosis with the contralateral ptosis masked by facial weakness.

Bilateral cerebral ptosis is not uncommon (Caplan, 1974; Nutt, 1977; Krohel and Griffin, 1978) (Fig. 55.171). In some cases, the ptosis is asymmetric, primarily because of the effect of associated facial weakness on the ipsilateral eyelid fissure. The duration of cerebral ptosis is highly variable. It may last from 2 weeks to 5 months or more (Caplan, 1974; Nutt, 1977). The anatomic basis of ptosis caused by a hemisphere infarct is unknown.

Eyelid Retraction. Elander et al. (1957) reported the unique occurrence of eyelid retraction in a patient with occlusion of the ipsilateral common carotid artery. The patho-

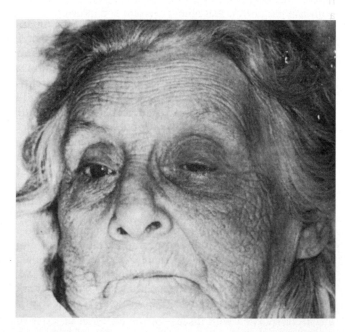

Figure 55.170. Unilateral cerebral ptosis. This elderly patient suffered a stroke characterized by acute left hemiparesis and unilateral, supranuclear, left ptosis. (From Caplan LR. Ptosis. J Neurol Neurosurg Psychiatry *37:* 1–7, 1974.)

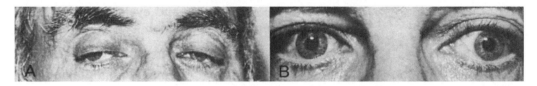

Figure 55.171. Bilateral cerebral ptosis. The patient suffered bilateral frontal lobe infarctions. *A*, At the time of the stroke, the patient had severe, bilateral ptosis. *B*, Two months later, the patient's ptosis has completely resolved. (From Krohel GB, Griffin JF. Cortical blepharoptosis. Am J Ophthalmol *85:* 632–634, 1978.)

physiology of the eyelid retraction is unclear. It may have been caused by irritation and consequent hyperactivity of the oculosympathetic pathway related to the occlusion, but unilateral pupillary dilation would be expected in such a setting, and this patient had isocoric pupils that reacted equally to both light and accommodative stimuli. A more plausible explanation is that the eyelid retraction was not, in fact, related to carotid occlusive disease but was a manifestation of otherwise asymptomatic thyroid disease (e.g., euthyroid Graves' disease).

Ocular Pain. Although eye pain is usually not considered a symptom of carotid occlusive disease unless it is associated with other symptoms and signs of vascular disease, Cohen and McNamara (1980) described a 63-year-old man who developed severe "knife-like" pain in the right eye and orbital region. The pain lasted 1 hour and was partially relieved by aspirin. Three hours later, the pain returned and was associated with nausea and vomiting. The next day, the patient became acutely confused and experienced an exacerbation of eye pain. He then complained of transient numbness of the left hand that lasted 10 minutes. Cerebral angiography showed 95% stenosis of the right internal carotid artery. Following an uncomplicated right carotid endarterectomy, the patient's eye pain resolved and did not return.

We followed a 65-year-old man with an otherwise classic idiopathic nonarteritic AION who had persistent ipsilateral periocular and hemicranial discomfort but no other neurologic symptoms or signs. Two months after the onset of visual loss, he developed a contralateral hemiparesis and was found to have an occluded internal carotid artery on the side of the optic neuropathy. Frequent, unaccustomed headache or eye pain may be a sign of generalized ischemia from ipsilateral carotid occlusive disease (Caplan, 1993).

Homonymous Visual Field Defects. Homonymous visual field defects contralateral to an occluded internal or common carotid artery and caused by ischemic changes in the territory of the carotid artery and its branches are almost always accompanied by other neurologic signs of carotid artery territory ischemia (Hollenhorst, 1962). Walsh and Smith (1952) observed that an incomplete homonymous hemianopia in this setting was most dense in the lower quadrant of the visual field, and they related this finding to the circulatory dependence of the upper part of the optic radiation on the middle cerebral artery. Hollenhorst (1962) could not confirm this finding and emphasized that incomplete homonymous field defects were as likely to be denser above as below in his patients. He also observed that when the hemianopia had sloping margins, improvement in the visual field usually occurred. As noted above, when the posterior cerebral artery originates from the internal carotid artery, atherosclerotic disease of the internal carotid artery may produce a homonymous hemianopia not only from infarction of the optic tract, lateral geniculate body, and optic radiation, but also from infarction of the ipsilateral striate cortex (Cohen, 1989; Pessin et al., 1989; Balcer et al., 1996). In such cases, the hemianopic field defect usually is the only abnormality present. Gasecki et al. (1994) described a 76-year-old man with bilateral occipital infarctions related to an ulcerated stenotic left internal carotid artery that presumably produced emboli to the occipital lobes through a persistent trigeminal artery. In patients with carotid artery occlusion, the risk of watershed infarction (and possible retrochiasmal visual field defects) is decreased when the posterior communicating arteries measure at least 1 mm in diameter (Schomer et al., 1994).

We saw an unusual case of a 45-year-old man who experienced a traumatic aortic valvular injury while waterskiing. When he awoke after valvular surgery, he had a dense right homonymous hemianopia, multiple cotton-wool spots in his left eye, and an RAPD. He had no other neurologic symptoms or signs. Neuroimaging revealed an infarction in the territory of the left anterior choroidal artery, involving the left optic tract (Fig. 55.172).

Bitemporal Visual Field Defects. Patients with occlusion or severe stenosis of the siphon of one or both internal carotid arteries may develop an optic chiasmal syndrome (Hughes, 1958; Lee and Schatz, 1975). In such patients, the blood supply to the optic chiasm from the affected internal carotid artery is reduced, producing an infarction of the chiasm. An ischemic chiasmal syndrome also may result from occlusion of small branches that originate from the internal carotid, anterior cerebral, and anterior communicating arteries (Hughes, 1958; Hilton and Hoyt, 1966) (Figs. 55.173 and 55.174). Such changes are particularly likely to occur in patients with fusiform dilation of the supraclinoid portion of the internal carotid arteries, the anterior cerebral arteries, or all of these structures (dolichoectasia—see Chapter 53).

Ocular Signs of Bilateral Carotid Artery Occlusive Disease. Although most patients with stenosis or occlusion of the internal carotid artery develop monocular or homonymous visual difficulties, bilateral carotid artery disease may produce bilateral ocular symptoms and signs that may occur simultaneously or nonsimultaneously. Sadun et al. (1983) described a 39-year-old man who complained of blurred vision in the left eye 4 months after he was involved in a motor vehicle accident that left him with clumsiness and

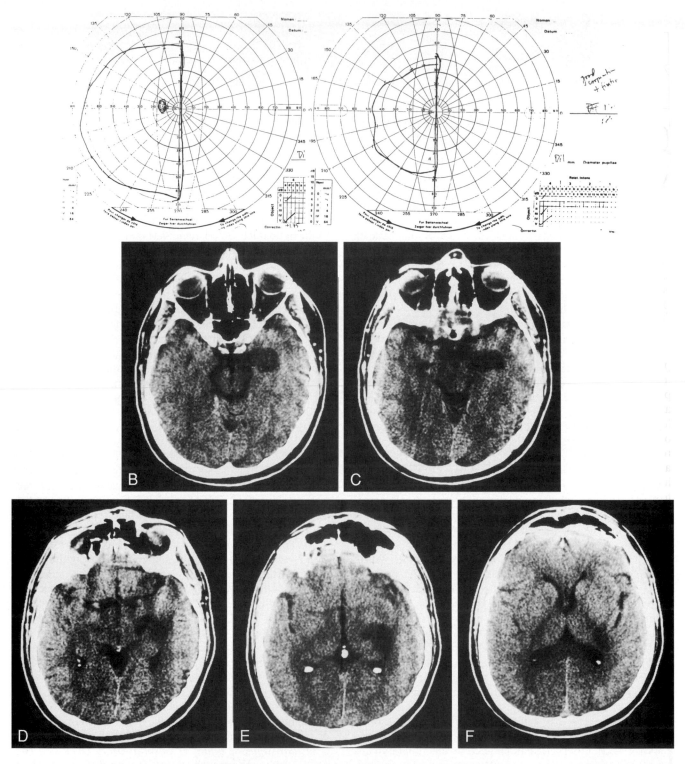

Figure 55.172. Left anterior choroidal artery infarction with resultant dense right homonymous hemianopia (*A*) in a 45-year-old man who suffered traumatic injury to his aortic valve and subsequent cerebral embolism. *B–F*, Axial computed tomographic scans, shown from most caudal (*B*) to most rostral (*F*), demonstrates lucency in the distribution of the left anterior choroidal artery.

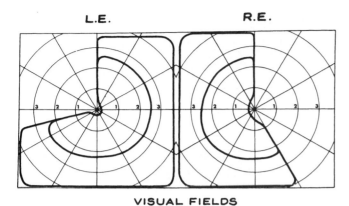

L.E.   R.E.

VISUAL FIELDS

ISOPTERS : 5W/1000 AND 25W/1000

Figure 55.173. The atherosclerotic optic chiasmal syndrome. The patient has an incomplete bitemporal hemianopia with reduction of central vision in both eyes. (From Hilton GF, Hoyt WF. An arteriosclerotic chiasmal syndrome: Bitemporal hemianopia associated with fusiform dilatation of the anterior cerebral arteries. JAMA *196*:1018–1020, 1966.)

paresthesias of the left hand thought to be caused by damage to the left brachial plexus. At the time of examination, the patient had an incongruous, incomplete homonymous hemianopia. He also had inability to reproduce spatial figures, left-arm weakness, and left-arm hypesthesia. Cerebral angiography revealed complete occlusion of **both** internal carotid arteries just distal to the carotid bifurcation. Hupp et al. (1984) described an 81-year-old woman with systemic hypertension who experienced an embolic branch retinal artery occlusion in the right eye followed within 24 hours by a CRAO in the left eye. The patient was found to have stenosis of the proximal portion of the right internal carotid artery and mild irregularity of the left internal carotid artery. Fisher and Yellin (1985) described a patient who experienced an episode of bilateral, asymmetric visual loss that resolved over 2–3 minutes. She denied other neurologic symptoms.

The patient's right eye had normal visual function; the left eye had visual acuity of 20/40 and pallor of the left optic disc but no RAPD. Cerebral angiography showed severe stenosis of both internal carotid arteries. The absence of an RAPD in this case may have been related to subclinical ischemia of the right eye or optic nerve.

Atherosclerosis and other diseases that predispose to bilateral carotid occlusion (e.g., moyamoya disease) may involve the distal portions of both internal carotid arteries, thus reducing perfusion to the optic chiasm and producing a chiasmal syndrome characterized by bitemporal hemianopia (Lee and Schatz, 1975; Ahmadi et al., 1984). Bilateral middle cerebral artery occlusion, usually nonsimultaneous, may occur in patients with bilateral carotid artery stenosis or occlusion. Such patients may develop complete or nearly complete cerebral blindness from bilateral destruction of the optic radiations (Fig. 55.175A). In other patients, an infarct in the distribution of one of the branches of the internal carotid artery may be associated with a contralateral infarct in the distribution of the posterior cerebral artery, producing complete or nearly complete loss of vision from bilateral destruction of the optic radiations, striate cortex, or both (Fig. 55.175B).

Ocular Symptoms and Signs of Ophthalmic Artery Occlusion. The ocular symptoms and signs of ophthalmic artery occlusion are much the same as those of internal carotid artery occlusion. Transient monocular loss of vision may occur (Weinberger et al., 1980), as may both AION and PION (Suzuki et al., 1983). The ocular ischemic syndrome can develop in patients with severe ophthalmic artery stenosis or occlusion (Bronner, 1961; Bronner and Lobstein, 1966; Madsen, 1966; Bettelheim, 1967; Bullock et al., 1972; Brown and Magargal, 1988; Brown, 1994b), as may various types of retinal strokes.

When both the retinal and choroidal circulations are compromised from ophthalmic artery occlusion, more dramatic clinical symptoms and signs occur than result from a CRAO or an ION alone. Visual loss is typically severe, with most eyes having no light perception or only bare perception of

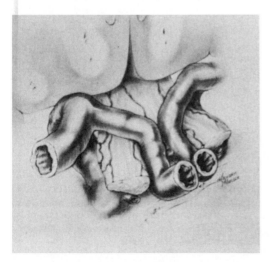

Figure 55.174. Artist's drawing of findings at surgery in the patient whose visual fields are depicted in Figure 55.173. The intracranial portions of both internal carotid arteries are diffusely enlarged, as are the A1 and proximal A2 segments of both anterior cerebral arteries. Note that the distal portions of the A1 segments and the proximal portions of the A2 segments extend between and slightly below both optic nerves. (From Hilton GF, Hoyt WF. An arteriosclerotic chiasmal syndrome: Bitemporal hemianopia associated with fusiform dilatation of the anterior cerebral arteries. JAMA *196*:1018–1020, 1966.)

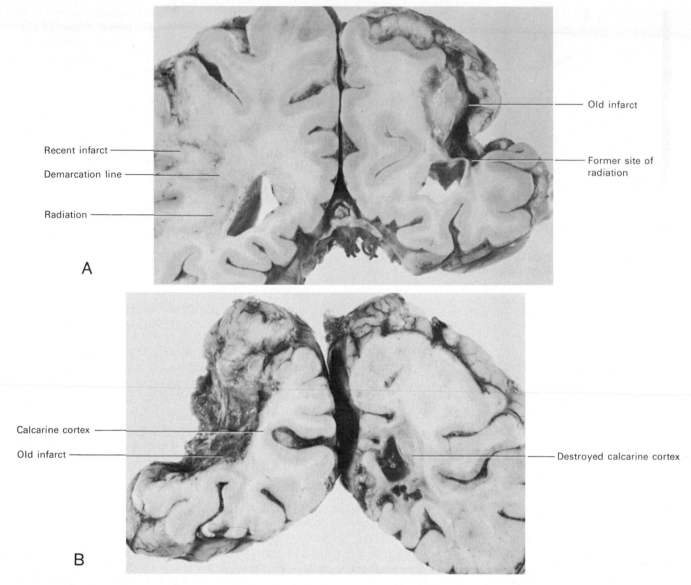

Figure 55.175. Cerebral blindness from bilateral infarctions related to carotid artery disease. *A*, A 70-year-old woman had experienced several strokes. She was nearly blind when she died. Coronal section through the posterior parietal lobes shows that an old, collapsed infarct in the supply territory of the angular branch of the middle cerebral artery destroyed nearly the entire optic radiation on the right side. A more recent, well-demarcated infarct affects the supply territory of the corresponding angular artery on the left side, including the left optic radiation. These lesions produced bilateral homonymous hemianopias. *B*, A 49-year-old man became confused, blind, and incoherent. He died from the effects of pulmonary embolism. Coronal section through the occipital lobes shows that the left radiation is totally destroyed by an old infarct in the supply territory of the angular and lower parietal branches of the middle cerebral artery. Equally old is an incomplete infarction of the right calcarine cortex and the territory supplied by the calcarine branch of the posterior cerebral artery. The lesion on the left extended rostrally into the posterior half of the temporal lobe and into the inferior parietal lobe. (From Lindenberg R, Walsh FB, Sacks JG. Neuropathology of Vision. An Atlas. Philadelphia, Lea & Febiger, 1973.)

light (Brown et al., 1986; Rafuse et al., 1997). There may be associated discomfort and pupillary dilation, the latter presumably from concurrent ischemia to the ciliary ganglion or iris sphincter. The eye may be hypotonous. The retinal vessels are markedly constricted, but there may not be a cherry-red spot. The optic disc may or may not be swollen. Visual loss is usually permanent, and most patients develop a characteristic fundus appearance characterized by optic

atrophy, arterial attenuation, and diffuse pigmentary changes (Rafuse et al., 1997) (Fig. 55.176).

The ophthalmic artery can become occluded in several ways: (*a*) by a thrombus originating within the artery itself; (*b*) by a thrombus propagating from an occluded internal carotid artery; (*c*) by an embolus from a distant site (most often the heart, the common carotid artery, or the extracranial portion of the internal carotid artery); or (*d*) by an extrinsic

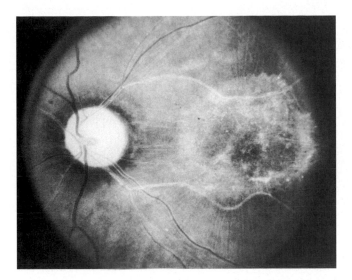

Figure 55.176. Funduscopic appearance of ophthalmic artery occlusion. The disc is pale, the arteries are mere ghost vessels, and pigmentary changes are notable, especially in the macular region. The patient's vision was no light perception.

process that compresses the vessel (e.g., a tumor or aneurysm). When only the proximal portion of the vessel is occluded, there may be no ocular symptoms or signs, because collateral channels from branches of the external carotid artery usually provide sufficient blood supply to the orbital and ocular vessels normally supplied by the ophthalmic artery. When the occlusion is more extensive, the ocular symptoms and signs are significant.

Symptoms and Signs of Vertebrobasilar Artery System Ischemia

The vertebrobasilar system is the posterior arterial system of the brain. Stenoses, occlusions, and reductions in blood flow at various locations in the system produce a vast array of neurologic and visual disturbances, most of which are caused by damage to the mesencephalon, pons, medulla, cerebellum, and occipital lobes (Tatu et al., 1996) (Fig. 55.177). These disturbances may be transient or persistent and inconsequential or catastrophic.

The vertebrobasilar arterial system supports the neural components of the entire brainstem ocular motor mechanism as well as those of the posterior visual sensory pathways and visual (striate) cortex. For this reason, ocular motor and visual symptoms and signs play a major role in the diagnosis of vascular insufficiency in the vertebrobasilar system (Bogousslavsky and Meienberg, 1987).

Transient Ischemic Attacks from Intermittent Insufficiency of the Vertebrobasilar Arterial System

Before 1940, minimal clinical attention was paid to thrombosis of the basilar artery because it was generally believed that death was an immediate and inevitable consequence. In 1946, however, Kubik and Adams described the effects of

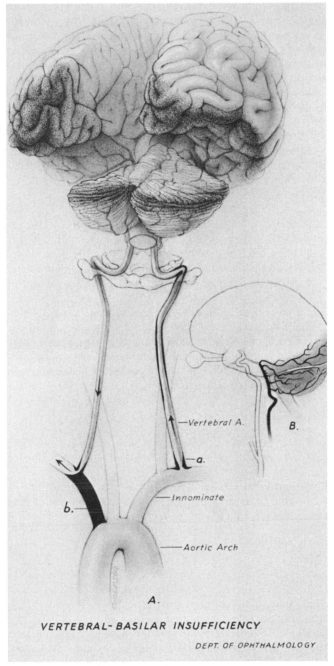

Figure 55.177. Vertebrobasilar arterial system ischemia. The *stippled areas* of A indicate the terminal areas of cerebral and cerebellar vascular supply served by the vertebrobasilar arterial system. *a,* Atheromatous stenosis at the origin of a vertebral artery. Stenosis or occlusion of the vertebral or basilar arteries or their branches may produce severe neurologic symptoms and signs. *b,* Occlusion of the proximal left subclavian artery may produce a subclavian steal syndrome in which blood flowing toward the brain in the right vertebral artery *(arrow)* is diverted back down the left vertebral artery and into the distal subclavian artery *(arrows)*. *B,* Lateral view of the brain shows distribution of the vertebrobasilar arterial system with respect to the cerebral hemispheres and cerebellum. (From Hoyt WF. Some neuro-ophthalmologic considerations in cerebral vascular insufficiency. Arch Ophthalmol *62:*260–272, 1959.)

occlusion of the basilar artery and showed that these neurologic deficits could be recognized during life. These investigators reported clinical and autopsy findings from 18 cases and described four patients with an occlusion of the basilar artery who had survived. As a result of the publication of this important article by Kubik and Adams (1946), physicians increasingly began to recognize premonitory symptoms of major occlusions of the vertebral and basilar arteries and their branches. Denny-Brown (1951) reported a case of basilar artery occlusion in which he attributed the fluctuating symptoms and signs to a state of episodic insufficiency in the circle of Willis. Fisher and Cameron (1953) reported a favorable response to anticoagulation in a 70-year-old woman with incipient basilar artery thrombosis, and they also emphasized the importance of transient warning phenomena as a prelude to the actual thrombotic event. Silversides (1954) described 22 cases of basilar artery thrombosis and suggested that premonitory symptoms might be the result of periodic insufficiency of blood flow to the brainstem.

In 1955, Millikan and Sickert introduced the concept of "intermittent insufficiency of the basilar arterial system." Eight years later, Bradshaw and McQuaid (1963) stated that "The syndrome of vertebrobasilar insufficiency is, in our experience, one of the most frequent diagnoses in neurologic practice; more common than disseminated sclerosis, and outnumbering the total of all other causes of disturbances in the posterior cranial fossa."

SYMPTOMS OF VERTEBROBASILAR ARTERIAL SYSTEM TIAS.

The symptoms of vertebrobasilar arterial system TIAs may be general, neurologic, visual, or a combination of these.

General Symptoms. The symptoms of TIAs in the territory of the vertebrobasilar system are much more varied than the symptoms of TIAs in the territory of the carotid system (Heyman et al., 1974; Whisnant et al., 1978; Naritomi et al., 1979; Heyman et al., 1984a). **Vertigo** is exceedingly common. This sensation of rotation of oneself or of the environment may occur as an isolated symptom (Gomez et al., 1996) or in association with other brainstem or visual symptoms, particularly tinnitus, loss of balance, transient deafness, diplopia, and vomiting. Ackerman et al. (1977) described a 10-year-old boy in whom vertigo and diplopia were the first symptoms of basilar artery occlusion. The patient had no neurologic abnormalities except for dysarthria when he was initially examined, even though arteriography revealed complete occlusion of the basilar artery proximal to the origins of the superior cerebellar arteries. Within 24 hours, he had a completely normal neurologic examination. Five days later, he again experienced vertigo, this time associated with headache and somnolence; the next day, he became mute and quadriplegic.

Vertigo may arise peripherally from ischemia in the territory of the internal auditory artery. It also may arise centrally from ischemia in the lateral tegmentum of the pons near the middle cerebellar peduncle or from ischemia of the temporoparietal cortex. Vertigo occurred at least once, and often repeatedly, in 42 of 54 cases (78%) of vertebrobasilar artery

insufficiency described by Bradshaw and McQuaid (1963). Vomiting out of proportion to dizziness is particularly suggestive of ischemic lesions in the brainstem vestibular system, helping to differentiate these central lesions from labyrinthine (end-organ) disorders (Fisher, 1996).

Transient **dysarthria** is a frequent symptom of vertebrobasilar insufficiency, and both **dysphagia** and **sensory symptoms over the face** are also common. **Circumoral numbness** is emphasized as an important symptom of vertebrobasilar insufficiency by many investigators, but it is an infrequent symptom in our patients.

Transient **weakness and sensory disturbances** of one side of the body often occur in patients with vertebrobasilar insufficiency (see Table 1 in Heyman et al., 1984a). Bilaterality or alternation of these symptoms from one side to the other in separate attacks is very suggestive of a vertebrobasilar origin of the TIA. Transient sensory symptoms on one side of the face and on the opposite side of the body also suggest focal brainstem ischemia.

A **drop attack** is one of the most spectacular forms of vertebrobasilar TIAs. The patient suddenly falls to the ground without warning. There is no loss of consciousness, nor is there any vertigo or unsteadiness. The patient can usually arise immediately, but he or she may find that the legs are too weak to allow this. The underlying pathophysiology of this rare phenomenon remains unknown. It should be noted that most drop attacks are not caused by vertebrobasilar disease, but are more often cardiac or syncopal in origin. In addition, drop attacks caused by verterbrobasilar disease are almost never isolated; thus, a careful history and examination will usually uncover other evidence of vertebrobasilar ischemia.

Headache is more common in patients who experience vertebrobasilar TIAs than in patients with carotid system TIAs (see Chapter 36). It may persist longer than other neurologic symptoms and may occasionally occur independently. Often occipital in location, it may be accentuated by stooping or straining.

Rarely, transient **confusion**, **loss of awareness**, and even **amnesia** are symptoms of vertebrobasilar insufficiency. When any of these symptoms occur in the absence of obvious brainstem symptoms, the patient may be thought to have frontal lobe disease.

Visual Symptoms. Episodes of **blurred, dim, or complete loss of vision** occur in patients with vertebrobasilar insufficiency almost as often as attacks of vertigo. Unlike the episodes of monocular transient visual loss that occur in patients with carotid system disease, the episodes of visual loss that occur in patients with vertebrobasilar insufficiency are always **bilateral**, with both eyes being affected simultaneously and symmetrically (Hoyt, 1959; Minor et al., 1959; Hollenhorst, 1962; Williams and Wilson, 1962; Olbert, 1985; Dennis et al., 1989). They are not associated with the sensations of color that often accompany retinal TIAs, and the episodes usually are unrelated to activity, time of day, or body position unless there is a fixed deficit with relative hypoperfusion.

A typical attack is characterized by sudden dimming or graying of vision that may cause the patient momentarily to stop what he or she is doing. The change in vision may be described as a "grayout of vision," "a sensation of looking through fog or smoke," or "the feeling that someone has turned down the lights." The patient may at first attribute such episodes to dirty or improperly fitted glasses, and he or she initially may spend much time cleaning and repositioning them. Patients who do not wear glasses may interpret such attacks as indicating a need for them, whereas patients who wear glasses may assume they need new ones. Another assumption made by some patients who experience these episodes of bilateral visual loss is that there is a film of tears or mucus over the eyes, and they may attempt to wipe the presumed film away. Other patients may assume that the visual episodes are caused by a faulty bulb in a reading lamp or room light, and they may change the bulb several times before they are convinced that this is not the case. We saw one elderly woman who had experienced one or two attacks of bilateral visual dimming every few days for several months. She had changed all the light bulbs in her house, and she had even had an electrician check the electric wiring in the house, berating him when he could not find anything wrong.

Some attacks of blurred vision that result from vertebrobasilar insufficiency last less than a minute (Dennis et al., 1989). Such attacks may be so short that the patient does not have time to appreciate fully what is happening. If the patient happens to be driving a car at the time of an attack, however, he or she will be acutely aware of the visual loss and may be forced to slow down or even pull over to the side of the road until vision returns. Attacks of visual dimming that last a minute or more are sufficiently long to cause the patient to worry. Although total visual loss is rare, the patient may be unable to distinguish faces or to see a chair or sofa on which to sit. These attacks of longer duration may be accompanied by flickering, flashing "stars" of silvery light in a homonymous or altitudinal field of vision. The flashing points of light may have a streaming effect resembling snowflakes rushing through the headlight beams of a moving automobile (Hoyt, 1963).

When patients with vertebrobasilar insufficiency have repetitive attacks of visual blurring, the attacks have the following characteristics: (*a*) they commonly last only a few seconds and rarely last more than 5 minutes; (*b*) they may vary in duration in the same patient; (*c*) they are usually much shorter in duration than are attacks of vertigo, dizziness, diplopia, dysphagia, dysarthria, or facial numbness; and (*d*) they may occur alone or in combination with other transient symptoms of vertebrobasilar insufficiency. It is not possible to predict the prognosis of a patient from the pattern of visual attacks (Fisher, 1962). An isolated episode may occur in one patient days or weeks before a stroke. Another patient may experience multiple attacks over a period of weeks or months before a stroke occurs. In some cases, a stroke never occurs.

The episodes of blurred vision that occur in patients with vertebrobasilar artery insufficiency must be differentiated from the blackouts of vision (transient monocular visual loss) associated with carotid insufficiency. As noted above, the latter attacks are almost always monocular, are often associated with abnormal color sensation, and may be characterized by complete loss of vision in the affected eye. Brief episodes of bilateral blurred or dimmed vision also may occur in patients with increased ICP. These attacks are clinically indistinguishable from those in patients with vertebrobasilar insufficiency, but patients with increased ICP who experience such attacks always have papilledema. Migraine can cause bilateral visual loss (Moen et al., 1988). However, migraine-induced visual loss usually lasts about 20 minutes, a period of time much longer than the typical vertebrobasilar TIA. Furthermore, migraine tends to have early positive symptoms with build-up over time and gradual clearing, often followed by headache (Fisher, 1980; Fisher, 1968b; Caplan, 1993). A past history of migraine attacks, a history of migraine in the family, and the age of the patient may also help to establish this diagnosis (see Chapter 56), but this is not always the case.

Transient visual symptoms other than visual blurring or dimming may result from vertebrobasilar insufficiency. Transient horizontal or vertical **diplopia** is a common manifestation of vertebrobasilar insufficiency, although it occurs less frequently than does transient blurred vision. The diplopia may result from transient ischemia of the ocular motor nerves or their nuclei (ocular motor nerve paresis) or from transient ischemia to supranuclear or internuclear ocular motor pathways (skew deviation, internuclear ophthalmoplegia [INO], gaze paresis) (see Chapter 29). Curiously, in addition to the sensation of diplopia, the patient often has the distinct "feeling" that the eyes are crossing or deviating apart (Fisher, 1967a; Coppeto, 1988). Most episodes of transient diplopia caused by vertebrobasilar insufficiency last 5–10 minutes, although some last for an hour or more (Hoyt, 1959). DeVivo and Farrell (1972) described a previously healthy 10-year-old boy who began to experience brief episodes of diplopia that were relieved by covering either eye. During some of the episodes, he was confused and unsteady. He also was "dizzy" during some of the episodes but denied headache or nausea. He subsequently had two or three episodes of numbness and tingling of the tongue and one episode of confusion and dysarthria. He eventually developed a stroke characterized by right-sided numbness and weakness of the body, ataxia, and Horner's syndrome.

Not all patients with transient misalignment of the eyes are aware of true diplopia. Some patients initially may refer to these disturbances as "blurred vision" until they are asked to describe them in detail, at which time it becomes clear either that the "blurred vision" is actually diplopia or that the patient has visual confusion, the superimposition of the different images seen with the fovea of each eye (see Chapter 27).

Transient, complete 90–180 degree inversion of the visual image occasionally occurs in patients with vertebrobasilar ischemia (Bender et al., 1983; Ropper, 1983; Steiner et al., 1987; Mehler, 1988a). This form of **visual allesthesia** probably is caused by transient ischemia of the vestibular-otolith pathways in the medulla. It occurs most often in patients with the lateral medullary syndrome of Wallenberg (see below).

Williams and Wilson (1962) emphasized that **formed visual hallucinations** may be produced by vertebrobasilar insufficiency. These hallucinations, which may last 30 minutes or more, may be associated with decreased consciousness, but they usually occur in an otherwise alert patient who is aware that the visual images are not real. The hallucinations are generally restricted to a hemianopic field, and they are often complex. One of the patients reported by Williams and Wilson (1962) described a tropical shore with white sands, blue sky, and brilliant flowers. Brust and Behrens (1977) reported two patients in whom formed visual hallucinations were the presenting symptoms of a posterior cerebral artery occlusion. One patient described a right-field hallucination of ''four or five men'' who were ''variably dressed (two or three in business suits, one in a cowboy suit and hat, one in a plaid shirt), moving about, not speaking, and not relating to one another.'' A patient reported by Mauskop et al. (1984) described ''little people dancing on the left side.''

Some of the visual hallucinations that occur in patients with posterior cerebral artery occlusion are **palinoptic**, with the hallucinations consisting of recently or previously seen images (Bender et al., 1968; Feldman and Bender, 1970; Brust and Behrens, 1977; Meadows and Munro, 1977; Trobe and Bauer, 1986). In most patients, any actions in the perseverated image progress at normal speed; however, Cleland et al. (1981) reported the case of a young woman who developed a right parietal infarct after an episode of complicated migraine and who experienced episodes of visual perseveration in which all movements seemed to be speeded up ''as though she was watching a film being shown at the wrong speed, that speed being about twice normal.'' Williams and Wilson (1962) attributed the visual hallucinations and visual perseveration that occur in patients with posterior cerebral artery occlusion to intermittent ischemia in the hippocampal gyrus, a structure supplied by part of the posterior cerebral artery. Some of these hallucinations may occur on the edge of the hemianopic field as the posterior cerebral artery ischemia is either developing or clearing.

Some patients describe episodic ''jumping of the eyes'' or ''jumping of vision'' (**oscillopsia**, see Chapter 27) during attacks of dizziness or vertigo.

PATHOPHYSIOLOGY OF VERTEBROBASILAR ARTERIAL SYSTEM TIAS

The cause of transient episodes of vertebrobasilar ischemia remains a subject of speculation. Comments made in this chapter concerning TIAs that result from carotid artery system ischemia would seem to be equally applicable to vertebrobasilar TIAs. A number of variables can play a role in an attack (Millikan and Siekert, 1955; Williams, 1964; Naritomi et al., 1979). These include:

1. Congenital aplasia or hypoplasia of one of the vertebral arteries, the basilar artery, one of the posterior communicating arteries, or any of their branches;
2. Persistent carotid-basilar anastomotic channels (see Chapter 52);
3. Sites of atheromatous or other arterial disease;
4. Efficiency of collateral circulation;
5. Changes in cardiac output;

6. Changes in regional blood flow;
7. Hypertensive vascular disease causing poor reactivity of brainstem and cortical arterioles to changes in mean blood pressure or increased pCO_2;
8. Microembolization from atheromata in the vertebral or basilar arteries;
9. Anemia, polycythemia, or other disorders affecting blood viscosity; and
10. Mechanical factors causing restriction of flow in vertebral arteries.

Thromboembolism from atherosclerotic disease of the vertebrobasilar arterial system is probably the most important initiating event and contributes to the pathogenesis of symptoms of vertebrobasilar ischemia, but hemodynamic factors and dysautoregulation are also important and frequently contributory phenomena.

Head Movement and Cervical Arthritis: Their Relation to Blood Flow in the Vertebrobasilar System. The vertebral arteries usually are unequal in size (see Chapter 52). Hutchinson and Yates (1956) emphasized this asymmetry and noted that one vertebral artery, usually the right, may even be absent. The importance of this finding is obvious. The entire vertebrobasilar system is dependent on a single cervical vessel in some patients. Atherosclerotic occlusion or mechanical compression of the principal (or only) vertebral artery may thus cause disproportionately severe effects. The effects of head movement (rotation or extension) on blood flow were demonstrated by a number of investigators, both in cadavers (de Kleyn and Nieuwenhuyse, 1927; Tatlow and Bammer, 1957; Toole and Tucker, 1960) and in patients using cerebral angiography (Sheehan et al., 1960; Bauer et al., 1961; Li et al., 1988). Even in normal patients, rotation of the head to one side may temporarily reduce or even abolish blood flow through the atlantoaxial segment of the contralateral vertebral artery. The vertebral artery passes through the transverse process of the atlas and therefore must move when the atlas moves. Rotation of the head to one side carries the atlas with it and puts traction on the contralateral vertebral artery, actually pulling it out of its canal in the cervical spine.

In a patient with cervical spondylosis and associated osteophytes, rotation of the head may diminish blood flow through the ipsilateral vertebral artery (Fig. 55.40). Sheehan et al. (1960) called this phenomenon ''spondylotic vertebral artery compression.'' These investigators demonstrated vertebral compression in 26 patients with this type of cervical arthritis and emphasized that the associated neurologic symptoms and signs included all the transient and permanent effects of vertebrobasilar insufficiency syndromes as well as those of cervical nerve root compression. Spondylotic vertebral artery compression is aggravated by atheromatous disease of the extracranial portion of the internal carotid artery and of the intracranial vessels (Bauer et al., 1961).

As noted in Chapter 53 and earlier in this chapter, chiropractic and other manipulation of the neck may precipitate symptoms of brainstem ischemia. Ford (1952) reported the case of a 17-year-old boy with congenital absence of the odontoid process and atlantoaxial instability in whom neck manipulation produced occipital and medullary ischemia, and Brain (1963) described an elderly woman with cervical spondylosis who became blind from occipital lobe ischemia after neck manipulation. Other investigators described similar cases (Mehalic and Farhat, 1974; Levy et al., 1980; Frumkin and Baloh, 1990). The immediate neurologic and visual disturbances produced by neck manipulation are most often the result of vascular compression with secondary reduction in blood flow, embolism, or both, whereas the delayed deficits are probably caused by intimal injury or dissection leading to thrombus formation and late embolism.

Reversal of Blood Flow in the Vertebral Artery (Subclavian Steal). Proximal occlusion of a subclavian artery produces an unusual alteration in the direction of flow in the ipsilateral vertebral artery. The lowered pressure in the distal segment of the subclavian artery may siphon (steal) blood from the vertebral artery on that side (Fig. 55.177) and so produce fluctuating symptoms of vertebrobasilar insufficiency (see section on aortocranial disease below). Patients with these symptoms may be thought to have primary occlusive disease of the vertebral or basilar arteries until it is appreciated that such symptoms are related to, or exacerbated by, physical activity such as arm raising. When such patients are then found to have a decreased or absent radial pulse and a reduction in blood pressure on one or both sides, the diagnosis becomes evident.

Neurologic and Ocular Signs of Occlusive Disease of the Vertebrobasilar Arterial System

Objective signs of occlusive disease in the vertebrobasilar system are caused by ischemic lesions located in the brainstem, cerebellum, thalamus, and occipital lobes. These signs indicate the location, and, to a lesser degree, the extent of a nonfunctioning area of brain tissue. Although neuroimaging studies, particularly MR imaging, can provide a reasonably accurate assessment of the pathologic process, clinical differentiation between focal hemorrhage in the brainstem and occlusion of small perforating arterioles is often impossible (Kempe, 1964; Kase et al., 1980; Ausman et al., 1985; Kase et al., 1985a; Dubin and Quencer, 1987). A history of previous TIAs in the vertebrobasilar territory or rapid onset of neurologic signs in a middle-aged or elderly patient suggests an ischemic lesion, and a history of pre-existing systemic hypertension, peripheral vascular occlusive disease, or cardiac abnormality further supports this diagnosis.

Localization of responsible occlusions in various portions of main trunks or branches of the vertebral and basilar arteries from clinical data is often inaccurate (Ausman et al., 1985). Thrombotic occlusion of a vertebral artery may produce no signs at all, but it is just as likely to cause signs of infarction in one or both occipital lobes (Fisher, 1970; Caplan, 1979).

Occlusion of the basilar artery also produces a wide variety of manifestations. For example, complete occlusion of a caudal segment of the basilar artery can cause immediate coma, pinpoint pupils, flaccid quadriplegia, complete anesthesia, progressive hyperpyrexia, and death, whereas occlusion of the rostral portion of the basilar artery often produces

severe neurobehavioral disturbances, ophthalmologic signs, motor signs, or a combination of these from damage to brainstem-diencephalic structures and to one or both posterior hemispheres (Caplan, 1980; Mehler, 1988b, 1988c, 1989). Basilar artery occlusion in other patients may produce an isolated hemiparesis that initially suggests a lesion in the cerebral hemisphere but within hours becomes a bilateral hemiplegia associated with coma or a locked-in syndrome (Mori et al., 1979; Fisher, 1988—see below). From a neuro-ophthalmologic standpoint, thrombosis of the basilar artery can produce an isolated homonymous hemianopia that suggests localized disease of the posterior cerebral artery or cortical blindness that initially may be mistaken for nonorganic visual loss (Kearns et al., 1955; Symonds and MacKenzie, 1957; Olbert, 1985). It also may produce only transient neurologic symptoms or isolated brainstem signs that indicate little more than malfunction of a few tiny paramedian arterioles (Pessin et al., 1987a; Labauge et al., 1989; Brandt et al., 1995). Hence, although basilar artery stenosis and occlusion can be associated with fatal or severe brainstem infarction, significant basilar disease may result in more limited stroke syndromes, presumably on the basis of local occlusion of the origin of paramedian perforating arteries (Bogousslavsky et al., 1993; Brandt et al., 1995).

Hutchinson and Yates (1956) discussed the importance of collateral blood flow from the posterior communicating arteries in vertebrobasilar occlusion. These investigators emphasized that life can continue if there is retrograde flow in the cephalic segment of the basilar artery (Fig. 55.178). Labauge et al. (1989) also emphasized that long-term sur-

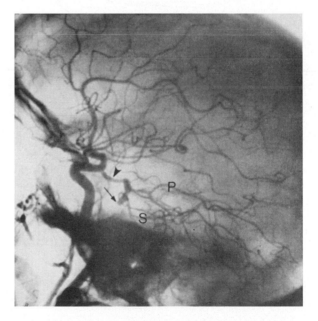

Figure 55.178. Occlusion of the basilar artery with development of collateral flow through the posterior communicating artery. Cerebral arteriogram, lateral view, shows occlusion of the basilar artery with reconstitution of the cephalic segment (*arrow*) from the internal carotid artery via the posterior communicating artery (*arrowhead*). Both posterior cerebral (*P*) and superior cerebellar (*C*) arteries are filled by this route.

vival with minimal or no neurologic deficit is possible in patients with occlusions restricted to the rostral or middle portion of the basilar artery, provided that such patients have good collateral blood supply from the carotid arterial system. The prognosis in patients with basilar artery occlusion thus seems to depend on many factors, including the location and extent of the occlusion, the rapidity with which the occlusion has occurred, and the extent of collateral circulation to the brainstem and subcortical structures (Brandt et al., 1995).

Specific effects of stenosis, failure of collateral circulation, hypertensive vascular disease, and embolism from mural thrombosis cannot be differentiated with any degree of certainty by history and clinical examination alone, although the patterns of clinical deficits and localization can

suggest the most likely mechanisms. Disabling lesions of the brainstem frequently are caused by lesions in tiny vessels that are too small to be demonstrated angiographically but may be visible by neuroimaging techniques, especially MR imaging. Nevertheless, angiography may detect other extracerebral or intracerebral occlusive changes that establish the presence of atheromatous disease, and angiography also may reveal the remarkable collateral vascular channels that circumvent total occlusion of the vertebrobasilar system (Ausman et al., 1985) (Fig. 55.178).

Despite the difficulties in differentiating large- from small-vessel disease in patients with vertebrobasilar insufficiency and in determining the precise location of a particular lesion producing a neurologic or visual deficit, it seems ap-

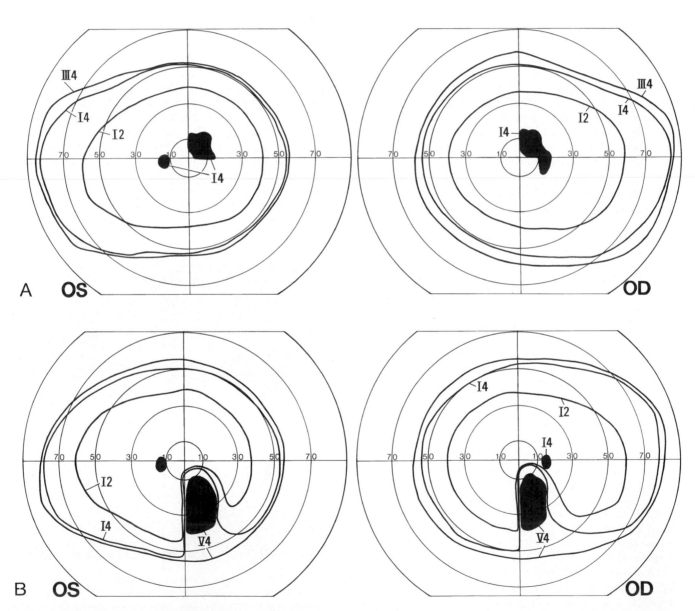

Figure 55.179. Incomplete homonymous hemianopic defects from occipital lobe infarction. *A*, Congruous homonymous hemianopic scotomas in a patient with an infarct of the inferior lip of the left calcarine cortex. Note the few degrees of macular sparing. *B*, Inferior homonymous hemianopic scotomas that break out to the periphery in a patient with an infarct of the left superior occipital cortex.

propriate to identify certain syndromes that result from verte-brobasilar occlusive disease (Gillilan, 1964). These syndromes vary in severity and may occur in various combinations in the same patient.

HEMIPARESIS FROM VERTEBROBASILAR ARTERIAL DISEASE

One of the most important concepts in the localization and diagnosis of cerebrovascular ischemic disease is that disease of the carotid arterial system usually produces **unilateral** neurologic deficits whereas disease of the vertebrobasilar system produces **bilateral** deficits. However, unilateral hemiparesis may be a prominent feature of several syndromes that result from occlusion in the vertebrobasilar system. Most of these syndromes result from lacunar infarction and include: (*a*) pure motor hemiparesis, (*b*) ataxic hemiparesis, and (*c*) the dysarthria-clumsy hand syndrome (Fisher, 1982a; Bamford and Warlow, 1988; Weisberg, 1988; Caplan, 1993). Other vertebrobasilar syndromes in which unilateral hemiparesis is prominent are the following: (*a*) proximal occlusion of the posterior cerebral artery with damage to the cerebral peduncle, (*b*) ipsilateral hemiplegia in the lateral medullary syndrome (of Wallenberg), and (*c*) pyramidal hemiparesis (Caplan et al., 1988; Hommel et al., 1990a).

Fisher (1988) described a phenomenon, called **herald hemiparesis**, that results from basilar artery occlusion. This unilateral hemiparesis occurs not infrequently within the first few hours of impending basilar artery occlusion. The hemiparesis may be mild when the patient is first evaluated, but within 6–12 hours a full syndrome of basilar artery thrombo-sis develops, with bilateral paralysis of the face, arms, and legs, associated with coma or the locked-in syndrome (Mori et al., 1979). According to Fisher (1988), the growing thrombus probably blocks the orifices of the paramedian basilar branches, first on one side of the pons and then on the other side.

INFARCTIONS IN THE TERRITORY OF THE POSTERIOR CEREBRAL ARTERIES

An infarction in the posterior cerebral artery territory commonly is usually caused by embolism, either cardiogenic or from a more proximal vertebrobasilar intra-arterial or unknown source (Fisher and Karnes, 1965; Fisher, 1968b; Castaigne et al., 1973; Fisher, 1980; Koroshetz and Ropper, 1987). It is caused less often by atherosclerosis of the posterior cerebral artery (Castaigne et al., 1973; Pessin et al., 1985, 1987b).

An isolated homonymous visual field defect of sudden onset is the hallmark of a vascular lesion in the occipital lobe (Smith, 1962b; Trobe et al., 1973; Kaul et al., 1974; McAuley and Ross Russell, 1979; Spector et al., 1981; Ross Russell, 1984; Miyamoto et al., 1986; Pessin et al., 1987c; Milandre et al., 1994). Such a lesion is usually the result of infarction in the territory supplied by the posterior cerebral artery. The field defect may be complete or incomplete, but when it is incomplete or scotomatous, it invariably is extremely congruous (Figs. 55.179 and 55.180). When there is a complete homonymous hemianopia, macular sparing is the rule rather than the exception (Safran et al., 1978), and

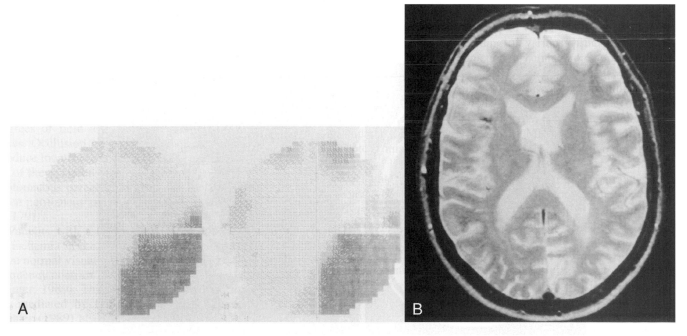

Figure 55.180. Incomplete right homonymous defect secondary to embolic left posterior cerebral artery infarction. The patient was a 45-year-old man with a history of coronary artery disease, tobacco abuse, and colon cancer, status-post curative pelvic exenteration. *A*, Six months earlier, he had noted trouble with his vision down and to the right. Static perimetry reveals an incomplete right homonymous hemianopia, denser below. *B*, T2-weighted magnetic resonance image, axial view, reveals a hypodense area consistent with a small infarction in the superior bank of the left calcarine cortex. An echocardiogram revealed a left ventricular apical clot.

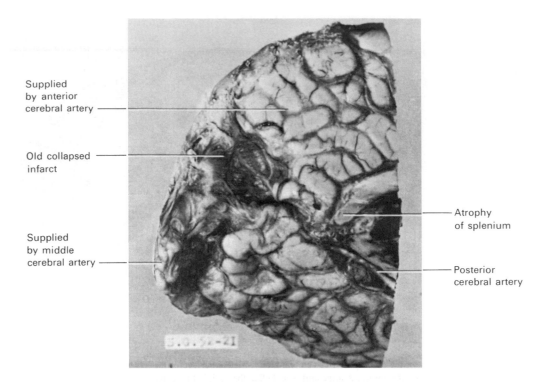

Supplied
by anterior
cerebral artery

Old collapsed
infarct

Supplied
by middle
cerebral artery

Atrophy
of splenium

Posterior
cerebral artery

Figure 55.184. Occipital lobe infarct causing a macular-sparing homonymous hemianopia. The patient was a 69-year-old man with systemic hypertension who experienced a stroke characterized by a macular-sparing right homonymous hemianopia. He died 7 years later. View of the medial surface of the left occipital lobe shows a collapsed infarct in the supply territories of the left calcarine and parieto-occipital branches of the posterior cerebral artery. The infarct destroyed the calcarine cortex except for its most rostral and caudal portions. This patient probably had sparing of the temporal crescent. (From Lindenberg R, Walsh FB, Sacks JG. Neuropathology of Vision. An Atlas. Philadelphia, Lea & Febiger, 1973.)

Pointer, 1989). These issues are discussed in detail in Chapter 9 of this text.

In rare patients, occlusion of a branch of the posterior cerebral artery produces a homonymous visual field defect quite different from the typical homonymous hemianopia or quadrantanopia. The defect consists of a *horizontal homonymous sectoranopia* that is relatively congruous (Figs. 55.134*A* and 55.134*B*). Although this defect occasionally can be caused by damage to the optic radiations in the anterior occipital lobe (Carter et al., 1985; Sato et al., 1986), it is usually caused by occlusion of the **lateral choroidal artery**, a branch of the posterior cerebral artery that supplies a portion of the **lateral geniculate nucleus** (Fig. 55.134*C*). Patients who develop a persistent, horizontal, homonymous sectoranopia from infarction of the portion of the lateral geniculate supplied by the lateral choroidal artery invariably develop bilateral, sectoral, optic atrophy that usually becomes visible within 4–6 weeks after infarction (Fig. 55.186).

In some cases of occipital lobe infarction, the anterior portion of the lobe is unaffected, resulting in sparing of part or all of the peripheral 30 of the contralateral, monocular temporal field—**temporal crescent** (Harris, 1897; Benton et al., 1980) (Fig. 55.181). In other cases, part or all of the temporal crescent is selectively impaired (Kronfeld, 1932; Bender and Kanzer, 1939).

Symptoms of posterior cerebral artery occlusion usually occur without warning. The patient may have a slight sensation of dizziness or light-headedness and then becomes aware of a homonymous visual field defect. Some patients initially experience **complete blindness**, with vision returning in the ipsilateral homonymous visual field within minutes. Pain in the ipsilateral eye or over the ipsilateral brow (contralateral to the hemianopia) is an important although inconstant symptom in such patients (Knox and Cogan, 1962; Safran and Roth, 1983) (see Chapter 36). According to Knox and Cogan (1962), this pain is referred from the tentorial branches of the trigeminal nerve. A midline strip of the tentorium receives its blood supply from small infratentorial meningeal branches arising directly from the posterior cerebral artery (Schnürer and Stattin, 1953). It is likely that ischemia in these branches produces the pain.

Improvement in the affected visual field is the rule rather than the exception after unilateral occipital lobe infarction (Kaul et al., 1974; Mauskop et al., 1984), particularly when the field defect has sloping margins. The ultimate degree of recovery may not be apparent for weeks or even several months, although almost all recovery occurs within 6 months. Recovery of visual field in the region of fixation indicates sparing of cortical tissue at the occipital pole and usually results from collateral blood flow from peripheral leptomeningeal branches of the middle cerebral artery. Residual homonymous field defects are characteristically congruous (Figs. 55.179–55.181). The defects may take many

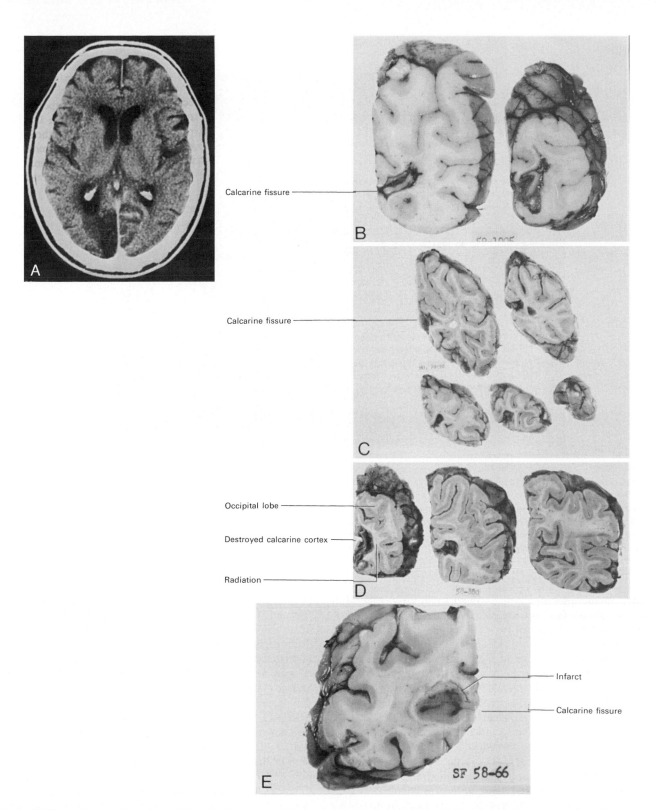

Figure 55.185. Infarcts in the territory of the calcarine branch of the posterior cerebral artery. These infarcts produced known or presumed incomplete, congruous homonymous hemianopias or homonymous hemianopic paracentral scotomas. *A*, CT scan shows typical appearance of infarct in the region of the calcarine artery. *B*, Infarct of the cortex and white matter of the caudal portion of the calcarine area. *C*, A cystic infarct selectively destroys most of the right calcarine cortex. The lower lip is more damaged than the upper lip, and some visual cortex at the occipital pole is intact. The infarct is medial to the ventricle, and it does not extend into the optic radiation. The patient was known to have a congruous left homonymous field defect, denser above. *D*, An old infarct has destroyed the most caudal portion of the calcarine cortex (*left photograph*). More rostrally (*middle photograph*), the infarct remains limited to the calcarine cortex but is smaller. Still further rostrally (*right photograph*), the infarct is not seen, and the most proximal portion of the calcarine cortex appears normal. *E*, There is a slightly hemorrhagic, well-demarcated infarct affecting only the upper lip of the calcarine cortex. (*B–E* from Lindenberg R, Walsh FB, Sacks JG. Neuropathology of Vision. An Atlas. Philadelphia, Lea & Febiger, 1973.)

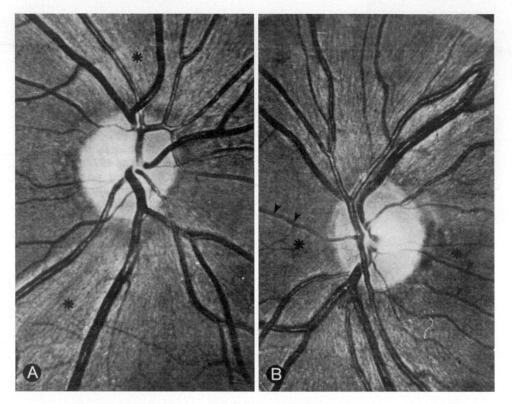

Figure 55.186. Sectoral retinal and nerve fiber layer atrophy in a patient with a homonymous, horizontal sectoranopia from damage to the lateral geniculate body in the territory of the lateral choroidal artery. The patient had a right-sided lesion and a left homonymous sectoranopia. *A,* The right optic disc shows mild diffuse atrophy and there is mild thinning of the superior and inferior arcuate nerve fiber bundles (*asterisks*). The nasal and papillomacular nerve fibers are normal. *B,* The left optic disc shows band pallor with sparing of its upper and lower poles. The superior and inferior arcuate nerve fiber bundles appear almost normal, but the nerve fiber layer in the nasal and papillomacular regions is thinned (*asterisks*). Note prominence of blood vessels in regions of thinned nerve fiber layer (*arrowheads*). (From Frisén L, Holmegaard L, Rosencrantz M. Sectorial optic atrophy and homonymous, horizontal sectoranopia: A lateral choroidal artery syndrome? J Neurol Neurosurg Psychiatry *41*:374–380, 1978.)

forms, including homonymous quadrantanopias, homonymous scotomas, or constriction of the affected homonymous field to within a degree or two of fixation (Wall, 1985) (see Chapter 8).

Patients with an occipital lobe infarction that produces a complete contralateral homonymous hemianopia have a disturbance of eye movements that reflects their inability to see into the contralateral hemifield. Saccades into the hemianopic visual field are dysmetric, and patients with such abnormalities usually develop a variety of compensatory strategies to increase saccadic accuracy. These strategies include staircases of "search saccades" with backward glissadic drifts, deliberate overshooting saccades to bring a target into the intact visual hemifield, and, with a predictable target, saccades using memory of previous target location (Meienberg et al., 1981; Meienberg, 1983).

Smooth pursuit usually remains intact with unilateral infarction of the occipital lobe (Kestenbaum, 1961; Daroff and Hoyt, 1971; Sharpe and Deck, 1978); however, unilateral infarction of the parietal lobe may produce a pursuit defect that is present primarily, but not exclusively, for tracking targets moving toward the side of the lesion and that is independent of both homonymous hemianopia and hemispatial

neglect (Larmande et al., 1980; Thurston et al., 1988; Morrow and Sharpe, 1990). This pursuit abnormality is reflected in an asymmetric response to a hand-held "optokinetic" drum or tape. There is a reduced response when the drum is rotated or the tape is moved toward the side of the lesion (Cogan and Loeb, 1949; Tos et al., 1972). Morrow and Sharpe (1990) suggested that the asymmetric pursuit deficit that occurs in patients with posterior hemisphere lesions (particularly those in the parietal lobe) results from damage to a pursuit pathway that originates in Brodmann areas 19 and 39 and descends to the brainstem through the posterior limb of the internal capsule. Unilateral parietal lobe infarction also may cause an increase in saccadic reaction time (latency) for refixations directed toward the side contralateral to the infarct, even when there is no visual field defect (Sundqvist, 1979).

Patients with a unilateral occipital infarction have a substantial risk of developing an infarction in the contralateral occipital lobe. Bogousslavsky et al. (1983a) studied 58 patients with unilateral occipital lobe infarction that produced homonymous hemianopia. Over a follow-up period ranging from 12–72 months with a mean of 39.6 months, 13 patients (22.4%) suffered an infarction in the contralateral occipital lobe. Advanced age, general vascular risk, a history of strokes, and, most importantly, an absence of improvement of the initial visual field defect were strongly associated with a subsequent contralateral infarction.

Infarction of the **thalamus** may result from proximal occlusion of the posterior cerebral artery, although it may also result from occlusion of the smaller arteries arising from this vessel and supplying the thalamus (Percheron, 1973, 1976a, 1976b, 1977) or from occlusion of the distal portion of the basilar artery (top of the basilar syndrome; rostral basilar artery syndrome—see below). Bogousslavsky et al. (1988c) described four distinct clinical syndromes caused by infarction of specific portions of the thalamus supplied by particular arteries.

Inferolateral infarction occurs from occlusion of the inferolateral arteries that primarily supply the ventral posterior nuclear group. Patients with inferolateral thalamic infarction experience sudden numbness and tingling and, less commonly, pain on the opposite side of the body. These sensations are usually followed by complete hemicorporeal sensory loss with occasional sparing of proprioception. About 75% of patients also have some weakness or ataxia. Disturbances of eye movements, visual loss, and behavioral disturbances are not part of this syndrome, but Toda and Matsumura (1989) described a patient who developed acute hemifacial spasm associated with numbness of the right hand, involuntary jerking movements of the right upper extremity, and weakness of the right lower extremity from a lacunar infarction of the ventrolateral nucleus of the thalamus. In addition, several investigators described contralateral hemiplegia in patients with proximal posterior cerebral artery occlusion that damages not only the lateral thalamus but also the cerebral peduncle in the lateral mesencephalon (Caplan et al., 1988; Hommel et al., 1990a; Hommel et al., 1991).

Tuberothalamic infarction occurs when there is interruption of the blood supply from the anterior thalamosubthalamic paramedian artery (polar artery of Percheron—see Chapter 52). This artery supplies the anterior region of the thalamus, including the ventral anterior nucleus and part of the ventral lateral nucleus. Patients with a tuberothalamic infarction have substantial neuropsychologic disturbances characterized primarily by aphasia in left-sided infarction and hemineglect and impaired visuospatial processing in right-sided infarction (Watson and Heilman, 1979, 1981; Bogousslavsky et al., 1988c; Cappa et al., 1989; Rapcsak et al. 1989). As with inferolateral infarction, disturbances of eye movements are rare in tuberothalamic infarction, although transient motor and sensory signs opposite the side of the infarct are common.

Posterior choroidal artery infarction produces a homonymous horizontal sectoranopia, as described above, with almost no other findings except an asymmetric optokinetic response. Occasionally there are hemisensory disturbances, neuropsychological dysfunction, and movement disorders. Rarely are ocular motility disturbances present (Neau and Bogousslavsky, 1996). This type of infarction is the least common in most series (Bogousslavsky et al., 1988c).

Paramedian infarction results from occlusion of the posterior thalamosubthalamic paramedian artery that supplies the paramedian part of the rostral mesencephalon and thalamus, including the intralaminar nuclear group and most of the dorsomedial nucleus (Percheron, 1973) (see Chapter 52). Patients with this syndrome have disturbances of behavior in addition to disturbances of ocular motility, ataxia, sensory disturbances, and mild pyramidal signs (Schuster, 1936, 1937; Castaigne et al., 1966; Segarra et al., 1974; Castaigne et al., 1981; Trimble and Commings, 1981; Guberman and Stuss, 1983; Graff-Radford et al., 1984; Wall et al., 1984; Biller et al., 1985; Graff-Radford et al., 1985; Lepore et al., 1985; Von Cramon et al., 1985; Kömpf and Oppermann, 1986; Gentilini et al., 1987; Katz et al., 1987; Bogousslavsky et al., 1988c; Beversdorf et al., 1995; Clark and Albers, 1995). Initially, these patients often have deficits in arousal, but they gradually improve to normal wakefulness. When awake, the patients have impaired attention, impaired mental control, and slowed verbal and motor responsiveness. They are apathetic and poorly motivated, and they have a flat or occasionally labile affect. A disturbance of memory, characterized by both anterograde and retrograde loss, is common. The cognitive deficits are often permanent. These behavioral disturbances are called **thalamic dementia**, and they are usually associated with substantial abnormalities of vertical eye movement and convergence caused by damage to ocular motor pathways in the mesencephalon (see below). Such patients may experience peduncular hallucinosis even though they have no evidence of mesencephalic dysfunction (Feinberg and Rapcsak, 1989). It should be noted that most paramedian and tuberothalamic infarctions occur with top of the basilar ischemia and occlusion of the penetrating paramedian arteries (see below) rather than with posterior cerebral artery occlusions.

Many patients with thalamic infarction have symptoms of more than one of the four groups described by Bogousslavsky et al. (1988c). For example, some patients have extensive sensory disturbances typical of inferolateral infarction combined with neuropsychological disturbances more commonly seen in patients with paramedian infarction. Other patients have hemisensory disturbances associated with contralateral homonymous hemianopia, a combination that is almost diagnostic of infarction in the posterior cerebral artery territory (Caplan, 1993).

Bassetti and Staikov (1995) described a syndrome caused by infarction in the superficial and deep territories of the posterior cerebral artery, called **hemiplegia vegetativa alterna**. In their patient, damage to the anterolateral midbrain, ventroposterolateral thalamic-subthalamic area, and temporo-occipital lobes caused ipsilateral Horner's syndrome and contralateral hemihyperhidrosis, homonymous hemianopia, hemihyperesthesia, and hemiparesis. The occurrence of sympathetic abnormalities on both sides of the body in a patient with a unilateral infarct argues for the existence of at least two antagonistic sympathetic pathways, one uncrossed and excitatory and the other crossed and inhibitory.

Gomez et al. (1987) described two patients who developed acute **esotropia**, stupor, and impaired upward gaze as the initial presentation of thalamic ischemia. Both patients had normal pupils and no ptosis. One patient regained conscious-

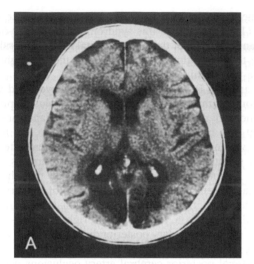

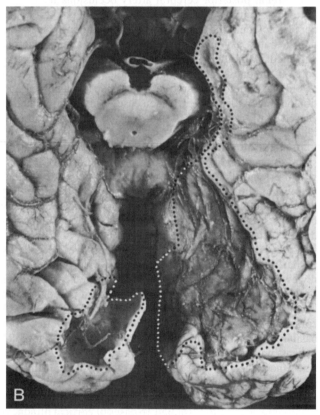

Figure 55.187. Bilateral simultaneous posterior cerebral artery occlusion. *A*, CT scan shows bilateral low density lesions in the occipital lobes. The patient had a history of cardiac disease and experienced the sudden onset of confusion and cortical blindness. *B*, Pathologic specimen from a patient who suffered simultaneous bilateral occipital lobe infarctions (*dots*). The cerebral hemispheres are viewed from below. There is a large cystic infarct in the territory of the left posterior cerebral artery and a smaller infarct in the territory of the right calcarine artery. Note sparing of both occipital poles. The patient probably had a complete right homonymous hemianopia with macular sparing and a left homonymous hemianopic scotoma or an incomplete homonymous hemianopia with macular sparing. (From Zülch KJ. The Cerebral Infarct. Berlin, Springer-Verlag, 1985.)

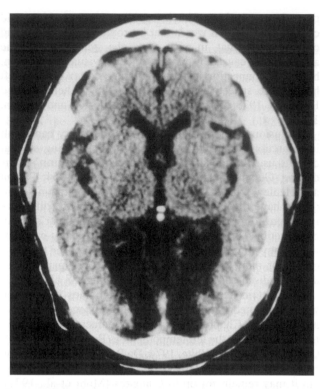

Figure 55.188. Bilateral simultaneous posterior cerebral artery occlusion secondary to embolic infarction from a cardiac arrhythmia. Axial computed tomographic scan shows symmetric areas of low density in both occipital lobes. Despite apparent involvement of both occipital poles on the scan, the patient had 20/30 vision in each eye because of five degrees of macular sparing.

tions. Denial of blindness or **Anton's syndrome** (Anton, 1899) was common, although not present in all cases. Indeed, Gloning et al. (1962) emphasized that Anton's syndrome is not specific for cortical blindness; it occurs in patients who are blind from other causes, including bilateral optic neuropathy. The only requirement for Anton's syndrome is a general reduction in cerebral function during any kind of blindness (Lessell, 1975a).

In the patients studied by Gloning et al. (1962), cortical blindness lasted only a few days (11 days in the most severe case) before a step-wise return of vision commenced. In most patients, vision returned in three stages. The first stage was characterized by return of perception of motion (the Riddoch phenomenon—Riddoch, 1917—see Chapter 8). Patients in whom this occurred saw objects only when the objects were moving, not when they were stationary. Light sense and light projection usually returned after perception of motion, followed by return of color perception. Color perception often returned in the following sequence: red, blue, yellow, and, finally, green. In the study by Gloning et al. (1962), return of visual field began in the center of the field in all but one of 16 cases (see also Walsh, 1966). Some patients who regained no more than a central island of vision had what the authors called "**inverse Anton's syndrome**." Such patients denied that they could see anything at all, even when it was emphasized to them that they had intact central vision and could accurately identify objects placed in their central visual field. After initial central clearing of vision, patients who recovered further visual function often became aware of a shimmering white light in the portion of the peripheral field that was about to recover.

The second stage of return of vision was characterized by frequent, brief periods of graying out of vision similar to the prodrome before vision was lost. The last stage of visual recovery consisted of recovery of binocular perception, and the disappearance of such symptoms as metamorphopsia, polyopia, visual agnosia, spatial disorientation, and prosopagnosia. Despite improvement, recovery was rarely complete, with the extent of improvement depending on the severity of permanent cortical damage. Vascular insufficiency or embolism in the vertebrobasilar system seemed to be responsible in all cases.

Cortical blindness caused by vascular disease differs in several ways from traumatic cortical blindness (Gloning et al., 1962). First, Anton's syndrome is common in patients with vascular cortical blindness but rare in patients with traumatic cortical blindness. Second, recovery is rapid with vascular lesions but usually extremely slow after trauma. Finally, the occipital tip and, thus, central vision are less affected by vascular lesions than by severe trauma.

Minor et al. (1959) identified nine cases of bilateral, simultaneous homonymous hemianopia among 144 patients with clinical evidence of vertebrobasilar insufficiency. Six of the nine patients had an INO, a sign that Minor et al. (1959) associated with atherosclerosis of the basilar artery and its penetrating branches.

Bilateral posterior cerebral artery occlusion may produce visual field defects other than cortical blindness. When bilateral homonymous hemianopias are complete except for macular sparing, the patient may have a small island of vision in each eye that mimics a constricted visual field (Fig. 55.189).

Whether the residual field is limited to one homonymous field or is bilateral, its hemianopic nature is usually clear if careful testing of the field along the vertical meridian is performed (Halpern and Sedler, 1980). Conversely, bilateral occipital infarctions can affect central vision and spare the temporal crescent on one side (Fig. 55.190). Bilateral infarctions that affect the superior occipital lobe on one side and the inferior occipital lobe on the other produce bilateral quadrantic defects that are called "checkerboard fields" or "crossed-quadrant homonymous hemianopia" (Felix, 1926; Cross and Smith, 1982; Dyer et al., 1990) (Fig. 55.191). Infarctions that affect the superior or inferior occipital lobes on both sides produce bilateral altitudinal field defects similar to those seen in patients with bilateral AION (Symonds and MacKenzie, 1957; Heller-Bettinger et al., 1976; McAuley and Ross Russell, 1979; Bogousslavsky et al., 1987c) (Figs. 55.192–55.196).

Bilateral occipital lobe infarction can produce decreased central visual acuity in both eyes without any obvious hemianopic defect. The loss of central vision probably results from generalized ischemia of the occipital lobes.

When there is bilateral posterior cerebral artery occlusion, the most common findings in addition to bilateral visual field loss or cortical blindness are amnesia and agitated delirium (Caplan and Stein, 1986). Amnesia caused by bilateral mesial temporal infarction may be permanent and closely resembles Korsakoff's syndrome. Infarction of the hippocampal, fusiform, and lingual gyri on both sides produces an agitated hyperactive state that is often confused with delirium tremens (Horenstein et al., 1962; Medina et al., 1974, 1977).

Bálint's syndrome can occur in patients who experience bilateral simultaneous or sequential posterior cerebral artery occlusions. Although this syndrome is discussed in detail in Chapter 9 of this text, we also describe it in this chapter for

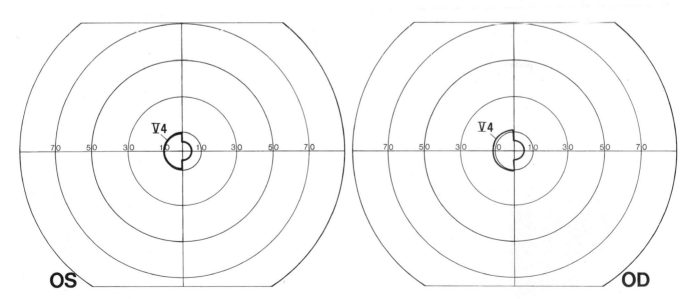

Figure 55.189. Bilateral "constricted" visual fields from bilateral homonymous hemianopia with bilateral macular sparing. Note that the macular sparing respects the vertical midline.

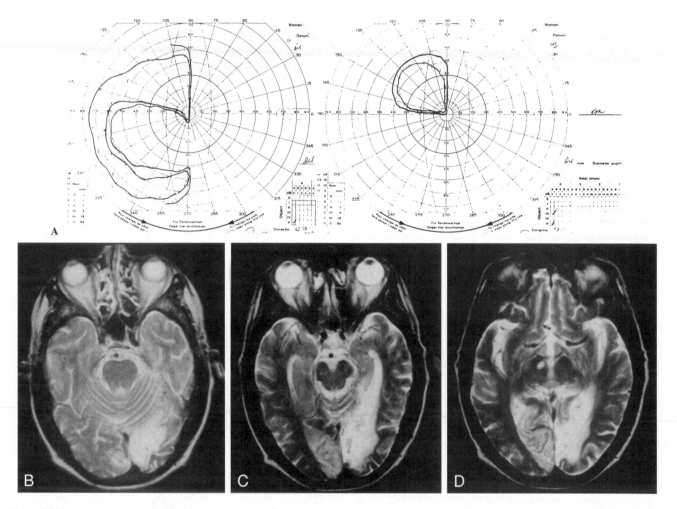

Figure 55.190.   Clinical and neuroimaging findings in a patient with bilateral posterior cerebral artery occlusion. *A*, Bilateral homonymous hemianopic defects secondary to bilateral posterior cerebral artery infarction. Note the dense right homonymous hemianopia combined with a left inferior homonymous quadrantanopia with sparing of the left temporal crescent. *B–D*, T2-weighted axial magnetic resonance images demonstrate infarctions in the territories of both posterior cerebral arteries, worse on the left than the right, and extending less inferiorly and less anteriorly on the right.

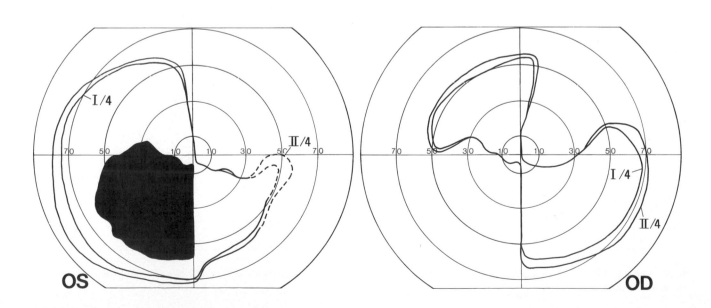

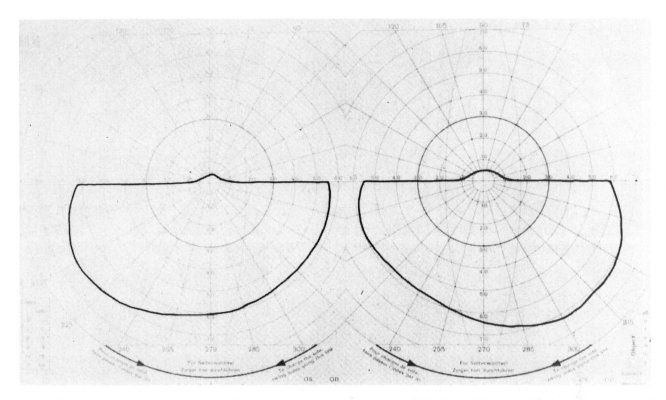

Figure 55.192. Visual field defects in a 73-year-old man with systemic hypertension, atrial fibrillation, and diabetes mellitus who developed acute loss of the visual field in both eyes associated with headaches. There is a macular-sparing, congruous, superior altitudinal hemianopia with complete preservation of the inferior visual field of both eyes. (From Bogousslavsky J, Miklossy J, Deruaz JP, et al. Lingual and fusiform gyri in visual processing: A clinico-pathologic study of superior altitudinal hemianopia. J Neurol Neurosurg Psychiatry 50:607–614, 1987.)

the sake of continuity. Bálint (1905, 1907, 1909) was the first to describe a patient with what seemed to be three specific visuomotor abnormalities. First, the patient had what Bálint (1905) called a "psychic paralysis of gaze." The patient's field of view seemed to be restricted so that he could attend to only one object at a time, regardless of the size of the object or the number of objects in the field of view. Second, the patient had a spatial disorder of attention. Bálint (1905) noted that the patient "does not take notice of things lying to either side of the object (of interest), but when he gets an impulse by being told to do so he is more attentive and sees other things." Curiously, "the attention of the patient is always directed (by approximately 35 to 40) to the right-hand side of space and when he is asked to direct his attention to another object after having fixed his gaze on a first one, he tends to the right-hand rather than the left-hand side." Finally, Bálint (1905) used the term "optic ataxia" to describe the misreaching, particularly with the right hand, by the patient that occurred "only when the movements are dependent on vision." This was in marked contrast to pa-tients with tabes dorsalis, who had difficulty in guiding movements using only proprioceptive information; i.e., with the eyes closed.

Bálint (1905) realized that his patient's deficits were not purely sensory. The patient had full visual fields, and he could name colors accurately. Nor were the deficits purely motor, because none of the voluntary muscles, including the extraocular muscles, was paralyzed. Instead, the patient seemed to suffer from a disruption of mechanisms that lay between sensation and movement; specifically, he seemed not to be able to use visual information to guide the eyes or the limbs (Hussain and Stein, 1988). The patient subsequently developed a right hemiplegia and aphasia; he died about 2 years after Bálint (1905) first examined him. At autopsy, the patient's brain showed bilateral parieto-occipital infarctions (Bálint, 1907, 1909) (Fig. 55.197).

Hecaen and Ajuriaguerra (1954) subsequently called this condition "Bálint's syndrome." These investigators reemphasized the triad of "psychic paralysis of visual fixation," "optic ataxia," and visuospatial disorientation. After this

◄———

Figure 55.191. Crossed quadrant (checkerboard) visual field defects. The patient was a 70-year-old woman who suffered bilateral simultaneous occipital lobe infarctions. An infarction in the superior portion of the right occipital lobe produced a left, inferior, congruous, homonymous quadrantanopia. Note complete preservation of the temporal crescent in the left eye, producing a quadrantic *scotoma* in that eye. An infarction in the inferior portion of the left occipital lobe produced a right, superior, congruous, homonymous quadrantanopia.

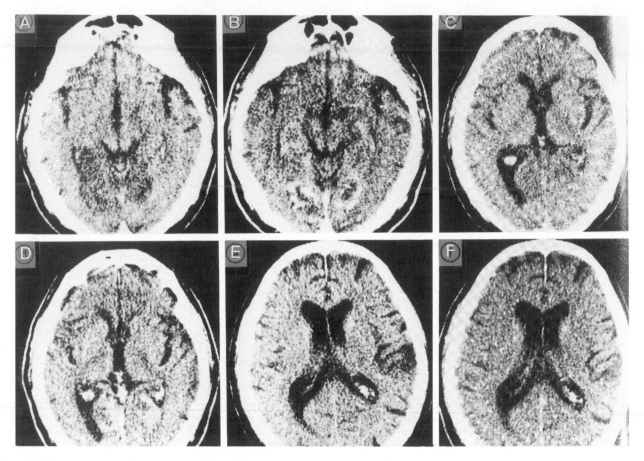

Figure 55.193. Appearance of CT scan in the patient described in Figure 55.192. Serial *slices A* to *F* are taken from inferior to superior. Bilateral medial occipital infarctions are seen in *slices A* to *D*, all of which are inferior to the calcarine fissure. (From Bogousslavsky J, Miklossy J, Deruaz JP, et al. Lingual and fusiform gyri in visual processing: A clinico-pathologic study of superior altitudinal hemianopia. J Neurol Neurosurg Psychiatry *50:*607–614, 1987.)

report, numerous complete and incomplete cases of Bálint's syndrome were described (Luria, 1959; Tyler, 1968; Eyssette, 1969; Kase et al., 1977; Rondot et al., 1977; Ross Russell and Bharucha, 1978; Hausser et al., 1980; Montero et al., 1982; De Renzi, 1985; Leigh and Tusa, 1985; Pierrot-Deseilligny et al., 1986; Trobe and Bauer, 1986; Perenin and Vighetto, 1988; Watson and Rapcsak, 1989) (Fig. 55.198).

Patients with Bálint's syndrome have a variety of abnormalities of fixation and tracking. They have great difficulty locating a stationary object in space, although they can maintain fixation on the object once they locate it. They can track a moving target, but if the target begins to move rapidly, it is lost and cannot be relocated. Patients with Bálint's syndrome can converge when their own finger or hand is used as a stimulus, but if some other object is used, they are unable to converge. Similarly, when an object is suddenly brought close to the eyes of a patient with Bálint's syndrome, the patient may not blink; however, the patient will blink if his or her finger suddenly is moved close to the face. Although patients with Bálint's syndrome can recognize that an object is moving, they are often unable to state in what direction

the object is moving. Despite these disturbances of eye movement, other types of eye movements are unaffected. For example, patients with Bálint's syndrome can make normal eye movements in response to sound or other sensory stimuli, and they have a normal vestibulo-ocular reflex. Watson and Rapcsak (1989) described a patient with Bálint's syndrome who lost the ability to blink spontaneously. Bálint's syndrome probably occurs much more frequently after bilateral watershed infarctions of the parieto-occipital regions from systemic hypotension than from thromboembolic carotid or vertebrobasilar disease.

Tsutsui et al. (1980) described a 51-year-old woman with bilateral infarctions in areas 17, 18, and 19. The patient had visual acuity of 20/200 OU associated with complete loss of the inferior field of vision and constriction of the superior visual field in both eyes. The patient could not make visually-guided pursuit or saccadic eye movements, but saccades were intact to verbal stimuli, and the vestibulo-ocular reflex was normal in all directions. This patient thus apparently had an atypical acquired ocular motor apraxia that differed from Bálint's syndrome in that neither optic ataxia nor disturbances of visual attention were present.

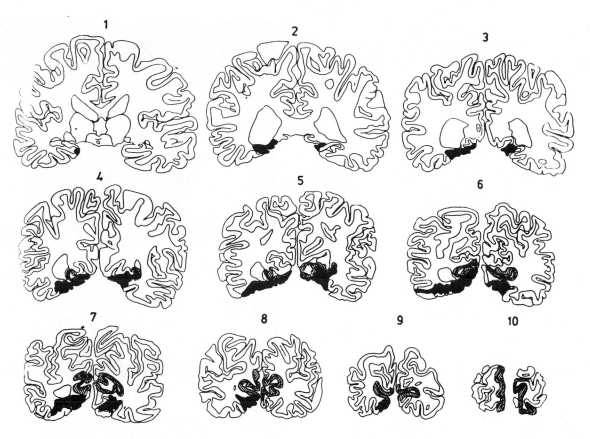

Figure 55.194. The patient whose fields are depicted in Figure 55.192 and whose CT scan is shown in Figure 55.193 died about 6 months after the onset of visual symptoms. Schematic representation of coronal brain sections with *slice 1* being the most rostral section and *slice 10* the most caudal shows bilateral occipitotemporal infarctions (*black areas*). *Hatched areas* correspond to spared calcarine cortex. Note that the infarctions are relatively symmetric and located inferior to the calcarine fissure. Also note complete sparing of both occipital poles. (From Bogousslavsky J, Miklossy J, Deruaz JP, et al. Lingual and fusiform gyri in visual processing: A clinico-pathologic study of superior altitudinal hemianopia. J Neurol Neurosurg Psychiatry *50:*607–614, 1987.)

Patients who experience bilateral superior occipital lobe strokes may develop **simultagnosia**. Such patients complain of piecemeal perception of the visual environment wherein objects may look fragmented or even appear to vanish from direct view (Damasio, 1985; Rizzo and Hurtig, 1987; Rizzo and Robin, 1990). Simultagnosia cannot be explained by simple visual field defects or by low visual acuity. Rizzo and Robin (1990) studied two patients with simultagnosia and found that the patients could orient attention to spatial targets in visual, auditory, and mixed-modal conditions, but when the patients were required to give an immediate response to the appearance or disappearance at unpredictable intervals of any element in a random-dot display, they could detect less than 50% of 1600 events, and they had increased "mirages" and prolonged reaction times compared with normal control subjects. These results support the contention that simultagnosia is caused by a defect in visual attention that results in an inability to sustain visuospatial processing across simultaneous elements in an array. Simultagnosia, like Bálint's syndrome and other higher disorders of visual processing and attention, occurs much more frequently after systemic hypotensive crises than from occlusion of the posterior cerebral arteries. Common causes include cardiac arrest and intraoperative hypotension.

When occipital lobe infarction is limited to the lower banks of the calcarine fissures on both sides, the major findings are prosopagnosia and defective color vision (Meadows, 1974; Albert et al., 1975; Green and Lessell, 1977; Pearlman et al., 1979; Damasio et al., 1980; Jaeger et al., 1988; Michel et al., 1989), although these disturbances are not invariably present (Bogousslavsky et al., 1987c). Tsutsui et al. (1980) described a patient with bilateral occipital lobe infarctions limited to the superior banks of the calcarine fissure who could make no visually-elicited eye movements despite having sufficient residual vision to do so. She made normal eye movements on command (except for upward gaze), and she had normal vestibulo-ocular reflexes. The patient thus had an atypical form of acquired ocular motor apraxia, possibly from bilateral damage to visual association areas.

Degos et al. (1987) described a patient in whom occlusion of terminal branches of both posterior cerebral arteries resulted in partial interhemispheric disconnection associated

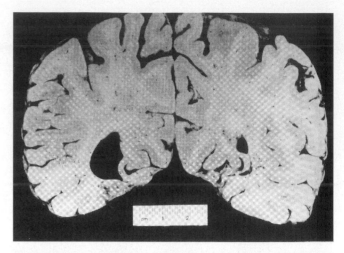

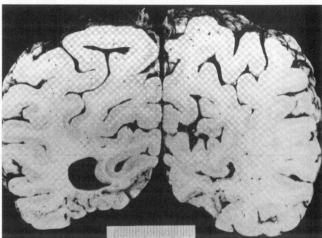

Figure 55.195. Coronal brain sections from patient described in Figures 55.192–55.194. The sections correspond to *levels 5* and *6* in Figure 55.194. Note bilateral infarctions of inferior occipital cortex. (From Bogousslavsky J, Miklossy J, Deruaz JP, et al. Lingual and fusiform gyri in visual processing: A clinico-pathologic study of superior altitudinal hemianopia. J Neurol Neurosurg Psychiatry *50:*607–614, 1987.)

with complete ischemic destruction of the splenium and of the posterior part of the body of the corpus callosum. The most prominent features of disconnection of the cerebral hemispheres in this patient were left tactile anomia (despite rather good tactile-motor integration between hemispheres), left visual anomia, agraphia of the left hand, and "diagonistic" apraxia.

Infarction of one or both occipital lobes may result from local atheromatous disease, or it may be an expression of vascular insufficiency or embolism originating more proximally in the vertebrobasilar arterial system (Hebel and von Cramon, 1987). In addition, when one or both posterior cerebral arteries arise anomalously from the carotid artery (see Chapter 52), occipital infarction may indicate insufficiency of the carotid vascular system, not the vertebrobasilar system (Pessin et al., 1989).

In patients with posterior cerebral artery occlusion, angiography may identify the site of occlusion (Hoyt and Newton, 1970) (Fig. 55.199). It must be emphasized, however, that nonfilling of a posterior cerebral artery during a vertebral arteriogram does not prove that the vessel is occluded. Because the posterior cerebral artery in question normally may fill from the carotid circulation and not from the vertebrobasilar circulation (Pessin et al., 1989), a selective ipsilateral carotid arteriogram must also be performed, and it is probably best to perform a four-vessel angiogram in such patients (Ausman et al., 1985).

ROSTRAL BASILAR ARTERY SYNDROME (TOP OF THE BASILAR SYNDROME)

Patients with occlusion of the rostral portion of the basilar artery—the top of the basilar syndrome—may experience extensive infarction of the mesencephalon, thalamus, hypothalamus, paramedian diencephalon, medial temporal lobes, and occipital lobes. Damage to these structures produces a variety of behavioral, neuro-ophthalmologic, and motor signs (Kubik and Adams, 1946; Caplan, 1980, 1984; Mehler, 1988b, 1988c, 1989). Disturbances in behavior caused by damage to posterior hemisphere structures include visual agnosia, color anomia and amnesia, topographic disorientation and agnosia, anosognosia, Klüver-Bucy syndrome, Anton's syndrome, Bálint's syndrome, or a combination of these. Disturbances of behavior caused by infarction of brainstem and diencephalic structures include changes in the normal sleep-wake cycle and peduncular hallucinosis characterized by vivid and well-formed visual hallucinations (Feinberg

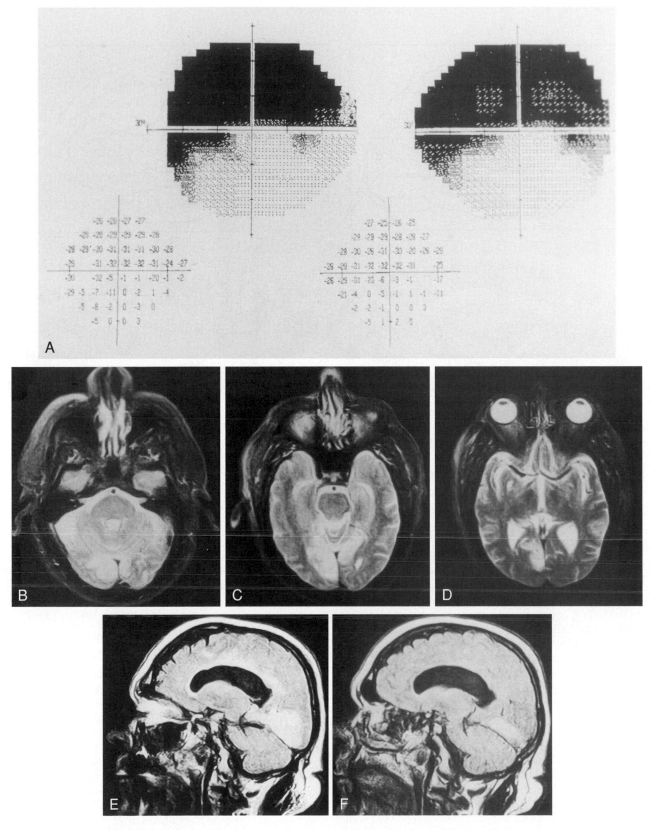

Figure 55.196. Bilateral posterior cerebral artery infarctions with superior altitudinal visual field defects. The patient was a 71-year-old man who had the acute onset of complete visual loss, followed by clearing inferiorly. *A*, Static perimetry reveals bilateral superior altitudinal defects. Note that the defects do not perfectly obey the horizontal midline, particularly on the left side. This suggests mild involvement of the superior lip of the right calcarine fissure. *B–F*, T2-weighted magnetic resonance imaging (*B–D,* Axial views; *E* and *F,* Sagittal views to the right and left of midline, respectively) demonstrate hyperintense areas consistent with infarcts primarily in the inferior portions of both occipital lobes.

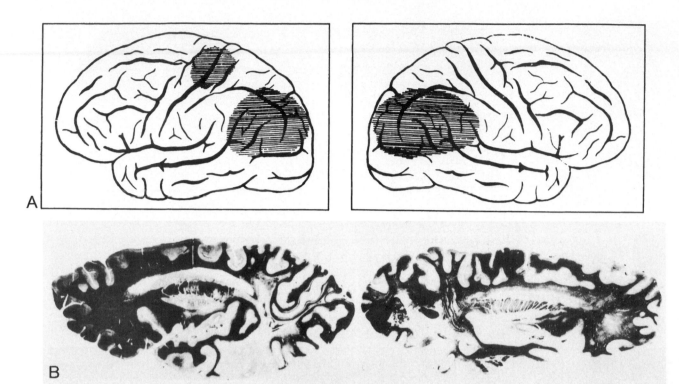

Figure 55.197.   Pathology of Bálint's syndrome of psychic paralysis of visual fixation, optic ataxia, and visuospatial distortion. *A,* Bálint's sketches of "softenings" of the brain found at postmortem examination. Note that the lesions include the posterior parietal lobes of both hemispheres. *B,* Near sagittal sections from corresponding parts of left (*left side of photograph*) and right (*right side of photograph*) hemispheres showing bilateral parieto-occipital infarctions. (From Husain M, Stein J. Rezsö Bálint and his most celebrated case. Arch Neurol *45:*89–93, 1988.)

and Rapcsak, 1989). A prominent feature of the top-of-the-basilar syndrome is an altered level of alertness with apathy, hypersomnolence, or even coma (Caplan, 1980).

The neuro-ophthalmologic abnormalities that occur in patients with a top of the basilar syndrome are caused by both hemispheric and brainstem infarction. Manifestations of hemispheric damage include homonymous visual field defects (including horizontal sectoranopia), cortical blindness, complex visual hallucinations, acquired cerebral dyschromatopsia, visual allesthesia, palinopsia, and polyopia. Damage to the brainstem causes disorders of ocular motility and alignment, including isolated disturbances of vertical gaze, complete or incomplete dorsal midbrain syndrome, and abnormalities of convergence and divergence (Caplan, 1980; Gomez et al., 1987; Mehler, 1988c). Pupillary abnormalities may reflect involvement of the oculomotor nuclear complex, the rostral descending sympathetic system, or both. Motor signs in addition to those affecting the extraocular muscles include hemiparesis and quadriparesis from damage to the corticobulbar and corticospinal tracts.

Some patients with the rostral basilar artery syndrome experience an acute stroke without premonitory symptoms. Others develop typical symptoms of posterior circulation ischemia, such as transient bilateral or hemianopic visual loss, vertigo, and numbness before the acute event occurs.

The rostral basilar artery syndrome may result from atherosclerotic thrombosis of the basilar artery or from emboli originating in the heart or in distal large arteries. It also may occur in patients with a giant aneurysm arising from the tip of the basilar artery, in patients with vasculitis, and after angiography (Mehler, 1989).

The outcome of patients with the rostral basilar artery syndrome varies considerably. Some patients recover substantially within several weeks, whereas others have an extremely poor outcome (Mehler, 1988b, 1988c, 1989).

VERTEBRAL ARTERY OCCLUSION

Whether or not vertebral artery occlusion produces neurologic findings depends primarily on the location of the occlusion (Caplan, 1984). When the **proximal** portion of the vessel gradually occludes, extensive collateral circulation develops, particularly from the ascending cervical and transverse cervical branches of the thyrocervical trunk and from the occipital branches of the external carotid arteries (Caplan, 1979, 1983, 1984). In such cases, the occlusion often produces no symptoms or signs unless the contralateral vertebral artery was previously occluded or is congenitally aplastic or hypoplastic, or unless there is downstream artery-to-artery embolism from the occluded arterial stump (Koroshetz and Ropper, 1985; Caplan, 1993).

When the **distal** portion of the extracranial vertebral artery becomes occluded, as may occur after neck trauma or chiropractic manipulation, ischemia is limited to the lateral me-

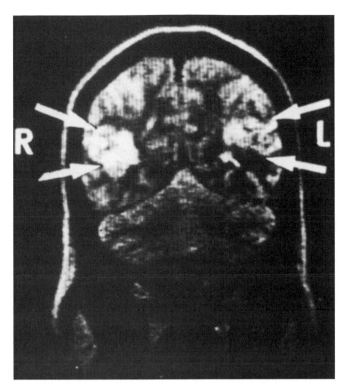

Figure 55.198. MR imaging in a patient with Bálint's syndrome. The patient was a 41-year-old woman with hypertensive encephalopathy who complained of bilateral loss of vision. Neurologic examination revealed element's of Bálint's syndrome. MR imaging shows bilateral parieto-occipital lesions consistent with infarctions. Cerebral angiography showed occlusion of the left parieto-occipital branch of the posterior cerebral artery and slow flow through the right parieto-occipital branch. *R*, Right hemisphere lesion; *L*, left hemisphere lesion. (From Watson RT, Rapcsak SZ. Loss of spontaneous blinking in a patient with Bálint's syndrome. Arch Neurol *46:* 567–570, 1989.)

dulla or pons and the ipsilateral cerebellum (Mueller and Sahs, 1976; Easton and Sherman, 1977; Caplan, 1979; Sherman et al., 1981; Caplan, 1984). When there are initial signs of bilateral brainstem dysfunction, the course is often progressive and fatal (Kreiger and Ozaki, 1980). Postmortem examination in such cases usually reveals extensive brainstem and cerebellar infarction.

Bilateral vertebral artery occlusion may produce few or no neurologic symptoms and signs, or it may produce a devastating neurologic catastrophe, depending on the location of the occlusions. Alexander (1882) ligated one or both vertebral arteries low in the neck in 21 young patients with epilepsy, none of whom developed any serious neurologic sequelae. Fisher (1970) described five patients with bilateral occlusion of the proximal vertebral arteries demonstrated by angiography. All patients had experienced TIAs, but only one patient had permanent neurologic dysfunction, and that person also had occlusion of the internal carotid artery at the siphon on the appropriate side to explain the findings. Bilateral vertebral artery occlusion, however, may produce a devastating neurologic syndrome when it affects the intracranial portions of the vessels (Caplan, 1983, 1984). Such

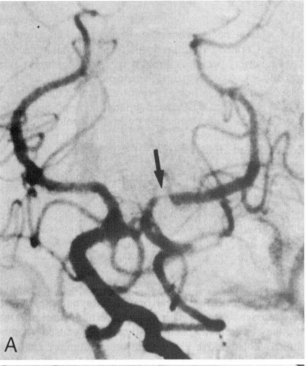

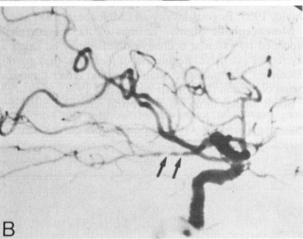

Figure 55.199. Stenosis of the posterior cerebral artery. *A*, Left vertebral arteriogram in a 68-year-old man who had experienced two TIAs. One was characterized by weakness and loss of vision to the right side. The right arm became clumsy, and speech was garbled. The episode lasted 2–3 hours. The second TIA was characterized by isolated weakness of the right hand. The arteriogram shows severe stenosis of the proximal left posterior cerebral artery just distal to its junction with the posterior communicating artery (*arrow*). *B*, Right common carotid arteriogram, lateral view, in a 69-year-old man with a history of three TIAs consisting of visual loss to the left side. During one of these episodes, he also experienced tingling of the left hand and face. Neurologic examination revealed a left, superior, homonymous quadrantanopia. The arteriogram shows a long, irregular, beaded appearance of the ambient segment of the right posterior cerebral artery (*arrows*). These lesions were thought to be primary stenotic regions, although emboli might have produced this appearance. (From Pessin MS, Kwan ES, DeWitt LD, et al. Posterior cerebral artery stenosis. Ann Neurol *21:*85–89, 1987.)

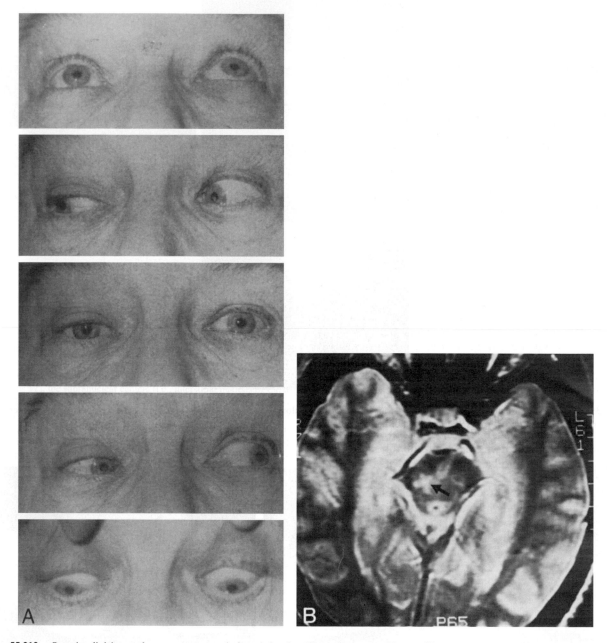

Figure 55.212. Superior division oculomotor nerve paresis from infarction. The patient was a 66-year-old woman who developed dizziness and binocular vertical diplopia. *A,* The patient has a paresis affecting the superior division of the right oculomotor nerve. Note right ptosis and limitation of upward gaze in the right eye unassociated with any other ocular motor deficit or pupillary inequality. *B,* MR image, T2-weighted axial section, shows an irregular zone of increased signal intensity (*arrow*) compatible with an infarct. (From Ksiazek SM, Repka MX, Maguire A, et al. Divisional oculomotor nerve paresis caused by intrinsic brainstem disease. Ann Neurol *26:*714–718, 1989.)

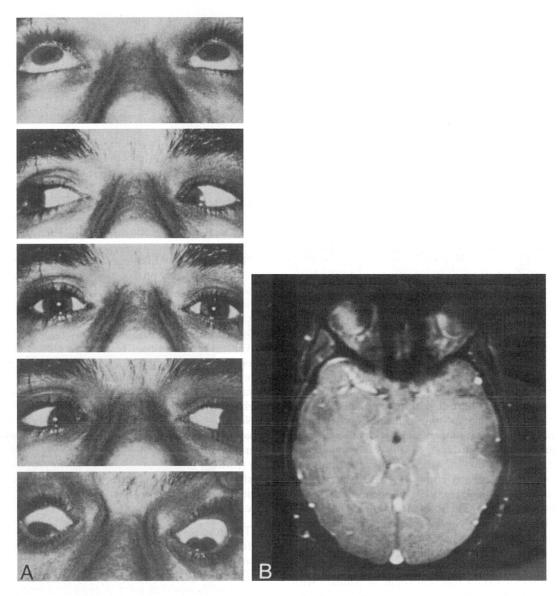

Figure 55.213. Inferior division oculomotor nerve paresis from mesencephalic infarct. The patient was a 30-year-old man who awoke with painless vertical diplopia. His examination was normal except for an abnormality of right eye movement and a dysconjugate torsional jerk nystagmus with the larger amplitude in the right eye. *A,* The patient has a right inferior division oculomotor nerve paresis. Note dilated right pupil and mild limitation of infraduction and adduction of the right eye with normal supraduction of the eye and absence of ptosis. *B,* MR image, T1-weighted fast scan (axial view), shows hypointense lesion in the mesencephalon consistent with a small hemorrhagic infarct. (From Ksiazek SM, Repka MX, Maguire A, et al. Divisional oculomotor nerve paresis caused by intrinsic brainstem disease. Ann Neurol *26:*714–718, 1989.)

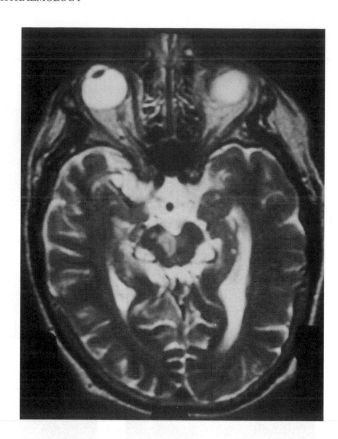

Figure 55.216. Neuroimaging in a patient with Weber's syndrome. The patient was 64 years old and had a complete right oculomotor palsy as well as a left hemiparesis. A T2-weighted axial magnetic resonance image shows a hyperintense area consistent with an infarct on the right side of the mesencephalon in the region of the right oculomotor nerve fascicle and the right corticospinal tract.

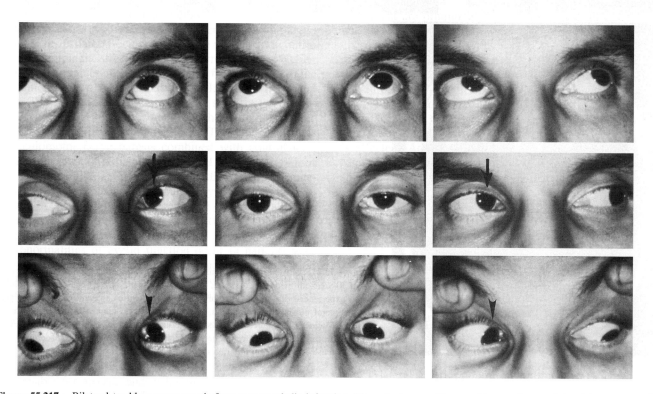

Figure 55.217. Bilateral trochlear nerve paresis from mesencephalic infarction. The patient was a 28-year-old man who was injured in a motorcycle accident. Neuroimaging studies confirmed damage to the dorsal mesencephalon. Note bilateral underaction of superior oblique muscles (*arrowheads*) and bilateral overaction of inferior oblique muscles (*arrows*).

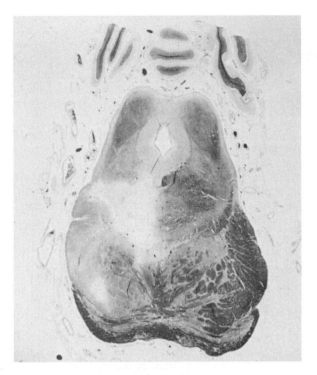

Figure 55.218. Coronal section through the caudal mesencephalon in a patient with a basilar artery occlusion shows an infarct affecting the right trochlear nerve nucleus. (Courtesy of Dr. Richard Lindenberg.)

dromes usually result from small vessel occlusion, but they may also result from occlusion of the entire basilar artery. A minimal expression of these syndromes is an **isolated abducens nerve paresis**. It was once assumed that any intrinsic brainstem lesion, particularly an infarction, that produced an abducens nerve paresis would also produce other brainstem signs. CT scanning and MR imaging show that this is not the case (Donaldson and Rosenberg, 1988; Bronstein et al., 1990a). Indeed, many cases of abducens nerve paresis previously assumed to be caused by microvascular occlusion along the peripheral portion of the nerve in the subarachnoid space or cavernous sinus, or that were designated "idiopathic," are caused by intrinsic vascular lesions in the pons. Similar small vascular lesions in the pons can cause isolated trigeminal sensory neuropathy, trigeminal neuralgia, facial paresis, or hemifacial spasm (Ambrosetto and Forlani, 1988).

Another minimal expression of a medial or paramedian pontine syndrome is a **unilateral internuclear ophthalmoplegia** (Smith and Cogan, 1959; Cogan, 1970). This condition is characterized by weakness of adduction of the eye on the side of the lesion (Fig. 55.207). The weakness may be manifest as: (*a*) inability to adduct the eye beyond the midline, (*b*) mild limitation of adduction with decreased adduction velocity, or (*c*) mild decrease in the velocity of adducting saccades without limitation of adduction. In the eye contralateral to the lesion, the primary abnormality is horizontal, abducting nystagmus that consists of a centripetal (inward) drift of the eye, followed by a corrected saccade. A unilateral INO is caused by damage to the MLF, and, as

is the case with mesencephalic (and medullary) lesions, it may be accompanied by a skew deviation with the higher eye on the side of the lesion (Keane, 1975a). Patients with an INO also have disturbances of vertical eye movement, particularly pursuit, because the MLF conveys bidirectional signals for vertical pursuit and vestibular smooth eye movements in humans (Ranalli and Sharpe, 1988).

A **horizontal gaze paresis** can be caused by a small, medial or paramedian infarct of the pons that damages either the ipsilateral abducens nucleus or the ipsilateral paramedian pontine reticular formation (PPRF) (Masucci, 1965; Masson et al., 1978; Pierrot-Deseilligny et al., 1978, 1981b; Bogousslavsky et al., 1984; Bronstein et al., 1990b; López et al., 1996) (Fig. 55.219). Such a paresis may be associated initially with conjugate deviation of the eyes away from the side of the lesion (Henn et al., 1982). Because fibers subserving horizontal vestibular function travel directly to the abducens nucleus (thus bypassing the PPRF), the eyes can still be moved to the paretic side using vestibular stimulation (e.g., oculocephalic maneuver), and convergence is usually intact in patients with a horizontal gaze paresis caused by a lesion of the PPRF (Pierrot-Deseilligny et al., 1981b; Bogousslavsky et al., 1984; Baker and Carr, 1987; Deleu et al., 1988). In patients with a horizontal gaze paresis caused by a lesion of the abducens nucleus, the eyes cannot be so moved.

Incomplete lesions of the PPRF, particularly those that affect only its caudal portion, do not produce a complete horizontal gaze paresis. Instead, they cause slowing or absence of all ipsilaterally directed saccades, with preservation of ipsilateral pursuit (Henn et al., 1982; Bogousslavsky et al., 1984; Kommerell et al., 1987; Pierrot-Deseilligny et al., 1989). This dissociation between saccades and pursuit is similar to that for upward gaze seen in patients with a dorsal mesencephalic syndrome (see above). Lesions of the abducens nucleus are essentially always associated with ipsilateral peripheral facial paresis caused by damage to the genu of the facial nerve fasciculus as it passes around the nucleus (Meienberg et al., 1981).

A vascular lesion of the medial pons may affect the abducens nerve nucleus or the PPRF, together with the ipsilateral MLF, after it has crossed the midline from the contralateral abducens nucleus. Such a lesion produces the **one-and-a-half syndrome** (Case Records of the Massachusetts General Hospital, 1953; Enoksson, 1965; Fisher, 1967a; Crevits et al., 1975; Masson et al., 1978; Pierrot-Deseilligny et al., 1981b; Prier et al., 1982; Wall and Wray, 1983; Bogousslavsky et al., 1984; Blondel et al., 1986; Deleu et al., 1988; Wolin et al., 1996; Yigit et al., 1996). This syndrome consists of a horizontal gaze paresis combined with an ipsilateral INO (Fig. 55.220). There is little or no movement of either eye when the patient attempts to look in one direction (toward the side of the lesion), and there is little or no movement of the adducting eye when the patient attempts to look in the opposite direction (away from the side of the lesion). As noted above, if the horizontal gaze paresis portion of the one-and-a-half syndrome is produced by a lesion of the abducens nerve nucleus, the eyes cannot be driven to the side of the lesion by oculocephalic or caloric testing. If, however, the responsible lesion damages the rostral portion of the PPRF, oculocephalic or caloric testing will reveal

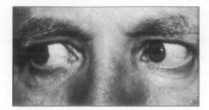
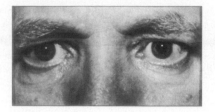
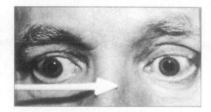

Figure 55.219. Left horizontal gaze palsy from infarction in the region of the left paramedian pontine reticular formation (PPRF). The patient was a 62-year-old man who could not voluntarily look to the left; however, we had full horizontal responses with oculocephalic testing.

intact horizontal eye movements toward the side of the lesion (in the direction of the horizontal gaze paresis) (Pierrot-Deseilligny et al., 1978; Wall and Wray, 1983; Deleu et al., 1988).

Lesions affecting the MLF and PPRF in the pons are not necessarily static. In Case Records of the Massachusetts General Hospital (1953), a patient was described with thrombosis of the basilar artery who had severe neurologic dysfunction indicating infarction of the pons. At one point during the course of his illness, the patient had a left one-and-a-half syndrome. When the patient attempted to look to the left, neither eye moved. When the patient attempted to look to the right, the left eye did not adduct, but the right eye moved fully. Three days later, however, the patient still had a complete left INO, but when he attempted to look to the left, both eyes moved well, although eccentric gaze to that side could not be maintained. The improvement in this patient's ophthalmoparesis, which occurred despite worsening of his overall neurologic status, was probably caused by infarction of the left MLF with only edema of the left PPRF. As the edema resolved, the eyes were able to move to the left, whereas the infarct affecting the left MLF prevented any improvement in eye movement on attempted right horizontal gaze.

In the acute phase of a one-and-a-half syndrome, there may be an exotropia of the eye opposite the lesion. This occurs because of the tendency of both eyes to deviate away from the direction of the gaze paresis, combined with the inability of the eye on the side of the lesion to deviate because of the INO. Thus, only the contralateral eye deviates outward, producing an exotropia. This phenomenon is called a **paralytic pontine exotropia** (Sharpe et al., 1974; Crevits et al., 1975; Bogousslavsky and Regli, 1983b; Blondel et al., 1986). Patients with a paralytic pontine exotropia may develop oculopalatal myoclonus months to years later if the central tegmental tract is also damaged (Wolin et al., 1996).

Extensive occlusion of midline perforating vessels may damage the MLF on both sides, producing a bilateral INO (Gonyea, 1974) (Figs. 55.221 and 55.222). Patients with this condition have abnormalities of vertical gaze, including gaze-evoked upbeat and downbeat nystagmus and absent vestibular vertical eye movements (Jenkyn et al., 1978; Bogousslavsky et al., 1984; Leigh and Zee, 1991).

Bilateral destruction of the PPRF can cause not only a bilateral horizontal gaze paresis but also a **vertical gaze paresis** (Bogousslavsky and Regli, 1984c; Henn et al., 1984). It is assumed that this condition results from damage to pontine afferents to the MRF, but the explanation for a complete ophthalmoplegia from a lesion limited to the pons remains questionable.

Small infarcts affecting the **ventromedial** pons may damage the abducens nerve fascicle and the corticobulbar and corticospinal tracts on the same side. This damage produces an abducens nerve paresis and a contralateral hemiparesis

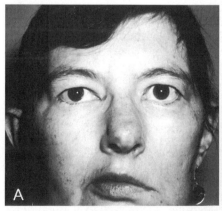
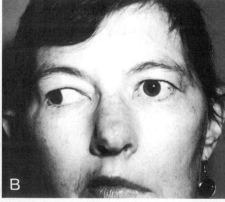
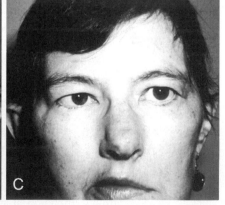

Figure 55.220. One-and-a-half syndrome caused by a hemorrhagic infarct in the pons. The patient was a 47-year-old woman who experienced sudden onset of dizziness, facial weakness, and double vision. *A,* The patient's eyes are relatively straight in primary position. *B,* On attempted right lateral gaze, the right eye abducts fully, but the left eye adducts poorly. *C,* On attempted left lateral gaze, neither eye moves much past the midline. Note profound left facial weakness.

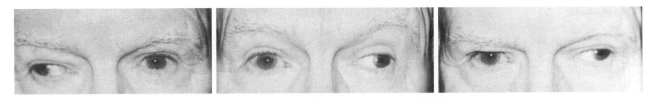

Figure 55.221. Bilateral internuclear ophthalmoplegia. The patient was a 70-year-old man who had a small-vessel infarction in the pons. Note the bilateral limitation of adduction and the exotropia in primary position (*center photograph*).

that often affects the face (Raymond's syndrome) (Raymond and Cestan, 1903; Silverman et al., 1995). An ipsilateral peripheral facial nerve paresis may also occur in such patients when the lesion extends sufficiently laterally to damage the fascicle of the facial nerve (Millard-Gubler syndrome) (Millard, 1856; Gubler, 1856; Silverstein, 1964; Silverman et al., 1995).

As noted above, medial pontine syndromes may be separated into those affecting primarily the superior (rostral), middle, or inferior (caudal) portions of the pons. The typical **medial superior pontine syndrome** produces a variety of neurologic signs, including: (*a*) ipsilateral cerebellar ataxia from damage to the superior cerebellar peduncle, middle cerebellar peduncle, or both; (*b*) oculopalatal myoclonus from damage to the central tegmental tract (Lapresle and Ben Hamida, 1970); (*c*) contralateral hemiparesis affecting face, arm, and leg from damage to the corticobulbar and corticospinal tracts; and, rarely, (*d*) decreased touch, vibration, and position senses from damage to the medial lemniscus. Because the lesion is confined to the rostral portion of the pons, neither the abducens nucleus nor the PPRF are usually affected; however, an INO is common.

The **medial midpontine syndrome** consists of: (*a*) ipsilateral ataxia of limbs and gait from damage to the middle cerebellar peduncle on the side of the lesion; and (*b*) contralateral paralysis of the face, arm, and leg from damage to the corticobulbar and corticospinal tracts. In rare cases, caudal extension of the lesion damages the medial lemniscus, producing variably impaired touch and proprioception. An INO is not uncommon in patients with medial midpontine infarction, but horizontal gaze paresis, abducens nerve paresis, and one-and-a-half syndrome do not usually occur unless the lesion extends caudally.

The **medial inferior pontine syndrome** produces: (*a*) ipsilateral ataxia of limbs and gait from damage to the middle cerebellar peduncle; (*b*) contralateral paralysis of the face, arm, and leg; (*c*) ipsilaterally impaired tactile and proprioceptive sense over half the body from damage to the medial lemniscus; and (*d*) various disturbances of horizontal eye movement from damage to the abducens nerve nucleus, abducens nerve fascicle, PPRF, MLF, or a combination of these structures. In addition, damage to vestibular nuclei and their connections to the ocular motor structures produces varieties of vestibular nystagmus.

Various involuntary, vertical bobbing motions of the eyes may be seen in patients with extensive, paramedian pontine lesions. The motions are usually conjugate and consist of a slow movement in one direction followed by a fast movement in the other, taking the eyes between midposition and upgaze or downgaze (Goldschmidt and Wall, 1987; Mehler, 1988d; Titer and Laureno, 1988). These movements are similar to vertical nystagmus; however, their frequency is irregular, their amplitude is quite large, and they usually occur in comatose patients. **Ocular bobbing** consists of an intermittent, usually conjugate, rapid downward movement of the eyes followed by a slower return to primary position (Fisher, 1964; Daroff and Waldman, 1965; Hameroff et al., 1969; Nelson and Johnston, 1970; Susac et al., 1970; Tijssen and Ter Bruggen, 1986). **Reverse bobbing** consists of rapid deviation of the eyes upward, followed by a slow return to primary position (Daroff et al., 1978; Brusa et al., 1983).

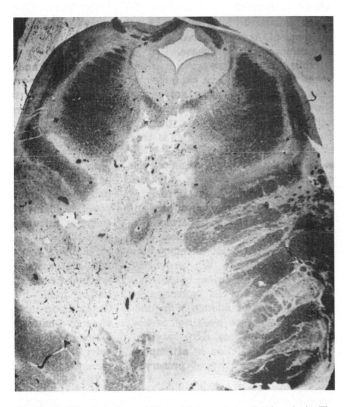

Figure 55.222. Pathology of bilateral internuclear ophthalmoplegia. The patient had severe cerebrovascular and cardiovascular disease. Section through the pontomesencephalic junction shows paramedian necrosis with areas of coalescing cavitation in the regions normally occupied by the medial longitudinal fasciculi. Note that the lesion damages structures on both sides of the midline. (From Gonyea EF. Bilateral internuclear ophthalmoplegia: Association with occlusive cerebrovascular disease. Arch Neurol *31:*168–173, 1974.)

Inverse ocular bobbing, also called ocular dipping, consists of a slow, downward movement of the eyes followed by a rapid return to midposition (Knobler et al., 1981; van Weerden and van Woerkom, 1982; Stark et al., 1984). **Converse ocular bobbing** (inverse-reverse bobbing; reverse ocular dipping) consists of a slow upward movement of the eyes followed by a rapid return to mid-position (Goldschmidt and Wall, 1987; Titer and Laureno, 1988). In the majority of cases, the patients with these movements are comatose, quadriplegic, and have complete bilateral horizontal gaze paresis from extensive infarction or hemorrhage.

Lateral pontine syndromes produce ocular motor disturbances less frequently than do medial pontine syndromes. The **lateral superior pontine syndrome** (syndrome of the superior cerebellar artery) consists of: (*a*) cerebellar ataxia from damage to the ipsilateral superior and middle cerebellar peduncles, superior surface of the cerebellum, and the dentate nucleus; (*b*) dizziness, nausea, and vomiting, probably from damage to vestibular connections in the brainstem; (*c*) impaired pain and thermal sense on the face, limbs, and trunk on the side opposite the lesion from damage to the spinothalamic tract; and (*d*) impaired touch, vibration, and position sense, more in the leg than in the arm, from damage to the lateral portion of the medial lemniscus (Guillain et al., 1928; Worster-Drought and Allen, 1929; Davison et al., 1935; Thompson, 1944; Amarenco and Hauw, 1990a). Patients with this syndrome often have a central Horner's syndrome from damage to descending sympathetic fibers in the lateral pons, and they may have a skew deviation and vestibular nystagmus from damage to vestibular pathways. If the lesion extends medially to any degree, an INO may occur, as may other disturbances of horizontal eye movements, including ipsilateral abducens nerve paresis, horizontal gaze paresis, and one-and-a-half syndrome (Kase et al., 1985a).

Patients with occlusion of the proximal or distal portions of the superior cerebellar artery often show a tendency of the eyes to drift horizontally during vertical saccades (Benjamin et al., 1986; Ranalli and Sharpe, 1986; Uno et al., 1989). This disturbance is similar to that seen in patients with Wallenberg's syndrome, but the eyes tend to deviate toward the side opposite the lesion, rather than toward the side of the lesion as occurs in Wallenberg's syndrome (see below). This phenomenon is therefore called **contrapulsion of saccades** to distinguish it from the lateropulsion of eye movements that occurs in patients with Wallenberg's syndrome.

The **lateral midpontine syndrome** produces: (*a*) ataxia of the limbs on the side of the lesion from damage to the ipsilateral middle cerebellar peduncle; (*b*) ipsilateral paralysis of the muscles of mastication from damage to the motor fibers or nucleus of the ipsilateral trigeminal nerve; and (*c*) impaired sensation of the side of the face ipsilateral to the lesion from damage to the sensory fibers or nucleus of the trigeminal nerve. Patients with this syndrome have disturbances of horizontal gaze only if the lesion extends sufficiently dorsomedially to damage the MLF and produce an INO or sufficiently caudally to damage the abducens nerve nucleus, PPRF, or both.

The **lateral inferior pontine syndrome** (syndrome of the anterior inferior cerebellar artery; Foville's syndrome) (Fo-

ville, 1858) is characterized by: (*a*) ipsilateral peripheral facial paralysis from damage to the facial nerve nucleus or fascicle; (*b*) ipsilateral deafness, tinnitus, or both from damage to the auditory nerve or cochlear nucleus; (*c*) ataxia from damage to the middle cerebellar peduncle and cerebellar hemisphere; (*d*) impaired sensation of the side of the face ipsilateral to the lesion from damage to the descending tract and nucleus of the ipsilateral trigeminal nerve; and (*e*) impaired pain and thermal sensation over half the body contralateral to the lesion from damage to the spinothalamic tract (Adams, 1943; Atkinson, 1949; Amarenco et al., 1990a; Silverman et al., 1995). In some patients, a central Horner's syndrome results from interruption of descending sympathetic fibers. In addition, patients with this syndrome usually have severe vertigo, nausea, vomiting, and oscillopsia associated with marked vestibular nystagmus from damage to the vestibular nerve or nuclei (Perneczky et al., 1981). They also have horizontal gaze paresis toward the side of the lesion from damage to the PPRF, and, if the lesion extends more medially, damage to the ipsilateral abducens nerve nucleus, abducens nerve fascicle, the MLF, or a combination of these structures may produce a variety of other horizontal gaze disturbances (Pierrot-Deseilligny et al., 1981b). In our experience, the lateral inferior pontine syndrome is almost always incomplete.

Fisher (1989b) described a 64-year-old hypertensive man who developed an ischemic infarct of the tegmentum of the caudal lateral pons in the region of the pontomedullary junction. The patient had dysarthria, a staggering gait, incoordination of handwriting, right facial weakness, horizontal nystagmus on attempted gaze away from the side of the lesion, ocular dysmetria, right appendicular ataxia, and left-sided dissociated sensory loss for pain and temperature. The patient's findings were similar to, but less severe than, those of patients with the lateral medullary syndrome of Wallenberg (see below).

Some patients develop a diffuse **ventral pontine infarction** from occlusion of the basilar artery or its short ventral penetrating pontine branches. The resulting lesion may damage the corticospinal and corticobulbar tracts but spare the ocular motor pathways. A patient in whom this phenomenon occurs may show the paradoxical signs of akinetic mutism (see below) with normal eye fixation and movement (Kemper and Romanul, 1967).

One of the most devastating syndromes that results from ventral pontine infarction is the **locked-in syndrome** (Cravioto et al., 1960; Nordgren et al., 1971; Hawkes, 1974; Dehaene and Martin, 1976; Britt et al., 1977; Masson et al., 1978; Gilroy, 1984; Marés et al., 1987; Rae-Grant et al., 1989). Although this condition occasionally occurs in patients with mesencephalic infarction (see above), it usually results from a large lesion in the ventral pons that spares the pathways for somatic sensation and the nonspecific ascending system of neurons and fibers that are responsible for arousal and wakefulness, but interrupts the corticobulbar, corticospinal, and horizontal ocular motor pathways, thus depriving the patient of speech and the capacity to respond in most other ways. Patients with the locked-in syndrome are alert, but they are totally paralyzed and unable to communicate unless they have intact eyelid and vertical eye movements (Plum and Posner, 1966; Rae-Grant et al., 1989). When one side of the pontine tegmentum is spared, such patients may demonstrate a one-and-a-half syndrome (Bogousslavsky et al., 1984). Tijssen and Ter Bruggen (1986) described a patient in whom a large infarction of the pons produced a locked-in syndrome associated with ocular bobbing.

Medullary Signs. The **medial medullary syndrome** (anterior spinal artery syndrome; alternating hypoglossal hemiplegia; syndrome of the pyramid; Déjerine's anterior bulb syndrome) results from damage to roots or nuclei of the hypoglossal nerves, the pyramids, and the medial lemnisci. Clinical signs include ipsilateral weakness of the tongue, gaze-evoked nystagmus, contralateral hemiplegia, and contralateral loss of both proprioception and tactile sensation from the trunk and extremities (Hauw et al., 1976; Gan and Noronha, 1995; Kim et al., 1995; Vuilleumier et al., 1995; Toyoda et al., 1996; Bassetti et al., 1997).

The **lateral medullary syndrome** (Wallenberg's syndrome; posterior inferior cerebellar artery syndrome) affects the roots, nuclei, or both of the vagus nerve, producing ipsilateral laryngeal or pharyngeal weakness (Wallenberg, 1895). The roots or nuclei (or both) of the glossopharyngeal nerve are also damaged in this syndrome, resulting in ipsilateral weakness and analgesia of the soft palate and loss of the gag reflex. Damage to the spinal tract and nucleus of the trigeminal nerve produces ipsilateral loss of pain and diminution of temperature sensation in the face. A central (first-order neuron) Horner's syndrome results from damage to descending reticulospinal tracts to the sympathetic centers in the spinal cord. Damage to the lateral spinothalamic tracts produces contralateral loss of pain and temperature sensation in the trunk and extremities, and damage to the ventral ascending tract of the trigeminal nerve produces contralateral loss of pain and temperature sensation in the face (Sacco et al., 1993; Kim et al., 1994b; Gan and Noronha, 1995; Vuilleumier et al., 1995) (Fig. 55.223).

Patients with the lateral medullary syndrome usually have ipsilateral **cerebellar** signs from damage to fibers travelling in the inferior cerebellar peduncle, but actual infarction of the cerebellum is rare (Sacco et al, 1993). The triad of a central Horner's syndrome, ipsilateral ataxia, and contralateral hypalgesia clinically identifies a lateral medullary infarction. Other common signs include ipsilateral facial weakness and ocular motor disturbances, such as ocular dysmetria, nystagmus, skew deviation, ocular tilt reaction, and a variety of disorders of visual-vestibular interaction (Isch, 1957; Silfverskiöld, 1965; Waespe and Wichmann, 1990). The ocular motor disturbances also may be produced by damage to the inferior and medial vestibular nuclei and to the vestibulospinal tract in the brainstem (Currier et al., 1961; Moberg et al., 1962; Silfverskiöld, 1965; Waespe and Wichmann, 1990). When there is a skew deviation, the lower eye is usually on the side of the lesion (Keane, 1975a).

In some cases of Wallenberg's syndrome, skew deviation is associated with ipsilateral head tilt and ocular torsion—the **ocular tilt reaction** (Westheimer and Blair, 1975a, 1975b; Brandt and Dieterich, 1987; Dieterich and Brandt, 1993). In

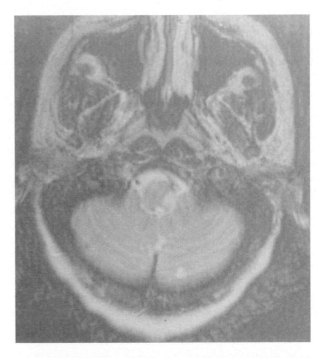

Figure 55.223. Neuroimaging appearance of a lateral medullary infarction. The patient was a 24-year-old woman with a history of migraine, who was taking oral contraceptives when she experienced sudden loss of her left visual field followed by severe left-sided headache, postural nausea, vertigo, and disorientation. Over the next day, she developed a left hemifacial and right hemicorporal sensory loss, vertical diplopia, oscillopsia, and altered balance. Examination 2 months later was notable for decreased sensation on the left face and right body, a left Horner's syndrome, left ocular tilt reaction, and left lateropulsion of saccades. T2-weighted axial magnetic resonance image shows left-sided hyperintense area consistent with an infarct in the lateral medulla.

such cases, the ocular torsion is dysconjugate and associated with a prominant excyclotropia of the ipsilateral hypotropic eye. Such patients often show a deviation of the subjective visual vertical midline in the direction of the spontaneous head tilt, indicating a pathologic shift of the internal representation of the gravitational vector.

The nystagmus that occurs in patients with Wallenberg's syndrome is usually positional (Hagström et al., 1969). Most often horizontal or torsional, it is of greatest amplitude during gaze toward the side of the lesion (Currier et al., 1961); however, downbeat, periodic alternating, and even see-saw nystagmus may occur in patients with Wallenberg's syndrome (Jensen, 1959; Moberg et al., 1962; Daroff, 1965; Mastaglia, 1974). Daroff et al. (1968) also described gaze-evoked eyelid and ocular nystagmus that were inhibited by the near reflex in a patient with Wallenberg's syndrome.

Bjerver and Silfverskiöld (1968) reported that some patients with infarctions of the lateral medulla experienced "lateropulsion of the body." These patients felt as though their bodies were being pulled to one side. Because of this, the patients attempted to counteract these feelings by leaning to the opposite side. They tended to fall toward the side of the lesion when walking with the eyes closed or the feet together.

A phenomenon similar to lateropulsion of the body affects eye movements. This condition, called **lateropulsion of eye movements**, is characterized by the feeling that the eyes are being pulled toward the affected side (Kommerell and Hoyt, 1973; Hörnsten, 1974a, 1974b; Frisén, 1978; Meyer et al., 1980; Baloh et al., 1981; Kirkham et al., 1981; Cambier et al., 1982; Uno et al., 1989; Waespe and Wichmann, 1990; Dieterich and Brandt, 1992; Solomon et al., 1995). If the patient is asked to fixate straight ahead and gently close the eyelids, the eyes deviate conjugately toward the side of the lesion. This deviation is reflected in the corrective saccades that the patient must make on reopening the eyelids and reaquiring the target. In some patients, lateropulsion of eye movements occurs during normal blinking. Lateropulsion of eye movements interferes with both saccadic and pursuit eye movements (Fig. 55.224).

Horizontal saccades are hypometric when directed against the bias (away from the side of the lesion) and hypermetric when directed with the bias (toward the side of the lesion). Quick phases of nystagmus are similarly affected. Those directed away from the side of the lesion are smaller than those toward the lesion. When attempting to make a purely vertical saccade, a patient with lateropulsion of eye movements makes an **oblique** saccade directed toward the side of the lesion and then must make one or more corrective saccades away from the side of the lesion to bring the eyes to the target (Kirkham et al., 1981). With time, vertical saccades may become even more abnormal. S-shaped saccadic trajectories may appear a week or more after the onset of the disorder. These may reflect an adaptive strategy to correct the saccadic abnormality.

Patients with lateropulsion of eye movements have severe impairment of smooth pursuit in addition to impairment of saccades. Pursuit away from the side of the lesion (opposite the direction of bias) is severely impaired, whereas pursuit toward the side of the lesion is normal or nearly so (Meyer et al., 1980).

Some patients with Wallenberg's syndrome experience an unusual visual distortion in which the environment appears tilted (Fig. 55.225). In most cases, tilting is not severe; however, some patients complain of 90 degree or even 180 degree tilting of images (Silfverskiöld, 1965; Bjerver and Silfv-

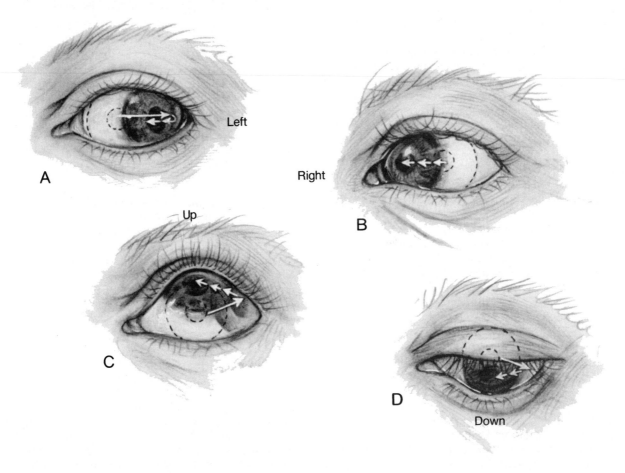

Figure 55.224. Lateropulsion of saccades in a patient with a left Wallenberg syndrome. *A*, On attempted left lateral gaze, the patient overshoots the target and must make a corrective saccade. *B*, On attempted right lateral gaze, the patient makes a series of hypometric saccades. *C* and *D*, On attempted upward and downward gaze, the eyes tend to move obliquely to the left, and several refixation movements to the right are needed to get them back to center. (Redrawn from Kommerell G, Hoyt WF. Lateropulsion of saccadic eye movements: Electro-oculographic studies in a patient with Wallenberg's syndrome. Arch Neurol 28:313–318, 1973.)

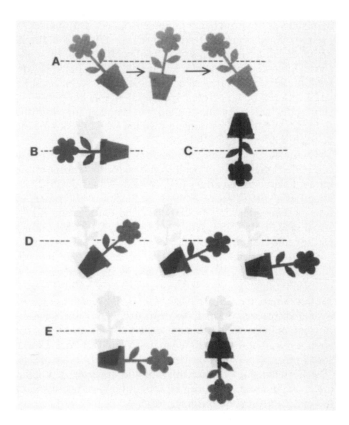

Figure 55.225. Schematic representation of the illusions of tilting experienced by five patients with presumed medullary or pontomedullary disease. *A*, Sudden tilting of the entire room counterclockwise 45 for 1 second, then slow return to normal position over 5–8 seconds overshooting 10 clockwise, followed by sudden return to 45 clockwise. *B*, Tilting precisely 90 clockwise with persistence of the tilted image for about 1 hour. *C*, All objects perceived as turned upside down for 5 minutes after awakening. *D*, Episodes of variable, sudden, clockwise tilting of images around a point in the right lower quadrant of the visual field. *E*, Most episodes were abrupt clockwise tilting to almost or exactly 90, with one episode of complete inversion of images. Turning occurred around a point in the left lower quadrant of the visual field. (From Ropper AH. Illusion of tilting of the environment: Report of three cases. J Clin Neuroophthalmol *3:*147–151, 1983.)

erskiöld, 1968; Hagström et al., 1969; Hörnsten, 1974a, 1974b; Ropper, 1983; López et al., 1995). This syndrome is thought to result from a disturbance of the vestibular-otolith apparatus or its central connections (Ropper, 1983).

Other symptoms that occur in patients with the lateral medullary syndrome of Wallenberg include ipsilateral pain in the face, contralateral pain and dysesthesia of the body, headache behind the eye or ear on the side of the lesion, weakness of the ipsilateral side of the face, hiccoughing, nausea, and vomiting. Contralateral hyperhidrosis may appear 6–8 months after the stroke, probably from dysfunction of sympathetic pathways (Rousseaux et al., 1996).

The lateral medullary syndrome is rarely complete. Freddo et al. (1989) reviewed the records of 28 patients with this condition and concluded that the most frequent symptoms at onset were paresthesias of the ipsilateral face,

contralateral body, or both, as well as ataxia and dysphagia. The most frequent signs were ipsilateral ataxia, contralateral hypesthesia, and Horner's syndrome.

The lateral medullary syndrome of Wallenberg is frequently a manifestation of thrombosis or dissection of the vertebral artery proximal to the origin of the posterior inferior cerebellar artery (Baker, 1961; Fisher et al., 1961; Currier et al., 1962; Escourolle et al., 1976; Freddo et al., 1989). It may also be caused by occlusion of the posterior inferior cerebellar artery itself (Gorelick et al., 1985; Caplan, 1993; Fisher and Tapia, 1987; Freddo et al., 1989), particularly in African-Americans (Gorelick et al., 1985). Variability in this syndrome is the rule rather than the exception, because the courses and sizes of the vertebral and posterior inferior cerebellar arteries are unpredictable (Currier et al., 1961, 1962; Moberg et al., 1962; Wolff et al., 1962).

Most patients with infarction of the lateral medulla have a good prognosis for recovery of neurologic function and return to normal activity (Currier et al., 1958). Signs and symptoms improve quickly except for ataxia (Currier et al., 1961), but most patients walk reasonably well in time. Bernat and Hunter (1978) described a particularly "benign" lateral medullary syndrome occurring in young, otherwise healthy men after substantial outdoor excercise. In all four cases reported by Bernat and Hunter (1978), the symptoms and signs resolved within 48 hours and did not recur. One of the patients was followed for almost 30 years without any evidence of recurrent cerebrovascular or cardiovascular disease.

Some patients have a particularly poor prognosis after infarction of the lateral medulla (Fisher et al., 1961; see Table in Caplan et al., 1986a). When there is a large infarction in the ipsilateral inferior cerebellar hemisphere, a posterior fossa pressure cone can develop and produce death from medullary compression (Lehrich et al., 1970; G.W. Duncan et al., 1975; Sypert and Alvord, 1975). Aspiration can occur in patients with severe dysphagia, resulting in pneumonia and death from intercurrent infection (Fisher et al., 1961). Other patients with lateral medullary infarcts experience cardiovascular and autonomic disturbances that can produce sudden death and that are probably caused by an acute increase in vagal tone resulting from damage to the dorsal motor nucleus of the vagus nerve (Khurana, 1982).

Ondine's curse, a failure to initiate breathing when asleep, occurs not only in patients with bilateral lateral pontine or medullary tegmental vascular and other lesions (Severinghaus and Mitchell, 1962; Devereaux and Keane, 1973; Devereaux et al., 1973; Dooling and Richardson, 1977; Beal et al., 1983; Caplan et al., 1986a), but also in patients with unilateral lesions (Levin and Margolis, 1977). This condition results from damage to the medullary center for automatic breathing control. It is named after Ondine (actually Undine, from the Latin, *undina,* a watersprite), a vengeful water nymph who killed her unfaithful human lover by depriving him of all automatic functions so that he suffocated during sleep (Rolak, 1996).

Other reasons for poor outcome after lateral medullary infarction include clot propagation from the vertebral artery to the basilar artery, clot embolization from the vertebral artery, and bilateral intracranial vertebral artery disease (Koroshetz and Ropper, 1985; Caplan et al., 1986a; Koroshetz and Ropper, 1987).

CEREBELLAR SIGNS OF OCCLUSIVE DISEASE OF THE VERTEBROBASILAR ARTERIAL SYSTEM

The diagnosis of a cerebellar stroke may be obvious: Sudden vomiting, ataxia, vertigo, and headache in a patient over 50 years of age with systemic hypertension or diabetes mellitus (Amarenco and Hauw, 1990a, 1990b; Amarenco, 1991; Kase, 1994). Unfortunately, this clinical picture is the exception rather than the rule. Macdonell et al. (1987) found that 80% of patients with cerebellar infarction presented with subtle, nonspecific symptoms of dizziness, vertigo, or both, and about 25% of these patients had no cerebellar signs when they were examined. Such patients may be thought to have labyrinthitis or a similar, benign labyrinthine disorder (G. W. Duncan et al., 1975). The cerebellar lesion may swell and compress the structures in the cerebellopontine angle, resulting in damage to the ipsilateral trigeminal, abducens, facial, and vestibulocochlear nerves. More importantly, it may also compress the caudal brainstem. When there is only minimal compression of the brainstem, few isolated neurologic signs may be present. For example, a horizontal gaze paresis unassociated with contralateral hemiparesis may occur (Caplan, 1993). In many cases, however, severe compression of the brainstem results after cerebellar infarction. In such patients, the plantar responses become extensor, systolic blood pressure rises, diastolic blood pressure falls, the pulse slows, and respirations may cease (Fairburn and Oliver, 1956; Lehrich et al., 1970; Savitz et al., 1977; Amarenco and Hauw, 1990a, 1990b; Amarenco, 1991). Prompt decompression in such cases may prevent death and result in eventual improvement in neurologic function (see Table VI in Schmidek and Guthikonda, 1979).

The ocular signs of cerebellar lesions are discussed in Chapters 29 and 31 of this text. It suffices here merely to emphasize that a wide variety of disturbances of eye movement occur in patients with cerebellar infarction, including:

1. Inaccurate horizontal and vertical saccades despite normal velocities and latencies (saccadic dysmetria);
2. Disturbances of fixation, especially square wave jerks and increased slow drift;
3. Impaired smooth pursuit with the head moving;
4. Gaze-evoked nystagmus;
5. Rebound nystagmus;
6. Downbeat nystagmus;
7. Positional nystagmus;
8. Skew deviation;
9. Impaired optokinetic nystagmus;
10. Impaired fixation suppression of caloric-induced nystagmus;
11. Increased gain of the vestibulo-ocular reflex.

Lesions that produce these disturbances usually affect the cerebellar hemispheres and vermis, and they often damage the brainstem; however, isolated lesions of the cerebellar hemispheres or vermis may produce isolated disturbances of eye movement (Pierrot-Deseilligny et al., 1990). In addition, large cerebellar infarctions with brainstem compression can cause hydrocephalus and resultant false localizing signs. Halkin et al. (1995) described a 73-year-old woman with a large left cerebellar stroke, ipsilateral brainstem compression, acute hydrocephalus and proptosis and chemosis of the right eye. Ventricular drainage resulted in regression of the ocular findings within 24 hours.

The most common vascular lesions found in patients with cerebellar infarction are occlusion or severe stenosis of the intracranial vertebral artery (Sypert and Alvord, 1975; Macdonell et al., 1987; Kase, 1994), occlusion of the posterior inferior cerebellar artery (Schmidek and Guthikonda, 1979; Amarenco et al., 1989; Amarenco, 1991; Kase, 1994), and cardiogenic emboli (Amarenco et al., 1990b). Most cerebellar infarcts occur in the distribution of the posterior inferior cerebellar artery (G.W. Duncan et al., 1975; Sypert and Alvord, 1976; Scotti et al., 1980; Amarenco et al., 1989, 1990b, 1990c; Amarenco, 1991; Kase, 1994). Nevertheless, some cerebellar infarcts occur in the territory of the anterior inferior cerebellar artery, the superior cerebellar artery, or the territories of both vessels (Amarenco and Hauw, 1990a, 1990b; Amarenco et al., 1990b; Amarenco, 1991; Kase, 1994). When only the territory of the superior cerebellar artery is infarcted, there is a high likelihood of occlusion of the distal third of the basilar artery.

Patients with cerebellar infarction limited to the territory of the superior cerebellar artery often present with acute gait ataxia with little or no vertigo, ipsilateral limb ataxia, and upbeat nystagmus (Kase et al., 1985a). Ho et al. (1981) reported that these patients tend to have a better prognosis, with less tendency to develop brainstem compression from swelling of infarcted cerebellar tissue, than patients with cerebellar infarction in the distribution of the posterior inferior cerebellar artery; however, Amarenco and colleagues (Amarenco et al., 1989; Amarenco and Hauw, 1990a, 1990b; Amarenco, 1991) found that patients with cerebellar infarction affecting only the territory of the posterior inferior cerebellar artery had the most benign prognosis.

Symptoms and Signs of Lacunar Infarction

The majority of strokes are apparently related to occlusion or stenosis of large extracranial and intracranial arteries; however, disease of microscopic-sized intracranial arteries may also cause stroke (Fisher, 1965a–c, 1967b, 1969, 1982a; Arboix et al., 1990). These **lacunar infarctions** have a predilection for anatomic sites nourished by penetrating vessels. Some of these deep lesions produce characteristic clinical syndromes, whereas others are clinically silent or produce findings difficult to distinguish from large-vessel disease (Fisher, 1982a; Bamford and Warlow, 1988; Weisberg, 1988; Tuszynski et al., 1989; Gan et al., 1997). Landau (1989) recommended that strokes be classified by size (small, medium, large), location (thalamus, pons, etc.), and type (ischemic, hemorrhagic) based on the results of clinical examination and neuroimaging studies. He argued that both the term "lacune" and the concept of a "lacunar infarct" are antiquated and should be discarded. He and others also emphasized that lacunar syndromes may be caused by occlusion or stenosis of large vessels, resulting in hemodynamic cerebral ischemia (Millikan and Futrell, 1990; Waterston et al., 1990), by local obstruction of the origin of deep perforating branches by disease in the larger parent vessel (Caplan, 1989b; Bogousslavsky et al., 1991b), and by nonischemic lesions (e.g., aneurysm rupture, cerebral abscess, multiple sclerosis, glioma, hemorrhage) (Anzalone and Landi, 1989). We nevertheless include lacunar strokes in our classification because they are too fixed in neurologic literature to be ignored.

The causes of true lacunar infarctions are diverse (Millikan and Futrell, 1990). The most common are atherosclerotic microvascular thrombosis, microembolism, microaneurysm, and arteritis (Fisher, 1979; Mohr, 1982; Miller, 1983; Mohr, 1986). Hypertension is present in about two-thirds of patients with lacunar stroke (Mohr et al., 1978; Pullicino et al., 1980; Donnan et al., 1982b; Weisberg, 1982; Tuszynski et al., 1989; Arboix et al., 1990; You et al., 1995). Lodder et al. (1990) studied risk-factor profiles in 102 consecutive patients with a lacunar infarct and 202 consecutive patients with an infarct in the distribution of the carotid arterial system and concluded that hypertension is no more important in the pathogenesis of a lacunar infarct than it is in the development of other types of ischemic stroke that are presumed to be caused by atherosclerotic thromboembolism in a major artery. However, You et al. (1995) found no association of lacunar infarction with heart disease, suggesting that there is a unique pathophysiologic mechanism for lacunar stroke apart from generalized atherosclerosis. Lodder et al. (1990) also found that cardioembolic occlusion is an unusual cause of lacunar infarction (see also van Merwijk et al., 1990). Other apparent risk factors for lacunar infarction are smoking and diabetes mellitus (Tuszynski et al., 1989; Arboix et al., 1990; You et al., 1995). In ophthalmologically asymptomatic patients with brain lacunar infarctions, fluorescein angiography demonstrated prolonged arteriovenous passage time, independent of hypertension or diabetes, supporting an underlying microcirculatory abnormality (Schneider et al., 1993).

Marie (1901) first emphasized isolated hemiplegia as a sign of lacunar infarction, but C. Miller Fisher and his colleagues (Fisher, 1965b; Fisher and Curry, 1965) popularized this concept. They called the syndrome of **isolated** weakness of face, arm, and leg **pure motor hemiplegia**, taught that it was almost always caused by a lacunar infarction in the pons or internal capsule rather than by large-vessel disease, and emphasized that it almost always occurred in patients with systemic hypertension. Pure motor hemiplegia is probably the most common syndrome caused by symptomatic lacunar stroke (Tuszynski et al., 1989). By definition, patients with pure motor hemiplegia have no sensory, visual, or intellectual abnormalities.

A second common lacunar syndrome is called **pure sensory stroke** (Fisher, 1965c, 1978a, 1982b). A patient with this condition has somatosensory complaints without other symptoms or signs. All hemicorporeal sensations are represented in the relatively small area occupied by the thalamic somatosensory relay nuclei. In the somatosensory cortex,

however, the hand and face have very large representations, whereas the trunk, scalp, and regions incapable of fine sensory distinctions have very little representation. Isolated numbness of the inner mouth, eye, ear, scalp, chest, back, abdomen, or genitalia thus do not usually result from a stroke affecting the parietal cortex, but from a lacunar infarct, hemorrhage, or other lesion in the posterior ventrolateral thalamic nucleus, in thalamocortical or subthalamic sensory pathways, or in the pons (Groothuis et al., 1977; Fisher, 1978a; Rosenberg and Koller, 1981; Fisher, 1982b; Tuttle and Reinmuth, 1984; Graveleau et al., 1986; Hommel et al., 1989). Azouvi et al. (1989) reported a pure sensory stroke in a patient with a hemorrhage in the mesencephalon that was limited to the spinothalamic pathway.

Most patients with pure sensory stroke describe numbness, tingling, or pins and needles sensations in the face, limbs, or trunk. These sensations may develop an unpleasant quality, characterized as burning, soreness, or tightness within a few days after onset. These painful sensory symptoms may mimic the symptoms of myocardial ischemia (Gorson et al., 1996). In patients with pure sensory stroke, subjective complaints are more impressive than objective loss of sensation. Indeed, many patients with this syndrome have no detectable loss of threshold to any sensory modality, whereas others have only a minimal qualitative or quantitative difference in the two sides of the body. By definition, all motor, visual, and intellectual functions are normal in patients with pure sensory stroke.

The **dysarthria-clumsy hand syndrome** is a distinct syndrome characterized by slurred speech, weakness of the tongue, face, and pharynx, and clumsiness of the ipsilateral hand (Fisher, 1967b). The lesion is located in the contralateral basis pontis, where it interrupts descending corticobulbar fibers (Glass et al., 1990).

Ataxic hemiparesis is characterized by a combination of weakness, pyramidal signs, and ataxia in the leg only or in the arm and leg on the same side of the body (Fisher and Cole, 1965; Fisher, 1978b). Weakness usually is less prominent than ataxia in such patients. The responsible lesion is usually in the contralateral basis pontis, base of the mesencephalon, or posterior limb of the internal capsule; however, Boiten and Lodder (1990) described a patient who developed ataxic hemiparesis from a lacunar infarct of the ventrolateral nucleus of the thalamus.

Combined sensory dysfunction and pyramidal signs with weakness on the same side of the body is called a **sensory-motor stroke** (Mohr et al., 1977). This syndrome was present in 11% of 169 patients with lacunar strokes whose autopsy reports were reviewed by Tuszynski et al. (1989). There is no accompanying visual field defect nor loss of higher cortical function in a patient with this syndrome, although the patient is not infrequently dysarthric (Arboix and Marti-Vilalta, 1990). The responsible lesion is usually a large infarct that straddles the lateral thalamus and the posterior limb of the internal capsule. Lee et al. (1989) described a patient who developed an acute **hypesthetic ataxic hemiparesis**—essentially a sensory-motor stroke—from such a lesion. The hypesthesia and hemiparesis were on the same side, and the lesion was a lacunar infarct bordering the medial portion of the posterior limb of the internal capsule.

A lacunar infarct may cause acute **hemichorea, hemiballismus,** or **hemiparkinsonian stiffness**. Patients with these conditions experience the sudden onset of abnormal movements or tone on one side of the body, often associated with slight weakness. The responsible lesion is in the subthalamus, striatum, globus pallidum, or thalamus (Kase et al., 1981; Mohr, 1982).

Lacunar infarcts can cause not only the well-known neurologic syndromes described above but also isolated ocular motor nerve pareses. For example, an isolated oculomotor nerve paresis can be caused by a lacunar infarction in the mesencephalon (Collard et al., 1990; Ferbert et al., 1990; Hriso et al., 1990). The paresis may consist of weakness of one muscle (e.g., the inferior rectus), one division (e.g., the superior or inferior division), or all the extraocular muscles innervated by the oculomotor nerve. The pupil may or may not be affected. Trochlear nerve paresis, both unilateral and bilateral, may also be caused by lacunar infarction in the dorsal caudal mesencephalon (Iwakiri and Yoshida, 1990), and isolated abducens nerve paresis may be caused by a small lacunar infarct in the pons (Bronstein et al., 1990a). Isolated horizontal or vertical gaze paresis, often with dissociation between saccadic and pursuit eye movements, can occasionally be caused by small lacunar infarcts in the brainstem (Bronstein et al., 1990b). The availability of MR imaging greatly improves the ability to diagnose lacunar infarcts (Arboix et al., 1990; Glass et al., 1990; Hommel et al., 1990b; Iwakiri and Yoshida, 1990).

Although the majority of lacunar infarctions are clinically silent, multiple lacunar infarcts may cause syndromes more complicated than simply the sum of their individual manifestations. Clinical syndromes include dementia, parkinsonism, hyperreflexia, motor and sensory signs, and pseudobulbar abnormalties of speech, swallowing, and emotional control (Caplan, 1993, 1995). These syndromes are usually associated with severe abnormalities of the cerebral white matter and ventricular enlargement (**Binswanger's disease**) that can be identified using CT scanning or MR imaging (Awad et al., 1986). The white matter changes are called leukoaraiosis; they probably correspond to widespread gliosis and atrophy secondary to chronic microvascular ischemia from diffuse small vessel disease (Hachinski et al., 1987). Hemorrheologic changes with hyperviscosity or amyloid angiopathy may contribute in some cases (Gray et al., 1985; Schneider et al., 1987; Caplan, 1993). The clinical manifestations of Binswanger's disease are variable and range from none to subtle abnormalities of cognition and behavior to severe abulia and dementia (Babikian and Ropper, 1987; Hachinski et al., 1987; Caplan, 1993, 1995; Pantoni and Garcia, 1995). Most patients have slowed responses, and many exhibit aphasic abnormalities, changes in personality, memory loss, and visuospatial difficulties. Gait abnormalities, pyramidal signs, hyperreflexia and pseudobulbar palsy are common. The clinical course is usually that of step-wise progression.

A syndrome resembling progressive supranuclear palsy (PSP) occurs in some patients with multiple infarcts (Schwab and England, 1968; Dubinsky and Jankovic, 1987; Moses and Zee, 1987; Tanner et al., 1987). PSP is usually caused by a degenerative process that affects subcortical structures, including the superior colliculus, substantia nigra, locus ceruleus, subthalamic nucleus, dentate nucleus, and globus pallidus, resulting in dementia, parkinsonism, and ophthalmoplegia that is supranuclear, at least until the late stages of the disease (Steele et al., 1964; Jankovic, 1984; Kristensen, 1985; Maher and Lees, 1986) (see Chapter 50). Nevertheless, a PSP-like syndrome may develop after episodes of systemic hypotension or from multiple, nonsimultaneous thrombotic or embolic occlusions of the small vessels supplying the structures normally damaged in patients with PSP. Patients with multi-infarct PSP usually have abrupt onset and rapid progression (less than 1 year) (Moses and Zee, 1987).

Symptoms and Signs of Aortocranial Disease: Combined Carotid and Vertebrobasilar Syndromes

The classification of symptoms and signs of occlusive cerebrovascular disease under the broad headings of carotid and vertebrobasilar disease is convenient and useful in clinical practice. The use of this classification should not, however, obscure the fact that atheromatous disease, syphilis, vasculitis, and other vascular occlusive disorders can affect one or both internal carotid arteries and the vertebral or basilar arteries in the same patient. Such disorders may also occlude the large arteries in the thorax from which the carotid and vertebrobasilar circulations originate. These combined occlusions of major cerebral arterial systems, which Fazekas et al. (1963) called "aortocranial disease," produce a variety of clinical symptoms and signs that may defy analysis from clinical data alone.

Generalized Disease of the Carotid and Vertebrobasilar Arteries

In a study of vertebral artery occlusion, Hutchinson and Yates (1956) mentioned that vertebral artery disease could play a role in the production of clinical syndromes normally associated with occlusion of the internal carotid arteries. These investigators described cases in which symptoms and signs of chronic vertebral artery occlusion were precipitated by acute occlusive events in the carotid arterial system. Indeed, four of their patients were found at autopsy to have infarctions both in the cerebral hemispheres and in the cerebellum.

Transient **monocular** visual loss is not an expected symptom of vertebrobasilar insufficiency. In a patient with carotid occlusive disease or agenesis of a carotid artery, however, collateral flow to the eye may arrive via the vertebrobasilar system through the posterior communicating arteries. In such a case, cervical compression of a vertebral artery could precipitate an attack of monocular visual loss, and occlusion of that vessel could cause complete monocular blindness from retinal or optic nerve ischemia and infarction.

Patients with occlusion of the carotid and the basilar (or vertebral) arteries may experience TIAs, some of which suggest carotid circulation disease and others vertebrobasilar disease (Miyamoto et al., 1986). Doniger (1963) reported the case of a 43-year-old woman who, during the preceding 10 years, experienced two transient episodes of right hemiparesis and numerous attacks of transient cortical blindness. Cerebral arteriography showed total occlusion of both carotid arteries and the basilar artery.

Aortic Arch Syndromes

Symptoms and signs suggesting combined carotid and vertebrobasilar arterial disease may result not only from direct occlusion of these vessels but also from occlusion of the vessels from which they originate. Chronic occlusion of the aortic arch or of one or more of its major trunks results in a variety of cephalic and brachial vascular insufficiency states that are called **aortic arch syndromes** (Ross and McKusick, 1953) (Fig. 55.226). These syndromes are most often caused by severe atherosclerosis, syphilis, and connective tissue disease.

The visual and neurologic effects of obstructions at the

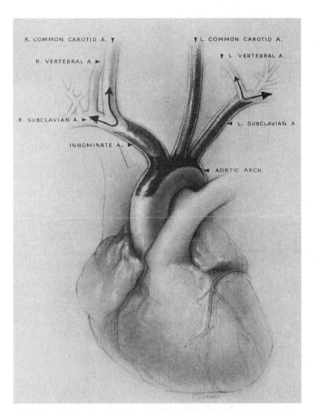

Figure 55.226. Anatomy of the aortic arch showing areas of obstruction that cause aortic arch syndromes. *Shaded* regions indicate areas of potential atherosclerotic occlusion. *Stippled* areas are potential sites of thrombotic occlusion. *Arrows* show directions of blood flow. Note that if the proximal portion of the left subclavian artery becomes occluded, blood still may reach the subclavian artery through reverse flow in the left vertebral artery. Similarly, if the proximal portion of the innominate artery becomes occluded, blood may reach the right subclavian artery through reverse flow in the right vertebral artery. In both cases, blood is "stolen" from the opposite vertebral artery. (From Tour RL, Hoyt WF. The syndrome of the aortic arch: Ocular manifestations of "pulseless disease" and a report of a surgically treated case. Am J Ophthalmol *47*:35–48, 1959.)

level of the aortic arch depend on: (*a*) the location of the obstruction, (*b*) the status of intracranial circulation, and (*c*) the efficiency of the aortocervical collateral circulation. A patient with occlusion of the aortic arch may have no symptoms of cerebrovascular insufficiency, occasional TIAs in either the carotid or the vertebrobasilar territory, or severe ischemic symptoms and signs with chronic trophic changes in the neck, face, orbit, and brain from impaired blood flow.

The visual and neurologic deficits that occur in patients with aortic arch syndromes are nonspecific. Any of the symptoms or signs that are described in the sections of this chapter concerned with carotid or vertebrobasilar insufficiency can occur in patients with these syndromes. There are, however, certain physical findings that characterize occlusions of the major trunks of the aortic arch. These include reduction or absence of pulses and blood pressure in one or both arms and the neck, a continuous murmur that is audible in the neck and over the upper thorax, and weakness and claudication in one or both extremities after brief manual exercise. When exercise of one arm produces an attack of cerebrovascular insufficiency, the diagnosis of occlusion of the ipsilateral, proximal subclavian artery is almost certain (see below).

SUBCLAVIAN STEAL SYNDROME (PROXIMAL OCCLUSION OF THE LEFT SUBCLAVIAN ARTERY)

Contorni (1960) first described the phenomenon of reversed flow in the left vertebral artery associated with proximal occlusion of the left subclavian artery; however, Reivich et al. (1961) first recognized the effect of this condition on the circulation to the brain. These investigators evaluated two patients with proximal occlusion of the left subclavian artery, both of whom had symptoms of vertebrobasilar insufficiency. Both patients had reversed blood flow in the left vertebral artery. Blood flow measurements showed that blood flowed up the right vertebral artery to the origin of the basilar artery and then returned back down the left vertebral artery into the circulatory bed of the left arm (Figs. 55.177 and 55.227). Reivich et al. (1961) found that the reduction in cerebral blood flow resulting from this siphoning effect was as much as 40%. An editorial by Fisher (1961a), which accompanied the article by Reivich et al.(1961), called this anterograde-retrograde vertebral-vertebral shunting the **subclavian steal syndrome** and correctly predicted that manual exercise on the side of the occluded subclavian artery might precipitate symptoms of insufficiency in the posterior cerebral circulation. North et al. (1962) subsequently reviewed 59 cases of proximal obstruction of the subclavian artery. Twenty-six of these patients (44%) had only symptoms of claudication in the arm on the side of the occlusion. The remaining 33 patients (56%), however, also had neurologic symptoms. Neurologic symptoms were present in eight of 13 patients with right-sided occlusion, 14 of 33 patients with left-sided occlusion, and 11 of 13 patients with bilateral occlusion. Similar figures were reported by Hennerici et al. (1988a), who found that among 324 patients with reversed vertebral artery blood flow, 115 (46%) had neurologic symptoms.

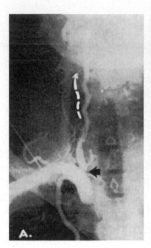
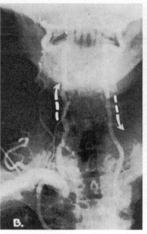
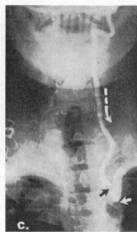

Figure 55.227. Angiography of the subclavian steal syndrome. The patient has an occlusion of the proximal portion of the left subclavian artery. *A,* The innominate and right subclavian arteries fill normally as does the right vertebral artery (*arrow*). Note that the blood in the right vertebral artery is flowing normally in a proximal to distal direction (*dashed arrow*). *B,* In a later phase of the arteriogram, blood in the right vertebral artery continues to flow in a proximal to distal direction; however, the left vertebral artery is now filled by blood that is flowing in a *retrograde* direction from distal to proximal (*dashed arrows*). This blood has been diverted from its normal course into the basilar artery to the contralateral vertebral artery. Note that there is no filling of the left subclavian artery in this phase of the arteriogram. *C,* Blood flowing in a retrograde fashion down the left vertebral artery (*dashed line*) now fills the left subclavian artery (*black arrow*) just distal to the site of occlusion (*white arrow*). (From Newton TH, Wylie EJ. Collateral circulation associated with occlusion of the proximal subclavian and innominate arteries. AJR *91:*394–405, 1964.)

Six of the 33 patients with neurologic symptoms evaluated by North et al. (1962) described and also demonstrated a clear association between exercise of an arm and episodic neurologic symptoms. One patient, a 46-year-old woman, described spinning dizziness, blurred vision, and weakness of the right side of the body, all of which first occurred shortly after she began to comb her son's hair with the left hand. Other symptoms experienced by this patient, all of short duration, included a sensation of burning around both eyes and a crawling sensation around the left ear. Examination revealed barely perceptible left radial, brachial, and subclavian pulses. Blood pressure was 160/70 mm Hg in the right arm and 110/70 mm Hg in the left arm. A loud murmur was audible over the right clavicle. Twelve rapid flexions of the left arm produced vertigo and blurred vision within 30 seconds. These symptoms lasted 1–2 minutes. Subsequent arteriography showed total proximal occlusion of the left subclavian artery with retrograde flow in the ipsilateral vertebral artery. The patient underwent a subclavian endarterectomy, and all symptoms disappeared.

As demonstrated by the patient described by North et al. (1962), the most frequent systemic symptoms of the subclavian steal syndrome relate to the ipsilateral arm and hand. Coolness, weakness, and pain during use of the arm are common, but they may not be sufficiently severe to stimulate the patient to consult a physician. Only two of 10 patients with subclavian steal syndrome evaluated by Spetzler et al. (1987) had ipsilateral arm weakness. Among the 324 patients evaluated by Hennerici et al. (1988a), pain, numbness, and fatigue of the arm were reported by about one-third of the patients, but only 15 patients had evidence of severe brachial ischemia or embolism in distal arterial branches of the upper limbs.

According to North et al. (1962), the most common neurologic symptom of the subclavian steal syndrome is **dizziness**, usually of a spinning or vertiginous character. Diplopia, blurred vision (which may be visual confusion from ocular misalignment—see Chapter 27), oscillopsia, and staggering all occur, but much less frequently, and usually in association with an episode of dizziness. Such episodes are usually quite brief and, as noted above, are usually precipitated by exercising the ischemic arm. Four of the 10 patients evaluated by Spetzler et al. (1987) complained of dizziness that was often postural in nature, four patients had experienced vertigo, and two patients complained of diplopia. Six of the patients had experienced syncopal episodes or drop attacks.

Hennerici et al. (1988a) reported that only 16 of 324 patients (5%) with subclavian steal syndrome had neurologic symptoms or signs consistent with vertebrobasilar ischemia. These 16 patients represented 14% of the number of patients with neurologic symptoms of signs. The remaining 99 patients with neurologic symptoms (31% of the total number of patients; 86% of the patients with neurologic symptoms or signs) had evidence of **hemispheric** ischemia related to associated atherosclerotic disease of one or both carotid arteries. Hennerici et al. (1988a) did not consider dizziness or tinnitus as neurologic events, however. Had they done so, the percentage of their patients with neurologic symptoms would have been considerably increased from the 46% they reported, and the percentage with vertebrobasilar symptoms also would have been increased.

Dwyer-Joyce (1972) described abnormal visual fields in a patient with subclavian steal syndrome. Both fields showed significant nasal defects. One optic disc was said to show "some pallor." These abnormalities probably were not directly related to the steal syndrome itself but rather to ischemia of the optic nerves caused by associated carotid vascular insufficiency.

North et al. (1962) recommended that the subclavian steal syndrome be called the "brachial-basilar insufficiency syndrome," noting that this type of vertebral-vertebral shunt requires two patent vertebral arteries with a reduced head of pressure at the origin of one of them. This shunt may be so active that additional collateral circulation is drawn into the vertebral siphon from the occipital branches of the external carotid artery. In addition, Couves et al. (1963) noted that retrograde flow from the internal carotid artery through the circle of Willis may also participate in the collateral blood supply to an arm with a proximally occluded subclavian trunk.

The diagnosis of subclavian steal syndrome is usually straightforward. Any patient with symptoms of cerebrovascular insufficiency, a bruit over the supraclavicular area, and a reduction in pulse and blood pressure in the ipsilateral arm should be considered to have a proximal occlusion of the subclavian artery until arteriography proves otherwise (Mannick et al., 1962). Bryant and Spencer (1966) emphasized, however, that the physical findings in patients with subclavian occlusion may be subtle. Among 14 patients with subclavian occlusion, 10 had a palpable radial pulse with only a mild reduction in blood pressure on the side receiving collateral blood from the vertebral artery. Nevertheless, the diagnosis of subclavian steal syndrome can usually be made by physical examination. There is invariably a difference in the wrist and antecubital pulses in the two arms. The pulse in the affected limb is smaller in amplitude and delayed compared with the other side. Blood pressure is also reduced asymmetrically, although in most cases, the pulse asymmetry is more obvious (Caplan, 1993). As noted above, a supraclavicular bruit may be present.

Although TIAs compatible with vertebrobasilar ischemia occur in patients with subclavian steal syndrome, a posterior circulation stroke is rare (Baker et al., 1974). Caplan (1993) could find only two documented examples of serious brainstem or cerebellar infarction in patients with subclavian steal syndrome, and both strokes followed episodes of severe hypotension. Only one of the 10 patients with subclavian steal syndrome treated by Spetzler et al. (1987) had a fixed neurologic deficit: an ataxic gait. Hennerici et al. (1988a) followed 54 patients with subclavian steal syndrome but without previous neurologic symptoms for up to 7 years (mean, 45 months). During the period of follow-up, eight patients (15%) experienced one or more TIAs, and one patient suffered a hemispheric stroke. No patient in this group experienced a posterior circulation stroke. During this period, 11 of the 54 patients died. Death was caused by cardiac dysfunction in eight patients and by the effects of a massive hemispheric stroke in another. Hennerici et al. (1988a) emphasized that the subclavian steal syndrome should be considered a marker for atherosclerotic vascular disease in general, rather than an indicator of a patient's risk to develop subsequent ischemic cerebrovascular events from hemodynamic insufficiency in the affected territory. The findings of Moran et al. (1988) support this conclusion. These investigators followed 55 patients with subclavian steal syndrome for

1–6 years (mean, 4.1 years). During this period, although three patients died, and 10 patients had a hemisphere TIA or stroke, no patient experienced a stroke in the territory of the vertebrobasilar arterial system.

OCCLUSION OF THE INNOMINATE ARTERY (THE INNOMINATE STEAL SYNDROME)

The anterior counterpart of the subclavian steal syndrome results from occlusion of the proximal portion of the innominate artery. In this setting, the blood supply of the right arm originates not only from blood that flows from the left vertebral artery directly to the right vertebral artery at the junction of these two vessels but also from blood that flows in a normal fashion in the left carotid arterial system, crosses to the contralateral side via the circle of Willis, and then flows retrograde through the right internal and common carotid artery to reach the distal innominate artery and its peripheral branches (Fig. 55.228). Patients with this syndrome thus have a pattern of blood flow that may compromise intracranial structures normally supplied by both the basilar and the right internal carotid arterial systems (Newton and Wylie, 1964), producing neurologic symptoms and signs

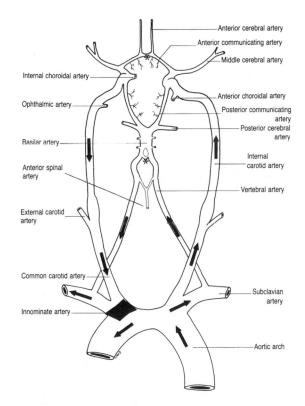

Figure 55.228. Pathophysiology of the innominate steal syndrome. There is occlusion of the proximal portion of the innominate artery. Blood flows from the aortic arch in normal fashion into the left subclavian, left common carotid, and left vertebral arteries (*arrows on the right*). Blood then crosses the midline at the junction of the vertebral arteries and through the anterior communicating artery (*asterisks*) and flows in retrograde fashion down the right vertebral and internal carotid/common carotid arteries (*arrows on the left*) to reach the distal portion of the innominate artery and its branches.

suggesting both carotid and vertebrobasilar disease. Blakemore et al. (1965) described a patient with occlusion of the innominate artery who had episodes of poor balance and blurred vision in the right eye during exercise of the right arm. These authors called this condition the **innominate steal syndrome**.

Patients with the innominate steal syndrome have reduced ocular blood flow and ophthalmic artery pressure on the right side. In such patients, the right eye may show ischemic changes ranging from mild stasis retinopathy to the complete ocular ischemic syndrome.

OCCLUSION OF THE INNOMINATE ARTERY AND THE LEFT SUBCLAVIAN ARTERY

Some patients have occlusion of both the innominate artery and the proximal portion of the left subclavian artery (Newton and Wylie, 1964). In such patients, blood flow to the head arrives exclusively via the left common carotid artery. The blood is then siphoned off to the distal portions of the right and left subclavian arteries by retrograde flow through the basilar and vertebral arteries and through the right common carotid artery (Fig. 55.229).

OCCLUSION OF MULTIPLE MAJOR BRANCHES OF THE AORTIC ARCH

Severe forms of the aortic arch syndrome are rare (Fig. 55.230), but they are of extreme importance because of the severe neurologic and visual symptoms and signs they produce. A variety of conditions can produce complete or nearly

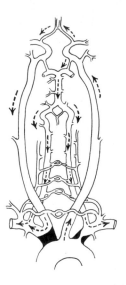

Figure 55.229. Collateral circulation in the combined left subclavian and innominate artery occlusion syndrome. Blood from the heart flows in normal fashion through the left carotid arterial system. Some blood then crosses the midline via the anterior communicating artery and proceeds in retrograde fashion down the right carotid arterial system to the distal innominate artery. Blood flow may also be directed from the left internal carotid artery into the left posterior communicating artery, down the basilar artery, and into both vertebral arteries. Retrograde flow in the vertebral arteries then supplies the left subclavian artery on the left and the innominate artery on the right. (From Newton TH, Wylie EJ. Collateral circulation associated with occlusiion of the proximal subclavian and innominate arteries. AJR *91*:394–405, 1964.)

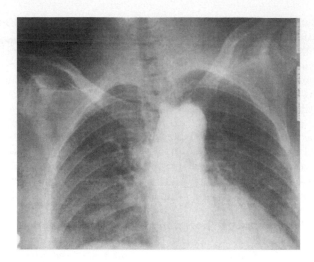

Figure 55.230. Aortogram shows complete occlusion of the major branches of the aortic arch. The patient complained mainly of recurrent episodes of monocular loss of vision.

complete occlusion of the aortic arch and its major branches. The most common cause, as might be expected, is severe atherosclerosis (Judge et al., 1962). Next in frequency are syphilitic aortitis, Takayasu's disease, congenital lesions, neoplastic occlusion, and embolism.

The complex patterns of collateral circulation around proximal obstructions of all the major trunks of the aortic arch defy detailed description. The head and upper extremities become mutually dependent on a diffuse, multichanneled thoracocervical network of small blood vessels containing a low-pressure pulseless blood column. Physiologic control mechanisms that normally insure adequate cerebral circulation are inactivated or greatly impaired. The large-caliber carotid, vertebral, and subclavian arteries distal to the aortic arch may act as interconnecting shunts, allowing blood to ebb and flow between the brachial and the cerebrovascular beds with changes in posture or extracerebral vascular demand.

Most of the protean symptoms and signs characteristic of the major aortic arch syndromes are caused by the drastically impaired blood flow to the head, neck, and upper extremities. Patients commonly experience claudication and paresthesias in the upper extremities after manual exercise, particularly arm raising (Jervell, 1954). Some patients complain of intermittent claudication in the jaw muscles when they attempt to eat food. This complaint may be mistaken for a symptom of giant cell arteritis (see Chapter 57). Neurologic symptoms, which emphasize the diffuse nature of the insufficiency, include syncope, transient paralysis, aphasia, dizziness, vertigo, and intractable headache.

Visual symptoms are the most constant clinical feature in patients with occlusion of the aortic arch and its major branches (Currier et al., 1954) (Fig. 55.230). These symptoms may be caused by insufficient blood flow in the carotid arterial circulation, vertebrobasilar arterial circulation, or both. Patients may have transient visual disturbances ranging from mild blurring of vision to complete loss of vision that may occur in one eye or both eyes simultaneously. When only one eye is affected, a disturbance in the carotid circulation is the cause; however, when both eyes lose vision simultaneously, either both carotid circulations or the vertebrobasilar circulation are at fault. In such cases, the pathophysiology of the visual loss may not be apparent unless the patient is examined during an episode. If the pupils are dilated and unreactive to light stimulation, anterior (carotid) circulation insufficiency is the cause, but if both pupils are reactive to light stimulation despite bilateral blindness, posterior (vertebrobasilar) insufficiency is the cause.

Frovig (1946) emphasized that monocular or bilateral loss of vision in patients with aortic arch disease may be related to physical activity. He called the phenomenon **visual claudication.** Shimizu and Sano (1951) also emphasized the relationship of visual loss and physical activity, but these investigators noted that the activity was often as seemingly insignificant as a change in posture, such as arising from a chair. Shimizu and Sano (1951) also noted that many patients with Takayasu's disease had a head posture characterized by flexion of the neck, because extension of the neck produced syncope, blindness, or both. They emphasized that transient monocular loss of vision was aggravated by wearing a necktie or a tight collar.

Some of the most prominent signs of a severe aortic arch syndrome are atrophy of the soft tissues of the face, disappearance of orbital fat, and wasting of the temporalis muscles. Heydenreich (1957) emphasized that many patients had a characteristic skeleton-head appearance that he called **Knochenschädel.** Other investigators described perforation of the nasal septum, ulceration of the palate, bleeding gums, loss of teeth, alopecia, trophic changes in the hands, and atrophy of arm muscles (Hirsch et al., 1964).

The early and late manifestations of chronically reduced orbital and ocular blood flow are described in detail in the earlier section in this chapter concerned with the ocular signs of carotid occlusive disease. Indeed, some of the most dramatic examples of chronic hypoxic ocular disease occur in patients with the major aortic arch syndromes (Font and Naumann, 1969; Kahn et al., 1986b). Some of these changes include retinal neovascularization, retinal detachment, retinal and vitreous hemorrhage, cataract, hypotony, and intractable neovascular glaucoma. A complete ocular ischemic syndrome is not uncommon (Brown, 1994b).

Tour and Hoyt (1959) described a 50-year-old woman with a history of syphilis treated by ''injections'' and a 3-year history of episodes of transient visual loss. The episodes, which occurred about every 3 weeks and lasted 5–10 minutes, were usually characterized by complete loss of vision, although sometimes vision was only blurred. The visual loss usually occurred only in the left eye, but it occasionally occurred just in the right eye, and sometimes it occurred in both eyes simultaneously. The episodes were never preceded by flashes of light or other aura, and initially they were not related to activity or time of day. The patient did, however, experience a dull bitemporal headache during some of the attacks. She also had three or four episodes of transient hemiplegia and a 3–4-minute episode of aphasia. About 3 months before the patient was first examined, her visual episodes became more frequent until they were occurring several

times a day. They were now precipitated by arising from bed quickly or from a chair. The patient also began to experience episodes of dizziness and giddiness.

During a general physical examination, neither radial nor carotid pulses were palpable on either side. The systolic blood pressure was 40 mm Hg in the right arm, 60 mm Hg in the left arm, and 140 mm Hg in both legs. A neurologic examination was normal. Ocular examination revealed visual acuity of 20/20 OU with normal central and peripheral visual fields in both eyes. The left pupil was larger than the right, and both pupils were nonreactive to light and accommodative stimuli. Extraocular movements were normal. Intraocular pressures were markedly reduced in both eyes. The pressure in the right eye was only 6 mm Hg; the pressure in the left eye was too low to be recorded. Ophthalmoscopic examination revealed markedly dilated retinal veins with peculiar segmentation in some areas in the midperiphery. The retinal arteries were irregular in caliber with areas of localized narrowing, but there were no aneurysmal dilations. The optic discs seemed normal, and there were no hemorrhages or exudates. Pulse pressure in the retinal arteries was almost nonexistent, and the entire arterial tree could be completely blanched by exerting minimal digital pressure on either globe. An arteriogram showed no filling of the innominate artery except for the first centimeter distal to its origin. There was also no filling of the proximal 4–5 cm of both common carotid arteries and the proximal one-third of both subclavian arteries (Fig. 55.230). There was delayed filling of the peripheral portions of the right carotid and both subclavian arteries, presumably via collateral channels.

The patient underwent surgery, at which time firm, localized obstructions could be palpated in the innominate, left carotid, and left subclavian arteries. A thromboendarterectomy of the innominate and left common carotid arteries was performed. At the conclusion of the procedure, a bounding pulse was present in the right brachial artery and in both carotid arteries. The patient recovered rapidly after surgery, and the visual and neurologic episodes did not recur. A postoperative ocular examination revealed that intraocular pressures had improved to 15 mm Hg in the right eye and 10 mm Hg in the left eye. The arterial circulation could no longer be occluded with light pressure on either globe. Pathologic examination of the material removed from the innominate artery showed a large, organized thrombus surrounded by a thin layer of intima with hyalinization and arteriosclerotic change.

DIAGNOSIS

In order to determine the natural history, appropriate treatment, and prognosis of patients with either transient or permanent symptoms and signs of ischemic cerebrovascular and ocular disease, it is essential to know the underlying cause (Caplan, 1988a; Cusimano and Ameli, 1989). A patient of any age who has transient monocular loss of vision and cardiac valvular disease requires a different treatment and has a much different prognosis than an elderly patient with the same symptom who has no evidence of heart disease but does have hypertension and stenosis or occlusion of the ipsilateral internal carotid artery, or a young patient also with the same symptom but with a history of migraine and no evidence of either carotid or cardiac disease.

A **history** from a patient with a presumed TIA or stroke must include the circumstances of onset, including activity being performed, physical position of the patient (i.e., lying down, standing, or sitting), quickness of development of symptoms, duration of symptoms, and a complete list of complaints. Most importantly, the physician must take the time to listen to what the patient says, as the history provides important information that will help define the pathophysiologic mechanism.

A complete family history should be obtained from any patient with presumed ischemic cerebrovascular disease. Such a history may contain significant information about hypertension, diabetes mellitus, cardiac disease, blood dyscrasias, or stroke.

A complete **physical examination** follows the history. In the general physical examination, the emphasis is directed toward detecting evidence of any pathologic condition in the cardiovascular system. The physician should pay attention to heart rate, rhythm, and sound. Blood pressure should be checked in both upper extremities. Peripheral pulses should be checked, and the patient should be examined for signs of congestive heart disease.

By definition, the neurologic examination will be normal in a patient after a TIA unless the patient has had a previous stroke or is having a TIA or stroke at the time of the examination. The examiner should pay particular attention to the patient's speech and use of language, ability to perform skilled hand movements, gait, and facial movement, all of which may reveal subtle defects. In a patient with a presumed stroke, specific combinations of neurologic signs—described in earlier sections of this chapter—will often help establish the site of the defect.

Auscultation of the cervical vessels may provide information concerning the pattern of blood flow and the presence of atherosclerotic disease (David et al., 1973; Wright, 1974; Kistler et al., 1978; Hurst et al., 1980; Kistler et al., 1984a; Ingall et al., 1989). David et al. (1973) found that only 14% of arteries over which bruits could be heard were angiographically normal in both asymptomatic patients and in patients with previous TIA. Indeed, over 50% of these vessels had more than 50% stenosis. Ingall et al. (1989) found angiographic evidence of ipsilateral extracranial carotid atherosclerosis in about 75% of patients with both symptomatic and asymptomatic cervical bruits. However, Sauve et al. (1994) found that one-third of patients with symptomatic carotid stenosis of greater than 70% had no bruits, making cervical bruits alone of poor predictive value in the selection of patients for angiography.

When listening for a bruit in the cervical region, the bell of the stethoscope is placed in the supraclavicular fossa, beginning in the region of the aortic valve and moved slowly upward. This progressive movement will help to distinguish transmitted cardiac sounds from bruits arising in the innominate, subclavian, common carotid, or internal carotid arteries (Allen and Mustian, 1962; Rennie et al., 1964; Sandok et

al., 1982; Chambers and Norris, 1985). Rigorous auscultation and palpation should be avoided, as there is a small but definite risk of precipitating carotid occlusion or embolization (Fig. 55.231). The patient should be examined in a sitting or lying position to reduce or eliminate any extraneous sounds related to an abnormal neck position. If respiratory sounds obscure auscultation, the patient should be asked to stop breathing for a few seconds. Most examiners grade bruits by loudness on a scale from 1 (barely audible) to 6 (loudest). The timing (systolic, diastolic, systolic-diastolic), duration (short, medium, long), quality (rough, soft, smooth), and pitch (high, low) should also be described, although there may be considerable disagreement among examiners in such descriptions (Chambers and Norris, 1985).

Some investigators suggest that because the appropriate treatment for some patients with asymptomatic carotid artery disease is still unclear and surgery of the carotid artery not without significant risk (see below), auscultation of the neck could subject a patient to an inappropriate health and cost risk (Kuller and Sutton, 1984). Furthermore, the bruit heard may reflect external or common, rather than internal, carotid artery disease and may simply be a marker of diffuse atherosclerotic disease. However, because patients with an asymptomatic bruit have a higher risk of stroke than do patients without a bruit, because patients with a history of TIA and a cervical bruit also have a significant risk of stroke, and because there is convincing evidence that patients with asymptomatic high-grade stenosis have a better prognosis after surgical intervention, it is reasonable for a patient and the patient's doctor to know whether or not a cervical bruit is present on one or both sides of the neck. The physician and the patient then can decide together the extent of further evaluation and the appropriate management of the patient's condition.

Auscultation of the eyes may provide information about blood flow in the carotid arterial system (Fisher, 1957). The patient is instructed to close both eyes, and the bell of the stethoscope is placed lightly over one of the eyes. The patient is then told to open the opposite eye and to stop breathing for a few moments. Hu et al. (1988) found that ocular bruits were the only auscultatory finding in 14 of 50 patients (28%) with confirmed atherosclerotic disease of the carotid arteries. An ocular bruit may suggest atherosclerotic disease of the carotid siphon, although it may also be a sign of an abnormal arterial-venous connection, such as a carotid-cavernous fistula (see Chapter 54).

As noted above, an **ophthalmologic examination** is often crucial in establishing a diagnosis of cerebrovascular disease. Of special significance are an abnormally low intraocular pressure or ocular pulse amplitude on one or both sides and a significant difference in intraocular pressures or pulses between the two eyes (Knox, 1973). Perkins (1985) found that an intraocular pressure of 10 mm Hg or less in one or both eyes or a difference of 3 mm Hg or more between the two eyes indicated reduced arterial flow to the eye with lower pressure, as did a difference between the two eyes in the size of the ocular pulse observed during routine tonometry. Ophthalmoscopy, in fact, may provide absolute evidence

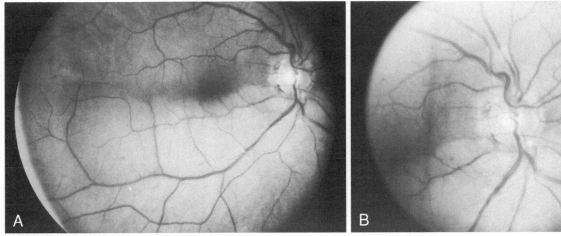

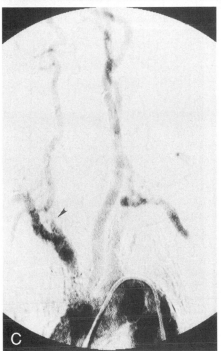

Figure 55.231. Branch retinal artery occlusion after carotid auscultation and palpation. The patient was a 59-year-old woman with coronary artery disease, mitral valve disease, and aortic insufficiency, who was admitted for elective mitral valve surgery. She also had a history of Hodgkin's disease, cured 30 years earlier with cobalt mantle irradiation. During the past year, she had experienced approximately 10 episodes of transient monocular visual loss in the right eye. The night before her surgery, her carotid arteries were auscultated and palpated by a cardiologist. Immediately thereafter, she complained of loss of vision in the superior portion of the visual field of the right eye. Visual acuity in the right eye was 20/40, and the visual field in that eye showed a superior altitudinal defect. *A* and *B*, An embolus is present in the proximal portion of the inferior branch artery of the right eye, and the inferior retina is edematous and white. *C*, An arch arteriogram reveals occlusion of the right common carotid artery at its origin (*arrow*), presumably a result of previous radiation combined with atherosclerotic disease. Palpation of the occluded carotid may have dislodged embolic material, a so-called stump embolus.(From Newman NJ. Evaluating the patient with transient monocular visual loss: The young versus the elderly. Ophthalmol Clin North Am 9:455–466, 1996.)

of vascular occlusive disease, particularly when emboli are identified in retinal arteries. In addition, retinal hemorrhage, soft exudates (cotton-wool spots), arterial narrowing, and venous stasis retinopathy (see above) may help establish a diagnosis of carotid arterial system disease. Fluorescein angiography may be used to document reduced ocular arterial blood flow, and it may also identify vascular disturbances of the retina and choroid that may not be apparent during ophthalmoscopy (David et al., 1961; Hollenhorst and Kearns, 1961; Pemberton and Britton, 1964; David et al., 1966; Choromokos et al., 1982; Rizzo, 1993).

When ischemic cerebrovascular disease is suspected from the results of a careful history and meticulous physical, neurologic, and ophthalmologic examinations, various tests may aid in establishing the diagnosis. In the following section on diagnostic techniques, we discuss: (*a*) imaging studies, (*b*) studies that measure cerebral blood flow or metabolism, (*c*) noninvasive tests of extracranial vascular anatomy and blood flow, (*d*) angiography, (*e*) tests of cardiac function, and (*f*) miscellaneous tests.

Imaging Studies

Brain imaging studies, particularly CT scanning and MR imaging, have revolutionized the diagnosis, if not the treatment, of stroke. These studies provide an excellent anatomic view of the various structures of the brain, and they are particularly useful in distinguishing ischemic from hemorrhagic stroke (Culebras et al., 1997; Saver et al., 1997).

Computed tomographic scanning has changed the study of cerebrovascular disease as it has the study of intracranial tumors (Kistler et al., 1975; Ringelstein et al., 1989; Caplan,

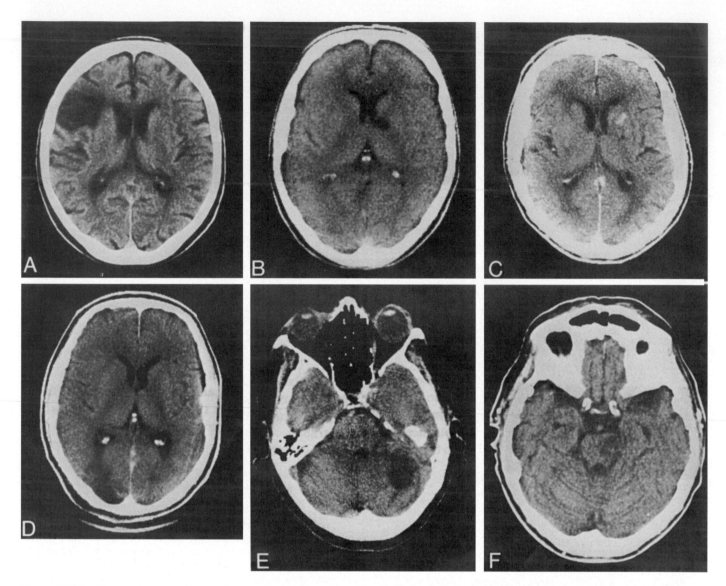

Figure 55.232. Computed tomographic scanning in patients with vasculopathic neurologic symptoms and signs. *A*, Axial view in patient with infarct in the territory of the middle cerebral artery. Note large area of low density. *B*, Small ischemic (lacunar) infarct affecting the internal capsule. *C*, Hemorrhagic infarct in the same location as *B*. *D*, Ischemic infarct in the territory of the posterior cerebral artery. *E*, Ischemic infarct in a cerebellar hemisphere. *F*, Infarct in the pons. The patient had an ipsilateral horizontal gaze paresis and facial weakness.

1993; Mohr et al., 1995; Davis and Newman, 1996) (Fig. 55.232). CT scanning can:

1. Confirm or exclude intracranial hemorrhage in a patient with a recent stroke;
2. Define the location, size, and mass effect of an intracranial hemorrhage;
3. Confirm or exclude a recent subarachnoid hemorrhage;
4. Directly image an intracranial aneurysm, AVM, or other abnormal vascular structure;
5. Define the vascular territory and size of an infarction, particularly when the infarct is within the cerebral hemisphere;
6. Detect unsuspected old or recent infarcts and hemorrhages;
7. Identify unsuspected nonvascular lesions, such as tumors or subdural hematomas;
8. Detect hydrocephalus;
9. Differentiate between an ischemic and a hemorrhagic stroke.

CT images obtained in patients during an acute infarction in the territory of the middle cerebral artery may be predictive of the ultimate size and severity of the infarction (Moulin et al., 1996). Early signs predictive of poor outcome include a hyperdense middle cerebral artery, early parenchymatous signs (specifically, attenuation of the lentiform nucleus, loss of the insular ribbon, and hemispheric sulcus effacement), and midline shift. Patients with asymptomatic stenosis of the carotid artery, transient monocular loss of vision, or TIAs have a high prevalence of asymptomatic cerebral infarction and cerebral atrophy on CT scanning (Goldenberg and Reisner, 1983; Calandre et al., 1984; Zukowski et al., 1984; Grigg et al., 1988), and patients with a history of a previous stroke often have a silent stroke elsewhere that can be identified by CT scanning (Grigg et al., 1988; Kase et al., 1988). CT is the imaging modality of choice in the critically ill or poorly cooperative patient, especially with the advent of fast techniques, such as spiral (also called helical) scanning (Davis and Newman, 1996). Spiral technology has also sparked a renewed interest in the use of CT for volumetric, dynamic, vascular, and cerebral perfusion imaging (see below).

There are, however, important limitations to conventional CT scanning. The CT scan may be normal in a patient with an acute infarction and of little help in patients experiencing TIAs, unless it identifies an unsuspected ''silent'' infarction.

In addition, CT scanning is not the optimum technique for imaging the structures in the posterior fossa, particularly the brainstem.

For patients with ischemic cerebrovascular disease, CT helps clarify the pathologic anatomy of the affected brain, but it is less helpful in determining the mechanism of TIA and stroke or the precise location and severity of an occlusive vascular lesion (Ringelstein et al., 1989). Overall, the usefulness of CT in an individual patient depends on two factors: the adequacy and completeness of available clinical data and the experience and neurologic sophistication of the physician caring for the patient (Caplan, 1993).

Magnetic resonance imaging provides superb axial, coronal, and sagittal views of the entire CNS. It is especially useful in imaging vascular and neural structures in the posterior fossa, particularly the cerebellum and brainstem (Pykett

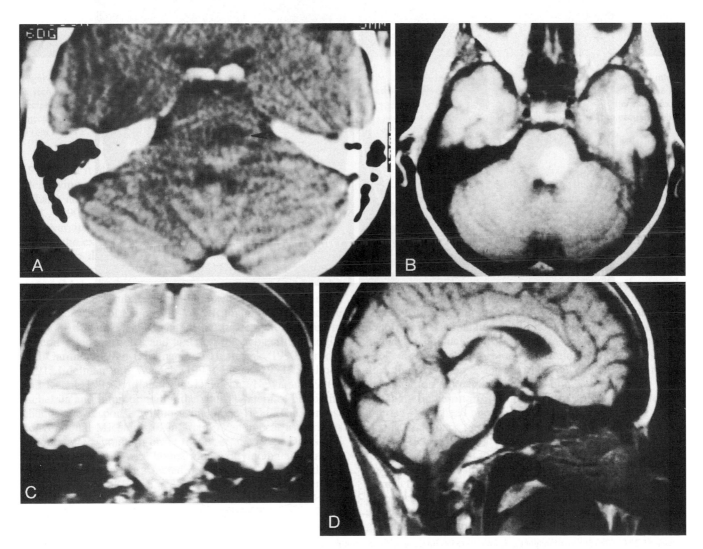

Figure 55.233.   Advantages of magnetic resonance imaging in localization of posterior fossa vascular lesions. The patient was a 47-year-old woman with acute onset of pontine signs and symptoms, including horizontal gaze paresis, facial paresis, and trigeminal sensory neuropathy. Her appearance is seen in Figure 58.220. *A*, CT scan, axial view, shows ill-defined lesion in the region of the pons (*arrowhead*). *B–D*, MR images show exact location of the lesion and identify it as a hemorrhagic infarct. *B*, Axial section; *C*, Coronal section; *D*, Sagittal section.

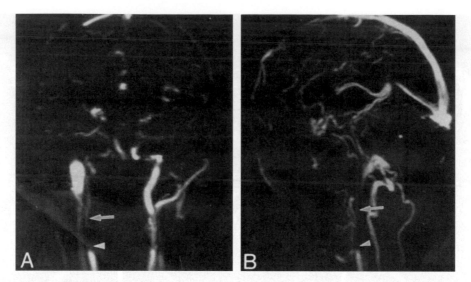

Figure 55.236. Magnetic resonance angiography showing stenosis of the right internal carotid artery. *A,* Coronal view shows region of stenosis (*arrowhead*). There is loss of distal signal for several centimeters because of complex patterns of flow in poststenotic segment (*arrow*). Flow can be detected distally, but it is not normal compared with the opposite side. *B,* Sagittal view of same patient also shows area of stenosis (*arrowhead*) and disordered poststenotic flow (*arrow*). MR angiography does not require the injection of intra-arterial or intravenous contrast material.

tion rather than simple imaging studies. These tests, which provide data about blood flow, brain metabolism, brain activity, and the blood-brain barrier, are described in the following section.

Tests That Measure Cerebral Blood Flow or Metabolism

In 1948, Kety and Schmidt devised a technique that measured average blood flow to the brain. The patient inhaled nitrous oxide, an inert gas, during which time samples of arterial blood going to the brain and jugular venous blood were analyzed for nitrous oxide concentration. Cerebral blood flow was then calculated from the difference in nitrous oxide concentration in arterial and venous blood during the 10-minute period of inhalation. Although this technique was used for many years, it was of limited usefulness because it was able to estimate only total or average blood flow to the brain; it provided no information regarding regional cerebral blood flow (rCBF). Ingvar and Lassen (1961) subsequently measured rCBF in humans by injecting radioactive isotopes into the extracranial vessels during angiography. Obrist and his colleagues (Obrist et al., 1967, 1975) introduced a method for measuring rCBF using inhaled xenon-133 and extracranial recording devices similar to those used by Ingvar and Lassen (1961). The **xenon inhalation technique** for measuring rCBF devised by Obrist et al. (1967, 1975) is safe and can be performed on multiple occasions, permitting sequential determinations in any patient. Unfortunately, the equipment needed to perform this study is expensive and cumbersome, and it is unclear the extent to which the technique is useful in the diagnosis and management of an individual stroke patient (Caplan, 1993).

Xenon-enhanced CT scanning is a technique in which a patient inhales xenon-133 during CT scanning (Gur et al.,

1982; Segawa et al., 1983). The xenon modifies or enhances the CT images, permitting visualization of relative blood flow in the regions imaged. Xenon inhalation can also be used in conjunction with SPECT scanning (Rootwelt et al., 1986; Delecluse et al., 1989; Kerty et al., 1989) (see below).

Positron emission tomographic scanning has revolutionized the study of cerebral blood flow and metabolism both in normal persons and in patients with cerebral ischemia (Kuhl et al., 1980; Ackerman et al., 1981; Baron et al., 1981; Phelps et al., 1982; Buonanno et al., 1983; Frackowiak and Wise, 1983; Martin and Raichle, 1983; Powers et al., 1984; Powers and Raichle, 1985; Frackowiak, 1986; Hennerici et al., 1988b; De Reuck, 1989; Powers et al., 1989a, 1989b; Sette et al., 1989; Yamauchi et al., 1990; Prichard and Brass, 1992; Sawle, 1995). PET scanning uses very expensive equipment capable of imaging positron particles. Positron-emitting radionuclides such as oxygen-15, fluorine-18, carbon-11, and nitrogen-13 can be synthesized by a cyclotron, attached (tagged) to physiologically active compounds, and given to a patient noninvasively at acceptably low doses of radiation. Two- or three-dimensional studies of the distribution of these radionuclides over time provide what might be called a physiologic or metabolic image of the brain. PET scanning can be used to study changes in rCBF and metabolism during various activities (e.g., eye movement, visual or auditory stimulation) in both normal and impaired subjects (Fig. 55.237). PET scanning has the potential to provide insight into the pathophysiology of acute stroke by providing information regarding the degree of hemodynamic and metabolic compromise. Unfortunately, the practical usefulness of PET scanning in patients with ischemic cerebrovascular disease is limited by the expense of the equipment and radionuclides, the extreme length of time required for testing, the cumulative radiation exposure, and the need for ancillary

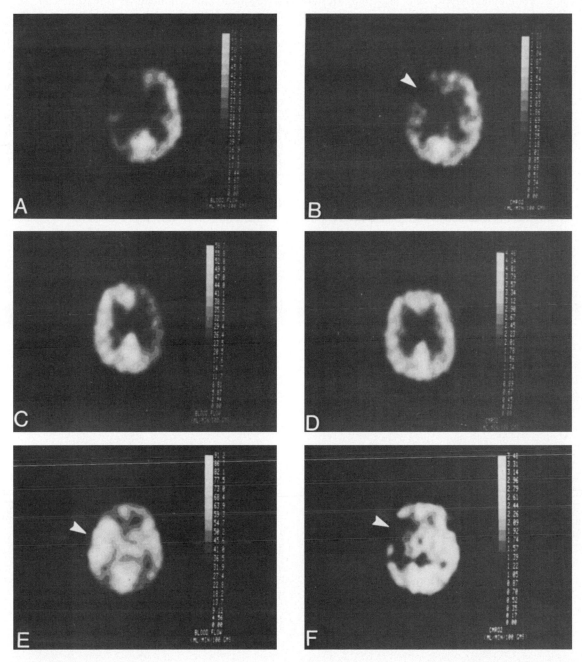

Figure 55.237. Positron emission tomography in patients with ischemic cerebrovascular disease. *A* and *B*, Axial images from a 53-year-old man who experienced a left frontal infarction about 5 months earlier. Within the region of the infarct, regional cerebral blood flow (*A*) and oxygen metabolism (*B*) are markedly decreased (*arrowheads*). *C* and *D*, Axial images from a 69-year-old man with occlusion of the right internal carotid artery who had experienced a right hemisphere TIA 6 weeks earlier. Regional blood flow is markedly decreased in the territory of the right middle cerebral artery (*C*), although oxygen metabolism is only slightly decreased. *E* and *F*, Axial images from a 55-year-old woman with occlusion of the right common carotid artery who experienced mild dysphasia during arteriography 7 days earlier. *E*, Cerebral blood flow is abnormally high in the left hemisphere (*arrowhead*), whereas it is normal in the right hemisphere. *F*, Metabolism is decreased in the left hemisphere (*arrowhead*). The increased flow in the left hemisphere is luxury perfusion in a 7-day-old infarct. (From Powers WJ, Raichle ME. Positron emission tomography in cerebrovascular disease. In Stroke: Pathophysiology, Diagnosis, and Management. Editors, Barnett HJM, Mohr JP, Stein BM, et al., Vol 1, pp 127–140. New York, Churchill Livingstone, 1986.)

physicists and chemists. Despite occasional clinical cases in which PET scanning has defined a brain lesion missed on conventional neuroimaging (Kiyosawa et al., 1996; Moster et al., 1996), this procedure is currently more useful as a research tool than as a practical diagnostic test in cerebrovascular disease (Caplan, 1993).

Single-photon emission computed tomographic scanning uses radionuclear camera equipment and does not require a cyclotron to generate the radionuclides (Stokely et al., 1980; Kuhl et al., 1982; Vorstrup et al., 1983; Ackerman, 1984; Hill et al., 1984; Hemmingsen et al., 1986; Chollet et al., 1989; Giubilei et al., 1990; Holman and Tumeh, 1990; Caplan, 1991b; Fayad and Brass, 1991; Prichard and Brass, 1992; Sawle, 1995; Report of the Therapeutics and Technology Assessment Subcommittee of the American Academy of Neurology, 1996). A flow tracer or a receptor-binding substance is tagged with a radionuclide and injected intravenously; the radiotracer is assumed to accumulate in different areas of the brain proportionately to the rate of regional cerebral perfusion. Computerized image reconstruction provides slices of radioactivity concentration in three planes, and abnormalities are revealed as regions of either low flow (hypoperfusion) or high flow (hyperperfusion). Hence, SPECT scanning can provide clinically useful information about brain perfusion with greater availability and at less cost than PET scanning, but the resolution, estimates of metabolic rates, and flexibility of application of SPECT scanning are less optimal than with PET scanning. Three brain perfusion radiopharmaceutical agents are used in SPECT scanning: iodine-123 *N*-isopropyl-p-iodoamphetamine, technetium-

99m hexamethylpropylenamine oxime, and ^{99m}Tc ethyl cysteinate dimer (Report of the Therapeutics and Technology Assessment Subcommittee of the American Academy of Neurology, 1996). Inhalation of the inert gas ^{133}Xe can also be used with SPECT scanning to study rCBF over time (Delecluse et al., 1989; Nabi Nemati, 1990). Other radiotracers can be used to determine biochemical interactions, such as receptor binding (Report of the Therapeutics and Technology Assessment Subcommittee of the American Academy of Neurology, 1996).

SPECT scanning, like PET scanning, is used primarily for research and in the occasional clinical setting in which conventional neuroimaging is unrevealing (Moster et al., 1996). It is not used routinely in the practical diagnosis and management of patients with known or suspected cerebrovascular disease (Rango et al., 1989; Holman and Tumeh, 1990; Caplan, 1991b). However, there are clinical settings in which functional imaging with SPECT may complement the anatomic imaging of standard CT or MR techniques (Report of the Therapeutics and Technology Assessment Subcommittee of the American Academy of Neurology, 1996) (Fig. 55.238). SPECT scanning is more sensitive in the early detection of acute ischemia than CT scanning or MR imaging. The pattern of radiotracer uptake may suggest the underlying stroke mechanism; i.e., embolic versus hemodynamically significant proximal large-vessel lesions. SPECT scanning of acute cerebral infarction in the patient in whom the causative vascular lesion has already been demonstrated by noninvasive techniques or conventional angiography may provide information regarding the ischemic penumbra and

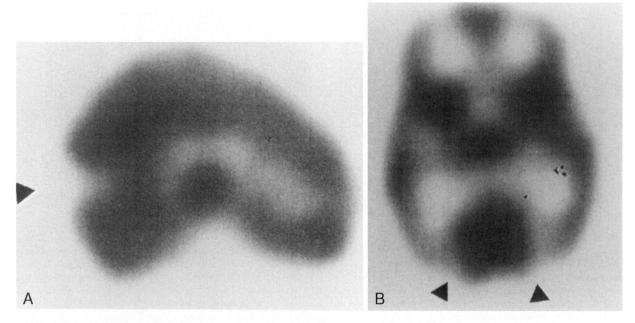

Figure 55.238.   Single-photon emission computed tomographic (SPECT) scan in a patient thought to have nonorganic visual loss demonstrates perfusion defects in the occipital regions bilaterally. The patient was a 20-year-old woman with carbon monoxide poisoning, who had bilateral homonymous congruous hemianopic central scotomas. CT scanning and MR imaging gave normal results. HMPAO-SPECT scan (*A*, Midsagittal; *B*, Axial) reveals decreased perfusion to the posterior portion of the occipital lobes bilaterally (*arrowheads*) (From Moster ML, Galetta SL, Schatz NJ. Physiologic functional imaging in ''functional'' visual loss. Surv Ophthalmol *40:*395–399, 1996.)

collateral flow, information that may aid in prognosis and therapy (Caplan, 1991b; Fayad and Brass, 1991). Some investigators believe that the extent and character of an abnormality on SPECT scanning can be used not only to predict the degree of neurologic recovery after stroke but also to determine which patients will develop a stroke after experiencing a TIA (Bushnell et al., 1989; Bogousslavsky et al., 1990; Giubilei et al., 1990).

MR imaging can be used to acquire functional information regarding various regions within the normal and diseased brain. Regional cerebral blood volume and flow can be demonstrated using diffusion, perfusion, and spectroscopy techniques (see above). Another MR technique that allows visualization of metabolic change within regions of the brain is **functional MR imaging** (Belliveau et al., 1991; Kaufman, 1994; Turner, 1994; Sawle, 1995). Functional MR imaging can be used to noninvasively map cerebral activation following a variety of stimuli. It is mostly an experimental tool, providing information regarding cerebral metabolism during normal human activity; however, clinical applications include surgical planning for treatment of seizure disorders and intracranial tumors, investigation of cognitive and psychiatric disorders, and monitoring the effects of drug therapy on brain function (Turner, 1994). Initial demonstrations of functional MR imaging in normal humans used the visual cortex, and abnormal responses were subsequently demonstrated in patients with homonymous hemianopia (Miki et al., 1996) (Fig. 55.239). The role of functional MR in the evaluation of patients with cerebrovascular disease has yet to be determined.

Noninvasive Tests of Extracranial Vascular Anatomy and Blood Flow

Diagnostic techniques for the evaluation of carotid and vertebrobasilar occlusive disease can be divided into noninvasive and invasive tests (Ackerman, 1979; Sanborn and Miller, 1980; Ackerman, 1983; Hershey et al., 1984; Kistler et al., 1984a; Becker and Burde, 1988; Duprez, 1989; Ackerman, 1995). Noninvasive tests are primarily useful in the diagnosis of carotid arterial system patency, but such techniques are also important in the evaluation of intracranial vascular patency of both the anterior and posterior circulations. Invasive tests are useful in patients with carotid artery disease, vertebrobasilar disease, or both.

In the sections that follow, noninvasive tests that specifically study the vascular anatomy and blood flow of the carotid arterial system are divided into two major groups: **direct** assessment of vascular anatomy, particularly at the carotid bifurcation, and **indirect** assessment of the hemodynamics of the internal carotid artery system distal to the bifurcation (Sandok, 1978; Ackerman, 1995). This is followed by a discussion of other noninvasive techniques, including transcranial Doppler, MRA, and spiral (dynamic) CT angiography, which have more broad cerebrovascular applications.

Direct Noninvasive Assessment of the Carotid Arterial System

Ultrasonography may be used to assess directly the patency of the carotid arterial system. Several types of ultraso-

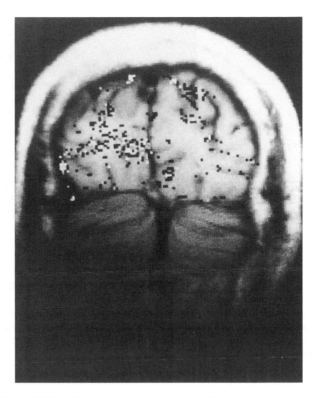

Figure 55.239. Functional magnetic resonance (MR) imaging in a patient with a complete right homonymous hemianopia. The MR image was obtained on a coronal slice, 8 mm rostral from the occipital pole along the calcarine fissure, in a 58-year-old man with a cerebral infarction causing a complete right homonymous hemianopia with macular splitting. An area of significant activation is observed predominantly on the right calcarine cortex (left side of photograph). (From Miki A, Nakajima T, Fujita M, et al. Functional magnetic resonance imaging in homonymous hemianopia. Am J Ophthalmol *121:*258–266, 1996.)

nographic instruments may be used (Ackerman, 1995). **Directional Doppler imaging** devices use a piezoelectric crystal that emits a high frequency ultrasound wave. When the transmitted ultrasound wave strikes a moving object such as a red blood cell within an artery or vein, a portion of the wave is reflected back toward the probe (Fig. 55.240). The reflected signal is detected by a receiving crystal and translated into an audible signal, the frequency of which is proportional to the velocity of flow of the red blood cells. The frequency of this reflected signal is either above or below the base frequency depending on whether the red blood cells are moving toward or away from the probe. A **continuous-wave Doppler** uses two piezoelectric crystals within the scanning probe. One is a sending crystal that transmits a continuous wave of high-frequency ultrasound into tissue. The other is a receiver that continuously detects reflected Doppler signals. A **pulsed Doppler** uses a single piezoelectric crystal that acts alternately as a sender and a receiver of ultrasonic waves. The crystal emits short bursts of high frequency ultrasound at very rapid intervals. By varying the time interval between the pulse of ultrasound and the time during which the crystal acts as a receiver, flow from varying

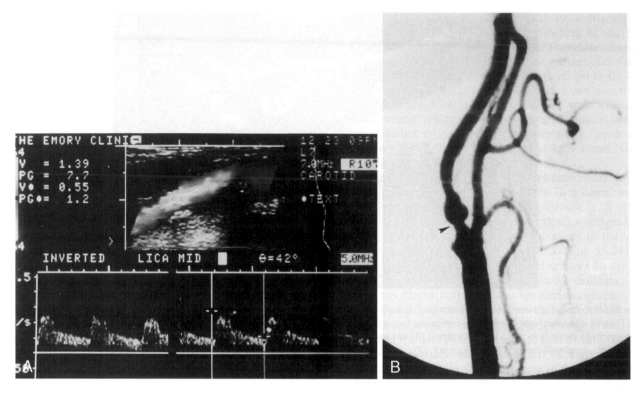

Figure 55.243. Duplex study of internal carotid artery stenosis compared with conventional arteriogram. *A*, Color Doppler display of the left internal carotid artery. *B*, Arteriogram from the same patient demonstrating the same stenotic segment (*arrowhead*). (Courtesy of Dr. William E. Torres.)

ing et al., 1996; Steinke et al., 1996). The power Doppler system generates images that resemble a map of the density and number of red blood cells in the vessels, without measuring the direction or velocity of blood flow. It may prove particularly helpful in the assessment of plaque morphology and the degree of carotid stenosis, although it is limited in assessing hemodynamics.

A number of difficulties limit the practical use and interpretation of tests using ultrasonography (Blackshear et al., 1980; Ackerman, 1983; Matsumoto and Rumwezzll, 1983; Zweibel et al., 1983; Bridgers, 1989). The instruments are expensive and their use requires carefully trained personnel. The tests take at least 40–60 minutes to perform. Interpretation relics heavily on the expertise of the person performing the test. The tests do not differentiate well between severe stenosis and occlusion of a common, internal, or external carotid artery (a limitation that may have significant implications for treatment). Some lesions are anatomically beyond the reach of the scanner, particularly when there is a high bifurcation of the common carotid artery. If there is calcium in a plaque, it may absorb the ultrasonic waves and degrade the image (Kistler et al., 1984a).

We agree with Becker and Burde (1988) that the best available noninvasive technique for routine detection of vascular abnormalities within the carotid arterial system is duplex scanning. It is an excellent way to identify hemodynamically significant lesions that may then be confirmed with angiography, and it is the only noninvasive test that can detect hemodynamically insignificant but potentially harm-

ful lesions, perhaps better than angiography (see also Goodson et al., 1987). Many investigators find that duplex scanning combined with one of the indirect noninvasive techniques (usually ocular pneumoplethysmography) increases the accuracy of diagnosis of carotid occlusive disease to over 95% (Lynch et al., 1981; Savino, 1989; Ackerman, 1995). Some investigators even argue that duplex scanning alone may be adequate for detection of surgically treatable carotid artery disease and that preoperative angiography is unnecessary (Ringelstein, 1995; Strandness, 1995). Others believe that the poor correlation between angiography and ultrasonography in some large studies performed at respected medical centers makes preoperative angiography essential (Barnett et al., 1995a; Eliasziw et al., 1995a; Hachinski, 1995; Srinivasan et al., 1995). As MR angiographic techniques are refined (see below), a combination of duplex scanning and MRA may preclude the need for conventional angiography, even when a potential surgical lesion is identified (Young et al., 1994; Blakeley et al., 1995; Kent et al., 1995; Patel et al., 1995). Kent et al. (1995) found that this combination of tests was associated with the lowest long-term morbidity and mortality and had the most favorable cost-effectiveness ratio for symptomatic patients with surgically amenable lesions.

Indirect Noninvasive Assessment of the Carotid Arterial System

Ophthalmodynamometry (ODM) is a noninvasive test that apparently measures pressure in the ophthalmic artery.

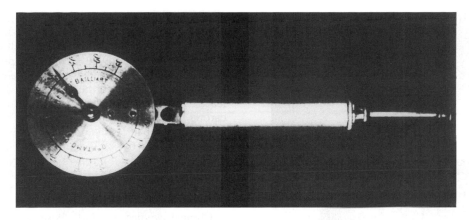

Figure 55.244. Baillart ophthalmodynamometer. Note the footplate that rests against the anesthethized eye at one end of the instrument and the gauge at other.

It determines the force applied to an eye that is necessary to raise intraocular pressure to a level at which the retinal arteries begin to pulsate and eventually collapse. The point at which the artery begins to pulsate is equivalent to systemic diastolic pressure, and the point at which retinal blood flow ceases is systolic pressure.

The technique and instrumentation for ODM were developed in 1906, but they were first popularized by Bailliart in 1917. Although Bailliart is frequently credited for having used ODM in patients with carotid artery disease, the relationship between ODM readings and carotid artery patency was not appreciated until 1936, when Baurmann first observed that ODM readings for an eye are decreased when the ipsilateral carotid artery is compressed. Subsequently, a number of investigators emphasized the importance of this technique in examining patients with carotid artery disease (Thomas and Petrohelos, 1953; Smith et al., 1959b; Kearns, 1979; Sanborn and Miller, 1980; Sanborn et al., 1981a).

The technique described by Bailliart (1917) is often called **compression ODM**, because the instrument used raises intra-ocular pressure by compressing the eye with a footplate attached to a gauge (Fig. 55.244). Compression ODM can be performed by one person, but it is more easily performed by two. When the test is performed by one person, the instrument is held against the eye with one hand, and the ocular fundus is viewed with a direct ophthalmoscope held with the other hand. This technique is quite cumbersome and difficult to master. When the test is performed by two persons, one person manipulates the ophthalmodynamometer, and the other person observes the ocular fundus using either a direct or an indirect ophthalmoscope (Hollenhorst, 1958; Smith, 1963, 1964; Sanborn et al., 1981a, 1981b) (Fig. 55.245). We prefer the two-person technique for its ease and accuracy.

In 1936, Kukan reported a technique for ODM in which the pressure applied to the eye is provided by the development of a vacuum rather than by compression. The vacuum is generated by a syringe attached to a suction cup placed at the limbus of the eye being tested. This technique, called **suction ODM**, was subsequently simplified to enable a single observer to observe and record both diastolic and systolic measurements (Linksz, 1942; Galin et al., 1969) (Fig. 55.246).

There are several theoretical advantages of suction ODM over compression ODM (Galin et al., 1969; Zaret et al., 1979). Suction ODM distorts the eye less than compression ODM, because the eye is not pushed into the orbit during the test. This may decrease the possibility of kinking or obstructing blood vessels in the orbit. In addition, the suction cup cannot slip off the sclera at higher pressures, as can the footplate of the compression ophthalmodynamometer. Finally, because the eye is not pushed into the orbit, patients are able to fixate a target more easily during the procedure.

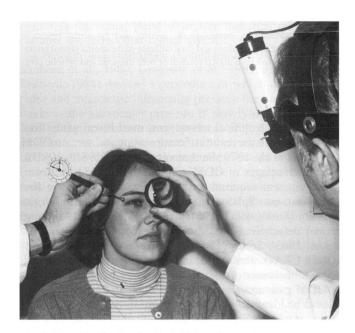

Figure 55.245. Two-person technique for compression ophthalmodynamometry. One person compresses the eye with the ophthalmodynamometer and reads the gauge. The second person observes the ocular fundus for initial pulsation (diastolic value) and final complete collapse (systolic value) of the central retinal artery.

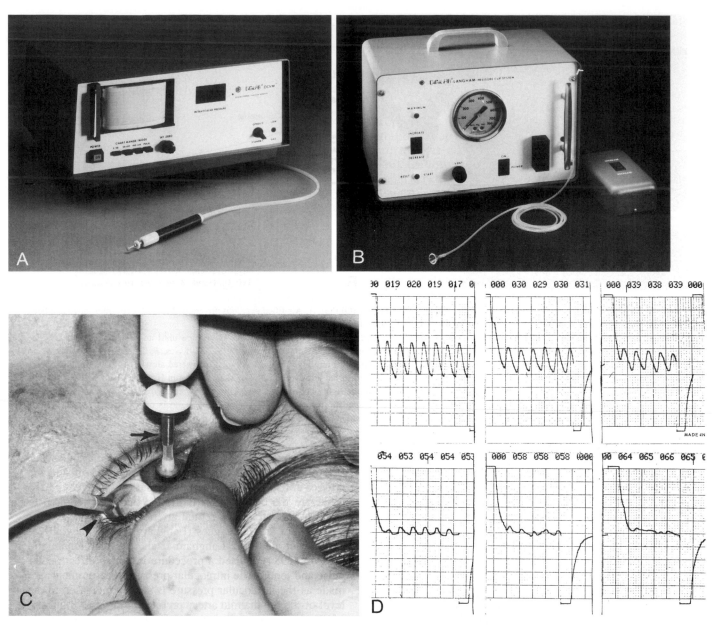

Figure 55.248. Oculocerebrovasculometry (OCVM). This technique uses a pneumotonometer to measure directly and simultaneously the intraocular pressure and the amplitude of the ocular pulse while intraocular pressure is gradually increased using an instrument that applies vacuum to the outside of the eye through a suction cup. The intraocular pressure is gradually increased until the ocular pulse disappears, and the relationship between the intraocular pressure at this point and the blood pressure is analyzed. *A,* Pneumotonometer used to measure the intraocular pressure and the amplitude of the ocular pulse. *B,* Instrument used to raise intraocular pressure. Note suction cup that attaches to outside of eye. *C,* Measurement of intraocular pressure and ocular pulse amplitude with pneumotonometer probe *(arrow)* as intraocular pressure is increased via vacuum applied through scleral suction cup *(arrowhead).* *D,* Series of simultaneous measurements of intraocular pressure and ocular pulse amplitude as the intraocular pressure is raised. Note digital readout of intraocular pressure average at top of each series of measurements. Also note gradual disappearance of ocular pulse as the intraocular pressure is raised from 19 mm Hg to 65 mm Hg.

Periorbital directional Doppler ultrasonography measures flow direction in the supratrochlear and supraorbital branches of the ophthalmic artery, thereby assessing changes in internal carotid artery flow and pressure (Ackerman, 1995). Reversal of flow in these arterial branches can be caused by lesions in any segment of the internal carotid ar-

tery, including the bifurcation, the siphon, and the ophthalmic artery. If there is disease in both the internal and external carotid arteries, the results may not be helpful. Operators must be skilled in performing this test for accurate results to be obtained.

Indirect tests that detect hemodynamic alterations cannot

be expected to be completely accurate in diagnosing carotid artery disease in view of the potential for hemodynamically insignificant lesions, such as ulcerated plaques, to produce significant transient and permanent neurologic and visual deficits (Moore and Hall, 1968; Maddison and Moore, 1969; Moore and Hall, 1970; Javid et al., 1971; Moore et al., 1978) as well as the tendency for significant collateral flow to develop in many patients with severe carotid artery disease. Other limitations of these tests are that: (*a*) patients must be fully cooperative; (*b*) the tests may not detect bilateral carotid arterial system disease; (*c*) the tests will not differentiate severe stenosis of the internal carotid artery from occlusion of that artery; (*d*) there may be wide variation in the results obtained by different examiners; (*e*) some of the tests that involve contact with the globe should not be performed or cannot be interpreted in patients with a variety of eye diseases, including conjunctivitis, glaucoma, acute retinal ischemia, and allergy to topical anesthetics, and in patients who have recently undergone eye surgery.

Indirect tests of carotid patency seem to provide reasona-ble diagnostic information when a stenosis of 60–75% is present, and such tests become quite accurate with a stenosis of 85–90% (Bone et al., 1981). With complete or nearly complete occlusion, the true-positive rate may be as high as 90–95% and the false-positive rate only 1–5% (Ackerman, 1979, 1983). Thus, if one simply is concerned about detecting high-grade carotid artery stenosis or occlusion, indirect tests that can be performed in the physician's office would seem to be appropriate (Strik, 1981). Almost all investigators agree, however, that indirect noninvasive studies should be combined with one or more direct studies, and that they cannot and should not replace arteriography in the diagnosis of carotid artery disease (Sanborn et al., 1980; Kapsch et al., 1981; Sanborn et al., 1981a, 1981b; Ackerman, 1995). We are not impressed with any major advantage of one indirect test over another.

Other Noninvasive Tests

Pulsed **transcranial Doppler** insonation of the intracerebral arteries is a method of indirect and direct noninvasive

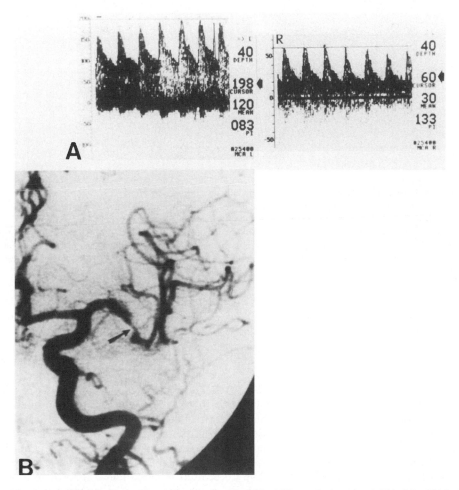

Figure 55.249. Transcranial Doppler findings in a patient with stenosis of the left middle cerebral artery. *A*, The right middle cerebral artery (*right*) is normal, with peak systolic velocity of 60 cm/s (*arrow*). The left middle cerebral artery (*left*) shows a peak systolic value of 198 cm/s (*arrow*). *B*, Conventional arteriography confirms a severe stenosis in the left middle cerebral artery (*arrow*). (From Ackerman RH. Neurovascular non-invasive evaluation. In Radiology. Editors, Taveras JM, Ferrucci JT, pp 1–28. Philadelphia, JB Lippincott, 1995.)

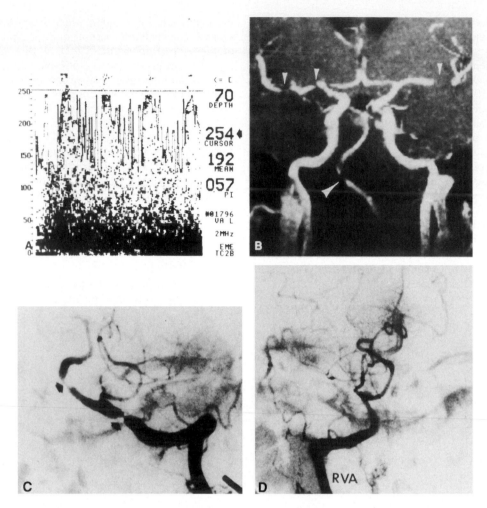

Figure 55.250. Markedly abnormal left vertebral artery transcranial Doppler findings (*A*) in a patient whose magnetic resonance angiogram (MRA) (*B*) showed vertebrobasilar-junction signal drop-out (*large arrowhead*) that initially was attributed to artifact. The transcranial Doppler tracing shows markedly increased velocities to 254 cm/s and severe turbulence. *C*, Conventional arteriography, performed because of the transcranial Doppler findings, confirms severe left vertebral artery stenoses (*arrows*). Although the transcranial Doppler found a normal right vertebral artery signal, the MRA (2D time-of-flight) failed to demonstrate the vessel, presumably because of slowed flow, because conventional arteriography (*D*) shows a normal right vertebral artery that ends as a posterior inferior cerebellar artery. The areas of signal drop-out in the middle cerebral arteries bilaterally (*B*, *upper arrowheads*) were normal by transcranial Doppler. (From Ackerman RH. Neurovascular non-invasive evaluation. In Radiology. Editors, Taveras JM, Ferrucci JT, pp 1–28. Philadelphia, JB Lippincott, 1995.)

investigation that may be helpful in both diagnosing and monitoring therapy in patients with stenosis or occlusion of extracranial or intracranial arteries (Aaslid et al., 1982; Arnolds and von Reutern, 1986; Aaslid, 1986; Becker and Burde, 1988; DeWitt and Wechsler, 1988; Zanette et al., 1989; Caplan et al., 1990b; Kelley et al., 1990; Norris, 1990; Tettenborn et al., 1990; Kushner et al., 1991; Babikian and Wechsler, 1993). In this procedure, the velocity of blood flow in the anterior, middle, and posterior cerebral arteries, and in the ophthalmic, vertebral, and basilar arteries is measured. There is a significant inverse correlation between blood flow in the ophthalmic, anterior cerebral, or middle cerebral arteries and the degree of internal carotid artery stenosis (Schneider et al., 1987; Kelley et al., 1990). A similar inverse correlation exists for posterior cerebral artery blood flow and vertebrobasilar stenosis. Severe stenosis or occlusion of intracranial arteries can also be demonstrated with this technique (Fig. 55.249). Directional Doppler testing at the occipital-nuchal junction near the atlas can detect a reversal of vertebral artery flow, thus indicating a low-pressure system in the vertebral arteries (Kaneda et al., 1978; Berguer et al., 1980). Continuous-wave Doppler analysis can also provide useful information about the patency of the extracranial and intracranial vertebral and basilar arteries (Fig. 55.250). The addition of an echocontrast agent can enhance image acquisition (Otis et al., 1995). Furthermore, transcranial Doppler can detect intracranial emboli and can be used as an indirect diagnostic test for paradoxical emboli in which air bubbles injected into the venous system are detected intracranially (see below). Finally, transcranial Doppler can be used in the direct detection of emboli within the intracranial vessels from more proximal sources, such as the internal carotid artery (i.e., during carotid endarterectomy) and the heart (i.e., during coronary artery bypass surgery).

Transcranial Doppler velocimetry has many advantages (Caplan et al., 1990b; Therapeutics and Technology Assessment Subcommittee, American Academy of Neurology, 1990). It is an effective, noninvasive test that uses small, portable, and relatively inexpensive equipment. The test can be repeated often and safely, thereby allowing detection of changes over time and after various physiologic, pharmacologic, and positional changes. It also can be used to monitor changes during surgery. The major disadvantage of transcranial Doppler velocimetry is that it is based upon the ability to find and identify a given vascular signal. It thus depends on the ability of the observer. The failure to detect a signal does not necessarily mean that the vessel is not present or patent.

As noted above, **magnetic resonance angiography** is a noninvasive technique for imaging vascular structures (Ross et al., 1989; Edelman et al., 1990a, 1990b; Keller and Drayer, 1992; Siebert et al., 1992; Pernicone et al., 1992; Anderson et al., 1993; Hamed et al., 1993; Potchen et al., 1993; Kaufman, 1994; Stock et al., 1995). Using this technique, the arterial or venous circulations can be selected and viewed in a variety of projections, without the need for intravenous contrast material. Stationary tissue signals from surrounding brain are decreased and moving tissue signals within the vessels are enhanced. A variety of MRA sequences can be applied, depending on the site and type of vascular pathology suspected. These include 2-dimensional or 3-dimensional time-of-flight and phase-contrast sequences. In time-of-flight imaging, T1-weighted brain anatomy is suppressed but is still detectable in the background, whereas phase-contrast images use a subtraction technique to remove essentially all signal from surrounding tissues. The advantage of 3-dimensional time-of-flight MRA is that signal loss from complex or nonlaminar flow is minimized. Its disadvantage is the loss of signal within longer blood vessels, a problem partially overcome by the use of the Multiple Overlapping Thin Slab Acquisition (MOTSA) technique (Blatter et al., 1992, 1993). Two-dimensional time-of-flight MRA is better able to detect slow flow and is less motion-sensitive. Phase-contrast MRA can quantify blood flow and differentiate recent clot from blood flow. Its disadvantage is that the blood velocities to be imaged must be preselected.

The advantage of MRA over conventional angiography is its noninvasive nature, its relatively rapid acquisition times, its ability to display the entire vascular anatomy in relation to the surrounding tissue, its ability to quantify flow, and its lack of reliance on skilled intervention (Fig. 55.251). It must be remembered, however, that MRA is not a simple display of vascular anatomy but rather an extrapolation of physiologic data obtained from the flow characteristics of protons to demonstrate vascular anatomy (Kaufman, 1994). Because of the physiology of blood flow, and particularly the laminar slow flow that typically occurs near the vessel walls, the diameter of blood vessels as shown on MRA may appear smaller than on contrast angiography (Fig. 55.252). Similarly, plaques and ulcerations may not be well visual-

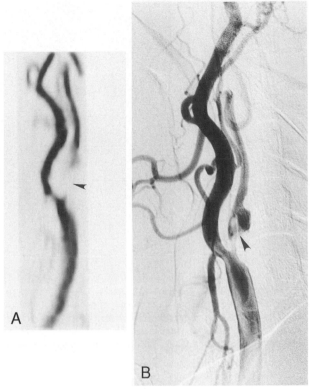

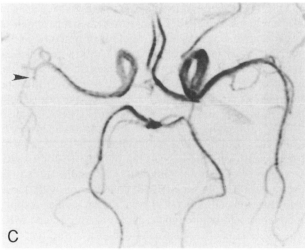

Figure 55.251. Magnetic resonance angiogram (MRA) of artery-to-artery embolus from internal carotid artery disease. The patient was a 49-year-old man who developed an acute left hemiparesis. Conventional MR imaging (not shown) showed ischemic changes in the distribution of the right middle cerebral artery. *A*, MRA (2D time-of-flight) of the right carotid bifurcation demonstrates a focal area of flow signal loss in the proximal internal carotid artery (*arrowhead*) with re-establishment of signal more distally indicating antegrade flow through high-grade stenosis. *B*, Conventional arteriography confirms the high-grade stenosis and also demonstrated a clot in the poststenotic segment (*arrowhead*). *C*, MRA (3D time-of-flight) of the circle of Willis demonstrates an abrupt cutoff of flow signal in the right proximal M2 segment of the middle cerebral artery (*arrowhead*), indicating embolic occlusion (Courtesy of Dr. Jay Cinnamon.)

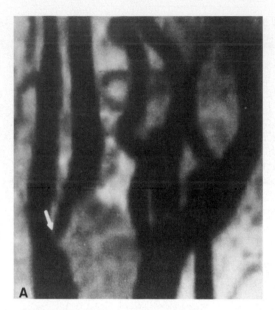
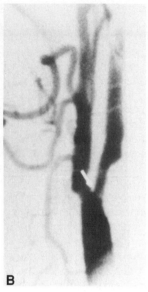

Figure 55.252.   Overestimation of the degree of stenosis in the internal carotid artery by magnetic resonance angiography (MRA). *A*, The MRA (2D time-of-flight) in this asymptomatic patient suggests a hairline residual lumen at the origin of the internal carotid artery (*arrow*). *B*, Intra-arterial digital subtraction arteriography shows a minimal area of stenosis (*arrow*). (From Ackerman RH. Neurovascular non-invasive evaluation. In Radiology. Editors, Taveras JM, Ferrucci JT, pp 1–28. Philadelphia, JB Lippincott, 1995.)

ized on MRA because of irregularities in flow that can occur in these regions. Hence, MRA may overestimate arterial stenosis and miss some vascular pathology of potential importance, especially in the evaluation of carotid artery disease. Nevertheless, MRA, using 3-dimensional time-of-flight combined with the MOTSA technique, is nearly 100% specific in detecting significant cervical carotid artery stenosis when the images are normal (Blatter et al., 1993; Mittle et al., 1994), although high degrees of carotid stenosis may be inaccurately read by MRA as showing complete occlusion, an important distinction given the indications for surgical intervention (see below). Although some studies already indicate a definite role for MRA in combination with duplex ultrasonography (Kent et al., 1995), further studies comparing conventional angiography, duplex scanning, and MRA for the evaluation of cervical carotid disease are needed (Mittle et al., 1994).

Another technique of vascular imaging is **spiral (dynamic) CT angiography** (Napel et al., 1992; Polacin et al., 1992; Schwartz et al., 1992; Bluemke and Chambers, 1995; Link et al., 1996). Advantages of spiral CT scanning over MRA include shorter examination times and true illustration of arterial caliber in stenotic regions. Maximum intensity projection CT angiography correlates well with conventional angiography in the depiction of both normal and abnormal carotid artery anatomy (Dillon et al., 1993; Marks et al., 1993; Leclerc et al., 1995) (Figs. 55.253 and 55.254). It also approaches the sensitivity of MRA for screening for intracranial vascular occlusive disease, although there may be some difficulty distinguishing the carotid siphon from the skull base (Katz et al., 1995).

Invasive Testing of Extracranial and Intracranial Vascular Disease: Angiography

Selective intra-arterial angiography remains the standard against which all other diagnostic tests of arterial patency and blood flow are judged (Kistler et al., 1984a; Cusimano and Ameli, 1989; Caplan and Wolpert, 1991; Barnett et al., 1995a). The preferred technique is by cannulation of the femoral artery and advancement of the catheter through the aortic arch and into the specific arteries to be studied. Contrast material is then injected under pressure into each of these arteries in turn. The entire cervical-cerebral circulation can be visualized with technically excellent films in almost every patient with this technique (Fig. 55.255).

This procedure is not without risk, however. The morbidity and mortality of conventional four-vessel angiography consists mainly of stroke, presumably caused by embolism or dye-induced vasospasm. Among large retrospective studies, the rate of permanent neurologic complications ranges from 0 to 5% (Kerber et al., 1978; Faught et al., 1979; Eisenberg et al., 1980; Earnest et al., 1983; Hankey et al., 1990; Heiserman et al., 1994), with a mortality rate of about 0.1% (Hankey et al., 1990). Some investigators believe that the risk is higher in elderly patients with substantial atheromatous disease who undergo longer procedures with greater volumes of radiographic contrast (Vitek, 1973; Faught et al., 1979; Heiserman et al., 1994), but Eisenberg et al. (1980) retrospectively evaluated 85 patients with angiographically demonstrable severe (more than 90%) stenosis of the internal carotid artery and found that **none** suffered either immediate or delayed complications from angiography. Other investigators also report that selective cerebral angiography is rela-

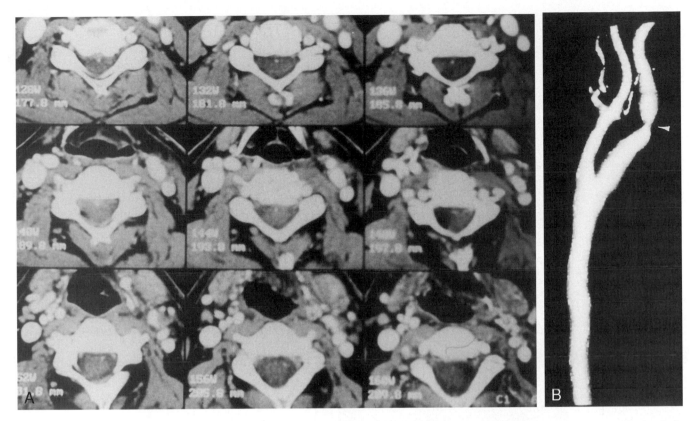

Figure 55.253. Spiral (dynamic) computed tomograhic (CT) angiography of a stenotic right internal carotid artery. *A*, Axial images acquired by standard CT imaging. *B*, Reformatted images show stenotic segment (*arrowhead*). (Courtesy of Dr. William E. Torres, M.D.)

tively safe in all settings when performed by experienced personnel (Robertson and Watridge, 1979; Buonanno and Toole, 1981; Heiserman et al., 1994). The risk of angiography obviously varies among institutions, depending on the experience and expertise of the angiographers (Gabrielsen, 1994). Although some institutions still perform angiography via direct needle puncture of the right brachial, left common carotid, or vertebral arteries, we do not believe that this technique is appropriate for most patients, nor do we advocate obtaining films that show only the cervical portion of the cerebral circulation.

Selective intra-arterial angiography not only allows quantification of the degree of extracranial stenosis but also demonstrates the degree of patency in the major vessels comprising the intracranial circulation (Gomensoro et al., 1973; Houser et al., 1974). On the other hand, angiography may have as low as a 50% accuracy in identifying small ulcerative plaques (Eikelboom et al., 1983b), and it thus may be less sensitive than real-time B-scan ultrasonography in detecting such lesions (Walsh et al., 1986).

Digital subtraction angiography (DSA) is performed with equipment that detects x-rays with an image-intensifying tube (Mistretta et al., 1981; Modic et al., 1982; Ackerman, 1983). The output of this tube is scanned with a video camera, and the video signal is logarithmically amplified and digitized for storage in the scanner. A computer is used for processing these data. Before contrast material is in-

jected, fluoroscopic images are obtained, converted to digital data, and stored in the computer memory. This image, in the form of digitized data, is subsequently subtracted from the images produced as contrast material passes through the region of interest. The resulting images are then viewed in real-time.

DSA can be performed by injecting iodinated contrast material into an arm vein in the anticubital fossa (intravenous DSA; IV-DSA) or by the same direct femoral approach used for conventional intra-arterial angiography (intra-arterial DSA; IA-DSA). Because of its many disadvantages, including a heavy volume load of contrast material risking renal failure and its relatively poor intracranial resolution, IV-DSA is used much less frequently than other forms of arteriography. On the other hand, IA-DSA is an excellent technique in evaluating patients with presumed extracranial and intracranial vascular disease (Brant-Zawadzki et al., 1983; Lipchik and Mewissen, 1990) (Fig. 55.256). The images produced using IA-DSA are equal in clarity to those obtained with conventional arteriography, although the spatial resolution is slightly less. The decision to use IA-DSA as opposed to conventional intra-arterial angiography thus is based on individual preferences. Either procedure may be appropriate in a particular patient.

Caplan (1993) emphasized several critical rules for angiography in patients with presumed ischemic cerebrovascular disease, the four most important are the following. First,

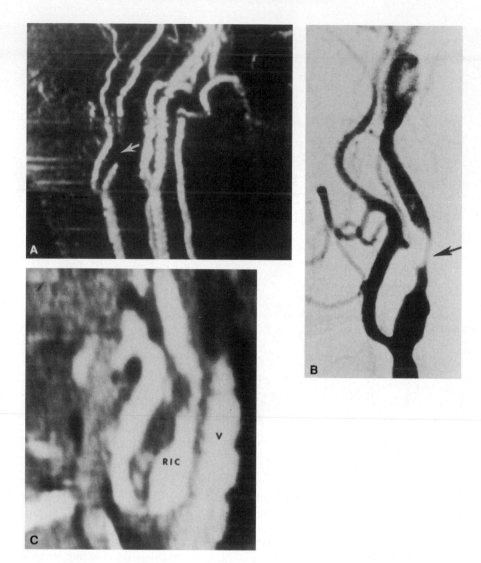

Figure 55.254. Correlation of magnetic resonance angiography (MRA)(*A*), conventional angiography (*B*), and spiral computed tomographic (CT) angiography (*C*). The patient was a 76-year-old man with an asymptomatic right carotid bruit in whom carotid Doppler studies were consistent with a residual lumen diameter of 1.75–2.0 mm in the right internal carotid artery (*RIC*), but indirect tests suggested a much more severe lesion in the carotid-ophthalmic system. To better document the severity of the bifurcation lesion and to assess for a siphon stenosis, MRA and then arteriography were done; an investigational spiral CT study was performed for correlative purposes. *A*, the MRA shows nonspecific signal drop-out in the proximal RIC (*arrow*). *B*, Conventional arteriography demonstrates a stenosis (*arrow*) that correlates with the Doppler estimate. *C*, The spiral CT images of the bifurcation correlate well with the findings on conventional arteriography. *V*, Jugular vein. Interestingly, MRA showed no evidence of stenosis of the carotid siphon, whereas conventional angiography showed tight stenosis. (From Ackerman RH. Neurovascular non-invasive evaluation. In Radiology. Editors, Taveras JM, Ferrucci JT, pp 1 –28. Philadelphia, JB Lippincott, 1995.)

tailor the procedure to the patient and the individual problem. Second, obtain information from the most critical area first. If a patient has clinical symptoms and signs of left internal carotid artery disease, this vessel should be studied first, so that if there are complications or other difficulties, the most important information has been obtained. Third, the clinician responsible for the patient and the angiographer should work together to determine the optimum procedure. Fourth, use the least amount of dye and the least number of injections that will provide sufficient information needed to determine optimum therapy.

Tests of Cardiac Function

Because cardiac disease plays a major role in the production of TIAs and stroke (Furlan, 1987), patients with symptoms and signs of ischemic cerebrovascular disease should be evaluated carefully for a possible cardiac disturbance (Sirna et al., 1990). In addition, numerous studies show that mortality from all forms of ischemic cerebrovascular disease is caused primarily from coronary artery disease (see below). The issue, therefore, is not whether to evaluate the heart, but how thoroughly (Cerebral Embolism Task Force, 1986a, 1986b; Sirna et al., 1990). An evaluation clearly begins with

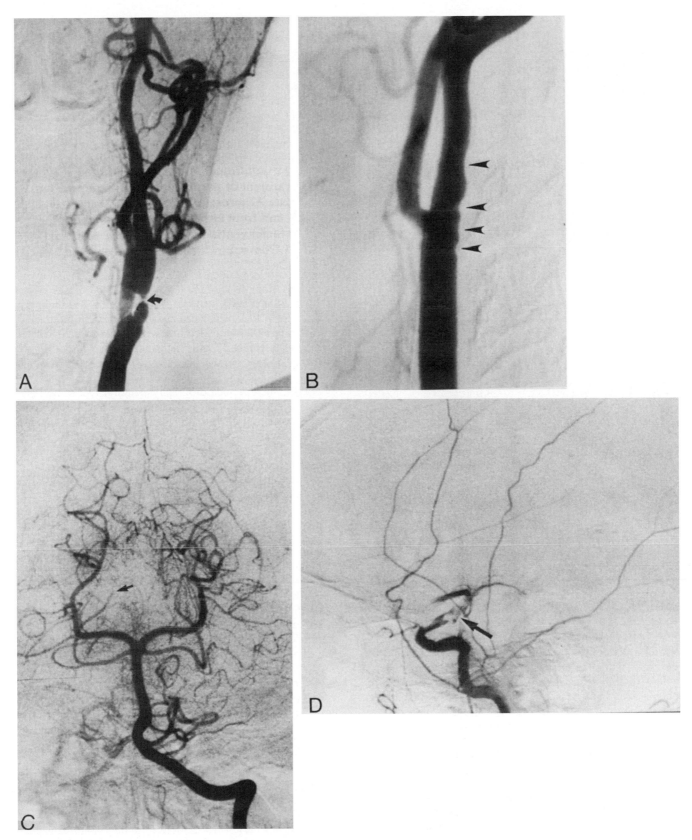

Figure 55.255. Cerebrovascular occlusive disease detected using conventional selective, intra-arterial, subtraction angiography. *A*, Severe stenosis just distal to the origin of the internal carotid artery (*arrow*) in a patient experiencing episodes of transient loss of vision in the ipsilateral eye. *B*, Multiple small ulcerative plaques (*arrowheads*) in the distal common and proximal internal carotid arteries in a patient experiencing TIAs affecting the contralateral arm and leg. *C*, Selective vertebral arteriogram shows embolic occlusion of the left superior cerebellar artery (*arrow*). *D*, Embolic occlusion of the internal carotid artery at the siphon (*arrow*).

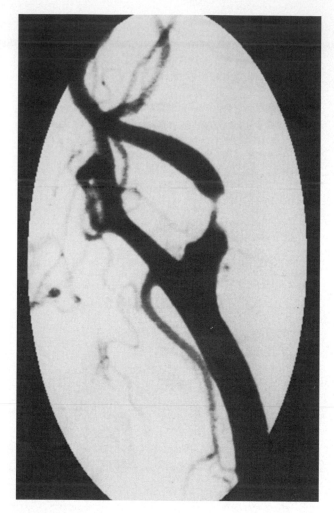

Figure 55.256. Intra-arterial digital subtraction angiography (IA-DSA). Severe stenosis of the right internal carotid artery at its origin in a 74-year-old woman with recurrent TIAs. Note that clarity of image is equal to that of conventional subtraction angiography, although spatial resolution is slightly less.

a careful **history** and **examination** performed by a cardiologist, internist, or family practioner. An **electrocardiogram** with a rhythm strip and a **chest x-ray** should probably be obtained routinely because of their low cost, safety, and high value as screening studies. A **Holter monitor**, a device that records the electrocardiogram over a 24-hour period, may be useful in those patients suspected of having intermittent arrhythmia. It should certainly be performed in any patient whose initial electrocardiogram suggests a rhythm disturbance.

Routine **transthoracic echocardiography** has a low yield in large, unselected series of stroke patients (Bergerson and Shah, 1981; Greenland et al., 1981; Larson et al., 1981; Lovett et al., 1981; Knopman et al., 1982; Come et al., 1983); however, two-dimensional echocardiography has a high yield in patients with ischemic stroke when there is: (*a*) known or suspected cardiac disease, particularly cardiac valvular disease; (*b*) a clinical course that suggests embolism;

(*c*) a history of peripheral embolism in the extremities, abdominal viscera, or both; or (*d*) absence of a clear thrombotic explanation for cerebral ischemia (Knopman et al., 1982; Caplan et al., 1983; Cerebral Embolism Task Force, 1989; Hofmann et al., 1990; Tegeler and Downes, 1991; Caplan, 1993). This last group of patients should not be overlooked. Young patients with no apparent reason for atherosclerosis may harbor unexpected cardiac sources of stroke, such as tumors, abnormal valves, right-to-left shunts through a PFO or cardiomyopathy. Other patients in whom intensive cardiac testing should be performed include those with findings highly suggestive of a more proximal source of embolus: (*a*) absence of extracranial vascular disease on noninvasive testing; (*b*) a superficial infarct on CT scanning or MR imaging in the distribution of a peripheral branch of the middle or posterior cerebral artery; (*c*) a neuroimaging study showing infarcts in multiple vascular territories; (*d*) normal arteriography in a patient whose clinical deficit and CT scanning or MR imaging are not consistent with lacunar infarction; or (*e*) arteriographic evidence of distal cutoff of a branch of a cerebral artery or a luminal filling defect without severe proximal stenosis or other vascular occlusive lesion (Caplan, 1993).

Transthoracic echocardiography cannot detect emboli that are very small, such as those occasionally seen in endocarditis and some mural thrombi, and those that have already left their cardiac place of origin (Caplan, 1991a). However, standard 2-dimensional transthoracic echocardiography is probably sufficient to detect most valvular lesions, large mural thrombi, and cardiac wall abnormalities (Fig. 55.97).

Transesophageal echocardiography, although more uncomfortable for the patient than transthoracic echocardiography, is more sensitive in detecting a PFO, atrial septal defect, cardiac aneurysm, subtle valvular lesions, and lesions of the proximal aorta (Hofmann et al., 1990; Cujec et al., 1991; Lee et al., 1991; Tegeler and Downes, 1991; Cabanes et al., 1993; Di Tullio et al., 1993; Amarenco et al., 1994; Comess et al., 1994; Hanna et al., 1994; Klotzsch et al., 1994; Daniel and Mugge, 1995; Leung et al., 1995; Mas et al., 1995; Ossemann et al., 1995; Di Tullio et al., 1996; French Study of Aortic Plaques in Stroke Group, 1996; Nighoghossian et al., 1996; Rauh et al., 1996; Stone et al., 1996) (Figs. 55.102, 55.106, and 55.257). In our experience, transthoracic echocardiography is sufficient as a screening test for a cardiac source of emboli in older patients with ischemic stroke who have no thrombotic explanation for cerebral ischemia. We reserve transesophageal echocardiography for patients at very high risk for cardiac embolism in whom transthoracic echocardiography was unrevealing and for young patients who have experienced a stroke without an obvious cause (Leung et al., 1995). In contrast, it is our experience that echocardiography, whether transthoracic or transesophageal, is of low yield in patients of any age with transient events and no permanent deficit. In particular, patients with transient monocular visual loss rarely have an underlying cardiac source.

Although transesophageal echocardiography is the "gold standard" for detecting a PFO, **transcranial Doppler sonography** after venous injection of an ultrasonic contrast

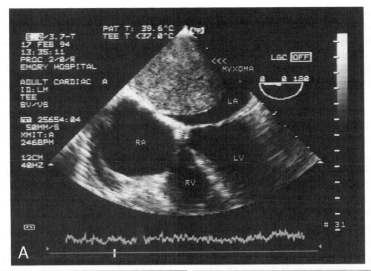

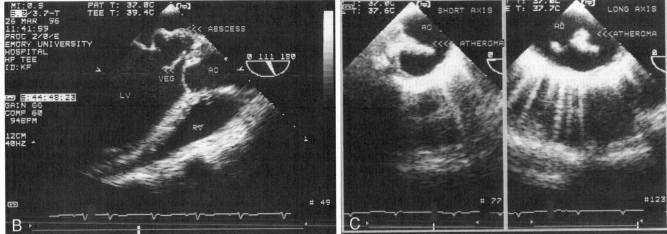

Figure 55.257. Transesophageal echocardiography. *A*, Left atrial myxoma. *B*, Aortic vegetation and abscess. *C*, Marked atheromatous disease in the thoracic aortic arch. *RA*, right atrium; *RV*, right ventricle; *LA*, left atrium; *LV*, left ventricle; *VEG*, vegetation; *AO*, aorta. (Courtesy of Dr. Randolph P. Martin.)

agent is also useful in the detection of right-to-left shunts (Chimowitz et al., 1991; Teague and Sharma, 1991; Di Tullio et al., 1993; Klotzsch et al., 1994). This technique is less costly, less invasive, and less sonographer-dependent than transesophageal echocardiography.

Miscellaneous Tests in Patients with Ischemic Cerebrovascular Disease

Thrombosis and embolism can be caused by a variety of disturbances detectable with routine screening of venous blood (Cusimano and Ameli, 1989). Although the yield from such studies is low (Rolak et al., 1990), the results, when abnormal, play a crucial role in the diagnosis and treatment of specific patients in the appropriate setting.

The level of the hematocrit clearly affects blood viscosity and the rheologic properties of blood. Fibrinogen also affects blood viscosity and is easily measured. Because thrombocytosis can cause abnormal clotting, a platelet count is an important test that should be performed in any patient with possible ischemic (or hemorrhagic) cerebrovascular disease (Mundall et al., 1972a, 1972b). Many patients without a high absolute platelet count nevertheless have increased platelet aggregability, often called the "sticky platelet syndrome." Tests of platelet function should be considered in patients with otherwise unexplained transient monocular visual loss, TIAs, or stroke, even when the platelet count is normal (Uchiyama et al., 1983). Assessment of protein C, protein S, and antithrombin III levels may prove informative. Tests for the Factor V Leiden mutation should also be performed. Immunoassay for antiphospholipid antibodies is also appropriate, because elevated concentrations of these antibodies are found in some patients with otherwise unexplained transient or permanent visual and neurologic vascular disturbances (see above). Such patients may subsequently be found to have cardiac valvular vegetations (Young et al., 1989).

Because vasculitis is a common cause of stroke, an eryth-

of stroke. The natural history of plaques has not been adequately studied; they may re-endothelialize and become less of a stroke risk. It is clear, however, that patients with ulcerated plaques and significant stenosis are at greater risk of stroke than those with plaques in a non-stenosed artery (Caplan, 1993; Hedera et al., 1996; Iannuzzi et al., 1995).

Prognosis of Patients with Transient Ischemic Attacks

The prognosis of a patient who experiences a TIA is directly related to the cause of the episode (Caplan, 1988a). Unfortunately, most articles that describe the prognosis of patients with TIAs do not identify the specific cause of the episode (Brust, 1977; Kistler et al., 1984a, 1984b; Warlow, 1984; Caplan, 1988a; Scheinberg, 1988; G. Howard et al., 1989; Sorensen et al., 1989). In such studies, the risk of stroke after TIA varies from 2 to 50%. This wide discrepancy results not only from patient classifications that overlook the different causes of TIAs but also from poor documentation of the severities and locations of causative atheromatous lesions and different durations of follow-up. Thus, some studies may have included patients whose neurologic symptoms resulted from seizures or the effects of migraine (Fisher, 1980; Cohen et al., 1984). Other studies fail to consider that the natural history of a single TIA caused by an embolus from the heart differs from that of recurrent, stereotyped TIAs associated with a tightly stenotic lesion at the origin of the internal carotid artery (Ziegler and Hassanein, 1973). Other problems in comparing studies of the natural history of patients with TIAs include: (a) differing age groups of patients studied; (b) variation in the temporal boundary between TIAs and subsequent stroke; (c) inclusion in some studies of patients with isolated vertigo; (d) inclusion in some studies of patients not only with previous TIAs but also with previous stroke leaving minimal neurologic residua; (e) differences among studies in referral patterns because some were hospital-based whereas others were community-based; and (f) the fact that some studies are retrospective, whereas others are prospective (Warlow, 1984).

Nevertheless, four results are possible in any patient who experiences a TIA (Committee on Health Care Issues, American Neurological Association, 1987; Becker and Burde, 1988):

1. No further TIAs will occur;
2. Further TIAs will occur without permanent neurologic sequelae;
3. A stroke will occur;
4. A major cardiac or other noncerebral vascular event will occur.

The risk of stroke in the normal population is about 1% or less per year (Cartlidge et al., 1977; Whisnant, 1983). After a TIA, the risk increases to 12–17% over the next 12 months (Whisnant, 1983; Trobe, 1987; Whisnant and Wiebers, 1987; Cusimano and Ameli, 1989; Hass et al., 1989; Dennis et al., 1990). Thereafter, the annual risk of stroke is about 3–6% (Heyman et al., 1974; Cartlidge et al., 1977; The Canadian Cooperative Study Group, 1978; Easton et

al., 1983; Whisnant, 1983; Heyman et al., 1984a; Trobe, 1987; Patterson, 1988; Sze et al., 1988; Sorensen et al., 1989; Dennis et al., 1990; Wilterdink and Easton, 1992). Multivariate analysis of data from the Dutch TIA study identified several independent risk factors for subsequent stroke, myocardial infarction or vascular death among TIA patients: age greater than 65 years, male sex, dysarthria, multiple attacks, diabetes, angina pectoris, intermittent claudication, CT evidence of any cerebral infarction, electrocardiographic evidence of an anteroseptal infarct, ST depression, left ventricular hypertrophy, or left atrial conduction delay (The Dutch TIA Trial Study Group, 1993; Pop et al., 1994). This trial also showed that 55% of the patients who experienced a recurrent ischemic stroke had infarctions in the same territory as their qualifying ischemic events (Cillessen et al., 1993). These recurrent infarctions from the same arterial lesion occurred sooner than strokes associated with other lesions. Patients with TIAs who have normal carotid angiograms still have an increased frequency of stroke when compared with the expected rate in the normal population (Marshall and Wilkinson, 1971).

Patients who experience one or more TIAs have an increased mortality rate compared with a normal age-matched population, although there is some evidence that this rate has decreased in recent years (G. Howard et al., 1989; Dennis et al., 1990). The 10-year survival rate in patients who experience one or more TIAs is only about 40%, compared with 60% in age-matched control subjects (Cartlidge et al., 1977). The annual mortality rate of patients with TIAs is about 6% per year (Whisnant et al., 1978; Heyden et al., 1980; Ramirez-Lassepas and Cipolle, 1988; Sorensen et al., 1989; Dennis et al., 1990). The vast majority of deaths after TIA result from cardiac dysfunction related to coronary artery disease rather than from the effects of stroke (Fields et al., 1970; Goldner et al., 1971; DeWeese et al., 1973; Whisnant et al., 1973; Heyman et al., 1974; Toole et al., 1975; Cartlidge et al., 1977; The Canadian Cooperative Study Group, 1978; Toole et al., 1978; Simonsen et al., 1981; Heyman et al., 1984a, 1984b; Cusimano and Ameli, 1989; Falke et al., 1989; Sorensen et al., 1989), and postmortem studies document the association of atherosclerosis in neck vessels with similar lesions in the coronary arteries (Young et al., 1960; Mitchell and Schwartz, 1962; Solberg et al., 1968).

Rokey et al. (1984) prospectively examined 50 consecutive patients with TIAs or mild stroke caused by atherosclerotic disease and found that 29 of the patients (58%) had significant coronary artery disease, compared with a 7% prevalence of coronary artery disease in other patients of similar age. This is particularly true in men and again emphasizes that cerebrovascular occlusive disease is a strong predictor of ischemic cardiac disease. Indeed, the mortality rate for patients with TIA exceeds by 2 1/2 times the annual mortality among patients without known heart disease and even exceeds the 3–4% annual mortality rate among patients with angina pectoris (Scheinberg, 1988).

The quality of life is significantly affected in patients who experience one or more TIAs, even when they do not experience a subsequent stroke or death. Sorensen et al. (1989) found that such patients had decreased capacity for work, general asthenia and fatigue, and impaired memory. Without a doubt, once a patient experiences a TIA and learns the significance of such an attack, his or her emotional and physical state can be profoundly affected even if he or she never experiences another ischemic event.

A number of investigators attempted to determine the natural history of patients with TIA related to proven atherosclerotic carotid artery disease. In a randomized United States cooperative study (Fields et al., 1977), 79 patients with TIAs in the distribution of the carotid arterial system and angiographically defined lesions of the appropriate carotid artery who did not undergo surgery had stroke after entry at a rate of slightly less than 6% per year for 3 years, after which the rate was less than 2% per year. In a Danish cooperative study, Sorensen et al. (1983) followed 102 patients who had experienced a TIA in the distribution of the carotid artery over a 25-month period, during which 11% suffered a stroke, and seven patients (7%) died, five from cardiac dysfunction and one from the effects of a stroke. Cote et al. (1983) followed 47 patients with occlusion of the internal carotid artery who either had experienced one or more TIAs without neurologic residua or had minor neurologic residua. During an average follow-up of 34.4 months, only seven patients (15%) experienced a stroke in the distribution of the occluded vessel. It must be noted, however, that this study excluded patients with coexisting conditions that might have caused the occlusion (e.g., patients with overt cardiogenic sources of emboli) and patients "likely to die from other illnesses within 12 months." Other studies report the annual combined risk of stroke, death, or both, in patients with angiographically or noninvasively proven carotid artery disease and TIAs in the appropriate distribution to be about 7–10% per year (Ruether and Dorndorf, 1978; The Canadian Cooperative Study Group, 1978; Whisnant and Wiebers, 1987). In the NASCET, the 2-year ipsilateral stroke rate in the medically treated group was 26% (North American Symptomatic Carotid Endarterectomy Trial Collaborators, 1991), whereas in the ECST, the 3-year ipilateral stroke rate in the medically treated group was 14% (European Carotid Surgery Trialists Collaborative Group, 1991). In both studies, the risk of subsequent stroke increased with the degree of ipsilateral carotid stenosis. In the NASCET, a silent infarction on CT scanning did not independently alter the prognosis for subsequent stroke (Eliasziw et al., 1995b). However, contralateral carotid artery stenosis increased the risk of ipsilateral stroke in patients with symptomatic severe stenosis (Gasecki et al., 1995). Indeed, the more severe the contralateral stenosis, the greater the risk of ipsilateral stroke (69.4% risk at 2 years if the contralateral internal carotid artery was occluded, 29.3% if the contralateral internal carotid artery had severe stenosis, and 26.2% if the contralateral internal carotid artery had mild-to-moderate stenosis). In addition, patients with significant carotid stenosis and recurrent ipsilateral ischemic events extending back more than 6 months are at more than twice the risk of stroke as those patients who are newly symptomatic (Paddock-Eliasziw et al., 1996).

The risk of stroke after a cardiogenic TIA is not known. Bogousslavsky et al. (1986c, 1986d) performed complete angiographic and cardiac evaluations on 205 patients who had experienced one or more TIAs. Six percent of these patients had an isolated potential cardiac source of emboli, and 19% had a potential cardiac source of emboli associated with carotid artery disease on the side corresponding to the TIA.

A number of investigators attempted to define the overall risk of stroke in patients with a variety of cardiac diseases (Mohr et al., 1978; Herman et al., 1982; Caplan et al., 1983; Cerebral Embolism Study Group, 1983; Chambers et al., 1983; Wolf et al., 1983a, 1983b; Cerebral Embolism Task Force, 1986a; Ramirez-Lassepas et al., 1987). The risk of stroke depends on the nature of the cardiac disease. Patients with chronic, nonrheumatic AF have a stroke risk of about 5% per year, whereas patients with a prosthetic heart valve have a risk of about 1–4% per year (Wolf et al., 1983b; Petersen, 1990). Patients with an acute myocardial infarction have a 3% risk of stroke over the first month, whereas patients with rheumatic heart disease (including AF) have a 20% stroke rate. It may be assumed that patients who experience a TIA caused by embolism from the heart have an even higher risk of stroke if no treatment is given.

Most of the discussion regarding prognosis in patients after a TIA refers primarily to TIAs that occur in the distribution of the carotid arterial system. Vertebrobasilar TIAs may be more benign than TIAs that occur in the distribution of the carotid arterial system. Marshall (1964) reported that patients who experienced vertebrobasilar TIAs had a better prognosis with respect to subsequent stroke and death than patients with carotid distribution TIAs, but he included patients with isolated, nonspecific symptoms such as vertigo in his series. Ziegler and Hassanein (1973) reported that three of 19 patients with carotid system TIAs experienced a stroke within 3 years of the onset of symptoms, whereas only three of 44 patients with vertebrobasilar TIA experienced a posterior circulation stroke over the same time period. The number of patients in this series is small, however, and the significance of the difference in stroke rate may therefore be questioned. In addition, the apparently favorable prognosis for patients with vertebrobasilar TIA may also reflect the inclusion of patients with isolated diplopia, dysphagia, vertigo, or numbness of the face. Using a more restricted definition of vertebrobasilar TIA, several investigators (Cartlidge et al., 1977; Whisnant et al., 1978; Heyman et al., 1984a) found **no difference** in the probability of stroke between patients with carotid TIA and patients with vertebrobasilar TIA. In addition, the frequency and causes of death in the two groups of patients were similar.

TIAs in young adults are generally believed to be benign, especially if the cause of the event remains unidentified (Ferro and Crespo, 1994). In one study of 13 patients aged 8 to 38 years who had suffered one or more transient attacks of bilateral blindness, often precipitated by exercise, stress, or postural change, none experienced a major vascular event during a mean follow-up of 10 years (Bower et al., 1994).

Prognosis of Patients with Transient Monocular Loss of Vision (Amaurosis Fugax)

The risk of permanent visual loss in patients who experience recurrent episodes of transient monocular loss of vision is unknown. Fisher (1951b) recorded permanent residual visual loss in 42% of 138 cases he collected from the literature; however, Marshall and Meadows (1968) described permanent visual loss in only nine of 80 patients (11%) during a follow-up period ranging from 3 months to more than 10 years, and the actual risk of a persistent visual deficit after an episode of transient visual loss in general may be as low as 3% per year (Editorial, 1982; Lethlean, 1983). We believe that the prevalence of persistent visual loss in patients after repeated episodes of monocular visual loss depends on the extent of the testing performed. The more extensive and sensitive the testing, the higher the percentage of patients likely to show persistent visual deficits.

Meaningful statistics concerning the systemic prognosis of patients with transient monocular visual loss are more sparse than those concerning patients with TIA. Retrospective studies of patients with transient monocular visual loss generally include patients studied for symptoms **in addition to visual loss** or for signs of carotid atheromatous disease, such as a cervical bruit. Such studies report an annual risk of stroke from 1 to 10% (David, 1977; Barnett, 1980; Parkin et al., 1982; Uggerhoj et al., 1983; Venables et al., 1984; Poole and Ross Russell, 1985; The Amaurosis Fugax Study Group, 1990; Wilterdink and Easton, 1992). On the other hand, patients with visual symptoms caused by vasospasm have an excellent visual and neurologic prognosis, even when the attacks occur at an advanced age (Cohen et al., 1984).

Retrospective data on the natural course of patients with retinal infarcts and emboli reveal an annual stroke rate of about 3%, compared with about 6% for patients with hemispheric TIAs (Liversedge and Smith, 1962; Lorentzen, 1969; Karjalainen, 1971; Pfaffenbach and Hollenhorst, 1973; Appen et al., 1975; Savino et al., 1977; Hankey et al., 1991). Few prospective studies, however, have addressed this subject. Marshall and Meadows (1968) performed a 6-year prospective follow-up of 80 patients, less than one-quarter of whom had undergone cerebral angiography. There was only a 1.4% annual incidence of stroke in this group. A study by Hurwitz et al. (1985) of 35 patients with transient monocular loss of vision **and** angiographic evidence of atheromatous ipsilateral carotid stenosis who were followed without treatment for an average of 7 years reported only four patients with stroke: an annual stroke rate of only 2%. Lemak et al. (1986) randomized 11 patients with isolated transient monocular loss of vision to the placebo arm of a controlled trial of aspirin. During a follow-up period of at least 6 months, five of the patients had an ''unfavorable'' response, indicating that they: (a) died, (b) survived but experienced a retinal or cerebral infarction during the period, or (c) had the same number or more episodes of transient monocular visual loss as they had experienced in the 3 months before randomization. Unfortunately, the specific nature of the ''unfavorable'' response was not stated for each case by these investigators. It therefore is impossible to know which of these five patients simply had further episodes of transient monocular loss of vision and which died or experienced a stroke. Using meta-analysis of a number of studies mostly from the 1980s, Wilterdink and Easton (1992) calculated an annual stroke rate of 2.2% for patients who experienced transient monocular blindness.

The best prospective data to date on this issue come from the subgroup analysis of the NASCET (North American Symptomatic Carotid Endarterectomy Trial Collaborators, 1991; Easton and Wilterdink, 1994; Streifler et al., 1995). In this study, the cumulative 2-year risk of stroke for patients with high-grade symptomatic carotid stenosis who were entered into the study with transient monocular visual loss was 17%, compared with 44% in those patients with hemispheric TIAs. The risk of ipsilateral stroke in patients with retinal TIAs increased in proportion to the degree of carotid stenosis: At 2 years, the risk of ipsilateral stroke was 11.2% in patients with 75% stenosis compared with 28.9% in patients with 95% stenosis (Streifler et al., 1995). Transient monocular visual loss alone was a predictor of comparatively good outcome with respect to subsequent stroke, myocardial infarction or vascular death in the Dutch TIA trial (The Dutch TIA Trial Study Group, 1993).

The discrepancy between the stroke rate in patients with ocular TIAs (i.e., transient monocular visual loss) and cerebral TIAs is bothersome. Both groups of patients have a similar prevalence of carotid atherosclerosis (Ramirez-Lassepas et al., 1973), although some of the clinical-angiographic studies that are said to show this did not, in fact, evaluate patients with isolated, transient monocular visual loss. In a study entitled ''Clinical-angiographic correlations in amaurosis fugax'' by Sandok et al. (1974), the authors stated that no patient underwent angiography for transient monocular visual loss alone. All patients had other symptoms in addition to transient visual loss or had signs of extracranial vascular disease such as an asymptomatic bruit. Nevertheless, Trobe (1987) suggested that the explanation for the difference in stroke rate between patients who experience transient monocular visual loss and those who experience a cerebral TIA may be that an ocular TIA occurs at a much lower threshold than a neurologic TIA. This may reflect a greater functional sensitivity to ischemia in ocular tissues and the smaller caliber of ocular vasculature. One must also be absolutely sure that the pathophysiology underlying an episode of transient monocular visual loss is indeed vascular and related to thromboembolic disease.

The mortality rate in patients with transient monocular loss of vision, like the stroke rate, is somewhat unclear. According to Marshall and Meadows (1968), patients with transient monocular visual loss have an increased risk of death compared with a normal age- and sex-matched population. Death usually results not from the effects of stroke but rather from coronary artery disease or other cardiac dysfunction, just as it does in patients with asymptomatic cervical bruits, asymptomatic carotid artery stenosis, and recurrent TIAs (Heyman et al., 1984b). The risk of myocardial infarction in patients who have transient monocular visual loss is about 30% over the 5 years following the first episode (Hurwitz et al., 1985), and the mortality rate during this period is 18% (Poole and Ross Russell, 1985).

Savino et al. (1977) concluded that patients with visible retinal emboli, presumably originating from the heart or the great vessels, had a mortality rate that was four to five times greater than that of an age- and sex-matched control population without visible emboli, even when the emboli were asymptomatic. Patients who experienced a retinal stroke but in whom a retinal embolus was not seen had a mortality rate similar to that of the control population. The implication of this study is that patients with visible emboli in retinal vessels have absolute evidence of atherosclerotic disease affecting the heart, great vessels, carotid arteries, or a combination of these. Such patients thus share the same increased mortality rate as patients who have asymptomatic bruits, asymptomatic carotid artery disease, or neurologic TIAs in the setting of atherosclerotic disease. On the other hand, patients with central or branch artery occlusions, but without visible emboli, constitute a nonspecific group of patients. Some have diffuse atherosclerotic disease, whereas others have localized atherosclerotic disease, vasospastic disease, or other disorders associated with a lower risk of death.

Prognosis of Patients After Initial Stroke

Acute Mortality

Although stroke is the third most common cause of death in most developed countries, the acute mortality from an initial stroke has been falling rapidly in the United States since 1950 (Acheson, 1966; Kuller et al., 1970; Soltero et al., 1978; Anderson and Whisnant, 1982; Whisnant, 1983; Shahar et al., 1995). Between the years 1950 and 1973, stroke mortality decreased by about 2% per year. Since 1973, stroke mortality has decreased by about 5–7% per year (Klag et al., 1989; Bonita et al., 1990; Shahar et al., 1995). In 1985, the stroke mortality for all patients in the United States was only 0.045% for men and 0.035% for women (Bonita et al., 1990) compared with 0.2% in 1981 and 0.5% in 1950 (Klag et al., 1989). Subsequent studies show a continued trend in improved survival of stroke patients (Shahar et al., 1995). This reduction in stroke mortality is probably related to a variety of factors. Although a declining incidence in stroke numbers probably contributed to the decline in stroke mortality during the 1970s and earlier, other factors, including better transportation services to local hospitals, an increase in the number of intensive care units available to monitor and treat patients who experience an acute stroke, improved monitoring devices, and more active treatment of stroke patients are responsible for the continued decline of stroke mortality (Whisnant, 1983; Shahar et al., 1995).

The acute mortality rate for an **individual** patient who has a stroke varies with the nature and severity of the stroke and is also dependent on other factors. Factors determining survival in the short-term (less than 30-day) period include depressed consciousness on admission, conjugate gaze paresis, extremity weakness, earlier deterioration, advanced age, and heart disease (Oxbury et al., 1975; Chambers et al., 1987; Bonita et al., 1988; Spitzer et al., 1989; Fiorelli et al., 1995; Toni et al., 1995). The best predictive model of short-term survival in the series by Chambers et al. (1987) used only three variables: level of consciousness, leg weakness, and age.

Within the first 2 weeks after a stroke, death usually results from cerebral edema, transtentorial herniation, or severe brainstem dysfunction (Whisnant et al., 1971; Norris et al., 1984; Chambers et al., 1987). After 2 weeks, death usually results from cardiac or pulmonary complications of the stroke. Obviously, it is crucial to try to reduce the medical complications of acute stroke, including pulmonary embolism, aspiration pneumonia, urinary tract infections, etc. (Caplan, 1993).

Macdonell et al. (1987) compared the short-term mortality rates in patients with ischemic stroke in various locations. These investigators concluded that the short-term (less than 1 month) mortality rate was lowest for patients who had a lacunar stroke (1.2%) and highest for patients who had a cerebellar infarction (23%). In this study, the acute mortality from a hemisphere or brainstem stroke was 13–17%. Other investigators reported similar findings. Chambers et al. (1987) found that patients with acute, ischemic, carotid territory stroke had a 17% mortality rate within the first 30 days, and patients with acute, ischemic, vertebrobasilar territory stroke had an 18% mortality within this same period of time.

Long-Term Mortality

Patients who survive the initial effects of a stroke nevertheless have a substantially increased mortality after the event. The mortality rate for patients who survive an acute, ischemic stroke is about 5–10% per year, regardless of the cause or the location of the stroke (Norris et al., 1984; Nicholls et al., 1986; Cote and Caron, 1989). Sacco et al. (1989c) reported that of 335 patients who survived at least 30 days after an initial stroke, 37 (11%) died within 1 year. Factors that adversely affect long-term mortality in stroke patients include level of activity at time of discharge, number of neurologic deficits at stroke onset, advanced age, concomitant cardiac disease, and diabetes mellitus (Chambers et al., 1987; Sacco et al., 1989; Lai et al., 1995). In addition, men have a higher mortality rate after stroke than women. Heart disease is the cause of the majority of deaths in patients who survive an initial stroke (Whisnant et al., 1971).

Risk of Subsequent Stroke

The risk of subsequent stroke in a patient who has already had a stroke is much higher than for an otherwise normal person. Sacco et al. (1989c) reported that of 335 patients who survived at least 30 days after an initial stroke, 20 (6%) experienced a second stroke within 1 year. Sacco et al. (1989d) subsequently reported that the risk for recurrent stroke within 30 days after initial stroke was greatest for atherothrombotic infarction (about 8%) and least for lacunar infarction (about 2%). These investigators found that patients with cardiogenic embolic stroke had a stroke rate of about 4% during the month after the initial stroke. These statistics are consistent with the findings of other investigators that the risk of subsequent stroke in a patient who suffers an initial stroke is 3–9% per year, regardless of cause (Sacquegna et al., 1982; Nicholls et al., 1986; Sze et al., 1988; Flegel and Hanley, 1989; Wilterdink and Easton, 1992; Jorgensen et al., 1997). This stroke rate is somewhat higher than for patients who have experienced one or more TIAs (Wilterdink and Easton, 1992).

The risk factors for recurrent stroke are the same as those for an initial stroke. These include systemic hypertension, diabetes mellitus, coronary artery disease, myocardial infarction, AF, cigarette smoking, alcohol abuse, obesity, and advanced age (Alter et al., 1987; Sacco et al., 1989d; van Latum et al., 1995; Jorgensen et al., 1997). Davis et al. (1996) reported that risk factors among 143 patients with acute stroke who had previous silent cerebral infarctions on CT scanning included advanced age, male sex, African-American race, and hypertension. Stroke in young adults is generally believed to be benign, with a low acute mortality and few recurrent strokes (Ferro and Crespo, 1994).

Functional Status

Most patients who survive an acute stroke eventually experience some improvement in neurologic status. Improvement usually begins within 3 weeks to 6 months after the stroke, with the extent of recovery being dependent on a number of variables, including age, associated illnesses such as diabetes mellitus and previous myocardial infarction, and the severity of the initial neurologic dysfunction, particularly the degree of motor loss (McDowell and Louis, 1971; Wade and Hewer, 1987; Lincoln et al., 1989; Shah et al., 1989, 1990; Skyhoj Olsen, 1990). About 60–75% of stroke survivors eventually become totally independent, and only 3–9% remain totally dependent on assisted care (Gresham et al., 1979; Weddell and Beresford, 1979; Aho et al., 1980; Sorensen et al., 1982; Wade and Hewer, 1987). Factors compromising functional independence include urinary incontinence, advanced age, perceptual difficulties, severe loss of motor function, and poststroke depression (Feigenson et al., 1977; Andrews et al., 1982; Prescott et al., 1982; Wade et al., 1983, 1984; Lincoln et al., 1989; Shah et al., 1989; Parikh et al., 1990; Shah et al., 1990). Most of these factors cannot be modified; however, the early recognition and treatment of poststroke depression may substantially improve eventual functional outcome (Parikh et al., 1980).

Although it is generally believed that the functional outcome in young patients with stroke is better than in the elderly population, some statistics on this issue are quite sobering. In one long-term follow-up study of ischemic stroke patients ages 15 to 45 years, only 49% of 296 patients were still alive, were not disabled, had not experienced recurrent vascular events, and had not undergone major vascular surgery (Kappelle et al., 1994). Only 42% of the survivors had returned to work, and the majority of survivors reported emotional, social, or physical sequelae that lessened their quality of life.

Norris et al. (1984) found that 1 year after a stroke, patients who survived an ischemic stroke had significantly better neurologic function than did patients who survived a hemorrhagic stroke. In addition, patients who survived an ischemic stroke in the vertebrobasilar arterial system had significantly better neurologic function than did patients who survived an ischemic stroke in the carotid arterial system (p < 0.005). The difference in the neurologic status between these two groups of patients was said by Norris et al. (1984) to be even more striking at 5 years, but it was statistically insignificant because the number of patients was small. The superior outcome of patients with vertebrobasilar territory stroke in this study did not seem to be related to differences in risk factors. Preliminary analysis of these patients showed no striking difference between groups for age, sex, hypertension, diabetes mellitus, cardiac disease, or peripheral vascular disease. Instead, the one factor that correlated with improved outcome was the severity of initial neurologic disability, which was significantly less in patients with vertebrobasilar stroke than in patients with carotid territory stroke in this series. It is unclear whether or not comprehensive inpatient or outpatient rehabilitation significantly improves eventual neurologic status after an ischemic or hemorrhagic stroke (see below).

MANAGEMENT

No area of medicine is more controversial than the management of patients with ischemic cerebrovascular disease (Scheinberg, 1988; Fisher, 1989). Enormous progress has been made in the understanding of the pathophysiology of cerebrovascular disease, identification of types and causes of strokes, recognition of stroke risk factors, neuroimaging and cerebral blood flow techniques, and medical and surgical treatment (WHO/MNH Task Force on Stroke and Other Cerebrovascular Disorders, 1989; Barnett et al., 1995b). Nevertheless, differences of opinion remain with regard to the interpretation of many important studies and extant data, and there is no consensus regarding stroke prophylaxis or treatment. This unsettled state is partly related to the expense and difficulty of required studies. Many published studies are inadequately controlled, or they are not controlled at all. Such studies are often largely retrospective and based on the personal beliefs of the investigators. They have little or no usefulness. Even studies that are planned according to "state of the art" statistical and epidemiologic guidelines may be flawed in execution if personal bias is allowed to interfere with study protocol (Marshall, 1990). Nevertheless, we agree with Barnett (1990) and Hachinski (1990) that controlled clinical trials offer the best chance of determining the appropriate means to prevent and treat ischemic cerebrovascular disease (Barnett, 1990; Hachinski, 1990; Barnett et al., 1995b).

In this section, we examine the different approaches to the prevention and treatment of ischemic cerebrovascular disease. Some of these approaches were developed through careful, unbiased, controlled studies, whereas others resulted from unfounded or limited clinical impressions and may eventually be proven to be inappropriate or ineffective.

Therapeutic Options

A variety of therapeutic options exist for most patients who experience a stroke or who are at risk of experiencing one. These options include both medical and surgical treatments (Kistler et al., 1984b; Grotta, 1987; Becker and Burde, 1988; Scheinberg, 1988; Cusimano and Ameli, 1989; Caplan, 1993; Sherman et al., 1995; Saver et al., 1997).

Medical Therapy

Medical therapy for patients with ischemic cerebrovascular disease includes both acute and chronic anticoagulation, substances that inhibit platelet aggregation, and—in patients with acute stroke—thrombolytic drugs.

Hemostasis is the spontaneous arrest of bleeding from damaged blood vessels (Bloom and Thomas, 1987). Precapillary vessels contract immediately when cut. Within seconds, thrombocytes or blood platelets bind to the exposed collagen of the injured vessel by a process called platelet adhesion. Platelets also stick to each other to form a viscous mass. This platelet plug can stop bleeding quickly, but it must be reinforced by fibrin for long-term effectiveness. This reinforcement is initiated by local stimulation of the coagulation process by the exposed collagen of the cut vessel and by the released contents and membranes of platelets (Kaplan, 1978; Nesheim et al., 1980; Del Zoppo, 1988; Coller, 1990). The coagulation process begins with the production of thrombin by activation of reactions at the site of the platelet mass (Fig. 55.258). Thrombin causes further platelet aggregation by stimulating the release of adenosine diphosphate (ADP) from the platelets and by stimulating the synthesis of prostaglandins. Two classes of prostaglandins with opposite effects on platelet aggregation and thrombogenesis are formed. **Thromboxane A_2** is synthesized by the aggregated platelets and stimulates further aggregation, whereas **prostacyclin** is synthesized by the vessel wall and inhibits thrombosis. The result of this reaction is the development of a fibrin scaffolding along which an ingrowth of fibroblasts eventually produces a fibrotic reaction (Bloom and Thomas, 1989; Coller, 1990).

ANTICOAGULATION

Heparin is a heterogeneous group of straight-chain anionic mucopolysaccharides called glycosaminoglycans that have molecular weights that average 15,000 daltons (Jaques, 1980). Commercial heparin is usually prepared from bovine lung and porcine intestinal mucosa but can also be obtained from sheep and whales. A semisynthetic form of heparin, heparinoid, is also produced.

Intravenously injected heparin impairs blood coagulation almost immediately by forming an irreversible complex with a plasma cofactor called antithrombin III, several clotting factors, and thrombin (Estol and Pessin, 1990). This complex prevents the production of fibrin (Björk and Lindahl, 1982). Low concentrations of heparin increase the activity of antithrombin III, forming the basis for the administration of **low doses of heparin** as a therapeutic regimen.

Purified commercial preparations of heparin are relatively nontoxic, and side effects from the drug are thus infrequent.

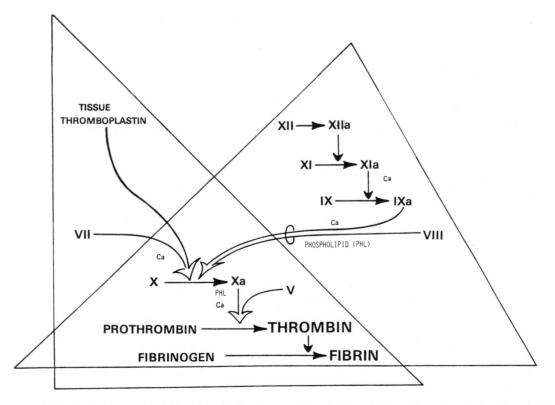

Figure 55.258. The blood coagulation sequence. This sequence can be activated either by the extrinsic pathway, through tissue thromboplastin (*triangle on left*) or by the intrinsic pathway, through activation of factor XII (*triangle on right*). The intrinsic and extrinsic pathways meet at a common point at the activation of factor X (*middle triangle*). It is at this point that prothrombin is converted to thrombin. (From Hirsh J. Anticoagulation and platelet antiaggregant agents. In Stroke: Pathophysiology, Diagnosis, and Management. Editors, Barnett HJM, Mohr JP, Stein BM, et al., Vol 2, pp 925–966. New York, Churchill Livingstone, 1986.)

Because heparin is obtained from animal tissue, it may produce a variety of hypersensitivity reactions, including chills, fever, urticaria, or anaphylactic shock. Increased loss of hair and reversible, transient, alopecia may also occur. Osteoporosis and spontaneous fractures occur in patients who receive 15,000 units or more of heparin daily for more than 3 months (Megard et al., 1982). Heparin causes transient mild thrombocytopenia in about 25% of patients and severe thrombocytopenia in rare patients. The mild reaction results from heparin-induced platelet aggregation, whereas severe thrombocytopenia is caused by formation of heparin-induced antiplatelet antibodies.

The chief complication of therapy with heparin is systemic (particularly retroperitoneal), intracranial, and even intraocular hemorrhage (Ramirez-Lassepas and Quinones, 1984; Putnam and Adams, 1985; see Table 6 in Keith et al., 1987; Estol and Pessin, 1990; Franke et al., 1990). Bleeding may be minimized by careful control of dosage, careful selection of patients, and avoidance of medications containing aspirin. Early anticoagulation with heparin, even after large cerebral infarction, is relatively safe, regardless of infarction size or clinical severity of the stroke (Chamorro et al., 1995; Chaves et al., 1996; Toni et al., 1996). The anticoagulant effect should be monitored by tests of blood clotting, such as the partial thromboplastin time (Hull and Hirsh, 1983; O'Reilly, 1985).

Sweet clover was planted in the Dakota plains and Canada in the late 1800s and early 1900s because it flourished on poor soil and could be used as a substitute for corn in silage. In 1924, Schofield described a hemorrhagic disorder in cattle that resulted from the ingestion of spoiled sweet clover silage. Campbell and Link (1941) subsequently identified the causative agent as bishydroxycoumarin (dicoumarol). Many cogeners of dicoumarol were subsequently synthesized, the most useful of which was racemic **warfarin** (Ikawa et al., 1944). The term, Warfarin, is an acronym for the patent holder of this cogener, **W**isconsin **A**lumni **R**esearch **F**oundation, plus the cou**marin**-derived suffix.

Dicoumarol and its cogeners were initially thought to be too toxic for humans, and the substance thus was used primarily as a rodenticide. In 1951, however, a man survived attempted suicide with large and repeated doses of a rodenticide containing warfarin. This led to clinical trials that established the safety of its use in humans (Link, 1959).

Warfarin sodium (coumadin) and similar substances inhibit blood clotting by interfering with the hepatic modification of the vitamin K-dependent clotting factors II, VII, IX, and X (Estol and Pessin, 1990; Hirsh, 1991). The therapeutic effect of these drugs does not occur until 8–12 hours after oral or intravenous administration because the effect is dependent on the half-lives of the affected clotting factors already in the circulation. These half-lives range from 6 to 60 hours.

Hemorrhage is the main untoward effect of coumadin and similar oral anticoagulants (Estol and Pessin, 1990; Hirsh, 1991; Fihn et al., 1993; van der Meer et al., 1993; Hylek and Singer, 1994; Hart et al., 1995). Hemorrhage may be generalized or focal, and it may be systemic, intracranial, intraocular, or a combination of these (Millikan, 1971;

Feman et al., 1972; Whisnant et al., 1978; Kelley et al., 1984). In order of decreasing frequency, hemorrhagic complications are ecchymoses, hematuria, uterine bleeding, melena, epistaxis, intracranial hematoma, gingival bleeding, hemoptysis, and hematemesis (O'Reilly, 1976). The risk of hemorrhagic complications with oral anticoagulants increases with duration of use and with variability of the prothrombin time ratio (Fihn et al., 1993).

Petitti et al. (1986) examined the courses of patients anticoagulated for venous thromboembolism. In their study, the cumulative risks for "major" hemorrhage were 10% at 3 months, 18% at 1 year, 26% at 2 years, and 41% at 5 years. Petty et al. (1988) used life-table techniques to determine risks of morbidity and mortality associated with long-term warfarin treatment in an anticoagulation clinic. Cumulative risks for life-threatening complications and warfarin-related death among all patients were 1% at 6 months, 5% at 1 year, and 7% at 2 and 3 years. Cox regression analysis using age as a continuous variable failed to show an effect of age on cumulative risks of complication. In this study, the occurrence of a minor complication during the course of therapy did not place a patient at higher risk for developing a major complication that would prompt discontinuation of therapy or cause death. There was no statistically significant difference between the cumulative risks of patients anticoagulated for cerebrovascular disease and the cumulative risks of patients anticoagulated for other indications. Long-term warfarin therapy thus does not appear to have a negative effect on quality of life, unless a bleeding episode has occurred (Lancaster et al., 1991).

Oral anticoagulant therapy must always be monitored by determination of one-stage prothrombin times, and the patient must be observed carefully for signs of bleeding, which often occurs even when the prothrombin time is within the expected therapeutic range (Loeliger and Lewis, 1982; Hirsh and Levine, 1986; Levine and Hirsh, 1986).

ANTIPLATELET THERAPY

Platelet-fibrin emboli originating from arteriosclerotic lesions in the extracranial and, to a lesser extent, in the intracranial arteries are responsible for a large number of strokes. In addition, platelets participate in the formation of thrombi that may occlude such vessels and also produce an ischemic stroke. The recognition of the important role played by platelets in the formation of both thrombi and emboli increased the interest in the use of drugs that inhibit platelet function (Fields and Hass, 1970; Thomas, 1972; Pedersen and FitzGerald, 1985; Frishman and Miller, 1986; Harker and Fuster, 1986; Coller, 1990; Patrono, 1994) (Fig. 55.259).

The antiplatelet effect of **acetylsalicylic acid (aspirin)** was first emphasized in the 1960s when it was discovered that aspirin prolongs bleeding time (Blatrix, 1963) and inhibits platelet aggregation (O'Brien, 1968). The effects of aspirin on platelet aggregation are mediated by inactivation of the enzyme **cyclooxygenase** (Roth and Majerus, 1975; Pedersen and FitzGerald, 1985; Frishman and Miller, 1986; Harker and Fuster, 1986) (Fig. 55.259). This enzyme, found primarily in platelets, controls the conversion of arachidonic

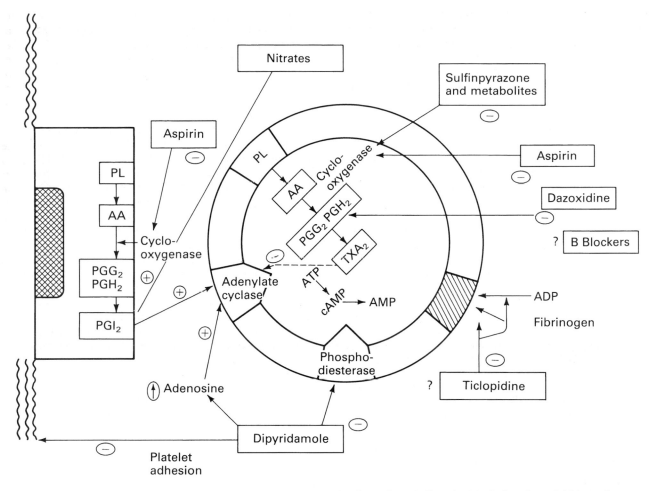

Figure 55.259. The sites of actions of various drugs that inhibit platelet function and metabolism. *Aspirin:* in low doses, inhibits cyclooxygenase irreversibly for the life span of the platelet. Higher doses inhibit endothelial cyclooxygenase, but the effect is transient. *Dipyridamole:* increases cyclic adenosine monophosphate (AMP) by inhibiting phosphodiesterase and by inhibiting uptake of adenosine by the platelet. It also inhibits adhesion of platelets to collagen. *Sulfinpyrazone:* inhibits platelet cyclooxygenase, although this effect is weak and reversible. *Ticlopidine:* may inhibit affinity of adenosine diphosphate (ADP) and fibrinogen for platelets. *Nitrates:* stimulate production of prostaglandins. *Dazoxidine:* inhibits production of thromboxane A_2. (From Hirsh J. Anticoagulation and platelet antiaggregant agents. In Stroke: Pathophysiology, Diagnosis, and Management. Editors, Barnett HJM, Mohr JP, Stein BM, et al., Vol 2, pp 925–966. New York, Churchill Livingstone, 1986.)

acid, a precursor common to many prostaglandins, into thromboxane A_2, a powerful **stimulator** of platelet aggregation. Cyclooxygenase also is found in endothelial cells of arteries and veins, where the endproduct is prostacyclin, a substance that strongly **inhibits** platelet aggregation (Moncada and Vane, 1979). Aspirin inhibits the production of both thromboxane A_2 and prostacyclin, thus inhibiting platelet aggregation by its effect on platelet cyclooxygenase and stimulating platelet aggregation by its effect on endothelial cell cyclooxygenase; however, the cyclooxygenase in platelets is more susceptible to aspirin than is cyclooxygenase in endothelial cells. Part of the explanation for this phenomenon is that endothelial cells can resynthesize cyclooxygenase, whereas platelets exposed to aspirin remain inactivated for their 10-day life (Marcus, 1983). In any event, the overall effect of aspirin is inhibition of platelet aggregation (Pedersen and FitzGerald, 1984).

The ideal antiplatelet dose of aspirin should completely suppress platelet cyclooxygenase but leave endothelial cyclooxygenase unaffected. To this end, a number of investigators have studied the biochemical effects of different daily doses of aspirin. The results are remarkably consistent, even though some doses were tested in volunteers, and others were tested in patients with cerebrovascular or cardiovascular disease. Bleeding time is prolonged markedly by daily doses between 30 and 50 mg (Preston et al., 1982; De Caterina et al., 1985a, 1985b; Weksler et al., 1985a; Kalmann et al., 1987; Toghi et al., 1992), only slightly by 20 mg (FitzGerald et al., 1983; Weksler et al., 1985b), and not at all by 10 mg (Kalmann et al., 1987). The production of active thromboxane is suppressed more than 90% by daily doses of aspirin ranging from 20 to 50 mg (FitzGerald et al., 1983; De Caterina et al., 1985a; Weksler et al., 1985b; Roberts et al., 1986; Toghi et al., 1992) but not by doses of 10 mg or less (Toivanen et al., 1984; Kalmann et al., 1987). At the same time, the urinary excretion of the primary metabolite of prostacyclin is unchanged with aspirin doses up to 35 mg (Patrignani et al., 1982; De Caterina et al., 1985a; Kalmann et al., 1987), and it is only partially suppressed by 50 mg (Roberts et al., 1986). Thus, 20 mg of aspirin per day is the minimum for inhibiting the synthesis of thromboxane and 30 mg for prolonging bleeding time. Both these low doses probably have a slight but transient effect on the production of prostacyclin.

Lorenz et al. (1989) explored the effect of timing on the antiplatelet effects of aspirin. These investigators studied platelet function and the formation of thromboxane and prostacyclin in healthy, nonsmoking volunteers during the administration of 40 mg of aspirin per day in three regimens: (a) as a split dose of 20 mg twice a day, (b) as a single dose of 40 mg/day, and (c) as an alternate day double dose of 80 mg. The results of this study indicate that maximum inactivation of platelets with sparing of prostacyclin formation is achieved by using low doses of aspirin in pulsed rather than split doses.

The side effects of aspirin are primarily gastrointestinal and dose-related (Levy, 1974). The main side effects are stomach pain, nausea, heartburn, and constipation. Some patients also develop occult gastrointestinal hemorrhage, and rare patients have melena or hematemesis (Hirsh, 1985). The side effects of aspirin are caused by gastric mucosal damage, which requires the presence of acid. They can thus be reduced or eliminated by neutralizing or preventing acid secretion by the use of enteric-coated aspirin or by using aspirin in a dose less than or equal to 325 mg per day (Hirsh, 1985). This dose is well within the theoretical range needed to insure maximum antiplatelet effects (Stuart, 1970). Buffered preparations of aspirin do not generally contain enough alkaline to neutralize the effects of aspirin and do not protect against aspirin-induced mucosal erosion (Leonards and Levy, 1972).

The discovery that aspirin has an antiplatelet effect led to the expectation that the drug might prevent stroke and other vascular complications in patients at risk. Numerous studies subsequently attempted to determine if aspirin has any effect in reducing the rate of stroke, TIAs, or death in patients thought to be at risk. As already emphasized in this chapter, most studies attempting to answer this question are flawed in design, execution, or both (Scheinberg, 1988). In addition, the dosage of aspirin used in these studies varies from 30 mg to 3000 mg per day, far in excess of the 20–30-mg dose that is considered to have an optimum antiplatelet effect (Patrono, 1994; and see above), although the experimental data on optimum dosage in normal subjects may not be clinically applicable to patients with vascular disease and damaged endothelium incapable of prostacyclin production (Caplan, 1993). Despite these concerns, there is evidence that aspirin is effective in reducing the incidence of stroke in selected patients (Fields et al., 1977; The Canadian Cooperative Study Group, 1978; Bousser et al., 1983; Miller and Lees, 1985; The American-Canadian Cooperative Study Group, 1985; A Swedish Cooperative Study, 1987; Riekkinen et al., 1987; Antiplatelet Trialists' Collaboration Group, 1994; Patrono, 1994). The mechanism of this beneficial ef-

fect may not be entirely a result of the antiplatelet action of aspirin, but it also may result from the anti-inflammatory properties of the drug (Ridker et al., 1997).

Dipyridamole (2,6-bis-diethanolamino-4,8-dipiperidino-pyrimido-[5,4-*d*]-pyrimidine; Persantine) is a pyrimidopyrimidine derivative that inhibits platelet function (Pedersen and FitzGerald, 1985; Frishman and Miller, 1986; Harker and Fuster, 1986; Coller, 1990). The mechanism by which this is accomplished in vivo is a subject of controversy (Fig. 55.259). According to FitzGerald (1987), the principal mechanisms by which dipyridamole inhibits platelet function are: (a) inhibition of the phosphodiesterase enzyme in platelets, resulting in an increase in intraplatelet cyclic adenosine monophosphate (AMP) and the consequent potentiation of the platelet-inhibiting actions of prostacylin (Moncada and Korbut, 1978; Kistler et al., 1984b); (b) direct stimulation of the release of prostacylin by vascular endothelial cells; and (c) inhibition of cellular uptake and metabolism of adenosine, thereby increasing its concentration at the platelet-vascular interface. In addition to these direct effects, dipyridamole may augment the platelet-inhibiting action of aspirin by a pharmacokinetic interaction. However, there are no data indicating that such an interaction leads to a synergistic antithrombotic effect (The American-Canadian Cooperative Study Group, 1985).

Large concentrations of dipyridamole are required to influence platelet aggregation in vitro, and, even in these concentrations, the inhibitory effect is quite weak (Emmons et al., 1965; Eliasson and Bygdeman, 1969; Cucuianu et al., 1971; Mills and Smith, 1971; Griguer et al., 1975). It is thus not surprising that it is difficult to demonstrate an inhibitory effect on platelet function in vivo (Emmons et al., 1965; Rajah et al., 1977). On the other hand, convincing evidence that platelet function is modified after oral administration of dipyridamole in humans is provided by studies of platelet survival (Harker and Slichter, 1972). Although these studies involved limited numbers of patients and were neither double-blinded nor placebo-controlled, they suggest that dipyridamole may modify the interaction of platelets with foreign surfaces and perhaps damaged blood vessels in humans. Kaiser et al. (1996) treated 23 patients with impaired ocular blood flow with dipyridamole and measured blood flow velocities in the extraocular vessels with CDFI before and after treatment. These investigators noted significantly improved blood flow in the ophthalmic and central retinal arteries of treated patients during treatment. Nevertheless, there are only a few clinical studies that suggest that this drug prevents stroke when used alone (Barnett et al., 1995b; Diener et al., 1996a).

Adverse effects associated with dipyridamole are generally mild, dose-related, and reversible. They include headache, dizziness, gastrointestinal discomfort, nausea, vomiting, diarrhea, peripheral vasodilation, flushing, weakness, syncope, rash, and pruritis. Most adverse effects of dipyridamole are transient, and they usually resolve during long-term therapy with the drug.

Sulfinpyrazone (Anturane) is a pyrazolone-derivative uricosuric agent. It competitively inhibits active reabsorption of uric acid at the proximal convoluted tubule, thus promoting urinary excretion of uric acid and reducing serum urate concentrations. Sulfinpyrazone also inhibits the release from platelets of AMP, ADP, adenosine triphosophate (ATP), and 5-hydroxytryptamine (5-HT) (Fig. 55.259). Inhibition of ADP and 5-HT results in decreased platelet adhesiveness and increases platelet survival time (Packham and Mustard, 1977; Kistler et al., 1984b; Pedersen and FitzGerald, 1985; Frishman and Miller, 1986; Harker and Fuster, 1986). There is no good clinical evidence to suggest that this agent alone prevents stroke (Barnett et al., 1995b).

Sulfinpyrazone has few side effects. Adverse gastrointestinal effects, particularly nausea, dyspepsia, and abdominal pain may occasionally occur, and some patients experience reactivation of previously quiescent peptic ulcer disease. Rash, dizziness, vertigo, and tinnitus may also occur in rare patients, as may blood dyscrasias. Because of its primary function, sufinpyrazone increases the concentration of uric acid in the renal tubules. It thus may promote the formation of uric acid stones that may cause renal colic and hematuria in patients with gout.

Ticlopidine is a thienopyridine that alters platelet membranes directly, independent of any effect on prostaglandins (Bruno and Molony, 1983; Panak et al., 1983; O'Reilly, 1985; Frishman and Miller, 1986; Harker and Fuster, 1986; Saltiel and Ward, 1987; Coller, 1990; Warlow, 1990) (Fig. 55.259). It inhibits platelet aggregation and secretion, reduces deposition of platelets and fibrin on artificial surfaces, and prolongs the bleeding time through its inhibitory effect on the ADP pathway of platelet aggregation (Feliste et al., 1987; Uchiyama et al., 1989; Heptinstall et al., 1995). It may also reduce fibrinogen levels and increase erythrocyte deformability (Editorial, 1991). Although ticlopidine is expensive, it is definitely effective in reducing the risk of stroke in selected patients (see below). Side effects are common, especially diarrhea, rash, and slight elevation of serum cholesterol (Gent et al., 1989; Hass et al., 1989). Serious neutropenia occurs in about 1% of patients, typically within the first 3 months of drug use. Although the neutropenia usually resolves once the drug is discontinued, this is not always the case (Barnett et al., 1995c; Shear and Appel, 1995; Shapiro and Walk, 1996; Haushofer et al., 1997). Thus, careful monitoring of the peripheral white blood cell count is required during the first few months of treatment.

Clopidogrel, an inhibitor of ADP that is chemically related to ticlopidine, is a promising drug for the prophylactic treatment of patients at risk for cerebrovascular disease (CAPRIE Steering Committee, 1996). Side effects of this medication are mostly of the "nuisance" variety, including rash and diarrhea. There is significantly less risk of gastrointestinal hemorrhage than with aspirin and less risk of neutropenia than with ticlopidine. The cost of this medication is high and thus may affect treatment decisions.

Substances that specifically inhibit thromboxane synthase, such as imidazole and similar compounds, might be expected to reduce platelet function substantially by preventing the production of thromboxane A_2 (Fisher et al., 1984; Pedersen and FitzGerald, 1985; Pettigrew et al., 1985; Harker and Fuster, 1986; Coller, 1990). **Picotamide** inhibits thromboxane synthase, antagonizes the thromboxane A_2 receptor, and enhances endothelial formation of prostacyclin (Gresele et al., 1989). In one study, long-term treatment of diabetic patients with picotamide slowed the evolution of early carotid atherosclerotic lesions compared with placebo (Cocozza et al., 1995). Further studies are indicated before thromboxane synthase inhibitors can be recommended for treatment of patients with ischemic cerebrovascular disease.

Platelet activating factor (PAF) is a potent inducer of platelet activation and thrombosis (Bourgain et al., 1985; Hanahan, 1986). This phosphoglyceride, derived from stimulated leukocytes, induces platelet activation within seconds (Joseph et al., 1989). It also causes direct neuronal damage (Kornecki and Ehrlich, 1988), cerebral vasoconstriction (Armstead et al., 1988), and cerebral hypoperfusion (Kochanek et al., 1988) in laboratory animals. Thus, PAF may play a role in the pathogenesis of cerebral thrombosis, and suppression of its effects on platelets and other intracranial structures could be of therapeutic value in patients with acute stroke or perhaps in patients with appropriate risk factors for development of stroke.

THROMBOLYTIC THERAPY

Anticoagulants and antiplatelet drugs prevent or reduce thrombosis. Other drugs may **reverse thrombosis** (Verstraete and Collen, 1986a, 1986b; Sloan, 1987; Del Zoppo, 1988; Saver et al., 1997) (Fig. 55.260). Some of these sub-

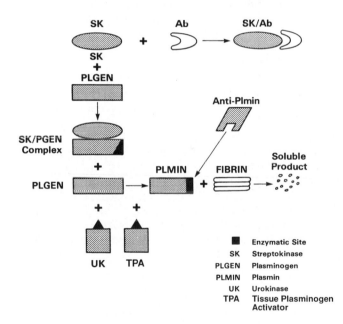

Figure 55.260. The mechanisms by which thrombolytic agents produce thrombolysis. Streptokinase (*SK*) is an indirect activator that initially combines with plasminogen (*PGEN*) to create an enzyme complex (*SK/PGEN Complex*) that cleaves plasminogen to plasmin (*PLMIN*). Plasmin then interacts with fibrin to break the latter down into soluble products. Streptokinase is neutralized by naturally occurring antibodies against plasmin (*Anti-Plmin*). A thrombolytic effect thus is not obtained until the antibodies are themselves neutralized by a loading dose of streptokinase. Urokinase (*UK*) is a direct activator of plasminogen. Tissue plasminogen activator (*TPA*) is also a direct activator of plasminogen. Its action is enhanced by the presence of fibrin. (Adapted from Hirsh J. Anticoagulation and platelet antiaggregant agents. In Stroke: Pathophysiology, Diagnosis, and Management. Editors, Barnett HJM, Mohr JP, Stein BM, et al., Vol 2, pp 925–966. New York, Churchill Livingstone, 1986.)

stances promote the dissolution of thrombi by stimulating the activation of endogenous plasminogen to plasmin (fibrinolysin), a proteolytic enzyme that hydrolyzes fibrin. Others induce local fibrinolysis without causing systemic fibrinolysis.

Streptokinase is a protein without known enzymatic activity that is obtained from group-C β-hemolytic streptococci. It interacts with and indirectly activates plasminogen. The complex of streptokinase and plasminogen has protease activity and catalyzes the conversion of plasminogen to plasmin (Fig. 58.260).

Urokinase is a proteolytic enzyme. Its only known natural substrate is plasminogen, which it activates directly to plasmin (Fig. 58.260). Urokinase was originally isolated from human urine, but it can be prepared from cultures of human renal cells.

Tissue plasminogen activator (TPA) preferentially activates plasminogen bound to fibrin. This confines fibrinolysis to a thrombus and thus avoids systemic activation of plasminogen. TPA initially was isolated from cultured human melanoma cells. It can be prepared using recombinant DNA technology (Pennica et al., 1983).

The thrombolytic drugs can cause hemorrhagic transformation of an ischemic infarction, formation of an intracerebral hematoma, systemic bleeding, and rethrombosis. They must be given with care, and patients to whom they are given must be carefully monitored.

AGENTS TO INCREASE PERFUSION

Theoretically, substances that increase cerebral perfusion at the time of an acute stroke should increase collateral circulation to the ischemic but viable tissue surrounding an infarction, thereby limiting the extent of functional compromise. Such agents include cerebral vasodilators (such as acetazolamide or the calcium channel blockers), volume expanders (such as dextrans), fibrinogen reducers (such as ancrod or ω-3 fatty acids), and perfluorochemicals (which increase oxygen delivery) (Caplan, 1993). Unfortunately, clinical studies are limited, and no consistent benefit has been demonstrated for any of these agents in stroke prevention or treatment. Similarly, the efficacy of hemodilution, which also increases cerebral perfusion, has yet to be proven.

AGENTS TO INCREASE BRAIN VIABILITY

Infarction may begin with impaired circulation to brain tissue, but neuronal death is a complex process with multiple contributing factors, including the level of cell activity, the presence of lactic acid and free radicals, the temperature of the system, the integrity of cell membranes, calcium homeostasis, and the presence of toxic neurotransmitters, including excitotoxins and nitric oxide (Pulsinelli, 1992; Caplan, 1993; Fisher et al., 1994; Iadecola et al., 1994; Lipton and Rosenberg, 1994; Saver et al., 1997). Theoretically, the modification of these factors could increase brain viability, especially in surrounding ischemic areas. Intense experimental research is underway in an attempt to develop agents which can target these specific factors influencing brain vulnerability to ischemic damage. Unfortunately, consistent, dramatic clinical applications have yet to be demonstrated.

Surgical Therapy

Several surgical procedures are used to treat patients with ischemic cerebrovascular disease (Auer et al., 1986). Patients with disease affecting but not occluding the common, internal, or external carotid arteries often undergo an **endarterectomy** or a percutaneous transluminal **angioplasty**. These procedures can also be performed on selected patients with symptomatic stenosis of one or both vertebral arteries (Allen et al., 1981; Ausman et al., 1984; Hopkins et al., 1987). For patients with complete occlusion of the common or internal carotid artery, severe stenosis of the intracranial portion of the internal carotid artery, occlusion or severe stenosis of the middle cerebral artery, and, occasionally, severe intracranial vertebrobasilar artery disease, an **extracranial to intracranial (EC-IC) bypass procedure** may be performed. Other vascular transposition techniques are advocated for patients with certain types of extracranial vertebrobasilar thrombo-occlusive disease.

ENDARTERECTOMY

In the early 1950s, Fisher (1951a, 1951b, 1952, 1954) and others (Webster et al., 1950; Johnson and Walker, 1951) described atherosclerotic disease of the common and the intracranial portion of the internal carotid arteries as a major cause of stroke. This led to the speculation that such lesions might be amenable to surgical therapy and that their removal **before** permanent neurologic or visual deficits occurred might prevent such events from occurring. Angiographic techniques to identify such lesions were subsequently improved, and a number of investigators published reports dealing with the potential risks and benefits of carotid endarterectomy (see Table A in Laws, 1988).

Although they were clearly not the first to perform a successful endarterectomy, Cooley et al. (1956) are usually given credit for popularizing this procedure. The patient described by Cooley et al. (1956) was a 71-year-old man with a subjective left-sided bruit who complained of dizziness on sitting or standing up. A loud bruit was audible under the angle of the left side of the mandible. Compression of the carotid artery obliterated the bruit. Temporary occlusion of the left common carotid artery for 30 seconds produced dizziness as well as weakness, numbness, and paresthesias in the entire right half of the body. Cerebral arteriography showed a tight stenosis at the bifurcation of the left common carotid artery. An endarterectomy was performed by placing a polyvinyl shunt with needle points at both ends above and below the region of pathology to bypass the carotid circulation during the period of occlusion. With the external carotid artery temporarily occluded, internal carotid blood flow was maintained by means of the shunt while the atheromatous plaque was removed from the vessel. The bypassed portion of the common and internal carotid artery was occluded by arterial clamps at both ends, and a transverse incision was made in the carotid bulb. The stenotic, partially calcified, atherosclerotic plaque was peeled out of the lumen by careful dissection, and the arteriotomy was closed. Arterial flow was restored after 9 minutes of carotid clamping during which period the shunt functioned satisfactorily.

Postoperatively, the patient had mild right-sided weakness and dysphasia that lasted about 12 hours and then began to resolve. At the time of discharge 6 days after surgery, the patient had only slight impairment of motion and sensation in the right hand. Within 1 month, right hand function was almost normal.

Carotid endarterectomy is one of the most common operations in the United States and Europe (Dyken and Pokras, 1984; North American Symptomatic Carotid Endarterectomy Study Group, 1987; Trobe, 1988). The precise technique used has changed little from the method reported by Cooley et al. (1956) and its subsequent, more detailed description by Murphey and Miller (1959) (see Loftus and Quest, 1995, for review of technical issues) (Fig. 55.261). Some physicians prefer to perform the procedure under local anesthesia, whereas others prefer general anesthesia (see Table 2 in Zuccarello et al., 1988). Some physicians use a shunt routinely (Thompson et al., 1970; Nunn, 1975; Haynes and Dempsey, 1979; Thompson, 1979; Whittemore, 1980; Gumerlock and Neuwelt, 1988). Most prefer to increase systemic blood pressure to improve cerebral perfusion pressure, isolate the portion of the artery to be manipulated between two clamps, and continuously monitor the patient's electroencephalographic findings. A shunt is placed only if there are electroencephalographic changes suggesting poor cerebral perfusion (Ojemann et al., 1975; Allen and Preziosi, 1981; Robertson and Auer, 1982; Browse and Ross Russell, 1984; Ferguson, 1986; Graham et al., 1986; Ojemann and Heros, 1986; Sundt et al., 1986; Spetzler, 1988). In most series, the average clamp time is about 20 minutes, although the range varies from 10 to 70 minutes (Tippett et al., 1985). Anticoagulation with heparin is begun just before clamping and is usually reversed after the arteriotomy is closed, although some physicians prefer to let coagulation return to normal naturally without pharmacologic reversal (Tippett et al., 1985).

The majority of patients who undergo endarterectomy do so because of symptomatic or asymptomatic atherosclerotic disease affecting the internal carotid artery. In most cases, the disease has produced stenosis or ulceration of the artery, and endarterectomy is associated with improvement in blood flow not only in the carotid artery but also in its branches, including the ophthalmic and central retinal arteries (Riihelä-inen et al., 1997). Patients with complete occlusion of the internal carotid artery are not usually considered candidates for endarterectomy unless it is thought that the occlusion is acute and that there are potentially reversible neurologic deficits (Meyer et al., 1986; Walters et al., 1987; see, however, Scheinberg, 1987). Occasionally, common or external carotid endarterectomies and even vertebral artery endarterectomies are performed (Jackson, 1967; Dieterich et al., 1968; Hopkins et al., 1987; Sterpetti et al., 1988; Ausman et al., 1990). Most patients in whom an external carotid endarterectomy is performed have occlusion of the ipsilateral internal carotid artery but have persistent symptoms of ipsilateral hemisphere ischemia. Intracranial vertebral endarterectomy can be performed in patients with severe stenosis proximal to the posterior inferior cerebellar artery.

Internal carotid endarterectomy poses definite risks. Besides the nonspecific risks of local hemorrhage and infection and the potential complications of anesthesia, patients who undergo carotid endarterectomy may develop perioperative complications that include stroke or death from embolization, carotid artery thrombosis, systemic hypotension, cerebral vasoconstriction, intracranial hemorrhage, and the postoperative hyperperfusion syndrome (Imparato et al., 1985; Krul et al., 1989; Sise et al., 1989; Brick et al., 1990; Breen et al., 1996). Death in the perioperative period usually results from heart attack or an ischemic or hemorrhagic stroke. Nonfatal heart attack, nonfatal stroke, angina, hemorrhage, infection, and seizures are all causes of potentially significant perioperative morbidity (Bruetman et al., 1963; Sundt et al., 1975; Solomon et al., 1986; Piepgras et al., 1988; Pomposelli et al., 1988; Kieburtz et al., 1989, 1990).

Perioperative mortality rates vary among series from 0 to 20% (average 2%), whereas morbidity ranges from about 1% to 25% (average 6%) (Thompson et al., 1978; West et al., 1979; Eriksson et al., 1981; Brott and Thalinger, 1984; Kistler et al., 1984b; Muuronen, 1984; Slavish et al., 1984; Warlow, 1984; Committee on Health Care Issues, American Neurological Association, 1987; Zurbruegg et al., 1987; Zuccarello et al., 1988; Cusimano and Ameli, 1989; Healy et al., 1989; Rosa, 1990; Easton and Wilterdink, 1994; Rothwell et al., 1996). In the NASCET, the morbidity and mortality rate attributable to surgery was 2.5% (North American Symptomatic Carotid Endarterectomy Trial Collaborators, 1991). The marked variation in mortality and morbidity rates among series is related to a number of factors, primarily surgical experience and patient selection (Hertzer et al., 1984; Zurbruegg et al., 1987; Cusimano and Ameli, 1989; Lyden et al., 1989; Easton and Wilterdink, 1994; Rothwell et al., 1996). In addition, much of the variability may reflect differences in methodology and authorship of various reports (Rothwell et al., 1996). In a systematic review of studies published since 1980, Rothwell et al. (1996) reported an overall risk of stroke, death, or both after carotid endarterectomy of 5.6%. Coronary artery disease (even when it is asymptomatic), recent myocardial infarction, hypertension (greater than 180/110 mm Hg), chronic obstructive pulmonary disease, obesity, previous history of stroke, recent symptoms, plaque ulceration, and age greater than 70 years are all risk factors for perioperative morbidity and mortality (Sundt et al., 1975; Fode et al., 1986; Trobe, 1988; North American Symptomatic Carotid Endarterectomy Trial Collaborators, 1991; Easton and Wilterdink, 1994). In addition, patients with recent, evolving, or multiple strokes have a higher risk of stroke or death in the perioperative period following carotid endarterectomy than do patients in whom angiography shows stenosis affecting the distal ipsilateral extracranial carotid artery, its siphon, or the contralateral carotid artery (Sundt et al., 1975; Toole et al., 1978; Lees and Hertzer, 1981; Muuronen, 1984; Brückmann et al., 1987).

Carotid endarterectomy may be associated with visual, as well as systemic, perioperative morbidity. Some patients experience loss of vision in the ipsilateral eye after endarterectomy (David et al., 1963; McBrien et al., 1963; Ross Russell, 1963; Shillito and Rockett, 1963; Blake, 1975; Treiman et al., 1977). In most patients, the visual loss is caused by

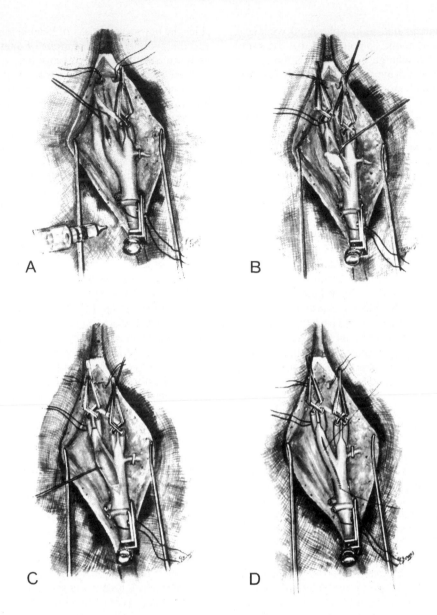

Figure 55.261.   Technique of carotid endarterectomy as described by Murphey and Miller. *A*, Exposure and incision of internal carotid artery showing a clot distally and the plaque proximally inside the artery. *B*, Method of removing the plaque. *C*, Lumen of the artery after endarterectomy. Note suture through distal intima. *D*, Closure of the artery. This technique has changed little since its original descriptions. (From Murphey F, Miller JH. Carotid insufficiency—Diagnosis and surgical treatment: A Report of twenty-one cases. J Neurosurg *16:*1–23, 1959.)

retinal or optic nerve emboli originating from the operative site. Other patients develop a homonymous visual field defect from embolic occlusion of arteries supplying the post-chiasmal visual sensory pathway. Diplopia occurs in some patients from embolic occlusion of small vessels supplying the ocular motor nerves in the cavernous sinus. A direct carotid-cavernous sinus fistula may also develop after attempted carotid endarterectomy using a Fogarty catheter or a similar device (Davie and Richardson, 1967; Barker et al., 1968; Kushner, 1981).

Even patients who do not seem to have any ill effects after carotid endarterectomy may be found to have experienced a silent cerebral infarction when neuroimaging studies are performed after surgery and compared with preoperative studies. Sise et al. (1989) found CT evidence of silent cerebral infarction in 17 of 97 patients (18%) after apparently uncomplicated carotid endarterectomy. In this study, patients with evidence by neuroimaging of preoperative cerebral infarction had the same incidence of new postoperative silent infarction as did patients with no evidence of preoperative infarction.

The reported results of carotid endarterectomy are affected not only by surgical experience and patient selection, but also by the circumstances under which patients are chosen. Prospective series are much more likely to have low morbidity and mortality rates, because the investigators are especially careful with patient selection and preoperative evaluation. In the series reported from the Johns Hopkins Hospital by Allen and Preziosi (1981), selection criteria were very stringent. All patients with any evidence of cardiac disease were evaluated extensively by a cardiologist before surgery, and several patients had preoperative implantation of a pacemaker. Indeed, 71% of patients entered into this study had an abnormal electrocardiogram, and 41% had a "significant" history of angina, congestive heart failure, or a previous myocardial infarction. Following completion of this prospective study, which quoted a mortality rate of less than 1% and a morbidity rate of about 3%, the selection criteria were relaxed, and the number of perioperative complications increased dramatically, although they were never reported. Similarly, the NASCET may not be directly applicable to the general population with TIA because some patients were denied entry into the study because they were thought to have too high a surgical risk secondary to coexistent systemic disease (North American Symptomatic Carotid Endarterectomy Trial Collaborators, 1991).

Many retrospective series consist of a group of patients, not always consecutive, in which the criteria for treatment may not always be consistent. Even though such series may have higher morbidity and mortality rates, they may more accurately reflect the risk of carotid endarterectomy in general than the rates reported in prospective studies.

Surgical bias also may affect the reporting of the outcome of carotid endarterectomy. Brott and Thalinger (1984) re-

viewed the outcome of all carotid endarterectomies performed in the greater Cincinnati area in 1980. In that year, 431 procedures were performed in 16 hospitals by 47 surgeons. The perioperative stroke rate was 8.6% and the death rate was 2.8%. Of the 37 perioperative strokes identified by Brott and Thalinger (1984), only 15 were listed by the surgeons in the discharge diagnosis. Based solely on the surgeon's reports, the stroke rate would have been only 3.5%.

When performed by an experienced surgeon who selects patients judiciously, the mortality rate of internal carotid endarterectomy should be 0–2%, and the morbidity rate should be less than 3% (Hass, 1980; see Table 2 in Tippett et al., 1985; Zeiger et al., 1987; Ferguson, 1988; Goldstein et al., 1997). The patency rate after this procedure is over 99%, with less than 1% of patients developing recurrent stenosis at the surgical site (French and Rewcastle, 1977). Recurrent stenosis may occur at any time, often more than 5 years after surgery (Fig. 55.262). External carotid endarterectomy, which also has an extremely high patency rate, is generally a safer operation than internal carotid endarterectomy. Sterpetti et al. (1988) summarized the results of 192 operations in 168 patients reported in the literature. None of the operations was associated with perioperative mortality, and only three patients experienced any perioperative neurologic deficits. The risk/benefit ratio of vertebral endarterectomy is unclear because so few cases have been reported (Allen et al., 1981; Ausman et al., 1984). Hopkins et al. (1987) performed intracranial vertebral endarterectomy on

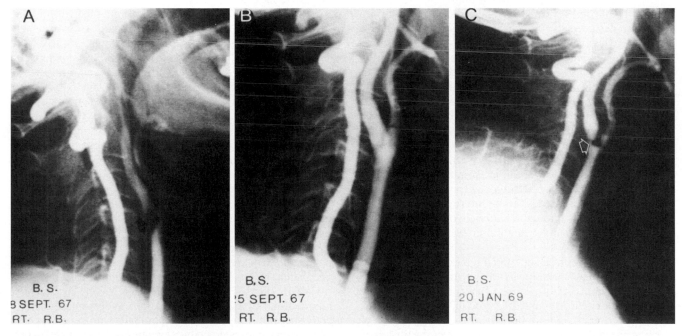

Figure 55.262. Recurrent stenosis after carotid endarterectomy. The patient was a 56-year-old woman with transient loss of vision in the right eye for 1 month. She had also experienced an episode of numbness and weakness of the left arm that cleared incompletely. *A*, Right brachial arteriogram, lateral view, shows severe stenosis of the right internal carotid artery at its origin (*arrow*). A right carotid endarterectomy was performed. *B*, Postoperative right brachial arteriogram, lateral view, performed 17 days after initial arteriogram and endarterectomy shows patent carotid bifurcation. The patient was well until 16 months later when she developed mild weakness of the left arm. A new, harsh bruit was heard over the right carotid bifurcation. *C*, Right brachial arteriogram, lateral view, shows recurrent stenosis at the bifurcation of the right common carotid artery (*arrow*). (From French BN, Rewcastle NB. Recurrent stenosis at site of carotid endarterectomy. Stroke *8*:597–605, 1977.)

two patients with 90–95% stenosis of the ipsilateral vertebral artery, occlusion of the contralateral vertebral artery, and vertebrobasilar circulation TIAs. One patient developed aseptic meningitis, and both patients developed communicating hydrocephalus that required a lumboperitoneal shunt. Nevertheless, both patients were asymptomatic 10 and 16 months after surgery, respectively.

PERCUTANEOUS TRANSLUMINAL ANGIOPLASTY

Percutaneous transluminal angioplasty became an established treatment of peripheral, renal, and coronary artery disease after the development of appropriate balloon dilation catheters. Angioplasty of the vessels supplying the intracranial circulation initially was not recommended because of concern about the risks of cerebral embolism following the procedure. Nevertheless, the procedure may be performed on stenotic carotid, vertebral, or intracranial arteries (Kerber et al., 1980; Mullan et al., 1980; Hasso et al., 1981; Motarjeme et al., 1981; Vitek, 1983; Wiggli and Gratzl, 1983; Théron et al., 1987; Brown et al., 1990; Clark et al., 1995; Higashida et al., 1995; Touho, 1995; Beebe et al., 1996; Clark and Barnwell, 1996; Ferguson, 1996; Ferguson and Ferguson, 1996; Terada et al., 1996). There are no large studies comparing the risk/benefit ratio of angioplasty with other surgical treatments or conventional medical therapy in any group of patients with cerebrovascular occlusive disease (Beebe et al., 1996).

EXTRACRANIAL TO INTRACRANIAL (EC-IC) BYPASS

In the late 1960s, several investigators described a surgical procedure designed to augment the collateral circulation to an ischemic hemisphere by the construction of an anastomosis between a branch of the ipsilateral external carotid artery (usually the posterior branch of the superficial temporal artery) and a cortical branch of the ipsilateral middle cerebral artery (Donaghy, 1967; Yaşargil, 1969; Yaşargil et al., 1970) (Figs. 55.160 and 55.161). This technique requires an operating microscope and microsuture technique to construct an end-to-side anastomosis between vessels whose diameters range from 1.0 to 1.5 mm (Yonekawa and Yasargil, 1976). Other types of bypass procedures, primarily designed for patients with intracranial vertebrobasilar ischemic disease, include occipital artery to posterior inferior cerebellar artery bypass and superficial temporal artery to either superior cerebellar artery or posterior cerebral artery bypass (Hopkins et al., 1987).

The patency rates of a superficial temporal artery to middle cerebral artery anastomosis range from 85 to 100% in most series (Gratzl et al., 1976; Chater, 1983; Andrews et al., 1985; The EC/IC Bypass Study Group, 1985b; Jack et al., 1988; Powers et al., 1989a). Intraoperative and postoperative cerebral blood flow studies in patients undergoing this procedure suggest that a successful anastomosis results in an augmentation of 15–20% in blood flow to the territory of the ipsilateral middle cerebral artery (Heilbrun et al., 1975; Crowell, 1976; Schmiedek et al., 1976; Spetzler and Chater, 1976), and postoperative angiography often demonstrates dramatic enlargement of both donor and recipient vessels

consistent with flow increases of 75–100% (Spetzler and Chater, 1976; Jack et al., 1988). Despite these improvements in cerebral blood flow, Drinkwater et al. (1984) were unable to detect any improvement in composite indices of cerebral function in any of 38 patients who underwent this type of bypass surgery for either ipsilateral carotid occlusion or distal stenosis not amenable to carotid endarterectomy.

The superficial temporal artery to middle cerebral artery bypass procedure is performed primarily in patients with symptomatic and, to a lesser extent, asymptomatic, occlusion of the internal carotid artery (Austin et al., 1974; Weinstein et al., 1984; Sundt et al., 1985; The EC/IC Bypass Study Group, 1985a, 1985b; Jack et al., 1988; Powers et al., 1989a; Kawaguchi et al., 1994), although it may also be performed in patients with symptomatic severe distal stenosis of the internal carotid artery (Drinkwater et al., 1984; The EC/IC Bypass Study Group, 1985a) and in patients with occlusion or severe stenosis of the middle cerebral artery (Andrews et al., 1985; Powers et al., 1989a). Kawaguchi et al. (1994) performed the procedure on 19 patients with occlusive internal carotid artery disease causing ischemic retinopathy. One month after the bypass, 12 patients had improvement in their ocular findings. The perioperative mortality and morbidity of this procedure are about the same as that of carotid endarterectomy. In most studies, the mortality rate of the procedure is less than 1%, and the morbidity rate varies from 2 to 12% (Samson et al., 1979; Weinstein et al., 1984; Andrews et al., 1985; Day, 1985; Sundt et al., 1985; The EC/IC Cooperative Study Group, 1985b; Whisnant et al., 1985; Jack et al., 1988; Powers et al., 1989a).

Bypass procedures involving vessels other than the middle cerebral artery are not regularly performed. Hopkins et al. (1987) reported on the results of arterial bypass surgery in 41 patients. Twenty-four of the patients (56%) underwent an occipital artery to posterior inferior cerebellar artery bypass, 12 patients underwent a superficial temporal artery to superior cerebellar artery bypass, and five patients underwent superficial temporal artery to posterior cerebral artery bypass. Postoperative angiography was performed in all but two patients (who refused angiography); those two patients underwent Doppler imaging. The bypass was found to be patent in 39 of 41 patients (95%). There was only one postoperative death (from delayed sepsis), but 16 patients (40%) developed postoperative complications that included pneumonia, communicating hydrocephalus, meningitis, respiratory insufficiency, and transient coma. Nevertheless, of the 40 patients who survived surgery, 38 became asymptomatic, one patient experienced a reduction in symptoms, and only one patient had no improvement over a mean follow-up period of 18 months. Hopkins and Budny (1989) subsequently reported that two of the patients who underwent an apparently successful superficial temporal artery to superior cerebellar artery bypass procedure eventually experienced major brainstem strokes.

EXTRACRANIAL VASCULAR TRANSPOSITION

A variety of vascular transposition procedures can be used to treat patients with extracranial vertebrobasilar thrombo-occlusive disease, such as subclavian steal syndrome. Most of these procedures involve transection of the affected vertebral artery near its origin, occlusion of the proximal stump of the vessel, and anastomosis of the vessel with the ipsilateral common carotid artery. This procedure is advocated for subclavian steal syndrome and for symptomatic stenosis of the proximal portion of the vertebral artery. Among 24 such procedures performed by Spetzler et al. (1987), there were no deaths and no major complications. Three patients developed an ipsilateral Horner's syndrome, however.

Management of Risk Factors

Perhaps the least controversial issue concerning the treatment of patients who have experienced, or are at risk for developing, stroke is the need to modify whenever possible the factors that predispose to atherosclerosis, heart disease, and stroke (Wolf et al., 1983a; Dyken et al., 1984; Bogousslavsky et al., 1986a; Becker and Burde, 1988; Patterson, 1988; Scheinberg, 1988; Cusimano and Ameli, 1989; Sacco et al., 1989a; WHO/MNH Task Force on Stroke and Other Cerebrovascular Disorders, 1989; Caplan, 1993; Bronner et al., 1995; Gorelick, 1995; Raps and Galetta, 1995; Sacco, 1995). **Hypertension** is probably the single most important controllable risk factor in almost all forms of both initial and recurrent stroke. It increases the overall incidence of thromboembolic stroke to four to eight times that of age-matched control subjects (Kannel et al., 1970, 1976a, 1976b), and its control reduces the risk of stroke 7-fold (Whisnant, 1977; Levy, 1979; Whisnant, 1983; Collins et al., 1990; MacMahon et al., 1990). It is clear from the results of several controlled clinical trials in the United States and elsewhere that patients whose hypertension is successfully treated, regardless of the pretreatment level of blood pressure, experience fewer strokes than untreated patients (Veterans Administration Cooperative Study Group on Antihypertensive Agents, 1967, 1970; Management Committee, 1980; Hypertension Detection and Follow-Up Program Cooperative Group, 1982; WHO/ISH Mild Hypertension Liaison Committee, 1982; Collins et al., 1990; MacMahon et al., 1990; SHEP Cooperative Research Group, 1991; Bronner et al., 1995; Gorelick, 1995; Sacco, 1995; Sacco et al., 1997).

Other modifiable risk factors for stroke are **cigarette smoking** and diet-induced **hyperlipidemia** (Abbott et al., 1986; Whisnant et al., 1990b; Robbins et al., 1994; Levine et al, 1995; Wannamethee et al., 1995). Both are difficult to modify, but the potential rewards of cessation of smoking and lowering of the concentration of cholesterol in the blood may be substantial.

The mechanism by which cigarette smoking is related to atherosclerosis and stroke is unclear, but smokers are five to six times more likely to experience an ischemic stroke than are nonsmokers (Donnan et al., 1989; Gill et al., 1989; Robbins et al., 1994; Wannamethee et al., 1995). After cessation of smoking, the relative risk of stroke declines substantially within 5 years, but a complete loss of risk is not seen in previously heavy smokers. Patients who smoke and who are at risk for stroke should be encouraged in the strongest

possible terms to stop smoking. Indeed, considering the adverse effects on health of cigarette smoking, it seems to us unconscionable that cigarettes continue to be manufactured legally and made available to men, women, and children around the world.

The risk of stroke can be substantially reduced by reducing the plasma cholesterol concentration, triglyceride concentration, or both (Duncan et al., 1977; Takeya et al., 1984; Iso et al., 1989; Bronner et al., 1995; Byington et al., 1995). Pooled results from four trials with a total of 1891 subjects investigating the efficacy of pravastatin, one of the HMG-coenzyme A reductase inhibitor class of lipid-lowering drugs, showed significant reductions in myocardial infarction, vascular death, and stroke in patients taking pravastatin compared with those taking placebo (Byington et al., 1995). The other statin drugs have similar effects (Herbert et al., 1997). The lower rates of stroke were similar to the reported effects of antiplatelet and antihypertensive therapies. We believe every effort should be made to reduce the cholesterol concentration in the blood to less than 200 mg/dL. Dietary modification may increase life expectancy, but not to as great an extent as smoking cessation (Grover et al., 1994). Greater intake of fruits and vegetables may protect against the development of stroke in men (Gillman et al., 1995).

As noted in an earlier section of this chapter, there is no conclusive data linking either acute or chronic **alcohol use** with ischemic stroke (Camargo, 1989; Gorelick, 1989; Gorelick, 1995). Nevertheless, we agree with Caplan (1993) that heavy alcohol consumption is an unhealthy habit, and that its cessation cannot but improve the quality, if not the length, of life. Similarly, the use of **illicit drugs**, particularly cocaine, can cause brain ischemia and hemorrhage and should be discontinued.

Perhaps the most controversial of all the modifiable risk factors is the use of **oral contraceptives**. It is not clear if the use of oral contraceptive agents is an independent risk factor for stroke and if so, to what degree. Furthermore, the compounds now used have a relatively lower estrogen content, which may make them less of a thrombotic risk. Nevertheless, because some retrospective studies suggest that the use of oral contraceptives increases the risk of both ischemic and hemorrhagic stroke from two to 13 times that of the normal population (Pullicino and Xuereb, 1989; Hannaford et al., 1994; WHO Collaborative Study of Cardiovascular Disease and Steroid Hormone Contraception, 1996a, 1996b), we believe that patients with other risk factors for stroke (e.g., hypertension, migraine, diabetes mellitus, hyperlipidemia, cigarette smoking) should not use oral contraceptives.

Some well-known risk factors for stroke are either not easily modifiable or their modification may not substantially alter stroke risk. These factors include diabetes mellitus, cardiac disease, and TIAs. Patients with **diabetes mellitus** should be kept in as good control as possible. There is, however, little evidence that patients whose diabetes is managed optimally have a significantly reduced risk of stroke. Sacco et al. (1989d) noted that an elevated blood sugar at the time of admission was one of the primary risk factors in patients with recurrent atherothrombotic, cardiogenic embolic, and lacunar stroke.

One of the major cardiac disorders that predisposes to stroke is chronic, nonrheumatic **atrial fibrillation** (Petersen, 1990). In the Framingham study (Wolf et al., 1978a, 1983b), patients with this condition had a stroke rate that was more than five times that of the normal population, corresponding to a yearly incidence of stroke of about 4.2%. Other studies report similar results (Flegel et al., 1987; Petersen et al., 1987; Boysen et al., 1988a; Aronow et al., 1989; D'Olhaberriague et al., 1989). In addition, Flegel and Hanley (1989) found that patients with nonrheumatic AF who experience a stroke are about twice as likely to have another stroke as are patients with the same condition who have never suffered a stroke, and they are 13.5 times more likely to have a recurrent stroke than the normal population. Because nonrheumatic AF is a major cause of fatal massive ischemic stroke (Yamanouchi et al., 1989), patients with chronic AF are usually placed on anticoagulant or antiplatelet therapy, particularly if they have already had a stroke (Fisher, 1972; Easton and Sherman, 1980; Hachinski, 1986; Sherman et al., 1986; Flegel and Hanley, 1989; Verheugt and Galema, 1989; Petersen, 1990; Albers et al., 1991).

Petersen et al. (1989) performed a placebo-controlled, randomized trial of warfarin (INR of 2.8–4.2) and aspirin (75 mg/day) for prevention of thromboembolic complications in 1007 patients with chronic AF. The incidence of both thromboembolic complications and vascular death were significantly lower in the group of patients treated with warfarin than in the groups treated with aspirin or placebo, which did not differ significantly. In the Boston Area Anticoagulation Trial for Atrial Fibrillation, warfarin prothrombin-time ratio (PT of 1.2–1.5 times control) was compared with the best medical therapy (which could include aspirin) in the prevention of stroke and death in 420 patients with AF (The Boston Area Anticoagulation Trial for Atrial Fibrillation Investigators, 1990). Warfarin proved effective, but the data on the effect of aspirin were inconclusive. Follow-up subgroup analysis from this study suggested that warfarin was significantly more effective than other therapy in preventing stroke (Singer et al., 1992). In the Veterans Affairs Stroke Prevention in Nonrheumatic Atrial Fibrillation Study, low-intensity anticoagulation with warfarin (PT of 1.2–1.5 times control) proved more effective than placebo in the prevention of cerebral infarction in 571 men, without producing an excess of major hemorrhage (Ezekowitz et al., 1992). In the European Atrial Fibrillation Trial, patients with nonrheumatic AF and a recent history of TIAs or minor stroke had a lower risk of recurrent stroke if they were treated with oral anticoagulation rather than aspirin or placebo (European Atrial Fibrillation Trial Study Group, 1993). In the Stroke Prevention in Atrial Fibrillation Study, 1644 patients with nonvalvular AF were randomized to receive warfarin (INR 1.7–4.6), aspirin (325 mg/day), or placebo (The Stroke Prevention in Atrial Fibrillation Investigators, 1990a, 1990b; Stroke Prevention in Atrial Fibrillation Investigators, 1991). Both warfarin and aspirin were superior to placebo in reducing systemic embolism, ischemic stroke, and TIAs. Aspirin reduced the occurrence of strokes categorized as noncardioembolic significantly more than it did strokes categorized as cardioembolic, emphasizing again the importance of considering the **pathogenesis** of a stroke when attempting to determine the appropriate therapy (Miller et al., 1993). In an extension of the Stroke Prevention in Atrial Fibrillation Study, called the Stroke Prevention in Atrial Fibrillation II Study, anticoagulation with warfarin was compared with aspirin 325 mg daily for prevention of ischemic stroke and systemic embolism (Stroke Prevention in Atrial Fibrillation Investigators, 1994). The study concluded that warfarin may be more effective than aspirin for prevention of ischemic stroke, but the absolute reduction in stroke rate by warfarin is small. In subgroup analysis, warfarin proved significantly more effective than aspirin in preventing cardioembolic strokes and strokes of uncertain pathophysiology but not strokes of noncardioembolic origin (Miller et al., 1996). Young patients without risk factors had a low rate of stroke and older patients had a substantial risk of stroke, regardless of which treatment was used. Similar conclusions were reached in a pooled analysis of five randomized controlled trials on the efficacy of antithrombotic therapy in AF (Atrial Fibrillation Investigators, 1994). Warfarin consistently decreased the risk of stroke in patients with AF (a 68% reduction in risk) with essentially no increase in the frequency of major bleeding. The efficacy of aspirin was less clear, with an overall pooled risk reduction of 36%. Patients with AF younger than 65 years and without a history of hypertension, previous stroke, TIAs, or diabetes mellitus were at very low risk of stroke even without treatment. In a decision and cost-effectiveness analysis including quality of life estimates, Gage and colleagues (1995) concluded that treatment with warfarin is cost-effective in patients with nonvalvular AF and one or more additional risk factors for stroke. However, in 65-year-old patients with AF but no other risk factors for stroke, treatment with warfarin instead of aspirin would affect quality-adjusted survival minimally but increase costs significantly. We currently recommend prophylactic anticoagulation treatment for older, high-risk AF patients and aspirin therapy as tolerated for younger, low-risk patients.

In one study, the optimum dose of anticoagulation with the lowest risk in patients with nonrheumatic AF and recent cerebral ischemia was that which produced an INR of 3.0 (European Atrial Fibrillation Trial Study Group, 1995). Hylek et al. (1996) found anticoagulant prophylaxis in patients with AF to be effective with INRs of 2.0 or greater and suggested tight control of anticoagulant therapy to maintain the INR between 2.0 and 3.0 (thereby limiting the increased risk of hemorrhage at higher INRs). A target value slightly higher (INR of 3.0–4.0) was suggested for patients with mechanical heart valves (Cannegieter et al., 1995).

About 2.5% of patients with acute **myocardial infarction** experience an ischemic stroke within 4 weeks, with the risk of stroke being highest within the first 2 weeks following the infarct (see Table 5 in Cerebral Embolism Task Force, 1986a; Cerebral Embolism Task Force, 1989). Three large, controlled clinical trials, individually and in aggregate, show that anticoagulation therapy in unselected patients with acute myocardial infarction reduces the likelihood of imminent ischemic stroke (Medical Research Council, 1969; Drapkin and Mersky, 1972; Veterans Administration Cooperative Study, 1973; Editorial, 1990). As might be expected, hemorrhagic complications are increased in such patients. Thus, the indications for prophylactic use of anticoagulants in the setting of an acute myocardial infarction remain controversial. Patients with mural thrombi, who are at particular risk for stroke, may be an identifiable subset who would potentially benefit from anticoagulant therapy (Cerebral Embolism Task Force, 1989; Editorial, 1990). A subsequent study of 3404 postmyocardial infarction patients followed for more than 3 years also confirmed that long-term anticoagulant therapy substantially reduces the risk of stroke and that the increased risk of bleeding complications in these patients is offset by a marked reduction in ischemic events (Azar et al., 1996). The efficacy of antiplatelet agents in such patients is unclear (Yanagihara and Whisnant, 1996).

Overall, about 20% of patients with **rheumatic mitral stenosis** have clinical embolism (Coulshed et al., 1970; Fleming and Bailey, 1971; Easton and Sherman, 1980; Beppu et al., 1984). The incidence of embolism is about 4% per year in such patients. Efforts were made to identify subgroups of patients who are at special risk of embolism (e.g., enlarged left atrium, severity of stenosis, associated cardiac failure) with inconclusive results except that patients with coexistent rheumatic mitral stenosis and AF have a risk of embolism that is three to seven times that of patients with mitral stenosis alone (Coulshed et al., 1970; Fleming and Bailey, 1971; Wolf et al., 1978a, 1978b; Fukuda and Nakamura, 1984). In view of these findings, prophylactic anticoagulation seems to be indicated in selected patients with rheumatic mitral stenosis, particularly those with AF (Szekely, 1964; Levine, 1981). In addition, because 30–75% of patients with rheumatic heart disease who experience an initial embolic stroke have another embolic cerebrovascular event at a rate of about 10% per year (Cerebral Embolism Task Force, 1986a), anticoagulation or surgical correction of the abnormal valve may be warranted in such patients. In patients with mechanical heart valves and high-risk patients with prosthetic tissue valves, the addition of aspirin to warfarin therapy can reduce the rate of major systemic embolism and the mortality from vascular causes (Turpie et al., 1993).

The overall risk of stroke in young adults with **mitral valve prolapse** is probably less than 1 in 6000 persons per year. Thus, no prophylactic treatment seems warranted in such patients as long as they are asymptomatic (Cerebral Embolism Task Force, 1986a). The treatment of patients who experience a stroke in the setting of MVP remains empiric. Based on the observation of platelet-fibrin emboli and platelet activation in such patients, the use of antiplatelet agents may be appropriate (Barnett, 1982; Fisher et al., 1982; Scharf et al., 1982).

Cerebral embolism is common in patients with **nonischemic dilated cardiomyopathies** of almost all types (Thomas et al., 1954; Segal et al., 1965; Parameswaran et al., 1969; Demakis et al., 1974; Shafii, 1977; Hodgman et al., 1982; See Table 6 in Cerebral Embolism Task Force, 1989). The common denominator in these cardiomyopathies seems to be a dilated, hypokinetic ventricle, with or without

secondary AF, that predisposes to thrombus formation and subsequent embolism. No controlled studies of antithrombotic therapy have been performed in such patients, but there is a general consensus that long-term anticoagulation is indicated even if there is no echocardiographically defined thrombus (Segal et al., 1978; Fuster et al., 1981; Cerebral Embolism Task Force, 1989).

Intra-atrial septal defects and **patent foramen ovale** are important risk factors for stroke in young adults (Lechat et al., 1985; Lechat et al., 1988; Gautier et al., 1989). There is some evidence to suggest that the risk is higher in those patients who also have atrial septal aneurysms. The optimum management of patients with these conditions is not clear and ranges from observation to antiplatelet agents, anticoagulants, and cardiac surgery (Devuyst et al., 1996).

Treatment of Specific Patient Groups

Management of Patients with Asymptomatic Cervical Bruit, Asymptomatic Carotid Disease, or Both

The rationale for treatment of a patient with an asymptomatic cervical bruit is based on the assumption that there is a significant prevalence of atherosclerotic or other occlusive disease of the internal or common carotid artery on the side of the asymptomatic bruit and that such disease will eventually produce permanent neurologic or visual disability through thromboembolic mechanisms. Some investigators thus recommend that patients with an asymptomatic cervical bruit who are considered to be candidates for endarterectomy undergo noninvasive testing of carotid patency. Patients found to have either large ulcerated plaques or hemodynamically significant stenosis may then be considered for endarterectomy in an effort to prevent subsequent stroke (Thompson et al., 1978; Moore et al., 1979; Quinones-Baldrich and Moore, 1985; Norris and Zhu, 1990; Moore et al., 1995).

The problem with this approach is that **less than 1%** of patients with an asymptomatic bruit experience a stroke in the territory of that vessel per year, and only 1–3% of patients with angiographically proven ipsilateral carotid artery disease experience any type of stroke each year (Whisnant, 1983; Chambers and Norris, 1984a, 1984b, 1986; The European Carotid Surgery Trialists Collaborative Group, 1995; Lanska and Kryscio, 1997). In addition, such patients have an increased risk of cardiovascular complications and related death compared with patients without a cervical bruit (Burke et al., 1982). Thus, the risk of stroke is quite low in patients with an asymptomatic cervical bruit, the risk of **directly related stroke** is exceptionally low, and the risk of cardiovascular death is substantial. Even carotid endarterectomy that is performed by an experienced surgeon in a center with an appropriately low operative and perioperative morbidity and mortality is unlikely to significantly improve the ultimate prognosis in many patients (Whisnant et al., 1983). An asymptomatic bruit should therefore be viewed primarily as evidence of **diffuse,** rather than focal, vascular disease (Heyman et al., 1980; Burke et al., 1982; Kuller and Sutton, 1984; Bogousslavsky et al., 1986a; Hennerici et al., 1987; White et al., 1990).

Several trials attempted to determine whether or not the

addition of carotid endarterectomy to aspirin plus risk factor modifications affects the incidence of ipsilateral TIAs, stroke, transient monocular loss of vision, or retinal infarction in patients with asymptomatic carotid stenosis in at least one artery (The CASANOVA Study Group, 1991; Mayo Asymptomatic Carotid Endarterectomy Study Group, 1992; Barnett and Haines, 1993; Hobson et al., 1993; Easton and Wilterdink, 1994; European Carotid Surgery Trialists Collaborative Group, 1995; The Executive Committee for the Asymptomatic Carotid Atherosclerosis Study, 1995). The results of three trials reported no statistically significant benefit for surgery in the prevention of stroke or death (The CASANOVA Study Group, 1991; Mayo Asymptomatic Carotid Endarterectomy Group, 1992; Hobson et al., 1993). However, none was sufficiently large to exclude such a benefit.

In 1994, a clinical advisory was issued from the National Institutes of Health regarding the interim results of the Asymptomatic Carotid Atherosclerosis Study (ACAS) (ACAS, 1994), followed by publication of these results in 1995 (Executive Committee for the ACAS, 1995). The interim results were based on 1662 patients with greater than 60% stenosis of the internal carotid artery who were randomized to either endarterectomy or observation, although all patients received aspirin and advice on modification of risk factors. After 4657 cumulative patient years of follow-up, the aggregate risk over 5 years for ipsilateral stroke and any perioperative stroke or death was 5.1% among patients assigned to surgery and 11.0% among those in the nonsurgical arm. Carotid endarterectomy was reported as beneficial with a relative reduction in the risk of stroke within 5 years of 53%. The success of the operation was dependent on a perioperative morbidity and mortality of less than 3%. Within 5 years after endarterectomy, men had a 66% relative risk reduction of stroke, whereas women had a 17% relative risk reduction. Excluding arteriographic and perioperative complications, the risk reduction after endarterectomy in this group of patients was 79% for men and 56% for women. There was no stratification by degree of stenosis provided, and patients were highly selected to avoid excessive surgical risk. The statistics were based on "intent to treat," meaning that randomization depended on carotid Doppler diagnosis, not angiography. Patients subsequently discovered on arteriography to have insignificant stenosis (7.4% of cases) were not endarterectomized but were analyzed like surgically treated patients. These interim results are at odds with the findings in the ECST in which 970 patients with asymptomatic stenosis ranging from 30 to 99% were found to have a risk of stroke or death at 3 years of only 3.9% (The European Carotid Surgery Trialists Collaborative Group, 1995). This is equivalent to an approximately 6.5% risk of stroke or death at 5 years, somewhat less than the 11.0% reported in the nonsurgical arm of the ACAS. However, even in the ECST, stroke risk increased with the degree of carotid stenosis: The 3-year risk of stroke was 5.7% for patients with 70–99% stenosis, 9.8% for patients with 80–89% stenosis, and 14.4% for patients with 90–99% stenosis.

Until the final results of these and other studies are made available, we agree with investigators who do not recommend surgical therapy for most patients with an asymptomatic cervical bruit without documented carotid artery disease or with hemodynamically insignificant carotid artery disease (Whisnant, 1983; Barnett et al., 1984; Chambers and Norris, 1984b; Yatsu and Fields, 1985; Sarasin et al., 1995; Warlow, 1995; Barnett et al., 1996b; Frey, 1996; Lanska and Kryscio, 1997; Mackey et al., 1997). Patients in whom a bruit is heard during a routine examination should undergo a careful search for potentially modifiable risk factors that increase the likelihood of stroke, vascular death, or both. Modification of such risk factors is probably the most important treatment that can be given to these patients. In view of the findings that the frequency of stroke in patients with an asymptomatic carotid bruit is maximum when carotid stenosis reaches 75–90% stenosis, it may be appropriate to examine all patients with an asymptomatic carotid bruit at regular intervals using Doppler duplex scanning. However, The European Carotid Surgery Trialists Collaborative Group (1995) argued that population screening for asymptomatic carotid stenosis cannot be justified from either a cost-effective or public health impact standpoint without a randomized, controlled trial to look specifically at this issue (see also Cronenwett et al., 1997 and Perry et al., 1997).

Although treatment of patients with asymptomatic cervical bruits, asymptomatic carotid artery disease, or both, with antiplatelet agents is likely to be without side effects, no evidence exists that such therapy is of long-term benefit in decreasing either the risk of subsequent stroke or vascular death. Indeed, Cote et al. (1995) reported that 325 mg per day of aspirin was not protective in patients with asymptomatic stenosis, but the dosage may not have been optimum. Similarly, there is no evidence that long-term anticoagulation, with its attendant risks, is useful in such patients.

Management of Patients with Transient Ischemic Attacks

The literature that pertains to the management of TIAs is, as noted above, confusing and contradictory. It contains numerous poorly controlled, retrospective, and nonrandomized studies purporting to show the effectiveness or lack thereof, of carotid endarterectomy, EC-IC bypass, aspirin, or other platelet antiaggregants, and anticoagulants in the prevention of stroke in patients with TIAs. Such studies are basically anecdotal and do not allow rational conclusions. In addition, most of these studies do not attempt to separate TIA patients by **cause**. Thus, patients who experienced an embolic event from a cardiac source are combined with patients who have symptomatic carotid occlusive disease and patients with complicated migraine. Despite these limitations, there are some guidelines for the management of patients with TIAs (Sandok et al., 1978; Matchar and Pauker, 1987a; Becker and Burde, 1988; Gorelick, 1995; Raps and Galetta, 1995). In the following sections, we review the data concerning optimum treatment of patients who experience carotid or vertebrobasilar arterial system TIAs.

MEDICAL TREATMENT OF PATIENTS WITH TIAS

A number of investigators attempted to determine if immediate anticoagulation, long-term anticoagulation, or treatment with antiplatelet agents is of any benefit in reducing the risk of vascular death or subsequent stroke in patients with one or more TIAs. Ramirez-Lassepas and Cipolle (1988) reviewed all 15 randomized studies published on the medical treatment of TIAs in which controls received no treatment or placebo and in which mortality was reported. These investigators used the odds ratio method to analyze the results to determine if treatment with either anticoagulation or antiplatelet agents had any effect on expected mortality. This meta-analysis showed that neither treatment modality significantly reduces mortality.

Because the risk of stroke may be highest in the first 30 days after a TIA, some investigators recommend **immediate anticoagulation** of patients with TIAs of increasing severity, frequency, or duration (Sandok et al., 1978). The potential benefit of such treatment must be compared with the potential risk of intracranial or systemic hemorrhage associated with heparin use in such patients. However, even in patients with large embolic stroke, acute anticoagulation, when carefully monitored, confers no substantially increased risk of hemorrhagic transformation of the infarction (Chamorro et al., 1995).

Biller et al. (1989) performed a prospective, randomized study in an attempt to ascertain the efficacy of intravenous heparin compared with aspirin in preventing an acute stroke in patients with a recent TIA. Fifty-five patients were entered into the study, of whom 45 underwent cerebral angiography as part of their evaluation. Most, but not all, of these patients had angiographic lesions in the distribution of the affected vessel. Patients randomized to the heparin group received an intravenous bolus injection of 5000 units of heparin sodium, followed by a constant maintenance infusion. Heparin was continued for a minimum of 3 days and a maximum of 9 days. Patients randomized to aspirin treatment were given 650 mg of aspirin twice a day (1300 mg/day) for a minimum of 3 and a maximum of 15 days. Both investigators and patients were aware of the treatment being given. In this study, one patient taking heparin experienced a stroke during the period of treatment, compared with four patients taking aspirin. In all cases, the stroke was in the distribution of the affected vessel. Although the results of this study suggest that heparin is more effective than aspirin (and, presumably, placebo) in preventing a related stroke in patients with an acute TIA, the differences are not statistically significant, possibly because of the small number of patients in the study. In addition, the investigators did not perform complete angiography on every patient, and they did not exclude nonatheromatous vascular diseases and potential cardiac sources of embolism in the patients they evaluated. Thus, no conclusions can therefore be drawn from the study of Biller et al. (1989) concerning the potential benefit of either acute anticoagulation or use of antiplatelet agents in patients with acute TIA. The results of the study do, however, emphasize the need for a prospective, randomized, clinical trial with an adequate number of patients to determine if either aspirin or heparin given immediately after an acute TIA is effective in preventing a permanent neurologic deficit in the immediate post-TIA period.

The results of several uncontrolled, nonrandomized studies suggest that **long-term anticoagulation** reduces the stroke rate in selected patients who experience one or more TIAs in the carotid or vertebrobasilar system (Frank, 1971), but the results of other studies do not support this conclusion (Jonas, 1988). In addition, any enthusiasm for the use of anticoagulant therapy in patients with TIA must be tempered by the realization that such therapy is potentially hazardous. Whisnant et al. (1978) showed that the risk of intracranial hemorrhage in patients aged 55–74 years who experience a TIA is eight times greater in patients on anticoagulant therapy than in untreated patients. Furlan et al. (1979b) also demonstrated the adverse effect of anticoagulant therapy on the incidence of intracerebral hemorrhage. In neither of these studies were the prothrombin times of patients who experienced an intracranial hemorrhage inappropriately prolonged. Both studies suggested that most patients who experience an intracranial hemorrhage while taking long-term anticoagulant therapy do so after a year or more of treatment. Elderly hypertensive patients seem to be at particular risk.

By far the most controversial aspect of medical management of TIA concerns the use of **long-term antiplatelet therapy**. In theory, the use of drugs that prevent platelet aggregation should reduce the probability of additional thrombotic and embolic events that result in stroke and myocardial infarction. Since 1969, randomized, controlled trials have analyzed the effectiveness of a variety of antiplatelet agents (i.e., aspirin, dipyridamole, and sulfinpyrazone), alone and in combination, against placebo, anticoagulants, or each other in the prevention of stroke after TIA or minor stroke (Acheson et al., 1969; Fields et al., 1977, 1978; The Canadian Cooperative Study Group, 1978; Ruether and Dorndorf, 1978; Olsson et al., 1980; Burén and Ygge, 1981; Roden et al., 1981; Candelise et al., 1982; Bousser et al., 1983; Garde et al., 1983; Sorensen et al., 1983; The American-Canadian Cooperative Study Group, 1985; European Stroke Prevention Study Group, 1987; Boysen et al, 1988b; The Dutch TIA Study Group, 1988; The Dutch TIA Trial Study Group, 1991; The SALT Collaborative Group, 1991; UK-TIA Study Group, 1991). As a result of these studies, a number of reviews and editorials expressed support for the use of antiplatelet agents, particularly aspirin, in patients who experience TIAs, regardless of cause (Dyken, 1983a; Fields, 1983; Quan et al., 1983; Gent, 1987; Cusimano and Ameli, 1989; Raps and Galetta, 1995).

Sze et al. (1988) performed a meta-analysis of seven randomized, controlled trials that compared aspirin, sulfinpyrazone, dipyridamole, or a combination of these drugs with placebo (Acheson et al., 1969; Fields et al., 1977; Ruether and Dorndorff, 1978; The Canadian Cooperative Study Group, 1978; Roden et al., 1981; Bousser et al., 1983; Sorensen et al., 1983). For aspirin compared with placebo, a nonsignificant reduction in stroke of 15% was found. For aspirin combined with sulfinpyrazone or dipyridamole compared with placebo, a 39% reduction in stroke was observed, but a 350% increase in gastrointestinal hemorrhage or peptic ulcer was noted. A trend in reduction of strokes for men was observed for all regimens containing aspirin. Sze et al. (1988) concluded from this analysis that an apparent benefit of aspirin-combination therapy on stroke in patients with one or more TIAs must be interpreted cautiously because of a number of possible biases. These investigators believed that aspirin alone may conceivably decrease the incidence of stroke after TIA by as much as 40%, but emphasized that a sample size of more than **13,000** patients would be needed to confirm such a benefit. It should also be noted that in all of the studies analyzed by Sze et al. (1988), the dose of aspirin used was 990–1500 mg per day, much more than the theoretically optimum dose for platelet antiaggregation (see above).

Another study, in which the protective effect of 300 mg of aspirin per day was compared with the effect of 1200 mg of aspirin per day and with placebo, showed no difference between the two doses of aspirin with regard to the occurrence of cerebrovascular, cardiovascular, or any other complications (UK-TIA Study Group, 1988, 1991). Compared with the placebo-treated patients, both aspirin groups together showed a significant reduction in death, nonfatal major stroke, and nonfatal myocardial infarction in this study. In the European Stroke Prevention Study (ESPS), aspirin 990 mg/day combined with dipyridamole 225 mg/day resulted in a significant reduction in stroke compared with placebo in patients at risk for stroke (European Stroke Prevention Study Group, 1987). Unlike an earlier Canadian study (The Canadian Cooperative Study Group, 1978), the ESPS demonstrated only a slightly greater therapeutic effect for men (Sivenius et al., 1991a). Aspirin and dipyridamole were particularly efficacious in reducing the incidence of stroke among those patients entered into the study with TIAs, especially those in the vertebrobasilar territory (Sivenius et al., 1991b). The beneficial effect of antiplatelet therapy was apparent in patients of all ages, including the elderly (Sivenius et al., 1995). In the European Stroke Prevention Study 2, low-dose aspirin (50 mg per day) and dipyridamole (400 mg per day) were effective individually and were additive in the secondary prevention of TIA and stroke (Diener et al., 1996a).

Other studies evaluated the effect of low doses of aspirin in the prevention of stroke in patients with TIAs. In a Swedish study of 1360 patients with recent TIAs or minor stroke, 75 mg/day of aspirin was associated with a significant reduction in the risk of stroke and death compared with placebo (The SALT Collaborative Group, 1991). In the Dutch TIA Trial, a randomized, controlled, double-blind clinical trial in patients with TIAs or nondisabling stroke, 30 mg of aspirin per day was as effective as 300 mg in the prevention of stroke and was better tolerated (The Dutch TIA Trial Study Group, 1991).

Pooling the results of several studies, the Antiplatelet Trialists' Collaboration Group concluded in 1988 that aspirin in the dose range of 300–1500 mg per day decreases the risk of vascular death, nonfatal stroke, or nonfatal myocardial infarction by 23–24%. A second analysis performed in 1994 reported similar results: With aspirin use, there was a 23% reduction in the risk of stroke, myocardial infarction, or vascular death, and a 22% reduction in the risk of stroke alone (Antiplatelet Trialists' Collaboration Group, 1994). The Stroke Council of the American Heart Association suggests aspirin in a dose range between 30 and 1300 mg/day as appropriate initial therapy for most patients after a TIA (Feinberg et al., 1994). Although most neurologists choose

an aspirin dose of 325 mg/day (Alberts et al., 1994), one retrospective study suggested a greater risk of recurrent stroke in patients taking less than 500 mg/day compared with patients on higher doses (Bornstein et al., 1994). In the Second European Stroke Prevention Study involving 6602 patients, treatment with a combination of low-dose aspirin (50 mg per day) and high-dose dipyridamole (400 mg per day) proved more effective in the secondary prevention of stroke than placebo or either agent alone (Sivenius et al., 1996). We agree with others that the optimum therapeutic dose of aspirin to prevent strokes in patients with TIAs has yet to be determined (Algra and van Gijn, 1996; Barnett et al., 1996a; Hart and Harrison, 1996).

The Ticlopidine Aspirin Stroke Study (TASS) was a randomized multicenter trial in which patients with recent TIAs or minor stroke were treated with aspirin 650 mg twice a day or ticlopidine 250 mg twice a day (Hass et al., 1989; Ticlopidine Aspirin Stroke Study Group, 1993). Ticlopidine proved more beneficial than aspirin in the reduction of stroke and death (21% risk reduction for stroke and 12% risk reduction for stroke and all causes of death), especially during the first year of treatment, although there were more side effects among the ticlopidine-treated patients. In a subgroup analysis, Grotta et al. (1992) identified patients with an especially favorable response to ticlopidine treatment: Women, patients with vertebrobasilar symptoms, patients who were aspirin failures or intolerant of aspirin or warfarin, and patients with diffuse atherosclerotic disease rather than high-grade carotid stenosis. Another subgroup analysis of TASS looked only at those patients with minor stroke as the entry event and concluded that ticlopidine was somewhat more effective than aspirin in the prevention of recurrent stroke (36% 1-year risk reduction) (Harbison, 1992). In later subgroup analyses, ticlopidine was shown to be more efficacious than aspirin in preventing strokes in whites (Weisberg et al., 1993) and in reducing the risk of subsequent TIAs in all patients (Bellavance et al., 1993). The Canadian American Ticlopidine Study (CATS) specifically chose mild-to-moderate stroke as entry criteria and also showed a reduction in the overall risk of stroke of approximately one-third with ticlopidine compared with placebo (Gent et al., 1989). In an analysis of ticlopidine use for the prevention of stroke in high-risk patients, Oster et al. (1994) concluded that ticlopidine-treated patients would suffer two fewer initial strokes per 100 than aspirin-treated patients, and that this benefit was cost-effective (but see editorial reply by van Gijn and Algra, 1994).

Because both aspirin and ticlopidine seem to reduce the risk of both fatal and nonfatal stroke, it might be assumed that combination therapy using **both aspirin and ticlopidine** would be associated with an even better prognosis in appropriately selected patients. Uchiyama et al. (1989) evaluated the effects on coagulation of 81 mg/day of aspirin and 100 mg/day of ticlopidine in 23 patients. These investigators found that combination therapy markedly inhibited platelet aggregation induced by ADP, PAF, and arachidonic acid, markedly reduced the plasma concentrations of β-thromboglobulin, platelet factor 4, and thromboxane B_2, and markedly increased the bleeding time in all patients. The results of this study suggest that the antiplatelet effects of aspirin and ticlopidine together are greater than the effects of either agent alone. It remains to be proven whether or not these effects would result in an improved outcome in selected patients with increased risk factors for stroke (Warlow, 1990).

In the Clopidogrel Versus Aspirin in Patients at Risk of Ischemic Events (CAPRIE) trial, 19,185 patients with recent myocardial infarction, stroke within the past 6 months, or current intermittent claudication were randomized to receive either clopidogrel 75 mg per day or aspirin 325 mg per day (CAPRIE Steering Committee, 1996). At the end of 3 years, the relative risk of ischemic stroke, myocardial infarction, or vascular-related death was 8.7% lower in patients taking clopidogrel. Side effects from clopidogrel were minimal.

Several investigators tried to combine data from many studies in order to generalize recommendations for medical therapy (Antiplatelet Trialists' Collaboration Group, 1994; Matchar et al., 1994; Barnett et al., 1995b). A collaborative overview summarized the data from 173 randomized trials of antiplatelet therapy (Antiplatelet Trialists' Collaboration Group, 1994). Among patients at high risk for occlusive vascular disease, antiplatelet therapy was definitely protective for subsequent myocardial infarction, nonfatal stroke, and vascular death, with risk reductions of one-third, one-third, and one-sixth, respectively. The most widely tested regimen was aspirin in a daily dosage of 75–325 mg. There was no clear evidence on the balance of risks and benefits of antiplatelet therapy in primary prevention among low-risk patients. From a pool of 900 articles dealing with medical treatment of stroke prevention, Matchar et al. (1994) identified 33 studies reporting the results of randomized controlled trials of antiplatelet agents or anticoagulants and combined the outcome data and follow-up. They concluded that warfarin should be given to patients with nonvalvular AF who are older than 60 years or who have additional risk factors for stroke (see above), that aspirin should be used as the initial therapy in patients with TIAs or minor stroke, that ticlopidine may be used in patients who do not tolerate or respond to aspirin or who have had a major stroke, and that aspirin should be given to patients who have a myocardial infarction to prevent a recurrent myocardial infarction, but that it only slightly reduces the risk of stroke in such patients. The optimum dose of aspirin has yet to be established, and the question remains whether the addition of other antiplatelet agents, such as dipyridamole, sulfinpyrazone, or even vitamin E (Steiner et al., 1995), enhances the protective role of aspirin in these patients.

Identifying the **cause** of the event is of utmost importance in the management of any patient with a TIA. In patients experiencing vertebrobasilar TIAs, especially patients who fail treatment with aspirin, ticlopidine may be particularly efficacious (Hass et al., 1989; Grotta et al., 1992). When antiplatelet agents fail, chronic anticoagulation is usually used empirically. In a retrospective multicenter study of patients with symptomatic intracranial large artery stenosis, Chimowitz et al. (1995) reported a favorable risk/benefit ratio for warfarin compared with aspirin for the prevention of major vascular events.

The efficacy of treatment in patients with TIAs can be measured in several ways, but almost all studies focus on the incidence of stroke or vascular death as endpoints. More difficult to measure, but equally important, is the severity of stroke. In most studies, minor strokes with little residual disability are considered the same as disabling strokes for purposes of determining prognosis. From the standpoint of disability, however, a RIND or minor stroke may be of no greater consequence than a TIA. Grotta et al. (1985) analyzed data from several studies (Fields et al., 1977, 1978; The Canadian Cooperative Study Group, 1978; Sorensen et al., 1983) in an effort to determine the effect of aspirin versus placebo on the **severity** of stroke that occurred in patients after TIAs. Analysis of the data suggested that strokes in patients treated with aspirin after TIAs are less severe than those in untreated patients.

SURGICAL TREATMENT OF PATIENTS WITH TIAS

The surgical treatment of patients who experience one or more TIAs depends largely on the distribution and cause of the attacks.

Surgical Treatment for Carotid Circulation TIAs. The central question is whether or not there is a favorable risk/benefit ratio for carotid endarterectomy in patients with carotid stenosis and focal TIAs in the distribution of the artery in which the lesion is present. The value of endarterectomy thus largely depends on whether or not the surgical mortality and morbidity are low enough to pose an advantage relatively early in follow-up over the cumulative rate of stroke occurrence in patients with unoperated carotid stenosis (Committee on Health Care Issues, American Neurological Association, 1987; Matchar and Pauker, 1987a, 1987b; Easton and Wilterdink; 1994; Nussbaum et al., 1996). Unfortunately, there is a great variation in surgical mortality and morbidity associated with endarterectomy. The surgeon performing the procedure must weigh the proposed advantage against the risk of surgery in the hospital where the operation is to be performed. Patient selection for endarterectomy also plays an important role in the results after surgery (Blaisdell et al., 1969; Toole et al., 1975). Carotid endarterectomy may precipitate stroke or death in those patients at greatest risk, leaving a select group of survivors who may have had a better prognosis, even without surgery (Muuronen, 1984; Hachinski, 1987). Patients who are more likely to benefit from carotid endarterectomy are thus those with symptomatic atherosclerotic carotid stenosis, few medical risk factors, no neurologic risk factors, and a life expectancy of at least 4 years (Zeiger et al., 1987).

Early randomized clinical trials assessing the efficacy of carotid endarterectomy in patients with TIAs were inconclusive (Fields et al., 1970; Shaw et al., 1984), but subsequent large, multicentered, randomized, controlled clinical trials helped define subgroups of patients who might benefit from the procedure (European Carotid Surgery Trialists Collaborative Group, 1991; Mayberg et al., 1991; North American Symptomatic Carotid Endarterectomy Trial Collaborators, 1991; Easton and Wilterdink, 1994; Goldstein et al., 1995; Moore et al., 1995). These studies assessed the effect of carotid endarterectomy on the stroke and vascular death rates in patients with carotid system TIAs (including transient monocular loss of vision) and minor stroke, with special attention to the degree of ipsilateral carotid stenosis. Maximum medical therapy in the NASCET was risk-factor modification and 1300 mg of aspirin per day; in the ECST, therapy was usually aspirin and modification of risk factors, and in the Veterans Administration Trial, it was 325 mg of aspirin daily. Combined surgical morbidity and mortality was 2.5% in NASCET patients with 70–99% stenosis and 4.7% in patients in the VA trial. The perioperative event rate for surgical patients with 70–99% stenosis in the ECST was 7.5%, but no comparable data for this time period were provided for medically treated patients. All three studies demonstrated efficacy for surgery in patients with symptomatic ipsilateral stenosis greater than 70% luminal narrowing. In this subgroup of patients, the NASCET demonstrated 2-year cumulative ipsilateral stroke rates of 26% among the 331 medically treated patients and 9% among the 328 surgically treated patients (relative risk reduction of 65%). In the ECST, the 3-year risk of stroke was 18% for the 323 medical patients and 11% for the surgical patients (relative risk reduction of 42%). Furthermore, in the NASCET, at an average follow-up of 18 months, patients with symptomatic high-grade stenosis randomized to surgery had the additional benefit of a greater reduction in functional impairment, including vision, than patients treated medically (Haynes et al., 1994).

Within the subgroup of symptomatic patients with 70–99% stenosis, there is evidence from the NASCET that the risk of subsequent stroke, and the relative risk reduction by performing surgery, is directly correlated to the severity of the ipsilateral carotid stenosis (Easton and Wilterdink, 1994; Morgenstern et al., 1997). Furthermore, there may be a need for urgency in considering carotid endarterectomy for patients in this subgroup who experience recurrent ipsilateral ischemic events extending back more than 6 months, because these patients are at particular risk for subsequent stroke (Paddock-Eliasziw et al., 1996). In addition, the risk of ipsilateral stroke in this high-risk subgroup directly correlated with the severity of the contralateral carotid stenosis (Gasecki et al., 1995). Carotid endarterectomy also reduced the stroke risk among patients with high-grade ipsilateral carotid stenosis and contralateral carotid stenosis, with a relative risk reduction of 68.2%. However, patients with contralateral internal carotid artery stenosis had a particularly significant perioperative rate of stroke and death that directly correlated with the severity of the contralateral stenosis. In a meta-analysis of these three major studies, adjusting for different primary endpoints and duration of follow-up, carotid endarterectomy had a similar benefit for symptomatic patients across trials and a similar benefit for men and women (Goldstein et al., 1995).

In the NASCET, although carotid endarterectomy in patients with high-grade stenosis was beneficial among those who presented with transient monocular visual loss (6% risk of stroke at 2 years in the surgical group versus 16.6% risk of stroke in the medical group), the cumulative risk for stroke at 2 years was only 17% in those patients entered into the trial with retinal TIAs, compared with 44% in patients with hemispheric TIAs (Streifler et al., 1995).

It is important to note that the NASCET excluded patients with significant heart disease and other significant medical risk factors. Furthermore applicability of these data to the community depends on comparably low surgical complication rates (Goldstein et al., 1997; Stukenborg, 1997; Wong et al., 1997).

In both the NASCET and the ECST, there was no proven benefit of carotid endarterectomy in patients with recent TIAs or minor stroke and less than 30% ipsilateral carotid artery stenosis (European Carotid Surgery Trialists Collaborative Group, 1991; North American Symptomatic Carotid Endarterectomy Trial Collaborators, 1991; Easton and Wilterdink, 1994). Results from the ECST suggest that among symptomatic patients with ipsilateral moderate stenosis, no benefit would be gained from endarterectomy over a period of 4–5 years in patients with 50–69% stenosis and 6–7 years in patients with 30–49% stenosis (European Carotid Surgery Trialists' Collaborative Group, 1996). The NASCET continues to evaluate the efficacy of the procedure in those symptomatic patients with 30–69% stenosis.

Percutaneous transluminal angioplasty has been performed in too few patients for any meaningful data to be collected and analyzed. There are both obvious benefits and obvious risks to the procedure, and these need to be addressed in a controlled, unbiased fashion before the procedure can be universally recommended or condemned (Beebe et al., 1996; Naylor et al., 1997). At this time, we can only agree with Terada et al. (1996) that it may be of benefit in certain carefully selected patients with carotid or vertebrobasilar arterial stenosis.

For patients with hemisphere TIAs or transient monocular loss of vision associated with occlusion of the ipsilateral internal carotid artery, two procedures are advocated. **External carotid endarterectomy** is a procedure that may significantly increase ipsilateral cerebral perfusion while at the same time offering an extremely low morbidity and mortality (Sterpetti et al., 1988). Although this procedure is safe and effective in reducing both transient monocular visual loss and hemisphere TIAs in patients with occlusion of the ipsilateral internal carotid artery (see Table II in Sterpetti et al., 1988), its efficacy in preventing subsequent stroke is unknown, and it almost certainly does not alter the increased risk of cardiac death in such patients.

A randomized trial of **superficial temporal artery to middle cerebral artery bypass**, designed to determine if the procedure reduces the rate of subsequent stroke among patients with occlusion or severe atherosclerotic narrowing of the internal carotid or middle cerebral artery and recent hemispheric or retinal strokes, TIAs, or both (The EC/IC Bypass Study Group, 1985a), failed to show any benefit from the procedure even though the bypass patency rate was 96%, and the 30-day surgical mortality and major stroke morbidity rates were 0.6% and 2.5%, respectively (The EC/IC Bypass Study Group, 1985b). In this study, both nonfatal and fatal stroke occurred more frequently and earlier in the patients who underwent surgery. Secondary survival analyses comparing the two groups for major strokes and all deaths, for all strokes and all deaths, and for ipsilateral ischemic strokes demonstrated a similar lack of benefit from surgery. Separate analyses of patients with different angiographic lesions did not identify any subgroup that benefited from surgery, but two subgroups of patients fared substantially worse in the surgical group: patients with severe stenosis of the middle cerebral artery and patients with symptomatic occlusion of the internal carotid artery. Although this study was criticized by some investigators for its methodology (Editorial, 1985; Ausman and Diaz, 1986; Awad and Spetzler, 1986; Day et al., 1986), it nevertheless stands as a model of its kind, and its results and conclusions should be accepted unless a similar controlled study invalidates them (Plum, 1985). At the present time, we recommend the procedure only for patients with the ocular ischemic syndrome associated with unilateral or bilateral occlusion of the internal carotid artery (Kawaguchi et al., 1994).

Surgical Treatment for Vertebrobasilar TIAs. Patients with vertebrobasilar TIAs are usually treated with antiplatelet agents or anticoagulation, even though less information regarding the efficacy of such treatment for vertebrobasilar TIAs exists than for carotid circulation TIAs (Dyken, 1983b; Kistler et al., 1984b; Sivenius et al., 1991b; Grotta et al., 1992). In addition, a number of surgical procedures are advocated for patients with symptomatic intracranial and extracranial thrombo-occlusive disease affecting the vertebrobasilar arterial system.

Carotid endarterectomy is occasionally performed for patients with vertebrobasilar TIAs who also have stenosis of one or both internal carotid arteries on the assumption that correction of associated carotid stenosis should improve total cerebral blood flow and thereby indirectly relieve symptoms caused by posterior circulation insufficiency and reduce the risk of vertebrobasilar stroke (Rosenthal et al., 1978). The rationale for such treatment is questionable at best, and the data supporting it are incomplete and inadequate. There is certainly no evidence that carotid endarterectomy prevents either subsequent stroke or vascular death in such patients. Although there is a role for carotid endarterectomy in selected patients with carotid system TIAs, we do not advocate this procedure for most patients with vertebrobasilar TIA.

Several investigators described their experience with **intracranial vertebral artery endarterectomy** for patients with vertebrobasilar TIAs and severe stenosis of the distal portion of one vertebral artery. Allen et al. (1981) performed the procedure on two patients, and Ausman et al. (1984) performed it on four patients. Of these six attempted endarterectomies, two were aborted because of lengthy plaque extension or erosion through the wall of the vertebral artery. Of the four procedures completed, three resulted in patent vessels. Hopkins et al. (1987) performed intracranial vertebral artery endarterectomy on two patients with severe (90–95%) but discrete stenotic lesions of the distal vertebral artery proximal to the posterior inferior cerebellar artery, associated with a hypoplastic contralateral vertebral artery in one case and an occluded contralateral vertebral artery in the other. One patient was experiencing episodes of syncope, dysarthria, ataxia, hemiparesis, and diplopia. The other patient had drop attacks, episodes of bilateral visual loss, diplopia, and dysarthria. Postoperative angiography showed a patent vessel in both patients, and although both developed communicating hydrocephalus requiring lumboperitoneal

shunt after surgery, they were asymptomatic within 1 year. Ausman et al. (1990) subsequently reported their experience with intracranial vertebral endarterectomy in six patients with vertebrobasilar insufficiency in whom medical therapy had failed. Four of the patients had 50–80% stenosis proximal to the posterior inferior cerebellar artery, one had 90% stenosis at the origin of this vessel, and one had 80% stenosis distal to the posterior inferior cerebellar artery. Significant complications occurred in four of the six patients, including leakage of CSF, medullary infarction, meningitis, cerebellar infarction, and death. Although three of the patients had improvement in symptoms after surgery, postoperative angiography showed an occluded endarterectomy in one of them. Intracranial vertebral endarterectomy may be appropriate for patients with vertebrobasilar TIAs when one vertebral artery is occluded or severely hypoplastic, and the other has a localized distal lesion. It must be emphasized, however, that this procedure is difficult to perform and has significant potential complications. We believe that it should be performed only by an experienced surgeon in an appropriate center.

An **occipital artery to posterior inferior cerebellar artery bypass procedure** may be performed for the treatment of significant diffuse stenosis proximal to the origin of the posterior inferior cerebellar artery that is thought to be producing symptoms of vertebrobasilar ischemia. Sundt and Piepgras (1985) described the results of the procedure in 39 patients. Two patients (5%) died in the perioperative period. Of the 37 surviving patients, 33 (89%) either became asymptomatic or experienced improvement in symptoms. Only four patients remained unchanged. Roski et al. (1982) treated 14 patients with this procedure and had no perioperative mortality or permanent morbidity, 100% graft patency, and neurologic improvement in all patients. Hopkins et al. (1987) treated 24 patients with this procedure, 14 of whom may have been those originally reported by Roski et al. (1982), because the authors are from the same institution. All 24 patients had patent bypasses. Although four patients had postoperative complications (meningitis in three, communicating hydrocephalus requiring shunting in one), all patients became asymptomatic.

Patients with vertebrobasilar circulation TIAs and angiographically demonstrated occlusive disease of the vertebral artery distal to the posterior inferior cerebellar artery, of the vertebrobasilar junction, or of the proximal or midbasilar artery may be treated with an **EC-IC bypass** distal to the stenotic lesion. Mortality rates from such procedures range from 6% (Hopkins et al., 1987) to 23% (El-Fiki et al., 1985). Similarly, bypass-patency rates range from 100% (Hopkins et al., 1987) to 3% (Sundt and Piepgras, 1985). In most series, over 90% of patients become asymptomatic or experience improvement in symptoms (Ausman et al., 1984; Hopkins et al., 1987). Nevertheless, major brainstem strokes may eventually occur in such patients (Hopkins and Budny, 1989).

It is clear that EC-IC bypass procedures in the posterior fossa can be performed with low perioperative mortality and morbidity, and that these procedures can reduce or eliminate pre-existing symptoms of vertebrobasilar ischemia. Nevertheless, such procedures are unlikely to affect the long-term mortality rate in such patients, and their efficacy in preventing subsequent vertebrobasilar stroke is unproven (Hopkins and Budny, 1989).

As noted above, **vertebral artery to common carotid artery transposition** is advocated for treatment of subclavian steal syndrome and symptomatic stenosis of the origin of the vertebral artery. Spetzler et al. (1987) performed this procedure on 10 patients with subclavian steal syndrome and 14 patients with stenosis of the proximal vertebral artery. There were no postoperative deaths, although five patients had mild postoperative complications. Three of the patients developed a postoperative Horner's syndrome, one patient developed a minor wound infection, and one patient developed occlusion of the ipsilateral subclavian artery. Over a follow-up period that ranged from 4 months to 4 years (mean, 19 months; median, 15 months), 20 patients (83%) became asymptomatic, three patients had reduction in the severity and frequency of symptoms, and one patient with a fixed deficit had no other symptoms and no progression of the deficit. This procedure, and similar ones performed in patients with extracranial vertebrobasilar disease, may be of benefit in selected patients when performed in a center with an appropriately low morbidity and mortality.

Percutaneous transluminal angioplasty using an intra-arterial balloon can be performed in patients with symptomatic stenosis at the origin of one of the verterbral arteries or the basilar artery. Numbers of patients are small and results are anecdotal, but there may be selected patients for whom the procedure should be considered (Terada et al., 1996).

Management of Patients with Transient Monocular Visual Loss

It is more difficult to judge the effects of medical treatment in patients with isolated, transient monocular loss of vision than in patients with other forms of TIAs. In the first place, there are many more causes for transient monocular visual loss than for transient neurologic dysfunction. It may be for this reason that patients with transient monocular visual loss do not necessarily have the same prognosis for either vascular death or stroke as do patients who experience a neurologic TIA (see above). Nevertheless, several investigators have attempted to determine the effect of medical therapy in patients with transient monocular visual loss.

Harrison et al. (1971) treated two patients with transient monocular visual loss with 600 mg of aspirin per day. One patient, a 67-year-old woman, had repeated episodes of transient visual loss in the right eye unassociated with any neurologic symptoms. An evaluation revealed a loud, high-pitched, right-sided cervical bruit and no evidence of cardiac disease. She was assumed to have right-sided carotid artery disease, which was subsequently substantiated when a right carotid angiogram showed ''marked'' stenosis at the origin of the right internal carotid artery. As soon as the patient began using aspirin, the frequency of the episodes of transient monocular visual loss markedly decreased. During a total of 62 days during which the patient took aspirin, she experienced only one episode of visual loss. The second patient reported by Harrison et al. (1971) was a 45-year-old man who experienced episodes of transient monocular visual

loss in the right eye about once or twice a week. Each episode lasted about 30–45 seconds. He had no other symptoms. A complete evaluation was unremarkable, although the patient did not undergo noninvasive diagnostic studies of carotid patency or angiography. After starting aspirin, he had only two episodes of transient monocular visual loss over 2 months. After switching to a placebo, he experienced seven attacks during 6 weeks.

Mundall et al. (1972a, 1972b) described a 63-year-old woman with idiopathic thrombocythemia (average platelet count—740,000/mm^3) who experienced 10–15 attacks of transient monocular visual loss a day in the left eye. She had previously undergone a left carotid endarterectomy. The patient was found to have abnormal spontaneous platelet aggregation. Aspirin, given in a dose of 600 mg four times a day (2400 mg per day), completely suppressed the abnormal platelet aggregability, and the patient had no further episodes of transient monocular visual loss.

Lemak et al. (1986) identified 26 patients who had been entered into the studies performed by Fields et al. (1977, 1978) because of one or more episodes of transient monocular visual loss and another 16 patients who had experienced both transient monocular visual loss and hemisphere TIAs, separately or concurrently. Fourteen patients with isolated transient monocular loss of vision and 13 patients with both transient monocular visual loss and hemisphere TIAs were treated with aspirin in a dose of 650 mg twice a day (1300 mg per day). Twelve patients with isolated, transient monocular visual loss and three patients with both transient visual loss and hemisphere TIAs were given placebo. After comparing the outcome of these patients with the outcome of other patients with hemisphere TIAs only, Lemak et al. (1986) concluded that patients with transient monocular visual loss responded as well to aspirin as did patients with hemisphere TIAs, particularly when there was evidence by angiography or noninvasive studies of ulceration or nonoccluding stenosis of the ipsilateral carotid artery.

At this time, there is no clear cut evidence that aspirin or any other drug that prevents or reduces platelet aggregation beneficially alters the ultimate visual or neurologic outcome in patients who experience transient monocular loss of vision. As with patients who experience neurologic TIAs, patients who experience one or more episodes of transient monocular visual loss should undergo a careful history and physical examination and a meticulous ocular examination. In some cases, noninvasive studies of carotid patency (e.g., duplex scanning and OPG) should be performed, whereas, in others, selective angiography may be appropriate (The Amaurosis Fugax Study Group, 1990). Young patients without obvious risk factors for atherosclerotic or other vascular disease should probably undergo a serum assay for antiphospholipid antibodies, tests for hematologic disorders, and possibly, a cardiac evaluation. Elderly patients may require an erythrocyte sedimentation rate. Treatment should be directed toward the underlying cause.

It may be appropriate to treat patients with transient monocular loss of vision with aspirin if there is evidence of stenotic or ulcerative disease in the carotid arterial system on the appropriate side (The Amaurosis Fugax Study Group,

1990). If there are elevated levels of antiphospholipid antibodies in the serum, antiplatelet agents may also be used, although oral anticoagulation may be the most efficacious method of preventing permanent thromboembolic events in such patients (Digre et al., 1989; Feldmann and Levine, 1995; Khamashta et al., 1995).

It is appropriate to consider carotid endarterectomy for patients with transient monocular visual loss and ipsilateral carotid artery stenosis greater than 70% (see above). In the NASCET, the cumulative risk for stroke at 2 years in patients with retinal TIAs and ipsilateral stenosis greater than 70% was 16.6% in patients treated medically and 6% in patients treated surgically (North American Symptomatic Carotid Endarterectomy Trial Collaborators, 1991; Streifler et al., 1995).

For patients with repeated attacks of transient monocular visual loss thought to be most consistent with a vasospastic pathophysiology, calcium-channel blocking drugs may be of benefit (Winterkorn et al., 1993).

Management of Patients with Retinal Stroke

Patients with retinal emboli have a substantially higher risk for stroke and a lower survival rate than normal patients, whether or not the embolus is symptomatic (Pfaffenbach and Hollenhorst, 1973; Savino et al., 1977; Eckardt et al., 1983). We agree with Becker and Burde (1988), Chawluk et al. (1988), and others who recommend that such patients undergo a complete systemic examination, evaluation of cardiac function, and noninvasive studies for carotid disease (duplex scanning) (De Potter and Zografos, 1990). Treatment should be directed at controllable risk factors, particularly systemic hypertension, smoking, and cardiac disease. Carotid endarterectomy may be appropriate therapy in selected patients with significant ipsilateral carotid stenosis, whereas others may benefit from aspirin.

We believe that patients who experience a retinal stroke but in whom a retinal embolus is not seen should at least be evaluated with a complete medical history and examination to identify potentially treatable diseases, such as giant cell arteritis, and to identify potentially modifiable risk factors. It may also be appropriate to perform noninvasive examination of the carotid arterial system using duplex scanning in specific patients (De Potter and Zografos, 1990). Patients with hemodynamically insignificant stenosis may be candidates for treatment with aspirin, whereas patients with stenosis greater than 70% on the side of the retinal stroke should be considered for carotid endarterectomy.

The management of acute retinal stroke, particularly CRAO, is discussed above. It suffices here to reiterate that there are no large, prospective, controlled clinical trials that show any particularly effective treatment. We recommend anterior chamber parecentesis, inhalation of carbogen, and reduction of intraocular pressure with acetazolamide or other osmotic agents, but we recognize that this treatment is of unproven efficacy (Atebara et al., 1995). Other agents proposed by investigators include sublingual nitroglycerin, oral warfarin, calcium-channel blocking drugs, vasodilators or antiplatelet agents, intravenous injection of heparin, uroki-

nase, or TPA, and intra-arterial infusion of urokinase or TPA (Mangat, 1995). Controlled trials will be necessary to determine if any of these regimens are of any benefit in restoring vision after a CRAO or branch retinal artery occlusion.

Management of Patients with Ischemic Optic Neuropathy

Whether anterior or retrobulbar, ION is only rarely associated with atheromatous disease of the ipsilateral common or internal carotid artery. Even when it is, the condition is more likely to be related to disease of the small vessels supplying the laminar and retrolaminar portions of the optic nerve than to emboli. Nevertheless, Guyer et al. (1985) found an increased incidence of cardiovascular and cerebrovascular events in patients after an attack of AION (although there was no difference in mortality), and both Sawle et al. (1990) and Hayreh et al. (1994) found a significantly increased mortality in such patients. We thus agree with Hayreh (1990) that patients with ION should undergo a careful history and medical examination to differentiate arteritic from nonarteritic ION. If a nonarteritic process is suspected, an attempt should be made to define any risk factors for atherosclerotic disease that may be controlled or modified. Patients with nonarteritic ION should be encouraged to obtain regular medical evaluations by their family physicians in the future. If the history or physical findings suggest occlusive disease of the common carotid artery or the extracranial portion of the internal carotid artery, the patient should undergo noninvasive testing using duplex scanning and oculopneumoplethysmography. If these tests reveal hemodynamically significant disease, it is appropriate to perform angiography and consider carotid endarterectomy in selected cases. If noninvasive testing does not reveal hemodynamically significant disease, angiography is probably not warranted, but such patients may be placed on aspirin.

The Ischemic Optic Neuropathy Decompression Trial (IONDT) demonstrated no benefit of optic nerve sheath decompression for nonarteritic AION compared with the natural history of the disorder (The Ischemic Optic Neuropathy Decompression Trial Research Group, 1995) (see Chapter 11). Both the efficacy and safety of thrombolytic agents and stellate ganglion block, advocated by Kajiwara et al. (1990) for the treatment of AION, are unknown.

Management of Patients with Acute Stroke

The immediate poststroke period is a vulnerable time of dynamic, complex change (Adams et al., 1994). Patients with a TIA or stroke onset of less than 48 hours previously should be hospitalized immediately (Lanska et al., 1994). Frequent TIAs, especially in a crescendo pattern, clinical features suggesting high-grade stenosis, or clinical features suggesting posterior circulation ischemia should also prompt hospital admission. Patients who experience an acute stroke may require a variety of supportive procedures to reduce the risk of subsequent death. Such patients also may be treated with a variety of medications in an attempt to reduce the severity of permanent neurologic dysfunction (Fisher, 1989; Scheinberg, 1991; Adams et al., 1994; Pessin et al., 1997).

ACUTE CARE

Acute stroke management has several goals: (*a*) to prevent aspiration, aspiration pneumonitis, pulmonary embolism, and cardiac dysfunction; (*b*) to improve regional blood flow in the periphery of the infarct in order to reduce the size of the infarct; (*c*) to reduce brain edema in order to improve circulation through compressed capillaries and to prevent herniation of brain tissue from one compartment to another; (*d*) to reduce energy requirements of brain tissue; and (*e*) to promote scavenging of cerebral free radicals produced by ischemia (Scheinberg, 1988; Brott and Reed, 1989; Schmidley, 1990; Scheinberg, 1991; Adams et al., 1994; Camarata et al., 1994; Wityk and Stern, 1994). The medical and nursing care provided in a neurologic critical care unit are likely crucial determinants in the ultimate outcome of patients with stroke (Adams et al., 1994) and probably explain the continued decline in mortality from acute ischemic stroke (see above).

Bounds et al. (1981) reported that 31% of deaths that occur after acute, ischemic stroke result from transtentorial herniation. The herniation is usually caused by progressive, uncontrolled edema in the damaged hemisphere. There is no evidence that the progression of such edema can be significantly reduced by treatment, even though mannitol and glycerol undoubtedly cause a temporary reduction in brain water (Larsson et al., 1976; Little, 1978; Bayer et al., 1987; Scheinberg, 1988). In fact, Sandercock (1987) analyzed eight published randomized, controlled trials of glycerol in acute stroke and concluded that because of wide confidence intervals, there was a distinct possibility that glycerol reduces the rate of early death by only 4% and **increases** the rate of later death by 28%. Nor is there any evidence that corticosteroid therapy beneficially affects cerebral infarction or edema (Dyken and White, 1955; Lee et al., 1974; Shubin and Fisher, 1989; Adams et al., 1994).

Studies using PET scanning demonstrate regions of low CBF but preserved oxygen metabolism after cerebral infarction (Frackowiak and Wise, 1983; Frackowiak, 1986; Frackowiak et al., 1987), suggesting that strategies aimed at increasing cerebral perfusion might salvage threatened tissue. Unfortunately, animal models of global ischemia and data from autopsy studies performed after cardiac arrest in humans demonstrate progression of neuron damage for at least 72 hours, despite rapid reperfusion (Pulsinelli et al., 1982b; Petito et al., 1987). Hemodilution therapy increases CBF in experimental studies with animals and in limited human studies (Matthews et al., 1976; Wood et al., 1982; Italian Acute Stroke Study Group, 1988; Heros and Korosue, 1989; Vorstrup et al., 1989), but there are no controlled studies in humans that convincingly demonstrate its efficacy in improving outcome after stroke. A study designed by The Hemodilution in Stroke Study Group (1989) to determine the outcome of patients given pentastarch to produce hypervolemic hemodilution after acute stroke suggested that such treatment might be beneficial in patients when treatment is begun within 12 hours, and satisfactory reduction of the hematocrit and increase in cardiac output is achieved. Unfortunately, this study was terminated prematurely to analyze possible excess mortality caused by cerebral edema in treated patients. Although some authors argue against performing any further trials of hemodilution (von Kummer et al., 1989), we and others (Grotta, 1989a, 1989b) believe that further study of the effect of hypervolemic hemodilution on the outcome of patients with acute stroke is needed.

Because neuron damage progresses despite restoration of adequate blood flow to ischemic cerebral tissue, treatment of patients with an acute stroke with substances that simply increase CBF may not result in neurologic improvement. Instead, therapy probably should be aimed at correcting abnormal ion fluxes and reducing or eliminating damaging cytotoxic byproducts of lipid metabolism, such as free radicals, that are released by even brief periods of ischemia (Wieloch et al., 1982; Raichle, 1983; Schmidley, 1990; Scheinberg, 1991; Pulsinelli, 1992; Adams et al., 1994). A massive influx of calcium into an ischemic neuron is thought to be the final metabolic insult that produces catabolism and cell necrosis from calcium overload (Gelmers, 1987; Wong and Haley, 1990); thus, calcium antagonists such as nimodipine are often given to patients with acute ischemic infarction in an attempt to prevent or reverse this calcium overload. The results of several studies are encouraging, but the data are both inconsistent and inconclusive (Gelmers, 1987; Sandercock, 1987; Gelmers et al., 1988; Coull et al., 1989; Eaton and Zweig, 1989; Oczkowski et al., 1989; Martínez-Vila et al., 1990; Wong and Haley, 1990). In addition, some studies report disappointing results, showing either no beneficial effect of nimodipine in acute ischemic stroke or some benefit only in severe cases treated early (Mohr et al., 1989; TRUST Study Group, 1990; The American Nimodipine Study Group, 1992). Nevertheless, meta-analysis of several of these studies, using pooled data from over 3700 patients, supports the view that early therapy with oral nimodipine (within 12 hours of stroke onset) may favorably influence the course of ischemic stroke (Mohr et al., 1994). Other calcium-channel blocking drugs may prove more efficacious, especially if they also stimulate selective cerebral vasodilation. However, a large double-blind, placebo-controlled trial of flunarazine, a blocker of the T-type calcium channels, demonstrated no beneficial effect in patients with acute ischemic stroke (Franke et al., 1996).

Clinical studies investigating a variety of other drugs that reduce brain energy requirements, scavenge free radicals, block opiate receptors in the brain, or antagonize excitatory amino acid function have been performed (Wise et al., 1972; Smith et al., 1974; Admani, 1978; Fallis et al., 1984; Steiner and Rose, 1986; Gelmers, 1987; Grotta, 1987; Sandercock, 1987; Fallis, 1989; Adams et al., 1994; Muir and Lees, 1995). To date, however, no modalities or drugs are clinically proven to prevent cerebral ischemia from progressing to infarction or to exert a beneficial effect upon the cerebral infarction itself (Grotta, 1987; Scheinberg, 1988, 1991; Adams et al., 1994). However, in a double-blind, placebo-controlled trial of lubeluzole in patients with acute ischemic stroke, a one-dosage regimen was not only safe but significantly reduced patient mortality at 28 days (Diener et al., 1996b). Lubeluzole exerts its neuroprotective action presumably by preventing the increase in extracellular glutamate and normalizing neuronal excitability in the peri-infarct region, as well as by inhibiting glutamate-induced nitric oxide-related neurotoxicity.

ANTICOAGULATION

Anticoagulation with heparin is often used in patients after an acute stroke (Easton, 1989; Marsh et al., 1989; Estol and Pessin, 1990). As is the case with TIAs, the efficacy of anticoagulation in such cases is unproven (Caplan, 1989a; Cerebral Embolism Task Force, 1989; Phillips, 1989a, 1989b; Scheinberg, 1989a, 1989b; Adams et al., 1994). Jonas (1988) reviewed the results of 16 acceptably randomized studies of anticoagulant therapy after cerebral or retinal infarct and analyzed the results from over 1000 anticoagulated patients and 1000 controls. He concluded that anticoagulant therapy is no better than other treatments after a **nonprogressive** (completed) stroke, regardless of whether or not the control (default) management is deliberately ineffective treatment or therapy with antiplatelet agents. Rothrock et al. (1989) also found no significant difference in the rate of early recurrent embolization among two groups of patients with acute, completed, cardioembolic stroke, one of which was immediately anticoagulated and the other of which was treated with aspirin, dipyridamole, or both. Other investigators reached similar conclusions (Cerebral Embolism Task Force, 1986b; Miller and Hart, 1988, 1989; Estol and Pessin, 1990; Adams et al., 1994). In a meta-analysis of randomized trials of antithrombotic therapy in patients with ishemic stroke, Sandercock et al. (1993) found a significant reduction in deep venous thrombosis but no reduction in pulmonary embolism or mortality. There is some evidence that patients with thrombosis in evolution may benefit from anticoagulation, but additional controlled data are needed (see also Sage, 1985).

The risk of CNS hemorrhage in patients who are treated with intravenous heparin after acute brain ischemia is estimated to range from 1% in patients who have had an acute partial stroke to about 2–4% in patients who have experienced a completed cardioembolic stroke (Miller and Hart, 1988, 1989; Rothrock et al., 1989). For years, stroke clinicians cautioned against the use of anticoagulation in patients with hemorrhagic infarctions as noted by neuroimaging and argued for the discontinuation of acute anticoagulation in the patient whose bland infarction becomes hemorrhagic during the course of treatment (Yatsu et al., 1988). However, Pessin et al. (1993) reported no major hemorrhagic complications among 12 patients at high risk for recurrent embolism and with CT evidence of hemorrhagic infarction who were anticoagulated. These findings were subsequently confirmed by others (Chamorro et al., 1995; Chaves et al., 1996; Toni et al., 1996).

Clearly, the timing and ultimate benefits from immediate anticoagulation for patients with fixed neurologic deficits, in whom no contraindication to heparin exists, are controversial (Caplan, 1989a; Miller and Hart, 1989; Scheinberg, 1989a, 1989b; Caplan, 1993). We agree with those investigators who believe that it is generally inappropriate to anticoagulate patients with an acute, completed, ischemic stroke, unless the patient is at high risk for recurrent embolism. It may be reasonable, however, to anticoagulate patients who are believed to be experiencing a **progressing** stroke, particularly when it is in the vertebrobasilar system (Udall, 1967; Kistler et al., 1984b; Sage, 1985; Grotta, 1987; Miller and Hart, 1988, 1989; Rothrock et al., 1989). In view of the difficulty in clinically differentiating primary intracerbral

hemorrhage from ischemic strokes (Udall, 1967), some type of neuroimaging study—either CT scanning or MR imaging—should almost always be performed to identify small (and occasionally large) intracerebral hemorrhages and subdural hematomas that may be diagnosed clinically as subcortical infarcts (Sage, 1985; Grotta, 1987; Miller and Hart, 1988, 1989). Patients being considered for acute anticoagulation, as well as their families, should be informed of the controversies, potential benefits, and potential risks of acute anticoagulation.

Most of the studies described above used standard unfractionated heparin administered intravenously. Clinical studies in patients with venous thrombosis suggest that low-molecular-weight heparin may be more effective than standard heparin, with no increase in the risk of bleeding. In a randomized, double-blind, placebo-controlled trial comparing two doses of subcutaneously administered low-molecular-weight heparin with placebo in the treatment of acute ischemic stroke, Kay et al. (1995) demonstrated better 6-month outcomes (reduced risk of death and functional dependency) in the heparin-treated groups. The treatment was safe, and the subcutaneous route of administration allowed for early mobilization of the patient and even for at-home treatment. Conventional low-dose heparin given subcutaneously may not be as efficacious (International Stroke Trial Collaboration Group, 1997), but combining it with aspirin may prove helpful (Bousser, 1997).

THROMBOLYTIC THERAPY

Substances that expedite clot lysis and restore normal circulation may limit ischemic damage and improve neurologic outcome. Various agents, including fibrinolysin, plasmin/plasminogen, streptokinase, urokinase, and recombinant TPA have been used both experimentally and clinically, and they have been given by both intravenous and intra-arterial routes (Del Zoppo, 1988; Adams et al., 1994; The National Institute of Neurological Disorders and Stroke r-TPA Stroke Study Group, 1995) (Fig. 55.263). Early trials were complicated by frequent intracerebral hemorrhages. Eight clinical trials evaluating the effect of late intravenous infusion of thrombolytic agents (fibrinolysin, plasmin/plasminogen, streptokinase, and urokinase) in patients with completed stroke were reviewed by Del Zoppo (1988–see Table 1). These studies showed that such agents did not substantially improve clinical outcome. Case reports and limited series suggested neurologic recovery following intra-arterial infusion of streptokinase or urokinase in patients with middle cerebral artery and vertebrobasilar circulation territory thrombotic occlusions, but hemorrhagic transformation was high (Del Zoppo, 1988; Zeumer et al., 1982, 1983a–c). Subsequent studies reported clot lysis and arterial recanalization in approximately 50% of patients treated with intra-arterial streptokinase or urokinase (Levine and Brott, 1992). Local intra-arterial administration of recombinant TPA may be efficacious in the treatment of acute embolic stroke (Sasaki et al., 1995).

The rates of recanalization are lower for intravenously delivered agents, but the safety margin may be better. However, two large, randomized trials of intravenous streptokinase were stopped early because of the high rate of symptomatic intracranial hemorrhage (Donnan et al., 1995;

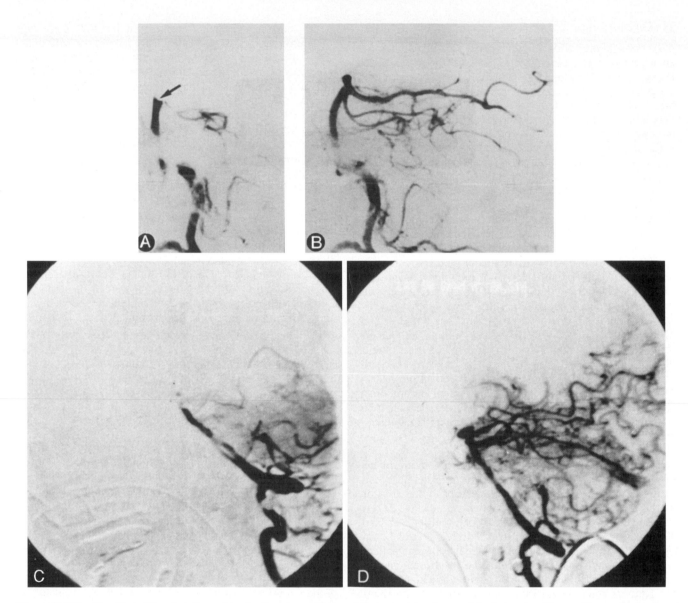

Figure 55.263.   The effect of thrombolytic agents on basilar artery occlusion. *A*, Pretreatment angiogram, lateral view, in a 43-year-old man who developed acute cortical blindness and bilateral oculomotor nerve pareses. The angiogram shows occlusion of the basilar artery at the origin of the superior cerebellar arteries (*arrow*). The patient was treated with local intra-arterial thrombolytic therapy. *B*, A repeat angiogram performed 24 hours after treatment with a fibrinolytic agent shows a patent basilar artery with normal filling of both superior cerebellar and posterior cerebral arteries. (From Kömpf D, Erbguth F, Kreiten K, et al. Bilateral third nerve palsy in basilar-vertebral artery disease: Report of three cases and review of the literature. Neuro-ophthalmology 7: 355–367, 1987.) *C*, Pretreatment digital subtraction angiogram, lateral view, in a 64-year-old woman with a history of a myocardial infarction who suddenly became comatose and was found to have a left hemiparesis and bilateral extensor plantar reflexes. The angiogram shows occlusion at the top of the basilar artery. The patient was treated with a bolus injection of tissue plasminogen activator (TPA) into the left vertebral artery, followed by a slow infusion of TPA over the next 90 minutes. *D*, 20 hours after infusion of TPA, a repeat angiogram shows a patent basilar artery with filling of the superior cerebellar and posterior cerebral arteries. (From Henze Th, Boeer A, Tebbe U, et al. Lysis of basilar artery occlusion with tissue plasminogen activator. Lancet 2: 1391, 1987.)

Hommel et al., 1995; Donnan et al., 1996; Multicenter Acute Stroke Trial—Europe Study Group, 1996). Similarly, the Multicenter Acute Stroke Trial (Multicenter Acute Stroke Trial—Italy MAST-I Group, 1995) was discontinued because of an increased incidence of early intracranial hemorrhage in patients receiving streptokinase, especially streptokinase and aspirin, compared with patients receiving aspirin or placebo. In preliminary studies, the safety of intravenous

recombinant TPA was demonstrated in patients with acute stroke, especially if given very early (within 90 and 180 minutes of stroke onset), and at low doses (less than 0.95 mg of TPA per kilogram of body weight) (Brott et al., 1992; Del Zoppo et al., 1992; Haley et al., 1992; von Kummer and Hacke, 1992). Two small, randomized studies of intravenous TPA for acute stroke found no demonstrable efficacy (Mori et al., 1992; Haley et al., 1993). A large placebo-controlled

European trial of 1.1 mg/kg of intravenous TPA given within 6 hours of stroke also showed no definitive benefit (Hacke et al., 1995). However, in a large multicentered trial supported by the National Institute of Neurological Disorders and Stroke (The National Institute of Neurological Disorders and Stroke rt-PA Stroke Study Group, 1995), treatment with intravenous TPA at a dose of 0.9 mg/kg within 3 hours of stroke onset improved clinical outcome at 3 months. Symptomatic intracerebral hemorrhage within 36 hours after stroke onset occurred in 6.4% of patients given TPA compared with 0.6% of patients given placebo, but mortality at 3 months was 17% in the TPA group and 21% in the placebo group. Treatment within 3 hours is likely critical when using these substances (Adams et al., 1996; Brott, 1996; Quality Standards Subcommittee of the American Academy of Neurology, 1996; Riggs, 1996).

ANTIHYPERTENSIVE THERAPY

Most patients with acute ischemic stroke are hypertensive (Hachinski and Norris, 1986), and a major dilemma is whether or not to treat their blood pressure at the time of admission. On the one hand, lowering blood pressure in such patients may further decrease arterial perfusion of an already ischemic brain, thus producing watershed infarction and facilitating formation of thrombi (Yatsu and Zivin, 1985; Miller and Hart, 1988; Brott and Reed, 1989). On the other hand, these risks may be outweighed by the hazards of not treating the hypertension (Spence and Del Maestro, 1985). In acute ischemic stroke, the brain commonly loses the ability to regulate its own blood supply. Cerebral perfusion thus varies with the systemic blood pressure. A high perfusion pressure promotes formation of edema, increased ICP, and ischemia.

Wallace and Levy (1981) studied 334 patients with acute stroke, half of whom had a history of hypertension. During the first 24 hours after admission, 84% of the patients showed hypertension (supine blood pressure greater than 150/90 mm Hg), but only one-third of the patients remained hypertensive after 10 days. In view of this natural history and the difficulty of knowing what effect lowering the pressure will have on unmeasurable intracranial factors, we agree with Hachinski (1985) that it would seem prudent not to treat hypertension in the acute phase but to identify the few situations in which treatment is warranted; e.g., hypertensive encephalopathy, myocardial insufficiency, and extreme hypertension (Brott and MacCarthy, 1989; Brott and Reed, 1989; Adams et al., 1994). Treatment of hypertension in acute stroke may also be warranted at lower levels in a young patient or in someone without a history or signs of hypertension.

The method of treating hypertension in a patient with an acute ischemic stroke may be as important as the decision to treat. Spence and Del Maestro (1985) emphasized that reduction of blood pressure should be **gradual and controlled**, stabilizing at lower but not necessarily normal levels. Brott and Reed (1989) provided an algorithm for emergency antihypertensive treatment in acute stroke that considers both systolic and diastolic levels and patient status.

Although available evidence dictates prudence in treating hypertension on admission for acute ischemic stroke, hypertension certainly should be treated once the patient is stable and ready for discharge. Indeed, chronic control of hypertension after stroke may be the single most important variable affecting the ultimate morbidity and mortality of such patients.

ANTIPLATELET THERAPY

The same issues raised above with respect to long-term antiplatelet treatment of patients who have experienced one or more TIAs also apply to patients who have experienced a thromboembolic stroke. Evidence demonstrating that the use of aspirin or other antiplatelet agents, such as ticlopidine, after ischemic stroke is associated with a lower rate of vascular death, subsequent stroke, or both, is increasing (see above). In the International Stroke Trial (IST), a large randomized open trial of up to 14 days of aspirin (300 mg daily) or subcutaneous heparin started as soon as possible after acute ischemic stroke, there was a small beneficial effect of aspirin on death and early recurrent stroke rates (International Stroke Trial Collaborative Group, 1997). Similarly, in the Chinese Acute Stroke Trial (CAST), a large randomized, placebo-controlled trial of aspirin (160 mg daily) begun within 48 hours of acute ischemic stroke and continued for up to 4 weeks, there was a 12% risk reduction with aspirin for death or stroke (CAST, 1997). Bousser (1997) emphasized that acute treatment with aspirin is clearly indicated after thrombotic infarction, but that anticoagulation is still the treatment of choice in patients with cardioembolic stroke. The role of combinations of antithrombotic agents and neuroprotective agents in the acute treatment of stroke remains to be determined. Ticlopidine may be particularly efficacious in preventing subsequent stroke in patients with previous stroke (Gent et al., 1989; Hass et al., 1989; Harbison, 1992; Ticlopidine Aspirin Stroke Study Group, 1993; Oster et al., 1994).

REHABILITATION

Few areas in neurology are in greater need of critical examination than stroke rehabilitation (Gresham et al., 1997). A prevalence of 600 per 100,000 population makes stroke a leading cause of serious disability (Kurtzke, 1982), but it remains unclear whether or not directed stroke rehabilitation is of benefit after stroke (Dobkin, 1989; Reding and McDowell, 1989; Ernst, 1990; Shah et al., 1990; Kalra et al., 1997). Hachinski (1989) emphasized that depression is a major factor in rehabilitation. About 50% of patients with stroke become depressed for at least 6 months and major depressive symptoms increasing with time (Robinson et al., 1984). Parikh et al. (1990) found that patients with poststroke depression were significantly more impaired in both physical activities and language function 2 years after stroke than were nondepressed patients. These investigators also suggested that early recognition and treatment of poststroke depression may substantially improve the ultimate functional outcome after stroke. Simple measures applied by family and unspecialized personnel may, however, be as effective as those provided by a specialized team (Ernst, 1990).

HEMORRHAGIC CEREBROVASCULAR DISEASE

Intracranial hemorrhage was first recognized as a cause of stroke by Morgagni in 1761. About 10% of strokes are caused by intracerebral hemorrhage (Whisnant et al., 1971; Matsumoto et al., 1973; Mohr et al., 1978; Caplan et al., 1983; Kunitz et al., 1984; Norris et al., 1984; Kase and Mohr, 1986; Warlow et al., 1987; Feldmann, 1991; Caplan, 1993; Kase and Caplan, 1994). There is a higher incidence of intracerebral hemorrhage in specific populations, such as African-American and Japanese patients, that have a high frequency of systemic hypertension (Wolf et al., 1975, 1977a, 1977b; Broderick et al., 1992; Kase and Caplan, 1994; Qureshi et al., 1997). Intracerebral hemorrhage occurs in patients of all ages, including children and adolescents (Higgins et al., 1989; Broderick et al., 1993a), middle-aged adults, and elderly patients in the 7th–9th decades of life (Mohr et al., 1978; Caplan et al., 1983; Kunitz et al., 1984). Intracerebral hemorrhage is a primary event in most patients, occurring at the time of neurologic symptoms and signs. Other patients experience hemorrhage into a previously ischemic lesion (Okada et al., 1989). Such late hemorrhage, which usually occurs within 1–2 weeks after an ischemic stroke (Yamaguchi et al., 1984; Hornig et al., 1986), is more common in patients with embolic stroke than in patients with nonembolic stroke (Fisher and Adams, 1951; Lodder et al., 1986).

PATHOPHYSIOLOGY

Intracerebral hemorrhage most often develops gradually. Bleeding into the brain usually originates from small, deep penetrating vessels under arteriolar or capillary pressure. This contrasts with the situation in subarachnoid hemorrhage, in which arteries on the brain surface leak blood under systemic arterial pressure (see Chapter 53). Symptoms in patients with subarachnoid hemorrhage usually begin instantaneously and consist of headache, loss of concentration, and vomiting. These symptoms are caused by the sudden increase in ICP that results when blood rapidly disseminates through the CSF around the substance of the brain. In patients with intracerebral hemorrhage, by contrast, the hematoma develops gradually over minutes or even hours. Fisher (1971b) examined serial sections of the brain after intracerebral hemorrhage. At the center of the lesion was a large mass of blood. At the periphery were many "fibrin globes"—little caps of fibrinous material plugging small vessels that had subsequently broken or leaked during life. As intracerebral hemorrhage develops, pressure within the central core of hemorrhage increases, compressing small vessels at the periphery of the hematoma. These peripheral arteries subsequently break, blood escapes, and the hematoma enlarges. As the lesion continues to increase in size, ICP increases, and tissue pressure surrounding the lesion also rises. Eventually, an equilibrium is reached, and bleeding stops. If the hematoma reaches the ventricle or surface of the brain, it may communicate with the CSF and discharge part of its hemorrhagic contents into the subarachnoid space.

GENERAL SYMPTOMS AND SIGNS

Because the brain is devoid of pain fibers, the initial release of blood into brain parenchyma does not cause headache. Instead, blood disrupts the function of a particular region of the brain. Clinical symptoms and signs usually evolve over a period of minutes to hours, but they may develop over days. Rarely (7%), transient neurologic deficits precede intracerebral hemorrhage (Gras et al., 1993). Analysis of the course of illness in 54 patients with well-documented intracerebral hemorrhage showed that 37 (69%) had gradual development of symptoms during a period of minutes or a few hours (Caplan and Mohr, 1978). Some patients stabilized during the first 24–48 hours after onset of symptoms but subsequently worsened 48–72 hours later. Herbstein and Schaumberg (1974) studied a group of patients with intracerebral hemorrhage to determine if progressive clinical decline was caused by continued bleeding or by edema around the lesion. These investigators tagged red blood cells with chromium-51 and injected the erythrocytes into the circulation 1–5 hours after an initial neurologic examination. Counts of radioactivity were made from the hematoma cavities at autopsies performed 1–15 days later. There was no increase in radioactivity within the hematomas, which were usually surrounded by edema. This finding suggests that it is the edema associated with an intracranial hematoma, rather than continued bleeding into surrounding tissue, that produces progressive neurologic deterioration after an acute intracranial hemorrhage.

Headache

The frequency of headache among patients with intracerebral hemorrhage varies widely depending on the size and location of the hemorrhage (Gorelick et al., 1986). In a study performed by Caplan and Mohr (1978), 17 of 48 patients (37%) who were able to provide a history described headache at the time of onset of neurologic symptoms. Another seven patients (15%) experienced headache later in the course of their illness. Twenty-four patients (50%) had no headache at any time. Gorelick et al. (1986) reported headache in 41 of 61 patients (67%). Eight of the patients experienced a headache before any other symptoms began (sentinal headache), whereas the remaining 33 patients experienced a headache at the time of onset of other symptoms of intracerebral hemorrhage. In the majority of these patients, the headache was unilateral, focal, and of mild or moderate severity. Similar results were reported by Vestergaard et al. (1993). Fisher (1968a) reported headache in 10 of 78 patients (13%) with putaminal hemorrhage. Ropper and Davis (1980) described headache in 12 of 26 patients (46%) with subcortical (lobar) hemorrhage, and Kase et al. (1982) described headache in 68% of such patients. Massaro et al. (1991) confirmed this increased frequency of severe headache among patients with lobar hemorrhage (60%) as opposed to patients with deep hemorrhage (30%).

Some studies suggest that patients with intracerebral hemorrhage are more likely to have a headache when the lesion is large. Hematomas near the surface are more likely to cause headache than those deep in the brain parenchyma. Headache is most frequent with cerebellar hemorrhages, followed by lobar hemorrhages (Hier et al., 1993; Melo et al., 1996). In addition, younger patients are more likely to experience headache than are older patients, probably because older patients tend to have more cerebral atrophy, thus providing more space for intracranial hematomas to expand before producing increased ICP. However, in a study of 289 patients with intracerebral hemorrhage (57% of whom had a headache at the onset of their stroke), Melo et al. (1996) found that hematoma location in the cerebellar or lobar regions, meningeal signs, and female gender were more predictive of headache than hematoma volume.

In patients with hemorrhagic stroke, headache probably results from escape of blood, which causes local distention, distortion, deformation, or stretching of pain-sensitive intracranial structures (Dalessio, 1972). Other mechanisms include raised ICP and irritation of meningeal pain fibers along the ventricular and CSF surfaces (Kase and Caplan, 1994). The results of the study by Melo et al. (1996) suggest that headache is related more to the activation of an anatomically distributed system in susceptible individuals and to subarachnoid bleeding than to intracranial hypertension.

Loss of Consciousness

Loss of consciousness usually occurs only in patients with large hematomas in the cerebral hemispheres or with hematomas in the brainstem, especially the pons. When a hematoma is located in the cerebral hemisphere, diminished consciousness is caused by the mass effect of the lesion and secondary increased ICP, especially if the hematoma has intraventricular extension (Massaro et al., 1991). Hematomas in the brainstem produce loss of consciousness through a direct effect on the reticular activating system. Of 60 patients with intracerebral hemorrhage evaluated by Caplan and Mohr (1978), 30 (50%) were alert when they were first examined. Only 16 patients (27%) were stuporous or comatose. Like headache, alterations in consciousness seem to occur with less frequency in older patients. Severe reduction in the level of consciousness in patients with intracerebral hemorrhage is a poor prognostic sign. In the study performed by Caplan and Mohr (1978), all 12 patients who presented stuporous or in coma after an intracerebral hemorrhage subsequently died despite treatment. An exception is thalamic hemorrhage, where stupor does not necessarily correlate with poor outcome (Kase and Caplan, 1994).

Vomiting

Vomiting is an especially important sign in patients with intracerebral hemorrhage. Few patients with ischemic lesions within the cerebral hemispheres vomit, but 25–50% of patients with hemorrhage in one or both cerebral hemispheres do (Mohr et al., 1978; Gorelick et al., 1986; Massaro et al., 1991). In such patients, vomiting is usually caused by increased ICP or secondary distortion of the 4th ventricle. Vomiting occurs in about one-third of patients with occlusive posterior circulation disease and over 50% of posterior circulation hemorrhages, presumably because of damage to structures in the floor of the 4th ventricle (Borison and Wang, 1953). Patients with cerebellar hemorrhage almost always experience vomiting early in the course of the lesion. Younger patients are more likely to experience vomiting (as well as headache and alterations in consciousness) than are older patients.

Seizures

Seizures are uncommon during the acute phase of any stroke, but they are more likely to occur in both young and old patients with an ischemic stroke caused by embolism (Clancy et al., 1985; Kilpatrick et al., 1990) and in patients with intracerebral hemorrhage (Mohr et al., 1978; Faught et al., 1989; Kilpatrick et al., 1990; Weisberg et al., 1991; Cervoni et al., 1994). Only 6% of patients with intracerebral hemorrhage evaluated by Mohr et al. (1978) experienced seizures at the onset or during the course of their illness. However, among 123 patients with primary intracerebral hemorrhage followed by Faught et al. (1989) for an average of 4.6 years or until death, 25% experienced one or more seizures. The seizures occurred within 24 hours after the hemorrhage in one-half of the cases and within 2 years after hemorrhage in the remainder. Faught et al. (1989) calculated that 50% of the patients would have experienced at least one seizure had all survived 5 years.

Subcortical hemorrhages (also called lobar or slit hemorrhages—see below) that are located near the junction of gray and white matter in the cerebral cortex and putaminal hemorrhages that undercut the cortex are especially epileptogenic (Caplan, 1993; Cervoni et al., 1994; Kase and Caplan, 1994). Interestingly, lobar hemorrhages in the frontal, parietal, or temporal regions are more commonly associated with seizures than similar hemorrhages in the occipital lobes (Weisberg et al., 1991). In the study by Faught et al. (1989), 54% of the patients who experienced seizures had hemorrhage into lobar subcortical structures. Faught et al. (1989) hypothesized that the overall prevalence of intracerebral hemorrhage-related seizures in their series was higher than that reported in other series (e.g., Mohr et al., 1978) because many small lobar hemorrhages that cause seizures could not be detected without thin-section CT scanning or MR imaging, procedures that were unavailable before the late 1970s and early 1980s. Seizures caused by such lesions would thus be ascribed to other causes or diagnosed as "idiopathic." Hemorrhages in the basal ganglia and putamen are occasionally associated with seizures, but seizures almost never occur in patients with isolated thalamic hemorrhage (Faught et al., 1989).

Intraocular Hemorrhage

Subhyaloid and retinal hemorrhages, often seen in patients with subarachnoid hemorrhage (see Chapter 53), are rare in patients with intracerebral hemorrhage. They are seen occasionally, however, in patients with intracerebral hematomas that are quite large and that have developed rapidly (Fisher, 1967a).

Other Symptoms and Signs

Neck stiffness occurs in approximately 17% of patients with intracerebral hemorrhage and is most commonly associated with lesions in the caudate (Mohr et al., 1978; Hier et al., 1993). This is probably because of the frequent release of blood into the ventricular and subarachnoid spaces from hemorrhage in this region. Other locations of hemorrhage associated with stiff neck include the putamen, thalamus, and cerebellum (Fisher, 1959b, 1967a; Walshe et al., 1977).

Stiff neck is uncommon in patients with pontine or lobar hemorrhage.

Some patients with intracerebral hemorrhage have electrocardiographic changes and arrhythmias suggestive of myocardial ischemia, especially patients with compression of the brainstem (Stober et al., 1988; Kase and Caplan, 1994). Central mechanisms are probably responsible, including increased catecholamine release and excitotoxin toxicity. Central mechanisms may also explain fever in patients who experience intracerebral hemorrhage, but a rigorous search for underlying infection or pulmonary embolism must always be performed in such patients (Kase and Caplan, 1994).

CAUSES

A few conditions are responsible for nearly all cases of intracerebral hemorrhage. These include systemic hypertension, blood dyscrasias, exogenous agents, amyloid angiopathy, vascular malformations, aneurysms, trauma, tumors, infective endocarditis, migraine, and alcohol abuse (McCormick and Rosenfield, 1973; Caplan and Stein, 1986; Hart et al., 1987; Warlow et al., 1987; Caplan, 1988b; Caplan, 1993; Kase and Caplan, 1994; Juvela et al., 1995).

Hypertension

The most common cause of intracerebral hemorrhage is systemic hypertension, present in 70–90% of patients with intracerebral hemorrhage (Mohr et al., 1978; Furlan et al., 1979b) and in over 90% of cases of massive intracerebral hemorrhage in autopsy series (Mutlu et al., 1963). Even in patients under 46 years of age, systemic hypertension is the third most common cause of intracerebral hemorrhage after rupture of an intracranial aneurysm or AVM (Bevan et al., 1990). Some patients with intracerebral hemorrhage have no previous history of hypertension but have high blood pressure at the time of initial examination. In such patients, it is often impossible to be certain how much, if any, of the blood pressure elevation is caused by raised ICP or what the level of blood pressure was just before the hemorrhage.

When systemic hypertension first develops, small intracranial arteries and capillaries are exposed to a high head of pressure. In some patients, the vessels rupture immediately, resulting in hemorrhage into brain tissue. Small arteries and arterioles that do not rupture eventually hypertrophy in an attempt to protect the capillary bed from the elevated pressure. When hypertension persists, degenerative changes, such as lipohyalinosis, fibrinoid necrosis, and microaneurysms, develop in vessel walls (Cole and Yates, 1967; Rosenblum, 1977; Wakai and Nagai, 1989). These changes predispose to later rupture of the vessel wall with subsequent intraparenchymal hemorrhage. Thus, the occurrence of intracerebral hemorrhage is actually biphasic: developing at the onset of hypertension as the result of acute effects on intracranial vessels and developing later from secondary degenerative changes in the walls of vessels exposed to chronically elevated blood pressure.

Older patients seem to develop intracerebral hemorrhage at relatively lower blood pressures than younger patients, perhaps because the degenerative vascular changes that result from chronic hypertension render the vessels more susceptible to rupture regardless of the eventual blood pressure.

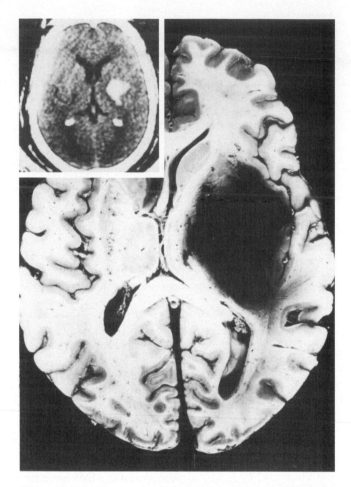

Figure 55.264. Hypertensive intracranial hemorrhage. Axial section through the brain of a 65-year-old man with untreated systemic hypertension who died after suffering an acute intracranial hemorrhage. The photograph shows a right-sided hemorrhage affecting the posterior half of the putamen, globus pallidus, posterior limb of the internal capsule, and claustrum. There is effacement of the ipsilateral lateral ventricle, and there is a significant midline shift from right to left. *Inset* shows the appearance of the CT scan in a similar case.

However, hypertension is still an important asociated condition for intracranial hemorrhage in the elderly (Broderick et al., 1993b). As noted above, symptoms and signs of increased ICP, such as headache, alteration in consciousness, vomiting, and papilledema, are less common in older patients, even those with sizable lesions. This makes the clinical differentiation between hemorrhagic and ischemic infarction extremely difficult.

The most common locations for hypertensive intracerebral hemorrhage are the putamen and thalamus (Fig. 55.264). These two regions account for over 50% of hypertensive hemorrhages (Caplan and Stein, 1986). Other regions of the brain that seem to be predisposed to hypertensive hemorrhage are the subcortical white matter, caudate nucleus, cerebellum, and pons (Moossy, 1984).

Bleeding Disorders

A variety of bleeding disorders can result in hemorrhage into the brain. In many such cases, systemic bleeding occurs

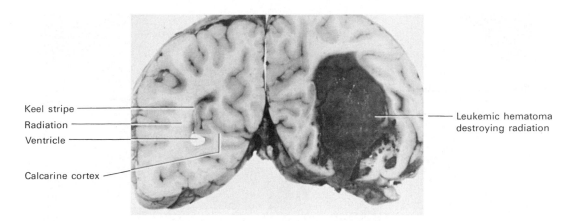

Keel stripe
Radiation
Ventricle
Calcarine cortex

Leukemic hematoma destroying radiation

Figure 55.265. Intracranial hematoma in a patient with acute leukemia. The patient was a 33-year-old man who complained of weakness of the arms and legs and of losing control of both arms. That night he awakened from sleep and vomited. The next morning he vomited again, and he then developed a severe headache. He was admitted to the hospital in coma at which time a diagnosis of acute lymphocytic leukemia was made. The patient died 2 hours after admission. The severely swollen brain showed a single hematoma in the posterior half of the right hemisphere. A coronal section through the brain shows that bleeding extends from the white matter of the lower temporal lobe into the white matter of the lower parietal lobe. The entire right optic radiation is destroyed. (From Lindenberg R, Walsh FB, Sacks JG. Neuropathology of Vision. An Atlas. Philadelphia, Lea & Febiger, 1973.)

simultaneously. Leukemia, hemophilia, thrombocytopenia, and DIC are important examples of such disorders (Fig. 55.265). Fluid-blood levels within the hematoma as identified by CT scanning or MR imaging can help differentiate intracerebral hematomas caused by coagulopathies (both intrinsic and exogenously induced) from those that are not (Pfleger et al., 1994).

Exogenous Agents

A variety of substances, taken internally, can produce intracerebral hemorrhage. By far the most common drugs that predispose to intracerebral hemorrhage are thrombolytic agents (Partanen and Nieminen, 1990; Kase et al., 1992; Wijdicks and Jack, 1993; Sloan et al., 1995) and the anticoagulants, particularly heparin and warfarin (Wintzen et al., 1984; Kase et al., 1985b; Kase and Mohr, 1986; Babikian et al., 1989; Mattle et al., 1989; Hirsh, 1991; Fihn et al., 1993; van der Meer et al., 1993) (Fig. 55.266). The single most important factor associated with anticoagulant-related intracerebral hemorrhage is prolongation of coagulation parameters beyond the recommended "therapeutic" range, a feature found in 75–85% of reported cases (see Table 27-1 in Kase and Mohr, 1986; see Table 1 in Babikian et al., 1989; Fihn et al., 1993). Most patients with anticoagulant-related intracerebral hemorrhage have systemic hypertension and are over 50 years of age (Babikian et al., 1989; Mattle et al., 1989; Wintzen et al., 1989). Such patients are usually being anticoagulated because of myocardial infarction, pulmonary embolism, and peripheral arterial disease. Other patients experience intracerebral hemorrhage during cardiac surgery. The hemorrhage in such patients may result from consumption of platelets and coagulation factors combined with the use of anticoagulation during extracorporeal circulation (Sila, 1989).

As opposed to intracerebral hemorrhage related to other causes, anticoagulant-related intracerebral hemorrhage often develops gradually and insidiously over many hours or even days. Anticoagulant-related intracerebral hemorrhage more frequently occurs in the cerebellum and cerebral lobes than does hypertensive intracerebral hemorrhage (Ott et al., 1974; Ropper and Davis, 1980). Finally, there appears to be a very high mortality and morbidity rate for patients with anticoagulant-related intracerebral hemorrhage, although asymptomatic hemorrhages may not be recognized (Chamorro et al., 1995).

Mattle et al. (1989) reported that there was no medical reason for one-third of the patients who developed anticoagulation-related intracerebral hemorrhage to have been anticoagulated in the first place. These authors suggested that the single most useful measure that can be taken to reduce the risk of anticoagulation-induced intracerebral hemorrhage is to discontinue the anticoagulants of patients who are being unnecessarily treated. We would add that the risk of anticoagulation-induced intracerebral hemorrhage can also be reduced simply by making certain that only those patients who truly require anticoagulation are anticoagulated in the first place.

A number of commonly abused substances may produce intracerebral hemorrhage. The most common is **amphetamine** (Delaney and Estes, 1980; Cahill et al., 1981b; D'Sousa and Shraberg, 1981; Lessing and Hyman, 1989; Imanse and Vanneste, 1990; Yen et al., 1994). This drug apparently produces fibrinoid necrosis and other degenerative changes in the walls of intracranial vessels, predisposing them to rupture (Citron et al., 1970; Rumbaugh et al., 1971a, 1971b). Amphetamine-induced intracerebral hemorrhage often presents within a few minutes of drug use, particularly when the drug is injected intravenously. Patients typically develop sudden headache, confusion, and seizures (Caplan et al., 1982a). In some patients, the amphetamine also induces systemic hypertension that may potentiate the intracerebral hemorrhage.

Cocaine may also induce a hemorrhagic stroke (see Table

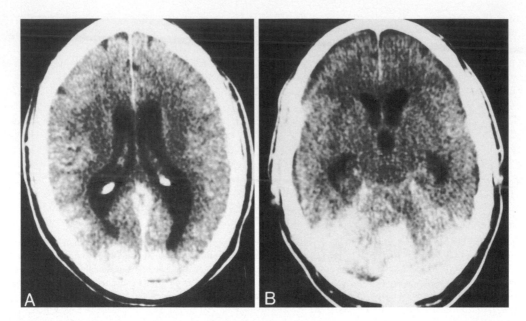

Figure 55.266. Intracranial hemorrhage caused by anticoagulation. The patient was a 62-year-old man who was being anticoagulated after a coronary artery angioplasty. The patient's coagulation parameters were well beyond the recommended "therapeutic" range when he developed the hemorrhage. *A,* Unenhanced CT scan, axial view, shows hyperintensity in both occipital lobes and in the cerebral sulci, particularly on the right side, consistent with intracerebral and subarachnoid hemorrhage. The lateral ventricles are moderately dilated. *B,* Unenhanced CT scan, axial view, at a slightly lower level, shows massive hyperintensity consistent with hemorrhage, throughout the posterior fossa.

2 in Klonoff et al., 1989; Deringer et al., 1990; Green et al., 1990; Levine et al., 1990b; Kibayashi et al., 1995; Nolte et al., 1996; Fessler et al., 1997). The stroke may occur following any route of administration, including inhalation, intranasal, intravenous, and intramuscular routes. Cocaine-induced stroke may be caused by a number of mechanisms (Fessler et al., 1997). Cocaine is a potent vasoconstrictor, and it thus causes dose-related elevations in blood pressure and pulse (Resnick et al., 1977). An increase in blood pressure and cardiac output after use of cocaine can result in rupture of a previously silent intracranial aneurysm or AVM (Fessler et al., 1997). Although cocaine can produce a cerebral vasculitis that can lead to intracerebral hemorrhage, this etiology appears to be uncommon. In a prospective autopsy study of 10 patients with cocaine-related intracranial hemorrhage, for example, Nolte et al. (1996) found no evidence of vasculitis. Aggarwal et al. (1996) performed an autopsy study of 14 cases of cocaine-related cerebrovascular disease and found no evidence of vasculitis in any of the cases. The results of these two studies suggest that the pharmacodynamic effects of cocaine, especially vasospasm and hypertensive surges, are the most likely mechanisms underlying fatal intracranial hemorrhages.

Other drugs capable of inducing systemic hypertension and acute intracerebral hemorrhage are the illegal substance **phencyclidine** (angel dust), and **phenylpropanolamine**, a sympathomimetic compound found in many over-the-counter appetite suppressants and decongestant medications (Citron et al., 1970; Eastman and Cohen, 1975; Stratton et al., 1978; Bessen, 1982; Caplan et al., 1982a; Mueller, 1983; Kase et al., 1987; Maher, 1987). As noted in an earlier sec-

tion of this chapter, intravenous injection of **Talwin** and **pyribenzamine** tablets that have been crushed and mixed with water or saline may cause an intracranial arteritis that leads to intracerebral hemorrhage (Caplan et al., 1982b).

Amyloid Angiopathy

Congophilic or **amyloid angiopathy** was first recognized as a cause of intracerebral hemorrhage in the late 1970s (Jellinger, 1977a, 1977b; Zenkevich, 1978). This disorder, which may be sporadic or inherited in an autosomal-dominant fashion, usually damages small arteries and arterioles in the leptomeninges and cerebral cortex (Haan et al., 1990a; Maeda et al., 1993) (Fig. 55.38). Lesions most commonly occur in the occipital and parietal regions, less often in the other cerebral lobes, and, rarely, in the deep basal gray matter, brainstem, or cerebellum. Hemorrhages often are quite large, and they often are multiple (Gilbert and Vinters, 1983; Finelli et al., 1984; Gilles et al., 1984; Haan et al., 1990a; Hendricks et al., 1990; Ohshima et al., 1990; Case Records of the Massachusetts General Hospital, 1991; Yong et al., 1992). Patients thus may develop acute focal neurologic deficits or diffuse neurologic dysfunction including dementia (Haan et al., 1990b; Case Records of the Massachusetts General Hospital, 1991).

Affected vessels are thickened by an acellular hyaline material that stains positively with PAS stain and has an apple-green birefringence with polarized Congo red stain (Vinters and Gilbert, 1983; Hendricks et al., 1990; Ohshima et al., 1990; Yong et al., 1992) (Fig 55.38). In some cases of amyloid angiopathy, the vessel wall seems to be reduplicated or split.

Hereditary amyloid angiopathy usually affects patients between 45 and 65 years of age (Haan et al., 1990a, 1990b). Two genetic defects can be identified in such persons: a mutation in the amyloid precursor protein in the Dutch form of hereditary cerebral hemorrhage with amyloidosis and a mutation in exon 2 of cystatin C in the Icelandic form (Graffagnino et al., 1994). These mutations do not appear to play a role in the more common sporadic form of the disease, however. Sporadic amyloid angiopathy predominantly affects persons over 65 years of age, and it has an extremely high frequency in the 8th and 9th decades of life (Vinters and Gilbert, 1983). Some series show a striking female predilection for the sporadic form of the disease (Lee and Stemmerman, 1978; Gilbert and Vinters, 1983). A genetic risk factor for Alzheimer's disease, the $\epsilon 4$ allele of the apolipoprotein E gene (see Chapter 50), is independently associated

with cerebral amyloid angiopathy and hemorrhage in nonfamilial cases (Greenberg et al., 1995) but not hereditary cases (Bornebroek et al., 1997).

Because the occipital lobe is a common site of hemorrhage in patients with amyloid angiopathy, the acute onset of a partial or complete homonymous field defect may be the first sign of the disease. We saw such a patient, a man who was well until age 59, when he experienced an acute stroke characterized by a right-sided headache, nausea, vomiting, and difficulty seeing to the left side. An examination revealed an incomplete, congruous, left homonymous hemianopia, and CT scanning showed a hemorrhagic lesion in the right occipitoparietal region. The patient was followed without treatment. The field defect improved over the next several months, and subsequent CT scans showed resolution of the hemorrhage. Eighteen months later, however, he had

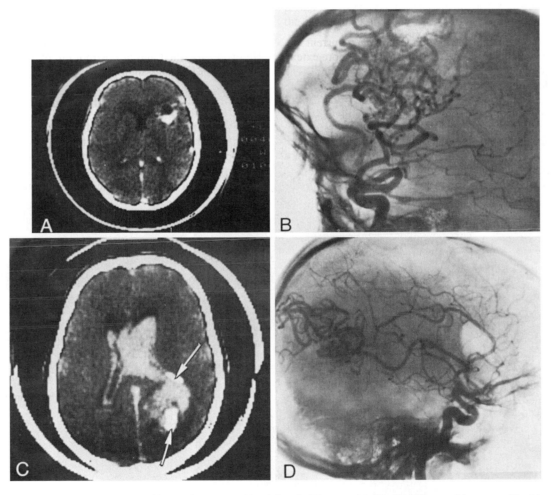

Figure 55.267. Intracranial hemorrhage caused by arteriovenous malformation. *A*, CT scan, axial view, in a 32-year-old woman with a history of seizures who developed a severe headache followed by a right hemiparesis and aphasia shows a left frontal lobe hemorrhage. *B*, Left internal carotid arteriogram, lateral view, shows a large arteriovenous malformation in the left frontal lobe. The malformation is fed by branches of the left anterior and middle cerebral arteries. *C*, CT scan, axial view, in a 38-year-old previously healthy man who developed a severe headache associated with loss of vision to the left side and then became comatose shows a massive intraventricular hemorrhage associated with a right occipital lobe hemorrhagic lesion that is surrounded by calcium (*arrows*). *D*, Right internal carotid arteriogram, lateral view, shows an arteriovenous malformation in the right occipital lobe. The malformation is fed by branches of the anterior and middle cerebral arteries. Vertebral angiography showed that the malformation was also fed by branches from the right posterior cerebral artery.

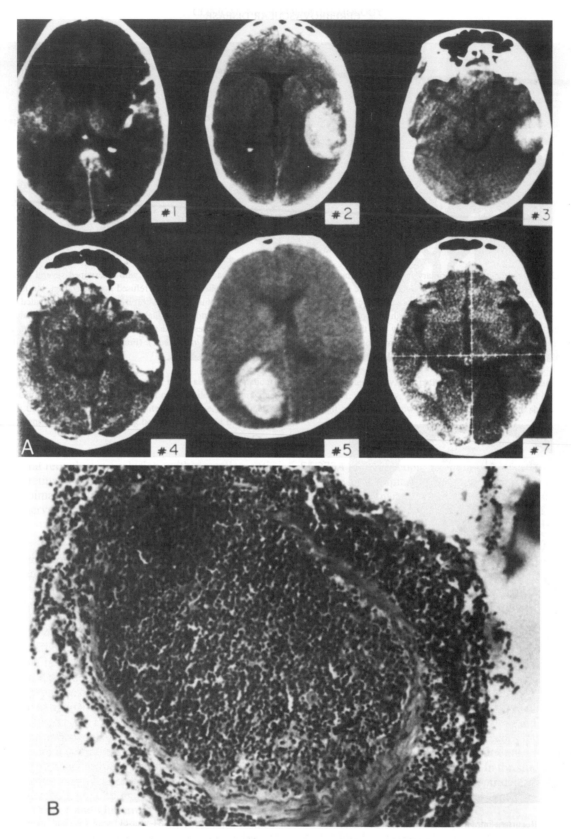

Figure 55.274. Infective endocarditis producing intracranial hemorrhage. *A,* Unenhanced CT scans, axial view, in 6 patients with intracranial hemorrhage from bacterial endocarditis caused by *Staphylococcus aureus.* Note varying locations of hemorrhages. *B,* Septic embolus in the middle cerebral artery with pyogenic arteritis in the patient whose CT scan is marked *#1.* (From Hart RG, Kagan-Hallet K, Joerns SE. Mechanisms of intracranial hemorrhage in infective endocarditis. Stroke *18:*1048–1056, 1987.)

during uncontrolled infection, particularly with virulent organisms, can cause acute, erosive arteritis with rupture; and (*c*) septic emboli during effective antimicrobial therapy or associated with nonvirulent organisms can injure the arterial wall, resulting in the subacute development of aneurysms that are often aseptic at the time of rupture. All three pathologies were demonstrated in a series of 16 patients with intracranial hemorrhage complicating infective endocarditis (Masuda et al., 1992).

Migraine

As noted in an earlier section of this chapter and in Chapter 56 of this text, some patients with migraine experience permanent neurologic deficits from stroke. In almost all cases, the stroke is ischemic; however, in some cases, an intracerebral hemorrhage occurs during an otherwise typical, common (without aura), or classic (with aura) migraine attack (Dunning, 1942; Cole and Aubé, 1987; Caplan, 1988b; Shuaib et al., 1989a). Caplan (1988b) suggested that intracerebral hemorrhage occurs in association with a migraine attack when cerebral tissue that has developed significant ischemia becomes reperfused. Alternatively, a sudden increase in ICP caused by protracted vomiting may produce or contribute to spontaneous intracerebral hemorrhage in such patients (Shuaib et al., 1989a).

Alcohol Abuse

Klatsky et al. (1989) studied the relationship between reported alcohol use and the incidence of hospitalization for several types of cerebrovascular disease. These investigators concluded that daily consumption of three or more drinks containing alcohol was related to higher hospitalization rates for hemorrhagic cerebrovascular disease, especially intracerebral hemorrhage. Juvela et al. (1995) found recent moderate and heavy alcohol intake to be an independent risk factor for intracerebral hemorrhage. Indeed, the amount of alcohol consumed within 1 week of intracerebral hemorrhage may be an independent determinant of subsequent outcome (Juvela, 1995). In addition, alcohol abuse is consistently found to be associated with systemic hypertension (Gleiberman and Harburg, 1986; Klatsky et al., 1986, 1989), and this association may further explain the higher risk of hemorrhagic cerebrovascular disease in patients who are heavy users of alcohol. Alcohol-induced bleeding tendency (Deykin et al., 1982; Laug, 1983; Mikhailidis et al., 1983; Friedman et al., 1996) and alcohol-related head trauma are other factors that may predispose a patient who abuses alcohol to intracerebral hemorrhage.

SIGNS AND SYMPTOMS BY LOCATION

The prognosis and treatment of an intracerebral hemorrhage often depend on the location of the hemorrhage. Certain locations, such as the cerebral lobes, the right putamen, and the cerebellum, are relatively accessible to surgical drainage, whereas others, such as the thalami and brainstem, are not. Although it is usually necessary to obtain a neuroimaging study to confirm the diagnosis and location of a hemor-

rhagic infarct, it is still valuable for the physician to know the symptoms and signs caused by hematomas in common intracranial locations (Fisher, 1961b; see Table 3 in Freeman et al., 1973; Caplan, 1993; Kase and Caplan, 1994).

Hemorrhages of the Lateral Basal Ganglia, Putamen, and Internal Capsule

Intracerebral hemorrhage that affects the basal ganglia, putamen, and internal capsule usually occurs in the setting of systemic hypertension. Indeed, this region is said to be the most commonly affected by hypertensive intracerebral hemorrhage (Caplan, 1993). Other causes of hemorrhage in this region are quite rare. Traumatic basal ganglia hemorrhage, observed in about 3% of closed head injuries (MacPherson et al., 1986), probably results from rupture of lenticulostriate or anterior choroidal arteries (Katz et al., 1989).

Hemorrhages that occur in the region of the lateral basal ganglia and internal capsule are usually called "**putaminal hemorrhages**," because they most often arise in the putamen and then spread to affect the internal capsule, basal ganglia, or both structures. Small putaminal hemorrhages may produce pure motor hemiparesis, thus mimicking an ischemic lacunar infarct (Weisberg, 1979; Tapia et al., 1983; Anzalone and Landi, 1989; Kim et al., 1994a); however, the usual findings in a patient with a "putaminal" hemorrhage are contralateral hemiparesis, contralateral hemisensory loss, contralateral homonymous hemianopia, and conjugate deviation of the eyes to the side of the hematoma (Fig. 55.275). The pupils are generally normal, and gait is hemiparetic. Patients with left putaminal hemorrhage usually have a nonfluent aphasia with relative preservation of the ability to repeat spoken language, whereas right-sided putaminal hem-

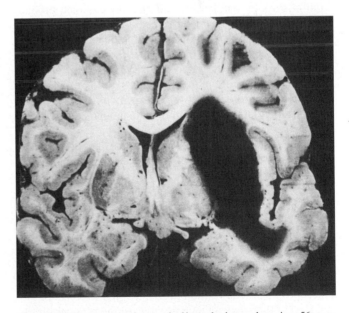

Figure 55.275. Large, left putaminal/capsular hemorrhage in a 56 year-old hypertensive woman. Note tracking into the white matter of the temporal lobe. The patient had a right, superior homonymous quadrantanopia from interruption of the optic radiation in the left temporal lobe.

orrhage often causes visual neglect in the left hemifield, motor impersistence, and constructional dyspraxia. These abnormalities of higher cortical function are probably caused by disconnection and undercutting of cortical zones. They usually are more transient in patients with intracerebral hemorrhage than in patients with cortical infarcts of equal size (Caplan, 1993). Some patients with putaminal hemorrhage develop ipsilateral adventitious movements that the family or observers call "tremor." These movements are probably caused by damage to ipsilateral descending projections of the extrapyramidal system.

Damage to fibers connecting the caudate, putamen, globus pallidum, and substantia nigra to the thalamus and prefrontal areas may be responsible for the development of a striking tendency to fall while standing, walking, or sitting in some patients with acute, unilateral, basal ganglia hemorrhage (Labadie et al., 1989). The problem in such patients is severe postural instability. The patients fall with a distinctly slow, tilting motion in a stereotypic lateral or diagonal trajectory. The falls occur with eyes opened but are exacerbated by eye closure.

As a hemorrhagic lesion of the putamen enlarges, it produces increasing stupor. The ipsilateral pupil at first becomes smaller and then larger than the contralateral pupil, the ipsilateral plantar response becomes extensor, and a horizontal gaze paresis develops. These signs are associated with a very poor prognosis because they are caused by compression of the brainstem (Hier et al., 1977; Caplan and Mohr, 1978).

The findings described above usually occur when a putaminal hemorrhage affects the medial and most anterior portion of the posterior putamen and the anterior two-thirds of the posterior limb of the internal capsule (Koba et al., 1977; Mizukami et al., 1981). Lesions that affect the anterior limb of the internal capsule and anterior putamen produce a milder syndrome, characterized by a transient hemiparesis unassociated with any sensory disturbance (Koba et al., 1977). When the hematoma is in the posterior third of the internal capsule and the far posterior extreme of the putamen, sensory abnormalities predominate with little or no hemiparesis. In such cases, an inferior homonymous quadrantanopia or an incomplete homonymous hemianopia that is denser below may be present. Lesions in the far posterior left putamen may produce a fluent aphasia because of undercutting of the temporal lobe or extension of the lesion into the temporal isthmus (see Chapter 9).

Putaminal hemorrhages vary greatly in size. In one series of 24 patients (Hier et al., 1977), the smallest hematoma volume was 20 mm³, whereas the largest was 225 mm³. Larger hemorrhages are more likely to rupture into the lateral ventricle, and they have a much higher mortality than do small putaminal hemorrhages (Hier et al., 1977; Stein et al., 1983). In most cases, the bleeding extends along the anteroposterior axis of the brain, but some lesions are globoid, and others extend laterally toward the cortical surface along white matter tracts. The source of bleeding in most patients with putaminal hemorrhage is the lateral lenticulostriate arteries (Mizukami et al., 1981).

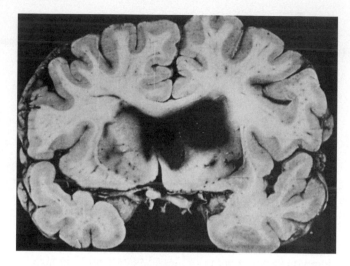

Figure 55.276. Hemorrhage originating from the head of the caudate nucleus in a 66-year-old hypertensive, diabetic man. Note involvement of the anterior limb of the internal capsule and extension into the lateral ventricle with formation of a ventricular cast.

Caudate Hemorrhage

Hemorrhage into the caudate nucleus accounts for only about 7% of intracerebral hemorrhage (Stein et al., 1984). Hematomas at this site often rapidly break into the adjacent lateral ventricle (Fig. 55.276). They also may spread laterally toward the internal capsule or inferiorly toward the hypothalamus. Early ventricular dilation by blood probably explains the most common symptoms of caudate hemorrhage: headache, vomiting, decreased alertness, and stiff neck (Stein et al., 1984; Weisberg, 1984). Patients with larger parenchymous lesions in this region develop contralateral hemiparesis, conjugate deviation of the eyes toward the side of the lesion, a conjugate gaze paresis to the side opposite the lesion, and an ipsilateral central Horner's syndrome (Stein et al., 1984). Sensory findings are usually minimal or absent.

The usual cause of caudate hemorrhage is hypertension, but AVMs are a particularly common cause in young, otherwise healthy patients. Caudate hematomas have a better prognosis than comparable-sized putaminal hemorrhages.

Thalamic Hemorrhage

Thalamic hematomas are usually located posterior to pyramidal tract fibers in the internal capsule, so that contralateral sensory abnormalities are usually more prominent than is hemiparesis (Caplan, 1993; Kumral et al., 1995). Sometimes, however, the contralateral limbs are ataxic or have choreic movements, and the contralateral hand may rest in a dystonic posture. The crucial findings that differentiate thalamic from caudate and putaminal hemorrhages are the **eye signs**. As noted above, patients with caudate or putaminal hemorrhage have conjugate deviation of the eyes toward the side of the lesion and a conjugate gaze paresis to the opposite side. The most common ocular motor disturbances observed in patients with thalamic hemorrhage are caused

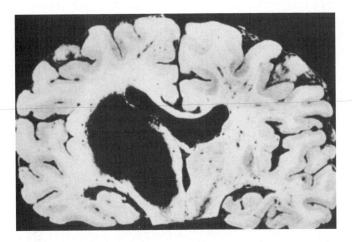

Figure 55.277. Right thalamic hemorrhage in a 71-year-old woman with systemic hypertension and cardiovascular disease. The patient had marked abnormalities of vertical eye movements. Note extension of the hemorrhage into the subthalamic area with compression of the dorsal mesencephalon.

by direct extension of the hematoma to the diencephalic-mesencephalic junction, by compression of the dorsal mesencephalon by the hematoma, or by secondary occlusion of perforating vessels supplying the dorsal midbrain (Fig. 55.277). These disturbances include: (*a*) paralysis of upward gaze; (*b*) tonic downward and medial deviation of the eyes as if they were looking at the tip of the nose; (*c*) acute esotropia caused by medial deviation of one or both eyes said to be caused by hyperconvergence; (*d*) dysconjugate gaze with limited abduction of one or both eyes (pseudo-sixth nerve paresis); (*e*) conjugate gaze deviation **away** from the side of the lesion (wrong-way deviation of the eyes); and (*f*) skew deviation (Fisher, 1959b, 1967a; Keane, 1975a, 1975b; Walshe et al., 1977; Caplan, 1980; Barraquer-Bordas et al., 1981; Tijssen, 1994; Kumral et al., 1995—see Chapter

29) (Fig. 55.278). A complete or incomplete dorsal mesencephalic (pretectal) syndrome is not uncommon (Keane, 1990).

Gilner and Avin (1977) described a 52-year-old woman with a right thalamic hemorrhage in whom tonic downward and medial deviation of the eyes occurred intermittently. The intermittent ocular deviation seemed to occur during transient, marked increases in ICP.

Brigell et al. (1984) measured saccadic and pursuit eye movements in a patient with a right thalamic hemorrhage using infrared oculography. The patient had full voluntary eye movements but tended to make spontaneous eye movements in the right hemifield of gaze. When the patient attempted to look toward the side of the lesion, saccades were normal, but pursuit was low in gain and interrupted by numerous small saccades. When the patient attempted to look away from the side of the lesion, saccades were hypometric, whereas pursuit was normal. Other authors reported similar results (Masdeu et al., 1980; Hirose et al., 1985; Hertle and Bienfang, 1990). Brigell et al. (1984) noted that this eye movement pattern resembles that seen in hemidecorticate patients. They postulated that the contraversive eye deviation that is often observed in patients with thalamic hemorrhage results from an interruption of the efferent pathways from the ipsilateral cerebral regions that mediate saccadic and pursuit eye movements.

Keane (1980) described a patient with a thalamic hemorrhage who developed opsoclonus. The opsoclonus lasted only a few days and then disappeared. Keane (1980) attributed this eye movement disturbance to traction on upper brainstem structures.

Patients with thalamic hemorrhage often have abnormalities of pupillary size and reactivity in addition to abnormalities of eye movement. The pupils tend to be small, anisocoric, and poorly reactive to light stimulation. These pupillary abnormalities are undoubtedly caused by damage to dorsal mesencephalic pupillomotor pathways and sympathetic pathways.

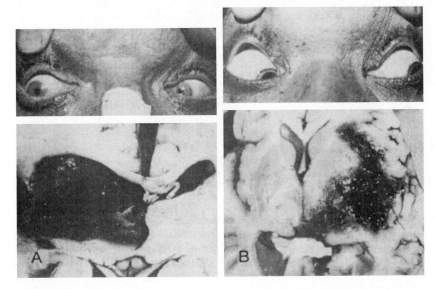

Figure 55.278. Contralateral ("wrong-way") deviation of the eyes caused by a thalamic-basal ganglia hemorrhage. *A, Above,* The patient's eyes are deviated to the right. *Below,* Coronal section immediately posterior to the mammillary bodies shows a left intracerebral hemorrhage affecting the thalamus, internal capsule, and basal ganglia. *B, Above,* In another patient with an intracranial hemorrhage, the eyes are deviated down and to the left. *Below,* Horizontal section through the mid-diencephalon shows a right intracerebral hemorrhage affecting the pretectum, thalamus, posterior limb of the internal capsule, globus pallidus, and putamen. (From Keane JR. Contralateral gaze deviation with supratentorial hemorrhage: Three pathologically verified cases. Arch Neurol *32:* 119–122, 1975.)

Homonymous field defects are common early in the course of thalamic hemorrhage but usually do not persist (Kase and Caplan, 1994). More frequently, patients manifest severe visual neglect.

Some findings in patients with thalamic hemorrhage depend on the side of the lesion. Patients with hemorrhage into the **left** thalamus often have an unusual type of aphasia. After beginning a conversation almost normally, they lapse into a remarkable fluent aphasia with many jargon or nonexistent words (i.e., neologisms) (Ciemins, 1970; Mohr et al., 1975; Samarel et al., 1976; Reynolds et al., 1978). The patients may repeat and duplicate words or syllables at the ends of words in both spoken and written language. They also commonly make paraphasic errors and are poor at naming objects. In contrast to patients with typical fluent aphasia, patients with thalamic aphasia have excellent comprehension of spoken language. The aphasia that occurs in patients with thalamic hemorrhage is thus a pure expressive aphasia with no receptive component. Patients with **right** thalamic hemorrhage often have neglect of the left visual hemifield and other visuospatial disturbances as well as anosognosia (Walshe et al., 1977; Watson and Heilman, 1979, 1981).

Decreased levels of consciousness and alertness with hypersomnolence are extremely common at the onset of a thalamic hemorrhage (Kumral et al., 1995). These disturbances result from damage to the rostral reticular activating system.

The prognosis for recovery from thalamic hemorrhage is not as good as from caudate or putaminal hemorrhages of comparable size, although depressed consciousness is not as dire a prognostic sign in thalamic lesions as it is in other supratentorial sites. Also, unlike putaminal hemorrhage, the severity of the deficit and mortality does not always correlate with ventricular extension for thalamic hemorrhage (Stein et al., 1983; Lampl et al., 1995; but see Kumral et al., 1995). Nevertheless, large thalamic hematomas over 3 cm in diameter are commonly associated with coma and death (Kwak et al., 1983; Kumral et al., 1995).

Subcortical (Lobar, Slit) Hemorrhages

Intracerebral hemorrhage may develop beneath the region of the junction between the gray and white matter of the cerebral cortex. Because such hemorrhages may be restricted to a single cerebral lobe, they are often called "lobar" hemorrhages; however, such lesions tend to undercut the cortex, and they often do not obey the strict divisions of the cerebral lobes. Subcortical hemorrhages usually spread in a linear direction along the white matter pathways. When the hematomas absorb, linear cavities remain. For this reason, these hemorrhages are often called **slit hemorrhages** (Caplan, 1993; Kase and Caplan, 1994).

Many subcortical hemorrhages are caused either by AVMs or by amyloid angiopathy; however, about 20% of hypertensive intracerebral hemorrhages are lobar (Kase and Caplan, 1994). The parietal and occipital lobes are affected more often than the frontal or temporal regions (Fig. 55.279).

The symptoms and signs of subcortical hemorrhages depend on the lobe or lobes that are primarily affected (Ropper and Davis, 1980; Kase et al., 1982), although all such hemorrhages may produce recurrent focal seizures. Anterior **fron-**

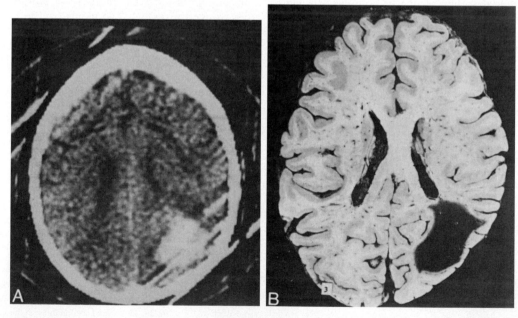

Figure 55.279. Lobar hemorrhage in the occipital lobe. The patient was a 64-year-old normotensive man who died from the effects of a pulmonary embolus 55 days after experiencing an intracranial hemorrhage. *A*, Unenhanced CT scan, axial view, performed 6 days after hemorrhage and 49 days before death, shows a lobar hemorrhage in the right occipital lobe. At autopsy, the cortical surface appeared normal, but on horizontal sectioning there was a 4.5 × 3 cm clot in the center of the right occipital lobe. *B*, Horizontal (axial) section through the brain at the level of the lateral ventricles shows a subcortical hematoma in the right occipital lobe. It may be assumed that the patient had a complete left homonymous hemianopia. (From Ropper AH, Davis KR. Lobar cerebral hemorrhages: Acute clinical syndromes in 26 cases. Ann Neurol 8:141–147, 1980.)

tal lobe hematomas usually cause abulia. Patients seem lethargic, and they have reduced spontaneity, prolonged latency in responding, and short, terse replies. If the hemorrhage extends toward the precentral gyrus or into the deep white matter of the frontal lobe, conjugate eye deviation toward the side of the lesion and contralateral hemiparesis usually occur, although Pessin et al. (1981) reported a patient with a large frontal-perisylvian hemorrhage from a ruptured aneurysm who developed conjugate horizontal eye deviation toward the side **opposite** the lesion. Autopsy examination confirmed the hemispheric locus of the hemorrhage and failed to disclose any lesion of the brainstem or thalamus to explain the ''wrong-way'' eye deviation. Sharpe et al. (1985) also described a patient with a discrete subcortical frontal lobe hematoma who had contralateral horizontal gaze deviation that persisted for 1 week. When the deviation resolved, ipsilaterally-directed saccades were hypometric, and saccadic latencies were prolonged in both horizontal directions. Smooth pursuit was paretic during tracking toward the side of the hematoma.

Lesions near the central sulcus produce contralateral motor and sensory signs. Aphasia occurs when the lesion is on the left side. If the frontal hematoma is large enough, it shifts the midline, causing compression of the contralateral oculomotor nerve associated with pupillary dilation on that side—a false localizing sign (Chen et al., 1994).

Temporal lobe hematomas produce agitation and delirium. They also are particularly prone to swell and may cause herniation without preceding hemiparesis. Brainstem compression may develop insidiously in such cases, with deepening stupor followed by an ipsilaterally dilated pupil indicating compression of the oculomotor nerve. Hallucinations, presumably epileptic in origin, occur in some cases (Cohen et al., 1992). Fluent aphasia can accompany a left temporal hemorrhage, whereas Fisher (1994) described a boy who experienced episodes of intense hunger coincident with bleeding into the right anterior temporal lobe.

Parietal lobe hemorrhage is usually associated with contralateral hemisensory loss. Complete or incomplete homonymous hemianopia may be present in the contralateral visual field. When the hemianopia is incomplete, it is usually incongruous and denser below. Patients with a parietal hematoma often have visual neglect of the contralateral hemifield. Differentiation between visual neglect and homonymous hemianopia in such cases may be difficult unless the proper technique for visual field testing is used. If each hemifield is tested separately, a patient with only visual neglect may seem to have normal visual fields unless double simultaneous stimulation is also performed. Conversely, a patient with only hemispatial visual neglect may seem to have a complete homonymous hemianopia if only double simultaneous stimulation is used and the hemifields are not tested separately (see Chapter 8). Asymmetry of ocular motor response to horizontally moving, repetitive targets is often seen in patients with a parietal lobe hematoma whether or not the lesion produces a homonymous field defect. In such patients, an abnormal response is observed when the optokinetic tape or drum is moved or rotated toward the side of the lesion.

A relatively normal response is seen when the target is moved or rotated toward the side opposite the lesion.

Occipital lobe hemorrhage usually produces a contralateral homonymous field defect that may be incomplete or complete. When incomplete, the field defect is congruous. Although most ischemic infarcts in the occipital lobe are unassociated with asymmetry of the optokinetic response, an occipital lobe hematoma may destroy sufficient surrounding tissue to produce the same type of asymmetry (abnormal response when the optokinetic tape or drum is moved or rotated toward the side of the lesion; relatively normal response when the tape or drum is moved or rotated toward the opposite side) as that seen with parietal lobe lesions. An occipital hematoma extending to the posterior parietal region may also produce mild contralateral hemisensory or motor signs as well as visual neglect.

Subcortical hemorrhages are important to diagnose, because the symptoms and signs they produce may be mistaken for those of an ischemic stroke, resulting in inappropriate therapy. In addition, large subcortical hemorrhages are usually relatively superficial and thus more accessible to surgical drainage than deeper lesions. Before the availability of neuroimaging techniques, such as CT scanning and MR imaging, the diagnosis of lobar hemorrhage was rarely made before death. Modern neuroimaging studies not only allow the diagnosis of subcortical hemorrhage to be made but also permit more accurate assessment of size and location, thus guiding appropriate management. These lesions generally are smaller than the hemorrhages that affect the putamen, caudate, and thalamus, and they have a lower mortality rate (Ropper and Davis, 1980). The functional outcome of patients with lobar intracerebral hemorrhage also is generally better than that of patients with intracerebral hematomas in other locations.

Primary Intraventricular Hemorrhage

Putaminal and caudate hemorrhages may extend into the lateral ventricle, producing secondary intraventricular hemorrhage (see above). In some cases, however, the principal locus of bleeding is within the ventricular cavity. Such ''primary'' ventricular hemorrhages usually originate from a small subependymal AVM or from extension of hemorrhage in the portion of the caudate nucleus just adjacent to the lateral ventricle.

The clinical syndrome of primary intraventricular hemorrhage is similar to that seen in subarachnoid hemorrhage. Patients experience a sudden headache associated with stiff neck, vomiting, and progressive lethargy. Some patients develop bilateral, symmetric hyperreflexia with extensor plantar responses.

In children, the most common cause of a primary intraventricular hemorrhage is an AVM arising from the choroid plexus (Butler et al., 1972). The lesion often obliterates itself as it ruptures. In adults, most intraventricular hemorrhages are caused by ventricular spread of primary hypertensive hemorrhage (Little et al., 1977).

Brainstem Hemorrhage

Primary brainstem hemorrhages most often affect the pons (Nakajima, 1983; Mangiardi and Epstein, 1988), although both mesencephalic and medullary hemorrhage occur more frequently than previously recognized before the availability of CT scanning and MR imaging. Pontine hemorrhage is most frequently caused by hypertension, whereas mesencephalic and medullary hemorrhage is most often associated with an AVM or some type of blood dyscrasia (Kase and Caplan, 1994). In addition, rapidly rising ICP can stretch median brainstem vessels and produce small hemorrhages (Duret hemorrhages—Duret, 1919) in the median or paramedian zones of the thalamus, mesencephalon, and pons (Caplan and Zervas, 1977).

Mangiardi and Epstein (1988) emphasized the distinction between a brainstem ''hemorrhage'' and a brainstem ''hematoma.'' These authors stressed that a hematoma is usually a subependymal, focal lesion caused by or associated with an intrinsic vascular malformation. It occurs in a younger age group than does a brainstem hemorrhage, rarely extends into the ventricular system, and may be evacuated with good result. Brainstem hemorrhage, however, tends to be a diffuse, deep, tegmentobasilar lesion that usually occurs in an older, hypertensive patient. It frequently extends into the ventricular system and is associated with a poor prognosis, regardless of treatment. In the following discussion, we use the terms hematoma and hemorrhage interchangeably, but we agree with Mangiardi and Epstein (1988) that a distinction between hematoma and hemorrhage may occasionally be useful from both diagnostic and therapeutic standpoints.

Mesencephalic Hemorrhage

Mesencephalic hemorrhages often produce disturbances of **eye movement**, particularly vertical gaze, and abnormalities of pupillary size and reactivity (Fig. 55.280). The severity of eye movement and pupillary signs depends on the size and location of the hematoma within the mesencephalon. Small lesions may produce isolated ocular motor deficits, whereas larger lesions tend to produce ocular motor and pupillary disturbances associated with other neurologic deficits (Scoville and Poppen, 1949; Caplan and Zervas, 1977; Humphreys, 1978; La Torre et al., 1978; see Table 1 in de Mendonca et al., 1990; Keane, 1990) (Fig. 55.281).

Durward et al. (1982b) described two patients with mesencephalic hematoma. In one patient, the cause was an AVM; the other patient was thought to have suffered a hypertensive hemorrhage. One patient had bilateral complete oculomotor and trochlear nerve pareses (Fig. 55.282), and the other patient had an ipsilateral complete right oculomotor nerve paresis and a partial right trochlear nerve paresis. Weisberg (1986) described six patients with spontaneous mesencephalic hemorrhage, all of whom had impaired upward gaze. Two of the patients had a tonic downward deviation of the eyes, and all had unequal pupils that reacted poorly to light stimulation.

All three patients described by Sand et al. (1986) had disturbances of vertical eye movements and pupillary abnormalities. One patient had a complete dorsal mesencephalic syndrome with light-near pupillary dissociation, as did a patient described by Lee et al. (1996). The second patient reported by Sand et al. (1986) had a vertical gaze paresis, a skew deviation, and bilateral Horner's syndrome. The third

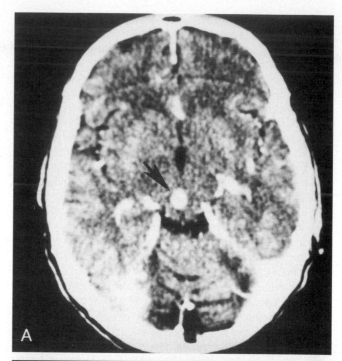

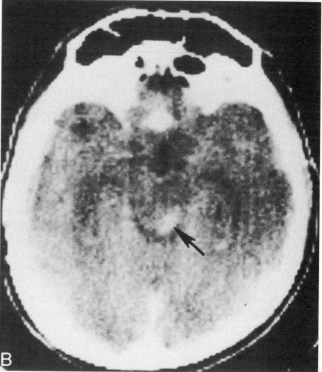

Figure 55.280. Mesencephalic hemorrhages producing abnormalities of eye movement. *A,* CT scan, axial view, in an elderly patient with a left nuclear oculomotor nerve paresis (see Figure 55.210). The scan shows a mesencephalic hematoma *(arrow). B,* CT scan, axial view, in a 56-year-old man with systemic hypertension who developed an acute headache associated with vertical diplopia. The patient had bilateral superior oblique pareses. The scan shows hemorrhage within the tectum of the mesencephalon *(arrow).* (From Wise J, Gomolin J, Goldberg LL. Bilateral superior oblique palsy: Diagnosis and treatment. Can J Ophthalmol *18:*28–32, 1983.)

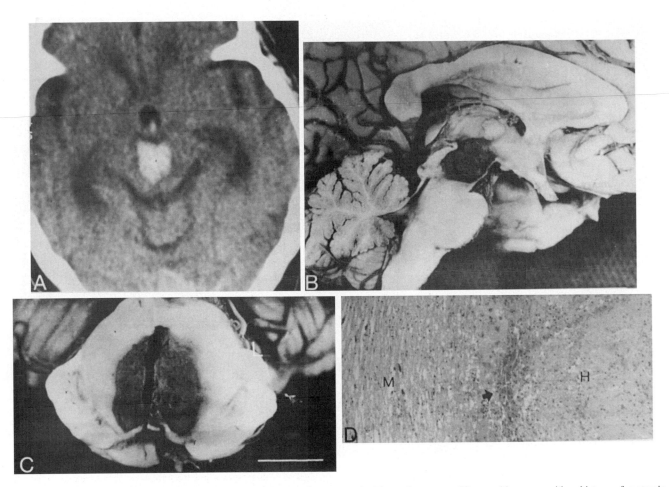

Figure 55.281. Mesencephalic hemorrhage producing bilateral ophthalmoparesis. The patient was a 70-year-old woman with a history of systemic hypertension and a previous stroke with right hemiparesis, from which she had partially recovered, who experienced acute diplopia while walking. Within a few minutes she was unable to open her eyes. On initial examination, the patient had bilateral ptosis, dilated unreactive pupils, absent vertical eye movements, and reduced horizontal gaze. She became comatose within several hours, and, despite supportive care, she died 5 weeks after the onset of diplopia. *A,* Unenhanced CT scan, axial view, shows large hyperintense lesion in the midline of the mesencephalon consistent with an acute hemorrhage. *B,* Sagittal section through the brainstem at autopsy shows a massive hemorrhage within the tegmentum of the mesencephalon. *C,* Coronal section through the mesencephalon shows the midline position of the tegmental hematoma. *D,* Histopathologic appearance of the mesencephalon shows a fairly discrete border *(arrow)* between the hematoma *(H)* and the parenchyma *(M).* (From de Mendonca A, Pimental J, Morgado F, et al. Mesencephalic haematoma: Case report with autopsy study. J Neurol *237:*55 58, 1990.)

patient had bilateral trochlear nerve paresis and an ipsilateral Horner's syndrome. Müri and Baumgartner (1995) also reported a patient with a left dorsal midbrain hematoma that caused a left Horner's syndrome, right trochlear nerve palsy, hypersomnia, and transient left trochlear nerve palsy. A patient described by Stern and Bernick (1986) had left inferior rectus weakness and bilateral ptosis, and two patients reported by Shuaib and Murphy (1987) had bilateral, complete oculomotor nerve pareses. Shuaib et al. (1989b) described a 35-year-old woman in whom a small hemorrhage in the mesencephalon caused a dilated, nonreactive pupil on the side of the lesion. The patient had no other general neurologic signs, but she did have minimal dysfunction of the right inferior and medial rectus muscles detected with a Hess screen. The hemorrhage subsequently resolved, and both the pupillary and ocular motor disturbances disappeared. Tachibana et al. (1990) reported the case of a 60-year-old man

who developed bilateral trochlear nerve paresis from a spontaneous mesencephalic hematoma (Fig. 55.283). The patient had no other disturbances of ocular motility, although he did have mild dysarthria, mild left hemiparesis, left hemiataxia, and an ataxic gait. Wise et al. (1983) reported a similar case (Fig. 55.280*B*) as did Dussaux et al. (1990). Mizuguchi et al. (1993) described a 7-year-old hemophiliac with recurrent intracerebral bleeding into the right cerebral peduncle causing **Weber's syndrome** (ipsilateral oculomotor nerve palsy and contralateral hemiparesis).

Horizontal gaze may be affected by mesencephalic hemorrhage. Bolling and Lavin (1987) described a 50-year-old man who developed horizontal diplopia in the setting of a transient right hemiparesis 15 years earlier. The patient had an exotropia in primary position. He was unable to look to the right voluntarily or when asked to fixate on a target to the right. Neither eye moved beyond the midline when the

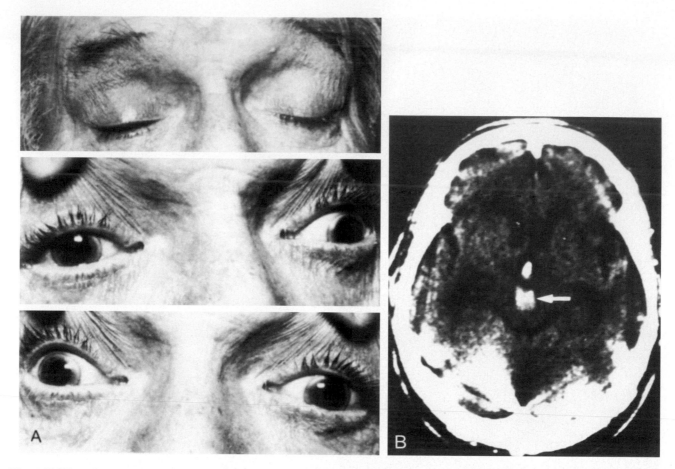

Figure 55.282. Bilateral oculomotor and trochlear nerve pareses in a 71-year-old man with a hypertensive mesencephalic hemorrhage. *A,* Appearance of the patient. *Top* photograph, the patient is attempting to open his eyes. He has a severe, bilateral ptosis. *Middle,* the patient is attempting to look to the left. Note marked limitation of adduction of the right eye with relatively normal abduction of the left eye. *Bottom,* the patient is attempting to look to the right. Note marked limitation of adduction of the left eye. The right eye has mild limitation of abduction, perhaps from hyperconvergence. The patient was unable to move the eyes up or down. *B,* CT scan, axial view, shows a hematoma within the mesencephalon (*arrow*). Blood is also visible within the inferior portion of the 3rd ventricle. (From Durward QJ, Barnett HJM, Barr HWK. Presentation and management of mesencephalic hematoma. J Neurosurg *56:*123–127, 1982.)

patient attempted to pursue a rightward moving target. The left eye was unable to look upward fully, but both eyes had normal saccadic and pursuit movements to the left. Oculocephalic testing produced full abduction in the right eye but no improvement in either adduction or elevation of the left eye. The pupils were anisocoric, with the right pupil being about 1 mm larger than the left. Both pupils reacted normally to light and near stimulation, and there was no ptosis. The patient was thought to have a partial left oculomotor paresis and a supranuclear right horizontal gaze paresis. CT scanning demonstrated a small, focal hemorrhage in the left mesencephalon. It was postulated by Bolling and Lavin (1987) that supranuclear descending pathways for horizontal gaze destined for the pons were damaged in the mesencephalon at a location where fibers serving both contralateral pursuit and saccades are located (Deleu, 1989; Lavin, 1989). Worthington and Halmagyi (1996) reported a 54-year-old woman with a midbrain hematoma and bilateral total ophthalmoplegia unassociated with other neurologic deficits.

After 5 days, she developed an alternating exotropia as abduction of each eye returned. The authors postulated that the lesion caused bilateral complete oculomotor nerve palsies, a bidirectional horizontal gaze palsy from disruption of descending pathways in the midbrain, and possibly a bidirectional vertical gaze palsy. Hertle and Bienfang (1990) described a patient with a thalamic hemorrhage who developed an acute esotropia. Neuroimaging studies showed that the hemorrhage extended into the midbrain (Fig. 55.284). Neuro-ophthalmologic examination revealed a 30–40 prism diopter esotropia that increased on attempted downward gaze. Testing of ductions and versions showed marked bilateral limitation of abduction, but normal vestibulo-ocular reflexes (Fig. 55.285). Both pupils were miotic, and they reacted poorly to both light and near stimulation. It was thought by Hertle and Bienfang (1990) that excessive convergence, perhaps caused by interruption of supranuclear inhibitory pathways, was the cause of the patient's esotropia. Other authors propose similar mechanisms for this so-called

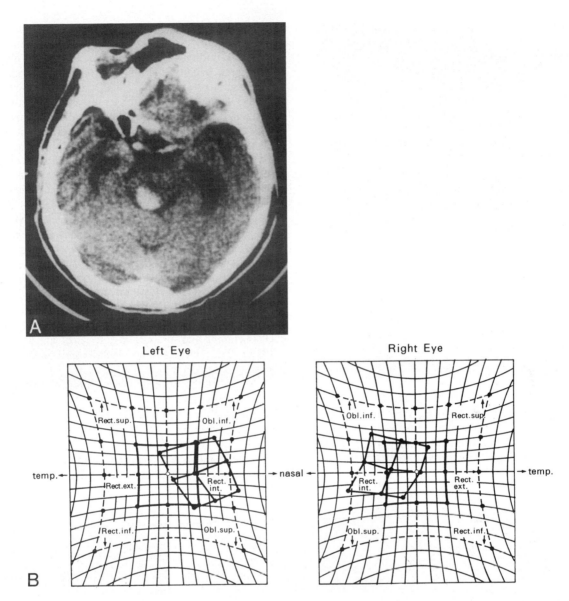

Figure 55.283. Bilateral trochlear nerve paresis from spontaneous mesencephalic hematoma. The patient was a 60-year-old man who suddenly collapsed while working outdoors. He was unconscious when he arrived at a local hospital. *A,* Unenhanced CT scan, axial view, shows a high density lesion in the tegmentum of the mesencephalon consistent with a hemorrhage. The lesion is predominantly on the left side at the level of the inferior colliculi, but it crosses the midline. The patient was treated conservatively. His level of consciousness gradually improved, and he began to complain of diplopia. Twelve days after onset of symptoms, neurologic examination revealed mild dysarthria, mild left hemiparesis, and ataxia. Neuro-ophthalmologic examination revealed an esotropia of 24 prism diopters associated with a left hypertropia of 4 prism diopters in primary position. Excyclotorsion exceeded 30 and increased on attempted downward gaze. *B,* Hess screen evaluation shows pattern consistent with bilateral trochlear nerve paresis. Note torsional aspect of strabismus. (From Tachibana H, Mimura O, Shiomi M, et al. Bilateral trochlear nerve palsies from a brainstem hematoma. J Clin Neuroophthalmol *10:*35–37, 1990.)

''thalamic esotropia'' (Gomez et al., 1987). The pathways involved may, in fact, be more mesencephalic.

Focal syndromes other than those affecting ocular motility may occur in patients with small hemorrhages in the mesencephalon. Azouvi et al. (1989) reported a case of pure sensory stroke from a hemorrhage in the mesencephalon that affected only the spinothalamic pathway, and other cases involve only the corticospinal tracts, producing pure motor hemiplegia (Kase and Caplan, 1994).

Pontine Hemorrhage

Pontine hemorrhage usually begins at the center of the pons at the junction of the tegmentum and the base (Silverstein, 1972). If it remains small and localized, the patient may have only minimal focal signs. Usually, however, the hematoma grows quickly and assumes a round or oval shape, destroying the center of the tegmentum and base of the pons (Figs. 55.233, 55.286, and 55.288). The blood may dissect

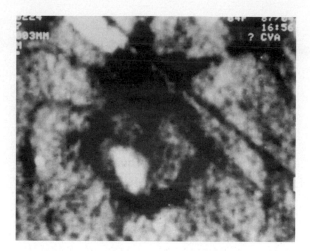

Figure 55.284. Acute esotropia from thalamic and mesencephalic hemorrhage. The patient was an 84-year-old woman with a history of coronary artery disease and hypertension who developed acute perioral numbness that spread to both sides of the body. She then experienced a severe right-sided headache, diplopia, dizziness, nausea, and left-sided weakness. CT scan, axial view, shows changes consistent with hemorrhage in the posterior medial thalamus and mesencephalon. (From Hertle RW, Bienfang DC. Oculographic analysis of acute esotropia secondary to a thalamic hemorrhage. J Clin Neuroophthalmol *10*:21–26, 1990.)

rostrally into the mesencephalon, superiorly into the 4th ventricle, or, less frequently, caudally into the medulla. Large pontine hemorrhages arise from the median pontine perforating vessels that originate from the basilar artery (see Chapter 52).

The signs that accompany large medial pontine hematomas are quadriparesis that is often associated with limb stiffness and rigidity, coma, pupils that are usually pinpoint and poorly reactive but that may be dilated and fixed, and rapid or irregular respirations (Steegman, 1951; Kushner and Bressman, 1985; Masiyama et al., 1985). Disturbances of horizontal and vertical eye movements are common. Many patients have a skew deviation; however, the most common abnormality is a horizontal gaze paresis that is usually bilateral. Patients with a bilateral horizontal gaze paresis, particularly those who are stuporous or comatose, often have continuous, involuntary, usually conjugate, vertical eye movements. Some of these abnormal vertical eye movements consist of a slow movement in one direction and a fast movement in the other, taking the eyes between upgaze or downgaze and midposition. These movements are named depending on whether the downward or upward movement is fast or slow and whether the movement is between upgaze and primary position or downgaze and primary position (e.g., ocular bobbing, ocular dipping, reverse ocular bobbing, etc.) (Fisher, 1964; Nelson and Johnston, 1970; Goldschmidt and Wall, 1987; Rosa et al., 1987; Mehler, 1988d; Titer and Laureno, 1988) (see above and Chapter 31).

Vertical, bobbing eye movements usually occur in patients with a large midline hemorrhage, but they were reported by Katz et al. (1982) in a patient with a unilateral pontine hematoma. Most patients in whom such movements develop die shortly thereafter.

Some conjugate, involuntary, vertical eye movements seen in patients with pontine hemorrhage consist of continu-

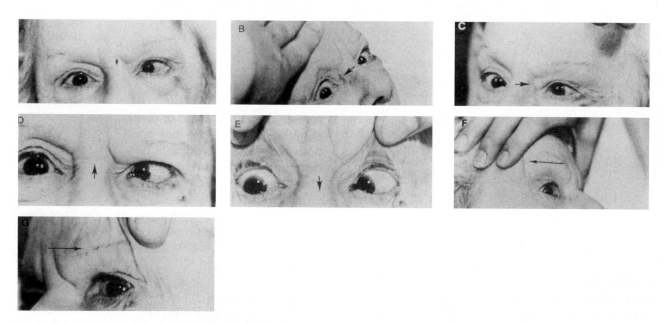

Figure 55.285. Ocular motility in the patient whose CT scan is shown in Figure 55.284. *A,* The patient prefers to fix with the right eye in primary position. With the right eye fixing, she has a large esotropia. *B,* The patient has marked limitation of abduction of the right eye when asked to look to the right. *C,* The patient has marked limitation of abduction of the left eye when asked to look to the left. *D,* The patient cannot elevate the eyes voluntarily. *E,* The patient can only minimally depress both eyes when asked to look downward. *F* and *G,* Abduction is full when tested with the Doll's head maneuver. (From Hertle RW, Bienfang DC. Oculographic analysis of acute esotropia secondary to a thalamic hemorrhage. J Clin Neuroophthalmol *10*:21–26, 1990.)

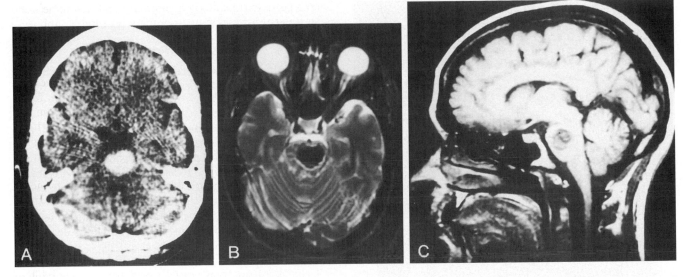

Figure 55.286. Pontine hemorrhage. Neuroimaging studies in a 25-year-old, previously healthy woman who experienced an acute headache and loss of consciousness. When she was examined initially, she had bilateral facial weakness, bilateral horizontal gaze paresis, and bilateral abducens nerve paresis. Corneal sensation was slightly reduced bilaterally as was facial sensation. *A*, Unenhanced CT scan, axial view, shows a large hemorrhage in the pons. *B*, T2-weighted MR image, axial view, shows massive low intensity lesion in the midpons, consistent with acute hemorrhage. *C*, T1-weighted MR image, sagittal view, shows more precise location of the pontine hemorrhage.

ous pendular oscillations. These movements, called **ocular myoclonus,** may persist for the rest of the patient's life, become synchronous with similar movements of the palate (oculopalatal myoclonus) (Lawrence and Lightfoote, 1975; see Chapter 31), be associated but asynchronous with palatal myoclonus (Stacy, 1982), or disappear (Cordonnier et al., 1985).

Larmande et al. (1982) described a patient with a massive pontine hemorrhage who had a locked-in syndrome but who never lost consciousness and was able to communicate by blink until her death several days later. In addition to a bilateral infranuclear paresis of horizontal gaze, she had a dissociated abnormality of vertical movements characterized by slowed vertical saccades with normal vertical pursuit. At autopsy, the mesencephalon was entirely normal despite the marked disturbance of vertical gaze (Fig. 55.288*A*). Most of the pontine tegmentum was destroyed by hemorrhage (Fig. 55.288*B–D*).

Headache and vomiting occasionally occur in patients with massive pontine hemorrhages, particularly when the hemorrhage extends into the 4th ventricle. Some pontine hemorrhages develop gradually (Kanyey, 1939), and early findings may be asymmetric. Deafness, dysarthria, facial numbness, asymmetric facial or limb weakness, and dizziness occasionally precede coma. Some patients have twitching, shivering, or spasmodic movements of the limbs, usually culminating in decerebrate rigidity.

Massive pontine hemorrhages are usually fatal, but not necessarily immediately. Death usually occurs 24–48 hours after onset, although survival for 7–10 days is not rare.

Small pontine hemorrhages, particularly those at the base or in the lateral tegmentum of the pons, are not only compatible with life but are also compatible with return of reason-

ably good neurologic function (Payne et al., 1978; Kase et al., 1980; Caplan and Goodwin, 1982; Tanaka et al., 1982; Kushner and Bressman, 1985; Masiyama et al., 1985). Many of these hemorrhages are probably caused by bleeding from a cavernous hemangioma. Lateral basal hematomas can cause pure motor hemiparesis (Weisberg, 1979; Gobernado et al., 1980; Shibagaki et al., 1983; Kameyama et al., 1989; Kim et al., 1994a) or ataxic hemiparesis (Schnapper, 1982; Kobatake and Shinohara, 1983), thus mimicking the findings in lacunar infarction (see above). Such lesions can spread into the adjacent tegmentum, causing unilateral cranial neuropathy, particularly abducens nerve paresis, horizontal gaze paresis, and facial nerve paresis. Raymond syndrome (ipsilateral abducens nerve palsy and contralateral hemiparesis) occurred in a 39-year-old man with a hemorrhage at the medial pontomedullary junction (Satake et al., 1995). Lateral tegmental hematomas arise from penetrating vessels that course from lateral to medial after branching from the lateral circumferential pontine arteries. These lesions affect the rostral pons and produce a variety of disturbances of horizontal eye movements, including ipsilateral horizontal gaze paresis, abducens nerve paresis, INO, or one-and-a-half syndrome (Fisher, 1967a; Caplan and Goodwin, 1982; Oommen et al., 1982; Dubin and Quencer, 1987; see Chapters 28 and 29) (Figs. 55.289 and 55.290).

Because the sensory lemniscus is located in the pontine tegmentum, patients with lateral tegmental hematomas usually have loss of pain, temperature, and position sense on the opposite side of the body (Caplan, 1993). Limb and truncal ataxia are usually present and may be bilateral or predominantly ipsilateral. Unilateral facial numbness or weakness, central Horner's syndrome, and transient deafness may also occur. Contralateral hemiparesis, when present, is usually

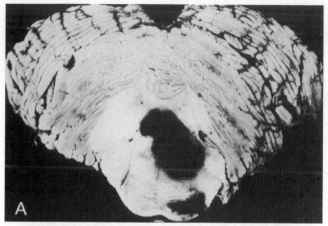

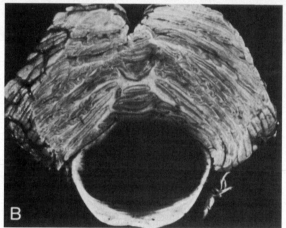

Figure 55.287. Pathologic specimens showing pontine hemorrhage. *A*, Hemorrhage primarily on the left side of the pons has ruptured into the 4th ventricle. *B*, Massive midline basal pontine hemorrhage has destroyed the basis and tegmentum of the pons on both sides.

mild and transient. Patients with such lesions usually recover with only minimal residual neurologic dysfunction, primarily disturbances of horizontal eye movements and facial nerve paresis.

Medullary Hemorrhage

Intramedullary hemorrhage is much less common than either pontine or mesencephalic hemorrhage. Following the first description of a primary medullary hemorrhage by Kempe in 1964, several other cases were described (see Table 21.3 in Kase and Caplan, 1994). The hemorrhages in this region are usually unilateral, tegmental or basal, and rarely lateral. Most cases have ipsilateral facial hypesthesia, limb ataxia, gait imbalance, palatal weakness, dysphonia, dysphagia, and horizontal nystagmus. Ipsilateral Horner's syndrome and contralateral hemisensory disturbances are reported less frequently. Contralateral hemiparesis and ipsilateral hypoglossal palsy occur more often in medullary hemorrhages than in lateral medullary infarctions (Kase and Caplan, 1994). Rousseaux et al. (1991) reported a patient

with a posterior medullary hemorrhage and first upbeat and later downbeat nystagmus in primary position.

Cerebellar Hemorrhage

Hemorrhage into the cerebellum probably accounts for about 10% of all intracerebral hemorrhages and 7% of hypertensive intracerebral hemorrhages (Caplan, 1993; Kase and Caplan, 1994). Conversely, about 60–75% of patients with cerebellar hemorrhage have chronic hypertension (McKissock et al., 1960; Freeman et al., 1973; Ott et al., 1974). These patients tend to be older than patients in whom the hemorrhage is caused by a vascular malformation (McKissock et al., 1960). Although the frequency of cerebellar hemorrhage is relatively low, the diagnosis is extremely important because of the good prognosis with prompt surgical treatment and the poor prognosis if treatment is delayed or not provided (Chawla, 1970; Ott et al., 1974; Brennan and Bergland, 1977; Freeman et al., 1978; Editorial, 1988).

Cerebellar hemorrhage usually originates in the region of the dentate nucleus, arising from distal branches of the supe-

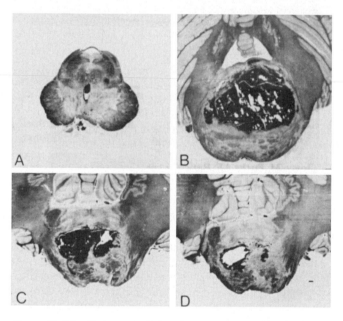

Figure 55.288. Brainstem pathology in a patient with abnormal vertical eye movements and a locked-in syndrome. The patient was a 50-year-old woman with chronic systemic hypertension who was admitted to the hospital after she developed an acute left hemiplegia without loss of consciousness. Her condition deteriorated rapidly immediately after admission. She became quadriplegic and developed complete respiratory paralysis that required tracheal intubation and assisted ventilation. The patient nevertheless remained conscious and communicated by blinking. The patient had complete paralysis of horizontal gaze. Vertical saccades were slowed, whereas vertical pursuit movements were normal. The patient subsequently died. *A*, Section through the midbrain shows no major lesions. There is blood in the cerebral aqueduct. *B*, Section through the rostral pons shows a massive hemorrhage that is mainly located in the tegmentum just beneath the intact 4th ventricle. *C* and *D*, The hemorrhage becomes less marked in successively more caudal sections through the pons. (From Larmande P, Hénin D, Jan M, et al. Abnormal vertical eye movements in the locked-in syndrome. Ann Neurol *11*:100–102, 1982.)

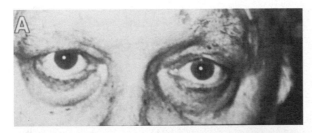
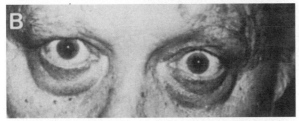
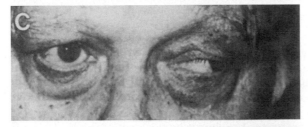
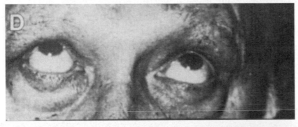
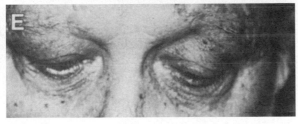

Figure 55.289. One-and-a-half syndrome associated with facial paresis in a patient with an acute pontine hemorrhage. The patient was a 58-year-old man with systemic hypertension who experienced sudden diplopia unassociated with other neurologic symptoms or signs. About 3 weeks later, he developed right facial weakness. *A-E,* The patient has a right one-and-a-half syndrome. *A,* The eyes are aligned in primary position. Note right lower lid laxity and ectropion caused by right facial weakness. *B,* On attempted right lateral gaze, neither eye moves past the midline. *C,* On attempted left lateral gaze, the left eye abducts fully with normal velocity, but the right eye abducts slowly and incompletely. *D* and *E,* Vertical eye movements are normal. (From Oommen KJ, Smith MS, Labadie EL. Pontine hemorrhage causing Fisher one-and-a-half syndrome with facial paralysis. J Clin Neuroophthalmol 2:129–132, 1982.)

rior cerebellar and posterior inferior cerebellar arteries. The hematoma collects around the dentate and spreads into the white matter of the cerebellar hemisphere, frequently rupturing into the 4th ventricle (Fig. 55.291). Occasionally, a primary vermian hemorrhage occurs (Kase and Caplan, 1994). The adjacent brainstem may be compressed from above by the lesion (Fig. 55.292).

One of the most consistent symptoms in patients with cerebellar hemorrhage is the inability to walk. Some patients even have difficulty remaining in a sitting or standing position, and they often lean or tilt toward the side of the hematoma. Patients have been known to crawl or slide to the bathroom or the telephone. Vomiting also is quite frequent, occurring in 60–90% of patients (Taneda et al., 1987; Kase and Caplan, 1994). The combination of vomiting and difficulty walking may initially suggest the diagnosis of an "inner ear" disturbance. We saw a patient with chronic hypertension and obesity who experienced the sudden onset of difficulty with balance and vomiting. He called his internist, described his symptoms, and was told he had "the flu" and should stay in bed until he felt better. Only when he developed other evidence of brainstem dysfunction was he examined and hospitalized, at which time the correct diagnosis was made.

Headache commonly occurs in patients with cerebellar hemorrhage and occasionally may be the most prominent symptom (Norris et al., 1969; Taneda et al., 1987). It usually is most severe in the occipital, neck, and frontal regions. Dysarthria, hiccups, and tinnitus occur, but they are much less frequent. Loss of consciousness at onset is distinctly unusual, but about one-third of patients are obtunded by the time they reach the hospital (Fisher et al., 1965b; Ott et al., 1974; Brennan and Bergland, 1977).

Many visual and neurologic signs in patients with cerebellar hemorrhage are caused by compression of the brainstem (Case Records of the Massachusetts General Hospital, 1962, 1967b), but others are caused by interruption of the normal pathways that connect the cerebellum with the other parts of the brain, particularly the brainstem. Most visual disturbances are related to dysfunction of the ocular motor system and include ipsilateral abducens nerve or horizontal gaze paresis toward the side of the hematoma, skew deviation, INO, various forms of nystagmus, ocular dysmetria, and macrosaccadic oscillations (Fisher et al., 1965b; Ott et al., 1974; Brennan and Bergland, 1977; Masson et al., 1986; Kattah and Dagi, 1990). Pupillary signs include small pupils that are poorly reactive and Horner's syndrome, which may be unilateral and ipsilateral to the hematoma or bilateral. Neurologic signs include gait ataxia and rebound overshoot of a rapidly elevated arm. Hemiparesis is rarely present.

As a cerebellar hematoma expands, the pons and medulla become increasingly compressed. Patients develop increasing stupor, bilateral horizontal gaze paresis, and bilateral extensor plantar responses. This state can develop rapidly. In the series reported by Fisher et al. (1965b), only two of 18 patients had a benign course. The other 16 patients developed coma, usually within a few hours after the onset of symptoms. Among those patients not comatose on admission in the series reported by Brennan and Bergland (1977),

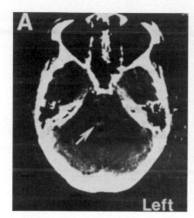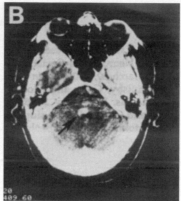

Figure 55.290. Appearance of CT scan in the patient whose eye movements are shown in Figure 55.289. *A,* Unenhanced image, axial view, shows a small hyperintense lesion consistent with a hemorrhage in the pons *(arrow). B,* Enhanced image, axial view, shows lesion in more detail *(arrow).* The patient's ocular motor disorder eventually resolved completely, and the CT scan became normal. (From Oommen KJ, Smith MS, Labadie EL. Pontine hemorrhage causing Fisher one-and-a-half syndrome with facial paralysis. J Clin Neuroophthalmol 2:129–132, 1982.)

80% deteriorated to coma with one-fourth of these patients doing so within **3 hours** of the onset of symptoms.

Some patients with cerebellar hemorrhage have a more indolent course, presenting with symptoms and signs of hydrocephalus that results from obstruction of the 4th ventricle by the hematoma (Shenkin and Zavala, 1982; Taneda et al., 1987). Abulia, dementia, incontinence, and a shuffling slow gait are common in these patients, who initially may be thought to have normal-pressure hydrocephalus if preceding symptoms such as dizziness, headache, and vomiting are not elicited during the history. Other patients with laterally placed cerebellar hematomas develop cranial neuropathies from compression of structures in the cerebellopontine angle. Such patients have dysfunction of the trigeminal, abducens, facial, and vestibulocochlear nerves as well as ataxia. Tinnitus and even hearing loss are rare presenting signs (Matsuda et al., 1993). Finally, rare patients have an acute hemorrhage into the vermis and 4th ventricle, resulting in severe headache, vomiting, and rapid development of coma (Kase and Caplan, 1994).

The course of cerebellar hematomas is unpredictable, with larger lesions frequently causing coma and death (Taneda et al., 1987). Although some authors stress the good functional

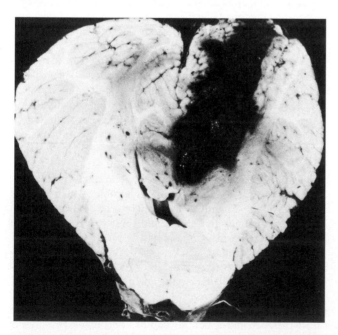

Figure 55.291. Cerebellar hemorrhage. The hemorrhage arose in the region of the dentate nucleus and tracked inferiorly, compressing and distorting the 4th ventricle.

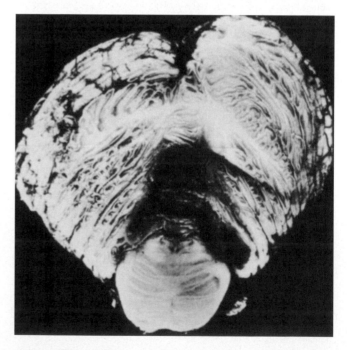

Figure 55.292. Bilateral vermian hemorrhage with compression of the 4th ventricle and dorsal pons.

recovery that is occasionally observed in patients with spontaneous cerebellar hemorrhage treated nonsurgically (Heiman and Satya-Murti, 1978; Melamed and Satya-Murti, 1984), it is probably wise to drain all lesions 3 cm or more in diameter, particularly when they cause an alteration of mental status (Ojemann and Heros, 1983) and are associated with evidence by neuroimaging of significant obliteration of the quadrigeminal cistern by rostral displacement of the vermis (Taneda et al., 1987). Some patients with small lesions can be successfully treated by medical decompression using systemic corticosteroids and osmotic diuretic agents, whereas others can be treated by ventricular drainage alone (Shenkin and Zavala, 1982). Mohadjer et al. (1990) reported good results using CT-guided stereotactic fibrinolysis and evacuation of cerebellar hemorrhages.

Optic Nerve and Optic Chiasmal Hemorrhage

As noted above, hemorrhage may occur within the substance of the optic nerves and optic chiasm, or it may occur between the orbital or intracranial portions of the nerves and the dural sheath that surrounds them (Figs. 55.269–55.271). Blunt **trauma** is the usual cause of such hemorrhage, although small vascular malformations and even aneurysms within the orbit may hemorrhage spontaneously.

When hemorrhage affects the proximal portion of the optic nerve adjacent to the globe, particularly when the hemorrhage is between the optic nerve sheath and the nerve itself, the ophthalmoscopic picture resembles that of a CRVO, probably because the hemorrhage compresses and occludes the central retinal vein as it exits from the optic nerve and traverses the space between the nerve and the sheath. The fundus of the affected eye shows mild to severe swelling of the optic disc, multiple retinal hemorrhages, and dilation of retinal veins. In this setting, CT scanning (with coronal views) or MR imaging may show the hemorrhage (Fig. 55.271), and immediate decompression of the sheath may allow recovery of vision.

When hemorrhage affects the posterior orbital, intracanalicular, or intracranial portions of one or both optic nerves, the picture is similar to that seen when the optic chiasm is affected. Visual loss occurs immediately or within a few hours after injury or spontaneous hemorrhage in one or both eyes. Any type of field defect may be present. If optic nerve damage is unilateral or sufficiently asymmetric, an RAPD is present on the side of the affected (or more severely affected) optic nerve. The optic disc appears normal for several weeks.

When the optic chiasm is affected, visual loss is almost always abrupt and bilateral (Maitland et al., 1982; Corboy and Galetta, 1989; see bibliography in Regli et al., 1989; Warner et al., 1996). When there is residual visual function, the field defect may have a bitemporal appearance (Fig. 55.293), but more often there is diffuse field loss. The pupils may have a relatively normal reaction, or they may be sluggishly reactive to light while retaining a normal response to near (or proprioceptive) stimulation. If all vision is lost in both eyes, the pupils are nonreactive to light stimulation. The optic discs usually appear normal for about 4–5 weeks, then optic atrophy becomes apparent. Neuroimaging studies, particularly MR imaging, are critical in the diagnosis of intrachiasmatic hemorrhage, especially if there is an underlying cavernous malformation (Fig. 55.294). In patients with severe visual loss, aspiration of the intrachiasmatic hematoma or excision of the angioma may result in significant visual recovery (Regli et al., 1989), although some patients improve spontaneously (Warner et al., 1996). Recurrent chiasmal hemorrhage probably indicates a chiasmal vascular malformation (Warner et al., 1996). Friedman et al. (1996) reported the remarkable case of a 41-year-old man with dif-

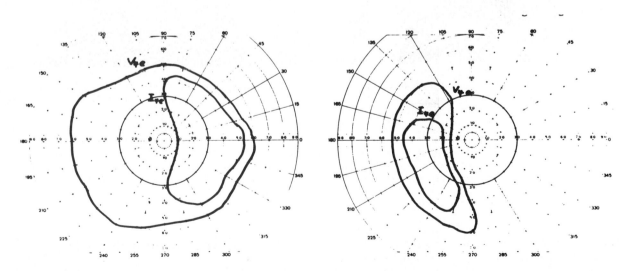

Figure 55.293. Bitemporal hemianopia in a patient with an intrachiasmatic hemorrhage caused by a cavernous angioma of the optic chiasm. The patient was a 28-year-old, previously healthy woman who complained of right-sided headache, blurred vision in the right eye, and a visual field defect in both temporal fields. Visual acuity was about 4/200 OD and 20/20 OS. There is a relative temporal defect in the visual field of the right eye and a complete temporal hemianopia with involvement of macular vision in the left visual field. (From Regli L, de Tribolet N, Regli F, et al. Chiasmal apoplexy: Haemorrhage from a cavernous malformation in the optic chiasm. J Neurol Neurosurg Psychiatry 52:1095–1099, 1989.)

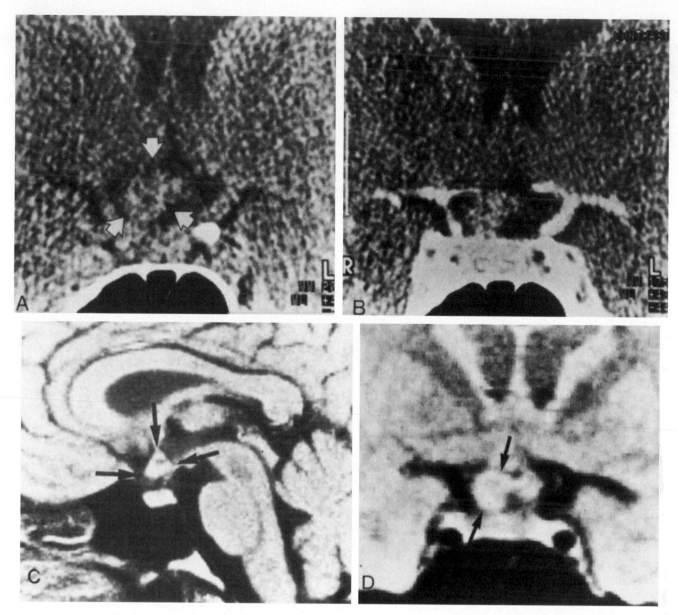

Figure 55.294. Neuroimaging studies performed in the patient whose visual fields are illustrated in Figure 55.293. *A,* Unenhanced CT scan, coronal view through the region of the optic chiasm, shows a high density mass in the suprasellar cistern *(arrows). B,* Enhanced CT scan, coronal view, shows that the lesion enhances poorly. *C,* MR image, sagittal view, shows enlargement of the optic chiasm *(arrows).* Within the chiasm there is mild peripheral hyperintensity with central hypointensity, consistent with intraparenchymal hemorrhage. *D,* MR image, coronal view, shows enlargement of the optic chiasm, particularly on the right side with a mixed hypo- and slightly hyperintense signal *(arrows).* Exploration of the optic chiasm revealed a hemorrhagic cavernous malformation that was excised. The patient's visual acuity improved to 20/20 OD and 20/10 OS after surgery. The visual field of the left eye became normal, and the visual field of the right eye improved until the patient had a relative temporal hemianopic defect, denser above. (From Regli L, de Tribolet N, Regli F, et al. Chiasmal apoplexy: Haemorrhage from a cavernous malformation in the optic chiasm. J Neurol Neurosurg Psychiatry *52:* 1095–1099, 1989.)

fuse hemorrhage of the intracranial optic nerves, optic chiasm, and optic tracts, attributed to alcohol-induced coagulopathy. The patient was followed without surgical intervention, and subsequent neuroimaging demonstrated complete resolution of the hemorrhage and atrophy of the visual pathways. The patient's vision improved substantially (55.295).

Lateral Geniculate Hemorrhage

Hemorrhage confined to the lateral geniculate body is unusual. Nakahashi et al. (1988) reported a 76-year-old man who experienced sudden loss of vision to the left side and was found to have a complete left homonymous hemianopia. CT scanning demonstrated a small hemorrhage in the right

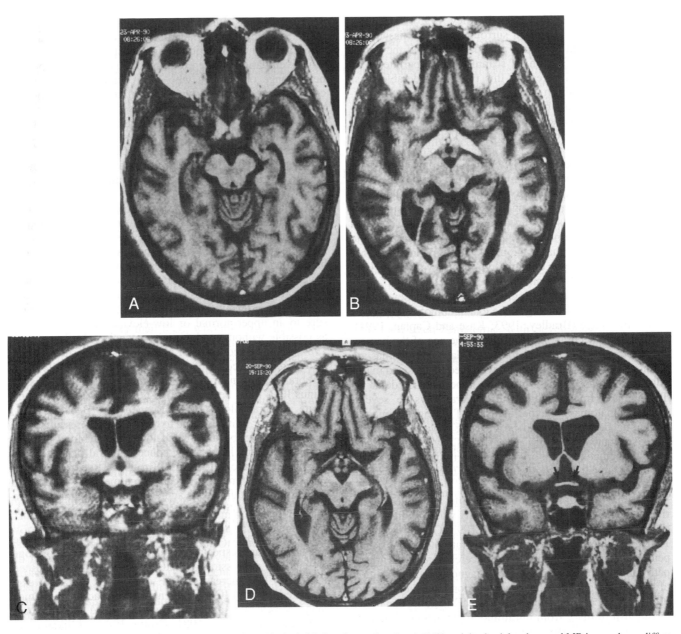

Figure 55.295. Visual pathway hemorrhage associated with alcohol-induced coagulopathy. *A-C,* T1-weighted axial and coronal MR image shows diffuse enlargement of the intracranial optic nerves, optic chiasm, and optic tracts, showing high signal intensity, and there was no significant enhancement after gadolinium. *D, E,* T1-weighted MR image 5 months later shows resolution of the visual pathway hemorrhage, with minimal hyperintensity of the optic chiasm and optic tract. The optic chiasm and optic tract appear somewhat thinner than normal (*arrows*). No vascular malformation is present. (From Friedman DI, Aravapalli RR, Shende MC. Visual pathway hemorrhage associated with alcohol-induced coagulopathy. J Neuroophthalmol *16:*124–133, 1996.)

lateral geniculate body. The field defect gradually improved until it became an incongruous homonymous horizontal sectoranopia, consistent with damage to the territory supplied by the lateral choroidal artery (see above).

DIAGNOSIS

Throughout this chapter, we have emphasized that it can be extremely difficult to differentiate clinically between an ischemic and a hemorrhagic stroke. For this reason, we rec-

ommend that all patients with any type of stroke undergo some type of neuroimaging study, either CT scanning or MR imaging. Both studies can identify the location of the lesion or lesions, differentiate between ischemic and hemorrhagic lesions, and determine the extent of associated brain edema.

In addition, neuroimaging studies can often help determine the **age** of an intracerebral hematoma (Gomori et al., 1985; Bradley, 1993). A hematoma initially has regular, smooth contours. During the first 48 hours, large hematomas may show fluid-blood levels, indicating that the hematoma

Bailliart P. La pression arterielle dan les branches de l'artère centrale de la retine; nouvelle technique pour la determiner. Ann Oculist *154*:648–666, 1917.

Baird AE, Benfield A, Schlaug G, et al. Enlargement of human cerebral ischemic lesion volumes measured by diffusion-weighted magnetic resonance imaging. Ann Neurol *41*:581–589, 1997.

Bakay L, Leslie EV. Surgical treatment of vertebral artery insufficiency caused by cervical spondylosis. J Neurosurg *23*:596–602, 1965.

Baker AB. The medullary blood supply and the lateral medullary syndrome. Neurology *11*:852–861, 1961.

Baker AB, Iannone A. Cerebrovascular disease. I. The large arteries of the circle of Willis. Neurology *9*:321–332, 1959.

Baker AB, Resch JA, Loewenson RB. Hypertension and cerebral atherosclerosis. Circulation *39*:701, 1969.

Baker R, Rosenbaum A, Caplan L. Subclavian steal syndrome. Contemp Surg *4*: 96–104, 1974.

Baker RS, Carr WA. Pontine infarction: Angiography and magnetic resonance imaging. Surv Ophthalmol *32*:141–143, 1987.

Bakey L, Sweet WH. Cervical and intracranial intra-arterial pressures with and without vascular occlusion. Surg Gynecol Obstet *95*:67–75, 1952.

Bakey L, Sweet WH. Intra-arterial pressures in the neck and brain. J Neurosurg *10*: 353–359, 1953.

Balcer LJ, Galetta SL, Hurst RW, et al. Occipital lobe infarction from a carotid artery embolic source. J Neuroophthalmol *16*:33–35, 1996.

Balcer LJ, Galetta SL, Yousem DM, et al. Pupil-involving third-nerve palsy and carotid stenosis: Rapid recovery following endarterectomy. Ann Neurol *41*: 273–276, 1997.

Bálint R. A figyelem zavara az agyfeltekek bantamainal (disorders of attention with disease of the cerebral hemispheres). Termeszettudomanyi Kozlony *1*:82, 1905.

Bálint R. A nezes lelki benulasa, optikai ataxia, a figyelem terbeli zavara (psychic paralysis of gaze, optic ataxia, and disturbance of spatial attention). Orvosi Hetilap *1*:209–236, 1907.

Bálint R. Seelenähmung des "Schauens," optische Ataxie, raumliche Störung der Aufmerksamkeit. Monatschr Psychiatr Neurol *25*:51–81, 1909.

Ball CJ. Atheromatous embolism to the brain, retina, and choroid. Arch Ophthalmol *76*:690–695, 1966.

Ballen PH, Fox MJ, Weissman GS. Ischemic optic neuropathy secondary to intestinal hemorrhage. Ann Ophthalmol *17*:486–488, 1985.

Baloh RW, Yee RD, Honrubia V. Eye movements in patients with Wallenberg's syndrome. Ann NY Acad Sci *374*:600–613, 1981.

Bamford JM, Warlow CP. Evolution and testing of the lacunar hypothesis. Stroke *19*:1074–1082, 1988.

Bamford J, Sandercock P, Dennis M, et al. A prospective study of acute cerebrovascular disease in the community: The Oxfordshire Community Project—1981–1986. 2. Incidence, case fatality rates and overall outcome at one year of cerebral infarction, primary intracerebral and subarachnoid haemorrhage. J Neurol Neurosurg Psychiatry *53*:16–22, 1990.

Bank H, Shibolet S, Gilat T, et al. Mucormycosis of head and neck structures. A case with survival. Br Med J *1*:766–768, 1962.

Baquis GD, Pessin MS, Scott RM. Limb shaking—A carotid TIA. Stroke *16*:444–448, 1985.

Barger AC, Beeuwkes R III, Lainey LL, et al. Hypothesis: Vasa vasorum and neovascularization of human coronary arteries. N Engl J Med *310*:175–177, 1984.

Barinagarrementeria F, Cantu-Brito C, De La Pena A, et al. Prothrombotic states in young people with idiopathic stroke: A prospective study. Stroke *25*:287–290, 1994.

Barinagarrementeria F, Figueroa T, Huebe J, et al. Cerebral infarction in people under 40 years: Etiologic analysis of 300 cases prospectively evaluated. Cerebrovasc Dis *6*:75–79, 1996.

Barker WF, Stern WE, Krayenbuhl H, et al. Carotid endarterectomy complicated by carotid cavernous sinus fistula. Ann Surg *167*:568–572, 1968.

Barlow JB, Bosman CK. Aneurysmal protrusion of the posterior leaflet of the mitral valve: An ausculatory-electrocardiographic syndrome. Am Heart J *71*:166–178, 1966.

Barlow JB, Pocock WA, Marchand P, et al. The significance of late systolic murmurs. Am Heart J *66*:443–452, 1963.

Barnes RW, Liebmann PR, Marszalek PB, et al. Natural history of asymptomatic carotid disease in patients undergoing cardiovascular surgery. Surgery *90*: 1075–1083, 1981.

Barnett HJM. Transient cerebral ischemia: Pathogenesis, prognosis and management. Ann R Coll Phys Surg Can *7*:153–173, 1974.

Barnett HJM. Progress towards stroke prevention. Neurology *30*:1212–1225, 1980.

Barnett HJM. Embolism in mitral valve prolapse. Ann Rev Med *33*:489–507, 1982.

Barnett HJM. The contribution of multicenter trials to stroke prevention and treatment. Arch Neurol *47*:441–444, 1990.

Barnett HJM, Aldis AE. Delayed cerebral ischemic episodes distal to occlusion of major cerebral arteries. Neurology *25*:370, 1975.

Barnett HJM, Haines SJ. Carotid endarterectomy for asymptomatic carotid stenosis. N Engl J Med *328*:276–279, 1993.

Barnett HJM, Jones MW, Boughner DR, et al. Cerebral ischemic events associated with prolapsing mitral valve. Arch Neurol *33*:777–782, 1976.

Barnett HJM, Peerless SJ, Wei M. The "stump" of the internal carotid artery: A source for further cerebral embolic ischemia. Stroke *8*:14–15, 1977.

Barnett HJM, Peerless SJ, Kaufmann JCE. "Stump" of internal carotid artery—A source for further cerebral embolic ischemia. Stroke *9*:448–456, 1978.

Barnett HJM, Boughner DR, Taylor DW, et al. Further evidence relating mitral valve prolapse to cerebral ischemic events. N Engl J Med *302*:139–144, 1980.

Barnett HJM, Plum F, Walton JN. Carotid endarterectomy—An expression of concern. Stroke *15*:941–943, 1984.

Barnett HJM, Stein BM, Mohr JP, et al. Stroke: Pathophysiology, Diagnosis, and Management. Vol 1. New York, Churchill Livingstone, 1986.

Barnett HJM, Stein BM, Mohr JP, et al. Stroke: Pathophysiology, Diagnosis, and Management. 2nd ed. New York, Churchill Livingstone, 1992.

Barnett HJM, Eliasziw M, Meldrum HE. The identification by imaging methods of patients who might benefit from carotid endarterectomy. Arch Neurol *52*: 827–831, 1995a.

Barnett HJM, Eliasziw M, Meldrum HE. Drugs and sugery in the prevention of ischemic stroke. N Engl J Med *332*:238–248, 1995b.

Barnett HJM, Eliasziw M, Meldrum HE. Prevention of ischemic stroke (reply). N Engl J Med *333*:460, 1995c.

Barnett HJM, Kaste M, Meldrum H, et al. Aspirin dose in stroke prevention: Beautiful hypotheses slain by ugly facts. Stroke *27*:588–592, 1996a.

Barnett HJM, Eliasziw M, Meldrum HE, et al. Do the facts and figures warrant a 10-fold increase in the performance of carotid endarterectomy on asymptomatic patients? Neurology *46*:603–608, 1996b.

Baron JC, Bousser MG, Comar D, et al. Noninvasive tomographic study of cerebral blood flow and oxygen metabolism in vivo: Potentials, limitations, and clinical applications in cerebral ischemic disorders. Eur Neurol *20*:273–284, 1981.

Barraquer-Bordas L, Illa I, Escartin A, et al. Thalamic hemorrhage: A study of 23 patients with diagnosis by computed tomography. Stroke *12*:524–527, 1981.

Bassetti C, Lovblad KO. Vertical gaze palsy from paramedian thalamic stroke without midbrain involvement. Stroke *27*:567, 1996.

Bassetti C, Staikov IN. Hemiplegia vegetativa alterna (ipsilateral Horner's syndrome and contralateral hemihyperhidrosis) following proximal posterior cerebral artery occlusion. Stroke *26*:702–704, 1995.

Bassetti C, Bogousslavsky J, Barth A, et al. Isolated infarcts of the pons. Neurology *46*:165–175, 1996.

Bassetti C, Bogousslavsky J, Mattle H, et al. Medial medullary stroke: Report of seven patients and review of the literature. Neurology *48*:882–890, 1997.

Basso A, Capitani E. Spared musical abilities in a conductor with global aphasia and ideomotor apraxia. J Neurol Neurosurg Psychiatry *48*:407–412, 1985.

Bathen J, Sparr S, Rokseth R. Embolism in sinoatrial disease. Acta Med Scand *203*: 7–11, 1978.

Batjer HH, Reisch JS, Allen BC, et al. Failure of surgery to improve outcome in hypertensive putaminal hemorrhage. A prospective randomized trial. Arch Neurol *47*:1103–1106, 1990.

Batko KA, Appen RE. Ophthalmodynamometry: A reappraisal. Ann Ophthalmol *11*: 1499–1508, 1979.

Baudrimont M, Dubas F, Joutel A, et al. Autosomal dominant leukoencephalopathy and subcortical ischemic stroke. Stroke *24*:122–125, 1993.

Bauer R, Sheehan S, Meyer JS. Arteriographic study of cerebrovascular disease. II. Cerebral symptoms due to kinking, tortuosity, and compression of the carotid and vertebral arteries in the neck. Arch Neurol *4*:119–131, 1961.

Bauer RB. Mechanical compression of the vertebral arteries. In Vertebrobasilar Arterial Occlusive Disease. Editors, Berguer R, Bauer RB, pp 45–71. New York, Raven Press, 1984.

Bauer RM, Rubens AB. Agnosia. In Clinical Neuropsychology. Editors, Heilman KM, Valenstein E, 2nd ed, pp 187–241. New York, Oxford University Press, 1985.

Baurmann M. Druckmessungen an der Netzhautzentralarterie. Berlin Dtsch Ophthalmol Ges *51*:228–239, 1936.

Bayer AJ, Pathy MSJ, Newcombe R. Double-blind randomized trial of intravenous glycerol in acute stroke. Lancet *1*:405–408, 1987.

Bayliss R, Clarke C, Oakley CM, et al. The microbiology and pathogenesis of infective endocarditis. Br Heart J *50*:513–519, 1983.

Bazin A, Peruzzi P, Baudrillard JC, et al. Myxome cardiaque avec métastases cérébrales. Neurochirurgie *33*:487–489, 1987.

Beal MF, Fisher CM. Neoplastic angioendotheliosis. J Neurol Sci *53*:359–375, 1982.

Beal MF, Park TS, Fisher CM. Cerebral atheromatous embolism following carotid sinus pressure. Arch Neurol *38*:310–312, 1981a.

Beal MF, Williams RS, Richardson EP Jr, et al. Cholesterol embolism as a cause of transient ischemic attacks and cerebral infarction. Neurology *31*:860–865, 1981b.

Beal MF, Richardson EP Jr, Brandstetter R, et al. Localized brainstem ischemic damage and Ondine's curse after near drowning. Neurology *33*:717–721, 1983.

Bean WB. Infarction of the heart. III. Clinical concern and morphological findings. Ann Intern Med *12*:71–94, 1958.

Becker WL, Burde RM. Carotid artery disease. A therapeutic enigma. Arch Ophthalmol *106*:34–39, 1988.

Beebe HG, Archie JP, Baker WH, et al. Concern about safety of carotid angioplasty. Stroke *27*:197–198, 1996.

Begg EJ, McGrath MA, Wade DN. Inadvertent intra-arterial injection. A problem of drug abuse. Med J Aust *2*:561–563, 1980.

Beghi E, Bogliun G, Cosso P, et al. Stroke and alcohol intake in a hospital population. A case-control study. Stroke 26:1691–1696, 1995.

Behrman S. Amaurosis fugax et amaurosis fulminans. Arch Ophthalmol 45:458–467, 1951.

Bellavance A, for the Ticlopidine Aspirin Stroke Study Group. Efficacy of ticlopidine and aspirin for prevention of reversible cerebrovascular ischemic events: The Ticlopidine Aspirin Stroke Study. Stroke 24:1452–1457, 1993.

Belliveau JW, Kennedy DN Jr, McKinstry RD, et al. Functional mapping of the human visual cortex by magnetic resonance imaging. Science 254:716–719, 1991.

Benassi G, Ricci P, Calbucci F, et al. Slowly progressive ischemic stroke as first manifestation of essential thrombocythemia. Stroke 20:1271–1272, 1989.

Bender MB. Disorders in visual perception. In Problems of Dynamic Neurology. Editor, Halpern L, pp 319–375. Jerusalem, Hebrew University Hadassah Medical School, 1963.

Bender MB. Brain control of conjugate horizontal and vertical eye movements. A survey of the structural and functional correlates. Brain 103:23–69, 1980.

Bender MB, Kanzer MG. Dynamics of homonymous hemianopias and preservation of central vision. Brain 62:404–442, 1939.

Bender MB, Feldman M, Sobin AJ. Palinopsia. Brain 91:321–338, 1968.

Bender MB, Rudolph SH, Stacy CB. The neurology of the visual and oculomotor systems. In Clinical Neurology. Editors, Baker AB, Baker LH, Vol 1, Chap 12, p 43. Philadelphia, Harper and Row, 1983.

Benedikt M. Tremlement avec paralysie croisée du moteur oculaire commun. Bull Med 3:547–548, 1889.

Benjamin EE, Zimmerman CF, Troost BT. Lateropulsion and upbeat nystagmus are manifestations of central vestibular dysfunction. Arch Neurol 43:962–964, 1986.

Benjamin EE, Plehn JE, D'Agostino RB, et al. Mitral annular calcification and the risk of stroke in an elderly cohort. N Engl J Med 327:374–379, 1992.

Benson DF, Marsden CD, Meadows JC. The amnesic syndrome of posterior cerebral artery occlusion. Acta Neurol Scand 50:133–145, 1974.

Benton S, Levy I, Swash M. Vision in the temporal crescent in occipital infarction. Brain 103:83–97, 1980.

Bentwich Z, Rosen Z, Ganor S, et al. Chronic rhinocerebral mucormycosis (phycomycosis) with occlusion of the left internal carotid artery. Israel J Med Sci 4: 977–981, 1968.

Beppu S, Park YD, Sakakibara H, et al. Clinical features of intracardiac thrombosis based on echocardiographic observation. Jpn Circ J 48:75–82, 1984.

Berciano J. Sneddon syndrome: Another Mendelian etiology of stroke. Ann Neurol 24:586–587, 1988.

Bergen RL, Cangemi FE, Glassman R. Bilateral arterial occlusion secondary to Barlow's syndrome. Ann Ophthalmol 14:673–675, 1982.

Berger JR, Harris JO, Gregorios J, et al. Cerebrovascular disease in AIDS: A case-control study. AIDS 4:239–244, 1990.

Bergeron TT, Rumbaugh CL. Air embolism associated with the use of malfitting plastic connectors in angiography. Radiology 98:689–690, 1971.

Bergerson G, Shah P. Echocardiography unwarranted in patients with cerebral ischemic events. N Engl J Med 304:489, 1981.

Berguer R, Higgins R, Nelson R. Noninvasive diagnosis of reversal of vertebral artery blood flow. N Engl J Med 302:1349–1351, 1980.

Berman SS, Devine JJ, Erdoes LS, et al. Distinguishing carotid artery pseudo-occlusion with color flow doppler. Stroke 26:434–438, 1995.

Bernat JL, Hunter RW. The benign lateral medullary syndrome. Arch Neurol 35: 112–113, 1978.

Bernstein EF. Amaurosis Fugax. New York, Springer-Verlag, 1988.

Bessen H. Intracranial hemorrhage associated with phencylidine abuse. JAMA 248: 585–586, 1982.

Besson G, Bogousslavsky J, Hommel M, et al. Patent foramen ovale in young stroke patients with mitral valve prolapse. Acta Neurol Scand 89:23–26, 1994.

Bethune JE, Landrigan PL, Chipman LD. Angiokeratoma corporis diffusum (Fabry's disease) in two brothers. N Engl J Med 264:1280–1285, 1961.

Bettelheim H. Zur atiologie der ischamischen Papillenschwellung. Ophthalmologica 150:241–251, 1965.

Bettelheim H. Obliteration of the ophthalmic artery. Klin Monatsbl Augenheilkd 150: 636–643, 1967.

Bevan H, Sharma K, Bradley W. Stroke in young adults. Stroke 21:382–386, 1990.

Beversdorf DQ, Jenkyn LR, Petrowski JT, et al. Vertical gaze paralysis and intermittent unresponsiveness in a patient with a thalamomesencephalic stroke. J Neuro-ophthalmol 15(4):230–235, 1995.

Beylot J, Vallat M, Pesme D. Nevrite optique apres hemorragie digestive. Sem Hop Paris 56:1921–1922, 1976.

Bickerstaff ER. Neurological Complications of Oral Contraceptives. Oxford, Clarendon Press, 1975.

Biller J, Mathews KD, Love BB. Stroke in Children and Young Adults. Boston, Butterworth-Heinemann, 1994.

Biller J, Challa VR, Toole JF, et al. Nonbacterial thrombotic endocarditis. A neurologic perspective of clinicopathologic correlations of 99 patients. Arch Neurol 39:95–98, 1982.

Biller J, Shapiro R, Evans LS, et al. Oculomotor nuclear complex infarction: Clinical and radiological correlation. Arch Neurol 41:985–987, 1984.

Biller J, Sand JJ, Corbett JJ, et al. Syndrome of the paramedian thalamic arteries:

Clinical and neuroimaging correlation. J Clin Neuro-ophthalmol 5:217–223, 1985.

Biller J, Adams HP Jr, Johnson MR, et al. Paradoxical cerebral embolism: Eight cases. Neurology 36:1356–1360, 1986.

Biller J, Johnson MR, Adams HP Jr, et al. Further observations on cerebral or retinal ischemia in patients with right-left intracardiac shunts. Arch Neurol 44:740–743, 1987.

Biller J, Bruno A, Adams HP Jr, et al. A randomized trial of aspirin or heparin in hospitalized patients with recent transient ischemic attacks: A pilot study. Stroke 20:441–447, 1989.

Biller J, Saver JL. Ischemic cerebrovascular disease and hormone therapy for infertility and transsexualism. Neurology 45:1611–1613, 1991.

Biousse V, Newman NJ, Sternberg P Jr. Retinal vein occlusion and transient monocular visual loss associated with hyperhomocystinemia. Am J Ophthalmol 124: 257–260, 1997.

Bird TD, Lagunoff D. Neurological manifestations of Fabry disease in female carriers. Ann Neurol 4:537–540, 1978.

Bisiach E, Geminiani G, Berti A, et al. Perceptual and premotor factors of unilateral neglect. Neurology 40:1278–1281, 1990.

Bitzer M, Topka H. Progressive cerebral occlusive disease after radiation therapy. Stroke 26:131–136, 1995.

Bjerver K, Silfverskiöld BP. Lateropulsion and imbalance in Wallenberg's syndrome. Acta Neurol Scand 44:91–100, 1968.

Björk I, Lindahl U. Mechanism of the anticoagulant action of heparin. Mol Cell Blochem 48:161–182, 1982.

Blackwell E, Merory J, Toole JF, et al. Doppler ultrasound scanning of the carotid bifurcation. Arch Neurol 34:145–148, 1977.

Blackshear WM, Phillips DJ, Chikos PM, et al. Carotid artery velocity patterns in normal and stenotic vessels. Stroke 11:67–71, 1980.

Blaine ES. Manipulative (chiropractic) dislocations of atlas. JAMA 85:1356–1359, 1925.

Blair DW, Irvine WT, Taylor RC. Recovery from neurological sequelae after cardiac arrest. Br Med J 1:1521–1522, 1958.

Blaisdell FW, Clauss RH, Galbraith JG, et al. Joint study of extracranial arterial occlusion. IV. A review of surgical considerations. JAMA 209:1889–1895, 1969.

Blaisdell FW, Glickman M, Trunkey DD. Ulcerated atheroma of the carotid artery. Arch Surg 108:491–496, 1974.

Blake J. Ocular embolism. Trans Ophthalmol Soc UK 95:88–93, 1975.

Blakeley DD, Oddone EZ, Hasselblad V, et al. Noninvasive carotid artery testing: A meta-analytic review. Ann Intern Med 122:360–367, 1995.

Blakemore WS, Hardesty WH, Berulacque JE, et al. Reversal of blood flow in right vertebral artery accompanying occlusion of the innominate artery. Ann Surg 161: 353–356, 1965.

Blatrix C. Allongement du temps de saignement sous l'influence de certains médicaments. Nouv Rev Fr Hematol 3:346–350, 1963.

Blatter DD, Parker DL, Ahn SS, et al. Cerebral MR angiography with multiple overlapping this slab acquisition. Part II. Early clinical experience. Radiology 183: 379–389, 1992.

Blatter DD, Bahr AL, Parker DL, et al. Cervical carotid MR angiography with multiple overlapping thin-slab acquisition: Comparison with conventional angiography. AJR 161:1269–1277, 1993.

Blauth C, Arnold J, Kohner EM, et al. Retinal microembolism during cardiopulmonary bypass demonstrated by fluorescein angiography. Lancet 2:837–839, 1986.

Blauth CI, Arnold JV, Schulenberg WE, et al. Cerebral microembolism during cardiopulmonary bypass. Retinal microvascular studies in vivo with fluorescein angiography. J Thorac Cardiovasc Surg 95:668–676, 1988.

Blondel M, Defoort S, Bouchez B, et al. Syndrome un et demi de Fisher. Atteinte du moyau du VI associée à une exotropie pontine paralytique. Acta Neurol. Belge 86:217–223, 1986.

Bloom AL, Thomas DP. Haemostasis and thrombosis. London, Churchill Livingstone, 1987.

Bluemke DA, Chambers TP. Spiral CT angiography: An alternative to conventional angiography[1]. Radiology 195:317–319, 1995.

Bluth E, Hughes RL. Importance of carotid artery plaque distribution and hemorrhage. Arch Neurol 45:602, 1988.

Bluth EI, Kay D, Merritt CR, et al. Sonographic characterization of carotid plaque: Detection of hemorrhage. AJR 146:1061–1065, 1986.

Bockenheimer SA, Mathias K. Percutaneous transluminal angioplasty in arteriosclerotic internal carotid artery stenosis. AJNR 4:791–792, 1983.

Boers GH, Smals AG, Trijbels FJ, et al. Heterozygosity for homocystinuria in premature peripheral and cerebral occlusive disease. N Engl J Med 313:709–715, 1985.

Bogen JE. The callosal syndrome. In Clinical Neuropsychology. Editors, Heilman KM, Valentstein E, pp 295–338. New York, Oxford University Press, 1985.

Boghen DR, Glaser JS. Ischaemic optic neuropathy. Brain 98:689–708, 1975.

Bogousslavsky J, Meienberg O. Eye-movement disorders in brain-stem and cerebellar stroke. Arch Neurol 44:141–148, 1987.

Bogousslavsky J, Regli F. Nuclear and prenuclear syndromes of the oculomotor nerve. Neuro-ophthalmology 3:211–216, 1983a.

Bogousslavsky J, Regli F. Exotropie pontine paralytique et non paralytique. Rev Neurol 139:219–223, 1983b.

Bogousslavsky J, Regli F. Upgaze palsy and monocular paresis of downgaze from ipsilateral thalamo-mesencephalic infarction: A vertical "one-and-a-half" syndrome. J Neurol 231:43–45, 1984a.

Bogousslavsky J, Regli F. Atteinte intra-axiale du nerf moteur oculaire commun dans les infarctus mésencéphaliques. Rev Neurol 140:263–270, 1984b.

Bogousslavsky J, Regli F. Convergence and divergence sykinesis: A recovery pattern in benign pontine hematoma. Neuro-ophthalmology 4:219–225, 1984c.

Bogousslavsky J, Regli F. Borderzone infarctions distal to internal carotid artery occlusion: Prognostic implications. Ann Neurol 20:346–350, 1986.

Bogousslavsky J, Regli F. Ischemic stroke in adults younger than 30 years of age. Cause and prognosis. Arch Neurol 44:479–482, 1987.

Bogousslavsky J, Regli F. Anterior cerebral artery territory infarction in the Lausanne Stroke Registry. Clinical and etiologic patterns. Arch Neurol 47:144–150, 1990.

Bogousslavsky J, Regli F, Van Melle G. Unilateral occipital infarction: Evaluation of the risks of developing bilateral loss of vision. J Neurol Neurosurg Psychiatry 46:78–80, 1983a.

Bogousslavsky J, Regli F, Ghika J, et al. Internuclear ophthalmoplegia, prenuclear paresis of contralateral superior rectus, and bilateral ptosis. J Neurol 230:197–203, 1983b.

Bogousslavsky J, Miklossy J, Regli F, et al. One-and-a-half syndrome in ischaemic locked-in state: A clinico-pathological study. J Neurol Neurosurg Psychiatry 47:927–935, 1984.

Bogousslavsky J, Vinuela F, Barnett HJM, et al. Amaurosis fugax as the presenting manifestation of dural arteriovenous malformation. Stroke 16:891–893, 1985a.

Bogousslavsky J, Regli F, Van Melle G. Risk factors and concomitants of internal carotid artery occlusion or stenosis. A controlled study of 159 cases. Arch Neurol 42:864–867, 1985b.

Bogousslavsky J, Despland PA, Regli F. Asymptomatic tight stenosis of the internal carotid artery: Long-term prognosis. Neurology 36:861–863, 1986a.

Bogousslavsky J, Miklossy J, Deruaz JP, et al. Unilateral left paramedian infarction of the thalamus and midbrain: A clinico-pathological study. J Neurol Neurosurg Psychiatry 49:686–694, 1986b.

Bogousslavsky J, Hachinski VC, Boughner DR, et al. Cardiac and arterial lesions in carotid transient attacks. Arch Neurol 43:223–228, 1986c.

Bogousslavsky J, Hachinski VC, Boughner DR, et al. Clinical predictors of cardiac and arterial lesions in carotid transient ischemic attacks. Arch Neurol 43:229–233, 1986d.

Bogousslavsky J, Despland PA, Regli F. Spontaneous carotid dissection with acute stroke. Arch Neurol 44:137–140, 1987a.

Bogousslavsky J, Regli F, Zografos L, et al. Optico-cerebral syndrome: Simultaneous hemodynamic infarction of optic nerve and brain. Neurology 37:263–268, 1987b.

Bogousslavsky J, Miklossy J, Deruaz JP, et al. Lingual and fusiform gyri in visual processing: A clinico-pathologic study of superior altitudinal hemianopia. J Neurol Neurosurg Psychiatry 50:607–714, 1987c.

Bogousslavsky J, Van Melle G, Regli F. The Lausanne stroke registry: Analysis of 1,000 consecutive patients with first stroke. Stroke 19:1083–1092, 1988a.

Bogousslavsky J, Regli F, Van Melle G, et al. Migraine stroke. Neurology 38:223–227, 1988b.

Bogousslavsky J, Regli F, Uske A. Thalamic infarcts: Clinical syndromes, etiology, and prognosis. Neurology 38:837–848, 1988c.

Bogousslavksy J, Gaio JM, Caplan LR, et al. Encephalopathy, deafness and blindness in young women: A distinct retinocochleocerebral arteriolopathy? J Neurol Neurosurg Psychiatry 52:43–46, 1989.

Bogousslavsky J, Delaloye-Bishof A, Regli F, et al. Prolonged hypoperfusion and early stroke after transient ischemic attack. Stroke 21:40–56, 1990a.

Bogousslavsky J, Van Melle G, Regli F, et al. Pathogenesis of anterior circulation stroke in patients with nonvalvular atrial fibrillation: The Lausanne Stroke Registry. Neurology 40:1046–1050, 1990b.

Bogousslavsky J, Regli F, Maeder P. Intracranial large-artery disease and 'lacunar' infarction. Cerebrovasc Dis 1:154–159, 1991a.

Bogousslavsky J, Cachin C, Regli F, et al. Cardiac sources of embolism and cerebral infarction—Clinical consequences and vascular concomitants: The Lausanne Stroke Registry Group. Neurology 41:855–859, 1991b.

Bogousslavsky J, Regli F, Maeder P. Intracranial large-artery disease and 'lacunar' infarction. Cerebrovasc Dis 1:154–159, 1991c.

Bogousslavsky J, Regli F, Maeder P, et al. The etiology of posterior circulation infarcts: A prospective study using magnetic resonance imaging and magnetic resonance angiography. Neurology 43:1528–2533, 1993.

Bogousslavsky J, Maeder P, Regli F, et al. Pure midbrain infarction: Clinical syndromes, MRI, and etiologic patterns. Neurology 44:2032–2040, 1994.

Bogousslavsky J, Garazi S, Jeanrenaud X, et al., for the Lausanne Stroke with Paradoxal Embolism Study Group. Stroke recurrence in patients with patent foramen ovale: The Lausanne study. Neurology 46:1301–1305, 1996.

Boiten J, Lodder J. Ataxic hemiparesis following thalamic infarction. Stroke 21:339–340, 1990.

Bolling JP, Beuttner H. Acquired retinal arteriovenous communications in occlusive disease of the carotid artery. Ophthalmology 97:1148–1152, 1990.

Bolling JP, Lavin PJM. Combined gaze palsy of horizontal saccades and pursuit contralateral to a midbrain hemorrhage. J Neurol Neurosurg Psychiatry 50:789–791, 1987.

Bone GE, Dickinson D, Pornajzl MJ. A prospective evaluation of indirect methods for detecting carotid atherosclerosis. Surg Gynecol Obstet 152:587–592, 1981.

Bonita R, Ford MA, Stewart AW. Predicting survival after stroke: A three-year follow-up. Stroke 19:669–673, 1988.

Bonita R, Stewart A, Beaglehole R. International trends in stroke mortality: 1970–1985. Stroke 21:989–992, 1990.

Bonnefoi B, Mesana T, Camilleri JF, et al. Troubles neurologiques révélateurs d'un myxome auriculaire: Trois cas. Rev Neurol 146:508–510, 1990.

Bon Tempo CP, Roman JA Jr, De Leon A Jr, et al. Radiographic appearance of the thorax in systolic click-late systolic murmur syndrome. Am J Cardiol 36:27–31, 1975.

Booy R. Amaurosis fugax in a young woman. Lancet 335:1538, 1990.

Borison H, Wang S. Physiology and pharmacology of vomiting. Pharmacol Rev 5:193–230, 1953.

Bornbroek M, Haan J, Van Duinen SG, et al. Dutch hereditary cerebral amyloid angiopathy: Structural lesions and apolipoprotein E genotype. Ann Neurol 41:695–698, 1997.

Bornstein NM, Norris JW. Benign outcome of carotid occlusion. Neurology 39:6–8, 1989.

Bornstein NM, Krajewski A, Lewis AJ, et al. Clinical significance of carotid plaque hemorrhage. Arch Neurol 47.958–959, 1990.

Bornstein NM, Karepov VG, Aronovich BD. Failure of aspirin treatment after stroke. Stroke 25:275–277, 1994.

Boros L, Thomas C, Weiner WJ. Large cerebral vessel disease in sickle cell anemia. J Neurol Neurosurg Psychiatry 39:1236–1239, 1976.

Borruat FX, Bogousslavsky J, Uffer S, et al. Orbital infarction syndrome. Ophthalmology 100:562–568, 1993.

Boudouresques J, Gosset A, Khalil R. Sténoses et occlusions de la carotide interne. Pp 17406-A-20. Encyclopédie Médico-chirurgicale, Paris, 1970.

Bounds JV, Weibers DO, Whisnant JP, et al. Mechanisms and timing of deaths from cerebral infarction. Stroke 12:474–477, 1981.

Bourgain RH, Maes L, Braquet P, et al. The effect of 1-0-alkyl-2-acetyl-sn-glycero-3-phosphocholine (PAF-acether) on the arterial wall. Prostaglandins 30:185–197, 1985.

Bourgeois J, Patorgis C. Internal carotid artery disease. J Am Optom Assoc 55:511–517, 1984.

Boushey CJ, Beresford SAA, Omenn GS, et al. A quantitative assessment of plasma homocysteine as a risk factor for vascular disease. Probably benefits of increasing folic acid intakes. JAMA 274:1049–1057, 1995.

Bousser MG. Aspirin or heparin immediately after stroke? Lancet 349:1564–1565, 1997.

Bousser MG, Touboul PJ, Cabanis E, et al. The significance of ocular bruits in ischaemic cerebro-vascular disease. Neuro-ophthalmology 1:211–218, 1981.

Bousser MG, Eschwege E, Haguenau M, et al. "AICLA" controlled trial of aspirin and dipyridamole in the secondary prevention of athero-thrombotic cerebral ischemia. Stroke 14:5–14, 1983.

Bower S, Dennis M, Warlow C, et al. Long-term prognosis of transient lone bilateral blindness in adolescents and young adults. J Neurol Neurosurg Psychiatry 57:734–736, 1994.

Boysen G, Nyboe J, Appleyard M, et al. Stroke incidence and risk factors for stroke in Copenhagen, Denmark. Stroke 19:1345–1353, 1988a.

Boysen G, Sorenson PS, Juhler M. Danish very low-dose aspirin after carotid endarterectomy trial. Stroke 19:211, 1988b.

Bradley WG Jr. MR appearance of hemorrhage in the brain. Radiology 189:15–26, 1993.

Bradshaw P, McQuaid P. The syndrome of vertebrobasilar insufficiency. Q J Med 32:279–296, 1963.

Brain L. Some unsolved problems of cervical spondylosis. Br Med J 1:771–777, 1963.

Brandt KD, Lessell S. Migrainous phenomena in systemic lupus erythematosus. Arthritis Rheum 2:7–16, 1978.

Brandt KD, Lessell S, Cohen AS. Cerebral disorders of vision in systemic lupus erythematosus. Ann Intern Med 83:1975a.

Brandt KD, Sumner RD, Ryan TJ, et al. Herniation of mitral leaflets in Ehlers-Danlos syndrome. Am J Cardiol 36:524–528, 1975b.

Brandt T, Dieterich M. Pathological eye-head coordination in roll: Tonic ocular tilt reaction in mesencephalic and medullary lesions. Brain 110:649–666, 1987.

Brandt T, Dieterich M. Vestibular syndromes in the roll plane: Topographic diagnosis from brainstem to cortex. Ann Neurol 36:337–347, 1994.

Brandt T, Pessin MS, Kwan ES, et al. Survival with basilar artery occlusion. Cerebrovasc Dis 5:182–187, 1995.

Brant-Zawadzki M, Gould R, Norman D, et al. Digital subtraction cerebral angiography by intra-arterial injection: Comparison with conventional angiography. AJR 140:347–353, 1983.

Brattstrom LE, Hardebo JE, Hultberg BJ. Moderate homocysteinemia—A possible risk factor for arteriosclerotic vascular disease. Stroke 15:1012–1016, 1984.

Breen JC, Caplan LR, DeWitt LD, et al. Brain edema after carotid surgery. Neurology 46:175–181, 1996.

Brekkan A, Lexow PE, Woxholt G. Glass fragments and other particles contaminating contrast media. Acta Radiol 16:600–608, 1975.

Brennan RW, Bergland RM. Acute cerebellar hemorrhage: Analysis of clinical findings and outcome in 12 cases. Neurology 27:527–532, 1977.

Brennan RW, Patterson RH, Kessler J. Cerebral blood flow and metabolism during cardiopulmonary bypass: Evidence of microembolic encephalopathy. Neurology 21:665–672, 1971.

Brey RL, Hart RG, Sherman DG, et al. Antiphospholipid antibodies and cerebral ischemia in young people. Neurology 40:1190–1196, 1990.

Brick JF, Dunker RO, Gutierrez AR. Cerebral vasoconstriction as a complication of carotid endarterectomy. Case report. J Neurosurg 73:151–153, 1990.

Brickner ME. Cardioembolic stroke. Am J Med 100:465–474, 1996.

Bridgers SL. Clinical correlates of Doppler/ultrasound errors in the detection of internal carotid artery occlusion. Stroke 20:612–615, 1989.

Brierley JB, Brown AW. The origin of lipid phagocytes in the central nervous system. J Comp Neurol 211:397–417, 1982.

Brierley JB, Graham EI. Hypoxia and vascular disorders of the central nervous system. In Greenfield's Neuropathology. Editors, Adams JH, Corsellis JAN, Duchen LW, pp 125–207. New York, John Wiley & Sons, 1984.

Brigell M, Babikian V, Goodwin JA. Hypometric saccades and low-gain pursuit resulting from a thalamic hemorrhage. Ann Neurol 15:374–378, 1984.

Bril V, Sharpe JA, Ashby P. Midbrain asterixis. Ann Neurol 6:362–364, 1979.

Briley DP, Coull BM, Goodnight SH Jr. Neurological disease associated with antiphospholipid antibodies. Ann Neurol 25:221–227, 1989.

Brillman J, Howieson J. Transient midbrain syndromes as a complication of vertebral angiography. Relationship to antecedent structural disease. J Neurosurg 41:71–74, 1974.

Brindley GS. The discrimination of after images. J Physiol 147:194–203, 1959.

Brion S, Jedynak CP. Trouble du transfert interhémisphérique à propos de trois observations de tumeurs du corps calleux: Le signe de la main étrangère. Rev Neurol 126:257–266, 1972.

Britt RH, Herrick MK, Hamilton RD. Traumatic locked-in syndrome. Ann Neurol 1:590 592, 1977.

Britton TC, Guiloff RJ. Carotid artery disease presenting as cough headache. Lancet 1:1406–1407, 1988.

Brockmeier LB, Adolph RJ, Gustin BW, et al. Calcium emboli to the retinal artery in calcific aortic stenosis. Am Heart J 101:32–37, 1981.

Broderick JP, Swanson JW. Migraine-related strokes. Clinical profile and prognosis in 20 patients. Arch Neurol 44:868–871, 1987.

Broderick JP, Brott T, Tomsick T, et al. The risk of subarachnoid and intracerebral hemorrhages in blacks as compared with whites. N Engl J Med 326:733–736, 1992.

Broderick JP, Talbot GT, Prenger E, et al. Stroke in children within a major metropolitan area: The surprising importance of intracerebral hemorrhage. J Child Neurol 8:250–255, 1993a.

Broderick JP, Brott T, Tomsick T, et al. Lobar hemorrhage in the elderly. The undiminishing importance of hypertension. Stroke 24:49–51, 1993b.

Brodmann K. Vergleichende Localisationslehre der Grosshirnrinde in ihren Prinzipien Dargestellt auf Grund des Zellenbaues. Leipzig, Barth, 1909.

Brodmann K. Individuelle Variationen der Sehsphäre und ihre Bedeutung fur die Klinik der Hinterhauptschüsse. Allgz Psychiatr 74:564–568, 1918.

Brody A. New perspectives in CT and MRI imaging. Neurology Clinics 9:273–286, 1991.

Bronner A. L'ischémie neuro-rétienne par oblitération de l'artère ophtalmique. Intérêt dynamométrique et périmétrique. Bull Soc Ophtalmol Fr 5–6:315–319, 1961.

Bronner A, Lobstein PA. The syndrome of occlusion of the ophthalmic artery. Doc Ophthalmol 20:660–667, 1966.

Bronner LL, Kanter DS, Manson JE. Primary prevention of stroke. N Engl J Med 333:1392–1400, 1995.

Bronstein AM, Morris J, Du Boulay G, et al. Abnormalities of horizontal gaze. Clinical, oculographic and magnetic resonance imaging findings. I. Abducens palsy. J Neurol Neurosurg Psychiatr 53:194–199, 1990a.

Bronstein AM, Rudge P, Gresty MA, et al. Abnormalities of horizontal gaze. Clinical, oculographic and magnetic resonance imaging findings. II. Gaze palsy and internuclear ophthalmoplegia. J Neurol Neurosurg Psychiatry 53:200–207, 1990b.

Brott T. Thrombolysis for stroke. Arch Neurol 53:1305–1306, 1996.

Brott T, MacCarthy EP. Antihypertensive therapy in stroke. In Medical Therapy of Acute Stroke. Editor, Fisher M, pp 117–142. New York, Marcel Dekker, 1989.

Brott T, Reed RL. Intensive care for acute stroke in the community hospital setting. Stroke 20:694–697, 1989.

Brott T, Thalinger K. The practice of carotid endarterectomy in a large metropolitan area. Stroke 15:950–955, 1984.

Brott T, Adams HP Jr, Olinger CP, et al. Measurements of acute cerebral infarction: A clinical examination scale. Stroke 20:864–870, 1989.

Brott TG, Haley EC Jr, Levy DE, et al. Urgent therapy for stroke. Part I. Pilot study of tissue plasminogen activator administered within 90 minutes. Stroke 23:632–640, 1992.

Brown GC. Anterior ischemic optic neuropathy occurring in association with carotid artery obstruction. J Clin Neuro-ophthalmol 6:39–42, 1986a.

Brown GC. Macular edema in association with severe carotid artery obstruction. Am J Ophthalmol 102:442–448, 1986b.

Brown GC. Retinal arterial obstructive disease. In Retina. Editors, Schachat AP, Murphy RP, 2nd ed, Vol 2, pp 1361–1377. St Louis, CV Mosby, 1994a.

Brown GC. The ocular ischemic syndrome. In Retina. Editors, Schachat AP, Murphy RP, 2nd ed, Vol 2, pp 1515–1527. St Louis, CV Mosby, 1994b.

Brown GC, Magargal LE. Central retinal artery obstruction and visual acuity. Ophthalmology 89:14–19, 1982.

Brown GC, Magargal LE. The ocular ischemic syndrome. Clinical, fluorescein angiographic and carotid angiographic features. Int Ophthalmol 11:239–251, 1988.

Brown GC, Shields JA. Cilioretinal arteries and retinal arterial occlusion. Arch Ophthalmol 97:84–92, 1979.

Brown GC, Magargal LE, Shields JA, et al. Retinal arterial obstruction in children and young adults. Ophthalmology 88:18–25, 1981.

Brown GC, Magargal LE, Simeone FA, et al. Arterial obstruction and ocular neovascularization. Ophthalmology 89:139–146, 1982.

Brown GC, Magargal LE, Schachat A, et al. Neovascular glaucoma. Etiologic considerations. Ophthalmology 91:315–320, 1984a.

Brown GC, Shah HG, Magargal LE, et al. Central retinal vein obstruction and carotid artery disease. Ophthalmology 91:1627–1633, 1984b.

Brown GC, Magargal LE, Sergott R. Obstruction of the retinal and choroidal circulation. Ophthalmology 93:1373–1382, 1986.

Brown MM, Thompson AJ, Wedzicha JA, et al. Sarcoidosis presenting with stroke. Stroke 20:400–405, 1989.

Brown MM, Butler P, Gibbs J, et al. Feasibility of percutaneous transluminal angioplasty for carotid artery stenosis. J Neurol Neurosurg Psychiatry 53:238–243, 1990.

Brown MS, Goldstein JL. Lipoprotein metabolism in macrophages: Implications for cholesterol deposition in atherosclerosis. Annu Rev Biochem 52:223–261, 1983.

Brown MS, Kovanen PT, Goldstein JL. Regulation of plasma cholesterol by lipoprotein receptors. Science 212:628–635, 1981.

Brown OR, Loster FE, DeMots H. Incidence of mitral valve prolapse in the asymptomatic normal. Circulation 52(Supp 2):77, 1975.

Brown OR, DeMots H, Kloster FE, et al. Aortic root dilatation and mitral valve prolapse in Marfan's syndrome: An echocardiographic study. Circulation 52:651–657, 1978.

Brown RH, Schauble JF, Miller NR. Anemia and hypotension as contributers to perioperative loss of vision. Anesthesiology 80:222–226, 1994.

Browne TR, Wray SH. Subconjunctival hemorrhage as a complication of ophthalmodynamometry in an anticoagulated patient. Am J Ophthalmol 76:981–983, 1973.

Brownstein S, Font RL, Alper MG. Atheromatous plaques of the retinal blood vessels. Histologic confirmation of ophthalmoscopically visible lesions. Arch Ophthalmol 90:49–52, 1973.

Browse NL, Ross Russell R. Carotid endarterectomy and the Javid shunt: The early results of 215 consecutive operations for transient ischemic attacks. Br J Surg 71:53–57, 1984.

Brucker AJ. Disk and peripheral retinal neovascularization secondary to talc and cornstarch emboli. Am J Ophthalmol 88:864–867, 1979.

Brückmann H, del Zoppo GJ, Ferbert A, et al. Carotid endarterectomy: Factors influencing perioperative complications. J Neurol 235:39–41, 1987.

Bruetman ME, Fields WS, Crawford ES, et al. Cerebral hemorrhage in carotid artery surgery. Arch Neurol 9:458–467, 1963.

Bruno A, Adams HP Jr, Biller J, et al. Cerebral infarction due to moyamoya disease in young adults. Stroke 19:826–833, 1988.

Bruno A, Graff-Radford NR, Biller J, et al. Anterior choroidal artery territory infarction: A small vessel disease. Stroke 20:616–619, 1989.

Bruno A, Corbett JJ, Biller J, et al. Transient monocular visual loss patterns and associated vascular abnormalities. Stroke 21:34–39, 1990.

Bruno A, Russell PW, Jones WL, et al. Concomitants of asymptomatic retinal cholesterol emboli. Stroke 23:900–902, 1992.

Bruno A, Jones WL, Austin JK, et al. Vascular outcome in men with asymptomatic retinal cholesterol emboli: A cohort study. Ann Intern Med 122:249–253, 1995.

Bruno JJ, Molony BA. Ticlopidine. In New Drugs Annual: Cardiovascular Drugs. Editor, Scriabine A, pp 295–316. New York, Raven Press, 1983.

Brusa A, Firpo MP, Massa S, et al. Typical and reverse bobbing: A case with localizing value. Eur Neurol 23:151–155, 1983.

Brusa A, Massa S, Piccardo A, et al. Le nystagmus palpébral. Rev Neurol 140:288–292, 1984.

Brust JCM. Transient ischemic attacks: Natural history and anticoagulation. Neurology 27:701–707, 1977.

Brust JCM, Behrens MM. "Release hallucinations" as the major symptom of posterior cerebral artery occlusion: A report of 2 cases. Ann Neurol 2:432–436, 1977.

Brust JCM, Richter R. Stroke associated with addiction to heroin. J Neurol Neurosurg Psychiatry 39:194–199, 1976.

Bruyn RPM, van der Veen JPW, Donker AJM, et al. Sneddon's syndrome. Case report and literature review. J Neurol Sci 79:243–253, 1987.

Bryant GL, Weinblatt ME, Rumbaugh C, et al. Cerebral vasculopathy: An analysis of sixteen cases. Semin Arthritis Rheum 15:297–302, 1986.

Bryant LR, Spencer FC. Occlusive disease of subclavian artery. JAMA 196:123–128, 1966.

Buge A, Escourolle R, Hauw J, et al. Syndrome pseudobulbaire aigu infarctus bilateral limité du territoire des artères choroïdiennes antérieures. Rev Neurol 135:313–318, 1979.

Bulens C, Meerwaldt JD, Van der Wildt GJ, et al. Spatial contrast sensitivity in unilateral cerebral ischaemic lesions involving the posterior visual pathway. Brain 112:507–520, 1989.

Bullock JD, Falter RT, Downing JE, et al. Ischemic ophthalmia secondary to an ophthalmic artery occlusion. Am J Ophthalmol 74:486–493, 1972.

Buonanno F, Toole JF. Management of patients with established ("completed") cerebral infarction. Stroke 12:7–16, 1981.

Buonanno F, Kistler JP, DeWitt LD, et al. Proton (IH) nuclear magnetic resonance (NMR) imaging in stroke syndromes. Neurol Clin 1:243–262, 1983.

Burchfiel CM, Curb JD, Rodriguez BJ, et al. Glucose intolerance and 22-year stroke incidence: The Honolulu Heart Program. Stroke 25:951–957, 1994.

Burde RM. Discussion of Cohen GR, Harbison JW, Blair CJ, et al. Clinical significance of transient visual phenomena in the elderly. Ophthalmology 91:441–442, 1984.

Burde RM. Amaurosis fugax: An overview. J Clin Neuro-Ophthalmol 9:185–189, 1989.

Burde RM, Smith ME, Black JT, et al. Retinal artery occlusion in the absence of a cherry red spot. Surv Ophthalmol 27:181–186, 1982.

Buréu A, Ygge J. Treatment program and comparison between anticoagulants and platelet aggregation inhibitors after transient ischemic attack. Stroke 12:578–580, 1981.

Burger PC, Burch JG, Vogel FS. Granulomatous angiitis, an unusual etiology of stroke. Stroke 8:29–35, 1977.

Burger SK, Saul RF, Selhorst JB, et al. Transient monocular blindness caused by vasospasm. New Engl J Med 325:870–873, 1991.

Buring JE, Hebert P, Romero J, et al. Migraine and subsequent risk of stroke in the Physician's Health Study. Arch Neurol 52:129–134, 1995.

Burke PA, Callow AD, O'Donnel TF Jr, et al. Prophylactic carotid endarterectomy for asymptomatic bruit: A look at cardiac risk. Arch Surg 117:1222–1227, 1982.

Burnbaum MD, Selhorst JB, Harbison JW, et al. Amaurosis fugax from disease of the external carotid artery. Arch Neurol 34:532–535, 1977.

Bushnell DL, Gupta S, Mlcoch AG, et al. Prediction of language and neurologic recovery after cerebral infarction with SPECT imaging using N-isopropyl-p-(I 123) iodoamphetamine. Arch Neurol 46:665–669, 1989.

Butler A, Partain R, Netsky M. Primary intraventricular hemorrhage. Neurology 22: 675–686, 1972.

Büttner-Ennever JA, Büttner U, Cohen B, et al. Vertical gaze palsy and the rostral interstitial nucleus of the medial longitudinal fasciculus. Brain 105:125–149, 1982.

Byers B. Blindness secondary to steroid injections into the nasal turbinates. Arch Ophthalmol 97:79–80, 1979.

Byington RP, Jukema JW, Salonen JT, et al. Reduction in cardiovascular events during pravastatin therapy: Pooled analysis of clinical events of the Pravastatin Atherosclerosis Intervention Program. Circulation 92:2419–2425, 1995.

Cabanes L, Mas JL, Cohen A, et al. Atrial septal aneurysm and patent foramen ovale as risk factors for cryptogenic stroke in patients less than 55 years of age: A study using transesophageal echocardiography. Stroke 24:1865–1873, 1993.

Cahill DW, Salcman M, Hirsch D, et al. Unilateral internuclear ophthalmoplegia due to angiographic embolism through a primitive trigeminal artery. Neurology 31: 751–753, 1981a.

Cahill DW, Knipp H, Mosser J. Intracranial hemorrhage with amphetamine abuse. Neurology 31:1058–1059, 1981b.

Calandre L, Gomara S, Bermejo F, et al. Clinical CT correlations in TIA, RIND, and strokes with minimum residua. Stroke 15:663–666, 1984.

Calderwood SB, Swinski LA, Waternaux CM, et al. Risk factors for the development of prosthetic valve endocarditis. Circulation 72:31–37, 1985.

Call GK, Abbott WM, Macdonald NR, et al. Correlation of continuous-wave Doppler spectral flow analysis with gross pathology in carotid stenosis. Stroke 19: 584–588, 1988a.

Call GK, Fleming MC, Sealfon S, et al. Reversible cerebral segmental vasoconstriction. Stroke 19:1159–1170, 1988b.

Calmettes L, Deodati F, Dupre A, et al. Manifestations oculaires du syndrome de Fabry. Bull Soc Ophtalmol Fr 6:513–517, 1959.

Calori G, D'Angelo A, Valle PD, et al. The effect of cigarette-smoking on cardiovascular risk factors: A study of monozygotic twins discordant for smoking. Thromb Haemost 75:14–18, 1996.

Caltrider ND, Irvine AR, Kline HJ, et al. Retinal emboli in patients with mitral valve prolapse. Am J Ophthalmol 90:534–539, 1980.

Camarata PJ, Heros RC, Latchaw RE. "Brain attack": The rationale for treating stroke as a medical emergency. Neurosurgery 34:144–158, 1994.

Camargo CA Jr. Moderate alcohol consumption and stroke: The epidemiologic evidence. Stroke 20:1611–1626, 1989.

Cambier J, Masson M, Poullot B, et al. Déviation tonique du regard au cours du syndrome de Wallenberg. Rev Neurol 138:839–844, 1982.

Cambier J, Graveleau P, Decroix JP, et al. Le syndrome de l'artère choroïdienne antérieure: Étude neuropsychologique de 4 cas. Rev Neurol 139:553–559, 1983.

Camerlingo M, Finazzi G, Casto L, et al. Inherited protein C deficiency and nonhemorrhagic arterial stroke in young adults. Neurology 41:1371–1373, 1991.

Cammarosano C, Lewis W. Cardiac lesions in acquired immune deficiency syndrome (AIDS). J Am Coll Cardiol 5:703–706, 1985.

Campbell HA, Link KP. Studies on the hemorrhagic sweet clover disease. IV. The isolation and crystallization of the hemorrhagic agent. J Biol Chem 138:21–33, 1941.

Campbell JK. Early diagnosis of an atrial myxoma with central retinal artery occlusion. Ann Ophthalmol 6:1207–1211, 1974.

Campion J, Latto R, Smith YM. Is blindsight an effect of scattered light, spared cortex, and near-threshold vision? Behav Brain Sci 6:423–486, 1983.

Campo RV, Reeser FH. Retinal telangiectasia secondary to bilateral carotid artery occlusion. Arch Ophthalmol 101:1211–1213, 1983.

Candelise L, Landi G, Perrone P, et al. Randomized trial of aspirin and sulfinpyrazone in patients with TIA. Stroke 13:173–179, 1982.

Cannegieter SC, Rosendaal FR, Wintzen AR, et al. Optimal oral anticoagulant therapy in patients with mechanical heart valves. N Engl J Med 333:11–17, 1995.

Canoso RT. Antiphospholipid antibodies. Basic mechanisms, clinical features, and animal models. Stroke 24:124–125, 1993.

Caplan LR. Ptosis. J Neurol Neurosurg Psychiatry 37:1–7, 1974.

Caplan LR. Stroke prevention—Early signs of the patient at risk. Resident Staff Phys. Pp 51–65, Sept, 1977.

Caplan LR. Occlusion of the vertebral or basilar artery. Stroke 10:277–282, 1979.

Caplan LR. "Top of the basilar" syndrome. Neurology 30:72–79, 1980.

Caplan LR. Bilateral distal vertebral artery occlusion. Neurology 33:552–558, 1983.

Caplan LR. Patterns of posterior circulation infarctions: Correlation with vascular pathology. In Vertebrobasilar Arterial Occlusive Disease. Editors, Berguer R, Bauer RB, pp 15–25. New York, Raven Press, 1984.

Caplan LR. TIAs: We need to return to the question, "What is wrong with Mr. Jones?" Neurology 38:791–793, 1988a.

Caplan LR. Intracerebral hemorrhage revisited. Neurology 38:624–627, 1988b.

Caplan LR. To heparinize or not: An unsettled issue. Stroke 20:968, 1989a.

Caplan LR. Intracranial branch atheromatous disease: A neglected, understudied, and underused concept. Neurology 39:1246–1250, 1989b.

Caplan LR. Of birds and nests and cerebral emboli. Rev Neurol 147:265–273, 1991a.

Caplan LR. Question-driven technology assessment: SPECT as an example. Neurology 41:187–191, 1991b.

Caplan LR. Migraine and vertebrobasilar ischemia. Neurology 41:55–61, 1991c.

Caplan LR. Brain embolism, revisited. Neurology 43:1281–1287, 1993.

Caplan LR. Binswanger's disease-revisited. Neurology 45:626–633, 1995.

Caplan LR, Goodwin JA. Lateral tegmental brainstem hemorrhage. Neurology 32: 252–260, 1982.

Caplan LR, Hedley-White T. Cueing and memory dysfunction in alexia without agraphia. Brain 97:251–262, 1974.

Caplan LR, Mohr JP. Intracerebral hemorrhage: An update. Geriatrics 33:42–52, 1978.

Caplan LR, Stein RW. Stroke: A Clinical Approach. London, Butterworths, 1986.

Caplan LR, Wolpert SM. Angiography in patients with occlusive cerebrovascular disease: Views of a stroke neurologist and neuroradiologist. AJNR 12:593–601, 1991.

Caplan LR, Hier DB, Banks G. Current problems in cerebrovascular disease: Stroke and drug abuse. Stroke 13:869–872, 1982a.

Caplan LR, Zervas NT. Survival with permanent midbrain dysfunction after surgical treatment of traumatic subdural hematoma: The clinical picture of a Duret hemorrhage? Ann Neurol 1:587–589, 1977.

Caplan LR, Chedru F, Lhermitte F, et al. Transient global amnesia and migraine. Neurology 31:1167–1170, 1981.

Caplan LR, Thomas C, Banks G. Central nervous system complications of T's and blues addiction. Neurology 32:623–628, 1982.

Caplan LR, Hier D, D'Cruz I. Cerebral embolism in the Michael Reese Stroke Registry. Stroke 14:530–536, 1983.

Caplan LR, Stein R, Patel D, et al. Intraluminal clot of the carotid arteries detected angiographically. Neurology 34:1175–1181, 1984.

Caplan LR, Babikian V, Helgason C, et al. Occlusive disease of the middle cerebral artery. Neurology 35:975–982, 1985.

Caplan LR, Pessin MS, Scott RM, et al. Poor outcome after lateral medullary infarcts. Neurology 36:1510–1513, 1986a.

Caplan LR, Gorelick PB, Hier DB. Race, sex, and occlusive cerebrovascular disease: A review. Stroke 17:648–655, 1986b.

Caplan LR, De Witt LD, Pessin MS, et al. Lateral thalamic infarcts. Arch Neurol 45: 959–964, 1988.

Caplan LR, Schmahmann JD, Kase CS, et al. Caudate infarcts. Arch Neurol 47: 133–143, 1990a.

Caplan LR, Brass LM, DeWitt LD, et al. Transcranial Doppler ultrasound: Present status. Neurology 40:696–700, 1990b.

Cappa SF, Vignolo LA, Papagno C, et al. Thalamic aphasia. Neurology 39:874, 1989.

CAPRIE Steering Committee. A randomised, blinded, trial of clopidogrel versus aspirin in patients at risk of ischaemic events (CAPRIE). Lancet 348:1329–1339, 1996.

Carlson MR, Pilger IS, Rosenbaum AL. Central retinal artery occlusion after carotid angiography. Am J Ophthalmol 81:103–104, 1976.

Carney JA. Differences between nonfamilial and familial cardiac myxoma. Am J Surg Pathol 9:53–55, 1985.

Carney JA, Gordon H, Carpenter PC, et al. The complex of myxomas, spotty pigmentation, and endocrine overactivity. Medicine 64:270–283, 1985.

Carney JA, Hruska LA, Beauchamp GD, et al. Dominant inheritance of the complex of myxomas, spotty pigmentation, and endocrine overactivity. Mayo Clin Proc 61:165–172, 1986.

Carolei A, Marini C, Ferranti E, et al. The National Reserach Council Study Group.

A prospective study of cerebral ischemia in the young. Analysis of pathogenic determinants. Stroke 24:362–367, 1993.

Carolei A, Marini C, De Matteis G, et al. History of migraine and risk of cerebral ischemia in young adults. Lancet 347:1503–1506, 1996.

Carpenter MB, Noback CR, Moss ML. The anterior choroidal artery. Its origins, course, distributions and variations. Arch Neurol Psychiatr 71:714–722, 1954.

Carter JE. Panretinal photocoagulation for progressive ocular neovascularization secondary to occlusion of the common carotid artery. Ann Ophthalmol 16:572–576, 1984.

Carter JE. Chronic ocular ischemia and carotid vascular disease. Stroke 16:721–728, 1985.

Carter JE. Carotid artery disease and its ocular manifestations. Ophthalmol Clin North Am 5:425, 1992.

Carter JE, O'Connor P, Shacklett D, et al. Lesions of the optic radiations mimicking lateral geniculate nucleus visual field defects. J Neurol Neurosurg Psychiatry 48:982–988, 1985.

Cartlidge NEF, Whisnant JP, Elveback LR. Carotid and vertebral-basilar transient cerebral ischemic attacks. A community study, Rochester, MN. Mayo Clin Proc 52:117–120, 1977.

Case Records of the Massachusetts General Hospital: Case 39451. N Engl J Med 249:776–780, 1953.

Case Records of the Massachusetts General Hospital: Case 69-1962. N Engl J Med 267:823–827, 1962.

Case Records of the Massachusetts General Hospital: Case 25-1967. N Engl J Med 276:1368–1377, 1967a.

Case Records of the Massachusetts General Hospital: Case 35-1967. N Engl J Med 277:423–428, 1967b.

Case Records of the Massachusetts General Hospital: Case 51-1973. N Engl J Med 289:1360–1366, 1973.

Case Records of the Massachusetts General Hospital: Case 46-1975. N Engl J Med 293:1138–1145, 1975.

Case Records of the Massachusetts General Hospital: Case 27-1991. N Engl J Med 325:42–54, 1991.

Caselli RJ, Hunder GG, Whisnant JP. Neurologic disease in biopsy-proven giant cell (temporal) arteritis. Neurology 38:352–359, 1988.

Cassady JV. Central retinal vein thrombosis. Am J Ophthalmol 36:331–335, 1953.

CAST (Chinese Acute Stroke Trial) Collaborative Group. CAST: Randomised placebo-controlled trial of early aspirin use in 20,000 patients with acute ischaemic stroke. Lancet 349:1641–1649, 1997.

Castaigne P, Lhermitte F, Gautier JC, et al. Corrélations cliniques et artériographiques dans 20 cas d'accidents ischémiques du cerveau d'origine athéroscléreuse. Rev Neurol 106:497–501, 1962.

Castaigne P, Buge A, Cambier J, et al. Demence thalamique d'origine vasculaire per ramollissement bilatéral limité au territoire du pedicule retro-mamillaire (a propos de deux observations anatomocliniques). Rev Neurol 114:89–108, 1966.

Castaigne P, Lhermitte F, Gautier JC, et al. Internal carotid artery occlusion. A study of 61 instances in 50 patients with post-mortem data. Brain 93:231–258, 1970.

Castaigne P, Lhermitte F, Gautier JC, et al. Arterial occlusions in the vertebro-basilar system. A study of 44 patients with post-mortem data. Brain 96:113–154, 1973.

Castaigne P, Brunet P, Derouesne C, et al. Atrophic optique post-hemorragique. Nouv Presse Med 5:1631–1633, 1976.

Castaigne P, Lhermitte F, Buge A, et al. Paramedian thalamic and midbrain infarcts. Clinical and neuropathological study. Ann Neurol 10:127–148, 1981.

Castaldo JE, Nicholas GG, Gee W, et al. Duplex ultrasound and ocular pneumoplethysmography: Concordance in detecting severe carotid stenosis. Arch Neurol 46:518–522, 1989.

Castanon C, Amigo MC, Banales JL, et al. Ocular vaso-occlusive disease in primary antiphospholipid syndrome. Ophthalmology 102:256–262, 1995.

Castro O, Johnson LN, Mamourian AC. Isolated inferior oblique paresis from brainstem infarction. Arch Neurol 47:235–237, 1990.

Celesia GG, Brigell MG, Vaphiades MS. Hemianopic anosognosia. Neurology 49:88–97, 1997.

Cerebral Embolism Study Group. Immediate anticoagulation of embolic stroke: A randomized trial. Stroke 14:668–676, 1983.

Cerebral Embolism Task Force: Cardiogenic brain embolism. Arch Neurol 43:71–84, 1986a.

Cerebral Embolism Task Force: Cerebral embolism. Chest 89(Suppl):82–98, 1986b.

Cerebral Embolism Task Force: Cardiogenic brain embolism. The second report of the Cerebral Embolism Task Force. Arch Neurol 46:727–743, 1989.

Cervoni L, Artico M, Salvati M, et al. Epileptic seizures in intracerebral hemorrhage: A clinical and prognostic study of 55 cases. Neurosurg Rev 17:185–188, 1994.

Chabriat H, Vahedi K, Iba-Zizen MT, et al. Clinical spectrum of CADASIL: A study of 7 families. Lancet 346:934–939, 1995.

Chabriat H, Joutel A, Vahedi K, et al. CADASIL (cerebral autosomal dominant arteriopathy with subcortical infarcts and leukoencephalopathy). J Mal Vasc 21:277–282, 1996.

Chace R, Hedges TR III. Retinal artery occlusion due to moyamoya disease. J Clin Neuro-Ophthalmol 4:31–34, 1984.

Chajek T, Fainaru M. Behçet's disease: Report of 41 cases and review of the literature. Medicine 54:179–196, 1975.

Challa VR, Moody DM. The value of magnetic resonance imaging in the detection of Type II hemorrhagic lacunes. Stroke 20:822–825, 1989.

Chambers BR, Norris JH. Stroke risk and asymptomatic carotid stenosis. Stroke 15:186, 1984a.

Chambers BR, Norris JW. The case against surgery for asymptomatic carotid stenosis. Stroke 15:964–967, 1984b.

Chambers BR, Norris JW. Clinical significance of asymptomatic neck bruits. Neurology 35:742–745, 1985.

Chambers BR, Norris JW. Outcome in patients with asymptomatic neck bruits. N Engl J Med 315:860–865, 1986.

Chambers BR, Donnan GA, Bladen PF. An analysis of the first 700 consecutive admissions to the Austin Hospital Stroke Unit. Aust NA J Med 13:57–64, 1983.

Chambers BR, Norris JW, Shurvell BL, et al. Prognosis of acute stroke. Neurology 37:221–225, 1987.

Chamorro A, Vila N, Saiz A, et al. Early anticoagulation after large cerebral embolic infarction: A safety study. Neurology 45:861–865, 1995.

Chan JL, Ross ED. Left-handed mirror writing following right anterior cerebral artery infarction: Evidence for nonmirror transformation of motor programs by right supplementary motor area. Neurology 38:59–63, 1988.

Chan RKT, Fleming L, Finan J, et al., for the NASCET Group. Clinical presentation of transient monocular visual loss in patients with extracranial internal carotid artery disease. Neurology 46:A392, 1996.

Chancellor AM, Glasgow GL, Ockelford PA, et al. Etiology, prognosis, and hemostatic function after cerebral infarction in young adults. Stroke 20:477–482, 1989.

Chandler PA, Trotter RT. Angle-closure glaucoma: Subacute types. Trans Am Ophthalmol Soc 52:265–290, 1954.

Chater N. Results of neurological microvascular extracranial-intracranial bypass for stroke: A decade of experience. West J Med 138:531–533, 1983.

Chaves CJ, Pessin MS, Caplan LR, et al. Cerebellar hemorrhagic infarction. Neurology 46:346–349, 1996.

Chawla JC. Spontaneous cerebellar hemorrhage. Br Med J 1:93–94, 1970.

Chawluk JB, Kushner MJ, Bank WJ, et al. Atherosclerotic carotid artery disease in patients with retinal ischemic syndromes. Neurology 38:858–863, 1988.

Cheitlin MD, Byrd RC. Prolapsed mitral valve: The commonest valve disease? Curr Probl Cardiol 8:1–54, 1984.

Chen R, Sahjpaul R, Del Maestrz RF, et al. Initial enlargement of the opposite pupil as a false localizing sign in intraparenchymal frontal haemorrhage. J Neurol Neurosurg Psychiatry 57:1126–1128, 1994.

Cherubin CE, Baden M, Kavaler F, et al. Infective endocarditis in narcotic addicts. Ann Intern Med 69:1091–1098, 1968.

Chester EM, Agamanolis DP, Banker BQ, et al. Hypertensive encephalopathy: A clinicopathologic study of 20 cases. Neurology 28:928–939, 1978.

Chiari H. Über das Verhalten des Teilungswinkels der Carotis communis bei der Endarteriitis chronica deformans. Verb Deutsch Path Ges 9:326–330, 1905.

Chievitz E, Thiede T. Complications and causes of death in polycythaemia vera. Acta Med Scand 172:513–523, 1962.

Chimowitz MI, Nemec JJ, Marwick TH, et al. Transcranial Doppler ultrasound identifies patients with right-to-left cardiac or pulmonary shunts. Neurology 41:1902–1904, 1991.

Chimowitz MI, Kokkinos J, Stong J, et al., for the Warfarin-Aspirin Symptomatic Intracranial Disease Study Group. The Warfarin-Aspirin Symptomatic Intracranial Disease Study. Neurology 45:1488–1493, 1995.

Chin JH. Recurrent stroke caused by spondylotic compression of the vertebral artery. Ann Neurol 33:558–559, 1993.

Chisholm IA. Optic neuropathy of recurrent blood loss. Br J Ophthalmol 53:289–295, 1969.

Chokroverty S, Rubino FA. "Pure" motor hemiplegia. J Neurol Neurosurg Psychiatry 38:896–899, 1975.

Chollet F, Celsis P, Clanet M, et al. SPECT study of cerebral blood flow reactivity after acetazolamide in patients with transient ischemic attacks. Stroke 20:458–464, 1989.

Chopra JS, Prabhakar S. Clinical features and risk factors in stroke in young. Acta Neurol Scand 60:289–300, 1979.

Choromokos EA, Raymond LA, Sacks JG. Recognition of carotid stenosis with bilateral simultaneous retinal fluorescein angiography. Ophthalmology 89:1146–1148, 1982.

Chumbley LC, Harrison EG, DeRemee RA. Allergic granulomatosis and angiitis (Churg-Strauss syndrome): Report and analysis of 30 cases. Mayo Clin Proc 52:477–484, 1977.

Chung SM, Gay CA, McCrary JA. Nonarteritic ischemic optic neuropathy. The impact of tobacco use. Ophthalmology 101:779–782, 1994.

Churg J, Strauss L. Allergic granulomatosis, allergic angiitis, and periarteritis nodosa. Am J Pathol 27:277–300, 1950.

Ciemins V. Localized thalamic hemorrhage: A cause of aphasia. Neurology 20:776–782, 1970.

Cillessen JPM, Kappelle LJ, van Swieten JC, et al. Does cerebral infarction after a previous warning occur in the same vascular territory? Stroke 24:351–354, 1993.

Citron BP, Halpern M, McCarron M, et al. Necrotizing angiitis associated with drug abuse. N Engl J Med 283:1003–1011, 1970.

Clancy R, Malin S, Laraque D, et al. Focal motor seizures heralding stroke in full-term neonates. Am J Dis Child 139:601–606, 1985.

Clark JM, Albers GW. Vertical gaze palsies from medial thalamic infarctions without midbrain involvement. Stroke 26:1567–1570, 1995.

Clark WM, Barnwell SL. Endovascular treatment for acute and chronic brain ischemia. Curr Opin Neurol 9:62–67, 1996.

Clark WM, Barnwell SL, Nesbit G, et al. Safety and efficacy of percutaneous transluminal angioplasty for intracranial atherosclerotic stenosis. Stroke 26:1200–1204, 1995.

Clarke EC, Harrison CV. Bilateral carotid artery obstruction. Neurology 6:705–715, 1956.

Clarkson JC. Central retinal vein occlusion. In Retina. Editors, Schachat AP, Murphy RP, 2nd ed, Vol 2, pp 1379–1386. St Louis, CV Mosby, 1994.

Cleland PG, Saunders M, Rosser R. An unusual case of visual perseveration. J Neurol Neurosurg Psychiatry 44:262–263, 1981.

Coakham HB, Duchen LW, Scaravilli F. Moyamoya disease: Clinical and pathological report of a case with associated myopathy. J Neurol Neurosurg Psychiatry 42:287–289, 1979.

Coats G. Obstruction of the central artery of the retina. Roy Lond Ophthal Hosp Rep 16:262–306, 1905.

Cocozza M, Picano T, Oliviero U, et al. Effects of Picotamide, an antithromboxane agent, on carotid atherosclerotic evolution. A two-year, double-blind, placebo-controlled study in diabetic patients. Stroke 26:597–601, 1995.

Cogan DG. Neurology of the Ocular Muscles. 2nd ed. Springfield, IL, Charles C Thomas, 1956.

Cogan DG. Blackouts not obviously due to carotid occlusion. Arch Ophthalmol 66:180–187, 1961.

Cogan DG. Internuclear ophthalmoplegia, typical and atypical. Arch Ophthalmol 84:583–589, 1970.

Cogan DG. Ophthalmic complications of systemic vascular disease. In Major Problems in Internal Medicine. Vol 3. Philadelphia, WB Saunders, 1974.

Cogan DG, Loeb DR. Optokinetic response and intracranial lesions. Arch Neurol Psychiatr 61:183–187, 1949.

Cogan DG, Wray SH. Vascular occlusions in the eye from cardiac myxomas. Am J Ophthalmol 80:396–403, 1975.

Cogan DG, Kuwabara T, Moser H. Fat emboli in the retina following angiography. Arch Ophthalmol 71:308–313, 1964.

Cohen GR, Harbison JW, Blair CJ, et al. Clinical significance of transient visual phenomena in the elderly. Ophthalmology 91:436–442, 1984.

Cohen JJ, Miller S. Eyeball bruits. N Engl J Med 255:459–464, 1956.

Cohen L, Verstichel P, Pierrot-Deseilligny C. Hallucinatory vision of a familiar face following right temporal hemorrhage. Neurology 42:2052, 1992.

Cohen MM, McNamara MF. Eye pain due to carotid stenosis. Ann Ophthalmol 12:1056–1057, 1980.

Cohen MM, Hemalatha CP, D'Addario RT, et al. Embolization from a fusiform middle cerebral artery aneurysm. Stroke 11:158–161, 1980.

Cohen SN. Occipital infarction with hemianopia from carotid occlusive disease. Stroke 20:1433–1434, 1989.

Colditz GA, Bonita R, Stamper MJ, et al. Cigarette smoking and risk of stroke in middle-aged women. N Engl J Med 318:937–941, 1988.

Cole A, Aubé M. Late onset migraine with intracerebral hemorrhage: A recognizable syndrome. Neurology 37(Suppl 1):238, 1987.

Cole F, Yates P. Intracerebral microaneurysms and small cerebrovascular lesions. Brain 90:759–768, 1967.

Collaborative Group for the Study of Stroke in Young Women. Oral contraception and increased risk of cerebral ischemia or thrombosis. N Engl J Med 288:871–878, 1973.

Collaborative Group for the Study of Stroke in Young Women. Oral contraceptives and stroke in young women. Associated risk factors. JAMA 231:718–722, 1975.

Collard M, Saint-Val C, Mohr M, et al. Paralysie isolée du nerf moteur oculaire commun par infarctus de ses fibres fasciculaires. Rev Neurol 146:128–132, 1990.

Coller BS. Platelets and thrombolytic therapy. N Engl J Med 322:33–42, 1990.

Coller BS, Owen J, Jesty J, et al. Deficiency of plasma protein S, protein C, or antithrombin III and arterial thrombosis. Arteriosclerosis 7:456–462, 1987.

Collice M, D'Angelo V, Areno O. Surgical treatment of common carotid artery occlusion. Neurosurgery 12:515–524, 1983.

Collins R, Peto R, MacMahon S, et al. Blood pressure, stroke, and coronary artery disease. Part 2, short-term reductions in blood pressure: Overview of randomised drug trials in their epidemiological context. Lancet 335:827–838, 1990.

Collins RC, Al-Mondhiry H, Chernik NL, et al. Neurologic manifestations of intravascular coagulation in patients with cancer: A clinicopathologic analysis of 12 cases. Neurology 25:795–806, 1975.

Come PC, Riley MF, Bivas NK. Roles of echocardiography and arrhythmia monitoring in the evaluation of patients with suspected systemic embolism. Ann Neurol 13:527–531, 1983.

Comerota AJ, Cranley JJ, Cook SE. Real-time B-mode carotid imaging in diagnosis of cerebrovascular disease. Surgery 6:718–729, 1981.

Comess KA, DeRook FA, Beach KW, et al. Transesophageal echocardiography and carotid ultrasound in patients with cerebral ischemia: Prevalence of findings and recurrent stroke risk. J Am Coll Cardiol 23:1598–1603, 1994.

Committee on Health Care Issues, American Neurological Association: Does carotid endarterectomy decrease stroke and death in patients with transient ischemic attacks? Ann Neurol 22:72–76, 1987.

Connett MC, Lansche JM. Fibromuscular hyperplasia of the internal carotid artery (report of a case). Ann Surg 162:59–62, 1965.

Connolly JE, Brownell DA, Levine EF, et al. Accuracy and indications of diagnostic studies for extracranial carotid disease. Arch Surg 120:1229–1232, 1985.

Contorni L. Il circolo collaterale vertebro-vertebrale nelle obliterazaione dell'arteria succlavia alla sua origine. Minerva Chir 15:268–271, 1960.

Cooley DA, Al-Naaman YD, Carton CA. Surgical treatment of arterio-sclerotic occlusion of common carotid artery. J Neurosurg 13:500–506, 1956.

Cooperman M, Martin EW, Evans WE. Significance of asymptomatic carotid bruits. Arch Surg 113:1339–1340, 1978.

Coppeto JR. Transient ischemic attacks and amaurosis fugax from Timolol. Ann Ophthalmol 17:64–665, 1985.

Coppeto JR. Vertebrobasilar degeneration and chronic visual migraine. Neuro-ophthalmology 8:1–7, 1988.

Coppeto JR, Currie JN, Monteiro MLR, et al. A syndrome of arterial-occlusive retinopathy and encephalopathy. Am J Ophthalmol 98:189–202, 1984a.

Coppeto JR, Lessell S, Lessell IM, et al. Diffuse disseminated atheroembolism. Three cases with neuro-ophthalmic manifestation. Arch Ophthalmol 102:225–228, 1984b.

Coppeto JR, Wand M, Bear L, et al. Neovascular glaucoma and carotid artery obstructive disease. Am J Ophthalmol 99:567–570, 1985.

Corbett JJ, Schatz NJ, Shults WT, et al. Slowly alternating skew deviation: Description of a pretectal syndrome in three patients. Ann Neurol 10:540–546, 1981.

Corboy JR, Galetta SL. Familial cavernous angiomas manifesting with an acute chiasmal syndrome. Am J Ophthalmol 108:245–250, 1989.

Cordonnier M, Goldman S, Zegers de Beyl D, et al. Reversible acquired pendular nystagmus after brainstem hemorrhage. Neuro-ophthalmology 5:47–50, 1985.

Coria F, Rebollo M, Quintana F, et al. Occipitoatlantal instability and vertebrobasilar ischemia: Case report. Neurology 32:303–305, 1982.

Corrigall D, Bolen J, Hancock EW, et al. Mitral valve prolapse and infective endocarditis. Am J Med 63:215–222, 1977.

Corse AM, Stern BJ. Neurosarcoidosis and stroke. Stroke 21:152–153, 1990.

Cosgrove G, Leblanc R, Meagher-Villemure K, et al. Cerebral amyloid angiopathy. Neurology 35:625–631, 1985.

Coslett HB. Neglect in vision and visual imagery: A double dissociation. Brain 120:1163–1171, 1997.

Coslett HB, Saffran EM. Preserved object recognition and reading comprehension in optic aphasia. Brain 112:1091–1110, 1989.

Cote R, Caron JL. Management of carotid artery occlusion. Stroke 20:123–126, 1989.

Cote R, Barnett HJM, Taylor DW. Internal carotid occlusion: A prospective study. Stroke 14:898–902, 1983.

Cote R, Battista RN, Abrahamowicz M, et al. Lack of effect of aspirin in asymptomatic patients with carotid bruits and substantial carotid narrowing. Ann Intern Med 123:649–655, 1995.

Cotineau J, Sorato M, Le Guelec M. Emboles migrateurs rétiniens au cours de l'angiographie carotidienne. J Fr Ophthalmol 1:119–123, 1978.

Coull BM, Goodnight SH. Antiphospholipid antibodies, prethrombotic states, and stroke. Stroke 21:1370–1374, 1990.

Coull BM, Mela-Riker L, Tan Y. Calcium entry blockers in ischemic stroke. In Medical Therapy of Acute Stroke. Editor, Fisher M, pp 143–164. New York, Marcel Dekker, 1989.

Coulshed N, Epstein EJ, McKendrick CS, et al. Systemic embolism in mitral valve disease. Br Heart J 32:26–34, 1970.

Countee RW, Gnanadev A, Chavis P. Dilated episcleral arteries—A significant physical finding in assessment of patients with cerebrovascular insufficiency. Stroke 9:42–45, 1978.

Couves CM, Hilliard JR, Pribram HFW. Abnormalities of vertebrobasilar circulation due to subclavian artery disease. Can Med Assoc J 88:343–346, 1963.

Cowan CL Jr, Butler G. Ischemic oculopathy. Ann Ophthalmol 15:1052–1057, 1983.

Cravioto H, Silberman J, Feigin I. A clinical study of akinetic mutism. Neurology 10:10–21, 1960.

Crawford ES, De Bakey ME, Blaisdell FW, et al. Hemodynamic alterations in patients with cerebral arterial insufficiency before and after operation. Surgery 48:76–94, 1960.

Crawford FA, Sethi GK, Scott SM, et al. Systemic emboli due to cloth wear in a Starr-Edwards Model 2320 aortic prosthesis. Ann Thorac Surg 16:614–619, 1973.

Crevits LE, Logue RB. Carotid artery murmurs; continuous murmur over carotid bulb—new sign of carotid artery insufficiency. JAMA 167:2177–2182, 1958.

Crevits L, de Reuck J, vander Eecken H. Paralytic pontine exotropia in subarachnoid hemorrhage: A clinicopathological correlation. Clin Neurol Neurosurg 78:269–276, 1975.

Crew JR, Dean M, Johnson JM, et al. Carotid surgery without angiography. Am J Surg 148:217–220, 1984.

Critchley M. The anterior cerebral artery, and its syndromes. Brain 53:120–165, 1930.

Cronenwett JL, Birkmeyer JD, Nackman GB, et al. Cost-effectiveness of carotid endarterectomy in asymptomatic patients. J Vasc Surg 25:298–311, 1997.

Cronqvist S, Efsing HO, Palcios E. Emboli complications in cerebral angiography with the catheter technique. Acta Radiol 10:97–107, 1970.

Cross SA, Smith JL. Crossed-quadrant homonymous hemianopsia. The "checkerboard" field defect. J Clin Neuro-Ophthalmol 10:219–222, 1982.

Crowe NW, Nickles TP, Troost BT, et al. Intrachiasmal hemorrhage: A cause of delayed post-traumatic blindness. Neurology 39:863–865, 1989.

Crowell RM. Electromagnetic flow studies of superficial temporal artery by-pass graft. In Microsurgical Anastomoses for Cerebral Ischemia. Pp 116–124. Springfield, IL, Charles C Thomas, 1976.

Cucuianu MP, Nishizawa EE, Mustard JF. Effect of pyrimido-pyrimidine compounds on platelet function. J Lab Clin Med 77:958–974, 1971.

Cujec B, Bolasek P, Voli C, et al. Transesophageal echocardiography in the detection of potential cardiac source of embolism in stroke patients. Stroke 22:727–733, 1991.

Culebras A, Kase CS, Masdeu JC, et al. Practice guidelines for the use of imaging in transient ischemic attacks and acute stroke. Stroke 28:1480–1497, 1997.

Cull RE. Internal carotid artery occlusion caused by giant cell arteritis. J Neurol Neurosurg Psychiatry 42:1066–1067, 1979.

Cullen JF. Visual field defects following cerebral angiography. Trans Ophthalmol Soc UK 89:47–55, 1969.

Cullen JF, Duvall J. Posterior ischemic optic neuropathy (P.I.O.N.). Neuro-ophthalmology 3:15–19, 1983.

Cummings JL, Gittinger JW Jr. Central dazzle. A thalamic syndrome? Arch Neurol 38:372–374, 1981.

Cupps TR, Moore PM, Fauci AS. Isolated angiitis of the central nervous system: A prospective diagnostic and therapeutic experience. Am J Med 74:97–105, 1983.

Curb JD, Abbott RD, MacLean CJ, et al. Age-related changes in stroke risk in men with hypertension and normal blood pressure. Stroke 27:819–824, 1996.

Currier RD, DeJong RN, Boles GG. Pulseless disease: Central nervous system manifestations. Neurology 4:818–830, 1954.

Currier R, Giles C, Westerberg M. The prognosis of some brainstem vascular syndromes. Neurology 8:664–668, 1958.

Currier RD, Giles CL, DeJong RN. Some comments on Wallenberg's lateral medullary syndrome. Neurology 11:778–791, 1961.

Currier RD, Schneider RC, Preston RE. Angiographic findings in Wallenberg's lateral medullary syndrome. J Neurosurg 19:1058–1067, 1962.

Cusimano MD, Ameli FM. Transient cerebral ischemia. Can Med Assoc J 140:27–33, 1989.

Dagi LR, Currie J. Branch retinal artery occlusion in the Churg-Strauss syndrome. J Clin Neuro-Ophthalmol 5:229–237, 1985.

Dalal PM. Strokes in the young in West Central India. Adv Neurol 25:339–348, 1979.

Dalessio DJ. Wolff's Headache and Other Head Pain. Pp 88–89, 189–212. New York, Oxford University Press, 1972.

Damasio AR. Disorders of complex visual processing: Agnosia, achromatopsia, Bálint's syndrome and related difficulties of orientation and construction. In Principles of Behavioral Neurology. Editor, Mesulam MM, pp 259–282, Philadelphia, FA Davis, 1985.

Damasio A, Yamada T, Damasio H, et al. Central acromatopsia: Behavioral, anatomic, and physiologic aspects. Neurology 30:1064–1071, 1980.

Damasio A, Damasio H, Van Hoesen G. Prosopagnosia: Anatomic basis and behavioral mechanisms. Neurology 32:331–341, 1982.

Danchin N, Voiriot P, Briancon S, et al. Mitral valve prolapse as a risk factor for infective endocarditis. Lancet 1:743–745, 1989.

Dandapani BK, Suzuki S, Kelley RE, et al. Relation between blood pressure and outcome in intracerebral hemorrhage. Stroke 26:21–24, 1995.

Daniel WG, Mugge A. Transesophageal echocardiography. N Engl J Med 332:1268–1279, 1995.

Daras M, Tuchman AJ, Marks S. Central nervous systemic infarction related to cocaine abuse. Stroke 22:1320–1325, 1991.

Dark AJ, Rizk SN. Progressive focal sclerosis of retinal arteries: As equal to impaction of cholesterol emboli. Br Med J 1:270–273, 1967.

Daroff RB. See-saw nystagmus. Neurology 15:874–877, 1965.

Daroff RB, Hoyt WF. Supranuclear disorders of ocular control systems in man: Clinical, anatomical and physiological correlations. In The Control of Eye Movements. Editors, Bach-y-Rita P, Collins CC, Hyde JE, pp 175–235. New York, Academic Press, 1971.

Daroff RB, Waldman AL. Ocular bobbing. J Neurol Neurosurg Psychiatry 28:375–377, 1965.

Daroff RB, Hoyt WF, Sanders MD, et al. Gaze-evoked eyelid and ocular nystagmus inhibited by the near reflex: Unusual ocular motor phenomena in a lateral medullary syndrome. J Neurol Neurosurg Psychiatry 31:362–367, 1968.

Daroff RB, Troost BT, Dell'Osso LF. Nystagmus and related ocular oscillations. In Neuro-Ophthalmology. Editor, Glaser JS, pp 219–240. Hagerstown, MD, Harper and Row, 1978.

Davenport J, Hart RG. Prosthetic valve endocarditis 1976–1987: antibiotics, anticoagulation, and stroke. Stroke 21:993–999, 1990.

David NJ. Neuro-ophthalmology of occlusive disease in the vertebral-basilar arterial system. In Neuro-ophthalmology Symposium of the University of Miami and the Bascom Palmer Eye Institute. Editor, Smith JL, Vol 2, pp 206–222. St Louis, CV Mosby, 1965.

David NJ. Amaurosis fugax—and after? In Neuro-Ophthalmology. Symposium of the University of Miami and the Bascom Palmer Eye Institute. Editor, Smith JL, Vol 9, pp 8–28. St Louis, CV Mosby, 1977.

David NJ, Saito Y, Heyman A. Arm to retina fluorescein appearance time. A new method of diagnosis of carotid artery occlusion. Arch Neurol 5:165–170, 1961.

David NJ, Klintworth GK, Friedberg SJ, et al. Fatal atheromatous cerebral embolism associated with bright plaques in the retinal arterioles. Report of a case. Neurology 13:708–713, 1963.

David NJ, Norton EWD, Gass JDM, et al. Fluorescein retinal angiography in carotid occlusion. Arch Neurol 14:281–287, 1966.

David TE, Humphries AW, Young JR, et al. A correlation of neck bruits and atherosclerotic arteries. Arch Surg 107:729–731, 1973.

Davidson SI. Reported adverse effects of oral contraceptives on the eye. Trans Ophthalmol Soc UK 91:561–574, 1971.

Davie JC, Richardson R. Distal internal carotid thrombo-embolectomy using a Fogarty catheter in total occlusion. J Neurosurg 27:171–177, 1967.

Davis DO, Rumbaugh CL, Gibson JM. Angiographic diagnosis of small-vessel emboli. Acta Radiol 9:264–271, 1969.

Davis PC, Newman NJ. Advances in neuroimaging of the visual pathways. Am J Ophthalmol 121:690–705, 1996.

Davis PH, Dambrosia JM, Schoenberg BS, et al. Risk factors for ischemic stroke: A prospective study in Rochester, MN. Ann Neurol 20.121, 1986.

Davis PH, Dambrosia JM, Schoenberg BS, et al. Risk factors for ischemic stroke: A prospective study in Rochester, MN. Ann Neurol 22:319–327, 1987.

Davis PH, Clarke WR, Bendixen BH, et al., and the TOAST Investigators. Silent cerebral infarction in patients enrolled in the TOAST study. Neurology 46:942–948, 1996.

Davis RH, Schuster B, Knobel SF, et al. Myxomatous degeneration of the mitral valve. Am J Cardiol 28:449, 1971.

Davison C, Goodhart SP, Savitsky N. The syndrome of the superior cerebellar artery and its branches. Arch Neurol Psychiatr 33:1143–1174, 1935.

Dawson DM, Fischer EG. Neurologic complications of cardiac catheterization. Neurology 27:496–497, 1977.

Day AL. EC-IC bypass for MCA obstruction. In Cerebral Revascularization. Editors, Spetzler RF, Carter LP, Selman WR, et al., pp 458–466. New York, Thieme-Stratton, 1985.

Day AL, Rhoton AL Jr, Little JR. The extracranial-intracranial bypass study. Surg Neurol 26:222–226, 1986.

De Bono DP, Warlow CP. Mitral-annulus calcification and cerebral or retinal ischemia. Lancet 2:383–385, 1979.

De Bono DP, Warlow CP. Potential sources of emboli in patients with presumed transient cerebral or retinal ischemia. Lancet 1:343–345, 1981.

de Bray JM, Galland F, Lhoste P, et al. Colour doppler and duplex sonography and angiography of the carotid artery bifurcations. Prospective, double-blind study. Neuroradiology 37:219–224, 1995.

De Caterina R, Gianessi D, Boem A, et al. Equal antiplatelet effects of aspirin 50 or 324 mg/day in patients after acute myocardial infarction. Thromb Haemost 54:528–532, 1985a.

De Caterina R, Gianessi D, Bernini W, et al. Selective inhibition of thromboxane related platelet function by low-dose aspirin in patients after myocardial infarction. Am J Cardiol 55:589–590, 1985b.

Decroix JP, Graveleau P, Masson M, et al. Infarction in the territory of the anterior choroidal artery. A clinical and computerized tomography study of 16 cases. Brain 109:1071–1085, 1986.

Degos JD, Gray F, Louarn F, et al. Posterior callosal infarction: Clinicopathological correlations. Brain 110:1155–1171, 1987.

Degos R. Malignant atrophic papulosis. Br J Dermatol 100:21–35, 1979.

Dehaene I, Dom R. A mesencephalic locked-in syndrome. J Neurol 227:255–259, 1982.

Dehaene I, Martin JJ. "Locked-in" syndrome: A clinico-pathological study of two cases. Eur Neurol 14:81–89, 1976.

Dehaene I, van Zandijcke M. See-saw jerk nystagmus. Neuro-Ophthalmology 4:261–263, 1984.

Déjerine J. Des différentes variétés de cécité verbale. Mém Soc Biol 4:1–30, 1892.

de Kleyn A, Nieuwenhuyse P. Schwindelanfälle und Nystagmus bei einer bestimmten Stellung des Kopfes. Acta Otolaryngol 11:155–157, 1927.

Delaney P, Estes M. Intracranial hemorrhage with amphetamine abuse. Neurology 30:1125–1128, 1980.

Delecluse F, Voordecker P, Raftopoulos C. Vertebrobasilar insufficiency revealed by xenon-133 inhalation SPECT. Stroke 20:952–956, 1989.

Deleu D. Combined gaze palsy of horizontal saccades and pursuit contralateral to a midbrain haemorrhage. J Neurol Neurosurg Psychiatry 52:144, 1989.

Deleu D, Solheid C, Michotte A, et al. Dissociated ipsilateral horizontal gaze palsy in one-and-a-half syndrome: A clinicopathologic study. Neurology 38:1278–1280, 1988.

Deleu D, Buisseret T, Ebinger G. Vertical one-and-a-half syndrome. Supranuclear downgaze paralysis with monocular elevation palsy. Arch Neurol 46:1361–1363, 1989.

Dellmann F. Metastische Prozesse am Auge bei Endocarditis lenta. Klin Monatsbl Augenheilkd 63:661–671, 1919.

Del Zoppo GJ. Thrombolytic therapy in cerebrovascular disease. Stroke 19:1174–1179, 1988.

Del Zoppo GJ, Poeck K, Pessin MS, et al. Recombinant tissue plasminogen activator in acute thrombotic and embolic stroke. Ann Neurol 32:78–86, 1992.

Demakis JG, Proskey A, Rahimtoola SH, et al. The natural course of alcoholic cardiomyopathy. Ann Intern Med 80:293–297, 1974.

de Mendonca A, Pimentel J, Morgado F, et al. Mesencephalic haematoma: Case report with autopsy study. J Neurol 237:55–58, 1990.

DeMonte F, Peerless SJ, Rankin RN. Carotid transluminal angioplasty with evidence of distal embolization. Case report. J Neurosurg 70:138–141, 1989.

Dempsey RJ, Diana AL, Moore RW. Thickness of carotid artery athero-sclerotic plaque and ischemic risk. Neurosurgery 27:343–348, 1990.

Dennis MS, Bamford JM, Sandercock PAG, et al. Lone bilateral blindness: A transient ischaemic attack. Lancet 1:185–188, 1989.

Dennis M, Bamford J, Sandercock PAG, et al. Prognosis of transient ischemic attacks in the Oxfordshire Community Stroke Project. Stroke 21:848–853, 1990.

Denny-Brown D. The treatment of recurrent cerebrovascular symptoms and the question of "vasospasm." Med Clin North Am 35:1457–1474, 1951.

De Potter P, Zografos L. Occlusions artérielles rétiniennes: Étiologie et facteurs de risque à propos de 151 cas. Klin Monatsbl Augenheilkd 196:360–363, 1990.

Deppisch L, Fayem A. Nonbacterial thrombotic endocarditis. Am Heart J 92:723–729, 1976.

De Renzi E. Disorders of spatial orientation. In Handbook of Clinical Neurology. Editor, Fredericks JAM, Vol 1, pp 405–422. Amsterdam, Elsevier Science Publishers, 1985.

De Renzi E, Colombo A, Faglioni P, et al. Conjugate gaze paresis in stroke patients with unilateral damage: An unexpected instance of hemispheric asymmetry. Arch Neurol 39:482–486, 1982.

De Renzi E, Zambolin A, Crisi G. The pattern of neuropsychological impairment associated with left posterior cerebral artery infarcts. Brain 110:1099–1116, 1987.

De Reuck J. Clinical and neuropsychological aspects of atherosclerotic carotid disease, studied by positron emission tomography. Bull Soc Belge Ophtalmol 231:15–20, 1989.

Deringer PM, Hamilton LL, Whelan MA. A stroke associated with cocaine use. Arch Neurol 47:502, 1990.

Desnick RJ, Sweeley CC. Fabry's disease: Alpha galactosidase A deficiency. In The Metabolic Basis of Inherited Disease. Editors, Stanbury JB, Wyngaarden JB, Frederickson DS, et al., 5th ed, pp 906–944. New York, McGraw-Hill. 1983.

de Veber G, Schwarting G, Kolodny E, et al. Fabry disease: Immunocytochemical characterization of neuronal involvement. Ann Neurol 28:15, 1990.

Devereaux MW, Keane JR. Ondine's curse—neuro-ophthalmologic considerations. In Neuro-ophthalmology Symposium of the University of Miami and the Bascom Palmer Eye Institute. Editors, Smith JL, Glaser JS, Vol 7, pp 128–130. St Louis, CV Mosby, 1973.

Devereaux MW, Keane JR, Davis RL. Automatic respiratory failure associated with infarction of the medulla: Report of two cases with pathologic study of one. Arch Neurol 29:46–52, 1973.

Devereux RB, Brown WT. Genetics of mitral valve prolapse. Prog Med Genet 5:139–161, 1983.

Devereux RB, Perloff JK, Reichek N, et al. Mitral valve prolapse. Circulation 54:3–14, 1976.

Devereux RB, Brown WT, Kramer-Fox R, et al. Autosomal dominant inheritance of symptomatic and asymptomatic mitral valve prolapse: Effect of age and sex on gene expression. Ann Intern Med 97:826–832, 1982.

Devinsky O, Bear D, Volpe BT. Confusional states following posterior cerebral artery infarction. Arch Neurol 45:160–163, 1988.

DeVivo DC, Farrell FW Jr. Vertebrobasilar occlusive disease in children. A recognizable entity. Arch Neurol 26:278–281, 1972.

Devuyst G, Bogousslavsky J, Ruchat P, et al. Prognosis after stroke followed by surgical closure of patent foramen ovale: A prospective follow-up study with brain MRI and simultaneous transesophageal and transcranial Doppler ultrasound. Neurology 47:1162–1166, 1996.

DeWeese JA, Rob CG, Satran R, et al. Results of carotid endarterectomy for transient ischemic attacks: Five years later. Ann Surg 178:258–264, 1973.

DeWitt LD, Caplan LR. Antiphospholipid antibodies and stroke. ANJR 12:454–456, 1991.

DeWitt LD, Wechsler LR. Transcranial Doppler. Stroke 19:915–921, 1988.

DeWitt LD, Buonanno FS, Kistler JP, et al. Nuclear magnetic resonance imaging in evaluation of clinical stroke syndromes. Ann Neurol 16:535–545, 1984.

Deykin D, Janson P, McMahon L. Ethanol potentiation of aspirin-induced prolongation of the bleeding time. N Engl J Med 306:852–854, 1982.

Dhooge M, De Laey JJ. The ocular ischemic syndrome. Bull Soc Belge Ophtalmol 231:1–13, 1989.

Diener HC, Cunha L, Forbes C, et al. European Stroke Prevention Study 2: Dipyridamole and acetylsalicylic acid in the secondary prevention of stroke. J Neurol Sci 143:1–13, 1996a.

Diener HC, Hacke W, Hennerici M, et al., for the Lubeluzole International Study Group. Lubeluzole in acute ischemic stroke: A double-blind, placebo-controlled Phase II trial. Stroke 27:76–81, 1996b.

Dienst EC, Gartner S. Pathologic changes in the eye associated with subacute bacterial endocarditis: Report of five cases with autopsy. Arch Ophthalmol 31:198–206, 1944.

Dieterich EB, Liddicoat JE, McCutchen JJ, et al. Surgical significance of the external carotid artery in the treatment of cerebrovascular insufficiency. J Cardiovasc Surg 15:213–223, 1968.

Dieterich M, Brandt T. Wallenberg's syndrome: Lateropulsion, cyclorotation, and subjective visual vertical in thirty-six patients. Ann Neurol 31:399–408, 1992.

Dieterich M, Brandt T. Ocular torsion and tilt of subjective visual vertical area sensitive brainstem signs. Ann Neurol 33:292–299, 1993.

Diggs LW, Jones RS. Clinicopathologic conference. Am J Clin Pathol 22:1194–1200, 1952.

Digre KB, Durcan FJ, Branch DW, et al. Amaurosis fugax associated with antiphospholipid antibodies. Ann Neurol 25:228–232, 1989.

Dillon EH, Van Leeuwen MS, Fernandez MA, et al. CT angiography: Application to the evaluation of carotid artery stenosis. Radiology 189:211–219, 1993.

Diringer MN. Intracerebral hemorrhage: Pathophysiology and management. (Review). Crit Care Med 21:1591–1603, 1993.

Di Tullio M, Sacco RL, Gopal A, et al. Patent foramen ovale as a risk factor for cryptogenic stroke. Ann Intern Med 117:461–465, 1992.

Di Tullio M, Sacco RL, Venketasubramanian N, et al. Comparison of diagnostic techniques for the detection of a patent foramen ovale in stroke patients. Stroke 24:1020–1024, 1993.

Di Tullio MR, Sacco RL, Gersony D, et al. Aortic atheromas and acute ischemic stroke: A transesophageal echocardiographic study in an ethnically mixed population. Neurology 46:1560–1566, 1996.

Dixon S, Pais SO, Raviola C, et al. Natural history of nonstenotic, asymptomatic ulcerative lesions of the carotid artery. A further analysis. Arch Surg 117:1493–1498, 1982.

Dobkin BH. Focused stroke rehabilitation programs do not improve outcome. Arch Neurol 46:701–703, 1989.

D'Olhaberriague L, Hernández-Vidal A, Molina L, et al. A prospective study of atrial fibrillation and stroke. Stroke 20:1648–1652, 1989.

Donaghy RMP. Patch and by-pass in microangial surgery. In Microvascular Surgery. Editors, Donaghy RMP, Yasargil MG, pp 75–86. St Louis, CV Mosby, 1967.

Donaldson D, Rosenberg NL. Infarction of abducens nerve fascicle as cause of isolated sixth nerve palsy related to hypertension. Neurology 38:1654, 1988.

Doniger DE. Bilateral complete carotid and basilar artery occlusion in a patient with minimal deficit: Case report and discussion of diagnostic implications. Neurology 13:673–678, 1963.

Donnan GA, Sharbrough FW, Whisnant JP. Carotid occlusive disease. Effect of bright light on visual evoked response. Arch Neurol 39:687–689, 1982a.

Donnan GA, Tress BM, Bladin PF. A prospective study of lacunar infarction using computerized tomography. Neurology 32:49–56, 1982b.

Donnan GA, Adena MA, O'Malley HM, et al. Smoking as a risk factor for cerebral ischemia. Lancet 2:643–647, 1989.

Donnan GA, Hommel M, Davis SM, et al. Streptokinase in acute ischaemic stroke. Lancet 346:56, 1995.

Donnan GA, Davis SM, Chambers BR, et al. Streptokinase for acute ischemic stroke with relationship to time of administration. JAMA 276:961–966, 1996.

Donoso LA, Magargal LE, Eiferman RA, et al. Recurrent vascular obstructions from left atrial myxoma. Neuro-ophthalmology 2:59–65, 1981.

Donzis PB, Factor JS. Visual field loss resulting from cervical chiropractic manipulation. Am J Ophthalmol 123:851–852, 1997.

Dooling EC, Richardson EP Jr. Ophthalmoplegia and Ondine's curse. Arch Ophthalmol 95:1790–1793, 1977.

Dorazio RA, Ezzet F, Nesbitt NJ. Long-term follow-up of asymptomatic carotid bruits. Am J Surg 140:212–213, 1980.

Dorfman LJ, Marshall WH, Enzmann DR. Cerebral infarction and migraine: Clinical and radiologic correlations. Neurology 9:317–322, 1979.

Douglas DJ, Schuler JJ, Buchbinder D, et al. The association of central retinal artery occlusion and extracranial carotid artery disease. Ann Surg 208:85–90, 1988.

Doyle PW, Gibson G, Dolman CL. Herpes zoster ophthalmicus with contralateral hemiplegia: Identification of cause. Ann Neurol 14:84–85, 1983.

Drapkin A, Mersky C. Anticoagulant therapy after acute myocardial infarction: Relation of therapeutic benefit to patient's age, sex and severity of infarction. JAMA 222:541–549, 1972.

Dreizen NG, Framm L. Sudden unilateral visual loss after autologous fat injection into the glabellar area. Am J Ophthalmol 107:85–87, 1989.

Drinkwater JE, Thompson SK, Lumley JSP. Cerebral function before and after extraintracranial carotid bypass. J Neurol Neurosurg Psychiatry 47:1041–1043, 1984.

Drummond GT, Wuebbolt G. Bilateral ophthalmoplegia during percutaneous transluminal coronary angioplasty. Can J Ophthalmol 25:152–155, 1990.

D'Sousa T, Shraberg D. Intracranial hemorrhage associated with amphetamine use. Neurology 31:922–923, 1981.

Duane TD. Observations on the fundus oculi during black-out. Arch Ophthalmol 51:343–355, 1954.

Duane TD, Osher RH, Green WR. White centered hemorrhages: Their significance. Ophthalmology 87:66–69, 1980.

Dubin L, Quencer RM. Brain stem infarct. J Clin Neuro-Ophthalmol 7:112–113, 1987.

Dubinsky RM, Jankovic J. Progressive supranuclear palsy and a multi-infarct state. Neurology 37:570–576, 1987.

Ducros A, Nagy T, Alamowitch S, et al. Cerebral autosomal dominant arteriopathy with subcortical infarcts and leukoencephalopathy, genetic homogeneity, and mapping of the locus within a 2-cM interval. Am J Hum Genet 58:171–181, 1996.

Duff TA, Ayeni S, Levin AB, et al. Nonsurgical management of spontaneous intracerebral hematoma. Neurosurgery 9:387–393, 1981.

Duke-Elder S. System of Ophthalmology. Diseases of the Outer Eye. Vol 8, p 873. St Louis, CV Mosby, 1971.

Duker JS, Belmont JB. Ocular ischemic syndrome secondary to carotid artery dissection. Am J Ophthalmol 106:750–752, 1988.

Duker JS, Brown GC. Neovascularization of the optic disc associated with obstruction of the central retinal artery. Ophthalmology 96:87–91, 1989.

Duker JS, Brown GC, Brooks L. Retinal vasculitis in Crohn's disease. Am J Ophthalmol 103:664–668, 1987.

Duncan G, Gruber J, Dewey CF Jr, et al. Evaluation of carotid stenosis by phonoangiography. N Engl J Med 293:1124–1129, 1975.

Duncan GW, Parker SW, Fisher CM. Acute cerebellar infarction in the PICA territory. Arch Neurol 32:364–368, 1975.

Duncan GW, Pessin MS, Mohr JP, et al. Transient cerebral ischemic attacks. Adv Intern Med 21:1–20, 1976.

Duncan GW, Lees RS, Ojemann RG, et al. Concomitants of atherosclerotic carotid artery stenosis. Stroke 8:665–669, 1977.

Dunning HS. Intracranial and extracranial vascular accidents in migraine. Arch Neurol Psychiatr 48:396–406, 1942.

Duprez D. Non-invasive diagnosis of carotid artery disease. Bull Soc Belge Ophtalmol 231:21–26, 1989.

Duquesnel J, Pouillaude JM, Froment JC, et al. De la presence de fragments de verre dans les opacifiants vasculaires. J Radiol 54:297–300, 1973.

Durand-Fardel M. Traite des ramollisements du cerveau. Paris, Baillière, 1843.

Duret H. Traumatismes Cranio-cérébraux. Paris, Librairie Félix Alcan, 1919.

Durward QJ, Ferguson GG, Barr HWK. The natural history of asymptomatic carotid bifurcation plaques. Stroke 13:459–464, 1982a.

Durward QJ, Barnett HJM, Barr HWK. Presentation and management of mesencephalic hematoma. J Neurosurg 56:123–127, 1982b.

Dussaux P, Plas J, Brion S. Parésie bilatérale du muscle grand oblique, par hématome de la calotte mésencéphalique. Rev Neurol 146:45–47, 1990.

Dutton GN, Craig G. Treatment of a retinal embolus by photocoagulation. Br J Ophthalmol 73:580–581, 1989.

Dwyer-Joyce P. The fields in subclavian steal. Trans Ophthalmol Soc UK 92:819–824, 1972.

Dyer JA, Hirst LW, Vandeleur K, et al. Crossed-quadrant homonymous hemianopsia. J Clin Neuro-Ophthalmol 10:219–222, 1990.

Dyken ML. Editorial: Transient ischemic attacks and aspirin, stroke and death; negative studies and type II error. Stroke 14:2–4, 1983a.

Dyken ML. Anticoagulant and platelet-antiaggregating therapy in stroke and threatened stroke. Neurol Clin 1:223–242, 1983b.

Dyken ML, Pokras R. The performance of endarterectomy for disease of the extracranial arteries of the head. Stroke 15:948–950, 1984.

Dyken ML, White PT. Evaluation of cortisone in the treatment of cerebral infarction. JAMA 162:1531–1534, 1955.

Dyken ML, Klatte E, Kolar OJ, et al. Complete occlusion of common or internal carotid arteries. Arch Neurol 30:343–346, 1974.

Dyken ML, Wolf PA, Barnett HJM, et al. Risk factors in stroke. Stroke 15:1105–1111, 1984.

Eadie MJ. Benign amaurosis fugax of uncertain cause. Proc Aust Assoc Neurol 5: 251–253, 1968.

Eadie MJ, Sutherland JM, Tyrer JH. Recurrent monocular blindness of uncertain origin. Lancet 1:319–321, 1968.

EAFT Study Group. Silent brain infarction in nonrheumatic atrial fibrillation. Neurology 46:159–165, 1996.

Eagling EM, Sanders MD, Miller SJH. Ischaemic papillopathy. Br J Ophthalmol 58: 990–1008, 1974.

Earnest F IV, Forbes G, Sandok BA, et al. Complications of cerebral angiography: Prospective management of the risk. AJNR 4:1191–1197, 1983.

Eastman J, Cohen S. Hypertensive crisis and death associated with phencyclidine poisoning. JAMA 231:1270–1271, 1975.

Easton JD. Anticoagulation in cerebral ischemia. In Medical Therapy of Acute Stroke. Editor, Fisher M, pp 59–72. New York, Marcel Dekker, 1989.

Easton JD, Sherman DG. Cervical manipulation and stroke. Stroke 8:594–597, 1977.

Easton JD, Sherman DG. Management of cerebral embolism of cardiac origin. Stroke 11:433–444, 1980.

Easton JD, Wilterdink JL. Carotid endarterectomy: Trials and tribulations. Ann Neurol 35:5–17, 1994.

Easton JD, Hart RG, Sherman DG, et al. Diagnosis and management of ischemic stroke: 1. Threatened stroke and its management. Curr Probl Cardiol 8:1–76, 1983.

Eaton JM, Zweig R. Treatment of stroke. Neurology 39:875, 1989.

Eckardt C, Gotze O, Utermann D. Über die Lebenserwartung von Patienten mit Zirkulationsstörungen am hinteren Bulbusabschnitt. Ophthalmologica 187:34–42, 1983.

Edelman RR, Hesselink JR. Clinical magnetic resonance imaging. WB Saunders, Philadelphia, 1990.

Edelman RR, Warach S. Magnetic resonance imaging. (First of two parts). N Engl J Med 328:708–716, 1993.

Edelman RR, Mattle HP, Atkinson DJ, et al. MR angiography. AJR 154:937–946, 1990a.

Edelman RR, Mattle HP, O'Reilly GV, et al. Magnetic resonance imaging of flow dynamics in the circle of Willis. Stroke 21:56–65, 1990b.

Editorial: Amaurosis fugax. Lancet 1:838–839, 1982.

Editorial: Extracranial to intracranial bypass and the prevention of stroke. Lancet 2: 1401–1402, 1985.

Editorial: Cerebellar stroke. Lancet 1:1031–1032, 1988.

Editorial: Mitral valve prolapse. Lancet 1:1173–1175, 1989a.

Editorial: Brain damage and open-heart surgery. Lancet 2:364–366, 1989b.

Editorial: Left ventricular thrombosis and stroke following myocardial infarction. Lancet 335:759–760, 1990.

Editorial: Ticlopidine. Lancet 337:459–460, 1991.

Edmeads J. Headache in cerebrovascular disease. In Handbook of Clinical Neurology. Editor, Rose FC, Vol 4, Chap 48, pp 273–290. Amsterdam, Elsevier, 1986.

Edmiston WA, Harrison EC, Duick GF, et al. Thromboembolism in mitral porcine valve recipients. Am J Cardiol 41:508–511, 1978.

Edwards MS, Chater NL, Stanley JA. Reversal of chronic ocular ischaemia by extracranial-intracranial arterial by-pass: Case report. Neurosurgery 7:480–483, 1980.

Egbert JE, Schwartz GS, Walsh AW. Diagnosis and treatment of an ophthalmic artery occlusion during an intralesional injection of corticosteroid into an eyelid capillary hemangioma. Am J Ophthalmol 121:638–642, 1996.

Eggleston TF, Bohling CA, Eggleston HC, et al. Photocoagulation for ocular ischemia associated with carotid artery occlusion. Ann Ophthalmol 12:84–87, 1980.

Ehrenfeld WK, Lord RSA. Transient monocular blindness through collateral pathways. Surgery 65:911–915, 1969.

Ehrenfeld WK, Hoyt WF, Wylie EJ. Embolization and transient blindness from carotid atheroma. Arch Surg 93:787–794, 1966.

Eikelboom BC, Ackerstaff RGA, Ludwig JW, et al. Digital video subtraction angiography and duplex scanning in assessment of carotid artery disease: Comparison with conventional angiography. Surgery 94:821–825, 1983a.

Eikelboom BC, Riles TR, Mintzer R, et al. Inaccuracy of angiography in the diagnosis of carotid ulceration. Stroke 14:882–885, 1983b.

Einsiedel-Lechtape M. Embolic intracranial occlusions following complete internal carotid thrombosis. In Cerebral Vascular Disease 2. Editors, Meyer JS, Lechner M, Reivich M, pp 325–330. Amsterdam, Excerpta Medica, 1979.

Eisenberg RL, Bank WO, Hedgcock MW. Neurologic complications of angiography in patients with critical stenosis of the carotid artery. Neurology 30:895–897, 1980.

Elander CR, Bedrossian RH, Schaerer JP. Unilateral lid retraction. Association with common carotid thrombosis. Arch Ophthalmol 57:37–38, 1957.

El-Fiki M, Chater NL, Weinstein PR. Extracranial-intracranial arterial bypass for vertebrobasilar insufficiency. In Cerebral Revascularization. Editors, Spetzler RF, Carter LP, Selman WR, et al., pp 483–489. New York, Thieme-Stratton, 1985.

Eliasson R, Bygdeman S. Effect of dipyridamole and two pyrimido-pyrimidine derivatives on the kinetics of human platelet aggregation and on platelet adhesiveness. Scand J Clin Lab Invest 24:145–151, 1969.

Eliasziw M, Rankin RN, Fox AJ, et al., and for the North American Symptomatic Carotid Endarterectomy Trial (NASCET) Group. Accuracy and prognostic consequences of ultrasonography in identifying severe carotid artery stenosis. Stroke 26:1747–1752, 1995a.

Eliasziw M, Streifler JY, Spence JD, et al., and for the North American Symptomatic Carotid Endarterectomy Trial (NASCET) Group. Prognosis for patients following a transient ischemic attack with and without a cerebral infarction on brain CT. Neurology 45:428–431, 1995b.

Ellenberger C Jr, Epstein AD. Ocular complications of atherosclerosis: What do they mean? Sem Neurol 6:185–193, 1986.

Ellis PP. Occlusion of the central retinal artery after retrobulbar Corticosteroid injection. Am J Ophthalmol 85:352–356, 1978.

Ellis SJ, Small M. Denial of eye closure in acute stroke. Stroke 25:1958–1962, 1994.

Elschnig A. Über den Einfluss des Verschlusses der Arteria ophthalmica und der Carotid auf das Sehorgan. Graefe Arch Ophthalmol 39:151–177, 1893.

Elster AD. Questions and answers in magnetic resonance imaging, St Louis. CV Mosby, 1994.

Elster AD, Moody DM. Early cerebral infarction: Gadopentetate dimeglumine enhancement. Radiology 177:627–632, 1990.

Emmons PR, Harrison MJG, Honour AJ, et al. Effect of dipyridamole on human platelet behaviour. Lancet 2:603–606, 1965.

Engstrom J, Lowenstein D, Bredesen D. Cerebral infarctions and transient neurologic deficits associated with aquired immunodeficiency syndrome. Am J Med 86: 528–532, 1989.

Enoksson P. Internuclear ophthalmoplegia and paralysis of horizontal gaze. Acta Ophthalmol 43:697–707, 1965.

Eriksson SE, Link H, Alm A, et al. Results from 88 consecutive prophylactic carotid endarterectomies in cerebral infarction and transitory ischemic attacks. Acta Neurol Scand 63:209–219, 1981.

Ernerudh J, Olsson JE, von Schenck H. Antithrombin-III deficiency in ischemic stroke. Stroke 21:967, 1991.

Ernst E. A review of stroke rehabilitation and physiotherapy. Stroke 21:1081–1085, 1990.

Escourolle R, Hauw JJ, der Agopian P, et al. Les infarctus bulbaires. J Neurol Sci 29:103–113, 1976.

Estol CJ. Dr. C. Miller Fisher and the history of carotid artery disease. Stroke 27:559–566, 1996.

Estol CJ, Pessin MS. Anticoagulation: Is there still a role in atherothrombotic stroke? Stroke 21:820–824, 1990.

European Atrial Fibrillation Trial Study Group. Secondary prevention in non-rheumatic atrial fibrillation after transient ischemic attacks or minor stroke. Lancet 342:1255–1262, 1993.

European Atrial Fibrillation Trial Study Group. Optimal oral anticoagulant therapy in patients with nonrheumatic atrial fibrillation and recent cerebral ischemia. N Engl J Med. 333:5–10, 1995.

European Carotid Surgery Trialists' collaborative group, MRC European Carotid Surgery Tial. Interim results for symptomatic patients with severe (70–99%) or with mild (0–29%) carotid stenosis. Lancet 337:1235–1243, 1991.

European Carotid Surgery Trialists' Collaborative Group. Endarectomy for moderate symptomatic carotid stenosis: Interim results from the MRC European Cartoid Surgery Trial. Lancet 347:1591–1593, 1996.

European Stroke Prevention Study Group. European stroke prevention study: Principal end points. Lancet 2:1351–1354, 1987.

Evans DE, Zahorchak JA, Kennerdell JS. Visual loss as a result of primary optic nerve neuropathy after intranasal corticosteroid injection. Am J Ophthalmol 90:641–644, 1980.

Evarts CM. The fat embolism syndrome: A review. Surg Clin North Am 50:493–507, 1970.

Executive Committee for the Asymptomatic Carotid Atherosclerosis Study: Endarterectomy for asymptomatic carotid artery stenosis. JAMA 273:1421–1428, 1995.

Eyssette M. Le syndrome pariéto-occipital bilatéral. Thése de doctorat. Lyon, France, 1969.

Ezekowitz MD, Bridgers SL, James KE, et al., for the Veterans' Affairs Stroke Prevention in Nonrheumatic Atrial Fibrillation Investigators. Warfarin in the prevention of stroke associated with nonrheumatic atrial fibrillation. N Engl J Med 327:1406–1412, 1992.

Fabian RH, Peters BH. Neurological complications of hemoglobin SC disease. Arch Neurol 41:289–292, 1984.

Faggiotto A, Ross R, Harker L. Studies of hypercholesterolemia in the nonhuman primate: I. Changes that lead to fatty streak formation. Arteriosclerosis 4:323–340, 1984a.

Faggiotto A, Ross R, Harker L. Studies of hypercholesterolemia in the nonhuman primate. II. Fatty streak conversion to fibrous plaque. Arteriosclerosis 4:341–356, 1984b.

Fairburn B, Oliver L. Cerebellar softening: a surgical emergency. Br Med J 1:1335–1336, 1956.

Fairfax AJ, Lambert CD. Neurological aspects of sinoatrial heart block. J Neurol Neurosurg Psychiatry 39:576–580, 1976.

Fairfax AJ, Lambert CD, Leatham A. Systemic embolism in chronic sinoatrial disorder. N Engl J Med 295:190–193, 1976.

Falke P, Stavenow L, Young M, et al. Differences in mortality and cardiovascular morbidity during a 3-year follow-up of transient ischemic attacks and minor strokes. Stroke 20:340–344, 1989.

Fallis RJ. Neuropeptides and cerebral ischemia. In Medical Therapy of Acute Stroke. Editor, Fisher M, pp 165–188. New York, Marcel Dekker, 1989.

Fallis RJ, Miller M, Lobo RA. A double-blind trial of naloxone in the treatment of acute stroke. Stroke 15:627–629, 1984.

Farah MG. Familial atrial myxoma. Ann Intern Med 83:358–360, 1975.

Faught E, Trader SD, Hanna GR. Cerebral complications of angiography for transient ischemia and stroke: Prediction risk. Neurology 29:4–15, 1979.

Faught E, Peters D, Bartolucci A, et al. Seizures after primary intracerebral hemorrhage. Neurology 39:1089–1093, 1989.

Fawcett IM, Barrie T, Sheldon C, et al. The prevalence of carotid artery disease in patients presenting with amaurosis fugax. Trans Ophthalmol Soc UK 104:787–791, 1985.

Fazekas JF, Paul RE, Callow AD, et al. Diagnosis of aortocranial disease. Am J Med 34:93–102, 1963.

Fayad PB, Brass LM. Single photon emission computed tomography in cerebrovascular disease. Curr Concepts Cerebrovasc Dis Stroke 26:7–12, 1991.

Featherstone HJ. Clinical features of stroke in migraine. A review. Headache 26:128–133, 1986.

Feigenson JS, McDowell FH, Meese P, et al. Factors influencing outcome and length of stay in a stroke rehabilitation unit. Stroke 8:651–656, 1977.

Feinberg WM, Rapcsak SZ. Peduncular hallucinosis after paramedian thalamic infarction. Ann Neurol 26:125, 1989.

Feinberg WM, Albers GW, Barnett HJM. Guidelines for the management of transient ischemic attacks. Stroke 25:1320–1335, 1994.

Feinglass EJ, Arnett SC, Dorsch CA, et al. Neuropsychiatric manifestations of systemic lupus erythematosus: Diagnosis, clinical spectrum, and relationship to other features of the disease. Medicine 55:323–339, 1976.

Feldman M, Bender MB. Visual illusions in parieto-occipital lesions of the brain. In Origin and Mechanisms of Hallucinations. Editor, Keup W, pp 23–26. New York, Plenum Press, 1970.

Feldmann E. Intracerebral hemorrhage. Stroke 22:684–691, 1991.

Feldmann E, Levine SR. Cerebrovascular disease with antiphospholipid antibodies: Immune mechanisms, significance, and therapeutic options. Ann Neurol 37:5114–5130, 1995.

Feldmann E, Daneault N, Kwan E, et al. Chinese-white differences in distribution of occlusive cerebrovascular disease. Neurology 40:1541–1545, 1990.

Feldon SE, Renna T, Weiss H. Amaurosis fugax due to isolated atherosclerotic carotid artery disease in a young woman. Ann Neurol 2:541–542, 1977.

Feliste R, Delebassee D, Simon MF, et al. Broad spectrum anti-platelet activity of ticlopidine and PCR 4099 involves the suppression of the effects of released ADP. Thromb Res 48:403–415, 1987.

Felix CH. Crossed quadrant hemianopsia. Br J Ophthalmol 10:191–195, 1926.

Feman SS, Bartlett RE, Roth AM, et al. Intraocular hemorrhage and blindness associated with systemic anticoagulation. JAMA 220:1354–1355, 1972.

Ferbert A, Müllges W, Biniek R. Fascicular third nerve palsy with decreased vertical saccade velocity of the contralateral eye. Neuro-ophthalmology 10:33–38, 1990.

Ferguson GG. Carotid endarterectomy: To shunt or not to shunt? Arch Neurol 43:615–617, 1986.

Ferguson GG. Comments on Zuccarello M, Yeh HS, Tew JM. Morbidity and mortality of carotid endarterectomy under local anesthesia: A retrospective study. Neurosurgery 23:449, 1988.

Ferguson GG. Angioplasty for carotid disease. Arch Neurol 53:698–700, 1996.

Ferguson RDG, Ferguson JG. Carotid angioplasty. In search of a worthy alternative to endarterectomy. Arch Neurol 53:696–698, 1996.

Fernex M, Fernex C. La degenerescence mucoide des valvules mitrales. Helv Med Acta 25:694–705, 1958.

Ferrand J. Essai sur l'hemiplégie des vieillards: Les lacunes de désintégration cérébrale. Paris, Thesis, 1902.

Ferro JM, Crespo M. Prognosis after transient ischemic attack and ischemic stroke in young adults. Stroke 25:1611–1616, 1994.

Ferry AP, Abedi H. Diagnosis and management of rhino-orbital mucormycosis. A report of 16 personally observed cases. Ophthalmology 90:1096–1104, 1983.

Fesenmeier JT, Kuzniecky R, Garcia JH. Akinetic mutism caused by bilateral anterior cerebral tuberculous obliterative arteritis. Neurology 40:1005–1006, 1990.

Fessler RD, Esshaki CM, Stankewitz RC, et al. The neurovascular complications of cocaine. Surg Neurol 47:339–345, 1997.

Fields WS. Aspirin for prevention of stroke: A review. Am J Med 74(Suppl 6A):61–65, 1983.

Fields WS, Hass WK. Aspirin, Platelets and Stroke: Background for a Clinical Trial. St Louis, Warren H Green, Inc, 1970.

Fields WS, Breutman ME, Weibel J. Collateral circulation of the brain. Monogr Surg Sci 2:183–259, 1965.

Fields WS, Maslenikov V, Meyer JS, et al. Joint study of extracranial arterial occlusion. V. Progress report of prognosis following surgery or nonsurgical treatment for transient cerebral ischemic attacks and cervical carotid artery lesions. JAMA 211:1993–2003, 1970.

Fields WS, Lemak NA, Frankowski RF, et al. Controlled trial of aspirin in cerebral ischemia. Stroke 8:301–316, 1977.

Fields WS, Lemak NA, Frankowski RF, et al. Controlled trial of aspirin in cerebral ischemia. Part II. Surgical group. Stroke 9:309–319, 1978.

Fihn SD, McDonnell M, Martin D, et al., for the Warfarin Optimized Outpatient Follow-up Study Group. Risk factors for complications of chronic anticoagulation. Ann Intern Med 188:511–520, 1993.

Filatov V, Tom D, Alexandrakis G, et al. Branch retinal artery occlusion associated with directional coronary atherectomy after percutaneous transluminal coronary angioplasty. AJO 120:391–393, 1995.

Finelli P, Kessimian N, Bernstein P. Cerebral amyloid angiopathy manifesting as recurrent intracerebral hemorrhage. Arch Neurol 41:330–333, 1984.

Fink ME, Drusin R, Lamb J, et al. Cerebrovascular complications of cardiac transplantation. Stroke 18:294, 1987.

Finkelstein S, Kleinman GM, Cuneo R, et al. Delayed stroke following carotid occlusion. Neurology 30:84–88, 1980.

Finnerty FA Jr, Witkin L, Fazekas JF. Cerebral haemodynamics during cerebral ischaemia induced by acute hypotension. J Clin Invest 33:1227–1232, 1954.

Fiorelli M, Alperovitch A, Argentino C, et al., and for the Italian Acute Stroke Study Group. Prediction of long-term outcome in the early hours following acute ischemic stroke. Arch Neurol 52:250–255, 1995.

Fischer GG, Anderson DC, Farber R, et al. Prediction of carotid disease by ultrasound and digital subtraction angiography. Arch Neurol 42:224–227, 1985.

Fischer-Williams M, Gottschalk PG, Browell JN. Transient cortical blindness. An unusual complication of coronary angiography. Neurology 20:353–355, 1970.

Fisher CM. Occlusion of the internal carotid artery. Arch Neurol Psychiatr 65:346–377, 1951a.

Fisher CM. Transient monocular blindness associated with hemiplegia. Trans Am Neurol Assoc 47:154–157, 1951b.

Fisher CM. Transient monocular blindness associated with hemiplegia. Arch Ophthalmol 47:167–203, 1952.

Fisher CM. Occlusion of the carotid arteries: Further experiences. Arch Neurol Psychiatr 72:187–204, 1954.

Fisher CM. Cranial bruit associated with occlusion of the internal carotid artery. Neurology 7:299–306, 1957.

Fisher CM. Observations of the fundus oculi in transient monocular blindness. Neurology 9:333–347, 1959a.

Fisher CM. The pathologic and clinical aspects of thalamic hemorrhage. Trans Am Neurol Assoc 84:56–59, 1959b.

Fisher CM. Editorial. A new vascular syndrome: "The subclavian steal." N Engl J Med 265:912–913, 1961a.

Fisher CM. Clinical syndromes in cerebral hemorrhage in pathogenesis and treatment of cerebrovascular disease. In Proceedings of the Annual Meeting of the Houston Neurological Society. Editor, Fields WS, pp 318–342. Springfield, IL, Charles C Thomas, 1961b.

Fisher CM. Concerning recurrent transient cerebral ischemic attacks. Can Med Assoc J 86:1091–1099, 1962.

Fisher CM. Ocular bobbing. Arch Neurol 11:543–546, 1964.

Fisher CM. Lacunes: Small deep cerebral infarcts. Neurology 15:774–785, 1965a.

Fisher CM. Pure motor hemiplegia of vascular origin. Arch Neurol 13:30–44, 1965b.

Fisher CM. Pure sensory stroke involving face, arm, and leg. Neurology 15:76–80, 1965c.

Fisher CM. Some neuro-ophthalmological observations. J Neurol Neurosurg Psychiatry 30:383–392, 1967a.

Fisher CM. A lacunar stroke, the dysarthric-clumsy hand syndrome. Neurology 17:614–617, 1967b.

Fisher CM. Headache in acute cerebrovascular disease. In Handbook of Clinical Neurology. Editors, Vinken PJ, Bruyn GW, Vol 5, pp 124–156. New York, John Wiley & Sons, 1968a.

Fisher CM. Migraine accompaniments versus arteriosclerotic ischemia. Trans Am Neurol Assoc 93:211–213, 1968b.

Fisher CM. The arterial lesions underlying lacunes. Acta Neuropathol 12:1–15, 1969.

Fisher CM. Occlusion of the vertebral arteries. Arch Neurol 22:13–19, 1970.

Fisher CM. Cerebral ischemia: Less familiar types. Clin Neurosurg 18:267–335, 1971a.

Fisher CM. Pathological observations in hypertensive cerebral hemorrhages. J Neuropathol Exp Neurol 30:536–550, 1971b.

Fisher CM. Treatment of chronic atrial fibrillation. Curr Probl Cardiol 1:1284, 1972.

Fisher CM. Clinical syndromes of cerebral thrombosis, hypertensive hemorrhage, and ruptured saccular aneurysm. Clin Neurosurg 22:117–147, 1975.

Fisher CM. Bilateral occlusion of basilar artery branches. J Neurol Neurosurg Psychiatry 40:1182–1189, 1977.

Fisher CM. Thalamic pure sensory stroke: A pathologic study. Neurology 28:1141–1144, 1978a.

Fisher CM. Ataxic hemiparesis. Arch Neurol 35:126–128, 1978b.

Fisher CM. Capsular infarcts. The underlying vascular lesions. Arch Neurol 36:65–73, 1979.

Fisher CM. Late-life migraine accompaniments as a cause of unexplained transient ischemic attacks. Can J Neurol Sci 7:9–17, 1980.

Fisher CM. The headache and pain of spontaneous carotid dissection. Headache 22:60–65, 1981.

Fisher CM. Lacunar strokes and infarcts: A review. Neurology 32:871–876, 1982a.

Fisher CM. Pure sensory stroke and allied conditions. Stroke 13:434–447, 1982b.

Fisher CM. Unusual vascular events in the territory of the posterior cerebral artery. Can J Neurol Sci 13:1–7, 1986.

Fisher CM. The "herald hemiparesis" of basilar artery occlusion. Arch Neurol 45:1301–1303, 1988.

Fisher CM. "Transient monocular blindness" versus "amaurosis fugax." Neurology 39:1622–1624, 1989a.

Fisher CM. Lacunar infarct of the tegmentum of the lower lateral pons. Arch Neurol 46:566–567, 1989b.

Fisher CM. Hunger and the temporal lobe. Neurology 44:1577–1579, 1994.

Fisher CM. Vomiting out of proportion to dizziness in ischemic brainstem strokes. Neurology 46:267, 1996.

Fisher CM, Adams RD. Observations on brain embolism with special reference to the mechanism of hemorrhagic infarction. J Neuropathol Exp Neurol 10:92–94, 1951.

Fisher CM, Cameron DG. Concerning cerebral vasospasm. Neurology 3:468–473, 1953.

Fisher CM, Caplan LR. Basilar artery branch occlusion: A cause of pontine infarction. Neurology 21:900–905, 1971.

Fisher CM, Cole M. Homolateral ataxia and crural paresis, a vascular syndrome. J Neurol Neurosurg Psychiatry 28:48–55, 1965.

Fisher CM, Curry HB. Pure motor hemiplegia of vascular origin. Arch Neurol 13:30–44, 1965.

Fisher CM, Karnes WE. Local embolism. J Neuropathol Exp Neurol 24:174, 1965.

Fisher CM, Tapia J. Lateral medullary infarction extending to the lower pons. J Neurol Neurosurg Psychiatry 50:620–624, 1987.

Fisher CM, Karnes WE, Kubik CS. Lateral medullary infarction—the pattern of vascular occlusion. J Neuropathol Exp Neurol 20:323–378, 1961.

Fisher CM, Gore I, Okabe N, et al. Atherosclerosis of the carotid and vertebral arteries—extracranial and intracranial. J Neuropathol Exp Neurol 24:455–476, 1965a.

Fisher CM, Picard EH, Polak A, et al. Acute hypertensive cerebellar hemorrhage: Diagnosis and surgical treatment. J Nerv Ment Dis 140:38–57, 1965b.

Fisher M. Medical Therapy of Acute Stroke. New York, Marcel Dekker, 1989.

Fisher M, Yellin A. Bilateral visual loss in carotid artery disease. J Clin Neuro-Ophthalmol 5:109–111, 1985.

Fisher M, Weiner BH, Ockene IS, et al. Platelet activation and mitral valve prolapse. Neurology 32:197–200, 1982.

Fisher M, Weiner B, Ockene IS, et al. Selective thromboxane inhibition: A new approach to antiplatelet therapy. Stroke 15:813–816, 1984.

Fisher M, Blumenfeld AB, Smith TW. The importance of carotid artery plaque disruption and hemorrhage. Arch Neurol 44:1086–1089, 1987.

Fisher M, Lingley JF, Blumenfeld A, et al. Anterior choroidal artery territory infarction and small-vessel disease. Stroke 20:1591–1592, 1989.

Fisher M, Sotak CH, Minematsu K, et al. New magnetic resonance techniques for evaluating cerebrovascular disease. Ann Neurol 32:115–122, 1992a.

Fisher M, Sotak CH, Minematsu K, et al. Innovative magnetic resonance technologies for evaluating cerebrovascular disease. Ann Neurol 32:115–122, 1992b.

Fisher M, Jones S, Sacco RL. Prophylactic neuroprotection for cerebral ischemia. Stroke 25:1075–1080, 1994.

Fisher M, Prichard JW, Warach S. New magnetic resonance techniques for acute ischemic stroke. JAMA 274:908–911, 1995

FitzGerald GA. Dipyridamole. N Engl J Med 316:1247–1257, 1987.

FitzGerald GA, Oates JA, Hawiger J, et al. Endogenous synthesis of prostacyclin and thromboxane and platelet function during chronic administration of aspirin in man. J Clin Invest 71:676–688, 1983.

Fleck BW, Cullen JF. Chronic ocular hypoxia associated with carotid insufficiency, presenting with hyphaema. Neuro-ophthalmology 5:9–11, 1985.

Flegel KM, Hanley J. Risk factors for stroke and other embolic events in patients with nonrheumatic atrial fibrillation. Stroke 20:1000–1004, 1989.

Flegel KM, Shipley MJ, Rose G. Risk of stroke in nonrheumatic atrial fibrillation. Lancet 1:526–529, 1987.

Fleming HA, Bailey SM. Mitral valve disease, systemic embolism and anticoagulants. Postgrad Med J 47:599–604, 1971.

Fode NC, Sundt TM Jr, Robertson TJ, et al. Multi-center retrospective review of results and complications of carotid endarterectomy in 1981. Stroke 17:370–376, 1986.

Fogelholm R, Aho K. Ischemic cerebrovascular disease in young adults. Acta Neurol Scand 49:415–427, 1973.

Fogelholm R, Nuutila M, Vuorela AL. Primary intracerebral haemorrhage in the Jyvaskyla region, Central Finland, 1985–1989: Incidence, case fatality rate, and functional. J Neurol Neurosurg Psychiatry 55:546–552, 1992.

Foix C, Hillemand P. Les syndromes de l'artère cerebrale antérieure. Encephale 20:209–232, 1925.

Foix C, Chavany JA, Hillemand P, et al. Oblitération de l'artère choroïdienne antérieure. Ramollissement de son territoire cérébral. Hémiplégie, hémianesthésie, hémianopsie. Bull Soc Ophtalmol Fr 27:221–223, 1925.

Folsom AR, Prineas RJ, Kaye SA, et al. Incidence of hypertension and stroke in relation to body fat distribution and other risk factors in older women. Stroke 21:701–706, 1990.

Folsom AR, Wu KK, Shahar E, et al., and for the Atherosclerosis Risk in Communities (ARIC) Study Investigators. Association of hemostatic vaiables with prevalent cardiovascular disease and asymptomatic carotid artery atherosclerosis. Arterioscler Thromb 13:1829–1836, 1993.

Font RL, Naumann G. Ocular histopathology in pulseless disease. Arch Ophthalmol 82:784–788, 1969.

Ford CS, Frye JL, Toole JF, et al. Asymptomatic carotid bruit and stenosis: A prospective follow-up study. Arch Neurol 43:219–222, 1986.

Ford FR. Diseases of the Nervous System in Infancy, Childhood and Adolescence. 3rd ed. Springfield, IL, Charles C Thomas, 1952.

Ford RG, Siekert RG. Central nervous system manifestations of periarteritis nodosa. Neurology 15:114–122, 1965.

Forsyth PD, Dolan G. Activated protein C resistance in cases of cerebral infarction [letter]. Lancet 354:795, 1995.

Foulkes MA, Wolf PA, Price TR, et al. The Stroke Data Bank: Design, methods, and baseline characteristics. Stroke 19:547–554, 1988.

Foville A. Note sur une paralysie peu connue de certains muscle de l'oeil, et sa liason avec quelques points de l'anatomie et la physiologie de la protuberance annulaire. Bull Soc Anat Paris 33:373–405, 1858.

Fox JC. Restoration of cerebral function after prolonged cardiac arrest. J Neurosurg 6:361–367, 1949.

Fox JL. Intracranial Aneurysms. Vol 1, pp 317–318. New York, Springer-Verlag, 1983.

Frackowiak RSJ. PET scanning: Can it help resolve management issues in cerebral ischemic disease? Stroke 17:803–807, 1986.

Frackowiak RSJ, Wise RJ. Positron tomography in ischemic cerebrovascular disease. Neurol Clin North Am 1:183–200, 1983.

Frackowiak RSJ, Wise RJ, Biggs JM, et al. Positron emission tomographic studies in aging and cerebrovascular disease at Hammersmith Hospital. Ann Neurol 15:S112–S118, 1987.

Fraga A, LaValle C. Takayasu's arteritis. Clin Rheum Dis 6:405–412, 1980.

Franceschetti A. Fabry's disease: Ocular manifestations. In The Eye and Inborn Errors in Metabolism. Editors, Bergsma D, Bron AJ, Cotlier E, Vol 12, No 3, pp 195–208. New York, AR Liss Co, 1976.

Francois J, Van Langenhone E. Embolisms of the central artery of the retina following a retrobulbar injection of methylprednisolone acetate. Bull Soc Belg Ophtalmol 155:517–523, 1970.

Francois J, Neetens A, Collette JM. Vascularization of the optic pathway. IV. Optic tract and geniculate body. Br J Ophthalmol 40:341–354, 1956.

Frank G. Comparison of anticoagulation and surgical treatments of TIA. A review and consolidation of recent natural history and treatment studies. Stroke 2: 369–377, 1971.

Franke CL, de Jonge J, van Swieten JC, et al. Intracerebral hematomas during anticoagulant treatment. Stroke 21:726–730, 1990.

Franke CL, van Swieten JC, Algra A, et al. Prognositc factors in patients with intracerebral haematoma. J Neurol Neurosurg Psychiatry 55:653–657, 1992.

Franke CL, Palm R, Dalby M, et al. Flunarizine in stroke treatment (FIST): A double-blind, placebo-controlled trial in Scandinavia and the Netherlands. Acta Neurol Scand 93:56–60, 1996.

Freddo L, Sacco RL, Bello JA, et al. Lateral medullary syndrome: Clinicoanatomical features studied by magnetic resonance and vascular imaging. Ann Neurol 26: 157, 1989.

Freeman JW, Kennedy RM, Petty SS. Prognosis of nonoperated cerebellar hemorrhage. Ann Neurol 4:389–399, 1978.

Freeman RE, Onofrio BM, Okazaki H, et al. Spontaneous intracerebellar hemorrhage: Diagnosis and surgical treatment. Neurology 23:84–90, 1973.

French Study of Aortic Plaques in Stroke Group. Atherosclerotic disease of the aortic arch as a risk factor for recurrent ischemic stroke. N Engl J Med 334:1216–1221, 1996.

French BN, Rewcastle NB. Recurrent stenosis at site of carotid endarterectomy. Stroke 8:597–605, 1977.

Freund CS. Ueber optische Aphasie und Seelenblindheit. Arch Pyschiatr Nervenkrankh 20:276–297, 1889.

Frey JL. Asymptomatic carotid stenosis: Surgery's the answer, but that's not the question. Ann Neurol 39:405–406, 1996.

Friberg TR, Gragoudas ES, Regan CDJ. Talc emboli and macular ischemia in intravenous drug abuse. Arch Ophthalmol 97:1089–1091, 1979.

Fricke M. Kompensationsmechanismen bei intra- und extrakraniellen Gefäßeverschlussen. Fortschr Roentgenstr 122:481–492, 1975.

Friedenwald JS, Rones B. Some ocular lesions in septicemia. Trans Am Ophthalmol Soc 28:286–300, 1930.

Friedenwald JS, Rones B. Ocular lesions in septicemia. Arch Ophthalmol 5:175–188, 1931.

Friedman DI, Aravapalli SR, Shende MC. Visual pathway hemorrhage associated with alcohol-induced coagulopathy. J Neuroophthalmol 16:124–133, 1996.

Frisén L. Lateropulsion of the eyes—a localizing brainstem sign. J Neurol 218: 171–177, 1978.

Frisén L. Quadruple sectoranopia and sectorial optic atrophy: A syndrome of the distal anterior choroidal artery. J Neurol Neurosurg Psychiatry 42:590–594, 1979.

Frisén L, Holmegaard L, Rosencrantz M. Sectorial optic atrophy and homonymous, horizontal sectoranopia: A lateral choroidal artery syndrome? J Neurol Neurosurg Psychiatry 41:374–380, 1978.

Frishman WH, Miller KP. Platelets and antiplatelet therapy in ischemic heart disease. Curr Prob Cardiol 11:71–122, 1986.

Frisoni GB, Anzola GP. Neck manipulation and stroke. Neurology 40:1910, 1990.

Fritz VU, Voll CL, Levien LJ. Internal carotid artery occlusion: Clinical and therapeutic implications. Stroke 16:940–944, 1985.

Fritz WL, Klein HJ, Schmidt K. Arteriovenous malformation of the posterior (sic) ethmoidal artery as an unusual cause of amaurosis fugax. The ophthalmic steal syndrome. J Clin Neuro-Ophthalmol 9:165–168, 1989.

Frohman LP, Rescigno R, Bielory L. Neuro-ophthalmologic manifestations of the antiphospholipid antibody syndromes. Ophthalmology 96(Suppl):105, 1989.

Frovig AG. Bilateral obliteration of the common carotid artery—thromboangiitis obliterans? Acta Psychiatr Neurol Scand 39(Suppl):7–79, 1946.

Frumkin LR, Baloh RW. Wallenberg's syndrome following neck manipulation. Neurology 40:611–615, 1990.

Fry CL, Carter JE, Kanter MC, et al. Anterior ischemic optic neuropathy is not associated with carotid artery atherosclerosis. Stroke 24:539–542, 1993.

Fryer DG, Crane R, Margolis MT. Angiographic changes in intracranial arteritis of ophthalmic herpes zoster. Ann Neurol 15:311–312, 1984.

Fryer JA, Myers PC, Appleberg M. Carotid intraplaque hemorrhage: The significance of neovascularity. J Vasc Surg 6:341–349, 1987.

Fujii K, Lenkey C, Rhoton AL Jr. Microsurgical anatomy of the choroidal arteries: Lateral and third ventricles. J Neurol 52:165–188, 1980.

Fujimoto T, Suzuki H, Tanoue K, et al. Cerebrovascular injuries induced by activation of platelets in vivo. Stroke 16:245–250, 1985.

Fujino T. The blood supply of the lateral geniculate body. Jpn J Ophthalmol 6:24–33, 1962.

Fujino T, Curtin VT, Norton EWD. Experimental central retinal vein occlusion: A comparison of intraocular and extraocular occlusion. Arch Ophthalmol 81: 395–406, 1969.

Fujino T, Akiya S, Takagi S, et al. Amaurosis fugax for a long duration. J Clin Neuro-Ophthalmol 3:9–12, 1983.

Fukuchi T, Tamura K, Seki R, et al. Internal carotid artery occlusion with neovascular glaucoma. Folia Ophthalmol Jpn 39:1531–1538, 1988.

Fukuda Y, Nakamura K. The incidence of thromboembolism and hemocoagulative background in patients with rheumatic heart disease. Jpn Cire J 48:59–66, 1984.

Furlan AJ. The Heart and Stroke. New York, Springer-Verlag, 1987.

Furlan AJ, Whisnant JP, Kearns TP. Unilateral visual loss in bright light. An unusual symptom of carotid artery occlusive disease. Arch Neurol 36:675–676, 1979a.

Furlan AJ, Whisnant JP, Elveback LR. The decreasing incidence of primary intracerebral hemorrhage: A population study. Ann Neurol 5:367–373, 1979b.

Furlan AJ, Cracuin AR, Salcedo E, Mellino M. Risk of stroke in patients with mitral annular calcification. Stroke 15:801–803, 1984.

Fuster V, Gersh BJ, Guiliani ER, et al. The natural history of idiopathic dilated cardiomyopathy. Am J Cardiol 47:525–531, 1981.

Futrell N, Millikan C. Frequency, etiology, and prevention of stroke in patients with systemic lupus erythematosus. Stroke 20:583–591, 1989.

Gabrielsen TO. Neurologic complications of cerebral angiography. AJNR 15: 1408–1411, 1994.

Gacs G, Fox A, Barnett HJM, et al. Occurrence and mechanisms of occlusion of the anterior cerebral artery. Stroke 14:952–959, 1983.

Gaffney JF, Kingston WJ, Metlay LA, et al. Left ventricular thrombus and systemic emboli complicating the cardiomyopathy of Duchenne's muscular dystrophy. Arch Neurol 46:1249–1252, 1989.

Gage BF, Cardinalli AB, Albers GW, et al. Cost-effectiveness of warfarin and aspirin for prophylaxis of stroke in patients with nonvalvular atrial fibrillation. JAMA 274:1839–1845, 1995.

Galetta SL, Wulc AE, Goldberg HI, et al. Rhinocerebral mucormycosis: Management and survival after carotid occlusion. Ann Neurol 28:103–107, 1990.

Galin MA, Baras I, Cavero R, et al. Compression and suction ophthalmodynamometry. Am J Ophthalmol 67:388–392, 1969.

Galle G, Lang GK, Ruprecht KW, et al. Die Bedeutung des orbitalen Kollateralkreislaufs für die Entsstehung ischämischer Ophthalmopathien bei stenosierenden Erkrankungen der Arteria carotis interna. Fortschr Neurol Psychiatr 51:261–269, 1983.

Galligioni F, Andrioli GC, Marin G, et al. Hypoplasia of the internal carotid artery associated with cerebral pseudoangiomatosis. AJR 112:251–262, 1971.

Galloway IR, Greitz T. The medial and lateral choroidal arteries. An anatomic and roentgenographic study. Acta Radiol 53:353–366, 1960.

Galve E, Candell-Riera J, Pigrau C, et al. Prevalence, morphologic types, and evolution of cardiac valvular disease in systemic lupus erythematosus. N Engl J Med 319: 817–823, 1988.

Gan R, Noronha A. The medullary vascular syndromes revisited. J Neurol 242: 195–202, 1995.

Gan R, Sacco RL, Kargman DE, et al. Testing the validity of the lacunar hypothesis: The Northern Manhattan Stroke Study experience. Neurology 48:1204–1211, 1997.

Garcia I, Fainstein V, Rios A, et al. Nonbacterial thrombotic endocarditis in a male homosexual with Kaposi's sarcoma. Arch Intern Med 143:1243–1244, 1983.

Garde A, Samuelson K, Fahlgren H, et al. Treatment after transient ischemic attacks: A comparison between anticoagulant drug and inhibition of platelet aggregation. Stroke 14:677–681, 1983.

Garland PE, Crandall AS, Creel DJ, et al. Visual disturbance resulting from intranasal steroid injection. Arch Ophthalmol 107:22–23, 1989.

Garvey GT, Neu HC. Infective endocarditis: An evolving disease. Medicine 57: 105–127, 1978.

Gasecki AP, Fox AJ, Lebrun LH, et al. Bilateral occipital infarctions associated with carotid stenosis in a patient with persistent trigeminal artery. Stroke 25: 1520–1523, 1994.

Gasecki AP, Eliasziw M, Ferguson GG, et al. Long-term prognosis and effect of endarterectomy in patients with symptomatic severe carotid stenosis and contralateral carotid stenosis or occlusion: Results from NASCET. J Neurosurg 83: 778–782, 1995.

Gass JDM. A fluorescein angiographic study of macular dysfunction secondary to retinal vascular disease. VI. X-ray irradiation, carotid artery occlusion, collagen vascular disease and vitritis. Arch Ophthalmol 80:606–617, 1968.

Gassmann A. Zur histologie der rontgenulcera. Fortschr Geb Roentgenstr Nuklearmed Erganzungsband 1:2199–2207, 1899.

Gauthier G, Rohr J, Wildi E, et al. L'hématome disséquant de l'artère carotide interne: Revue géneérale de 205 cas publiés dont dix personnels, Schweiz. Arch Neurol Neurochir Psychiatr 136:53–74, 1985.

Gautier JC, Pradat-Diehl P, Loron PL, et al. Accidents vasculaires cerebraux des sujets jeunes. Une etude de 133 patients ages de 9 á 45 ans. Rev Neurol 145:437–442, 1989.

Gee W, Smith CA, Hinson CE, et al. Ocular pneumoplethysmography in carotid artery disease. Med Instrum 8:244–248, 1974.

Gee W, Oller DW, Wylie EJ. Noninvasive diagnosis of carotid occlusion by ocular pneumoplethysmography. Stroke 7:18–21, 1976.

Gee W, Oller DW, Homer LD, et al. Simultaneous bilateral determination of the systolic pressure of the ophthalmic arteries by ocular pneumoplethysmography. Invest Ophthalmol Visual Sci 16:86–89, 1977a.

Gee W, Oller DW, Amundsen DG, et al. The asymptomatic carotid bruit and the ocular pneumoplethysmograph. Arch Surg 112:1381–1388, 1977b.

Gelmers HJ. Effects of calcium antagonists on the cerebral circulation. Am J Cardiol 59:173B–176B, 1987.

Gelmers HJ, Gorter K, Weerdt CJ, et al. A controlled trial of nimodipine in acute ischemic stroke. N Engl J Med *318*:203–207, 1988.

Genee E, Honegger H. Netzhaut Arterienverschlusb bei Angiographie der arteria carotis interna. Med Welt *18*:1066–1068, 1969.

Gent M. Single studies and overview analyses: Is aspirin of value in cerebral ischemia? Stroke *18*:541–544, 1987.

Gent M, Blakely JA, Easton JD, et al., and the CATS Group. The Canadian American Ticlopidine Study (CATS) in thromboembolic stroke. Lancet *1*:1215–1220, 1989.

Gentilini M, De Renzi E, Crisi G. Bilateral paramedian thalamic artery infarcts: Report of eight cases. J Neurol Neurosurg Psychiatry *50*:900–909, 1987.

Gerber SL, Cantor LB. Progressive optic atrophy and the primary antiphospholipid antibody syndrome. Am J Ophthalmol *110*:443–444, 1990.

Gerrity RG. The role of the monocyte in atherogenesis. I. Transition of blood-borne monocytes into foam cells in fatty lesions. Am J Pathol *103*:181–190, 1981.

Gerstmann J. Syndrome of finger agnosia, disorientation for right and left, agraphia and acalculia. Local diagnostic value. Arch Neurol Psychiatr *44*:398–408, 1940.

Geschwind DH, FitzPatrick M, Mischel PS, et al. Sneddon's syndrome is a thrombotic vasculopathy: Neuropathologic and neuroradiologic evidence. Neurology *45*: 557–560, 1995.

Geschwind N. Disconnection syndromes in animals and man. Brain *88*:237–294, 585–644, 1965.

Geschwind N, Fusillo M. Color-naming defects in association with alexia. Arch Neurol *15*:137–146, 1966.

Geschwind N, Kaplan E. A human cerebral disconnection syndrome. Neurology *12*: 675–685, 1962.

Geyer JJ, Franzini DA. Myxomatous degeneration of the mitral valve complicated by nonbacterial thrombotic endocarditis with systemic embolization. Am J Clin Pathol *72*:489–492, 1979.

Ghanchi FD, Williamson TH, Lim CS, et al. Colour Doppler imaging in giant cell (temporal) arteritis: Serial examination and comparison with non-arteritic anterior ischaemic optic neuropathy. Eye *10*:459–464, 1996.

Ghika J, Bogousslavsky J, Regli F. Infarcts in the territory of the deep perforators from the carotid system. Neurology *39*:507–512, 1989.

Gibson JM, Cullen JF. Blindness and visual field defects following cerebral angiography. Neuro-ophthalmology *2*:297–303, 1982.

Gilbert J, Vinters H. Cerebral amyloid angiopathy: Incidence and complications in the aging brain. I. Cerebral hemorrhage. Stroke *14*:915–923, 1983.

Giles WH, Kittner SJ, Anda RF, et al. Serum folate and risk for ischemic stroke. First National Health and Nutrition Examination survey. Epidemiologic follow-up study. Stroke *26*:1166–1170, 1995.

Gill JS, Zezulka AV, Shipley MJ, et al. Stroke and alcohol consumption. N Engl J Med *315*:1041–1046, 1986.

Gill JS, Shipley MJ, Tzementzis SA, et al. Cigarette smoking: A risk factor for hemorrhagic and nonhemorrhagic stroke. Arch Intern Med *149*:2053–2057, 1989.

Gilles C, Brucher J, Khoubesserian P, et al. Cerebral amyloid angiopathy as a cause of multiple intracerebral hemorrhages. Neurology *34*:730–735, 1984.

Gillilan LA. The correlation of the blood supply to the human brain stem with clinical brain stem lesions. J Neuropathol Exp Neurol *23*:78–108, 1964.

Gillman MW, Cupples LA, Gagnon D, et al. Protective effect of fruits and vegetables on development of stroke in men. JAMA *273*:1113–1117, 1995.

Gilman S. Cerebral disorders after open-heart operations. N Engl J Med *272*:489–498, 1965.

Gilman S. Neurological complications of open heart surgery. Ann Neurol *28*:475–476, 1990.

Gilner LI, Avin B. A reversible ocular manifestation of thalamic hemorrhage: A case report. Arch Neurol *34*:715–716, 1977.

Gilroy J. The "locked-in" syndrome. In Vertebrobasilar Arterial Occlusive Disease. Editors, Berguer R, Bauer RB, pp 73–776. New York, Raven Press, 1984.

Gilroy J, Meyer JS. Auscultation of the neck in occlusive cerebrovascular disease. Circulation *25*:300–310, 1962.

Ginsberg MD, Greenwood SA, Goldberg HI. Noninvasive diagnosis of extracranial cerebrovascular disease: Oculoplethysmography-phonoangiography and directional Doppler ultrasonography. Neurology *29*:623–631, 1979.

Giovannoni G, Fritz VU. Transient ischemic attacks in younger and older patients: A comparative study of 798 patients in South Africa. Stroke *24*:947–953, 1993.

Giubilei F, Lenzi GL, Di Piero V, et al. Predictive value of brain perfusion single-photon emission computed tomography in acute ischemic stroke. Stroke *21*: 895–900, 1990.

Glancy DL, O'Brien K, Gold H, et al. Atrial fibrillation in patients with idiopathic hypertrophic subaortic stenosis. Br Heart J *32*:652–659, 1970.

Glass JD, Levey AI, Rothstein JD. The dysarthria-clumsy hand syndrome: A distinct clinical entity related to pontine infarction. Ann Neurol *27*:487–494, 1990.

Gleiberman L, Harburg E. Alcohol usage and blood pressure: A review. Hum Biol *58*:1–31, 1986.

Gloning I, Gloning K, Tschabitscher H. Die occipitale Blindheit auf vasculärer Basis: Untersuchungsergebnisse von 16 eigenen Fällen. Albrecht v Graefes Arch Ophthalmol *165*:138–177, 1962.

Gobernado J, de Molina A, Gineno A. Pure motor hemiplegia due to hemorrhage in the lower pons. Arch Neurol *37*:393, 1980.

Goerlitz M. Histologische Untersuchung eines Falles von Erblindung nach schwerem Blutverlust. Klin Monatsbl Augenheilkd *64*:763–782, 1920.

Goldberg G, Meyer NH, Toglia JU. Medial frontal cortex infarction and the alien hand sign. Arch Neurol *38*:683–686, 1981.

Golden GS. Stroke syndromes in childhood. Neurol Clin *3*:59–75, 1985.

Goldenberg G, Reisner TH. Angiographic findings in relation to clinical course and results of computed tomography in cerebrovascular disease. Eur Neurol *22*: 124–130, 1983.

Goldner JC, Whisnant JP, Taylor WF. Long-term prognosis of transient cerebral ischemic attacks. Stroke *2*:160–167, 1971.

Goldschmidt TJ, Wall M. Slow-upward ocular bobbing. J Clin Neuro-Ophthalmol *7*: 241–243, 1987.

Goldstein LB, Bertels C, Davis JN. Interobserver reliability of the NIH stroke scale. Arch Neurol *46*:660–662, 1989.

Goldstein LB, Hasselblad V, Matchar DB, et al. Comparison and meta-analysis of randomized trials of endarterectomy for symptomatic carotid artery stenosis. Neurology *45*:1965–1970, 1995.

Goldstein LB, Moore WS, Robertson JT, et al. Complication rates for carotid endarterectomy: A call to action. Stroke *28*:889–890, 1997.

Golub BM, Sibony PA, Coller BS, et al. Protein S deficiency associated with central retinal artey occlusion. Arch Ophthalmol *108*:918, 1990.

Gombos GM, Moreno DH, Bedrossian PB. Retinal vascular occlusion induced by oral contraceptives. Ann Ophthalmol *7*:215–217, 1975.

Gomensoro JB, Maslenikov V, Azambuja N, et al. Joint study of extracranial arterial occlusion. VIII. Clinical-radiographic correlation of carotid bifurcation lesions in 177 patients with transient cerebral ischemic attacks. JAMA *224*:985–991, 1973.

Gomez CR. Carotid plaque morphology and risk for stroke. Stroke *21*:148–151, 1990.

Gomez CR, Cruz-Flores S, Malkoff MD, et al. Isolated vertigo as a manifestation of vertebrobasilar ischemia. Neurology *47*:94–97, 1996.

Gomez SM, Gomez CR, Selhorst JB. Acute esotropia: A sign of thalamic ischemia. Neurology *37*(Suppl 1):289, 1987.

Gomori JM, Grossman RI, Hackney DB, et al. Intracranial hematomas: Imaging by high-field MR. Radiology *157*:87–93, 1985.

Gonyea EF. Bilateral internuclear ophthalmoplegia: Association with occlusive cerebrovascular disease. Arch Neurol *31*:168–173, 1974.

Goodson SF, Flanigan DP, Bishara RA, et al. Can carotid duplex scanning supplant arteriography in patients with focal carotid territory symptoms? J Vasc Surg *5*: 551–557, 1987.

Goodwin JA, Kansu T. Vulpian's sign: Conjugate eye deviation in acute cerebral hemisphere lesions. Neurology *36*:711–712, 1986.

Goodwin JA, Gorelick P, Helgason C. Transient monocular visual loss: Amaurosis fugax versus migraine. Neurology *34*(Suppl 1):246, 1984.

Goodwin JA, Gorelick PB, Helgason CM. Symptoms of amaurosis fugax in atherosclerotic carotid artery disease. Neurology *37*:829–832, 1987.

Gorelick PB. The status of alcohol as a risk factor for stroke. Stroke *20*:1607–1610, 1989.

Gorelick PB. Stroke prevention. Arch Neurol *52*:347–355, 1995.

Gorelick PB, Caplan L, Hier D, et al. Racial differences in the distribution of occlusive cerebrovascular disease. Neurology *34*:54–59, 1984.

Gorelick PB, Caplan L, Hier D, et al. Racial differences in the distribution of posterior circulation disease. Stroke *16*:785–790, 1985.

Gorelick PB, Hier DB, Caplan LR, et al. Headache in acute cerebrovascular disease. Neurology *36*:1445–1450, 1986.

Gorelick PB, Rodin MB, Langenberg P, et al. Is acute alcohol ingestion a risk factor for ischemic stroke? Results of a controlled study in middle-aged and elderly stroke patients at three urban medical centers. Stroke *18*:359–364, 1987.

Gorelick PB, Caplan LR, Langenberg P, et al. Clinical and angiographic comparison of asymptomatic occlusive cerebrovascular disease. Neurology *38*:852–858, 1988.

Gorelick PB, Rodin MB, Langenberg P, et al. Weekly alcohol consumption, cigarette smoking, and the risk of ischemic stroke: Results of a case-control study at three urban medical centers in Chicago, IL. Neurology *39*:339–343, 1989.

Gorson KC, Pessin MS, DeWitt LD, et al. Stroke with sensory symptoms mimicking myocardial ischemia. Neurology *46*:548–551, 1996.

Gorvai D. Insufficiency of the vertebral artery treated by decompression of its cervical part. Br Med J *2*:233–234, 1964.

Goulet Y, Mackay CG. Atheromatous embolism: An entity with polymorphous symptomatology. Can Med Assoc J *88*:1067–1070, 1963.

Goulon M, Barois A, Grosbuis S, et al. Fat embolism after repeated infusions of fat emulsions. Nouv Presse Med *3*:13–18, 1974.

Gowers WR. On a case of simultaneous embolism of central retinal and middle cerebral arteries. Lancet *2*:794–796, 1875.

Graffagnino C, Herbstreith MH, Roses AD, et al. A molecular genetic study of intracerebral hemorrhage. Arch Neurol *51*:981–984, 1994.

Graff-Radford NR, Eslinger PJ, Damasio AR, et al. Nonhemorrhagic infarction of the thalamus: Behavioral, anatomical and physiological correlates. Neurology *34*:14–23, 1984.

Graff-Radford NR, Damasio AR, Yamada T, et al. Nonhaemorrhagic thalamic infarction: Clinical, neuropsychological and electrophysiological findings in four anatomical groups defined by computerized tomography. Brain *108*:485–516, 1985.

Graham AM, Gewertz BL, Zarins CK. Predicting cerebral ischemia during carotid endarterectomy. Arch Surg 121:595–598, 1986.

Graham DI, Adams H. "Idiopathic" thrombosis in the vertebrobasilar arterial system in young men. Br Med J 1:20–28, 1972.

Graham EM, Spaltron DJ, Barnard RO, et al. Cerebral and retinal vascular changes in systemic lupus erythematosus. Ophthalmology 92:444–448, 1985.

Graham IM, Daly LE, Refsum HM, et al. Plasma homocysteine as a risk factor for vascular disease: The European Concerted Action Project. JAMA 277:1775–1781, 1997.

Gras P, Grosmaire N, Fayolle H, et al. Transient neurologic deficit preceding intracerebral hemorrhage. Physiopathological hypotheses. Rev Neurol (Paris) 149:224–226, 1993.

Gratzl O, Schmiedek P, Spetzler R, et al. Clinical experience with extra-intracranial arterial anastomosis in 65 cases. J Neurosurg 44:313–324, 1976.

Grauer K, Grauer MC. Familial atrial myxoma with bilateral recurrence. Heart Lung 12:600 602, 1983.

Gravanis MB, Campbell WB. The syndrome of prolapse of the mitral valve: An etiologic and pathogenic enigma. Arch Pathol Lab Med 106:369–374, 1982.

Graveleau P, Decroix JP, Samson Y, et al. Déficit sensitif isolé d'un hémicorps par hématome du pont. Rev Neurol 142:788–790, 1986.

Gray F, Dubas F, Roullet E, et al. Leukoencephalopathy in diffuse hemorrhagic cerebral amyloid angiopathy. Ann Neurol 18:54–59, 1985.

Green D, Joynt RJ. Vascular accidents to the brain stem associated with neck manipulation. JAMA 170:522–524, 1959.

Green GJ, Lessell S. Acquired cerebral dyschromatopsia. Arch Ophthalmol 95:121–128, 1977.

Green JP, Newman NJ, Winterkorn JS. Paralysis of downgaze in two patients with clinical-radiologic correlation: Arch Ophthalmol 111:219–222, 1993.

Green RM, Kelly KM, Gabrielsen T, et al. Multiple intracerebral hemorrhages after smoking "crack" cocaine. Stroke 21:957–962, 1990.

Green WR. Histopathologic studies of hypotensive retinopathy. In Management of Retinal Vascular and Macular Disorders. Editors, Fine SL, Owens SL, pp 5–27. Baltimore, Williams & Wilkins, 1983.

Green WR. Retina. In Ophthalmic Pathology. An Atlas and Textbook. Editor, Spencer WH, 4th ed, Vol 2, pp 749–751. Philadelphia, WB Saunders, 1996.

Greenberg J, Massey EW. Cerebral infarction in sickle cell trait. Ann Neurol 18:354–355, 1985.

Greenberg SM, Rebeck GW, Vonsattel JPG, et al. Apolipoprotein E4 and cerebral hemorrhage associated with amyloid angiopathy. Ann Neurol 38:254–259, 1995.

Greenberg SM, Finklestein SP, Schaefer PA. Petechial hemorrhages accompanying lobar hemorrhage: Detection by gradient-echo MRI. Neurology 46:1751–1754, 1996.

Greenfield DS, Hefferick PA, Hedges TR III. Color doppler imaging of normal orbital vasculature. Ophthalmology 102:1598–1605, 1995.

Greengard JS, Eichinger S, Griffin JH, et al. Brief report: Variability of thrombosis among homozygous siblings with resistance to activated protein C due to an Arg→Gln mutation in the gene for factor V. N Engl J Med 331:1559–1562, 1994.

Greenland P, Knopman DS, Mikell FL, et al. Echocardiography in diagnostic assessment of stroke. Ann Intern Med 95:51–53, 1981.

Greer M, Schotland D. Abnormal hemoglobins as a cause of neurologic disease. Neurology 12:114–123, 1962.

Gresele P, Deckmyn H, Arnout J, et al. Characterization of N,N'-bis(3-picolyl)-4-methoxy-isophtalamide (picotamide) as a dual thromboxane synthase inhibitor/thromboxane A2 receptor antagonist in human platelets. Thromb Haemost 61:479–484, 1989.

Gresham GE, Phillips TF, Wolf PA, et al. Epidemiologic profile of long-term stroke disability: The Framingham study. Arch Phys Med Rehab 60:487–591, 1979.

Gresham GE, Alexander D, Bishop DS, et al. Rehabilitation. Stroke 28:1522–1526, 1997.

Greven CM, Slusher MM, Weaver RG. Retinal arterial occlusions in young adults. Am J Ophthalmol 120:776–783, 1995.

Greven CM, Weaver RG, Owen J, et al. Protein S deficiency and bilateral branch retinal artery occlusion. Ophthalmology 98:33–34, 1991.

Griewing B, Morgenstern C, Driesner F, et al. Cerebrovascular disease assessed by color-flow and power doppler ultrasonography. Comparison with digital subtraction angiography in internal carotid artery stenosis. Stroke 27:95–100, 1996.

Griffin MR, Wilson WR, Edwards WD, et al. Infective endocarditis: Olmstead County, Minnesota, 1950 through 1981. JAMA 254:1199–1202, 1985.

Grigg MJ, Papadakis K, Nicolaides AN, et al. The significance of cerebral infarction and atrophy in patients with amaurosis fugax and transient ischemic attacks in relation to internal carotid stenosis: A preliminary report. J Vasc Surg 7:215–222, 1988.

Griguer P, Brochier M, Raynaud R. Étude de l'effet inhibiteur du dipyridamole sur l'adhésivité et l'agrégation plaquettaires "in vitro" et "in vivo." Ann Cardiol Angeiol 24(Suppl):2–36, 1975.

Grindal AB, Cohen RJ, Saul RF, et al. Cerebral infarction in young adults. Stroke 9:39–42, 1978.

Grizzard WS, Blackshear WM, Rush JA, et al. Noninvasive carotid evaluation using pulsed Doppler imaging for patients with ophthalmic disorders. Ophthalmology 89:1235–1240, 1982.

Groothuis DR, Duncan GW, Fisher CM. The human thalamocortical sensory path in the internal capsule: Evidence from a small capsular hemorrhage causing a pure sensory stroke. Ann Neurol 2:328–331, 1977.

Grosset DG, Ebrahim S, Bone I, et al. Stroke in pregnancy and the puerperium: What magnitude of risk? J Neurol Neurosurg Psychiatry 58:129–131, 1995.

Grossling HR, Pelligrini VD. Fat embolism syndrome: A review of the pathophysiology and physiological basis of treatment. Clin Orthop 165:68–82, 1982.

Grotta JC. Current medical and surgical therapy for cerebrovascular disease. N Engl J Med 317:1505–1516, 1987.

Grotta JC. Stroke, hemodilution, and mortality. Stroke 20:1286–1287, 1989.

Grotta JC, Bigelow RH, Hu H, et al. The significance of carotid stenosis or ulceration. Neurology 34:437–442, 1984.

Grotta JC, Lemak NA, Gary H, et al. Does platelet antiaggregant therapy lessen the severity of stroke? Neurology 35:632–636, 1985.

Grotta JC, Norris JW, Kamm B, et al. Baseline and Angiographic Data Subgroup. Prevention of stroke with ticlopidine: Who benefits most? Neurology 42:111–115, 1992.

Grover SA, Gray-Donald K, Joseph L, et al. Life expectancy following dietary modification or smoking cessation: Estimating the benefits of a prudent lifestyle. Arch Intern Med 154:1697–1704, 1994.

Growdon JH, Winkler GF, Wray SH. Midbrain ptosis. A case with clinicopathologic correlation. Arch Neurol 30:179–181, 1974.

Guberman A, Stuss D. The syndrome of bilateral paramedian thalamic infarction. Neurology 33:540–546, 1983.

Gubler A. Hemiplegie alternée d'une lésion du pont et la documentation de la preuve de la décussation. Gaz Hebd Med Chirurg 3:749–754, 789–792, 811–816, 1856.

Guerry D, Wiesinger H. Ocular complications in carotid angiography. Am J Ophthalmol 55:241–243, 1963.

Guest IA, Woolf AL. Fatal infarction of brain in migraine. Br Med J 1:225–226, 1964.

Guillain G, Bertrand I, Peron N. Le syndrome de l'artère cérébelleuse supérieure. Rev Neurol 2:835–843, 1928.

Gumerlock MK, Neuwelt EA. Carotid endarterectomy: To shunt or not to shunt. Stroke 19:1485–1490, 1988.

Gunderson CH, Hoyt WF. Geniculate hemianopia: Incongruous homonymous field defects in two patients with partial lesions of the lateral geniculate nucleus. J Neurol Neurosurg Psychiatry 34:1–6, 1971.

Guntheroth WG, Motulsky AG. Inherited primary disorders of cardiac rhythm and conduction. Prog Med Genet 5:381–402, 1971.

Gur D, Wolfson S, Yonas H, et al. Progress in cerebrovascular disease: Local cerebral blood flow by xenon-enhanced CT. Stroke 13:750–758, 1982.

Gutman FA, Zegarra H. Ocular complications in cardiac surgery. Surg Clin North Am 51:1095–1103, 1971.

Guyer DR, Miller NR, Auer CL, et al. The risk of cerebrovascular and cardiovascular disease in patients with anterior ischemic optic neuropathy. Arch Ophthalmol 103:1136–1142, 1985.

Haan J, Algra PR, Roos RAC. Hereditary cerebral hemorrhage with amyloidosis-Dutch type. Clinical and computed tomographic analysis of 24 cases. Arch Neurol 47:649–653, 1990a.

Haan J, Lanser JBK, Zijderveld I, et al. Dementia in hereditary cerebral hemorrhage with amyloidosis—Dutch type. Arch Neurol 47:965–967, 1990b.

Hachinski VC. Hypertension in acute ischemic strokes. Arch Neurol 42:1002, 1985.

Hachinski VC. Atrial fibrillation and recurrent stroke. Arch Neurol 43:70, 1986.

Hachinski VC. Carotid endarterectomy. Arch Neurol 44:654, 1987.

Hachinski VC. Stroke rehabilitation. Arch Neurol 46:703, 1989.

Hachinski VC. Multicenter trials in stroke. Arch Neurol 47:445, 1990.

Hachinski VC. The issue is standards, not techniques. Arch Neurol 52:834, 1995.

Hachinski VC, Potter P, Merskey H. Leuko-araiosis. Arch Neurol 44:21–23, 1987.

Hachinski VC, Norris JW. The Acute Stroke. Philadelphia, FA Davis, 1986.

Hachinski VC, Graffagnino C, Beaudry M, et al. Lipids and stroke. Arch Neurol 53:303–308, 1996.

Hacke W, Kaste M, Fieschi C, et al., for the ECASS Study Group. Intravenous thrombolysis with recombinant tissue plasminogen activator for acute hemispheric stroke. JAMA 274:1017–1025, 1995.

Hacke W, Schwab S, Horn M, et al. "Malignant" middle cerebral artery territory infarction. Clinical course and prognostic signs. Arch Neurol 53:309–315, 1996.

Haerem AT. Blindness following massive gastrointestinal hemorrhage. Ann Intern Med 36:883–888, 1952.

Hager H. Die Diagnose der Karotisthrombose durch den Augenarzt. Klin Monatsbl Augenheilkd 141:801–840, 1962.

Hagley SR. The fulminant fat embolism syndrome. Anaesth Intens Care 11:162–165, 1983a.

Hagley SR. Fulminant fat embolism—Case reports. Anaesth Intens Care 11:167–170, 1983b.

Hagström L, Hörnsten G, Silfverskiöld BP. Oculostatic and visual phenomena occurring in association with Wallenberg's syndrome. Acta Neurol Scand 45:568–582, 1969.

Hahn HH, Schweid AI, Beatty HN. Complications of injecting dissolved methylphenidate tablets. Arch Intern Med 123:656–659, 1969.

Halbmayer WM, Haushofer A, Schon R, et al. The prevalence of poor anticoagulant response to activated protein C (APC resistance) among patients suffering from stroke or venous thrombosis and among healthy subjects. Blood Coag Fibrinol 5:51–57, 1994.

Haley EC Jr, Levy DE, Brott TF, et al. Urgent therapy for stroke. Part II. Pilot study of tissue plasminogen activator administered 91–180 minutes from onset. Stroke 23:641–645, 1992.

Haley EC, Brott TG, Sheppard GL, et al., and for the TPA Bridging Study Group. Pilot randomized trial of tissue plasminogen activator in acute ischemic stroke. Stroke 24:1000–1004, 1993.

Halkin A, Ablin J, Steiner I. Unilateral proptosis due to cerebellar stroke. Letters to the Editor. JNNP 643–645, 1995.

Hall S, Barr W, Lie JT, et al. Takayasu's arteritis: A study of 32 North American patients. Medicine 64:89–99, 1985.

Hallermann D, Singh G. Iatrogenic central retinal artery embolization: A complication of cardiac catheterization. Ann Ophthalmol 16:1025–1027, 1984.

Halmagyi GM, Brandt T, Dieterich M, et al. Tonic contraversive ocular tilt reaction due to unilateral mesodiencephalic lesion. Neurology 40:1503–1509, 1990.

Halperin JJ, Luft BJ, Anand AK, et al. Lyme neuroborreliosis: central nervous system manifestations. Neurology 39:753–759, 1989.

Halpern JI, Sedler RR. Traumatic bilateral homonymous hemianopic scotomas. Ann Ophthalmol 12:1022–1026, 1980.

Halperin JL, Hart RG. Atrial fibrillation and stroke: New ideas, persisting dilemmas. Stroke 19:937–941, 1988.

Hamed LM, Silbiger J, Silbiger M, et al. Magnetic resonance angiography of vascular lesions causing neuro-ophthalmic deficits. Surv Ophthalmol 37:425–434, 1993.

Hameroff SB, Garcia-Mullin R, Eckholdt J. Ocular bobbing. Arch Ophthalmol 82:774–780, 1969.

Hanahan DJ. Platelet activating factor: A biologically active phosphoglyceride. Annu Rev Biochem 55:483–509, 1986.

Handler CE, Perkins GD. Sickle cell trait and multiple cerebral infarctions. J R Soc Med 75:550–553, 1982.

Haney WP, Preston RE. Ocular complications of carotid arteriography in carotid occlusive disease. Arch Ophthalmol 67:33–43, 1962.

Hankey GJ. Isolated angiitis/angiopathy of the central nervous system. Cerebrovasc Dis 1:2–15, 1991.

Hankey GJ, Warlow CP, Sellar RJ. Cerebral angiographic risk in mild cerebrovascular disease. Stroke 21:209–222, 1990.

Hankey GJ, Slattery JM, Warlow CP. Prognosis and prognostic factors of retinal infarction: A prospective cohort study. BMJ 302:499–504, 1991.

Hanna JP, Sun JP, Furlan AJ, et al. Patent foramen ovale and brain infarct: Echocardiographic predictors, recurrence, and prevention. Stroke 25:782–786, 1994.

Hannaford PC, Croft PR, Kay CR. Oral contraception and stroke: evidence from the Royal College of General Practitioners' oral contraception study. Stroke 25:935–942, 1994.

Hansen PE, Damgard-Jensen L, Nehen AM. Retinale emboljer efter carotisarteriografi. To tilfaelde af eksogene fremmedlegemer. Ugeskr Laeger 140:3059–3061, 1978.

Hanson MR, Hodgman JR, Conomy JP. A study of stroke associated with prolapsed mitral valve. Neurology 28:341, 1978.

Hanson MR, Conomy JP, Hodgman JR. Brain events associated with mitral valve prolapse. Stroke 11:490–505, 1980.

Hanson MR, Conomy JP, Capraro J. Mitral valve prolapse, cerebral ischemia, and bacterial endocarditis. Neurology 32(Suppl 2):A88, 1982.

Hanson MR, Tomsak RL, Kosmorsky GS. Neuro-ophthalmologic complications of cardiac catheterization. Neurology 36(Suppl 1):193, 1986.

Harbison JW. Ticlopidine versus aspirin for the prevention of recurrent stroke: Analysis of patients with minor stroke from the Ticlopidine Aspirin Stroke Study. Stroke 23:1723–1727, 1992.

Harbison JW, Palmer K, Ochs A. Migrainous amaurosis fugax. Presented at the 7th Annual International Society of Neuro-Ophthalmology Meeting. Vancouver, Canada, May 12, 1988.

Harbridge DF. Spasm of the central retinal artery. Ophthalmic Rev 25:282–284, 1906.

Hardin CA. Vertebral artery insufficiency produced by cervical osteoarthritic spurs. Arch Surg 90:626–664, 1963.

Hardin CA, Williamson WP, Steegman AT. Vertebral artery insufficiency produced by cervical osteoarthritic spurs. Neurology 10:855–858, 1960.

Hardy WG, Lindner DW, Thomas LM, et al. Anticipated clinical course in carotid artery occlusion. Arch Neurol 6:138–150, 1962.

Harker LA, Fuster V. Pharmacology of platelet inhibitors. J Am Coll Cardiol 8:21B–32B, 1986.

Harker LA, Slichter SJ. Platelet and fibrinogen consumption in man. N Engl J Med 287:999–1005, 1972.

Harker LA, Slichter SJ, Scott CR, et al. Homocystinemia: vascular injury and arterial thrombosis. N Engl J Med 291:537–543, 1974.

Harris W. Hemianopia with special reference to its transient varieties. Brain 20:308–364, 1897.

Harrison MJG, Marshall J. Evidence of silent cerebral embolism in patients with amaurosis fugax. J Neurol Neurosurg Psychiatry 40:651–654, 1977.

Harrison MJG, Marshall J. Atrial fibrillation, TIAs, and completed strokes. Stroke 15:441–442, 1984.

Harrison MJG, Marshall J. The variable clinical and CT findings after carotid occlusion: The role of collateral blood supply. J Neurol Neurosurg Psychiatry 51:269–272, 1988.

Harrison MJG, Meadows JC, Marshall J, et al. Effect of aspirin in amaurosis fugax. Lancet 2:743, 1971.

Hart RG. Comparison of ticlopidine and aspirin for the prevention of stroke. N Engl J Med 322:404, 1990.

Hart RG, Easton JD. Mitral valve prolapse and cerebral infarction. Stroke 13:429–430, 1982.

Hart RG, Harrison MJG. Aspirin wars: The optimal dose of aspirin to prevent stroke. Stroke 27:585–587, 1996.

Hart RG, Haworth S. Bilateral common carotid occlusion with hypoxic ocular sequelae. Br J Ophthalmol 55:383–388, 1971.

Hart RG, Miller VT. Cerebral infarction in young adults: A practical approach. Stroke 14:110–114, 1983.

Hart RG, Kanter MC. Hematologic disorders and ischemic stroke. A selective review. Stroke 21:1111–1121, 1990.

Hart RG, Miller VT, Coull B, et al. Cerebral infarction associated with lupus anticoagulants: Preliminary report. Stroke 15:114–118, 1984.

Hart RG, Kagan-Hallet K, Joerns SE. Mechanisms of intracranial hemorrhage in infective endocarditis. Stroke 18:1048–1056, 1987.

Hart RG, Foster JW, Luther MF, et al. Stroke in infective endocarditis. Stroke 21:695–700, 1990.

Hart RG, Boop BS, Anderson DC. Oral anticoagulants and intracranial hemorrhage. Facts and hypotheses. Stroke 26:1471–1477, 1995.

Hartel WC, Spoor TC, Hammer ME. Retinal embolism following percutaneous femoral cerebral angiography. J Clin Neuro-Ophthalmol 2:49–54, 1982.

Hartnett ME, Pruett RC, Dasilva KC, et al. Antiphospholipid antibody syndrome associated with microscotomata. Am J Ophthalmol 118:397–398, 1994.

Harvey JR, Teague SM, Anderson JL, et al. Clinically silent septal defects with evidence for cerebral embolization. Ann Intern Med 105:695–697, 1986.

Harward TRS, Kroener JM, Wickbom IG, et al. Natural history of asymptomatic ulcerative plaques of the carotid bifurcation. Am J Surg 146:208–212, 1983.

Hass WK. Caution falling rock zone: An analysis of the medical and surgical management of threatened stroke. Proc Inst Med Chic 33:80–84, 1980.

Hass WK, Fields WS, North RR, et al. Joint study of extracranial arterial occlusions. II. Arteriography, techniques, sites and complications. JAMA 203:961–968, 1968.

Hass WK, Easton JD, Adams HP Jr, et al. A randomized trial comparing ticlopidine hydrochloride with aspirin for the prevention of stroke in high-risk patients. N Engl J Med 321:501–507, 1989.

Hasso AN, Bird CR, Zinke DE, et al. Fibromuscular dysplasia of the internal carotid artery: Percutaneous transluminal angioplasty. AJNR 2:175–180, 1981.

Haugland JM, Asinger RW, Mikell FL, et al. Embolic potential of left ventricular thrombi detected by two-dimensional echocardiography. Circulation 70:588–594, 1984.

Hauser RA, Lacey M, Knight MR. Hypertensive retinopathy. Magnetic resonance imaging demonstration of reversible cortical and white matter lesions. Arch Neurol 45:1078–1083, 1988.

Haushofer A, Halbmayer WM, Prachar H. Neutropenia with ticlopidine plus aspirin. Lancet 349:474–475, 1997.

Hausmann N, Richard G. Effect of high dose steroid bolus on occlusion of ocular central artery: angiographic study. Br Med J 303:1445–1446, 1991.

Hausser CO, Robert F, Giard N. Balint's syndrome. Can J Neurol Sci 7:157–161, 1980.

Hauw J, Der Agopian P, Trelles L, et al. Les infarctes bulbaires. J Neurol Sci 28:83–102, 1976.

Havel RJ. Classification of the hyperlipidemias. Annu Rev Med 28:195–209, 1977.

Hawkes CH. "Locked-in" syndrome: Report of seven cases. Br Med J 4:379–382, 1974.

Haynes CD, Dempsey SL. Carotid endarterectomy: Review of 276 cases in a community hospital. Ann Surg 189:258–261, 1979.

Haynes RB, Taylor DW, Sackett DL, et al. Prevention of functional impairment by endarterectomy for symptomatic high-grade carotid stenosis. JAMA 271:1256–1259, 1994.

Hayreh SS. Occlusion of the central retinal vessels. Br J Ophthalmol 49:626–645, 1965.

Hayreh SS. Pathogenesis of occlusion of the central retinal vessels. Am J Ophthalmol 72:998–1011, 1971.

Hayreh SS. Anterior ischaemic optic neuropathy. I. Terminology and pathogenesis. Br J Ophthalmol 58:955–963, 1974a.

Hayreh SS. Anterior ischaemic optic neuropathy. III. Treatment, prophylaxis, and differential diagnosis. Br J Ophthalmol 58:981–989, 1974b.

Hayreh SS. Anterior Ischemic Optic Neuropathy. Berlin, Springer-Verlag, 1975.

Hayreh SS. Central retinal vein occlusion. In The Eye and Systemic Disease. Editor, Mausolf FA, 2nd ed, pp 223–275. St Louis, CV Mosby, 1980.

Hayreh SS. Anterior ischemic optic neuropathy. Arch Neurol 38:675–678, 1981a.

Hayreh SS. Anterior ischemic optic neuropathy. V. Optic disc edema as early sign. Arch Ophthalmol 99:1030–1040, 1981b.

Hayreh SS. Posterior ischemic optic neuropathy. Ophthalmologica 182:29–41, 1981c.

Hayreh SS. Classification of central retinal vein occlusion. Ophthalmology 90:458–474, 1983.

Hayreh SS. Discussion of Brown GC, Shah HG, Magargal LE, et al. Central retinal vein obstruction and carotid artery disease. Ophthalmology 91:1631–1633, 1984.

Hayreh SS. Anterior ischemic optic neuropathy. Differentiation of arteritic from non-aneritic type and its management. Eye 4:25–41, 1990.

Hayreh SS, Podhajsky BSN. Ocular neovascularisation with retinal vascular occlusion. Arch Ophthalmol 100:1585–1596, 1982.

Hayreh SS, Joos KM, Podhajsky PA, et al. Systemic diseases associated with nonarter-itic anterior ischemic optic neuropathy. Am J Ophthalmol 118:766–780, 1994.

Hayreh SS, Piegors DJ, Heistad DD. Serotonin-induced constriction of ocular arteries in atherosclerotic monkeys: Implications for ischemic disorders of the retina and optic nerve head. Arch Ophthalmol 115:220–228, 1997.

Healy DA, Clowes AW, Zierler RE, et al. Immediate and long-term results of carotid endarterectomy. Stroke 20:1138–1142, 1989.

Hebel N, von Cramon DY. Der Posteriorinfarkt. Fortschr Neurol Psychiatr 55:37–53, 1987.

Hecaen H, Ajuriaguerra J. Balint syndrome (psychic paralysis of visual fixation) and its minor forms. Brain 77:373–400, 1954.

Hedera P, von Maravic M, Bruckmann H. Effect of collateral flow patterns on outcome of carotid occlusion. Stroke 27:160, 1996.

Hedges TR. Ophthalmoscopic findings in internal carotid occlusion. Bull Johns Hop-kins Hosp 3:89–97, 1962.

Hedges TR. Ophthalmoscopic findings in internal carotid occlusion. Am J Ophthalmol 55:1007–1012, 1963.

Hedges TR, Weinstein JD. Ophthalmic artery pressure response to carotid occlusion. Neurology 14:192–201, 1964.

Hedges TR Jr, Giliberti O, Magargal LE. Intravenous digital subtraction angiography and its role in ocular vascular disease. Arch Ophthalmol 103:666–669, 1985.

Heeney DJ, Koo AH. Bilateral cortical blindness associated with carotid stenosis in a patient with a persistent trigeminal artery. Case report. J Neurosurg 52:709–711, 1980.

Heick A, Birket-Smith M, Fedders O, et al. Dilatation of pupils in a "top of the basilar" stroke. Ophthalmic Res 19:292–297, 1987.

Heilman KM, Watson RT. The neglect syndrome—A unilateral defect in the orienting response. In Lateralization in the Nervous System. Editors, Harnard S, Doty RW, Goldstein L, et al. New York, Academic Press, 1977.

Heilbrun MP, Reichman OH, Anderson RE, et al. Regional cerebral blood flow studies following superficial temporal-middle cerebral artery anastomosis. J Neurosurg 43:706–716, 1975.

Heiman TD, Satya-Murti S. Benign cerebellar hemorrhages. Ann Neurol 3:366–368, 1978.

Heimburger RF, Demyer W, Reitan RM. Implications of Gerstmann's syndrome. J Neurol Neurosurg Psychiatry 27:52–57, 1964.

Heiserman JE, Dean BL, Hodak JA, et al. Neurologic complications of cerebral angi-ography. Am J Neuroradiol 15:1401–1407, 1994.

Heiskala H, Somer H, Kovanen J, et al. Microangiopathy with encephalopathy, hearing loss and retinal aneriolar occlusions: Two new cases. J Neurol Sci 86:239–250, 1988.

Helgason C, Caplan LR, Goodwin J, et al. Anterior choroidal artery-territory infarc-tion. Report of cases and review. Arch Neurol 43:681–686, 1986.

Helgason CM. Blood glucose and stroke. Stroke 19:1049–1053, 1988.

Heller-Bettinger I, Kepes JJ, Preskorn SH., et al. Bilateral altitudinal anopia caused by infarction of the calcarine cortex. Neurology 26:1176–1179, 1976.

Helweg-Larsen S, Sommer W, Strange P, et al. Prognosis for patients treated conserva-tively for spontaneous intracerebral hematomas. Stroke 15:1045–1048, 1984.

Hemmingsen R, Mejsholm B, Vorstrup S, et al. Carotid surgery, cognitive function, and cerebral blood flow in patients with transient ischemic attacks. Ann Neurol 20:13–19, 1986.

Hendricks HT, Franke CL, Theunissen PHMH. Cerebral amyloid angiopathy: Diagno-sis by MRI and brain biopsy. Neurology 40:1308–1310, 1990.

Henkes HE. Electroretinography in circulatory disturbances of the retina. II. The electroretinogram in cases of occlusion of the central retinal artery or one of its branches. Arch Ophthalmol 51:42–53, 1954.

Henn V, Büttner-Ennever JA, Hepp K. The primate oculomotor system. I. Motoneu-rons. II. Premotor system: A synthesis of anatomical, physiological, and clinical data. Hum. Neurobiol. 1:77–95, 1982.

Henn V, Lang W, Hepp K, et al. Experimental gaze palsies in monkeys and their relation to human pathology. Brain 107:619–636, 1984.

Hennerici M, Rautenberg W, Trockel U, et al. Spontaneous progression and regression of small carotid atheroma. Lancet 1:1415–1419, 1985.

Hennerici M, Hülsbömer HB, Hefter H, et al. Natural history of asymptomatic extra-cranial arterial disease. Results of a long-term prospective study. Brain 110:777–791, 1987.

Hennerici M, Klemm C, Rautenberg W. The subclavian steal phenomenon: A common vascular disorder with rare neurologic deficits. Neurology 38:669–673, 1988a.

Hennerici M, Herzog H, Rautenberg W, et al. Intracranial Doppler and positron emis-sion tomography in patients with asymptomatic carotid artery occlusion. Ann Neurol 24:127, 1988b.

Heptinstall S, May JA, Glenn JR, et al. Effects of ticlopidine administered to healthy volunteers on platelet function in whole blood. Thromb Haemost 74:1310–1315, 1995.

Herald S, Kummer R, Jaeger C. Follow-up of spontaneous intracerebral hemorrhage by computed tomography. J Neurol 228:267–276, 1982.

Herbert PR, Gaziano JM, Chan KS, et al. Cholesterol lowering with statin drugs, risk of stroke, and total mortality: An overview of randomized trials. JAMA 278:313–321, 1997.

Herbstein D, Schaumberg H. Hypertensive intracerebral hemorrhage: An investigation of the initial hemorrhage and rebleeding using chromium-Cr51-labeled erythro-cytes. Arch Neurol 30:412–414, 1974.

Herman B, Leyten ACM, Luijk JH, et al. Epidemiology of stroke in Tilburg, The Netherlands. Stroke 13:629–634, 1982.

Herman P. Migraine, large pupils, mitral valve prolapse, and emotional disturbances: An autonomic disorder. Headache 27:340–344, 1987.

Herman P. Migraine and mitral valve prolapse. Arch Neurol 46:1165, 1989.

Heros RC. Comment on Mehdorn HM, Nau HE, Förster M. Carotid artery occlusion and ocular ischemia: Therapy control with evoked potentials. Neurosurgery 19:1034, 1986.

Heros RC, Korosue K. Hemodilution for cerebral ischemia. Stroke 20:423–427, 1989.

Hershey FB, Barnes RW, Sumner DS. Noninvasive Diagnosis of Vascular Disease. Pasadena, CA, Appleton Davies, 1984.

Herskovitz S, Lipton RB, Lantos G. Neuro-Behçet's disease: CT and clinical corre-lates. Neurology 38:1714–1720, 1988.

Hertle RW, Bienfang DC. Oculographic analysis of acute esotropia secondary to a thalamic hemorrhage. J Clin Neuro-Ophthalmol 10:21–26, 1990.

Hertzer NR, Beven EG, Benjamin SP. Ultramicroscopic ulcerations and thrombi of the carotid bifurcation. Arch Surg 112:1394–1402, 1977.

Hertzer NR, Avellone JC, Farrell CJ, et al. The risk of vascular surgery in a metropoli-tan community, with observations on surgeon experience and hospital size. J Vasc Surg 1:13–21, 1984.

Hess RF, Pointer JS. Spatial and temporal contrast sensitivity in hemianopia. A com-parative study of the sighted and blind hemifields. Brain 112:871–894, 1989.

Heubner D. Die Luetische Erkrankung der Hirnarterien. Leipzig, Vogel-Verlag KG, 1874.

Heuer DK, Gager WE, Reeser FH. Ischemic optic neuropathy associated with Crohn's disease. J Clin Neuro-Ophthalmol 2:175–181, 1982.

Heyden S, Heiss G, Heyman A, et al. Cardiovascular mortality in transient ischemic attacks. Stroke 11:252–255, 1980.

Heydenreich A. Die Durchblutungestörungen am Auge bei der "Pulseless Disease." Z Aerztl Fortbild 51:199–204, 1957.

Heyman A, Leviton A, Millikan CH, et al. Report of the Joint Committee for Stroke Facilities. XI. Transient focal cerebral ischemia: Epidemiological and clinical aspects. Stroke 5:277–287, 1974.

Heyman A, Wilkinson WE, Heyden S, et al. Risk of stroke in asymptomatic persons with cervical arterial bruits: A population study in Evans County, Georgia. N Engl J Med 302:838–841, 1980.

Heyman A, Wilkinson WE, Hurwitz BJ, et al. Clinical and epidemiologic aspects of vertebrobasilar and nonfocal cerebral ischemia. In Vertebrobasilar Arterial Occlusive Disease. Medical and Surgical Management. Editors, Berguer R, Bauer RB, pp 27–36. New York, Raven Press, 1984a.

Heyman A, Wilkinson WE, Hurwitz BJ, et al. Risk of ischemic heart disease in patients with TIA. Neurology 34:626–630, 1984b.

Hicks PA, Leavitt JA, Mokri B. Opthalmic manifestations of vertebral artery dissec-tion: Patients seen at the Mayo Clinic from 1976 to 1992. Ophthalmology 101:1786–1792, 1994.

Hier DB, Davis K, Richardson EP Jr, et al. Hypertensive putaminal hemorrhage. Arch Neurol 1:152–159, 1977.

Hier DB, Babcock DJ, Foulkes MA. Influence of site on course of intracerebral hemorrhage. J Stroke Cerebrovasc Dis 3:65–74, 1993.

Higashida RT, Tsai FY, Halbach VV, et al. Interventional neurovascular techniques in the treatment of stroke—state-of-the-art therapy. J Intern Med 237:105–115, 1995.

Higgins JJ, Kammerman LA, Fitz CK. Stroke in children: A ten-year experience at a children's hospital. Ann Neurol 26:480, 1989.

Higgins RA. Neovascular glaucoma associated with ocular hypoperfusion secondary to carotid artery disease. Aust J Ophthalmol 12:155–162, 1984.

Hill TC, Magistretti PL, Holman BL, et al. Assessment of regional cerebral blood flow [rCBF] in stroke using SPECT and N-isopropyl [I-122]-p-iodoamphetamine [IMP]. Stroke 15:40–45, 1984.

Hillbom M, Haapaniemi H, Juvela S, et al. Recent alcohol consumption, cigarette smoking, and cerebral infarction in young adults. Stroke 26:40–45, 1995.

Hilton GF, Hoyt WF. An arteriosclerotic chiasmal syndrome. Bitemporal hemianopia associated with fusiform dilatation of the anterior cerebral arteries. JAMA 196:200–202, 1966.

Hilton-Jones D, Ponsford JR, Graham N. Transient visual obscurations, without papill-oedema. J Neurol Neurosurg Psychiatry 45:832–834, 1982.

Hindfelt B, Nilsson O. Brain infarction in young adults. Acta Neurol Scand 55:145–157, 1977.

Hinton RC, Kistler JP, Fallon JT, et al. Influence of etiology of atrial fibrillation on incidence of systemic embolism. Am J Cardiol 40:509–513, 1977.

Hirose G, Kin T, Murakami E. Alexia without agraphia associated with right occipital lesion. J Neurol Neurosurg Psychiatry 40:225–227, 1977.

Hirose G, Kosoegawa H, Saeki M, et al. The syndrome of posterior thalamic hemor-rhage. Neurology 35:998–1002, 1985.

Hirsch MS, Aikat BK, Basu AK. Takayasu's arteritis: Report of five cases with immunologic studies. Bull Johns Hopkins Hosp 115:29–64, 1964.

Hirsh J. The optimal antithrombotic dose of aspirin. Arch Intern Med 145:1582–1583, 1985.

Hirsh J. Oral anticoagulant drugs. N Engl J Med 324:1865, 1991.

Hirsh J, Levine M. Therapeutic range for the control of oral anticoagulant therapy. Arch Neurol 43:1162–1164, 1986.

Ho SU, Kim KS, Berenberg RA, et al. Cerebellar infarction: A clinical and CT study. Surg Neurol 16:350–352, 1981.

Hoare AM, Keogh AJ. Cerebrovascular moyamoya disease. Br Med J 1:430–432, 1974.

Hobson RW II, Weiss DG, Fields WS, et al. Efficacy of carotid endarterectomy for asymptomatic carotid stenosis. N Engl J Med 328:221–227, 1993.

Hodgman MT, Pessin MS, Homans DC, et al. Cerebral embolism as the initial manifestation of preipartum cardiomyopathy. Neurology 32:668–671, 1982.

Hoefnagels KLJ. Rubeosis of the iris associated with occlusion of the carotid artery. Ophthalmologica 148:196–200, 1964.

Hoffman WF, Wilson CB, Townsend JJ. Recurrent transient ischemic attacks secondary to an embolizing saccular middle cerebral artery aneurysm. Case report. J Neurosurg 51:103–106, 1979.

Hofmann T, Kasper W, Meindertz T, et al. Echocardiographic evaluation of patients with clinically suspected arterial emboli. Lancet 336:1421–1424, 1990.

Hogan MJ, Kimura SJ, Thygeson P. Uveitis in association with rheumatism. Arch Ophthalmol 57:400–413, 1957.

Holladay JT, Arnoult JB, Ruiz RS. Comparative evaluation of current ophthalmodynamometers. Am J Ophthalmol 87:665–674, 1979.

Hollenhorst RW. Ophthalmodynamometry and intracranial vascular disease. Med Clin North Am 48:951–958, 1958.

Hollenhorst RW. Ocular manifestations of insufficiency or thrombosis of the internal carotid artery. Am J Ophthalmol 47:753–767, 1959.

Hollenhorst RW. Significance of bright plaques in the retinal arterioles. JAMA 178:23–29, 1961.

Hollenhorst RW. Carotid and vertebral-basilar arterial stenosis and occlusion: Neumophthalmologic considerations. Trans Am Acad Ophthalmol Otolaryngol 66:166–180, 1962.

Hollenhorst RW. The neuro-ophthalmology of strokes. In Neuro-Ophthalmology Symposium of the University of Miami and the Bascom Palmer Eye Institute. Editor, Smith JL, Vol 2, pp 109–121. St Louis, CV Mosby, 1965.

Hollenhorst RW. Embolic retinal phenomena. In Symposium on Neuro-Ophthalmology. Transactions of the New Orleans Academy of Ophthalmology. Pp 168–190. St Louis, CV Mosby, 1976.

Hollenhorst RW, Kearns TP. The fluorescein dye test of circulation time in patients with occlusive disease of the carotid arterial system. Mayo Clin Proc 36:457–465, 1961.

Hollenhorst RW, Wagener HP. Loss of vision after distant hemorrhage. Am J Med Sci 218:209–218, 1950.

Hollenhorst RW, Brown JR, Wagener HP, et al. Neurologic aspects of temporal arteritis. Neurology 10:490–498, 1960.

Holley KE, Bahn RC, McGoon DC, et al. Spontaneous calcific embolization associated with calcific aortic stenosis. Circulation 27:197–202, 1963a.

Holley KE, Bahn RC, McGoon DL, et al. Calcific embolization associated with valvotomy for calcific aortic stenosis. Circulation 28:175–181, 1963b.

Holman BL, Tumeh SS. Single-photon emission computed tomography (SPECT). Applications and potential. JAMA 263:561–564, 1990.

Hommel M, Besson G, Pollak P, et al. Pure sensory stroke due to a pontine lacune. Stroke 20:406–408, 1989.

Hommel M, Besson G, Pollak P, et al. Hemiplegia in posterior cerebral artery occlusion. Neurology 40:1496–1499, 1990a.

Hommel M, Besson G, Le Bas JF, et al. Prospective study of lacunar infarction using magnetic resonance imaging. Stroke 21:546–554, 1990b.

Hommel M, Moreaud O, Besson G, et al. Site of arterial occlusion in the hemiplegic posterior cerebral artery syndrome. Neurology 41:604–605, 1991.

Hommel M, Boissel JP, Cornu C, et al. Termination of trial of streptokinase in severe acute ischaemic stroke. Lancet 345:57, 1995.

Hopkins LN, Budny JL. Complications of intracranial bypass for vertebro-basilar insufficiency. J Neurosurg 70:207–211, 1989.

Hopkins LN, Martin NA, Hadley MN, et al. Vertebrobasilar insufficiency. Part 2. Microsurgical treatment of intra-cranial vertebrobasilar disease. J Neurosurg 66:662–674, 1987.

Horenstein S, Chamberlain W, Conomy J. Infarction of the fusiform and calcarine regions: Agitated delirium and hemianopsia. Trans Am Neurol Assoc 92:357–367, 1962.

Horenstein S, Hambrook G, Roat GW, et al. Arteriographic correlates of transient ischemic attacks. Trans Am Neurol Assoc 97:132–136, 1972.

Hornig CR, Dorndorf W, Agnoli AL. Hemorrhagic infarction—A prospective study. Stroke 17:179–185, 1986.

Hörnsten G. Wallenberg's syndrome. Part I. General symptomatology, with special reference to visual disturbances and imbalance. Acta Neurol Scand 50:434–446, 1974a.

Hörnsten G. Wallenberg's syndrome. Part II. Oculomotor and oculostatic disturbances. Acta Neurol Scand 50:447–468, 1974b.

Horowitz DR, Tuhrim S, Budd J, et al. Aortic plaque in patients with brain ischemia: Diagnosis by transesophageal echocardiography. Neurology 42:1602–1604., 1992.

Horwitz NH, Wener L. Temporary cortical blindness following angiography. J Neurosurg 40:583–586, 1974.

Hotson JR, Pedley TA. The neurological complications of cardiac transplantation. Brain 99:673–694, 1976.

Hougaku H, Matsumoto M, Handa N, et al. Asymptomatic carotid lesions and silent cerebral infarction. Stroke 25:566–570, 1994.

Houser OW, Sundt TM Jr, Holman CB, et al. Atheromatous disease of the carotid artery. Correlation of angiographic, clinical, and surgical findings. J Neurosurg 41:321–331, 1974.

Howard G, Brockschmidt JK, Rose LA, et al. Changes in survival after transient ischemic attacks: Observations comparing the 1970s and 1980s. Neurology 39:982–985, 1989.

Howard RS, Ross Russell RW. Prognosis of patients with retinal embolism. J Neurol Neurosurg Psychiatry 50:1142–1147, 1987.

Howard VJ, Howard G, Harpold GJ, et al. Correlation of carotid bruits and carotid atherosclerosis detected by B-mode real-time ultrasonography. Stroke 20:1331–1335, 1989.

Hoyt CS. Acquired "double elevator" palsy and polycythemia vera. J Pediatr Ophthalmol Strabis 15:362–365, 1978.

Hoyt WF. Some neuro-ophthalmologic considerations in cerebral vascular insufficiency. Arch Ophthalmol 62:260–272, 1959.

Hoyt WF. Vascular lesions of the visual cortex with brain herniation through the tentorial incisura. Arch Ophthalmol 64:44–57, 1960.

Hoyt WF. Transient bilateral blurring of vision. Arch Ophthalmol 70:746–751, 1963.

Hoyt WF. Retinal ischemic symptoms in cardiovascular diagnosis. Postgrad Med 52:85–90, 1972.

Hoyt WF, Beeston D. The Ocular Fundus in Neurologic Disease. A Diagnostic Manual and Stereo Atlas. P 114. St Louis, CV Mosby, 1966.

Hoyt WF, Newton TH. Angiographic changes with occlusion of arteries that supply the visual cortex. NZ Med J 72:310–317, 1970.

Hoyt WF, Walsh FB. Cortical blindness with partial recovery following acute cerebral anoxia from cardiac arrest. Arch Ophthalmol 60:1061–1069, 1958.

Hriso E, Miller A, Masdeu JC. Monocular elevation weakness and ptosis. Neurology 1(Suppl):309, 1990.

Hu HH, Liao KK, Wong WJ, et al. Ocular bruits in ischemic cerebrovascular disease. Stroke 19:1229–1233, 1988.

Hu HH, Sheng WY, Yen MY, et al. Color doppler imaging of orbital arteries for detection of carotid occlusive disease. Stroke 24:1196–1203, 1993.

Huckman MS, Haas J. Reversed flow through the ophthalmic artery as a cause of rubeosis iridis. Am J Ophthalmol 74:1094–1099, 1972.

Hughes B. Blood supply of the optic nerves and chiasm and its clinical significance. Br J Ophthalmol 42:106–125, 1958.

Hull R, Hirsh J. Long-term anticoagulant therapy in patients with venous thrombosis. Arch Intern Med 143:2061–2063, 1983.

Hultquist GT. Über Thrombose und Embolie der Arteria carotis und hierbei vorkommende Gehirnveränderungen. Eine pathologische-anatomische Studie. Stockholm, Gustav Fischer Verlag, 1942.

Humphrey JG, Newton TH. Internal carotid artery occlusions in young adults. Brain 83:565–578, 1960.

Humphrey WT. Central retinal artery spasm. Ann Ophthalmol 11:877–881, 1979.

Humphreys RP. Computerized tomographic definition of mesencephalic hematoma with evacuation through pedunculotomy. Case report. J Neurosurg 49:749–752, 1978.

Humphries AW, Young JR, Santilli PH, et al. Unoperated, asymptomatic significant internal carotid artery stenosis: A review of 182 instances. Surgery 80:695–698, 1976.

Hunt JR. The role of the carotid arteries and causation of vascular lesions of the brain with remarks on certain special features of the symptomatology. Am J Med Sci 147:704–713, 1914.

Hupp SL, David NJ, Glaser JS. Consecutive bilateral retinal artery occlusion. Neuroophthalmology 4:137–140, 1984.

Hupperts RMM, Lodder J, Heuts-van Raak EPM, et al. Infarcts in the anterior choroidal artery territory: Anatomical distribution, clinical syndromes, presumed pathogenesis and early outcome. Brain 117:825–834, 1994.

Hurst JW, Hopkins LG, Smith RB III. Noises in the neck. N Engl J Med 302:862–863, 1980.

Hurwitz BJ, Heyman A, Wilkinson WE, et al. Comparison of amaurosis fugax and transient cerebral ischemia: A prospective clinical and arteriographic study. Ann Neurol 18:698–704, 1985.

Hussain M, Stein J. Rezsö Bálint and his most celebrated case. Arch Neurol 45:89–93, 1988.

Hutchinson EC, Yates PO. The cervical portion of the vertebral artery: A clinical pathological study. Brain 79:319–331, 1956.

Hutton WL, Snyder WB, Fuller D, et al. Focal parafoveal retinal telangiectasia. Arch Ophthalmol 96:1361–1367, 1978.

Hylek EM, Singer DE. Risk factors for intracranial hemorrhage in outpatients taking warfarin. Ann Intern Med 120:897–902, 1994.

Hylek EM, Skates SJ, Sheehan MA, et al. An analysis of the lowest effective intensity

dent whom we examined was an All-American college lacrosse player who began to experience episodes of monocular visual loss during both practice and lacrosse games. There was significant debate regarding whether or not the young man should be allowed to continue playing lacrosse, particularly because the episodes of visual loss began just before the start of the National College Athletic Association lacrosse tournament. When we saw him, he was agitated and depressed because of the possibility that he would not be able to compete in the upcoming tournament or continue playing lacrosse or other sports. He was afraid that he would have to quit college because of this. After evaluating the patient, it was our opinion that he was experiencing exercise-induced migraine. We recommended that he be allowed to play, and he did so without incident. He continued to play lacrosse the following year, occasionally experiencing brief episodes of visual loss in one or the other eye. Five years later, the patient experienced the first of several typical migraine headaches, some of which were preceded by visual aura.

Although allergy is considered by some investigators to be a precipitant of migraine, migraine itself is not usually considered an allergic condition (Diamond and Medina, 1980; Davidoff, 1995). Medina and Diamond (1976) determined the serum concentration of immunoglobulin E (IgE) in 99 patients with migraine and compared the results with the concentration in 27 patients with muscle contraction headaches. Elevated IgE concentrations were found in 5.7% of patients with migraine and in 3.7% of patients with muscle contraction headaches. Medina and Diamond (1976) also questioned 504 patients about personal and family history of atopy. Seventy-three of these patients had muscle contraction headaches, 55 had cluster headaches, 259 had migraine, and 117 had both muscle contraction headaches and migraine. The prevalence of atopy in these patient groups did not differ significantly from each other or from the prevalence in the general population.

Some investigators believe that cerebral angiography can induce an attack of migraine with permanent neurologic, visual, or systemic sequelae (Patterson et al., 1964; Diamond and Dalessio, 1982). In some of these patients, angiography shows evidence of arterial vasospasm (Dukes and Vieth, 1964; Kwentus et al., 1985). To assess the risk of angiography-induced migraine, Shuaib and Hachinski (1988) reviewed the charts of 142 patients with a final diagnosis of migraine who had undergone a total of 149 angiograms for a variety of reasons, including acute headache, exertional headache, and new focal symptoms. Six patients had basilar artery migraine, five had ophthalmoplegic migraine, and three had hemiplegic migraine. The remainder of the patients had either migraine headaches with typical aura or migraine headaches without aura. Transient cerebral events, including amnesia, hemisensory changes, hemiparesis, and global confusion, occurred in only five patients (3.5%) during or shortly after cerebral angiography. Three of these patients also developed a migraine headache, but no patient experienced a permanent neurologic or visual deficit following angiography. One patient experienced an attack of angina that lasted 3 minutes, and one patient with a history of severe ischemic heart disease developed a myocardial infarction 2 hours after angiography. Over the same period, 2.8% of 1002 consecutive patients who underwent angiography at the same institute experienced temporary focal symptoms after angiography, and another 0.4% of patients experienced permanent sequelae (Dion et al., 1987). The findings of Shuaib and Hachinski (1988) suggested that cerebral angiography that is performed in a patient with known or suspected migraine can occasionally induce a typical migraine attack but rarely produces a permanent visual or neurologic sequela.

CLINICAL CHARACTERISTICS OF MIGRAINE BY TYPE

MIGRAINE WITHOUT AURA (COMMON MIGRAINE)

Migraine without aura has been generally accepted to replace the term **common migraine** and is defined by a set of criteria developed by the Headache Classification Committee of the International Headache Society (1988) (Tab. 56.3). Whether one refers to this condition as common migraine or migraine without aura, the basic features of a migraine headache without preceding, well-defined visual symptoms, neurologic symptoms, or both are well-documented (Selby and Lance, 1960; Lance and Anthony, 1966; Olesen, 1978; Tfelt-Hansen and Olesen, 1985; Solomon et al., 1988; Hupp et al., 1989; Davidoff, 1995; Silberstein, 1995).

Migraine headaches without aura affect at least 10% of the population (Troost, 1988) and probably are much more prevalent, because many patients have mild headaches that undoubtedly are a form of migraine but that go unreported because they occur infrequently, are of a mild nature, or are simply accepted by the patient as a part of life (Waters and O'Connor, 1971).

Migraine headaches without aura are responsible for about 60% of all types of migraine attacks (Troost, 1988). They are unilateral in adults about 60–70% of the time (Diamond, 1987; Solomon et al., 1988; Davidoff, 1995; Silberstein, 1995), but only 20% to 30% of the time in children (Davidoff, 1995). They vary greatly from person to person, and they and may also differ in frequency, duration, and intensity at different times in the same person.

The frequency of attacks of migraine without aura is unpredictable. Most sufferers of this condition experience one to four headaches a month, but some persons complain of headache every few days, and others experience only one or two a year (Diamond and Medina, 1980). Migraine headaches rarely occur on a daily basis; however, Medina and Diamond (1977, 1981) described a group of patients with migraine whose headaches occurred in groups separated by headache-free periods. The attacks occurred in cycles that lasted an average of 6 weeks. During each cycle, severe headaches occurred several times per week and lasted about 24 hours. The cycles were accompanied by depression in

Table 56.3
Diagnostic Criteria for Migraine Without Aura (Common Migraine)

At least five attacks lasting 4–72 hours
Headache has at least two of the following characteristics:
   Unilateral location
   Pulsating quality
   Moderate or severe intensity
   Aggravation by routine physical activity
At least one of the following during headache:
   Nausea and/or vomiting
   Photophobia and phonophobia
Normal neurologic exam and no evidence of organic disease that could
   cause headaches

Adapted from the Headache Classification Committee of the International Headache Society, 1988.

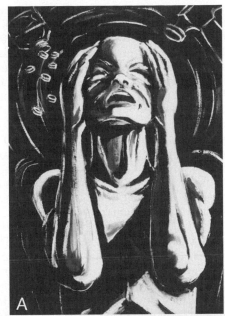

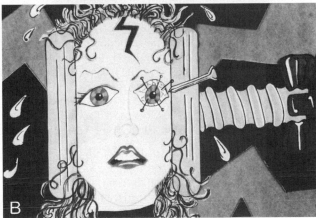

Figure 56.2. Artists' depictions of their own migraine headaches. *A*, By Gerard MacKay Jr.; *B*, By Lisa Lamotte. (Courtesy of Sandoz Pharmaceutical Company.)

many patients. The cycles recurred an average of five times a year.

Most migraine headaches last a minimum of 4 hours, with many lasting 1 or 2 days (Diamond and Medina, 1980). Very severe attacks may last for several weeks (Diamond, 1987).

A migraine headache usually begins as a dull ache that gradually develops into a pulsating or throbbing type of pain. The pulsating or throbbing sensation is thought to be a feature that can be used to distinguish migraine headaches from nonmigraine headaches (Solomon et al., 1988). The pain, which initially may come and go, eventually becomes constant. It can vary in intensity from a barely perceptible ache to a severity causing prostration (Fig. 56.2). When the headache is severe, it may be worsened by sudden changes in position, walking, or bodily effort. Bright lights and loud noises also may increase the intensity of a migraine headache, as may any mental effort. On the other hand, pressure on the superficial scalp arteries in the region of the pain may reduce the severity of the headache (Graham, 1979; Drummond and Lance, 1983; Davidoff, 1995).

Nausea usually accompanies severe migraine headaches, although vomiting does not usually occur unless the headaches are of long duration. Lewis et al. (1988) described a patient with common migraine who had episodes of syncope that occurred only in association with the nausea and vomiting of a migraine attack. An evaluation revealed that the patient had paroxysmal sinus bradycardia and atrioventricular block apparently caused by increased vagal activity associated with vomiting (Talwar et al., 1985). Anorexia also may occur in association with a migraine headache, with a severity corresponding to that of the headache. When the headache is mild, anorexia tends to be minimal and may even be absent. When the headache is severe, however, anorexia is always present, usually severe, and associated with nausea, vomiting, or both. Nausea, vomiting, anorexia, or a combination of these occur in about 90% of cases (Selby and Lance, 1960; Lance and Anthony, 1966; Olesen, 1978; Diamond, 1987; Solomon et al., 1988; Davidoff, 1995).

Photophobia often occurs in patients during a migraine headache (Selby and Lance, 1960; Olesen, 1978; Solomon et al., 1988; Davidoff, 1995). The pathophysiology of photophobia in patients with migraine is unknown, although Eck-

ardt et al. (1943) suggested that it is caused by vascular irritation of the trigeminal nerve (see Chapter 36).

Minor disturbances in sympathetic dysfunction occur in some patients during an attack of migraine without aura. Drummond (1990) evaluated 80 patients with unilateral migrainous headache and found that during and between episodes of headache, the pupil on the symptomatic side dilated more slowly and less extensively in darkness than the opposite pupil, suggesting that the oculosympathetic pathway was compromised. Drummond (1990) used thermography to show that patients with this apparent oculosympathetic dysfunction also had a warmer upper forehead and orbit on the side of the headache. These findings suggested that extracranial vascular changes and oculosympathetic dysfunction during migraine without aura are caused by activation of trigeminal-vascular reflexes or by antidromic release of vasoactive substances from trigeminal nerve terminals.

Rare patients with migraine without aura develop periorbital ecchymosis associated with a typical attack (Brasch and Levinsohn, 1898; DeBroff and Spierings, 1990; Troost, 1996). The cause of the ecchymosis, which accompanies the headache and resolves over several days, is unknown. Vascular fragility may play a role in some patients; however, other patients have an undiscovered vascular lesion, such as an orbital varix or lymphangioma, that is responsible for the hemorrhage.

Most patients who suffer from migraine without aura do not appear to have any permanent deficits. This may not be true. Hooker and Raskin (1986) administered a number of neuropsychologic tests to 15 patients with common migraine and compared the results with those from 15 matched volunteers without headache. Subjects with migraine were required to have a 2-year or longer history of 1–10 attacks per month, each lasting no longer than 24 hours. The group of patients with common migraine demonstrated significantly greater neuropsychologic impairment and more self-reported cognitive difficulties than the nonheadache group. On the basis of these findings, Hooker and Raskin (1986) speculated that common migraine, like classic migraine (see below), may produce a disturbance of cerebral function that persists beyond the attack itself. Other investigators have not been able to corroborate these findings (Leijdekkers et al., 1990), and they have speculated that the findings of Hooker and Raskin (1986) may only be valid for a small number of patients with common migraine.

MIGRAINE WITH AURA (CLASSIC MIGRAINE)

Migraine with aura, the new term replacing classic migraine, has three distinct parts: the aura, the headache, and the post-headache period. It therefore tends to be a more well defined clinical syndrome than is migraine without aura. Migraine with aura is defined by the Headache Classification Committee of the International Headache Society (1988) as at least two attacks, each of which includes three of the four features listed in Tab. 56.4. The criteria also include a normal neurologic exam and no evidence of organic disease that could cause headaches (Headache Classification Committee of the International Headache Society, 1988). This form of migraine is responsible for about 10–35% of migraine at-

Table 56.4
Diagnostic Criteria for Migraine With Aura (Classic Migraine)

At least two attacks
Aura must exhibit at least three of following characteristics:
　Fully reversible and indicative of focal cerebral cortical and/or brain stem dysfunction
　Gradual onset
　Duration less than 60 minutes
　Followed by headache with a free interval of less than 60 minutes, or headache may begin before or simultaneously with the aura
Normal neurologic exam and no evidence of organic disease that could cause headaches

Adapted from the Headache Classification Committee of the International Headache Society, 1988.

Table 56.5
Visual Phenomena of Migraine

Silver streaks
White lights
Light objects appear excessively bright
All objects appear gray or yellow
Photophobia
Distortion of all linear objects
Dancing and moving cobwebs
Moving black veils
Scintillating picket fences
Silver stars
Wavy perpendicular lines
Flashing gold lights
Fourth-of-July sparklers (prevent reading)
Pinwheels
Welder's sparks
Sparkling starlike objects
Rotating gears
Visual field interference (multiple)
Diplopia
Zigzag streaks of light
Shimmering spots of light
Small pinpoint circles of light (red, yellow, blue)
Varicolored circles
Green spots (partial loss of vision)
Central bright-red flashing lights
Shimmering gray-brown spots (partial loss of vision)
Corrugated lines of light
Irregular reddish areas
Shimmering reddish circles (enlarge and interfere with vision)
Black spaces surrounded by shimmering triangles
Rotating black or dark gray spots
Halo vision (without glaucoma)
Herringbone pattern
Narrowed peripheral fields (prevent reading)

tacks (Diamond and Medina, 1980; Diamond, 1987) and may be preceded by nonspecific premonitory or prodromal symptoms (see above).

Aura

The syndrome of classic migraine begins with a brief period of visual disturbance, neurologic dysfunction, or both called an **aura** (from the Latin, meaning a breeze, odor, or gleam of light). The aura of classic migraine usually lasts 5–60 minutes, although it may last longer. When the aura of classic migraine lasts only a few minutes, it usually terminates before the headache begins. Between the visual or neurologic disturbance and the headache, there may be a symptom-free interval during which the patient feels relatively well. The headache then begins and gradually worsens. When an aura lasts 30–60 minutes, there is usually an overlap between the aura and the headache, with the visual or neurologic symptoms diminishing as the headache begins. In some cases, the aura persists for a few minutes or even hours during the headache phase.

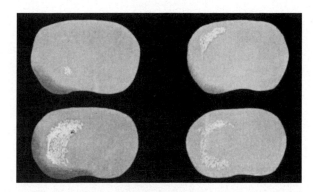

Figure 56.3. Progressive visual aura of migraine. The four drawings depict successive stages of the visual aura of an attack of migraine. In this case, an initial dimness began peripherally in the left lower portion of the visual field of both eyes. This was followed immediately by the appearance of a stellate sphere that was adjacent to the region of dimness but separate from it (*top left*). The sphere disappeared, but from its neighborhood came a luminous zigzag that developed suddenly and expanded superiorly still in the left homonymous hemifield (*bottom left*). Noncolored circles of light were seen between the zigzag lines. With time, the disturbed visual field began to clear (*bottom right*). Complete clearing occurred first in the inferior left quadrant, where the disturbance had begun (*top right*). The visual field eventually returned to normal, at which time an intense headache began in the opposite temple. (From Gowers WR. Subjective visual sensations. Trans Ophthalmol Soc UK *15*:1–38, 1895.)

Visual Aura

The visual disturbances that comprise the aura of classic migraine are many and varied, because they can arise from any part of the visual sensory pathway (Tab. 56.5) (Speed, 1964; Hachinski et al., 1973). These abnormal visual sensations originate from the striate cortex in most cases, but

sometimes they originate from the retina, optic nerve, or even the optic chiasm.

VISUAL DISTURBANCES ORIGINATING IN THE STRIATE CORTEX

Transient Visual Disturbances. Most patients with classic migraine experience an aura that consists of binocular scotomas associated with impressions of glittering lights or shimmering, silvery, wave-like phenomena much like the heat waves that one sees driving on the highway on a hot summer day (Hachinski et al., 1973; Miyazaki et al., 1976; Melen et al., 1978) (Fig. 56.3). The subjective details of

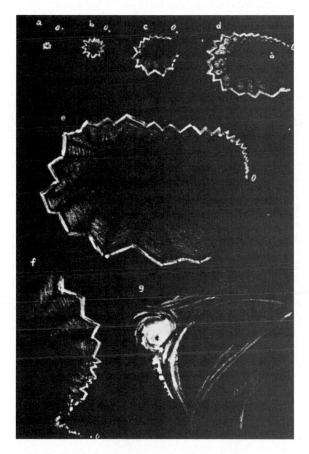

Figure 56.5. Left-sided fortification aura of migraine. This illustration by the astronomer Dr. Hubert Airy is a copy of a colored drawing that depicted Dr. Airy's own scotoma. (*a*), A bright stellate object suddenly appeared below and to the left side of fixation (*o*). It enlarged rapidly, first as a circular reduplicated zigzag, with the inner duplications being seen more faintly than the outer ones (*b*). As the arc of the circle increased, the circle opened centrally toward fixation (*c*). It then became more oval in shape (*d*), and the lines that made up the fortification spectrum became longer as the process extended toward the periphery of the visual field (*e*). When the spectrum had extended through the greater portion of the visual field away from fixation, the upper portion began to expand (*f*). At this time, the lower part of the spectrum disappeared. The phenomenon ended in a whirling beam of light (*g*) 20 minutes after it began. At this time, Dr. Airy developed a right-sided headache. (From Airy H: Phil Trans Roy Soc *160*:247–264, 1870.)

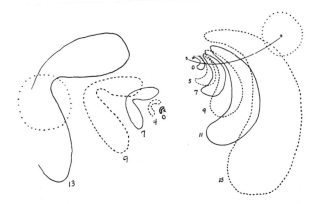

Figure 56.4. Spread of a migrainous scotoma from the center of the visual field to the periphery. Two maps depicting the shape and rate of the drift of negative scotomas observed and recorded by K.S. Lashley in 1941. The numbers indicate the number of minutes that it took before the scotoma expanded to a new position. *O* indicates the center of the visual field. The dotted circle indicates the position of the normal blind spot. Lashley noted that the form of the scotomas remained constant as they drifted toward the periphery of the visual field. (From Lashley KS. Patterns of cerebral integration indicated by the scotomas of migraine. Arch Neurol Psychiatr *46*:331–339, 1941.)

migrainous scotomas have been described by numerous medical and nonmedical writers. Some of the most detailed descriptions were those of Gowers (1888, 1893, 1895) and of Jolly (1902). These authors emphasized that the scotoma is usually restricted to the right or left half of the visual field and ranges in size from a scarcely noticeable blind spot to a complete homonymous hemianopia. The scotoma may appear suddenly near the center of vision, or it may gradually develop. In most cases, the scotoma begins as a disturbance of central vision that steadily spreads into the peripheral field (Fig. 56.4). As the scotoma enlarges, the disturbed area moves or drifts across the visual field so that its central border moves away from the center of fixation as its peripheral margin invades the temporal or nasal field (Figs. 56.5 and 56.6). However, spread from the peripheral field toward the central field also may occur. This pattern is often associated with development of a complete homonymous hemianopia.

Scotomas that originate from the visual cortex may be negative (i.e., the region is completely dark) or positive (i.e., the region is light). Positive scotomas are often associated with brilliantly colored shimmering lights. These lights often present as a curtain across a portion of the visual field, preventing the patient from seeing clearly (Fig. 56.7). This visual sensation is called **teichopsia** (from the Greek, "teichos," meaning wall, and "opsia," meaning vision).

Whether or not they are associated with teichopsia, homonymous scotomas that occur as a visual aura in classic migraine often have a shimmering border (Fig. 56.8). These scintillating scotomas are perhaps the most common visual disturbance experienced by patients with classic migraine (Walsh, 1951; Manzoni et al., 1985; Hupp et al., 1989). The border of a scintillating scotoma is illuminated and seems to flicker and undulate. The outline is often that of a series of reduplicated, parallel, silvery or colored lines that form angles or polygons along the leading edge of the scotoma

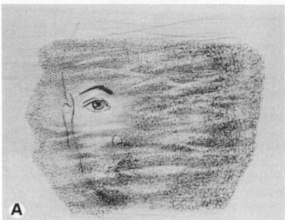

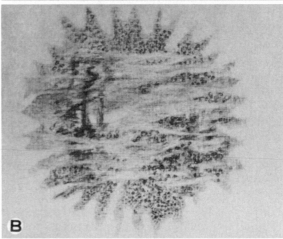

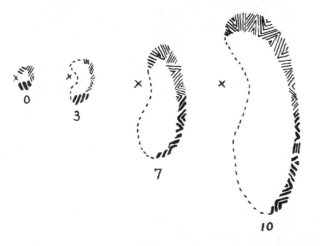

Figure 56.6. Successive maps of a scintillating scotoma showing gradual enlargement of fortification figures and gradual movement away from fixation (*x*). These drawings were made by Lashley as he observed his own scotomas. (From Lashley KS: Patterns of cerebral integration indicated by the scotomas of migraine. Arch Neurol Psychiatr *46*:331–339, 1941.)

Figure 56.7. Two examples of the visual aura of migraine drawn by a 50-year-old artist who had suffered from migraine since adolescence. Following a prodromal period marked by a feeling of apprehension, the patient's visual symptoms began. The patient first noted horizontal wavering images, as if everything were being observed through a "sheet of water." *A*, This drawing depicts the areas of her son's face that were visible and those that were blurred out. The blurred area included the entire right side of the visual field and the inferior left visual field. The patient stated that everything that she could see looked "fluid." "Pinpoint-like globules were present in the area of visual loss . . . it was like snow on a TV screen . . . contours of objects seemed to waver and move like reflections in water . . . there were no zigzags in the periphery . . . it was as if something was wrong with the horizontal adjustment of the TV set . . . all color was gone . . . the attack lasted about 30 minutes and then I could see again but my face on the right side and my right hand became numb, and then my headache started." *B*, On another occasion, the same patient experienced what she described as a "sunburst attack." It occurred as she was driving down a wooded road. It started as did her usual attacks, and she quickly stopped her car. She remembered that the color green (trees) could be seen only in the central portion of the left field of vision. "Zigzag bright light surrounded the central area, and tiny molecular droplets danced aimlessly through the image. All forms that could be perceived seemed to wobble like reflections in water. Horizontal ripples passed back and forth across the central field of vision. The periphery of vision was blind and seemed like a silvery haze that pulsated in and out at the zigzag zone." This visual aura cleared in 35 minutes and was followed by a right-sided headache and severe nausea.

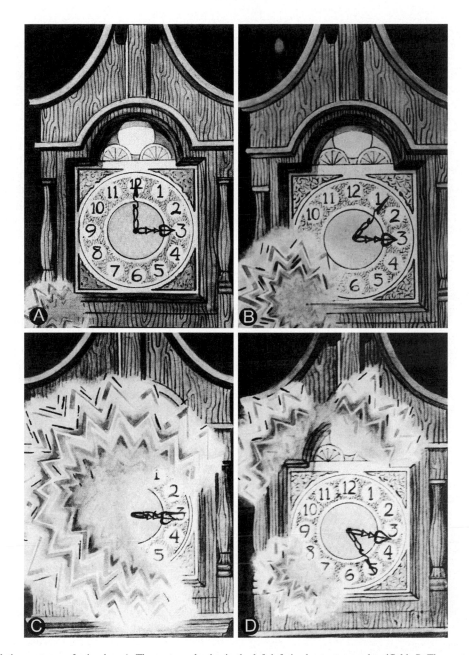

Figure 56.8. Scintillating scotoma of migraine. *A,* The scotoma begins in the left inferior homonymous hemifield. *B,* The scotoma expands within the next few minutes. It still is localized to the left inferior quadrant of the visual field. *C,* Within 15 minutes after onset, the scotoma has expanded into the center of the visual field, obscuring all but the right paracentral region. *D,* Within 25 minutes after the onset of symptoms, the scotoma has begun to break up. Note fortification figure that is part of the scintillating scotoma. (From Hupp SL, Kline LB, Corbett JJ: Visual disturbances of migraine. Surv Ophthalmol *33*:221–236, 1989.)

(Figs. 56.5–56.8). This pattern is called a **fortification figure** because of its similarity to a map of the bastions surrounding a castle or town (Richards, 1971) (Fig. 56.9). Field defects that have such a characteristic pattern are often called **fortification scotomas**. Scintillations and fortification figures may occur in the absence of a true scotoma; however, they, like the scotomas, are usually congruous in the homonymous fields (Fig. 56.10). Although they are usually seen with both eyes, they may seem more pronounced in one eye, and rare patients describe them in one eye only (see the section on visual aura originating in the retina or optic nerve, below).

The homonymous scotomas of migraine seldom persist for more than 15–20 minutes. The patient may not appreciate the hemianopic character of the scotoma, but he or she frequently states that the right or left half of viewed objects was absent or blurred during the episode. Some patients are unable to describe the sensation except by shaking their fore-

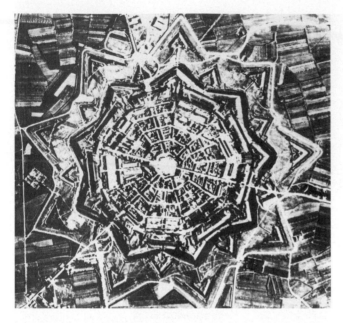

Figure 56.9. Aerial photograph of an early Italian military fortification demonstrating the angulation often seen in the visual aura of migraine with and without headache. Note similarity of figure to the scotomas depicted in Figures 56.4–56.7. (From Hupp SL, Kline LB, Corbett JJ: Visual disturbances of migraine. Surv Ophthalmol *33*:221–236, 1989.)

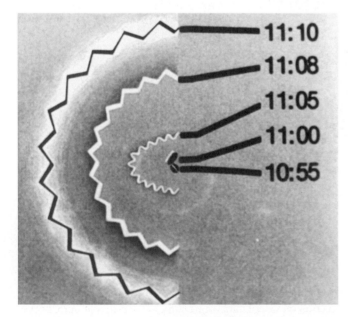

Figure 56.10. Hemianopic nature of a fortification scotoma. Note gradual enlargement of the scotoma over 15 minutes. Also note that the scotoma remains localized to the left homonymous hemifield. (From Hupp SL, Kline LB, Corbett JJ: Visual disturbances of migraine. Surv Ophthalmol *33*: 221–236, 1989.)

arm and hand in the periphery of the field of vision. Most patients are able to describe the exact dates, times, and circumstances of each attack.

In 1941, Lashley applied his training as a neurophysiologist to an analysis of his own migrainous scotomas and made a number of observations that have enhanced the understanding of scintillating scotomas. He noted that his scotoma usually began as a small blind or scintillating spot less than 1 in diameter that would drift away from the fovea toward one side or the other (Figs. 56.4 and 56.6). The right and left sides were affected with equal frequency. In most instances, the upper and lower quadrants of the affected side were both involved, but occasionally the scotoma was confined to either the homonymous upper or lower quadrant. A complete homonymous hemianopia rarely occurred. On one occasion out of more than 100 attacks, Lashley (1941) experienced complete blindness in both lower quadrants, with sparing of the macula. Symonds (1952) subsequently commented on the occasional occurrence of scotomas and other visual disturbances in both upper or both lower visual fields, emphasizing that such a disturbance could originate from the supra- or infra-calcarine cortex of both sides or from the upper or lower halves of both retinas (see also Heyck, 1962).

Lashley (1941) charted his scotomas as they drifted peripherally and discovered that each had a distinct shape that was roughly preserved as the area drifted across the visual field. Not only did the form of the scotoma remain constant during its drift, but when there were fortification figures, these also maintained their characteristic pattern in each part of the affected area. The size of the fortification figures did not increase with enlargement of the scotoma, but additional figures became visible as the area grew (Fig. 56.6). Lashley (1941) could not sketch the figures accurately, because the rate of scintillation was almost 10 per second, and the form changed rapidly. He was, however, able to distinguish small figures that ranged from large and simple angles to polygons (Fig. 56.11).

Lashley (1941) also noted that the rate of propagation and drift of his scotomas was fairly uniform. About 10–12 minutes were required for the outer margin to spread from fixation to the blind spot of the ipsilateral eye. The rate of spread beyond this point was rapid and difficult to estimate, but the total time required for the disturbance to spread from fixation to the peripheral field was about 20 minutes. The negative area of the scotoma persisted for about 5 minutes. The development and recovery of complete hemianopia each required about 15–20 minutes.

Lashley (1941) described the phenomenon of "completion of figure" in the negative scotomas of migraine that he experienced. Fuchs (1920) previously had emphasized that in traumatic hemianopias, geometric patterns are seen as complete, even though a part of the figure falls within the blind hemifield. Lashley (1941) observed this same phenomenon when the migrainous scotoma was present without scintillations. He cited two instances, one of which is repeated here.

Talking with a friend I glanced just to the right of his face whereon his head disappeared. His shoulders and necktie were still visible

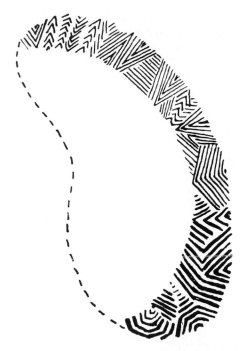

lasted for a few minutes and was then followed by a sensation as if looking through steam or hot air. After a further time, a zigzag C-shaped figure appeared in front of each eye. It was composed of dazzling white and gold colors in unbroken but irregular lines that were in constant motion. Each spectrum appeared to be about 30 cm in diameter when projected into space, and each contained rows of irregular lines with colored lines at the periphery. The vibrations seemed to occur at the rate of 8–12 per second. These sensations lasted from a few minutes to 1/2 hour at most. They then gradually disappeared, and the visual acuity and field became normal.

Wolff (1948) reported the observations of Dr. A.M. Cahan regarding his visual sensations during attacks of classic migraine. Dr. Cahan's visual auras were of predictable duration and lasted long enough for him to attempt to modify them using drugs (Fig. 56.12). The scotomas normally lasted 40–45 minutes. To ascertain whether or not dysfunction of the cerebral vasculature was responsible for the visual symptoms, Cahan inhaled a vasodilator, amyl nitrite. On several occasions, Cahan inhaled just enough amyl nitrite to produce a flushed sensation in the head without an appreciable change in blood pressure. The scotoma immediately disappeared but recurred about 6 minutes after inhalation. On one occasion, Cahan experienced an inferior homonymous quadrantic scotoma. He inhaled a large amount of amyl nitrite, felt a head flush, and his vision cleared completely. Three seconds later, he experienced complete loss of vision in both eyes associated with faintness. Two minutes after this, the visual field was normal, but 5 minutes later, the left upper field contained scintillating scotomas that progressed to become a complete left superior homonymous quadrantanopia over 12 minutes.

Figure 56.11. Lashley's sketch to show apparent differences among fortification figures. The coarser and more complicated figures are generally in the lower part of the visual field. The fortification figures appear as a series of parallel white or colored scintillating lines that form angles or polygons along the margins of the scotomatous area. The parallel lines cannot be counted, but they give the impression of groups of five or more. These seem to sweep across the figure toward the advancing margin and are constantly renewed at the inner margin "like the illusion of movement of a revolving screw." (From Lashley KS: Patterns of cerebral integration indicated by the scotomas of migraine. Arch Neurol Psychiatr *46*:331–339, 1941.)

but the vertical stripes in the wall paper behind him seemed to extend down to the necktie. Quick mapping revealed an area of total blindness covering about 30 just off the macula. It was quite impossible to see this as a blank area when projected on the striped wall or other uniformly patterned surface, although any intervening object failed to be seen.

On another occasion, with complete hemianopsia, including the macula, it was possible to divide a complex object on any line of fixation. A human face was sharply divided by fixating the tip of the nose, so that half, including one nostril only, was visible. At the same time it was impossible to fixate a circular object so that only half was seen. Fixating a chalk mark on the middle of a billiard ball failed to make any part of the ball invisible, although the ball was considerably larger than the readily divided nose.

Other investigators provided interesting and detailed accounts of their visual auras as well. G.L. Johnson (1936) described initial indistinctness of vision in each eye associated with a quivering sensation in front of the eyes. Print was blurred and tremulous, and the central field of vision seemed greatly contracted, although the peripheral field remained intact. Reading was difficult but not impossible. The pupils were dilated, but they reacted to light. This phase

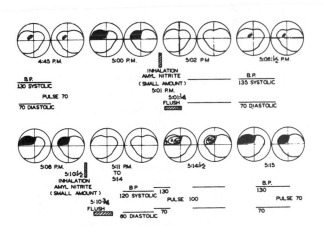

Figure 56.12. The influence of inhalation of amyl nitrite on a migrainous scotoma. The scotoma begins at 4:45 PM and progresses to affect the upper left homonymous quadrant by 5:00 PM. Amyl nitrite is inhaled at 5:01 PM. Immediately after inhalation, the scotoma disappears (5:02 PM), but it reappears centrally 4 minutes later (5:06 PM), and in 2 minutes, it affects the entire superior left homonymous quadrant. Another inhalation of amyl nitrite at this time (5:10 PM) again causes the field to clear for 3 minutes, but the field defect returns within 5 minutes (5:14 PM). (From Wolff HG: Headache and Other Head Pain. 2nd ed. New York, Oxford University Press, 1963.)

Creditor (1982) beautifully described the typical visual aura of his own migraine attacks. The initial symptom was usually a scotoma on one or the other side of the visual field. Occasionally, he experienced a visual symptom that preceded the scotoma. This symptom consisted of a visual distortion in which the halves of peoples' faces were vertically displaced in the midline in such a way that one eye appeared to be a centimeter or two lower than the other. Whether or not the scotoma was preceded by visual distortion, it always had the visual quality of the images in "kaleidoscopes," with the only difference being that the scotoma was silvery rather than multicolored. The scotoma sometimes began as a tiny circular area in the paracentral region of the field on one side or the other. At other times, the scotoma began as a narrow rectangle that moved rapidly in one direction or the other. On still other occasions, the scotoma had no specific geometric shape. Whether geometric or otherwise, the defect tended to enlarge and drift laterally in the visual field, gradually losing its "scintillating, shimmering quality as it was subtly replaced by a homonymous hemianopia." The visual aura usually lasted 15–30 minutes, although longer and shorter durations "were not infrequent."

Unequivocal evidence that some visual auras originate in the brain rather than in the eye is provided by patients who experience typical migrainous visual aura despite having undergone previous bilateral enucleations. Alvarez (1960) summarized the visual auras of 618 patients with visual aura associated with classic migraine. One of these patients experienced typical scintillating scotomas although she had undergone bilateral enucleations because of painful blindness, probably resulting from glaucoma. The patient had typical classic migraine attacks that began with a visual aura characterized by scotomas consisting of a dark, egg-shaped area having in its center two shining dots, one white and one black. Around the edges of the "egg" was an irregular black border that faded to nothingness. At the base was a "sand dune" with many brilliant grains of sand in constant motion.

A similar patient was described by Peatfield and Rose (1981). The patient was a 38-year-old woman who had undergone bilateral enucleations when she was 2 years old because of bilateral retinoblastoma. When she was 9 years old, she experienced severe migraine headaches with a visual aura characterized by bright flashes of light passing across the visual fields from right to left. She described the shapes of the flashes as circles, squares, triangles, oblongs, and snakes of different colors. The visual aura was followed by a headache that was strictly unilateral, most often left-sided, and about 24 hours in duration. The patient stated that the visual hemifield on the side of the headache seemed much blacker than usual.

In some patients with classic migraine, typical scintillating scotomas can be induced by light. Heyck (1966) reported that several patients with a typical history of migraine headache preceded by scintillating scotoma told him that their attacks could be provoked by a flashing bright light. Others stated that they could induce an attack by staring at the glittering surface of water or at a field covered with snow. Still others could experience an attack while driving if they looked at the flickering light transmitted through a picket fence or a row of roadside trees. Some patients experienced visual aura if they watched a flickering television set. We have seen two patients in whom flashing or flickering lights could induce a classic migraine attack. One of these patients experienced an attack while he was undergoing a static perimetric examination.

Vertebrobasilar artery disease can produce occipital ischemia that mimics migraine with aura. We examined the records of a 65-year-old man who experienced several episodes of scintillating scotomas followed by severe headaches. He was evaluated by an ophthalmologist who found no abnormalities and suspected that the patient had migraine; however, the patient subsequently experienced episodes of vertigo and then had a major stroke that resulted in a locked-in syndrome.

One of the most dramatic and frightening forms of migrainous visual aura is total blindness. The patient who suffers this type of visual loss may experience symptoms similar to those described above, but the scotomas and scintillations are present in both the right and left fields of vision. Some patients describe a gradual contraction of both fields from the nasal and temporal periphery inward. Recovery usually occurs within 10 to 15 minutes, at which time there is often an initial sensation of bright light immediately in front of the patient. The visual fields then begin to widen from the center outward as if a curtain were being pulled away. Dr. Frank Walsh (Walsh and Hoyt, 1969a) experienced such an episode as the initial attack of classic migraine while he was giving a conference on neuro-ophthalmology. He subsequently experienced numerous episodes of scintillating scotomas in one or both homonymous hemifields, but he never again experienced complete blindness. We examined several patients who experienced episodes of transient complete blindness during the course of an attack of classic migraine, one of whom suffered permanent partial visual loss (see below). We agree with Walsh (1951) that a visual aura characterized by complete bilateral loss of vision almost always originates in the visual cortex and consists of a bilateral homonymous hemianopia, although bilateral simultaneous visual loss may occasionally originate more anteriorly in the optic chiasm, optic nerves, or retinas.

DIFFERENTIAL DIAGNOSIS OF SCINTILLATING SCOTOMA

Scintillating scotomas may be produced by disorders other than migraine that affect any portion of the visual sensory pathway. The most common locations for such lesions are the retina and vitreous and the striate cortex.

Disorders of Retina and Vitreous. Patients with various disorders of the retina and vitreous may experience sparks or flashes of light that mimic the scintillating scotomas that occur during the visual aura of migraine. Perhaps the most common setting in which such sparks or flashes occur is during acute vitreous or retinal detachment (Coppeto, 1988a). Klein (1988) described two patients in whom such symptoms occurred after retinal detachment surgery in which subretinal fluid either could not be completely drained

(Case 1) or was not drained at all (Case 2). As the fluid resorbed, the patients experienced scintillations in the field of vision corresponding to the region of elevated retina. Both patients' visual symptoms disappeared once the fluid had completely resorbed.

The visual symptoms of patients with vitreous or retinal disease that mimic the visual aura of migraine consist mainly of flashes and sparks of white light rather than colored light, although we examined a patient in whom the onset of a retinal detachment was heralded by a flash of violet light in the superior visual field. Other characteristic features of the visual symptoms of patients with vitreoretinal disease are that they are clearly uniocular, last longer than typical migrainous visual aura, and occur without any associated headache. We have also examined numerous patients with such symptoms in whom the vitreous was extremely syneretic but not detached. The symptoms were rather constant and clearly monocular. When the vitreous finally detached, the symptoms abruptly stopped (see also Verhoeff, 1941).

Lesions of the Occipital Lobe. Tumors affecting the visual cortex occasionally produce scintillating scotomas that mimic those of migraine. Pepin (1990) described a 44-year-old woman who began to experience severe, intermittent, bifrontal and left hemicranial, pulsating headaches accompanied by nausea and vomiting. The headaches occurred about three times a week, lasted 4–6 hours, and were sometimes preceded by a photopsia of colored stars moving in the right visual field. The patient initially was thought to have migraine, but she developed papilledema, and an evaluation revealed a metastatic adenocarcinoma in the left parietal lobe with surrounding edema.

We examined a woman with a history of breast cancer, treated with radical mastectomy, who experienced the onset of episodes of scintillating scotomas in the left homonymous visual field, unassociated with headache. After experiencing several of these episodes, she noted a persistent field defect. The patient had no previous history of migraine. When we first examined her, we found a small, congruous, left homonymous hemianopic scotoma. A computed tomographic (CT) scan was unrevealing. Over the next 2 weeks, the patient continued to experience scintillating scotomas in the left homonymous hemifield, and when she was examined at the end of this period, the visual field defect had increased in size. A repeat CT scan was normal; however, a third CT scan performed 2 weeks after the second showed a small mass in the right occipital lobe that was biopsied and found to be metastatic carcinoma. After treatment with radiation and chemotherapy, the patient experienced no further visual episodes, although she had a permanent homonymous field defect.

Donin and Keane (1981) reported a 38-year-old man who experienced brief episodes of scintillating scotoma. The visual episodes were initially unassociated with headache, but within 2 weeks, a headache regularly followed an episode. The patient was initially thought to have migraine; however, he subsequently developed papilledema and was ultimately found to have a medulloblastoma that had diffusely infiltrated the brain.

Selhorst et al. (1981) described a 47-year-old man who experienced stereotyped episodes of visual dysfunction since he was a teenager. The episodes were characterized by a flash of light in the right homonymous hemifield "as if a light bulb went off." The sudden photopsia consisted of "crinkling, jagged bars of blue lights" just to the right and inferior to central fixation. This positive scotoma initially measured about 4–5, but it gradually tripled in size over 15–30 minutes as its borders enlarged into an oval. As the scotoma expanded, the patient noted sensations of turbulence, shimmering, or rolling at its margins. He was unable to see through the scotoma because its center was filled with small lines that "wiggled like the surface of lightly boiling water." After about 30 minutes, the patient noted a faint, yellow glow to the scotoma, and his vision began to clear. As the vision cleared, the patient developed a nonspecific headache. These episodes initially occurred about once a month. After age 20, however, the patient experienced the episodes only once or twice a year, and they were not followed by a headache. When the patient was 45 years old, the episodes increased in frequency until they occurred about 1–2 times a week. After one such episode, the patient noted persistent blurred vision. An examination at this time revealed a small, relative, homonymous hemianopic scotoma in the right inferior field. Neuroimaging studies revealed a left-sided occipital convexity meningioma associated with prominent dural arteriovenous shunts. The patient underwent complete excision of the tumor, after which he had no further visual episodes over a follow-up period of more than 1 year.

Arteriovenous malformations (AVMs) located in the occipital lobe may also produce visual symptoms and headaches that may be confused with migraine (Fig. 56.13). Troost and Newton (1975) emphasized that the visual symptoms that occur in patients with occipital lobe AVMs are usually brief, episodic, unformed, and unassociated with the angular, scintillating figures that usually distinguish migrainous cortical visual phenomena. Nevertheless, the complete clinical symptom complex of classic migraine may occasionally be mimicked by an AVM in the occipital lobe (Sacks, 1970; Weiskrantz et al., 1974; Troost et al., 1979; Kattah and Luessenhop, 1980).

The patient described by Weiskrantz et al. (1974) was a 34-year-old man who had experienced headaches since age 14. The headaches were always preceded by a flashing light that appeared in an oval-shaped area immediately to the left of fixation. The oval enlarged, primarily by downward extension, over several minutes. About 15 minutes after the onset of visual symptoms, the flashing lights were replaced by a white scotoma covering the oval area with a crescent of colored lights around its lateral and lower margins. At this point, the headache occurred. It was always on the right side and was followed by vomiting about 15 minutes later, by which time the scotoma had extended to include the crescent of colored lights. The headache persisted for up to 48 hours. These attacks occurred about every 6 weeks until the patient was in his twenties, at which time they increased in frequency to about once every 3 weeks. After one attack at age 25, he noted a persistent defect in the visual field, smaller than the scotoma of previous attacks and situated to the left of fixation. An angiogram revealed an AVM at the tip of

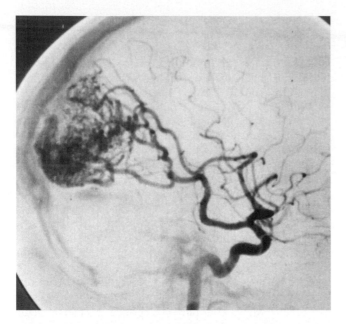

Figure 56.13. Occipital lobe arteriovenous malformation apparently responsible for attacks of typical migraine with visual aura in a 20-year-old patient who had experienced stereotyped migraine attacks characterized by right homonymous hemianopic visual symptoms since age 7. Carotid arteriogram, lateral view, shows a large AVM within the right occipital lobe that is fed by branches of the middle and posterior cerebral arteries. The patient's "migraine attacks" completely stopped after the malformation was removed. (From Troost BT, Mark LE, Maroon JC: Resolution of classic migraine after removal of an occipital lobe AVM. Ann Neurol 5: 199–201, 1979.)

the right occipital lobe. The malformation was removed, following which the patient had a homonymous hemianopia that split the macula but spared a bit of the superior field, primarily the temporal crescent of the left eye. In addition, he experienced flashing lights and well-formed visual hallucinations in the blind left hemifields that occurred over about 5 weeks and then disappeared. The patient had no further headaches after surgery (see also Sanders et al., 1974).

Troost et al. (1979) described a 20-year-old woman who reported stereotyped "migraine attacks" beginning at 7 years of age, with a frequency that gradually increased from twice a year to once a day. Each episode was characterized by the appearance of an angular, colorful, luminous, pulsating visual disturbance. A scotoma with a brilliant scintillation slowly expanded over 30 minutes to affect the central and right homonymous visual fields. The disturbed area then would seem to move or "drift" to the right inferiorly and then back to the left, diminishing in size and intensity. Forty minutes after onset, a single "zigzag" luminescent line would remain in the left visual field. It then blended into a "fog" and disappeared within the next 5 minutes. Inevitably, the disappearance of the visual spectra was followed by an intense, throbbing, right temporoparietal headache accompanied by nausea and vomiting. The headache lasted 5–6 hours. Between attacks, the patient had completely normal neurologic and neuro-ophthalmologic examinations.

Because of the strict unilaterality of the patient's symptoms, and the lack of any success in treating the patient, a CT scan was performed. This demonstrated a lesion in the right occipital lobe that was found by angiography to be an AVM (Fig. 56.13. After resection of the AVM, the patient had a left homonymous field defect, but she had no further episodic visual symptoms or headaches during the next 10 years.

The patient reported by Kattah and Luessenhop (1980) was a 38-year-old woman who developed headaches during her teens, shortly after delivery of her first child. Attacks usually began with a visual aura consisting of scintillating bright lights that moved from the center to the periphery of the left visual field and lasted about 30 minutes. As the visual phenomena disappeared, the patient developed a severe headache associated with nausea and often with vomiting. Medical treatment failed to relieve the symptoms, and the headaches eventually increased in frequency until they were occurring every day. An evaluation revealed an AVM in the right occipital lobe. After resection of this lesion, the patient had no further headaches.

A few patients have been reported in whom cerebral venous sinus thrombosis produced damage to one or both occipital lobes, thereby causing positive visual phenomena resembling those of migraine aura. Montiero et al. (1984) described a 33-year-old woman who developed multicolored photopsias and a relative left homonymous hemianopia 3 days postpartum. A CT scan showed hypodensities in both occipital lobes, and angiography showed cerebral venous sinus thrombosis. The symptoms resolved completely. D.S. Newman et al. (1989) described two patients who developed visual symptoms that were consistent with the aura of migraine, but without an associated headache, in the setting of cerebral venous sinus thrombosis. One patient was a 30-year-old woman who experienced the sudden onset of vividly colored photopsias in the central field of vision of both eyes. The photopsias slowly spread outward over minutes to affect the entire visual field. These positive visual phenomena resolved over 30 minutes and were replaced by a dense scotoma. The second patient developed frequent episodes of visual blurring associated with vertical wavy lines and teichopsia. The episodes lasted 10–30 minutes and were associated with a sensation of "pressure" in the vertex region. Neuroimaging studies revealed cerebral venous thrombosis in both patients.

Scintillating scotomas occasionally may occur in patients with systemic vascular disorders, such as systemic lupus erythematosus (SLE) (Atkinson and Appenzeller, 1975; Friedman, 1976; Brandt and Lessell, 1978; Lessell, 1979; Isenberg et al., 1982; Honda, 1985, 1987). Some of these patients may have two separate diseases: migraine and SLE, whereas in others, SLE produces changes in the vessels that in turn produce the scotomas. We examined two young women who experienced recurrent scintillating scotomas in the setting of SLE. Neither patient had either a family history of migraine or a personal history of previous attacks of migraine. The scotomas disappeared in both patients when they were placed on an increased dose of systemic corticosteroids.

OTHER VISUAL DISTURBANCES ORIGINATING FROM THE CEREBRAL HEMISPHERES

Several investigators described in detail some of the minor disturbances of visual perception experienced by patients with migraine (Klee and Willanger, 1966; Hachinski et al., 1973; Ardila and Sanchez, 1988; Liu et al., 1995). These disturbances are less spectacular than the fortification spectra. They may occur as part of the visual aura preceding a typical migraine headache, but they also occur during the headache, or even between attacks of headache if the condition is severe and chronic. Liu et al. (1995) described 10 patients with migraine who developed persistent positive visual phenomena lasting months to years. The phenomena involved the entire field of vision of both eyes and were variously described as "snow," "rain," "lines of ants," "dots," and "TV static." Neurologic and ophthalmologic examinations were normal in all patients.

Micropsia and macropsia may cause the patient to note that objects seem abnormally small or large and yet do not seem to be abnormally near or far away (Fig. 56.14A). Sometimes only the image of the object of interest seems unusually small or large, whereas the surrounding objects in the field of vision retain their normal relative sizes.

Visual allesthesia may occur during some episodes of migraine. Some viewed objects may be inverted 45, 90, or even 180 (Fig. 56.14B). (See also "Alice in Wonderland" below).

Metamorphopsia may cause the linear components of viewed objects to seem displaced or wavy. Surfaces may seem to bend upward or downward. Horizontal or vertical lines may seem wavy and appear to be in constant motion. Objects with complex contours may appear distorted.

Monocular diplopia or polyopia may occur (Drake, 1983). The secondary images often seem to originate from the main image of the object of interest after a short period of fixation. Kosmorsky (1987) described doubling of images within a typical scintillating hemianopic scotoma. When either eye was covered, the images remained doubled. This doubling of images was the same whether an object was viewed with either eye alone or both eyes together. When polyopia is present, images may be adjacent to each other with variable overlap in a linear, diagonal, or even circular pattern. Sinoff and Rosenberg (1990) described a patient with persistent monocular diplopia after several attacks of migraine with visual aura consisting of a right homonymous hemianopic scotoma.

Binocular diplopia is a rare visual symptom in patients with migraine. Liveing (1873) mentioned it, and Symonds (1952) described a friend and colleague, examined "over a period of many years," who began at age 24 to have attacks of classic migraine, "beginning with dimness of vision and scintillating figures followed after half an hour by dull headache." At age 34, the patient experienced episodes during which he had "diplopia with one image appearing obliquely above the other, lasting only for a minute and followed by headache of the same type with which he was familiar in his other attacks." Symonds (1952) emphasized that diplopia that occurs as part (or all) of the aura of a migraine attack

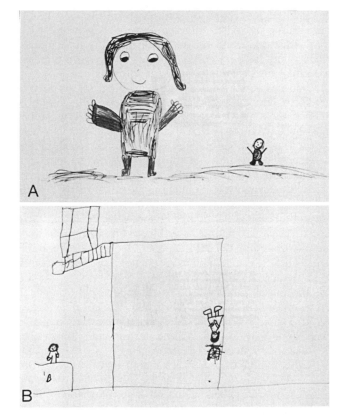

Figure 56.14. Drawings of abnormal visual phenomena observed by children during an attack of migraine. *A*, Drawing of micropsia as observed by a child who suffered from migraine with visual aura. Other children (*right*) appeared unusually small to the patient (*left*) during some of her attacks. *B*, Drawing by a 9-year-old girl who had episodes that began with double vision. Colors of objects then changed, and a bitemporal headache developed. On one occasion before the headache began, the child saw a picture as being upside down and her mother as walking upside down. In this drawing, a picture in the room (*upper left corner*) is upside down as is the patient's mother (*right*). (From Hachinski VC, Porchawka J, Steele JC: Visual symptoms in the migraine syndrome. Neurology 23:570–579, 1973.)

is distinct from the diplopia of ophthalmoplegic migraine (see below). Slavin (1989) reported a 10-year-old boy with migraine who had two episodes of typical migraine headache, each associated with the development of a comitant esotropia. The first episode lasted 20 minutes. During this episode, the patient had 10 prism diopters of esotropia at near, although he was orthophoric at distance, and he had full ductions and versions. The second episode occurred about 18 months later, at which time the patient developed a small comitant esotropia that was present at both distance and near. The episode lasted 20 minutes. It has been suggested that patients who develop binocular diplopia in association with migraine have a limited form of basilar artery migraine (see below), but there is no evidence to support this contention.

Halos and other corona phenomena may occur. The patient may observe color borders or a shiny, shimmering, silvery halo around objects.

Apparent movement of stationary objects may be observed. The movement may be upward, downward, backward, forward, or a combination of these. Some stationary objects may seem to recede, whereas others seem to be approaching the patient at a slow rate of speed.

Abnormal rate of movement of moving objects may be noted. In such instances, a moving object will seem to be moving too slowly or too quickly. Patients may complain that the movement is like that of a movie that has been speeded up to twice or three times normal speed, or that moving objects seem to be traveling in slow motion.

Generalized dimming of vision may affect the entire visual field of both eyes, the homonymous left or right hemifields, the upper or lower fields of both eyes, or the central portions of both visual fields (Symonds, 1952; Heyck, 1962; Speed, 1964). Sometimes an object will seem clear when initially observed, but the image will fade after several seconds. These phenomena may originate in the striate cortex, in the retinas, or in both locations.

Pulsation phenomena may be described by the patient as cyclic blurring of images, cyclic changes in apparent size, or cyclic doubling of contours. Peripheral portions of a blurred visual field may seem to pulsate inward and outward or to fluctuate in brightness.

Changes in color, contrast, or both may be noted (Fig. 56.15) (Lawden and Cleland, 1993). Some objects become colorless or gray. Others seem to change color. Some objects become faded and difficult to see.

Visual perseveration causes objects, particularly those with a light color, to be seen in the central field after gaze has been directed elsewhere.

Formed visual hallucinations may occasionally occur during the visual aura of migraine. Walsh (1951) described a minister who had suffered from migraine for many years. He experienced transient homonymous hemianopia on many occasions, and he finally developed a permanent homony-

mous quadrantanopia. Thereafter, he occasionally experienced visual aura consisting of seeing large numbers of skunks, most of which had their tails cocked in the "ready" position, in the blind fields. Corbett (1983) described a 52-year-old woman with a 37-year history of predominantly right-sided headaches that were always preceded by blurring of the left visual field lasting 20 minutes. After one such attack, she had a permanent left superior homonymous quadrantanopia. For the next several days, she reported seeing "the same woman walking across the street with her dog" repeatedly over 30 minutes and other palinopic images in the left visual field. CT scanning demonstrated a right occipital lobe infarct, a small infarct in the left occipital lobe, and a large infarct in the right frontal lobe.

VISUAL SYMPTOMS ORIGINATING IN THE OPTIC CHIASM

Butler (1933) reported bitemporal hemianopia lasting about 2 1/2 hours in a patient who also had polyuria during a severe attack of migraine. Drs. V. De Groot and Frank Walsh (Walsh and Hoyt, 1969b) examined a 30-year-old man who had an attack of unilateral headache preceded by a brief episode of bitemporal hemianopia. The man was subsequently migraine-free for 8 years and then, over the course of 1 year, suffered several transient episodes of visual loss characterized by bitemporal hemianopia without headache. Other authors have reported patients with migraine in whom the visual aura was characterized by a bitemporal visual disturbance (Hedges, 1979; Shiogai et al., 1988). We have examined several such patients. In all cases, the deficit was described as an area of blurred vision, often preceded by scintillations or fortification spectra, that began in the temporal periphery of both visual fields and gradually moved centrally over 3–7 minutes, until the entire temporal field of both eyes was affected by the process. In some cases, there was a true bitemporal hemianopia; in others, the temporal fields were affected by scintillations but there was no definite field loss. In some cases, visual acuity seemed clear, whereas in others, central vision seemed to be affected. In all cases, the defect cleared completely within 30 minutes. Some of these patients subsequently suffered a hemicranial or bifrontal headache; others did not. In four patients who underwent complete neurologic evaluation including CT scanning, magnetic resonance (MR) imaging, or both, no abnormalities were noted.

The differential diagnosis of transient bitemporal hemianopia with and without subsequent headache includes both extrinsic and intrinsic mass lesions affecting the optic chiasm. In particular, one must consider the possibility of a vascular malformation within the optic chiasm that has bled. Such a lesion should be easily detectable using MR imaging (see Chapter 43).

VISUAL SYMPTOMS ORIGINATING IN THE OPTIC NERVE

The visual aura of migraine may be characterized by sudden monocular loss of vision absolutely identical with that experienced by patients with amaurosis fugax (see Chapter 55). In most cases, visual loss is transient and is caused by retinal ischemia (see below and retinal migraine). In some

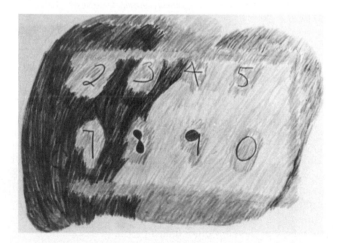

Figure 56.15. Drawing of abnormal contrast as observed by a child who suffered from migraine with visual aura. A number chart viewed by the patient during an attack was obscured on the left side and was unusually bright on the right side. (From Hachinski VC, Porchawka J, Steele JC: Visual symptoms in the migraine syndrome. Neurology *23*:570–579, 1973.)

instances, however, optic nerve ischemia is responsible for transient monocular visual loss in the setting of migraine. In such cases, monocular visual loss occurs without any change in the appearance of the retinal vessels. If visual loss persists, there may be optic disc swelling in the affected eye (anterior ischemic optic neuropathy) or the optic disc initially may appear normal, only to become pale within 4 to 6 weeks (posterior ischemic optic neuropathy; see below and Chapter 11).

VISUAL SYMPTOMS ORIGINATING IN THE RETINA (SEE ALSO RETINAL MIGRAINE, BELOW)

Most visual symptoms in patients with migraine originate in the striate cortex and are binocular. Even most monocular symptoms are actually binocular and hemianopic because the patient is ignoring the smaller homonymous nasal hemifield. Truly monocular visual symptoms occur in approximately 1 in 200 migraineurs (Troost, 1996), originating from the ipsilateral retina in the majority of cases. Rarely, visual symptoms arise from both retinas. Fisher (1959) reviewed 138 cases of transient monocular blindness (i.e., amaurosis fugax) and concluded that 24 (17%) were caused by migraine. Other investigators agree that transient monocular visual loss in young, otherwise healthy adolescents and adults is most often related to migraine, even when there is no associated headache (Goodwin et al., 1984; Booy, 1990; O'Sullivan, 1992; Davidoff, 1995).

PHOTOPHOBIA

This is a prominent symptom in the majority of cases. It may occur as part of the visual aura, resolving at the time of headache, or it may persist during the entire migraine attack. Eckardt et al. (1943) suggested that photophobia arises from irritation of the trigeminal nerve.

Pupillary Signs

Unilateral pupillary dilation occurs in patients with migraine (Hallett and Cogan, 1970; Edelson and Levy, 1974; Miller et al., 1986; Jacobson, 1995). In some patients, the pupillary dilation occurs just before or during a migraine attack (Fig. 56.16), whereas in others, it seems to occur independently from such attacks. In rare cases, pupillary dilation may be bilateral and associated with blurred vision (Parrish and Todorov, 1981). Some authors describe the affected pupils as being nonreactive or poorly reactive to light or near stimulation despite normal visual function in the eye (Poos, 1934; Alpers and Yaskin, 1951; Corbett, 1983; Woods et al., 1984). Lesions affecting any portion of the oculomotor nerve could conceivably produce such a phenomenon (Sunderland, 1952). For example, Lee and Lance (1977) described three children with basilar artery migraine (see below) who developed transient, unilaterally dilated pupils in association with their stupor. It is likely that the transient pupillary dilation in these patients was caused by damage to parasympathetic pupillary fibers in the brainstem or in the proximal portion of the oculomotor nerve. In most patients, however, it seems likely that the site of damage is the ciliary ganglion or short ciliary nerves (Loewenfeld, 1980).

Other unilaterally dilated pupils that occur in the setting of migraine do, in fact, react rather well to both light and near stimulation (Woods et al., 1984; Jacobson, 1995). Patients with such pupils invariably have normal accommodation. We and others believe that the sympathetic, not the parasympathetic, pupillary fibers are affected in such cases (Herman, 1983; Jacobson, 1995). Thompson et al. (1983) described 26 patients with episodic eccentric pupillary dilation thought to be caused by segmental spasm of the pupillary dilator muscle. Although 11 of the 26 patients had definite (8) or probable (3) migraine headaches, the episodes of pupillary distortion that occurred in these patients were said to be unrelated to their headaches. We have seen several patients in whom segmental dilation of the pupil occurred during the aura of classic migraine. Such patients must have transient hyperfunction of the sympathetic fibers travelling to the pupillary dilator, producing dilation of the pupil without affecting its ability to constrict and without affecting accommodation. Interestingly, Woods et al. (1984) rejected this conclusion because none of the patients that they examined (all of whom had normal accommodation and reactive pupils) had eyelid retraction, conjunctival blanching, or hyperhidrosis, even though they accepted the hypothesis that a lesion affecting the intracranial portion of the oculomotor nerve could produce isolated pupillary dilation without ptosis or ophthalmoparesis. It must be remembered that unilateral pupillary mydriasis associated with ipsilateral visual loss and orbital or ocular pain may be caused not only by migraine but also by intermittent acute angle closure glaucoma (Ravits and Seybold, 1984; Sarkies et al., 1985; Woods et al., 1985).

Drummond (1987) measured pupillary diameter in darkness and in dull and bright illumination in 39 patients with migraine. Mean pupil diameter measured between attacks in patients with migraine did not differ significantly from mean pupil diameter measured in control subjects without migraine; however, mean pupil diameter measured in migraine sufferers during an episode of migraine was significantly smaller ($p < 0.05$) at every level of illumination than in control subjects.

Neurologic Aura

The most common auras of classic migraine are visual, but transient neurologic symptoms may also occur, either in isolation or associated with visual symptoms. These neurologic symptoms include disturbances of sensation, aphasia, vertigo, and complex neuropsychologic phenomena.

The most common neurologic aura are unilateral, cortically-evoked sensory changes such as paresthesias, numbness, objective analgesia of a hand and the corresponding circumoral area, and limb pain (Liveing, 1873; Bruyn, 1986; Guiloff and Fruns, 1988). These sensory changes usually do not spread, but pain may occasionally radiate from the side of the head to the neck and arm (Gowers, 1888), and numbness of the hand may ascend up the arm to the neck and then to the side of the tongue, or it may descend to affect the ipsilateral leg. Most sensory changes, like visual aura, recur in stereotyped fashion for many years. They usually

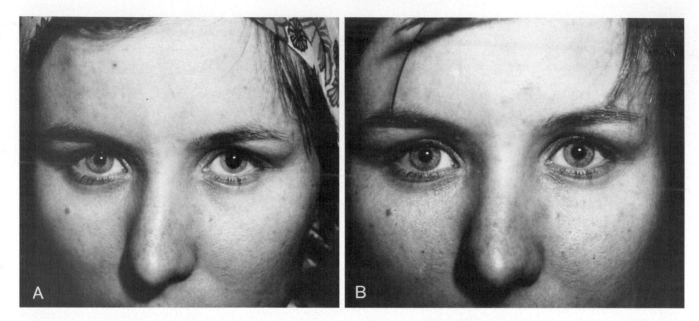

Figure 56.16. Transient, unilateral pupillary dilation during an attack of migraine. The patient is a 25-year-old nurse with a long history of attacks of migraine without aura. During a typical attack she noted some mild blurred vision in the left eye and was observed to have anisocoria. *A*, There is anisocoria with the left pupil larger than the right. The patient had normal distance and near visual acuity in the left eye. Constriction of the left pupil was both incomplete and slow. *B*, 30 minutes after resolution of headache, the patient's pupils are equal and normally reactive.

last 5–20 minutes, and they usually affect the side opposite the headache.

Transient aphasia, occasionally associated with agraphia, is probably the next most common nonvisual, neurologic aura of migraine after sensory disturbances. The aphasia is usually of the expressive (nonfluent, motor) type. The patient suddenly is unable to find the proper words or cannot speak at all. The sensorium is normal in other respects, and the patient understands questions even though he or she cannot answer them. Disturbances of speech are usually brief, rarely lasting more than 20 minutes. Patients with aphasia as part of a migrainous aura may experience simultaneous paresthesias of the right hand.

Patients may experience alexia as a transient neurologic symptom of migraine. Fleishman et al. (1983) described a 60-year-old woman with a 45-year history of migraine headaches without aura who experienced a single episode of alexia without agraphia, associated with nausea and a typical migraine headache. The episode lasted 30 minutes. The patient went to sleep, and when she awoke later in the day, she was "okay" but she "felt funny." A complete neurologic evaluation performed 7 days later was unremarkable. A similar case was reported by Bigley and Sharp (1983). Their patient was a 35-year-old physician who had previously experienced three attacks of right homonymous hemianopia lasting 20–30 minutes, each followed by a bifrontal throbbing headache lasting 12–24 hours. During the third attack, the patient also experienced numbness and decreased coordination of the right hand that lasted 5 minutes. About 2 years later, the patient developed a right homonymous hemianopia that lasted 45 minutes and was followed by a bifrontal, dull, throbbing headache. The patient attempted to read and found

that although he could see individual letters and words, he could not understand what they meant. He could understand spoken words, and he could write normally. About 30 minutes after the onset of neurologic symptoms, the patient regained the ability to comprehend words and sentences. He then experienced numbness of the right hand that lasted 5 minutes. The headache lasted about 24 hours. The day after this attack, the patient underwent a complete neurologic examination that was normal except for mild slowing of rapid alternating movements on the right side. The results of a variety of serologic studies were normal as were the results of an electrocardiogram, electroencephalogram, and CT scan. The patient was thought to have experienced an attack of alexia without agraphia as part of the aura of a migraine attack.

Although others before him had recorded episodes of transient hemiparesis during an attack of migraine, Charcot (1892) is usually credited with the first comprehensive essay on the subject. Whitty (1953) emphasized that there are two forms of "hemiplegic migraine": familial and sporadic. The familial form is characterized by weakness, always on the same side, that persists for days, outlasting the headache. (See also Familial Hemiplegic Migraine below). Consciousness is impaired in some patients. In the sporadic form, weakness with and without hemisensory symptoms occurs on one side or the other as part of the aura and improves slowly as the headache develops. The sporadic form may worsen or occur for the first time during pregnancy (Mandel, 1988). Rosenbaum (1960) agreed with the classification proposed by Whitty's (1953). He hypothesized that the underlying mechanism of the hemiparetic aura was transient vasospasm followed by reversible cerebral edema. Importantly, vasospasm has been documented in retinal migraine (see below) and in some cases of nonembolic amaurosis fugax (Burger et al., 1991; Winterkorn and Teman, 1991).

Vertigo is a common symptom in patients with basilar artery migraine (see below), but it also occurs as part of the neurologic aura of classic migraine. It is thought that patients with migraine have hypersensitive vestibular systems that predispose them to vertigo, dizziness, and motion sickness (Kuritzky et al., 1981a, 1981b).

Complex neuropsychologic symptoms can occur as part of the aura of classic migraine (Ardila and Sanchez, 1988). Some of these symptoms are visual, such as macropsia, micropsia, palinopsia, pelopsia, and teleopsia (see above). Nonvisual symptoms include anomia, depersonalization, olfactory hallucinations, gustatory hallucinations, and acalculia.

Neurologic and visual aura can occur simultaneously. Bradshaw and Parsons (1965) reported that 88% of 77 patients with sensory or motor neurologic aura had visual changes. About half of these patients had teichopsia that started in the homonymous field on the side of the motor or sensory disturbance, and 13 patients (17%) probably experienced a homonymous hemianopia. In no case did a homonymous visual disturbance occur on the side opposite the motor or sensory disturbances, although two patients had generalized diminution of vision in both eyes, amounting almost to total blindness, and two patients had transient, bilateral, central scotomas.

Headache

The headache that occurs in patients after a typical visual or neurologic aura is identical with that which occurs without aura. As noted above, it usually begins as the aura resolves, although it may occur concurrently with the aura, or it may even precede the aura. Most patients experience unilateral headache, but the side of the headache is not constant. Sjaastad et al. (1989) evaluated 31 patients with migraine headaches that followed visual or neurologic aura to determine how often the headaches were unilateral and if they tended to alternate sides or occur on the same side each time there was an attack. These investigators reported that 84% of the patients had completely or predominantly unilateral headaches. Other authors report the frequency of bilateral headache to be as high as 40% (Silberstein et al., 1995). The headaches in all of these patients are sometimes right-sided and sometimes left-sided. The same issues that we have discussed regarding the duration, frequency, and intensity of common migraine headaches (i.e., migraine without aura) apply to migraine headaches that are associated with an aura.

Migraine headaches that are preceded by aura account for about 30% of all types of migraine attacks. They vary greatly from person to person, and they may also differ in frequency, duration, and intensity at different times in the same person.

The frequency of attacks of migraine with aura are unpredictable. They generally occur less frequently than do common migraines. Most sufferers of this condition experience about one attack a month, but some persons have only one or two attacks a year, and others have one attack each week (Diamond and Medina, 1980). Medina and Diamond (1977,

1981) described a group of patients with migraine whose attacks occurred in clusters, separated by symptom-free periods. The attacks occurred in cycles that lasted an average of 6 weeks. During each cycle, severe headaches, preceded by visual symptoms and associated with nausea, vomiting, and photophobia, occurred several times a week and lasted about 24 hours. In many patients, the cycles were accompanied by depression. The cycles recurred an average of five times a year.

Most headaches that follow a visual or neurologic aura last 1–6 hours (Graham, 1979). In general, such headaches do not last as long as headaches that occur without aura (Diamond and Medina, 1980).

Like migraine headaches without aura, migraine headaches that follow or occur concurrently with aura are often associated with anorexia, nausea, vomiting, and photophobia. When the headache is severe, anorexia and nausea are almost always present, although vomiting does not usually occur unless the headache is of long duration. Anorexia, nausea, and vomiting occur in about 90% of cases of classic migraine (Diamond, 1987).

The neurologic dysfunction of the classic migraine attack is usually transient and completely reversible. Disturbances of sensory, motor, cognitive, and amnestic function are paroxysmal, typically resolving within 60 minutes (Hooker and Raskin, 1986). Despite the apparent clinical clearing of these deficits, evidence has accumulated suggesting that subtle higher cortical dysfunction may persist after repeated attacks of migraine with aura. Klee and Willanger (1966) reported that 75% of patients with classic migraine whom they studied demonstrated mild impairment in abstraction ability and verbal memory. These authors suggested that the impairment developed gradually in association with the increasing severity of the attacks. In a controlled study, Schuchman and Thetford (1970) found that patients with classic migraine scored significantly lower on the Wechsler Adult Intelligence Scale Digit Span subtest, a measure of attention and immediate memory, than did control subjects. In another controlled study, Zeitlin and Oddy (1984) found that patients with severe classic migraine demonstrated significantly slower reaction times, less efficient processing of information, and poorer verbal memory performance, than did patients without migraine. In a questionnaire study, patients with classic migraine reported significantly more memory problems than did medical and psychiatric patients without headache (Mahrer et al., 1966). Hooker and Raskin (1986) administered a number of neuropsychologic tests to 16 outpatients with classic migraine and compared the results with those from 15 matched volunteers without headache. Subjects with classic migraine were required to have a 2-year or longer history of 1–10 attacks per month, each lasting no longer than 24 hours. The group of patients with classic migraine demonstrated significantly greater than average neuropsychologic impairment and more self-reported cognitive difficulties than the nonheadache group. On the basis of these findings, Hooker and Raskin (1986) concluded that classic migraine produces a disturbance of cerebral function that persists beyond the attack itself. Other investigators failed to corroborate these findings (Leijdekkers et al.,

1990), and they speculated that permanent neuropsychologic disturbances develop only in a small number of patients with classic migraine.

MIGRAINE WITH PROLONGED AURA (COMPLICATED MIGRAINE)

General Concepts

Before 1988, the term **complicated migraine** was used for migraine that was accompanied or followed by prolonged visual or neurologic deficits or by mental aberrations (Kunkel, 1987). Lance (1982) and others suggested that the symptoms must outlast the headache by more than 24 hours in order for an attack of migraine to be called "complicated." Subsequently, this disorder was reclassified as **migraine with prolonged aura** (Headache Classification Committee of the International Headache Society, 1988).

An excellent example of migraine with prolonged aura was described by Dr. Frank Walsh (Walsh and Hoyt, 1969c). With Dr. V.O. Eareckson, he examined an 18-year-old girl who was unable to read after a severe headache. She perseverated and exhibited nominal aphasia. All her symptoms disappeared by the next day.

Familial Hemiplegic Migraine

In 1910, Clarke described a family in which 11 relatives from four generations experienced recurrent attacks of hemicranial headache associated with transient contralateral hemiparesis. Subsequent authors further characterized this condition, which should be distinguished from a sporadic form that consists solely of migraine with a hemiplegic aura (see above) (Symonds, 1952; Whitty, 1953; Rosenbaum, 1960; Bradshaw and Parsons, 1965; Ohta et al., 1967; Young et al., 1970; Whitty, 1971; Heyck, 1973; Dooling and Sweeney, 1974; Zifkin et al., 1980; Gastaut et al., 1981; Joutel et al., 1995; Athwal and Lennox, 1996). In most cases of familial hemiplegic migraine, motor impairment—either hemiplegia or hemiparesis—precedes the headache, but it may occasionally follow it. Other symptoms may be present, including paresthesias, aphasia, prosopagnosia, visual disturbances, impaired mentation, confusion, and even coma. The symptoms and signs may last for days rather than hours. The headache is usually contralateral to the hemiplegia. It is usually severe, pulsating, and almost always associated with nausea, vomiting, or both. Like the neurologic symptoms and signs, it may persist for hours to days.

Familial hemiplegic migraine is an autosomal-dominant genetically heterogeneous condition with about half of the affected families expressing a specific locus on chromosome 19 (Joutel et al., 1993, 1994; Ophoff et al., 1994; Hutchinson et al., 1995; Joutel et al., 1995). Some genetic studies also link familial hemiplegic migraine to nearby gene loci for cerebral autosomal-dominant arteriography with subcortical infarcts (CADASIL) (Joutel et al., 1993, 1994; Hutchinson et al., 1995; Weller et al., 1996) and for a familial form of cerebellar atrophy with nystagmus (Joutel et al., 1995; Elliott et al., 1996). Although some of the patients who suffer from the condition are otherwise normal between attacks, others have a variety of persistent neurologic and visual disturbances that predate the onset of the migraine attacks. These disturbances include retinal pigmentary degeneration, deafness, ataxia, and asymmetric tremor in varying combinations. Severe disturbances of eye movement are often present in patients with familial hemiplegic migraine, including inability to generate smooth eye movements, gaze-paretic nystagmus, rebound nystagmus, failure of fixation suppression of the vestibulo-ocular reflex both horizontally and vertically, and low gain of the optokinetic system (Ohta et al., 1967; Young et al., 1970; Codina et al., 1971; Zifkin et al., 1980; Elliott et al., 1996). These abnormalities are believed to be caused by primary degenerative changes in the brainstem and cerebellum (Elliott et al., 1996) rather than by the effects of repeated ischemic migrainous episodes. The presence of retinal pigmentary changes in some patients with familial hemiplegic migraine supports this view.

Migraine Aura Without Headache (Acephalgic Migraine)

Although migraine headache preceded by visual aura was described several thousand years ago, it was not until the 12th century that the Abbess Hildegard of Bingen wrote the first report of a patient who experienced typical visual auras that were not followed by headache (Singer, 1928). Subsequent authors described anecdotal reports of similar cases (Gill, 1890). In 1895, Gowers delivered the Bowman lecture on the visual scotomas of migraine in which he presented several drawings of typical visual aura described by patients who had never experienced any headache. Subsequently, numerous investigators emphasized that patients with a history of typical migraine headaches preceded by aura or migraine headaches without aura may at times experience visual or neurologic aura that are not followed by headache (Alvarez, 1960; Whitty, 1967; Friedman, 1971; Whitty, 1971; Aring, 1972; Fisher, 1980, 1986; Mathew, 1987; Coppeto, 1988b) (Fig. 56.17). Creditor (1982) described his gradual transition over about 30 years from having attacks of migraine headache preceded by visual aura, neurologic aura, or both, to a symptom-free period that lasted about 20 years, to rare episodes of visual or neurologic aura unassociated with headache. Alvarez reported that 13% of 618 patients with otherwise typical migraine attacks experienced acephalgic migraine, usually in later life. In addition, some patients who have never had a significant headache nevertheless experience occasional or recurrent, stereotyped, isolated, visual or neurologic aura (G.L. Johnson, 1936; Carroll, 1970; Whitty, 1971; Wolter and Burchfield, 1971; Hedges, 1972; Wiley, 1979; Fisher, 1980, 1986; Mathew, 1987; Hupp et al., 1989). In some of these patients, the aura only occurs under specific circumstances, such as during or after exercise (Atkinson and Appenzeller, 1981; O'Connor and Tredici, 1981; Thompson, 1987; Imes and Hoyt, 1989).

O'Connor and Tredici (1981) identified and evaluated 61 patients with acephalgic migraine. The age of these patients ranged from 21 to 61 years. Visual symptoms were identical with those experienced by patients with classic migraine and included scintillating scotomas, transient hemianopias, bilat-

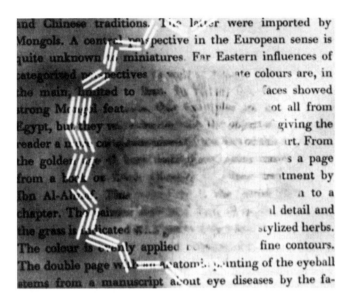

Figure 56.17. Visual aura without headache (acephalgic migraine). Photographic representation of a scintillating scotoma that occurred in a patient without headache. Note darkening of the left homonymous visual field associated with blurring of central vision and a fortification figure in the left hemifield. (From Wiley RG: The scintillating scotoma without headache. Ann Neurol *11*:581–585, 1979.)

eral central scotomas, transient monocular loss of vision, altitudinal visual field loss, tunnel vision, and extreme peripheral field (temporal crescent) loss. Visual symptoms lasted from 15 seconds to 3 hours. A positive family history was obtained in only 24% of patients, and only two patients had a previous history of common or classic migraine headache. Other visual symptoms that may be experienced by patients with acephalgic migraine include "sparkling," "dancing," or "dazzling" lights, bursts of light "as if a flash bulb went off," and rainbow-colored arches that are shades of red, green, gold, yellow, blue, or purple (Gowers, 1895; Fisher, 1980; Hupp et al., 1989).

An attack of migraine aura without headache may be characterized by transient neurologic symptoms instead of transient visual symptoms (Fisher, 1980, 1986). Such symptoms include paresthesias, dysarthria, aphasia, brainstem symptoms, and hemiparesis. Vertigo is often a prominent symptom (Bramwell and McMullen, 1926; Slater, 1979; Moretti et al., 1980; Behan and Carlin, 1982; Mathew, 1987). A patient with these symptoms may be thought to have experienced a transient ischemic attack from thrombotic or embolic cerebrovascular disease, particularly when the patient is over 40 years old (Fisher 1980, 1986). There are, however, some features of migrainous transient neurologic symptoms that distinguish them from the symptoms produced by cerebrovascular disease (Fisher 1980, 1986). Transient neurologic dysfunction associated with scintillating scotomas is almost never caused by cerebrovascular disease, particularly when there is a gradual buildup of the scintillations. Another reliable sign of migrainous paresthesias is the "march" of numbness as it gradually spreads over the face or fingers and hand and migrates from face to limb or vice versa or crosses to

the face and hand on the opposite side. The evolution usually occurs over 15–25 minutes. This gradual spread is unusual in thrombotic or embolic cerebrovascular disease. Patients with migrainous aura unassociated with headache often experience a progression from one symptom to another without a delay. A patient may thus experience paresthesias followed immediately by aphasia or paralysis, with one symptom disappearing as the next develops. The occurrence of two or more similar or identical neurologic episodes helps to exclude embolism, although thrombosis could produce such episodes. The history of a similar "spell" associated with a headache suggests migraine rather than cerebrovascular disease and finally, one may be reassured by the presence of a generally benign course without permanent neurologic sequelae.

A diagnosis of acephalgic migraine should not be made in any patient unless embolic and thrombotic cerebrovascular disease and a seizure disorder have been excluded by appropriate examinations and diagnostic tests (Hedges and Lackman, 1976; Fisher, 1980; O'Connor and Tredici, 1981; Schatz, 1981). Selected patients may need to undergo a thorough neurologic examination, a cardiac evaluation that includes echocardiography and Holter monitoring, rheologic studies, serologic studies for evidence of connective tissue (collagen vascular) disease, cerebral angiography, or a combination of these (Fisher, 1980; Schatz, 1981). In addition, Mortimer et al. (1990b) believed that acephalgic migraine can be differentiated from other conditions, such as transient ischemic attacks, demyelinating disease, and simple partial epilepsy, by the results of flash and pattern visual-evoked potentials (see below).

Acephalgic migraine should be a diagnosis of exclusion in most patients, especially older patients without a history of migraine who experience a transient neurologic episode, and children who experience episodes of transient monocular loss of vision (see Chapter 55).

We examined a 15-year-old girl who experienced episodes of transient monocular visual loss in the left eye. She had no history of motion sickness, somnambulism, or migraine in the past, and she appeared to be perfectly healthy. The episodes of visual loss were sudden and unassociated with scintillations, fortification scotomas, etc. They consisted of painless, rapid blurring of vision as if a curtain were being pulled down over the left eye. Vision was poor for about 15 minutes, after which the "curtain would rise" rapidly, and vision would return to normal. The patient could not tell when an episode of visual loss was about to begin, nor did she ever experience a headache during or after an episode. A complete neuro-ophthalmologic examination, including static perimetry, was normal. The patient underwent a complete systemic evaluation that culminated in cerebral angiography. The results of all studies were normal, and a diagnosis of acephalgic migraine was made. About 6 months later, the patient experienced a severe, right-sided headache associated with nausea and vomiting, but without visual symptoms. The headache lasted 24 hours. She subsequently had several other right- and left-sided headaches, some of which were preceded by monocular and binocular visual loss with and without scintillations.

and may alternate sides with attacks; extraocular muscle paralysis may occur with the first attack of headache or, rarely, precede it. Usually, however, the paralysis appears subsequent to an established migraine pattern.

3. Exclusion of other causes, by arteriography, surgical exploration, or autopsy.

Walsh and O'Doherty (1960) applied the above criteria to about 200 cases previously recorded as ophthalmoplegic migraine. They excluded all patients with associated disease capable of producing the clinical picture, all patients without a history of headache, and all patients who had a single attack without a previous history of headache. An autopsy was performed in only eight cases, and only one of these cases was subsequently classified as true ophthalmoplegic migraine. This case, originally reported by Alpers and Yaskin (1951), fulfilled all three of the criteria established by Walsh and O'Doherty: (*a*) the patient initially had typical attacks of migraine with and without aura; (*b*) subsequent episodes were associated with oculomotor nerve paresis; and (*c*) no evidence was found, either clinically or at autopsy, of another organic cause for the symptom complex. Subsequent investigators reported similar cases (Ford, 1952; Ver Brugghen, 1955; Lincoff and Cogan, 1957).

Friedman et al. (1962) studied the records of 5000 patients with a diagnosis of migraine and found eight examples (0.16%) of ophthalmoplegic migraine. All eight patients had recurrent attacks of headache, usually accompanied by nausea and vomiting, and ipsilateral oculomotor nerve paresis. In all cases, the headache was located, at least in part, in the orbital region. It tended to be continuous and intense. The oculomotor nerve paresis reached a maximum as the headache began to resolve. The paresis persisted for 1–4 weeks before resolving.

Unlike most other forms of migraine, ophthalmoplegic migraine does not occur more often in women than in men (Corbett, 1983). Instead, it occurs equally in both sexes, perhaps because it almost always begins in childhood, and the incidence of migraine is the same in both sexes until menarche (Bille, 1962).

The majority of patients with ophthalmoplegic migraine experience their initial attack in the 1st decade of life, usually before 5 years of age (Fig. 56.20). In fact, ophthalmoplegic migraine may occur in infants (Charcot, 1892; Suckling, 1888; Ford, 1952; van Pelt and Andermann, 1964; Woody and Blaw, 1986; Vollrath-Junger, 1988).

Because ophthalmoplegic migraine most often occurs in infancy or early childhood, the first attack may be incorrectly ascribed to some other process, such as trauma, aneurysm, infection, or even a recent immunization. Only when the condition resolves and then recurs is the correct diagnosis made. Such a case was reported by Chan et al. (1980), who initially described a 17-month-old boy with an isolated right oculomotor nerve paresis that developed 2 weeks after he was given measles vaccine. Two years later, Thompson (1982) suggested that, in fact, it was more likely that this patient had ophthalmoplegic migraine. Hassin (1987) subsequently reported that the patient experienced a severe right-sided headache associated with pallor, nausea, vomiting, and

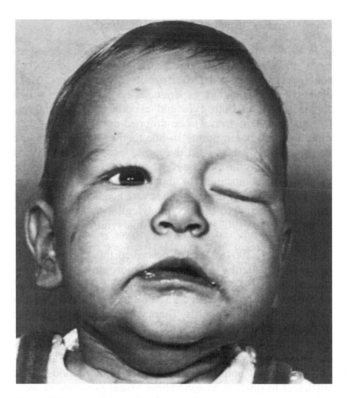

Figure 56.20. Ophthalmoplegic migraine in a 10-month-old child. Note complete left ptosis. Most cases of ophthalmoplegic migraine begin within the first decade of life, usually before 5 years of age. (From Vollrath-Junger C. Rezidivierende OKulomotoriusolähmungen: Ein Fall von ophthalmoplegisher migräne? Klin Monatsbl Augenheilkd *192*:154–156, 1988.)

crying when he was 3 1/2 years of age. Three days later, he developed a right-sided ophthalmoparesis and ptosis. The ptosis resolved within several days, and the ophthalmoparesis resolved over 8–9 weeks. At age 5, the patient had two episodes of right-sided oculomotor nerve paresis, and, at age 6, he experienced a right-sided headache associated with vomiting, nausea, and insomnia. MR imaging and a complete neurologic examination gave normal results. Angiography was not permitted by the patient's parents.

Rare patients experience their first attack of ophthalmoplegic migraine in adulthood, but such patients almost always have a history of typical migraine headaches with and without aura since childhood, a family history of migraine, or both (Fenichel, 1968; see Table in Cruciger and Mazow, 1978). We are thus reluctant to make a diagnosis of ophthalmoplegic migraine in an adult unless: (*a*) there is a strong family history of migraine; (*b*) the patient has had other types of migraine in the past; and (*c*) other causes of painful ophthalmoplegia have been excluded by appropriate laboratory and neuroimaging studies (see also Smith and Quencer, 1984).

The headache that occurs in patients with ophthalmoplegic migraine is not invariably severe. Whitty (1970) stated that the headache was often "insignificant," and it may even be absent in rare cases (Durkan et al., 1981—see below). We examined one child in whom recurrent oculomo-

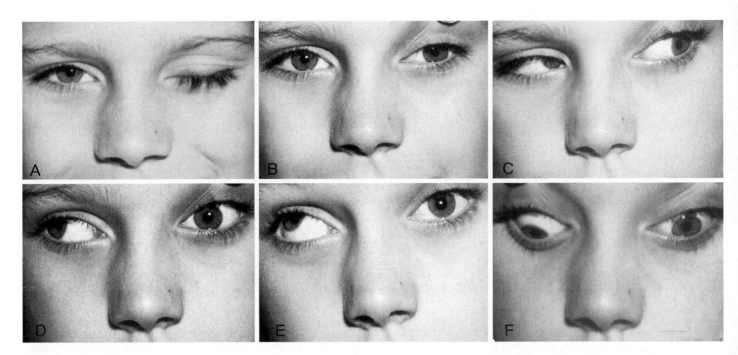

Figure 56.21. Ophthalmoplegic migraine in a 10-year-old child. Note complete left oculomotor nerve paresis. The left pupil is not dilated, but it was sluggishly reactive.

tor nerve paresis was associated with a mild aching sensation around and behind the ipsilateral orbit. Until we examined him in the midst of an attack, it was not clear if he was experiencing ophthalmoplegic migraine or recurrent orbital pseudotumor.

As noted above, ophthalmoplegic migraine usually affects the oculomotor nerve. Initially, the paresis may be characterized by ptosis and minimal limitation of eye movement. Within a few hours, however, the oculomotor nerve paresis becomes complete or nearly so (Fig. 56.21), although Katz and Rimmer (1989) described a 13-year-old girl who experienced recurrent attacks of ophthalmoplegic migraine initially characterized by paresis of only the muscles supplied by the superior division of the oculomotor nerve (Fig. 56.22).

In our experience and in that of others (Friedman et al., 1962; Pearce and Foster, 1965; Loewenfeld, 1980; Corbett, 1983), the pupil is almost always affected, although in many cases it is only mildly dilated and reacts sluggishly to light and near stimulation. Nevertheless, some patients with ophthalmoplegic migraine have a complete oculomotor nerve paresis except for total sparing of the pupil (Friedman et al., 1962). Vijayan (1980) described such a patient, and he concluded from a review of the literature that the pupil is unaffected in about 40% of cases. This has not been our experience.

When the oculomotor nerve paresis recovers, ptosis may begin to improve before there is evidence of improved ocular motility or pupillary constriction to light or near stimulation.

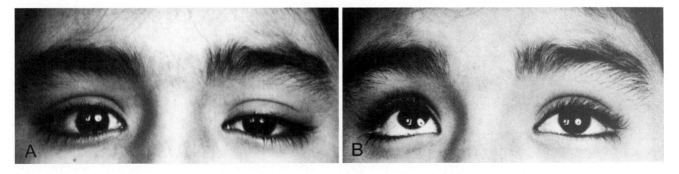

Figure 56.22. Ophthalmoplegic migraine characterized by paresis of the superior division of the oculomotor nerve. The patient was a 13-year-old girl who previously had experienced three episodes of painless left ptosis without diplopia at ages 9, 10, and 11. Each of these episodes lasted 48 hours and then resolved. The patient was examined 6 days after the onset of a fourth attack. *A,* The patient has a moderate left ptosis. There is no exotropia, nor is there anisocoria. *B,* There is marked limitation of elevation of the left eye. (From Katz B, Rimmer S: Ophthalmoplegic migraine with super ramus oculomotor paresis. J Clin Neuro-ophthalmol *9*:181–183, 1989.)

In most cases, however, there is a generalized, rapid improvement. Complete resolution of the paresis usually occurs (Miller, 1977; Harley, 1980; Keith, 1987), but some patients with repeated attacks have persistent ophthalmoparesis, ptosis, anisocoria with the affected pupil having a sluggish reaction to light, or a combination of these (Friedman et al., 1962; Vollrath-Junger, 1988). In rare instances, reported attacks of ophthalmoplegic migraine lead to secondary oculomotor nerve synkinesis (aberrant regeneration) (Walsh and Hoyt, 1969d; Lepore and Glaser, 1980; O'Day et al., 1980).

The trochlear and abducens nerves are affected in ophthalmoplegic migraine much less often than is the oculomotor nerve. Walsh and Hoyt (1969d) reported cases of isolated trochlear nerve paresis in ophthalmoplegic migraine, and a few other cases have also been reported (Ostfeld and Wolff, 1957). We have seen one such case, an 8-year-old boy whose mother and father both had severe migraine. The child initially was noted to have spells of head holding and irritability at about 2 years of age. When he was 4 years old, he began to experience severe headaches that occurred about three to four times a year and were associated with nausea and occasional vomiting. During these episodes, the child complained that light hurt his eyes. He would go to his room, turn off the lights, and lie down. The headache usually resolved within 24 hours. When he was 7 years old, the child complained of double vision during a typical migraine attack, although the parents did not notice anything wrong with the child's eyes. The double vision lasted about 1 week and then resolved. The child subsequently had several more attacks of migraine during which he experienced diplopia. We examined him in the midst of one attack. At that time, he had a right hypertropia of about 12 prism diopters in primary position at distance. The hypertropia increased on left gaze, and it was greatest when the patient looked down and to the left. The hypertropia decreased when the head was tilted toward the left shoulder, and it increased when the head was tilted toward the right shoulder. The patient also had 4 prism diopters of excyclotorsion when measured using double Maddox rods (see Chapter 27). A diagnosis of ophthalmoplegic migraine affecting the right trochlear nerve was made. The patient underwent a complete neurologic examination, Prostigmin test, and MR imaging. No abnormalities were found. The trochlear nerve paresis resolved completely over the next 3 weeks.

Isolated abducens nerve paresis occurs as part of ophthalmoplegic migraine more often than trochlear nerve paresis but not as often as oculomotor nerve paresis. Walsh and Hoyt (1969d) stated that the ratio of abducens nerve paresis to oculomotor nerve paresis was about 1:10, and we would agree (see also Harris, 1976). Osuntokun and Osuntokun (1972) identified only one case of ophthalmoplegic migraine with abducens nerve paresis compared with 18 cases of oculomotor nerve paresis. We have seen only two patients with isolated abducens nerve paresis as part of the ophthalmoplegic migraine syndrome. One patient was a 5-year-old boy with stereotyped attacks since 3 years of age. The other patient was a 25-year-old man with a long history of typical migraine headaches preceded by scintillating scotomas. He also had occasional migraine headaches without aura. During an otherwise typical migraine headache unassociated with visual aura, the patient developed severe horizontal diplopia that persisted after the headache resolved. He was admitted to the Johns Hopkins Hospital at which time the neurologic examination was normal except for a left abducens nerve paresis. With the right eye fixing, the patient had an esotropia of 24 prism diopters; the right eye could abduct only about 30 beyond the midline. The patient underwent lumbar puncture and four-vessel cerebral angiography. He also underwent a variety of serologic studies, including tests for vasculitis. All results were negative or normal. The patient's abducens nerve paresis began to improve about 10 days after onset and completely resolved within 6 weeks.

More than one ocular motor nerve may be affected during an attack of ophthalmoplegic migraine. Dr. Frank Walsh (Walsh and Hoyt, 1969d) stated that he had seen two cases of total unilateral ophthalmoplegia. One of the patients had experienced five attacks that consisted of left-sided headache, immobility of the left eye, ptosis, and a dilated fixed pupil. After each attack, the ophthalmoplegia persisted for about 2 weeks. After the fifth attack, there was a persistent paresis of the left inferior rectus muscle. The patient underwent cerebral angiography and pneumoencephalography with examination of the cerebrospinal fluid. Both studies were normal.

As noted above, almost all cases of ophthalmoplegic migraine are unilateral. Hutchinson and Donaldson (1989) described a 37-year-old woman who experienced typical migraine attacks about twice a month since age 12. The attacks were characterized by an aura of scintillating photopsias followed within 2 hours by a left frontal headache associated with vomiting, diarrhea, and occasional tingling of the hands and feet. After a typical attack, the patient awoke with what the authors stated was "moderate left ptosis" but which photographically appeared to be bilateral ptosis, left greater than right. There was also bilateral, generalized limitation of eye movement, and both pupils were dilated and nonreactive to light or near stimulation. The ophthalmoplegia did not improve during oculocephalic testing. The patient underwent a complete neurologic evaluation that included serologic studies, CT scan, cerebral angiography, and lumbar puncture. The results of all studies were normal except for an elevated protein content and an increased IgG: albumin ratio in the cerebrospinal fluid. Within 1 week, the patient's ptosis almost completely resolved, eye movements were asymmetrically improved, and both pupils reacted to light and near stimulation. Ten weeks after the onset of the condition, the patient had no evidence of internal or external ophthalmoplegia. Over the next 5 years, she had no further attacks of ophthalmoplegia. Hutchinson and Donaldson (1989) postulated that the ophthalmoplegia in this patient resulted from simultaneous damage to the ocular motor nerves in both cavernous sinuses.

Increased intracranial pressure can cause herniation of the hippocampal gyrus, producing an oculomotor nerve paresis that occasionally may be transient, recurrent, and associated with severe headache, thus mimicking ophthalmoplegic migraine, at least superficially. Harrington and Flocks (1953) described a 50-year-old man with a 50 lb weight loss over the previous 6 months who complained of generalized headache, periodic dizziness, episodes of urinary incontinence, and a marked diminution in sense of smell. Neurologic examination revealed that the patient had slight deviation of the tongue to the left, hypalgesia of the left face, weakness of the left masseter muscle, plantar reflexes that were equivocally extensor, and bilateral papilledema. Over a period of 16 days, the patient had six attacks of transient paresis of the right oculomotor nerve associated with a right frontal headache. Each attack lasted only about 5 minutes, and there was complete resolution of the ophthalmoplegia until the last attack, following which the patient had persistent oculomotor nerve paresis that was still present 4 days later when the patient died. Autopsy revealed bronchogenic carcinoma with metastasis to the right frontal and right temporal lobes. There was marked herniation of the right hippocampal gyrus over the edge of the tentorium with pressure on and stretching of the right oculomotor nerve. Although this case emphasizes that recurrent, painful oculomotor nerve paresis may result from herniation of the hippocampal gyrus, it is doubtful that anyone would mistake this case for true ophthalmoplegic migraine. First, the patient was an adult who had never had migraine in the past. Second, the patient had numerous other chronic systemic and neurologic symptoms and signs, including papilledema. Finally, the patient's episodes of oculomotor nerve paresis were much shorter than normal ophthalmoplegic migraine.

Diabetic ophthalmoparesis can produce a clinical picture similar to that of ophthalmoplegic migraine, but diabetic ophthalmoparesis rarely occurs in children. In addition, the ophthalmoparesis that occurs in patients with diabetes mellitus, hypertension, giant cell arteritis, and other systemic vasculopathies usually persists longer than the ophthalmoplegia associated with migraine.

The differential diagnosis of ophthalmoplegic migraine is the differential diagnosis of painful ophthalmoplegia affecting one or more of the ocular motor nerves. When only the oculomotor nerve is affected, the primary concern is an intracranial aneurysm, even in a young child (Miller, 1977; Gabianelli et al., 1989). Such an aneurysm may be located at the junction of the internal carotid and posterior communicating arteries, at the junction of the basilar and superior cerebellar arteries, at the tip of the basilar artery, or within the cavernous sinus (see Chapter 53). It has been suggested that thin-section CT scanning, MR imaging, MR angiography (MRA) or spiral contrast-enhanced CT scanning (also called dynamic CT scanning) have sufficient resolution to permit identification of any aneurysm producing a painful oculomotor nerve paresis and that cerebral angiography is not necessary when one of these studies gives normal results, particularly in children (Bailey et al., 1984; Smith and Quencer, 1984; Woody and Blaw, 1986; Teasdale et al., 1989; Tomsack et al., 1991). This may be true for infants and young children with a typical presentation (Bailey et al., 1984; Smith and Quencer, 1984; Woody and Blaw, 1986; Gabianelli et al., 1989), but we still believe that conventional angiography should be considered in selected children and adults with painful oculomotor nerve paresis and normal results with CT scanning, MR imaging, or both, particularly

when the pupil is affected, and there is no other obvious explanation for the paresis (see also Fox, 1989).

Mucocele of the sphenoid sinus can produce painful ophthalmoplegia as can a variety of inflammatory lesions and tumors that invade the cavernous sinus. In most cases, such lesions can be detected using MR imaging, particularly when some type of paramagnetic contrast agent is used to enhance the images.

The pathogenesis of ophthalmoplegic migraine is unclear. The unilateral nature of the headache and the oculomotor nerve paresis that begins with ptosis and ends with complete paresis suggests a lesion in the peripheral portion of the oculomotor nerve. Rapid onset of the paresis could result from compression, ischemia, or both. Ehlers (1928) reported two patients with episodes of headache and oculomotor nerve paresis who experienced a visual aura consisting of a contralateral homonymous scotoma before each attack. Because of this combination of symptoms and signs, Ehlers (1928) postulated that changes in the caliber of the posterior cerebral artery were responsible for the oculomotor nerve paresis. Other investigators (Walsh and O'Doherty, 1960; Wolff, 1963; Vollrath-Junger, 1988) ascribed ophthalmoplegic migraine to compression of one or more of the ocular motor nerves by a dilated or edematous cavernous portion of the internal carotid artery (Fig. 56.23). Support for the compression theory of ophthalmoplegic migraine came from the results of angiographic studies performed in three patients during an attack and from some experimental pharmacologic studies. In one patient reported by Walsh and O'Doherty (1960), angiography showed narrowing of the intracavernous portion of the right internal carotid artery during an attack of right-sided ophthalmoplegic migraine. The left internal carotid artery appeared normal. Repeat angiography was performed in this patient during a second attack

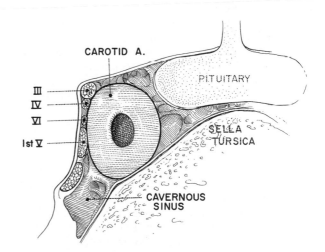

Figure 56.23. Illustration showing the possible pathogenesis of ophthalmoplegic migraine. An edematous carotid artery compresses or renders ischemic one or more of the ocular motor nerves within the cavernous sinus. One might expect more cases of ophthalmoplegic migraine affecting the abducens nerve than the oculomotor nerve if this mechanism were correct, however. (From Walsh JP, O'Doherty DS: A possible explanation of the mechanism of ophthalmoplegic migraine. Neurology *10*:1079–1084, 1960.)

on the left side. The right internal carotid artery appeared normal, but there was narrowing of the cavernous portion of the left internal carotid artery. A second patient described by Walsh and O'Doherty (1960) had a "suggestion of narrowing of the internal carotid artery ipsilateral to the oculomotor nerve paresis." Friedman et al. (1962) reported segmental narrowing of the basilar artery between the origins of the superior cerebellar and posterior cerebral arteries in one patient with ophthalmoplegic migraine.

In addition to these reports, Imes et al. (1984) described a 31-year-old man with a history of episodes of typical ophthalmoplegic migraine that began at age 5. Each episode was characterized by severe, right-sided headache, nausea, vomiting, and right oculomotor nerve paresis. The headache typically lasted about 5 days, and recovery of the oculomotor nerve paresis usually occurred over 1–2 weeks. Beginning at age 7, the patient had residual oculomotor nerve paresis that increased with subsequent attacks. By the time the patient was seen by Imes et al. (1984), he experienced 60–70 episodes, and he had a significant oculomotor nerve paresis with a right exotropia and hypotropia, 4 mm of right ptosis, inability to elevate or depress the right eye, poor adduction of the right eye, and a right pupil that was 3 mm in diameter and nonreactive. An evaluation revealed a small, perimesencephalic vascular anomaly involving the peduncular and ambient segments of the right posterior cerebral artery. The anomaly filled from both the basilar artery and the right internal carotid artery through a large posterior communicating artery. Imes et al. (1984) suggested that the patient's chronic oculomotor nerve paresis was directly related to the vascular anomaly; however, they could not explain why the paresis should be aggravated by typical migraine headaches, nor did they discuss the absence of aberrant regeneration in this patient. If the anomaly were related to the oculomotor nerve paresis, it was probably on a vascular rather than a compressive basis (see below).

In an attempt to elucidate the mechanism of paresis of ocular motor nerves in migraine, Ostfeld and Wolff (1957) administered norepinephrine solution (4 cc of a 0.2% solution in a liter of 5% dextrose in water) intravenously to three patients relatively early in an attack of ophthalmoplegic migraine. The doses were sufficient to raise systolic blood pressure in all three patients by 20–30 mm Hg. The oculomotor nerve paresis was unaffected in one patient. In the other two patients, one with an oculomotor nerve paresis and one with a trochlear nerve paresis, ocular motor function returned almost to normal within 70–90 minutes. Since norepinephrine has the capacity to constrict large and small arteries and to reduce edema, these observations also support the hypothesis that at least some cases of ophthalmoplegic migraine are caused by compression of affected nerves by thickened or edematous arterial walls and periarterial edema.

Although there is circumstantial angiographic and experimental evidence that favors the compression theory of ophthalmoplegic migraine, certain clinical and angiographic features of the condition support an ischemic cause. In the first place, the angiographic changes observed by Walsh and O'Doherty (1960) and by Friedman et al. (1962) have not been observed in other patients with ophthalmoplegic mi-

graine in whom angiography was performed during the attack (see Table 1 in Vijayan, 1980). If the vascular anomaly of the right posterior cerebral artery detected by Imes et al. (1984) in a patient with typical right-sided ophthalmoplegic migraine and a persistent right oculomotor nerve paresis was directly related to the paresis, it must have been on a vascular basis, since we would have expected chronic compression to produce some evidence of aberrant regeneration of the oculomotor nerve, which was not present. In the second place, if compression were the cause of most cases of ophthalmoplegic migraine, we would expect the abducens nerve to be affected more often than the oculomotor nerve, since it is located within the cavernous sinus between the lateral wall of the intracavernous portion of the carotid artery and the lateral wall of the sinus rather than in the deep layer of the lateral wall away from the artery as are the oculomotor and trochlear nerves (see Chapters 25 and 52).

A more plausible explanation for ophthalmoplegic migraine is that during the attack, a reduction in the flow of blood through the internal carotid artery, and perhaps occasionally through the posterior cerebral or basilar artery, reduces flow to one or more of the ocular motor nerves, producing an ischemic ocular motor nerve paresis. Vijayan (1980) argued that since about two-thirds of patients with ophthalmoplegic migraine characterized by oculomotor nerve paresis have a pupil that is completely spared or incompletely affected, an ischemic process is more likely than a compressive one. Although we agree that ischemic neuropathy is more likely to be the cause of the ophthalmoparesis in ophthalmoplegic migraine than compression from an enlarged, edematous artery, the data provided by Vijayan (1980) do not prove the case, because intracranial aneurysms and other lesions that compress the oculomotor nerve do, in fact, occasionally produce oculomotor nerve paresis with relative or complete pupillary sparing. This is particularly true when the aneurysm is in the cavernous sinus (see Chapters 28 and 53).

Further evidence supporting the theory of ischemia is the association of ophthalmoplegic migraine with an abnormal hemoglobin in Nigerians (Osuntoken et al., 1972), and reports of Gadolinium-enhanced MR imaging showing enhancement of the affected oculomotor nerve with no evidence of a compressive process (Stommel et al., 1993; Straube et al., 1993). We observed similar MR imaging findings in a 5-year-old girl with a history of headaches who presented with a painful pupil-involving oculomotor nerve paresis consistent with an attack of ophthalmoplegic migraine. Gadolinium-enhanced MR imaging demonstrated enhancement of the involved oculomotor nerve (Fig. 56.24).

Clearly, some patients with migraine experience only visual aura unassociated with headache (see below). It thus is not surprising that ophthalmoplegic migraine rarely may occur without associated headache. Durkan et al. (1981) reported two children with isolated, recurrent, painless oculomotor nerve paresis in whom a diagnosis of painless ophthalmoplegic migraine was suspected. One patient experienced her first episode at 1 year of age. A neurologic examination, CT scan, and serologic studies all gave normal results. The child experienced a second attack at age 2½. A repeat neuro-

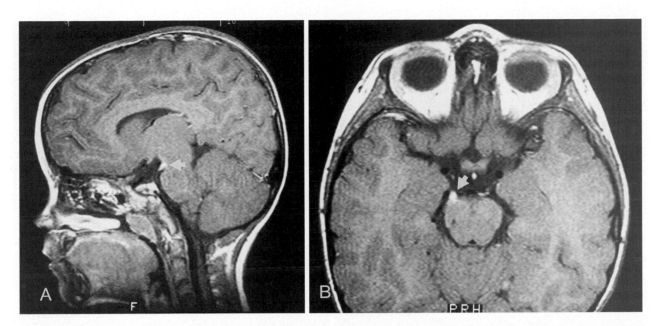

Figure 56.24. Gadolinium-enhanced T1 images of a 5-year-old girl with a history of migraine headaches presenting with a painful pupil-involving right 3rd paresis consistent with an attack of ophthalmoplegic migraine. *A,* Sagittal gadolinium-enhanced T1 image demonstrating enhancement (*arrow*) of the right 3rd cranial nerve as it exits the brainstem. *B,* T1-weighted gadolinium-enhanced axial image with enhancement (*arrow*) of the 3rd cranial nerve exiting the brainstem.

logic examination was normal, as were the results of a CT scan, edrophonium (Tensilon) test, lumbar puncture, cerebral angiography, and serologic studies. About 8 months after the second attack, the patient experienced a severe, generalized headache associated with vomiting. A neurologic examination was normal, and the headache resolved within 24 hours. The second patient reported by Durkan et al. (1981) was 5 years old at the time he developed an acute, complete, right oculomotor nerve paresis with a dilated and fixed pupil. A neurologic examination and CT scan gave normal results. The condition improved spontaneously. Two months later, the only abnormality detected was 1 mm of anisocoria.

RETINAL MIGRAINE

Retinal migraine was briefly mentioned under visual aura (see above) but deserves further discussion because it is more common than ophthalmoplegic migraine, affecting as many as 1 in 200 migraineurs (Troost, 1988, 1996). The Headache Classification Committee of the International Headache Society (1988) defined this migraine type as: repeated attacks of monocular scotoma or blindness lasting less than one hour and associated with headache. Embolic, structural, or other vascular disorders must be ruled out. Manifestations of retinal migraine were reviewed by Hupp et al. (1989) and are discussed below.

Transient monocular visual loss, usually in young adults under 40 years old, is the most frequent clinical presentation and may occur as altitudinal field to loss, concentric constriction, or total blindness (Wilbrand and Saenger, 1901; Moore, 1922; Hachinski et al., 1973; Goodwin et al., 1984; Tomsak and Jergens, 1987; Appleton et al., 1988; Hupp et al., 1989; Tippin et al., 1989; O'Sullivan, 1992). There is often a history of migraine or, more rarely, cluster headache. The visual loss may be associated with sparkling showers of flickering specks of light (retinal photopsias), or it may occur without any other associated visual phenomena. The episode rarely lasts more than 5–10 minutes, and it is often followed by an ipsilateral headache that may be constant or intermittent. Long-lasting amaurotic attacks with recovery are more likely to be migrainous then short attacks; one report described recovery of vision after $7\frac{1}{2}$ hours (Fujino et al, 1983). When headaches occur, they are usually ipsilateral and may occur before, during, or after a headache. Some patients experience repeated attacks of this type, whereas others experience only one such attack amidst attacks of homonymous scintillating scotomas.

If the retina is examined ophthalmoscopically during an attack of monocular visual loss in the setting of migraine, the retinal vessels usually appear constricted (Rosenstein, 1925; Gronvall, 1938; Heyck, 1962; Joffe, 1973; Kline and Kelly, 1980; O'Sullivan, 1992), and the color of the choroid is pale, suggesting constriction of choroidal vessels (Fig. 56.25). In some patients, one or more cotton wool spots (soft exudates) may be seen, indicating a permanent anatomic defect that may or may not be appreciated clinically by the patient after the attack abates. Patients with bilateral, altitudinal visual loss may show constriction of the retinal arteries in the portion of the retina of both eyes corresponding to the affected visual field (Wilbrand and Saenger, 1906).

Wolter and Burchfield (1971) described the unusual case of a 20-year-old man with an 8-year history of what was

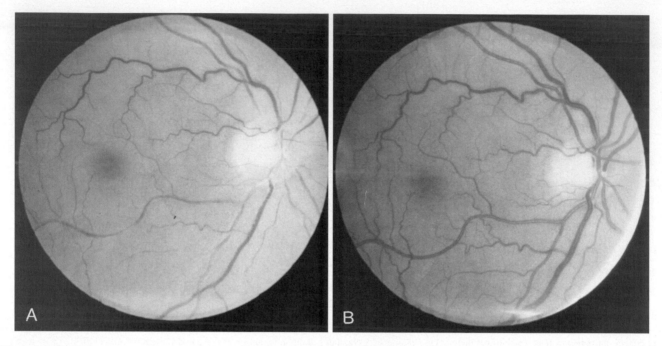

Figure 56.25. Appearance of the retina of the right eye during an attack of migraine in which the visual aura consisted of transient loss of vision in the right eye only. *A*, The retinal vessels are constricted, and the choroid appears pale during the period of visual loss. *B*, After vision has recovered, the retinal vessels seem normal or perhaps slightly dilated. The choroid has a normal appearance. (Courtesy of Dr. Richard Saul.)

thought to be acephalgic migraine characterized by episodes of painless, complete blindness in the right eye. The attacks occurred about once a month and lasted 20–30 minutes. They were never associated with headache, nausea, or neurologic symptoms. One such attack occurred while the patient was being seen for a routine eye examination. Fifteen minutes after the onset of visual loss, the patient had no light perception in the right eye. The right pupil was nonreactive to direct light stimulation, although it reacted when light was shined in the left eye. The left pupil reacted normally to light, but it did not react when light was shined in the right eye. Ophthalmoscopic examination revealed diffuse retinal edema with a "cherry-red" macular spot, but the retinal arteries appeared normal. Three hours after the onset of visual loss, the right ocular fundus appeared normal with no evidence of retinal edema. Subsequent examination revealed normal visual acuity, visual field, pupillary responses, and ophthalmoscopic appearance in both eyes. It is likely that retinal arterial spasm occurred at the time of initial visual loss and lasted only a very short time, just long enough to produce retinal edema but not long enough to produce clinical evidence of permanent visual dysfunction. Such spasm would almost certainly not last longer than a few minutes and perhaps substantially less. Although this patient had no clinical evidence of visual dysfunction and thought his visual function was normal between attacks, an electroretinogram may have shown persistent abnormalities consistent with retinal ischemia.

Retinal vasospasm can cause transient monocular blindness in both young (O'Sullivan et al., 1992) and older (Burger et al., 1991; Winterkorn and Teman, 1991) patients.

Winterkorn and Teman (1991) treated their patient with a calcium channel blocker, and the amaurotic episodes resolved. Miller and Santoro (1981) likewise reported resolution of recurrent monocular amaurosis in a 26-year-old patient after treatment with a calcium channel blocker. Retinal migraine was thought to be causative in most of the amaurotic attacks of the younger group, but the visible retinal vasospasm present in the six patients (ages 59–78 years) reported by Burger et al. (1991) and Winterkorn and Teman (1991) probably was not caused by migraine. Two of the patients reported by Burger et al. (1991) had biopsy-proven giant cell arteritis, and all of the elderly patients probably had proximal atherosclerotic cerebrovascular disease which Williams et al. (1989) suggested predisposes to vasospasm by increasing the vasculature sensitivity to vasoconstrictors such as serotonin. These observations suggest that the retinal and choroidal circulations can constrict in response to a chemical or neural stimulus initiated not only by migraine, but also by conditions remote to the retinal circulation, such as athersclerosis and giant cell arteritis.

Most attacks of partial or complete loss of vision that originate in the retina as part of retinal migraine are transient. Nevertheless, permanent monocular or binocular loss of visual acuity, visual field, or both may develop. When the visual defect is substantial, there is almost always ophthalmoscopic evidence of a central or branch retinal artery occlusion (Galezowski, 1882; Löhlein, 1922; Wegner, 1926; Riley et al., 1935; Vallery-Radot, 1937; Gronvall, 1938; Graveson, 1949; Symonds, 1952; Baron and Chavannes, 1958; Connor, 1962; Heyck, 1962; Krapin, 1964; Pearce and Foster, 1965; Fisher, 1971; Joffe, 1973; Brown et al., 1981; Gray and Car-

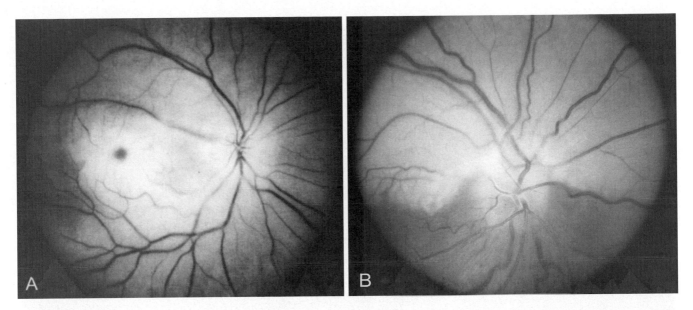

Figure 56.26. Retinal arterial occlusions in migraine. *A*, Central retinal artery occlusion in a 29-year-old man who was experiencing episodes of migraine associated with transient loss of vision in the right eye. The occlusion developed coincident with the initiation of propranolol therapy. (From Katz B. Migrainous central retinal artery occlusion. J Clin Neuro-ophthalmol 6:69–71, 1986). *B*, Branch artery occlusion in a 34-year-old woman with migraine attacks that were often associated with loss of vision in either the right or the left eye but never both eyes simultaneously. During a typical attack, visual acuity was completely lost in the right eye for 15 minutes. The superior visual field then cleared, but an inferior field defect remained.

roll, 1985; Katz, 1986; see Table 3 in Hupp et al., 1989; Inan et al., 1994) (Fig. 56.26). A few cases of permanent visual loss have occurred during or immediately after beginning treatment for migraine (Katz, 1986; N.J. Newman et al., 1989), suggesting that the cause of the retinal vascular occlusion may have been related to the treatment rather than to the migraine itself (Burde, 1986; Katz, 1986). Nevertheless, most occur in patients with untreated migraine. We and others believe that migraine is the most common cause of branch or central retinal artery occlusion in otherwise healthy patients under 40 years of age (Brown et al., 1981).

N.J. Newman et al. (1989) described a woman with presumed migraine headaches without aura who experienced a central retinal artery occlusion in the left eye unassociated with headache. A complete evaluation revealed only bilateral optic disc drusen. About 3 weeks after loss of vision in the left eye, the patient experienced episodes of visual blurring in the right eye. The episodes occurred about once a week, and they lasted 2–5 seconds. Over the next 8 years, the episodes of transient loss of vision in the right eye continued. Although the patient still had headaches, the headaches and the episodes of visual loss were never associated temporally. Eight years after losing vision in the left eye, the patient abruptly lost vision in the right eye and was found to have an acute central retinal artery occlusion in that eye. The bilateral, nonsimultaneous central retinal artery occlusions in this patient may have been caused by the synergistic effects of migraine and optic disc drusen, which are said by some authors to occur together more frequently than would be expected by chance alone (Webb and McCrary, 1977).

Patients in whom a mild visual field defect remains after a typical migraine attack initially may have a small cotton-wool spot (soft exudate) in the region of the retina corresponding to the field defect (Corbett, 1983) (Fig. 56.27). The cotton-wool spot usually disappears within several days, after which a nerve fiber bundle defect may be observed in the affected area, or the area may appear normal despite the persistent field defect (Fig. 56.28). We have examined several patients in whom small paracentral or arcuate scoto-

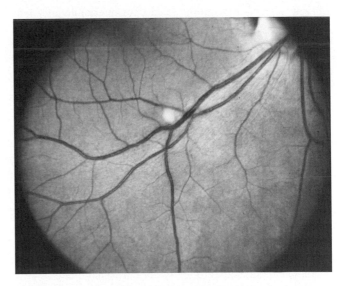

Figure 56.27. Cotton wool spot in a patient with a small superonasal defect in the visual field of the right eye after an attack of migraine that was associated with blurred vision in the right eye. There is a small cotton wool spot along the inferior temporal branch artery.

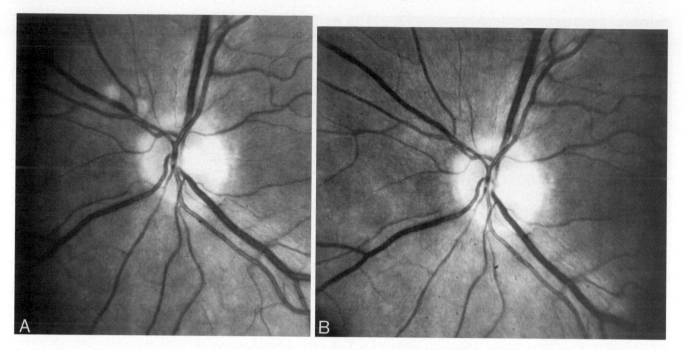

Figure 56.28. Clearing of a cotton wool spot in a 34-year-old woman who developed a persistent visual field defect in the left eye after an attack of migraine with visual aura consisting of blurred vision in the left eye. *A,* Appearance of the left ocular fundus 36 hours after the attack shows a small peripapillary cotton wool spot in the superonasal region. *B,* 1 month after the visual episode, the cotton wool spot has resolved, leaving mild loss of the nerve fiber layer. The patient had a small persistent scotoma adjacent to the blind spot.

mas remained after an attack of otherwise typical migraine. In some of these patients, ophthalmoscopic examination disclosed abnormalities of the arteries, nerve fiber layer, and optic disc corresponding to the field defect, whereas in others, no obvious abnormality could be detected even when fluorescein angiography was performed.

DuBois et al. (1988) described a 38-year-old man with a 28-year history of migraine headaches, predominantly left-sided, preceded by visual aura. During one of these attacks, the patient experienced photosensitivity, impaired night vision, and constriction of the peripheral visual field of both eyes that persisted after the headache resolved. A neuro-ophthalmologic examination revealed a possible hemianopic depression of the visual field of the right eye and a paracentral scotoma in the visual field of the left eye. Ophthalmoscopy disclosed mild narrowing of the retinal vessels, although fluorescein angiography gave normal results. An electroretinogram showed a mildly abnormal a-wave and markedly abnormal photopic and scotopic b-wave function in both eyes. Multilocus dark adaptometry yielded a threshold that was elevated 1 log unit in the right eye and 3 log units in the left eye at 120 minutes. Contrast sensitivity was depressed in both eyes at all spatial frequencies. These findings were thought to be most consistent with severe impairment of retinal function (DuBois, 1988; Dubois et al., 1988).

Some patients with clinically normal visual function after recurrent attacks of migraine with visual aura or after recurrent visual aura without headache, probably have subclinical evidence of retinal ischemia, optic nerve ischemia, or both. In an earlier section of this chapter, we mentioned the 20-year-old patient reported by Wolter and Burchfield (1971) who had monthly attacks of complete blindness in the right eye since 12 years of age. The attacks were never associated with headache, nausea, or neurologic symptoms, and they usually lasted about 20–30 minutes. The patient was examined about 15 minutes after the onset of a typical attack and was found to have no perception of light in the right eye and no direct pupillary response to light in that eye. Although the ocular fundus showed no narrowing or spasm of retinal arteries, there was photographically demonstrable retinal edema and a "cherry-red" spot in the macula. Although this patient had perfectly normal visual function in the right eye after resolution of the attack, neither static perimetry nor contrast sensitivity testing were performed, and he did not undergo any electrophysiologic studies. In view of the finding of transient retinal edema in this patient, and the likelihood that such edema occurred on a regular basis, it seems likely that more sensitive studies of retinal function would have shown evidence of permanent retinal ischemia even though standard examination techniques did not.

Scattered pigmentary changes in the retina resembling unilateral retinitis pigmentosa are observed in patients with migraine who experience repeated attacks of uniocular visual loss (Hupp et al., 1989). These changes were attributed by Connor (1962) to retinal and choroidal ischemia. Gronvall (1938) described a patient who developed a serous retinal detachment, apparently from ischemia of the posterior segment of the eye during an attack of migraine. Walsh and Hoyt (1969f) reported having seen patients who developed typical central serous retinopathy after an attack of migraine.

None of these patients described episodes of transient monocular visual loss. Instead, their symptoms included blurred vision, micropsia, and slow adaptation to changes in light intensity.

Retinal and vitreous hemorrhage may occur during attacks of retinal migraine (Löhlein, 1922; Gronvall, 1938; Dunning, 1942; Wolff, 1963; Victor and Welch, 1977; see Table 3 in Hupp et al., 1989). In some of these cases, the hemorrhage is related to vomiting. In others, it may indicate venous stasis retinopathy (Victor and Welch, 1977; Corbett, 1983).

Branch and central retinal vein occlusion occasionally occur in patients with migraine (Löhlein, 1922; Vallery-Radot, 1937; Friedman, 1951; Coppeto et al., 1986). Coppeto et al. (1986) suggested that patients with retinal venous occlusion in the setting of migraine usually have some additional systemic vasculopathy (e.g., hypertension, collagen vascular disease) and that the retinal vascular occlusion may result from the synergistic effect of this other vascular disorder with the migraine.

Generally, the prognosis for retinal migraine is the same as that of migraine with aura; i.e., very good. Recurrent attacks occur at varying intervals, and if attacks are frequent (several per month), prophylactic therapy may be warranted. Many medications can be used, including amyl nitrate, nitroglycerin, propranolol, calcium channel blockers, isoproterenol, aspirin, napronen, and pentoxyphilline (Corbett, 1983). Vasoconstrictive compounds such as ergots, sumatriptan, and perhaps even propranolol (Burde, 1986) should be avoided.

Retinal or ocular migraine as a cause of transient monocular visual loss is a diagnosis of exclusion. There are no distinguishing symptoms to separate retinal migraine from amaurosis fugax caused by retinal microembolism (Goodwin et al., 1987).

MIGRAINE WITH AURA AND PERMANENT VISUAL OR NEUROLOGIC DEFICIT

Most permanent visual and neurologic deficits in patients with migraine result from ischemia to the brain, eye, or both. In rare cases, intracerebral hemorrhage may produce neurologic and visual deficits (Cole and Aubé, 1990). In some of these cases, permanent deficits seem to be induced by the migraine attack and thus are true migraine-related strokes. In other instances, factors other than migraine, such as hypertension, mitral valve prolapse, oral contraceptive agents, diabetes mellitus, smoking, and the presence of antiphospholipid antibodies seem to be responsible (Welch and Levine, 1990). In the section that follows, we discuss migraine-related permanent visual loss and stroke.

Permanent Visual Deficits

Permanent visual deficits may occur in any patient who experiences the visual aura of migraine (Corbett, 1983; Hupp et al., 1989). The deficits may be severe or minimal. They range from total blindness in one or both eyes to a small scotoma in the visual field of one eye (Ferroir et al., 1981; Vignat et al., 1982; Lewis et al., 1989). Permanent visual deficits, like transient ones, may result from damage to any part of the visual sensory system, including the striate cortex,

optic chiasm, optic nerve, retina, and choroid (Kupersmith et al., 1979; Safran, 1985; Kupersmith et al., 1987).

Permanent Homonymous Visual Field Defects from Ischemia of the Striate Cortex

The homonymous field defects that occur as part of the classic migraine syndrome almost always are transient, but occasionally they persist. The patient with a permanent defect usually has experienced recurrent, transient scintillating scotomas in the same region of visual space before the permanent event occurs (Ormond, 1913; Hunt, 1915; Symonds, 1952). These transient episodes have often occurred in a crescendo fashion, becoming more and more frequent and perhaps lasting longer and longer over the preceding several days to weeks.

A permanent homonymous field defect may be complete or partial. When partial, the defects in the two eyes are almost always exquisitely congruous as would be expected from a lesion in the striate cortex (Figs. 56.29 and 56.30). Symonds (1952) described a 54-year-old man who had experienced attacks of migraine since childhood. The attacks were stereotyped. They were always characterized by the occurrence of wavy lines in rapid movement that would appear on one or other side of the visual field and spread gradually across the whole field. This visual aura would last 30–40 minutes, followed by severe frontal headache with nausea and, when he was younger, vomiting. The headache would last all day, but after he had slept, the headache would disappear. One morning, he awoke with the usual wavy lines in the right field of vision, and he expected the usual sequence. This time, however, the wavy lines remained at the right periphery instead of travelling across the field, and no headache developed. The vision of wavy lines persisted over the next 6 months, at which time he was examined by Symonds, who found a right homonymous hemianopia with macular sparing. Left carotid and vertebral angiography showed no abnormalities.

Hollenhorst (1953) described a residual homonymous hemianopia in four patients after an attack of migraine with visual aura, and Connor (1962) described six patients with isolated, permanent, homonymous hemianopia as a sequela of migraine. Kupersmith et al. (1987) reported 17 patients with cerebral infarcts related to migraine, 16 of whom had residual homonymous field defects (Fig. 56.30), and Lewis et al. (1989) reported three patients who developed a homonymous hemianopia after experiencing recurrent migraine headaches that were predominantly unilateral and located on the side contralateral to the field defect. We and others (Elmaleh et al., 1987) have observed permanent homonymous hemianopia with sparing of the macula after an otherwise typical migraine attack, as well as several patients in whom a permanent, congruous, hemianopic scotoma persisted after an otherwise typical attack of classic migraine.

A permanent homonymous quadrantanopia or quadrantic scotoma may be present after an attack of migraine (Schiff-Wertheimer, 1926; T.H. Johnson, 1936; Rich, 1948) (Fig. 56.29B). Walsh (1951) reported a patient who developed a permanent homonymous quadrantanopia after experiencing a transient homonymous hemianopia on many occasions be-

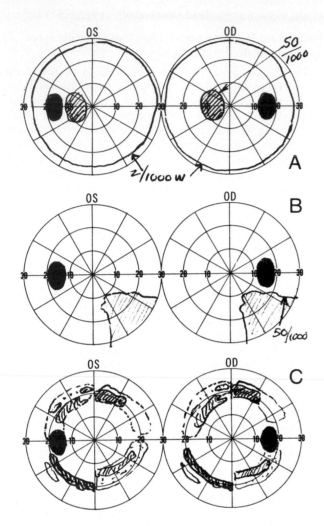

Figure 56.29. Permanent defects in the visual field from damage to the striate cortex during an attack of migraine with visual aura. *A*, Dense, left, homonymous hemianopic scotoma in a 13-year-old boy who was experiencing episodes of transient homonymous hemianopia and scintillating scotoma separately affecting either the left or the right homonymous visual field followed by headache and nausea. His first symptoms began when he was 6 years old. Note apparent sparing of the macula and marked congruity of the scotoma that must have resulted from damage to both occipital poles just above and below the calcarine fissure. *B*, Congruous right inferior homonymous quadrantanopia that remained after an episode of transient homonymous hemianopia in a 28-year-old man who had experienced attacks of migraine with aura since he was 14 years old. Again note exquisite congruity of the defects and sparing of the macula that typically results from a posterior occipital infarct. *C*, Unusual, scattered, bilateral congruous homonymous scotomas in a 45-year-old woman who for years had experienced attacks of bilateral loss of vision that lasted 15–20 minutes. The visual loss was associated with a luminous, shimmering, silvery sensation in both the right and the left halves of the field of vision. The patient had normal appearing ocular fundi and a normal electroretinogram. Although the visual field defects seem as though they should be retinal or optic nerve in origin, they obey the vertical midline and are quite congruous.

fore a migraine headache. The patient subsequently experienced visual hallucinations in the blind quadrantic regions (see above). Corbett (1983) reported a similar patient. One of the patients with migraine-related stroke reported by Rothrock et al. (1988a) initially presented with stupor, weakness of the right arm, and cortical blindness. CT scanning eventually demonstrated bilateral occipital infarcts. The patient's condition gradually improved, but she had persistent memory loss and a left inferior homonymous quadrantanopia (see also Rothrock et al., 1988b).

Although some patients with migraine experience cortical blindness as part of the visual aura (see above), the blindness almost always resolves completely. When it does not, it usually leaves the patient with a homonymous visual field defect, as in the case described by Rothrock et al. (1988a, 1988b). Nevertheless, some patients are left with bilateral, homonymous visual field defects that reflect damage to both occipital lobes (Fig. 56.29C). Dr. Walter Dandy examined a patient who suffered permanent bilateral homonymous hemianopia with macular sparing after an attack of classic migraine (Walsh and Hoyt, 1969e). We have seen a patient who experienced transient cortical blindness during an attack of migraine, following which the patient became aware of defects in both the right and left hemifields. When examined 24 hours after the onset of visual loss, she had bilateral homonymous hemianopic scotomas that were unchanged 3 months later when the patient was re-examined.

Dr. William F. Hoyt (Walsh and Hoyt, 1969e) examined a patient who experienced simultaneous, permanent loss of the superior half of the visual field of both eyes after an attack of migraine. The patient had no optic disc swelling in either eye at the time of visual loss and never developed optic atrophy. The field defects probably were caused by infarcts of the infracalcarine portions of both occipital lobes. Moen et al. (1988) reported a 37-year-old man with a history of migraine who experienced bilateral occipital lobe infarctions and was left with a residual bilateral superior quadrantanopia. Ford (Walsh and Hoyt, 1969e) examined a patient who lost vision permanently in the inferior quadrants of both eyes after a migraine attack. The findings were most consistent with bilateral occipital lobe infarctions. The superior portions of the cortex were affected in this case.

Most of the cases of permanent homonymous hemianopia that occur in the setting of migraine do so in patients with untreated disease. Nevertheless, Gilbert (1982) reported a patient who experienced a crescendo in the number and severity of her classic migraine attacks and was treated with propranolol, 20 mg tid. Two weeks later, she developed dysarthria, left hemiplegia, a left sensory defect, and a dense left homonymous hemianopia. This stroke may have been caused not by the migraine itself but by the vasoconstrictive effects of propranolol. For this reason, Burde (1986) recommended using β-blocking agents with extreme caution in patients with any form of migraine other than migraine headache without aura (common migraine).

Permanent Bitemporal Hemianopia from Optic Chiasmal Ischemia

It is surprising how few patients develop permanent bitemporal field loss after a migraine attack, considering the

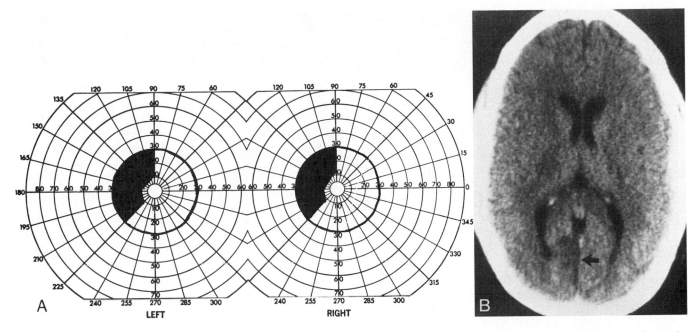

Figure 56.30. Appearance and pathophysiology of permanent cortical visual field defects in a patient with migraine associated with visual aura. *A,* Permanent, dense, left homonymous scotoma in a patient who was experiencing typical migraine headaches with visual aura consisting of a transient left homonymous hemianopia. On one occasion, the field defect did not clear completely. Note macular sparing and marked congruity of the defects. *B,* CT scan performed in the patient shows a region of low density in the right occipital lobe consistent with an infarct (*arrow*). (From Kupersmith MJ, Warren FA, Hass WK: The non-benign aspects of migraine. Neuro-ophthalmology 7:1–10, 1987.)

large number of patients in whom the visual aura of migraine is characterized by a scintillating bitemporal hemianopia or scotoma that eventually becomes complete. We are unaware of any reports in the literature of such cases, although we have experience with one case. We examined a 38-year-old man with a persistent visual field defect after a typical attack of classic migraine. For many years, the patient experienced attacks of migraine that began with a visual aura characterized by the appearance of scintillating scotomas in the temporal periphery of both eyes. The visual deficits would expand and drift toward fixation over 15–20 minutes. At the end of this time, the patient would be unable to see to the left of fixation with the left eye and to the right of fixation with the right eye. The deficit would last for 5–10 minutes and would then begin to clear slowly and simultaneously in both temporal hemifields. Vision became normal within 30 minutes after the onset of visual symptoms. At about the time the bitemporal field defect became complete, the patient would develop a progressively severe headache that became excruciating within 1–2 hours. The headache was associated with anorexia, nausea, and occasional vomiting, and it lasted 6–12 hours. These attacks occurred about 2–3 times a year. During one such attack, the patient noted that the visual field defect had cleared incompletely at the time the headache began and had not cleared further by the time the patient had visual had resolved. When examined by us, the patient had visual acuity of 20/15 OU with normal color perception; however, there was an incomplete bitemporal hemianopia that was denser above. Neither CT scanning nor MR imaging demonstrated any abnormalities. The patient underwent diet modification, and he was also placed on propranolol. He had no

further attacks of migraine over the next 3 years, during which time his visual field defect remained stable.

Permanent Visual Defects from Ischemic Optic Neuropathy

Pasteur et al. (1937) described a patient who experienced acute monocular visual loss as part of the aura of an attack of migraine. The visual loss did not resolve, and an ophthalmologic examination disclosed optic disc swelling with surrounding peripapillary hemorrhages in the affected eye. Other investigators described similar cases of anterior ischemic optic neuropathy occurring as part of an otherwise classic migraine syndrome (McDonald and Sanders, 1971; Victor and Welch, 1977; Cowan and Knox, 1982; Weinstein and Feman, 1982; Corbett, 1983; see Figure 4 in O'Hara and O'Connor, 1984; see Table 3 in Hupp et al., 1989) (Fig. 56.31).

Katz (1985) described a 49-year-old woman who experienced bilateral, sequential attacks of anterior ischemic optic neuropathy associated with migraine. The patient experienced attacks of severe migraine headaches preceded by scintillating scotoma since she was a teenager. At age 49, she developed acute loss of vision in the right eye associated with a typical migraine headache. Examination at this time revealed that the left eye was normal. The right eye had vision of counting fingers, decreased color vision, an "altitudinal" field defect, a relative afferent pupillary defect, and a swollen optic disc. Six months later, the patient experienced an identical event in the left eye that resulted in decreased central vision, an inferior field defect, and optic disc

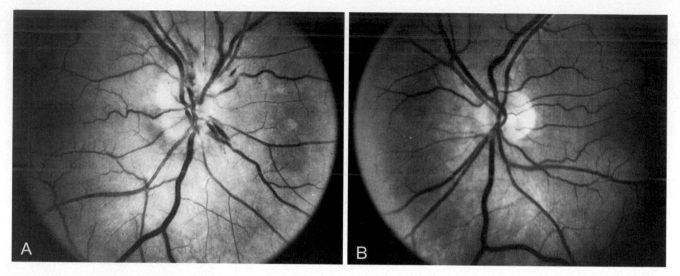

Figure 56.31.   Anterior ischemic optic neuropathy in a 44-year-old man with typical migraine headaches often associated with blurred vision in one eye, usually the right. After a typical episode during which visual acuity was diminished in the right eye, the vision in that eye did not improve. When the patient was examined 24 hours later, the right eye had visual acuity of 20/200, an inferior altitudinal field defect, and a relative afferent pupillary defect. The left eye was normal. *A*, Ophthalmoscopic appearance in the right eye is that of a typical anterior ischemic optic neuropathy with hyperemic swelling of the optic disc and several flame-shaped hemorrhages on the surface of the disc and in the superficial peripapillary retina. *B*, The left optic disc is normal except that it is somewhat small and has virtually no cup.

swelling. Visual acuity in the left eye eventually recovered to 20/30; however, vision in the right eye remained counting fingers. Both optic discs eventually became pale. The patient suffered no further attacks of visual loss over the next 6 years. In our experience, patients who develop an anterior ischemic optic neuropathy in the setting of migraine all have "disc at risk;" i.e., small optic disc with small or no cups.

Posterior (retrobulbar) ischemic optic neuropathy occasionally occurs in patients with migraine. (Lee et al., 1996). In some patients, it is associated with other evidence of a middle cerebral artery stroke (Rothrock et al., 1988a), but in most cases it occurs as an isolated phenomenon. Pelosse and Saraux (1987) reported the case of a 26-year-old man with migraine who developed a visual field defect in the right eye during a typical episode of migraine. He was found to have visual acuity of 20/20 in the eye, but there was an inferior nasal quadrantic defect. The ocular fundus initially seemed normal, but mild optic disc pallor eventually developed. O'Hara and O'Connor (1984) described two patients with classic migraine who had evidence of a unilateral optic neuropathy, including pallor of the optic disc in the affected eye, when they were examined 2 months and 12 months after visual loss, respectively. Because neither patient underwent ophthalmoscopic examination at the time of initial loss of vision, it is possible that one or both patients experienced an attack of retrobulbar, rather than anterior, ischemic optic neuropathy in association with migraine. Lee et al. (1996) reported three patients who experienced posterior ischemic optic neuropathy after well documented migraine attacks.

Permanent Visual Defects from Retinal and Choroidal Ischemia

These are discussed in the section on Retinal Migraine above.

Permanent Diplopia

Binocular diplopia that persists after an attack of migraine is unusual, even in cases of ophthalmoplegic migraine. Nevertheless, rare patients experience permanent, binocular diplopia after basilar artery migraine, ophthalmoplegic migraine, or simple classic migraine. The diplopia may result from ischemia of one or more of the ocular motor nerves or the brainstem ocular motor pathways.

Permanent monocular diplopia was reported in a patient by Sinoff and Rosenberg (1990). The patient was a 35-year-old man with a 1-year history of hemicranial headaches associated with a migratory crescent-shaped scotoma in the right, superior, homonymous field. The patient stated that he saw two "real-looking" images, equal in size and side by side with a slight vertical offset. The images were seen both monocularly and binocularly. The diplopia was not affected by pinhole or slit viewing. MR imaging showed bilateral areas of increased signal in frontal, parietal, and occipital cerebral white matter on T2-weighted images.

Tonic Pupil from Ischemia of the Ciliary Ganglion or the Short Posterior Ciliary Nerves

Massey (1981) emphasized that migraine and tonic pupils occur in the same general population. They both are more common in young women. Among 22 patients with a tonic pupil, Massey identified eight (36%) with a history of migraine (with and without typical aura). Although there was no obvious temporal association between an attack of migraine and the observation of a persistently dilated pupil in any of the eight patients, there is no reason that a tonic pupil could not result from ischemia of the ciliary ganglion, short ciliary nerves, or both. We are aware of a patient with biopsy-proven giant cell arteritis (see Chapter 57) who developed an acute tonic pupil that was undoubtedly caused by such ischemia. A similar process could produce a tonic pupil in a patient with migraine.

Permanent Neurologic Deficits

The prognosis in patients who experience neurologic aura before a migraine headache is surprisingly benign. Some patients experience more than 100 attacks of transient hemiplegia or sensory disturbance without permanent dysfunction. Of 4874 patients age 50 years or younger who were diagnosed as having migraine at the Mayo Clinic, only 20 (0.4%) subsequently had a migraine-related stroke (Broderick and Swanson, 1987). In only eight cases was the stroke in a distribution other than the posterior cerebral artery, and four of these patients had a reversible ischemic neurologic deficit that lasted more than 24 hours but less than 1 week. Thus, only 4 of 4874 patients with migraine (< 0.1%) had permanent, migraine-related, neurologic but nonvisual dysfunction. Kupersmith et al. (1987) also emphasized that the majority of patients with migraine-related stroke have a visual field defect as the main, and often the only, neurologic disturbance.

Nevertheless, death caused by the effects of massive cerebral infarction can occur in patients with migraine (Whitty, 1953; Guest and Woolf, 1964; Rothrock et al., 1988a) (Fig. 56.32), as can residual aphasia, hemiparesis, hemiplegia, and hemisensory disturbances (Critchley and Ferguson, 1933; Dunning, 1942; Murphy, 1955; Connor, 1962; Fisher, 1971; Davis-Jones et al., 1972; O'Connor, 1972; Boisen, 1975; Cohen and Taylor, 1979; Dorfman et al., 1979; Rascol et al., 1980; Featherstone, 1986; Broderick and Swanson, 1987; Couch, 1987; Kupersmith et al., 1987; Bogousslavsky et al., 1988; Rothrock et al., 1988a, Tzourio et al., 1993; Rothrock et al., 1994). Henrich (1989) found that patients with classic migraine have an increased incidence of ischemic stroke compared with the general population. In many of these cases, there also is a permanent ipsilateral homonymous field defect or contralateral monocular visual loss (Connor, 1962; Dorfman et al., 1979; Broderick and Swanson, 1987; Elmaleh et al., 1987; Kupersmith et al., 1987; Rothrock et al., 1988a). Neurologic deficits are usually caused by ischemic damage to a portion of the one or both cerebral hemispheres, but they may also result from brainstem infarction in rare cases. In still other cases, an intracerebral hemorrhage occurs in association with an attack of migraine (Dunning, 1942; Cole and Aubé, 1987; Caplan, 1988; Shuaib et al., 1989; Cole and Aubé, 1990) (Figs. 56.33 and 56.34). In such cases, the hemorrhage may result from reperfusion of ischemic tissue, from rupture of the wall of a previously spastic vessel, from increased intracranial pressure caused by prolonged vomiting, or from a combination of these mechanisms (Caplan, 1988; Shuaib et al., 1989; Cole and Aubé, 1990).

Although the overall incidence of stroke associated with migraine attacks is low, migraine is a common cause of stroke in young, otherwise healthy adults (Hart and Miller, 1983; Spaccavento and Solomon, 1984; Hilton-Jones and Warlow, 1985). Broderick and Swanson (1987) concluded

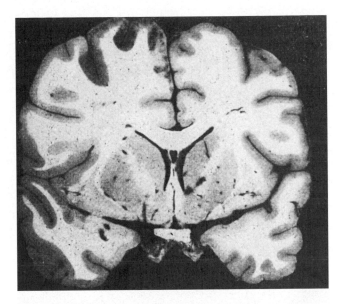

Figure 56.32. Fatal infarction of the brain in migraine. The patient was a 28-year-old man with a 2-year history of migraine headaches. The attacks were characterized by severe bifrontal headaches and nausea. They usually lasted 2–3 hours. He was eating a meal when he suddenly became unresponsive, slumped onto a couch, and became cold and pale. On admission to a local hospital, he was semicomatose with a right hemiparesis. He died 20 hours after the onset of neurologic symptoms and signs. At autopsy, the brain was hyperemic, and there were pial hemorrhages. A coronal section through the cerebral hemispheres shows hemorrhagic infarction of the left superior and middle frontal convolutions. Small hemorrhages are present in the internal capsule. (From Guest IA, Woolf AL: Fatal infarction of brain in migraine. Br Med J *1*:225–226, 1964.)

that migraine caused 25% of all strokes in patients 50 years of age or younger in Rochester, Minnesota between 1976 and 1979, and Bogousslavsky et al. (1988) reported that migraine accounted for 10.4% of all strokes in patients under 45 years of age in Lausanne, Switzerland. Rothrock et al. (1994) noted that migrainous stroke is more common in migraine with aura and in patients with a history of a previous migraine-associated stroke. Most of these patients are women. This may simply be related to the increased incidence of migraine in women in general, but Tzourio et al. (1993) reported an independent association between migraine and the risk of ischemic stroke in a case control study. Some young patients with apparent migraine-related stroke also have mitral valve prolapse (Procacci et al., 1975, 1976; Herman, 1987, 1989). It is impossible to know if the stroke was caused by vasospasm (see discussion of vasospasm in Retinal Migraine section above) or embolism in these patients. Some patients with stroke apparently caused by migraine have elevated concentrations of antiphospholipid antibodies in the serum (Shuaib and Barcley, 1989; Frohman et al., 1989; Silvestrini et al., 1993, 1994). These antibodies may cross-react with platelets to produce thrombosis (Briley et al., 1989; Digre et al., 1989; Levine and Welch, 1989; Young et al., 1989; Brey et al., 1990; Kushner, 1990; Levine et al., 1990).

As noted above, there is some evidence that patients with

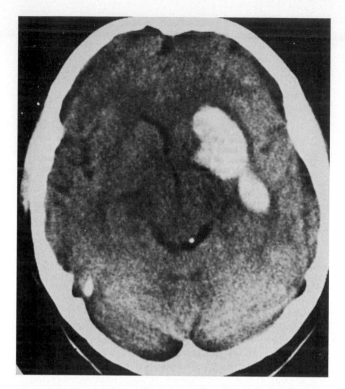

Figure 56.33. Intracerebral hemorrhage in migraine. The patient was a 41-year-old woman with a 25-year history of migraine with visual aura. Attacks were characterized by severe, unilateral headache that affected either side of the head, were accompanied by nausea, sonophobia, and photophobia, and lasted 12–24 hours. Most headaches were preceded by scintillating scotomas that lasted 10–15 minutes. The patient experienced a typical attack of migraine except that the headache persisted for 36 hours and then became generalized. The patient developed severe vomiting, became drowsy, and developed slurred speech. She was admitted to a local hospital where she was found to have a global aphasia and a right hemiparesis affecting the face, arm, and leg. A CT scan, axial view, performed 36 hours after the onset of symptoms and signs, shows a hemorrhage in the basal ganglia on the left side. An arteriogram was normal, and the patient slowly improved over the next week. At the time of discharge, her only deficit was slightly decreased dexterity in the right hand. (From Shuaib A, Metz L, Hing T: Migraine and intracerebral hemorrhage. Cephalalgia *9*: 59–61, 1989.)

common migraine (migraine without aura) and patients with classic migraine (migraine with typical aura) have subtle neuropsychologic dysfunction even though they seem to be neurologically and visually normal. Klee and Willanger (1966) reported that 75% of patients with classic migraine whom they studied demonstrated mild impairment in abstraction ability and verbal memory. These authors suggested that the impairment developed gradually in association with the increasing severity of the attacks. In a controlled study, Schuchman and Thetford (1970) found that patients with classic migraine scored significantly lower on the Wechsler Adult Intelligence Scale Digit Span subtest, a measure of attention and immediate memory, than did control subjects. In another controlled study, Zeitlin and Oddy (1984) found that patients with severe classic migraine demonstrated significantly slower reaction times, less efficient

processing of information, and poorer verbal memory performance, than did patients without migraine. In a questionnaire study, patients with classic migraine reported significantly more memory problems than did medical and psychiatric patients without headache (Mahrer et al., 1966). Hooker and Raskin (1986) administered a number of neuropsychologic tests to 16 patients with classic migraine between attacks, 15 patients with common migraine between attacks, and 15 matched volunteers without headache. Both migraine groups demonstrated significantly greater than average neuropsychologic impairment and more self-reported cognitive difficulties than did the nonheadache control group. On the basis of these findings, Hooker and Raskin (1986) concluded that both common and classic migraine produce a disturbance of cerebral function that persists beyond the attack itself. This conclusion is consistent with the findings of other authors that a substantial percentage of patients with severe, recurrent migraine, but without permanent focal visual or neurologic deficits, have evidence by neuroimaging techniques of diffuse cerebral atrophy, focal infarctions, or both (Hungerford et al., 1976; Pavese et al., 1994). (See MR imaging Section in Diagnostic Tests below).

The prevalence of major risk factors in patients who experience migraine-related stroke is no higher than that for an age-matched general population (Bogousslavsky et al., 1988; Rothrock et al., 1988a). For this reason, most investigators believe that persistent vasospasm affecting the extracranial vessels, intracranial vessels, or both is responsible for the occurrence of stroke in patients with migraine (Bogousslavsky et al., 1988; Rothrock et al., 1988a). In this regard, it is important to emphasize that cerebral infarction, both ischemic and hemorrhagic, can occur shortly after patients are placed on propranolol, a beta-adrenergic blocking agent (Prendes, 1980; Gilbert, 1982; Shuaib et al., 1989; Cole and Aubé, 1990). Because of these cases and others in which isolated retinal artery occlusion has occurred in the setting of migraine recently treated with propranolol (Katz, 1986), it was suggested by Burde (1986) that beta-adrenergic blocking agents be used with extreme caution in any patients with forms of migraine other than migraine headache without aura (common migraine) and that initial prophylactic treatment of all forms of migraine be with calcium channel blocking agents rather than with beta-adrenergic blockers (see, however, Smith, 1986).

CHILDHOOD MIGRAINE

All forms of migraine, with the possible exception of cluster headache, occur in children (Vahlquist, 1955; Burke and Peters, 1956; Bille, 1962; Deubner, 1977; Sparks, 1978; Cogdon and Forsyth, 1979; Prensky and Sommer, 1979; Shinnar and D'Souza, 1982; Sillanpää, 1983; Fenichel, 1985; Rothner, 1987; Troost, 1996). Children experience symptoms similar to those found in adults, but attacks may be more frequent and abdominal complaints more prominent (Holguin and Fenichel, 1967). Indeed, certain forms of migraine with aura (e.g., basilar artery migraine, ophthalmoplegic migraine) occur most often in childhood. It is probable that most migrainous episodes begin in childhood

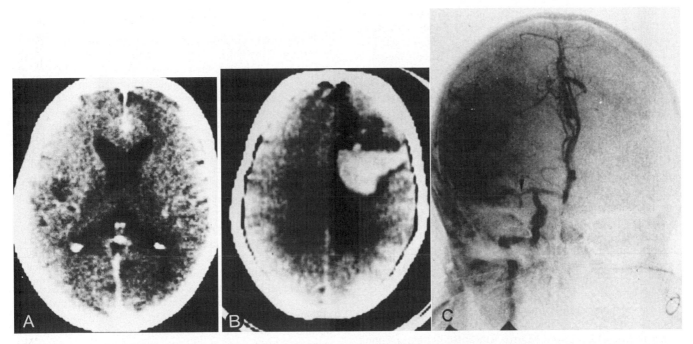

Figure 56.34. Intracranial hemorrhage with arterial vasospasm in a patient with migraine. The patient was a 61-year-old woman with a 4-year history of migraine headaches preceded by an aura of left-sided paresthesias. She initially was evaluated because of worsening headache. A neurologic examination was normal as were the results of a CT scan (*A*) and a lumbar puncture. One day after the CT scan, the patient's headache worsened, and she became lethargic. On admission to the hospital she had a left hemiplegia, a left homonymous hemianopia, and a right gaze preference. *B*, Repeat unenhanced CT scan, axial view, now shows a large, right frontoparietal hematoma. *C*, Right internal carotid arteriogram, anteroposterior view, shows focal spasm of the initial segment of the right middle cerebral artery (*arrowhead*). The hematoma was evacuated, and the patient made a slow recovery. (From Cole AJ, Aubé M: Migraine with vasospasm and delayed intracerebral hemorrhage. Arch Neurol *47*:53–56, 1990.)

(Krupp and Friedman, 1933; Michael and Williams, 1952), but the diagnosis is not made because the child cannot adequately describe the symptoms.

Certain disturbances that occur in children may portend the eventual development of typical migraine in later life. These include the Alice in Wonderland syndrome, motion sickness, episodes of vertigo, proxysmal torticollis, somnambulism, gastrointestinal distress, and acute confusion.

Alice in Wonderland Syndrome

An unusual migraine syndrome encompassing alterations of time sense, body image, and analysis of the environment, was labeled the "Alice in Wonderland" syndrome (Todd, 1955; Hachinski et al., 1973). Golden (1979) reported the syndrome in two children and an excerpt from the description by an 11-year-old girl is given below:

> As I started to go into Mommy's room I grabbed my door—it felt about one foot thick in my hand. As I went through the hall, it felt as if as I was going too fast. (Like you want to stop but energy is keening up inside you. You feel like you are going to burst and your eyes are going to pop out—like you're going to explode.) Things were going too fast. I felt like my hands were made of tiny twigs with a little mushy flesh on the outside. I felt like I was holding things in my hands.

Motion Sickness

The most common migraine equivalent is probably motion sickness (Graham, 1979). We and others obtain a history of motion sickness in 60–80% of patients who eventually experience typical migraine attacks with and without aura (Pearce, 1971; Kuritzky et al., 1981a). Among patients without migraine, the prevalence of motion sickness in childhood is only about 10%.

Benign Paroxysmal Vertigo

Children both with and without a history of motion sickness may experience recurrent episodes of vertigo. The episodes occur suddenly and without warning. They usually last several minutes, but they may last several hours or even days in rare cases (Eeg-Olofsson et al., 1982). Patients with such episodes may also experience nausea, vomiting, and oscillopsia (Dunn and Snyder, 1976). They may become pale, and they may develop nystagmus, but they do not lose consciousness. Most attacks occur within the first 4 years of life. They may occur as frequently as several times a week or as rarely as once a year. They often stop spontaneously after several months or years. Benign paroxysmal vertigo in childhood is thought by many authors to be a migraine equivalent (Mira et al., 1984; Hockaday, 1987; Abu-Arefeh et al., 1995). Children with this syndrome often have an increased prevalence of dizzy spells and vertiginous episodes between attacks of migraine later in life (Basser, 1964; Fenichel, 1967; Watson and Steele, 1974). Such patients (as well as those with motion sickness) may have hypersensitive or otherwise abnormal vestibular systems (Koenigsberger et al., 1970; Kuritzky et al., 1981a, 1981b; Mira et al., 1984).

Benign Paroxysmal Torticollis

Benign paroxysmal torticollis in children is a periodic disorder initially described by Snyder (1969). It usually begins during the first year of life, and it usually disappears before 5 years of age. The condition is characterized by recurrent spells of torticollis that may be accompanied by other symptoms and signs, including irritability, drowsiness, ataxia, nystagmus, pallor, and vomiting (Snyder, 1969; Raab, 1970; Chutorian, 1974; Lipson and Robertson, 1978; Deonna and Martin, 1981; see Table 2 in Hanukoglu et al., 1984; Roulet and Deonna, 1988). The periodicity and duration of the neck symptoms resemble those of benign paroxysmal vertigo, and they may have the same origin (Sanner and Bergström, 1979; Eeg-Olofsson et al., 1982). Infants who experience benign paroxysmal torticollis often have relatives with typical migraine, and they may themselves develop typical migraine later in life (Deonna and Martin, 1981; Roulet and Deonna, 1988). For these reasons, benign paroxysmal torticollis is considered by many authors to be a migraine equivalent (Hockaday, 1987).

Somnambulism

Another portend of migraine is somnambulism (Barabas et al., 1983; Giroud and Dumas, 1984). Barabas et al. (1983) reported that 30% of children with migraine headaches also suffered from somnambulism, whereas only about 5% of children with nonmigraine headaches sleepwalked. Giroud et al. (1986) performed a retrospective study in which they looked for a history of somnambulism in childhood in 122 patients with migraine and 110 patients with nonmigraine headaches. These investigators reported findings similar to those reported by Barabas et al. (1983). About 29% of patients with migraine had childhood somnambulism, whereas only about 5% of patients with nonmigraine headaches sleepwalked as a child.

It is unclear why migraine and somnambulism are related. Migraine is thought to be caused in part by a disturbance in the metabolism of serotonin. There may also be an association between serotonin and of sleep disorders. Jouvet (1967, 1969) introduced the "monoaminergic theory of the sleep states." This theory implicates serotonin as both the inducer and maintainer of slow-wave sleep. Several studies demonstrated that somnambulism occurs during stages III and IV sleep and in transition to lighter stages (Kales and Kales, 1970; Anders and Weinstein, 1972). Dexter (1979) showed that in patients with migraine, there is a relative instability of the concentration of platelet-bound serotonin during stages III and IV of rapid eye movement (REM) and non-REM sleep. This instability may cause a derangement in the smooth transition through various sleep stages, resulting in the increased frequency of somnambulism in children who either have or ultimately develop migraine.

Cyclic Vomiting

Some young children experience stereotyped episodes of vomiting in the absence of other symptoms of gastrointestinal disease. Although such children initially may be thought to have some type of primary gastrointestinal disorder, they probably have a migraine equivalent, and they are more prone to develop typical attacks of migraine later in life (Waters, 1972; Symon et al., 1995). Lance and Anthony (1966) found a past history of vomiting attacks in childhood in 23% of adults with migraine compared with 12% of adults with tension headache.

A variant of cyclic vomiting in childhood may be the syndrome of abdominal migraine. Bille (1962, 1964) found that 20% of children with typical migraine experienced episodes of abdominal pain compared with 3% of the control group. In many of these children, the attacks of abdominal pain are associated with nausea, vomiting, pallor, and sweating. We examined an otherwise healthy 5-year-old boy who experienced such episodes about once every 8 weeks. The episodes were always the same. The child would awaken at about 7 a.m. in obvious discomfort. He would complain that he had a "tummyache." He would then retch for several minutes, during which time he would become quite pale. As soon as he stopped retching, his appearance returned to normal, and he became completely comfortable. He was not losing weight, his appetite was normal, and he had neither diarrhea nor constipation. His mother had severe motion sickness, and both his aunt and his maternal grandmother had severe migraines. The patient subsequently developed migraine headaches without aura at age 12.

According to Lundberg (1978), adults with migraine are 12 times more likely to have experienced abdominal migraine in childhood than adults with other types of headaches. A diagnosis of abdominal migraine can be made in the following setting: (a) recurrent, stereotyped attacks of abdominal pain lasting from one to several hours, usually located in the upper part of the abdomen, beginning in early childhood; (b) no abdominal symptoms between attacks; (c) no other evidence of gastrointestinal disease; and (d) a personal or family history of typical migraine or migraine equivalent (Lundberg, 1978).

Acute Confusional Migraine

A variant of migraine that occurs almost exclusively in children and adolescents is acute confusional migraine (Gascon and Barlow, 1970; Emery, 1977; Ehyai and Fenichel, 1978; Tinuper et al., 1985; Bruyn, 1986; Parrino et al., 1986; Pietrini et al., 1987; Haan et al., 1988; Sheth et al., 1995). Most of these patients initially develop acute confusion and vomiting, after which they exhibit phobic, hysteriform, stereotyped behavior associated with impairment of consciousness and agitation. The combination of confusion and agitation seems to be quite typical. The attacks usually last no longer than 12 hours, and they almost always end with sleep, after which the patient awakens free of symptoms and signs. There is often global or partial retrograde and anterograde amnesia. The EEG typically shows diffuse, marked slow-wave activity and frontal intermittent rhythmic delta activity during the acute stage, both patterns disappearing within 24–72 hours.

Acute confusional migraine occasionally occurs in patients without any preceding attacks of any other form of migraine, but most patients who develop this syndrome have both a personal history (83%) and a family history (75%) of some type of migraine (Pietrini et al., 1987). It may also occur after mild head trauma, in which case the patient may be thought to have a cerebral concussion (Haan et al., 1988). Other disorders that produce a clinical picture similar to that of acute confusional migraine include toxic or metabolic encephalopathies, encephalitis, seizures, right middle cerebral artery infarction, and basilar artery migraine (Gascon and Barlow, 1970; Mori and Yamadori 1987; Haan et al., 1988).

Alternating Hemiplegia of Childhood

Alternating hemiplegia of childhood, a rare condition characterized by repeated attacks of hemiplegia involving alternate sides or both sides of the body with onset before 18 months, may be a form of complicated migraine (Davidoff, 1995). The episodes of hemiplegia can last minutes to days and may be accompanied by dystonic posturing, choreoathetoid movements, nystagmus, tachycardia, mydriasis, and sweating (Dittrich et al., 1979; Krägeloh and Aicardi, 1980; Andermann et al., 1994; Gordon, 1995). The previously normal child may later show signs of developmental delay and neurologic deficits.

OTHER MIGRAINE EQUIVALENTS

Cardiac Migraine

Some migraineurs experience recurrent episodes of angina-type chest pain accompanied by a headache unassociated with physical exertion (Leon-Sotomayor, 1974). The electrocardiograms show typical ST segment abnormalities during the episode, and the chest pain, which is often referred to as Prinzmetal's angina, is relieved by sublingual nitroglycerine, suggesting that arterial spasm (see discussion of vasospasm in retinal migraine above) is the etiology (Miller et al., 1981; Wayne, 1986).

Transformed Migraine (Chronic Daily Headache)

An important advance in headache understanding is recognition of the phenomenon of episodic migraine evolving into a pattern of daily or almost-daily headache with superimposed periodic typical attacks of migraine. This headache evolution is called **transformed migraine**. The persistent daily headache is often unassociated with typical migraine symptoms and resembles a traditional tension-type headache (Silberstein et al., 1995). Symptoms of chronic depression are often present as is a history of excessive use of analgesics or ergotamine tartrate (Young and Silberstein, 1993).

Mathew (1990a) studied a group of hospitalized patients with daily headache after withdrawal from ergotamine analgesics, or both. Daily headache eventually ceased in over 60% of patients, but acute withdrawal symptoms of headache, nausea, vomiting, nervousness, and sleep disturbance occurred for up to 10 days. The treatment of transformed migraine includes prophylactic drugs such as tricyclic antidepressants and divalproex (Rothrock et al., 1994).

RELATIONSHIP BETWEEN MIGRAINE, CLUSTER HEADACHE, AND EPISODIC PAROXYSMAL HEMICRANIA

The condition called cluster headache (or histaminic cephalgia) is discussed in Chapter 36 of this text. Some investigators believe that this condition is a variant of migraine (Wolff, 1963; Bickerstaff, 1968; Friedman, 1968; Duvoisin, 1972; Friedman, 1972; Pearce, 1980; Hupp et al., 1989), whereas others consider it to be a completely separate condition (Horton et al., 1939; Robinson, 1958; Ekbom, 1970; Sjaastad, 1976; Diamond, 1979; Graham, 1979; Russell, 1984; Silberstein, 1994). The Headache Classification Committee of the International Headache Society (1988) defined cluster headache as at least five prior attacks of severe, unilateral, orbital, suborbital, and/or temporal pain lasting 15–180 minutes if untreated, and associated with at least one of the following: conjunctival injection, lacrimation, nasal congestion, rhinorrhea, forehead and facial sweating, miosis, ptosis, or eyelid edema, all ipsilateral to the side of repetitive headache (Headache Classification Committee of the International Headache Society, 1988). Those who link migraine and cluster headache emphasize their similarities, whereas those who separate them stress their differences.

Migraine occurs most often in women, whereas cluster headache is much more common in men (Sjaastad et al., 1988). Migraine begins more often in childhood or adolescence, although it may produce symptoms at any age. Cluster headache almost always occurs in middle age or later. As a general rule, the location of head pain is similar in both migraine and cluster headache. It tends to be unilateral, with the temple, forehead, and orbit being common sites. Migraine headaches usually last several hours, and patients who experience them often require medication to relieve the attacks. Cluster headaches usually last less than an hour and terminate spontaneously and abruptly. Migraine usually begins during the day, whereas cluster headache often commences at night. In both conditions, there may be flushing of the face, but increased pulsation of the temporal artery is a more prominent feature of migraine than of cluster headache. Autonomic dysfunction, usually mild, occurs in some patients with migraine (Appenzeller, 1969; Havanka-Kanniainen et al., 1988; Drummond, 1990), but it is an almost universal feature of cluster headache (Sjaastad, 1988; Raskin, 1989).

Lacrimation may occur in both conditions, but it is more prominent and bothersome in patients with cluster headache than in patients with migraine. Other signs of oculosympathetic dysfunction that occur more commonly in cluster headache than in migraine are rhinorrhea and postganglionic Horner's syndrome (Horton et al., 1939; Kunkle and Anderson, 1960; Nieman and Hurwitz, 1961; Riley and Moyer,

1971; Fanciullacci et al., 1982; Vijayan and Watson, 1982; Watson and Vijayan, 1982; Drummond, 1988; Sjaastad, 1988).

Most cluster headaches are unassociated with visual or neurologic symptoms; however, Medina and Diamond (1977) described seven patients with headaches that had a cluster pattern but were preceded or accompanied by scotomas, photopsias, weakness contralateral to the side of the headache, or contralateral paresthesias.

Vascular instability apparently plays a role in the development of cluster headache as it does in the occurrence of migraine; however, although the vascular disturbances in migraine seem to affect primarily the external carotid arterial system, the vascular disturbances that occur in patients with cluster headache apparently affect the internal carotid arterial system. Northfield (1938) and Wolff (1955) reported that injections of histamine into the common or internal carotid artery almost always produced a headache that was usually ipsilateral, whereas injection of histamine into the external carotid artery rarely produced a headache. Horven et al. (1972) performed ''dynamic tonometry'' in patients with both migraine and cluster headache. These investigators demonstrated an increase in intraocular pressure synchronous with the pulse during cluster headache. Horven and Sjaastad (1977) subsequently reported that during a cluster headache, there is an increase in intraocular pressure, ocular pulse amplitude, and corneal temperature in the ipsilateral eye. All of these findings are consistent with an increase in blood flow in and around the affected eye during a cluster headache, and they are also consistent with the angiographic observation of Ekbom and Greitz (1970) of dilation of the ophthalmic artery in patients during a cluster headache. Such findings are not observed in patients with migraine.

The results of thermography also suggest that patients experience an increase in blood flow in the internal carotid arterial system during a cluster headache. Using this technique, Friedman et al. (1973) demonstrated hypothermic islands in the periorbital skin in 85% of patients with cluster headache but in only 2% of patients with migraine. These hypothermic regions were usually located in areas of skin supplied by branches of the internal carotid artery. In 11 patients examined thermographically during spontaneous attacks of cluster headache, heat loss from the affected orbit and cheek was up to 1.5 C greater than heat loss from the opposite side (Drummond and Lance, 1984).

Other signs of unilateral extracranial vasodilation during cluster headache include increases in extracranial and intracranial blood flow measured by the rate of clearance of radioactive xenon (Henry et al., 1978; Sakai and Meyer, 1978), increases in temporal pulse amplitude (Drummond and Anthony, 1985), and increases in velocity of blood flow through the supratrochlear artery on the symptomatic side (Schroth et al., 1983). Finally, Messert and Black (1978) documented the postoperative development of cluster headache in patients who have undergone ipsilateral carotid endarterectomy.

Studies by Goadsby and Edvinsson (1994) linked activation of the trigeminovascular system to the pain and vasodilation of cluster. These reasearchers found elevation of both calcitonin gene-related polypeptide (CGRP)—a marker for trigeminovascular activation—and vasoactive intestinal polypeptide (VIP)—a parasympathetic marker—in the external jugular vein ipsilateral to the headache of cluster patients.

Like migraine, cluster headache may be induced by certain substances, particularly nitrates. Ekbom (1968) described typical attacks of cluster headache in patients taking nitroglycerin, and Bernat (1979) described a patient who developed cluster headaches after taking isosorbide dinitrate for angina. Mueller and Meienberg (1983) reported a 54-year-old man who developed a severe, unilateral headache accompanied by ipsilateral ptosis and miosis that began about 2 months after beginning isosorbide dinitrate and that resolved a few days after stopping the drug. When treatment was restarted with the informed consent of the patient, the headaches recurred.

Certain biochemical abnormalities may permit differentiation between patients with migraine and patients with cluster headache. Anthony and Lance (1971) found reduced concentrations of serotonin in platelets during the headache phase of a migraine attack but not during an episode of cluster headache. On the other hand, patients experiencing a cluster headache had increased concentrations of histamine in the serum compared with patients experiencing a migraine headache. Ziegler et al. (1976) attempted to confirm these findings but could not do so.

Some drugs that are used to treat migraine can also be used to treat cluster headache. In particular, ergotamine, sumatriptan, and methysergide—drugs that are often used to treat migraine headache—may also be effective against cluster headache (Duvoisin, 1972; Lance, 1978; Silberstein, 1994). Calcium channel blocking agents such as verapamil may be useful in preventing cluster headache as they are in preventing migraine (see below) (Gabai and Spierings, 1989; Silberstein, 1994). On the other hand, some drugs that do not affect attacks of migraine can abort attacks of cluster headache. Inhalation of 100% oxygen often produces pain relief (Kudrow, 1981; Friedman and Mikropoulos, 1958; Fogan, 1985), and prednisone may result in satisfactory relief of pain in 70–80% of patients with cluster headache (Jammes, 1975; Couch and Ziegler, 1978; Kudrow, 1978, 1980). Lithium has been used in some patients with cluster headaches with good results (Ekbom, 1974, 1977; Kudrow, 1977; Mathew, 1978; Ekbom, 1981), although the side effects of this drug limit its usefulness. Caviness and O'Brien (1980) used chlorpromazine in doses ranging from 75 to 700 mg per day to treat 13 patients with cluster headache who had experienced no improvement with other medicines. The drug produced complete relief of headache in 12 of the 13 patients, and in nine of these patients, withdrawal of the drug 2–3 weeks later did not result in return of symptoms. Hering and Kuritzky (1989) studied the effect of sodium valproate on cluster headache in 15 patients who participated in an open pilot study. Two of the patients described marked reduction in pain, and nine reported complete disappearance of pain. Thus, 11 of 15 patients (73%) responded favorably to the drug. Patients with severe cluster headache that is refractory to all medical therapy may experience relief after sphenopalatine ganglionectomy (Meyer et al., 1970), a procedure that is not recommended for patients with migraine.

Some investigators recognize two uncommon variants of cluster headache—chronic and episodic paroxysmal hemicrania. (Russell, 1984; Kudrow et al., 1987; Blau and Engel, 1990). These conditions are similar to cluster headache except that the attacks are shorter in duration (less than 45 minutes) and occur more frequently (6–12 times per day). In addition, chronic and episodic paroxysmal hemicrania respond dramatically to indomethacin, whereas typical cluster headaches do not (Geaney, 1983; Blau and Engel, 1990).

Whether one believes that cluster headache is a variant of migraine or a separate entity, in most cases a careful history and examination are sufficient to distinguish these two entities from each other and from other disorders that cause head or face pain (Ekbom, 1970). Once the correct diagnosis is made, appropriate treatment can be started.

RELATIONSHIP BETWEEN MIGRAINE AND SEIZURES

Migraine both causes and mimics seizures. Seizures may arise from a stroke of any type (see Chapter 55). Stroke-related seizures can occur at the time of the stroke, or they may develop years later. Alternatively, seizures may be triggered by transient cortical ischemia from any source, including migraine (Andermann, 1987). Some patients with basilar artery migraine may initially be thought to have seizures, as may patients whose migrainous aura are characterized by migratory paresthesias. Similarly, patients with migraine-induced transient global amnesia may have symptoms similar to those experienced by patients with complex partial (temporal lobe) seizures. This diagnostic confusion is further complicated by a high incidence of electroencephalographic disturbances, often paroxysmal, in patients with migraine (Prensky and Sommer, 1979). These changes probably reflect migrainous neuronal dysfunction, but they may be interpreted erroneously as epileptogenic activity (Basser, 1969). Lai et al. (1989) performed electroencephalography on 38 patients with a history of diet-induced migraine. Electroencephalography was performed on an initial baseline day and on a second day after challenge with chocolate, red wine, cheese, or fasting. Not only did a unilateral headache occur in 16 patients (42%) after dietary challenge, but the EEG became abnormal in 12 of these patients (32%). Those wishing to learn more about the relationship of migraine and epilepsy should consult the excellent text edited by Andermann and Lugaresi (1987).

PATHOGENESIS

There is no aspect of migraine that is more confusing or controversial than its actual pathogenesis (Amery et al., 1984; Dexter, 1987; Edmeads, 1987; Lance, 1987; Hupp et al., 1989). It is not even clear whether migraine is a single entity or multiple disorders (Hachinski, 1985; Ziegler, 1985). Neither the cause of the aura nor the cause of the headache have been clearly delineated, although many theories have been advanced (Olesen, 1987; Welch, 1987; Spierings, 1988; Silberstein et al., 1995; Noack and Rothrock, 1996).

VASOGENIC THEORY OF MIGRAINE

The classic theory of the pathogenesis of migraine, first propounded by Wolff (1963), is that vasoconstriction is responsible for cerebral ischemia and the focal visual and neurologic symptoms of the migraine aura, whereas vasodilation evokes the headache phase (Diamond and Dalessio, 1982; Dalessio, 1985) (Fig. 56.35). The release of serotonin from platelets is thought to produce these changes (Anthony and Lance, 1975; Muck-Seler et al., 1979; D'Andrea et al., 1982; Pradalier and Launay, 1982; Waldenlind et al., 1985; Malmgren and Hasselmark, 1988; D'Andrea et al., 1989a, 1989b). Different exogenous and endogenous factors initially trigger the sudden release of serotonin from the dense bodies within platelets. Serotonin then produces dilation of capillaries and constriction of extracranial and some intracranial arteries (Lance et al., 1967). Serotonin is absorbed by the blood vessels and nearby tissues where it is rapidly metabolized, causing a marked drop in circulating serotonin (Anthony et al., 1969). This drop causes a rebound effect that results in vasodilation of the arteries and constriction of the capillaries. Both arterial distention and inflammation then produce the headache phase of migraine (Ostfeld, 1962; Moskowitz, 1984).

Several clinical features of classic migraine support vasospasm as a contributing factor in the aura of migraine. These features include the production of a migraine scotoma by infusion of noradrenaline with resolution of the scotoma when the infusion is stopped (Tunis and Wolff, 1953), abolition of the scotoma with low-dose amyl nitrate and carbon dioxide (Schumacher and Wolff, 1941), and increased scotoma with high-dose amyl nitrate (Schumacher and Wolff, 1941).

The vasoconstriction/vasodilation theory of the pathogenesis of migraine advanced by Wolff (1963) was accepted largely without question until the 1970s when various techniques, primarily inhalation or intra-arterial injection of [133]Xe (see Chapter 55), were used to measure both general and regional cerebral blood flow (rCBF). Initial studies supported Wolff's theory by showing both a reduction of rCBF during the aura of classic migraine (Simard and Paulson, 1973) and an increase in rCBF in patients during the headache phase of migraine (Skinhoj and Paulson, 1969; O'Brien, 1971; Skinhoj, 1973; Mathew et al., 1976; Henry et al., 1978). In a particularly elegant study, Sakai and Meyer (1978) found regional reductions in CBF in gray matter during the aura of an attack of classic migraine. During the headache phase, however, and during an attack of common migraine, CBF in gray matter was uniformly increased and only returned to baseline levels slowly over several days after the attack ended. These studies were criticized by some

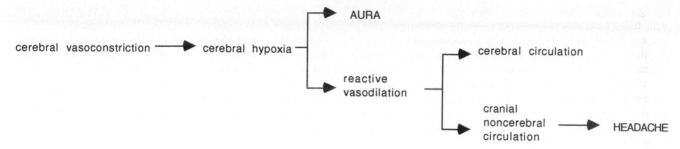

Figure 56.35. Schematic representation of Wolff's vasoconstriction/vasodilation theory of migraine. According to this theory, cerebral vasoconstriction produces cerebral hypoxia that produces the aura of migraine and also produces reactive vasodilation. The vasodilation affects not only the cerebral circulation but also the cranial noncerebral circulation, thus producing headache. (From Spierings ELH: Recent advances in the understanding of migraine. Headache 28:655–658, 1988.)

authors who believed that the changes in blood flow were not sufficient to explain the significant clinical symptoms and signs in patients with migraine. In particular, Olesen (1987) stated that no study had shown convincing evidence of substantial cerebral hypoperfusion during the aura of a classic migraine attack (see, however, Simard and Paulson, 1973), nor had any study shown substantial cerebral hyperperfusion during the headache phase of migraine. Indeed, the results of a number of studies by Olesen and his colleagues (Olesen et al., 1981a, 1982; Lauritzen et al., 1983a) in patients with both spontaneously occurring and angiographically-induced migraine contradicted the traditional theory of vasoconstriction followed by vasodilation as the cause of migraine.

Olesen et al. (1982) produced migraine headache without aura by percutaneous puncture of the internal carotid artery and then injected ^{133}Xe into the vessel to measure CBF during the headache. These investigators found no significant changes in regional or general CBF during the resting state, at the time of onset of headache, or at the height of the headache. Olesen et al. (1981a) and Lauritzen et al. (1983a) also studied CBF in patients with angiographically-produced migraine headache preceded by aura. These patients showed a change in CBF described by the investigators as "spreading oligemia." This phenomenon generally began in the occipital region, and it spread anteriorly at a speed of about 2 mm/min over the hemisphere. However, the oligemia did not cross the rolandic or Sylvian sulci; it reached the primary sensorimotor area after symptoms produced from that region had already begun; and it persisted long after any focal symptoms resolved. Olesen, Lauritzen, and their colleagues suggested, therefore, that the visual and neurologic aura of migraine are not secondary to observed oligemia. Rather, the oligemia was thought to be merely an epiphenomenon occurring in some patients with migraine. In addition, Olesen et al. (1981a, 1982) and Lauritzen et al. (1983a) found no change in CBF to explain the headache phase of the induced migraine attack.

The studies of CBF performed by Olesen and his colleagues (Olesen et al., 1981a, 1982; Lauritzen et al., 1983a) on patients with angiographically-induced migraine were dismissed by some investigators, partly because they dealt only with healthy patients who developed angiographically-

induced migraine and not with patients who had spontaneous migraine with or without aura, and partly because a major drawback of measurements of CBF with ^{133}Xe is a considerable overestimation of CBF in low-flow regions because of scattered radiation from unaffected parts of the brain (e.g., Compton scatter) (Hanson et al., 1975; Skyhoj Olsen et al., 1987; Skyhoj Olsen and Lassen, 1989). Similar findings were reported in patients with spontaneous migraine, however.

Olesen et al. (1981b) evaluated patients whose migraine headaches could be induced by red wine or certain foods. Studies in six such patients using inhalation of ^{133}Xe showed only slight, nonsignificant global increases in rCBF during attacks and complete absence of focal or global reduction in CBF just before the onset of the attack. Lauritzen and Olesen (1984) studied 12 patients with spontaneous attacks of migraine headache without aura during the attack, after treatment, and after 7 migraine-free days. These investigators found no focal or generalized abnormalities of rCBF during attacks, nor was there any difference in CBF during attacks, after treatment, or between attacks. In view of these findings, it is not surprising that Olesen (1987) concluded that the cause of migraine attacks (particularly the headache phase) was "essentially unexplained."

Studies using more sophisticated techniques to detect alterations in rCBF have subsequently suggested that changes in rCBF are, indeed, associated with both the aura and the headache of migraine attacks (Juge and Gauthier, 1980; Gulliksen and Enevoldsen, 1984; Skyhoj Olsen et al., 1987; Juge, 1988; Skyhoj Olsen and Lassen, 1989; Olesen et al., 1990; Friberg, 1991; Woods et al., 1994). Andersen et al. (1988) found evidence of delayed cerebral hyperemia following cerebral hypoperfusion using single photon emission computed tomography (SPECT) in patients with migraine headaches with preceding aura. This article was of significance not only because of its findings but also because one of its authors was Olesen, one of the leading authorities to challenge the vasogenic theory of migraine, initially postulated by Wolff (1963). The article by Andersen et al. (1988) did not support the entire vasogenic theory of Wolff (1963), however. These investigators found that the headache that occurred in their patients often disappeared even though the CBF hyperemia persisted. They therefore concluded that although cerebral hypoperfusion followed by hyperperfusion may trigger an attack of classic migraine, there is still no evidence to support the contention that the headache phase of migraine is specifically related to hyperperfusion. Skyhoj Olsen and Lassen (1989) measured CBF in 11 patients during attacks of migraine headache with aura using the ^{133}Xe intra-arterial technique. These investigators also found initial focal decreases in CBF consistent with mild cerebral ischemia during the aura of the attack. In a later study, Olesen et al. (1990) reported statistically significant changes in rCBF correlated with the aura and headache of angiographically induced migraine. The aura phase was associated with decreased rCBF that persisted well into the headache phase. Cerebral hyperperfusion then began as the headache continued and persisted 1–2 hours after the headache abated. These findings support the theory that the aura of migraine may be a manifestation of a primary neuronal event (see section below) and that changes in rCBF occur mainly in response. Woods et al. (1994) substantiated the presence of spreading oligemia during a migraine attack using positron emission tomography (PET). Kobari et al. (1989) performed prospective, color-coded, cross-sectional imaging of rCBF in 22 patients with migraine headaches using the stable xenon-enhanced CT method. These investigators found evidence of substantial cerebral hyperperfusion in these patients compared with control subjects, although they did not detect any initial hypoperfusion. The hyperperfusion affected not only the cerebral cortex but also subcortical structures including the thalamus, basal ganglia, and subcortical white matter. Robertson et al. (1989) studied CBF using the ^{133}Xe inhalation technique during the headache-free period in 92 patients with migraine and found age-related differences in cerebrovascular resistance and CBF that they thought might be of significance in determining the threshold for an attack of migraine.

Despite continued arguments from various investigators (see, for example, Kronberg et al., 1990), it would seem from the above data and from the clinical reports of patients with persistent visual and neurologic deficits after otherwise straightforward attacks of migraine, that changes in rCBF do occur in patients with classic, and to a lesser extent common, migraine and that these changes may cause cerebral ischemia (Skyhoj Olsen et al., 1981; Skyhoj Olsen, 1990; Skyhoj Olsen and Friberg, 1990). However, it is likely that these rCBF changes, and the ischemia that they may produce, are epiphenomena associated with neuronal dysfunction (see below) and not the cause of a migraine attack.

THEORY OF SPREADING DEPRESSION

In 1941, Carl Lashley emphasized the drift of the scintillating scotoma of migraine across the visual field. He believed that the scintillations were caused by a phase of intense cortical excitation that advanced along the area of the cerebral cortex corresponding to the scotoma. Lashley (1941) calculated that the rate of propagation of the wave of excitation was about 3 mm/min or less. He concluded that this wave of excitation was followed by a period of total cortical inactivity or inhibition. At about the same time, Leao (1944) described an unusual neurophysiologic phenomenon in the cortex of experimental animals. The disturbance, which he called **spreading cortical depression,** could be initiated by systemic administration of potassium chloride, direct focal brain injury, anoxia, and tetanic stimulation of the corpus callosum. It consisted of a slowly moving wave of cortical inactivity that was preceded by a wave of excitation and that was propagated at a rate of 2–3 mm per minute (Leao and Morrison, 1945). A marked wave of dilation of pial arteries accompanied the wave of cortical neuronal excitation.

Milner (1958) first emphasized the striking similarity in the clinical observations in humans by Lashley (1941) and the experimental observations in animals by Leao (1944). Milner (1958) theorized that migraine scotomas are manifestations of spreading depression triggered in susceptible persons and that other symptoms of migraine are caused by spread of depression to other areas of the cerebral cortex. Kunkle (1963) extended the concept developed by Milner (1958) by suggesting that the aura of a migraine attack was not simply a preliminary phenomenon but, in fact, was the main event in an attack of "classic" migraine. It subsequently was suggested that an attack of migraine originates in the central nervous system with a burst followed by a depression of neuronal activity (Olesen et al., 1981a). This, in turn, produces the spreading oligemia observed by measurement of rCBF during attacks of classic migraine (Olesen et al., 1981a; Lauritzen et al., 1983a, 1983b; see above).

Experimental studies in animals have shown changes in high-energy phosphates during spreading depression (Quistorf et al., 1979). Similar changes occur in patients during an attack of migraine. Welch et al. (1989) measured brain energy phosphate metabolism and intracellular pH in patients with migraine with and without aura using in vivo phosphorus-31 nuclear magnetic resonance (NMR) spectroscopy. During an attack of migraine preceded by aura, there was evidence of disordered energy phosphate metabolism, whereas no such disturbance was detected during an attack of migraine without aura. No changes in intracellular pH were detected in any patient during an attack of either common migraine or classic migraine. Welch et al. (1989) interpreted these findings as being consistent with spreading depression as the cause of classic migraine. Welch et al. (1993) subsequently recorded the cortical activity of migraineurs using magnetoencephalography and found changes that appear to represent spreading depression.

THEORY OF DISTENTION AND PULSATION OF THE EXTERNAL CAROTID ARTERY AS A CAUSE OF MIGRAINE HEADACHES

Wolff and associates (Graham and Wolff, 1938; Sutherland and Wolff, 1940; Schumacher and Wolff, 1941) related the headache phase of the migraine attack to distention and increased amplitude of pulsation—not blood flow—of the branches of the external carotid artery. The internal carotid, vertebral, and basilar arteries, and the first few centimeters of the main cerebral arteries arising from the circle of Willis were considered by these investigators to be possible, but probably minor, participants in the headache phase of the migraine attack.

These opinions were based on experiments that showed that the amplitude of pulsation of the intracranial vessels was not increased significantly during the headache phase of the migraine attack, nor could the headache be relieved by dampening of the intracranial pulsations by increasing cerebrospinal fluid pressure from 800 to 900 mm H_2O. On the other hand, reduction of the amplitude of pulsation of the branches of the external carotid artery by medication (especially ergotamine), physical compression, or denervation with a local anesthetic could decrease or completely eliminate the headache. Subsequent studies of blood flow, pulsation, or both in the external carotid artery and its branches confirmed the hyperperfusion of that system during at least some of the headache phase of a migraine attack (Spierings, 1979; Drummond and Lance, 1983; Schroth et al., 1983; Spierings and Graham, 1989; Iversen et al., 1990). Indeed, even Andersen et al. (1989) agreed that the pain of a migraine headache may be caused by abnormalities in and around extracerebral, cranial arteries. Nevertheless, it seems unlikely that dilation of the extracerebral cranial vessels alone is responsible for migraine headaches (Drummond and Lance, 1983; Noack and Rothrock, 1996).

Graham and Wolff (1938) realized that dilation of blood vessels alone was not sufficient to cause the often excruciating pain of migraine headache (see also Drummond and Lance, 1983). They found that experimental dilation of cranial arteries was painful but not to the extent generally observed during a typical migraine headache. They therefore postulated that a decrease in pain threshold occurred at the same time as dilation of the external carotid artery and its branches. Wolff et al. (1953) subsequently observed that the pain threshold is decreased at the site of the pain during a migraine headache compared with the headache-free interval. Chapman et al. (1960) attributed this decrease in pain threshold to the accumulation in the affected tissues of a substance, initially called "headache stuff" and later called "neurokinin." Chapman et al. (1960) isolated this substance from perfusates of the skin at the site of the pain, and they demonstrated its ability to produce pain when administered to volunteers. They also showed that the activity of neurokinin markedly decreases after administration of ergotamine and that this decrease in activity is associated with a decrease in intensity of pain. It is likely that "neurokinin" is similar to or identical with substance P, a protein released during stimulation of the trigeminovascular system (see below) and which may be modulated by the inhibitory receptors that respond to serotonin agonists such as ergotamine and sumatriptan.

ROLE OF THE TRIGEMINAL NERVE IN THE PATHOGENESIS OF MIGRAINE

It is believed that the trigeminal nerve participates in the pathogenesis of migraine headaches (Moskowitz et al., 1979; Moskowitz, 1984, 1991, 1992). Fibers of the trigeminal

nerve are situated at the interface between the circulation and the brain. These fibers apparently sample continuously the microenvironment of the blood vessel wall. Neural activation releases vasoactive neurotransmitters from their afferent processes (Lembeck, 1983), and these neurotransmitters in turn provoke inflammatory changes in the cerebral blood vessels. At the same time, these nerves transmit nociceptive signals to the central nervous system. Moskowitz (1992) identified parts of the trigeminovascular system of both an excitatory and inhibitory nature. Activation of unmyelinated C-fibers stimulates sensory neurons within the brainstem, but neuronal activity may be inhibited by stimulation of a specific presynaptic receptor within the trigeminovascular network that resembles a type 1 serotonin receptor. Substance P, a vasoactive peptide and putative transmitter, is released from perivascular nerve fibers by noxious stimuli. It mediates both vasodilation and increases in vascular permeability. Thus, the brain not only regulates its own blood flow but to some extent also controls its molecular and chemical environment.

Moskowitz (1992) suggested that the headache that occurs during an attack of migraine is related to an inflammatory reaction of the extracranial blood vessels (Fig. 56.36). He postulated that headache triggers activate or depolarize perivascular axons. Depolarization is accompanied by the local release of neurotransmitters (such as substance P) from axon varicosities and by orthodromic and antidromic conduction. Reaching the brainstem and higher centers, orthodromic impulses mediate the perception of pain and provide the afferent limb for trigeminal reflexes. Antidromic conduction is associated with depolarization-induced release of substance P into the blood vessel wall. Released substance P increases vascular permeability and dilates blood vessels. It also activates macrophages to synthesize thromboxanes, activates lymphocytes, and degranulates mast cells causing local release of histamine. These phenomena may all interact to produce local inflammation and a hyperalgesic response that prolongs head pain (Moskowitz, 1992).

The relationship between peripheral trigeminovascular activity in migraine and the central nervous system is linked by expression of a phosphoprotein encoded by the C-fos gene in neurons of the brainstem and dorsal horn of the spinal cord (Sagar et al., 1988; Moskowitz et al., 1993). C-fos activity increases with stimulation by growth factors and neurotransmitters (Sagar et al., 1988). Moskowitz (1993) noted increased C-fos activity in the brainstem and spinal cord after noxious stimuli were applied to the meninges but found decreased levels of C-fos when trigeminal afferents were severed or serotonin agonists, including sumatriptan (see below), were administered to the meninges prior to the noxious stimulation. Moskowitz et al. (1993) further demonstrated that central C-fos expression was increased by recurrent spreading depression, thus identifying spreading depression as a brain cortex event capable of activating the trigeminovascular system with its brainstem connections and possibly initiating a headache (Silberstein, 1995; Noack and Rothrock, 1996).

The importance of brainstem participation in a migraine attack was also supported by the work of Weiller et al.

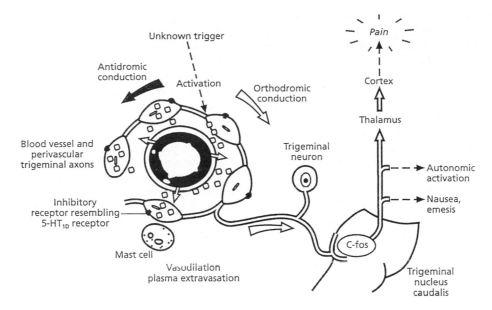

Figure 56.36. Vascular headache mechanisms. Headache triggers activate (depolarize) perivascular trigeminal axons, which release vasoactive neuropeptides to promote neurogenic inflammation (vasodilation, plasma extravasation, mast cell degranulation). Depolarization is accompanied by local release of neurotransmitters, such as substance P, from axonal varicosities. Orthodromic and antidromic conduction along trigeminovascular fibers spread the inflammatory response to adjacent tissues and transmits nociceptive information towards the trigeminal nucleus caudalis and higher brain centers for the perception of pain. Sumatriptan activates an inhibitory 5-HT1D receptor and blocks neuropeptide release and impulse conduction. Neurogenic inflammation and C-fos expression in the nucleus caudalis is blocked. (Adapted from Moskowitz MA. Neurogenic vs. vascular mechanisms of sumatriptan and ergot alkaloids in migraine. Trends Pharmacol Sci *12*:307–311, 1992.)

(1995). The authors used PET to evaluate changes in rCBF during a migraine attack. Increased rCBF was found in cingulate, auditory, and visual cortices and in the brainstem. After injection of sumatriptan, a serotonin agonist (see below), there was complete relief of headache, photophobia, and phonophobia as well as normalization of rCBF in the corresponding cortices. The brainstem increase of rCBF persisted, suggesting that its continued activation may account for recurrence of symptoms including headache (Silberstein et al., 1995).

The research described above suggests that stimuli for the headache of migraine may be generated centrally as well as peripherally. Centrally generated stimuli may then be transmitted peripherally through pathways such as the trigeminovascular system. Stimulated perivascular trigeminal axons release vasoactive neuropeptides and promote neurogenic inflammation. Orthodromic and antidromic conduction along trigeminovascular fibers spreads the inflammatory reaction to adjacent tissues and transmits nociceptive information toward the trigeminal nucleus caudalis and higher brain centers that recognize the sensation of pain (Fig. 56.36) (Moskowitz 1993).

ROLE OF SEROTONIN IN MIGRAINE

Serotonin (5-hydroxytryptamine, 5-HT) is a biogenic amine that is important in the control of feeding behavior, thermoregulation, sexual behavior, and sleep, and that is often linked to migraine activity (Sicuteri et al., 1961; Curran et al., 1965; Anthony et al., 1967; Anthony and Lance, 1975;

Somerville, 1976; Silberstein, 1994). Evidence for involvement of 5-HT in migraine is based in part on the observation that reserpine, which enhances 5-HT release and therefore depletes central nervous system 5-HT stores, may precipitate a migraine attack (Kimball et al., 1960; Anthony et al., 1967; Lance et al., 1967). The attack may then be aborted by administration of 5-HT, its precursors, or agonists such as sumatriptan. Thus, the serotonergic system, with at least seven classes of receptors, may act as a modulator of neural systems, such as the trigeminal and spinal pain pathways, (see above) thought to be involved in migraine (Moskowitz, 1992; Silberstein, 1994a).

A UNIFYING THEORY OF MIGRAINE

It is clear from the above discussion that multiple phenomena are responsible for both the aura and the headache that occur as part of the migraine syndrome. Spierings (1988) believed that spreading depression produces the aura of migraine as Lashley (1941), Milner (1958), and Kunkle (1963) first suggested (see also Pearce, 1985). The headache may be triggered from stimuli generated centrally or peripherally and which are then transmitted via pathways such as the trigeminovascular network with modulation in part by serotonergic receptors (Silberstein et al., 1995). Changes in cerebral blood flow are secondary phenomena produced as a result of initial neuronal dysfunction and perpetuated by vascular inflammation related to neurotransmitter release and activity of trigeminovascular fibers.

Migraine seems to be a reaction pattern to a number of factors. This reaction pattern is apparently caused by an interaction between inherited traits and exogenous or endogenous factors (Diamond and Medina, 1980; Moskowitz, 1984; Welch, 1987, 1993). The inherited traits include neurovascular instability and platelet changes (Malmgren and Hasselmark, 1988). Neurovascular instability is shown in the high frequency of electroencephalographic abnormalities and disturbances in the autonomic system of patients with migraine (Appenzeller, 1969; Havanka-Kanniainen et al., 1988; Lance, 1993). Alterations in monoamine oxidase (MAO) type B in platelets make these cells more prone to release serotonin and other biochemical substances that are stored within them (Hilton, 1971; Corbett, 1983; D'Andrea et al., 1989a, 1989b; D'Andrea et al., 1995a). In addition, platelets in patients with migraine seem to demonstrate hyperaggregability when compared with platelets from patients without migraine (Hilton and Cummings, 1972; Kalendovsky and Austin, 1975; Couch and Hassanein, 1977; D'Andrea et al.,

1995b). Other abnormalities of blood, such as the presence of hemoglobin AS, may also predispose to migraine (Osuntokun and Osuntokun, 1972).

Welch (1987, 1993) proposed a unifying model of the cerebral mechanisms that initiate an attack of migraine. In this model, a stressful event is transduced, projected through the thalamus to the primary cortex, and then relayed to the orbitofrontal cortex where a cellular process occurs that initiates activity in neurons that form the orbitofrontal-brainstem pathway to the intrinsic noradrenergic system. The activation of this pathway is related to a set of event-related electrochemical responses that involve shifts of extracellular potassium, release of norepinephrine, and activation of cyclic adenosine monophosphate (see also Pearce, 1985). Noack and Rothrock (1996) described a unified model for migraine (Fig. 56.37) that combines the central aspects of migraine pathogenesis as delineated by Welch (1993) with the trigeminovascular model of Moskowitz et al. (1993).

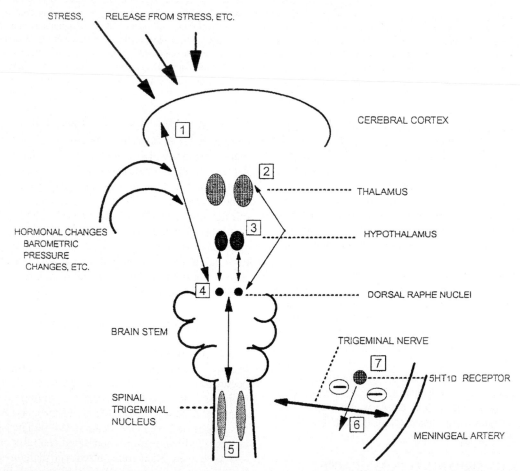

Figure 56.37. A unified model of migraine genesis. Various internal and external migraine triggers may affect the cortex (*1*), thalamus (*2*) and hypothalamus (*3*), further agitating inherently unstable serotoninergic transmission in the midbrain dorsal raphe (*4*) and the spinal trigeminal nucleus (*5*). Spreading depression may be triggered initiating the aura while neuropeptide release at the junction of the trigeminal nerve and the meningeal artery (*6*) results in perivascular inflammation and acute head pain. Reciprocal communication between this peripheral trigeminovascular system and central pain pathways perpetuates the migraine attack. Activation of the presynaptic 5HT1D receptor at the trigeminovascular junction (*7*) may inhibit neuropeptide release and relieve acute migraine pain. (Adapted from Noack H, Rothrock JF. Migraine: Definitions, mechanisms and treatment. South Med J *89*:762–769, 1996.)

EXAMINATION OF THE MIGRAINE PATIENT

HISTORY

When examining a patient complaining of headache, recurrent transient visual loss, or other neurologic phenomena, age and history are of major significance (Smith, 1977; Hupp et al., 1989; Davidoff, 1995; Troost, 1996). The history must include questions regarding the occurrence of migraine equivalents in childhood, the precise nature of any visual or neurologic symptoms, and the presence or absence of any predisposing factors. Premenopausal women specifically should be asked if they are taking an oral contraceptive agent, because most women do not consider this a medicine. The characteristics of the headache that are important to learn include onset, duration, periodicity, timing, localization, intensity, character, precipitating factors, accompanying symptoms and signs, and response to therapy.

When considering transient visual loss, the examiner must localize the source of visual dysfunction as either anterior or posterior visual pathway. As mentioned above, even an astute observer may often ignore the smaller nasal field and report a binocular event as monocular. During an attack, each eye should be occluded and the field of the uncovered eye examined. When visual phenomena occur in the peripheral visual field, an occipital source is likely. Retinal visual disturbances tend to produce alterations in central vision. Also, displacing one eyeball with a finger will move the visual disturbance if it originates in the retina, but the disturbance will remain fixed if it originates in the occipital cortex.

Often the description of the nature, duration, and timing of the episode permits the correct diagnosis. Certain distinctive characteristics of migraine include: build-up and migration of scintillating scotoma, march of paresthesias, progression from one symptom to another, recurrence of similar episodes, duration of episodes usually 15–30 minutes, history of similar "spells" with headache, and benign course.

A previous history of migraine symptoms is helpful but may be absent in up to 25% of patients (Bille, 1962). A positive family history is less likely to be obtained in acephalgic migraineurs than in those with headache (Schatz, 1981).

DIFFERENTIAL DIAGNOSIS

In an earlier section of this chapter, we discussed lesions that may produce scintillating scotomas similar to those of migraine. In addition, other types of transient visual and neurologic dysfunction with and without associated or subsequent headache that are compatible with migraine occasionally occur in patients with other disorders, including aneurysms, AVMs, cardiac valvular disease (particularly mitral valve prolapse), congenital vascular anomalies, tumors, connective tissue disease, and severe atherosclerotic and nonatherosclerotic vascular disease (Mackenzie, 1953, 1954; Sabra, 1959; Lees, 1962; Duvoisin and Yahr, 1965; Fisher, 1967; Troost et al., 1979; Fisher, 1980; Kattah and Luessenhop, 1980; Donin and Keane, 1981; Selhorst et al.,

1981; Feldmann and Posner, 1986; Coppeto and Greco, 1987; Dulli et al., 1987; Benrabah et al., 1988; Coppeto, 1988b; Herman, 1989). Manor et al. (1985) reported migraine-like headaches in three middle-aged patients without a history of migraine but in whom myelography had been previously performed. In all three cases, drops of contrast material were detected in the basal cisterns, and it was suggested by the authors that an allergic or toxic reaction to this material may have produced the symptoms. Primary ocular disturbances such as acute angle closure glaucoma and hyphema may produce visual symptoms and headache that mimic migraine (Ravits and Seybold, 1984; Sarkies et al., 1985; Woods et al., 1985; Coppeto and Kawalick, 1986). Finally, increased concentrations of antiphospholipid antibodies may be present in patients who experience migraine-like visual and neurologic phenomena (Frohman et al., 1989; Shuaib and Barcley, 1989). Systemic, intracranial, and ocular lesions thus must always be considered in patients with new-onset migraine, even when the attacks seem typical. Some of these patients may, of course, have two separate disorders: migraine and another process (Coppeto and Greco, 1987); in others, the structural lesion or systemic disorder is probably responsible for the attacks (Troost et al., 1979; Kattah and Luessenhop, 1980; Donin and Keane, 1981; Selhorst et al., 1981; Dulli et al., 1987).

DIAGNOSTIC TESTS

Indications

Most patients with migraine, regardless of the age of onset, have a history so typical (see above), combined with a normal physical examination, that they can be managed without the need for any diagnostic studies. Only if the episodes continue despite aggressive therapy, should these patients receive further evaluation. Other patients with atypical histories or abnormal physical examinations, particularly those over 40 years old who develop isolated acephalgic visual and/or neurologic symptoms, headache always on the same side preceded by visual symptoms, or visual complaints associated with other neurologic abnormalities, require complete evaluation (Fisher, 1980; Schatz, 1981; Hupp et al., 1989). Such an evaluation may include an evaluation of cardiac function, hematologic and serologic evaluation including assay for antiphospholipid antibodies, noninvasive blood flow studies, neuroimaging, and other studies discussed below.

Cerebral Angiography

Before CT scanning and MR imaging were available, angiography was used to investigate patients with presumed migraine, particularly patients with unusual visual or neurologic aura or persistent deficits. It became clear that between attacks of migraine, angiography showed no abnormalities

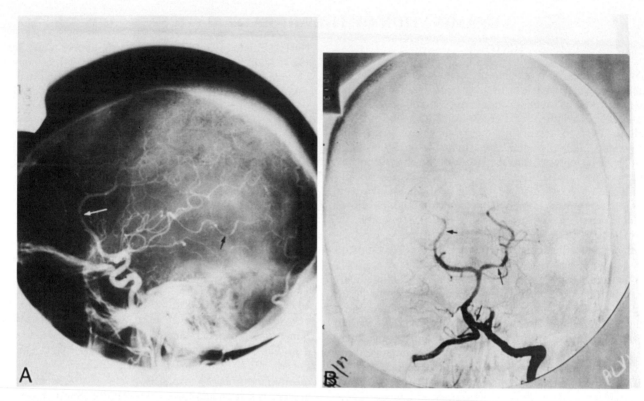

Figure 56.38. Multiple areas of stenosis or spasm in a 36-year-old woman with a history of migraine headaches without aura since early adolescence. The headaches usually were hemicranial, more often on the right, and associated with nausea, photophobia, and osmophobia. They lasted 24–48 hours and occurred several times a month. Precipitating factors included menstruation, relaxation after stress, and exposure to a hot environment. About 6 months after beginning propranolol, the patient developed a severe headache that was much worse than her usual headache. The headache persisted for 3 days and then worsened. Results of CT scanning and lumbar puncture were normal. *A,* Left internal carotid arteriogram, lateral view, shows focal areas of stenosis or spasm of the pericallosal and middle cerebral arteries (*arrows*). *B,* Vertebral arteriogram, anteroposterior view, shows focal areas of spasm or stenosis in the left vertebral artery and in both posterior cerebral arteries (*arrows*). The patient was treated with analgesics, and the headache gradually resolved. (From Solomon S, Lipton RB, Harris PY: Arterial stenosis in migraine: Spasm or arteriopathy? Headache *30*:52–61, 1990.)

(Pearce and Foster, 1965). Even during attacks of migraine, most angiograms are normal (Bruyn, 1968). Nevertheless, some patients with presumed migraine have generalized or focal constriction of intracranial arteries, usually the internal carotid artery or its branches (Garnic and Schellinger, 1983; Masuzawa et al., 1983; Lieberman et al., 1984; Serdaru et al., 1984; Kwentus et al., 1985; Schon and Harrison, 1987; see Table 1 in Solomon et al., 1990) (Fig. 56.38). The arterial constriction seen in some of these patients may be induced by the angiogram itself; in others, it may be caused by the underlying migraine (Solomon et al., 1990).

MR Imaging and CT Scanning

MR imaging is the diagnostic imaging modality of choice in the patient with an atypical history, abnormal physical examination, or unexpected response to appropriate therapy (see indications above). Previously, CT scanning was used as the primary method of screening, usually yielding normal results, although atrophy, ischemic changes, and cerebral edema were reported.(Cuetter and Aita, 1983; Du Boulay et al., 1983). The techniques of MR angiography and spiral CT scanning may replace the need for cerebral angiography in

patients suspected of harboring an aneurysm or arterio-venous malformation (Tomsak et al., 1991).

MR imaging of ''ordinary'' migraineurs is not diagnostic. Nevertheless, migraineurs, particularly those over 40 years of age, have an increased incidence of foci of high signal intensity involving the white matter on long TR sequences (Osborne et al., 1991; Pavese et al., 1994; De Benedittis et al., 1995) (Fig. 56.39). The normal incidence of these white matter changes is very low in young patients and increases to as high as 80% in the elderly. There still remains the issue whether young migraineurs, under the age of 40, would show this same increased incidence of white matter abnormalities (Osborne et al., 1991; De Benedittis et al., 1995). Interestingly, an increased incidence of these same white matter lesions occurs in patients with tension headaches, suggesting that both migraine and tension headaches share some common pathogenic mechanisms (De Benedittis et al., 1995).

The abnormal high intensity white matter signals observed on MR imaging in patients with migraine can be divided into two groups: (*a*) periventricular, and (*b*) those found in the deep white matter away from the ventricular system. Pavese et al. (1994) found that of 129 migraineurs, 20% had abnormal deep white matter foci that were not periventricu-

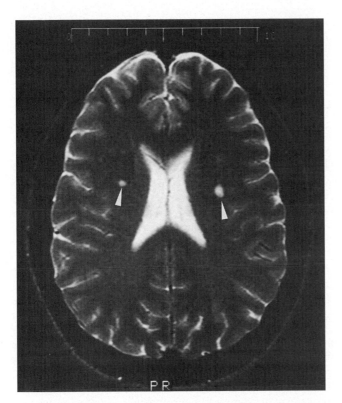

Figure 56.39. T2-weighted magnetic resonance image in a 45-year-old man with a history of migraine without aura. Note two deep white matter intensities (*arrows*) that may represent a normal nonspecific finding but are noted more frequently in patients with migraine.

lar. These deep white matter lesions are associated with an increased risk of cerebrovascular accidents, thus giving weight to the assumption that migraine represents a cerebrovascular risk factor (Rothrock et al., 1988a, 1988b).

EEG

Certainly, some migrainous phenomena closely resemble seizure activity and this relationship is discussed above (see Migraine and Seizures). Many authors report an increased frequency of EEG abnormalities in the interictal period of migraineurs (Davidoff, 1995), but none of the abnormalities are exclusively found in patients with migraine. Unless syncope or epilepsy occurs in connection with headache, EEG evaluation is unnecessary.

Visual-Evoked Potentials

The significance of abnormalities of the visual-evoked response in patients with migraine is unclear; some authors postulate an increased response to sensory stimuli, possibly from central activation (Tsounis et al., 1993; Woestenburg et al., 1993), whereas others consider a generalized disturbance of transmission in the central nervous system caused by recurrent cerebral ischemia (Raudino, 1988), much like the findings of permanent, subtle, neuropsychologic dysfunction that have been reported in patients with migraine (see Permanent Neurologic Deficits above).

Several investigators have described disturbances in the visual-evoked potential in visually asymptomatic adults and children with classic, common, and acephalgic migraine (Regan and Heron, 1970; MacLean et al., 1975; Gawel et al., 1983; Mortimer et al., 1990a, 1990b; Tagliati et al., 1995; Tsounis et al., 1993; Woestenburg et al., 1993), whereas others have found no such disturbances (Mariani et al., 1988; Raudino, 1988). Kennard et al. (1978) used a checkerboard stimulus and found that the latency of the major positive wave was greater and the amplitude larger in patients with migraine headaches with and without aura than in a group of age-matched control subjects. Connolly et al. (1982) reported similar findings using unpatterned flashes. Marsters et al. (1988) used both flash and pattern light stimulation to evoke the visual potential in adults with a diagnosis of common or classic migraine and in a group of control patients without migraine. These investigators then calculated a "fast wave coefficient" that appeared to correlate well with the medical diagnosis. Similar results were obtained by the same group of investigators in children with migraine with or without aura (Mortimer et al., 1990a) and in patients with acephalgic migraine (Mortimer et al., 1990b). Marsters, Mortimer, and their colleagues believe that the visual-evoked potential can be used to provide a fast, reliable, and accurate diagnosis for migraine on an individual basis in both adults and children.

TREATMENT

Before beginning treatment of migraine of any kind, the physician must first ascertain from the patient the length to which the patient is willing to go in order to control the attacks. Patients with rare attacks that occur only once or twice a year or whose attacks consist only of brief visual aura without headache often refuse to consider any therapy that they believe would alter their lifestyle in an unacceptable manner. Thus, many patients who suffer from attacks of migraine may nevertheless refuse to change their approach to stress, to alter their diet, or to begin taking any medicine. Only when a patient clearly accepts a comprehensive approach to migraine can the physician formulate a treatment plan.

MODIFICATION OF PREDISPOSING FACTORS

Proper treatment of any disorder begins with basic issues. The first step in the treatment of a patient with migraine is to identify specific factors that trigger an attack and attempt to avoid or eliminate them by an alteration of the patient's lifestyle (Diamond and Medina, 1980; Wilkinson, 1988; see Table 5 in Hupp et al., 1989). This begins by insuring that the patient has a regular sleep-wake cycle with adequate sleep, a well-balanced diet, and regular exercise. Patients with migraines that are triggered by certain substances in the diet (e.g., caffeine, aspartame, tyramine, etc.) should initially avoid all foods containing these substances until the migraines are under control. Certain foods may then be added back to the diet, one-by-one, to assess their impact on the migraine attacks. Medicinal trigger factors such as oral contraceptives, estrogen replacement therapy, caffeine-containing drugs, decongestant medications, and overusage of analgesics and ergots should be eliminated if possible.

MANAGEMENT OF STRESS

Because stress is the primary trigger of migraine attacks (see above), stress management, biofeedback therapy, psychotherapy, and even acupuncture may be helpful in the control of migraine in selected patients (Adler and Adler, 1976; Diamond et al., 1978; Libo and Arnold, 1983; Philipp et al., 1983; Loh et al., 1984; Daly et al., 1985; Sorbi and Tellegen, 1986, 1988; Wilkinson, 1988; Sorbi et al., 1989).

DIGITAL TEMPLE MASSAGE

In an earlier section of this chapter, we emphasized that the pain of a migraine headache may occasionally be relieved by pressure on the superficial scalp arteries in the region of the pain (Graham, 1979; Drummond and Lance, 1983). In addition, Lipton (1986) reported that the headache phase of migraine attacks preceded by visual aura can occasionally be prevented by digital massage of the superficial temporal arteries during the aura.

MEDICAL THERAPY

Medical therapy of migraine is of three types: (a) symptomatic, (b) abortive, and (c) prophylactic (Friedman, 1972; see Table 5 in Hupp et al., 1989; Peroutka, 1990). Some patients need only one type of drug, whereas others require a combination of two or even three types to adequately control their migraine attacks (Mathew, 1990b).

Symptomatic Treatment

Drugs that may be used to reduce or eliminate symptoms during an attack of migraine include analgesics, anti-inflammatory agents, antiemetics, and sedatives (Wilkinson, 1988; Backonja et al., 1989; Silberstein et al., 1995). These drugs are usually effective only for infrequent, mild attacks.

Abortive Treatment

Some drugs can be used to abort an attack of migraine, particularly a migraine headache. These drugs are most useful when the headache is preceded by an aura, and the drugs are taken during this aura before the headache begins. Most of these drugs are not as effective once a headache has begun, but they may still abort a headache even when taken in the late phase of an attack (Graham, 1979). Dihydroergotamine (DHE) and sumatriptan are important first line abortive drugs that work almost as well in the middle as in the beginning of a migraine attack (Silberstein et al., 1995). Judicious use of abortive drugs may prevent a patient with migraine from requiring prophylactic therapy, thus reducing the risk of side effects from chronic medical therapy (Mathew, 1990b). Those patients best suited to abortive therapy have relatively few attacks, minor disability from attacks, no med-

ical contraindication to abortive drug therapy, and excellent response to abortive drugs (Mathew, 1990). The most successful abortive drugs are ergotamine tartrate and similar agents, sumatriptan, nonsteroidal anti-inflammatory drugs (NSAIDs), and calcium channel blocking agents.

Ergotamine preparations probably are one of the drugs most commonly used to abort an attack of migraine (Friedman, 1972). Ergotamine tartrate was first recognized as being useful in the treatment of migraine in 1883 (Liveing). Its estimated effectiveness ranges from 90% when used parenterally, to 80% when given in suppository form, to 50% when given orally (Dalessio, 1980). Ergotamine stimulates smooth muscle, producing vasoconstriction. It also produces a sympatholytic reaction in medullary tissue, and it acts as an α-adrenergic blocking agent in peripheral tissue (Rall and Schleifer, 1980).

Numerous authors have attested to the ability of ergotamine preparations to abort attacks of migraine, particularly those that begin with an aura (Whitty, 1971; Friedman, 1972; Creditor, 1982). Wilkinson et al. (1978) used ergotamine given in suppository form (1 mg ergotamine tartrate) to treat 310 patients with migraine headaches. All of the patients had some improvement. Forty percent of the patients became free of symptoms, usually within 180 minutes, 51% of the patients had improvement in symptoms but retained a slight residual headache, and 9% of the patients had slight improvement in symptoms. Unfortunately, ergotamine can produce a variety of side effects, including nausea, vomiting, muscle aches, diarrhea, and difficulty swallowing (Diamond, 1976; Pradalier et al., 1985; Saper and Jones, 1986; Sargent et al., 1988). In addition, regular usage of ergotamine may result in recurrent, rebound headaches (Friedman, 1972; Saper, 1987b) (see Chapter 36). This usually occurs as a consequence of excessive dosage, but serious reactions have also been reported at acceptable treatment concentrations or when the drug has been taken in the setting of peripheral vascular disease, systemic hypertension, or ischemic heart disease (Enge and Silvertssen, 1965). Patients with ergotamine-induced, rebound headaches experience: (a) increasing frequency of headaches, (b) loss of feeling of well-being, (c) fatigue, and (d) depression (Friedman, 1972). Diamond and Medina (1975, 1980) recommended the mild vasoconstricting agent isomethoptene in combination with an antiemetic agent for those patients whose headaches occur so often that ergotamine cannot be taken.

Sumatriptan, a selective 5HT-1 receptor agonist, was developed as an acute treatment for migraine (Baar et al., 1989; Brion et al., 1989; Doenicke et al., 1989; Humphrey et al., 1989; Perrin et al., 1989; Tfelt-Hansen et al., 1989; Humphrey et al., 1990; Peroutka, 1990). Clinical trials indicate that sumatriptan reduces or relieves migraine symptoms in approximately 70% of patients within 1 hour after administration (Cady et al., 1991). It is available in both oral and subcutaneous forms, but the time of onset is slightly delayed and efficacy is mildly diminished when sumatriptan is used orally (Plosker and McTavish, 1994; Silberstein, 1995). Sumatriptan is contraindicated in patients with ischemic heart disease, angina, uncontrolled hypertension, and vertebrobasilar migraine (Plosker and McTavish, 1994). The most frequent side effects of this drug are pain at the injection site, flushing, burning, and warm or hot sensations. In patients at risk for angina, the first dose should be administered under medical supervision after a normal electrocardiogram (Silberstein et al., 1995).

Subcutaneous sumatriptan was compared with subcutaneous DHE and found to have a faster onset of action, although by 4 hours both were equally effective. Sumatriptan does have a higher 24-hour headache recurrence rate (40% vs. 20%) than DHE (Silberstein et al., 1995).

A number of nonsteroidal, anti-inflammatory drugs (NSAIDs) can be used to abort migraine attacks. These drugs include aspirin, ketoprofen, tolfenamic acid, naproxen, and indomethacin. The rationale for using NSAIDs is based on the painful nature of the migraine attacks, the hypothesis of sterile inflammation in the pathophysiology of the attacks, and the role played by platelets in the onset of the attacks (see above). Pradalier et al. (1988) reviewed the literature concerning controlled trials of NSAIDs versus placebo or reference substances for the treatment of migraine. These authors found convincing evidence that a number of NSAIDs, particularly aspirin, naproxen, and tolfenamic acid, were better than placebo, and as good as or better than, ergotamine tartrate in reducing both the severity and the duration of an attack of migraine (Hakkarainen et al., 1979, 1980; Tfelt-Hansen and Olesen, 1984; Johnson et al., 1985a; Nestvold et al., 1985; Pradalier et al., 1985). Subsequent controlled trials clearly established the efficacy of NSAIDs in the treatment of acute migraine attacks (Kinnunen et al., 1988; Sargent et al., 1988; Andersson et al., 1989; Havanka-Kanniainen, 1989), although there is some variability among these studies in the amount of benefit derived from some of the drugs. Among these agents, naproxen and ibuprofen seem to be the most efficacious of the NSAIDs in aborting attacks of migraine. Pearce et al. (1983) compared the efficacy of ibuprofen with that of aspirin in aborting migraine attacks and concluded that ibuprofen was superior to aspirin in its reduction of both the severity and the duration of an attack of migraine.

Calcium channel blocking agents are usually used to prevent migraine attacks (see below); however, they also may be of benefit in aborting an attack of migraine. Soyka et al. (1988, 1989) performed a double-blind trial that compared the effect of intravenously administered flunarizine with placebo in reducing the severity and frequency of migraine attacks. Seventy-four percent of patients who received flunarizine reported complete relief of pain or marked reduction of intensity of pain within 60 minutes, whereas complete relief or marked reduction of pain occurred in 28% of patients who received placebo. Apart from a sedative effect reported by nine patients, there were no side effects from flunarizine. Based on these findings, Soyka et al. (1928, 1989) concluded that flunarizine is an acceptable alternative to ergotamine for the treatment of migraine headaches with and without aura.

Prophylactic Treatment

The best medicinal approach to recurrent migraine attacks is prophylactic. Several types of drugs are used to prevent attacks of migraine (Silberstein et al., 1995):

1. Agents that block β-adrenergic sympathetic receptors (β-blocking agents);
2. Drugs that inhibit or block the normal calcium channels (calcium channel blocking agents);
3. Tricyclic antidepressants (Peroutka, 1990);
4. Anticonvulsants (divalproex);
5. Antiserotonin (methysergide);
6. Ergot alkaloids and mixtures (ergonovine maleate, ergotamine with phenobarbital);
7. Aspirin and NSAIDS, and
8. Others.

Drug categories 1–4 are considered "first-line" agents.

The most common β-blocking agent in use is propranolol (Inderal) (Smith, 1977; Frishman, 1981). This drug was first recommended for the prevention of migraine by Bekes et al. in 1968, but it was not until 1972, when Weber and Reinmuth reported the results of a double-blind, controlled study comparing the effects of propranolol to placebo, that the effectiveness of this drug became clear. Subsequently, numerous reports attested to its efficacy in preventing migraine attacks (Malvea et al., 1973; Wideroe and Vigander, 1974; Diamond and Medina, 1976; Behan and Reid, 1980; Olsson et al., 1984; Nadelmann et al., 1986; Ziegler et al., 1987). Propranolol can be used in gradually increasing amounts beginning at a dose of 20 mg bid and increasing as needed or tolerated to as much as 160 mg bid. It is most helpful in preventing migraine headaches without aura (common migraine) (Raskin and Schwartz, 1980; Lance, 1981; Diamond et al., 1982; Rosen, 1983; Stellar et al., 1984; Tfelt-Hansen et al., 1984). It can also be used to treat migraine with visual aura (Kupersmith et al., 1979), but several patients have developed permanent visual or neurologic complications after propranolol was used to treat attacks of migraine preceded by aura (Prendes, 1980; Gilbert, 1982; Katz, 1986). In view of these findings, Burde (1986) recommended that propranolol and other β-adrenergic blocking agents be used primarily for the prevention of migraine without aura and not for other forms of migraine except with "extreme caution." β-Adrenergic blocking agents other than propranolol may be useful in preventing migraine, particularly timolol (Stellar et al., 1984) and nadolol, both of which have a long plasma half-life (20–24 hours compared with 4–6 hours for propranolol) and fewer side effects than propranolol (Sudilovsky et al., 1987). Contraindications to the use of propranolol and other β-adrenergic blocking agents include asthma, chronic obstructive lung disease, congestive heart failure, atrioventricular conduction disturbances, and insulin or monoamine oxidase therapy (Diamond and Medina, 1980).

Calcium channel blocking agents are generally well tolerated except for their tendency to produce chronic constipation. Such agents are especially helpful in preventing attacks of migraine preceded by neurologic aura, familial hemiplegic migraine, and basilar artery migraine. Calcium channel blocking agents may also be helpful in preventing migraine headaches that are not preceded by aura, migraine headaches preceded by visual aura, and migraine aura without headaches when treatment with β-blocking agents is unsuccessful or thought not to be warranted because of potential vasoconstrictive side effects (see above). The most commonly used agents are verapamil and diltiazem. Verapamil is a papaverine-derived calcium entry blocking agent that has significant effects on cerebral blood flow, arterial dilation, and release of serotonin from both brain and platelets (Solomon, 1989). Since Solomon et al. first described the efficacy of verapamil in the prophylaxis of migraine in 1983, numerous controlled and uncontrolled studies have confirmed that it is a safe, well-tolerated, and effective agent for prevention of migraine (Markley et al., 1984; Jonsdottir et al., 1987; Prusinski and Kozubski, 1987; Solomon and Diamond, 1987; Solomon, 1989). Nifedipine is also effective in preventing migraine, both in adults (Meyer et al., 1983, 1985; McArthur et al., 1989) and in children (Roddy and Giang, 1989). Nifedipine is not, however, as effective as propranolol for the initial prophylaxis of migraine (Albers et al., 1989). Other calcium channel blocking agents that can prevent migraine in both adults and children include flunarizine (Louis, 1981; Amery, 1983; Diamond and Schenbaum, 1983; Frenken and Nuijten, 1984; Mentenopoulos et al., 1985; Sorensen et al., 1986; Amery, 1988; Lücking et al., 1988; Martinez-Lage, 1988; Sorge et al., 1988; Spierings and Messinger, 1988; Ludin, 1989; Albani et al., 1990) and nimodipine (Havanka-Kanniainen et al., 1982; Meyer and Hardenberg, 1983; Havanka-Kanniainen et al., 1985; Meyer et al., 1985; Ansell et al., 1988; Migraine-Nimodipine European Study Group, 1989a, 1989b; Battistella et al., 1990; Leone et al., 1990), but these drugs are either less effective—or no more effective—than propranolol in the initial prophylaxis of migraine with or without aura. In addition, Dalla Volta et al. (1990) reported insomnia and disturbances of perception in two patients taking oral flunarizine for migraine prophylaxis. The symptoms resolved when the drug was stopped, and in one patient, they recurred when the drug was restarted. Albani et al. (1990) described sleepiness and sedation in 13 of 40 patients (32.5%) and weight gain in 11 of 40 patients (20.8%) taking flunarizine for migraine prophylaxis. Such side effects may be unacceptable when compared with the side effects of other drugs used to prevent migraine.

The tricyclic antidepressant drugs, particularly nortriptyline, may be used to prevent attacks of migraine. Nortriptyline is the major metabolite of amitriptyline, but it has less sedative and anticholinergic effects. Other effective antidepressant agents include amitriptyline, imipramine, and doxepin (Couch et al., 1976; Couch and Hassanein, 1979; Ziegler et al., 1987). The efficacy of the tricyclic antidepressive agents in preventing migraine does not seem to be related to their effect on anxiety or depression, but instead to their ability to reduce platelet aggregability (Ziegler et al., 1987).

Divalproex, a γ-amino butyric acid (GABA) agonist, is a relatively safe and common anticonvulsant that is efficacious in the prophylaxis of migraine (Jensen et al., 1994; Rothrock et al., 1994; Mathew et al., 1995). Side effects include sedation, hair loss, tremor, weight gain, gastrointestinal complaints, and changes in cognitive performance. Hepatotoxicity, found almost exclusively in children, is the most serious complication (Silberstein et al., 1995).

Each of the "first-line" medicines used to prevent migraine attacks (categories 1–4 above) has a two-thirds chance of being tolerated and effective in any given patient. Thus, several trials of different medication may be needed before success is achieved. Patients must therefore be informed of the complex nature of the treatment and the need for patience during the treatment trials. In addition, the concept of successful treatment must be defined before starting medication. For most physicians and their patients, the goal is adequate control, rather than complete eradication, of migraine attacks.

Certain mistakes are commonly made by physicians attempting to treat migraine with preventive medicines. Foremost is the tendency to give up too soon. This is particularly apt to occur when patients are given too little medication. Each trial of medication should be continued for at least 1 month. This provides for adequate time to increase the dosage to therapeutic levels and to allow for therapeutic benefit. Patients should be advised that improvement probably will not occur immediately and that because of the side effects of the drug, some patients feel worse before they begin to feel better.

In general, it is usually best to use only one preventive drug at a time. Some patients, however, seem to respond only when a combination of drugs, such as nortriptyline and verapamil or naldolol, are used.

Patients whose migraines do not respond to the β-blocking agents, calcium channel blockers, or antidepressants described above may nevertheless show response to other drugs. Potential "second-line" drugs for migraine prophylaxis include cyproheptadine, methysergide, and various NSAIDs such as naproxen (Graham, 1979).

Cyproheptidine (periactin) structurally resembles the phenothiazine antihistaminic drugs, and it has both antihistamine and antiserotonin properties (Diamond et al., 1972; Douglas, 1975). Cyproheptidine may be quite effective in the prophylactic treatment of migraine, although patients using it may gain a considerable amount of weight (Wilkinson, 1988). Other side effects of cyproheptidine include drowsiness (often transient), dry mouth, anorexia, nausea, and dizziness. Children seem to tolerate cyproheptidine better than adults (Diamond and Medina, 1980).

Methysergide (Sansert) has a chemical structure similar to serotonin (Curran et al., 1967). At some receptor sites, it acts like serotonin; at others, it neutralizes the effects of serotonin. It provides excellent prophylaxis against migraine (Friedman and Elkind, 1963; Penderson and Moller, 1966; Kabler, 1967; Smith, 1977; Graham, 1979; Silberstein, 1994); however, it has a number of significant side effects that limit its usefulness. These include nausea, vomiting, muscle weakness, and myalgias. Retroperitoneal, pleuropulmonary, and endocardial fibrosis is a rare (1/500) but major complication (Carr and Biswas, 1966; Graham et al., 1966; Schwartz and Kark, 1966; Elkind et al., 1968; Graham, 1979; Wilkinson, 1988; Silberstein, 1994). Nevertheless, methysergide may be used for short periods without significant risk in selected patients.

Ergonovine maleate is an ergot derivative with oxytocic and vasoconstrictive properties. Commonly used in the treatment of postpartum hemorrhage, it may prevent attacks of migraine during menstruation in some patients who are unresponsive to other drugs (Gallagher, 1989). It seems to be most effective when taken several times a day during menses.

Pradalier et al. (1988) analyzed the literature concerning controlled trials of NSAIDs versus placebo or reference drugs in the long-term prevention of migraine. These investigators concluded that there were ample data from controlled trials that NSAIDs such as ketoprofen, aspirin, indomethacin, tolfenamic acid, naproxen, and fenoprofen calcium were superior to placebo in the long-term prevention of migraine (Stensrud and Sjaastad, 1974; O'Neill and Mann, 1978; Lindegaard et al., 1980; Mikkelsen and Viggo Falk, 1982; Sargent et al., 1985; Welch et al., 1985; Ziegler and Ellis, 1985; Johnson et al., 1986; Diamond et al., 1987); however, there was no evidence that these drugs were superior to β-adrenergic blocking agents (Baldrati et al., 1983; Sargent et al., 1985; Behan and Connelly, 1986; Johnson et al., 1986). The results of the Physicians' Health Study, a randomized, double-blind, placebo-controlled trial that studied low-dose aspirin (325 mg every other day) therapy among over 22,000 male physicians aged 40–84 years, also suggest that low doses of aspirin may be effective in preventing or reducing the frequency of migraine with and without aura (Buring et al., 1990; Dalessio, 1990).

For many years, the leaves of the aromatic plant *Tanacetum parthenium,* also called "feverfew" because of its use as an antipyretic, have been used as a lay remedy for the prevention of migraine. Feverfew extract inhibits the release of serotonin from platelets in vitro (Heptenstall et al., 1985), and this mechanism may be responsible for the clinical benefit in patients with migraine (Johnson, 1983). Johnson et al. (1985b) conducted a double-blind study in which some patients who were using feverfew to prevent migraine were switched to a placebo preparation. An increase in the frequency and severity of migraine attacks in patients switched to placebo provided indirect evidence of the efficacy of this remedy. Subsequently, Murphy et al. (1988) reported the results of a randomized, double-blind, placebo-controlled study in which 72 patients with migraine were randomly allocated to receive either one capsule of feverfew leaves or matching placebo for 4 months. The patients were then switched to the other treatment arm of the study for another 4 months. Treatment with feverfew was associated with a reduction in the mean number and severity, but not the duration, of migraine attacks. There were no serious side effects of the substance. It would seem that effective prophylaxis of migraine may not be limited to expensive commercial products but may also be found in nature and in health food shops.

REFERENCES

Abu-Arefeh I, Russell G. Paroxysmal vertigo as a migraine equivalent in children: A population-based study. Cephalalgia *15*(1):22–25, 1995.

Ad Hoc Committee on Classification of Headache: Classification of headache. JAMA *179*:717–718, 1962.

Adler CS, Adler SM. Biofeedback therapy for the treatment of headaches: A 5-year follow-up. Headache *16*:189–191, 1976.

Albani M, Baldrati A, Cortelli P, et al. Flunarizine plasma concentrations and side effects in migraine patients. Headache *30*:369–370, 1990.

Albers GW, Simon LT, Hamik A, et al. Nifedipine versus propranolol for the initial prophylaxis of migraine. Headache *29*:214–217, 1989.

Alpers BJ, Yaskin HE. Pathogenesis of ophthalmoplegic migraine. Arch Ophthalmol *45*:555–566, 1951.

Alvarez WC. The migrainous personality and constitution; the essential features of the disease: A study of 500 cases. Am J Med Sci *213*:1–8, 1947.

Alvarez WC. The migrainous scotoma as studied in 618 patients. Am J Ophthalmol *49*:489–504, 1960.

Amery WK. Flunarizine, a calcium channel blocker: A new prophylactic drug in migraine. Headache *23*:70–74, 1983.

Amery WK. Onset of action of various migraine prophylactics. Cephalalgia *8*(8): 11–14, 1988.

Amery WK, Van Neuten JM, Wauquier A (Editors). The Pharmacological Basis of Migraine Therapy. London, Pitman Ltd, 1984.

Andermann E, Andermann F, Silver K, et al. Benign familial nocturnal alternating hemiplegia of childhood. Neurology *44*(10):1812–1814, 1994.

Andermann F. Migraine and epilepsy: An overview. In Migraine and Epilepsy. Editors, Andermann F, Lugaresi E, pp 405–422. Boston, Butterworths, 1987.

Andermann F, Lugaresi E (Editors). Migraine and Epilepsy. Boston, Butterworths, 1987.

Anders TF, Weinstein P. Sleep and its disorders in infants and children: A review. Pediatrics *50*:312–324, 1972.

Andersen AR, Friberg L, Skyhoj Olsen T, et al. Delayed hyperemia following hypoperfusion in classic migraine: Single photon emission computed tomographic demonstration. Arch Neurol *45*:154–159, 1988.

Andersen AR, Olesen J, Skyhoj Olsen T, et al. Cerebral hypoperfusion followed by hyperperfusion in classic migraine (Reply). Arch Neurol *46*:606, 1989.

Anderson PG: Ergotamine headache. Headache *15*:118–121, 1975.

Andersson PG, Hinge HH, Johansen O, et al. Double-blind study of naproxen vs. placebo in the treatment of acute migraine attacks. Cephalalgia *9*:29–32, 1989.

Ansell E, Fazzone T, Festenstein R, et al. Nimodipine in migraine prophylaxis. Cephalalgia *8*:269–272, 1988.

Anthony M, Lance JW. Histamine and serotonin in cluster headache. Arch Neurol *25*:225–231, 1971.

Anthony M, Lance JW. The role of serotonin in migraine. In Modern Topics in Migraine. Editor, Pearce J, pp 107–123. London, Heineman, 1975.

Anthony M, Hinterberger H, Lance JW. Plasma serotonin in migraine and stress. Arch Neurol *16*:544–552, 1967.

Anthony M, Hinterberger H, Lance JW. The possible relationship of serotonin to the migraine syndrome. Res Clin Stud Headache *2*:29–59, 1969.

Appenzeller O. Vasomotor function in migraine. Headache *9*:147–155, 1969.

Appleton R, Farrell K, Buncic JR, et al. Amaurosis fugax in teenagers: a migraine variant. Am J Dis Child *142*:331–333, 1988.

Ardila A, Sanchez E. Neuropsychologic symptoms in the migraine syndrome. Cephalalgia *8*:67–70, 1988.

Aring CD. The migrainous scintillating scotoma. JAMA *220*:519–522, 1972.

Athwal BS, Lennox GG. Acetazolamide responsiveness in familial hemiplegic migraine. Ann Neurol *40*:820–821, 1996.

Atkinson RA, Appenzeller O. Headache in small vessel disease of the brain: A study of patients with systemic lupus erythematosus. Headache *15*:198–201, 1975.

Atkinson RA, Appenzeller O. Headache in sports. Semin Neurol *1*:334–343, 1981.

Baar HA, Brand J, Doenicke A, et al. Treatment of acute migraine with subcutaneous GR43175 in West Germany. Cephalalgia *9*(9):83–88, 1989.

Backonja M, Beinlich B, Dulli D, et al. Haloperidol and lorazepam for the treatment of nausea and vomiting associated with the treatment of intractable migraine headaches. Arch Neurol *46*:724, 1989.

Bailey TD, O'Connor PS, Tredici TJ, et al. Ophthalmoplegic migraine. J Clin Neuroophthalmol *4*:225–228, 1984.

Baldrati A, Cortelli P, Procaccianti G, et al. Propranolol and acetylsalicylic acid in migraine prophylaxis. Acta Neurol Scand *67*:181–186, 1983.

Barabas G, Ferrari M, Matthews WS. Childhood migraine and somnambulism. Neurology *33*:948–949, 1983.

Baron A, Chevannes H. Migraine ophtalmique et obliteration d'une branche de l'artere centrale de la retine. Bull Soc Ophtalmol Fr *58*:81–86, 1958.

Basser LS. Benign proxysmal vertigo of childhood. Brain *87*:141–152, 1964.

Basser LS. The relation of migraine and epilepsy. Brain *92*:285–300, 1969.

Battistella PA, Ruffilli R, Moro R, et al. A placebo-controlled crossover trial of nimodipine in pediatric migraine. Headache *30*:264–268, 1990.

Behan PO, Carlin J. Benign recurrent vertigo. In Advances in Migraine, Research and Therapy. Editor, Rose FC, pp 49–55. New York, Raven Press, 1982.

Behan PO, Connolly K. Prophylaxis of migraine: A comparison between naproxen sodium and Pizotifen. Headache *26*:237–239, 1986.

Behan PO, Reid M. Propranolol in the treatment of migraine. Practitioner *224*: 201–204, 1980.

Bekes M, Matos L, Rausch J, et al. Treatment of migraine with propranolol. Lancet *2*:980, 1968.

Bennett DR, Fuenning SI, Sullivan G, et al. Migraine precipitated by head trauma in athletes. Am J Sports Med *8*:202–205, 1980.

Benrabah R, Cabanis E-A, Haut J, et al. Migraine ophtalmique et malformations arterielles cervico-cephaliques: A propos d'une observations. Bull Soc Ophtalmol Fr *88*:27–31, 1988.

Bernat JL. Cluster headaches from isosorbide dinitrate. Ann Neurol *6*:554–555, 1979.

Bernsen HJJA, Van de Vlasakker C, Verhagen WIM, et al. Basilar artery migraine stroke. Headache 30:142–144, 1990.

Bickerstaff ER. Basilar artery migraine. Lancet 1:15–17, 1961a.

Bickerstaff ER. Impairment of consciousness in migraine. Lancet 2:1057–1059, 1961b.

Bickerstaff ER. The basilar artery and the migraine-epilepsy syndrome. Proc R Soc Med 55:167–169, 1962.

Bickerstaff ER. Cluster headaches. In Handbook of Clinical Neurology. Editors, Vinken PJ, Bruyn GW, Vol 5, pp 111–118. Amsterdam, Elsevier, 1968.

Bickerstaff ER. Basilar artery migraine. In Controversies and Clinical Variants of Migraine. Editor, Saper JR, pp 81–86. New York, Pergamon Press, 1987.

Bigley GK, Sharp FR. Reversible alexia without agraphia due to migraine. Arch Neurol 40:114–115, 1983.

Bille BO. Migraine in school children. Acta Paediatrica 51(Supp 136):74–145, 1962.

Bille BO. Migraine in school children. Acta Paediatr 64:499–508, 1964.

Blau JN. Migraine prodromes separated from the aura: Complete migraine. Br Med J 281:658–660, 1980.

Blau JN. Resolution of migraine attacks: Sleep and the recovery phase. J Neurol Neurosurg Psychiatry 45:223–226, 1982.

Blau JN (Editor). Migraine. Clinical and Research Aspects. Baltimore, Johns Hopkins University Press, 1987.

Blau JN. Migraine postdromes: Symptoms after attacks. Cephalalgia 11:229–231, 1991.

Blau JN, Engel H. Episodic paroxysmal hemicrania: A further case and review of the literature. J Neurol Neurosurg Psychiatr 53:343–344, 1990.

Blau JN, Thavapalan M. Preventing migraine: A study of precipitating factors. Headache 28:481–483, 1988.

Bogousslavsky J, Regli F, Van Melle G, et al. Migraine stroke. Neurology 38:223–227, 1988.

Boisen E. Strokes in migraine: Report on seven strokes associated with severe migraine attacks. Dan Med Bull 22:100–106, 1975.

Booy R. Amaurosis fugax in a young woman. Lancet 335:1538, 1990.

Bradshaw P, Parsons M. Hemiplegic migraine. A clinical study. Q J Med 34:65–85, 1965.

Bramwell E, McMullen WH. Discussion on migraine. Br Med J 2:765–775, 1926.

Brandt KD, Lessell S. Migrainous phenomena in systemic lupus erythematosus. Arthritis Rheum 21:7–16, 1978.

Brasch M, Levinsohn G. Ein Fall yon Migraene mit Blutungen in die Augenhohle waehrend des Anfalls. Klin Wschr 35:1146–1150, 1898.

Brey RL, Hart RG, Sherman DG, et al. Antiphospholipid antibodies and cerebral ischemia in young people. Neurology 40:1190–1196, 1990.

Briley DP, Coull BM, Goodnight SH Jr. Neurological disease associated with antiphospholipid antibodies. Ann Neurol 25:221–227, 1989.

Brion N, Bons J, Plas J, et al. Initial clinical experience with the use of subcutaneous GR43175 in treating acute migraine. Cephalalgia 9(9):79–82, 1989.

Broderick JP, Swanson JW. Migraine-related strokes. Clinical profile and prognosis in 20 patients. Arch Neurol 44:868–871, 1987.

Brown GC, Magargal LE, Shields JA, et al. Retinal arterial obstruction in children and young adults. Am J Ophthalmol 88:18–25, 1981.

Bruyn GW. Complicated migraine. In Handbook of Clinical Neurology. Editors, Vinken PJ, Bruyn GW, Vol 15, pp 66–68. Amsterdam, North Holland, 1968.

Bruyn GW. Migraine equivalents. In Handbook of Clinical Neurology. Editors, Vinken PJ, Bruyn GW, Klawans HL, Rose FC, Vol 4, pp 155–171. Amsterdam, Elsevier Science Publishers, 1986.

Burde RM. Migraine. J Clin Neuroophthalmol 6:72–73, 1986.

Burger SK, Saul RF, Selhorst JB, et al. Transient monocular blindness caused by vasospasm. N Engl J Med 325(12):870–873, 1991.

Buring JE, Peto R, Hennekens CH. Low-dose aspirin for migraine prophylaxis. JAMA 264:1711–1713, 1990.

Burke EC, Peters GA. Migraine in childhood. Am J Dis Child 92:330–336, 1956.

Butler TH. Scotomata in migrainous subjects. Br J Ophthalmol 17:83–87, 1933.

Butler TH. Uncommon symptoms of migraine. Trans Ophthalmol Soc UK 61:205–222, 1941.

Cady RK, Wendt JK, Kirchner JR, et al. Treatment of acute migraine with subcutaneous sumatriptan. JAMA 265(21):2831–2835, 1991.

Callaghan N. The migraine syndrome in pregnancy. Neurology 18:197–201, 1968.

Capildeo R, Rose FC. Towards a new classification of migraine. In Advances in Migraine Research and Therapy. Editor, Rose FC, pp 1–6. New York, Raven Press, 1982.

Caplan LR. Intracerebral hemorrhage revisited. Neurology 38:624–627, 1988.

Carr RJ, Biswas BK. Methysergide and retroperitoneal fibrosis. Br Med J 2:1116–1117, 1966.

Carroll D. Retinal migraine. Headache 10:9–13, 1970.

Caviness VS, O'Brien P. Current concepts: Headache. N Engl J Med 302:446–449, 1980.

Chan CC, Sogg RL, Steinman L. Isolated oculomotor palsy after measles immunization. Am J Ophthalmol 89:446–448, 1980.

Chancellor AM, Wroe SJ, Cull RE. Migraine occurring for the first time during pregnancy. Headache 30:224–227, 1990.

Chapman LF, Ramos AO, Goodell H, et al. A humoral agent implicated in vascular headache of the migraine type. Arch Neurol 3:223–229, 1960.

Charcot JM. Sur un cas de migraine ophthalmoplegique: (paralysie oculo-matrice periodique). Progr Med 1:83–86; 91–102, 1890.

Charcot JM. Clinique des Maladies du Système Nerveux. p 71. Paris, Veuve Babé et Cie, 1892.

Chu ML, Shinnar S: Headaches in children under 7 years of age. Ann Neurol 28:433, 1990.

Chutorian AM. Benign paroxysmal torticollis, tortipelvis and retrocollis of infancy. Neurology 24:366–367, 1974.

Clarke JM. On recurrent motor paralysis in migraine: With report of a family in which recurrent hemiplegia accompanied the attacks. Br Med J 1:1534–1538, 1910.

Codina A, Acarin PN, Miguel F, et al. Migraine hémiplégique associée à un nystagmus. Rev Neurol 124:526–530, 1971.

Cogdon PJ, Forsyth WI. Migraine in childhood: A study of 300 children. Dev Med Child Neurol 21:209–216, 1979.

Cohen RJ, Taylor JR. Persistent neurologic sequelae of migraine: A case report. Neurology 29:1175–1177, 1979.

Cole AJ, Aubé M. Late onset migraine with intracerebral hemorrhage: A recognizable syndrome. Neurology 37(1):238, 1987.

Cole AJ, Aubé M. Migraine with vasospasm and delayed intracerebral hemorrhage. Arch Neurol 47:53–56, 1990.

Collaborative Group for the Study of Stroke in Young Women: Oral contraceptives and stroke in young women: Associated risk factors. JAMA 231:718–722, 1975.

Connolly JF, Gawel M, Rose FC. Migraine patients exhibit abnormalities in the visual evoked potential. J Neurol Neurosurg Psychiatry 45:464–467, 1982.

Connor RCR. Complicated migraine. A study of permanent neurological and visual defects caused by migraine. Lancet 2:1072–1075, 1962.

Coppeto JR. Migraine-like accompaniments of vitreous detachment. Neuroophthalmol 8:197–203, 1988a.

Coppeto JR. Vertebrobasilar degeneration and chronic visual migraine. Neuroophthalmol 8:1–7, 1988b.

Coppeto JR, Greco P. Unilateral internuclear ophthalmoplegia, migraine, and supratentorial arteriovenous malformation. Am J Ophthalmol 104:191–192, 1987.

Coppeto JR, Kawalick M. Ocular pseudomigraine after posterior chamber intraocular lens implantation. Am J Ophthalmol 102:393–394, 1986.

Coppeto JR, Lessell S, Sciarra R, et al. Vascular retinopathy in migraine. Neurology 36:267–270, 1986.

Corbett JJ. Neuro-ophthalmologic complications of migraine and cluster headaches. Neurol Clin 1:973–995, 1983.

Couch JR. Stroke and migraine. In Controversies and Clinical Variants of Migraine. Editor, Saper JR, pp 69–80. New York, Pergamon Press, 1987.

Couch JR, Hassanein RS. Platelet aggregability in migraine. Neurology 27:843–848, 1977.

Couch JR, Hassanein RS. Amitriptyline in migraine prophylaxis. Arch Neurol 36:695–699, 1979.

Couch JR, Ziegler DK. Prednisone therapy for cluster headache. Headache 18:219–221, 1978.

Couch JR, Ziegler DK, Hassanein RS. Amitriptyline in the prophylaxis of migraine: Effectiveness and relationship of anti-migraine and anti-depressant effects. Neurology 26:121–127, 1976.

Cowan CL, Knox DL. Migraine optic neuropathy. Ann Ophthalmol 14:164–166, 1982.

Creditor MC. Me and migraine. N Engl J Med 307:1029–1032, 1982.

Critchley M, Ferguson FR. Migraine. Lancet 1:123–126, 1933.

Cruciger MP, Mazow ML. An unusual case of ophthalmoplegic migraine. Am J Ophthalmol 86:414–417, 1978.

Cuetter AC, Aita JF. CT scanning in classic migraine. Headache 23:195, 1983.

Curran DA, Hinterberger H, Lance JW. Total plasma serotonin, 5-hydroxyindoleacetic acid and p-hydroxy-m-methoxymandelic acid excretion in normal and migrainous subjects. Brain 88:997–1010, 1965.

Curran DA, Hinterberger H, Lance JW. Methysergide. Res Clin Stud Headache 1:74–122, 1967.

Curzon G, Barrie M, Wilkinson M. Headache and amine changes after administration of reserpine to migrainous patients. In Background to Migraine. Editor, Cochran AL, pp 127–132. London, Heinemann, 1970.

Dalessio DJ. Is there a difference between classic and common migraine? What is migraine, after all? Arch Neurol 42:275–276, 1985.

Dalessio DJ. Aspirin prophylaxis for migraine. JAMA 264:1721, 1990.

Dalla Volta G, Magoni M, Cappa S, et al. Insomnia and perceptual disturbances during flunarizne treatment. Headache 30:62–63, 1990.

Dalsgaard-Nielsen T, Bryndum B, Fog-Moller F, et al. The effect of percutaneous nitroglycerine upon the concentration of serotonin, epinephrine and norepinephrine in venous blood from migrainous subjects during attack-free intervals. Headache 14:231–234, 1974.

Daly EJ, Zimmerman JS, Donn PA, et al. Psychophysiological treatment of migraine and tension headaches: A 12-month follow-up. Rehab Psychol 30:3–10, 1985.

D'Andrea G, Toldo M, Cortellazzo S, et al. Platelet activity in migraine. Headache 22:207–212, 1982.

D'Andrea G, Welch KMA, Riddle JM, et al. Platelet serotonin metabolism and ultrastructure in migraine. Arch Neurol 46:1187–1189, 1989a.

D'Andrea G, Welch KMA, Grunfeld S, et al. Platelet norepinephrine and serotonin balance in migraine. Headache 29:657–659, 1989b.

D'Andrea G, Cananzi AR, Perini F, et al. Platelet models and their possible usefullness in the study of migraine pathogenesis. Cephalalgia 15(4):265–271, 1995a.

D'Andrea G, Hasselmark L, Cananzi AR, et al. Metabolism and menstrual cycle rhythmicity of serotonin in primary headaches. Headache 35(4):216–221, 1995b.

Daroff RB. New headache classification. Neurology 38:1138–1139, 1988.

Davidoff RA. Migraine: Manifestations, pathogenesis, and management. Philadelphia, FA Davis Company, 1995.

Davis-Jones A, Gregory MC, Whitty CWM. Permanent sequelae in the migraine attack. In Background to Migraine (Fifth Symposium). Editor, Cummings JN, pp 25–27. New York, Springer-Verlag, 1972.

De Benedittis G, Lorenzetti A, Sina C, et al. Magnetic resonance imaging in migraine and tension-type headache. Headache 35(5):264–268, 1995.

DeBroff BM, Spierings ELH. Migraine associated with periorbital ecchymosis. Headache 30:260–263, 1990.

Deonna T, Martin D. Benign paroxysmal torticollis in infancy. Arch Dis Child 56:956–959, 1981.

DeRomanis F, Buzzi MG, Assenza S, et al. Basilar migraine with electroencephalographic findings of occipital spike-wave complexes: A long-term study in seven children. Cephalalgia 13(3):192–196, June 1993.

Deubner DC. An epidemiologic study of migraine and headache in 10–20 year olds. Headache 17:173–180, 1977.

Dexter JD. The relationship between Stage III & IV & REM sleep and arousals with migraine. Headache 19:364–369, 1979.

Dexter JD. Pathogenesis of migraine: Neurogenic and Endocrine/Humoral Phenomena. In Controversies and Clinical Variants of Migraine. Editor, Saper JR, pp 105–110. New York, Pergamon Press, 1987.

Diamond S. Treatment of migraine with isometheptene, acetaminophen, and dichloralphenazone combination: A double-blind crossover trial. Headache 15:282–287, 1976.

Diamond S. Cluster headache: Relation to and comparison with migraine. Postgrad Med 66:87–91, 1979.

Diamond S. Clinical features in migraine. In Controversies and Clinical Variants of Migraine. Editor, Saper JR, pp 11–20. New York, Pergamon Press, 1987.

Diamond S, Dalessio DJ. The Practicing Physician's Approach to Headache. 3rd ed, p 39. Baltimore, Williams & Wilkins, 1982.

Diamond S, Medina JL. Isometheptene: A non-ergot drug in the treatment of migraine. Headache 15:211–213, 1975.

Diamond S, Medina JL. Double blind study of propranolol for migraine prophylaxis. Headache 16:24–27, 1976.

Diamond S, Medina JL. Review article: Current thoughts on migraine. Headache 20:208–212, 1980.

Diamond S, Schenbaum H. Flunarizine, a calcium channel blocker in the prophylactic treatment of migraine. Headache 23:39–42, 1983.

Diamond S, Baltes BJ, Levine HW. A review of the pharmacology of drugs used in the therapy of migraine. Headache 12:37–43, 1972.

Diamond S, Diamond-Falk J, De Veno T. The value of biofeedback in the treatment of chronic headache: A five-year retrospective study. In Proceedings of the Biofeedback Research Society Annual Meeting, 1978.

Diamond S, Kudrow L, Stevens J, et al. Long-term study of propranolol in the treatment of migraine. Headache 22:268–271, 1982.

Diamond S, Solomon G, Freitag F, et al. Fenoprofen in the prophylaxis of migraine: A double-blind placebo controlled study. Headache 27:246–249, 1987.

Digre KB, Durcan FJ, Branch DW, et al. Amaurosis fugax associated with antiphospholipid antibodies. Ann Neurol 25:228–232, 1989.

Dion JE, Gates PC, Fox AJ, et al. Clinical events following neuroangiography: A prospective study. Stroke 18:997–1004, 1987.

Dittrich J. Havlová M, Nevsimalová S. Paroxysmal hemiparesis in childhood. Dev Med Child Neurol 21:800–807, 1979.

Doenicke A, Melchart D, Bayliss EM. Effective improvement of symptoms in patients with acute migraine by GR43175 administered in dispersible tablets. Cephalalgia 9(9):89–92, 1989.

Donin JF, Keane JR. Migraine, pseudotumor cerebri, blindness and death. Presented at the 13th Annual Frank B. Walsh Society Meeting. Houston, February 27–28, 1981.

Dooling EC, Sweeney VP. Migrainous hemiplegia during breast-feeding. Am J Obstet Gynecol 118:568–570, 1974.

Dorfman LJ, Marshall WH, Enzmann DR. Cerebral infarction and migraine: Clinical and radiologic correlations. Neurology 29:317–322, 1979.

Douglas WW. Histamine and antihistamines: 5-hydroxytryptamine and antagonists. In The Pharmacological Basis of Therapeutics. Editors, Goodman LS, Gilman A, 5th ed, pp 590–629. New York, McMillan Publishing Co, 1975.

Drake ME. Migraine as an organic cause of monocular diplopia. Psychosomatics 24:1024–1027, 1983.

Drummond PD. Pupil diameter in migraine and tension headache. J Neurol Neurosurg Psychiatry 50:228–230, 1987.

Drummond PD. Autonomic disturbances in cluster headache. Brain 111:1199–1209, 1988.

Drummond PD. Disturbances in ocular sympathetic function and facial blood flow in unilateral migraine headache. J Neurol Neurosurg Psychiatry 53:121–125, 1990.

Drummond PD, Anthony M. Extracranial vascular responses to sublingual nitroglyc-

erin and oxygen inhalation in cluster headache patients. Headache 25:70–74, 1985.

Drummond PD, Lance JW. Extracranial vascular changes and the source of pain in migraine headache. Ann Neurol 13:32–37, 1983.

Drummond PD, Lance JW. Thermographic changes in cluster headache. Neurology 34:1292–1298, 1984.

DuBois L. Peripheral and central neurologic loss in complicated migraine. Am Orthopt J 38:177–181, 1988.

DuBois LG, Sadun AA, Lawton TB. Inner retinal layer loss in complicated migraine. Arch Ophthalmol 106:1035–1037, 1988.

DuBoulay GH, Ruiz JS, Rose FC, et al. CT changes associated with migraine. AJNR 4:472–473, 1983.

Dukes HT, Vieth RG. Cerebral arteriography during migraine prodrome and headache. Neurology 14:636–639, 1964.

Dulli DA, Levine RL, Chun RW, et al. Migrainous neurologic dysfunction in Hodgkin's disease. Arch Neurol 44:689, 1987.

Dunn DW, Snyder CH. Benign proxysmal vertigo of childhood. Am J Dis Child 130:1099–1100, 1976.

Dunning HS. Intracranial and extracranial vascular accidents in migraine. Arch Neurol Psychiatr 48:396–406, 1942.

Durkan GP, Troost BT, Slamovits TL, et al. Recurrent painless oculomotor palsy in children. A variant of ophthalmoplegic migraine? Headache 21:58–62, 1981.

Duvoisin RC. Clinical survey. Part 2: The cluster headache. JAMA 222:1403–1406, 1972.

Duvoisin RC, Yahr MD. Posterior fossa aneurysms. Neurology 15:231–241, 1965.

Eagling EM, Sanders MD, Miller SJH. Ischaemic papillopathy: Clinical and fluorescein angiographic review of 40 cases. Br J Ophthalmol 58:990–1007, 1974.

Eckardt LB, McLean JM, Goodell H. Experimental studies on headache: Genesis of pain from eye. Res Nerv Ment Dis 23:209–227, 1943.

Edelson R. Menstrual migraine and other hormonal aspects of migraine. Headache 25:376–379, 1985.

Edelson RN, Levy DE. Transient benign pupillary dilation in young adults. Arch Neurol 31:12–14, 1974.

Edmeads J. Pathogenesis of migraine: Traditional vs. current vascular theories. In Controversies and Clinical Variants of Migraine. Editor, Saper JR, pp 97–104. New York, Pergamon Press, 1987.

Eeg-Olofsson O, Ödkvist L, Lindskog U, et al. Benign paroxysmal vertigo in childhood. Acta Otolaryngol 93:283–289, 1982.

Ehlers H. On pathogenesis of ophthalmoplegic migraine. Acta Psychiatr Neurol Scand 3:219–225, 1928.

Ehyai A, Fenichel GM. The natural history of acute confusional migraine. Arch Neurol 35:368–369, 1978.

Ekbom K. Nitroglycerin as a provocative agent in cluster headache. Arch Neurol 19:487–493, 1968.

Ekbom K. A clinical comparison of cluster headache and migraine. Acta Neurol Scand 46(41):1–48, 1970.

Ekbom K. Lithium vid kroniska symptom av cluster headache. Opusc Med 19:148–156, 1974.

Ekbom K. Lithium in the treatment of chronic cluster headache. Headache 17:39–40, 1977.

Ekbom K. Lithium for cluster headache: Review of the literature and preliminary results of long-term treatment. Headache 21:132–139, 1981.

Ekbom K, Greitz T. Carotid angiography in cluster headache. Acta Radiol Diagn 10:177–186, 1970.

Eldridge P, Punt JAG, Clarke S, et al. Transient traumatic cortical blindness in children—A type of classical migraine in childhood. J Neurol Neurosurg Psychiatry 52:1458, 1989.

Elkind AH. Provoking influences of migraine: The controversies. In Controversies and Clinical Variants of Migraine. Editor, Saper JR, pp 87–96. New York, Pergamon Press, 1987.

Elkind AH, Friedman AP, Bachman A, et al. Silent retroperitoneal fibrosis associated with methysergide therapy. JAMA 206:1041–1044, 1968.

Elliott MA, Peroutka SJ, Welch S, et al. Familial hemiplegic migraine, nystagmus, and cerebellar atrophy. Ann Neurol 39(1):100–106, 1996.

Elmaleh C, Dubuisson C, Fouret C, et al. A propos de cas de migraine ophtalmique ayant entraine une hemianopsie laterale definitive chez une jeune fille de 19 ans. Bull Soc Ophtalmol Fr 87:1223–1226, 1987.

Elser JM, Woody RC. Migraine headache in the infant and young child. Headache 30:366–368, 1990.

Emery S. Acute confusional state in children with migraine. Pediatrics 60:110–114, 1977.

Enge I, Silvertssen E. Ergotism due to therapeutic doses of ergotamine tartrate. Am Heart J 70:665–670, 1965.

Epstein M, Hockaday J, Hockaday T. Migraine and reproductive hormones throughout the menstrual cycle. Lancet 1:553–556, 1975.

Fanciullacci M, Pietrini U, Gatto G, et al. Latent dysautonomic pupillary lateralization in cluster headache: A pupillometric study. Cephalalgia 2:135–144, 1982.

Featherstone HJ. Clinical features of stroke in migraine. A review. Headache 26:128–133, 1986.

Feldmann E, Posner JB. Episodic neurologic dysfunction in patients with Hodgkin's disease. Arch Neurol 43:1227–1233, 1986.

Fenichel GM. Migraine as a cause of benign paroxysmal vertigo of childhood. J Pediatr 71:114–115, 1967.

Fenichel GM. Migraine in childhood. Brief review of this inherited disorder which strikes five per cent of school-age children. Clin Pediatr 7:192–194, 1968.

Fenichel GM. Migraine in children. Neurol Clin 3:77–94, 1985.

Ferroir J-P, Ruszniewski P, Reignier A, et al. Déficit visuel monoculaire permanent, complication exceptionnelle de la migraine. Nouv Presse Med 10:2042–2043, 1981.

Fisher CM. Observations of the fundus oculi in transient monocular blindness. Neurology 9:333–347, 1959.

Fisher CM. Some neuro-ophthalmological observations. J Neurol Neurosurg Psychiatry 30:383–392, 1967.

Fisher CM. Cerebral ischemia—Less familiar types. Clin Neurosurg 18:267–336, 1971.

Fisher CM. Late-life migraine accompaniments as a cause of unexplained transient ischemic attacks. Can J Neurol Sci 7:9–17, 1980.

Fisher CM. An unusual case of migraine accompaniments with permanent sequela—A case report. Headache 26:266–270, 1986.

Fleishman JA, Segall JD, Judge FP. Isolated transient alexia. A migrainous accompaniment. Arch Neurol 40:115–116, 1983.

Fogan L. Treatment of cluster headache. A double-blind comparison of oxygen vs. air inhalation. Arch Neurol 42:362–363, 1985.

Ford FR. Diseases of the Nervous System in Infancy, Childhood and Adolescence. 3rd ed, pp 1183–1184. Springfield, IL, Charles C Thomas Publisher, 1952.

Fothergill J. Remarks on that complaint commonly known under the name of sick headache. Med Obs Soc Phys Lond 6:103–137, 1784.

Fox AJ. Angiography for third nerve palsy in children. J Clin Neuroophthalmol 9:37–38, 1989.

Frenken CWGM, Nuijten STM: Flunarizine, a new preventive approach to migraine. Clin Neurol Neurosurg 86:17–20, 1984.

Friberg L. Cerebral blood flow changes in migraine: Methods, observations and hypotheses. J Neurol 238:S12–S17, 1991.

Friedman AP. Clinical survey. Part 1: Migraine Headaches. JAMA 222:1399–1402, 1972.

Friedman AP. Headache. Clin Neurol 2:1–28, 1976.

Friedman AP. The migraine syndrome. Bull NY Acad Med 44:45–62, 1968.

Friedman AP. Migraine: Historical perspectives. In Controversies and Clinical Variants of Migraine. Editor, Saper JR, pp 1–4. New York, Pergamon Press, 1987.

Friedman AP, Elkind AH. Appraisal of methysergide in the treatment of vascular headaches of the migraine type. JAMA 184:125–128, 1963.

Friedman AP, Merritt HH. Headache: Diagnosis and Treatment. pp 218–219. Philadelphia, FA Davis, 1959.

Friedman AP, Mikropoulos MD. Cluster headaches. Neurology 8:653–663, 1958.

Friedman AP, Harter DH, Merritt HH. Ophthalmoplegic migraine. Arch Neurol 7:320–327, 1962.

Friedman AP, Wood EH, Rowan AS. Observations on vascular headache of the migraine type. In Background to Migraine: Fifth Migraine Symposium. Editor, Cumings JN, pp 1–17. New York, Springer-Verlag, 1973.

Friedman B. Migraine: With special reference to scintillating scotomata. EENT Monthly 50:52–58, 1971.

Friedman MW. Occlusion of central retinal vein in migraine. Arch Ophthalmol 45:678–682, 1951.

Frishman WH. Beta-adrenoceptor antagonists: New drugs and new indications. N Engl J Med 305:500–506, 1981.

Frohman LP, Rescigno R, Bielory L. Neuro-ophthalmologic manifestations of the antiphospholipid antibody syndromes. Ophthalmol 96(Suppl):105, 1989.

Fuchs W. Untersuchungen über das Sehen der Hemianopiker und Hemiamblyopiker. II. Die totalisierende Gestaltauffassung. In Psychologische Analysen Hirnpathologischer Falle. Editors, Gelb A, Goldstein K, pp 419–561. Leipzig, Johann Ambrosius Barth, 1920.

Fujino T, Akiya S, Takagi S, et al. Amaurosis fugax for a long duration. J Clin Neuroophthalmol 3:9–12, 1983.

Gabai IJ, Spierings ELH. Prophylactic treatment of cluster headache with verapamil. Headache 29:167–168, 1989.

Gabianelli EB, Klingele TG, Burde RM. Acute oculomotor nerve palsy in childhood: Is arteriography necessary? J Clin Neuroophthalmol 9:33–36, 1989.

Galezowski X. Ophthalmic megrim. Lancet 1:176–177, 1882.

Gallagher RM. Menstrual migraine and intermittent ergonovine therapy. Headache 29:366–367, 1989.

Ganji S. Basilar artery migraine: EEG and evoked potential patterns during acute stage. Headache 26:220–223, 1986.

Garnic JD, Schellinger D. Arterial spasm as a finding intimately associated with the onset of vascular headache. Neuroradiology 24:273–276, 1983.

Gascon G, Barlow C. Juvenile migraine, presenting as an acute confusional state. Pediatrics 45:628–635, 1970.

Gastaut JL, Yermenos E, Bonnefoy M, et al. Familial hemiplegic migraine: EEG and CT scan study of two cases. Ann Neurol 10:392–395, 1981.

Gawel M, Connolly JF, Rose FC. Migraine patients exhibit abnormalities in the visual evoked potential. Headache 23:49–52, 1983.

Geaney DP. Indomethacin-responsive episodic cluster headache. J Neurol Neurosurg Psychiatry 46:860–861, 1983.

Gilbert GJ. An occurrence of complicated migraine during propranolol therapy. Headache 21:81–83, 1982.

Gill JW. Transient recurrent attacks of lateral hemianopsia. Br Med J 1:233, 1890.

Giroud M, Dumas R. Fréquence du somnambulisme chez l'enfant migraineux. Presse Méd 7:443, 1984.

Giroud M, D'Athis P, Guard O, et al. Migraine et somnambulisme: Une enquete portant sur 122 migraineux. Rev Neurol 142:42–46, 1986.

Goadsby PG, Edvinsson L. Human in vivo evidence for trigeminovascular activation in cluster headache. Neuropeptide changes and effects of acute attacks therapies. Brain 117(3):427–434, 1994.

Golden GS. The "Alice in Wonderland Syndrome" in juvenile migraine. Pediatrics 63:517, 1979.

Golden GS, French JH. Basilar artery migraine in young children. Pediatrics 56:722–726, 1975.

Goodwin JA, Gorelick P, Helgason C. Transient monocular visual loss: Amaurosis fugax versus migraine. Neurology 34(1):246, 1984.

Goodwin JA, Gorelick PB, Helgason CM. Symptoms of amaurosis fugax in atherosclerotic carotid artery disease. Neurology 37:829–832, 1987.

Gordon N. Alternating hemiplegia of childhood. Dev Med Child Neurol 37(5):464–468, 1995.

Gowers WR. A Manual of Diseases of the Nervous System. Philadelphia, Blakiston, 1888.

Gowers WR. A Manual of Diseases of the Nervous System. Vol 2, p 838. Philadelphia, Blakiston, 1893.

Gowers WR. Subjective visual sensations. Trans Ophthalmol Soc UK 15:1–38, 1895.

Gowers WR. The Borderlands of Epilepsy: Faints, Vagal Attacks, Vertigo, Migraine, Sleep Symptoms and Their Treatment. London, Churchill, 1907.

Graham JR. Migraine headache: Diagnosis and management. Headache 19:133–141, 1979.

Graham JR, Wolff HG. Mechanism of migraine headache and action of ergotamine tartrate. Arch Neurol Psychiatr 39:737–763, 1938.

Graham JR, Suby HL, LeCompte PR, et al. Fibrotic disorders associated with methysergide therapy for headache. N Engl J Med 274:359–363, 1966.

Graveson GS. Retinal arterial occlusion in migraine. Br Med J 2:838–840, 1949.

Gray JA, Carroll JD. Retinal artery occlusion in migraine. Postgrad Med J 61:517–518, 1985.

Greenblatt SH. Posttraumatic transient cerebral blindness. Association with migraine and seizure diatheses. JAMA 225:1073–1076, 1973.

Gronvall A. On changes in the fundus oculi and persisting injuries to the eye in migraine. Acta Ophthalmol 16:602–611, 1938.

Gubler M. Des paralysies de la troisieme paire droit, recidivant pour la troisieme fois. Gaz Hop 33:65, 1860.

Guest IA, Woolf AL. Fatal infarction of brain in migraine. Br Med J 1:225–226, 1964.

Guiloff RJ, Fruns M. Limb pain in migraine and cluster headache. J Neurol Neurosurg Psychiatry 51:1022–1031, 1988.

Gulliksen G, Enevoldsen E. Prolonged changes in rCBF following attacks of migraine accompagnée. Acta Neurol Scand 69(98):270–271, 1984.

Haan J, Ferrari MD, Brouwer OF. Acute confusional migraine: Case report and review of the literature. Clin Neurol Neurosurg 90:275–278, 1988.

Haas DC, Lourie H. Trauma-triggered migraine: An explanation for common neurological attacks after mild head injury. J Neurosurg 68:181–188, 1988.

Haas DC, Sovner RD. Migraine attacks triggered by mild head trauma, and their relation to certain post-traumatic disorders of childhood. J Neurol Neurosurg Psychiatry 32:548–554, 1969.

Haas DC, Pineda GS, Lourie H. Juvenile head trauma syndromes and their relationship to migraine. Arch Neurol 32:727–730, 1975.

Hachinski V. Common and classic migraine. One or two entities? Arch Neurol 42:277, 1985.

Hachinski VC, Porchawka J, Steele JC. Visual symptoms in the migraine syndrome. Neurology 23:570–579, 1973.

Hakkarainen H, Vapaatalo H, Gothoni G, et al. Tolfenamic is as effective as ergotamine during migraine attacks. Lancet 2:326–328, 1979.

Hakkarainen H, Quiding H, Stockman O. Mild analgesic as an alternative to ergotamine in migraine. A comparative trial with acetylsalicylic acid, ergotamine tartrate and dextropropoxphene compound. J Clin Pharmacol 20:590–595, 1980.

Hallett M, Cogan DG. Episodic unilateral mydriasis in otherwise normal patients. Arch Ophthalmol 84:130–136, 1970.

Hanington E. Monoamine oxidase and migraine. Lancet 2:1148–1149, 1974.

Hanson EJ, Anderson RE, Sundt TM. Comparison of 85krypton and 133xenon cerebral blood flow measurements before, during, and following incomplete ischemia in the squirrel monkey. Circ Res 36:18–26, 1975.

Hanukoglu A, Somekh E, Fried D. Benign paroxysmal torticollis in infancy. Clin Pediatr 23:272–274, 1984.

Harley RD. Paralytic strabismus in children. Ophthalmol 87:24–43, 1980.

Harrington DO, Flocks M. Ophthalmolegic migraine. Pathogenesis: Report of pathological findings in a case of recurrent oculomotor paralysis. Arch Ophthalmol 49:643–655, 1953.

Harris M. Ophthalmoplegic migraine and periodic migrainous neuralgia: Migraine variants with ocular manifestations. Ophthal Semin 1:413–450, 1976.

Hart RG, Miller VT. Cerebral infarction in young adults: A practical approach. Stroke 14:110–114, 1983.

Hassin H. Ophthalmoplegic migraine wrongly attributed to measles immunization. Am J Ophthalmol 104:192–193, 1987.

Havanka-Kanniainen H. Treatment of acute migraine attack: Ibuprofen and placebo compared. Headache 29:507–509, 1989.

Havanka-Kanniainen H, Myllylä VV, Hokkanen E. Nimodipine in the prophylaxis of migraine, a double blind study. Acta Neurol Scand 65(90):77–78, 1982.

Havanka-Kanniainen H, Kokkanen E, Myllylä VV. Efficacy of nimodipine in the prophylaxis of migraine. Cephalalgia 5:39–43, 1985.

Havanka-Kanniainen H, Tolonen U, Myllylä VV. Autonomic dysfunction in migraine: A survey of 188 patients. Headache 28:465–470, 1988.

Hawkes CH. Dipyridamole in migraine. Lancet 2:153, 1978.

Headache Classification Committee of the International Headache Society: Classification and diagnostic criteria for headache disorders, cranial neuralgias and facial pain. Cephalalgia 8(7):1–96, 1988.

Hedges TR. Isolated ophthalmic migraine: Its frequency, mechanisms, and differential diagnosis. In Neuro-Ophthalmology Symposium of the University of Miami and the Bascom Palmer Eye Institute. Editor, Smith JL, Vol 6, pp 140–150. St. Louis, CV Mosby, 1972.

Hedges TR. An ophthalmologist's view of headache. Headache 19:151–155, 1979.

Hedges TR, Lackman RD. Isolated ophthalmic migraine in the differential diagnosis of cerebro-ocular ischemia. Stroke 7:379–381, 1976.

Henrich JB. A controlled study of ischemic stroke risk in migraine patients. J Clin Epidemiol 42:773–780, 1989.

Henry PY, Vernhiet J, Orgogozo JM, et al. Cerebral blood flow in migraine and cluster headache. Res Clin Stud Headache 6:81–88, 1978.

Heptinstall S, White A, Williamson L, et al. Extracts of feverfew inhibit granule secretion in blood platelets and polymorphonuclear leucocytes. Lancet 1: 1071–1074, 1985.

Hering R, Kuritzky A. Sodium valproate in the treatment of cluster headache: An open clinical trial. Cephalalgia 9:195–198, 1989.

Herman P. Severe headaches, large pupils, and mitral valve prolapse in young women. Neurology 33(2):144, 1983.

Herman P. Severe headaches, large pupils, mitral valve prolapse, and emotional disturbances: An autonomic disorder. Headache 27:340–344, 1987.

Herman P. Migraine and mitral valve prolapse. Arch Neurol 46:1165, 1989.

Heyck H. Die Neuroligischen Begleiterscheinungen der Migräne und das Problem des "angiospastischen Hirninsults." Nervenarzt 33:193–203, 1962.

Heyck H. Kopfschmerz und vegetatives Nervensystem (Migräne und verwandte Kopfschmerzformen). Akt Fragen Psychiatr Neurol 4:167–201, 1966.

Heyck H. Varieties of hemiplegic migraine. Headache 12:135–142, 1973.

Hilton BP. Blood platelets: A pathological difference between migrainous and control subjects. Hemicrania 2:3–5, 1971.

Hilton BP, Cummings JN. 5-Hydroxytryptamine levels and platelet aggregation responses in subjects with acute migraine headache. J Neurol Neurosurg Psychiatry 35:505–509, 1972.

Hilton-Jones D, Warlow CP. The causes of stroke in the young. J Neurol 232:137–143, 1985.

Hockaday JM. Problems in childhood migraine. Neuroepidemiol 6:234–238, 1987.

Hockaday JM (Editor). Migraine in Childhood. London, Butterworth, 1988.

Hockaday JM, Whitty CWM. Factors determining the electroencephalogram in migraine: A study of 560 patients according to clinical type of migraine. Brain 92: 769–788, 1969.

Holguin J, Fenichel GM. Migraine. J Pediatr 70:290–297, 1967.

Hollenhorst RW. Ocular manifestations of migraine, report of 4 cases of hemianopia. Mayo Clin Proc 28:686–693, 1953.

Honda Y. Scintillating scotoma as the first symptom of systemic lupus erythematosus. Am J Ophthalmol 99:607, 1985.

Honda Y. Scintillating scotoma as the first symptom of systemic lupus erythematosus. Metab Pediatr Systemic Ophthlmol 10:22–23, 1987.

Hooker WD, Raskin NH. Neuropsychologic alterations in classic and common migraine. Arch Neurol 43:709–712, 1986.

Horton BT, MacLean AR, Craig WM. A new syndrome of vascular headache: Results of treatment with histamine. Preliminary report. Proc Staff Meet Mayo Clin 14: 257–260, 1939.

Horven I, Sjaastad O. Cluster headache syndrome and migraine: Ophthalmological support for a two-entity theory. Acta Ophthalmol 55:35–51, 1977.

Horven I, Nornes H, Sjaastad O. Different corneal indentation pulse pattern in cluster headache and migraine. Neurology 22:92–98, 1972.

Horwitz D, Lovenberg W, Engelman K, et al. Monoamine oxidase inhibitors, tyramine and cheese. JAMA 188:1108–1110, 1964.

Humphrey PPA, Feniuk W, Perren MJ, et al. The pharmacology of the novel 5-HT1-like receptor agonist, GR43175. Cephalalgia 9(9):23–34, 1989.

Humphrey PPA, Feniuk W, Perren MJ. Anti-migraine drugs in development: Advances in serotonin receptor pharmacology 30(Suppl):12–16, 1990.

Hungerford GD, du Boulay GH, Zilkha KJ. Computerised axial tomography in patients with severe migraine: A preliminary report. J Neurol Neurosurg Psychiatry 39: 990–994, 1976.

Hunt JR. A contribution to the paralytic and other persistent sequelae of migraine. Am J Med Sci 150:313–314, 1915.

Hupp SL, Kline LB, Corbett JJ. Visual disturbances of migraine. Surv Ophthalmol 33:221–236, 1989.

Hutchinson DO, Donaldson IM. Ophthalmoplegic migraine with bilateral involvement. J Neurol Neurosurg Psychiatry 52:807–808, 1989.

Hutchinson M, O'Riordan J, Javed M, et al. Familial hemiplegic migraine and autosomal dominant arteriopathy with leukoencephalopathy (CADASIL). Ann Neurol 38(5):817–824, 1995.

Imes RK, Hoyt WF. Exercise-induced transient visual events in young healthy adults. J Clin Neuroophthalmol 9:178–180, 1989.

Imes RK, Monteiro MLR, Hoyt WF. Ophthalmoplegic migraine with proximal posterior cerebral artery vascular anomaly. J Clin Neuroophthalmol 4:221–223, 1984.

Inan LE, Uysal H, Ergun U, et al. Complicated retinal migraine. Headache 34(1): 50–52, 1994.

Isenberg DA, Meyrick-Thomas D, Snaith ML, et al. A study of migraine in systemic lupus erythematosus. Ann Rheum Dis 41:30–32, 1982.

Isler H. Retrospect: The history of thought about migraine from Aretaeus to 1920. In Migraine. Clinical and Research Aspects. Editor, Blau JN, pp 659–674. Baltimore, Johns Hopkins University Press, 1987.

Iversen HK, Nielsen TH, Olesen J, et al. Arterial responses during migraine headache. Lancet 336:837–839, 1990.

Jacobson DM. Benign episodic unilateral mydriasis: Clinical characteristics. Ophthalmol 102:1623–1627, 1995.

Jacome DE, Leborgne J. MRI studies in basilar artery migraine. Headache 30:88–90, 1990.

Jammes JJ. The treatment of cluster headaches with prednisone. Dis Nerv Syst 36: 375–376, 1975.

Jensen R, Brinck T, Olesen J. Sodium valproate has a prophylactic effect in migraine without aura: A triple-blind, placebo-controlled crossover study. Neurology 44: 647–651, 1994.

Joffe SN. Retinal blood vessel diameter during migraine. EENT Monthly 52:338–342, 1973.

Johns DR. Migraine provoked by aspartame. N Engl J Med 315:456, 1986.

Johnson ES. Patients who chew chrysanthemum leaves. MIMS Magazine, pp 32–35. May 15, 1983.

Johnson ES, Ratcliffe DM, Wilkinson M. Naproxen sodium in the treatment of migraine. Cephalalgia 5:5–10, 1985a.

Johnson ES, Kadam NP, Hylands DM, et al. Efficacy of feverfew as prophylactic treatment of migraine. Br Med J 291:569–573, 1985b.

Johnson GL. Subjective visual sensations. Arch Ophthalmol 16:1–4, 1936.

Johnson RH, Hornabrook RW, Lambie DG. Comparison of mefenamic acid and propranolol with placebo in migraine prophylaxis. Acta Neurol Scand 76:490–492, 1986.

Johnson TH. Homonymous hemianopia. Practical points in interpretation, with report of forty-nine cases in which the lesion in the brain was verified. Arch Ophthalmol 15:604–616, 1936.

Jolly F. Ueber Flimmerskotom und Migrane. Berl Klin Wochenschr 39:973–976, 1902.

Jonsdottir M, Meyer J, Rodgers R. Efficacy, side effects and tolerances compared during headache—Treatment with three different calcium blockers. Headache 27:364–369, 1987.

Joutel A, Tournier Lasserve E, Bousser MG. Hemiplegic migraine. Presse Med 24(8): 411–414, 1995.

Joutel A, Bousser MG, Biousse V, et al. A gene for familial hemiplegic migraine maps to chromosome 19. Nat Genet 5(1):40–45, 1993.

Joutel A, Bousser MG, Biousse V, et al. Familial hemoplegic migraine. Localization of a responsible gene on chromosome 19. Rev Neurol (Paris) 150(5):340–345, 1994.

Jouvet M. Neurophysiology of the sleep states. Physiol Rev 47:117–177, 1967.

Jouvet M. Biogenic amines and the states of sleep. Science 163:32–41, 1969.

Juge O. Regional cerebral blood flow in the different clinical types of migraine. Headache 28:537–549, 1988.

Juge O, Gauthier G. Mesures de débit sanguin cérébral regional (DSCR) par inhalation de Xénon-133: Application cliniques. Bull Schweiz Akad Med Wiss 36:101–115, 1980.

Kabler JD. Methysergide maleate (Sansert) and the prevention of migraine. Wisc Med J 66:435–436, 1967.

Kalendovsky Z, Austin JH. "Complicated migraine:" Its association with increased platelet aggregability and abnormal plasma coagulation factors. Headache 15: 18–35, 1975.

Kales A, Kales J. Evaluation, diagnosis, and treatment of clinical conditions related to sleep. JAMA 213:2229–2235, 1970.

Kattah JC, Luessenhop AJ. Resolution of classic migraine after removal of an occipital lobe AVM. Ann Neurol 7:93, 1980.

Katz B. Bilateral sequential migrainous ischemic optic neuropathy. Am J Ophthalmol 99:489, 1985.

Katz B. Migrainous central retinal artery occlusion. J Clin Neuroophthalmol 6:69–71, 1986.

Katz B, Rimmer S. Ophthalmoplegic migraine with superior ramus oculomotor paresis. J Clin Neuroophthalmol 9:181–183, 1989.

Keith CG. Oculomotor nerve palsy in childhood. Aust NZ J Ophthalmol 15:181–184, 1987.

Kennard C, Gawel M, Rudolph N de M, et al. Visual evoked potentials in migraine subjects. Res Clin Stud Headache 6:72–80, 1978.

Kimball RW, Friedman AP, Vallejo E. Effect of serotonin in migraine patients. Neurology (NY) 10:107–111, 1960.

Kinnunen E, Erkinjuntti T, Färkkilä M, Palomäki H, Porras J, Teirmaa H, Freudenthal Y, Andersson P: Placebo-controlled double-blind trial of pirprofen and an ergotamine tartrate compound in migraine attacks. Cephalalgia 8:175–179, 1988.

Klee A, Willanger R. Disturbances of visual perception in migraine. Review of the literature and a report of eight cases. Acta Neurol Scand 42:400–414, 1966.

Klein RM. Scintillating scotoma after retinal detachment surgery. Am J Ophthalmol 105:94–95, 1988.

Kline LB, Kelly CL. Ocular migraine in a patient with cluster headaches. Headache 20:253–257, 1980.

Kobari M, Meyer JS, Ichijo M, et al. Hyperperfusion of cerebral cortex, thalamus and basal ganglia during spontaneously occurring migraine headaches. Headache 29:282–289, 1989.

Koehler SM. A new dietary caution for migraine sufferers. Dir Appl Nutr 1:1–7, 1986.

Koehler SM, Glaros A. The effect of aspartame on migraine headache. Headache 28:10–13, 1988.

Koenigsberger MR, Chutorian AM, Gold AP, et al. Benign paroxysmal vertigo in childhood. Neurology 20:1108–1113, 1970.

Kohlenberg RJ. Tyramine sensitivity in dietary migraine: A critical review. Headache 22:30–34, 1982.

Kosmorsky G. Unusual visual phenomenon during acephalgic migraine. Arch Ophthalmol 105:613, 1987.

Krägeloh I, Aicardi J. Alternating hemiplegia in infants: Report of five cases. Develop Med Child Neurol 22:784–791, 1980.

Krapin D. Occlusion of the central retinal artery in migraine. N Engl J Med 270:359–360, 1964.

Kronberg D, Dalgaard P, Lauritzen M. Ischemia may be the primary case of neurological deficits in classic migraine. Arch Neurol 47:124–125, 1990.

Krupp GR, Friedman AP. Recurrent headache in children: A study of 100 clinical cases. NY State J Med 53:43, 1933.

Kudrow L. The relationship of headache frequency to hormone uses in migraine. Headache 15:36–40, 1975.

Kudrow L. Lithium prophylaxis for chronic cluster headache. Headache 17:15–18, 1977.

Kudrow L. Comparative results of prednisone, methysergide, and lithium therapy in cluster headache. In Current Concepts of Migraine Research. Editor, Green R, pp 159–163. New York, Raven Press, 1978.

Kudrow L. Cluster Headache: Mechanisms and Management. Oxford, Oxford University Press, 1980.

Kudrow L. Response of cluster headache attacks to oxygen inhalation. Headache 21:1–4, 1981.

Kudrow L, Kudrow DB. Inheritance of cluster headache and its possible link to migraine. Headache 34(7):400–407, 1994.

Kudrow L, Esperanca P, Vijayan N. Episodic paroxysmal hemicrania? Cephalalgia 7:197–201, 1987.

Kunkle EC. Mechanisms of headache with particular reference to vascular headache. Trans Am Acad Ophthalmol 67:758–765, 1963.

Kunkle EC, Anderson WB. Dual mechanisms of eye signs of headache in cluster pattern. Trans Am Neurol Assoc 85:75–79, 1960.

Kunkel RS. Controversies in classification of migraine. In Controversies and Clinical Variants of Migraine. Editor, Saper JR, pp 5–10. New York, Pergamon Press, 1987.

Kupersmith MJ, Hass WK, Chase NE. Isoproterenol treatment of visual symptoms in migraine. Stroke 10:299–305, 1979.

Kupersmith MJ, Warren FA, Hass WK. The non-benign aspects of migraine. Neuro-ophthalmol 7:1–10, 1987.

Kuritzky A, Ziegler DK, Hassanein R. Vertigo, motion sickness and migraine. Headache 21:227–231, 1981a.

Kuritzky A, Toglia UJ, Thomas D. Vestibular function in migraine. Headache 21:110–112, 1981b.

Kushner MJ. Prospective study of anticardiolipin antibodies in stroke. Stroke 21:295–298, 1990.

Kwentus J, Kattah J, Koppicav M, et al. Complicated migraine and cerebral angiography: A report of an unusual adverse reaction. Headache 25:240–245, 1985.

Lai C-W, Dean P, Ziegler DK, et al. Clinical and electrophysiological responses to dietary challenge in migraineurs. Headache 29:180–186, 1989.

Lance JW. The Mechanism and Management of Headache. 3rd ed. London, Butterworths, 1978.

Lance JW. Headache. Ann Neurol 10:1–10, 1981.

Lance JW. Mechanisms and Management of Migraine. 4th ed, pp 122–123. London, Butterworths, 1982.

Lance JW. A personal perspective on the pathogenesis of migraine. In Controversies and Clinical Variants of Migraine. Editor, Saper JR, pp 111–118. New York, Pergamon Press, 1987.

Lance JW. Current concepts of migraine pathogenesis. Neurology 43(3):S11–S15, 1993.

Lance JW, Anthony M. Some clinical aspects of migraine—A prospective study of 500 patients. Arch Neurol 15:356–361, 1966.

Lance JW, Anthony M, Gonski A. Serotonin, the carotid body, and cranial vessels in migraine. Arch Neurol 16:553–558, 1967.

Lapkin ML, Golden GS. Basilar artery migraine. A review of 30 cases. Am J Dis Child 132:278–281, 1978.

Lapkin ML, French JH, Golden GS, et al. The electroencephalogram in childhood basilar artery migraine. Neurology 27:580–583, 1977.

Lashley KS. Patterns of cerebral integration indicated by the scotomas of migraine. Arch Neurol 46:331–339, 1941.

Lauritzen M, Olesen J. Regional cerebral blood flow during migraine attacks by xenon-133 inhalation and emission tomography. Brain 107:447–461, 1984.

Lauritzen M, Skyhoj Olsen T, Lassen NA, et al. Changes in regional cerebral blood flow during the course of classic migraine attacks. Ann Neurol 13:633–641, 1983a.

Lauritzen M, Skyhoj Olsen T, Lassen NA, et al. Regulation of regional cerebral blood flow during and between migraine attacks. Ann Neurol 14:569–572, 1983b.

Lawden MC, Cleland PG. Achromatopsia in the aura of migraine. J Neurol Neurosurg Psychiatry 56(6):708–709, 1993.

Leao AAP. Spreading depression of activity in cerebral cortex. J Neurophysiol 7:359–390, 1944.

Leao AAP, Morrison RS. Propagation of spreading cortical depression. J Neurophysiol 8:33–45, 1945.

Lee AG, Brazis PW, Miller NR. Posterior ischemic optic neuropathy associated with migraine. Headache 36:506–509, 1996.

Lee CH, Lance JW. Migraine stupor. Headache 17:32–38, 1977.

Lees F. The migrainous symptoms of cerebral angiomata. J Neurol Neurosurg Psychiatry 25:45–50, 1962.

Lees F, Watkins SM. Loss of consciousness in migraine. Lancet 2:647–649, 1963.

Leijdekkers MLA, Passchier J, Goudswaard P, et al. Migraine patients cognitively impaired? Headache 30:352–358, 1990.

Lembeck F. Peripheral substance P neurones: Afferent, efferent or both functions? In Substance P. Editors, Skrabanek P, Powell D, pp 81–85. Dublin, Boole, 1983.

Leone M, Frediani F, Patruno G, et al. Is nimodipine useful in migraine prophylaxis? Further considerations. Headache 30:363–365, 1990.

Leon-Sotomayor LA. Cardiac migraine—Report of twelve cases. Angiology 25:161–171, 1974.

Lepore FE, Glaser JS. Misdirection revisited. A critical appraisal of acquired oculomotor nerve synkinesis. Arch Ophthalmol 98:2206–2216, 1980.

Lessell S. The neuro-ophthalmology of systemic lupus erythematosus. Doc Ophthalmol 47:13–42, 1979.

Lessell S, Kylstra J. Exercise-induced visual hallucinations, a symptom of occipital lobe tumors. J Clin Neuroophthalmol 8:81–83, 1988.

Levine SR, Welch KMA. Antiphospholipid antibodies. Ann Neurol 26:386–389, 1989.

Levine SR, Deegan MJ, Futrell N, et al. Cerebrovascular and neurologic disease associated with antiphospholipid antibodies: 48 cases. Neurology 40:1181–1189, 1990.

Lewis NP, Fraser AG, Taylor A: Syncope while vomiting during migraine attack. Lancet 2:400–401, 1988.

Lewis RA, Vijayan N, Watson C, et al. Visual field loss in migraine. Ophthalmol 96:321–326, 1989.

Libo LM, Arnold GE. Relaxation practice after biofeedback therapy: A long-term follow-up study of utilization and effectiveness. Biofeedback Self Regul 8:217–227, 1983.

Lieberman AN, Jonas S, Hass WK, et al. Bilateral cervical carotid and intracranial vasospasm causing cerebral ischaemia in a migrainous patient: A case of "diplegic migraine." Headache 24:246–248, 1984.

Lincoff HA, Cogan DG. Unilateral headache and oculomotor paralysis not caused by aneurysm. Arch Ophthalmol 57:181–189, 1957.

Lindegaard KF, Ovrelio L, Sjaastad O. Naproxen in the prevention of migraine attacks: A double-blind placebo-controlled cross-over study. Headache 20:96–98, 1980.

Lipson EH, Robertson WC. Paroxysmal torticollis of infancy: Familial occurrence. Am J Dis Child 132:422–423, 1978.

Lipton RB, Newman LC, Cohen JS, et al. Aspartame as a dietary factor in headache. Neurology 38:356, 1988a.

Lipton RB, Newman LC, Solomon S. Aspartame and headache. N Engl J Med 318:1200, 1988b.

Lipton RB, Newman LC, Cohen JS, et al. Aspartame as a dietary trigger of headache. Headache 29:90–92, 1989.

Lipton SA. Prevention of classic migraine headache by digital massage of the superficial temporal arteries during visual aura. Ann Neurol 19:515–516, 1986.

Liu GT, Schatz NJ, Galetta SL, et al. Persistent positive visual phomenia in migraine. Neurology 45:664–668, 1995.

Liveing E. On Megrim, Sick-Headache, and Some Allied Disorders. London, Churchill, 1873.

Loewenfeld IE. Pupillary defect in "ophthalmoplegic migraine." In Symposium of the Bascom Palmer Eye Institute and the University of Miami. Editor, Glaser JS, Vol 10, pp 180–200. St Louis, CV Mosby, 1980.

Loh L, Nathan PW, Schott GD, et al. Acupuncture versus medical treatment for migraine and muscle tension headaches. J Neurol Neurosurg Psychiatry 47: 333–337, 1984.

Löhlein W. Erblindung durch Migräne. Dtsch Med Wschr 48:1408–1409, 1922.

Louis P. A double-blind placebo controlled prophylactic study of flunarizine (Sibelium) in migraine. Headache 21:235–239, 1981.

Lücking CH, Oestreich W, Schmidt R, et al. Flunarizine vs. propranolol in the prophylaxis of migraine: Two double-blind comparative studies in more than 400 patients. Cephalalgia 8(8):21–26, 1988.

Ludin H-P. Flunarizine and propranolol in the treatment of migraine. Headache 29: 218–223, 1989.

Lundberg PO. Abdominal migraine. Triangle 17:81–84, 1978.

Mackenzie ICK. Clinical presentation of cerebral angioma: Review of 50 cases. Brain 76:184–214, 1953.

Mackenzie ICK. Diagnosis of cerebral angioma. Postgrad Med J 30:631–639, 1954.

MacLean C, Appenzeller O, Cordardo JT, et al. Flash evoked potentials in migraine. Headache 14:193–198, 1975.

Mahrer AR, Mason DJ, Rosenshine MA. A headache syndrome in psychiatric patients. J Clin Psychol 33:411–414, 1966.

Malmgren R, Hasselmark L. The platelet and the neuron: Two cells in focus in migraine. Cephalalgia 8:7–24, 1988.

Malvea BP, Gwon N, Graham JR. Propranolol prophylaxis of migraine. Headache 12:163–167, 1973.

Mandel S. Hemiplegic migraine in pregnancy. Headache 28:414–416, 1988.

Manor RS, Dubnov B, Kott E, et al. Presumed post-myelography migraine-like phenomena. Neuroophthalmol 5:169–174, 1985.

Manzoni GC, Farina S, Lanfranchi M, et al. Classic migraine—Clinical findings in 164 patients. Eur Neurol 24:163–169, 1985.

Mariani E, Moschini V, Pastorino G, et al. Pattern-reversal visual evoked potentials and EEG correlations in common migraine patients. Headache 28:269–271, 1988.

Markley H, Cheronis J, Piepho R. Verapamil prophylactic therapy of migraine. Neurology 34:973–976, 1984.

Marsters JB, Good PA, Mortimer MJ. A diagnostic test for migraine using the visual evoked potential. Headache 28:526–530, 1988.

Martinez-Lage JM. Flunarizine (Sibelium) in the prophylaxis of migraine. An open, long-term, multi-center trial. Cephalalgia 8(8):15–20, 1988.

Massey EW. Migraine during pregnancy. Ob Gyn Surv 32:693–696, 1977.

Massey EW. Pupillary dysautonomia and migraine: Is Adie's pupil caused by migraine? Headache 21:143–146, 1981.

Masuzawa T, Shinoda S, Furuse M, et al. Cerebral angiographic changes on serial examination of a patient with migraine. Neuroradiol 24:277–281, 1983.

Mathew NT. Clinical subtypes of cluster headache and response to lithium therapy. Headache 18:26–30, 1978.

Mathew NT. The borderlands of migraine: Migraine equivalents and migraine accompaniments. In Controversies and Clinical Variants of Migraine. Editor, Saper JR, pp 43–58. New York, Pergamon Press, 1987.

Mathew NT. Drug-induced headache. Neurol Clin 8:903–912, 1990a

Mathew NT. Abortive versus prophylactic treatment of migraine—A reappraisal. Headache 30:238–239, 1990b.

Mathew NT, Hrastnik F, Meyer JS. Regional cerebral blood flow in the diagnosis of vascular headache. Headache 15:252–260, 1976.

Mathew NT, Saper J, Silberstein S, et al. Migraine prophylaxis with divalproex. Arch Neurol 52:281–286, 1995.

Mathews WB. Footballer's migraine. Br Med J 2:326–327, 1972.

McArthur JC, Marek K, Pestronk A, et al. Nifedipine in the prophylaxis of classic migraine: A crossover, double-masked, placebo-controlled study of headache frequency and side effects. Neurology 39:284–286, 1989.

McDonald JV. Basilar artery migraine. Case report. J Neurosurg 72:289–291, 1990.

McDonald WI, Sanders MD. Migraine complicated by ischaemic papillopathy. Lancet 2:521–523, 1971.

Mears E, Grant ECG. "Anoviar" as an oral contraceptive. Br Med J 2:75–79, 1962.

Medina JL, Diamond S. Migraine and atopy. Headache 15:271–274, 1976.

Medina JL, Diamond S. The clinical link between migraine and cluster headache. Arch Neurol 34:470–472, 1977.

Medina JL, Diamond S. Cyclical migraine. Arch Neurol 38:343–344, 1981.

Melen O, Olson SF, Hodes BL. Visual disturbance in migraine. Postgrad Med 64: 139–143, 1978.

Mentenopoulos G, Manafi T, Logothetis J, et al. Flunarizine in the prevention of classical migraine: A placebo-controlled evaluation. Cephalalgia 5(2):135–140, 1985.

Messert B, Black JA. Cluster headache, hemicrania, and other head pains: Morbidity of carotid endarterectomy. Stroke 9:559–562, 1978.

Meyer JS, Hardenberg J. Clinical effectiveness of calcium entry blockers in prophylactic treatment of migraine and cluster headaches. Headache 23:266–277, 1983.

Meyer JS, Binns PM, Ericsson AD, et al. Sphenopalatine ganglionectomy for cluster headache. Arch Otolaryngol 92:475–484, 1970.

Meyer JS, Nance M, Walker M, et al. Migraine and cluster headache treatment with calcium antagonists supports a vascular pathogenesis. Headache 25:358–367, 1985.

Michael MI, Williams JM. Migraine in children. J Pediatr 41:18, 1952.

Migraine-Nimodipine European Study Group (MINES): European multicenter trial of nimodipine in the prophylaxis of common migraine (migraine without aura). Headache 29:633–638, 1989a.

Migraine-Nimodipine European Study Group (MINES): European multicenter trial of nimodipine in the prophylaxis of classic migraine (migraine with aura). Headache 29:639–642, 1989b.

Mikkelsen BM, Viggo Falk J. Prophylactic treatment of migraine with tolfenamic acid. Acta Neurol Scand 66:105–111, 1982.

Miller D, Waters DD, Warnica W, et al. Is variant angina the coronary manifestation of a generalized vasospastic disorder? N Engl J Med 304:763–771, 1981.

Miller FW, Santoro TJ. Nifedipine in the treatment of migraine headache and amaurosis fugax in patients with systemic lupus erythematosis. N Engl J Med 311:921, 1981.

Miller NR. Solitary oculomotor nerve palsy in childhood. Am J Ophthalmol 83: 106–111, 1977.

Miller NR, Keltner JL, Gittinger JW, et al. Intermittent pupillary dilation in a young woman. Surv Ophthalmol 31:65–68, 1986.

Milner PM. Note on a possible correspondence between the scotomas of migraine and the spreading depression of Leao. Electroencephalogr Clin Neurophysiol 10: 705, 1958.

Mira E, Piacentino G, Lanzi G, et al. Benign paroxysmal vertigo in childhood: A migraine equivalent. ORL 46:97–104, 1984.

Miyazaki T, Notani M, Kawabatake H, et al. Visual aura in migraine. Folia Psychiatr Neurol Jpn 30:343–348, 1976.

Moen M, Levine SR, Newman DS, et al. Bilateral posterior cerebral artery strokes in a young migraine sufferer. Stroke 19:525–528, 1988.

Montiero LR, Hoyt WF, Imes RK. Puerperal cerebral blindness. Arch Neurol 41: 1300–1301, 1984.

Moore RF. Medical Ophthalmology. pp 237–242. London, J and A Churchill Ltd, 1922.

Moretti G, Manzoni GC, Daffara P, et al. Benign recurrent vertigo and its connection with migraine. Headache 20:344–346, 1980.

Mori E, Yamadori A. Acute confusional state and acute agitated delirium: Occurrence after infarction in the right middle cerebral artery territory. Arch Neurol 44: 1139–1143, 1987.

Morimoto Y, Nakajima S, Nishioka R, et al. Basilar artery migraine with transient MRI and EEG abnormalities. Rinsho Shinkeigaku 33(1):61–67, Jan 1993.

Mortimer MJ, Good PA, Marsters JB: The VEP in acephalgic migraine. Headache 30:285–288, 1990a.

Mortimer MJ, Good PA, Marsters JB, et al. Visual evoked responses in children with migraine: A diagnostic test. Lancet 335:75–77, 1990.

Moskowitz MA. The neurobiology of vascular head pain. Ann Neurol 16:157–168, 1984.

Moskowitz MA. The visceral organ brain: Implications for the pathophysiology of vascular headache. Neurology 41:182–186, 1991.

Moskowitz MA. Neurogenic versus vascular mechanisms of sumatriptan and ergot alkaloids in migraine. Trends Pharmacol Sci 13:307–311, 1992.

Moskowitz MA, Reinhard JF, Romero J, et al. Neurotransmitters and the fifth cranial nerve: Is there a relation to the headache phase of migraine? Lancet 2:883–884, 1979.

Moskowitz MA, Nozaki K, Kraig RP. Neocortical spreading depression provokes the expression of c-fos protein-like immunoreactivity within trigeminal nucleus caudalis via trigeminovascular mechanisms. J Neurosci 13(3):1167–1177, 1993.

Muck-Seler D, Degnovic Z, Dupelj M. Platelet serotonin (5-HT) and 5-HT-releasing factor in plasma of migrainous patients. Headache 19:14–17, 1989.

Muellbacher W, Mamoli B. Prolonged impaired consciousness in basilar artery migraine. Headache 34(5):282–285, May 1994.

Mueller RA, Meienberg O. Hemicrania with oculosympathetic paresis from isosorbide dinitrate. N Engl J Med 308:458, 1983.

Murphy JJ, Heptinstall S, Mitchell JRA. Randomised double-blind placebo-controlled trial of feverfew in migraine prevention. Lancet 2:189–192, 1988.

Murphy PJ. Cerebral infarction in migraine. Neurology 5:359–361, 1955.

Murray JB. Psychophysiological aspects of migraine headaches. Psych Rep 48: 139–162, 1981.

Nadelmann JW, Stevens J, Saper JR. Propranolol in the prophylaxis of migraine. Headache 26:175–182, 1986.

Nestvold K, Kloster R, Partinen M, et al. Treatment of acute migraine attack: Naproxen and placebo compared. Cephalalgia 5:115–119, 1985.

Newman DS, Levine SR, Curtis VL, et al. Migraine-like visual phenomena associated with cerebral venous thrombosis. Headache 29:82–85, 1989.

Newman NJ, Lessell S, Brandt EM. Bilateral central retinal artery occlusions, disk drusen, and migraine. Am J Ophthalmol 107:236–240, 1989.

Nieman EA, Hurwitz LJ. Ocular sympathetic palsy in periodic migrainous neuralgia. J Neurol Neurosurg Psychiatry 24:369–373, 1961.

Noack H, Rothrock JF. Migraine: Definitions, mechanisms and treatment. South Med J 89:762–769, 1996.

Northfield DWC. Some observations on headache. Brain 61:133–162, 1938.

O'Brien MD. Cerebral blood changes in migraine. Headache 10:139–143, 1971.

O'Connor PJ. Strokes in migraine. In Background to Migraine (Fifth Symposium). Editor, Cummings JN, pp 40–44. New York, Springer-Verlag, 1972.

O'Connor PS, Tredici TJ. Acephalgic migraine. Fifteen years experience. Ophthalmol 88:999–1002, 1981.

O'Day J, Billson F, King J. Ophthalmoplegic migraine and aberrant regeneration of the oculomotor nerve. Br J Ophthalmol 64:534–536, 1980.

O'Hara M, O'Connor PS. Migrainous optic neuropathy. J Clin Neuroophthalmol 4: 85–90, 1984.

Ohta M, Araki S, Kuroiwa Y. Familial occurrence of migraine with a hemiplegic syndrome and cerebellar manifestations. Neurology 17:813–817, 1967.

Olesen J. Some clinical features of the acute migraine attack. An analysis of 750 patients. Headache 18:268–271, 1978.

Olesen J. Significance of trigger factors in migraine. In Progress in Migraine Research. Editor, Rose FC, Vol 2, pp 18–20. London, Pitman Books, 1984.

Olesen J. The ischemic hypothesis of migraine. Arch Neurol 44:321–322, 1987.

Olesen J, Larsen B, Lauritzen M. Focal hyperemia followed by spreading oligemia and impaired activation of rCBF in classic migraine. Ann Neurol 9:344–352, 1981a.

Olesen J, Tfelt-Hansen P, Henriksen L, et al. The common migraine attack may not be initiated by cerebral ischemia. Lancet 2:438–440, 1981b.

Olesen J, Lauritzen M, Tfelt-Hansen P, et al. Spreading cerebral oligemia in classical and normal blood flow in common migraine. Headache 22:242–249, 1982.

Olesen J, Friberg L, Olsen TS, et al. Timing and topography of cerebral blood flow, aura, and headache during migraine attacks. Ann Neurol 28(6):791–798, Dec 1990.

Olsson JE, Behring HC, Forssman B, et al. Metoprolol and propranolol in migraine prophylaxis: A double-blind multicentric study. Acta Neurol Scand 70:160–168, 1984.

O'Neill BP, Mann JD. Aspirin prophylaxis in migraine. Lancet 2:1179–1181, 1978.

Ophoff RA, van Eijk R, Sandkuijl LA, et al. Genetic heterogeneity of familial hemiplegic migraine. Genomics 22(1), 21–26, 1994.

Ormond AW. Two cases of permanent hemianopsia following severe attacks of migraine. Ophthal Rev 32:193–201, 1913.

Osborn RE, Alder DC, Mitchell CS. MR imaging of the brain in patients with migraine headaches. AJNR 12:521–524, 1991.

Ostfeld AM. The Common Headache Syndromes: Biochemistry, Pathophysiology and Therapy. Springfield, IL, Charles C Thomas, 1962.

Ostfeld AM, Wolff HG. Studies on headache participation of ocular structures in the migraine syndrome. Bibl Ophthalmol 1:634–647, 1957.

O'Sullivan F, Rossor M, Elston JS. Amaurosis fugax in young people. Br J Ophthalmol 76(11):660–662, 1992.

Osuntokun O, Osuntokun BO. Ophthalmoplegic migraine and hemoglobinopathy in Nigerians. Am J Ophthalmol 74:451–455, 1972.

Parrino L, Pietrini V, Spaggiari MC, et al. Acute confusional migraine attacks resolved by sleep: Lack of significant abnormalities in post-ictal polysomnograms. Cephalalgia 6:95–100, 1986.

Parrish DO, Todorov AB. Transient bilateral visual reduction and mydriasis after propranalol treatment. Ann Neurol 10:583, 1981.

Pasteur V-R, Blamoutier P, Mawas L, et al. Accès de migraine ophtalmique suivis d'une hémorrhagie rétinienne. Ann Med 42:132–137, 1937.

Patterson RH, Goodell H, Dunning HS. Complications of cerebral angiography. Arch Neurol 10:513–520, 1964.

Pavese N, Canapicchi R, Nuti A, et al. White matter MRI hyperintensities in 129 consecutive migraine patients. Cephalalgia 14(5):342–345, 1994.

Pearce I, Frank GJ, Pearce JMS. Ibuprofen compared with paracetamol in migraine. Practitioner 227:465–467, 1983.

Pearce JMS. General review: Some etiological factors in migraine. In Background to Migraine. Editor, Cummings JN, pp 1–7. London, Heinemann, 1971.

Pearce JMS. Chronic migrainous neuralgia: A variant of cluster headache. Brain 103: 149–159, 1980.

Pearce JMS. Is migraine explained by Leao's spreading depression? Lancet 2: 763–766, 1985.

Pearce JMS. Historical aspects of migraine. J Neurol Neurosurg Psychiatry 49: 1097–1103, 1986.

Pearce JMS, Foster JB. An investigation of complicated migraine. Neurology 15: 333–340, 1965.

Peatfield RC, Rose FC. Migrainous visual symptoms in a woman without eyes. Arch Neurol 38:466, 1981.

Pelosse B, Saraux H. Deficit monoculaire definitif apres migraine ophtalmique. Bull Soc Ophtalmol Fr 87:19–21, 1987.

Penderson E, Moller CE. Methysergide in migraine prophylaxis. Clin Pharmacol Ther 7:520–526, 1966.

Pepin EP. Cerebral metastasis presenting as migraine with aura. Lancet 336:127–128, 1990.

Perkin JE, Hartje JC. Diet and migraine: A review of the literature. J Am Dietetic Assoc 83:459–463, 1983.

Peroutka SJ. The pharmacology of current anti-migraine drugs. Headache 30(Suppl.): 5–11, 1990.

Perrin VL, Färkkilä M, Goasguen J, et al. Overview of initial clinical studies with intravenous and oral GR43175 in acute migraine. Cephalalgia 9(9):63–72, 1989.

Philipp M, Schäffer ML, Peters UH. 3-Jahres Katamnese bei psychosomatisch behandelten chronischen Kopfschmerzsyndromen. Zeitschr Psychosom Med 29: 270–275, 1983.

Phillips BM: Oral contraceptive drugs and migraine. Br Med J 2:99, 1968.

Pietrini V, Terzano MG, D'Andrea G, et al. Acute confusional migraine: Clinical and electroencephalographic aspects. Cephalalgia 7:29–37, 1987.

Plosker GL, McTavish D. Sumatriptan. A reappraisal of its pharmacology and therapeutic efficacy in the acute treatment of migraine and cluster headache. Drugs 47(4):622–651, 1994.

Polyak S. The Vertebrate Visual System. pp 735–747. Chicago, University of Chicago Press, 1957.

Poos F. Klinische Beobachtungen bei der Hemicrania vasomotoria mit Ausfallserscheinungen im Bereiche des Schorgans. Klin Monatsbl Augenheilkd 92: 58–74, 1934.

Pradalier A, Launay JM. 5-Hydroxytryptamine uptake by platelets from migrainous patients. Lancet 1:862, 1982.

Pradalier A, Rancurel G, Dordain G, et al. Acute migraine attack therapy: Comparison of naproxen sodium and an ergotamine tartrate compound. Cephalalgia 5: 107–113, 1985.

Pradalier A, Clapin A, Dry J. Treatment review: Non-steroid anti-inflammatory drugs in the treatment and long-term prevention of migraine attacks. Headache 28: 550–557, 1988.

Prendes JL. Considerations on the use of propranolol in complicated migraine. Headache 20:93–95, 1980.

Prensky AL, Sommer D. Diagnosis and treatment of migraine in children. Neurology 29:506–510, 1979.

Procacci PM, Savran SV, Schreiter SL, et al. Clinical frequency and implications of mitral valve prolapse in the female population. Circulation 52(2):78, 1975.

Procacci PM, Savran SV, Schreiter SL, et al. Prevalence of clinical mitral valve prolapse in 1169 young women. N Engl J Med 249:1086, 1976.

Prusinski A, Kozubski W. Use of verapamil in the treatment of migraine. Wiad Lek 40:734–738, 1987.

Quistorf B, Gjedde A, Hansen AJ. Spatial analysis of the freeze trapped brain provides for temporal resolution of an event: Metabolic-electrical and blood flow changes during spreading depression. Acta Physiol Scand 105:42A, 1979.

Raab EL. Paroxysmal torticollis in infancy. Am J Dis Child 119:378, 1970.

Raj Gupta D, Strobos RJ. Bilateral papillitis associated with Cafergot therapy. Neurology 22:793–797, 1972.

Rall TW, Schleifer LS. Drugs affecting uterine motility. In The Physiological Basis of Therapeutics. Editors, Goodman LS, Gilman A, 6th ed, pp 935–950. New York, MacMillan, 1980.

Rascol A, Cambier J, Guiraud B, et al. Accidents ischémiques cérébraux au cours de crises migraineuses. A propos de migraines compliquées. Rev Neurol 135: 867–884, 1980.

Raskin NH. Cluster headache: Localization. Headache 29:579–580, 1989.

Raskin NH, Schwartz RK. Interval therapy of migraine: Long-term results. Headache 20:336–340, 1980.

Raudino F. Visual evoked potential in patients with migraine. Headache 28:531–533, 1988.

Ravits J, Seybold ME. Transient monocular visual loss from narrow-angle glaucoma. Arch Neurol 41:991–993, 1984.

Regan D, Heron JR. Simultaneous recording of visual evoked and neutrals from the left and right hemisphere in migraine. In Background to Migraine. Editor, Cochrane T, p 66. London, Heinemann, 1970.

Rich WM. Permanent homonymous quadrantanopia after migraine. Br Med J 1: 592–594, 1948.

Richards W. The fortification illusions of migraines. Sci Am 224:89–96, 1971.

Riley FC Jr, Moyer NJ. Oculosympathetic paresis associated with cluster headaches. Am J Ophthalmol 72:763–768, 1971.

Riley HA, Brickner RM, Soltz SE: Unusual types of migraine. Bull Neurol Inst NY 4:403–421, 1935.

Robertson WM, Welch KMA, Levine SR, et al. The effects of aging on cerebral blood flow in migraine. Neurology 39:947–951, 1989.

Robinson BW. Histaminic cephalgia. Medicine 37:161–180, 1958.

Roddy SM, Giang DW. Nifedipine prophylaxis of migraines in children. Ann Neurol 26:456–457, 1989.

Rosen JA. Observations on the efficacy of propranolol for the prophylaxis of migraine. Ann Neurol 13:92–93, 1983.

Rosenbaum HE. Familial hemiplegic migraine. Neurology 10:164–170, 1960.

Rosenstein AM. Beitrag zu den beidersteitigen Verdunkelungen des Sehvermögens mit vorübergehendem ophthalmoskopischen Befund bei Herzklappenfehler. Klin Monatsbl Augenheilkd 75:357–363, 1925.

Ross RT. Hemiplegic migraine. Can Med Assoc J 78:10–16, 1958.

Rothner AD. The migraine syndrome in children and adolescents. In Controversies and Clinical Variants of Migraine. Editor, Saper JR, pp 59–68. New York, Pergamon Press, 1987.

Rothrock JF, Walicke P, Swenson MR, et al. Migrainous stroke. Arch Neurol 45: 63–67, 1988a.

Rothrock JF, Swenson MR, Lyden PD. Migrainous stroke. Stroke 19:1306, 1988b.

Rothrock JF, North J, Madden K, et al. Migraine and migrainous stroke: Risk factors and prognosis. Neurology 43(12):2473–2476, 1993.

Rothrock JF, Kelly NM, Brody ML, et al. A differential response to treatment with divalproex sodium in patients with intractable headache. Cephalalgia 14(3): 241–244, 1994.

Roulet E, Deonna T. Benign paroxysmal torticollis in infancy. Dev Med Child Neurol 30:409–410, 1988.

Rowsell AR, Neylan C, Wilkinson M. Ergotamine-induced headaches in migrainous patients. J Headache 13:65–67, 1973.

Russel D. Chronic paroxysmal hemicrania: severity, duration and time of occurrence of attack. Cephalalgia 4:53–56, 1984.

Ryan RE. A controlled study of the effects of oral contraceptives on migraine. Headache 17:250–252, 1978.

Sabra F. Observations on 100 cases of cerebral angioma. JAMA 170:1522–1524, 1959.

Sacks OW. Migraine: Evolution of a Common Disorder. Los Angeles, University of California Press, 1970.

Safran AB. Les complications vasculaires de la migraine au niveau oculaire. Klin Monatsbl Augenheilkd 186:491–494, 1985.

Sagar SM, Sharp FR, Curran T. Expression of c-fos protein in brain: Metabolic mapping at the cellular level. Science 240(4857):1328–1331, 1988.

Sakai F, Meyer JS. Regional cerebral hemodynamics during migraine and cluster headaches measured by the 133Xe inhalation method. Headache 18:122–132, 1978.

Salmon ML, Winkelman JZ, Gay AJ. Neuro-ophthalmic sequelae in users of oral contraceptives. JAMA 206:85–91, 1968.

Sanchez-Precioso S, Garcia-Canto E, Villaescusa O, et al. A retrospective study of infant headache. Rev Neurol 23(122):764–768, 1995.

Sanders MD, Warrington EK, Marshall J, et al. "Blindsight": Vision in a field defect. Lancet 1:707–708, 1974.

Sandler M, Youdim MBH, Hanington E. A phenylethylamine oxidising defect in migraine. Nature 250:335–337, 1974.

Sanner G, Bergström B. Benign paroxysmal torticollis in infancy. Acta Paediatr Scand 68:219–223, 1979.

Saper JS (Editor). Controversies and Clinical Variants of Migraine. New York, Pergamon Press, 1987a.

Saper JR. Ergotamine dependency—A review. Headache 27:435–438, 1987b.

Saper JR, Jones JM. Ergotamine tartrate dependency: features and possible mechanisms. Clin Neuropharmacol 9:244–256, 1986.

Sargent JD, Baumel B, Peters K, et al. Aborting a migraine attack: Naproxen sodium vs. ergotamine plus caffeine. Headache 28:263–266, 1988.

Sargent JD, Solbach P, Damasio H, et al. A comparison of naproxen sodium to propranolol hydrochloride and a placebo control for the prophylaxis of migraine headache. Headache 25:320–324, 1985.

Sarkies NJC, Sanders MD, Gautier-Smith PC. Episodic unilateral mydriasis and migraine. Am J Ophthalmol 99:217–218, 1985.

Saundby R. A case of megrim, with paralysis of third nerve. Lancet 2:345, 1882.

Schatz NJ. Discussion of O'Connor PS, Tredici TJ: Acephalgic migraine. Fifteen years experience. Ophthalmol 88:1002–1003, 1981.

Schiffman SS, Buckley CE III, Sampson HA, et al. Aspartame and susceptibility to headache. N Engl J Med 317:1181–1185, 1987.

Schiff-Weretheimer S. Thèse Paris, No 66, 1926.

Schon F, Harrison MJH. Can migraine cause multiple segmental cerebral artery constrictions? J Neurol Neurosurg Psychiatry 50:492–494, 1987.

Schroth G, Gerber WD, Langohr HD. Ultrasonic Doppler flow in migraine and cluster headache. Headache 23:284–288, 1983.

Schuchman H, Thetford WN. A comparison of personality traits in ulcerative colitis and migraine patients. J Abnorm Psychol 76:443–452, 1970.

Schumacher GA, Wolff HG. Experimental studies on headache: A. Contrast of histamine headache with the headache of migraine and that associated with hypertension. B. Contrast of vascular mechanisms in preheadache and in headache phenomena of migraine. Arch Neurol Psychiatr 45:199–215, 1941.

Schwartz FD, Kark RM. Methysergide and retroperitoneal fibrosis. Am Heart J 72:843–844, 1966.

Selby G, Lance JW. Observations on 500 cases of migraine and allied vascular headache. J Neurol Neurosurg Psychiatry 23:23–32, 1960.

Selhorst JB, Slatkin N, Waybright EA, et al. Thirty years of visual migraine. Presented at the 13th Annual Frank B. Walsh Society Meeting. Houston, February 27–28, 1981.

Sentor HG, Lieberman AN, Pinto R. Cerebral manifestations of ergotism: Report of a case and review of the literature. Stroke 7:88–92, 1976.

Serdaru M, Chiras J, Cugas M, et al. Isolated benign cerebral vasculitis or migrainous vasospasm? J Neurol Neurosurg Psychiatry 47:73–76, 1984.

Shafey S, Scheinberg P. Neurological syndromes occurring in patients receiving synthetic steroids (oral contraceptives). Neurology 16:205–211, 1966.

Shapiro SL. The anatomy of migraine. EENT Monthly 53:78–83, 1974.

Sheth RD, Riggs JE, Bodensteiner JB. Acute confusional migraine: A variant of transient global amnesia. Pediatr Neurol 12(2):129–131, 1995.

Shinnar S, D'Souza BJ. Migraine in children and adolescents. Pediatr Rev 3:257–262, 1982.

Shiogai T, Takeuchi K, Akiyama R. Bitemporal hemianopsia as a prodromal symptom of ophthalmic migraine. A report of three cases. Neuroophthalmol 8:131–140, 1988.

Shuaib A, Barcley LL. Migraine-stroke and antiphospholipid antibody. Ann Neurol 26:131, 1989.

Shuaib A, Hachinski VC. Migraine and the risks from angiography. Arch Neurol 45:911–912, 1988.

Shuaib A, Metz L, Hing T. Migraine and intracerebral hemorrhage. Cephalalgia 9:59–61, 1989.

Sicuteri F, Testi A, Anselmi B. Biochemical investigations in headache; increase in hydroxyindoleacetic acid excretion during migraine attacks. Int Arch Allergy Appl Immunol 19:55–58, 1961.

Silberstein SD. Serotonin (5-HT) and migraine. Headache 34(7):408–417, 1994a.

Silberstein SD Pharmacologic management of cluster headache. CNS Drugs 2(3):199–207, 1994b.

Silberstein SD, Lipton RB. Epidemiology of migraine. Neuroepidemiol 12:179–194, 1993.

Silberstein SD, Lipton RB. Overview of diagnosis and treatment of migraine. Neurology 44:S6–S16, 1994.

Silberstein SD, Lipton RB, Saper JR, et al. Headache and facial pain. Continuum 1(5), 1995.

Sillanpää M. Changes in the prevalence of migraine and other headaches during the first seven school years. Headache 23:15–19, 1983.

Sillanpää M, Hillevi A. Epidemiology of headache in childhood and adolescence. In Gallai V and Guidotti V (eds): Juvenile headache. Elsevier, Amsterdam, pp 99–104, 1991.

Silvestrini M, Matteis M, Troisi E, et al. Migrainous stroke and the antiphospholipid antibodies. Eur Neurol 34(6):316–319, 1994.

Silvestrini M, Cupini LM, Matteis M, et al. Migraine in patients with stroke and antiphospholipid antibodies. Headache 33(8):421–426, 1993.

Simard D, Paulson OB. Cerebral vasomotor paralysis during migraine attack. Arch Neurol 29:207–209, 1973.

Singer CJ. From Magic to Science: Essays on the Scientific Twilight. New York, Liverwright, 1928.

Sinoff SE, Rosenberg M. Permanent cerebral diplopia in a migraineur. Neurology 40:1138–1139, 1990.

Sjaastad O. So-called "vascular headache of migraine type": One or more nosological entities? Acta Neurol Scand 54:125–139, 1976.

Sjaastad O. Cluster headache: On the inadequacy of existing hypotheses concerning the origin of the autonomic phenomena. Cephalalgia 8:133–137, 1988.

Sjaastad O, de Souza Carvalho D, Fragoso YD. The cluster phenomenon: An unspecific feature? Cephalalgia 8:61–65, 1988.

Sjaastad O, Fredricksen TA, Sand T, et al. Unilaterality of headache in classic migraine. Cephalalgia 9:71–77, 1989.

Skinhoj E. Hemodynamic studies within the brain during migraine. Arch Neurol 29:95–98, 1973.

Skinhoj E, Paulson OB. Regional blood flow in internal carotid distribution during migraine attack. Br Med J 3:569–570, 1969.

Skyhoj Olsen T. Migraine with and without aura: The same disease due to cerebral vasospasm of different intensity. A hypothesis based on CBF studies during migraine. Headache 30:269–272, 1990.

Skyhoj Olsen T, Friberg L. Ischemia may be the primary cause of neurological deficits in classic migraine. Arch Neurol 47:125–127, 1990.

Skyhoj Olsen T, Lassen NA. Blood flow and vascular reactivity during attacks of classic migraine—Limitations of the Xe-133 intraarterial technique. Headache 29:15–20, 1989.

Skyhoj Olsen T, Larsen B, Bech Skriver E, et al. Focal cerebral ischemia measured by the intra-arterial 133xenon method. Stroke 12:736–746, 1981.

Skyhoj Olsen T, Friberg L, Lassen NA. Ischemia may be the primary cause of the neurologic deficits in classic migraine. Arch Neurol 44:156–161, 1987.

Slater R. Benign recurrent vertigo. J Neurol Neurosurg Psychiatry 42:363–367, 1979.

Slatter KH. Some clinical and EEG findings in patients with migraine. Brain 91:85–98, 1968.

Slavin ML. Transient comitant esotropia in a child with migraine. Am J Ophthalmol 107:190–191, 1989.

Smith CH. Recurrent vomiting in children: Its etiology and treatment. J Pediatr 10:719–742, 1937.

Smith JL. Migraine. In Neuro-ophthalmology Update. Editor, Smith JL, pp 345–349. New York, Masson, 1977.

Smith JL. Permanent infarctions complicating migraine. J Clin Neuroophthalmol 6:74–75, 1986.

Smith JL, Quencer RM. Practical questions in the neuroradiologic workup of ophthalmoplegic migraine. J Clin Neuroophthalmol 4:219–220, 1984.

Snyder CH. Paroxysmal torticollis in infancy. Am J Dis Child 117:458–460, 1969.

Solomon GD. Verapamil in migraine prophylaxis—A five-year review. Headache 29:425–427, 1989.

Solomon GD, Diamond S. Verapamil in migraine prophylaxis-comparison of dosages. Clin Pharmacol Ther 1:202, 1987.

Solomon GD, Steel JG, Spaccavento LJ. Verapamil prophylaxis of migraine: A double-blind, placebo-controlled study. JAMA 250:2500–2502, 1983.

Solomon S, Cappa KG, Smith CR. Common migraine: Criteria for diagnosis. Headache 28:124–129, 1988.

Solomon S, Lipton RB, Harris PY. Arterial stenosis in migraine: Spasm or arteriopathy? Headache 30:52–61, 1990.

Somerville BW. A study of migraine in pregnancy. Neurology 22:824–828, 1972.

Somerville BW. Estrogen withdrawal migraine: 1. Duration of exposure required and attempted prophylaxis by premenstrual estrogen administration. Neurology 25: 239–255, 1975.

Somerville BW. Platelet-bound and free serotonin levels in jugular and forearm venous blood during migraine. Neurology 26:41–45, 1976.

Sorbi M, Tellegen B. Differential effects of training in relaxation and stress-coping in patients with migraine. Headache 26:473–481, 1986.

Sorbi M, Tellegen B. Stress-coping in migraine. Soc Sci Med 26:351–358, 1988.

Sorbi M, Tellegen B, Du Long A. Long-term effects of training in relaxation and stress-coping in patients with migraine: A 3-year follow-up. Headache 29: 111–121, 1989.

Sorensen PS, Hansen K, Olesen J. A placebo controlled, double blind, cross-over trial of flunarizine in common migraine. Cephalalgia 6:7–14, 1986.

Sorge F, De Simone R, Marano E, et al. Flunarizine in prophylaxis of childhood migraine. Cephalalgia 8:1–6, 1988.

Soyka D, Taneri Z, Oestreich W, et al. Flunarizine iv in the acute treatment of the migraine attack. A double-blind placebo-controlled study. Cephalalgia 8(8): 35–40, 1988.

Soyka D, Taneri Z, Oestreich W, et al. Flunarizine iv in the acute treatment of common or classical migraine attacks—A placebo-controlled double blind trial. Headache 29:21–27, 1989.

Spaccavento LJ, Solomon GD. Migraine as an etiology of stroke in young adults. Headache 24:19–22, 1984.

Sparks JP. The incidence of migraine in school children: A surbey by the medical officers of school associations. Practitioner 221:407–411, 1978.

Speed WG. A few interesting neurologic manifestations of migraine. Headache 3: 128–133, 1964.

Spierings ELH. Craniovascular accompaniments of the vascular headache of the migraine type. Headache 19:397–399, 1979.

Spierings ELH. Recent advances in the understanding of migraine. Headache 28: 655–658, 1988.

Spierings ELH, Graham JR. Cerebral hypoperfusion followed by hyperperfusion in classic migraine. Arch Neurol 46:605–606, 1989.

Spierings ELH, Messenger HB. Flunarizine vs pizotifen in migraine prophylaxis: A review of comparative studies. Cephalalgia 8(8):27–30, 1988.

Spierings ELH, Reinders MJ, Hoogduin CAL. The migraine aura as a cause of avoidance behavior. Headache 29:254–255, 1989.

Stellar S, Ahrens SP, Meibohm AR, et al. Migraine prevention with timolol. A double-blind crossover study. JAMA 252:2576–2580, 1984.

Stensrud P, Sjaastad O. Clinical trial of a new anti-bradykinin, anti-inflammatory drug, ketoprofen, in migraine prophylaxis. Headache 14:96–100, 1974.

Stewart WF, Lipton RB, Celentano DD, et al. Prevalence of migraine headache in the United States. Relation to age, income, race, and other sociodemographic factors. JAMA 267:64–69, 1992.

Stommel EW, Ward TN, Harris RD. MRI findings in a case of ophthalmoplegic migraine. Headache 33:234–237, 1993.

Straube A, Bandmann O, Buttner U, et al. A contrast enhanced lesion of the III nerve on MR of a patient with ophthalmoplegic migraine as evidence of Tolosa-Hunt syndrome. Headache 33:446–448, 1993.

Sturzenegger MH, Meienberg O. Basilar artery migraine: A follow-up study of 82 cases. Headache 25:408–415, 1985.

Suckling CW. Ophthalmolegia and migraine. Brain 10:241–242, 1888.

Sudilovsky A, Elkind AH, Ryan RE Sr, et al. Comparative efficacy of nadolol and propranolol in the management of migraine. Headache 27:421–426, 1987.

Sunderland S. Mechanism responsible for changes in the pupil unaccompanied by disturbances of extraocular muscle function. Br J Ophthalmol 36:638–644, 1952.

Sutherland AM, Wolff HG. Experimental studies on headache: Further analysis of the mechanism of headache in migraine, hypertension, and fever. Arch Neurol Psychiatr 44:929–949, 1940.

Swanson JW, Vick NA. Basilar artery migraine: 12 patients, with an attack recorded electroencephalographically. Neurology 28:782–786, 1978.

Symon DN, Russell G. The relationship between cyclic vomiting syndrome and abdominal migraine. J Pediatr Gastroenterol Nutr 21(1):S42–S43, 1995.

Symonds C. Migrainous variants. Trans Med Soc Lond 67:238–249, 1952.

Tagliati M, Sabbadini M, Bernardi G, et al. Multichannel visual evoked potentials in migraine. Electroencephalogr Clin Neurophysiol 96(1):1–5, 1995.

Talwar KK, Edvardsson N, Varnauskas E. Paroxysmal vagally mediated AV block with recurrent syncope. Clin Cardiol 8:339–340, 1985.

Tarnower A, Alguire P. Ergotism masquerading as arteritis. Postgrad Med 85: 103–108, 1989.

Teasdale E, Macpherson P, Statham P. Non-invasive investigation for oculomotor palsy due to aneurysm. J Neurol Neurosurg Psychiatry 52:929, 1989.

Tfelt-Hansen P, Olesen J. Effervescent metoclopramide and aspirin (Migravess) versus effervescent aspirin or placebo for migraine attacks: A double-blind study. Cephalalgia 4:107–111, 1984.

Tfelt-Hansen P, Olesen J. Methodological aspects of drug trials in migraine. Neuroepidemiology 4:204–236, 1985.

Tfelt-Hansen P, Standnes B, Kangasneimi P, et al. Timolol and propranolol for common migraine prophylaxis. Acta Neurol Scand 69(98):264–265, 1984.

Tfelt-Hansen P, Brand J, Dano P, et al. Early clinical experience with subcutaneous GR43175 in acute migraine: An overview. Cephalalgia 9(9):73–78, 1989.

The Medical Letter: Foods potentially harmful to patients taking MAO inhibitors. March 26, 1976.

Thompson HS: The pupil. In Neuro-Ophthalmology. Editors, Lessell S, van Dalen JTW, Vol 2, pp 226–229. Amsterdam, Excerpta Medica, 1982.

Thompson HS, Zackon DH, Czarnecki JSC. Tadpole-like pupils: Presumed segmental spasms of the iris dilator muscle. Am J Ophthalmol 96:467–477, 1983.

Thompson JK. Exercise-induced migraine prodrome symptoms. Headache 27: 250–251, 1987.

Tinuper P, Cortelli P, Sacquegna T, et al. Classic migraine attack complicated by confusional state: EEG and CT study. Cephalalgia 5:63–68, 1985.

Tippin J, Corbett JJ, Kerber RE, et al. Amaurosis fugax and ocular infarction in adolescents and young adults. Ann Neurol 26:69–77, 1989.

Todd J. The syndrome of Alice in Wonderland. Can Med Assoc J 73:701–704, 1955.

Tomsak RL, Jergens PB. Benign recurrent transient monocular blindness: A possible variant of acephalgic migraine. Headache 27:66–69, 1987.

Tomsak RL, Masaryk TJ, Bates JH. Magnetic resonance angiography (MRA) of isolated aneurysmal third nerve palsy. J Clin Neuroophthalmol 11:16–18, 1991.

Troost BT. Migraine. In Clinical Ophthalmology. Editors, Duane TD, Jaeger EA, Vol 2, Chap 19. Philadelphia, Harper & Row, 1988.

Troost BT. Migraine and other headaches. In Clinical Ophthalmology. Editor, Duane TD, Vol 3. Philadelphia, JB Lippincott, 1996.

Troost BT, Newton, TH. Occipital lobe arteriovenous malformations. Clinical and radiologic features in 26 cases with comment on the differentiation from migraine. Arch Ophthalmol 93:250–256, 1975.

Troost BT, Mark LE, Maroon JC. Resolution of classic migraine after removal of an occipital lobe AVM. Ann Neurol 5:199–201, 1979.

Tsounis S, Milonas J, Gilliam F. Hemi-field pattern reversal visual evoked potentials in migraine. Cephalalgia 13(4):267–271, 1993.

Tunis MM, Wolff HG. Treatment of headache. Med Clin North Am 37:1251–1270, 1953.

Tzourio C, Iglesias S, Hubert J, et al. Migraine and risk of ischemic stroke: A case-controlled study. Br Med J 307:289–292, 1993.

Udenfriend S, Lovenberg W, Sjoerdman A. Physiological active amines in common fruits and vegetables. Arch Biochem 85:487–490, 1959.

Uhthoff W. Untersuchungen über die bei der multiplen herdsklerose vorkommenden augenstorungen. Arch Psychiatr Nervenkr 21:55–116, 303–410, 1890.

Vahlquist B. Migraine in children. Int Arch Allergy Appl Immunol 7:348–355, 1955.

Vahlquist B, Hackzell G. Migraine of early onset. Study of thirty-one cases in which disease first appeared between one and four years of age. Acta Paediatr 38: 622–636, 1949.

Vallery-Radot P. Une figure originale, le Docteur Véron Progr Med (Suppl):41–46, 1937.

van Pelt W, Andermann F. On the early onset of ophthalmoplegic migraine. Am J Dis Child 107:628–631, 1964.

Ver Brugghen A. Pathogenesis of ophthalmoplegic migraine. Neurology 5:311–318, 1955.

Verhoeff FH. Moore's subjective "lightning streaks." Trans Am Ophthalmol Soc 39: 220–226, 1941.

Victor DI, Welch RB. Bilateral retinal hemorrhages and disk edema in migraine. Am J Ophthalmol 84:555–558, 1977.

Vignat J-P, Bourgeois H, Goasquen J, et al. Manifestations campimétriques irréversibles au décours de crises migraineuses. Bull Soc Ophtalmol Fr 82:995–999, 1982.

Vijayan N. Ophthalmoplegic migraine: Ischemic or compressive neuropathy? Headache 20:300–304, 1980.

Vijayan N, Watson C. Evaluation of oculocephalic sympathetic function in vascular headache syndromes. II. Oculocephalic sympathetic function in cluster headache. Headache 22:200–202, 1982.

Vollrath-Junger C. Rezidivierende Okulomotoriuslähmungen: Ein Fall von ophthalmoplegisher Migräne? Klin Monatsbl Augenheilkd 192:154–156, 1988.

Waldenlind E, Ross SB, Saaf J, et al. Concentration and uptake of 5-hydroxytryptamine in platelets with cluster headache and migraine patients. Cephalalgia 5: 45–54, 1985.

Walsh FB. The ocular symptoms of migraine. N Carolina Med J 12:271–273, 1951.

Walsh FB, Hoyt WF. Clinical Neuro-Ophthalmology. 3rd ed, Vol 2, p 1662. Baltimore, Williams & Wilkins, 1969a.

Walsh FB, Hoyt WF. Clinical Neuro-Ophthalmology. 3rd ed, Vol 2, p 1674. Baltimore, Williams & Wilkins, 1969b.

Walsh FB, Hoyt WF. Clinical Neuro-Ophthalmology. 3rd ed, Vol 2, p 1667. Baltimore, Williams & Wilkins, 1969c.

Walsh FB, Hoyt WF. Clinical Neuro-Ophthalmology. 3rd ed, Vol 2, p 1675. Baltimore, Williams & Wilkins, 1969d.

Walsh FB, Hoyt WF. Clinical Neuro-Ophthalmology. 3rd ed, Vol 2, p 1663. Baltimore, Williams & Wilkins, 1969e.

Walsh FB, Hoyt WF. Clinical Neuro-Ophthalmology. 3rd ed, Vol 2, p 1673. Baltimore. Williams & Wilkins, 1969f.

Walsh JP, O'Doherty DS. A possible explanation of the mechanism of ophthalmoplegic migraine. Neurology 10:1079–1084, 1960.

Waters WE. Migraine and symptoms in childhood: Bilious attacks, travel sickness and eczema. Headache 12:55–61, 1972.

Waters WE, O'Connor PJ. Epidemiology of headache and migraine in women. J Neurol Neurosurg Psychiatry 34:148–153, 1971.

Waters WE, O'Connor PJ. Prevalence of migraine. J Neurol Neurosurg Psychiatry 38:613–616, 1975.

Watson C, Vijayan N. Evaluation of oculocephalic sympathetic function in vascular headache syndromes: Part I. Methods of evaluation. Headache 22:192–199, 1982.

Watson P, Steele JC. Proxysmal dysequilibrium in the migraine syndrome of childhood. Arch Otolaryngol 99:177–179, 1974.

Wayne VS. A possible relationship between migraine and coronary artery spasm. Aust N Z J Med 16:708–710, 1986.

Webb NR, McCrary JA III. Hyaline bodies of the optic disc and migraine. In Neuro-ophthalmology Update. Editor, Smith JL, pp 155–162. New York, Masson, 1977.

Weber RB, Reinmuth OM. The treatment of migraine with propranolol. Neurology 22:366–369, 1972.

Wegner W. Augenspiegelbefunde bei Migräne. Klin Monatsbl Augenheilkd 76:194–202, 1926.

Weiller C, May A, Limmroth V, et al. Brain stem activation in spontaneous human migraine attacks. Nat Med 1(7):658–660, 1995.

Weinstein JM, Feman SS. Ischemic optic neuropathy in migraine. Arch Ophthalmol 100:1097–1100, 1982.

Weiskrantz L, Warrington EK, Sanders MD, et al. Visual capacity in the hemianopic field following a restricted occipital ablation. Brain 97:709–728, 1974.

Welch KMA. Migraine. A biobehavioral disorder. Arch Neurol 44:323–327, 1987.

Welch KMA, Levine SR. Migraine-related stroke in the context of the International Headache Society classification of head pain. Arch Neurol 47:458–462, 1990.

Welch KMA, Ellis DJ, Keenan PA. Successful migraine prophylaxis with naproxen sodium. Neurology 35:1304–1310, 1985.

Welch KMA, Barkley GL, Tepley N, et al. Central neurogenic mechanisms of migraine. Neurology 43(6 Suppl 3):S21–S25, 1993.

Welch KMA, Levine SR, D'Andrea G, et al. Preliminary observations on brain energy metabolism in migraine studied by in vivo phosphorus 31 NMR spectroscopy. Neurology 39:538–541, 1989.

Weller M, Petersen D, Dichgans J, et al. Cerebral angiography complications link cerebral autosomal dominant arteriopathy with subcortical infarcts and leukoencephalopathy to familial hemiplegic migraine. Neurology 46(3):844, 1996.

Whitty CWM. Familial hemiplegic migraine. J Neurol Neurosurg Psychiatry 16:172–177, 1953.

Whitty CWM. Migraine without headache. Lancet 2:283–285, 1967.

Whitty CWM. Migraine variants. Br Med J 1:38–40, 1971.

Whitty CM, Hockaday JM, Whitty MM. The effect of oral contraceptives on migraine. Lancet 1:856–859, 1966.

Wideroe T-E, Vigander T. Propranolol in the treatment of migraine. Br Med J 2:699–701, 1974.

Wilbrand H, Saenger A. Die Neurologie des Auges. Vol 2, pp 71–73. Wiesbaden-München, JF Bergmann, 1901.

Wilbrand H, Saenger A. Die Neurologies des Auges, Vol 3, Pt 2, pp 968–1005. Wiesbaden-München, JF Bergmann, 1906.

Wiley RG. The scintillating scotoma without headache. Ann Ophthalmol 11:581–585, 1979.

Wilkinson M. Treatment of migraine. Headache 28:659–661, 1988.

Wilkinson M, Williams K, Leyton M. Observations on the treatment of the acute attack of migraine. Res Clin Stud Headache 6:141–146, 1978.

Williams JK, Baumbach GL, Armstrong ML, et al. Hypothesis: Vasoconstriction contributes to amaurosis fugax. J Cereb Blood Flow Metab, 9(1):111–116, 1989.

Wilson SAK. Neurology. Arnold, London, 1940.

Winterkorn JM, Teman AJ. Recurrent attacks of amaurosis fugax treated with calcium channel blocker. Ann Neurol 30(3):423–425, 1991.

Winterkorn JMS, Odel JG, Behrens MM. Ergotamine headache mistaken for temporal arteritis. Ann Neurol 28:396, 1990.

Woestenburg JC, Kramer CJ, Orlebeke JF, et al. Brain potential differences related to spatial attention in migraineurs with and without aura symptoms support supposed differences in activation. Headache 33(8):413–416, 1993.

Wolff HG. Headache and Other Head Pain. 1st ed., London, Oxford University Press, 1948.

Wolff HG. Headache mechanisms. Int Arch Allerg 7:210–278, 1955.

Wolff HG. Headache and Other Head Pain. 2nd ed, New York, Oxford University Press, 1963.

Wolff HG, Dalessio DJ. Wolff's Headache and Other Head Pain. 4th ed. New York, Oxford University Press, 1980.

Wolff HG, Tunis MM, Goodell H. Studies on headache: Evidence of tissue damage and changes in pain sensitivity in subjects with vascular headaches of the migraine type. Arch Int Med 92:478–484, 1953.

Wolter JR, Burchfield WJ. Ocular migraine in a young man resulting in unilateral transient blindness and retinal edema. J Pediatr Ophthalmol 8:173–176, 1971.

Woods D, O'Connor PS, Fleming R. Episodic unilateral mydriasis and migraine. Am J Ophthalmol 98:229–234, 1984.

Woods D, O'Connor PS, Fleming R. Episodic unilateral mydriasis and migraine (Reply). Am J Ophthalmol 99:218, 1985.

Woods RP, Iacoboni M, Mazziotta A. Brief report: Bilateral spreading cerebral hypoperfusion during spontaneous migraine headache. N Engl J Med 331(25):1691, 1994.

Woody RC, Blaw ME. Ophthalmoplegic migraine in infancy. Clin Pediatr 25:82–84, 1986.

World Federation of Neurology's Research Group on Migraine and Headache: Migraine. Hemicrania 1:3–4, 1969.

Young GF, Leon-Barth CA, Green J. Familial hemiplegic migraine, retinal degeneration, deafness, and nystagmus. Arch Neurol 23:201–209, 1970.

Young SM, Fisher M, Sigsbee A, et al. Cardiogenic brain embolism and lupus anticoagulant. Ann Neurol 26:390–392, 1989.

Young WB, Silberstein SD. Hemicrania continua and symptomatic medication overuse. Headache 33(9):485–487, 1993.

Zeitlin C, Oddy M. Cognitive impairment in patients with severe migraine. Br Med J Clin Psychol 23:27–35, 1984.

Ziegler DK. The headache symptom: How many entities? Arch Neurol 42:273–274, 1985.

Ziegler DK, Ellis DJ: Naproxen in prophylaxis of migraine. Arch Neurol 42:582–584, 1985.

Ziegler DK, Stephenson HR, Ward DF. Migraine, tyramine and blood serotonin. Headache 16:53–57, 1976.

Ziegler DK, Hurwitz A, Hassanein RS, et al. Migraine prophylaxis. A comparison of propranolol and amitriptyline. Arch Neurol 44:486–489, 1987.

Zifkin B, Andermann E, Andermann F, et al. An autosomal dominant syndrome of hemiplegic migraine, nystagmus, and tremor. Ann Neurol 8:329–332, 1980.

CHAPTER 57

Vasculitis

Steven L. Galetta

PATHOPHYSIOLOGY
SPECIFIC DISORDERS AND THEIR NEURO-
 OPHTHALMOLOGIC FEATURES
 Vasculitides
 Behçet's Disease

Connective Tissue Diseases
Arthritides
Malignant Atrophic Papulosis (Degos' Disease, Köhlmeier-Degos'
 Disease)
Idiopathic Retinal Vasculitis

In this chapter, we consider disorders that produce neuro-ophthalmologic symptoms and signs from inflammation of blood vessels. We have chosen to limit the discussion to **noninfectious** conditions. Infectious causes of vasculitis (e.g., syphilis) are discussed in Chapter 60 of this text.

Most of the major disorders discussed in this chapter are often classified as **rheumatic diseases** (Jabs, 1994). These disorders apparently result from an external or internal challenge to an abnormal or disturbed immunogenetic system. Some of the rheumatic diseases are characterized entirely by vasculitis (e.g., giant cell arteritis [GCA]). These diseases are called the **vasculitides** (Fauci et al., 1978; see Table 5 in Sigal, 1987; Jennette et al., 1994; Lie, 1994a). Some investigators include Behçet's disease in this group, whereas others, including ourselves, consider it a distinct entity. Other rheumatic diseases, characterized by diffuse inflammation of connective tissue, including blood vessels (e.g.,

systemic lupus erythematosus [SLE]), are called the **connective tissue diseases.** Finally, some of the rheumatic diseases only occasionally have a significant vasculitic component (e.g., rheumatoid arthritis). Jabs (1994) classifies these disorders as the **arthritides.** They include rheumatoid arthritis, juvenile rheumatoid arthritis, and the seronegative spondyloarthropathies. The condition known as malignant atrophic papulosis (Degos' disease) may also be a form of vasculitis and, therefore, is discussed in this chapter. There is no perfect classification of these disorders, and various authors differ in exactly which category to place some of them (see, for example, Table 1 in Moore and Cupps, 1983; Table 5 in Sigal, 1987; Jabs, 1994; Lie, 1994a). The reader interested in pursuing the subject of rheumatic diseases in more detail should read the superb *Textbook of Rheumatology,* edited by Kelley et al. (1997), and the comprehensive chapter by Jabs (1994).

PATHOPHYSIOLOGY

Immunologic processes mediate the localization and destruction of substances that, if disseminated, could disrupt the host's complex internal milieu (Snyderman, 1988). The immune system has several unique features that permit it to combat microbial invasion and provide resistance against the spread of cancer. Unlike other tissues, the immune system consists not only of fixed structures (i.e., thymus, spleen, and lymph nodes) but also of motile cells that wander throughout the body, performing surveillance. It also is the only tissue that is able to destroy other components of the host. Both the protective and the destructive abilities of the immunologic processes depend largely on their potential to produce inflammation. Therefore, understanding how inflammation is initiated is essential to understanding immu-

nologically mediated resistance and comprehending how tissue destruction occurs in the rheumatic disorders.

The immune system, as defender of the host, must differentiate ''self'' from ''nonself'' and then rapidly destroy or otherwise render harmless any substances recognized as ''nonself.'' A progression of immunologic recognition, amplification of the immune reaction, accumulation of inflammatory cells, and, finally, destruction of the inciting agent is an ongoing process.

Inflammatory reactions can be initiated by either specific or nonspecific **recognition.** Antibodies and receptors on lymphocytes can recognize unique determinants (epitopes) on antigens, whereas nonspecific recognition can be initiated by components of the immune system that bind to materials based on their charge, their reaction to the external environment, or their composition. Nonspecific recognition is mediated in part by phagocytic cells, such as polymorphonuclear leukocytes (PMNs) and macrophages, and by substances such as C3b and the Hageman factor.

After recognition of "nonself," the immune system activates **amplification** systems that continue the process of inflammation. The type of amplifier depends on the recognition component and the nature and location of the inciting material (Snyderman, 1988). Amplification components of the immune system such as complement cleavage products, cytokines, and other phlogistic factors magnify the initial response to "nonself." Inflammatory reactions also can be initiated by nonimmunologic means. Inflammation that follows tissue necrosis results from the direct cleavage of complement components by lysosomal proteases released by injured cells. Lysosomal proteases and hydrolases also may be released by PMNs that have phagocytosed certain substances such as the monosodium urate or calcium pyrophosphate dihydrate crystals of gout and pseudogout.

Regardless of the type of inflammatory response, the **accumulation** of granulocytes and macrophages can result in phagocytosis and degradation of the material that initiated the inflammatory event. The factors that determine if an inflammatory response will be protective or destructive depend in part on the nature, location, quantity, and digestibility of the inciting agent and in part on the genetic makeup and the immunoregulatory competency of the host. In general, when the antigen or other inciting agent is rapidly destroyed, the inflammatory process is self-limited. When the antigen persists or is excessive in amount, the inflammatory response can be extensive and prolonged.

Immunologically mediated inflammatory reactions are generally separated into four types, although it is not unusual for a disease to be associated with more than one and even all of them. The four types of reactions are: (a) inflammation initiated by reagenic immunoglobulin (Ig) E antibodies, (b) tissue destruction mediated by cytotoxic antibodies, (c) inflammation initiated by immune complexes, and (d) inflammation initiated by lymphocytes (Snyderman, 1988).

IgE antibodies can bind to mast cells and basophils with one portion of their structure and to specific antigens with another portion. Shortly after an antigen binds to an IgE antibody that is already bound to a mast cell or basophil, the cell degranulates and secretes its intracellular products, including histamine, heparin, and eosinophil chemotactic factors. Release of these substances causes an increase in local vascular permeability within seconds, producing vascular stasis and smooth muscle contraction. These types of reactions are responsible for such allergic phenomena as urticaria, seasonal rhinitis, asthma, and systemic anaphylaxis. They do not play a role in the diseases under consideration in this chapter.

The development of **antibodies to antigens on the surface of a host's own cells** can result in tissue destruction. When these antibodies bind to the cells, a destructive reaction develops that begins with the release of inflammatory mediators and the accumulation of inflammatory cells. Release of lysosomal enzymes and toxic oxygen radicals by inflammatory cells and direct cytolysis of target cells contribute to tissue destruction. Spontaneous development of antibody to apparently normal tissues characterizes certain connective tissue diseases such as SLE.

The formation or deposition of certain types of **immune complexes** in local tissues produces an inflammatory response characterized by the accumulation of PMNs within hours, followed by an influx of macrophages. Immune complexes initiate this reaction in several ways. The combination of IgM or IgG antibodies with antigen leads to binding and activation of the first component of the complement system, a complex series of proteins that are found primarily in the plasma and that act together as an important amplifier of inflammatory events (Fearon, 1988; Moxley and Ruddy 1993). As a result of this activation, several other proteins in the complement system are cleaved and activated. One of the protein fragments (C3a) enhances vascular permeability, contracts smooth muscle, and degranulates both mast cells and basophils. Another fragment (C5a) becomes a potent inflammatory polypeptide that induces migration of PMNs and macrophages to the site of deposition of the immune complex, where they bind to the complex and begin the process of phagocytosis.

If the amount of immune complex deposited locally is not great, the material can be phagocytosed and digested without tissue destruction. If the amount is large, or if a significant portion is lodged in vessel walls, permanent tissue destruction may occur. PMNs and macrophages contain abundant lysosomal enzymes, and they are capable of producing oxygen free radicals that are toxic to tissue. The lysosomal enzymes and free radicals are released during phagocytosis of immune complexes, particularly when these complexes are numerous or large. The lysosomal enzymes are capable of cleaving more C5, producing more C5a, and thus attracting more leukocytes and macrophages to the site of inflammation. When these processes occur within vessel walls, they produce vasculitis that can lead to hemorrhagic necrosis and local tissue destruction (Parums, 1994). Immune complex deposition is the most commom purported cause of systemic vasculitis and occurs in entities such as polyarteritis nodosa (PAN) and rheumatoid arthritis (Somer, 1993).

Lymphocyte-initiated inflammatory reactions are called "delayed hypersensitivity" reactions because maximum accumulation of inflammatory cells does not occur for 48–72 hours after secondary exposure to the inciting antigen. The antigen is encountered initially by macrophages that partially digest it. The altered antigen is subsequently recognized by lymphocytes that contain specific surface receptors for it. Interaction between the lymphocytes and the altered antigen initiates the synthesis and release of substances called cytokines from the lymphocytes. The cytokines diffuse to areas of vessel walls closest to the immunologic reaction. Increased vascular permeability develops, during which chemotactic gradients attract macrophages and other lymphocytes. At the same time, the cytokines also activate the macrophages, which become more metabolically active, develop higher levels of hydrolytic enzymes, and become better able to destroy antigen.

Lymphocytes at the inflammatory site also release cytokines that recruit nonsensitized lymphocytes, thus expanding the clones of cells capable of recognizing and responding to the specific antigen. If the inflammatory response is able to destroy the antigen completely, the response resolves and produces little or no tissue necrosis. If there is a large amount of antigen, the antigen is difficult to digest, or both, the inflammatory process continues. New cells continually arrive to replace dying cells, thus providing a continuous release of proteolytic enzymes and toxic oxygen free radicals. Cell-mediated immunity plays a role in most granulomatous inflammatory disorders, including Wegener's granulomatous, Churg-Strauss syndrome, and GCA (Somer, 1993).

SPECIFIC DISORDERS AND THEIR NEURO-OPHTHALMOLOGIC FEATURES

VASCULITIDES

Two main categories of vasculitis may produce neuro-ophthalmologic manifestations: (a) primary central nervous system (CNS) vasculitides, and (b) systemic necrotizing vasculitides that often affect the CNS. Strict classification of vasculitis is difficult because the etiology and pathogenesis of many vasculitic entities remain unknown (Lie, 1992; Tervaert and Kallenberg, 1993; Lie, 1994a). The main disorders that compose the primary CNS vasculitides are granulomatous angiitis of the nervous system (GANS), microangiopathy of the eye and brain (Susac's syndrome), and Cogan's syndrome. Eales' disease and acute posterior multifocal placoid pigment epitheliopathy (APMPPE) also may be placed in this category. The disorders that compose the group of systemic necrotizing vasculitides that often affect the CNS are PAN, Churg-Strauss disease, GCA, Takayasu's arteritis (pulseless disease), Wegener's granulomatosis, lymphomatoid granulomatosis, Henoch-Schönlein purpura, and mixed cryoglobulinemia (Moore and Fauci, 1981; Moore and Cupps, 1983; Sigal, 1987; Jabs, 1994). In the following section, we discuss each of these disorders as they pertain to neuro-ophthalmology. A condition called **nonsystemic vasculitic neuropathy** produces isolated peripheral neuropathy without evidence of associated systemic or CNS vasculitis (Torvik and Berntzen, 1968; Dyck et al., 1984; Kissel et al., 1985; Dyck et al., 1987; Said et al., 1988). The clinical pattern of the neuropathy is variable and includes multiple mononeuropathy (mononeuritis multiplex), asymmetric neuropathy, distal polyneuropathy, and sensory polyneuropathy. The pathologic features are those of an ischemic neuropathy caused by a necrotizing vasculitis affecting small epineural arterioles that is indistinguishable from that which affects patients with systemic necrotizing vasculitides (Dyck et al., 1987; Said et al., 1988; see below). This condition has no significant neuro-ophthalmologic or ocular manifestations and therefore is not discussed further in this text.

Primary Central Nervous System Vasculitides

Isolated Granulomatous Angiitis of the Central Nervous System

Isolated granulomatous angiitis of the central nervous system is an idiopathic, recurrent vasculitis confined to the vessels of the brain and spinal cord (Cravioto and Feigin, 1959; Nurick et al., 1972; Harrison, 1976; Vincent, 1977; Cupps et al., 1983; Moore and Cupps, 1983; Kattah et al., 1987; Sigal, 1987; Moore, 1989; Calabrese et al., 1992; Ozawa et al., 1995; Rhodes et al., 1995). It usually occurs in young adults, but it occasionally occurs in children (Levin et al., 1989) and in older adults (Kattah et al., 1987; Zimmerman et al., 1990). The condition, which affects primarily small, and sometimes medium-sized, blood vessels, is also called "granulomatous angiitis" because the affected vessels are surrounded by an infiltrate composed of lymphocytes, macrophages, and giant cells (Kolodny et al., 1968; Younger et al., 1986; Vanderzant et al., 1988; Younger et al., 1988; Moore, 1989) (Figs. 57.1 and 57.2). These vessels can thrombose, causing microinfarction.

Significant vasculitis rarely is seen outside the cranium in patients with GANS, although the spinal cord and temporal arteries occasionally may be affected (Sigal, 1987). A few cases show pathologic abnormalities outside the nervous system, most notably in the lung and kidney, but none of the cases have clinical manifestations referable to these organs (see Table 3 in Sigal, 1987). Arteritic involvement of the temporal arteries, systemic vessels, and the large intracranial vessels in some reported cases of GANS makes its relationship to GCA uncertain, and overlap between these two entities may exist. In a review of autopsy cases of GANS, patients with angiitis confined to the small vessels did not show temporal artery involvement (Rhodes et al., 1995). Furthermore, systemic vasculitis was mainly associated with cases demonstrating large vessel involvement. This report emphasizes that GANS is a disorder that primarily affects small cerebral vessels.

GANS usually begins with diffuse cerebral dysfunction characterized by headache, seizures, lethargy, and confusion (Cravioto and Feigin, 1959; Cupps and Moore, 1983; Moore, 1989). Cortical visual disturbances and visual hallucinations often occur (Nurick et al., 1972; Zimmerman et al., 1990). In some cases, there is evidence of intracerebral or subarachnoid hemorrhage (Clifford-Jones et al., 1985; Biller et al., 1987; Zimmerman et al., 1990; Kumar et al., 1997). Other patients present with focal symptoms and signs of an acute stroke (Burger et al., 1977), and still others present with the clinical picture of multiple infarcts (Sigal, 1987; Koo and Massey, 1988). The malaise, fever, myalgias, and arthralgias that are frequent in systemic vasculitides (see below) characteristically are absent in patients with this condition (Moore and Cupps, 1983).

As GANS progresses, focal deficits become increasingly prominent. Eventually, about 75% of patients develop multiple, localized lesions of the cerebrum, cerebellum, or brainstem (Moore, 1989). Cranial neuropathies may occur late in the course of the disease. The nerves most commonly affected are the ocular motor, trigeminal, and facial nerves. Sigal (1987) described the findings in 61 patients with GANS. Five patients developed oculomotor nerve paresis, corticosteroids will suffice (Calabrese et al., 1993; Calabrese and Duna, 1995).

Microangiopathy of Brain, Retina, and Inner Ear

An unusual but apparently distinct form of vasculitis that affects the brain and retina initially was described in two patients by Pfaffenbach and Hollenhorst (1973), who ascribed the process to SLE of the CNS despite inconclusive laboratory tests. Susac et al. (1979) subsequently recognized the unique features of the disease and called it **microangiopathy of brain and retina.** The condition is similar to GANS; however, it specifically causes obliteration of the retinal arteries in both eyes in addition to the arteries of the brain and meninges. The condition occurs predominantly in women 18–40 years of age (Coppeto et al., 1984; Monteiro et al., 1985; Swanson et al., 1985; McFadyen et al., 1987; Heiskala et al., 1988; Mass et al., 1988; Bogousslavsky et al., 1989; Schwitter et al., 1992; Susac, 1994; Vila et al., 1995; Li et al., 1996; Wildemann et al., 1996; Ballard et al., 1997).

The clinical features of microangiopathy of brain and retina, also called Susac's syndrome, include multiple branch retinal arterial occlusions (Figs. 57.5 and 57.6) and an en-

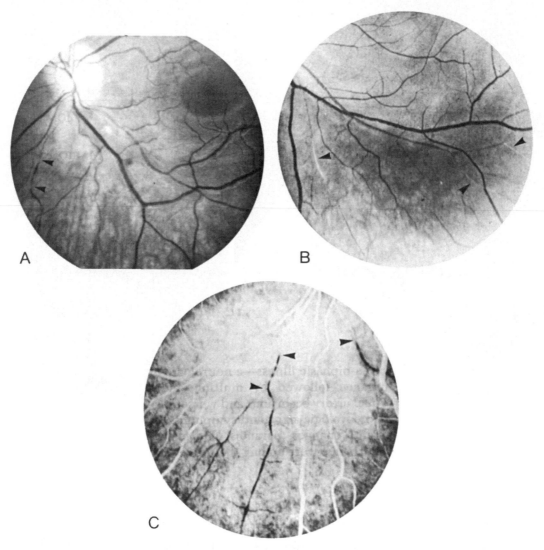

Figure 57.5. Retinal branch arterial occlusions in the syndrome of microangiopathy of the brain and retina. *A,* Appearance of left ocular fundus of a 21-year-old woman with tinnitus, progressive hearing loss, and vertigo. The patient subsequently developed numerous neurologic deficits. About 6 months after the onset of neurologic symptoms and signs, the patient awoke with loss of the upper field of vision in the left eye. Note focal occlusions of a branch retinal arteriole *(arrowheads). B,* Appearance of left ocular fundus in a 21-year-old woman who developed transient diplopia, photophobia, headache, nausea, and vomiting. She then developed ''personality changes.'' The only laboratory abnormalities were a nonspecifically abnormal electroencephalogram and an elevated concentration of protein in the cerebrospinal fluid. The patient improved spontaneously. About 1 year later, however, she developed headache, hearing loss, and a change in her personality shortly after giving birth to an anencephalic child. She was found to be confused and euphoric, with poor memory and a labile mood. Although the patient had no visual complaints, several peripheral retinal arterioles are occluded *(arrowheads). C,* Fluorescein angiogram in the right eye of the same patient shows several branch arterial occlusions *(arrowheads).* (From Coppto JR, Currie JN, Monteiro MLR, et al. A syndrome of arterial-occlusive retinopathy and encephalopathy. Am J Ophthalmol 98:189–202, 1984.)

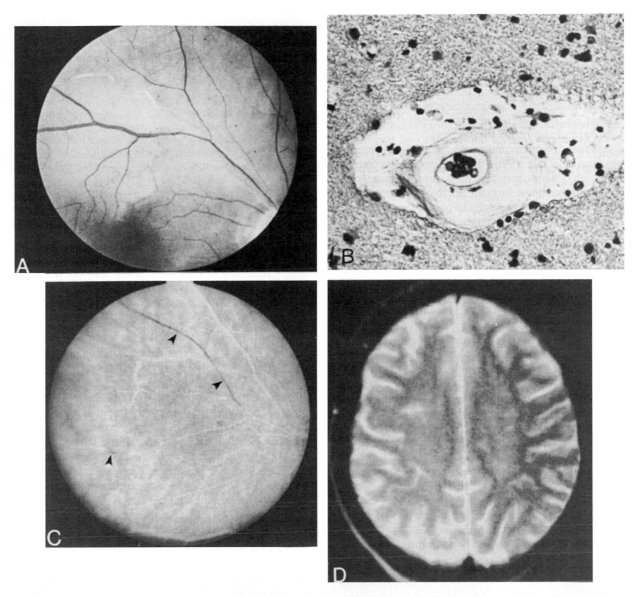

Figure 57.6. Microangiopathy of brain and retina. *A*, Ophthalmoscopic appearance of the right ocular fundus in a 40-year-old woman with headache, confusion, inappropriate behavior, generalized hyperactive deep-tendon reflexes, ankle clonus, and bilateral extensor plantar reflexes. Note narrowed superior temporal retinal artery and subtle nerve fiber layer infarcts. The distal portion of the artery has a "silver streak" appearance. *B*, Brain biopsy from right frontal cortex in the same patient shows sclerosis of media and adventitia of a small cortical blood vessel. Similar changes were seen in small pial vessels. (From Susac JO, Hardman JM, Selhorst JB. Microangiopathy of the brain and retina. Neurology *29*:313–316, 1979.) *C*, Fluorescein angiogram of the right ocular fundus in a 19-year-old woman with headaches, confusion, an unsteady gate, hearing loss, and loss of visual acuity in the right eye. The patient was ataxic, incontinent, and had bilateral extensor plantar reflexes. Visual acuity was 20/50 OD and 20/20 OS. The angiogram shows marked distal arteriolar sheathing and occlusions (*arrowheads*). *D*, T2-weighted axial magnetic resonance image in the same patient shows areas of increased signal intensity in the white matter of both cerebral hemispheres. (From Bogousslavsky J, Gaio J-M, Caplan LR, et al. Encephalopathy, deafness and blindness in young women: A distinct vestibulocochleocerebral arteriolopathy? J Neurol Neurosurg Psychiatry *52*:43–46, 1989.)

cephalopathy characterized by early disturbances in behavior and memory. Hearing loss is so common that the condition was called a "retinocochleocerebral" arteriolopathy by Bogousslavsky et al. (1989). Except for minimal CSF pleocytosis and an increased concentration of protein in the CSF, there are no consistent laboratory or radiographic abnormalities. The condition is not associated with interstitial keratitis,

which differentiates it from Cogan's syndrome (Sigal, 1987). Nonperfused retinal arteriolar segments may contain a white material that stains on fluorescein angiography. Notis et al. (1995) noted retinal vessel wall hyperfluorescence 5 days before retinal infarction, suggesting an underlying endothelial defect. The pathogenesis of this microangiopathic condition remains unclear, but antibody-mediated endothelial

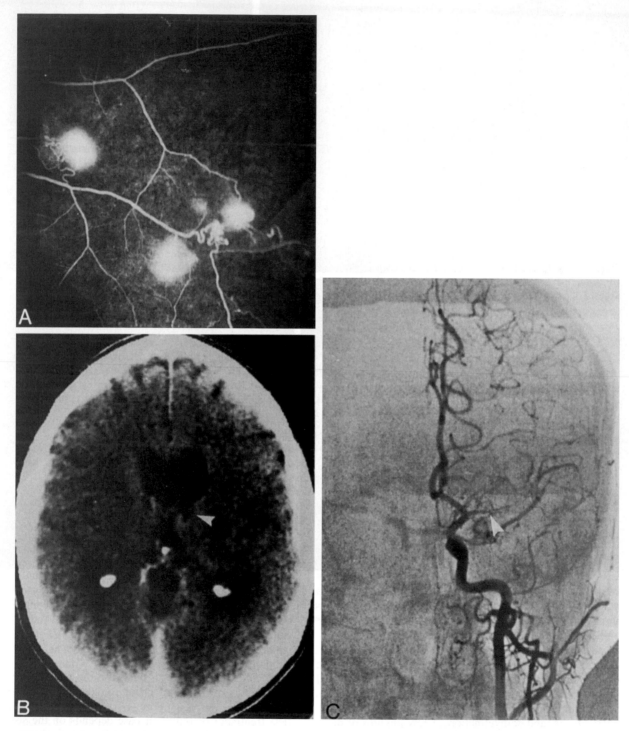

Figure 57.12.   Stroke in Eales' disease. The patient was a 38-year-old man with acute hemiparesis and dysarthria who had noted decreased vision in the left eye 6 months earlier. Visual acuity was 20/40 OD and 20/400 OS with a left relative afferent pupillary defect. *A*, Fluorescein angiogram, late arteriovenous phase, shows leakage from retinal neovascularization posterior to a peripheral zone of nonperfusion. Note multiple arteriovenous shunts and beading of retinal veins. *B*, Enhanced CT scan, axial view, shows hypodensities in the right basal ganglia and left anterior thalamus (*arrowhead*) consistent with cerebral infarctions. *C*, Cerebral arteriogram, anteroposterior view, shows occlusion of the left middle cerebral artery (*arrowhead*). (From Gordon MF, Coyle PK, Golub B. Eale's disease presenting as stroke in the young adult. Ann Neurol *24:*264–266, 1988.)

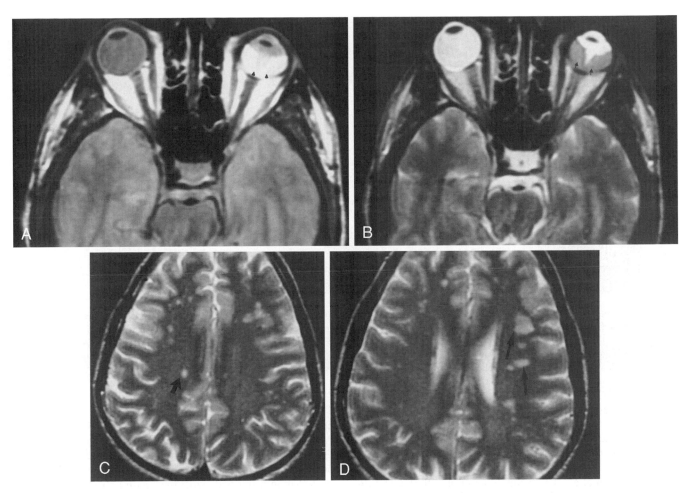

Figure 57.13. Neuroimaging in Eales' disease. Axial magnetic resonance (MR) images of the orbits show intraocular high signal intensity on proton density-weighted images (*A*) and low signal intensity on T2-weighted images (*B*). The shape and density of the signals suggests a complete hemorrhagic retinal detachment (*arrows*). *C* and *D*, Axial T2-weighted MR images at two levels through the cerebral hemispheres show numerous areas of high signal intensity in the supratentorial white matter (*arrows*).

sion itself, nor is there any definitive treatment of the cerebral vasculitis, although systemic corticosteroids are used with mixed results.

Acute Posterior Multifocal Placoid Pigment Epitheliopathy

Acute posterior multifocal placoid pigment epitheliopathy was first described by Gass in 1968 (Gass, 1968a). It is an acute ocular condition, occurring in both men and women from 20 to 50 years of age, that is characterized by loss of central vision associated with the appearance of multiple pale lesions at the level of the retinal pigment epithelium (Gass, 1968a; Bird, 1994). Both eyes usually are affected. Spontaneous recovery occurs within 3 weeks of the onset of the disease. Between 80 and 97% of affected eyes eventually recover visual acuity of 20/40 or better (Lewis and Martonyi, 1975; Damato et al., 1983; Gass, 1983; Saraux and Pelosse, 1987; Williams and Mieler, 1989). Older patients with markedly reduced visual acuity and foveal involvement may have a less favorable prognosis (Pagliarini et al., 1995).

The characteristic change seen in the ocular fundus of a patient with APMPPE consists of multifocal, yellow-white lesions in the posterior pole at the level of the retinal pigment epithelium (Fig. 57.14). The lesions are typically round and discrete. Within 1 week after the appearance of the lesions, the opacification of the pigment epithelium resolves, and within another 2 weeks, a well-defined scar replaces the original lesion (Bird, 1994) (Fig. 57.15). Additional lesions may be seen in the peripheral fundus weeks to months after the onset of the original lesions in the posterior pole.

Patients with APMPPE occasionally have ocular manifestations in addition to the typical chorioretinal placoid lesions. These include iridocyclitis (Savino et al., 1974; Holt et al., 1976), peripheral corneal thinning (Jacklin, 1977), retinal vasculitis with serous detachment of the retina (Bird and Hamilton, 1972; Isashiki et al., 1986), central retinal vein occlusion (Charteris et al., 1989), and anterior optic neuritis or papillitis (Van Buskirk et al., 1971; Kirkham et al., 1972; Savino et al., 1974; Holt et al., 1976; Jacklin, 1977; Miller and Fine, 1977; Priluck et al., 1981) (Fig. 57.16).

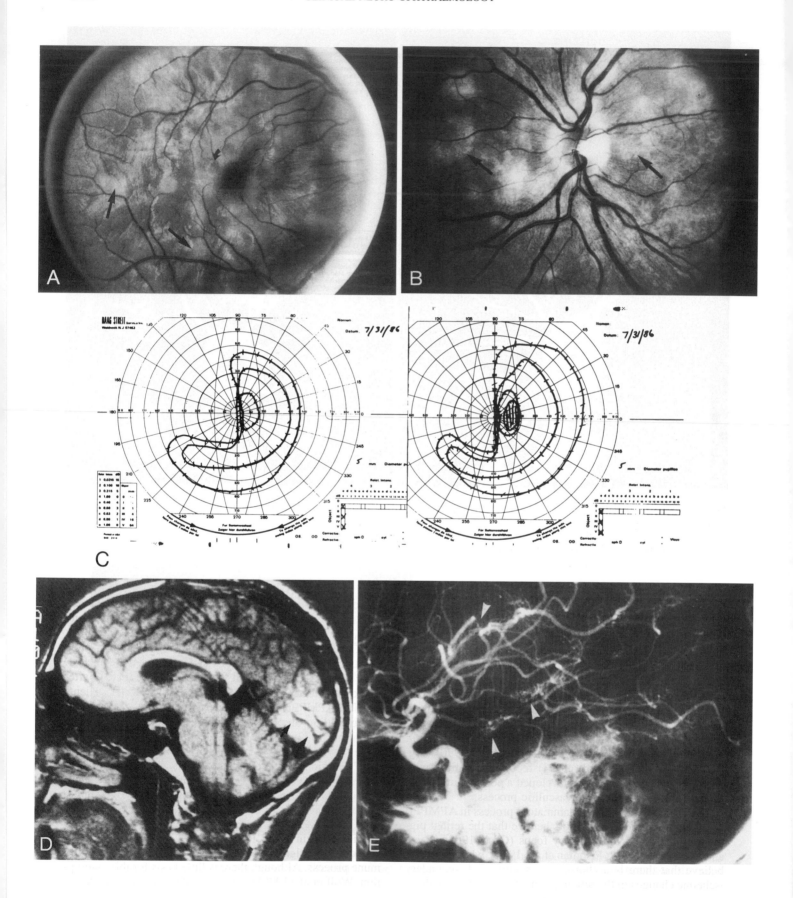

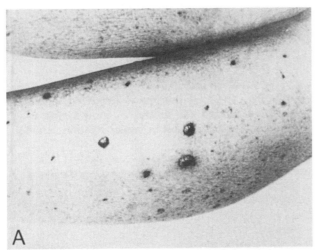

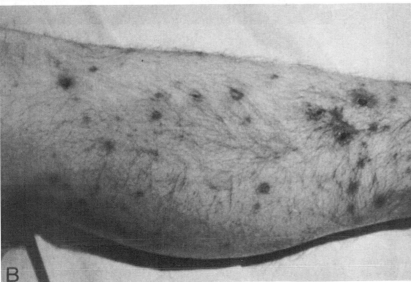

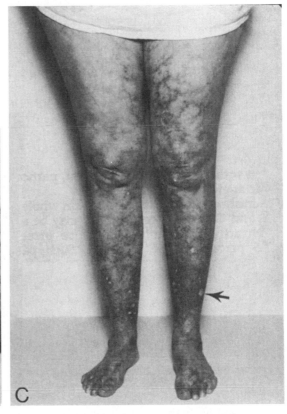

Figure 57.18. Skin lesions of polyarteritis nodosa. *A*, Painful, nodular, hemorrhagic purpura affecting the left leg of a patient with PAN. (From Purcell JJ Jr. Polyarteritis nodosa. In The Eye in Systemic Disease. Editors, Gold DH, Weingeist TA, pp 51–53. Philadelphia, JB Lippincott, 1990.) *B*, Sharply circumscribed infarcts of the skin. The lesions are 1–1.5 cm in diameter and are in various stages of healing. *C*, Livido reticularis of the lower extremities, most marked over the anterior region of the left thigh but also visible over the right thigh, legs below the knees, and dorsa of feet. Petechiae and ulcers (*arrow*) are present on anterior and medial portions of both legs. (From Conn DL, Hunder GG. Vasculitis and related disorders. In Textbook of Rheumatology. Editors, Kelley WN, Harris ED Jr, Ruddy S, et al. 3rd ed, pp 1167–1199. Philadelphia, WB Saunders, 1989.)

oped optic neuritis and a daughter who developed APMPPE within a 6-month period. All three patients had the human leukocyte antigens (HLA) B7 and DR2, suggesting that the patients may have been immunogenetically predisposed to

inflammation in the optic nerve or choroid. In another report, two cousins with recurrent APMPPE had HLA-DR2 but not B7 (Kim et al., 1995). Data from several indocyanine green angiographic studies support an ischemic etiology for APM-

◄───

Figure 57.17. APMPPE associated with cerebral vasculitis. The patient was a 23-year-old man who developed an acute left homonymous hemianopia 2 months after the onset of typical APMPPE. Visual acuity was 20/25 OD and 20/20 OS. *A*, Right ocular fundus shows multiple white-yellow opacities (*long arrows*) in the posterior pole. Several lesions near the fovea show early pigmentation consistent with healing (*short curved arrow*). *B*, Left ocular fundus shows multiple yellow, white, and pigmented lesions (*arrows*) surrounding the optic disc. *C*, The visual field shows an incomplete, congruous, left homonymous hemianopia that is denser above than below. *D*, Unenhanced T1-weighted MR image, sagittal view, shows hyperintensity of the right occipital lobe (*arrows*) consistent with a hemorrhagic infarction. *E*, Right internal carotid arteriogram, lateral view, shows multiple areas of vascular irregularity with evidence of neovascularization (*arrows*). (From Weinstein JM, Bresnick GH, Bell CL, et al. Acute posterior multifocal placoid pigment epitheliopathy associated with cerebral vasculitis. J Clin Neuroophthalmol *8*:195–201, 1988.)

PPE. These studies show areas of early and late hypofluorescence corresponding with regions of choroidal hypoperfusion (Dhaliwal et al., 1993; Yuzawa et al. 1994; Howe et al., 1995).

Most patients with APMPPE do not require treatment for the condition because it is of short duration, associated with visual recovery, and limited to the eye. Systemic corticosteroids and other immunosuppressive agents are usually given to patients with extremely poor visual acuity or evidence of associated cerebral vasculitis. Corticosteroids in combination with cyclophosphamide for 6–12 months is one proposed regimen for patients with cerebral arteritis (Comu et al., 1996). A recurrence of the disorder after withdrawal of systemic corticosteroids was reported by Lewis and Martonyi (1975), and Charteris et al. (1989) reported a central retinal vein occlusion in the eye of a patient with APMPPE 1 week after steroids were stopped.

Systemic Necrotizing Vasculitides

Polyarteritis Nodosa (Periarteritis Nodosa)

Polyarteritis nodosa is a disease of small and medium-sized arteries. It may damage any organ, but the skin, joints, peripheral nerves, gastrointestinal tract, and kidney are most often affected (Conn et al., 1993). The disorder ranges in severity from a limited to a progressive fulminant disease.

DEMOGRAPHICS

PAN is an uncommon disorder, with an annual rate of incidence of about 0.2–0.7 per 100,000 (Masi, 1967; Kurland et al., 1969) and an overall prevalence of 2–6 per 100,000 (Kurland et al., 1969, 1984). The disease is more common in men, with a sex ratio of about 2 to 1. Persons of all ages are affected, but the condition is more common in patients 40–60 years of age. PAN is usually a sporadic condition, but it may occasionally be familial (Schneider and Goldman, 1962; Reveille et al., 1989).

SYSTEMIC MANIFESTATIONS

PAN has a varied presentation, ranging from mild, limited disease to a fulminating and rapidly fatal condition (Cohen et al., 1980). Most patients experience **constitutional symptoms** of fever, malaise, and weight loss. These symptoms are associated with manifestations of multiple system damage, including skin lesions, a peripheral neuropathy, and asymmetric polyarthritis.

The **skin lesions** are many and varied. They include palpable purpura, ulcerations, livedo reticularis, and ischemic changes of the distal digits (Figs. 57.18 and 57.19).

The **peripheral neuropathy** may be the initial manifestation of PAN and eventually occurs in about 50–60% of patients with the condition (Moore and Cupps, 1983). It may affect the upper or lower extremities. The onset may be sudden, with pain and paresthesias radiating in the distribution of a peripheral nerve, followed in hours or days by a motor deficit of the same nerve. This may progress asymmetrically to affect other peripheral nerves and produce a mononeuritis

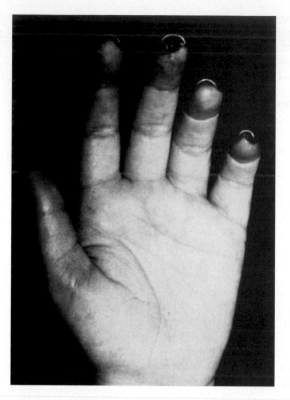

Figure 57.19. Ischemia of the distal digits in a patient with polyarteritis nodosa. (Courtesy of Dr. Douglas Jabs.)

multiplex or a multiple mononeuropathy. As progressive damage occurs, a symmetric polyneuropathy develops that is characterized by diffuse motor and sensory dysfunction. Healing occurs with time and appropriate therapy. Residual symptoms are more frequent in the legs than in the arms, and such symptoms are more likely to be sensory than motor (Moore and Cupps, 1983). Histologic studies of affected nerves show occlusion of the vasa nervorum (Dyck et al., 1972; Wees et al., 1982).

An asymmetric, episodic, nondeforming **polyarthritis** affecting the larger joints of the lower extremity develops in 20% of cases and is common in the early stages of the disease.

Evidence of damage to visceral organs such as the kidneys, gastrointestinal tract, heart, and lungs may occur at the time of onset of the disease or later (Conn et al., 1993; Valente et al., 1997) (Fig. 57.20). Clinical evidence of **renal damage** includes proteinuria and microscopic hematuria. In one series, progressive renal failure was the cause of death in 65% of cases (Rose, 1957). Acute renal failure may also occur but is rare (Ladefoged et al., 1969). **Systemic hypertension** not infrequently results from the chronic effects of persistent renal disease. **Abdominal pain** is the most common gastrointestinal symptom. Localized pain may indicate involvement of the gallbladder or appendix, whereas diffuse abdominal pain may indicate mesenteric thrombosis with or without peritonitis, particularly when there is associated abdominal distention. Hematemesis and melena are caused by vasculitis of the upper and lower gastrointestinal tracts, respectively. **Cardiac damage** is more common pathologically than clinically. Nevertheless, patients with PAN may develop symptomatic or silent myocardial infarction, congestive heart failure, or arrythmia (Fig. 57.21). Clinical **involvement of the lung** is rare in patients with PAN. When it occurs, however, it tends to be characterized by a diffuse infiltration that may precede evidence of involvement of other organs.

CENTRAL NERVOUS SYSTEM MANIFESTATIONS

Clinically apparent damage to the CNS occurs in about 23–53% of patients with PAN (Sheehan et al., 1958; Ford and Siekert, 1965; Travers et al., 1979; Moore and Fauci, 1981; Moore and Cupps, 1983). It is less common than peripheral nervous system disease, and it usually is a late manifestation of PAN (Sigal, 1987). Patients with PAN experience a variety of different neurologic disturbances. Two common presentations are: (*a*) a diffuse encephalopathy that affects cognitive function or level of altertness and (*b*) focal or multifocal disturbances of the brain or spinal cord (Moore and Cupps, 1983). Both are caused by vasculitis, either of the intracranial vessels or of the vessels of the head and neck. The diffuse encephalopathy usually is insidious in onset but can evolve within a single day. Focal or generalized seizures may occur. Hypertension may accompany or follow the de-

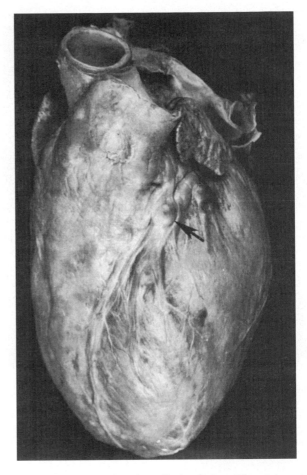

Figure 57.21. Polyarteritis nodosa affecting the heart. Necrotizing arteritis affecting the coronary arteries has produced an aneurysm arising from the proximal portion of the left anterior descending coronary artery (*arrow*). (From Conn DL, Hunder GG. Vasculitis and related disorders. In Textbook of Rheumatology. Editors, Kelley WN, Harris ED Jr, Ruddy S, et al. 3rd ed, pp 1167–1199. Philadelphia, WB Saunders, 1989.)

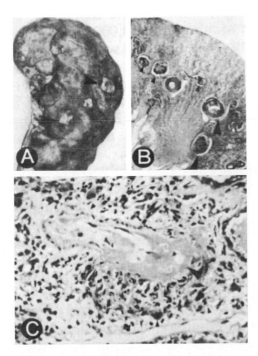

Figure 57.20. Kidney damage in a patient with polyarteritis nodosa. *A*, External surface of kidney shows multiple infarcts (*arrowheads*). *B*, There is aneurysmal dilation of interlobar (*large arrowheads*) and arcuate (*small arrowheads*) arteries. *C*, An arcuate artery shows severe necrotizing inflammation with fibrinoid necrosis (*arrowhead*). (From Wagoner RD, Holly KE. Parenchymal renal disease: Clinical and pathologic features. In Textbook of Renal Pathophysiology. Editor, Knox FG, pp 226–253. Hagerstown, MD, Harper & Row, 1978.)

velopment of the encephalopathy. In such cases, therapy must be directed at both the vasculitis and the hypertension. The symptoms of encephalopathy associated with PAN may resolve spontaneously over days to weeks, and recurrence is unusual.

Focal neurologic dysfunction other than peripheral neuropathy is caused by stroke, and it usually is sudden in onset (Moore and Cupps, 1983). The dysfunction may result from damage to cerebral cortex, brainstem, cerebellum, or a combination of these (Maitland et al., 1986; Sedwick and Margo, 1989). Isolated homonymous hemianopia may occur in this setting. Strokes that occur in the setting of PAN may be hemorrhagic or ischemic (see Chapter 55).

Lomeo et al. (1989) described a patient with PAN and systemic hypertension who developed a spontaneous dissection of the internal carotid artery characterized by left-sided headache and neck pain that were worsened by a change of head position. It is unclear if the dissection was caused by vasculitis, was related to the patient's hypertension, or was an unrelated fortuitous event.

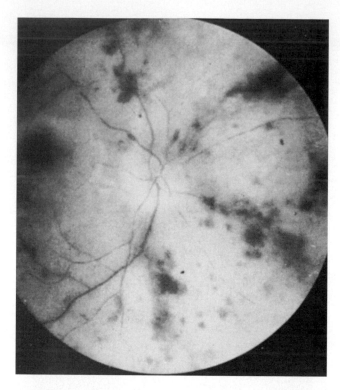

Figure 57.22. Retinal vasculitis in polyarteritis nodosa. Diffuse retinal edema, retinal hemorrhages, and markedly narrowed retinal vessels in a 71-year-old man with biopsy-proven PAN, a right homonymous hemianopia, and decreased vision in the right eye. (From Haskjold E, Froland S, Egge K. Ocular polyarteritis nodosa: Report of a case. Acta Ophthalmol *65:*749–751, 1987.)

OCULAR AND NEURO-OPHTHALMOLOGIC MANIFESTATIONS

Ocular manifestations occur in 10–20% of patients with PAN (Jabs, 1994). Intraocular findings include hypertensive retinopathy associated with chronic or acute renal failure, cotton-wool spots, and branch and central retinal artery occlusions related to intraocular vasculitis (Gaynon and Asbury, 1943; Goar and Smith, 1952; Wise, 1952; Duguid, 1954; Böck, 1956; Sheehan et al., 1958; Blodi and Sullivan, 1959; Rosen, 1968; Solomon and Solomon, 1978; Kincaid and Schatz, 1983; Morgan et al., 1986; Haskjold et al., 1987; Graham et al., 1989) (Fig. 57.22). In rare cases, retinal veins are affected (Morgan et al., 1986). Marginal corneal ulceration, episcleritis, keratitis, uveitis, necrotizing scleritis, and nonrhegmatogenous retinal detachment from choroidal ischemia can also occur (Goldsmith, 1946; Herbert and McPherson, 1947; Ingalls, 1951; Cogan, 1955; Moore and Sevel, 1966; Walsh and Hoyt, 1969a; Kielar, 1976; Stefani et al., 1978; Purcell et al., 1984; Brown et al., 1985; Morgan et al., 1986; Kinyoun et al., 1987; Purcell, 1990) (Fig. 57.23).

Both anterior optic neuropathy (with optic disc swelling) and posterior or retrobulbar optic neuropathy (without optic disc swelling) occur in patients with PAN (Goldstein and Wexler, 1937; Kimbrell and Wheliss, 1967; Saraux et al., 1982a, 1982b; Denis et al., 1984; Hutchinson, 1984; Haskjold et al., 1987). The acute, painless onset of visual loss in such patients is most compatible with an ischemic process, presumably resulting from inflammatory occlusion of the posterior ciliary arteries (Fig. 57.24). Nevertheless, some cases of optic neuropathy may result from inflammation of the nerve itself (Goldstein and Wexler, 1937) (Fig. 57.25). The optic neuropathy of PAN may be unilateral or bilateral. When bilateral, it may affect both eyes simultaneously, or one eye may be affected days, weeks, or even months before the second eye (Kimbrell and Wheliss, 1967). Saraux et al. (1982b) reported a patient with PAN who developed an acute anterior optic neuropathy in the right eye. One week later, she developed a visual field defect in the left eye from a retrobulbar optic neuropathy.

Patients with PAN may experience transient monocular

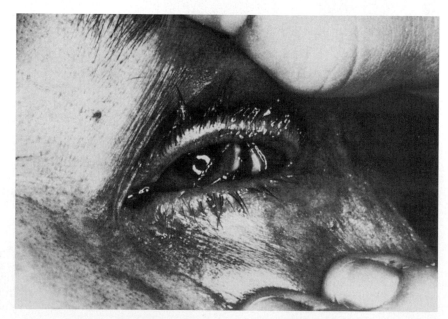

Figure 57.23. Necrotizing scleritis in a patient with polyarteritis nodosa. (From Purcell JJ Jr. Polyarteritis nodosa. In The Eye in Systemic Disease. Editors, Gold DH, Weingeist TA, pp 51–53. Philadelphia, JB Lippincott, 1990.)

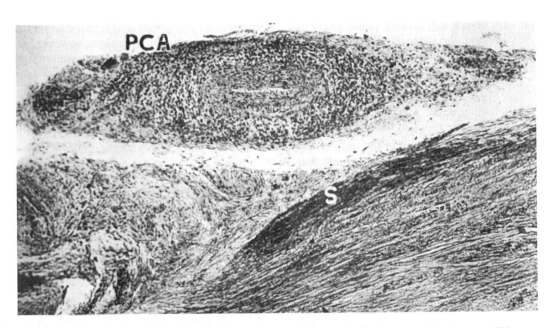

Figure 57.24. Inflammatory occlusion of a posterior ciliary artery in a 45-year-old man who died 4 months after the onset of biopsy-proven PAN. The patient had lost vision in both eyes shortly before death. Cross-section through a short posterior ciliary artery (*PCA*) shows that the adventitia, media, and intima of the vessel are infiltrated with chronic inflammatory cells that have occluded the lumen. *S*, sclera. (From Goldstein I, Wexler D. Bilateral atrophy of the optic nerve in periarteritis nodosa. Arch Ophthalmol *18:*767–773, 1937.)

visual loss. The episodes result from transient ischemia to the retina, optic nerve, or both. The ischemia may be caused by arteritis with thrombosis of any of the arteries that supply the eye, including the common carotid, internal carotid, ophthalmic, central retinal, or posterior ciliary arteries. Newman

et al. (1974) reported the case of a 48-year-old man with biopsy-proven PAN who began to experience transient monocular loss of peripheral vision. The episodes of visual loss were characterized by concentric narrowing of the visual field over 1–2 minutes until there remained only a central

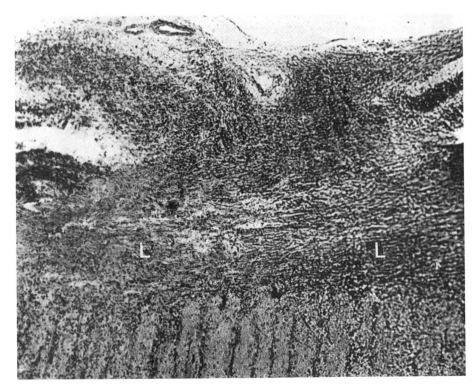

Figure 57.25. Inflammation of the optic nerve in polyarteritis nodosa. The patient was a 25-year-old man who died 4 months after developing biopsy-proven PAN. The patient lost vision in both eyes shortly before death. Histopathologic appearance of the proximal portion of the optic nerve shows diffuse infiltration by chronic inflammatory cells. *L*, lamina cribrosa. (From Goldstein I, Wexler D. Bilateral atrophy of the optic nerve in periarteritis nodosa. Arch Ophthalmol *18:*767–773, 1937.)

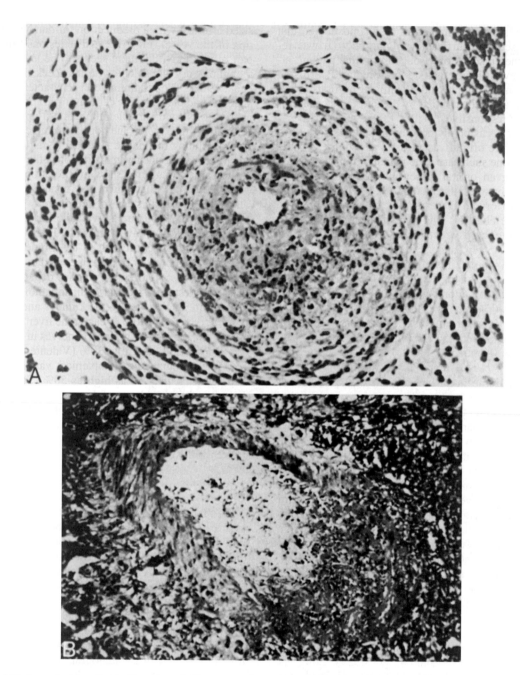

Figure 57.27. Pathology of acute polyarteritis nodosa. *A,* Numerous polymorphonuclear leukocytes and lymphocytes are infiltrating the adventitia and media of an orbital artery, producing necrosis of the vessel wall. *B,* The right lower portion of the wall of another artery shows fibrinoid necrosis with formation of a microaneurysm. There is marked infiltration of the vessel wall by polymorphonuclear leukocytes. (Courtesy of Dr. JT Lie.)

17-year-old girl who gradually developed an unsteady gait and visual blurring associated with a 15-pound weight loss, weakness, and episodes of incoherent speech. Physical examination showed apathy, blunted affect, and severe cognitive defects. The patient had generalized ataxia, increased deep tendon reflexes, and downbeat nystagmus. A variety of serologic studies were normal or gave negative results except for an elevated ESR. CT scans, cerebral arteriography, and analysis of CSF gave normal results. The patient subsequently developed mononeuritis multiplex. At this time, renal, celiac, and mesenteric arteriograms revealed multiple abnormalities consistent with vasculitis, and a diagnosis of PAN was made.

PAN is not the same entity as a disorder called **microscopic polyangiitis**. Microscopic polyangiitis tends to affect small vessels such as capillaries, venules, and arterioles, and it has a propensity to produce lung hemorrhage. In addition, microscopic polyangiitis is associated with antineutrophilic cytoplasmic antibodies (ANCAs), but not hepatitis B infection (Guillevin and Lhote, 1995).

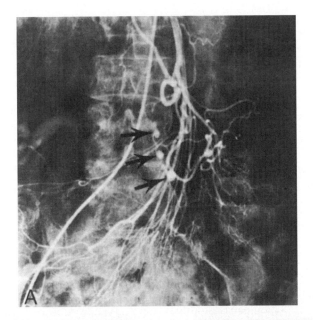

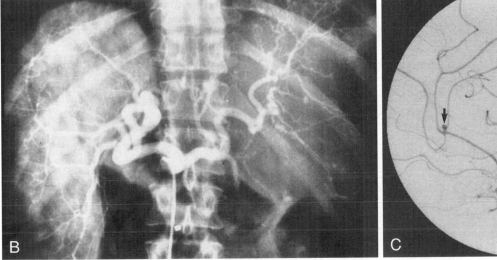

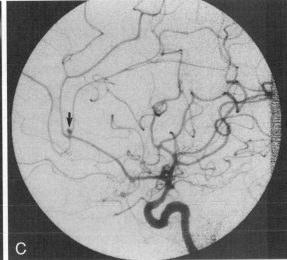

Figure 57.28. Results of arteriography in polyarteritis nodosa. *A*, Superior mesenteric arteriogram shows several small aneurysms (*arrows*) in branches of the superior mesenteric artery in a patient with PAN. (Courtesy of Dr. AW Stanson.) *B*, Celiac arteriogram in another patient with PAN shows arterial irregularity and aneurysm formation that is especially severe on the left side. (Courtesy of Dr. Douglas Jabs.) *C*, Cerebral arteriogram in patient with polyarteritis nodosa. Lateral view shows tapered supraclinoid internal carotid artery and a distal aneurysm (*arrow*). (From Hurst RW, Grossman RI. Neuroradiology of central nervous system vasculitis. Semin Neurol *14:*32–340, 1994).

PROGNOSIS AND TREATMENT

Untreated patients with PAN have a 5-year survival rate of only 13% (Moore and Cupps, 1983; Conn and Hunder, 1989). The use of systemic corticosteroids improves survival to about 48% (Fauci et al., 1978), and when corticosteroids are given in combination with cytotoxic agents such as cyclophosphamide or azathioprine, the overall rate of survival is about 80% (Frohnert and Sheps, 1967; Leib et al., 1979; Moore and Cupps, 1983). In the series reported by Moore and Fauci (1981), no patient showed progression or experienced new neurologic dysfunction while receiving cyclophosphamide. In patients with normal renal function and no major organ involvement, it may be reasonable to begin treatment only with corticosteroids (Hoffman and Fauci, 1994); however, patients with renal, cardiac, or neurologic manifestations typically require the addition of a cytotoxic agent. Patients with PAN isolated to the skin have a benign prognosis but may suffer chronic relapses (Siberry et al., 1994). Some of these patients go on to develop systemic PAN requiring aggressive immunosuppressive therapy.

Despite treatment, death may occur in patients with PAN from the effects of the disease or from the effects of its treatment. PAN commonly follows an acute course, and most deaths occur within the first year (Sack et al., 1975; Cohen et al., 1980). These deaths are usually caused by uncontrolled vasculitis or by the infectious complications of treatment, particularly when cyclosphosphamide is used (Bradley et al., 1989). Deaths that occur later in the course of the disease usually result from vascular complications of the disease, such as myocardial infarction or renal disease, or from complications of treatment (Fortin et al., 1995). Patients with PAN associated with hepatitis B infection are best treated with steroids, α-interferon, and plasma exchange (Guillevin et al., 1992, 1994).

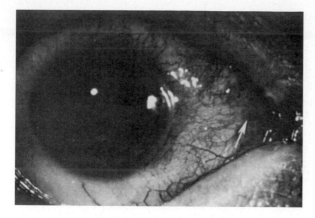

Figure 57.29. Conjunctival involvement in Churg-Strauss syndrome. The patient was a 64-year-old man with a 2-month history of rhinitis, bronchitis, and otitis media who developed a swollen right upper eyelid. Note diffuse injection of conjunctiva and area of conjunctival thickening near the plica semilunaris (*arrow*). (From Shields CL, Shields JA, Rozanski TI. Conjunctival involvement in Churg-Strauss syndrome. Am J Ophthalmol *102:* 601–605, 1986.)

Allergic Angiitis and Granulomatosis (Churg-Strauss Vasculitis)

In 1951, Churg and Strauss described 13 patients with severe bronchial asthma and disseminated necrotizing vasculitis. All 13 patients had fever, eosinophilia, and clinical evidence of multisystem damage associated with a histologic pattern of necrotizing arteritis, eosinophilic infiltration of tissue, and extravascular granulomas. Churg and Strauss (1951) considered this condition an entity distinct from PAN and called it ''allergic granulomatosis.''

DEMOGRAPHICS

Allergic angiitis and granulomatosis, also called the Churg-Strauss syndrome or Churg-Strauss vasculitis, affects men twice as often as women. The age at onset varies from 15 to 70 years, with a mean of about 40 years (Chumbley et al., 1977; Conn et al., 1993; Valente et al., 1997). The cause of this condition is unknown. There is no direct evidence to suggest an infectious agent, although immunoglobulins and complement were demonstrated in vessel walls in one case (Hunder and Lie, 1983), and elevated concentrations of serum IgE were demonstrated in several cases (Conn et al., 1976).

SYSTEMIC MANIFESTATIONS

Respiratory manifestations are usually the first feature of the disease (DeRemee et al., 1980). Asthma is the most frequent disorder, although some patients develop bronchitis or pneumonitis. Isolated respiratory disease is usually present for many years before there is evidence of systemic disease (Chumbley et al., 1977).

Cutaneous lesions develop in about two-thirds of patients with Churg-Strauss syndrome (Finan and Winkelmann, 1983). Subcutaneous nodules are the most common lesions, but petechiae, purpura, and infarction of the skin may occur (Conn et al., 1993; Valente et al., 1997).

Peripheral neuropathy, usually mononeuritis multiplex, is found in most patients. It usually develops late in the course of the disease.

Cardiac damage occurs in some patients with Churg-Strauss syndrome. It usually causes congestive heart failure but may cause myocardial infarction.

Abdominal symptoms occur in some patients from granulomatous vasculitis affecting the vessels of the gastrointestinal tract. Patients may experience infarction, ulceration,

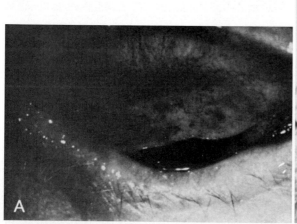
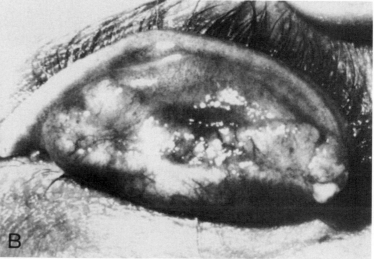

Figure 57.30. Eyelid involvement in Churg-Strauss syndrome. *A*, In a 64-year-old man with rhinitis, bronchitis, and otitis media who developed swelling of the right upper eyelid, the tarsus is thickened and has increased vascularity. A biopsy established the diagnosis of Churg-Strauss syndrome. (From Shields CL, Shields JA, Rozanski TI. Conjunctival involvement in Churg-Strauss syndrome. Am J Ophthalmol *102:*601–605, 1986.) *B*, Numerous nodules of the superior tarsal conjunctiva are seen in another patient with biopsy-proven Churg-Strauss syndrome. (From Robin JB, Schanzlin DJ, Meisler DM, et al. Ocular imvolvement in the respiratory vasculitides. Surv Ophthalmol *30:*127–140, 1985.)

and even perforation of the stomach, small intestine, or large intestine. Granulomatous involvement of the bowel, liver, or omentum may produce a palpable abdominal mass.

Renal disease develops in a variable number of patients with Churg-Strauss syndrome, although renal failure is uncommon (Lanham et al., 1984). Eosinophilic granulomas of the prostate and lower urinary tract are a unique feature of this disease, and they may cause urinary retention.

CNS manifestations of Churg-Strauss syndrome are rare. Seizures may occasionally occur (Valente et al., 1997), and some patients develop focal cerebral or brainstem signs, such as individual or multiple cranial nerve pareses (Rackemann and Greene, 1939; Harkavy, 1941; Chumbley et al., 1977).

OCULAR AND NEURO-OPHTHALMOLOGIC MANIFESTATIONS

Ocular involvement in Churg-Strauss syndrome is uncommon (Robin et al., 1985; Alberts et al., 1994). Eosinophilic granulomas may develop on the eyelids or conjunctiva (Ashton and Cook, 1978; Meisler et al., 1981; Nissim et al., 1982; Shields et al., 1986) (Figs. 57.29 and 57.30), and similar lesions may develop on or within the eye itself, producing episcleritis, scleritis, and panuveitis (Cury et al., 1955). Chumbley et al. (1977) described the findings in 30 patients with Churg-Strauss syndrome, one of whom developed a marginal corneal ulcer. Neuro-ophthalmologic disturbances in Churg-Strauss syndrome include episodes of transient monocular visual loss, retinal ischemia, branch and central retinal artery occlusion, ischemic optic neuropathy, and various cranial neuropathies including ocular motor nerve pareses (Rackemann and Greene, 1939; Harkavy, 1941; Weinstein et al., 1983; Dagi and Currie, 1985; Lanham and Churg, 1991) (Fig. 57.31). Alberts et al. (1994) described a 76-year-old woman who developed asthma, peripheral neuropathy, jaw claudication, and visual loss in one eye from anterior ischemic optic neuropathy (AION). A temporal artery biopsy revealed an eosinophilic vasculitis without giant cells. The patient's vision improved from hand motions to 20/60 with high-dose corticosteroid treatment. This case emphasizes that the clinical presentation of Churg-Strauss and other vasculitides may occasionally mimic the profile of GCA.

PATHOLOGY

The characteristic pathologic changes in Churg-Strauss syndrome include small necrotizing granulomas and necrotizing vasculitis that affect primarily small arteries and venules (Churg and Strauss, 1951) but also damage capillaries (Lichtig et al., 1989). The granulomas are typically about 1 mm or more in diameter, and they are commonly located near small arteries or veins (Fig. 57.32). They are composed of a central eosinophilic core surrounded radially by macrophages and giant cells (Fig. 57.33). Inflammatory cells are also present in the granulomas, with eosinophils predominating in the early stages of development. Macrophages and giant cells predominate in the more chronic lesions.

The vascular lesions of Churg-Strauss syndrome may be seen in all stages of development. Acutely, there is segmental fibrinoid necrosis with a leukocytic infiltration characterized primarily by eosinophils in the vessel walls and perivascular

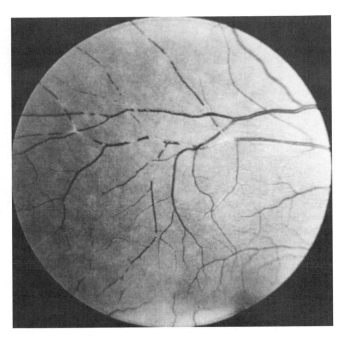

Figure 57.31. Branch retinal artery occlusion in a patient with Churg-Strauss syndrome. The patient was a 46-year-old Asian woman with Churg-Strauss syndrome characterized by a history of adult-onset asthma, intermittent petechial and purpuric vesicular rashes, fevers, recurrent sinusitis, mononeuritis multiplex, an elevated erythrocyte sedimentation rate, an eosinophilia in the peripheral blood that ranged from 10 to 70%, and a biopsy from several tissues showing acute and chronic vasculitis with a prominent eosinophilic component. Onset of visual loss in the right eye was sudden; visual acuity was 20/200 in the right eye, and there was a relative afferent pupillary defect on the right. The right ocular fundus shows multiple branch retinal arterial occlusions with white intraluminal material in the superior retinal arterial arcade. The patient was treated with low molecular weight dextran, heparin, and systemic corticosteroids with improvement in vision. (From Dagi LR, Currie J. Branch retinal artery occlusion in Churg-Strauss syndrome. J Clin Neuroophthalmol 5:229–237, 1985.)

spaces. Aneurysms or thrombosis may occur. Chronic changes of endothelial proliferation, narrowing of the lumen, and reparative fibrosis of affected vessels all occur during healing. An important feature in many arterial lesions is the presence of macrophages and giant cells around necrotic areas (Conn et al., 1993; Valente et al., 1997).

DIAGNOSIS

The diagnosis of Churg-Strauss syndrome is made on the basis of both clinical and pathologic features. The development of systemic disease in a middle-aged patient with a history of asthma should alert the physician to the possible diagnosis. Diagnostically helpful features are noncavitary lung infiltrates, nodular skin lesions, heart failure, and significant eosinophilia that often accounts for 50% of the white blood cell count. Perinuclear ANCAs (P. ANCAs) are found in about 70% of patients (Guillevin et al., 1993; Valente et al., 1997). The diagnosis is substantiated by biopsy of affected tissues, such as the lung, skin, or prostate, revealing the characteristic eosinophilic necrotizing extravascular granulomas and vasculitis affecting small vessels. The American College

SYSTEMIC MANIFESTATIONS

The mean age at onset of GCA is 70 years, with a range of about 50 to more than 90 years of age (Hunder, 1996). This is also the mean age of onset of polymyalgia rheumatica (PMR), a disorder characterized by aching and morning stiffness in the proximal portions of the extremities and torso and an elevated ESR that is believed by some authors to be a manifestation or limited form of GCA (Sumkin and Healey, 1969; Rynes et al., 1977; Papadakis and Schwartz, 1986; Hunder, 1993; Turnbull, 1996; Hunder, 1997). Whereas GCA affects men and women equally, PMR affects women about twice as often as men (Hunder and Allen, 1978–1979).

The onset of GCA may be abrupt or insidious. Visual and neurologic symptoms usually begin acutely, whereas systemic symptoms are most often slowly progressive. In most instances, GCA begins with systemic symptoms that may be present for weeks or months before the diagnosis is established. However, there is no specific set of clinical features that absolutely predicts a positive temporal artery biopsy (Gabriel et al., 1995).

Constitutional symptoms, including fatigue, anorexia, and weight loss, occur in most patients and may be the only evidence of the disease (Klein et al., 1975; Healey and Wilske, 1977, 1978; Jabs, 1994; Hunder, 1996). Other patients develop nonspecific arthralgias and myalgias (Keltner, 1982).

Alterations in mental status, including depression, delusional thinking, impairment of memory, malaise, and frank dementia, may occur (Shenberger et al., 1981; Pascuzzi et al., 1989). These symptoms may be the earliest manifestations of the disease, although they may be ignored or misinterpreted by both the patient and the physician, especially when the patient is elderly (Paulley and Hughes, 1960; Hamilton et al., 1971). Neuroimaging studies performed in patients with GCA-related dementia often show evidence of multiple cerebral infarcts (Caselli and Hunder, 1993).

Headache is the most common symptom of GCA, being present in 40–90% of patients (Hamilton et al., 1971; Hunder et al., 1975; Huston et al., 1978; Goodman, 1979; Keltner, 1982; McDonnell et al., 1986; Machado et al., 1987, 1988), and it is also the most common initial symptom (Calamia and Hunder, 1980). The pain is frequently marked and lancinating in quality. It is often localized to the regions along the arteries of the scalp but may be much less well defined (Hunder, 1993).

Scalp tenderness is a common symptom in patients with GCA, particularly those with headache (Keltner, 1982; Hunder, 1993, 1996, 1997). The tenderness is usually localized to the temporal or occipital arteries (Fig. 57.35), but in some cases it is diffuse. We examined a 72-year-old woman who was correctly diagnosed as having GCA after she complained of a single spot of tenderness in the right superior parietal region that she discovered when she attempted to brush her hair. Tender spots or nodules may develop over any part of the scalp, particularly over the course of the superficial temporal artery (Fig. 57.36). We saw a 67-year-old man with diplopia who was thought to have myasthenia gravis. The patient initially denied any systemic or focal symptoms, but during the examination, which was performed in the early evening, he seemed to be extremely tired. When asked about this, he admitted that he had not been sleeping well because his right temple was so tender that he could not tolerate any pressure on it. He tried to sleep on his left side, but whenever he inadvertently turned over in his sleep, he developed pain that would awaken immediately. We have examined other patients who first noted severe tenderness of the temples when they attempted to put on glasses.

Intermittent claudication may occur in the muscles of the jaw, the neck, the extremities, and, rarely, the tongue or throat. Patients not infrequently complain of jaw, ear, or neck pain when they chew or swallow. The pain is thought to arise from ischemic damage to the muscles of mastication supplied by the facial artery. It is often more severe on one side, and is one of the strongest predictors of GCA (Hayreh et al., 1997). In severe cases, there also may be trismus and dysphagia (Desser, 1969). Similar pain may occur when moving an extremity supplied by an affected artery. In extreme cases, inflammatory thrombosis of an artery causes gangrene of the scalp, an extremity, or even the tongue (Hunder, 1993, 1997).

Facial swelling can occur in patients with GCA (Cohen et al., 1982; Manganelli et al., 1992; Ghanchi et al., 1996a).

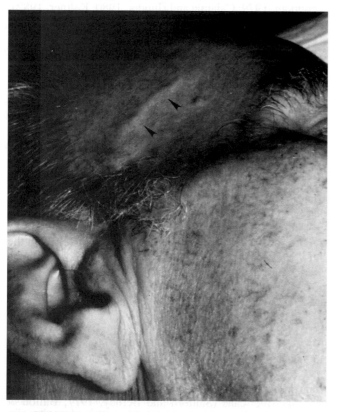

Figure 57.35. Tender, prominent temporal artery (*arrowheads*) in a 65-year-old man with sudden loss of vision in the right eye, a swollen right optic disc, and an elevated erythrocyte sedimentation rate. Biopsy of this artery revealed evidence of giant cell arteritis.

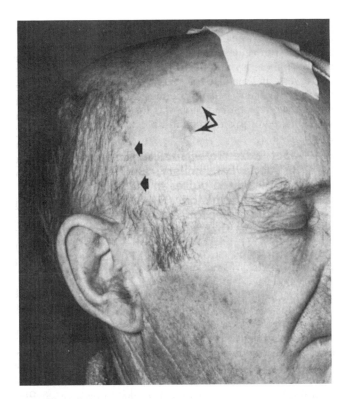

Figure 57.36.   Giant cell arteritis affecting the temporal artery. Short segments of the anterior branch of the vessel were tender and erythematous (*long arrows*). Biopsy of the posterior branch of the vessel (*short arrows*) has been performed. (From Hunder GG. Giant cell arteritis and polymyalgia rheumatica. In Textbook of Rheumatology. Editors, Kelley WN, Harris ED Jr, Ruddy S, et al. 3rd ed, pp 1200–1208. Philadelphia, WB Saunders, 1989.)

This sign develops because of occlusion of the facial artery by the disease and may be a predictor of visual loss in the ipsilateral eye (Ghanchi et al., 1996a).

Prominent **respiratory tract symptoms** occur in about 10% of patients with GCA (Karam and Fulmer, 1982; Larson et al., 1984; Kramer et al., 1987; Ladanzi and Fraser, 1987). These symptoms include productive and nonproductive cough, sore throat, and hoarseness. They occur because of ischemia of the trachea and bronchial tree caused by systemic vasculitis (Paice, 1989).

Cardiovascular manifestations occur in patients with GCA from the effects of vasculitis upon the coronary arteries or aorta. Affected patients may experience angina pectoris, or they may develop congestive heart failure or myocardial infarction that may prove fatal (Crompton, 1959; Spencer and Hoyt, 1960; McKusick, 1962; Harrison and Bevan, 1967; Harris, 1968; Lie et al., 1986; Hupp et al., 1990; Morris and Scheib, 1994). There is also an increased incidence of aortic aneurysms and dissection in patients with GCA (Evans et al., 1995).

Gastrointestinal manifestations of GCA are extremely rare. Harrison (1948) reported microscopic evidence of arteritis in the mesenteric arteries of a patient with GCA, and Russell (1959) described a 75-year-old woman who devel-

oped severe abdominal pain and vomiting during the course of her illness and was found at laparotomy to have a gangrenous segment of small bowel. The affected segment of bowel was excised, and histopathologic examination of the tissue revealed evidence of a necrotizing arteritis.

About 15% of patients with GCA initially develop a **fever** for which no obvious cause can be found (Ghose et al., 1976). This "fever of unknown origin" is often higher than 39 C, and it may be associated with shaking chills (Paulley and Hughes, 1960; Healey and Wilske, 1977, 1978; Calamia and Hunder, 1981).

NEUROLOGIC MANIFESTATIONS

Neurologic disturbances occur in about 30% of patients with GCA (Andrews, 1966; Cochran et al., 1978; Lipton et al., 1987; Caselli et al., 1988a, 1988b; Hunder, 1996). These are diverse, but the most common are peripheral neuropathies, TIAs, and strokes.

The **peripheral neuropathies** include mononeuropathies and polyneuropathies that may affect the upper or lower extremities (Paulley and Hughes, 1960; Warrell et al., 1968; Mulcahy et al., 1984; Feigal et al., 1985; Caselli et al., 1988a; Caselli and Hunder, 1993). The median nerve seems to be most frequently affected, but other nerves, including the ulnar, radial, peroneal, tibial, and sciatic, may also be affected. Spinal nerves may be involved, and the fifth cervical nerve appears to be particularly vulnerable (Caselli and Hunder, 1993). Significant abnormalities in both nerve action-potential amplitudes and conduction velocities of affected limbs indicate that the neuropathies are caused by both axonal destruction and demyelination. Angiographic and pathologic studies of affected extremities confirm widespread arteritis of the vessels supplying the affected nerves. Most patients improve after treatment with systemic corticosteroids (see below).

Cerebral, cerebellar, and brainstem syndromes indistinguishable from those caused by other vasculopathies may occur in patients with GCA, either as the initial manifestation of the disease or during its course. The CNS manifestations of GCA usually result from stenosis or occlusion of—or embolization from—affected carotid, vertebral, or basilar arteries or, rarely, from their branches (Cardell and Hanley, 1951; McCormick and Neubuerger, 1958; Crompton, 1959; Hollenhorst et al., 1960; Hinck et al., 1964; Andrews, 1966; Wilkinson and Russell, 1972; Hirsch et al., 1974; Chisholm, 1975; Cohen and Damaske, 1975; Enzmann and Scott, 1977; Healey and Wilske, 1977; Cochran et al., 1978; Healey and Wilske, 1978; Huston et al., 1978; Goodman, 1979; Wang and Henkind, 1979; Goodwin, 1980; Shenberger et al., 1981; Howard et al., 1984; Monteiro et al., 1984; Lipton et al., 1987; Caselli et al., 1988b; Crompton et al., 1989; Imakita et al., 1993; Buttner et al., 1994) (Figs. 57.37 and 57.38). Patients with GCA and diffuse cerebral ischemia develop an organic brain syndrome, confusion, or nonspecific disturbances of mentation (Keltner, 1982; Caselli et al., 1988b, Caselli and Hunder, 1993). Some authors believe that involvement of the vertebrobasilar arterial system is more common than is involvement of the carotid arterial system in GCA and that the lateral medullary syndrome of Wallenberg

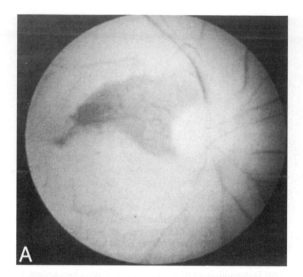

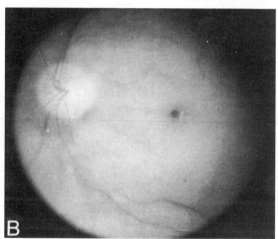

Figure 57.39. Bilateral central retinal artery occlusion in giant cell arteritis (GCA). The patient was a 65-year-old man who developed acute loss of vision in the right eye. *A,* The right ocular fundus shows a central retinal artery occlusion with sparing of a portion of the retina supplied by a cilioretinal artery. Three days later, the patient suddenly lost vision in the left eye. *B,* The left ocular fundus shows a complete central retinal artery occlusion with narrowed retinal arteries, diffuse retinal edema, and a cherry-red spot in the macula. Although the patient had no symptoms of GCA and had a normal erythrocyte sedimentation rate on two occasions, biopsy of the left temporal artery revealed GCA. (From Mohan K, Gupta A, Jain IS, et al. Bilateral central retinal artery occlusion in occult temporal arteritis. J Clin Neuroophthalmol *9:*270–272, 1989.)

tected by treating patients in the supine position (Cullen and Coleiro, 1976). Systemic hypotension, reduced cardiac output, and mechanical pressure on the carotid arteries were also considered to be possible mechanisms for visual loss in the second eye of a patient with GCA during recovery from general anesthesia for a laryngectomy (McGowan, 1967), and Wessels (1987) reported a 72-year-old man who developed a posterior ischemic optic neuropathy (PION) in the right eye immediately after undergoing successful aorto-femoral bypass surgery that was uncomplicated by hypotension or substantial blood loss. In view of these cases, it is generally recommended that elective surgery be postponed in patients with GCA until there is no evidence of active disease (McGowan, 1967).

Although most patients with choroidal ischemia from GCA have no clinical symptoms, **acute choroidal ischemia** characterized by nonrhegmatogenous retinal detachment and pigmentary changes may occasionally occur and produce decreased vision (Spolaore et al., 1984; Quillen et al., 1993).

Anterior ischemic optic neuropathy is the most common cause of visual loss in patients with GCA (Palm, 1958; Cohen, 1973; Jonassen et al., 1979; Graham, 1980; Keltner,

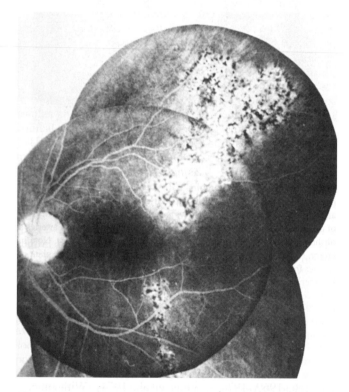

Figure 57.40. Sectoral choroidal ischemia in a patient with giant cell arteritis. The patient was a 79-year-old woman who suddenly lost vision in the left eye. Visual acuity was counting fingers in the eye. There was optic disc swelling consistent with an anterior ischemic optic neuropathy. Two weeks after the onset of visual loss, the left optic disc is pale, the retinal arteries are narrow, and there is a large, triangular choroidal scar with both hyper- and hypopigmentation in the superotemporal region. A smaller region of scarring is present inferotemporally. (From Spolaore R, Gaudric A, Coscas G, et al. Acute sectorial choroidal ischemia. Am J Ophthalmol *98:*707–716, 1984.)

Winkler, 1983). Signs of retinal ischemia include cotton-wool spots and intraretinal hemorrhages (Melberg et al., 1995) (Fig. 57.42). The effect of posture on retinal ischemia in patients with GCA was described by Hollenhorst (1967). Vision may be significantly reduced by changing position from lying down to standing or sitting, by bending over, or by excercising. Visible sludging of blood is observed when patients sit or stand, with recovery to normal when they lie down. It is important to recognize this phenomenon because vision compromised by poor retinal blood flow may be pro-

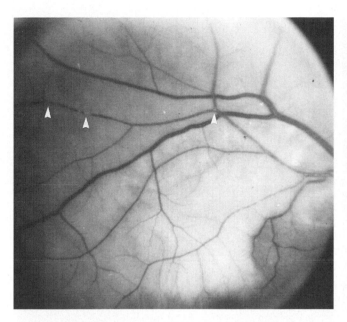

Figure 57.41. Branch retinal artery occlusion in giant cell arteritis. The patient was a 75-year-old woman with a 3-month history of intermittent fevers and jaw claudication who suddenly lost vision in the right eye. Visual acuity was 20/400 OD and there was a dense inferior altitudinal field defect in the right eye. The ocular fundus shows occlusion of the superior temporal retinal branch artery with diffuse retinal edema. Multiple emboli are seen in the occluded artery (*arrowheads*). An erythrocyte sedimentation rate was markedly elevated, and a temporal artery biopsy confirmed the diagnosis of GCA.

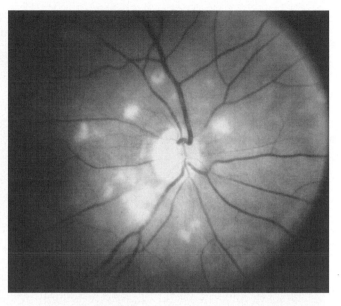

Figure 57.42. Retinal ischemia in giant cell arteritis (GCA). The patient was a 73-year-old woman with acute loss of vision in the right eye. She had a 2-month history of headache and pain in the left temple. The left eye had evidence of a retrobulbar ischemic optic neuropathy. The right ocular fundus shows multiple cotton-wool spots surrounding a normal optic disc. Visual acuity in this eye was 20/20. An erythrocyte sedimentation rate was elevated, and a temporal artery biopsy confirmed the diagnosis of GCA. Treatment with systemic corticosteroids was associated with disappearance of the cotton-wool spots, although visual acuity in the left eye did not recover.

1982), although only about 5% of patients with AION have GCA (Guyer et al., 1985). Arteritic AION usually is unilateral (Fig. 57.43), but it may be bilateral and simultaneous (Fig. 57.44), or the second eye may become affected days, weeks, or even months after the first eye, particularly if treatment is not begun immediately or is stopped while the disease is still active (Wagener and Hollenhorst, 1958; Russell, 1959; Cullen, 1963; Egge et al., 1966; Cohen, 1973; Cohen and Damaske, 1975; Miller et al., 1979; Graham, 1980; Bronster et al., 1983; Brownstein et al., 1983) (Fig. 57.45). In fact, it is estimated that bilateral blindness will develop in 25–50% of untreated patients who originally present with loss of vision in one eye (Birkhead et al., 1957; Johnston, 1973). Visual loss caused by AION may occur abruptly, or it may be preceded by episodes of transient monocular loss of vision that occasionally may be induced by activity or changes in posture (Hollenhorst et al., 1960; Raymond et al., 1980; Wykes et al., 1984; Caselli et al., 1988b) or that may alternate between eyes (Finelli, 1997). Loss of vision is usually profound, with over 80% of patients having visual acuity of less than hand motions. The affected optic disc usually shows milky or pale swelling, indicating infarction (Figs. 57.43–57.45), although hyperemic disc swelling occasionally may occur. Cotton-wool spots and flame-shaped intraretinal hemorrhages may be present in the peripapillary region (Melberg et al., 1995) (Fig. 57.43).

Unlike the optic discs of patients who develop nonarteritic

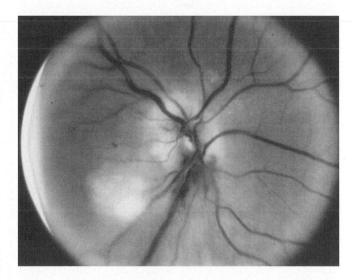

Figure 57.43. Anterior ischemic optic neuropathy in a patient with giant cell arteritis (GCA). The patient was an elderly woman with a history of headaches who suddenly lost vision in the right eye. Visual acuity was bare light perception in the right eye. Visual acuity in the left eye was normal. The right optic disc shows pale swelling. Note the inferior peripapillary hemorrhage and cotton-wool spot. An erythrocyte sedimentation rate was elevated, and a temporal artery biopsy confirmed the diagnosis of GCA.

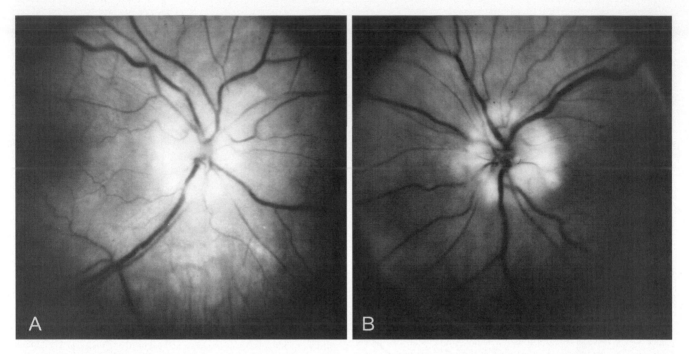

Figure 57.44. Bilateral simultaneous anterior ischemic optic neuropathy in a patient with giant cell arteritis. The patient was an 81-year-old woman with a 4-month history of headaches, malaise, and scalp tenderness who suddenly lost vision in both eyes. When initially examined, she had no light perception in either eye. *A* and *B*, The right and left optic discs show marked pale swelling. An erythrocyte sedimentation rate was markedly elevated. The patient refused a temporal artery biopsy.

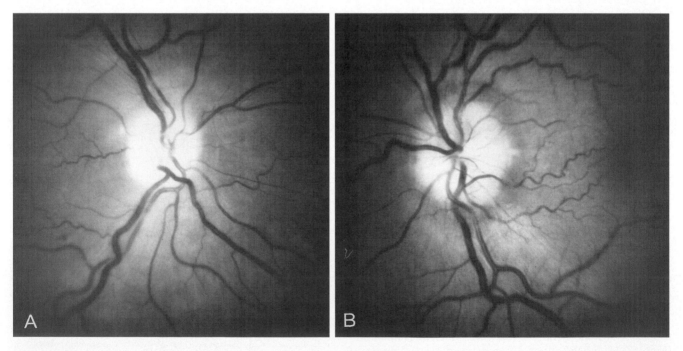

Figure 57.45. Bilateral sequential anterior ischemic optic neuropathy in a patient with giant cell arteritis. The patient was a 77-year-old woman with a 2-week history of headache and jaw pain who suddenly lost vision in the right eye. The right optic disc was noted to be swollen. A diagnosis of anterior ischemic optic neuropathy was made, but no evaluation was performed. Six weeks later, the patient lost vision in the left eye. Visual acuity was 20/100 OD and 20/400 OS. *A*, The right optic disc is pale and still slightly swollen. *B*, The left optic disc is moderately swollen and pale. Note that neither disc has a large optic cup. An erythrocyte sedimentation rate was elevated, and a temporal artery biopsy confirmed the diagnosis of GCA.

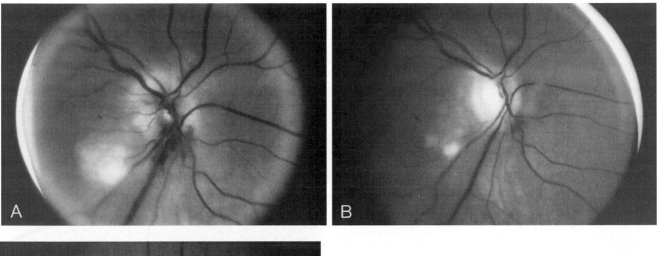

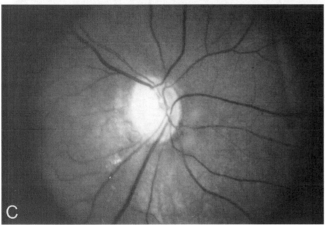

Figure 57.46. Progression to optic atrophy in a patient with arteritic anterior ischemic optic neuropathy. *A,* Right optic disc at the time of initial visual loss. Note pale optic disc swelling, peripapillary hemorrhage, and cotton-wool spot. The retinal arteries are not especially narrow. The diagnosis of GCA was confirmed by biopsy in this patient, and she was treated with systemic corticosteroids. *B,* 8 weeks after visual loss, the optic disc swelling has resolved, and both the hemorrhage and the cotton-wool spot are resolving. Note narrowing of retinal vessels. *C,* 4 months after visual loss, the optic disc is pale (note large optic cup), the peripapillary hemorrhage is no longer visible, and the cotton-wool spot has almost resolved. Note that the retinal vessels, especially the arteries, are markedly narrowed.

AION, which are invariably somewhat small and have a small cup-to-disc ratio (see Chapter 11), the optic discs of patients with arteritic AION may be of any size and shape. Thus, a small disc and cup may be associated with **either** nonarteritic or arteritic AION, whereas a normal or large cup in a patient with AION suggests an arteritic process until proven otherwise. After an attack of arteritic AION, the disc swelling gradually resolves, the optic disc becomes pale, and the retinal arteries become narrow (see Chapter 11) (Fig. 57.46).

Arteritic AION is caused by inflammatory occlusion of the short posterior ciliary arteries that supply the immediate retrolaminar and laminar portions of the optic disc (Kreibig, 1953; Crompton, 1959; Manschot, 1965a; Wolter and Phillips, 1965; Henkind et al., 1970; Macmichael and Cullen, 1972; Hinzpeter and Naumann, 1976) (Figs. 57.47 and 57.48). The inflammation may also produce sectoral areas of choroidal ischemia (McLeod et al., 1978; Spolaore et al., 1984).

Posterior (retrobulbar) ischemic optic neuropathy is responsible for acute visual loss in some patients with GCA (Spencer and Hoyt, 1960; Cohen, 1973; Johnston, 1973; Cohen and Damaske, 1975; Hayreh, 1981; Wessels, 1987). Although PION is generally much less common than is AION, it occurs with increasd frequency in patients with the

systemic vasculitides and especially in patients with GCA. In our opinion, GCA should be considered in any elderly patient who loses vision acutely and is found to have a normal-appearing fundus in the affected eye associated with a relative afferent pupillary defect (RAPD) (Haddad and Winkler, 1983) (Fig. 57.49). The visual loss need not be profound. Gladstone (1982) described a 76-year-old man who complained of slightly decreased visual acuity in the left eye. Vision was correctable to 20/20 in the right eye and to 20/25 in the left eye, but he had a significant visual field defect in the left eye, and there was a definite left RAPD, although both fundi appeared normal. A diagnosis of retrobulbar optic neuropathy was made, and an evaluation was begun. Within 2 weeks, the patient developed temple pain and jaw claudication, and he was found to have a markedly elevated ESR of 90 mm/hr. A temporal artery biopsy confirmed the diagnosis of GCA. PION occurs from interruption of blood flow to the retrolaminar portion of the optic nerve. The infarction may affect the orbital, intracanalicular, or intracranial portions of the nerve, or a combination of these. In most cases of GCA-associated PION, histopathologic examination reveals inflammatory occlusion of the ophthalmic and short posterior ciliary arteries (Spencer and Hoyt, 1960) (Fig. 57.50). As in patients with arteritic central retinal artery

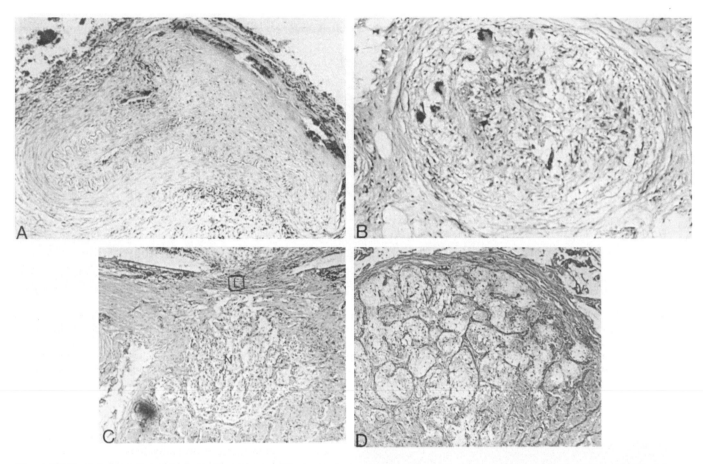

Figure 57.50. Pathology of posterior ischemic optic neuropathy in a patient with giant cell arteritis (GCA). The patient was a 77-year-old man with a 1-month history of bitemporal headaches and transient monocular visual loss in both eyes who suddenly lost vision in both eyes. On examination, he could not perceive light in either eye. Both pupils were moderately dilated, and neither pupil reacted to light stimulation. Ophthalmoscopic examination showed normal-appearing optic discs without pallor or swelling, and there were no retinal hemorrhages or exudates in either eye. The patient's erythrocyte sedimentation rate was elevated, and a temporal artery biopsy showed changes consistent with GCA. Eight days after beginning treatment, the patient became comatose, and an electrocardiogram showed changes consistent with a myocardial infarction. The patient died 14 days after the onset of permanent visual loss. Autopsy revealed a large infarct in the left ventricular wall of the heart associated with granulomatous inflammation of the coronary arteries and thrombosis of the left circumflex artery. Inflammatory changes also were present in the aorta, the iliac arteries, and both internal carotid arteries. *A,* The right ophthalmic artery near its origin from the internal carotid artery shows intimal thickening with narrowing of the lumen. Numerous chronic inflammatory cells including giant cells surround the artery and infiltrate its wall. *B,* A short posterior ciliary artery is occluded by a severe granulomatous inflammation. Note numerous multinucleated giant cells. Many short posterior ciliary arteries in both orbits were occluded or narrowed by granulomatous inflammation. *C,* Longitudinal section through the proximal portion of the right optic nerve shows a well-defined zone of ischemic necrosis (*N*) immediately behind the lamina cribrosa (*L*). *D,* Cross-section through the ischemic zone shows complete destruction of the nerve fiber and glial elements with preservation of the fibrovascular pial septae. (From Spencer WH, Hoyt WF. A fatal case of giant-cell arteritis (temporal or cranial arteritis) with ocular involvement. Arch Ophthalmol *64:*862–867, 1960.)

is most often affected, and in such cases, the paresis often spares the pupil (Fisher, 1959; Meadows, 1968; Walsh and Hoyt, 1969c; Graham, 1980) (Fig. 57.52). Nevertheless, GCA-related oculomotor nerve pareses occur in which the pupil is affected (Rush and Kramer, 1979; Rabinowich and Mehler, 1988). A patient with GCA described by Sibony and Lessell (1984) developed transient aberrant regeneration of the oculomotor nerve following an acute oculomotor nerve paresis presumably caused by the ischemic effects of the systemic disease. Diplopia may also result from damage to the ocular motor system in the brainstem. Monteiro et al. (1984) reported two patients with GCA whose primary initial

findings were truncal ataxia, upbeat nystagmus, and limited upward gaze. Crompton et al. (1989) described a 63-year-old man who developed horizontal diplopia and was found to have a **bilateral internuclear ophthalmoplegia** (INO) (Fig. 57.53). He also had constitutional symptoms and an elevated ESR. A temporal artery biopsy confirmed the diagnosis of GCA, and the patient was treated with prednisone. After 2 weeks of treatment, the patient's ocular motility had returned to normal. Trend and Graham (1990) reported two patients who developed diplopia from a **unilateral INO** associated with biopsy-proven GCA. Both patients experienced improvement in eye movement after treatment with systemic corticosteroids. We examined two patients with GCA who developed brainstem strokes characterized in part by a **skew deviation** and one patient who developed a horizontal one-and-a-half syndrome from a pontine infarction.

Some patients with diplopia have strabismus that does not correspond either to a typical ocular motor nerve paresis or to an intrinsic brainstem ocular motor disturbance (Lockshin, 1970). Such patients apparently have damage to individual or multiple extraocular muscles from vasculitis affecting the small arteries that supply these muscles (Barricks et al., 1977; Dimant et al., 1980; Goldberg, 1983) (Figs. 57.54 and 57.55).

Pupillary disturbances may occur in patients with GCA. The most common abnormality is an RAPD that results from ischemic damage to the retina, optic nerve, or both (see Chapter 24). Patients who develop bilateral complete blindness from retinal or optic nerve damage have bilateral dilated pupils that do not react to light stimulation but do react when proprioception is used to test the near response. This is probably the most common form of **light-near pupillary dissociation** that occurs in clinical practice (see Chapter 24). Unilateral or bilateral **tonic pupils** occur in some patients with GCA (Davis et al., 1968; Bronster et al., 1983; Coppeto and Greco, 1989) (Fig. 57.56). They presumably result from ischemia of the ciliary ganglion, short posterior ciliary nerves, or both. **Horner's syndrome** may occur in patients with GCA (Desser, 1969; Bell et al., 1980; Dimant et al., 1980; Bromfield and Slakter, 1988; Trend and Graham, 1990; Askari et al., 1993). The syndrome may be central,

preganglionic, or postganglionic, depending on where along the sympathetic pathway the ischemic damage occurs. In our experience, Horner's syndrome occurs most often in patients with GCA either as a central process associated with other signs of brainstem dysfunction or as a postganglionic condition in patients with oculomotor or abducens nerve paresis from ischemia in the cavernous sinus (see Chapters 24 and 28).

The **ocular ischemic syndrome** may develop in patients with GCA who develop inflammatory occlusion of the common carotid, internal carotid, or ophthalmic arteries (Zion and Goodside, 1974; Cullen and Coleiro, 1976; Hamed et al, 1992). Affected patients develop a typical syndrome of ocular ischemia that cannot be distinguished from that caused by atherosclerotic occlusion of the carotid or ophthalmic arteries (see Chapter 55). Such patients develop some or all of the following: (*a*) venous stasis retinopathy, (*b*) red eye, (*c*) mild uveitis, (*d*) progressive cataract, and (*e*) initially low intraocular pressure (Fig. 57.57).

Rare patients with GCA develop generalized ischemia not only of the eye but of all of the tissues in the orbit. Such patients may develop a clinical syndrome that suggests orbital pseudotumor or orbital cellulitis, characterized by proptosis, chemosis of the conjunctiva, limitation of eye movement, and reduced visual acuity (Bernard et al., 1951; Fisher, 1959; Zion and Goodside, 1974; Barricks et al., 1977; Stein et al., 1980; Karsenti et al., 1985; Clark and Victor, 1987; Laidlaw et al., 1990; Nassani et al., 1995). Treatment with systemic corticosteroids may result in resolution of the pro-

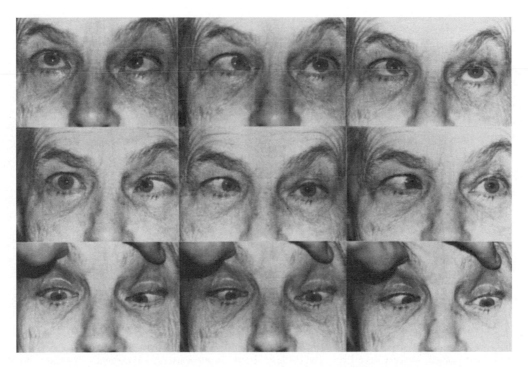

Figure 57.51. Bilateral abducens nerve paresis in a patient with giant cell arteritis (GCA). The patient was a 78-year-old woman with a 1-month history of neck and shoulder pain and a 12-day history of horizontal diplopia. The composite photograph shows bilateral weakness of abduction consistent with bilateral abducens nerve paresis. A temporal artery biopsy confirmed the diagnosis of GCA. (From Jay WM, Nazarian SM. Bilateral sixth nerve pareses with temporal arteritis and diabetes. J Clin Neuroophthalmol 6:91–95, 1986.)

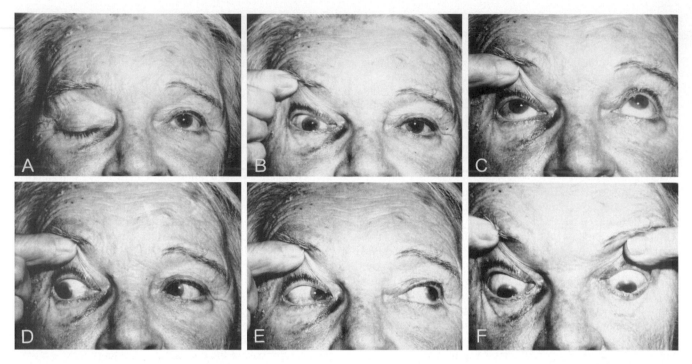

Figure 57.52. Superior division oculomotor nerve paresis in a patient with giant cell arteritis (GCA). The patient was an 80-year-old woman who had developed a right ptosis over 1 week. She had mild vertical diplopia, and she complained of constant pain over the right temple. *A,* The patient has a complete right ptosis. *B,* When the right upper eyelid is elevated manually, the pupil can be seen to be normal. *C,* There is limitation of elevation of the right eye. *D–F,* The right eye has normal abduction, adduction, and depression. An erythrocyte sedimentation rate was elevated, the patient was treated with systemic corticosteroids, and a temporal artery biopsy was performed that confirmed the diagnosis of GCA. The patient's oculomotor nerve paresis resolved completely over the next 3 months.

cess. This condition may also result from acute thrombosis of the superior ophthalmic vein (see Chapter 58). Although venous inflammation is unusual in GCA, it does occur in rare cases (Östberg, 1973).

Acute **ocular hypotony** is a rare complication of GCA (Haimböck, 1961; Bettelheim, 1968; Daicker and Keller, 1971; Nagy and Juhasc, 1971; Verdich and Nielsen, 1975; Radda et al., 1981a). It results from decreased production

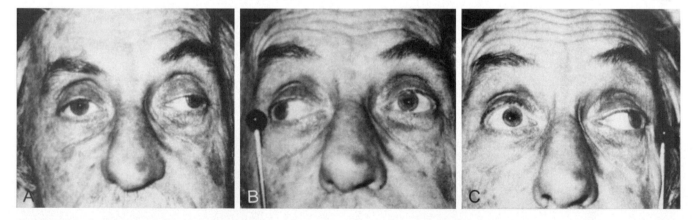

Figure 57.53. Bilateral internuclear ophthalmoplegia in a patient with giant cell arteritis (GCA). The patient was a 63-year-old man with a 2-month history of scalp tenderness and a 1-month history of malaise and pain in the left shoulder that radiated to the mastoid region who developed acute horizontal diplopia. *A,* The patient has a marked exotropia when fixing with the right eye. *B,* On attempted right gaze, there is limitation of adduction of the left eye. *C,* On attempted left gaze, the right eye does not adduct beyond the midline. An erythrocyte sedimentation rate was markedly elevated, and a temporal artery biopsy confirmed the diagnosis of GCA. The patient was treated with systemic corticosteroids. His pain and malaise improved dramatically shortly after he began treatment, and the internuclear ophthalmoplegia resolved over the next 3 weeks. (From Crompton JL, Burrow DJ, Iyer PV. Bilateral internuclear ophthalmoplegia: An unusual initial presenting sign of giant cell arteritis. Aust N Z J Ophthalmol *17:*71–74, 1989.)

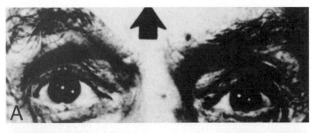

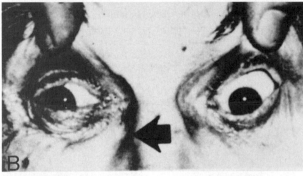

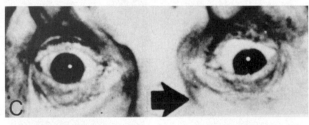

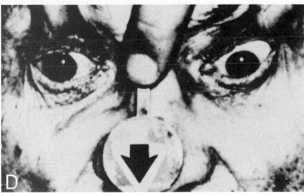

Figure 57.54. Ophthalmoparesis from vasculitis affecting the arteries supplying the extraocular muscles in a patient with giant cell arteritis (GCA). The patient was an 80-year-old man with a 6-month history of weight loss, a 2-month history of severe bifrontal headaches, a 6-week history of tenderness of the tongue and pain on mastication, and bilateral nonsimultaneous visual loss. The patient could not perceive light in either eye, and neither pupil reacted to light stimulation. There was no ptosis. Ophthalmoscopy revealed changes consistent with bilateral central retinal artery occlusions. *A–D,* There is generalized limitation of eye movement in all directions of gaze. The patient was treated with systemic corticosteroids, and a temporal artery biopsy was performed that confirmed the diagnosis of GCA. The patient died 9 days after admission to the hospital. (From Barricks ME, Traviesa DB, Glaser JS, et al. Ophthalmoplegia in cranial arteritis. Brain *100:*209–221, 1977.)

of aqueous humor caused by insufficient arterial blood flow to the ciliary body through the long posterior ciliary arteries (Daicker and Keller, 1971; Radda et al., 1981a).

Bilateral **marginal corneal ulceration** was reported in a patient with GCA by Gerstle and Friedman (1980). The patient also complained of severe orbital pain, and she subsequently developed conjunctival ulceration, scleral thinning, swelling over the bridge of the nose, and painful necrotic lesions of the fingernail beds. The skin and ocular lesions resolved when the patient was treated with systemic corticosteroids.

PATHOGENESIS

A variety of pathogenetic mechanisms have been suggested for both GCA and PMR, but no etiology is substantiated. The increasing incidence of both GCA and PMR after the age of 50 suggests that these disorders may be related to the aging process, although the precise relationship is unclear. GCA can occur in family members, including pairs of twins (Liang et al., 1974a; Granato et al., 1980; Novak et al., 1984; Tanenbaum and Tenzel, 1985; Mathewson and Hunder, 1986; Novak et al., 1986). This suggests a possible genetic factor in the development of GCA, and, in fact, several investigators reported that HLA-DR4 and Cw3 occur more commonly in affected patients than would be expected by chance alone (Calamia et al., 1981; Armstrong et al., 1983; Hunder et al., 1993). On the other hand, reports of conjugal GCA also raise the possibility of an environmental trigger (Galetta et al., 1990).

Both the humoral and cellular immune systems are implicated in the pathogenesis of GCA (Weyand and Bartley, 1997). The granulomatous histopathology of the disease (see below) suggests a cell-mediated immune reaction directed at antigens in or near elastic tissue or smooth muscle cells in arterial walls (Kimmelstiel et al., 1952; Wilkinson and Russell, 1972; Liang et al., 1974b; Albert et al., 1982; Chess et al., 1983); however, tests of cellular immunity in patients with GCA and in patients with PMR show no consistent abnormality (Papaioannou et al., 1979). Deposits of immunoglobulins and complement can be demonstrated intracellularly and adjacent to the internal elastic lamina in some affected temporal arteries (Liang et al., 1974b; Waaler et al., 1976; Park and Hazleman, 1978). Wells et al. (1989) evaluated 100 consecutive temporal artery biopsies using both light and direct immunofluorescence microscopy. These investigators found antibodies to IgG, IgM, IgA, C3, fibrinogen, or a combination of these in 93% of specimens with histopathologic characteristics of GCA. No such antibodies were detected in 87% of specimens without histopathologic features of GCA. These findings provide further evidence for the role of humoral immunity in the pathogenesis of GCA.

Increased numbers of circulating lymphoblasts are present in patients with active PMR (Egtedari et al., 1976), and reduced numbers of circulating cytotoxic/suppressor T-cells occur in similar patients (Benlahrache et al., 1983). Sera from patients with GCA and from patients with PMR contain increased concentrations of circulating immune complexes

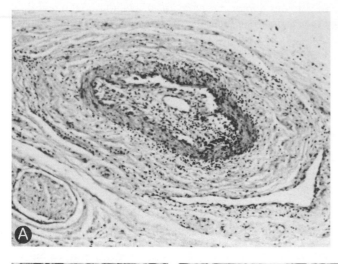

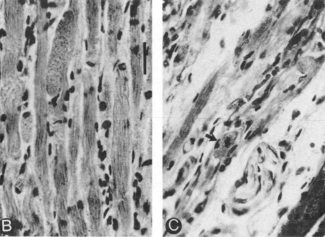

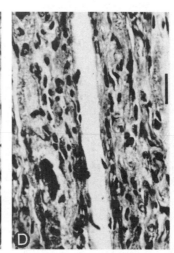

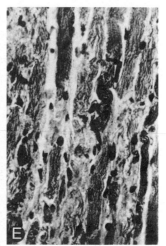

Figure 57.55. Pathology of nonspecific ophthalmoparesis in a patient with giant cell arteritis whose clinical appearance is shown in Figure 57.54. *A,* Inflammatory thrombosis of a small orbital branch of the ophthalmic artery. *B–E,* Sections through the extraocular muscles. *B,* Moderate coagulation necrosis and hyaline degeneration in the left inferior rectus muscle. Note large, nucleated macrophages in necrotic fibers. *C,* A pigment-laden macrophage (*arrow*) is seen in a necrotic fiber of the left lateral rectus muscle. *D,* Marked coagulation necrosis in the left lateral rectus muscle. *E,* Marked coagulation necrosis in the right superior rectus muscle. *Bars* = 0.05 mm. (From Barricks ME, Traviesa DB, Glaser JS, et al. Ophthalmoplegia in cranial artenitis. Brain *100:*209–221, 1977.)

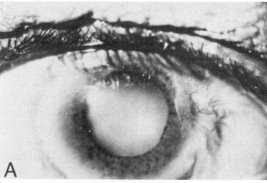

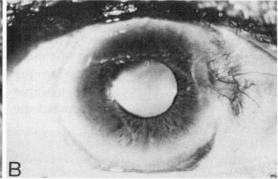

Figure 57.56. Tonic pupil in giant cell arteritis (GCA). The patient was a 75-year-old man with biopsy-proven GCA whose vision was diminished in both eyes because of ischemic optic neuropathy. Both pupils were dilated, and slit lamp biomicroscopy showed that only isolated segments of the iris sphincter constricted during light stimulation. Pupillary constriction to near stimulation was poor. There was no ptosis, and extraocular movements were full. *A,* The right pupil is moderately dilated. *B,* 30 minutes after instillation of 0.1% pilocarpine into the conjunctival sac, the pupil is constricted, suggesting denervation supersensitivity. (From Bronster DJ, Rudolph SH, Shanzer S. Pupillary ligh-near dissociation in cranial arteritis: A case report. Neuro-ophthalmology *3:*65–70, 1983.)

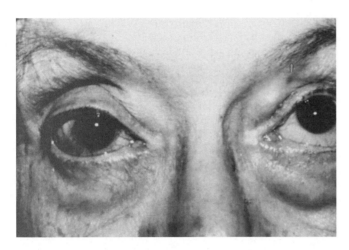

Figure 57.57. Ocular ischemic syndrome in a patient with giant cell arteritis. The patient was a 78-year-old woman who developed diplopia associated with decreased vision and pain in the right eye. The right eye is injected, hypotropic, and somewhat enophthalmic. The cornea is slightly hazy and there is a mild cataract. The ocular fundus on this side showed venous stasis retinopathy. The patient had an elevated erythrocyte sedimentation rate, and a temporal artery biopsy established the diagnosis. (Courtesy of Dr. David Knox.)

during active disease according to some investigators (Papaioannou et al., 1980) but not others (Radda et al., 1981b). When such complexes are present, their concentration seems to correlate positively with both the ESR and the concentration of γ-globulin in the serum. The findings described above suggest an ongoing immune response in patients with active GCA and PMR.

Molecular advances provide further insights into the potential pathogenesis of GCA. Of 42 patients with biopsy-proven GCA, 60% were shown to harbor the HLA-DRB1 gene, and the sequence demonstrated by most patients involved the amino acid positions 28–31 (Weyand et al., 1992, 1994a). A similar distribution of the HLA-DRB1 alleles was also found in patients with PMR (Weyand et al., 1994a).

Weyand et al. (1994b) isolated preactivated helper T-cells from biopsy specimens of untreated patients with GCA. These investigators found that a small number of these T-cells had undergone clonal proliferation. The discovery of identical proliferating T-cells in biopsy specimens and not in peripheral blood suggests that these cells are recognizing an in situ antigen (Weyand et al., 1994b).

An elevation of the cytokine interleukin 6 occurs in patients with GCA (Roche et al., 1993), and patients treated with corticosteroids experience a dramatic drop of the interleukin 6 level within hours. Furthermore, patients given only a single dose of 60 mg of prednisone have a gradual elevation of their interleukin 6 level 24 hours after the dose is administered. This finding may explain why some patients with GCA fail alternate-day steroid regimens. Even after a year of therapy, interleukin 6 levels quickly rise after discontinuation of steroids. Tissue-infiltrating macrophages and circulating monocytes are the major source of interleukin 6. Patients with PMR, but without vasculitis have only circula-

tory monocytes secreting interleukin 6 (Wagner et al., 1994). Furthermore, patients with GCA and not PMR have transcripts for interferon-γ cytokine mRNA. This finding suggests that GCA patients have a special type of CD4 helper T-cell called a Th-1 cell. Th-1 cells are not found in patients with PMR unless the patients also have active vasculitis (Weyand et al., 1994c).

PATHOLOGY

GCA is typically characterized by inflammation of the arteries that originate from the arch of the aorta, but almost any artery of the body, including the ophthalmic, central retinal, and posterior ciliary arteries, may be affected (Östberg, 1971, 1973; Klein et al., 1975) (Figs. 57.47, 57.48, 57.50, 57.55, and 57.58). The inflammation tends to affect the arteries in a segmental or patchy fashion (Fig. 57.59), but long portions of arteries may be affected (Klein et al., 1976; Lie, 1994b). In patients who die during the active phase of GCA, inflammation is most often seen in the superficial temporal, vertebral, ophthalmic, and posterior ciliary arteries, with the internal carotid, external carotid, and central retinal arteries being somewhat less commonly affected (Wilkinson and Russell, 1972). Other postmortem studies demonstrate inflammation in the proximal and distal aorta and in the subclavian, brachial, and abdominal arteries (Cardell and Hanley, 1951; Östberg, 1971; Pollock et al., 1973; Hyman, 1979) (Fig. 57.60). Intracranial arteries other than those supplying the orbit are affected infrequently (Wilkinson and Russell, 1972).

In mild cases of GCA, collections of T-lymphocytes may be confined to the region of the internal or external elastic lamina or to the adventitia (Albert et al., 1982; Chess et al., 1983). Intimal thickening without prominent cellular infiltration is usually present. In areas of more marked inflammation, all layers are affected (Albert et al., 1982). Necrosis of portions of the arterial wall, including the elastic laminae, and granulomas containing multinucleated histiocytic and foreign-body giant cells, histiocytes, lymphocytes (both T-helper and T-suppressor cells), and some plasma cells and fibroblasts are found (Hamilton et al., 1971; Parker et al., 1975; Banks et al., 1983; Chess et al., 1983; Wells et al., 1989). Some fibrinoid necrosis may be seen in biopsy specimens of patients with GCA, but diffuse fibrinoid necrosis and panarteritis should suggest the possibility of PAN or another systemic vasculitis. (Lie, 1994b). The pathologic diagnosis of GCA is also questionable when the infiltrate is nongranulomatous and does not contain a predominance of lymphocytes and histiocytes. Thrombosis may develop at sites of inflammation, but these areas may recanalize after the inflammation subsides. The inflammatory process is usually most marked in the inner portion of the media adjacent to the internal elastic lamina. Fragmentation and disintegration of elastic fibers occur, closely associated with an accumulation of giant cells; however, giant cells are not always seen in tissue sections, and they are **not required** for the diagnosis if other features, particularly fragmentation of the elastic lamina, are present (Wells et al., 1989; Lie, 1994b) (Fig. 57.61). In a study of 85 GCA biopsy specimens, giant cells were present in 50.7%. The presence of giant cells did not correlate with visual manifestations or the frequency of pain and jaw claudication (Schmidt and Laffler, 1994).

LABORATORY STUDIES

Patients with GCA usually have a mild to moderate **normochromic normocytic anemia,** with a normal leukocyte and differential count (Healey and Wilske, 1971; Love et al., 1986; Jacobson and Slamovits, 1987; Love et al., 1987). Rarely, it is the only abnormality. In other cases, however, a **thrombocytosis** is present and may predict an increased likelihood of subsequent visual or neurologic ischemic events (Krishna and Kosmorsky, 1997).

The **erythrocyte sedimentation rate** is measured by placing anticoagulated blood in a vertical cylindrical tube and

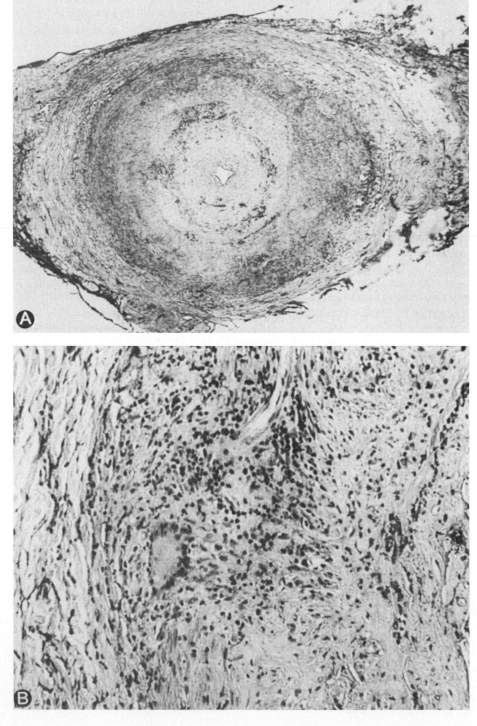

Figure 57.58. Pathology of giant cell arteritis. *A,* Lumen of the temporal artery has been markedly reduced in diameter by a diffuse inflammatory process that infiltrates the wall and produces subintimal proliferation. *B,* High-power photomicrograph of a portion of the vessel shows that the inflammation consists of lymphocytes, plasma cells, and giant cells.

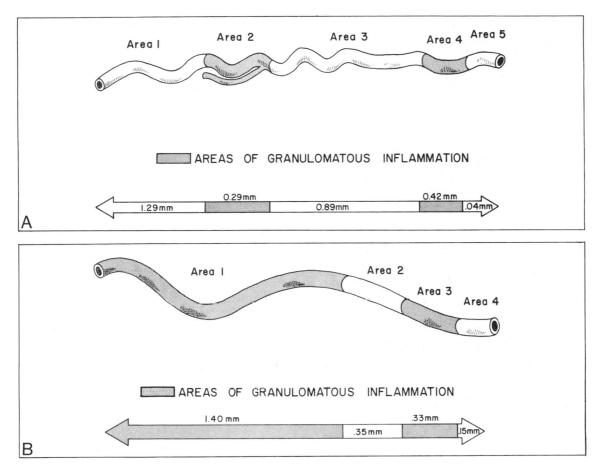

Figure 57.59. Schematic illustrations of the segmental involvement of a portion of the superficial temporal artery in two patients with giant cell arteritis. Note that unaffected areas range in size from 0.35 to 1.29 mm. *A*, From a 76-year-old woman who experienced sudden loss of vision in the right eye associated with right-sided temporal headaches. The right optic disc was swollen. *B*, From a 68-year-old man who suddenly lost vision in the left eye after a 2-month history of malaise and weight loss. The left retina showed evidence of ischemia with intraretinal hemorrhages and cotton-wool spots. (From Albert DM, Ruchman MC, Keltner JL. Skip areas in temporal arteritis. Arch Ophthalmol *94*:2072–2077, 1976.)

determining the rate of sedimentation of the red blood cells (Fig. 57.62). It has been known since the time of the ancient Greeks that the ESR may be altered in a variety of diseases. The major influence on the rate of sedimentation of red cells suspended in plasma is the degree to which they aggregate with one another (Bedell and Bush, 1985), and the three major factors that influence aggregation of erythrocytes are (*a*) the surface free energy of the cells, (*b*) the charge on the cells, and (*c*) the dielectric constant (Pollack, 1965). The first two forces attract and repel the cells, respectively. The dielectric constant is a property of the plasma related to the concentration of asymmetric molecules such as fibrinogen. An increase in fibrinogen or a similar molecule in the serum thus leads to greater cohesion of erythrocytes, with resulting aggregation and stacking (rouleaux) and a more rapid rate of fall (Kushner, 1989).

A markedly elevated ESR is found in more than 95% of patients with biopsy-proven GCA (Sox and Liang, 1986; Kyle et al., 1989), although the degree of elevation does not predict which patients are at increased risk for the development of ocular complications of the disease (Jacobson and Slamovits, 1987). In addition, some patients with clinical symptoms suggesting GCA and a positive temporal artery biopsy have an ESR that is well within normal limits (Cullen, 1963; Eagling et al., 1974; Cohen and Damaske, 1975; Kansu et al., 1977; Weintraub, 1978; Biller et al., 1982; Verin et al., 1985; Wong and Korn, 1986; Nevyas and Nevyas, 1987). Indeed, it is estimated that about 2% of patients with biopsy-proven GCA have a normal ESR (Healey and Wilske, 1980; Keltner, 1982). Jacobson and Slamovits (1987) separated 24 patients with biopsy-proven giant GCA into three groups based on the ESR at clinical presentation: low, 1–40 mm/hr; high, 41–80 mm/hr; and very high, >80 mm/hr. The presence of anemia in the very high ESR group, compared with the low ESR group, was the only statistically identified difference. These authors emphasized that in the setting of a normal hemoglobin, one cannot rely on the ESR to suggest the diagnosis of GCA. Therefore, it is clear that the finding of a normal ESR in a patient with symptoms or signs suggesting GCA should not dissuade the physician from proceeding with a temporal artery biopsy (Wong and Korn, 1986; Jacobson and Slamovits, 1987).

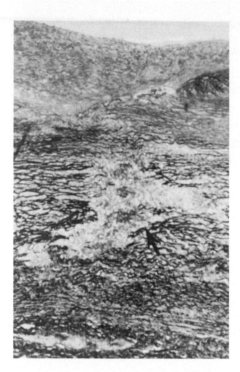

Figure 57.60. Giant cell arteritis affecting the proximal aorta in a patient who died after rupture of the descending aorta. This section of the ascending aorta is distal to the ruptured portion and shows destruction of elastic fibers (*arrow*). Neighboring sections showed infiltration of the vessel wall with lymphocytes and plasma cells. (From Hunder GG. Giant cell arteritis and polymyalgia rheumatica. In Textbook of Rheumatology. Editors, Kelley WN, Harris ED Jr, Ruddy S, et al. 3rd ed, pp 1200–1208. Philadelphia, WB Saunders, 1989.)

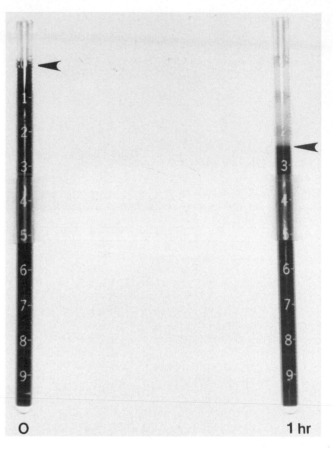

Figure 57.62. Erythrocyte sedimentation rate (Wintrobe method). Tube at *left side* of photograph shows level of red cells at beginning of test (*arrowhead*). Tube at *right side* of photograph shows level of red cells after 1 hour (*arrowhead*). Reading is about 25 mm/hr.

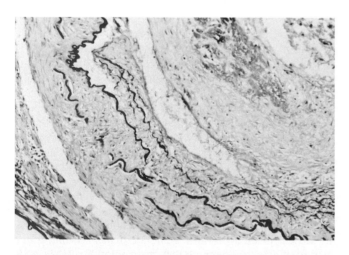

Figure 57.61. Pathology of giant cell arteritis (GCA). Temporal artery biopsy shows marked fragmentation and reduplication of the elastic lamina associated with mild chronic inflammation. Although no giant cells are present, a diagnosis of GCA can be made on the basis of chronic inflammation associated with fragmentation of the elastic lamina.

The concentration of **fibrinogen** in the serum is frequently increased in patients with GCA, whereas it is usually normal in other conditions that produce an elevated ESR (Holdstock and Mitchell, 1977). It may therefore be a helpful sign in patients with unexplained elevation of the ESR. Bates et al. (1989) measured the concentration of fibrinogen in the serum of 176 patients with biopsy-proven GCA before treatment and compared it with the ESR. These investigators found that a concentration of serum fibrinogen greater than 450 mg/dL was not as sensitive a predictor of a positive temporal artery biopsy as was an ESR over 30 mm/hr (82% versus 96%), but it was more specific (32% versus 68% false-positive rate). In our opinion, the greater specificity of the serum fibrinogen concentration in patients with possible GCA is not sufficient to warrant its use in place of the ESR to decide whether or not to perform a temporal artery biopsy.

C-reactive protein (CRP) is a substance present in human serum. It was first detected because of its ability to precipitate with the somatic C-polysaccharide of *Streptoccocus pneumoniae* in the presence of calcium ions (McCarty, 1982). CRP is present in trace amounts in normal persons, but its concentration rises dramatically after tissue injury (Kushner, 1989). Eshaghian and Goeken (1980) evaluated the concentration of CRP in 11 patients with biopsy-proven GCA and found that it was elevated in 10 of them (91%). It was also elevated, however, in 14 of 32 control patients (44%) with various ocular and systemic disturbances and negative temporal artery biopsies. Kyle et al. (1989) reported an elevated concentration of CRP in 49 of 55 (89%) patients with GCA. All of these patients also had an elevated ESR, however. Hayreh et al. (1997) studied 363 patients who had a temporal artery biopsy for suspected GCA, 223 of whom also had measurement of their CRP. These investigators found that the odds of a positive biopsy were over 3 times greater when the CRP was above 2.45 mg/dL. In fact, an elevated CRP was more sensitive (100%) for detection of GCA (as indicated by a positive temporal artery biopsy) than an elevated ESR (92%).

DIAGNOSIS

The diagnosis of GCA should be considered in any patient over 50 years of age who develops the new onset of headache, scalp tenderness, jaw claudication, ear pain, migratory arthralgias, unexplained prolonged fever or anemia, permanent or transient visual loss, or diplopia. Patients who complain of transient or permanent monocular or binocular loss of vision or diplopia should be questioned specifically about systemic symptoms of GCA. Such patients may not volunteer such information to the ophthalmologist because they do not recognize the relationship of any systemic difficulties they may be experiencing to their visual difficulties (Keltner, 1982).

A small percentage of patients with biopsy-proven GCA have no systemic symptoms at the time they first develop visual disturbances (Cohen and Damaske, 1975; Mohan et al., 1989). Such patients are said to have **occult giant cell arteritis** (Simmons and Cogan, 1962; Cullen, 1963; Friedman, 1965; Cullen, 1967a; Mohan et al., 1989; Glutz von Blotzheim and Borruat, 1996). GCA therefore must be included in the differential diagnosis of an elderly patient with visual loss or diplopia even when the patient has no constitutional or systemic symptoms.

Patients with a suspected diagnosis of GCA should undergo a careful examination of the arteries of the head and neck. These vessels should be evaluated for tenderness, enlargement, nodularity, and bruits. Goodman (1979) emphasized that about 50% of patients with GCA have at least one pulseless temporal artery. By comparison, Curran (1986) examined by palpation the frontal branches of both superficial temporal arteries of 100 patients 65 years of age or older, none of whom had symptoms or signs of GCA. Only four of the patients had a nonpalpable artery, and all four patients had a palpable artery on the contralateral side. Taken together, the data of Goodman (1979) and Curran (1986) suggest that a nonpalpable artery should be considered circumstantial evidence of GCA in a patient in whom the diagnosis is being considered.

An ESR should be performed immediately by either the Westergren (Westergren, 1924, 1926) or the Wintrobe (Wintrobe and Landsberg, 1935) method in any patient suspected of having GCA. The Westergren method requires a 4 to 1 dilution of blood. It thus must be performed in a laboratory and is therefore susceptible to laboratory error; however, it provides extremely accurate values when the ESR is elevated (Schrader, 1963). The Wintrobe method does not require any dilution of blood (Fig. 57.62), so it can be performed in any physician's office, and it provides extremely accurate values when the ESR is normal. A third method of measuring the ESR, the zeta method, is said to have several advantages over both the Westergren and Wintrobe methods (Bull and Brailsford, 1972; Love et al., 1988). It is unaffected by anemia, and it responds in a linear manner to increases in concentration of fibrinogen, γ-globulin, or both. Unfortunately, it is a somewhat complicated process that requires a special centrifuge. Most authors recommend that the Westergren method be used to determine the ESR in patients with suspected GCA (International Committee for Standardization in Hematology, 1977; Keltner, 1982), but we find the Wintrobe method to be just as helpful and more easily performed. We have no experience with the zeta method.

As noted above, most patients with GCA have a markedly elevated ESR (Kyle et al., 1989); however, a normal ESR does not eliminate the disease from consideration. A patient with clinical features of GCA and a normal ESR should still be considered to have GCA until proven otherwise, and that patient should probably be treated with systemic corticosteroids pending the outcome of a unilateral or bilateral temporal artery biopsy (see below).

There are no definitive studies regarding the range of the ESR in normal persons (Boyd and Hoffbrand, 1966; Böttiger and Svedberg, 1967; Kulvin, 1972; Milne and Williamson, 1972; Hayes and Stinson, 1976; Griffiths et al., 1984). In our opinion, the best data were provided by Miller et al. (1983), who indicated that the top normal ESR may be calculated by dividing the age by 2 for men and adding 10 to the age before dividing by 2 for women. Using this formula, the top normal ESR for a man of 80 is 40 mm/hr, whereas the top normal ESR for a woman of the same age is 45 mm/hr. Based on the results of a survey of 194 elderly subjects, Hanger et al. (1991) recommended that 3 be used instead of 2 as the dividing factor. Using their formula, the top normal ESR for a man of 80 is 26.7 mm/hr and the top normal ESR for a woman of the same age is 30 mm/hr. We believe that using this formula increases the sensitivity of the ESR in the diagnosis of GCA but significantly decreases the specificity of the test. We prefer the formula by Miller et al. (1983).

A CRP should also be performed in any patient in whom GCA is suspected. Hayreh et al. (1997) found that the CRP was more sensitive (100%) than the ESR (92%) in detecting GCA. In addition, the combination of the ESR and CRP gave the best specificity (97%).

The ocular pulse is diminished when the blood flow to the eye and orbit becomes reduced. Several investigators (Horven, 1970; Bienfang, 1989) emphasized that the amplitude of the ocular pulse often disappears or becomes markedly decreased in eyes with ischemic ocular damage (e.g., central retinal artery occlusion, ischemic optic neuropathy) caused by GCA, whereas the ocular pulse is generally unaffected in eyes with ischemic ocular damage from other causes such as atherosclerosis unless the ophthalmic or internal carotid arteries are completely occluded. The change in the ocular pulse amplitude occurs in patients with GCA because the disease affects the internal carotid artery, ophthalmic artery, or both. Thus the blood flow to the entire eye, not just to the optic nerve or retina, is reduced. Because the ocular pulse is dependent on ocular blood flow, particularly that to the choroid, it is generally unaffected by diseases such as atherosclerosis that may occlude only the central retinal artery or some of the short posterior ciliary arteries. The amplitude of the ocular pulse can easily be measured using a number of instruments such as the pneumotonograph. This device records the amplitude and shape of the ocular pulse using a gas tonometer probe with a soft plastic tip that rests on the anesthetized corneal surface (Walker et al., 1975; Langham and To'mey, 1978) (Fig. 57.63).

Bosley et al. (1989) found that ocular pneumoplethysmography (OPG-Gee) is useful in diagnosing GCA because of the generalized reduction of ocular blood flow that occurs in patients with the disorder. In their limited study, OPG-Gee had a sensitivity of 100% and a specificity of 93.4%, for a combined diagnostic accuracy of 94%. Although we agree with Bosley et al. (1989) that OPG-Gee is an extremely accurate method of determining reduction of ocular blood flow, we and others are concerned about the potential risk of visual loss in an eye whose blood flow may already be compromised when the intraocular pressure is raised significantly during the OPG-Gee technique (Bates, 1989). We believe that it is preferable to measure the amplitude of the ocular pulse as recommended by Bienfang (1989; see above) because it does not require artificially elevating or otherwise manipulating the intraocular pressure.

Color Doppler flow imaging in patients with GCA shows reduced velocities in the central retinal and posterior ciliary arteries (Ho et al., 1994; Ghanchi et al., 1996b; Kraft et al., 1996) and a characteristic hypoechoic halo around the perfused lumen of a stenosed or occluded artery (Kraft et al., 1996). Clinically unaffected eyes in such patients also show similar findings. This technique requires further study to verify its value in the diagnosis and management of GCA.

Fluorescein angiography may be helpful in distinguishing arteritic from nonarteritic AION. Mack et al. (1991) found a significant delay of choroidal filling times in patients with arteritic AION compared with filling times in patients with nonarteritic AION and with filling times in normal control subjects. Furthermore, several patients with GCA had improved choroidal filling times after treatment with systemic corticosteroids. These observations were confirmed by Siatkowski et al. (1993), who retrospectively studied angiograms of 19 patients with nonarteritic AION and 16 patients with arteritic AION. Patients with GCA had delayed dye appearance and delayed choroidal filling times. The mean dye-appearance time in these patients was 20.3 seconds compared with 11.29 seconds in patients without arteritis (p < 0.001), and the mean choroidal filling time in patients with GCA was 29.7 seconds compared with 12.9 seconds in patients without GCA (p < 0.002). When 18 seconds was used as a cutoff for total choroidal filling time, the sensitvity of fluoresein angiography for the diagnosis of GCA was 93%

and the specificity of 94%. However, the confidence limits on these percentages were wide, ranging from 69 to 100%, reflecting the small sample size.

A temporal artery biopsy should be performed in all patients suspected of having GCA. It is the most sensitive and specific diagnostic test for GCA, with at least a 95% sensitivity and a 100% specificity (Hall et al., 1983; Hedges et al., 1983; Vilaseca, 1987; Wells et al., 1989). Although some authors believe that a temporal artery biopsy is not needed in an elderly patient who develops headache, scalp tenderness, and visual loss, and who has an elevated ESR (Allsop and Gallagher, 1981; Paice, 1989), a positive temporal artery biopsy absolutely establishes the diagnosis. We agree with Kearns (1988) that it would seem prudent to have a tissue diagnosis whenever possible, for both medical and legal reasons, in view of the potential side effects of treatment for GCA. In addition, a tissue diagnosis helps to focus management in patients who are having difficulty tolerating systemic corticosteroids or who cannot be weaned off them (Stuart, 1989).

The technique used to perform a temporal artery biopsy is straightforward (Cohen and Smith, 1974; Brennan and McCrary, 1975; Miller and Aroichane, 1995). In most cases, the course of the artery can be identified by palpation even if it is not pulsating. When the artery cannot be palpated, Doppler ultrasonography may be used to locate it (Kelley, 1978) (Fig. 57.64). We have performed over 300 temporal artery biopsies and have always been able to identify the vessel using either palpation or ultrasonography. Once the artery has been localized and marked (Fig. 57.65A), the skin and subcutaneous tissue adjacent to it are anesthetized (Fig. 57.65B), and the area is prepped and draped. A skin incision is carried down through soft subcutaneous tissue until the artery, which lies on the surface of the fascia of the temporalis muscle, is identified by direct visualization (Fig. 57.65C). A portion of the artery is cleaned from its attachments to surrounding tissue (Fig. 57.65D) and isolated between two 4-0 or 6-0 silk sutures that are tightened around the vessel, tied, and cut (Figs. 57.65E and 57.65F). The portion of the artery between the two sutures is excised, using care not to crush the specimen (Fig. 57.65G). The skin incision is closed, using any standard technique (Fig. 57.65H), and a light pad is placed over the incision site. The skin sutures are removed in about 7 days.

There is almost no risk to a temporal artery biopsy (Stuart, 1989). Fisher (1971) reported a patient who experienced a stroke after biopsy of a temporal artery that was providing circulation to the brain in the setting of a carotid artery occlusion. Vollrath-Junger and Gloor (1989) described three patients with suspected GCA in whom a temporal artery biopsy might have produced major complications. In one case, there was severe stenosis of the ipsilateral internal carotid artery, and the cerebral perfusion to the ipsilateral hemisphere was primarily dependent on the temporal artery. If that artery had been biopsied, the patient might have suffered a major hemisphere stroke. In two other cases, there was proximal stenosis of the ophthalmic artery, and biopsy of the ipsilateral temporal artery might have resulted in blindness in the ipsilateral

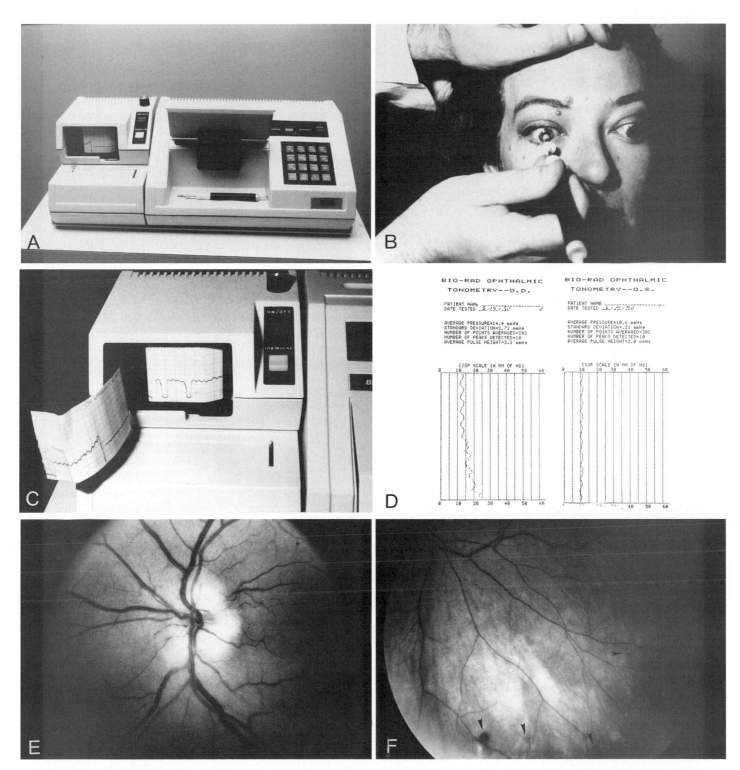

Figure 57.63. The use of the pneumotonograph to measure the amplitude of the ocular pulse in patients suspected of having giant cell arteritis. *A*, The machine simultaneously records the intraocular pressure and the amplitude of the ocular pulse in each eye. *B*, Measurements are obtained using a probe with a soft plastic tip that rests on the anesthetized corneal surface. *C*, The machine produces a real-time display of the intraocular pressure and ocular pulse. *D*, Pulse asymmetry in a patient with loss of vision in the left eye associated with an ophthalmoscopic picture of a combined anterior ischemic optic neuropathy and venous stasis retinopathy. Note that the average pulse height in the normal right eye is 3.2 mm Hg but only 2.0 mm Hg in the left eye. *E*, The left optic disc is pale and swollen. Note dilation of retinal veins. *F*, A few blot retinal hemorrhages are present in the retinal periphery (*arrowheads*). The clinical picture is compatible with combined anterior ischemic optic neuropathy and venous stasis retinopathy associated with occlusion of the carotid or ophthalmic artery.

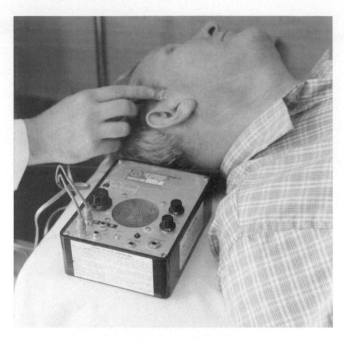

Figure 57.64. A portable Doppler ultrasonogram machine can be used to determine course of the superficial temporal artery before temporal artery biopsy.

eye. Vollrath-Junger and Gloor (1989) recommend that a Doppler ultrasonographic evaluation be performed on every patient before a temporal artery biopsy is performed to try to prevent such potential complications. Other reported complications of temporal artery biopsy are minimal. Foged (1981) reported chronic skin ulceration in the temporal region several months after biopsy. Slavin (1986) reported a brow droop after a temporal artery biopsy, and we are aware of a similar case. We are also aware of a case in which a severe hematoma occurred after biopsy when the proximal ligature slipped off the end of the artery. The patient required emergency surgery to stop the hemorrhage.

We agree with Coppeto and Monteiro (1990) that indurated or tender branches of the superficial temporal arteries should be biopsied preferentially and that biopsy of the artery on the side of visual symptoms or signs should be performed initially. Because of the common segmental involvement of the artery (Fig. 57.59), the specimen should be of sufficient length to reduce the risk of biopsying a normal portion of vessel that is sandwiched between two areas of inflammation. Although such ''skip areas'' are quite rare and often only a few millimeters in length (Goder, 1968; Cohen and Smith, 1974; Albert et al., 1976; Klein et al., 1976; McDonnell et al., 1986; Chambers and Bernardino, 1988), they occur with sufficient frequency that they must be taken into consideration when performing a temporal artery biopsy and when evaluating the specimen (Fig. 57.66). Chambers and Bernardino (1988) calculated the probability of finding an area of inflammation as small as 0.29 mm in various-sized biopsy specimens depending on the way they were processed and examined. These

authors concluded that there was a 99% probability of finding such an area when a biopsy at least 4 mm in length was divided into 1-mm segments with each segment being cut into at least nine sections, each of which was examined. Although we do not dispute the findings of Chambers and Bernardino (1988), we feel more confident in recommending that a specimen substantially longer than 4 mm be removed at the time of temporal artery biopsy. A biopsy specimen at least **2 cm in length** should be sufficient to provide an accurate assessment of any temporal artery, provided that it is examined appropriately (Errlinger et al., 1978; Keltner, 1982). The specimen should be embedded on end, and serial sections should be cut until the specimen is exhausted. The sections should be stained with hematoxylin and eosin and with a stain for elastin so that the status of the elastic lamina of the vessel can be determined. The sections should then be examined by an experienced pathologist who not only can recognize the features of acute GCA but also can identify ''healed'' GCA, which is characterized by mild lymphocytic infiltration and scarring (McDonnell et al., 1986; Wells et al., 1989) (Fig. 57.67). As emphasized by Chambers and Bernardino (1988), all of these sections need to be examined because some arteritic segments are only 0.3 mm long (Klein et al., 1976).

It is generally recommended that patients in whom the diagnosis of GCA is strongly suspected but in whom a temporal artery biopsy on one side is negative undergo biopsy of the contralateral temporal artery. A contralateral biopsy is said to be positive in the face of a negative biopsy on the first side in 8–13% of cases (Klein et al., 1976; Sorensen and Lorenzen, 1977; Hall and Hunder, 1984; Hayreh et al., 1997). Thus, a negative unilateral temporal artery biopsy does not eliminate the diagnosis of GCA (Reinecke, 1970; Keltner, 1982; Brownstein et al., 1983), although a patient in whom GCA is suspected and in whom bilateral temporal artery biopsies are negative should certainly be evaluated for other causes of his or her systemic symptoms and elevated ESR, such as systemic cancer, infection, or connective tissue disease (Keltner, 1982; Hedges et al., 1983; Roth et al., 1984; Bedell and Bush, 1985; Sox and Liang, 1986). It may also be appropriate in such a patient to pursue the diagnosis of GCA by biopsying the occipital artery (Kattah et al., 1990).

Although it seems clear that performing bilateral temporal artery biopies increases the likelihood of a positive result to some extent, it is by no means clear if such biopsies should be simultaneous or sequential. Some physicians routinely advise performing simultaneous temporal artery biopsies on both sides in all patients suspected of having GCA. In a study by Hayreh et al. (1997), a sequential biopsy was performed on the second side only when the results for the first side were equivocal or negative despite a strong clinical index of suspicion of GCA. Of 76 patients who underwent a second biopsy, the second biopsy was positive in seven (9.2%). Boyev et al. (1997) reviewed the pathologic results of 904 temporal artery specimens from the Eye Pathology of the Wilmer Eye Institute received over a 28-year period. A total of 182

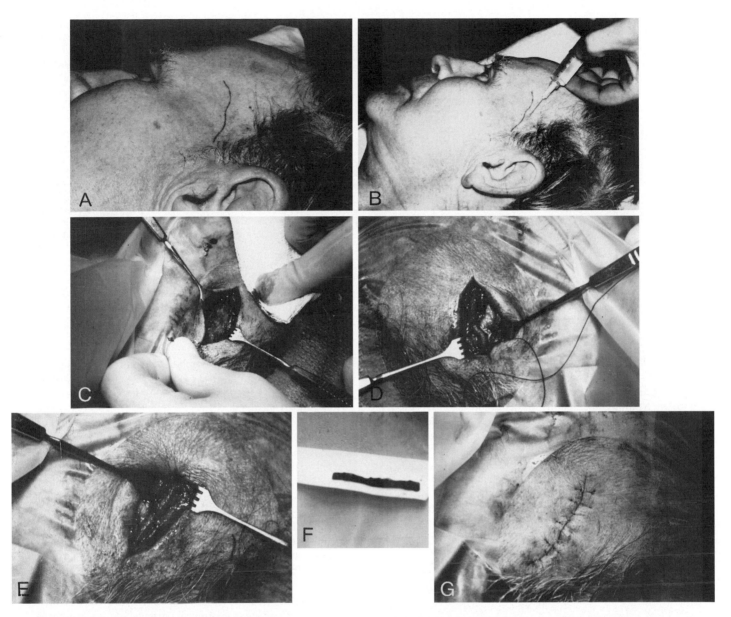

Figure 57.65. Technique of temporal artery biopsy. *A*, The course of the artery is determined by direct visualization, palpation, or Doppler ultrasonography (see Fig. 57.64) and is marked with brilliant green ink or a sterile marking pen. *B*, The skin and subcutaneous tissue on each side of the artery is anesthetized with a mixture of xylocaine and epinephrine. *C*, An incision is made in the skin along the course of the artery and is carried down through subcutaneous tissue. The artery can be identified on the surface of the fascia of the temporalis muscle (*arrowhead*). *D* and *E*, The connective tissue overlying the artery is removed, and a segment of the vessel is isolated between two 4-0 or 6-0 black silk sutures. *F*, The artery is excised. *G*, The incision is closed using interrupted 6–0 nylon sutures.

patients had either simultaneous (146 patients) or sequential (36 patients) bilateral biopsies. In only six of the 182 patients (3.3%) who underwent a bilateral biopsy, was the pathology on one side different from the other. All six had one side read as arteriosclerotic change. In three of the cases, the other side was thought to be consistent with healed arteritis; in the other three cases, the pathology was reported as possible early arteritis. In none of the six cases, whether the second biopsy was performed simultaneous with the first or sequentially, was one side read as unequivocal active arteritis. The results of this study suggest that when only a unilateral temporal artery biopsy is possible, the clinician can be reasonably confident in the pathologic results of that specimen.

TREATMENT AND PROGNOSIS

The only medication that is clearly effective in the treatment of GCA is systemic corticosteroids (Mosher, 1948;

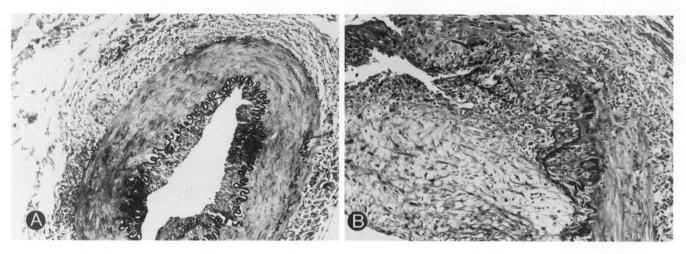

Figure 57.66. Skip area in a patient with giant cell arteritis. A 25-mm piece of temporal artery was removed for evaluation from a 75-year-old woman with headache, arthralgias, and confusion. *A,* One end of the artery shows normal architecture with no evidence of inflammation. *B,* The opposite end of the artery shows an intensive inflammation infiltrating the wall of the vessel, producing fragmentation of the elastic lamina, and narrowing the lumen. The infiltrate consists of lymphocytes, plasma cells, and giant cells. This arteritic portion of the vessel was only a few millimeters in length; the rest of the vessel showed no evidence of inflammation.

Hunder, 1993; Hoffman and Fauci, 1994; Hunder, 1996, 1997). Once the diagnosis of GCA is suspected, treatment with systemic corticosteroids should begin immediately, without awaiting the results of a temporal artery biopsy (Cohen and Smith, 1974; Albert et al., 1976; Klein et al., 1976). If the temporal artery is inflamed, evidence of active inflammation will be microscopically visible for at least 7–14 days after the start of steroid therapy (Fauchald et al., 1972; Fulton et al., 1976; Achkar et al., 1994). In the meantime, prompt initiation of treatment may prevent further damage from the disease, particularly loss of vision in what may be the patient's only seeing eye (Cullen, 1967a, 1967b;

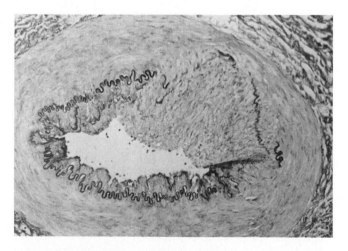

Figure 57.67. Pathology of healed giant cell arteritis. Section through the temporal artery of a patient with systemic symptoms and signs suggesting GCA who had been treated with systemic corticosteroids for several months and who had recently complained of blurred vision shows a region of fragmentation of the elastic lamina with proliferation of the intima but without evidence of inflammation.

Cohen, 1973). It must be emphasized that once vision is lost from central retinal artery occlusion or ischemic optic neuropathy in a patient with GCA, dramatic recovery of vision is rare (Russell, 1959; Egge et al., 1966; Cullen, 1967a, 1967b; Kearns, 1973; Diamond, 1991; Matzkin et al., 1992; Myles et al., 1992; Postel and Pollock, 1993; Liu et al., 1994). Therefore, the primary goal of therapy is to prevent visual loss in the opposite eye and to prevent ischemic damage to other organs in the body. The benefit of systemic corticosteroids in preventing both initial and further visual complications of GCA was first demonstrated by Birkhead et al. (1957), who reported a 3-fold decrease in the chance of involvement of a normal eye in a patient with GCA once treatment was begun compared with no treatment. Russell (1959) reported that among 13 patients with GCA treated with salicylates before the availability of systemic corticosteroids, five (38%) developed visual failure related to the disease, whereas among 10 patients who were treated with corticosteroids, none developed visual failure over the course of the disease. Cullen (1967a) reported that only one of 16 patients with GCA and unilateral loss of vision developed involvement of the second eye when corticosteroid treatment was started at the time of diagnosis in the first eye, and Palm (1958) reported loss of vision in the second eye in 15 of 17 patients (88%) with untreated GCA, compared with only one of eight eyes (13%) in patients with treated GCA. Other authors reported similar findings (Bennett, 1956; Meadows, 1968; Cohen, 1973). Nevertheless, we and others have seen patients in whom visual loss occurred in a previously unaffected eye several days and even weeks after apparently adequate treatment with oral corticosteroids was begun (Palm, 1958; Russell, 1959; Meadows, 1968; Smith, 1965; Cohen, 1973; Boghen and Glaser, 1975; Sorensen and Lorenzen, 1977; Huston et al., 1978; Hugod and Scheibel, 1979; Calamia and Hunder, 1980; Liu et al., 1994).

Many rheumatologists advocate beginning treatment with prednisone or prednisolone at a dose of about 1 mg/kg/day (Delecoeullerie et al., 1988; Kyle and Hazleman, 1989a); however, having frequently found this dose to be inadequate, we advocate a somewhat higher starting dose of 1.5–2.0 mg/kg/day. If the patient's symptoms do not respond within 24–72 hours, we and others recommend increasing the dosage. Some investigators recommend immediate hospitalization and treatment with **intravenous** systemic corticosteroids for several days before switching to oral corticosteroids. Although there is no definitive evidence that this method of treatment is more efficacious than oral treatment, it may be appropriate in selected patients with acute visual loss. Indeed, reversal of ischemic optic neuropathy with recovery of vision may occur after immediate institution of high-dose methylprednisolone at 1 g/day in divided doses for 1–3 days (Model, 1978; Rosenfeld et al., 1986; Matzkin et al., 1992; Liu et al., 1994; Ghanchi et al., 1996b). Liu et al. (1994) evaluated 45 patients with biopsy-proven GCA and visual symptoms. Forty-one of these patients had persistent visual loss. AION accounted for the visual loss in 88% of the affected eyes. Twenty-five patients received intravenous methylprednisolone, and 20 patients received oral prednisone. Visual improvement in this study was defined as a recovery of two or more lines of acuity and a final acuity of better than 20/80. Using this definition, 39% of affected eyes improved after intravenous therapy compared with 28% of eyes after oral treatment. This difference was not statistically significant, possibly because of the small number of patients in the study. Of more significance was that subsequent involvement of the fellow eye by GCA occurred only in patients treated with oral therapy. The results of this study are similar to those of Aiello et al. (1993), who reported visual improvement in 15% of affected eyes after high-dose intravenous steroid therapy. Most visual deterioration occurs within days of initiation of therapy, but some patients lose vision even after a year of therapy (Aiello et al., 1993; Wolin and Kent, 1995). Many of these patients are on very low dose prednisone at the time of their visual loss. We and others, however, have observed progression or new onset of visual loss **during treatment with high-dose corticosteroids** (Slavin and Margolis, 1988; Cornblath and Eggenberger, 1997). We believe that there is a small group of patients with active GCA who continue to deteriorate regardless of the dosage and route of administration of systemic corticosteroids (see also Palm, 1958; Wang and Henkind, 1979). For this group of patients, some other medication that acts more rapidly is clearly needed (see below).

Once an effective dose of steroid is identified, this dose should be maintained until symptoms resolve and the ESR returns to normal. Improvement in symptoms usually occurs within 24–72 hours after initiation of therapy, whereas the ESR may take several weeks to return to normal (Turner et al., 1974; Paice, 1989). Even if symptoms immediately resolve, and the ESR immediately returns to normal, the starting dose should be maintained for 2–4 weeks before beginning a slow taper of no more than 10% of the total daily dose every 1–2 weeks (Goodman, 1979; Hunder, 1993). The efficacy of the reduction program is then gauged by the pa-

tient's symptoms and ESR. The patient should be evaluated every 1–2 weeks, at which time an ESR should be obtained. Steroid reduction should not be continued unless both the symptoms and the ESR indicate that the disease is under control.

Patients with GCA should be given the required systemic corticosteroids in **daily** doses. Alternate-day administration of steroids is less effective than daily administration, and it cannot be depended upon to control the activity of the disease (Hunder et al., 1975; Paice, 1989). We have seen several patients with GCA who lost vision in their only remaining eye when their physicians switched them from daily to alternate-day prednisone therapy.

At some point in the course of reducing the dosage of steroids for a patient with GCA, the patient's ESR may begin to rise. If this occurs, it is important to verify that the rise is not artifactitious, and an additional ESR should therefore be performed immediately before any major change in the treatment regimen is made. If the rise is confirmed, further reduction should be stopped or the dosage increased until the ESR returns to normal and again stabilizes. Reduction in steroids can then be resumed, although it may need to be smaller or made at longer intervals. It is not uncommon for patients with GCA to require low daily maintenance doses of prednisone for many months or even years (Evans et al., 1994).

It must be emphasized that a rise in the ESR of a patient with GCA being treated with systemic corticosteroids is not always caused by persistence or reactivation of GCA. It may be caused by an intercurrent infection, especially one caused by an **opportunistic organism.** For example, we saw a 72-year-old man with diplopia, bilateral visual loss, tenderness of the right temple, and increasing fatigue. The patient had an elevated ESR and was immediately placed on oral prednisone. Within 24 hours, his temple pain, fatigue, and diplopia had resolved. A temporal artery biopsy, performed within 48 hours after prednisone was started, showed changes consistent with GCA. The patient was continued on prednisone at a dose of about 1.5 mg/kg/day for 1 month, during which time he continued to be free of symptoms, and his ESR dropped to normal. His internist then began to taper steroids at the rate of about 2.5–5 mg/day every 1–2 weeks. Within 6 months, the patient's dose of prednisone had been tapered to about 10 mg/day. At this time, he began to complain of increasing fatigue, confusion, and mild myalgias, and his ESR, which had been stable at about 20 mm/hr, began to increase. The dosage of prednisone was increased, but the patient's symptoms worsened, and the ESR continued to increase. The patient subsequently was evaluated and found to have cryptococcal meningitis. Another patient was a 70-year-old man with idiopathic CD4+ T-lymphocytopenia (see Chapter 69) who developed severe headaches and was found to have an elevated ESR. A tentative diagnosis of GCA was made, the patient was placed on oral prednisone, and bilateral temporal artery biopsies were performed. The day after the biopsies were performed, the patient abruptly lost vision in the left eye and was found to have a central retinal artery occlusion. A repeat ESR was even higher than before the patient was placed on prednisone. Accordingly, his prednisone dosage was increased; however,

24 hours later, the patient experienced a massive cerebral infarct. He died shortly thereafter. Postmortem examination revealed extensive aspergillosis with vascular invasion. There was no evidence of GCA.

GCA runs a self-limited course that may last only a few months but is more commonly **1–2 years** (Beevers et al., 1973; Huston et al., 1978; Kyle and Hazelman, 1990), and it may remain active for as long as 5–14 years after recognition of the disease (Östberg, 1971; Cullen, 1972; Cohen, 1973; Graham, 1980; Andersson et al., 1986; Gouet et al., 1986; Evans et al., 1994). Monitoring for relapse should continue for 6–12 months after stopping steroids, and patients should be instructed to contact a physician immediately if symptoms recur (Kyle and Hazelman, 1990). Most patients eventually can be completely withdrawn from steroids, although a small percentage seem to need low doses for several years or more to control musculoskeletal or visual symptoms (Cullen, 1972; Fulton et al., 1976; Graham, 1980; Kyle and Hazelman, 1990).

Because of the potentially significant side effects of both short- and long-term treatment with systemic corticosteroids (Sorensen and Lorenzen, 1977; Huston et al., 1978; Graham et al., 1981; Rubinow et al., 1984; Gouet et al., 1986; see Table 1 in Kyle and Hazleman, 1989b), physicians have attempted to find some other medicine to control GCA. To date, all efforts have had limited success. Dapsone, a drug used to treat leprosy, may be used in conjunction with systemic corticosteroids in an attempt to allow a more rapid reduction of medicine, but it cannot be used as a substitute for corticosteroids, and it has the potential side effect of severe anemia (Doury et al., 1983a, 1983b, 1984; Liozon et al., 1986; Reinitz and Aversa, 1988; Demaziere and Reinitz, 1989). Other agents, including nonsteroidal anti-inflammatory drugs and cytotoxic agents, have not been shown to be effective in treating GCA alone (Chuang et al., 1982; Wendling et al., 1985; De Silva and Hazleman, 1986) or in combination with systemic corticosteroids (Wilke and Hoffman, 1995), but a controlled clinical trial using methotrexate in conjunction with systemic corticosteroids is being performed.

Although the prognosis for vision that has been lost as a result of GCA is usually poor, regardless of treatment (Schneider et al., 1971), the prognosis for life is quite good when appropriate treatment is initiated early in the course of the disease. Hauser et al. (1971) found no evidence of reduced survival when patients with treated GCA were compared with a normal age- and sex-matched population, and other investigators have reported similar findings (Hamilton et al., 1971; Huston et al., 1978, Huston and Hunder, 1980; Nordborg and Bengtsson, 1989). Nevertheless, patients with GCA may die from the effects of the disease on the coronary or cranial arteries in the early stages of the disease, or from thromboembolic complications affecting the pulmonary, intracerebral, and cardiac arteries in the absence of histologic evidence of vasculitis (Wadman and Werner, 1972; Uriu and Reinecke, 1973). The proposed mechanism for this latter complication is hypercoagulability of blood with a decreased clotting time related to use of systemic corticosteroids. Graham et al. (1981) found an increased mortality in patients with GCA who required a maintenance dose of prednisone of more than 10 mg/day. The long-term side effects of steroids in GCA are highlighted by the study of Nesher et al. (1994). In a series of 43 patients, 58% suffered major complications including fractures and serious infections. Age over 75 and a starting dose of 40 mg of prednisone per day were associated with an increased frequency of complications. The authors conclude that the dose of corticosteroids should be individualized depending on the patient's age, severity of symptoms, and coexisting medical problems.

Hypersensitivity Vasculitis

The term **hypersensitivity vasculitis** is used to describe a group of conditions that are characterized by damage to small blood vessels of the skin and occasionally of other organs (Conn et al., 1993). These conditions are also called "leukocytoclastic vasculitides," because the pathologic process is infiltration of the small blood vessels by PMNs, destruction of the vessel walls, and fragmentation of the leukocytes (Zeek et al., 1948; Winkelmann and Ditto, 1964; Cream, 1976) (Fig. 57.68).

The pathogenesis of hypersensitivity vasculitis seems to be a reaction to one or more antigens, often drugs. Both immune complexes and cell-mediated reactions have been implicated in the development of necrotic vascular skin le-

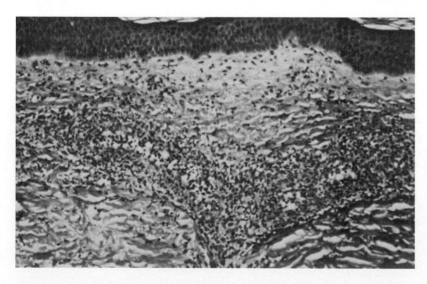

Figure 57.68. Hypersensitivity (leukocytoclastic) vasculitis. Dermal vessels show intense infiltration by inflammatory cells, primarily polymorphonuclear leukocytes. The inflammatory reaction has caused necrosis of the walls of the vessels and narrowing or occlusion of their lumens. Fragments of degenerated leukocyte nuclei ("nuclear dust") are visible in perivascular areas. (From Conn DL, Hunder GG. Vasculitis and related disorders. In Textbook of Rheumatology. Editors, Kelley WN, Harris ED Jr, Ruddy S, et al. 3rd ed, pp 1167–1199. Philadelphia, WB Saunders, 1989.)

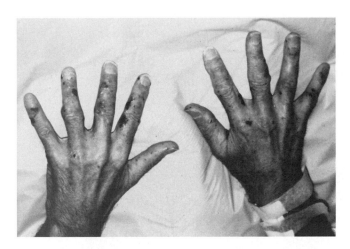

Figure 57.69. Hypersensitivity vasculitis affecting the hands. Note erythematous purpuric macules and papules that primarily involve the digits. (Courtesy of Dr. Douglas Jabs.)

sions (Soter, 1976). The inflammatory process is initiated by deposition of immune complexes derived from the circulation that have activated complement and generated chemotaxis of PMNs. The tissue necrosis results from the release of lysosomal enzymes and other noxious agents such as free radicals from the leukocytes (Sams et al., 1976).

The clinical manifestations in this group of disorders usually appear abruptly, beginning with skin lesions. In cases that are drug-induced, the symptoms usually develop within a few days after initiation of drug treatment. The reaction is neither time-predictable nor dose-dependent (Mullick et al., 1979).

The **skin lesions** are flat, erythematous, purpuric macules that progress to papules (Cream, 1976). The papular quality is important because it distinguishes these lesions from noninflammatory purpura. The eruption may occur on any part of the skin, but it is most common over dependent areas such as the lower extremities, the back, and the gluteal regions. Lesions may also appear on the forearms and hands (Fig. 57.69) but almost never on the upper portion of the trunk or on the face. Crops of lesions may develop at irregular intervals. The lesions last 1–4 weeks and then resolve, leaving hyperpigmentation and sometimes atrophic scars (Conn et al., 1993). The size of the lesions varies from a millimeter to several centimeters when individual lesions coalesce. Vesicles and bullae may develop in more severe cases.

Constitutional symptoms, including fever, may accompany the appearance of the skin lesions of hypersensitivity vasculitis. Arthralgias occur in the majority of patients, and other organs, including the kidneys, gastrointestinal tract, lungs, and brain, may be affected by vasculitis. Ophthalmic manifestations are rare but include uveitis, iridocyclitis, chemosis, retinal vasculitis, and optic neuropathy (Tsai et al., 1993).

The main disorders that are included under the heading of hypersensitivity vasculitis and that may have CNS manifestations, neuro-ophthalmologic manifestations, or both, are Henoch-Schönlein purpura and mixed cryoglobulinemia. These disorders are discussed in the sections that follow. It should be emphasized, however, that not all hypersensitivity

vasculitis syndromes fit into these categories. For example, Pless and Sandson (1997) described a patient with hypersensitivity vasculitis induced by D-penicillamine who developed a cerebral vasculitis characterized in part by upbent nystagmus and an INO.

HENOCH-SCHÖNLEIN PURPURA

The syndrome of Henoch-Schönlein purpura seems to be a distinct entity. Persons of any age may be affected, but the condition occurs most often in children, with a peak incidence at 4–11 years of age (Allen et al., 1960; Ansell, 1970; Valente et al., 1997). The disease occurs most often in the spring, and it often follows an upper respiratory tract infection. A classic triad of palpable purpura, arthritis, and abdominal pain occurs in about 50% of patients (Conn and Hunder, 1989; Cassidy, 1993). Skin lesions are similar to those described above, with some tendency for larger purpuric lesions to develop over the buttocks and lower extremities (Fig. 57.70). Edema of the feet and lower legs is common, and edema may also develop on the hands, scalp, and in the periorbital regions. The ankle and knee joints are affected most commonly, and they become swollen, warm, and tender. Gastrointestinal lesions may cause severe cramping, abdominal pain, intussusception, hemorrhage, protein-losing enteropathy, or, rarely, perforation. Renal damage, which occurs in about 50% of patients, may be associated with persistent renal insufficiency (Koskimies et al., 1974).

Patients with Henoch-Schönlein purpura may develop neurologic or visual dysfunction. In some cases, the neurologic symptoms and signs are caused by accompanying hypertension, whereas in others, they are produced by cerebral arteritis (Green, 1946; Gardner, 1948; Lewis and Philpott, 1956). Subarachnoid hemorrhage, ischemic and hemorrhagic strokes, and seizures can all occur. Some patients develop visual loss from intraorbital or intraocular hemorrhage (Benedict, 1930; Clark, 1932; Walsh and Hoyt, 1969d). In such cases, one or both eyes may be lost from intractable glaucoma (Clark, 1932).

Supportive treatment alone is usually adequate for mild cases of Henoch-Schönlein purpura, but more severe cases may require the use of systemic corticosteroids, intravenous immunogloblin therapy, or both (Rostoker et al., 1994) The disease is generally self-limited, resolving within 6–16 weeks. Most patients have no further difficulties, although 5–10% of patients relapse within a few weeks or months (Conn et al., 1993).

MIXED CRYOGLOBULINEMIA

In 1933, Wintrobe and Buell described a case of multiple myeloma in which a substance in the patient's serum precipitated at reduced temperatures and redissolved on heating. Lerner and Watson (1947) subsequently used the term **cryoglobulin** to describe a similar substance that precipitated from the serum of a patient with purpura, urticaria, and glomerulonephritis under similar circumstances. It is now clear that cryoglobulins—immunoglobulins that precipitate at 4 C and redissolve after warming to 37 C—occur in the serum of patients with a variety of clinical conditions (Barnett et al., 1970).

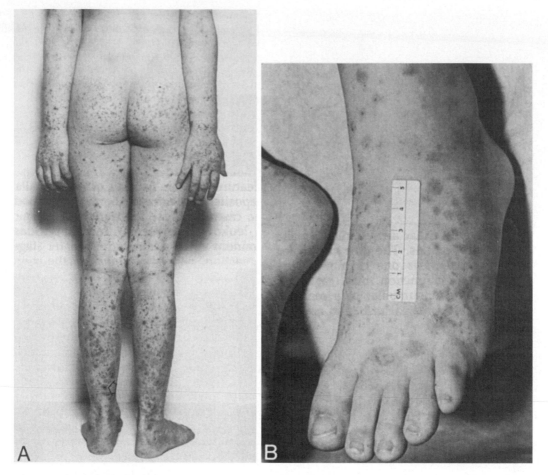

Figure 57.70. Cutaneous manifestations of Henoch-Schönlein purpura. *A*, Erythematous purpuric macules and papules are most prominent over the extensor surfaces of the distal regions of the upper and lower extremities and over the buttocks. A few small infarcts of the skin are visible (*arrow*). (From Conn DL, Hunder GG. Vasculitis and related disorders. In Textbook of Rheumatology. Editors, Kelley WN, Harris ED Jr, Ruddy S, et al. 3rd ed, pp 1167–1199. Philadelphia, WB Saunders, 1989.) *B*, Erythematous purpuric macules and papules on the foot and ankle of a 6-year-old boy with Henoch-Schönlein purpura. (From Schaller JG, Szer IS. Systemic lupus erythematosus, dermatomyositis, scleroderma, and vasculitis in childhood. In Textbook of Rheumatology. Editors, Kelley WN, Harris ED Jr, Ruddy S, et al. 3rd ed, pp 1325–1354. Philadelphia, WB Saunders, 1989.)

Cryoglobulins can be single-component and monoclonal, in which case they are usually composed of either IgG or IgM, or they may be mixed, composed of two different immunoglobulins, most frequently a combination of IgG and IgM. Single-component cryoglobulins are most often found in patients with blood dyscrasias such as multiple myeloma, whereas mixed cryoglobulins are most often found in patients with connective tissue diseases and in the systemic vasculitic syndrome called **mixed cryoglobulinemia**. There is also an association between hepatitis C virus infection and mixed cryoglobulinemia (Petty et al., 1996).

The syndrome of mixed cryoglobulinemia is characterized by purpura, arthralgia, weakness, and mixed cryoglobulinemia (LoSpalluto et al., 1962; Meltzer and Franklin, 1966). Patients with this condition develop a cutaneous vasculitis associated with evidence of widespread systemic vasculitis and progressive renal failure from glomerulone-

phritis (Fig. 57.71). The condition most often affects middle-aged women. As with other forms of hypersensitivity vasculitis, this disorder appears to be immune complex-mediated. Immune deposits containing complement can be demonstrated in skin vessel walls and along the glomerular basement membrane (Golde and Epstein, 1968; Cream, 1971). The cryoglobulins are present in small amounts, usually less than 100 mg/dL. They contain IgG and IgM, both of which are required for cryoprecipitation (Conn et al., 1993).

A peripheral neuropathy frequently occurs in patients with mixed cryoglobinemia. Both motor and sensory neuropathy occur at some time during the course of the disease in 7–17% of patients (Abramsky and Slavin, 1974; Brouet et al., 1974; Chad et al., 1982). Immunologically mediated demyelination and nerve ischemia, the latter a result of vasa nervorum obstruction by cryoglobulins or vasculitis, are the mechanisms that cause this neuropathy (Chad et al., 1982) (Fig. 57.72).

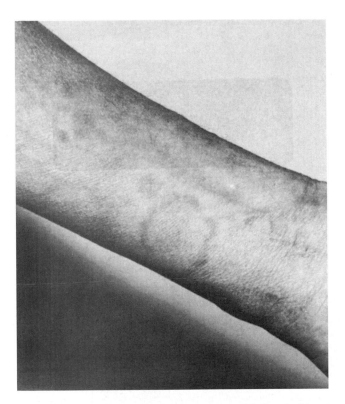

Figure 57.71. Cutaneous vasculitis in mixed cryoglobulinemia. There is a large, resolving urticarial lesion on the flexor surface of the forearm. Other smaller lesions also are present. (From Conn DL, Hunder GG. Vasculitis and related disorders. In Textbook of Rheumatology. Editors, Kelley WN, Harris ED Jr, Ruddy S, et al. 3rd ed, pp 1167–1199. Philadelphia, WB Saunders, 1989.)

CNS dysfunction occurs in 2–5% of patients with mixed cryoglobulinemia (Sigal, 1987). When the cerebral hemispheres are affected, patients may develop hemiparesis, hemisensory loss, aphasia, homonymous visual field defects, or a combination of these deficits. When the brainstem or cerebellum are damaged, patients may develop ataxia, dysarthria, diplopia, or crossed paralyses. Gorevic et al. (1980) described two patients in whom seizures occurred and one patient who suffered a stroke. Abramsky and Slavin (1974) reported four patients with symptoms referable to both the peripheral and the central nervous systems. In one of these patients, the neurologic manifestations were the first evidence of the systemic disease. Other authors subsequently described similar cases (Ristow et al., 1976; Chad et al., 1982; Petty et al., 1996). Cerebral angiography in such cases may demonstrate focal narrowing, vessel irregularities, or occlusion (Petty et al., 1996).

The cutaneous appearance of a patient with mixed cryoglobulinemia may be identical to that of a patient with Henoch-Schönlein purpura, but the presence of cryoglobulins, a positive rheumatoid factor, and low concentrations of complement in the serum allow these two conditions to be distinguished with relative ease. Distinguishing mixed cryoglobulinemia from SLE may be more difficult, but the absence of antibodies to deoxyribonucleic acid (DNA) and the absence of immunoglobulins at the dermal-epidermal junction of biopsy specimens in the latter condition permit the correct diagnosis to be made.

The treatment of mixed cryoglobulinemia depends on the severity of the disease. Patients with extensive disease may require high doses of systemic corticosteroids, cytotoxic drugs, or intravenously administered γ-globulin (Valente et al., 1997). In some cases, plasmapheresis is benefi-

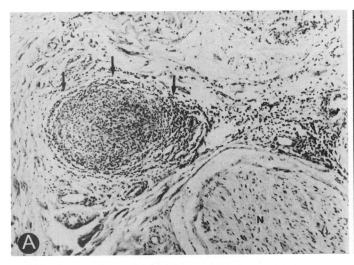

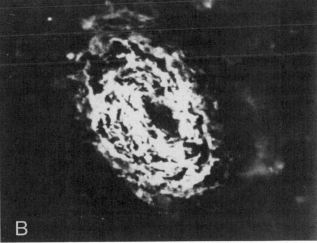

Figure 57.72. Pathology and immunology of mixed cryoglobulinemia. The patient was a 65-year-old woman with pain and paresthesias in the feet. She subsequently developed a bilateral foot drop, nonfluent dysphasia, and weakness of the right hand. A complete laboratory evaluation revealed a cryoglobulin concentration in the serum of 1.76 mg/ml (normal, <0.1 mg/ml). The cryoglobulins consisted of monoclonal IgM (kappa) and polyclonal IgG. *A*, Sural nerve biopsy shows inflammatory cells surrounding and infiltrating a medium-sized epineurial vessel (*arrows*). *N*, nerve fascicle. *B*, Cross-section through a medium-sized artery in the gastrocnemius muscle stained with fluorescein isothiocyanate-conjugated antiserum to human fibrinogen shows marked immunofluorescence in the wall of the vessel. (From Chad D, Pariser K, Bradley WG, et al. The pathogenesis of cryobulinemic neuropathy. Neurology *32*:725–729, 1982.)

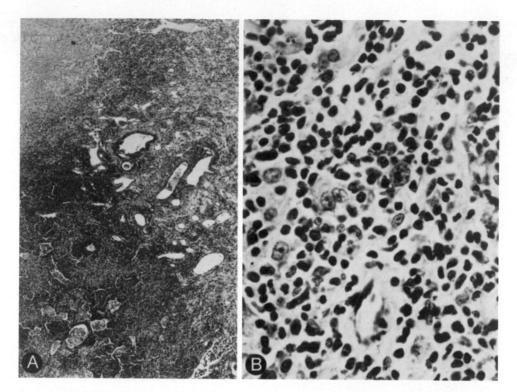

Figure 57.73. Pathology of lymphomatoid granulomatosis. *A*, Low magnification shows infiltration of a pulmonary arteriole (*center*) with extension of the infiltrate into the surrounding lung (*bottom left*). An area of necrosis is also visible (*top left*). *B*, High magnification of the same region shows that the infiltrate is composed primarily of small lymphocytes with only a few plasma cells, histiocytes, and atypical lymphoreticular cells (*center*). (From Katzenstein A-L, Carrington CB, Liebow AA. Lymphomatoid granulomatosis: A clinicopathologic study of 152 cases. Cancer *43:*360–373, 1979.)

cial. In patients with associated hepatitis C virus infection, interferon-α may be used (Petty et al., 1996).

Lymphomatoid Granulomatosis (Angiocentric T-Cell Lymphoma)

This rare disease was initially described by Liebow et al. (1972). It is characterized by an angiocentric and angiodestructive infiltration of various organs with atypical lymphocytoid and plasmacytoid cells (Cupps and Fauci, 1981a) (Fig. 57.73). The arteries and veins are infiltrated to such an extent that their morphology may be unrecognizable. Immunohistologic techniques using monoclonal antibodies to specific T- and B-cell surface antigens show that cases classified morphologically as lymphomatoid granulomatosis are, in fact, angiocentric T-cell lymphomas (Weis et al., 1986; Kleinschmidt-Demasters et al., 1992; Brazis et al., 1995).

The mean age of onset of this disease is 48 years, with a range of 7–85 years (Fauci et al., 1982). Men are affected slightly more often than women. Patients most often present with constitutional symptoms, including fever, malaise, and weight loss, and accompanying myalgias and arthralgias. The lungs are commonly affected, with respiratory symptoms consisting of cough, chest pain, and shortness of breath. Skin involvement occurs in 40% of patients and is characterized by the development of erythematous macules and indurated plaques (Conn and Hunder, 1989). Enlargement of the liver, spleen, or lymph nodes is uncommon.

Neurologic manifestations occur in about 30% of patients with lymphomatoid granulomatosis and are the presenting features of the disease in up to 21% of cases (Katzenstein et al., 1979). Neurologic disease can antedate other systemic manifestations by as much as 5 years, and it may progress even as lung and other systemic manifestations respond to therapy (Liebow et al., 1972; Verity and Wolfson, 1976; Katzenstein et al., 1979; Hogan et al., 1981; Patton and Lynch, 1982; Sigal, 1987). Patients may develop CNS manifestations, peripheral neuropathy, or both. Central neurologic manfestations are protean and include mental confusion, seizures, ataxia, and hemiparesis. Katzenstein et al. (1979) described peripheral facial nerve paresis, diplopia, transient blindness, deafness, and vertigo in their patients but gave no further details. The patient reported by Hogan et al. (1981) complained of oscillopsia and had a bilateral INO, indicating intrinsic damage to the brainstem. Some patients develop cranial neuropathies, including ocular motor nerve pareses, facial nerve paresis, and deafness. When the disease occurs as a mass lesion, intracranial pressure (ICP) may become increased, and patients may develop papilledema (Schmidt et al., 1984). Optic neuropathies occur in some patients with lymphomatoid granulomatosis. Kokmen et al. (1977) reported a patient in whom optic disc swelling occurred and then resolved spontaneously over several weeks. Brazis et al. (1995) reported a patient with multiple cranial nerve palsies and a retrobulbar optic neuropathy. MR imaging revealed an enhancing mass medial and inferior to the left optic nerve. There was also a separate enhancing mass in the region of the right cavernous sinus. The precise mechanism of the retrobulbar optic neuropathy is unclear; it may have resulted from either ischemia or direct compression.

The CNS pathology of lymphomatoid granulomatosis consists of a triad of (*a*) angiitis; (*b*) infiltration of tissue by lymphocytoid and plasmacytoid cells; and (*c*) necrosis of the meninges, parenchyma, and vessels (Verity and Wolfson, 1976; Pena, 1977) (Fig. 57.74). These features are often found in patients without clinical evidence of CNS involvement (Liebow et al., 1972). Conversely, some cases of lymphomatoid granulomatosis are apparently confined to the CNS (Kokmen et al., 1977; DeRemee et al., 1978; Schmidt et al., 1984).

Patients with lymphomatoid granulomatosis have no characteristic ocular manifestations; however, occasional patients develop uveitis, retinitis, eyelid involvement, or a combination of these findings (Katzenstein et al., 1979; Nichols et al., 1982; Robin et al., 1985; Rootman et al., 1988). We have never encountered the disease as an inflammatory process in the orbit, but we agree with Jakobiec and Jones (1979) that there is no reason why this could not occur. Haider (1993) reported a patient who developed a tonic pupil

shortly before the systemic features of lymphomatoid granulomatosis appeared.

Lymphomatoid granulomatosis lacks characteristic laboratory features. About 50% of patients have an elevated ESR, and a small percentage have leukopenia (Conn and Hunder, 1989). A chest X-ray may be helpful when it shows bilateral nodular densities, cavitation, or pleural effusion without hilar adenopathy. Cerebral angiography may show a pattern of narrowing consistent with vasculitis in patients with neurologic dysfunction (Liebow et al., 1972). A definitive diagnosis is made by biopsy of affected tissue with demonstration of characteristic histopathologic features.

Lymphomatoid granulomatosis usually is treated with high doses of systemic corticosteroids and cyclophosphamide (Moore and Cupps, 1983); however, many patients develop a malignant lymphoma that is unresponsive to therapy. Saldana et al. (1977) reported an 83% mortality rate among 24 patients treated with a combination of systemic corticosteroids and a single cytotoxic agent, and Israel et al. (1977) treated five patients with combination chemotherapy consisting of cyclophosphamide, vincristine, and prednisone with no survivors. Nevertheless, Fauci et al. (1982) achieved long-term remissions in seven of 15 patients, 13 of whom were treated with prednisone and cyclophosphamide, and other authors reported similar results (Drasga et al., 1984;

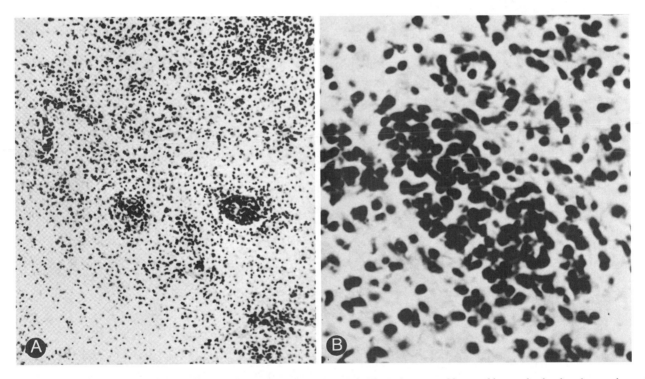

Figure 57.74. Central nervous system involvement in lymphomatoid granulomatosis. The patient was a 30-year-old man who developed a maculopapular rash, interstitial pneumonia, and generalized weakness of the extremities. An open lung biopsy was positive for lymphomatoid granulomatosis. The patient was treated with systemic corticosteroids. Three years later, the patient was found comatose at home. Lumbar puncture revealed increased intracranial pressure. The patient died several hours later. *A*, Diffuse small cell infiltration of the putamen. The adjacent neuropil shows patchy coagulative necrosis, demyelination, and petechiae. *B*, Higher magnification of the affected region shows mixed atypical histiocytic and plasmacytoid cells infiltrating the parenchyma and vessels of the brain. (From Verity MA, Wolfson WL. Cerebral lymphomatoid granulomatosis: A report of two cases, with disseminated necrotizing leukoencephalopathy in one. Acta Neuropathol *36:*117–124, 1976.)

Jenkins and Zaloznik, 1989). The development of CNS disease in a patient with lymphomatoid granulomatosis is associated with an especially poor prognosis. The 3-year survival rate may be as high as 40% in the absence of CNS disease, but it is only 6–13% when CNS disease is present (Katzenstein et al., 1979). It seems clear that patients with lymphomatoid granulomatosis should be treated with aggressive combination chemotherapy at the time of initial diagnosis in an effort to improve the grim prognosis of the disease.

Takayasu's Arteritis (Pulseless Disease)

HISTORY

In 1839, John Davy described progressive obliteration of the main branches of the aortic arch in a 55-year-old man. The patient had symptoms and signs of diffuse cerebrovascular insufficiency, and pulses were absent in both upper extremities. A diagnosis of syphilitic aortitis, made initially by history, was confirmed by postmortem findings. Seventeen

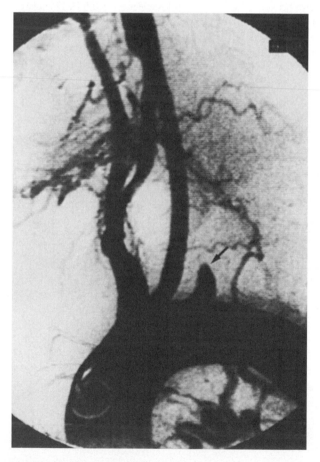

Figure 57.75. Arch aortogram in a patient with Takayasu's arteritis. The study shows a tapered occlusion of the left subclavian artery (*arrow*) and no filling of the right subclavian artery. Multiple dilated collateral channels are present at the base of the neck and in the upper thoracic region. (From Goldberg HI. Cerebral angiography. In Stroke: Pathophysiology, Diagnosis, and Management. Editors, Barnett HJM, Mohr JP, Stein BM, et al., Vol 1, pp 221–244. New York, Churchill Livingstone, 1986.)

years later, Savory (1856) described a young woman in whom the main arteries of both upper extremities and the left side of the neck were completely occluded. There was no evidence of syphilis in the patient, although the pathologic appearance of the occluded vessels was that of an obliterative arteritis.

The reports of Davy (1839) and Savory (1856) were more or less ignored, with subsequent investigators making no distinction between the two conditions, until 1908, when Takayasu described peculiar retinal changes consistent with chronic hypoxia in a young Japanese woman. He had no explanation for these changes, but in a discussion of the case, two of his colleagues stated that they had noted similar retinal alterations in two young women in whom radial pulses could not be detected (Walsh and Hoyt, 1969e). Other cases were subsequently published in Japan, and gradually a clinical picture emerged. The disease seemed to be an arteritis of unknown cause that occurred predominantly in young women. It affected the aortic arch and its branches, causing symptoms and signs of vascular insufficiency of the head, neck, and upper extremities. It was thought initially that this condition, called **pulseless disease** by Shimizu and Sano (1951), might be endemic in Japan. Indeed, in the Western hemisphere, the disease was not recognized as a separate entity and was simply confused with other types of aortic arch syndromes (Ross and McKusick, 1953). In 1956, however, Ask-Upmark presented the first clear classification of the aortic arch syndromes and emphasized that ''young female arteritis'' was a distinct entity. His study was published nearly 100 years after Savory's original description (Savory, 1856). It subsequently became clear that this condition, now called **Takayasu's arteritis**, is a systemic necrotizing vasculitis (Conn et al., 1993; Valente et al., 1997).

Most cases of Takayasu's arteritis are characterized by severe occlusive disease of the aortic arch and its branches (Park et al., 1989; Kerr et al., 1994) (Figs. 57.75 and 57.76). Varying degrees of narrowing, occlusion, and poststenotic dilation develop in the affected vessels, resulting in a wide variety of symptoms and signs.

DEMOGRAPHICS

The prevalence and incidence of Takayasu's arteritis are unknown. Cases occur throughout the world, although the largest number of case reports are from Japan. Nasu (1975) found 100 cases in about 300,000 autopsies registered in Japan over a period of 16 years (0.03%). Eighty to 90% of cases occur in women, and the onset of the disease is usually between the ages of 10 and 30 years (Lupi-Herrera et al., 1977; Ishikawa, 1978; Kerr et al., 1994).

Takayasu's arteritis may affect the entire aorta, the abdominal aorta, the ascending aorta, or just the aortic arch and its branches (Judge et al., 1962; Nakao et al., 1967; Lupi-Herrera et al., 1977). Arteries commonly affected include the innominate, common carotid, and subclavian arteries as well as the celiac, mesenteric, renal, pulmonary, iliac, and coronary arteries (Committee on Study of Arteritis, 1968; Cipriano et al., 1977).

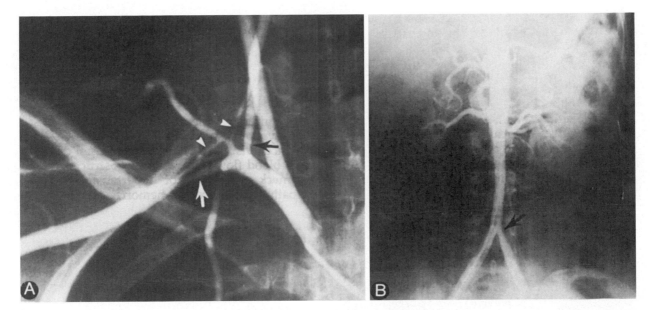

Figure 57.76. Results of angiography in Takayasu's arteritis. *A*, Aortic angiogram shows smooth-walled, tapered narrowing of the right subclavian artery (*white arrow*), right vertebral artery (*black arrow*), and arteries of the thyrocervical trunk (*arrowheads*). *B*, Abdominal aorta shows smooth-walled tubular narrowing of middle and lower portions and constriction of the left common iliac artery at its origin (*arrow*). (From Conn DL, Hunder GG. Vasculitis and related disorders. In Textbook of Rheumatology. Editors, Kelley WN, Harris ED Jr, Ruddy S, et al. 3rd ed, pp 1167–1199. Philadelphia, WB Saunders, 1989.)

SYSTEMIC MANIFESTATIONS

Takayasu's arteritis is usually separated into three clinical phases: (*a*) an acute stage characterized by symptoms and signs of a nonspecific systemic inflammation, (*b*) a phase of acute inflammation of the affected vessels, and (*c*) a chronic phase characterized by symptoms and signs of vascular occlusion (Moore and Cupps, 1983). In the initial phase of Takayasu's arteritis, patients develop nonspecific constitutional symptoms such as fatigue, weight loss, and low-grade fever (Ask-Upmark, 1954; Strachan, 1964). About 50% of patients also develop arthralgias or mild arthritis (Ishikawa, 1978). Evidence of vascular insufficiency caused by narrowing of large arteries becomes apparent with time. Important findings in such patients include tenderness, diminished pulses, and bruits over one or more brachial, subclavian, or carotid arteries (Kerr et al., 1994). The upper extremities may become cool. Patients in whom the entire aorta or just the abdominal portion of the aorta is affected may have femoral or abdominal bruits and decreased pulses in the lower extremities. Claudication of the extremities occurs in many patients, and affected extremities may develop ischemic ulcers.

Systemic hypertension develops in at least 50% of patients with Takayasu's arteritis (Moore and Cupps, 1983). It may be caused by narrowing of the aorta, decreased elasticity in the aortic wall, renal artery stenosis, or a combination of these mechanisms (Ask-Upmark, 1961; Kerr et al., 1994) (Fig. 57.77). Blood pressure may be difficult to assess, however, because of the diminished blood flow to the arms (Spencer et al., 1980). It may be measured by a wide cuff on the legs or by direct measurements in the ascending aorta (Conn et al., 1993).

As the disease progresses, the skin over the face may become atrophic, with loss of teeth and hair and with ulcers on the lips and the tip of the nose. If the pulmonary arteries are affected, the patient may develop dyspnea, hemoptysis, and pulmonary hypertension (Lupi-Herrera et al., 1975). Abdominal pain, diarrhea, and gastrointestinal hemorrhage may result from mesenteric artery ischemia. Angina pectoris occurs from narrowing of the coronary arteries (Fig. 57.78).

NEUROLOGIC MANIFESTATIONS

Neurologic symptoms and signs often develop in patients with Takayasu's arteritis. They may be the initial manifestation of the disease (Hall et al., 1985; Shelhamer et al., 1985), but they more often develop later in the course of the disease (Shimizu and Sano, 1951; Currier et al., 1954; Strachan et al., 1966). Occlusion of the carotid or vertebral arteries may result in generalized stroke or focal neurologic deficits (Currier et al., 1954; Lupi-Herrera et al., 1977; Ishikawa, 1978; Fraga and LaValle, 1980; Wolfe, 1989) (Fig. 57.79). Headache, dizziness, syncope, and blurred vision are common in such patients (Kerr et al., 1994). Patients with Takayasu's arteritis also may develop neurologic symptoms and signs from both ruptured and unruptured intracranial aneurysms (see Chapter 53), but it is unclear if the aneurysms occur independently or are a manifestation of the disease (see Table 1 in Masuzawa et al., 1984).

OCULAR MANIFESTATIONS

The most characteristic ocular findings are retinal arteriovenous anastomoses (Tanaka and Shimizu, 1987; Jabs, 1994;

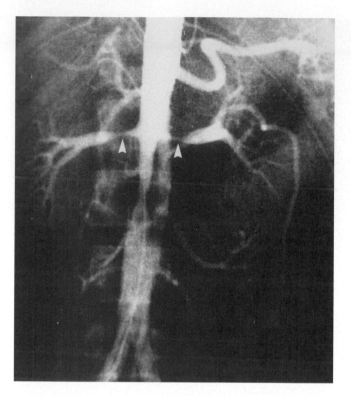

Figure 57.77. Renal artery stenosis in Takayasu's arteritis. Abdominal aortogram performed in a 21-year-old woman with severe systemic hypertension shows marked stenosis of the proximal portions of both renal arteries (*arrowheads*). Also note smooth segmental narrowing of the infrarenal abdominal aorta. (From Park JH, Han MC, Kim SH, et al. Takayasu arteritis: Angiographic findings and results of angiography. AJR *153*:1069–1074, 1989.)

Kishi et al., 1997) (Fig. 57.80). These lesions, generally seen around the optic disc and in the midperipheral retina, are thought to be caused by ocular ischemia. Other retinal vascular abnormalities include dilation of small retinal vessels, retinal microaneurysms, and intraretinal hemorrhages (Caccamise and Okuda, 1954; Pinkham, 1955; Ostler, 1957; Tour and Hoyt, 1959; Hirose, 1963; Hedges, 1964; Spencer et al., 1980; Lewis et al., 1993) (Fig. 57.80). In severe cases, a more complete ocular ischemic syndrome develops, characterized by peripheral retinal nonperfusion, neovascularization, and vitreous hemorrhage. Optic atrophy may develop from unilateral or bilateral ischemic optic neuropathies (Kalmansohn and Kalmansohn, 1957; Schmidt et al., 1997). Pathologic examination of such eyes reveals changes consistent with severe retinal, choroidal, and optic nerve ischemia (Dowling and Smith, 1960; Font and Naumann, 1969) (Fig. 57.81).

Patients with Takayasu's arteritis may develop loss of vision from occlusion of the common or internal carotid artery. Such patients may develop monocular blindness that may be associated with contralateral hemiparesis or other evidence of a hemisphere stroke (see Chapter 55). When the common carotid or external carotid arteries become occluded, hemifacial atrophy may develop (Kalmansohn and Kalmansohn, 1957).

PATHOLOGY

The earliest pathologic changes of Takayasu's arteritis are found in the adventitia and the outer part of the media. These changes consist of granulomatous inflammation with infiltration of lymphocytes, plasma cells, histiocytes, and occasional PMNs and multinucleated giant cells. As the disease progresses, a panarteritis develops. The elastic fibers and smooth muscles in the media undergo fragmentation and necrosis, and pronounced intimal thickening occurs in areas with inflamed outer layers (Fig. 57.82). The thickened intima and the contraction of the fibrotic media and adventitia cause narrowing and obliteration of the arterial lumen, which may be further compromised by endothelial proliferation. Thrombosis commonly occurs in the stenotic areas, and dissections or aneurysms may form in areas where the arterial wall has been weakened by the inflammatory process (Ueda et al., 1968; Nasu, 1975). Many asymptomatic patients have histologically active disease as determined by surgical biopsy specimens (Kerr et al., 1994).

PATHOGENESIS

The cause of Takayasu's arteritis is unknown. Infections with spirochetes, tubercle bacilli, and even *Streptococcus* species have been suggested as causes, but there is no solid evidence for any of them as inciting agents (Wolfe, 1989). Evidence of connective tissue disease, elevated concentrations of immunoglobulins in the serum, and antibodies

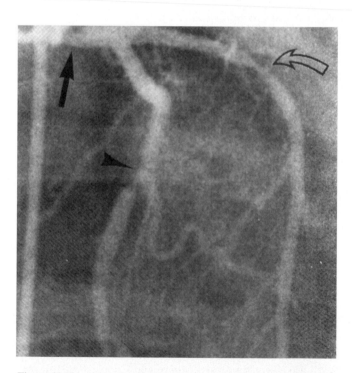

Figure 57.78. Coronary artery involvement in a 29-year-old woman with Takayasu's arteritis and angina pectoris. Left coronary arteriogram, anteroposterior view, shows irregular stenosis of the left main coronary artery (*straight arrow*), the middle left anterior descending coronary artery (*curved arrow*), and the left circumflex coronary artery (*arrowhead*). (From Park JH, Han MC, Kim SH, et al. Takayasu arteritis: Angiographic findings and results of angiography. AJR *153*:1069–1074, 1989.)

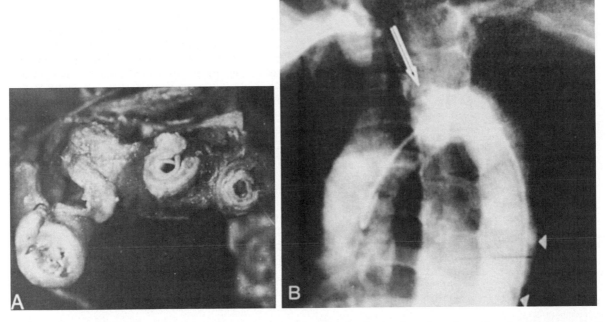

Figure 57.79. Carotid and vertebral artery stenosis in Takayasu's arteritis. *A*, Photograph taken from above the aortic arch in a patient who died from the effects of Takayasu's arteritis shows severe thickening of the walls with marked stenosis or occlusion of all of the vessels arising from the arch. The occluded innominate artery is on the left. (From Graham DI, Brierley JB. Hypoxia and vascular disorders of the central nervous system. In Greenfield's Neuropathology. Editors, Adams JH, Corsellis JAN, Duchen LW. 4th ed, pp 125–207. New York, John Wiley & Sons, 1984.) *B*, Thoracic aortogram, anteroposterior view, in a 27-year-old woman with Takayasu's arteritis and cerebral ischemia, shows occlusion of the left common carotid artery (*arrow*). Note irregularities in the wall of the descending aorta (*arrowheads*). (From Park JH, Han MC, Kim SH, et al. Takayasu arteritis: Angiographic findings and results of angiography. AJR *153:*1069–1074, 1989.)

against aortic tissue in some patients suggest an immunologic cause (Ueda et al., 1971). HLA studies indicate an increased frequency of HLA-Bw52 in Asians (Isohisa et al., 1978) and of MB3 and DR4 in North Americans (Volkman et al., 1982). These findings suggest that there may be an inherited susceptibility to Takayasu's arteritis.

DIAGNOSIS

The diagnosis of Takayasu's arteritis should be suspected in any patient, particularly a young woman, with symptoms of vascular ischemia and the finding of bruits, decreased or absent pulses, or a combination of these. The diagnosis is

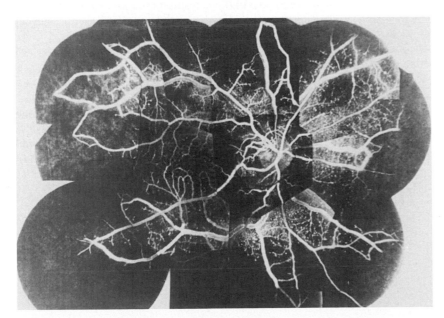

Figure 57.80. Fluorescein angiogram of the right ocular fundus in a patient with Takayasu's arteritis shows numerous retinal arteriovenous shunts and microaneurysms. Note also marked peripheral retinal nonperfusion. (From Shimizu K. Fluorescein Microangiography of the Ocular Fundus. pp 45–52. Baltimore, Williams & Wilkins, 1973.)

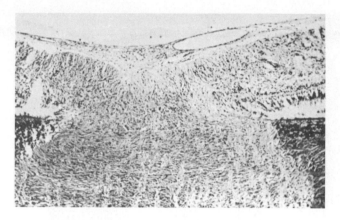

Figure 57.81. Optic atrophy in a patient with Takayasu's arteritis. The patient was a 35-year-old woman with a 1-month history of blurred vision, redness of both eyes, and photophobia. Physical examination revealed absent pulsations of radial, brachial, and carotid arteries. No blood pressure could be measured in either arm. Blood pressure in the lower extremities was 230/120 mm Hg. The patient underwent retrograde aortogram that failed to visualize the major branches of the aortic arch. The patient died 2 days after the aortogram from bacterial sepsis. At autopsy, there was complete thrombotic occlusion of the innominate, the left subclavian, and both common carotid arteries. Longitudinal section through the proximal portion of the left optic nerve shows diffuse atrophy. There is a thin, fibrovascular membrane overlying the optic disc and juxtapapillary retina. (From Font RL, Naumann G. Ocular histopathology in pulseless disease. Arch Ophthalmol *82:*784–788, 1969.)

confirmed by angiography, which shows vascular segments, some occluded, some dilated, and some with smooth-walled, tapered, focal or generalized narrowing (Sano et al., 1970; Lande and Berkmen, 1976; Park et al., 1989) (Figs. 57.75–57.79). The arteritis tends to affect the proximal portions of large vessels such as the aortic arch and subclavian and carotid arteries (Hurst and Grossman, 1994). Although histologic proof of vasculitis is preferred, the size of the affected vessels makes diagnostic biopsies difficult to perform. The National Institutes of Health criteria for active disease include a worsening or a new onset of at least two of the following: (*a*) clinical evidence of ischemia (e.g., extremity claudication or absent pulse), (*b*) systemic symptoms, (*c*) elevated ESR, (*d*) angiographic abnormalities (Kerr et al., 1994).

TREATMENT AND PROGNOSIS

Systemic corticosteroids suppress the systemic symptoms of Takayasu's arteritis, and they may be helpful in reversing arterial stenoses in the early stages of the disease (Fraga et al., 1972; Moore and Cupps, 1983; Hall et al., 1985). Pulses may improve dramatically, and ischemic symptoms such as claudication may disappear. Kulkarni et al. (1974) reported a case in which secondary hypertension resolved. Once fibrous tissue is laid down or after thrombosis occurs, the response to systemic corticosteroids is diminished, although long-term, low-dose steroids may still prevent progression of the disease (Valente et al., 1997). Patients requiring long-term, high-dose steroids for remission may benefit from cy-

totoxic agents such as cyclophosphamide or methotrexate (Hoffman et al., 1994; Hoffman, 1995). Nevertheless, approximately 20% of patients continue to progress despite medical therapy (Kerr et al., 1994). Surgical bypass of obstructed arteries or percutaneous transluminal angioplasty may be beneficial in selected patients (Warren and Friedman, 1957; Inada et al., 1970; Kimoto, 1979; Yagura et al., 1984; Park et al., 1989; Rao et al., 1993; Kerr et al., 1994) (Fig. 57.83), and panretinal photocoagulation may be used to treat severe retinal ischemia (Kishi et al., 1997).

The course of Takayasu's arteritis tends to be prolonged, with intermittent exacerbations and increasing impairment of the circulation. A few patients have spontaneous remissions, but most have progressive disease for many years (Strachan, 1964; Kerr et al., 1994). Death occurs most often from congestive heart failure or stroke. Nevertheless, the 5-year survival rate is 80–98% (Nakoa, 1967; Ishikawa, 1978; Hall et al., 1985; Conn and Hunder, 1989; Kerr et al., 1994), and the 10-year survival rate is 75–85% (Subramanyan et al., 1989). Severe hypertension, severe functional disability, and evidence of cardiac dysfunction are associated with a poor prognosis (Subramanyan et al., 1989).

Wegener's Granulomatosis

Wegener's granulomatosis was initially described in the 1930s (Wegener, 1936, 1939). It is characterized by necrotizing granulomatous lesions of the respiratory tract, glomerulonephritis, and systemic vasculitis (Godman and Churg, 1954; Fauci and Wolff, 1973; Wolff et al., 1974; DeRemee et al., 1976; Brandwein et al., 1983; Fauci et al., 1983; Robin et al., 1985; Allen, 1996). A form of the disease characterized by pulmonary involvement without renal involvement is called "limited Wegener's granulomatosis" (Carrington and Liebow, 1966; Cassan et al., 1970a; Marumo et al., 1990), and this form of the disease may be associated in particular with orbital manifestations (Cassan et al., 1970b; Spalton et al., 1981) (see below). In some patients, neuro-ophthalmologic findings resulting from meningeal and cerebral inflammation are the earliest manifestation of Wegener's granulomatosis (Newman et al., 1995) (Fig. 57.84). These patients may show no initial pulmonary, sinus, or renal involvement.

DEMOGRAPHICS

The disease is uncommon, but specific incidence and prevalence data have never been calculated. It seems to occur slightly more often in men than in women, however, and the age range is extensive, from 8 to 80 years of age, with a mean of about 45 years (Valente et al., 1997).

SYSTEMIC MANIFESTATIONS

The earliest manifestations of Wegener's granulomatosis are usually related to the upper respiratory tract (Hoffman et al., 1992). They include chronic rhinitis, chronic sinusitis, nasal ulceration, and serous otitis media. These disturbances may be accompanied by systemic symptoms of fever, weight loss, and anorexia. In addition, a suppurative otitis, saddle-nose defect, and hearing loss may occur (Fig. 57.85).

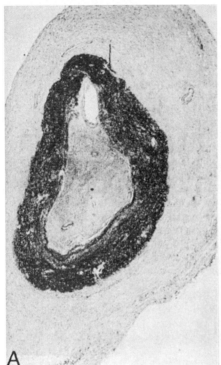

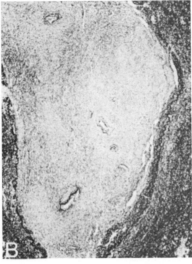

Figure 57.82. Pathology of Takayasu's arteritis. *A,* One of the large vessels arising from the aortic arch in a patient with Takayasu's arteritis is almost occluded by subintimal fibrosis. The remaining lumen is small and displaced eccentrically. There is focal scarring and destruction of elastic fibers in the media and marked sclerosis and thickening of the adventitia. *B,* High-power view of occluded lumen shows areas of recanalization. There is focal destruction of the internal elastic lamina. (From Font RL, Naumann G. Ocular histopathology in pulseless disease. Arch Ophthalmol *82:*784–788, 1969.)

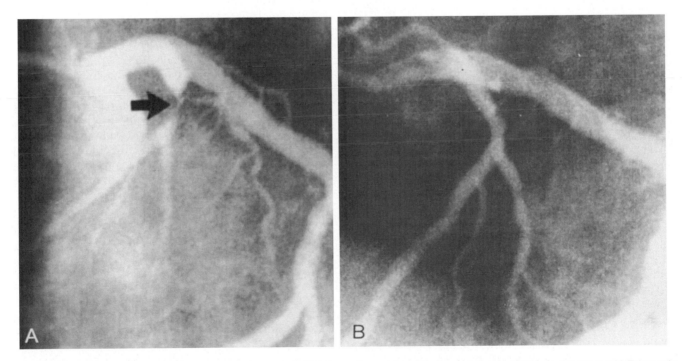

Figure 57.83. Percutaneous transluminal angioplasty in a patient with Takayasu's arteritis. *A,* Coronary arteriogram in 46-year-old woman with Takayasu's arteritis shows severe stenosis of the proximal portion of the left anterior descending artery (*arrow*). *B,* After two percutaneous transluminal angioplasties, the lumen is patent, and there is improved blood flow in the diagonal arteries. (From Park JH, Han MC, Kim SH, et al. Takayasu arteritis: Angiographic findings and results of angiography. AJR *153:*1069–1074, 1989.)

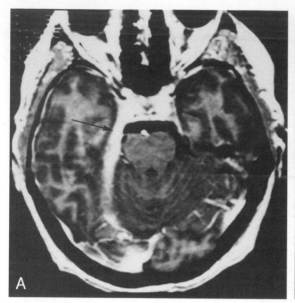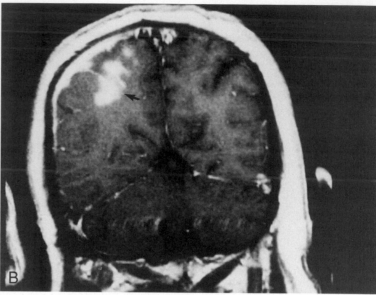

Figure 57.84. Neuroimaging in Wegener's granulomatosis. *A*, T1-weighted axial magnetic resonance (MR) image after intravenous injection of gadolinium-DTPA demonstrates prominent dural enhancement extending along the right tentorium (*arrow*) in a patient with Wegener's granulomatosis. *B*, Enhanced T1-weighted coronal MR image demonstrates parenchymal enhancement without mass effect within the right parieto-occipital region (*arrow*) and overlying meningeal enhancement. (From Newman NJ, Slamovits TL, Friedland S, et al. Neuro-ophthalmic manifestations of meningocerebral inflammation from the limited form of Wegener's granulomatosis. Am J Ophthalmol *120:*613–621, 1995.)

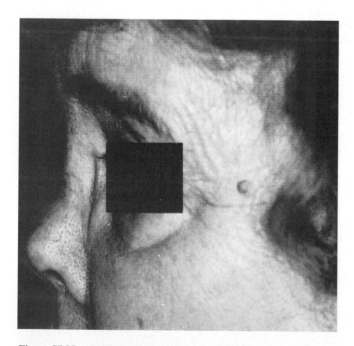

Figure 57.85. Saddle-nose deformity in a 57-year-old woman with nasal septal perforation from Wegener's granulomatosis. (From Bullen CL, Liesegang TJ, McDonald TJ, et al. Ocular complications of Wegener's granulomatosis. Arch Ophthalmol *90:*279–290, 1983.)

The lower respiratory tract is usually affected at some time during the course of the disease. The initial symptoms are cough, hemoptysis, and dyspnea. As the condition worsens, patients may develop pleuritic chest pain, cavitary lesions of the lung, and tracheal obstruction (Fig. 57.86).

Symptoms and signs of kidney dysfunction usually develop during the course of Wegener's granulomatosis, but they are rarely the initial manifestation of the disease. Evidence of kidney disease includes proteinuria, hematuria, red blood cell casts, and renal insufficiency (Conn et al., 1993; Valente et al., 1997). Hypertension is common.

The skin is affected in about 50% of patients with Wegener's granulomatosis. Purpura, the most common dermatologic abnormality, usually occurs over the lower extremities, but the trunk, upper extremities, and face may occasionally be affected (Fig. 57.87). In rare patients, the skin lesions become nodular or ulcerating (Hu et al., 1977) (Fig. 57.88).

Joint pains and myalgias occur in about 70% of patients with Wegener's granulomatosis (Hoffman et al., 1992). They usually occur early in the course of the disease, and they usually resolve without residual sequelae. A nondeforming arthritis affecting the large joints of the lower extremities also may occur, although synovitis is uncommon (Conn et al., 1993; Valente et al., 1997).

Clinical manifestations related to cardiac lesions are uncommon in patients with Wegener's granulomatosis. Nevertheless, arrhythmias and angina from coronary arteritis may occur as may pericarditis and congestive heart failure from cardiomyopathy (Valente et al., 1997).

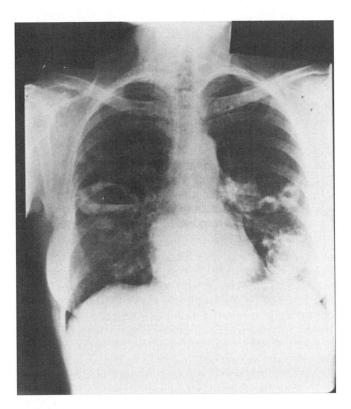

Figure 57.86. Chest X-ray in a 50-year-old woman with Wegener's granulomatosis shows bilateral, multiple, cavitating pulmonary nodules located mainly in the lower lobes. (From Bullen CL, Liesegang TJ, McDonald TJ, et al. Ocular complications of Wegener's granulomatosis. Arch Ophthalmol 90:279–290, 1983.)

NEUROLOGIC MANIFESTATIONS

Twenty to 50% of patients with Wegener's granulomatosis develop neurologic manifestations of the disease (Drachman, 1963; Anderson et al., 1975; Cupps and Fauci, 1981b; Hoffman et al., 1992; Nishino et al., 1993a). About half of these patients develop a vasculitis that affects the peripheral nerves, resulting in multiple recurrent mononeuropathies and symmetric polyneuropathy (Drachman, 1963; Kirker et al., 1989; Dickey and Andrews, 1990; Chalk et al., 1993; Nishino et al., 1993b; Sheldon, 1994). The rest of the patients with neurologic manifestations have evidence of CNS dysfunction, including cranial neuropathies and nonspecific evidence of cerebral vasculitis, such as aphasia, hemiparesis, and homonymous visual field defects (Drachman, 1963; Desnos et al., 1975; Sahn and Sahn, 1976; Kay and McCrary, 1979). The cranial neuropathies usually result from spread of primary lesions in the nasopharynx through the walls of the nasal cavity and paranasal sinuses or from the spread of primary lesions in the middle ear to the posterior fossa (Drachman, 1963). Granulomas also may extend from the paranasal sinuses to damage the pituitary gland and its stalk, producing diabetes insipidus, panhypopituitarism, or both (Haynes and Fauci, 1978). Primary granulomas of neural tissue are less common, but intracerebral granulomas occasionally occur as do primary granulomas of various cranial nerves (Nishino et al., 1993b; Weinberger et al., 1993; Newman et al., 1995). Some patients experience mild alterations in cognitive function, particularly memory (Moore and Cupps, 1983). Neurologic symptoms and signs are the initial or major manifestation of the disease in some patients. Seizures, strokes, and encephalopathy are late complications of untreated disease (Moore and Cupps, 1983). Hammans and Ginsberg (1989) reported a patient with Wegener's granulo-

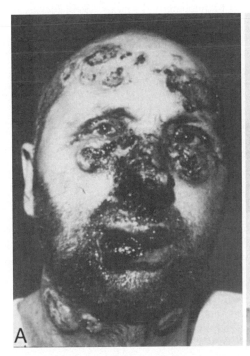
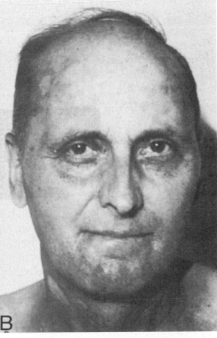

Figure 57.87. Skin involvement in Wegener's granulomatosis. *A*, The head and neck are covered by numerous hemorrhagic purpura and bullae, some of which are necrotic and ulcerating. *B*, Same patient after 2 months of treatment with cyclophosphamide and corticosteroids. (From Conn DL, Hunder GG. Vasculitis and related disorders. In Textbook of Rheumatology. Editors, Kelley WN, Harris ED Jr, Ruddy S, et al. 3rd ed, pp 1167–1199. Philadelphia, WB Saunders, 1989.)

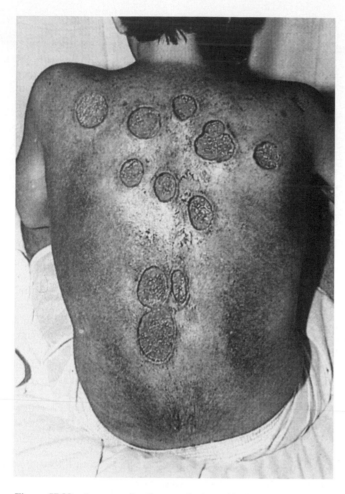

Figure 57.88. Large, nonhealing, punched-out skin lesions in a 36-year-old man. Skin biopsy confirmed the diagnosis of Wegener's granulomatosis. (From Bullen CL, Liesegang TJ, McDonald TJ, et al. Ocular complications of Wegener's granulomatosis. Arch Ophthalmol 90:279–290, 1983.)

matosis who developed obscurations of vision and was found to have bilateral papilledema. CSF pressure was 300 mm of water. The concentration of protein in the fluid was markedly elevated to 1.77 g/liter, and there were seven white blood cells/mm³. A CT scan showed findings consistent with sagittal sinus thrombosis, and angiography confirmed the diagnosis. The authors postulated that the thrombosis resulted from vasculitis, either by extension of thrombus from inflamed small vessels or from the effects of a chronic aseptic meningitis.

OCULAR AND NEURO-OPHTHALMOLOGIC MANIFESTATIONS

The ocular structures are affected in 30–60% of patients with both generalized and limited Wegener's granulomatosis (Straatsma, 1957; Fauci and Wolff, 1973; Coutu et al., 1975; Haynes et al., 1977; Kornblut et al., 1980; Spalton et al., 1981; Duncker et al., 1982; Bullen et al., 1983; Fauci et al., 1983; Liesegang et al., 1983; Marumo et al., 1990; Hoffman et al., 1992; Stavrou et al., 1993; Allen, 1996; Valente et al., 1997). The three main categories of ocular involvement

are orbital disease, scleritis with or without peripheral keratitis, and vascular complications from vasculitis (Jabs, 1994).

Orbital granulomas usually result from extension of disease from the paranasal sinuses (Fig. 57.89), but they may arise de novo within one or both orbits, and they may be the first clinical manifestation of the disease (Faulds and Wear, 1960; Blodi and Gass, 1968; Weiter and Farkas, 1972; Allen and France, 1977; Jakobiec and Jones, 1979; Duncker et al., 1982; Coppeto et al., 1985; Parelhoff et al., 1985; Robin et al., 1985; Rootman et al., 1988; Nishino et al., 1993a; Perry et al., 1997). Patients with such lesions may present with orbital swelling, redness, pain, proptosis, and ophthalmoparesis, suggesting a diagnosis of orbital pseudotumor, orbital cellulitis, or dacryocystitis (Montecucco et al., 1993; Yamashita et al., 1995) (Figs. 57.90–57.92). When orbital involvement is mild, patients may complain solely of diplopia, and they may have no other evidence of orbital disease (Pinchoff et al., 1983). A 62-year-old woman described by Kirker et al. (1989) developed an almost complete right external ophthalmoparesis without ptosis or proptosis during the course of her illness. The condition resolved within 5 days after she began treatment with prednisolone in a dose of 100 mg/day. It seems most likely that the limitation of eye movement was caused by inflammation affecting the ocular motor nerves either in the cavernous sinus or orbital apex rather than in the brainstem or subarachnoid space.

The **scleritis** that occurs in patients with Wegener's granulomatosis may be of any type, particularly diffuse anterior or necrotizing (Fig. 57.93). Jaben and Norton (1982) reported a patient who developed posterior scleritis that produced an exudative retinal detachment. Conjunctivitis, episcleritis, corneoscleral ulceration, and uveitis may accompany the scleritis of Wegener's granulomatosis or occur as isolated findings (Cogan, 1955; Straatsma, 1957; Frayer, 1960; Duncker et al., 1982; Bullen et al., 1983; Coppeto et al., 1985; Robin et al., 1985; Samuelson and Margo, 1990; Florine et al, 1993; Jordan and Addison, 1994; Power et al., 1995) (Figs. 57.94 and 57.95).

Retinal vascular and optic nerve complications of Wegener's granulomatosis result from the effects of vasculitis on the blood vessels of the retina and optic nerve. They occur in 10–18% of patients (Straatsma, 1957; Greenberger, 1967; Haynes et al., 1977; Bullen et al., 1983; Robin et al., 1985). Asymptomatic cotton-wool spots with and without intraretinal hemorrhages may occur, but some patients develop retinal artery occlusions, retinal vein occlusions, or both. Others develop severe retinal vasculitis characterized by widespread retinal vascular occlusions and perivascular sheathing leading to neovascularization, vitreous hemorrhage, and rubeotic glaucoma (Austin et al., 1978; Duncker et al., 1982; Bullen et al., 1983; Liesegang et al., 1983) (Fig. 57.96). Both anterior and retrobulbar optic neuropathy occur in this disease (Straatsma, 1957; Arruga et al., 1990). Although visual loss from optic neuropathy usually is permanent, the patient described by Kirker et al. (1989) developed an acute left retrobulbar optic neuropathy during the course of her disease, was treated with 30 mg of prednisolone per day, and experienced complete recovery of visual function within 1 week. A similar patient with bilateral retrobulbar

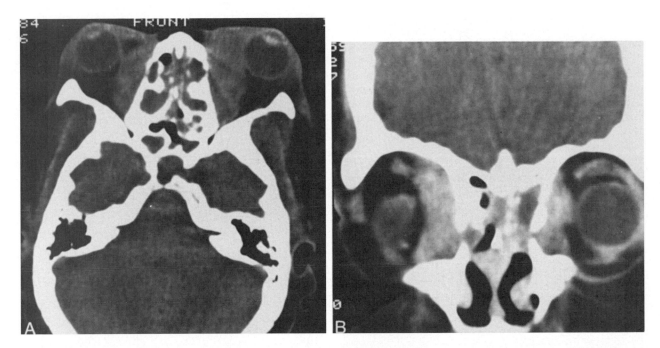

Figure 57.89. Paranasal sinus with extension into the orbits in Wegener's granulomatosis. The patient was a 54-year-old woman with recurrent sinusitis who developed bilateral proptosis. *A,* Unenhanced computed tomographic (CT) scan, axial view, shows almost complete opacification of the ethmoid and sphenoid sinuses with large masses in both orbits. *B,* CT scan, coronal view, after intravenous injection of iodinated contrast material shows opacification of the ethmoid sinuses on both sides with destruction of the medial orbital walls and masses in the medial portions of both orbits.

optic neuropathy was reported by Arruga et al. (1990). Optic neuropathy in Wegener's granulomatosis may result from ischemia or from compression by contiguous granulomatous masses arising within the orbit or sinuses. Belden et al. (1993) reported a patient with bilateral consecutive retrobulbar optic neuropathies associated with severe visual loss in Wegener's granulomatous. MR imaging showed enhancement of the intracanicular optic nerve sheaths. Vision improved only slightly to the count fingers range with immunosuppressive therapy.

Papilledema also occasionally develops in patients with Wegener's granulomatosis. It may be associated with meningitis, dural venous sinus thrombosis, or intracerebral granulomas (Fahey et al., 1954; Hammans and Ginsberg, 1989; Nishino et al., 1993a).

Nishino and Rubino (1993) reported four patients with Horner's syndrome and active Wegener's granulomatosis (Nishino and Rubino, 1993). There were no other neurologic symptoms to support a brainstem localization in these patients, but postganglionic involvement was suggested in two patients by the presence of orbital granulomatous inflammation. The other two patients may have had vasculitic involvement of the vasa nervorum supplying the sympathetic plexus.

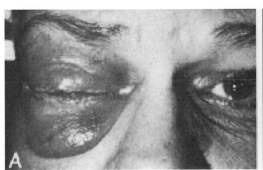
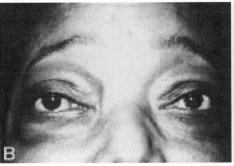
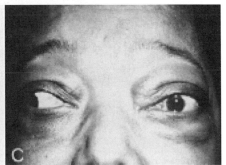

Figure 57.90. Orbital involvement in Wegener's granulomatosis. *A,* Right proptosis associated with marked edema and swelling of the eyelids in a patient with Wegener's granulomatosis. (From Jakobiec FA, Jones IS. Orbital inflammations. In Diseases of the Orbit. Editors, Jones IS, Jakobiec FA. pp 187–262. Hagerstown, MD, Harper & Row, 1979.) *B* and *C,* Bilateral proptosis and ophthalmoparesis in a woman with Wegener's granulomatosis whose CT scans are seen in Figure 57.89.

PATHOLOGY

Wegener's granulomatosis is characterized pathologically by the concurrence of (*a*) necrotizing granulomatous lesions of the upper airway, the lower respiratory tract, or both; (*b*) generalized and focal necrotizing vasculitis affecting both small arteries and veins in the lung; and (*c*) glomerulonephritis that is usually focal and segmental (Godman and Churg,

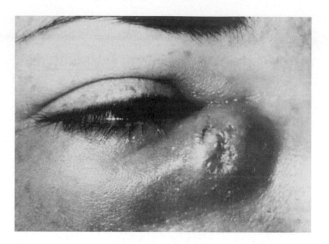

Figure 57.92. Apparent dacryocystitis in a patient with Wegener's granulomatosis. (From Grove AS Jr. Wegener's disease. In The Eye in Systemic Disease. Editors, Gold DH, Weingeist TA. pp 74–78. Philadelphia, JB Lippincott, 1990.)

1954; Wolff et al., 1974). The affected vessels are small, and they are often located adjacent to a granuloma. The vascular lesions consist of a mononuclear cell infiltration associated with fibrinoid necrosis (Fig. 57.97). The walls of the vessels become thickened, and there is focal destruction of the elastic lamina. The arterial lumen may become narrowed or occluded. The granulomas contain a central area of necrosis surrounded by granulation tissue with palisades of fibroblasts and scattered multinucleated giant cells of both the foreign-body and Langhans types (Fig. 57.97). Biopsies of orbital tissues may not show the classic triad of vasculitis, tissue necrosis, and granulomatous inflammation (Kalina et al., 1992; Perry et al., 1997). In such instances, one should rely on clinical features, biopsy material from extraorbital tissue, or serologic studies.

Granulomas and vasculitis may affect a variety of organs in patients with Wegener's granulomatosis. The most common renal lesion in patients with Wegener's granulomatosis is focal necrotizing glomerulonephritis (Fauci and Wolff, 1973). Nevertheless, renal lesions range from diffuse prolif-

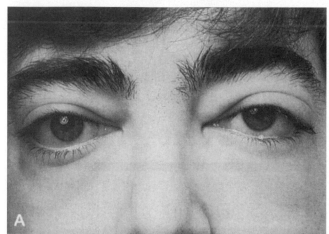

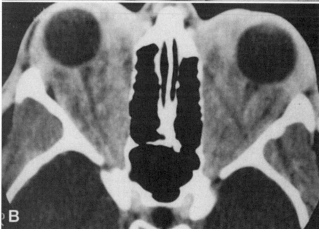

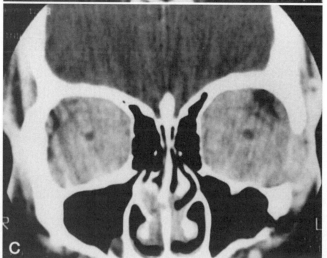

Figure 57.91. Wegener's granulomatosis mimicking bilateral diffuse orbital pseudotumor. The patient was a 21-year-old man with a 1-year history of recurrent bilateral eyelid swelling associated with injection of both eyes and bilateral proptosis. Visual acuity was 20/20 OU. *A*, External appearance of patient. Note moderate swelling and redness of both eyes. *B*, Axial computed tomographic (CT) scan shows evidence of a diffuse infiltrative process filling both orbits and completely surrounding the optic nerves. Note that the ethmoid and sphenoid sinuses appear to be normal. *C*, Coronal CT scan in same patient shows diffuse nature of the infiltrative process. The optic nerves are seen in cross-section as circular hypodensities surrounding by the hyperdense tissue. Note mild swelling of the nasal turbinates. The ethmoid and maxillary sinuses are clear. (From Perry SR, Rootman J, White VA. The clinical and pathologic constellation of Wegener granulomatosis of the orbit. Ophthalmology *104*:683–694, 1997.)

erative glomerulonephritis and interstitial nephritis to hyalinization of glomeruli. Granulomatous inflammation around glomeruli and a necrotizing vasculitis affecting small renal arteries occur but are uncommon. Granulomatous involvement of the paranasal sinuses, on the other hand, is common and may spread to contiguous structures, particularly the orbit (Haynes et al., 1977; see above). The pathologic changes found in skin lesions range from nonspecific acute and chronic inflammation to necrotizing granulomatous vasculitis (Hu et al., 1977). Granulomas or vasculitis are identified in the heart in 30% of autopsy cases. The pericardium, myocardium, and coronary arteries may all be affected (Fauci and Wolff, 1973). As noted above, the CNS may be involved by contiguous spread of granulomatous inflammation from the paranasal sinuses, nasopharynx, or middle ear, but primary granulomas may develop intracerebrally, within the cranial nerves, or in the meninges (Drachman, 1963; Sahn and Sahn, 1976). Vasculitis of the vasa nervorum of the peripheral nerves may cause mononeuritis multiplex

(MacFadyen, 1960; Stern et al., 1965). Inflammation of a medium-sized intracranial artery resulted in a stroke from thrombosis and hemorrhage in one reported case (Drachman, 1963). Granulomatous vasculitis rarely may be found in other sites, including the trachea, larynx, parotid gland, mastoid bone, and temporal bone (Conn et al., 1993).

PATHOGENESIS

The cause of Wegener's granulomatosis is unknown, but hypersensitivity mechanisms are suspected. The clinical course, with initial involvement of the respiratory tract followed by glomerulonephritis, suggests a possible chain of events in which a pathogenic agent gains entry to the respiratory tract and elicits an inflammatory response that later extends to other organs. The findings of subepithelial deposits adjacent to the basement membrane of the glomeruli in some renal biopsies suggest that the inflammation of Wegener's granulomatosis may be induced by immune complexes;

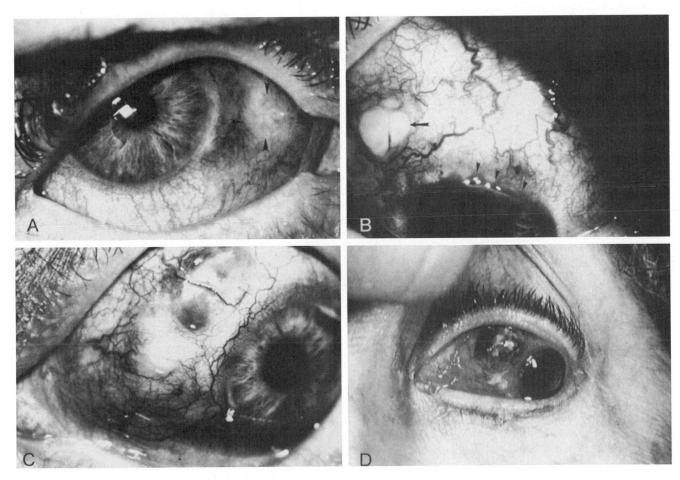

Figure 57.93. Necrotizing scleritis in Wegener's granulomatosis. *A–C*, Different stages of scleritis in a woman with Wegener's granulomatosis. *A*, Early stage in right eye is characterized by ischemic yellow-white appearance of the affected sclera (*arrowheads*). *B*, Left eye, an area of sclera has become white and thin (*arrow*). Note that the lesion is almost completely avascular. Also note the presence of a peripheral corneal ulcer (*arrowheads*). *C*, Progressive thinning of sclera produces severe ectasia with appearance of dark uveal tissue beneath intact but thin sclera. (Courtesy of Dr. Douglas Jabs.) *D*, Severe necrotizing scleritis in a 60-year-old woman with Wegener's granulomatosis. Note severe ectasia with perforation of sclera and protrusion of uveal tissue. (From Bullen CL, Liesegang TJ, McDonald TJ, et al. Ocular complications of Wegener's granulomatosis. Ophthalmology *90:*279–290, 1983.)

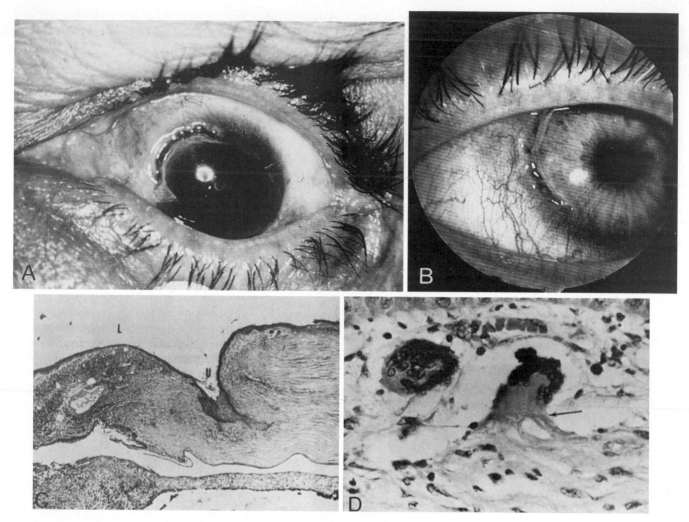

Figure 57.94. Peripheral corneal ulceration in Wegener's granulomatosis. *A*, In a 50-year-old man with Wegener's granulomatosis and pulmonary embolism. (From Bullen CL, Liesegang TJ, McDonald TJ, et al. Ocular complications of Wegener's granulomatosis. Ophthalmology *90:*279–290, 1983.) *B*, In a patient with previously undiagnosed Wegener's granulomatosis, there is a deep peripheral ulcer adjacent to an area of episcleritis. Necrotizing scleritis developed within several weeks after this photograph was obtained, and the eye was eventually enucleated. *C*, Histopathologic section through the ulcerated area seen in *B* shows that the ulcer (*U*) has re-epithelialized. Epithelioid cells and giant cells are present in the severely necrotic limbal tissues (*L*) and in the anterior portion of the sclera (*far left side of photograph*). *D*, Higher magnification of the superficial portion of the ulcer reveals two large giant cells. One of them is apposed to the interrupted collagen fibers (*arrow*) in the wall of the ulcer. (From Ferry AP. The eye and rheumatic diseases. In Textbook of Rheumatology. Editors, Kelley WN, Harris Jr ED, Ruddy S, et al. 3rd ed, pp 579–596. Philadelphia, WB Saunders, 1989.)

however, immunohistologic studies generally do not support this theory (Howell and Epstein, 1976; Ronco et al., 1983). Instead, an alteration of cell-mediated immunity may be responsible for Wegener's granulomatosis because the chemotactic response of PMNs from patients with the disease is decreased (Niinaka et al., 1977), and antibodies to cytoplasmic antigens in PMNs are found in such patients (van der Woude et al., 1985; Kallenberg et al., 1994).

The beneficial effect of antimicrobial agents in some patients with Wegener's granulomatosis provides indirect evidence that a specific pathogen is responsible for the disease, whereas the beneficial effect of cyclophosphamide in most patients provides indirect evidence that immunologic factors are important in the pathogenesis of the disease. Genetic susceptibility also may be a factor because there is an increased frequency of HLA-DR2, and perhaps HLA-B8, in patients with the disease (Katz et al., 1979; Elkon et al., 1983).

LABORATORY TESTS

Normochromic normocytic anemia, moderate leukocytosis without eosinophilia, an elevated ESR, thrombocytosis, and hypergammaglobulinemia (particularly IgA) are common abnormalities found in patients with Wegener's granulomatosis (Cupps and Fauci, 1981b; Fauci et al., 1983). The CRP is also elevated, and its concentration in the serum may be used to monitor the activity of the disease (Hind et al.,

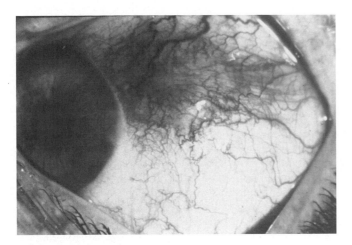

Figure 57.95. Nodular episcleritis in a patient with Wegener's granulomatosis. This lesion was the patient's only ocular abnormality. (Courtesy of Dr. Douglas Jabs.)

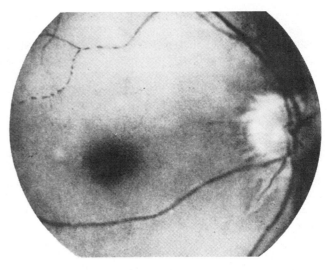

Figure 57.96. Vascular retinal and optic nerve complications of Wegener's granulomatosis. The patient was a 59-year-old man with known Wegener's granulomatosis who suddenly lost vision in the right eye. The patient could count fingers at 5 feet with the right eye. Left eye vision was 20/25. The right ocular fundus shows evidence of a mixed anterior ischemic optic neuropathy and a central retinal artery occlusion, with pale swelling of the optic disc, diffuse retinal edema, a cherry-red spot in the macula, and segmentation of blood in the superior temporal artery. The patient had no other risk factors for the development of a retinal vascular occlusion. (From Greenberger MH. Central retinal artery closure in Wegener's granulomatosis. Am J Ophthalmol 63:515–516, 1967.)

1984). Antinuclear antibodies (ANAs) and cryoglobulins are usually absent, but ANCAs are often present, and their concentration correlates with the severity of the disease and the effectiveness of treatment. Two major forms of ANCAs can be distinguished (Nolle et al., 1993). Wegener's granulomatosis is most closely associated with ''classic'' or ''cytoplasmic'' ANCAs (C-ANCAs). Perinuclear ANCAs (P-ANCAs) are nonspecific markers for the disease and may occur in a variety of inflammatory conditions such as microscopic polyangiitis, rheumatoid arthritis, and inflammatory bowel disease (Gross et al., 1993; Nolle et al., 1993; Kallenberg et al., 1994; Specks and Homburger, 1994). Although C-ANCAs have a high specificity for Wegener's granuloma-

tosis, patients with the limited form of the disease may be seronegative (Nolle et al., 1989; Newman et al., 1995). For instance, about 65% of patients with disease limited to the pulmonary tree have C-ANCAs, 90% of patients with exten-

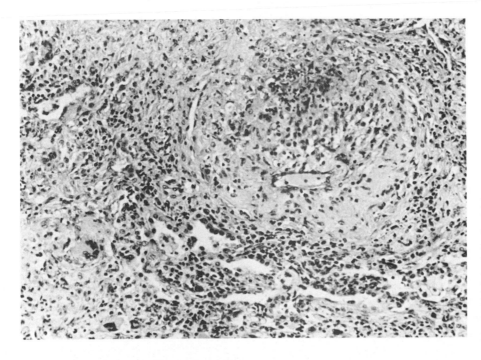

Figure 57.97. Pathology of Wegener's granulomatosis. Pulmonary biopsy specimen from a patient with orbital involvement shows a granuloma adjacent to a blood vessel that is almost obliterated by the inflammation. The granuloma consists of numerous mononuclear cells and multinucleated giant cells. (From Jakobiec FA, Jones IS. Orbital inflammations. In Diseases of the Orbit. Editors, Jones IS, Jakobiec FA. pp 187–262. Hagerstown, MD, Harper & Row, 1979.)

sive systemic disease harbor these antibodies, and C-ANCAs are detectable in 30% of patients in remission (Nolle et al., 1989; Specks and Homburger, 1994). Failure of C-ANCA titers to return to normal after treatment may predict patients at risk for recurrent ocular complications (Power et al., 1995).

DIAGNOSIS

The diagnosis of Wegener's granulomatosis may be established on the basis of the clinical features of the patient, the presence of C-ANCAs in the serum, and the histopathologic demonstration of necrotizing granulomas with vasculitis. The American College of Rheumatology established diagnostic criteria for Wegener's granulomatosis before the value of ANCA testing was fully realized (Leavitt et al., 1990). By American College of Rheumatology criteria, a patient must have two of the following: (a) nasal discharge or ulcers; (b) chest radiograph demonstrating nodules, fixed infiltrates, or cavities; (c) microhematuria with more than five erythrocytes per high-power field or red cell casts; or (d) granulomatous inflammation on biopsy. The diagnosis of Wegener's granulomatosis should be suspected in any patient with a systemic illness characterized in part by prominent repiratory tract symptoms. Nasal mucosal ulceration, proptosis, lung infiltrates or cavitation, proteinuria, and abnormalities of urine sediment should also suggest the diagnosis. Anemia, an elevated ESR, and leukocytosis confirm the systemic nature of the patient's illness. Because most patients with Wegener's granulomatosis have involvement of the upper respiratory tract early in the course of the illness, a biopsy of nasal mucosal or affected sinus tissues offers the best opportunity for securing a histologic diagnosis. A generous portion of tissue must be obtained to permit adequate pathologic examination (Conn et al., 1993; Valente et al., 1997). Evaluation of the patient with suspected Wegener's granulomatosis and rhino-orbital or cerebral involvement requires neuroimaging. CT scanning is superior to MR imaging in detecting the bone thickening or focal erosive changes seen with Wegener's granulomatosis. Granulomatous masses on T2-weighted MR imaging images show increased signal intensity and enhance after intravenous injection with a paramagnetic contrast agent such as gadolinium-DTPA (Hurst and Grossman, 1994; Newman et al., 1995).

TREATMENT AND PROGNOSIS

Before the 1960s, Wegener's granulomatosis was almost always fatal, with renal failure being the main cause of death (Walton, 1958). The mean untreated survival was only 5 months, and 1-year mortality was 82% (Jabs, 1994). Systemic steroid therapy produced clinical improvement in some cases, but the effect was transient; mean survival was increased to only about 12.5 months, and overall mortality was not affected (Hollander and Manning, 1967). The use of cytotoxic drugs has altered the course of the disease significantly. Cyclophosphamide, azathioprine, methotrexate, chlorambucil, and nitrogen mustard are all used to treat Wegener's granulomatosis with some degree of success, with cyclophosphamide being the most successful of these agents

for the systemic, neurologic, and ocular complications of the disease (Fahey et al., 1954; Brubaker et al., 1971; Fauci and Wolff, 1971; Fauci et al., 1971; Novack and Pearson, 1971; Raitt, 1971; Fauci and Wolff, 1973; Haynes et al., 1977; Moorthy et al., 1977; Jampol et al., 1978; Foster, 1980; Conn and Hunder, 1989; Hoffman et al., 1992; Hoffman and Fauci, 1994) (Fig. 57.87). Patients with mild disease occasionally may benefit from treatment with antimicrobial agents such as trimethoprim-sulfamethoxazole (DeRemee et al., 1985). Patients with significant systemic symptoms and signs usually are treated with a combination of prednisone and cyclophosphamide. When the systemic symptoms improve, the prednisone is tapered slowly, converted to an alternate-day regimen, and eventually stopped. Maintenance cyclophosphamide is usually continued for about 1 year after control of symptoms and then gradually tapered. Response to treatment can be judged not only by improvement in clinical symptoms and signs, but also by reduction in the ESR, serum concentration of CRP, and C-ANCAs (Cohen Tervaert et al., 1990; Valente et al., 1997).

Patients with significant renal insufficiency from Wegener's granulomatosis generally have a poor prognosis regardless of treatment (Pinching et al., 1983), and other patients may develop significant complications not only from the disease but also from its treatment. Hemorrhagic cystitis, bone marrow depression, an increased incidence of neoplasms, and infection are among the most significant complications of cyclophosphamide (Jampol et al., 1978; Bradley et al., 1989; Hoffman et al., 1992), whereas prednisone may predispose the patient to sepsis, osteoporosis, hypertension, and diabetes mellitus (see Chapter 48). Nevertheless, up to 90% of patients with Wegener's granulomatosis successfully achieve a remission with combined therapy (Reza et al., 1975; Fauci et al., 1983; Hoffman et al., 1992). Although some patients relapse when cyclophosphamide is discontinued, a second remission may be achieved with reinstitution of the drug (Steinman et al., 1980).

Lethal Midline Granuloma

The subject of lethal midline granuloma, a disease group that affects central facial structures and causes progressive necrosis and cavitation, is very confusing (Cutler, 1955; Duke and Naquin, 1957; Walton, 1960; Friedman, 1964; Eichel et al., 1966; Byrd et al., 1969; Kassel et al., 1969; Kay and McCrary, 1979; Berrenti et al., 1993) (Fig. 57.98). If patients with this condition are followed long enough, they usually develop other evidence of Wegener's granulomatosis. Nevertheless, there are many other disorders that can produce this clinical picture, including carcinomas of the paranasal sinuses or nasopharynx and lymphoma (Jakobiec and Jones, 1979). In such cases, there is no evidence of associated vasculitis.

BEHÇET'S DISEASE

In 1937, Hulusi Behçet, a Turkish professor of dermatology, described a chronic relapsing syndrome characterized by oral ulceration, genital ulceration, and uveitis. The condition probably had been described previously by Hippocrates (Adams, 1849), but Behçet (1937) emphasized its existence

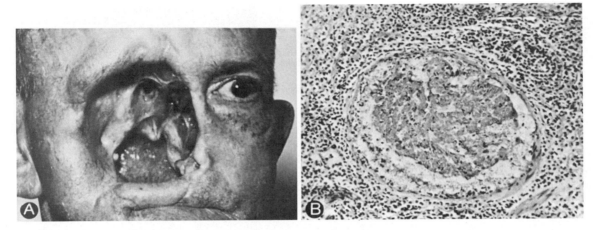

Figure 57.98. Lethal midline granuloma. The patient was a 44-year-old coal miner who had been treated for syphilis in the distant past and who had negative serologic tests for syphilis. He initially developed redness and swelling of the right side of the nose and of the right upper and lower eyelids. He then developed an ulcer in the region of the right caruncle that gradually enlarged. He subsequently required multiple operations to remove abnormal tissue and to attempt to repair the resulting defects. A diagnosis of lethal midline granuloma finally was made. At final operation, the right maxilla and all necrotic material were removed, and the patient was treated with systemic corticosteroids. The condition did not progress over the following 2 years, after which the patient was not seen again. *A*, Appearance of the patient after the final operation. *B*, Orbital tissue from the patient shows dense cellular infiltration by chronic inflammatory cells and multinucleated giant cells with thrombosis and recanalization of a central vessel. (From Duke JR, Naquin HA. Lethal midline granuloma. Trans Am Acad Ophthalmol Otolaryngol *61:*464–474, 1957.)

to the world, and the condition was ultimately called **Behçet's disease.** Additional features of Behçet's disease were subsequently reported by Behçet and others, including synovitis, cutaneous vasculitis resembling erythema nodosum, meningoencephalitis, aneurysms affecting large arteries, phlebitis, and discrete ulcers in the gastrointestinal tract (Behçet, 1939, 1940; Chajek and Fainaru, 1975; Chamberlain, 1977; Uthoff, 1986). Although Behçet's disease shares some clinical and pathologic features with the systemic necrotizing vasculitides, it is usually considered a separate entity (O'Duffy, 1990). The reader interested in learning more about Behçet's disease than is contained in this section should consult the authoritative text by Plotkin et al. (1988).

Demographics

The prevalence of Behçet's disease has a peculiar distribution. Most cases are reported from the eastern Mediterranean countries (O'Duffy et al., 1984) and from Japan (Oshima et al., 1963). The prevalence of Behçet's disease in Japan, where it is one of the leading causes of blindness, is about 1 per 1,000 (Shikano et al., 1966; Hirohata et al., 1975). Although several series of cases were reported from the United States (Mason and Barnes, 1968; O'Duffy et al., 1971; Wright and Chamberlain, 1978–1979; Denman et al., 1980; Hunder, 1985), there are no clear prevalence data from the country. The prevalence in Olmstead County, Minnesota, however, was estimated at about 1 per 16,000 (O'Duffy, 1989). Although men and women seem to be affected equally in most studies, men are affected more often than women in both North America and Australia (O'Duffy et al, 1971; Cooper and Penny, 1974; Hunder, 1985; Wakefield and McCluskey, 1990).

Clinical Manifestations

Recurrent **aphthous stomatitis** is virtually a sine qua non of Behçet's disease (O'Duffy, 1990; Valente et al., 1997). The aphthous oral ulcers are usually the first manifestation of the disease. They resemble the lesions of uncomplicated chancre sores, but they are more numerous. They usually occur on the buccal mucosa, lips, tongue, and pharynx, like chancre sores, but they may also develop throughout the gastrointestinal tract (Griffin et al., 1982). The oral ulcers are usually multiple, occur in groups, and are exceedingly painful (Valente et al., 1997). A typical, well-developed ulcer is 2–10 mm in diameter, has a central yellow base, and is surrounded by a vivid red halo (Fig. 57.99). Most ulcers heal in 3–30 days without residual scarring (Francis, 1970; Lehner, 1977; Rogers, 1977).

Recurrent **genital ulcers** affecting the vulva and vagina in women and the scrotum or penis in men resemble the oral aphthous ulcers (Fig. 57.100). Vulvar ulcers are painful, and they usually cause dyspareunia. Vaginal and cervical ulcers may be asymptomatic except for discharge (O'Duffy et al., 1971). Genital ulcerations recur much less frequently than do oral ulcers in most patients. In some patients, however, they are multiple, persistent, and heal with scarring.

Blindness caused by **anterior uveitis with hypopyon** was emphasized by Behçet in his initial report (Behçet, 1937), and this form of uveitis is particularly common in patients from the Middle East (Benezra and Cohen, 1986) and from Australia (Wakefield and McCluskey, 1990) (Fig. 57.101). Most patients, however, develop a posterior uveitis (Mamo and Baghdassarian, 1964; Colvard et al., 1977; Kishi et al., 1981; Michelson and Chisari, 1982; Horiuchi et al., 1983; Martenet, 1988; Jacobs et al., 1989; Wakefield and

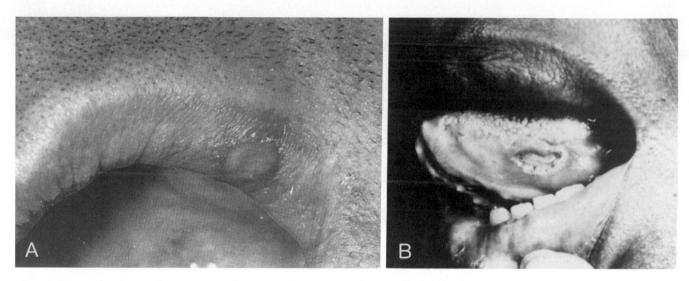

Figure 57.99. Oral aphthous ulcers in Behçet's disease. *A*, Painful oral aphthous ulcer of the upper lip. An erythematous border surrounds a necrotic, yellow ulcer. (From O'Duffy JD. Behçet's disease. In Textbook of Rheumatology. Editors, Kelley WN, Harris ED Jr, Ruddy S, et al. 3rd ed, pp 1209–1214. Philadelphia, WB Saunders, 1989.) *B*, Aphthous ulcer on the undersurface of the tongue in another patient with Behçet's disease. Note deep ulceration and rounded edges. (Courtesy of Dr. Douglas Jabs.)

McCluskey, 1990). Whether anterior or posterior, the uveitis of Behçet's disease tends to be bilateral, and it is seldom the initial manifestation of the disorder. In fact, the average length of time between the onset of initial symptoms (usually aphthous ulcers) and the onset of uveitis is 6 years (O'Duffy, 1989). Uveitis ultimately develops in about 70% of patients, however, and it is more likely to occur in men than in women.

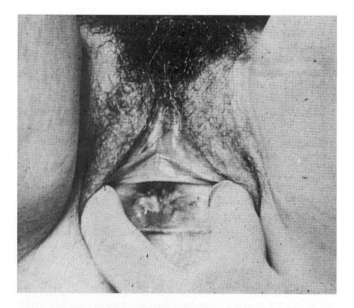

Figure 57.100. Genital aphthous ulcer in Behçet's disease. This asymptomatic vaginal ulcer was discovered during a routine pelvic examination of a patient who presented with polyarthritis, oral aphthous ulcers, and uveitis. (From O'Duffy JD, Carney JA, Deodhar S. Behçet's disease. Report of 10 cases, 3 with new manifestations. Ann Intern Med *75:*561–570, 1971.)

Ocular manifestations other than uveitis occur in patients with Behçet's disease, including conjunctivitis, keratitis, scleritis, and retinal vasculitis (Colvard et al., 1977; Jabs, 1994). In fact, retinal vasculitis may occur more frequently than uveitis and may be the initial manifestation of the disease. Between 1973 and 1987, Atmaca (1989) examined 300 patients with Behçet's disease who had retinal vascular disturbances. In 254 of these cases (85%), the retinal abnormalities were the first evidence of the disease. Horiuchi et al. (1983) reported retinal lesions in 81% of 525 eyes of 264 patients with Behçet's disease. The retinal changes of Behçet's disease, like the uveitis, are usually bilateral and may affect both arteries and veins (Graham et al., 1989; Kasp et al., 1989; Charteris et al., 1992). The earliest changes are hyperpermeability of vessels, which cannot be detected unless fluorescein angiography is performed (Shimizu, 1973; Horiuchi et al., 1983; Atmaca, 1989). More severe changes are manifest by vascular occlusion and retinal necrosis that can easily be seen with an ophthalmoscope (Shimizu, 1973; Dinning and Perkins, 1975; Colvard et al., 1977; Willerson et al., 1977; Cotticelli et al., 1980; Donoso et al., 1981; Horiuchi et al., 1983; Atmaca, 1989; Graham et al., 1989; Jacobs et al., 1989; Schilling et al., 1990) (Fig. 57.102). Massive hemorrhage, exudates, secondary neovascularization, and retinal detachment occasionally develop (Nakagawa et al., 1990) (Fig. 57.103). The end stage of this process is a blind, painful eye caused by the effects of neovascular glaucoma, hemorrhagic necrotizing retinitis, and obliterative vasculitis of the retina and choroid (Ikui, 1960; Fenton and Easom, 1964; Shikano, 1966; Naumann, 1973; Uga et al., 1977; Horiuchi et al., 1983; Miyake et al., 1997) (Fig. 57.103*D*). Kasp et al. (1989) found antiretinal antibodies in 21 of 38 patients (55%) with Behçet's disease who had retinal vascular abnormalities. These investigators found elevated concentrations

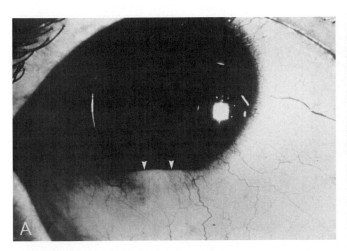
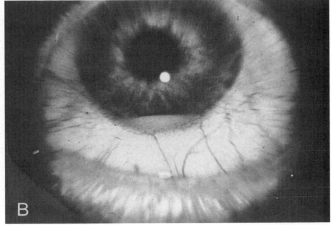

Figure 57.101. Anterior uveitis with hypopyon in Behçet's disease. *A*, Note quiet appearance of eye despite moderate hypopyon (*arrowheads*). (Courtesy of Dr. Douglas Jahs.) *B*, In another patient with Behçet's disease, the hypopyon is associated with mild injection of the eye. (Courtesy of Dr. Dennis Robertson.)

of circulating immune complexes in the serum of 12 of the 38 patients (32%). Nine patients in this series had both antiretinal antibodies and circulating immune complexes in their serum.

Neuro-ophthalmologic manifestations of Behçet's disease affect both the visual sensory and ocular motor systems. **Papilledema** may develop in association with increased ICP (Fig. 57.104). The raised ICP usually results from vasculitic occlusion of the superior sagittal or other intracranial dural venous sinuses, producing the syndrome of pseudotumor cerebri (Kalbian and Challis, 1970; Kozin et al., 1977; Reza and Demanes, 1978; Pamir et al., 1981; Bank and Weart, 1984; Bousser et al., 1985; Schell and Rathe, 1988; El-Ramahi and Al-Kawi, 1991; Wechsler et al., 1992; Fujikado and Imagawa, 1994) (see Chapter 58). It also may occur in the setting of diffuse meningoencephalitis (Wolff et al., 1965). **Optic atrophy** may occur as a consequence of chronic papilledema, or it may develop after an attack of anterior or posterior ischemic optic neuropathy or optic neuritis (Wolff et al., 1965; Scouras and Koutroumanos, 1976; Colvard et al., 1977; Cotticelli et al., 1980; Horiuchi et al., 1983; Fukuoka et al., 1987; Jacobs et al., 1989; Kansu et al., 1989) (Fig. 57.105). **Homonymous visual field defects** may develop in patients with Behçet's disease who experience a cerebral infarction that interrupts the postchiasmal visual pathway. **Ocular motor system abnormalities** that occur in patients with Behçet's disease include nystagmus and other disturbances of eye movement caused by brainstem or cerebellar ischemia (e.g., INO, and single or multiple ocular motor nerve pareses) (Colvard et al., 1977; Ishikawa et al., 1986; Saribas et al., 1991; Masai et al., 1996) (Fig. 57.106).

Synovitis occurs in about 50–60% of patients with Behçet's disease. It is oligoarticular or monoarticular, affects both large and small joints, usually affects the ankles and knees, and rarely causes joint destruction (Mason and Barnes, 1969; O'Duffy et al., 1971; Yurdakul et al., 1983).

A variety of skin lesions occurs in patients with Behçet's disease, including pustules, nodules, and papules (O'Duffy,

1989). Nodular cutaneous lesions confined to the lower extremities resemble erythema nodosum, but they differ from this condition in that they may occur in groups and also ulcerate. Some of these nodules are actually areas of vasculitis affecting superficial veins (O'Duffy et al., 1971). Some patients with Behçet's disease seem to have a nonspecific skin sensitivity to minor trauma such as a needle-stick, particularly when the disease is active (Nazarro, 1966). This finding is called the **pathergy phenomenon** (Yazici et al., 1984).

Neurologic dysfunction in patients with Behçet's disease may be separated into three patterns: (*a*) meningitis, (*b*) meningoencephalitis, and (*c*) focal parenchymal damage (Pallis and Fudge, 1956). **Meningitis or meningoencephalitis,** characterized by headache, fever, stiff neck, and CSF pleocytosis, occurs in 4–29% of patients with Behçet's disease (Kawakita et al., 1969; Chajek and Fainaru, 1975; O'Duffy and Goldstein, 1976; Shimizu et al., 1979; Serdaroglu et al., 1989). As is the case with uveitis, the meningoencephalitis of Behçet's disease is rarely the initial manifestation of the disease. It usually develops about 1.3 years after initial symptoms and signs of the condition (O'Duffy, 1989). Nevertheless, about 5% of patients develop neurologic symptoms and signs weeks to months before they develop any other features of the disease. Such patients, and those in whom neurologic features predominate, often are said to have "neuro-Behçet's disease" (Shimizu et al., 1979).

Patients with **parenchymal damage** in Behçet's disease may have a variety of deficits, including hemi- or quadriparesis, ataxia, pseudobulbar palsy, homonymous visual field defects, and ocular motor nerve pareses (Herrmann, 1953; Bienenstock and Margulies, 1961; Schotland et al., 1963; Wolff et al., 1965; Chajek and Fainaru, 1975; Colvard et al., 1977; Kozin et al., 1977; Shimizu et al., 1979; Bousser et al., 1985; Serdaroglu et al., 1989). The brainstem is the most frequent site of focal disease (Moore and Cupps, 1983), and, as noted above, eye movement abnormalities consistent with

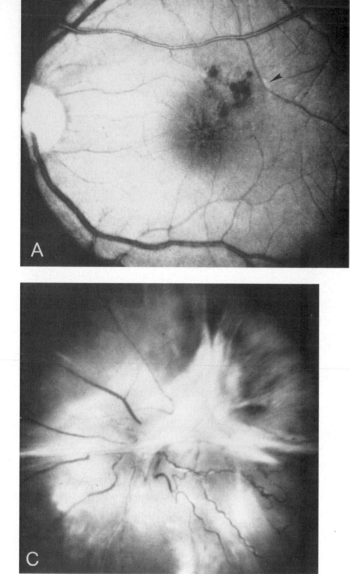

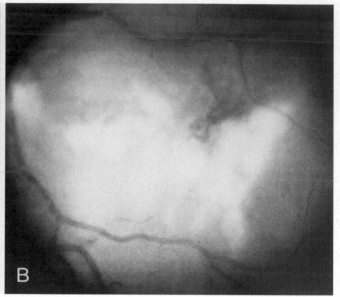

Figure 57.102. Progressive retinopathy in Behçet's disease. *A*, Early stage is characterized by mild intraretinal hemorrhage and small area of retinal arterial sheathing (*arrowhead*). *B*, With time, a hemorrhagic, exudative retinopathy develops that obscures the view of the macula. *C*, Chronic retinopathy has produced a severe fibrous reaction in the vitreous, obscuring the view of the optic disc and producing traction detachment of the retina. (Courtesy of Dr. Douglas Jabs.)

ischemic damage to intrinsic supranuclear and internuclear pathways are not uncommon in patients with brainstem lesions (Masai et al., 1996) (Fig. 57.106). In many cases, affected patients develop symptoms and signs referable to multiple lesions throughout the CNS, and the severity of neurologic dysfunction fluctuates considerably.

The CSF in most patients with neuro-Behçet's disease shows a lymphocytosis associated with an elevated concentration of protein but a normal concentration of γ-globulin (Kawakita et al., 1969). The electroencephalogram demonstrates mild slowing in more than half the patients. Cerebral angiography is usually normal but may show an avascular mass (Bienenstock and Margolies, 1961). Neuroimaging studies may occasionally be helpful in identifying CNS involvement in patients with Behçet's disease, particularly in patients with venous occlusive disease (Williams et al.,

1979; Rosenberger et al., 1982; Harper et al., 1985; Willeit et al., 1986; Miller et al., 1987; Herskovitz et al., 1988). MR imaging is preferred over CT scanning because of its ability to detect cerebral venous thrombosis and white matter abnormalities (Banna et al., 1991; El-Ramahi and Al-Kawi, 1991; Wechsler et al., 1992).

Recurrent attacks of meningitis are usually tolerated well by patients with Behçet's disease, and they cause no permanent deficits, but recurrent attacks of meningoencephalitis almost always cause neurologic residua, and they are associated with an increased mortality (Wolff et al., 1965; O'Duffy, 1978–1979). Pathologic examination in such cases shows lymphocytic perivascular infiltrates associated with diffuse demyelination, axonal degeneration, and foci of necrosis (Rubinstein and Urich, 1963; O'Duffy and Goldstein, 1976).

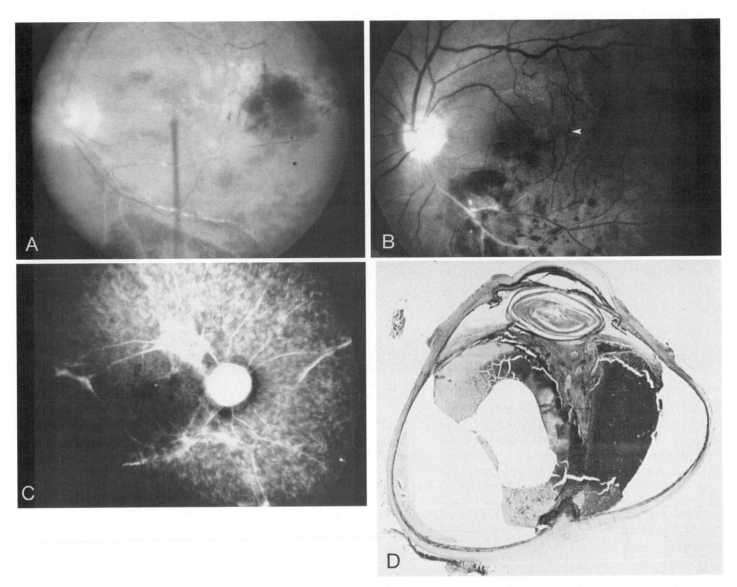

Figure 57.103. Severe retinopathy in four patients with Behçet's disease. *A*, The right ocular fundus shows a vitreous reaction, blurring details. Nevertheless, moderate intraretinal hemorrhage and exudate can be observed in the posterior pole, primarily temporal to the macula. The inferior temporal branch arteries are occluded and sheathed. *B*, Combined inferior temporal branch artery and vein occlusion in a patient with Behçet's disease. Note shunt vessels crossing macular region (*arrowhead*). *C*, Endstage retinopathy in Behçet's disease. The optic disc is atrophic and all retinal vessels are occluded. (Courtesy of Dr. Douglas Jabs.) *D*, Complete hemorrhagic retinal detachment in a blind, painful eye in a patient with Behçet's disease. (From Fenton RH, Easom HA. Behçet's syndrome: A histopathologic study of the eye. Arch Ophthalmol *72:*71–81, 1964.)

Arterial aneurysms and thrombosis of both veins and arteries may occur in patients with Behçet's disease (Enoch et al., 1968; Bank, 1973; Chajek and Fainaru, 1975; Imaizumi et al., 1980; Wechsler et al., 1987). Indeed, Behçet's disease is almost alone among the vasculitides as a frequent cause of fatal aneurysms of the pulmonary arterial tree (Davies, 1973; Grenier et al., 1981; Efthimiou et al., 1986). Aneurysms of other large arteries may cause life-threatening or fatal illness by rupture or thrombosis (Shimizu et al., 1979). Vasculitis of major veins, including the dural venous sinuses, can result in such divergent conditions as Budd-Chiari syndrome, occlusion of the vena cava, and, as noted above, pseudotumor cerebri (Kalbian and Challis, 1970; Reza and

Demanes, 1978; Shimizu et al., 1979; Graham et al., 1980; Pamir et al., 1981; Wilkey et al., 1983; Bank and Weart, 1984; Ben-Itzhak et al., 1985; Bousser et al., 1985; Schell and Rathe, 1988; El-Ramahi and Al-Kawi, 1991; Wechsler et al., 1992; Fujikado and Imagawa, 1994). Thrombosis of major arteries may produce myocardial infarction, limb ischemia, renovascular hypertension, or stroke (Koc et al., 1992). Overall, venous disease is much more common than arterial involvement.

Some patients with Behçet's disease develop inflammatory bowel disease that is clinically and pathologically identical with Crohn's disease (O'Duffy, 1978–1979). The ulcerations of the lower ileum and right side of the colon that occur in

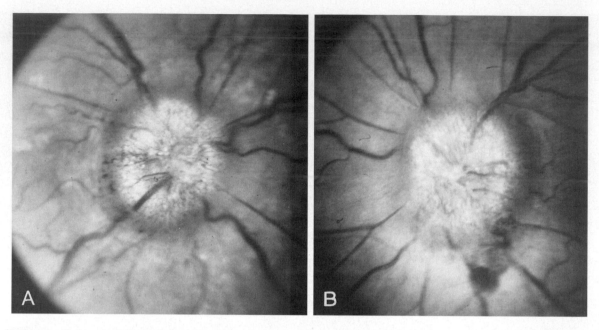

Figure 57.104. Papilledema in Behçet's disease. The patient was a 28-year-old man with known Behçet's disease and a 3-month history of severe headaches who became progressively lethargic and confused. *A* and *B*, The patient has chronic papilledema. Neuroimaging studies showed no evidence of an intracranial mass, and the ventricles were normal in size; however, there was occlusion of the superior sagittal sinus. Lumbar puncture confirmed increased intracranial pressure, and the patient was treated with acetazolamide.

such patients may perforate and require hemicolectomy and resection of the distal ileum (Baba and Moriota, 1982). Other findings reported in some patients with Behçet's disease include pericarditis and mild nephritis (Herreman et al., 1982). Additionally, a syndrome with features of both Behçet's disease and relapsing polychondritis, characterized by mouth ulcers, genital ulcers, and inflamed cartilage (MAGIC syndrome), has been described (Firestein et al., 1985).

Pathology

The oral and genital ulcers that occur in Behçet's disease show a chronic inflammatory reaction with aggregations of lymphocytes and monocytes infiltrating the basal and prickle cell layers of the epidermis and occasionally surrounding the vessels in the dermis (Lehner, 1969; Muller and Lehner, 1982). Similar perivascular inflammation, at times with frank necrosis of vessels, occurs in the skin, retinal vessels, and brain (McMenemey and Lawrence, 1957; Rubinstein and Urich, 1963; Shikano, 1966; Kawakita et al., 1969; O'Duffy et al., 1971) (Fig. 57.107). Other histopathologic abnormalities that may be seen in the CNS of patients with Behçet's disease include venous thrombosis, meningeal inflammation, and areas of isolated demyelination (Kawakita et al., 1969).

Pathogenesis

The pathogenesis of Behçet's disease is, like so many of the syndromes characterized by systemic vasculitis, unknown. Behçet (1937) described inclusion bodies in both the oral exudates and the hypopyons from his patients, and Sezer (1953) maintained that a virus was responsible, but subse-

quent efforts to isolate the virus from a variety of lesions, CSF, and lymphocytes were and continue to be unsuccessful (O'Duffy and Goldstein, 1976; Yananouchi et al., 1982).

Numerous immunologic abnormalities occur in patients with Behçet's disease. These include circulating antibodies to human mucosal and endothelial cells, lymphocytotoxicity to autologous oral mucous membrane cells and to heterologous oral epithelial cells, and blastic transformation of patient lymphocytes by human oral epithelial cells (Oshima et al., 1963; Lehner, 1967; Mason and Barnes, 1968; Lehner, 1972; Rogers et al., 1974; Reimer et al., 1982; Valente et al., 1997). As noted above, Kasp et al. (1989) found antiretinal antibodies in the serum of more than half of their patients with Behçet's disease who had retinal vascular abnormalities. Also, the similarity of the histologic lesions to those of delayed hypersensitivity suggests a disordered cellular immunity, even though studies of T-lymphocytes are normal in most patients (O'Duffy, 1989). In fact, Sakane et al. (1982) showed that the ratio of OK-T4 (helper) T-lymphocytes and OK-T8 (suppressor) T-lymphocytes in patients with Behçet's disease, which is normally 2:1, changes to 1:1 just before reactivation of the disease. Circulating immune complexes are found in the sera of 30–60% of patients with Behçet's disease (Gupta et al., 1978; Kasp et al., 1989), and C3 is present in subepithelial vessels within aphthous ulcers (Reimer et al., 1983). Many patients with Behçet's disease also have increased serum concentrations of IgA, IgG, IgM, C9, and cryoglobulins (Mason and Barnes, 1968; Cooper and Penny, 1974; Kawachi-Takahashi et al., 1974; Adinolfi and Lehner, 1976). Despite all of these immunologic findings, the putative antigen that may trigger an ''autoimmune'' response remains unidentified.

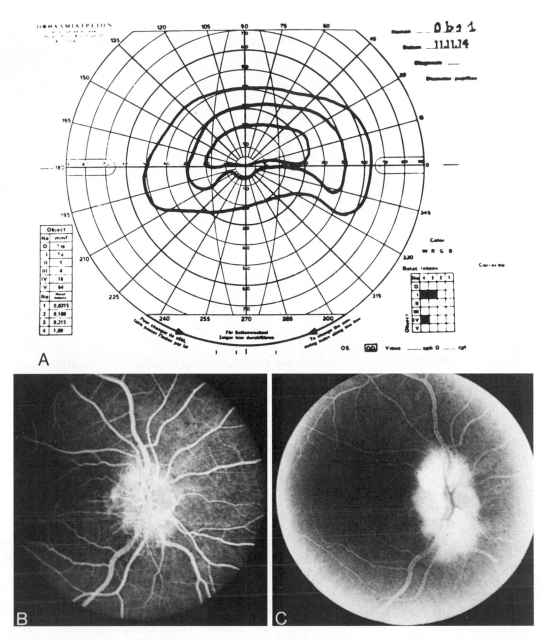

Figure 57.105. Anterior ischemic optic neuropathy in Behçet's disease. The patient was a 39-year-old man with a 5-year history of aphthous ulcers of the mucous membrane of the mouth and genitals who experienced sudden loss of vision in the right eye. The visual loss was most profound in the inferior field of vision. Visual acuity was 20/100 OD. *A*, Kinetic perimetry shows a marked inferior altitudinal defect in the visual field of the right eye. *B*, Fluorescein angiogram, early arteriovenous phase, shows swelling of the right optic disc with dilation of vessels on the surface of the disc. *C*, Fluorescein angiogram, late venous phase, shows marked leakage of dye from disc vessels. (From Scouras J, Koutroumanos J. Ischaemic optic neuropathy in Behçet's syndrome. Ophthalmologica *173:*11–18, 1976.)

Like many other disorders related to an altered immune response, there may be a genetic susceptibility to Behçet's disease, at least in some patient groups. Investigators have reported a 3- to 4-fold increased association of HLA-B5 in Japanese, Turkish, Mexican, Israeli and Italian patients with Behçet's disease compared with controls (Ohno et al., 1975; Yazici et al., 1980; Lavelle et al., 1981; Ohno et al., 1982; Baricordi et al., 1986; Arber et al., 1991), but not in British, German, or American patients (O'Duffy et al., 1976; Yazici

et al., 1980; Djawari et al., 1984; Moore and O'Duffy, 1986). According to O'Duffy (1989), a putative immune-associated antigen with linkage disequilibrium to HLA-B5 in some, but not in other, races would explain this discrepancy.

Diagnosis

The diagnosis of Behçet's disease is based on clinical findings. O'Duffy and Goldstein (1976) recommended that

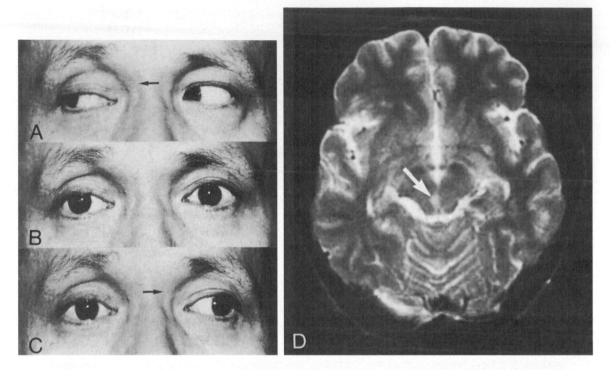

Figure 57.106.   Right internuclear ophthalmoplegia (INO) and skew deviation in a patient with Behçet's disease. *A*, Both eyes move fullly on attempted right gaze. *B*, In primary position, the patient prefers to fix with the right eye and has a mild left hypertropia and a marked right exotropia. *C*, On attempted left gaze, the left eye moves fully, but the right eye does not adduct beyond the midline. *D*, Axial T2-weighted magnetic resonance image shows a focal area of hyperintensity *(arrow)* along the midline of the right aspect of the mesencephalon in the location of the medial longitudinal fasciculus. (From Masai H, Kashii S, Kimura H, et al. Neuro-Behçet disease presenting with internuclear ophthalmoplegia. Am J Ophthalmol *122:*897–898, 1996.)

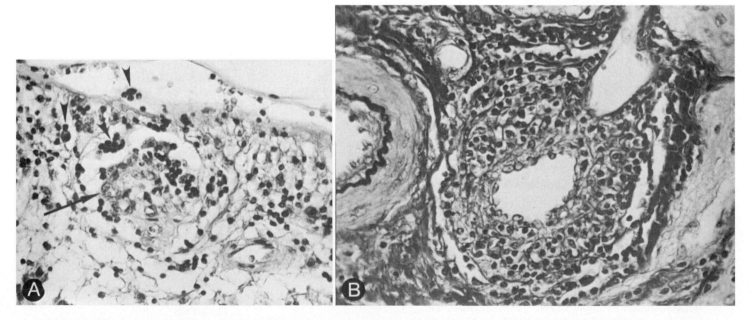

Figure 57.107.   Pathology of Behçet's disease. *A*, Cellular thrombus in retinal vessel *(arrow)*. Inflammatory cells are present in the thrombus and in the surrounding retina *(arrowheads)*. *B*, Severe phlebitis of the central retinal vein in the retrolaminar portion of the optic nerve. (From Fenton RH, Easom HA. Behçet's syndrome: A histopathologic study of the eye. Arch Ophthalmol *72:*71–81, 1964.)

the diagnosis be made only when recurrent aphthous stomatitis, genital aphthous ulcers, or both are associated with two or more of the following manifestations: (*a*) uveitis, (*b*) synovitis, (*c*) cutaneous vasculitis, (*d*) meningoencephalitis. According to these authors, an incomplete form of the disease is present when recurrent aphthous ulceration is associated with only one other criterion. Other authors suggested alternative diagnostic formulas based on combinations of "major" and "minor" criteria (Mason and Barnes, 1969; Shimizu et al., 1979), and the International Study Group for Behçet's Disease (1990) recommends that the diagnosis be made when oral ulceration is associated with at least two of four other features: genital ulceration, eye lesions, positive pathergy test, and either folliculitis or erythema nodosum.

Treatment and Prognosis

The natural history of untreated Behçet's disease is poor. Most patients lose all or part of their vision within 5 years (Mamo, 1970; Jabs, 1994), with the risk of visual loss being greatest in the first 2 years after diagnosis (Demiroglu et al., 1997). When eye disease remains confined to the anterior chamber, vision is usually not threatened, and the inflammation usually can be treated successfully with topical corticosteroids (Mimura et al., 1983; Chamberlain et al., 1988); however, when the posterior segment of the eye is affected, urgent and aggressive treatment is needed (Editorial, 1989), particularly in the early stage of the disease (Demiroglu et al., 1997). The use of systemic corticosteroids may delay the progression of such disease, but it probably does not alter the eventual visual or systemic outcome (Mimura et al., 1983; Benezra and Cohen, 1986). Photocoagulation may be of some benefit in preventing patients with retinal capillary nonperfusion from developing vitreous hemorrhage and neovascular glaucoma (Atmaca, 1990). Patients with vascular complications such as thrombophebitis may benefit from anticoagulation.

The severe systemic and ocular manifestations of Behçet's disease are best treated with a combination of systemic corticosteroids and cytotoxic agents, particularly cyclosporine (Chavis et al., 1992; Yilmaz et al., 1992; Nussenblatt, 1992; Atmaca and Batioglu, 1994), chlorambucil (Mamo and Azzam, 1970; Tricoulis, 1976; Bonnet, 1981; Mimura et al., 1983; O'Duffy et al., 1984; Schilling et al., 1990; Valente et al., 1997) and azathioprine (Yazici et al., 1990). The posterior uveitis and meningoencephalitis are particularly responsive to both of these drugs, although treatment may need to be continued for several years, and relapses may require temporary increases in dose (Abdalla and Bahgat, 1973; Dinning and Perkins, 1975; Mamo, 1976; O'Duffy et al., 1985; O'Duffy, 1989). Other cytotoxic agents that are effective in some patients with Behçet's disease include cyclophosphamide and methotrexate, but these drugs seem to be somewhat less effective than cyclosporine, chlorambucil, or azathioprine (Nussenblatt et al., 1985; Benezra and Cohen, 1986; Masuda et al., 1989; O'Duffy, 1989; Chavis et al., 1990; O'Duffy, 1990; Pahlitzsch et al., 1990; Hashimoto and Takeuchi, 1992; Chavis et al., 1992; Conn et al., 1993). FK 506 was effective in a small series of patients with Behçet's

disease and uveitis reported by Ishioka et al. (1994). Although all of the immunosuppressive agents have a significant oncogenic and cytotoxic potential, the complications that can result from using these drugs must be compared with the potential for blindness from uveitis and retinal vasculitis and the permanent disability or death from meningoencephalitis and other neurologic and systemic complications of the disease.

Colchicine, a drug that interferes with the mobilization of leukocytes, can be used in conjunction with systemic corticosteroids and cytotoxic agents to treat Behçet's disease (Horiuchi et al., 1983; Mimura et al., 1983). It seems to be particularly effective in controlling posterior uveitis and retinitis.

Plasmapheresis produces variable improvement in patients with Behçet's disease (Baudelot et al., 1979; Saraux et al., 1982c, 1982d; Aoi et al., 1983; Ozawa et al., 1983; Wizemann and Wizemann, 1984; Fukutomi et al., 1985; Bonnet et al., 1986; Raizman and Foster, 1989). This treatment may be of particular value in selected patients who are unresponsive to, or cannot tolerate, standard medical therapy.

Patients with Behçet's disease who develop pseudotumor cerebri from cerebral venous sinus thrombosis generally have a benign prognosis when the condition is recognized and treated early. Some patients, however, develop postpapilledema optic atrophy with permanent visual dysfunction, and a few die from the effects of the thrombosis (Bousser et al., 1985). In a series of 250 patients with Behçet's disease, 25 developed angiographically proven cerebral venous thrombosis (Wechsler et al., 1992). Most of these patients were treated with a combination of anticoagulation and corticosteroids, and neurologic symptoms improved in all of them.

CONNECTIVE TISSUE DISEASES

The connective tissue diseases are characterized by inflammation, in multiple organ systems, associated with antibody reactions to nuclear, cytoplasmic, and cell membrane antigens. These diseases include systemic lupus erythematosus, polymyositis, and scleroderma.

Systemic Lupus Erythematosus

SLE is a chronic inflammatory disease of unknown cause that may affect the skin, joints, kidneys, lungs, nervous system, serous membranes, and other organs of the body (Decker et al., 1975; Case Records of the Massachusetts General Hospital., 1990; Schur, 1993; Lahita, 1997). Patients with SLE have distinct immunologic abnormalities, particularly ANAs (Reichlin, 1989). Because of the diffuse, multisystemic nature of this disease, the American Rheumatism Association committee developed a set of diagnostic criteria in 1975, which were revised in 1982 (Cohen et al., 1975; Tan et al., 1982).

History

The term **lupus erythematosus** (from the Latin word, *lupus,* meaning "wolf" and the Greek word, *erythema,* meaning "flush") was initially used by Cazenave in 1851 to refer to an apparent dermatologic disorder characterized by severe skin rash of the face and extremities. It was subsequently recognized that the disorder known as "lupus" was often a systemic disease, not just a skin problem. Because autopsy studies in patients with SLE showed pathologic abnormalities of collagen-containing tissue, particularly blood vessels, it initially was classified as a "collagen vascular disease" (Klemperer et al., 1942; Manschot, 1961); however, the immunologic basis of the disease was subsequently recognized (Hargraves et al., 1948; Friou, 1957), and the term "collagen vascular disease" was replaced by "connective tissue disease," a term that correctly emphasizes that SLE is not a disorder of collagen alone.

Demographics

The prevalence of SLE is 4–250 cases per 100,000 population (Schur, 1993). It is more common in women than in men, and it may be more common in African-Americans than in Caucasians, at least in some cities (Fessel, 1974; Hochberg, 1985). Symptoms and signs of SLE may occur at any age, but the peak onset occurs in the 2nd–4th decades of life (Harvey et al., 1954; Estes and Christian, 1971), with 65% of affected patients experiencing the onset of symptoms from the ages of 16–55 (Rothfield, 1981). SLE also seems to be more common in urban than in rural areas (Schur, 1993).

Multiple independent segregating genes are implicated in SLE (Christian, 1987). These genes may affect immune regulation, immune responses, concentration of circulating complement proteins, function of the mononuclearphagocytic (reticuloendothelial) system, concentration and function of immunoglobulins, and metabolism of hormones. Evidence for the existence of such genes includes a high concordance rate (14–57%) in monozygotic twins (Block et al., 1975; Deapen et al., 1986) and a high prevalence of SLE in relatives of patients with SLE (Arnett et al., 1984). In addition, patients with SLE are more likely to have the HLA molecules DR2 and DR3 than are normal persons (Black et al., 1982; Schur et al., 1982; Arnett et al., 1984; Howard et al., 1986).

Clinical Manifestations

The clinical manifestations of SLE are extensive. They include nonspecific constitutional symptoms as well as symptoms and signs referable to almost every organ system in the body.

CONSTITUTIONAL SYMPTOMS

Fatigue is the most common complaint, occurring in 80–100% of patients with SLE (Dubois and Wallace, 1987; Reeves and Lahita, 1987; Schur, 1993, 1996), and it is often the first symptom of the disease (Liang et al., 1981). Fatigue may be so severe that the patient is unable to maintain a normal life-style, even when other manifestations of the disease are absent.

Weight loss of more than 5 pounds occurs in more than half of the patients with SLE (Rothfield, 1981) and is generally associated with other constitutional symptoms. It may be caused by lack of appetite, gastrointestinal disease, or the effects of medication. **Weight gain** may also occur in patients with active SLE, either from water retention associated with kidney disease or from the effects of the corticosteroids used to treat the disease.

Fever without concomitant infection occurs in more than 80% of patients with SLE at some time during the course of the disease (Dubois and Wallace, 1987; Reeves and Lahita, 1987; Schur, 1993, 1996). The fever of SLE, generally unassociated with chills or other clinical evidence of infection, is usually accompanied by a low, rather than an elevated, white blood cell count.

Constitutional symptoms other than those described above occur with variable frequency in patients with SLE. These symptoms include anorexia, nausea, vomiting, headache, and depression.

MUSCULOSKELETAL SYMPTOMS AND SIGNS

Musculoskeletal complaints are frequent in patients with SLE (Schur, 1993, 1996). Myalgia, arthralgia, and arthritis occur in up to 95% of patients, and they may precede the diagnosis of SLE by months to years (Stevens, 1983; Buyon and Zuckerman, 1987). The features of musculoskeletal involvement that suggest a diagnosis of SLE include a migratory nature, with symptoms in a particular joint disappearing spontaneously within 24 hours, symmetry, and a predilection for the knees, carpal joints, and the joints of the fingers (Schur, 1993) (Fig. 57.108). The wrists, ankles, elbows, shoulders, and hips are less frequently affected. The arthritis

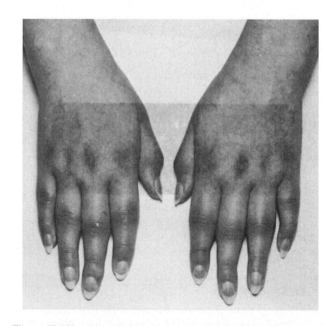

Figure 57.108. Musculoskeletal signs in systemic lupus erythematosus. The patient has symmetric, proximal, interphalangeal joint swelling. (From Michet CJ, Hunder GG. Examination of the joints. In Textbook of Rheumatology. Editors, Kelley WN, Harris ED Jr, Ruddy S, et al. 3rd ed, pp 425–441. Philadelphia, WB Saunders, 1989.)

is usually nondeforming and nonerosive, and the degree of pain often overshadows any objective physical findings. Muscular weakness associated with clinical and laboratory evidence of myopathy also occurs in patients with SLE (Mellgren et al., 1987).

MUCOCUTANEOUS LESIONS

The skin and mucous membranes are symptomatically affected in more than 80% of patients with SLE (Provost and Dore, 1983; Gilliam, 1987). More than 50% of patients develop a rash after exposure to ultraviolet (UV) light (Dubois and Wallace, 1987; Schur, 1996). The mechanism by which this **photosensitivity** occurs is unclear. UV light may damage the DNA or proteins in the skin, altering their structure to make them antigens to which antibodies are made. Antigen-antibody reactions may then produce a local inflammatory reaction. UV light may also significantly alter phospholipid metabolism in the cellular membranes of the skin, thus producing a rash. Finally, UV light may induce an increase in the production and release of cytokines from cutaneous keratinocytes and Langerhans cells. These cytokines may cause local inflammation and increased production of antibodies.

A typical **butterfly rash** occurs across the face in about 50% of patients with SLE (Schur, 1993) (Fig. 57.109). Its name is based on the shape of the erythema over the cheeks and the bridge of the nose. The rash usually occurs after exposure to UV light, lasts for hours to days, and may recur spontaneously without further exposure to sunlight or artificial UV light. The rash may precede other symptoms of SLE by months to years, or its appearance may be accompanied by other symptoms and signs of acute SLE. The affected skin appears red and slightly edematous, and it feels warm. Application of alcohol to the skin may actually increase the redness by increasing circulation to the skin. Histopathologic examination of affected skin is usually unremarkable except for mild abnormalities in the basal cell layer of the epidermis, although immunofluorescent staining may show immunoglobulins and complement at the dermal-epidermal junction (Provost and Dore, 1983) (Fig. 57.110).

Discoid skin lesions occur in some patients with SLE, but they are more common in patients who have the purely cutaneous form of the disease. They usually occur on the face, neck, and scalp (Fig. 57.111), but they also may develop on the ears (Fig. 57.112) and, infrequently, on the upper torso. The lesions are discrete, round, annular, erythematous, slightly thickened plaques that are covered by a well-formed adherent scale that plugs hair follicles (Gilliam, 1987; Laman and Provost, 1994). They generally enlarge slowly, leaving depressed central scars, telangiectasias, and depigmentation. Pathologic examination of discoid skin lesions reveals hyperkeratosis, follicular plugging, and changes in the basal cell layer consisting of loss of normal organization and orientation of basal cells, intracellular edema and vacuole formation, and mononuclear cell infiltration of the dermal-epidermal junction (Gilliam, 1987). A mononuclear cell infiltrate consisting primarily of T-lymphocytes may also be present in the dermis around blood

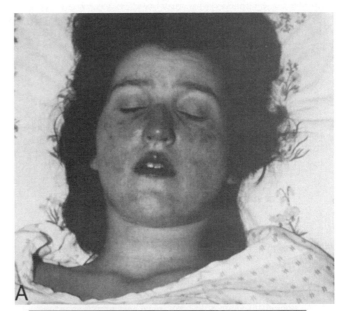

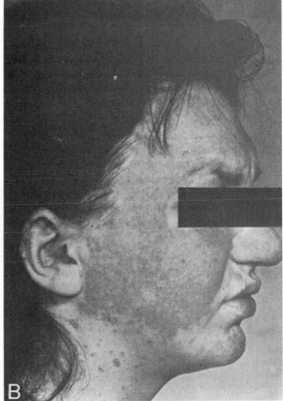

Figure 57.109. Malar "butterfly" rash in systemic lupus erythematosus. *A*, The patient was a 15-year-old girl who developed an acute febrile illness. (From Schaller JG, Szer IS. Systemic lupus erythematosus, dermatomyositis, scleroderma, and vasculitis in childhood. In Textbook of Rheumatology. Editors, Kelley WN, Harris ED Jr, Ruddy S, et al. 3rd ed, pp 1325–1354. Philadelphia, WB Saunders, 1989.) *B*, More extensive rash with slight scale over the malar regions and forehead. The distribution is determined by exposure to light. (From Soter NA. The skin and rheumatic diseases. In Textbook of Rheumatology. Editors, Kelley WN, Harris ED Jr, et al. 3rd ed, pp 597–610. Philadelphia, WB Saunders, 1989.)

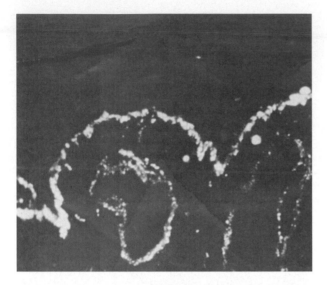

Figure 57.110. Immunofluorescent staining of the skin in a patient with systemic lupus erythematosus. Note bright intensity of granular deposits of IgM along the junction of the dermis and epidermis. Vascular staining also is present. (Courtesy of Dr. Terrence J Harrist.)

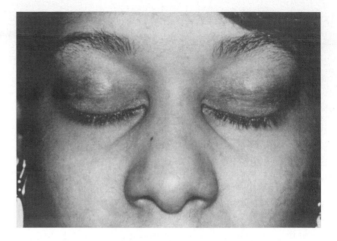

Figure 57.111. Discoid lupus erythematosus. Diffuse rash affecting both upper eyelids in a 35-year-old woman with chronic discoid lupus erythematosus. (From Insler MS, Boulware DW. Discoid lupus erythematosus. In The Eye in Systemic Disease. Editors, Gold DH, Weingeist TA. pp 48–50. Philadelphia, JB Lippincott, 1990.)

vessels. Immunofluorescent staining reveals immunoglobulin and complement components along the dermal-epidermal border (Smith et al., 1984).

About 10% of patients with SLE develop **subacute cuta-** **neous skin lesions** (Gilliam, 1987). These lesions begin as small, erythematous, slightly scaly papules that evolve into either a psoriaform or an annular form. The lesions often coalesce. They typically have erythematous edges, and they may be associated with telangiectasias, but they do not show the follicular plugging, hyperkeratosis, dermal atrophy, or

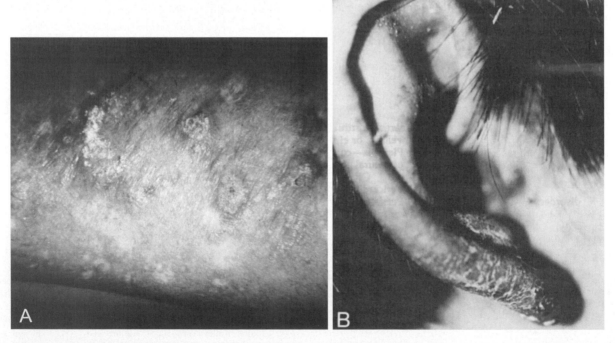

Figure 57.112. Discoid skin lesions in systemic lupus erythematosus (SLE). *A*, The lesions are discrete, round, annular, erythematous, slightly thickened plaques that are covered by a well-formed, adherent scale. Note other areas of hypopigmentation. (Courtesy of Dr. Douglas Jabs.) *B*, Discoid rash on the ear of a 10-year-old boy with SLE. The rash initially was mistaken for seborrheic dermatitis. (From Schaller JG, Szer IS. Systemic lupus erythematosus, dermatomyositis, scleroderma, and vasculitis in childhood. In Textbook of Rheumatology. Editors, Kelley WN, Harris ED Jr, Ruddy S, et al. 3rd ed, pp 1325–1354. Philadelphia, WB Saunders, 1989.)

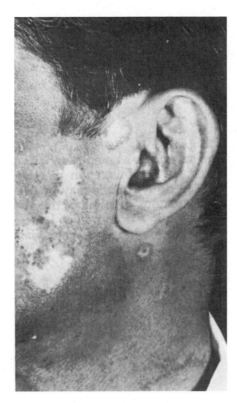

Figure 57.113. Chronic skin lesions in discoid lupus erythematosus. Note circumscribed, atrophic patches with hypopigmentation and hyperpigmentation on the face. (From Soter NA. The skin and rheumatic diseases. In Textbook of Rheumatology. Editors, Kelley WN, Harris ED Jr, Ruddy S, et al. 3rd ed, pp 597–610. Philadelphia, WB Saunders, 1989.)

pigment changes seen in discoid lesions. They most frequently develop on the shoulders, forearms, palms, neck, and upper torso (Fig. 57.113). The face usually is spared.

Rare patients with SLE develop firm nodules that may occur underneath cutaneous lesions (**lupus profundus**) or as isolated lesions (**lupus panniculitis**) (Gilliam, 1987). The nodules may develop in the mid-dermal, deep dermal, or subcutaneous layer (Fig. 57.114). They consist of perivascular infiltrates of mononuclear cells, and they may occur on the scalp, face, arms, chest, back, thighs, and buttocks (Diaz-Jouanen et al., 1975). They usually resolve spontaneously, but they may leave a depressed area, and they occasionally ulcerate.

Alopecia occurs in up to 71% of patients with SLE at some time during their illness (Rothfield, 1981; Dubois and Wallace, 1987). The hair loss may affect the scalp, eyebrows, eyelashes, beard, body hair, or a combination of these (Provost and Dore, 1983). It may or may not be associated with scarring of the skin. When scarring of skin is present, the hair loss is usually permanent. SLE patients may develop an unusual form of alopecia with hair loss along the periphery of the scalp. This form of hair loss is not permanent and usually signifies active disease (Laman and Provost, 1994). Alopecia may precede other manifestations of SLE.

The **mucous membranes** are affected in 25–40% of pa-

tients with SLE. Characteristic discoid lesions with erythema, atrophy, and depigmentation may occur on the lips, and irregularly shaped raised white plaques, silvery white scarred lesions, or areas of erythema may appear on the soft or hard palate. Punched-out erosions or ulcers with erythema around them may also occur. All of these lesions are painless, and they may be the first sign of SLE. Patients with SLE also may develop gingivitis, nasal ulcers, and damage to the mucosa of the upper airway, resulting in hoarseness (Schur, 1993, 1996).

Vascular cutaneous lesions develop in about 50% of patients with SLE (Schur, 1993). Different lesions may occur, depending on the type of blood vessel affected. These lesions include periungual erythema, livedo reticularis, telangiectasia, Raynaud's phenomenon, and various forms of vasculitis.

PULMONARY MANIFESTATIONS

Damage to the lung, its vasculature, the pleura, and the diaphragm occurs in about 50% of patients with SLE (Hunninghake and Fauci, 1979; Rothfield, 1983a; Pines et al., 1985) (Fig. 57.115). Lung damage in patients with SLE may be asymptomatic and only discovered during routine chest X-ray examination or performance of pulmonary function testing, or it may cause chest pain during breathing, coughing, dyspnea, or a combination of these. Progressive lung damage in patients with SLE may produce pulmonary edema, acute and chronic pneumonitis, and even pulmonary hypertension.

CARDIOVASCULAR MANIFESTATIONS

The most common cardiac abnormality in SLE is damage to the pericardium (Rothfield, 1983a; Stevens, 1987). Pa-

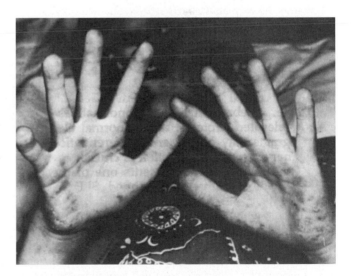

Figure 57.114. Subacute cutaneous skin lesions in systemic lupus erythematosus (SLE). The patient was an 8-year-old boy with SLE. Note palmar rash consisting of small, erythematous, slightly scaly papules. (From Schaller JG, Szer IS. Systemic lupus erythematosus, dermatomyositis, scleroderma, and vasculitis in childhood. In Textbook of Rheumatology. Editors, Kelley WN, Harris ED Jr, Ruddy S, et al. 3rd ed, pp 1325–1354. Philadelphia, WB Saunders, 1989.)

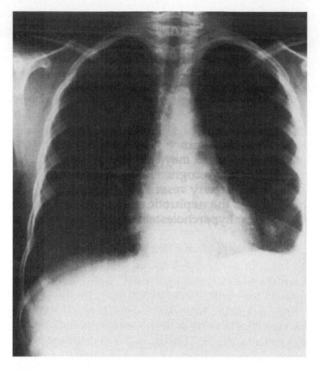

Figure 57.115. Pulmonary manifestations of systemic lupus erythematosus (SLE). The patient was a 10-year-old girl with SLE who developed difficulty breathing and chest pain. Chest X-ray, anteroposterior view, shows a left pleural effusion. (From Schaller JG, Szer IS. Systemic lupus erythematosus, dermatomyositis, scleroderma, and vasculitis in childhood. In Textbook of Rheumatology. Editors, Kelley WN, Harris ED Jr, Ruddy S, et al. 3rd ed, pp 1325–1354. Philadelphia, WB Saunders, 1989.)

tients may develop **acute pericarditis,** characterized by positional substernal chest pain, and symptomatic pericardial effusion also may occur. The pericardial fluid is a fibrinous exudate, and the pericardium itself may show foci of inflammation with mononuclear cells predominating.

Myocarditis may occur in patients with SLE (Stevens, 1987). Acute myocarditis may accompany other manifestations of acute SLE, particularly pericarditis. As the myocardium heals, fibrosis may occur, resulting in persistent cardiac dysfunction. Patients with lupus myocarditis may experience episodes of tachycardia, congestive heart failure, arrhythmias, and even cardiogenic shock (Disla et al., 1993).

Coronary artery disease occurs as a direct consequence of SLE in about 2–8% of patients, and it may cause a myocardial infarction with or without congestive heart failure (Harvey et al., 1954; Estes and Christian, 1971; Barker et al., 1989; Schur, 1993, 1996). Arteritis of the coronary arteries with accompanying deposition of immune complexes may predispose to atherosclerosis and subsequent occlusion of these vessels (Bonfiglio et al., 1972; Heibel et al., 1976).

Cardiac valvular disease is uncommon in patients with SLE. Some patients, however, develop marantic endocarditis (Devinsky et al., 1987, 1988). The lesions are usually located near the edge of the valve and consist of accumulations of immune complexes, mononuclear cells, necrosis, and both

fibrin and platelet thrombi (Fig. 57.116). The most common valves affected in SLE are the mitral valve, followed by the aortic and tricuspid valves (Stevens, 1987). Cardiac valvular disease is a common cause of TIAs and stroke in patients with SLE.

Gomez et al. (1988) studied 28 consecutive patients with SLE using two-dimensional echocardiography and Doppler ultrasonography. The results were correlated with titers of anticardiolipin antibody, one of the antiphospholipid antibodies (Levine and Welch, 1989) (see Chapters 55 and 58). The findings in this study suggested a strong association between myocardial and cardiac valvular involvement in SLE and raised anticardiolipin antibodies. Similar findings were reported by Khamashta et al. (1990).

HEMATOLOGIC MANIFESTATIONS

Abnormalities of the formed elements of the blood and of the coagulation system are common in patients with SLE. **Anemia** is the most common disturbance, occurring in about 50% of patients (Shoenfeld and Schwartz, 1983; Laurence and Nachman, 1987). The most frequent cause is suppressed erythropoiesis from chronic inflammation, uremia, or both, but other causes include blood loss, dietary insufficiency, hemolysis, and medication (Schur, 1993, 1996). **Leukope-**

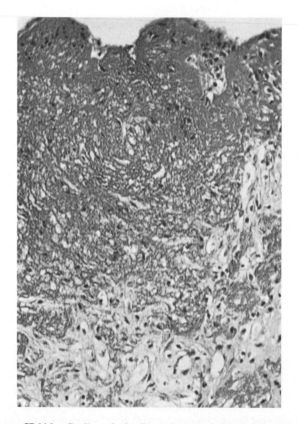

Figure 57.116. Cardiac valvular disease in systemic lupus erythematosus. Section through affected cardiac valves in a patient with marantic endocarditis shows a vegetation composed largely of fibrinoid material with trapped chronic inflammatory cells and fibroblasts. (From Robbins SL. Pathology, 3rd ed, p 259. Philadelphia, WB Saunders, 1967.)

nia may result from immune mechanisms, medications, and bone marrow dysfunction, and **lymphocytopenia** is particularly common during periods of active disease (Budman and Steinberg, 1977). **Thrombocytopenia** occurs in about 25–50% of patients with SLE, usually from enhanced destruction of platelets by antiplatelet antibodies (Schur, 1993, 1996).

A circulating anticoagulant, the "lupus anticoagulant," is demonstrated in some, but not all, patients with SLE. Despite its name, this antiphospholipid antibody does not induce bleeding diatheses in vivo; it was named because of its anticoagulant effects in vitro. In fact, the antiphospholipid antibodies are associated with **thrombotic disorders,** such as deep vein thrombophlebitis, myocardial infarction, cerebral venous sinus thrombosis, and stroke, and not with systemic or intracranial hemorrhage. Thromboembolism occurs in up to 50% of patients with SLE who possess the lupus anticoagulant (Bick and Baker, 1994). There is also evidence that an increased concentration of serum anticardiolipin antibody, another type of antiphospholipid antibody, correlates with both the systemic and ocular activity of SLE, particularly with the prevalence of thrombotic complications (Harris et al., 1983, 1985; Isenberg et al., 1986; Kalunian et al., 1988; Raz et al., 1988; Shergy et al., 1988; Alarcón-Segovia et al., 1989; Asherson et al., 1989a, 1989b; Buchanan et al., 1989; Lie, 1989; Maaravi et al., 1989; Out et al., 1989; Case Records of the Massachusetts General Hospital, 1990; Matsushima et al., 1997). The risk of thrombotic events also appears to correlate not only with the presence of antiphospholipid antibodies but also specifically with the degree of titer elevation and the IgG isotype (Bick and Baker, 1994; Feldmann and Levine, 1995). The mechanism by which antiphospholipid antibodies produce thrombosis is unknown, but possibilities include induction of platelet aggregation by the antibodies, inhibition of prostacylin production by the vascular endothelium, and neutralization of naturally occurring anticoagulants such as protein C and protein S (Boey et al., 1983; Harris et al., 1983; Glueck et al., 1985; Petri et al., 1987; Levine and Welch, 1989; Feldmann and Levine, 1995). A variety of therapies are used to treat the complications of the antiphospholipid syndrome, including warfarin, aspirin, prednisone, plasmapheresis, immunoglobin transfusion, and other immunosuppressive agents such as azathioprine, cyclophosphamide, and methotrexate (Feldmann and Levine, 1995). A large, retrospective nonrandomized study found that treatment with warfarin that produced an international normalized ratio greater than 3 was significantly more effective than treatment with aspirin or low-dose warfarin in preventing recurrent thrombosis (Khamashta et al., 1995).

RENAL MANIFESTATIONS

Renal disease is a frequent complication of SLE, occurring in about 50% of patients at some time during the course of the disease (Rothfield, 1983b; Pollak and Kant, 1987; Schur, 1996). Four types of renal disease can develop: (*a*) focal proliferative nephritis, (*b*) diffuse proliferative nephritis, (*c*) membranous nephritis, and (*d*) mesangial nephritis (see Table 61-5 in Schur, 1993).

Focal proliferative nephritis produces proteinuria and also may cause gross hematuria, but affected patients rarely develop the nephrotic syndrome, and they do not develop systemic hypertension or renal insufficiency. Light microscopic examination in patients with this condition shows segmental proliferation and necrosis in glomerular tufts and in the mesangial area (Schur, 1993) (Fig. 57.117). Electron microscopic examination in conjunction with immunofluorescent staining shows immunoglobulins (especially IgG) and C3 in the mesangium and scattered granular deposits in the subendothelial, subepithelial, and intrabasement membrane areas (Pollak and Kant, 1987).

Diffuse proliferative nephritis produces more severe renal dysfunction than does focal proliferative nephritis. Affected patients develop proteinuria and gross hematuria. Almost all patients develop symptoms and signs of renal insufficiency, and most eventually develop the nephrotic syndrome. Systemic hypertension is common. The condition may remit, but if it does not do so, about 50% of affected patients die of renal failure within 2 years (Austin et al., 1983, 1984). Pathologic examination of the kidneys of patients with diffuse proliferative nephritis shows hypercellularity, especially of mesangial and endothelial cells. Hyaline thrombi, consisting of IgG, IgM, complement, and fibrin, often occlude the capillary lumens, and tubular degenerative changes with interstitial accumulation of mononuclear cells are common (Pollak and Kant, 1987). Immunofluorescent staining reveals extensive granules and lumpy deposits of

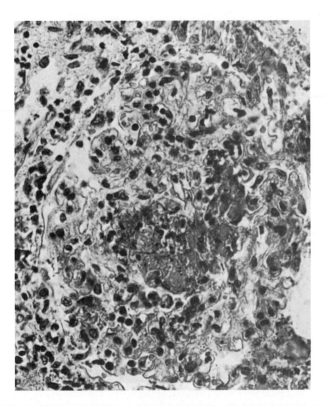

Figure 57.117. Pathology of focal proliferative nephritis in systemic lupus erythematosus. A glomerular tuft shows focal necrosis. (From Robbins SL. Pathology. 3rd ed, p 259. Philadelphia, WB Saunders, 1967.)

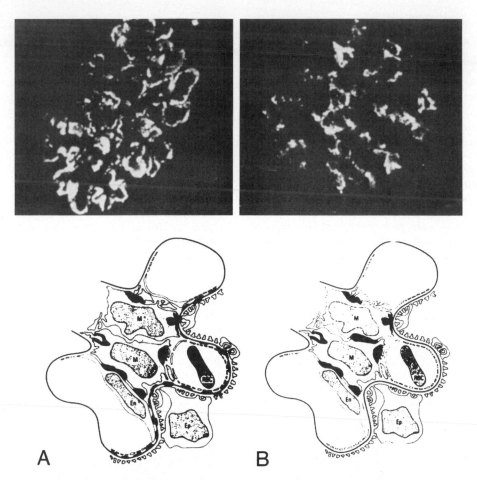

Figure 57.118. Schematic and immune fluorescent demonstration of immune complexes in two types of nephritis in systemic lupus erythematosus. *A*, In a patient with diffuse proliferative nephritis, the complexes are deposited in the mesangium and diffusely along the basement membrane, primarily in the subendothelial region. *B*, In a patient with mesangial nephritis, the complexes are limited to the mesangial region. In both cases, the tissue is stained with a fluoresceinated antibody to IgG. (From Woods VL Jr, Zvaifler NJ. Pathogenesis of systemic lupus erythematosus. In Textbook of Rheumatology. Editors, Kelley WN, Harris ED Jr, Ruddy S, et al. 3rd ed, pp 1077–1100. Philadelphia, WB Saunders, 1989.)

immunoglobulins and complement in the mesangial area, particularly along the glomerular basement membrane and especially on the endothelial side (Fig. 57.118*A*).

Membranous nephritis generally causes proteinuria without gross hematuria, although microscopic hematuria may be present. About 50% of patients present with the nephrotic syndrome, and about 80% of patients eventually develop it. Renal insufficiency, initially mild, worsens slowly with time. Pathologic examination of affected kidneys shows very little, if any, cellular proliferation or infiltration. Rather, there is diffuse, fairly uniform thickening of the glomerular basement membrane (Fig. 57.119). Electron microscopic examination of immunofluorescent-stained tissue discloses immunoglobulins and complement components all along the glomerular basement membrane in a fine granular pattern, especially in the subendothelial region. Intramembranous and mesangial deposits are also common.

Mesangial nephritis is the most common and least severe type of renal disease that affects patients with SLE. Patients with minimal disease have no clinical or laboratory evidence of renal dysfunction; other patients have minimal proteinuria, microscopic hematuria, or both. Systemic hypertension is characteristically absent, with neither significant renal insufficiency nor the nephrotic syndrome developing unless the patient develops the diffuse proliferative or membranous forms of nephritis (Schur, 1993, 1996). Light microscopic examination of kidney tissue from patients with minimal mesangial nephritis reveals no abnormalities, although deposition of immune complexes in the mesangial area can be detected by electron microscopy (Fig. 57.118*B*). Kidneys from patients with more advanced mesangial nephritis demonstrate immune deposits and hypercellularity in the mesangial area (Pollak and Kant, 1987).

GASTROINTESTINAL MANIFESTATIONS

Patients with SLE often have **nonspecific gastrointestinal complaints** (Brown et al., 1956; Hoffman and Katz, 1980; Zizic, 1983; Mayer, 1987; Schur, 1993, 1996). Some patients complain of difficulty swallowing, particularly during periods of stress. Dysphagia may result from damage to the esophagus, reflux of gastric acid, hiatal hernia, esophageal candidiasis, and even esophageal ulceration. Dyspepsia, abdominal pain, nausea, and vomiting may all occur in patients with SLE. When they occur in patients taking systemic corticosteroids, it is often assumed that they are caused by the irritant effect of the medicine and not by the disease itself; however, they may also occur in patients with SLE who are not taking medicine, and in such patients, response of the symptoms to steroids confirms an inflammatory cause.

Mesenteric vasculitis may develop in patients with SLE. It usually is characterized by lower abdominal pain that is insidious in onset and initially intermittent. Eventually, however, the patient may develop an acute abdomen with rebound tenderness from generalized ischemia and perforation (Zizic, 1983).

Pancreatitis occurs in about 8% of patients with SLE (Reynolds et al., 1982). Symptoms include upper abdominal pain, nausea, and vomiting. Laboratory studies show an increased concentration of amylase in the serum. The pancreatitis that occurs in patients with SLE is usually associated with other clinical evidence of active disease and is probably caused by vasculitis.

NEUROLOGIC AND PSYCHIATRIC MANIFESTATIONS

A variety of neurologic and psychiatric symptoms and signs may occur in patients with SLE (O'Connor and

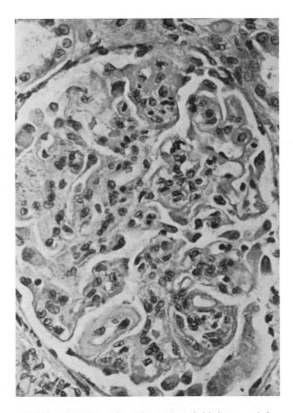

Figure 57.119. Pathology of membranous nephritis in systemic lupus erythematosus. A glomerulus shows diffuse thickening of the basement membranes. The capillary network is patent with no evidence of cellular proliferation or infiltration. (From Robbins SL. Pathology. 3rd ed, p 259. Philadelphia, WB Saunders, 1967.)

Musher, 1966; Johnson and Richardson, 1968; Devinsky et al., 1987; Mellgren et al., 1987; Sigal, 1987; Devinsky et al., 1988; Jongen et al., 1990; Liu et al., 1990; Stoppe et al., 1990; Lahita, 1997). Indeed, neurologic disease is the second or third leading cause of death in most series of patients with SLE (Ellis and Verity, 1979; Rosner et al., 1982). Neurologic disturbances may antedate the diagnosis of SLE, but they more often occur a few years after other manifestations of the disease develop (Johnson and Richardson, 1968; Estes and Christian, 1971; Gibson and Myers, 1976; Sigal, 1987). The frequency of CNS disease in patients with SLE increases with the duration of the systemic disease (Sigal, 1987).

Some disturbances are primarily psychiatric, and they usually are related to the effect of the disease on the patient's life-style (O'Connor and Musher, 1966; Feinglass et al., 1976). **Depression** is by far the most common of these symptoms (Miquel et al., 1994). It is the consequence not only of being sick but of realizing that one is never again going to be well and of having to deal with limitations on aspects of life that previously have been taken for granted, such as having and raising children, excercising strenuously, etc. Most patients eventually recover, but others incorporate the depression into their personality, resulting in many concurrent psychosomatic complaints. Still others become **psychotic.** Such patients exhibit increasing despair, loss of hope, and suicidal tendencies.

Some patients with SLE develop severe **anxiety** instead of, or in addition to, depression. Symptoms of anxiety usually develop during the first few years of illness. The anxious state may deteriorate into obsessive-compulsive behavior, phobias, hypochondriasis, and disturbances of sleep (Schur, 1993, 1996). Other disturbances commonly seen in patients with SLE include conversion reactions, affective disorders, and mood swings.

Headache is a frequent symptom in patients with SLE. The causes of headache in such patients are numerous (Vázquez-Cruz et al., 1990). For most patients, tension is the primary triggering factor, whereas other patients seem to have typical migraine headaches that are triggered by a variety of factors (see Chapter 56).

Seizures occur in about 15–20% of patients with SLE (Zvaifler, 1983). The seizures are usually of the grand mal type but may be of the petit mal, temporal lobe, focal, and jacksonian variety (Meagher et al., 1961; Bilaniuk et al., 1977; Gonzalez-Scarano et al., 1979; Jongen et al., 1990; Schur, 1993, 1996). Seizures may antedate the onset of SLE, be among its first signs, or develop during the course of the illness. There are many potential causes for seizures in patients with SLE, including damage from an acute inflammatory episode, old cortical damage with scar formation, metabolic imbalances, uremia, hypertension, infection, tumor, head trauma, and vasculopathy. Although some patients with seizures have angiographically proven CNS vasculitis (Graham et al., 1985; Bryant et al., 1986; Sakaki et al., 1990) (Fig. 57.120), postmortem examination of brain specimens from SLE patients with seizures usually reveals no evidence of vasculitis but, instead, evidence of nonvasculitic thrombosis and infarction.

About 10–15% of patients with SLE develop a **peripheral**

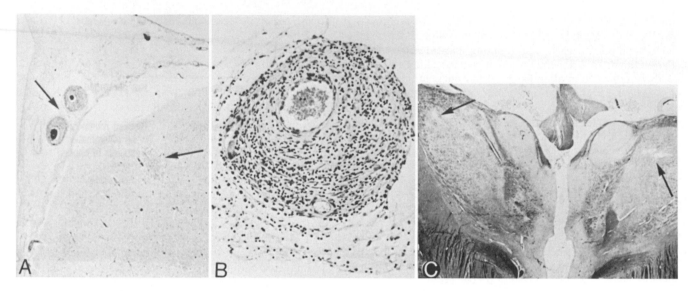

Figure 57.120. Cerebral vasculitis in systemic lupus erythematosus (SLE). The patient was a 16-year-old boy with SLE who developed severe kidney disease, myocardial dysfunction, and mental deterioration. He subsequently died from left ventricular failure and pulmonary embolism. *A*, Section through the cerebral meninges shows two arterioles surrounded by intense inflammation (*left arrow*). A microinfarct is seen in adjacent cerebral cortex (*right arrow*). *B*, Higher power of one of the arterioles shows marked perivascular inflammation infiltrating the walls of the vessel. Note that the lumen is not compromised. *C*, Small infarcts are present in the thalami (*arrows*). (From Graham EM, Spalton DJ, Barnard RO, et al. Cerebral and retinal vascular changes in systemic lupus erythematosus. Ophthalmology *92:*444–448, 1985.)

neuropathy, cranial neuropathy, or both (Bluestein, 1987; Schur, 1996). Peripheral neuropathies are usually asymmetric and mild, and they may affect more than one nerve. Sensory nerves are affected more often than motor nerves, but peripheral motor neuropathies, such as recurrent laryngeal palsy, occur (Espana et al., 1990). Some patients develop an autonomic neuropathy (Hoyle et al., 1985; Arruda et al., 1989), and others develop a progressive neuropathy that resembles the Guillain-Barré syndrome (Millette et al., 1986; Chaudhuri et al., 1989) (see Chapter 72).

The most common cranial nerve affected in SLE is the facial nerve, but the ocular motor and trigeminal nerves are not infrequently affected (see below). Facial and trigeminal neuropathies can occur during the course of SLE or as the initial manifestation of the disease (Johnson and Richardson, 1968; Estes and Christian, 1971; Bennett et al., 1972; Lundberg and Werner, 1972; Hagen et al., 1990).

The peripheral and cranial neuropathies of SLE are thought to be caused primarily by occlusion of small arteries supplying the affected nerves. The response of some of these neuropathies to systemic corticosteroids suggests that in such cases, the cause of the occlusion may be inflammatory. In some patients, however, the cause of the neuropathy seems to be primary demyelination (Rechthand et al., 1984; Chaudhuri et al., 1989). Such patients may respond dramatically to immunosuppressive therapy, plasmapheresis, or intravenously administered immune globulin.

Patients with SLE may experience both **TIAs and strokes** (Caplan and Stein, 1986; Devinsky et al., 1987, 1988; Futrell and Millikan, 1989). Some patients experience transient neurologic or visual symptoms similar to those experienced by patients with migraine (Brandt et al., 1975; Brandt and Les-

sell, 1978; Lessell, 1979; Honda, 1985, 1987; Mellgren et al., 1987). These symptoms probably are caused by vasospasm (Brandt et al., 1975; Brandt and Lessell, 1978; Shaw et al., 1979). Permanent visual or neurologic deficits that occur in patients with SLE are not related to intracranial vasculitis. Most patients with such deficits have little or no evidence of inflammation of intracranial arteries (Johnson and Richardson, 1968; Devinsky et al., 1988; Schur, 1993, 1996). Instead, the deficits are caused by one of three mechanisms: (*a*) large and medium-sized vessels become occluded or obliterated by thrombosis caused by an associated coagulopathy (Trevor et al., 1972; Hart et al., 1984; Shiozawa et al., 1986; Futrell and Millikan, 1989); (*b*) associated hypertensive renal disease results in occlusion of small vessels (Feinglass et al., 1976); or (*c*) cerebral or ocular embolism results from associated cardiac valvular disease (Devinsky et al., 1988; Galve et al., 1988; Futrell and Millikan, 1989).

In view of the different causes of CNS damage in patients with SLE, it is not surprising that neuroimaging studies performed in such patients show nonspecific findings, including enlargement of sulci, ventricular enlargement, and evidence of ischemic or hemorrhagic infarction (Gonzalez-Scarano et al., 1979; Miller et al., 1979; Asherson et al., 1989a, 1989b; Sibbitt et al., 1989) (Fig. 57.121). MR imaging provides more information than CT scanning, even in patients with acute neuropsychiatric manifestations (Sibbitt et al., 1989), but there are no pathognomonic MR imaging findings for CNS SLE. Indeed, patients with and without clinical evidence of CNS SLE may show nonspecific high-signal abnormalities of varying sizes in the white matter (Stimmler et al., 1993; Taccari et al., 1994; Ishikawa et al., 1994; Jarek et al., 1994). In one case, confluent and progressive white matter changes mimicked the MR imaging findings of progressive multifocal leukoencephalopathy (Kaye et al., 1992) (see Chapter 68). Positron emission tomographic (PET) scanning and MR spectroscopy are noninvasive tests that provide quantitative information about metabolic activity in the brain. Both tests give abnormal results in patients with neurologic or psychiatric manifestations of SLE, characteristically showing decreased oxygen ultilization, decreased glucose uptake, increased lactate, and decreased high-energy phosphates (Stoppe et al., 1990; Sibbitt and Sibbitt, 1993).

Kushner et al. (1987, 1990) used xenon-133 and single-photon emission CT (SPECT) scanning to study the patterns of cerebral blood flow (CBF) over time in patients with SLE unassociated with neurologic disease and in patients with SLE and various neurologic manifestations, including headache, stroke, psychosis, and encephalopathy. CBF was normal in patients with SLE who did not have neurologic manifestations or whose neurologic disease was in remission, but it was significantly reduced during exacerbations of neurologic symptoms and signs, with the magnitude of the reduction varying with the neurologic syndrome. CBF was least affected in patients with nonspecific symptoms such as headache or malaise, whereas patients with encephalopathy or psychosis exhibited the greatest reductions in CBF. The results of the studies performed by Kushner et al. (1987, 1990) suggest that measurements of CBF may provide a useful marker for the degree of disease activity in the CNS in patients with SLE; however, other studies using SPECT scanning in SLE patients have not found a correlation between abnormal findings and disease activity (Nossent et al., 1991).

Patients who experience a stroke in the setting of SLE are at high risk for a recurrent stroke (Futrell and Millikan, 1989), particularly patients with high titers of antiphospholipid antibodies. Such patients may benefit from chronic anticoagulation.

Meningitis may occur in patients with SLE. In most cases, the meningitis is caused by an infectious agent, but some patients develop an aseptic meningitis characterized by headache, nuchal rigidity, and lymphocytic pleocytosis in the CSF (Canoso and Cohen, 1975).

Transverse myelitis occurs in some patients with SLE (Penn and Rowan, 1968; Andrianakos et al., 1975; Gonzalez-Scarano et al., 1979; Warren and Kredich, 1984; Rubin and De Horatius, 1989). Affected patients initially develop

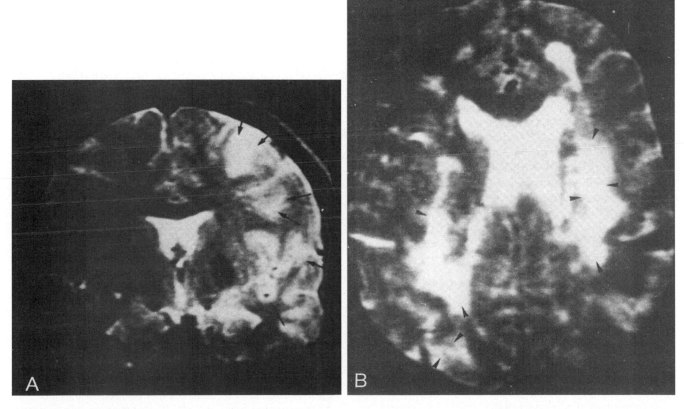

Figure 57.121. Neuroimaging in systemic lupus erythematosus (SLE). *A*, T2-weighted MR image, coronal view, in a 17-year-old woman with SLE, generalized seizures, ataxia, headache, and an organic brain syndrome. The scan shows several large, high-intensity lesions in the left cerebral cortex (*arrows*). The left side of the brain is brighter than the right because of a positioning artifact that resulted from a seizure during imaging. *B*, T2-weighted MR image, axial view, in a 56-year-old man with SLE, generalized seizures, headache, and an organic brain syndrome. Cortical and deep white matter lesions (*arrowheads*) are seen on both sides of the brain. (From Sibbitt WL Jr, Sibbitt RR, Griffey RH, et al. Magnetic resonance and computed tomographic imaging in the evaluation of acute neuropsychiatric disease in systemic lupus erythematosus. Ann Rheum Dis *48:*1014–1022, 1989.)

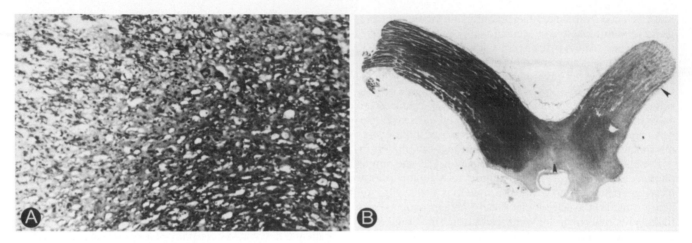

Figure 57.122. Devic's disease in systemic lupus erythematosus (SLE). The patient was a 21-year-old woman who was thought to have multiple sclerosis. Subsequent evaluations revealed evidence of SLE. During the course of her illness, the patient experienced a severe myelopathy and loss of vision in both eyes. She died of respiratory failure 4 years after the onset of paraparesis. *A,* Section through the cervical spinal cord shows rarefaction of white matter with dilation and vacuolation of nerve fibers. *B,* Section through the optic chiasm and the intracranial portions of the optic nerves shows severe atrophy and demyelination of the right optic nerve and part of the chiasm (*arrowheads*). (From April RS, Vansonnenberg E. A case of neuromyelitis optica (Devic's syndrome) in systemic lupus erythematosus: Clinicopathologic report and review of the literature. Neurology 26:1066–1070, 1976.)

sudden lower extremity weakness, sensory loss, or both, associated with loss of rectal and urinary bladder sphincter control. Some patients become quadriplegic. The onset of the myelitis usually occurs at the same time as other clinical evidence of active SLE. The syndrome is thought to be caused by arteritis that produces ischemic necrosis of the spinal cord (Schur, 1993, 1996); however, in some cases, an acute transverse myelitis is associated with bilateral optic neuritis (Devic's syndrome, neuromyelitis optica) (April and Vansonnenberg, 1976; Kinney et al., 1979), and in such cases, the major pathologic finding is demyelination in both the spinal cord and the optic nerves (Fig. 57.122). The mortality rate in patients with SLE-related transverse myelitis is high, and full recovery is rare for those who survive.

Although transverse myelitis is by far the most common form of myelopathy that occurs in patients with SLE, Liu et al. (1990) described a patient in whom a **Brown-Séquard syndrome** was the initial manifestation of the disease. The patient was a previously healthy 56-year-old man who developed over 3 weeks a warm feeling in the left foot spreading to the left buttock, numbness over the left arm and body below the clavicle, and weakness of the right arm and leg. Examination revealed a right hemiparesis that included the trapezius but spared the facial muscles and the sternocleidomastoid, diminished temperature and pain sensation on the left below C4, decreased vibration sensation bilaterally, increased deep-tendon reflexes on the right, and equivocal plantar responses. MR imaging and myelography showed enlargement of the cervical spinal cord. The patient was treated with systemic corticosteroids with rapid improvement in strength that was steroid-sensitive. Three months later, the patient was found to have laboratory evidence of SLE. It was thought by Liu et al. (1990) that the Brown-Séquard syndrome in this patient was caused by occlusion

of one or more sulcal arteries supplying the anterolateral spinal cord.

OCULAR MANIFESTATIONS

The **skin of the eyelids** may be affected by SLE (Fig. 57.111). In most cases, discoid lesions are located at the margins of the eyelids (Huey et al., 1983; Frith et al., 1990).

The eyes of patients with SLE are often dry from secondary **Sjögren's syndrome** (Steinberg and Talal, 1971). This condition, which develops in about 20% of patients with SLE, is indistinguishable from the dry eye syndrome that occurs in other patients with connective tissue disease (Hochberg et al., 1985).

Both **episcleritis** and **scleritis** occur in patients with SLE (Watson and Hayreh, 1976; Watson and Hazelman, 1976; Doherty et al., 1985; Turgeon and Slamovits, 1989; Frith et al., 1990). Some of the patients have idiopathic SLE, whereas others have SLE that has been induced by various medications (see Table 1 in Turgeon and Slamovits, 1989, and Table 240-6 in Schur, 1996).

Retinal vascular manifestations are the most common form of ocular involvement in patients with SLE (Jabs, 1994). In some patients, these abnormalities are minimal, consisting only of single or multiple microaneurysms and dilated retinal capillaries that can be detected only using fluorescein angiography (Santos et al., 1975). Patients with such defects usually are visually asymptomatic. The most common retinal vascular lesions observed in patients with SLE are cotton-wool spots (soft exudates), with and without intraretinal hemorrhages (Maumenee, 1940) (Fig. 57.123). The prevalence of cotton-wool spots in patients with SLE varies considerably depending on the population studied, the number of observations performed, and the experience of the observers. Gold et al. (1972) reported seeing cotton-wool spots in only 3% of outpatients with SLE, whereas Shearn and Pirofsky (1952) and Lanham et al. (1982a) observed these lesions in almost 30% of hospitalized patients. Cotton-wool spots that occur in patients with SLE do so independently of systemic hypertension. Instead, they correlate with disease activity (Klinkhoff et al., 1986) and are thought to be caused by the underlying microangiopathy of the disease. Pathologic studies demonstrate immune complexes, primarily immunoglobulin and complement, in the walls of the retinal vessels (Graham et al., 1985; Karpik et al., 1985).

Severe retinal vaso-occlusive disease occurs in some patients with SLE. Unilateral and bilateral central retinal artery occlusion, branch artery occlusion, central retinal vein occlusion, and diffuse retinal vaso-occlusive disease all are potential causes of visual loss (Goldstein and Wexler, 1932; Bishko, 1972; Gold et al., 1972; Appen et al., 1975; Coppeto and Lessell, 1977; Gold et al., 1977; Silverman et al., 1978; Kayazawa and Honda, 1981; Wong et al., 1981; Dougal et al., 1983; Hall et al., 1984; Laroche and Saraux, 1984; Vine

and Barr, 1984; Graham et al., 1985; Jabs et al., 1986a; Kameda et al., 1988; Asherson et al., 1989a, 1989b; Graham et al., 1989; Rubin and De Horatius, 1989; Kojima et al., 1990; Matsushima et al., 1997) (Fig. 57.124). In some cases, the retinopathy is the first manifestation of the disease (Wong et al., 1981). Asherson et al. (1989a) suggested that patients with SLE and increased concentrations of anticardiolipin antibody, have a higher risk of developing occlusive ocular vascular disease than do other patients with SLE.

Less common than retinopathy in patients with SLE is **choroidopathy.** Affected eyes show serous elevation of the sensory retina, elevation of the retinal pigment epithelium, or both (Gass, 1968b; Coppeto and Lessell, 1977; Diddie et al., 1977; Bankhurst et al., 1984; Kinyoun and Kalina, 1986; Klinkhoff et al., 1986; Jabs et al., 1988) (Fig. 57.125). Graham et al. (1985) reported the autopsy findings in a 16-year-old boy with acute SLE, chorea, and bilateral retinopathy. Many retinal and meningeal vessels were occluded by amorphous hyaline material without evidence of vasculitis. In

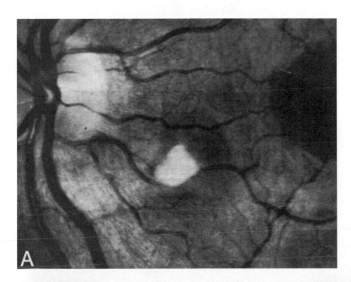

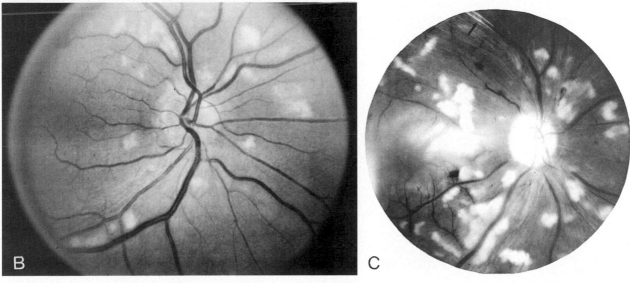

Figure 57.123. Retinopathy in systemic lupus erythematosus (SLE). *A,* Single cotton-wool spot in a woman with SLE. (From Ferry AP. The eye and rheumatic diseases. In Textbook of Rheumatology. Editors, Kelley WN, Harris ED Jr, Ruddy S, et al. 3rd ed, pp 579–596. Philadelphia, WB Saunders, 1989.) *B,* Multiple cotton-wool spots without hemorrhage in a patient with SLE. *C,* Multiple cotton-wool spots, intraretinal hemorrhages, arterial occlusion, and vascular sheathing (*arrow*) in another patient with SLE. (*B* and *C,* from Jabs DA, Fine SL, Hochberg MC, et al. Severe retinal vaso-occlusive disease in systemic lupus erythematosus. Arch Ophthalmol *104:*558–563, 1986.)

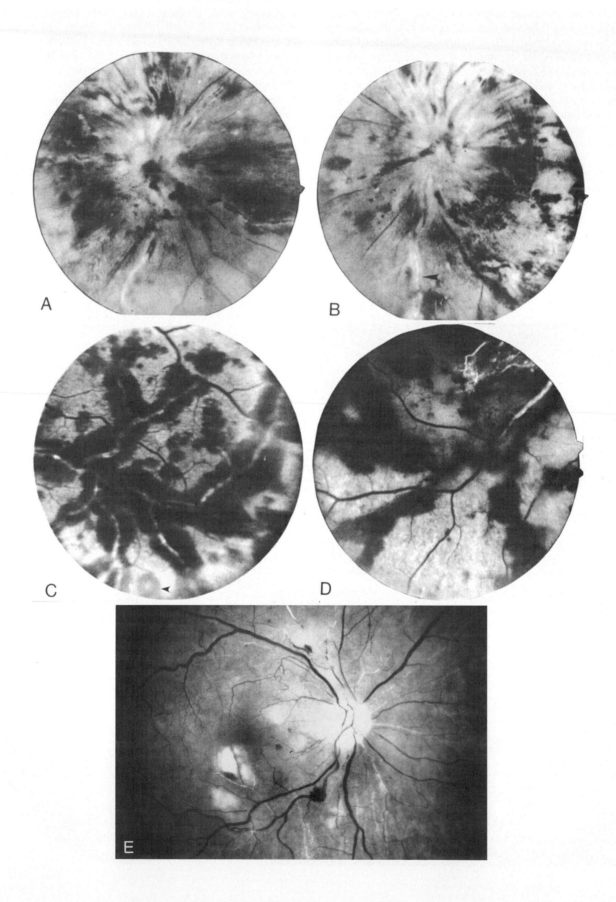

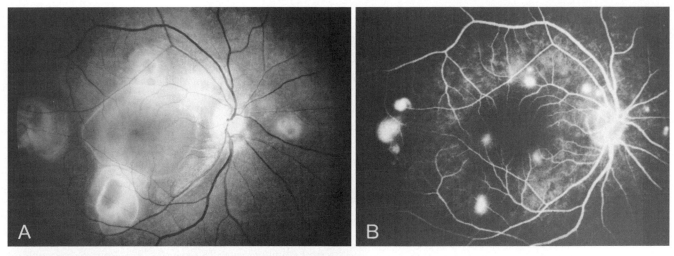

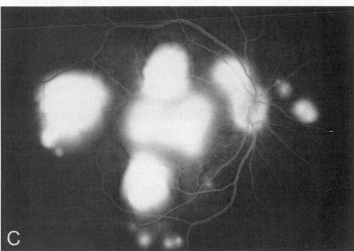

Figure 57.125. Choroidopathy in systemic lupus erythematosus (SLE). The patient was a 48-year-old woman with SLE who had systemic hypertension, nephritis, and Raynaud's phenomenon. Visual acuity was 20/200 OD and 20/25 OS. *A,* The right ocular fundus shows multiple serous elevations of the sensory retina, some of which are associated with small underlying detachments of the retinal pigment epithelium. *B,* Fluorescein angiogram, arteriovenous phase, shows multiple areas of slow accumulation of fluorescein in the subretinal fluid. *C,* Fluorescein angiogram, late phase, shows continued accumulation of fluorescein in the subretinal fluid. (From Jabs DA, Hanneken AM, Schachat AP, et al. Choroidopathy in systemic lupus erythematosus. Arch Ophthalmol *106:*230–234, 1988.)

addition, although the patient had no clinical evidence of choroidopathy, some choroidal vessels showed evidence of vasculitis with fibrinoid necrosis (Fig. 57.126).

ORBITAL MANIFESTATIONS

Bilateral periorbital edema without other orbital signs may be a manifestation of SLE (Norden et al., 1993). Proptosis also may develop in patients with SLE. The proptosis may be unilateral or bilateral (Grimson and Simons, 1983; Bankhurst et al., 1984) (Fig. 57.127). It is often associated with orbital pain, ophthalmoparesis, and signs of inflammation in the orbit or cavernous sinus (Brenner and Shock, 1974; Wilkinson and Panush, 1975; Evans and Lexow, 1978), although in some patients, unilateral proptosis occurs as an isolated phenomenon (Burkhalter, 1973).

Figure 57.124. Severe vaso-occlusive retinopathy in systemic lupus erythematosus (SLE). *A–D,* In a 32-year-old woman with SLE who lost vision abruptly in both eyes. When she initially was evaluated, visual acuity was hand motions at 1/3 meter in the right eye. The left eye could not perceive light. *A,* Appearance of right ocular fundus. The optic disc is markedly swollen, and there are numerous peripapillary intraretinal hemorrhages and soft exudates. Note extensive sheathing of retinal vessels. *B,* Appearance of left ocular fundus. The optic disc is markedly swollen, and there are numerous intraretinal hemorrhages and cotton-wool spots. Vascular sheathing is present (*arrowhead*), but it is not as prominent as in the right eye. *C,* A retinal vein and its branches show extensive sheathing. Note the surrounding cuff of hemorrhage that accompanies the vein and its tributaries. Also note other dot and blot hemorrhages, some of which have white centers (*arrowhead*). *D,* Fluorescein angiogram of right ocular fundus at 30 seconds shows slow filling of retinal arterioles, irregular vessel lumens, lack of venous filling, and persistence of fluorescence in retina and choroid. (From Coppeto J, Lessell S. Retinopathy in systemic lupus erythematosus. Arch Ophthalmol *95:*794–797, 1977.) *E,* The right ocular fundus from another patient with SLE shows cotton-wool spots, intraretinal hemorrhage, and multiple occluded retinal arteries. (From Jabs DA, Fine SL, Hochberg MC, et al. Severe retinal vaso-occlusive disease in systemic lupus erythematosus. Arch Ophthalmol *104:*558–563, 1986.)

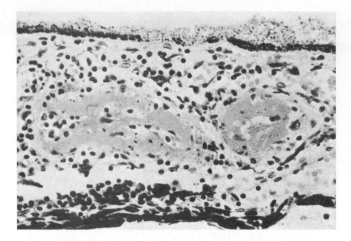

Figure 57.126. Pathology of the choroid in a patient with systemic lupus erythematosus and retinopathy. The patient had no clinical evidence of choroidopathy. Section through the choroid shows arterioles whose walls have become thickened and whose lumens have become occluded by vasculitis and fibrinoid necrosis. Note moderate inflammatory infiltrate throughout the choroid. (From Graham EM, Spalton DJ, Barnard RO, et al. Cerebral and retinal vascular changes in systemic lupus erythematosus. Ophthalmology *92*:444–448, 1985.)

Neuroimaging studies of the orbit performed in patients with SLE who have unilateral or bilateral proptosis often reveal enlargement of one or more extraocular muscles consistent with myositis (Grimson and Simons, 1983). In many cases, however, no specific abnormalities are seen, and it is assumed that a diffuse inflammatory process is present in the orbit.

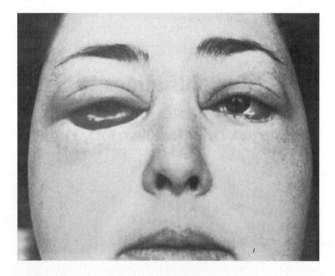

Figure 57.127. Proptosis in systemic lupus erythematosus (SLE). Note bilateral proptosis, chemosis, and injection of the conjunctiva in a 31-year-old woman with SLE. The condition improved after a course of plasmapheresis. (From Bankhurst AD, Carlow TJ, Reidy RW. Exophthalmos in systemic lupus erythematosus. Ann Ophthalmol *16*:669–671, 1984.)

NEURO-OPHTHALMOLOGIC MANIFESTATIONS

SLE may damage the visual sensory system from the optic nerve to the occipital lobe and the ocular motor system from the cerebral cortex to the extraocular muscles. As noted above, the ocular motor nerves may be individually damaged from lupus microangiopathy. We and others have examined patients with SLE who have one or more **ocular motor nerve pareses,** including complete and incomplete oculomotor nerve paresis (both pupil-sparing and pupil-affected), trochlear nerve paresis, and abducens nerve paresis (Johnson and Richardson, 1968; Lessell, 1979). In some patients, an isolated ocular motor nerve paresis is the initial manifestation of the disease (Sedwick and Burde, 1983; Rosenstein et al., 1989). Ocular motor nerve pareses may occur as isolated phenomena or associated with other cranial neuropathies, most often facial nerve paresis or trigeminal sensory neuropathy (Lundberg and Werner, 1972). Other components of the ocular motor system may be affected in SLE. Damage to ocular motor pathways within the brainstem may produce a variety of disturbances of vertical and horizontal gaze, including a unilateral or bilateral INO, skew deviation, and one-and-a-half syndrome (Fig. 57.128) (Cogan et al., 1950; Bailey et al., 1956; Meyer and Wild, 1975; Lessell, 1979; Jackson et al., 1986; Cogen et al., 1987; Yigit et al., 1996). Keane (1995) reviewed his inpatient experience with 33 SLE patients who had eye movement abnormalities and found that 48% of them had evidence of a brainstem infarction to account for their ocular motility impairment. Other causes included both infectious and aseptic meningitis, pseudotumor cerebri, ocular myositis, hypoxic encephalopathy, and the Guillain-Barré syndrome.

In patients with SLE, **ptosis** may be a manifestation of an oculomotor nerve palsy, a Horner's syndrome, the Guillain-Barré syndrome, orbital inflammation, or even coexisting myasthenia gravis. In some patients, the cause of the ptosis is difficult if not impossible to elucidate (Lanham et al., 1982b; Keane, 1995).

Nystagmus may occur in patients with SLE from damage to central or peripheral vestibular pathways. Vestibular nystagmus may be an isolated finding, but it is usually associated with other evidence of brainstem dysfunction, including diplopia. In one SLE patient, continuous **ocular flutter** led to the discovery of a hyperosmolar state (Keane, 1995).

Isolated **pupillary disturbances** are uncommon in patients with SLE. Most are relative afferent defects associated with an underlying optic neuropathy (see below). Although a dilated pupil may occur as part of an SLE-related oculomotor nerve paresis, but in our experience most such pareses spare the pupil. Lessell (1979) described a patient with SLE in whom Horner's syndrome occurred as part of a brainstem syndrome, and we have observed patients in whom disturbances of pupillary size and function developed in association with severe brainstem dysfunction in the terminal stages of the disease.

About 1–2% of patients with SLE develop an **optic neuropathy** at some point during the course of the disease (Hollenhorst and Henderson, 1951; Estes and Christian, 1971; Feinglass et al., 1976; Hochberg et al., 1985). The optic

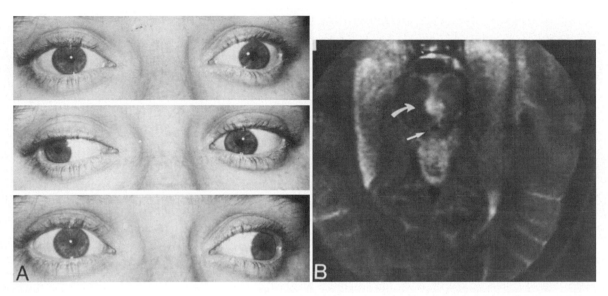

Figure 57.128. Internuclear ophthalmoplegia (INO) in systemic lupus erythematosus (SLE). The patient was a 23-year-old woman with SLE who developed headaches and diplopia. *A*, The patient has a bilateral INO. *B*, Unenhanced, T2-weighted MR image, axial view, shows increased intensity in the center of the mesencephalon in the region of the medial longitudinal fasciculi (*curved arrow*). The cerebral aqueduct appears as a low signal area (*straight arrow*). (From Cogen MS, Kline LB, Duvall ER. Bilateral internuclear ophthalmoplegia in systemic lupus erythematosus. J Clin Neuroophthalmol 7:69–73, 1987.)

neuropathy has extremely variable clinical features (see Table 2 in Jabs et al., 1986b). In some cases, it mimics an acute optic neuritis, in that there is sudden loss of central vision, an ipsilateral RAPD, and either a swollen or a normal optic disc (Vitale et al., 1973; Hackett et al., 1974; Shepherd et al., 1974; Cinefro and Frenkel, 1978; Contamin et al., 1978; Allen et al., 1979; Lessell, 1979; Dutton et al., 1982; Saraux et al., 1982b; Smith and Pinals, 1982; Stoudemire et al., 1982; Jabs et al., 1986b; Deutsch and Corwin, 1988) (Fig. 57.129). In such cases, there may be pain on movement of the affected eye (Oppenheimer and Hoffbrand, 1986). The visual loss may be unilateral or bilateral (Ninomiya et al., 1990; Ahmadieh et al., 1994), and it may be associated with a transverse myelitis (April and Vansonnenberg, 1976; Kinney et al., 1979; Jabs et al., 1986b) (Fig. 57.122). Patients with acute, unilateral visual loss and a normal optic disc in the affected eye may be misdiagnosed as having nonorganic visual loss if the RAPD is not appreciated by the examiner (Stoudemire et al., 1982). In other cases, the optic neuropathy is characterized by acute, painless loss of vision associated with an altitudinal visual field defect, an RAPD, and either a swollen or a normal optic disc (Henkind and Gold, 1973; Lessell, 1979; Hayreh, 1981) (Fig. 57.130). This presentation is more suggestive of an ischemic process. In still other cases, there is slowly progressive unilateral or bilateral visual loss, initially suggesting a compressive or toxic optic neuropathy (Jabs et al., 1986b). Some patients have no clinical evidence of optic neuropathy but have an abnormal visual-evoked response consisting of an increased latency in one or both eyes, indicating a subclinical optic neuropathy (Billingsley et al., 1985). MR imaging in some patients with SLE-associated optic neuropathy reveals enlargement and enhancement of the affected optic nerve. In others, the af-

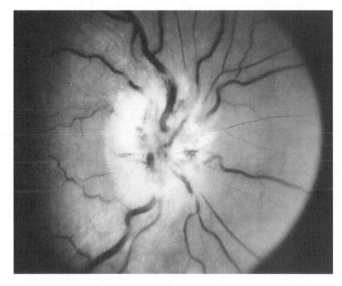

Figure 57.129. Acute anterior optic neuropathy suggesting optic neuritis in systemic lupus erythematosus. The patient was a 32-year-old woman with a history of Raynaud's phenomenon who experienced acute loss of vision in the right eye associated with pain behind the eye. The pain was exacerbated somewhat by eye movement. Visual acuity was 20/200 OD and 20/15 OS. Color vision was diminished in the right eye, and there was a right afferent pupillary defect. The visual field in the right eye showed a dense central/arcuate defect. The left eye had normal visual function, and the left ocular fundus was normal. The right optic disc is markedly swollen, and there are associated hemorrhages and soft exudates (cotton-wool spots) present. The patient was thought to have optic neuritis; however, serologic testing showed an elevated erythrocyte sedimentation rate, elevated titers of antinuclear antibody, and LE cells. The patient was placed on systemic corticosteroids with return of visual function to near normal.

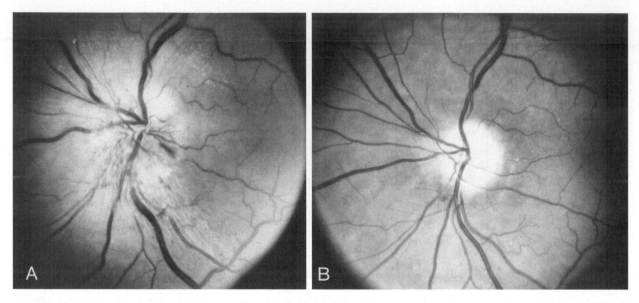

Figure 57.130.   Acute anterior optic neuropathy suggesting ischemic optic neuropathy in systemic lupus erythematosus (SLE). The patient was a 23-year-old woman with known SLE who experienced acute, painless loss of vision in the left eye during an exacerbation of her illness. Visual acuity was 20/20 OD and 20/100 OS. There was reduced color perception in the left eye, a left relative afferent pupillary defect, and loss of the inferior field of vision in the left eye. *A*, The left optic disc is hyperemic and swollen. Note several small flame-shaped hemorrhages on and adjacent to the optic disc. The patient was treated with increased doses of systemic corticosteroids without improvement in vision. *B*, 1 month after visual loss, the left optic disc is pale, the nerve fiber layer is diminished, and the retinal arteries are narrowed, especially superiorly. The patient had a persistent inferior visual field defect in the left eye.

fected nerve appears normal in size and shape but enhances after intravenous injection of gadolinium-DTPA or a similar paramagnetic contrast agent (Sklar et al., 1996).

The pathogenesis of the optic neuropathy that occurs in SLE is variable, and this explains the variable clinical presentation. In some cases, the condition results from microangiopathic disease within the optic nerve, whereas in others, there is evidence of demyelination (Hackett et al., 1974; Shepherd et al., 1974; April and Vonsonnenberg, 1976; Kinney et al., 1979) (Fig. 57.122). Some patients with SLE who develop optic neuropathy have normal serology when loss of vision develops (Dutton et al., 1982; Deutsch and Corwin, 1988). It is impossible to determine if the optic neuropathy that occurs in such patients is related to the underlying systemic disease or is an independent entity. Other patients develop unilateral or bilateral optic neuropathy without clinical evidence of SLE but with laboratory evidence that suggests an underlying connective tissue disorder (Kupersmith et al., 1988). An assay for ANAs is the most consistently abnormal blood study in such patients.

The **optic chiasm** is only rarely affected in patients with SLE (Lessell, 1979). It is probably affected more often in patients with neuromyelitis optica in the setting of SLE (April and Vansonnenberg, 1976). We examined a 35-year-old woman with clinical and laboratory evidence of SLE who noted the abrupt onset of bitemporal field loss. Examination revealed visual acuity of 20/20 OD and 20/30 OS. Color vision was normal bilaterally. Visual fields showed relative bitemporal field defects. Ophthalmoscopy showed a single cotton-wool spot in the retina of the right eye and

several spots associated with intraretinal hemorrhage in the left eye. Both optic discs appeared normal. An ESR was 67, and there was a positive ANA of 1:512. A CT scan showed a low-density lesion consistent with a silent infarction in the right frontal lobe. MR imaging showed no other lesions. Lumbar puncture gave normal results. The patient was treated with systemic corticosteroids for 2 months, over which time her visual field defects improved but did not completely disappear. Over this period, the patient's ESR returned to normal, and her ANA titer decreased to 1:80. It was thought that the patient had experienced an ischemic chiasmal syndrome caused by the microangiopathy of SLE.

Visual sensory difficulties in patients with SLE may originate from damage to the **retrochiasmal** portion of the visual sensory pathway. Some patients experience transient homonymous field defects identical with those experienced by patients with migraine (Atkinson and Appenzeller, 1975; Brandt and Lessell, 1978; Lessell, 1979; Isenberg et al., 1982; Honda, 1985, 1987). Such defects are scintillating and progressive, usually beginning on one side of the visual field and slowly expanding toward the center. Some of these patients may have two separate disorders, SLE and migraine, but in others, SLE is undoubtedly the cause of the transient visual disturbance.

Some patients with SLE develop permanent, homonymous visual field defects. Brandt et al. (1975) reported 12 patients with SLE who had permanent retrochiasmal visual disturbances, including homonymous hemianopic scotomas, complete or incomplete homonymous hemianopias, and cortical blindness. These authors emphasized that such disturbances may be the most prominent and disabling feature of the disorder. They may develop slowly and insidiously or occur suddenly. Trevor et al. (1972) reported a 32-year-old woman with SLE who developed a right homonymous hemianopia, a right hemiparesis, and aphasia over several days. Angiography showed occlusion of the supraclinoid segment of the left internal carotid artery. Traboulsi et al. (1985) described a 23-year-old woman with SLE who developed an acute, complete, right homonymous hemianopia with macular splitting (Fig. 57.131*A*). A CT scan showed changes consistent with a recent infarct of the left calcarine cortex (Fig. 57.131*B*). Rubin and De Horatius (1989) reported a 24-year-old woman who suddenly lost vision in both eyes and was found to have bilateral occipital lobe infarctions. The patient was subsequently discovered to have SLE. Patients with homonymous visual field defects or cortical blindness may have signs or symptoms of brainstem dysfunction if the affected artery is the vertebrobasilar territory.

Patients with SLE may experience **visual hallucinations** that may be formed or unformed (Lessell, 1979). Eight of the 12 patients in the series reported by Brandt et al. (1975) had visual hallucinations that were unaccompanied by auditory, tactile, or olfactory sensations. Formed hallucinations and visual allesthesia were associated with temporal lobe seizures in one patient. None of the patients was psychotic, nor were any of them using hallucinogenic drugs at the time. Two of the patients were confused and disoriented at the time they experienced single episodes of transient, unformed visual hallucinations.

Some patients with SLE develop increased ICP, and **pap-illedema** may occur in such patients (Lessell, 1979). There are many causes for increased ICP in patients with SLE, including sterile or infectious meningitis, meningoencephalitis, intraparenchymal or subarachnoid hemorrhage, elevated protein in the CSF, and cerebral edema associated with massive infarction (Lessell, 1979). In some patients, there is no obvious explanation for the increased ICP. Such patients have small or normal-sized ventricles by neuroimaging studies, and CSF that contains no cells and has a normal concentration of both protein and glucose. The clinical picture thus is that of **pseudotumor cerebri** (Bettman et al., 1968; Abramsky et al., 1972; Carlow, 1973; Silberberg and Laties, 1973; Carlow and Glaser, 1974; Li and Ho, 1989). In at least some of these cases, this syndrome is caused by obstruction of the superior sagittal or lateral sinus (Gibson and Myers, 1976; Kaplan et al., 1985; Shiozawa et al., 1986). This is one of the few settings in which pseudotumor cerebri may respond dramatically to treatment with systemic corticosteroids.

Associations

Some patients with SLE, who also have features of other connective tissue diseases, are said to have a **mixed connective tissue disease** (MCTD) (Bennett, 1989). In addition, patients with SLE may develop other autoimmune diseases, suggesting that a common or related immunologic disturbance may have triggered both disorders. Autoimmune disorders reported in patients with SLE include rheumatoid arthritis, myasthenia gravis, the Lambert-Eaton myasthenic

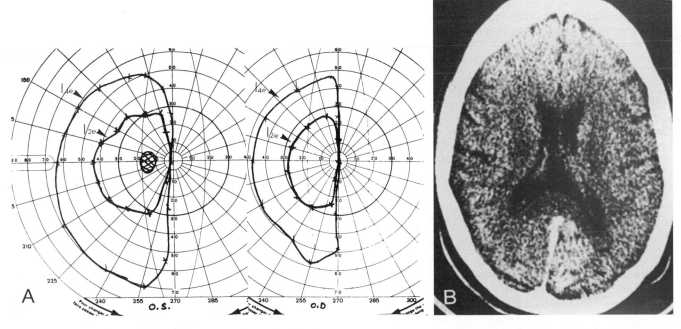

Figure 57.131. Homonymous hemianopia in systemic lupus erythematosus (SLE). The patient was a 23-year-old woman with known SLE who experienced acute loss of the right homonymous visual field. *A,* There is a complete, right, homonymous hemianopia with splitting of the macula. *B,* Enhanced CT scan, axial view, shows an area of increased density in the left occipital lobe consistent with a hemorrhagic infarction (*arrowheads*). (From Traboulsi EI, Mansour AM, Aswad MI, et al. Homonymous hemianopia and systemic lupus erythematosus. J Clin Neurophthalmol *5:*63–66, 1985.)

syndrome, and multiple sclerosis (MS) (Harvey et al., 1954; Rowland, 1955; Simpson, 1960; Denney and Rose, 1961; White and Marshall, 1962; Galbraith et al., 1964; Mäkelä et al., 1964; Piemme, 1964; Kissel et al., 1966; Wolff and Barrows, 1966; Branch and Swift, 1978; Lessell, 1979; Hughes and Katirji, 1986).

Drug-Induced Lupus

It is uncertain if medications can exacerbate preexisting SLE, but a variety of medications can produce a clinical and immunologic syndrome quite similar to idiopathic or spontaneous SLE (Weinstein, 1983, 1987; see Table 240-6 in Schur, 1996). The data are strongest for hydralazine and procainamide, both of which have been the subject of large prospective studies.

Drug-induced lupus usually begins a few months after the medication is begun. The symptoms are quite similar to those of idiopathic SLE, but there are some significant differences (see Table 240-7 in Schur, 1996). First, drug-induced lupus is reversible; when the drug is stopped, the symptoms gradually resolve. Second, the symptoms tend to be mild, with constitutional, joint, and pleuropericardial symptoms predominating. Renal and CNS disease, leukopenia, and anemia are uncommon. Third, the sex ratio is about equal in patients with drug-induced lupus. Finally, drug-induced lupus seems to occur rarely in African-Americans (Hess, 1987).

Pathogenesis

It is unclear why investigators have been unable to identify the cause of SLE. Although insufficient technology is one possibility, there are several others (Woods and Zvaifler, 1989). First, SLE may not be a single disease but rather a constellation of symptoms and signs produced by a variety of etiologic agents. Second, SLE may require the interaction of several factors to produce it (e.g., contact with a specific pathogen in a genetically predisposed host). Finally, SLE may simply be the clinical manifestation of a common pathogenetic mechanism that can be initiated by a variety of factors. Viral, genetic, and hormonal etiologies have all been proposed, but perhaps no single factor can independently produce the disease.

Although the cause of SLE is unknown, it is clear that much of the tissue damage, especially in the blood vessels and kidney, is caused by the deposition of antigen-antibody complexes (Zvaifler and Bluestein, 1982) (Figs. 57.118 and 57.132). Indeed, SLE is generally considered to be the prototype human immune complex disease. It is characterized by B-cell hyperreactivity, polyclonal B-cell activation, hypergammaglobulinemia, and multiple autoantibodies (Petz et al., 1971; Eisenberg et al., 1985; Rubin et al., 1986; Antes et al., 1988; Winkler et al., 1988; Uwatoko and Mannik, 1989). The autoantibodies found in the serum of patients with SLE include ANAs, antibodies to both single-stranded and double-stranded DNA, and antibodies to cytoplasmic components. The interaction of antigen with antibodies in the circulation causes the formation of soluble macromolecular complexes that can induce both acute and chronic inflammation (see above). The neuropsychiatric manifestations of SLE may be produced by multifocal cerebral infarcts or result from autoantibody-induced neuronal cell destruc-

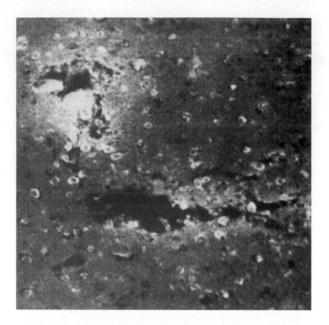

Figure 57.132. Immunofluorescent staining of cerebral cortex of a young woman who died with active systemic lupus erythematosus-related organic brain syndrome. This photomicrograph of anti-IgM immunofluorescence shows a ring pattern of staining of the neuronal cells clustered around a cerebral blood vessel. IgG staining (not shown) showed a similar ring pattern on cells throughout the field. (From Zvaifler NJ, Bluestein HG. The pathogenesis of central nervous system manifestations of systemic lupus erythematosus. Arthritis Rheum *25:*862–866, 1982.)

tion. In a small study of brain pathology in SLE, multifocal cerebral microinfarction was the predominant histopathologic change (Hanly et al., 1992).

Diagnosis

As noted above, the American Rheumatism Association developed a classification system for SLE in 1975 (Cohen et al., 1975), revised in 1982 (Tan et al., 1982), which includes 11 criteria: malar rash, discoid rash, photosensitivity, oral ulcers, arthritis, serositis, renal dysfunction, neurologic dysfunction, hematologic dysfunction, immunologic dysfunction, and presence of ANAs. The sensitivity and specificity of these criteria to diagnose SLE are about 96% when the disease is diagnosed by the presence of four or more criteria (Schur, 1996) (Table 57.1).

An assay for ANAs is the best screening test for SLE because it is positive in almost all patients with the disease (Schur, 1996). If the ANA assay is negative, the patient has a less than 0.14% probability of having SLE, whereas a positive ANA assay has a 35% positive predictive value (Griner et al., 1981). It must be remembered, however, that the ANA test is positive in 68% of patients with primary Sjögren's syndrome, in 40–75% of patients with scleroderma, in 16% of patients with juvenile rheumatoid arthritis, and in 25–50% of patients with the adult form of rheumatoid arthritis (Schur, 1993). Unfortunately, no gold standard exists for the diagnosis of CNS SLE. Based on a 10-year prospective study of SLE patients with neuropsychiatric disease, West et al. (1995) devised a battery of tests useful in the diagnosis of focal and diffuse CNS SLE. The three tests

Table 57.1.
Criteria for Classification of Systemic Lupus Erythematosus

Criterion	Definition
1. Malar rash	Fixed erythema, flat or raised, over the malar eminences, tending to spare the nasolabial folds.
2. Discoid rash	Erythematous raised patches with adherent keratotic scaling and follicular plugging; atrophic scarring may occur in older lesions.
3. Photosensitivity	Skin rash as a result of unusual reaction to sunlight, by patient history or physician observation.
4. Oral Ulcers	Oral or nasopharyngeal ulceration, usually painless, observed by a physician.
5. Arthritis	Nonerosive arthritis involving two or more peripheral joints, characterized by tenderness, swelling, or effusion.
6. Serositis	a. Pleuritis–Convicing history of pleuritic pain or rub heard by a physician or evidence of pleural effusion.
	OR
	b. Pericarditis–Documented by electrocardiogram or rub or evidence of pericardial effusion.
7. Renal disorder	a. Persistent proteinuria >0.5 g/day or >3+ if quantitiation not performed.
	OR
	b. Cellular casts–may be red cell, hemoglobin, granular, tubular, or mixed.
8. Neurologic disorder	a. Seizures–in the absence of offending drugs or known metabolic derangements, e.g., uremia, ketoacidosis, or electrolyte imbalance.
	OR
	b. Psychosis–in the absence of offending drugs or known metabolic derangements, e.g., uremis, ketoacidosis, or electrolyte imbalance.
9. Hematologic disorder	a. Hemolytic anemia, with reticulocytosis
	OR
	b. Leukopenia–<4000/mm^3 total on two or more occasions.
	OR
	c. Lymphopenia–<1500/mm^3 on two or more occasions.
	OR
	d. Thrombocytopenia–<100,000/mm^3 in the absense of offending drugs.
10. Immunologic disorder	a. Positive LE cell preparation
	OR
	b. Anti-DNA–antibody to native DNA in abnormal titer
	OR
	c. Anti-SM–presence of antibody to Sm nuclear antigen.
	OR
	d. False-positive serologic text for syphilis known to be positive for at least 6 months and confirmed by *Trepinema pallidum* immobilization or fluorescent treponemal antibody absorption test.
11. Antinuclear	An abnormal titer of antinuclear antibody by immunofluorescence or an equivalent assay at any point in time and in the absence of drugs known to be associated with "drug-induced lupus" syndrome.

(From Schur PH. Systemic lupus erythematosus. In Cecil Textbook of Medicine. Editors, Bennett JC, Plum F, 20th ed, pp 1475–1483. Philadelphia, WB Saunders, 1996.)

most useful in the diagnosis of diffuse CNS disease were: (*a*) elevated CSF immunoglobulin index and oligoclonal bands; (*b*) CSF antineuronal antibodies; and (*c*) serum antiribosomal antibodies. One of these tests was abnormal in every patient with diffuse CNS SLE, yielding a sensitivity of 100%, a specificity of 86%, and a positive predictive value of 95%. Serum antiribosomal antibodies were particularly likely to be present in patients with psychiatric manifestations. Patients with focal CNS manifestations of SLE usually had: (*a*) peripheral vasculitis or livedo reticularis, (*b*) antiphospholipid antibodies, and (*c*) an abnormal brain MR image showing changes consistent with focal lesions in the white matter. One abnormal finding yielded a sensitivity of 95%, a specificity of 86%, and a positive predictive value of 90% for the diagnosis of focal CNS SLE. Antibodies to the Sm antigen are highly specific for SLE and are particularly common in patients with CNS involvement (Lahita, 1997). Unfortunately, these antibodies are present in only 35% of all patients with SLE.

Frith et al. (1990) evaluated 18 patients with SLE and found a high incidence of deposition of immunoreactants in a linear pattern at the basement membrane zone in apparently normal bulbar conjunctiva. These investigators hypothesized that direct immunofluorescence of a bulbar conjunctival biopsy specimen might be helpful in diagnosing a patient with suspected SLE.

Prognosis

Although CNS manifestations of SLE may be quite dramatic, most are self-limited and reversible. Patients do not have a poor prognosis unless they have associated multisystem disease activity (Sibley et al., 1992). Indeed, the overall 10-year survival rate for patients with SLE is about 90% (Abu-Shakra et al., 1995a). Nevertheless, despite improved survival rates, a cohort of SLE patients still die at rates three times those of the general population (Abu-Shakra et al., 1994b; Gladmann, 1995). Death may result from refractory vasculitis involving the CNS, gastrointestinal tract, kidneys, heart, or pulmonary tree. Fulminant bleeding may occur from thrombocytopenia or hemolytic anemia. Death may also be a complication of therapy, with infection remaining a prominent cause (Abu-Shakra et al., 1995b).

Treatment

SLE is a disease without a cure (Steinberg, 1989). Treatment thus is directed toward relief of symptoms, suppression of certain presymptomatic abnormalities, and prevention of future pathology. A number of medicines are capable of suppressing symptoms and signs of SLE, but almost all have side effects (Fig. 57.133). In general, nonsteroidal drugs are typically used as first-line therapy for the arthritic manifestations, whereas antimalarial drugs are effective for refractory joint symptoms. Immunosuppressive agents are reserved for patients with major organ involvement (Fox and McCune, 1994). For patients with suspected diffuse CNS SLE, pulsed intravenous methylprednisolone for 3 days followed by a prolonged course of oral corticosteroids and a slow taper is extremely helpful. Patients with focal CNS manifestations should be evaluated for a source of emboli and should undergo an assay for antiphospholipid antibodies, following

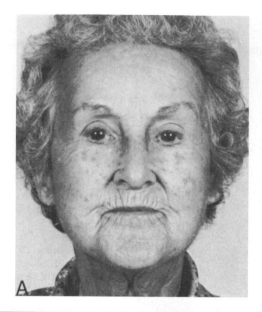

Figure 57.137.   Telangiectasia and calcinosis in scleroderma. *A*, The face of a woman with long-standing scleroderma shows multiple telangiectasias with exaggerated radial furrowing about the lips. (From Seibold JR. Scleroderma. In Textbook of Rheumatology. Editors, Kelley WN, Harris ED Jr, Ruddy S, et al. 3rd ed, pp 1215–1244. Philadelphia, WB Saunders, 1989.) *B*, Telangiectases and telangiectatic macules over the palms in a patient with scleroderma. (From Soter NA. The skin and rheumatic diseases. In Textbook of Rheumatology. Editors, Kelley WN, Harris ED Jr, Ruddy S, et al. 3rd ed, pp 597–610. Philadelphia, WB Saunders, 1989.) *C*, X-ray of the fingers of a patient with scleroderma shows resorption and dissolution of the phalangeal tufts and multiple areas of punctate subcutaneous calcinosis. (From Seibold JR. Scleroderma. In Textbook of Rheumatology. Editors, Kelley WN, Harris ED Jr, Ruddy S, et al. 3rd ed, pp 1215–1244. Philadelphia, WB Saunders, 1989.)

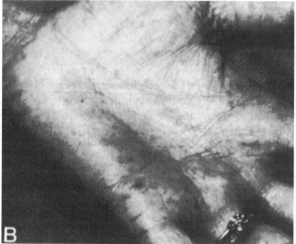

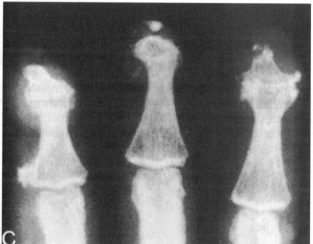

and calcinosis are common (Fig. 57.137). The disease usually begins peripherally, initially affecting the fingers and hands. It gradually spreads centripetally up the arms to affect the face and trunk.

About 95% of patients with scleroderma develop **Raynaud's phenomenon,** which is the initial complaint in about 70% of patients (Campbell and LeRoy, 1975; Rodnan et al., 1980). Raynaud's phenomenon is characterized initially by blanching of the nail beds, fingers, and toes with accompanying pain. The ears, nose, and tongue also may be affected. This phase, caused by vasospasm of small to medium-sized arteries, is induced by exposure to cold, cigarette smoke, stress, or a combination of these. As the vasospasm progresses, cyanosis develops, and the appearance of the affected skin changes to red and then to blue. During this period, there is local anoxia associated with an increase in the concentration of carbon dioxide at the site. When the concentration reaches a critical level, vasodilation occurs, producing severe pain and erythema. Persistent Raynaud's

phenomenon may cause gangrene or digital ulceration (Fig. 57.138). Raynaud's phenomenon occurs not only in patients with scleroderma, but also in patients with other types of connective tissue disease, and in patients who never develop any other evidence of connective tissue disease (Silman et al., 1990).

Scleroderma may damage almost every organ in the body. The esophagus may be affected, resulting in reduced or absent esophageal motility with gastroesophageal reflux (Seibold, 1993; LeRoy, 1996; Seibold, 1997) (Fig. 57.139). Damage to the upper and lower intestines may cause decreased motility, malabsorption, and diverticulosis. Cardiopulmonary disease is characterized primarily by pulmonary fibrosis that produces restrictive lung disease (Fig. 57.140). The consequences of this interstitial fibrosis include pulmonary hypertension and right-sided heart failure. In addition, fibrosis of cardiac muscle produces disturbances of conduction and arrhythmias. Musculoskeletal features of scleroderma include polyarthralgias, calcification, tendon friction

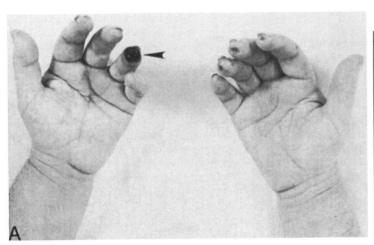

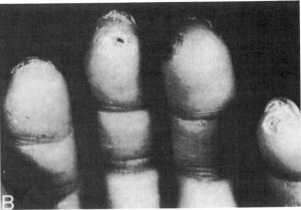

Figure 57.138. The consequences of persistent Raynaud's phenomenon. *A,* Multiple ischemic ulcerations of the tips of the digits with one digit showing sharply demarcated dry gangrene (*arrowhead*) in a patient with long-standing scleroderma. (From Seibold JR. Scleroderma. In Textbook of Rheumatology. Editors, Kelley WN, Harris ED Jr, Ruddy S, et al. 3rd ed, pp 1215–1244. Philadelphia, WB Saunders, 1989.) *B,* Ischemic ulcerations of the tips of the fingers in another patient with scleroderma and persistent Raynaud's phenomenon. (From Soter NA. The skin and rheumatic diseases. In Textbook of Rheumatology. Editors, Kelley WN, Harris ED Jr, Ruddy S, et al. 3rd ed, pp 597–610. Philadelphia, WB Saunders, 1989.)

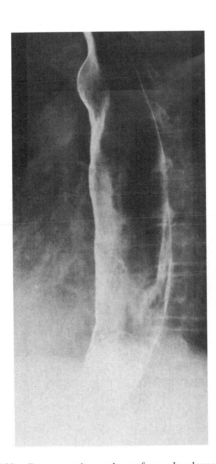

Figure 57.139. Damage to the esophagus from scleroderma. Barium esophagram in a patient with scleroderma shows dilation and aperistalsis of the distal esophagus and a patulous lower esophageal sphincter. (From Seibold JR. Scleroderma. In Textbook of Rheumatology. Editors, Kelley WN, Harris ED Jr, Ruddy S, et al. 3rd ed, pp 1215–1244. Philadelphia, WB Saunders, 1989.)

rubs, and myositis (Seibold, 1993, 1997) (Fig. 57.141). Renal failure, often associated with malignant hypertension, is a major cause of death in patients with scleroderma.

Scleroderma can be separated into several categories depending on the extent and severity of the disease. The **CREST syndrome** is named for its features of **c**alcinosis, **R**aynaud's phenomenon, **e**sophageal dysmotility, **s**clerodactyly, and **t**elangiectasia. This syndrome seems to have a slow, benign course compared with other forms of the disorder (McCarty et al., 1983; Seibold, 1993, 1997). **Diffuse systemic sclerosis** is the name given to the form of scleroderma characterized by more rapidly progressive skin disease and more severe damage to the viscera (Seibold, 1993, 1997). Some patients develop syndromes with symptoms and signs of scleroderma and other connective tissue or autoimmune diseases. The best known "overlap" syndrome is **mixed connective tissue disease,** which has clinical and laboratory features of SLE (see above), scleroderma, and myositis. Patients with this disorder usually have antibodies to ribonuclear protein. Long-term follow-up studies in patients with MCTD suggest that these patients eventually develop fairly typical systemic sclerosis, and some authorities thus argue that MCTD is not a true disease (Nimelstein et al., 1980). Searles et al. (1978) described a 38-year-old woman with MCTD in whom an isolated trigeminal sensory neuropathy was an early manifestation of the disease, and Hagen et al. (1990) reported trigeminal sensory neuropathy in 21 patients with MCTD and 15 patients with scleroderma. Wyble and Schimek (1962) reported a patient with scleroderma who developed GCA, and Hupp (1989) described a similar case. It is possible that the two disorders were somehow immunologically related, but it is more likely that GCA, a relatively common disease (see above), fortuitously occurred in a patient with an uncommon disease (scleroderma).

Scleroderma generally spares the CNS (Seibold, 1993, 1997). Although some patients with scleroderma experience

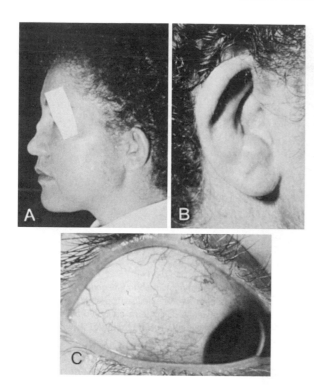

Figure 57.151. Features of relapsing polychondritis. *A,* Saddle-nose deformity with distorted "floppy" ear from auricular chondritis. *B,* Magnified view of inflamed ear shows inferior swelling from chondritis. *C,* Mild episcleritis is present. (Courtesy of Dr. Ernest W Smith.)

tibular dysfunction. Auditory impairment can also result from inflammation in the middle ear, obstruction of the eustachian tube caused by chondritis of the nasopharyngeal segment, and vasculitis affecting the internal auditory artery or its cochlear branch.

Recurrent arthropathy is the second most common clinical manifestation of relapsing polychondritis. It eventually develops in about 70% of patients (Herman, 1993; Hochberg, 1997). It varies from transient arthralgias, to a mono-, pauci-, or polyarticular, symmetric or asymmetric synovitis affecting both large and small peripheral joints and parasternal articulations. It typically presents as an episodic, asymmetric, nonerosive, and nondeforming arthritis lasting several days to several weeks, which resolves spontaneously or in response to anti-inflammatory agents (O'Hanlan et al., 1976). Occasionally, there is cervical, dorsal, or lumbar spine pain.

Nasal chondritis occurs in about 60% of patients with relapsing polychondritis (Herman, 1993; Hochberg, 1997). Affected patients develop nasal stuffiness or fullness, crusting, rhinorrhea, pain, and epistaxis. Typical episodes last only a few days, but repeated attacks eventually cause collapse of cartilage with retraction of the columella, resulting in a saddle-nose deformity (Figs. 57.151 and 57.152).

Laryngotracheal bronchial damage is a poor prognostic sign (Gibson and Davis, 1974). Hoarseness and tenderness over the thyroid cartilage and anterior trachea are common symptoms of such damage, and a nonproductive cough, dyspnea, aphonia, inspiratory stridor, and hemoptysis may de-

velop. Glottic, subglottic, and laryngeal inflammation with concomitant edema may necessitate tracheostomy in severe cases. Recurrent attacks may cause permanent loss of structural support, and death can occur from asphyxiation.

Cardiovascular complications occur in 30% of patients with relapsing polychondritis. Aortic insufficiency occurs primarily in men. It results from progressive dilation of the aortic ring and ascending aorta or from destruction of the valve cusps without dilation of the annulus. Mitral and tricuspid valvular insufficiency occur less frequently. Clinical evidence of cardiac valvular disease may develop as early as 6 months or as late as 15–20 years after the onset of systemic symptoms. Patients with such dysfunction may benefit from valvuloplasty or valve replacement. Patients with relapsing polychondritis may also develop aneurysms of the subclavian artery and of the ascending, thoracic, and abdominal aorta. Rupture of such aneurysms may lead to death (Cipriano et al., 1976). Other cardiovascular complications of relapsing polychondritis include pericarditis, myocarditis with conduction disturbances, endocarditis, and myocardial infarction.

Ocular manifestations are common in patients with relapsing polychondritis, occurring in about 59% of patients (Jabs,

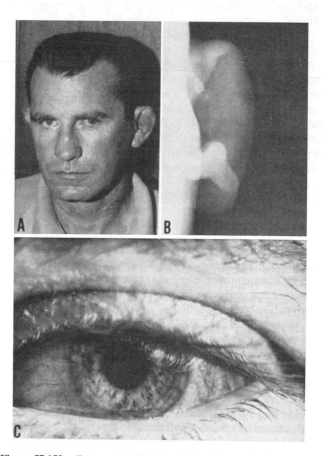

Figure 57.152. Features of relapsing polychondritis. *A,* Saddle-nose deformity; *B,* Calcification of ear seen by soft-tissue x-ray; *C,* Mild injection of left eye from episcleritis. (From Dolan DL, Lemmon GB, Teitelbaum SL. Relapsing polychondritis: Analytical literature review and studies on pathogenesis. Am J Med *41:*285–299, 1966.)

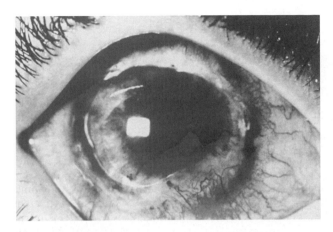

Figure 57.153. Ocular manifestations of relapsing polychondritis. The patient has marginal keratitis with thinning of the peripheral cornea. (Courtesy of Dr. Alice Matoba.)

1994). The most common manifestations are conjunctivitis, keratitis with and without marginal corneal ulceration, uveitis, episcleritis, and scleritis (Rucker and Ferguson, 1965; Anderson, 1967; Barth and Berson, 1968; Bergaust and Abrahamsen, 1969; Matas, 1970; McKay et al., 1974; Zion et al., 1974; Magargal et al., 1981; Matoba et al., 1984; Michelson, 1984; Isaak et al., 1986; Hoang-Xuan et al., 1990; Massry et al., 1995) (Figs. 57.151–57.153). Scleritis may be unilateral or bilateral and diffuse, nodular, or necrotizing (Hoang-Xuan et al., 1990). Posterior scleritis is often associated with chorioretinitis, exudative retinal detachment, proptosis, chemosis, ophthalmoparesis, optic disc swelling, or a combination of these. Retinopathy may occur in patients with relapsing polychondritis in the absence of scleritis. The retinopathy usually consists of a few cotton-wool spots and some intraretinal hemorrhages, but Isaak et al. (1986) reported a branch retinal vein occlusion in one patient and a central retinal vein occlusion in another.

Patients with relapsing polychondritis accompanied by systemic vasculitis may develop a variety of neurologic and neuro-ophthalmologic disturbances (Sundaram and Rajput, 1983; Massry et al., 1995). As noted above, vasculitis affecting the cochlear branch of the internal auditory canal may produce hearing loss. Arteritis of the vestibular branch of the internal auditory artery may produce episodes of vertigo, ataxia, nausea, and vomiting. Such patients may develop vestibular nystagmus. Other cranial neuropathies, including ocular motor nerve pareses, may also occur in patients with relapsing polychondritis and systemic vasculitis, as may hemiparesis, cerebellar signs, seizures, and dementia. Typical AION may occur (Sundaram and Rajput, 1983; Herman, 1993; Jabs, 1994) and may even be bilateral (Massry et al., 1995).

Relapsing polychondritis is often associated with other forms of connective tissue disease (see Table 81-2 in Herman, 1993). In most cases, these diseases antedate the onset of polychondritis by months to years. There is also an association of relapsing polychondritis with a variety of types of dysthyroidism, including hyperthyroidism, nontoxic goiter, hypothyroidism, and Hashimoto's disease. Ulcerative colitis may occur in association with relapsing polychondritis, as may a variety of myeloproliferative diseases, including acute and chronic myelogenous leukemia, aplastic anemia, and Hodgkin's disease (Michet et al., 1986).

There are no laboratory tests for diagnosing relapsing polychondritis. The diagnosis is made clinically and verified by biopsy of affected cartilage from the ear, nose, or respiratory tract (McAdam et al., 1976). Nevertheless, most patients with active disease have an elevated ESR and a modest leukocytosis. Thrombocytosis and eosinophilia may also occur, and a normocytic, normochromic anemia is often present. Other than biopsy, the most helpful diagnostic tests are radiographs or other imaging studies that show destruction of cartilage.

Patients with relapsing polychondritis may be treated with systemic corticosteroids, cytotoxic drugs, or nonsteroidal anti-inflammatory agents. The majority of patients respond to corticosteroid therapy with only a small number requiring immunosuppressive therapy (Willis et al., 1984; Huang-Xuan et al., 1990; Priori et al., 1993; Massry et al., 1995).

ARTHRITIDES

The arthritides are diseases that are primarily characterized by an inflammatory polyarthritis. Of all the disorders described in this chapter, they are least likely to produce either CNS or neuro-ophthalmologic complications.

Rheumatoid Arthritis

Rheumatoid arthritis is the most common rheumatic disease, affecting about 1–2% of adults (Jabs, 1994). It is an additive, symmetric, deforming, peripheral polyarthritis. Although any joint may become affected, the disease primarily attacks the small joints of the hands and feet (Figs. 57.154 and 57.155). Eighty percent of patients with rheumatoid arthritis have an autoantibody directed against IgG in their serum: the **rheumatoid factor** (Jabs, 1994). The ESR often is increased in patients with rheumatoid arthritis (Harris, 1993, 1997), and some investigators suggest that the ESR is the laboratory test that best correlates with disease activity (Bull et al., 1989; Pawlotsky et al., 1989); others disagree, however (Pullar and Capell, 1989; Scott and Spector, 1989).

Extra-articular disease is common in rheumatoid arthritis, and it may affect a wide variety of nonarticular tissues. Rheumatoid nodules occur in about 25% of patients with rheumatoid arthritis (Fig. 57.156). They are located subcutaneously on extensor surfaces and have a characteristic histologic appearance consisting of central necrosis with a surrounding palisade of inflammatory cells. The lungs may be affected with rheumatoid pleural effusions, pleural nodules, pulmonary nodules, and interstitial fibrosis (Fig. 57.157). Cardiac involvement is characterized by pericarditis and by rheumatoid nodules that are located in the conducting system, on the heart valves, or both (Hurd, 1979; Harris, 1993, 1997).

Rheumatoid **arteritis** affects fewer than 1% of patients with rheumatoid arthritis. It usually becomes manifest as either a peripheral polyneuropathy or as refractory skin ulcers. Patients may develop gangrene of the extremities (Fig.

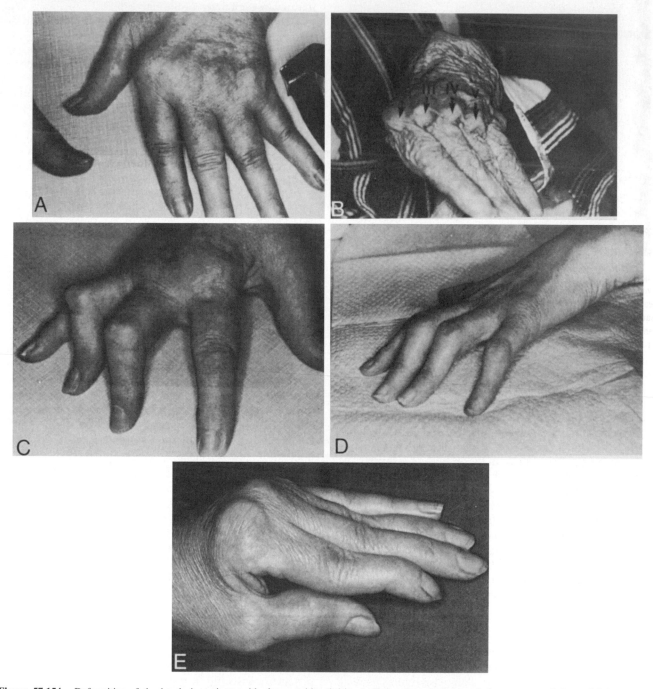

Figure 57.154. Deformities of the hands in patients with rheumatoid arthritis. *A,* Early ulnar deviation of the metacarpophalangeal joints without subluxation. Extensor tendons have slipped to the ulnar side. The fifth finger, in particular, is compromised with weak flexion, causing loss of power grip. *B,* Complete subluxation with marked ulnar deviation at the metacarpophalangeal joints in a 90-year-old woman with rheumatoid arthritis. *Numbered arrows* mark the heads of the metacarpals, now in direct contact with the joint capsule instead of the proximal phalanges. *C* and *D,* Early and late boutonnière deformity of the phalanges in rheumatoid arthritis. In *D,* Moderate soft tissue swellings are visible at the 2nd and 3rd metacarpophalangeal joints. *E,* Early swan neck deformity in rheumatoid arthritis. Synovial proliferation and early subluxation of the metacarpophalangeal joints also are present. (From Harris ED Jr. The clinical features of rheumatoid arthritis. In Textbook of Rheumatology. Editors, Kelley WN, Harris ED Jr, Ruddy S, et al. 3rd ed, pp 943–981. Philadelphia, WB Saunders, 1989.)

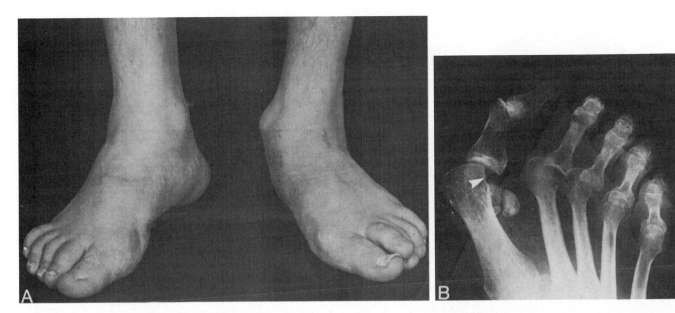

Figure 57.155. Foot deformities in rheumatoid arthritis. *A,* Valgus of ankle, pes planus, and forefoot varus deformity of the left foot caused by painful synovitis of the ankle, forefoot, and metatarsophalangeal joint in a 24-year-old man with severe rheumatoid arthritis. (From Harris ED Jr. The clinical features of rheumatoid arthritis. In Textbook of Rheumatology. Editors, Kelley WN, Harris ED Jr, Ruddy S, et al. 3rd ed, pp 943–981. Philadelphia, WB Saunders, 1989.) *B,* X-ray of the forefoot in another patient with severe rheumatoid arthritis shows subluxation and fibular deviation at the metatarsophalangeal joints and prominent marginal erosions of the first metatarsal head (*arrowhead*). (From Resnick D, Sartoris D, Cone RO III. Imaging. In Textbook of Rheumatology. Editors, Kelley WN, Harris ED Jr, Ruddy S, et al. 3rd ed, pp 650–708. Philadelphia, WB Saunders, 1989.)

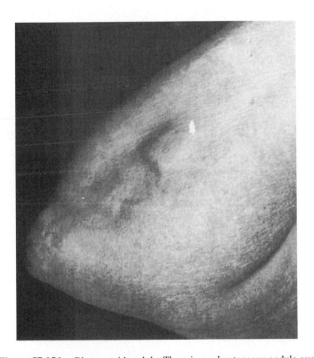

Figure 57.156. Rheumatoid nodule. There is a subcutaneous nodule over the ulnar aspect of the forearm in a patient with rheumatoid arthritis. (From Soter NA. The skin and rheumatic diseases. In Textbook of Rheumatology. Editors, Kelley WN, Harris ED Jr, Ruddy S, et al. 3rd ed, pp 597–610. Philadelphia, WB Saunders, 1989.)

57.158) or, occasionally, visceral ischemia (Scott et al., 1981; Harris, 1993, 1997). Crompton et al. (1980) reported the case of a 68-year-old woman with a 15-year history of rheumatoid arthritis, who developed cutaneous vasculitis, acute ischemic optic neuropathy, and progressive cardiac failure. She died about 10 months after onset of symptoms and signs. At autopsy, the patient had acute necrotizing vasculitis affecting the coronary arteries, periadrenal arteries, vasa nervorum of the sural nerve, and posterior ciliary arteries.

Rheumatoid arteritis may affect the CNS in a variety of ways (Nakano, 1975; Hurd, 1979; Chang and Paget, 1993). In nearly all cases, the neurologic symptoms and signs develop after the arthritis. The duration is variable, ranging from 1 to 30 years (Sigal, 1987). The manifestations of the disease are similarly diverse. They include seizures, dementia, hemiparesis, cranial neuropathies, Gerstmann syndrome, and cerebellar ataxia (Schmid et al., 1961; Ramos and Mandybur, 1975; Watson et al., 1977; Mandybur, 1979; Markenson et al., 1979; Watson, 1979; Beck and Corbett, 1983; Hagen et al., 1990). In many of these cases, histopathologic examination of affected neural tissue shows an extensive necrotizing vasculitis resulting in numerous infarcts. Severe amyloidosis of cerebral arterioles and senile plaques may be seen in areas with severe vasculitis (Ramos and Mandybur, 1975). Peripheral neuropathy and myositis also may occur in patients with rheumatoid vasculitis (Steinberg, 1960; Scott et al., 1981; Puechal et al., 1993, 1995).

Neurologic symptoms and signs occasionally develop in patients with rheumatoid arthritis who do not have evidence of arteritis. In these cases, intracranial rheumatoid nodules

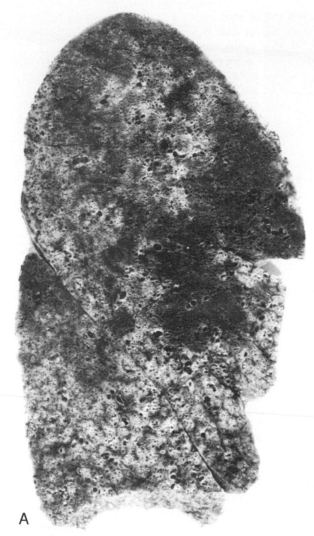

A

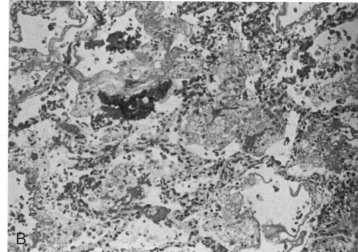

B

Figure 57.157. Lung involvement in rheumatoid arthritis. The patient was a 66-year-old woman with severe rheumatoid arthritis who died from the effects of interstitial pneumonitis. *A*, Gross appearance of the left lung shows dense interalveolar thickening by a fibrofibrinous exudate. The air sacs are becoming obliterated. *B*, Microscopic section through an affected area shows thickened alveolar septa associated with a marked fibrinous exudate. (Courtesy of Dr. Charles Faulkner III.)

or bony abnormalities affecting the leptomeninges, brain parenchyma, or both, are usually responsible (Maher, 1954; Steiner and Gelbloom, 1959; Kim, 1980). We examined a 54-year-old woman who developed bilateral abducens nerve pareses in the setting of rheumatoid arthritis. Neuroimaging studies suggested that multiple rheumatoid nodules on the clivus were responsible for the pareses. She was treated with systemic corticosteroids and immunosuppressive agents with resolution of the abducens nerve pareses. Myelopathy is also common in rheumatoid arthritis and is usually produced by compression rather than ischemia of the spinal cord (Henderson et al., 1993). Cranial nerve palsies and nystagmus rarely occur from brainstem compression by bony abnormalities. The presence of nystagmus, in particular, should suggest the presence of a coexisting Chiari I malformation (Rogers et al., 1994).

The ocular manifestations of rheumatoid arthritis most often result from damage to the anterior segment of the eye. These include dry eyes from Sjögren's syndrome, scleritis, episcleritis, and marginal corneal ulcers (Smith, 1957; Williamson, 1974; Crompton et al., 1980; Zierhut et al., 1989;

Liegner et al., 1990; Whitson and Krachmer, 1990; Ferry, 1993; Jifi-Bahlool et al., 1995; Messmer and Foster, 1995) (Fig. 57.159). About one-third of patients with anterior scleritis have an associated nongranulomatous uveitis (Smith, 1957; Ferry, 1993). The scleritis associated with rheumatoid arthritis is usually of the necrotizing variety and tends to be more severe than idiopathic scleritis. Patients with the scleritis of rheumatoid arthritis tend to be older and have significantly decreased vision (Sainz de la Maza et al., 1994). The anterior segment complications of rheumatoid arthritis usually are treated with systemic and topical corticosteroids, although severe ulcerative keratitis and nonhealing marginal corneal ulcers may require more aggressive therapy with topical cytotoxic agents, such as cyclosporine (Zierhut et al., 1989; Liegner et al., 1990).

Posterior segment ocular complications of rheumatoid arthritis include posterior scleritis that may or may not be associated with an exudative retinal detachment (Johnson and Vine, 1987; Jabs, 1994). Retinal vasculitis is unusual but occurs (Scherbel et al., 1965; Andrews et al., 1977; Meyer et al., 1978). This vasculitis is responsive to systemic corticosteroids. Retinal branch artery occlusion can also occur in patients with rheumatoid arthritis (Crompton et al., 1980).

Optic neuropathy may occur in the setting of rheumatoid arthritis. Kolmokova (1965) described ''interstitial degenerative changes'' in the optic nerve and chiasm in patients who died from the effects of rheumatoid arthritis, and McGavin et al. (1976) described a patient with rheumatoid arthritis who developed optic disc swelling, possibly ischemic in origin. Crompton et al. (1980) reported a beautifully documented case of rheumatoid arthritis, arteritis, and ischemic optic neuropathy. The patient, a 68-year-old woman with a 15-year history of rheumatoid arthritis, developed a flare-up of the disease associated with evidence of cutaneous vasculitis. She then developed sudden loss of vision in the left eye associated with pale swelling of the optic disc, and, 16 days later, blurred vision in the right eye associated with occlusion of a cilioretinal artery. The patient died from progressive heart failure about 2 months after the onset of visual symptoms. At autopsy, she had a diffuse necrotizing vasculitis affecting the coronary, periadrenal, and sural nerve arteries. In addition, necrotizing vasculitis affected one of the right posterior ciliary arteries, and lymphocytic vasculitis and perivasculitis were present in one of the left posterior ciliary arteries and several ciliary arterioles within the sclera of the left eye. In this case, rheumatoid arteritis was clearly responsible for the development of an AION and a retinal branch artery occlusion.

We examined a 58-year-old man with rheumatoid arthritis who developed sudden loss of vision in the right eye. Visual acuity was 20/400 OD and 20/20 OS. The patient had an altitudinal field defect in the right eye, a right RAPD, and a swollen right optic disc. He did not have any risk factors for AION other than rheumatoid arthritis, and a complete systemic evaluation, including tests of cardiac function and noninvasive studies of carotid artery patency, was unrevealing. On the other hand, the patient's rheumatoid arthritis seemed to be inactive, both clinically and by laboratory studies, at the time the optic neuropathy developed, and the opposite optic disc was slightly small with almost no central cup, consistent with the findings in most cases of nonarteritic AION.

An acquired superior oblique tendon sheath syndrome (Brown's syndrome) (Brown, 1950, 1958, 1962, 1973, 1974) may develop in patients with rheumatoid arthritis (Bielschowsky, 1904; Smith, 1965; Sanford-Smith, 1969; Sims, 1971; Scott and Knapp, 1972; Killian et al., 1977; Beck and Hickling, 1980; Knopf, 1989) (Fig. 57.160). The condition may be unilateral or bilateral, and it may be associated with orbital pain that is generalized or localized to the superior nasal region. Thought to be caused by stenosing tenosynovitis of the superior oblique tendon (Sanford-Smith, 1969; Mein, 1971; Wilson et al., 1989), it often resolves spontaneously but may require treatment with corticosteroids. The corticosteroids may be injected into the region of the trochlea or given systemically.

Patients with rheumatoid arthritis occasionally develop evidence of orbital inflammation. Konishi et al. (1986) reported the case of a 58-year-old woman with severe rheumatoid arthritis who developed an acute, progressive, left orbital apex syndrome characterized by visual loss, proptosis, chemosis, orbital and eye pain, and limitation of movement of the left eye. Corneal and facial sensation were reduced

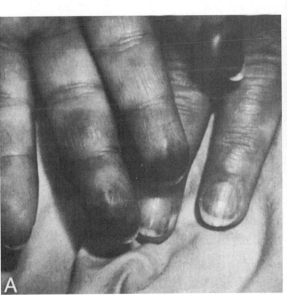
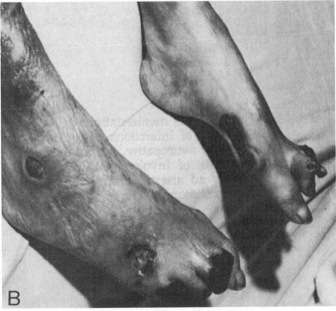

Figure 57.158. Rheumatoid vasculitis. *A*, Necrosis of the fingers in a patient with rheumatoid arthritis. (From Soter NA. The skin and rheumatic diseases. In Textbook of Rheumatology. Editors, Kelley WN, Harris ED Jr, Ruddy S, et al. 3rd ed, pp 597–610. Philadelphia, WB Saunders, 1989.) *B*, Gangrene of the toes with ulcerations of the feet from rheumatoid vasculitis. (From Conn DL, Hunder GG. Vasculitis and related disorders. In Textbook of Rheumatology. Editors, Kelley WN, Harris ED Jr, Ruddy S, et al. 3rd ed, pp 1167–1199. Philadelphia, WB Saunders, 1989.)

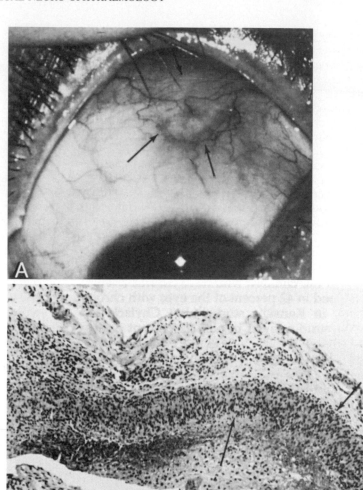

Figure 57.159. Episcleritis in rheumatoid arthritis. The patient was a 63-year-old woman with a 20-year history of rheumatoid arthritis. *A*, A slightly elevated, yellow-white episcleral lesion (*arrows*) is surrounded by dilated blood vessels. *B*, Histopathologic section through the lesion shows fibrinoid necrosis of episcleral collagen fibers in the lower and central portions of the field. Epithelioid cells (*arrows*) are palisaded in planes perpendicular to the central zone of necrosis, and they are sharply demarcated from the surrounding episcleral connective tissue, which is infiltrated by lymphocytes and plasma cells. (From Ferry AP. The eye and rheumatic diseases. In Textbook of Rheumatology. Editors, Kelley WN, Harris ED Jr, Ruddy S, et al. 3rd ed, pp 579–596. Philadelphia, WB Saunders, 1989.)

on the left side. A CT scan was normal, but cerebral angiography showed segmental narrowing of the left ophthalmic artery in the region of the orbital apex. The patient was treated with systemic corticosteroids with only slight improvement. She died from acute cardiac failure about 2 months after the onset of visual symptoms in the left eye, and 1 week after developing a "visual disturbance" of the right eye associated with deep eye pain. At autopsy, the periorbita at both orbital apices was thickened, and multiple rheumatoid nodules were present within the connective tissue of the posterior orbits between the cranial nerves. There was no evidence of vasculitis in either orbit or in the rest of the body.

An unusual case of apparently acquired Duane's retraction syndrome was reported by Baker and Robertson (1980) in a patient with active rheumatoid arthritis. The mechanism by which this occurred is unclear, because most cases of acquired Duane's syndrome result from orbital trauma that disrupts the sheaths of the oculomotor and abducens nerve, resulting in misregeneration. We do not understand how ischemia or mild inflammation could produce such a syndrome. Indeed, it is possible that this patient had a congenital Duane's syndrome that was recognized only after she became ill.

Juvenile Rheumatoid Arthritis

Juvenile rheumatoid arthritis (JRA) is defined as an arthritis of greater than 3 months' duration with an onset in a patient younger than 16 years of age (Jabs, 1994). The traditional classification of JRA depends on the pattern of presentation of the arthritis, and consists of polyarthritis, pauciarthritis, and systemic disease. Polyarthritis is said to be present when more than five joints are affected, whereas pauciarthritis affects four or fewer. Both forms of the disease are more common in girls than in boys by a 2:1 ratio.

Systemic JRA, the disorder originally described by Diamantberger (1891) and later by Still (1897), is characterized by a variable arthritis associated with systemic (and occasionally neurologic) features. The male to female ratio is about 1:1, and it usually affects children younger than 5 years of age (Jabs, 1994). The clinical features of systemic JRA include fever, a salmon-colored evanescent maculopapular rash, lymphadenopathy, splenomegaly, hepatitis, and serositis.

Patients with the systemic form of JRA may develop neurologic symptoms and signs (Sigal, 1987). Sievers et al. (1968) described a 17-year-old boy who developed lower extremity weakness and dysphasia 7 years after the onset of polyarticular JRA. Angiography demonstrated a mass effect without evidence of vasculitis. The patient subsequently experienced several seizures, and he therefore was treated with systemic corticosteroids. Shortly after starting steroid therapy, the patient's seizures stopped, and his angiogram returned to normal. In a series of 170 patients reported by Jan et al. (1972), eight developed meningismus, and three experienced seizures.

The primary ocular manifestation of JRA is iridocyclitis, which occurs in 10–20% of patients during the course of the disease (Chylack et al., 1975; Kanski, 1990; Jabs, 1994). Acute iridocyclitis usually occurs in a subset of patients with HLA-B27, whereas chronic iridocyclitis is more common in a subset of patients with ANA-positive pauciarticular disease (Stewart and Hill, 1967; Pietrowa and Duchowska, 1968; Schaller et al., 1969; Calabro et al., 1970; Chylack et al., 1975; Key and Kimura, 1975; Malaise-Stals, 1989). The uveitis of JRA typically occurs without the eye pain and

redness usually associated with intraocular inflammation and thus is often called "white iritis" (Giles, 1990). Patients with chronic iridocyclitis are more likely to develop other ocular complications, including posterior synechiae, cataract, and glaucoma (Chylack et al., 1975; Key and Kimura, 1975; Kanski, 1977; Cabral et al., 1994). Such patients also may develop band keratopathy, a disorder characterized by deposition of calcium in Bowman's layer of the cornea (Ferry, 1993) (Fig. 57.161). Iridocyclitis associated with JRA may produce insidous visual loss, and 12% of patients are eventually blinded by the inflammatory sequalae (Foster and Barrett, 1993). Both the acute and the chronic forms of uveitis that occur in patients with JRA usually are treated with topical corticosteroids and dilating agents. Systemic corticosteroids may be used to treat eyes that fail to respond to topical medications, and other immunosuppressive drugs may be beneficial in patients with JRA whose uveitis is unresponsive to topical or parenteral corticosteroids.

Diplopia from an acquired superior oblique tendon sheath syndrome may develop in patients with JRA as it does in patients with rheumatoid arthritis (Killian et al., 1977; Jacobs, 1983; Kemp et al., 1984; Wang et al., 1984; Moore and Morin, 1985; Roifman et al., 1985). The syndrome may be unilateral or bilateral, is often transient, and may respond dramatically to treatment with systemic or local corticosteroids.

Posterior segment lesions, other than macular edema related to iridocyclitis, are rare in patients with JRA. Chylack et al. (1975) reported that one of their patients with JRA and acute iridocyclitis developed papillitis, but these investiga-

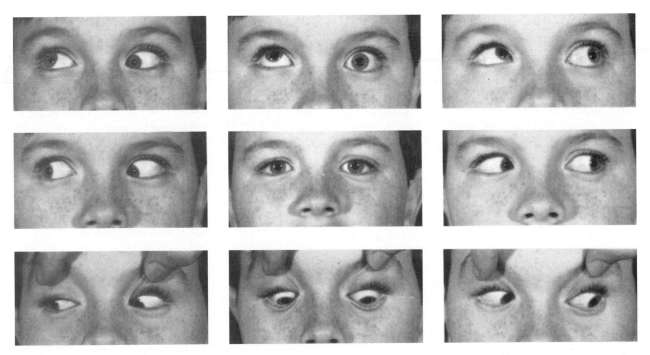

Figure 57.160. Superior oblique tendon sheath syndrome (Brown's syndrome). The patient has limitation of elevation of the left eye, particularly in adduction. Note that the eyes are relatively straight in primary position and downgaze. (From Wilson ME, Eustis HS Jr, Parks MM. Brown's syndrome. *Surv Ophthalmol 34:*153–172, 1989.)

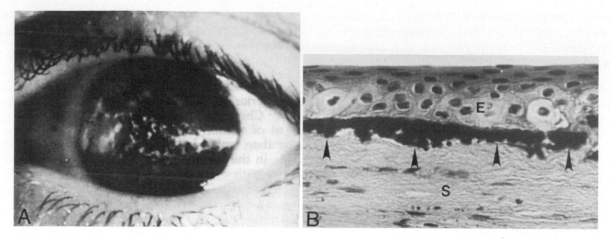

Figure 57.161. Band keratopathy in juvenile rheumatoid arthritis. *A*, In a 12-year-old girl with JRA, there is a horizontal band of calcium across the cornea that scatters the normal corneal light reflex. (Courtesy of Dr. Torrance A Makley.) *B*, Histopathologic appearance of band keratopathy. Note calcification and fragmentation of Bowman's layer beneath the corneal epithelium *(arrowheads)*. *E*, corneal epithelium; *S*, corneal stroma.

tors did not provide details of the examination findings except to state that the patient regained visual acuity of 20/20 in the affected eye after treatment with systemic corticosteroids.

Semple et al. (1990) reported a 4-year-old girl with JRA and chronic iridocyclitis who developed neovascularization of the optic disc. The neovascularization was probably caused by chronic intraocular inflammation, because the patient also had evidence of cystoid macular edema. The patient was treated with two periocular injections of aqueous triamcinolone, following which there was complete regression of the neovascularization.

Orbital inflammation with evidence of vasculitis occasionally occurs in patients with JRA. In addition, Littlewood and Lewis (1963) reported a 7-year-old boy who developed a Holmes-Adie syndrome, characterized by a tonic right pupil and absent knee and ankle deep-tendon reflexes, concurrent with his initial attack of JRA. It is possible that vasculitis affecting the ciliary ganglion or the short posterior ciliary nerves caused the tonic pupil and that a similar process, occurring in the cell bodies of the dorsal columns, was responsible for the absent deep-tendon reflexes.

Seronegative (HLA-B27-Associated) Spondyloarthropathies

The seronegative spondyloarthropathies include ankylosing spondylitis, Reiter's syndrome, psoriatic arthritis, and arthritis with inflammatory bowel disease (Jabs, 1994). Although linked by a statistical association with HLA-B27 and somewhat overlapping features, they nevertheless may be separated on the basis of specific clinical patterns (Arnett, 1987).

Ankylosing Spondylitis

Ankylosing spondylitis, a rare disorder that affects about 0.1–0.2% of the population (van der Linden et al., 1984), is characterized by damage to the axial skeleton causing

bony fusion (ankylosis). The cause is unknown. About 90% of patients with this condition possess HLA-B27, which is present in only 6–8% of the normal population (Schlosstein et al., 1973; Calin et al., 1983). Ankylosing spondylitis affects men more often than women, and it is much more common in Caucasians than in dark-skinned races (Arnett, 1987; Wollheim, 1993a; van der Linden, 1997).

The classic features of ankylosing spondylitis are chronic low back pain, fusion of the axial skeleton, and sacroiliitis (Calin, 1989a) (Fig. 57.162). Patients may also develop arthritis of the shoulders and hips, limited chest expansion, and restrictive lung disease. Other extra-articular features of ankylosing spondylitis include apical pulmonary fibrosis, aortic insufficiency caused by aortitis, and heart block.

Neurologic dysfunction may occur in patients with ankylosing spondylitis. It can be caused by a variety of lesions but most often develops in the late stages of the disease when the cauda equina becomes affected (Mathews, 1968; Gordon and Yudell, 1973; Russell et al., 1973; Thomas et al., 1974; Tullous et al., 1990). Affected patients develop progressive leg or buttock pain with sensory and motor impairment associated with bowel and bladder dysfunction. In some patients, progressive arachnoiditis and advanced bony disease affect the cervical spine. When this happens, the vertebral arteries may be affected, and patients may experience TIAs or strokes caused by vertebrobasilar insufficiency (see Chapter 55). Similar neurologic manifestations may develop in patients in whom the disease produces atlantoaxial subluxation (Coste et al., 1960; Davidson and Tyler, 1974) or spinal fracture (Hunter and Dubo, 1978) (Fig. 57.163). In all such cases, neurologic disease occurs in the setting of advanced spondylarthropathy (Sigal, 1987). Finally, MS appears to occur with a higher frequency in patients with ankylosing spondylitis than in the normal population (Thomas et al., 1974; Pillay and Hunter, 1976; Khan and Kushner, 1979). Although this association is considered unproven by some authors (Calin, 1989b; Dolan and Gibson, 1994), we believe that MS should be considered in any patient with ankylosing spondylitis who develops neurologic dysfunction that seems to be unrelated or out of proportion to the effect of the disease on the spinal cord or vertebral arteries.

The primary ocular manifestation of ankylosing spondylitis, ultimately affecting 25–33% of patients with the disease, is recurrent, acute, nongranulomatous **uveitis** (Wilkinson and Bywaters, 1958; Lenoch et al., 1959; Haarr, 1960; Malaise-Stals, 1989; Linssen and Meenken, 1995). One eye usually is affected at a time, although both eyes may experience attacks. Rare patients with ankylosing spondylitis develop a vitritis, but this almost always is associated with an anterior uveitis (Perkins, 1966; Belmont and Michelson, 1982; Rodriquez et al., 1994). Patients with posterior segment ocular involvement may occasionally develop retinal vasculitis and optic disc swelling associated with vitritis (Rodriquez et al., 1994). Other neuro-ophthalmologic complications of ankylosing spondylitis are usually caused either by vertebrobasilar insufficiency (see Chapter 55) or by concomitant MS (see Chapter 71).

The diagnosis of ankylosing spondylitis is made by physical examination and radiographic imaging. There are no laboratory studies that are typically abnormal in this disease,

even though the ESR is often elevated, especially early in the disease, and there may be a mild anemia. Tests for rheumatoid factor and ANAs are usually negative, although the concentration of alkaline phosphatase in the serum may be increased (Kendall et al., 1973).

Patients with ankylosing spondylitis usually are treated with analgesics and nonsteroidal anti-inflammatory drugs (Lisse, 1989). Patients in whom the disease is refractory to these agents may benefit from phenylbutazone. Systemic corticosteroids usually are not effective. Physical therapy is usually encouraged early in the course of the disease to keep the spine as straight as possible (Arnett, 1984). The iridocyclitis that develops in ankylosing spondylitis responds to topical corticosteroids and mydriatics, although rare patients require a short course of systemic corticosteroids. Patients with severe posterior segment involvement may require more aggressive immunosuppressive therapy (Rodriquez et al., 1994). Kelly and Storey (1989) described a patient with ankylosing spondylitis whose ability to ambulate was severely impaired by flexion contracture of the spine with loss of all neck movements. This resulted in a head-down position from which he could not see beyond about 1.5 m with

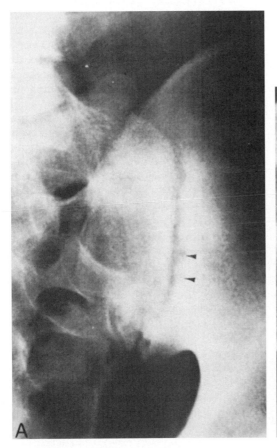
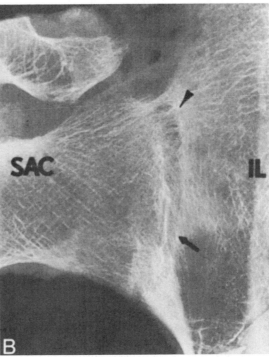

Figure 57.162. Sacroiliitis in ankylosing spondylitis. *A,* Plain X-ray of the sacroiliac joint shows an ill-defined band of sclerosis and prominent erosions of the subchondral bone plate that are most prominent on the iliac side of the articulation *(arrowheads). B,* Radiograph from a cadaver with ankylosing spondylitis shows complete intra-articular ankylosis of the ligamentous *(arrowhead)* and synovial *(arrow)* portions of the joint. *SAC,* sacrum; *IL,* ilium. (From Resnick D, Sartoris D, Cone RO III. Imaging. In Textbook of Rheumatology. Editors, Kelley WN, Harris ED Jr, Ruddy S, et al. 3rd ed, pp 650–708. Philadelphia, WB Saunders, 1989.)

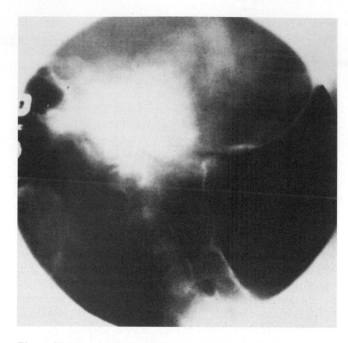

Figure 57.163. Atlanto-occipital subluxation causing bulbar symptoms and signs in ankylosing spondylitis. The patient was a 55-year-old man with severe ankylosing spondylitis who developed episodes of dizziness, dysphagia, and loss of voice. Lateral cervical tomogram shows upper cervical ankylosis with marked atlanto-occipital subluxation. (From Davidson RI, Tyler HR. Bulbar symptoms and episodic aphonia associated with atlanto-occipital subluxation in ankylosing spondylitis. J Neurol Neurosurg Psychiatry *37*:691–695, 1974.)

maximum upgaze. He was treated with a spectacle frame in which a 45-prism diopter plastic prism was placed base up in each opening and secured with cement and straps. This allowed the patient to see 6 m ahead with comfort when his eyes were in the primary position of gaze, and he was able to resume walking outdoors unaided. Other authors treat patients with ankylosing spondylitis with similar optical devices (Bennett, 1962; Gostin, 1971; Storey, 1973; Richer and Hall, 1986).

The prognosis for life in patients with ankylosing spondylitis is close to normal (Schlosstein et al., 1973; Wollheim, 1993a; van der Linden, 1997). Death usually is caused by cardiac dysfunction or by fracture of the cervical spine. Significant disability from progressive spinal disease develops in about 20% of patients regardless of treatment (Arnett, 1987).

Reiter's Syndrome

On August 21, 1916, a lieutenant in the Prussian army developed acute abdominal pain and diarrhea. The episode lasted 48 hours. Seven days later, the patient developed urethritis and conjunctivitis, and the next day he developed polyarthralgias and arthritis of the knees, ankles, elbows, wrists, and several interphalangeal joints. The symptoms and signs remitted within a few days, and the patient was well for 3 weeks. He then experienced recurrence of both the urethritis and the conjunctivitis. These events were recorded by Professor Hans Reiter (Reiter, 1916). The triad of arthri-

tis, urethritis, and conjunctivitis is now called **Reiter's syndrome.** Like ankylosing spondylitis, Reiter's syndrome has a definite genetic disposition in that HLA-B27 is found in 60–95% of affected patients (Fan and Yu, 1993; Jabs, 1994; Fan and Yu, 1997.

Reiter's syndrome exists in two forms: epidemic and endemic. **Epidemic** Reiter's syndrome occurs after infectious gastroenteritis caused by certain organisms such as Shigella, Salmonella, and Yersinia. The subsequent arthritis, which develops after the infectious gastroenteritis has resolved, is sterile. It seems to be an immunologic response to the organism, but the pathways by which the response occurs and the precise nature of the response are unknown (Arnett, 1987).

The cause of **endemic** Reiter's syndrome is also unknown. Both venereal disease and chlamydial infection have been suggested as possible causes, but there are no data supporting either process (Arnett, 1987; Fan and Yu, 1993, 1997). Weyand and Goronzy (1989) demonstrated circulating antibodies and proliferative T-cell responses to *Borrelia burgdorferi* in 18% of patients with Reiter's syndrome who came from an area of the Federal Republic of Germany where Lyme disease is endemic. Similar antibodies were found in only 3% of asymptomatic control subjects from the same area. Thus, at least some cases of endemic Reiter's syndrome are caused by *B. burgdorferi,* particularly in certain areas of the world (Arnett, 1989).

The **arthritis** of Reiter's syndrome is an asymmetric oligoarthritis that affects primarily the lower extremities, particularly the large joints such as the knees or ankles. Other articular features include periostitis, interphalangeal arthritis, and sacroiliitis (Fig. 57.164).

Mucocutaneous lesions include urethritis in men and cervicitis in women, painless oral ulcers, lesions of the fingernails and toenails, balanitis, and keratoderma blenorrhagicum (Figs. 57.165–57.167). Balanitis is characterized by painless, superficial erosions on the glans penis (Fan and Yu, 1993, 1997) (Fig. 57.166). The condition begins as small vesicles that can rupture to form a painless superficial ero-

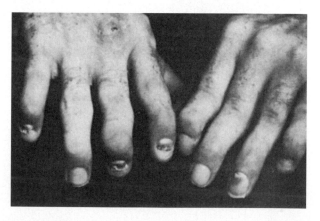

Figure 57.164. Arthritis in Reiter's syndrome. Swan neck deformities of the phalanges in a patient with chronic Reiter's syndrome. (From Michet CJ, Hunder GG. Examination of the joints. In Textbook of Rheumatology. Editors, Kelley WN, Harris ED Jr, Ruddy S, et al. 3rd ed, pp 425–441. Philadelphia, WB Saunders, 1989.)

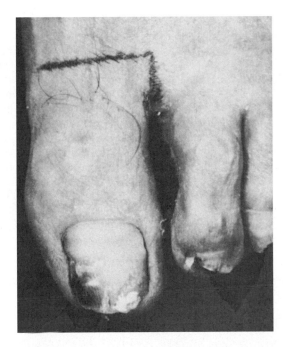

Figure 57.165. Lesions of the nails in Reiter's syndrome. Note typical destructive nature of change with subungual hyperkeratotic accumulation of material. (From Calin A. Reiter's syndrome. In Textbook of Rheumatology. Editors, Kelley WN, Harris ED Jr, Ruddy S, et al. 3rd ed, pp 1038–1052. Philadelphia, WB Saunders, 1989.)

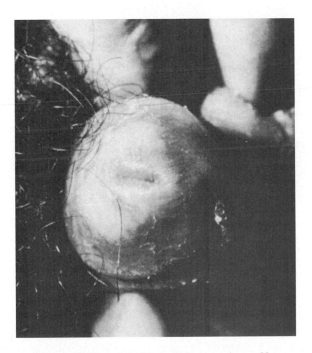

Figure 57.166. Circinate balanitis in Reiter's syndrome. Note opaque superficial ulceration. (From Calin A. Reiter's syndrome. In Textbook of Rheumatology. Editors, Kelley WN, Harris ED Jr, Ruddy S, et al. 3rd ed, pp 1038–1052. Philadelphia, WB Saunders, 1989.)

sion with little surrounding erythema. The lesions often coalesce to form a circular pattern (circinate balanitis). Keratoderma blenorrhagicum occurs most often on the soles of the feet, glans penis, and toes, although discrete lesions may develop on the limbs, scrotum, trunk, scalp, and palms (Calin, 1989c). These skin lesions begin as discrete vesicles that become opaque as their walls thicken. They eventually become hyperkeratotic nodules that may coalesce, resulting in a crust that may last for days, weeks, or months (Fig. 57.167). They eventually may disappear without a trace, although they frequently recur.

Conjunctivitis is one of the hallmarks of Reiter's syndrome. It tends to be a feature of early disease, particularly the initial attack (Jabs, 1994) (Fig. 57.168). A more serious ocular manifestation is **uveitis.** The uveitis is acute, nongranulomatous, and recurrent (Malaise-Stals, 1989). It is identical to that which occurs in patients with ankylosing spondylitis (see above). Acute anterior uveitis occurs in 5–10% of patients at the time of development of the other symptoms of Reiter's syndrome, and it develops at some time during the course of the disease in about 50% of patients (Jabs, 1994). An unusual **keratitis** characterized by subepithelial infiltrates and punctate epithelial lesions that progress until there is central loss of corneal epithelium is observed in some patients (Ostler et al., 1971; Saari et al., 1980; Lee et al., 1986). **Vitritis** occurs in some patients with Reiter's syndrome (Perkins, 1966) and may be associated with cystoid macular edema producing decreased central vision. Generalized uveitis also may be associated with **swelling of the optic disc** (Zewi, 1947; Rodriquez et al., 1994), but such cases usually are unassociated with other evidence of optic nerve dysfunction such as an RAPD. On the other hand, some patients with Reiter's syndrome develop true **optic neuritis** (Lindsay-Rea, 1947; Zewi, 1947; Oates and Hancock, 1959). The optic neuritis may be anterior or retrobulbar and unilateral or bilateral. Patients with Reiter's syndrome may also develop a **retinal vasculitis** associated with uveitis (Nolan and Cullen, 1967; Rodriquez et al., 1994).

Neurologic complications occur infrequently in Reiter's syndrome. Findings reported in such patients include peripheral neuropathy, transient hemiplegia, and cranial neuropathy (Csonka and Oates, 1957; Oates and Hancock, 1959). Good (1974) described neurologic dysfunction in 46 of 164 patients (28%) with Reiter's syndrome. Twenty patients developed neurologic symptoms and signs only during acute attacks of the disease, 14 patients developed neurologic disturbances shortly after flare-ups, and in 12 patients, neurologic symptoms and signs seemed to be unrelated to underlying disease activity. Only one of the patients experienced a cranial neuropathy: a 52-year-old man who experienced a transient glossopharyngeal neuralgia. The rest of the patients developed diverse neurologic manifestations, including loss of consciousness, depression, psychosis, seizures, and a peripheral neuropathy. None of the patients experienced loss of vision or diplopia. It would appear that in some patients with Reiter's syndrome, neurologic dysfunction is caused by cerebral vasculitis.

Reiter's syndrome is a major chronic rheumatic disease. Some patients have recurrent episodes with asymptomatic periods between exacerbations; however, most patients have

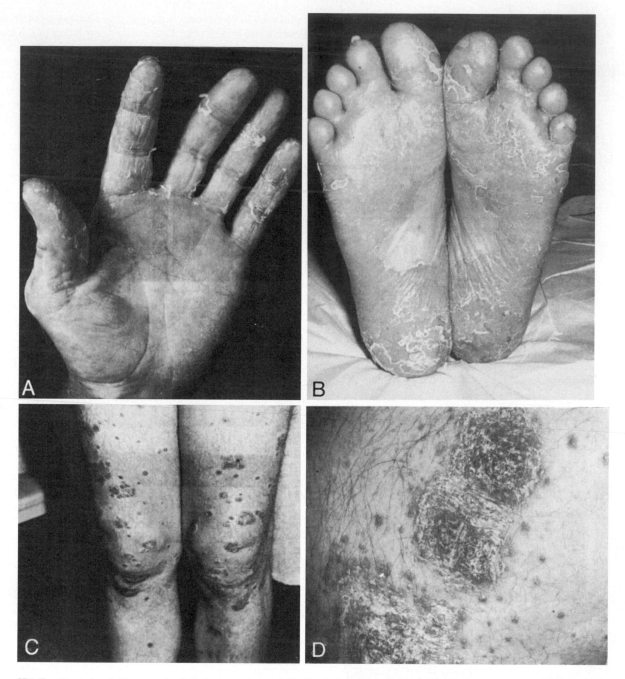

Figure 57.167. Keratodermia blenorrhagica in Reiter's syndrome. *A*, Scaling lesions are present on the palm. *B*, Scaling lesions are present on the soles of the feet. *C*, Keratotic plaques have developed over the lower extremities. *D*, Magnified view of keratotic plaques and nodules over the lower extremities. (*A* and *C*, from Calin A. Reiter's syndrome. In Textbook of Rheumatology. Editors, Kelley WN, Harris ED Jr, Ruddy S, et al. 3rd ed, pp 1038–1052. Philadelphia, WB Saunders, 1989. *B*, from Holland EJ. Reiter's syndrome. In The Eye in Systemic Disease. Editors, Gold DH, Weingeist TA. pp 56–58. Philadelphia, JB Lippincott, 1990. *D*, from Soter NA. The skin and rheumatic diseases. In Textbook of Rheumatology. Editors, Kelley WN, Harris ED Jr, Ruddy S, et al. 3rd ed, pp 597–610. Philadelphia, WB Saunders. 1989.)

persistent discomfort (Fan and Yu, 1993, 1997). There is no cure for the condition. The joint and soft tissue manifestations seem to respond reasonably well to nonsteroidal antiinflammatory agents such as indomethacin and phenylbutazone. The ocular manifestations can be treated with topical corticosteroids, although severe uveitis may require subcon-

junctival or systemic administration of steroids. Those patients with posterior segment ocular involvement may require more aggressive immunosuppressive therapy with agents such as methotrexate and azathioprine (Rodriquez et al., 1994). The neurologic manifestations of Reiter's syndrome are so uncommon that it is difficult to recommend a

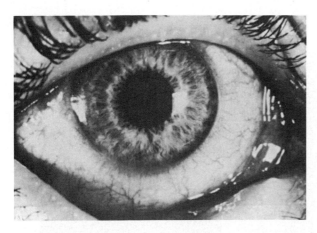

Figure 57.168. Conjunctivitis in Reiter's syndrome. Appearance of affected eye in a 25-year-old man with Reiter's syndrome shows a mucopurulent, papillary conjunctivitis.

specific form of treatment. Nonsteroidal anti-inflammatory agents may be tried, and if these are not helpful, systemic corticosteroids may be given.

Psoriatic Arthritis

Psoriatic arthritis is a syndrome in which psoriasis is associated with an inflammatory arthritis in patients with a negative test for rheumatoid factor (Michet, 1993; Jabs, 1994; Gladman, 1997). About 60% of patients with this condition test positively for the histocompatibility antigen HLA-B27 (Moll, 1984; Arnett, 1987).

Psoriasis is a cutaneous disorder characterized by erythematous, well-demarcated macules with silvery scales (Fig. 57.169). The lesions occur on extensor surfaces, partic-

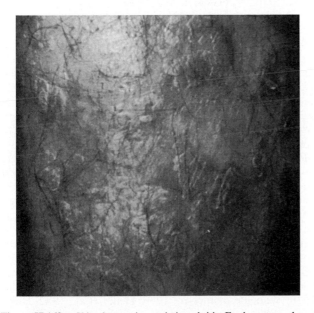

Figure 57.169. Skin changes in psoriatic arthritis. Erythematous plaques with layers of scale are evident. (From Soter NA. The skin and rheumatic diseases. In Textbook of Rheumatology. Editors, Kelley WN, Harris ED Jr, Ruddy S, et al. 3rd ed, pp 597–610. Philadelphia, WB Saunders, 1989.)

ularly the elbows and scalp, but they may also appear on the chest and back. The skin disease generally precedes the onset of arthritis by several years, but 16% of patients develop arthritis first (Jabs, 1994).

Most patients with psoriatic arthritis develop a monoarthritis or an asymmetric oligoarthritis that affects distal interphalangeal, proximal interphalangeal, or metatarsal interphalangeal joints (Fig. 57.170). Other forms of the arthritis are (*a*) disease that affects only the distal interphalangeal joints; (*b*) a severely deforming, widespread arthritis with ankylosis (arthritis mutilans); (*c*) a symmetric, additive, deforming polyarthritis similar to that seen in patients with rheumatoid arthritis; and (*d*) spondylitis (Michet, 1993; Jabs, 1994; Gladman, 1997).

Ocular and neurologic manifestations of psoriatic arthritis are both mild and uncommon. About 20% of patients have conjunctivitis, 7% develop uveitis, and 2% develop scleritis (Lambert and Wright, 1976; Jabs, 1994). The uveitis occurs primarily in patients with the spondylitic form of the disease. It is identical with the uveitis that occurs in patients with ankylosing spondylitis and Reiter's syndrome in that it is acute, nongranulomatous, and recurrent. Papillitis and retinal vasculitis may rarely complicate this condition (Rodriquez et al., 1994; Rechichi et al., 1997). The neurologic manifestations of psoriatic arthritis are usually caused either by atlantoaxial subluxation (Kaplan et al., 1964; Todoroki et al., 1981; Buskila and Gladman, 1989) or by progressive damage to the lower spinal cord in patients with the spondylitic form of the disease.

Most patients with psoriatic arthritis have minimal disability and require little treatment. Patients with the more aggressive forms of the disease may require intermittent treatment with nonsteroidal anti-inflammatory agents or systemic corticosteroids. Patients with severe skin lesions may benefit from methotrexate, retinoic acid derivatives, or psoralen plus ultraviolet light treatment (Gladman, 1997). The ocular disease of psoriatic arthritis usually is well controlled with topical corticosteroid preparations.

Arthritis with Inflammatory Bowel Disease (Enteropathic Arthritis)

Two main forms of inflammatory bowel disease occur in association with arthritis: ulcerative colitis and Crohn's disease. **Ulcerative colitis** is an inflammatory disorder of the gastrointestinal mucosa with diffuse involvement of the colon (Fig. 57.171). **Crohn's disease** is a focal granulomatous disease affecting various areas of both the small and the large bowel (Crohn et al., 1932) (Fig. 57.172). Crohn's disease also is called regional enteritis, granulomatous ileocolitis, and granulomatous colitis (Jabs, 1994). Some forms of enteropathic arthritis are caused by infectious agents (e.g., Whipple's disease). These disorders are discussed in Chapter 60 of this text.

Arthritis does not occur in every patient with either ulcerative colitis or Crohn's disease. The prevalence of arthritis is about 30% in ulcerative colitis and 25% in Crohn's disease (Wollheim, 1993b; Jabs, 1994; Wollheim, 1997). There are two main types of arthritis. Colitic arthritis is a nondeforming oligoarthritis that usually affects the large joints of the lower extremities. The activity of this arthritis parallels

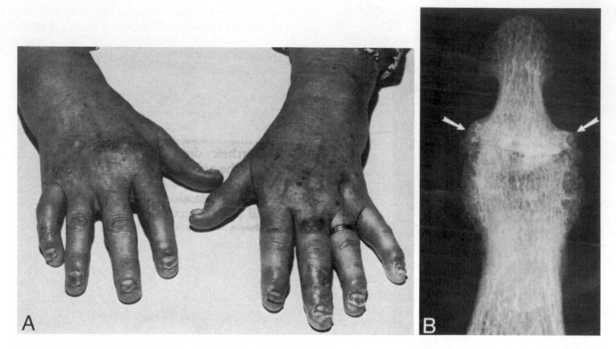

Figure 57.170. Psoriatic arthritis. *A*, Psoriasis of the hands and nails associated with symmetric swelling of the distal interphalangeal joints, proximal interphalangeal joints, metacarpophalangeal joints, and wrists. (From Michet CJ, Conn DL. Psoriatic arthritis. In Textbook of Rheumatology. Editors, Kelley WN, Harris ED Jr, Ruddy S, et al. 3rd ed, pp 1053–1063. Philadelphia, WB Saunders, 1989.) *B*, Plain X-ray of a finger of a patient with psoriatic arthritis shows narrowing of the distal interphalangeal joint associated with bony erosions (*arrows*). (From Metcalf RW. Arthroscopy. In Textbook of Rheumatology. Editors, Kelley WN, Harris ED Jr, Ruddy S, et al. 3rd ed, pp 709–718. Philadelphia, WB Saunders, 1989.)

the activity of the bowel disease. It is the most common form of arthritis that occurs in the setting of inflammatory bowel disease, eventually developing in about 25% of patients with ulcerative colitis and 20% of patients with Crohn's disease (Jabs, 1994). The second type of arthritis associated with inflammatory bowel disease is ankylosing spondylitis. This form of arthritis occurs in only about 4% of patients with inflammatory bowel disease, and its activity is unrelated to the activity of the bowel disease. About half of the patients with inflammatory bowel disease and spondylitis are HLA-B27-positive, and these patients are most likely to develop ocular manifestations (Wright et al., 1965; Greenstein et al., 1976; Arnett, 1987; Wollheim, 1993b, 1997).

Ocular inflammation occurs in about 4–6% of patients with inflammatory bowel disease (Edwards and Truelove, 1964; Billson et al., 1967; Hopkins et al., 1974; Knox, 1990). The ocular manifestations include episcleritis, scleritis, uveitis, and keratitis (Knox et al., 1980; van Vliet and van Balen, 1985; Knox, 1990; Soukiasian et al., 1994) (Fig. 57.173). Episcleritis and acute, nongranulomatous, recurrent uveitis are the most common ocular manifestations. All types of scleritis may develop, including necrotizing and posterior forms (Crohn, 1925; Ellis and Gentry, 1964; Billson et al., 1967; Evans and Eustace, 1973; Hopkins et al., 1974; Knox et al., 1984). Vitritis, choroidal infiltrates, retinitis, and retinal vascular disease may occur in patients with enteropathic arthritis, and such patients also may develop exudative retinal detachment, retrobulbar neuritis, anterior optic neuritis, or neuroretinitis (Ellis and Gentry, 1964; Macoul, 1970; Knox et al., 1980, 1984; Sedwick et al., 1984; Miura et al.,

1990; Ruby and Jampol, 1990; Ernst et al., 1991; Garcia-Diaz et al., 1995; Hutnik et al., 1996) (Fig. 57.174). Orbital myositis may develop and produce diplopia, pain, conjunctival swelling, and other signs of orbital disease (Greenstein et al., 1976; Weinstein et al., 1984).

Patients with inflammatory bowel disease may develop ocular complications from nutritional deficiency. Iansek and Edge (1985) reported a 62-year-old woman with a 9-year history of Crohn's disease who had developed a bowel obstruction for which she underwent resection of the ileum and ascending colon. Although the disease was quiescent, she had persistent steatorrhea characterized by passing 7–10 pale and greasy stools each day. The patient subsequently developed blurred vision and was found to have a bilateral optic neuropathy with profoundly impaired color perception and bilateral cecocentral scotomas. Evaluation revealed an iron deficiency anemia and reduced serum carotene, with normal serum vitamin B_{12} and red blood cell folate concentrations. The patient was treated with intramuscular injections of vitamins, and her visual function improved substantially over the next month.

Patients with inflammatory bowel disease, with and without arthritis, may develop ischemic visual loss, neurologic deficits, or both (Hogan et al., 1957; Kehoe and Newcomber, 1964; Silverstein and Present, 1971; Mayeux and Fahn, 1978; Schneiderman et al., 1979; Heuer et al., 1982; Duker et al., 1987). Ischemic ocular complications include central retinal artery occlusion, recurrent retinal branch artery occlusion, ischemic optic neuropathy, homonymous visual field defects, and ocular motor nerve paresis (Figs. 57.175 and

57.176). Neurologic complications include cerebral thromboembolism, cerebral venous thrombosis, transient brainstem ischemia, and massive cerebral and brainstem infarction (Greenstein et al., 1976) (Fig. 57.177). The cause of the cerebral and retinal vascular complications of inflammatory bowel disease is thought to be a hypercoagulable state characterized by thrombocytosis, short partial thromboplastin time, and elevated serum fibrinogen and factor VIII concentrations.

Patients with ulcerative colitis or Crohn's disease may be treated with systemic corticosteroids, cytotoxic agents, surgery, or a combination of these (Truelove and Jewell, 1974; Baker and Jewell, 1989; Bianchi et al., 1990; Lichtiger and Present, 1990). Platelet counts and coagulation factors become normal in some patients when the intestinal inflammation is successfully treated (Schneiderman et al., 1979).

MALIGNANT ATROPHIC PAPULOSIS (DEGOS' DISEASE, KÖHLMEIER-DEGOS' DISEASE)

Malignant atrophic papulosis (MAP), also called **Degos' disease,** is a rare, cutaneovisceral occlusive disease that occurs predominantly in young adults and is almost always fatal when neurologic involvement occurs (Köhlmeier, 1941; Degos et al., 1942; Degos, 1979; Subbiah et al., 1996). Affected patients develop a characteristic **skin rash**, most prominent on the trunk and arms, consisting of small papules that initially have a pale rose color. The papules subsequently become umbilicated and flattened to form irregular patches with a porcelain white center surrounded by a thin, red area. The rash usually spares the palms, soles, head, and oral mucosa. It almost always antedates the visceral lesions, often by weeks to years (Nomland and Layton, 1960; Degos, 1979).

Gastrointestinal complications occur in 61% of patients with MAP (Case Records of the Massachusetts General Hospital, 1980). The small intestine is most often affected, with patients developing signs and symptoms of perforation, obstruction, or pancreatitis. Laparotomy in such patients usually reveals a small intestine covered with yellow-white patches. More than 50% of patients die from intestinal perforation, usually within 2 years of the onset of the disease. Other gastrointestinal complications include hemorrhage of the upper and lower bowel, gastric ulceration, and malabsorption (Degos, 1979).

About 17–19% of patients with MAP develop **neurologic complications** (Culicchia et al., 1962; Gever et al., 1962; Winklemann et al., 1963; Degos, 1979; Dastur et al., 1981; Label et al., 1983). Skin manifestations usually precede the neurologic illness by 3–4 years, but neurologic signs and symptoms occasionally are the first evidence of the disease

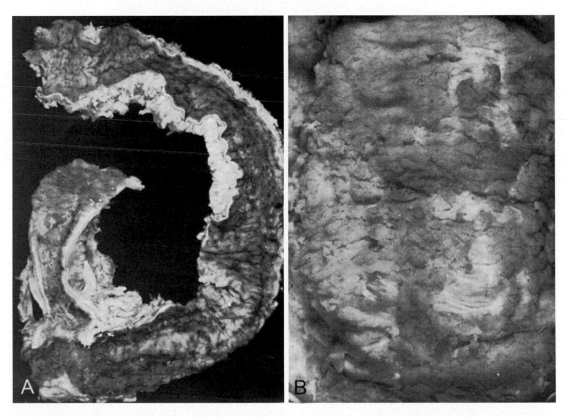

Figure 57.171. Ulcerative colitis. *A,* A view of the entire colon shows darker ulcerated lesions mainly in the cecal region. The pale areas are preserved mucosa. Note the accompanying disease in the terminal ileum. *B,* Magnified view of the ulcerations in chronic ulcerative colitis. The coalescence of numerous small ulcers has isolated islands of normal light-colored mucosa. (From Robbins SL. Pathology. 3rd ed, p 871. Philadelphia, WB Saunders, 1967.)

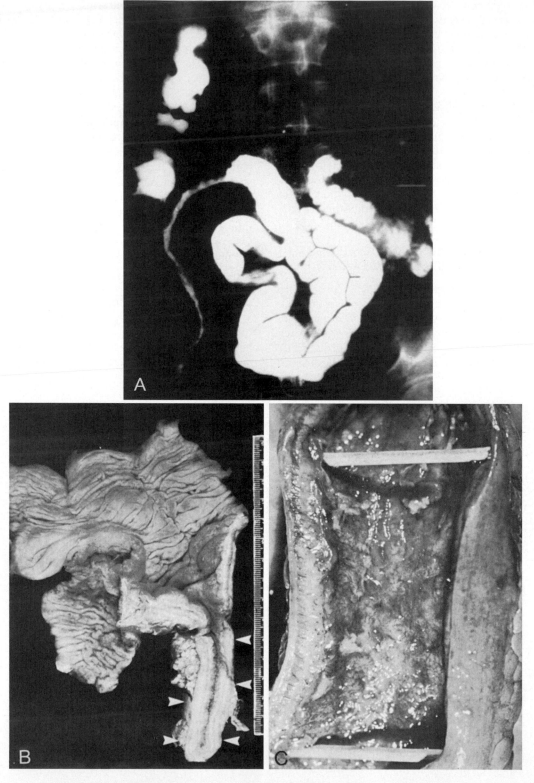

Figure 57.172. Crohn's disease (regional enteritis). *A*, Radiocontrast study shows typical "string" sign from narrowing of the lumen of the terminal ileum. (From Knox DL, Schachat AP, Mustonen E. Primary, secondary, and coincidental ocular complications of Crohn's disease. Ophthalmology *91:* 163–173, 1984.) *B*, Pathologic appearance of a specimen of bowel from a patient with Crohn's disease shows that the disease affects only the appendix and demonstrates the sharply delineated, marked thickening of the wall that is characteristic of the disorder *(arrowheads)*. *C*, Magnified view of a segment of affected bowel shows a markedly thickened wall associated with ulceration of the mucosa. Note that wooden pegs have been inserted to keep the lumen exposed. (*B* and *C*, from Robbins SL. Pathology. 3rd ed, p 851. Philadelphia, WB Saunders, 1967.)

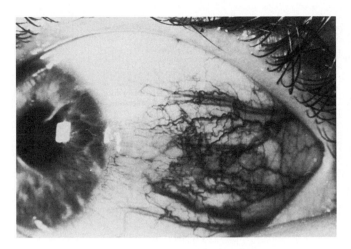

Figure 57.173. Episcleritis in Crohn's disease. (From Knox DL. Inflammatory bowel disease. In The Eye and Systemic Disease. Editors, Gold DH, Weingeist TA. pp 103–105. Philadelphia, JB Lippincott, 1990.)

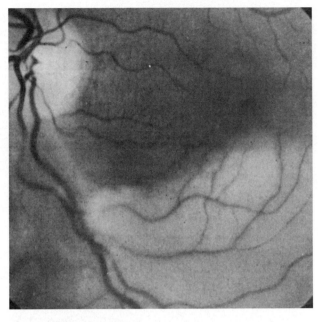

Figure 57.175. Branch retinal artery occlusion in inflammatory bowel disease. The patient was a 34-year-old man with a history of Crohn's disease affecting the jejunum, ileum, and colon who experienced acute visual loss in the left eye. The left ocular fundus shows retinal edema in the territory of the inferior temporal branch retinal artery. The patient had no other risk factors for retinal vascular occlusive disease. (From Schneiderman JH, Sharpe JA, Sutton DMC. Cerebral and retinal vascular complications of inflammatory bowel disease. Ann Neurol 5:331–337, 1979.)

(Burrow et al., 1991; Subbiah et al., 1996). Both the central and peripheral nervous systems may be affected, and monoparesis, hemiparesis, paraparesis, dysphasia, dementia, ataxia, cranial neuropathies, and polyradiculopathy can all

occur. The CSF in patients with neurologic manifestations of MAP consistently shows a markedly increased concentration of protein and a mild lymphocytosis; neuroimaging studies show nonspecific changes consistent with infarction, hemorrhage, or both; and cerebral angiography may show occlusion of distal arteries, arterial beading consistent with vasculitis, or normal findings (Petit et al., 1982).

Ophthalmologic signs and symptoms are uncommon in patients with MAP but may result from occlusion of ocular, orbital, or intracranial arteries and veins (Case Records of the Massachusetts General Hospital, 1980; Lee et al., 1984). Infarction of the bulbar conjunctiva is probably the most common ocular disturbance, but choroidal infarction, ischemic optic neuropathy, papilledema, ophthalmoparesis from ocular motor nerve paresis, ptosis, and homonymous visual field defects all occur (Köhlmeier, 1941; Culicchia et al., 1962; Winkelmann et al., 1963; Burrow et al., 1991; Subbiah et al., 1996).

The manifestations of MAP result from occlusion of small and medium-sized arteries and veins. Occluded regions are characterized by endothelial cell swelling, intimal proliferation, and fibrin thrombi (Su et al., 1985; Molenaar et al., 1987; Subbiah et al., 1996). Some affected vessels also show evidence of a necrotizing vasculitis, but this is an unusual finding.

The cause of MAP is unknown. It may be an immune disorder because similar skin lesions are occasionally ob-

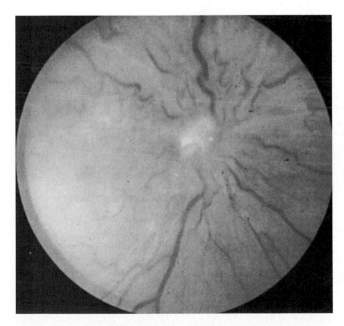

Figure 57.174. Anterior optic neuritis in inflammatory bowel disease. The patient was a 32-year-old woman with gastrointestinal symptoms for 12 years associated with intermittent blurred vision in the right eye. Ileal resection for intestinal obstruction confirmed the diagnosis of Crohn's disease. Visual acuity was 8/200 OD. The right optic disc is swollen, and there is exudative detachment of the peripapillary retina. The optic neuritis resolved when the patient's gastrointestinal disease was treated with a combination of systemic corticosteroids, sulfasalazine (Azulfidine), and diphenoxylate (Lomotil). (From Knox DL, Schachat AP, Mustonen E. Primary, secondary, and coincidental ocular complications of Crohn's disease. Ophthalmology 91:163–173, 1984.)

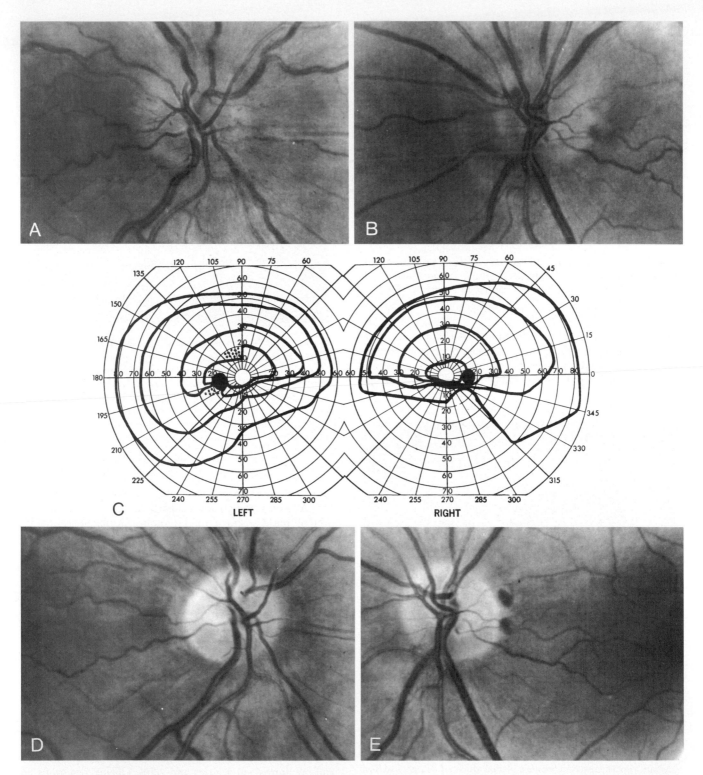

Figure 57.176. Bilateral anterior ischemic optic neuropathy in inflammatory bowel disease. The patient was a 24-year-old man with Crohn's disease who experienced sudden blurred vision in the inferior field of the right eye. Visual acuity was 20/30 OD and 20/25 OS. Color vision was mildly diminished in the right eye but was normal in the left eye. There was a right relative afferent pupillary defect. *A*, The right optic disc is hyperemic and swollen. A few nerve fiber layer hemorrhages are seen in the peripapillary region. *B*, The left optic disc also is mildly hyperemic and swollen. *C*, Kinetic perimetry demonstrates bilateral inferior altitudinal visual field defects. *D*, 3 weeks after the onset of visual symptoms, the right optic disc is pale, especially superiorly. There is mild periarteriolar and venular sheathing. *E*, The left optic disc also is pale superiorly. Note slight narrowing of the superior retinal arteries and generalized loss of the superior nerve fiber layer. (From Heuer DK, Gager WE, Reeser FH. Ischemic optic neuropathy associated with Crohn's disease. J Clin Neuroophthalmol 2:175–181, 1982.)

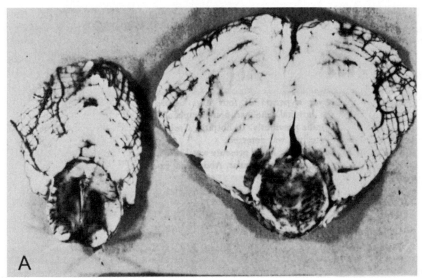

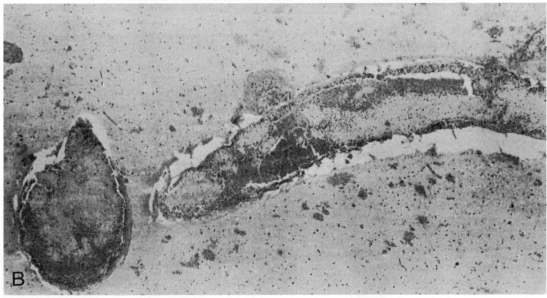

Figure 57.177. Ischemic neurologic complications of inflammatory bowel disease. The patient was a 12-year-old girl with ulcerative colitis who developed a generalized seizure followed by nausea and vomiting. She had a right homonymous hemianopia that cleared within 24 hours. Cerebral angiography showed a filling defect in the distal basilar artery extending into the left posterior cerebral artery. She died 11 days later after experiencing a grand mal seizure followed by a cardiorespiratory arrest. *A*, Hemorrhagic infarction of mesencephalic tegmentum and peduncles (*left*) and pons (*right*). *B*, Section through affected cerebral cortex shows thrombus in the cerebral veins, with infarction and hemorrhage of the cortex. The vessel walls are normal. (From Schneiderman JH, Sharpe JA, Sutton DMC. Cerebral and retinal vascular complications of inflammatory bowel disease. Ann Neurol 5:331–337, 1979.)

served in patients with connective tissue diseases such as SLE and scleroderma (Doutre et al., 1987); however, most of the skin lesions of MAP show no immunofluorescence when tested for immune complexes. In addition, most patients have no hematologic abnormalities, a normal ESR, and no ANAs (Molenaar et al., 1987). The observation of structures resembling the nucleocapsids of myxoviruses in endothelial cells and fibroblasts using electron microscopy suggests that at least some cases of MAP are caused by infection with one or more viruses (Degos, 1979; Case Records of the Massachusetts General Hospital, 1980).

There is no effective treatment for MAP. A variety of antibiotics, anticoagulants, platelet inhibitors, and immunosuppressive agents have been used with little or no effect on the progression of the disease. The median survival of patients with MAP is less than 2 years, although some women with isolated skin lesions may live 10 years or longer. Most deaths are caused by perforation of the small intestine. Other causes of death include respiratory failure, pericarditis, and stroke (Case Records of the Massachusetts General Hospital, 1980).

IDIOPATHIC RETINAL VASCULITIS

Retinal vasculitis may be a manifestation of most of the systemic disorders discussed in this chapter. In many of these cases, the patients are known to have an underlying systemic disease at the time the retinal vasculitis is discovered; in others, the retinal findings are the initial manifestation of the systemic disease. In some patients, however, retinal vasculitis occurs as an isolated phenomenon unassociated with any systemic or neurologic disease (Orzalesi and Ricciardi, 1971; Blumenkrantz et al., 1988; Souza Ramalho et al., 1988; Graham et al., 1989) (Fig. 57.178).

Idiopathic retinal vasculitis occurs in both men and women. There is a wide age range, but most patients are 15–50 years old (Blumenkrantz et al., 1988; Graham et al., 1989). The vasculitis usually affects both eyes, although the involvement may be asymmetric.

Graham et al. (1989) described 150 patients with retinal vasculitis, of whom 83 (55%) had evidence of underlying systemic disease, including Behçet's disease, sarcoidosis, uveomeningitis, seronegative spondyloarthropathy, polyarteritis nodosa, SLE, and Wegener's granulomatosis. The remaining 67 patients had no evidence of systemic or neuro-logic disease, either at the time the retinal vasculitis developed or over a follow-up period. The characteristics of the retinal vasculitis in these patients included peripheral vascular sheathing, macular edema, and diffuse capillary leakage. Venous and arterial occlusions, macular edema, and retinal infiltrates were less common. Most of the patients retained good vision. About two-thirds retained visual acuity of 20/60 or better in at least one eye, and only 22% had visual acuity worse than 20/60 in both eyes.

Blumenkrantz et al. (1988) reported seven patients with a more severe retinal vasculitis than that generally seen in the patients reported by Graham et al. (1989). The patients described by Blumenkrantz et al. (1988) had mild anterior uveitis, multifocal retinal vasculitis, retinal capillary nonperfusion, retinal hemorrhages, vitritis, and optic disc swelling. Blumenkrantz et al. (1988) suggested that these patients had a localized ocular form of Behçet's disease, infection with a herpes group virus other than varicella zoster virus, or a manifestation of an undefined infectious agent.

Many patients with presumed idiopathic retinal vasculitis may actually have an underlying systemic infectious or inflammatory disorder that simply has not been diagnosed at the time of the onset of the vasculitis and that remains undiagnosed throughout the period of follow-up. A relationship to MS may also exist, particularly in patients with purely venous involvement. Among 10 patients with a positive family history of MS or the HLA-B7 hapolotype who underwent

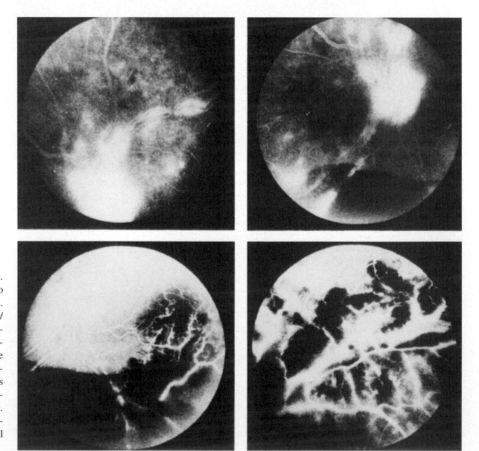

Figure 57.178. Idiopathic retinal vasculitis. The patient was a 56-year-old healthy man who developed severe loss of vision in both eyes. Visual acuity was light perception OD and 20/200 OS. Fluorescein angiography shows evidence of retinal vasculitis, with staining of vessel walls, areas of fluorescein leakage, multiple branch vessel occlusions, and areas of nonperfusion of the retina. A complete evaluation in this patient revealed nonspecific hematologic disturbances but no evidence of systemic disease. (From de Souza Ramalho P, Hormigo A, Martins R, et al. Hematological changes in retinal vasculitis. Eye 2:278–282, 1988.)

brain MR imaging, three had abnormal findings, with two patients showing extensive white matter changes (Gass et al., 1995). In another study, 32 of 67 patients with isolated idiopathic retinal vasculitis followed for 5 years developed systemic disease (Palmer et al., 1995). Thirteen patients in this group were diagnosed with MS. Thus, a small but potentially significant percentage of patients with presumed idiopathic retinal vasculitis demonstrate the same MR imaging changes that are observed in patients with MS (see Chapter 71).

Some patients with idiopathic retinal vasculitis harbor anticardiolipin antibodies, autoantibodies to endothelial cells, or both types of antibodies. It is unclear what role (if any) these autoantibodies play in the pathogenesis of this condition (Edelstein et al., 1992; Klok et al., 1992). In other patients, however, there is strong evidence that idiopathic retinal vasculitis is a localized, immune-mediated disorder. Kasp et al. (1989) found antiretinal antibodies in the serum of 33 of 63 patients (52%) with idiopathic retinal vasculitis, circulating immune complexes in 25 of these 63 patients (40%), and both antiretinal antibodies and circulating immune complexes in 14 patients (22%).

There is no standard treatment regimen for idiopathic retinal vasculitis. Most patients who require therapy respond to high-dose corticosteroids, whereas others need the addition of an immunosuppressive agent (Howe et al., 1994).

REFERENCES

Abdalla MI, Bahgat NED. Long-lasting remission of Behçet's disease after chlorambucil therapy. Br J Ophthalmol 57:706–711, 1973.

Abramsky O, Slavin S. Neurologic manifestations in patients with mixed cryoglobulinemia. Neurology 24:245–249, 1974.

Abramsky O, Melemed E, Sofer S. Involvement of nervous system in lupus erythematosus. Harefuah 83:313–316, 1972.

Abu-Shakra M, Khraishi M, Grosman H, et al. Primary angiitis of the CNS diagnosed by angiography. Q J Med 87:351–358, 1994a.

Abu-Shakra M, Urowitz MD, Gladmann DD. Improved survival in a cohort of SLE patients compared to the general population over a 25 year period of observation. Arthritis Rheum 37(suppl 9) (letter):S216, 1994b.

Abu-Shakra M, Urowitz MB, Gladmann DD, et al. Mortality studies systemic studies in systemic lupus erythematosus: Results from a single center. II. Predictor variables for mortality. J Rheumatol 22:1265–1270, 1995a.

Abu-Shakra MD, Urowitz MB, Gladmann DD, et al. Mortality studies in SLE: Results from a single center. I. Cases of death. J Rheumatol 22:1259–1264, 1995b.

Achkar AA, Lie JT, Hunder GG, et al. How does previous corticosteroid treatment affect the biopsy findings in giant (temporal) cell arteritis? Ann Intern Med 120:987–992, 1994.

Adams S. The genuine works of Hippocrates. Translated from Greek. A preliminary discourse and annotations. Epidemics III. 403, 1849.

Adamson TC III, Fox RI, Frisman DM, et al. Immunohistologic analysis of lymphoid infiltrates in primate Sjögren's syndrome using monoclonal antibodies. J Immunol 130:203–208, 1983.

Adinolfi M, Lehner T. Acute phase proteins and C9 in patients with Behçet's syndrome and aphthous ulcers. Clin Exp Immunol 25:36–39, 1976.

Agatston HJ. Scleroderma with retinopathy. Am J Ophthalmol 36:120–121, 1953.

Ahmadieh H, Roodpeyma S, Azarmina M, et al. Bilateral simultaneous optic neuritis in childhood systemic lupus erythematosus. J Neuroophthalmol 14:84–86, 1994.

Aiello PD, Trautman JD, McPhee TJ, et al. Visual prognosis in giant cell arteritis. Ophthalmology 100:550–555, 1993.

Alarcón-Segovia D, Delezé M, Oria CV, et al. Antiphospholipid antibodies and the antiphospholipid syndrome in systemic lupus erythematosus. A prospective analysis of 500 consecutive patients. Medicine 68:353–365, 1989.

Albert DM, Ruchman MC, Keltner JL. Skip areas in temporal arteritis. Arch Ophthalmol 94:2072–2077, 1976.

Albert DM, Searl SS, Craft JL. Histologic and ultrastructural characteristics of temporal arteritis. The value of the temporal artery biopsy. Ophthalmology 89:1111–1126, 1982.

Alberts AR, Lasonde R, Ackerman KR, et al. Reversible monocular blindness complicating Churg-Strauss syndrome. J Rheumatol 21:363–365, 1994.

Albrite JP, Resnick DM. Cogan's syndrome: Case presentations. Arch Otolaryngol 74:501–506, 1961.

Alexander EL. Neurologic disease in Sjögren's syndrome: mononuclear inflammatory vasculopathy affecting central/peripheral nervous system and muscle: A clinical review and update of immunopathogenesis. Rheum Dis Clin North Am 19:869–908, 1993.

Alexander EL, Alexander GE. Central nervous system (CNS) disease in primary Sjögren's syndrome (SS): Association with vasculitis and antibodies to Ro (SS-A). Arthritis Rheum. 25:S15, 1982.

Alexander EL, Alexander GE. Aseptic meningoencephalitis in primary Sjögren's syndrome. Neurology 33:593–598, 1983.

Alexander EL, McFarland H. Sjögren's syndrome mimicking multiple sclerosis. Ann Neurol 27:587, 1990.

Alexander EL, Provost TT, Stevens MB, et al. Neurologic complications of primary Sjögren's syndrome. Medicine 61:247–257, 1982a.

Alexander EL, Craft C, Dorsch C, et al. Necrotizing arteritis and spinal subarachnoid hemorrhage in Sjögren syndrome. Ann Neurol 11:632–635, 1982b.

Alexander EL, Beall SS, Provost TT, et al. Magnetic resonance imaging (MRI) in primary Sjögren's syndrome with CNS disease (CNS-SS). New clues to pathogenesis. Arthritis Rheum 29:S63, 1986a.

Alexander EL, Malinow K, Lejewski JE, et al. Primary Sjögren's syndrome with central nervous system disease mimicking multiple sclerosis. Ann Intern Med 104:323–330, 1986b.

Alexander GE, Provost TT, Stevens MB, et al. Sjögren syndrome: Central nervous system manifestations. Neurology 31:1391–1396, 1981.

Alhalabi M, Moore PM. Serial angiography in isolated angiitis of the CNS. Neurology 44:1221–1226, 1994.

Allen DM, Diamond LK, Howell DA. Anaphylactoid purpura in children (Schönlein-Henoch syndrome): Review with a follow-up of the renal complications. Am J Dis Child 99:833–854, 1960.

Allen IV, Miller JHD, Kirk J, et al. Systemic lupus erythematosus clinically resembling multiple sclerosis and with unusual pathological and ultrastructural features. J Neurol Neurosurg Psychiatr 42:392–401, 1979.

Allen JC, France TD. Pseudotumor as presenting sign of Wegener's granulomatosis in a child. J Pediatr Ophthalmol 14:158–159, 1977.

Allen NB. Wegener's granulomatosis: In Cecil Textbook of medicine. Editors, Bennett JC, Plum F, 20th ed, pp 1495–1498. Philadelphia, WB Saunders, 1996.

Allsop CJ, Gallagher PJ. Temporal artery biopsy in giant-cell arteritis: A reappraisal. Am J Surg Pathol 5:317–323, 1981.

Althaus C, Unsold R, Figge C, et al. Cerebral complications in acute posterior multifocal placoid pigment epitheliopathy. Germ J Ophthalmol 2:150–154, 1993.

Amalric P. Le territoire chooriorétininen de l'artère cilaire 1ongue postérieure. Etude clinique. Bull Soc Ophtalmol Fr 63:342, 1963.

Amalric P. Acute choroidal ischemia. Trans Ophthalmol Soc UK 91:305–322, 1971.

Anderson B. Ocular lesions in relapsing polychondritis and other rheumatoid syndromes. Am J Ophthalmol 64:35–50, 1967.

Anderson JM, Jamieson DG, Jefferson JM. Non-healing granuloma and the nervous system. Q J Med 44:309–323, 1975.

Andersson R, Malmvall B-E, Bentsson B-A. Long-term survival in giant cell arteritis including temporal arteritis and polymyalgia rheumatica. Acta Med Scand 220:361–364, 1986.

Andrews RS, McIntosh J, Petts V, et al. Circulating immune complexes in retinal vasculitis. Clin Exp Immunol 29:23–29, 1977.

Andrews JM. Giant cell (temporal) arteritis. Neurology 16:963–967, 1966.

Andrianakos AA, Duffy J, Suzuki M, et al. Transverse myelopathy in systemic lupus erythematosus. Ann Intern Med 83:616–624, 1975.

Ansell BM. Henoch-Schönlein purpura with particular reference to the prognosis of the renal lesion. Br J Dermatol 82:211–215, 1970.

Ansell BM. Management of polymyositis and dermatomyositis. Clin Rheum Dis 10:205–213, 1984.

Antes U, Heinz H-P, Loos M. Evidence for the presence of autoantibodies to the collagen-like portion of C1q in systemic lupus erythematosus. Arthritis Rheum 31:457–464, 1988.

Aoi K, Kurata N, Yamana S. Beneficial effects of plasma exchange on ocular lesions of a patient with Behçet's disease. Ther Plasmapheresis 3:425–428, 1983.

Appen RE, Wray SH, Cogan DG. Central retinal artery occlusion. Am J Ophthalmol 79:374–381, 1975.

April RS, Vansonnenberg E. A case of neuromyelitis optica (Devic's syndrome) in systemic lupus erythematosus. Clinicopathologic report and review of the literature. Neurology 26:1066–1070, 1976.

Arber N, Klein T, Meiner Z, et al. Case association of HLA B51 and B52 in Israeli patients with Behçet's syndrome. Ann Rheum Dis 50:351–353, 1991.

Armstrong RD, Behn A, Myles A, et al. Histocompatibility antigens in polymyalgia rheumatica and giant cell arteritis. J Rheumatol 10:659–661, 1983.

Arnett FC. The spondylarthropathies. In Rheumatic Diseases: Rehabilitation and Management. Editors, Riggs GK, Gall EP, pp 429–437. Woburn, MA, Butterworth, 1984.

Arnett FC. Seronegative spondylarthropathies. Bull Rheum Dis 37:1–12, 1987.

Arnett FC. The Lyme spirochete: Another cause of Reiter's syndrome? Arthritis Rheum 32:1182–1184, 1989.

Arnett FC, Reveille JD, Wilson RW, et al. Systemic lupus erythematosus. Current state of the genetic hypothesis. Semin Arthritis Rheum 14:24–35, 1984.

Arruda WO, Teive HAG, Ramina R, et al. Autonomic neuropathy in systemic lupus erythematosus. J Neurol Neurosurg Psychiatry 52:539–547, 1989.

Arruga J, Vidaller A, Carrera M, et al. Bilateral retrobulbar optic neuritis in Wegener's granulomatosis. Presented at the VIIIth International Neuro-Ophthalmology Symposium. Winchester, England. June 23–29, 1990.

Arthur G, Margolis G. Mycoplasma-like structures in granulomatous angiitis of the central nervous system. Case reports with light and electron microscopic studies. Arch Pathol Lab Med 101:382–387, 1977.

Asherson RA, Merry P, Acheson JF, et al. Antiphospholipid antibodies: A risk factor for occlusive ocular vascular disease in systemic lupus erythematosus and the primary antiphospholipid syndrome. Ann Rheum 48:358–361, 1989a.

Asherson RA, Baguley E, Khamashta MA, et al. Multiple small-vessel occlusions in systemic lupus erythematosus. Stroke 20:127–128, 1989b.

Ashton N, Cook C. Allergic granulomatous nodules of the eyelid and conjunctiva. The XXXVth Edward Jackson Memorial Lecture. Am J Ophthalmol 87:1–28, 1978.

Ashton N, Coomes EN, Garner A, et al. Retinopathy due to progressive systemic sclerosis. J Pathol Bacteriol 96:259–268, 1968.

Ashworth B, Tait GBW. Trigeminal neuropathy in connective tissue disease. Neurology 21:609–614, 1971.

Ask-Upmark E. On the pulseless disease outside of Japan. Acta Med Scand 149:161–178, 1954.

Ask-Upmark E. On the pathogenesis of hypertension in Takayasu's syndrome. Acta Med Scand 169:467–477, 1961.

Askari A, Jolobe OMP, Shepherd DI. Internuclear ophthalmoplegia and Horner's syndrome due to presumed giant cell arteritis. J R Soc Med 86:362, 1993.

Atkinson RA, Appenzeller O. Headache in small vessel disease of brain: A study of patients with systemic lupus erythematosus. Headache 15:198–201, 1975.

Atmaca LS. Fundus changes associated with Behçet's disease. Graefe's Arch Clin Exp Ophthalmol 227:340–344, 1989.

Atmaca LS. Experience with photocoagulation in Behçet's disease. Ophthalmic Surg 21:571–576, 1990.

Atmaca LS, Batioglu F. The efficacy of cyclosporin-a in the treament of Behçet's disease. Ophthalmic Surg 25:321–327, 1994.

Attwood W, Poser CM. Neurologic complications of Sjögren's syndrome. Neurology 11:1034–1041, 1961.

Austin HA III, Muenz LR, Joyce KM, et al. Prognostic factors in lupus nephritis. Contribution of renal histologic data. Am J Med 75:382–391, 1983.

Austin HA III, Muenz LR, Joyce KM, et al. Diffuse proliferative lupus nephritis: Identification of specific pathologic features affecting renal outcome. Kidney Int 25:689–695, 1984.

Austin P, Green WR, Salyer DC, et al. Peripheral corneal degeneration and occlusive vasculitis in Wegener's granulomatosis. Am J Ophthalmol 85:311–317, 1978.

Azar P Jr, Gohd RS, Waltman D, et al. Acute posterior multifocal placoid pigment epitheliopathy associated with an adenovirus type 5 infection. Am J Ophthalmol 80:1003–1005, 1975.

Baba S, Moriota S. Treatment of intestinal Behçet's disease. In Behçet's Disease: Pathogenetic Mechanism and Clinical Future. Editor, Inaba G, pp 559–570. Tokyo, University of Tokyo Press, 1982.

Bachmeyer C, Zuber M, Dupont S, et al. Adie syndrome as the initial sign of primary Sjögren syndrome. Am J Ophthalmol 123:691–692, 1997.

Bailey A, Sayer GT, Clark EC. Neuritis associated with systemic lupus erythematosus. Arch Neurol Psychiatr 75:251–259, 1956.

Baker K, Jewell DD. Cyclosporin for the treatment of severe inflammatory bowel disease. Aliment Pharmacol Ther 3:143–149, 1989.

Baker RS, Robertson WC Jr. Acquired Duane's retraction syndrome in a patient with rheumatoid arthritis. Ann Ophthalmol 12:269–272, 1980.

Ballard E, Butzer J, Donders J. Susac's syndrome: Neuropsychological characteristics in a young man. Neurology 47:266–268, 1996.

Ballou SP, Muhammad AK, Kushner I. Giant-cell arteritis in a black patient. Ann Intern Med 88:659–660, 1978.

Bank H. Thrombotic pulmonary manifestations in Behçet's syndrome. Israel J Med Sci 9:955, 1973.

Bank I, Weart C. Dural sinus thrombosis in Behçet's disease. Arthritis Rheum 27:816–818, 1984.

Bankhurst AD, Carlow TJ, Reidy RW. Exophthalmos in systemic lupus erythematosus. Ann Ophthalmol 16:669–671, 1984.

Banks PM, Cohen MD, Ginsburg WW, et al. Immunohistologic and cytochemical studies of temporal arteritis. Arthritis Rheum 26:1201–1207, 1983.

Banna A, El-Ramahi K. Neurologic involvement in Behçet disease: Imaging findings in 16 patients. AJNR. 12:791–796, 1991.

Baricordi OR, Sensi A, Pivetti-Pezzi P, et al. Behçet's disease associated with HLA-B51 and DRw52 antigens in Italians. Hum Immunol 17:297–301, 1986.

Barker RA, Bloom SR, Oakley CM, et al. The heart in systemic lupus erythematosus. A cause of myocardial infarction in a man of 20. Br Med J 299:245–247, 1989.

Barnett EV, Bluestone R, Cracchiolo A, et al. Cryoglobulinemia and disease. Ann Intern Med 73:95–107, 1970.

Baron M, Small P. Polymyositis/dermatomyositis: Clinical features and outcome in 22 patients. J Rheumatol 12:283–286, 1985.

Barricks MR, Travisa DB, Glaser JS, et al. Ophthalmoplegia in cranial arteritis. Brain 100:209–221, 1977.

Barrier J, Pion P, Massari R, et al. Epidemiologic approach to Horton's disease in Department of Loire-Atlantique: 110 cases in 10 years (1970–1979). Rev Med Interne 3:13–20, 1983.

Barth WF, Berson EL. Relapsing polychondritis, rheumatoid arthritis and blindness. Am J Ophthalmol 66:890–896, 1968.

Bates JH. Ocular pneumoplethysmography in giant-cell arteritis. Arch Ophthalmol 107:1279, 1989.

Bates JH, Tomsak RL, Spedick MJ, et al. Serum fibrinogen concentration in the diagnosis and management of biopsy-proven giant-cell arteritis. Ophthalmology 96(suppl):105, 1989.

Baudelot J, Esteves A, Leroux G, et al. Exchange plasmatique chez une maladie de Behçet. Nouv Presse Med 8:3563–3564, 1979.

Beck DO, Corbett JJ. Seizures due to central nervous system rheumatoid meningovasculitis. Neurology 35:1058–1061, 1983.

Beck M, Hickling P. Treatment of bilateral superior oblique tendon sheath syndrome complicating rheumatoid arthritis. Br J Ophthalmol 64:358–361, 1980.

Bedell SE, Bush BT. Erythrocyte sedimentation rate. From folklore to facts. Am J Med 78:1001–1009, 1985.

Beevers DG, Harpur JE, Turk KAD. Giant cell arteritis—the need for prolonged treatment. J Chron Dis 26:571–584, 1973.

Behçet H. Über rezidivierende aphthöse, durch ein Virus verursachte Geschwüre am Mund, am Auge und an den Genitalien. Dermatol Monatsschr Wochenschr 105:1152–1157, 1937.

Behçet H. Einige Bemerkungen zu meinen Beobachtungen über den Tri-Symptomenkomplex. Med Welt 13:1222–1227, 1939.

Behçet H. Some observations on the clinical picture of the so-called triple symptom complex. Dermatologica 81:73–83, 1940.

Beighton P, Gumpel JM, Kornes NGM. Prodromal trigeminal sensory neuropathy in progressive systemic sclerosis. Ann Rheum Dis 27:367–369, 1968.

Belden CJ, Hamed LM, Mancuso AA. Bilateral isolated retrobulbar optic neuropathy in limited Wegener's granulomatosis. J Clin Neuroophthalmol 13:119–123, 1993.

Bell TAG, Gibson RA, Tullo AB. A case of giant-cell arteritis and Horner's syndrome. Scott Med J 25:302, 1980.

Belmont JB, Michelson JB. Vitrectomy in uveitis associated with ankylosing spondylitis. Am J Ophthalmol 94:300–304, 1982.

Benbassat J, Gefel D, Larholt K, et al. Prognostic factors in polymyositis/dermatomyositis: A computer-assisted analysis of ninety-two cases. Arthritis Rheum 28:249–255, 1985.

Benedict WL. Schönlein-Henoch's purpura with intraocular hemorrhage and iritis. Report of a case. JAMA 95:1577–1579, 1930.

Benezra D, Cohen E. Treatment and visual prognosis in Behçet's disease. Br J Ophthalmol 70:589–592, 1986.

Bengtsson BA, Malmvall BE. The epidemiology of giant cell arteritis including temporal arteritis and polymyalgia rheumatica: Incidences of different clinical presentations and eye complications. Arthritis Rheum 24:899–904, 1981.

Ben-Itzhak J, Keren S, Simon J. Intracranial venous thrombosis in Behçet's syndrome. Neuroradiology 27:450–451, 1985.

Benlahrache C, Segond P, Anquier L, et al. Decrease of OKT8 positive T cell subset in polymyalgia rheumatica. Lack of correlation with disease activity. Arthritis Rheum 26:1472–1480, 1983.

Bennett AG. An unusual ophthalmic appliance. The Optician 144:291, 1962.

Bennett G. Cortisone therapy at visual loss in temporal arteritis. Br J Ophthalmol 40:430–433, 1956.

Bennett R, Hughes GR, Bywaters EG, et al. Neuropsychiatric problems in systemic lupus erythematosus. Br Med J 4:342–345, 1972.

Bennett RM. Mixed connective tissue disease and other overlap syndromes. In Textbook of Rheumatology. Editors, Kelley WN, Harris ED Jr, Ruddy S, et al, 3rd ed, pp 1147–1166. Philadelphia, WB Saunders, 1989.

Bergaust B, Abrahamsen AM. Relapsing polychondritis: Report of a case presenting multiple ocular complications. Acta Ophthalmol 47:174–181, 1969.

Bernard H, Rambert P, Pestel M. Arterite temporale et complications oculaire. Bull Mem Soc Med Paris 65:1271–1274, 1951.

Berrenti S, Segini G, Bruschini P, et al. Lethal midline granuloma: Rev Laryngol Otol Rhinol 114:37–42, 1993.

Bethlenfalvay NC, Nusynowitz ML. Temporal arteritis: A rarity in the young adult. Arch Intern Med 114:487–489, 1964.

Bettelheim A. Die acute Ophthalmomalacia eine Folgerscheinung der arteriitis cranialis. Graefe's Arch Klin Exp Ophthalmol 174:359–366, 1968.

Bettman JW Jr, Daroff RB, Sanders MD, et al. Papilledema and asymptomatic intracranial hypertension in systemic lupus erythematosus. A fluorescein angiographic study of resolving papilledema. Arch Ophthalmol 80:189–193, 1968.

Bewermeyer H, Nelles G, Huber M, et al. Pontine infarction in acute posterior multifocal placoid pigment epitheliopathy. J Neurol 241:22–26, 1993.

Bianchi Porro G, Petrillo M, Ardizzone S. Cyclosporin treatment for severe active ulcerative colitis. Lancet 336:439, 1990.

Bick RL, Baker WF. The antiphospholipid and thrombosis syndromes. Med Clin North Am 78:667–682, 1994.

Bicknell JM, Holland JV. Neurologic manifestations of Cogan syndrome. Neurology 28:278–281, 1978.

Bielschowsky A. Über Lahmungen des Musculus oblique inferior. Graefes Arch Ophthalmol 58:369–390, 1904.

Bienenstock H, Margulies ME. Behçet's syndrome: Report of a case with extensive neurologic manifestations. N Engl J Med 264:1342–1345, 1961.

Bienfang DC. Loss of the ocular pulse in the acute phase of temporal arteritis. Acta Ophthalmol 67(suppl 191):35–37, 1989.

Bilaniuk LT, Patel S, Zimmerman RA. Central nervous system disease in systemic lupus erythematosus. Radiology 124:119–121, 1977.

Biller J, Asconapé J, Weinblatt ME, et al. Temporal arteritis associated with a normal sedimentation rate. JAMA 247:486–487, 1982.

Biller J, Loftus CM, Moore SA, et al. Isolated central nervous system angiitis first presenting as spontaneous intracranial hemorrhage. Neurosurgery 20:310–315, 1987.

Billingsley LM, Yannakakis GD, Stevens MB. Evoked potentials (EPs): A sensitive test for CNS-SLE. Arthritis Rheum 28:S22, 1985.

Billson FA, DeDombal FT, Watkinson G, et al. Ocular complications of ulcerative colitis. Gut 8:102–106, 1967.

Bird AC. Acute multifocal placoid pigment epitheliopathy. In Retina. Editors, Schachat AP, Murphy RP, Patz A, Vol 2, pp 1713–1720. St Louis, CV Mosby, 1994.

Bird AC, Hamilton AM. Placoid pigment epitheliopathy presenting with bilateral serous retinal detachment. Br J Ophthalmol 56:881–886, 1972.

Birkhead NC, Wagener HP, Shick RM. Treatment of temporal arteritis with adrenal corticosteroids. JAMA 163:821–827, 1957.

Bishko F. Retinopathy in systemic lupus erythematosus: A case report and review of the literature. Arthritis Rheum 15:57–63, 1972.

Bitnum S, Daeschner CW, Travis LB, et al. Dermatomyositis. J Pediatr 64:101–131, 1964.

Black CM, Welsh KI, Fielder A, et al. HLA antigens and Bf allotypes in SLE: Evidence for the association being with specific haplotypes. Tissue Antigens 19:115–120, 1982.

Bloch KJ, Buchanan WW, Wohl MJ, et al. Sjögren's syndrome: A clinical, pathological, and serological study of sixty-two cases. Medicine 44:187–231, 1965.

Block SR, Winfield JB, Lockshin MD, et al. Twin studies in systemic lupus erythematosus. A review of the literature and presentation of 12 additional sets. Am J Med 59:533–552, 1975.

Blodi FC, Gass JDM. Inflammatory pseudotumor of the orbit. Br J Ophthalmol 52:79–93, 1968.

Blodi FC, Sullivan PB. Involvement of the eyes in periarteritis nodosa. Trans Am Acad Ophthalmol Otolaryngol 63:161–165, 1959.

Bluestein HG. Neuropsychiatric disorders in systemic lupus erythematosus. In Systemic Lupus Erythematosus. Editor, Lahita RG, pp 593–614. New York, John Wiley & Sons, 1987.

Blumenkranz MS, Kaplan HJ, Clarkson JG, et al. Acute multifocal hemorrhagic retinal vasculitis. Ophthalmology 95:1663–1672, 1988.

Böck J. Ocular changes in periarteritis nodosa. Am J Ophthalmol 42:567–577, 1956.

Boesen P, Sorensen SF. Giant cell arteritis, temporal arteritis and polymyalgia rheumatica in a Danish county: A prospective investigation, 1982–1985. Arthritis Rheum 30:294–299, 1987.

Boey ML, Colaco CB, Gharavi AE, et al. Thrombosis in SLE: Striking association with the presence of circulating lupus anticoagulant. Br Med J 287:1021–1023, 1983.

Boghen DR, Glaser JS. Ischemic optic neuropathy. Brain 98:689–708, 1975.

Bogousslavksy J, Gaio J-M, Caplan LR, et al. Encephalopathy, deafness and blindness in young women: A distinct retinocochleocerebral arteriolopathy? J Neurol Neurosurg Psychiatry 52:43–46, 1989.

Bohan A, Peter JB, Bowman RL, et al. A computer-assisted analysis of 153 patients with polymyositis and dermatomyositis. Medicine 56:255–286, 1977.

Bonfiglio TA, Bolti RE, Hagstrom JWC. Coronary arteritis, occlusion and myocardial infarction due to lupus erythematosus. Am Heart J 83:153–158, 1972.

Bonnet M. Immunosuppressive therapy of Behçet's syndrome. Long-term follow-up evaluation. J F Ophtalmol 4:455–464, 1981.

Bonnet M, Ouzan D, Trepo Ch. Exchanges plasmatiques et acyclovir dans la maladie de Behçet. J Fr Ophtalmol 9:15–22, 1986.

Bosley TM, Savino PJ, Sergott RC, et al. Ocular pneumoplethysmography can help in the diagnosis of giant-cell arteritis. Arch Ophthalmol 107:379–381, 1989.

Böttiger LE, Svedberg CA. Normal erythrocyte sedimentation rate and age. Br Med J 2:85–87, 1967.

Bousser M-G. Cerebral vein thrombosis in Behçet's syndrome. Arch Neurol 39:322, 1982.

Bousser M-G, Chiras J, Bories J, et al. Cerebral venous thrombosis—a review of 38 cases. Stroke 16:199–213, 1985.

Boyd RV, Hoffbrand BI. Erythrocyte sedimentation rate in elderly hospital in-patients. Br Med J 1:901–902, 1966.

Boyev LR, Harris LL, Miller NR, et al. Efficacy of unilateral versus bilateral temporal artery biopsies in detecting temporal arteritis. Invest Ophthalmol Vis Sci 38:S382, 1997.

Bradley JD, Brandt KD, Katz BP. Infectious complications of cyclophosphamide treatment for vasculitis. Arthritis Rheum 32:45–53, 1989.

Branch CE Jr, Swift TR. Systemic lupus erythematosus, myasthenia gravis, and Ehlers-Danlos syndrome. Ann Neurol 4:374–375, 1978.

Brandt KD, Lessell S. Migrainous phenomena in systemic lupus erythematosus. Arthritis Rheum 21:7–16, 1978.

Brandt KD, Lessell S, Cohen AS. Cerebral disorders of vision in systemic lupus erythematosus. Ann Intern Med 83:163–169, 1975.

Brandwein S, Easdaile J, Danoff D, et al. Wegener's granulomatosis: Clinical features and outcome in 13 patients. Arch Intern Med 143:476–479, 1983.

Brazis DF, Menke DM, McLeish WM, et al. Angiocentric T cell lymphoma presenting with multiple cranial nerve palsies and retrobulbar optic neuropathy. J Neuroophthalmol 15:152–157, 1995.

Brennan J, McCrary JA III. Diagnosis of superficial temporal arteritis. Ann Ophthalmol 7:1125–1129, 1975.

Brenner EH, Shock JP. Proptosis secondary to systemic lupus erythematosus. Arch Ophthalmol 91:81–82, 1974.

Brezin AP, Massin-Korobelnik P, Boudin M, et al. Acute posterior placoid pigment epitheliopathy after hepatitis B vaccine. Arch Ophthalmol 113:297–300, 1995.

Bromfield EB, Slakter JS. Horner's syndrome in temporal arteritis. Arch Neurol 45:604, 1988.

Bron KM, Gajaraj A. Demonstration of hepatic aneurysms in polyarteritis nodosa by arteriography. N Engl J Med 282:1024–1025, 1970.

Bronster DJ, Rudolph SH, Shanzer S. Pupillary light-near dissociation in cranial arteritis. A case report. Neuro-ophthalmology 3:65–70, 1983.

Brouet JC, Clauvel JP, Danon F, et al. Biologic and clinical significance of cryoglobulins. A report of 86 cases. Am J Med 57:775–788, 1974.

Brown CH, Shirey EK, Haserick JR. Gastrointestinal manifestations of systemic lupus erythematosus. Gastroenterology 31:649–666, 1956.

Brown GC, Brown MM, Hiller T, et al. Cotton-wool spots. Retina 5:206–214, 1985.

Brown HV. Congenital structural muscle anomalies. In Symposium on Strabismus. Transactions of the New Orleans Academy of Ophthalmology, pp 205–236. St Louis, CV Mosby, 1950.

Brown HV. Congenital structural anoamlies of the muscles. In Strabismus: Ophthalmic Symposium II, pp 391–427. St Louis, CV Mosby, 1958.

Brown HV. Strabismus in the adult: Superior oblique tendon sheath syndrome. In Symposium on Strabismus: Transactions of the New Orleans Academy of Ophthalmology, pp 252–255. St Louis, CV Mosby, 1962.

Brown HV. True and simulated superior oblique tendon sheath syndromes. Doc Ophthalmol 34:123–136, 1973.

Brown HV. True and simulated superior oblique tendon sheath syndromes. Aust J Ophthalmol 2:12–19, 1974.

Brownstein S, Nicolle DA, Codère F. Bilateral blindness in temporal arteritis with skip areas. Arch Ophthalmol 101:388–391, 1983.

Brubaker R, Font RL, Shepherd EM. Granulomatous sclero-uveitis: Regression of ocular lesions with cyclophosphamide and prednisone. Arch Ophthalmol 86:517–524, 1971.

Bruce GM. Retinitis in dermatomyositis. Trans Am Ophthalmol Soc 36:282–297, 1938.

Bryant GL, Weinblatt ME, Rumbaugh C, et al. Cerebral vasculopathy: An analysis of sixteen cases. Semin Arthritis Rheum 15:297–302, 1986.

Buchanan RRC, Wardlaw JR, Riglar AG, et al. Antiphospholipid antibodies in the connective tissue diseases: Their relation to the antiphospholipid syndrome and forme fruste disease. J Rheumatol 16:757–761, 1989.

Budman DR, Steinberg AD. Hematologic aspects of systemic lupus erythematosus: Current concepts. Ann Intern Med 86:220–229, 1977.

Bugg EI, Coonrad RW, Grimm KB. Giant cell arteritis and acute hand syndrome. J Bone Joint Surg 45:1269, 1963.

Bull BS, Brailsford JD. The zeta sedimentation rate. Blood 40:550–559, 1972.

Bull BS, Westengard JC, Farr M, et al. Efficacy of tests used to monitor rheumatoid arthritis. Lancet 2:965–967, 1989.

Bullen CL, Liesegang TJ, McDonald TJ, et al. Ocular complications of Wegener's granulomatosis. Ophthalmology 90:279–290, 1983.

Bullock JD, Thomas ER, Fletechur RL. Cerebrospinal fluid abnormalities in acute posterior multifocal placoid pigment epitheliopathy. Am J Ophthalmol 84:45–49, 1977.

Bunch TW, Worthingon JW, Combs JJ, et al. Azathioprine with prednisone for polymyositis. A controlled, clinical trial. Ann Intern Med 92:365–369, 1980.

Burger PC, Burch JG, Vogel FS. Granulomatous angiitis, an unusual etiology of stroke. Stroke 8:29–35, 1977.

Burkhalter E. Unique presentation of systemic lupus erythematosus. Arthritis Rheum 16:428, 1973.

Burrow JN, Blumberg P, Iyer P, et al. Kohlmeier-Degos disease: A multisystem vasculopathy with progressive cerebral infarction. Aust NZ J Med 21:49–51, 1991.

Buskila D, Gladman D. Atlantoaxial subluxation in a patient with psoriatic arthritis. Arthritis Rheum 32:1338–1339, 1989.

Buttner T, Heye N, Pazuntek H. Temporal arteritis with cerebral complications: Report of four cases. Eur Neurol 34:162–167, 1994.

Buyon JP, Zuckerman JD. Articular manifestations of systemic lupus erythematosus. In Systemic Lupus Erythematosus. Editor, Lahita RG, pp 791–820. New York, John Wiley & Sons, 1987.

Byrd L, Shearn M, Tu WH. Relationship of lethal midline granuloma to Wegener's granulomatosis. Arthritis Rheum 12:247–253, 1969.

Cabral DA, Petty RE, Malleson PN, et al. Visual prognosis in children with chronic anterior uveitis and arthritis. J Rheumatol 21:2370–2375, 1994.

Caccamise WC, Okuda K. Takayasu or pulseless disease. Am J Ophthalmol 37: 784–786, 1954.

Calabrese LH, Duna GF. Evaluation and treatment of central nervous system vasculitis. Curr Opin Rheum 7:37–44, 1995.

Calabrese LH, Furlan AJ, Gragg LA, et al. Primary angiitis of the central nervous system: Diagnostic criteria and clinical approach. Cleve Clin J Med 59:293–306, 1992.

Calabrese LH, Gragg LA, Furlan AJ. Benign angiopathy: A distinct subset of angiographically defined primary angiitis of the central nervous system. J Rheumatol 20:2046–2050, 1993.

Calabro JJ, Parrino GR, Atchoo PD, et al. Chronic iridocyclitis in juvenile rheumatoid arthritis. Arthritis Rheum 13:406–413, 1970.

Calamia KT, Hunder GG. Clinical manifestations of giant cell (temporal) arteritis. Clin Rheum Dis 6:389–403, 1980.

Calamia KT, Hunder GG. Giant cell arteritis (temporal arteritis) presenting as fever of undetermined origin. Arthritis Rheum 24:1414–1418, 1981.

Calamia KT, Moore SB, Elveback LR, et al. HLA-DR locus antigens in polymyalgia rheumatica and giant cell arteritis. J Rheumatol 8:993–996, 1981.

Calin A. Ankylosing spondylitis. In Textbook of Rheumatology. Editors, Kelley WN, Harris ED Jr, Ruddy S, et al, 3rd ed, pp 1021–1037. Philadelphia, WB Saunders, 1989a.

Calin A. Is there an association between ankylosing spondylitis and multiple sclerosis? Ann Rheum Dis 48:971–972, 1989b.

Calin A. Reiter's syndrome. In Textbook of Rheumatology. Editors, Kelley WN, Harris ED Jr, Ruddy S, et al, 3rd ed, pp 1038–1052. Philadelphia, WB Saunders, 1989c.

Calin A, Marder A, Becks E, et al. Genetic differences between B27 positive patients with ankylosing spondylitis and B27 positive healthy controls. Arthritis Rheum 26:1460–1464, 1983.

Callen JP, Hyla JF, Bole GG Jr, et al. The relationship of dermatomyositis and polymyositis to internal malignancy. Arch Dermatol 116:295–298, 1980.

Campbell PM, LeRoy EC. Pathogenesis of systemic sclerosis: A vascular hypothesis. Semin Arthritis Rheum 4:351–368, 1975.

Canoso JJ, Cohen AS. Aseptic meningitis in systemic lupus erythematosus. Arthritis Rheum 18:369–374, 1975.

Caplan LR, Stein RW. Stroke: A Clinical Approach. London, Butterworths, 1986.

Cardell BS, Hanley T. A fatal case of giant-cell or temporal arteritis. J Pathol Bacteriol 63:587–597, 1951.

Carlow TJ. Papilledema in lupus erythematosus. In Neuro-ophthalmology Symposium of the University of Miami and the Bascom Palmer Eye Institute. Editors, Smith JL, Glaser JS, pp 124–125. St Louis, CV Mosby, 1973.

Carlow TJ, Glaser JS. Pseudotumor cerebri syndrome in systemic lupus erythematosus. JAMA 228:197–200, 1974.

Carrington CB, Liebow AA. Limited forms of angiitis and granulomatosis of Wegener's type. Am J Med 41:497–527, 1966.

Case records of the Massachusetts General Hospital. Weekly clinicopathologic exercises: Case 42211. N Engl J Med 254:998–1002, 1956.

Case records of the Massachusetts General Hospital. Weekly clinicopathologic exercises: Case 44-1980. N Engl J Med 303:1103–1111, 1980.

Case records of the Massachusetts General Hospital. Weekly clinicopathologic exercises: Case 11-1990. N Engl J Med 322:754–769, 1990.

Caselli RJ. Giant cell (temporal) arteritis: A treatable cause of multi-infarct dementia. Neurology 40:753–755, 1990.

Caselli RJ, Hunder GG. Neurologic aspects of giant cell (temporal) arteritis. Rheum Dis Clin North Am 19:941–953, 1993.

Caselli RJ, Daube JR, Hunder GG, et al. Peripheral neuropathic syndromes in giant cell (temporal) arteritis. Neurology 38:685–689, 1988a.

Caselli RJ, Hunder GG, Whisnant JP. Neurologic disease in biopsy-proven giant cell (temporal) arteritis. Neurology 38:352–359, 1988b.

Cassan SM, Coles DT, Harrison EG Jr. The concept of limited forms of Wegener's granulomatosis. Am J Med 49:366–379, 1970a.

Cassan SM, Divertie MB, Hollenhorst RW, et al. Pseudotumor of the orbit and limited Wegener's granulomatosis. Ann Intern Med 72:687–693, 1970b.

Casselman W, Majoor MHJM, Albers FW. MR of the inner ear in patients with Cogan syndrome. AJNR 15:131–138, 1994.

Cassidy JT. Systemic lupus erythematosis, juvenile dermatomyositis, scleroderma, and vasculitis. In Textbook of Rheumatology. Editors, Kelley WN, Harris ED Jr, Ruddy S, et al, 4th ed, pp 1077–1102. Philadelphia, WB Saunders, 1993.

Cazenave PLA. Lupus Erythemateux (Erythème Centrifuge). Ann Malad Peau Syph 3:297–299, 1851.

Chad D, Pariser K, Bradley WG, et al. The pathogenesis of cryoglobulinemic neuropathy. Neurology 32:725–729, 1982.

Chajek T, Fainaru M. Behçet's disease: Report of 41 cases and a review of the literature. Medicine 54:179–196, 1975.

Chalk CH, Homburger HA, Dyck PJ. Anti-neutrophil cytoplasmic antibodies in vasculitic peripheral neuropathy. Neurology 43:1826–1827, 1993.

Chamberlain MA. Behçet's syndrome in 32 patients in Yorkshire. Ann Rheum Dis 36:491–499, 1977.

Chamberlain MA. Behçet's disease. Br Med J 2:1969–1970, 1978.

Chamberlain MA, Noble B, Clarke MA. A combined ophthalmic-rheumatological clinic for Behçet's disease. Br J Rheumatol 27(suppl 1):64, 1988.

Chambers WA, Bernardino VB. Specimen length in temporal artery biopsies. J Clin Neuroophthalmol 8:121–125, 1988.

Chang DJ, Paget SA. Neurologic complications of rheumatoid arthritis. Rheum Dis Clin North Am 19:955–973, 1993.

Char DH, Cogan DG, Sullivan WR Jr. Immunologic study of nonsyphilitic interstitial keratitis with vestibuloauditory symptoms. Am J Ophthalmol 80:491–494, 1975.

Charteris DG, Khanna V, Dhillon B. Acute posterior multifocal placoid pigment epitheliopathy complicated by central retinal vein occlusion. Br J Ophthalmol 731: 765–768, 1989.

Charteris DG, Clamp C, Rosenthal AR, et al. Behçet's disease: Activated T lymphocytes in retinal perivasculitis. Br J Ophthalmol 76:499–501, 1992.

Chaudhuri KR, Taylor IK, Niven RM, et al. A case of systemic lupus erythematosus presenting as Guillain-Barré syndrome. Br J Rheumatol 28:440–442, 1989.

Chavis PS, Antonios S, Tabbara K. Effects of cyclosporin on the retinal and optic nerve vasculitis of Behçet's disease. Presented at the VIIIth International Neuro-Ophthalmology Symposium. Winchester, England. June 23–29, 1990.

Chavis PS, Antonios SR, Tabbara KF. Cyclosporine effects on optic nerve and retinal vasculitis in Behçet's disease. Doc Ophthalmol 80:133–142, 1992.

Cherin P, Herson S, Wechsler B, et al. Intravenous immunoglobulin for polymyositis and dermatomyositis. Lancet 336:116, 1990.

Cheson BD, Bluning WZ, Alroy J. Cogan's syndrome: A systemic vasculitis. Am J Med 60:549–555, 1976.

Chess J, Albert DM, Bhan AK, et al. Serologic and immunopathologic findings in temporal arteritis. Am J Ophthalmol 96:283–289, 1983.

Chisholm IH. Cortical blindness in cranial arteritis. Br J Ophthalmol 59:332–333, 1975.

Chow C-C, Li EKM, Lai FM-M. Allergic granulomatosis and angiitis (Churg-Strauss syndrome): Response to pulse intravenous cyclophosphamide. Ann Rheum Dis 48:605–608, 1989.

Christian CL. Etiologic hypotheses for systemic lupus erythematosus. In Systemic Lupus Erythematosus. Editor, Lahita RG, pp 65–80. New York, John Wiley & Sons, 1987.

Chuang TY, Hunder GG, Ilstrup DM, et al. Polymyalgia rheumatica: A 10-year epidemiological clinical study. Ann Intern Med 97:672–680, 1982.

Chumbley LC, Harrison EG, DeRemee RA. Allergic granulomatosis and angiitis (Churg-Strauss syndrome): Report and analysis of 30 cases. Mayo Clin Proc 52: 477–484, 1977.

Churg J, Strauss L. Allergic granulomatosis, allergic angiitis, and periarteritis nodosa. Am J Pathol 27:277–301, 1951.

Chylack LT Jr, Bienfang DC, Bellows AR, et al. Ocular manifestations of juvenile rheumatoid arthritis. Am J Ophthalmol 79:1026–1033, 1975.

Cinefro RJ, Frenkel M. Systemic lupus erythematosus presenting as optic neuritis. Ann Ophthalmol 10:559–563, 1978.

Cipoletti JF, Buckingham RB, Barnes EL, et al. Sjögren's syndrome in progressive systemic sclerosis. Ann Intern Med 87:535–541, 1977.

Cipriano PR, Alonso DR, Baltaxe HA, et al. Multiple aortic aneurysms in relapsing polychondritis. Am J Cardiol 37:1097–1102, 1976.

Cipriano PR, Silverman JF, Perlroth MG, et al. Coronary arterial narrowing in Takayasu's aortitis. Am J Cardiol 39:744–750, 1977.

Citron BP, Halpern M, McCarron M, et al. Necrotizing angiitis associated with drug abuse. N Engl J Med 283:1003–1011, 1970.

Clark AE, Victor WH. An unusual presentation of temporal arteritis. Ann Ophthalmol 19:343–346, 1987.

Clark JS. Purpura hemorrhagica of the Schönlein-Henoch type. Report of a case. Arch Ophthalmol 8:649–653, 1932.

Clearkin LG, Hung SO. Acute posterior multifocal placoid pigment epitheliopathy associated with transient hearing loss. Trans Ophthalmol Soc UK 103:562–564, 1983.

Clifford-Jones RE, Love S, Gurusinghe N. Granulomatous angiitis of the central nervous system: A case with recurrent intracerebral haemorrhage. J Neurol Neurosurg Psychiatry 48:1054–1056, 1985.

Clyde WA, Thomas L. Pathogenesis studies in experimental mycoplasma disease: M. gallisepticum infections in turkeys. Ann NY Acad Sci 225:413–424, 1973.

Cobo LM, Haynes BF. Early corneal findings in Cogan's syndrome. Ophthalmology 91:903–907, 1984.

Cochran JW, Fox JH, Kelly MD. Reversible mental symptoms in temporal arteritis. J Nerv Ment Dis 166:446–447, 1978.

Cody DTR, Sones DA. Relapsing polychondritis: Audiovestibular manifestations. Laryngoscope 81:1208–1222, 1971.

Cogan DG. Syndrome of nonsyphilitic interstitial keratitis and vestibulo-auditory symptoms. Arch Ophthalmol 33:144–149, 1945.

Cogan DG. Nonsyphilitic keratitis with vestibuloauditory symptoms. Arch Ophthalmol 42:42–49, 1949.

Cogan DG. Corneoscleral lesions in periarteritis nodosa and Wegener's granulomatosis. Trans Am Ophthalmol Soc 53:321–344, 1955.

Cogan DG. Visual hallucinations as release phenomena. Graefes Arch Klin Exp Ophthalmol 188:139–150, 1973.

Cogan DG. Discussion of Cobo L, Haynes BF. Early corneal findings in Cogan's syndrome. Ophthalmology 91:907, 1984.

Cogan DG, Dickersin GR. Non-syphilitic interstitial keratitis with vestibulo-auditory symptoms—a case with fatal aortitis. Trans Am Ophthalmol Soc *61*:113–121, 1963.

Cogan DG, Kubik CS, Smith JL. Unilateral internuclear ophthalmoplegia. Arch Ophthalmol *44*:783–796, 1950.

Cogen MS, Kline LB, Duvall ER. Bilateral internuclear ophthalmoplegia in systemic lupus erythematosus. J Clin Neuroophthalmol *7*:69–73, 1987.

Cohen AS, Reynolds WE, Franklin EC, et al. Preliminary criteria for the classification of systemic lupus erythematosus. Bull Rheum Dis *21*:643–648, 1975.

Cohen BH, Sedwick LA, Burde RM. Retinopathy of dermatomyositis. J Clin Neuroophthalmol *5*:177–179, 1985.

Cohen DN. Temporal arteritis: Improvement in visual prognosis and management with repeat biopsies. Trans Am Acad Ophthalmol Otolaryngol *77*:74–85, 1973.

Cohen DN, Damaske MM. Temporal arteritis: A spectrum of ophthalmic complications. Ann Ophthalmol *7*:1045–1054, 1975.

Cohen DN, Smith TR. Skip areas in temporal arteritis: Myth versus fact. Trans Am Acad Ophthalmol Otolaryngol *78*:772–783, 1974.

Cohen MD, Ginsburg WW, Allen GL. Facial swelling and giant cell arteritis. J Rheumatol *9*:325–327, 1992.

Cohen RD, Conn DL, Ilstrup DM. Clinical features, prognosis, and response to treatment in polyarteritis. Mayo Clin Proc *55*:146–155, 1980.

Cohen Tervaert JW, Huitema MG, Hené RJ, et al. Prevention of relapses in Wegener's granulomatosis by treatment based on antineutrophil cytoplasmic antibody titre. Lancet *336*:709–711, 1990.

Colvard DM, Robertson DM, O'Duffy JD. The ocular manifestations of Behçet's disease. Arch Ophthalmol *95*:1813–1817, 1977.

Committee on Study of Arteritis: Clinical and pathological studies of aortitis syndrome. Jpn Heart J *9*:76–87, 1968.

Comu S, Verstraeten T, Rinkoff JS, et al. Neurological manifestations of acute posterior multifocal placoid pigment epitheliopathy. Stroke *27*:996–1001, 1996.

Conn DL, Hunder GG. Vasculitis and related disorders. In Textbook of Rheumatology. Editors, Kelley WN, Harris ED Jr, Ruddy S, et al, 3rd ed, pp 1167–1199. Philadelphia, WB Saunders, 1989.

Conn DL, McDuffie FC, Holley KE, et al. Immunologic mechanisms in systemic vasculitis. Mayo Clin Proc *51*:511–518, 1976.

Conn DL, Hunder GG, O'Duffy JD. Vasculitis and related disorders. In Textbook of Rheumatology. Editors, Kelley WN, Harris ED Jr, Ruddy S, et al, 4th ed, pp 1077–1102. Philadelphia, WB Saunders, 1993.

Contamin F, Singer B, Mignot B, et al. Sur un cas de lupus érythémateux disséminé avec atteinte de la moelle épinière et des deux nerfs optiques. Ann Med Interne *129*:463–469, 1978.

Cooke WT, Cloake PCP, Govan ADT, et al. Temporal arteritis: A generalized vascular disease. Q J Med *15*:47–76, 1946.

Cooper DA, Penny R. Behçet's syndrome: Clinical, immunological, and therapeutic evaluation of 17 patients. Med J Austr *4*:585–596, 1974.

Coppeto JR, Greco T. Mydriasis in giant-cell arteritis. J Clin Neuroophthalmol *9*:267–269, 1989.

Coppeto JR, Lessell S. Retinopathy in systemic lupus erythematosus. Arch Ophthalmol *95*:794–797, 1977.

Coppeto JR, Miller D. Polyarteritis nodosa diagnosed by temporal artery biopsy. Am J Ophthalmol *102*:541, 1986.

Coppeto JR, Monteiro M. Diagnosis of highly occult giant cell arteritis by repeat temporal artery biopsies. Neuro-ophthalmology *10*:217–218, 1990.

Coppeto JR, Currie JN, Monteiro MLR, et al. A syndrome of arterial-occlusive retinopathy and encephalopathy. Am J Ophthalmol *98*:189–202, 1984.

Coppeto JR, Yamase H, Monteiro MLR. Chronic ophthalmic Wegener's granulomatosis. J Clin Neuroophthalmol *5*:17–25, 1985.

Cornblath WT, Eggenberger ER. Progressive visual loss from giant cell arteritis despite high-dose intravenous methylprednisolone. Ophthalmology *104*:854–858, 1997.

Coste F, Merle d'Aubigné R, Garcin R. Troubles bulbaires paroxystiques par luxation antérieure atloido-occipitale dans un spondylarthrite ankylosante. Résultat favorable d'une greffe postérieure. Sem Hop Paris *36*:1130–1133, 1960.

Cotticelli L, Apponi-Battini G, Federico A, et al. Behçet's disease: An unusual case with bilateral obliterating retinal panarteritis and ischemic optic atrophy. Ophthalmologica *180*:328–332, 1980.

Coutu RE, Klein M, Lessell S, et al. Limited form of Wegener granulomatosis. Eye involvement as a major sign. JAMA *233*:868–871, 1975.

Cox NH, Lawrence CM, Langtry JAA, et al. Dermatomyositis. Disease associations and an evaluation of screening investigations for malignancy. Arch Dermatol *126*:61–65, 1990.

Cravioto H, Feigin I. Noninfectious granulomatous angiitis with a predilection for the nervous system. Neurology *9*:599–609, 1959.

Cream JJ. Immunofluorescent studies of the skin in cryoglobulinemic vasculitis. Br J Dermatol *84*:48–53, 1971.

Cream JJ. Clinical and immunological aspects of cutaneous vasculitis. Q J Med *45*:255–276, 1976.

Crohn BB. Ocular lesions complicating ulcerative colitis. Am J Med Sci *169*:260–267, 1925.

Crohn BB, Ginzburg L, Oppenheimer GD. Regional enteritis: Pathologic and clinical entity. JAMA *99*:1323–1329, 1932.

Crompton JL, Iyer P, Begg MW. Vasculitis and ischaemic optic neuropathy associated with rheumatoid arthritis. Aust NZJ Ophthalmol *8*:219–230, 1980.

Crompton JL, Burrow DJ, Iyer PV. Bilateral internuclear ophthalmoplegia—an unusual initial presenting sign of giant cell arteritis. Aust NZ J Ophthalmol *17*:71–74, 1989.

Crompton MR. The visual changes in temporal (giant-cell) arteritis. Brain *82*:377–390, 1959.

Csonka GW, Oates JK. Pericarditis and electrocardiographic changes in Reiter's syndrome. Br Med J *1*:866–869, 1957.

Culicchia CF, Gol A, Erickson EE. Diffuse central nervous system involvement in papulosis atrophicans maligna. Neurology *12*:503–509, 1962.

Cullen JF. Occult temporal arteritis. Trans Ophthalmol Soc UK *83*:725–736, 1963.

Cullen JF. Occult temporal arteritis. A common cause of blindness in old age. Br J Ophthalmol *51*:513–525, 1967a.

Cullen JF. Ischaemic optic neuropathy. Trans Ophthalmol Soc UK *87*:759–774, 1967b.

Cullen JF. Temporal arteritis: Occurrence of ocular complications 7 years after diagnosis. Br J Ophthalmol *56*:584–588, 1972.

Cullen JF, Coleiro JA. Ophthalmic complications of giant cell arteritis. Surv Ophthalmol *20*:247–260, 1976.

Cupps TR, Fauci AS. Lymphomatoid granulomatosis. In The Vasculitides. Editors, Cupps TR, Fauci AS, pp 88–98. Philadelphia, WB Saunders, 1981a.

Cupps TR, Fauci AS. Wegener's granulomatosis. In The Vasculitides. Editors, Cupps TR, Fauci AS, pp 72–87. Philadelphia, WB Saunders, 1981b.

Cupps TR, Moore PM, Fauci AS. Isolated angiitis of the central nervous system. Prospective diagnostic and therapeutic experience. Am J Med *74*:97–105, 1983.

Curran RE. Palpation of the superficial temporal artery in normal persons. Arch Ophthalmol *104*:1756, 1986.

Currier RD, Dejong RN, Bole GG. Pulseless disease. CNS manifestations. Neurology *4*:818–830, 1954.

Cury D, Breakey AS, Payne BF. Allergic granulomatosis angiitis associated with uveoscleritis and papilledema. Arch Ophthalmol *55*:261–266, 1955.

Cutler WM. The ocular manifestations of lethal midline granuloma: Two cases. Univ Mich Med Bull *21*:220–228, 1955.

Dagi LR, Currie J. Branch retinal artery occlusion in the Churg-Strauss syndrome. J Clin Neuroophthalmol *5*:229–237, 1985.

Daicker B, Keller HH. Riesencellarteriitis mit endookulärer Ausbreitung und Hypotonia bulbi dolorosa. Klin Monatsbl Augenheilkd *158*:358–372, 1971.

Damato BE, Nanjiana M, Foulds WS. Acute posterior multifocal placoid pigment epitheliopathy. A follow-up study. Trans Ophthalmol Soc UK *103*:517–522, 1983.

Dastur DK, Sinhal BS, Shroff HJ. CNS involvement in malignant atrophic papulosis (Kohlmeier-Degos disease): Vasculopathy and coagulopathy. J Neurol Neurosurg Psychiatry *44*:1256–1260, 1981.

Dau PC. Plasmapheresis in idiopathic inflammatory myopathy. Arch Neurol *38*:544–552, 1981.

Davidson RI, Tyler HR. Bulbar symptoms and episodic aphonia associated with atlanto-occipital subluxation in ankylosing spondylitis. J Neurol Neurosurg Psychiatry *37*:691–695, 1974.

Davies JD. Behçet's syndrome with haemoptysis and pulmonary lesions. J Pathol *109*:351–360, 1973.

Davis RH, Daroff RB, Hoyt WF. Tonic pupil after temporal arteritis. Lancet *1*:822, 1968.

Davy J. Researches, Physiological and Anatomical. Vol 1, p 426. London, Smith Elder and Co, 1839.

Deapen DM, Weinrib L, Langholz B, et al. A revised estimate of twin concordance in SLE: A survey of 138 pairs. Arthritis Rheum *29*:S26, 1986.

Decker JL, Steinberg AD, Gershwin ME, et al. Systemic lupus erythematosus. Contrasts and comparisons. Ann Intern Med *82*:391–404, 1975.

Degos R. Malignant atrophic papulosis. Br J Dermatol *100*:21–35, 1979.

Degos R, Delort J, Tricot R. Dermatite papulosquameuse atrophiante. Bull Soc Fr Dermatite Syph *49*:148–150, 1942.

Delecoeullerie G, Joly P, Cohen de Lara A, et al. Polymyalgia rheumatica and temporal arteritis: A retrospective analysis of prognostic features and different corticosteroid regimens. Ann Rheum Dis *47*:733–739, 1988.

Demaziere A, Reinitz E. Dapsone in the long-term treatment of temporal arteritis. Am J Med *87*:3, 1989.

Demiroglu H, Barişta I, Dündar S. Risk factor assessment and prognosis of eye involvement in Behçet's disease in Turkey. Ophthalmology *104*:701–705, 1997.

de Monteynard MS, Bodard-Rickelman E. Neuropathie optique ischemique bilaterale evoquant une maladie de Horton chez une femme de 40 ans. Bull Soc Ophtalmol Fr *86*:31–34, 1986.

Denis G, Fantin J, Grandon M, et al. Neuropathie ischémique aiguë bilatérale dans le carde d'une péri-art'aaerite noueuse. Bull Soc Ophtalmol Fr *84*:909–911, 1984.

Denman AM, Fialkow PJ, Pelton BK, et al. Lymphocyte abnormalities in Behçet's syndrome. Clin Exp Immunol *42*:175–185, 1980.

Denney D, Rose RL. Myasthenia gravis followed by systemic lupus erythematosus. Neurology *11*:710–713, 1961.

DeRemee RA, McDonald TJ, Harrison EG Jr, et al. Wegener's granulomatosis: Anatomic correlates, a proposed classification. Mayo Clin Proc *51*:777–781, 1976.

DeRemee RA, Weiland LH, McDonald TJ. Polymorphic reticulosis, lymphomatoid granulomatosis. Two diseases or one? Mayo Clin Proc 53:634–640, 1978.

DeRemee RA, Weiland LH, McDonald TJ. Respiratory vasculitis. Mayo Clin Proc 55:492–498, 1980.

DeRemee RA, McDonald TJ, Weiland LH. Wegener's granulomatosis: Observations on treatment with antimicrobial agents. Mayo Clin Proc 60:27–32, 1985.

De Silva M, Hazleman BL. Azathioprine in giant cell arteritis/polymyalgia rheumatica. A double blind study. Ann Rheum Dis 45:136–138, 1986.

Desnos J, Freeinaud L, Bigorgne JC, et al. Maladie de Wegener: Maniféstations oto-neuro-ophtalmologiques rélévatrices. Rev Otoneuroophtalmol 47:269–274, 1975.

Desser EJ. Miosis, trismus, and dysphagia. An unusual presentation of temporal arteritis. Ann Intern Med 71:961–962, 1969.

Deutman AF, Lion F. Choriocapillaris nonperfusion in acute multifocal placoid pigment epitheliopathy. Am J Ophthalmol 84:652–657, 1977.

Deutman AF, Oosterhuis JA, Boen-Tan TN, et al. Acute posterior multifocal placoid pigment epitheliopathy. Br J Ophthalmol 56:863–874, 1972.

Deutsch TA, Corwin HL. Lupus optic neuritis with negative serology. Ann Ophthalmol 20:383–384, 1988.

Devinsky O, Petito CK, Alonso DR. Clinical and neuropathologic findings in 50 patients with systemic lupus erythematosus (SLE). Neurology 37(suppl 1):323, 1987.

Devinsky O, Petito CK, Alonso DR. Clinical and neuropathological findings in systemic lupus erythematosus: The role of vasculitis, heart emboli, and thrombotic thrombocytopenic purpura. Ann Neurol 23:380–384, 1988.

Diamantberger MS. Du Rhumatisme Noueux (Polyarthrite Déformante), Chez les Enfants. Paris, Lecrosmier et Badé, 1891.

Dhaliwal RS, Maguire AM, Flower RW, et al. Acute posterior multifocal placoid epitheliopathy. An indocyanine green angiographic study. Retina 13:317–325, 1993.

Diamond JP. Treatable blindness in temporal arteritis. Br J Ophthalmol 75:432, 1991.

Diaz-Jouanen E, DeHoratius RJ, Alárcon-Segovia D, et al. Systemic lupus erythematosus presenting as panniculitis (lupus profundus). Ann Intern Med 82:376–379, 1975.

Dickey W, Andrews WJ. Wegener's granulomatosis presenting as peripheral neuropathy: Diagnosis confirmed by serum anti-neurophil antibodies. J Neurol Neurosurg Psychiatry 53:269–270, 1990.

Diddie KR, Aronson AJ, Ernest JT. Chorioretinopathy in a case of systemic lupus erythematosus. Trans Am Ophthalmol Soc 75:122–131, 1977.

Dimant J, Farmer PM, Sobol N. Giant cell arteritis in a black person. Arthritis Rheum 21:391–393, 1978.

Dimant J, Grob D, Brunner NG. Ophthalmoplegia, ptosis, and miosis in temporal arteritis. Neurology 30:1054–1058, 1980.

Dinning WJ, Perkins ES. Immunosuppressives in uveitis: A preliminary report of experience with chlorambucil. Br J Ophthalmol 59:397–403, 1975.

Disla E, Rhim HR, Reddy A, et al. Reversible cardiogenic shock in a patient with lupus myocarditis. J Rheumatol 20:2174, 1993.

Djawari D, Lang B, Horstein OP. HLA typing in patients of German origin with recurrent benign aphthosis and Behçet's disease. Z Hautkr 59:1005–1009, 1984.

Doherty M, Maddison PJ, Grey RHB. Hydralazine induced lupus syndrome with eye disease. Br Med J 290:675, 1985.

Dolan AL, Gibson T. Intrinsic spinal cord lesions in 2 patients with ankylosing spondylitis. J Rheumatol 21:1160–1161, 1994.

Donoso LA, Magargal LE, Eiferman RA, et al. Recurrent retinal vascular obstructions in Behçet's syndrome. Neuro-ophthalmology 1:191–197, 1981.

Dostrovsky A, Sagher F. Dermatomyositis and malignant tumor. Br J Dermatol 58:52–61, 1946.

Dougal MA, Evans LS, McClellan KR, et al. Central retinal artery occlusion in systemic lupus erythematosus. Ann Ophthalmol 15:38–40, 1983.

Doury P, Pattin S, Eulry F, et al. The use of dapsone in the treatment of giant cell arteritis and polymyalgia rheumatica. Arthritis Rheum 26:689–690, 1983a.

Doury P, Pattin S, Eulry F, et al. Interet de la dapsone dans le traitement de la maladie de Horton et de la pseudopolyarthrite rhizomelique. Rev Rheum Mal Osteoartic 50:277–280, 1983b.

Doury P, Fabresse FX, Patten S. La place de la dapsone dans le traitement de la maladie de Horton et de la pseudopolyarthrite rhizomelique. Ann Med Interne 135:31–35, 1984.

Doutre MS, Beylot C, Bioulac P, et al. Skin lesions resembling malignant atrophic papulosis in lupus erythematosus. Dermatologica 175:45–46, 1987.

Dowling JL, Smith TR. An ocular study of pulseless disease. Arch Ophthalmol 64:236–243, 1960.

Drachman DA. Neurological complications of Wegener's granulomatosis. Arch Neurol 8:145–155, 1963.

Drasga RE, Williams SD, Wills ER, et al. Lymphomatoid granulomatosis: Successful treatment with CHOP combination chemotherapy. Am J Clin Oncol 6:75–80, 1984.

Dubois EL, Wallace DJ. Clinical and laboratory manifestations of systemic lupus erythematosus. In Lupus Erythematosus. Editors, Wallace DJ, Dubois EL, pp 317–449. Philadelphia, Lea & Febiger, 1987.

Duffy J, Lidsky MD, Sharp JT, et al. Polyarthritis, polyarteritis, and hepatitis B. Medicine 55:1937, 1976.

Duguid JB. Periarteritis nodosa. Trans Ophthalmol Soc UK 74:25–40, 1954.

Duke JR, Naquin HA. Lethal midline granuloma. Trans Am Acad Ophthalmol Otolaryngol 61:464–474, 1957.

Duke-Elder WS, Dobree JH. Diseases of the retina. In System of Ophthalmology. Editor, Duke-Elder WS, Vol 10. St Louis, CV Mosby, 1967.

Duker JS, Brown GC, Brooks L. Retinal vasculitis in Crohn's disease. Am J Ophthalmol 103:664–668, 1987.

Duncker G, Beigel A, Lehmann H. Wegenersche Granulomatose: Okuläre Manifestationen, Diagnose und Therapie. Klin Monatsbl Augenheilkd 181:184–187, 1982.

Dutton JJ, Burde RM, Klingele TG. Autoimmune retrobulbar optic neuritis. Am J Ophthalmol 94:11–17, 1982.

Dyck PJ, Conn DL, Okazaki H. Necrotizing angiopathic neuropathy: Three-dimensional morphololgy of fiber degeneration related to sites of occluded vessels. Mayo Clin Proc 47:461–475, 1972.

Dyck PJ, Karnes J, Lais A, et al. Pathologic alterations of the peripheral nervous system in humans. In Peripheral Neuropathy. Editors, Dyck PJ, Lambert EH, Bunge R, Vol 1, pp 760–870. Philadelphia, WB Saunders, 1984.

Dyck PJ, Benstead TJ, Conn DL, et al. Nonsystemic vasculitic neuropathy. Brain 110:843–854, 1987.

Eagling EM, Sanders MD, Miller SJH. Ischaemic papillopathy. Clinical and fluorescein angiographic review of forty cases. Br J Ophthalmol 58:990–1008, 1974.

Eales H. Cases of retinal hemorrhage associated with epistaxis and constipation. Birmingham Med Rev 9:262–273, 1880.

Edelstein C, D'Cruz D, Hughes GR, et al. Anti-endothelial cell antibodies in retinal vasculitis. Curr Eye Res 11(suppl):203–208, 1992.

Editorial. Behçet's disease. Lancet 1:761–762, 1989.

Edwards FC, Truelove SC. The course and prognosis of ulcerative colitis. III. Complications. Gut 5:1–15, 1964.

Efthimiou J, Johnston C, Spiro SG, et al. Pulmonary disease in Behçet's syndrome. Q J Med 58:259–280, 1986.

Egge K, Midtbo A, Westby R. Arteritis temporalis. Acta Ophthalmol 44:49–56, 1966.

Egtedari AA, Esselinckx W, Bacon PA. Circulating immunoblasts in polymyalgia rheumatica. Ann Rheum Dis 35:158–162, 1976.

Ehsan T, Hasan S, Powers JM, et al. Serial magnetic resonance in isolated angiitis of the central nervous system. Neurology 45:1462–1465, 1995.

Eichel B, Harrison E, Devine K, et al. Primary lymphoma of the nose, including a relationship to lethal midline granuloma. Am J Surg 112:597–605, 1966.

Eisenberg RA, Dyer K, Craven SY, et al. Subclass restriction and polyclonality of the systemic lupus erythematosus marker antibody anti-Sm. J Clin Invest 75:1270–1277, 1985.

Elkon KB, Sutherland DC, Rees AJ, et al. HLA antigen frequencies in systemic vasculitis: Increase in HLA-DR2 in Wegener's granulomatosis. Arthritis Rheum 26:102–105, 1983.

Elliot AJ. Thirty-year observation of patients with Eales' disease. Am J Ophthalmol 80:404–408, 1975.

Elliot AJ, Harris GS. The present status of the diagnosis and treatment of periphlebitis retinae (Eales' disease). Can J Ophthalmol 4:117–122, 1969.

Ellis CJ, Hamer DB, Hunt RW, et al. Medical investigation of retinal vascular occlusion. Br Med J 2:1093–1098, 1964.

Ellis PP, Gentry JH. Ocular complications of ulcerative colitis. Am J Ophthalmol 58:779–785, 1964.

Ellis SG, Verity MA. Central nervous system involvement in systemic lupus erythematosus: A review of neuropathologic findings in 57 cases, 1955–1977. Semin Arth Rheum 8:212–221, 1979.

El-Ramahi KM, Al-Kawi MZ. Papilloedema in Behçet's disease: Value of MRI in diagnosis of dural sinus thrombosis. J Neuro Neurosur Psychiatry 54:826–829, 1991.

Emslie-Smith AM, Engel AG. Microvascular changes in early and advanced dermatomyositis: A quantitative study. Ann Neurol 27:343–356, 1990.

Enoch BA, Castillo-Olivares JD, Khoo TCL, et al. Major vessel complication in Behçet's syndrome. Postgrad Med J 44:453, 1968.

Enzmann D, Scott WR. Intracranial involvement of giant-cell arteritis. Neurology 27:794–797, 1977.

Ernst BB, Lowder CY, Meisler DM, et al. Posterior segment manifestations of inflammatory bowel disease. Ophthalmology 98:1272–1280, 1991.

Errlinger RE, Hunder GG, Ward LE. Polymyalgia rheumatica and giant cell arteritis. Annu Rev Med 29:15–22, 1978.

Escudero D, Latorre P, Codina M, et al. Central nervous system disease in Sjögren's syndrome. Ann Med Int 146:239–242, 1995.

Eshaghian J, Goeken JA. C-reactive protein in giant cell (cranial, temporal) arteritis. Ophthalmology 87:1160–1166, 1980.

Espana A, Gutierrez JM, Soria C, et al. Recurrent laryngeal palsy in systemic lupus erythematosus. Neurology 40:1143–1144, 1990.

Estes D, Christian CL. The natural history of systemic lupus erythematosus by prospective analysis. Medicine 50:85–95, 1971.

Estey E, Lieberman A, Pinto R, et al. Cerebral arteritis in scleroderma. Stroke 10:595–597, 1979.

Evans JM, Batts KP, Hunder GG. Persistent giant cell arteritis despite corticosteroid treatment. Mayo Clin Proc 69:1060–1061, 1994.

Evans JM, O'Fallon WM, Hunder GG. Increased incidence of aortic aneurysm and dissection in giant cell (temporal arteritis–a population based study). Ann Intern Med 122:502–507, 1995.

Evans OB, Lexow SS. Painful ophthalmoplegia in systemic lupus erythematosus. Ann Neurol 4:584–585, 1978.

Evans PJ, Eustace P. Scleromalacia perforans associated with Crohn's disease treated with sodium versenate (EDTA). Br J Ophthalmol 57:330–335, 1973.

Fahey JL, Leonard E, Churg J, et al. Wegener's granulomatosis. Am J Med 17:168–179, 1954.

Fan PT, Yu DTY. Reiters syndrome. In Textbook of Rheumatology. Editors, Kelley WN, Harris ED Jr, Ruddy S, et al, 4th ed, pp 961–973. Philadelphia, WB Saunders, 1993.

Fan PT, Yu DTY. Reiter's syndrome. In Textbook of Rheumatology. Editors, Kelley WN, Harris ED Jr, Ruddy S, et al. 5th ed, pp 983–997. Philadelphia, WB Saunders, 1997.

Fan PT, Davis JA, Somer T, et al. A clinical approach to systemic vasculitis. Semin Arthritis Rheum 9:248–304, 1980.

Farkas TG, Sylvester V, Archer D. The choroidopathy of progressive systemic sclerosis (scleroderma). Am J Ophthalmol 74:875–886, 1972.

Farrell DA, Medsger TA Jr. Trigeminal neuropathy in progressive systemic sclerosis. Am J Med 73:57–62, 1982.

Fauchald P, Rygvold O, Oystese B. Temporal arteritis and polymyalgia rheumatica: Clinical and biopsy findings. Ann Intern Med 77:845–852, 1972.

Fauci AS, Wolff SM. Treatment of Wegener's granulomatosis with cyclophosphamide. J Clin Invest 50:28a, 1971.

Fauci AS, Wolff SM. Wegener's granulomatosis: Studies in eighteen patients and a review of the literature. Medicine 52:535–561, 1973.

Fauci AS, Wolff SM, Johnson JS. Effect of cyclophosphamide upon the immune response in Wegener's granulomatosis. N Engl J Med 285:1493–1496, 1971.

Fauci AS, Haynes BF, Katz P. The spectrum of vasculitis: Clinical pathologic, immunologic, and therapeutic considerations. Ann Intern Med 89:660–676, 1978.

Fauci AS, Haynes BF, Costa J, et al. Lymphomatoid granulomatosis: Prospective clinical and therapeutic experience over ten years. N Engl J Med 306:68–75, 1982.

Fauci AS, Haynes BF, Katz P, et al. Wegener's granulomatosis: Prospective clinical and therapeutic experience with 85 patients for 21 years. Ann Intern Med 98:76–85, 1983.

Faulds JS, Wear AR. Pseudotumor of the orbit and Wegener's granuloma. Lancet 2:955–957, 1960.

Fearon DT. Complement. In Cecil Textbook of Medicine. Editors, Wyngaarden JB, Smith LH Jr, 18th ed, pp 1938–1940. Philadelphia, WB Saunders, 1988.

Feigal DW, Robbins DL, Leek JC. Giant cell arteritis associated with mononeuritis multiplex and complement-activating 19S IgM rheumatoid factor. Am J Med 79:495–500, 1985.

Feinglass EJ, Arnett FC, Dorsch CA, et al. Neuropsychiatric manifestations of systemic lupus erythematosus: Diagnosis, clinical spectrum, and relationship to other features of the disease. Medicine 55:323–339, 1976.

Feldmann E, Levine SR. Cerebrovascular disease with antiphospholipid antibodies: Immune mechanisms, significance, and therapeutic options. Ann Neurol 37:S114–S130, 1995.

Fenton RH, Easom HA. Behçet's syndrome. A histopathologic study of the eye. Arch Ophthalmol 72:71–81, 1964.

Ferry AP. The eye and rheumatic diseases. In Textbook of Rheumatology. Editors, Kelley WN, Harris ED Jr, Ruddy S, et al, 4th ed, pp 507–518. Philadelphia, WB Saunders, 1993.

Fessel WJ. Systemic lupus erythematosus in the community: Incidence, prevalence, outcome, and first symptoms; the high prevalence in black women. Arch Intern Med 134:1027–1035, 1974.

Finan MC, Winkelmann RK. The cutaneous extravascular necrotizing granuloma (Churg-Strauss granuloma) and systemic disease: A review of 27 cases. Medicine 62:142–158, 1983.

Finelli PF. Alternating amaurosis fugax and temporal arteritis. Am J Ophthalmol 123:850–851, 1997.

Fineman MS, Savino PJ, Federman JL, et al. Branch retinal artery occlusion as the initial sign of giant cell arteritis. Am J Ophthalmol 122:428–430, 1996.

Firestein GS, Gruber HE, Weisman MH, et al. Mouth and genital ulcers with inflamed cartilage: MAGIC syndrome. Five patients with features of relapsing polychondritis and Behçet's disease. Am J Med 79:65–72, 1985.

Fisher CM. Ocular palsy in temporal arteritis. Minn Med 42:1258–1268, 1959.

Fisher CM. Discussion of Schlezinger NS, Schatz NJ. Giant cell arteritis (temporal arteritis). Trans Am Neurol Assoc 96:12, 1971.

Fisher RG, Graham DY, Granmayeh M, et al. Polyarteritis nodosa and hepatitis-B surface antigen: Role of angiography in diagnosis. AJR 129:77–81, 1977.

Fishman GA, Rabb MF, Kaplan J. Acute posterior multifocal placoid pigment epitheliopathy. Arch Ophthalmol 92:235–238, 1974.

Fishman GA, Baskin M, Jednick N. Spinal fluid pleocytosis in acute posterior placoid pigment epitheliopathy. Ann Ophthalmol 9:33–36, 1977.

Florine CW, Dwyer M, Holland EJ. Wegener's granulomatosis presenting with sclerokeratitis diagnosed by antineutrophil cytoplasmic autoantibodies (ANCA). Surv Ophthalmol 37:373–376, 1993.

Foged EK. Chronic ulceration following biopsy of the temporal artery. Hautarzt 32:647, 1981.

Font RL, Naumann G. Ocular histopathology in pulseless disease. Arch Ophthalmol 82:784–788, 1969.

Ford RG, Siekert RG. Central nervous system manifestations of periarteritis nodosa. Neurology 15:114–122, 1965.

Fortin PR, Larson MG, Watters AK, et al. Prognostic factors in systemic necrotizing vasculitis of the polyarteritis nodosa group. A review of 45 cases. J Rheumatol 22:78–84, 1995.

Foster CS. Immunosuppressive therapy for external ocular inflammatory disease. Ophthalmology 87:140–150, 1980.

Foster CS, Barrett F. Cataract development and cataract surgery in patients with juvenile rheumatoid arthritis-associated iridocyclitis. Ophthalmology 100:809–817, 1993.

Fox DA, McCune WJ. Immunosuppressive drug therapy of systemic lupus erythematosus. Rheum Dis Clin North Am 20:265–299, 1994.

Fox GM, Heilskov T, Smith JL. Cogan's syndrome and seroreactivity to Lyme borreliosis. J Clin Neuroophthalmol 10:83–87, 1990.

Fox RI. Sjögren's syndrome. In Textbook of Rheumatology. Editors, Kelley WN, Harris ED Jr, Ruddy S, et al. 5th ed, pp 955–968. Philadelphia, WB Saunders, 1997.

Fox RI, Carstens SA, Fong S, et al. Use of monoclonal antibodies to analyze peripheral blood and salivary gland lymphocyte subsets in Sjögren's syndrome. Arthritis Rheum 25:419–426, 1982.

Fox RI, Kang H-I. Sjögrens syndrome. In Textbook of Rheumatology. Editors, Kelley WN, Harris ED Jr, Ruddy S, et al, 4th ed, pp 931–942. Philadelphia, WB Saunders, 1993.

Fraga A, LaValle C. Takayasu's arteritis. Clin Rheum Dis 6:405–412, 1980.

Fraga A, Mintz G, Valle L, et al. Takayasu's arteritis: Frequency of systemic manifestations (study of 22 patients) and favorable response to maintenance steroid therapy with adrenocorticosteroids (12 patients). Arthritis Rheum 15:617–624, 1972.

Francis TC. Recurrent aphthous stomatitis and Behçet's disease. Oral Surg 30:476–486, 1970.

Frayer WC. The histopathology of perilimbal ulceration in Wegener's granulomatosis. Arch Ophthalmol 64:58–64, 1960.

Friedman G, Friedman B, Benbassat J. Epidemiology of temporal arteritis in Israel. Israel J Med Sci 18:241–244, 1986.

Friedman I. Midline granuloma. Proc R Soc Med 57:289–297, 1964.

Friedman JJ. Occult temporal arteritis. Am J Ophthalmol 60:333–335, 1965.

Friou GJ. Clinical application of lupus serum nucleoprotein reaction using fluorescent antibody technique. J Clin Invest 36:890, 1957.

Frith P, Burge SM, Millard PR, Wojnarowska F. External ocular findings in lupus erythematosus: A clinical and immunopathological study. Br J Ophthalmol 74:163–167, 1990.

Froehlich F, Fried M, Gonvers JJ, et al. Association of Crohn's disease and Cogan's syndrome. Dig Dis Sci 39:1134–1137, 1994.

Frohnert PP, Sheps SG. Long-term follow-up study of periarteritis nodosa. Am J Med 43:8–14, 1967.

Fujikado T, Imagawa K. Dural sinus thrombosis in Behçet's disease: A case report. Jpn J Ophthalmol 38:411–416, 1994.

Fukuoka Y, Nakagawa Y, Tada R, et al. Visual disturbance probably due to optic nerve lesion in Behçet's disease. Folia Ophthalmol Jpn 38:1619–1625, 1987.

Fukutomi T, Katayama T, Fujiwara H. Plasma exchange therapy for intractable uveitis. Jpn J Clin Ophthalmol 39:1023–1027, 1985.

Fulton AB, Lee RV, Jampol LM, et al. Active giant cell arteritis with cerebral involvement. Findings following four years of corticosteroid therapy. Arch Ophthalmol 94:2068–2071, 1976.

Futrell N, Millikan C. Frequency, etiology, and prevention of stroke in patients with systemic lupus erythematosus. Stroke 20:583–591, 1989.

Gabriel SE, O'Fallon WM, Achkar AA, et al. The use of clinical characteristics to predict the results of temporal artery biopsy among patients with suspected giant cell arteritis. J Rheumatol 22:93–96, 1995.

Galbraith RF, Summerskill WHJ, Murray J. Systemic lupus erythematosus, cirrhosis, and ulcerative colitis after thymectomy for myasthenia gravis. N Engl J Med 270:229–232, 1964.

Galetta SL, Raps EC, Wulc AE, et al. Conjugal temporal arteritis. Neurology 40:1839–1842, 1990.

Galve E, Candell-Riera J, Pigrau C, et al. Prevalence, morphologic types, and evolution of cardiac valvular disease in systemic lupus erythematosus. N Engl J Med 319:817–823, 1988.

Garcia-Diaz M, Mira M, Nevado L, et al. Retinal vasculitis associated with Crohn's disease. Postgrad Med J 71:170–172, 1995.

Gardner D. The Schönlein-Henoch syndrome (anaphylactoid purpura). Q J Med 41:95–122, 1948.

Gass A, Graham E, Moseley IF, et al. Cranial MRI in idiopathic retinal vasculitis. J Neurol 242:174–177, 1995.

Gass JDM. Acute posterior multifocal placoid pigment epitheliopathy. Arch Ophthalmol 80:177–185, 1968a.

Gass JDM. A fluorescein angiographic study of macular dysfunction secondary to retinal vascular disease. VI. X-ray irradiation, carotid artery occlusion, collagen vascular disease, and vitritis. Arch Ophthalmol 80:606–617, 1968b.

Gass JDM. Acute posterior multifocal placoid pigment epitheliopathy: Long-term follow-up. In Management of Retinal Vascular and Macular Disorders. Editors, Fine SL, Owens SL, pp 176–181. Baltimore, Williams & Wilkins, 1983.

Gaynon IE, Asbury MK. Ocular findings in a case of periarteritis nodosa: A case report. Am J Ophthalmol 26:1072–1076, 1943.

Gerstle CC, Friedman AH. Marginal corneal ulceration (limbal guttering) as a presenting sign of temporal arteritis. Ophthalmology 87:1173–1176, 1980.

Gever SG, Freeman RG, Knox JM. Degos disease (papulosis atrophicans maligna): Report of a case with degenerative disease in the central nervous system. South Med J 55:56–60, 1962.

Ghanchi FD, Weir C, Dudgeon J. Facial swelling in giant cell (temporal) arteritis. Eye 10:747–749, 1996a.

Ghanchi FD, Williamson TH, Lim CS, et al. Colour Doppler imaging in giant cell (temporal) arteritis: Serial examination and comparison with non-arteritic anterior ischaemic optic neuropathy. Eye 10:459–464, 1996.

Ghose MK, Shensa S, Lerner PI. Arteritis of the aged (giant cell arteritis) and fever of unexplained origin. Am J Med 57:429–436, 1976.

Gibson GJ, Davis P. Respiratory complications of relapsing polychondritis. Thorax 29:726–731, 1974.

Gibson T, Myers AR. Nervous system involvement in systemic lupus erythematosus. Ann Rheum Dis 35:398–406, 1976.

Gieser SC, Murphy RP. Eales disease. In Retina. Editors, Ryan J, Schachat AP, Murphy RP, Vol 2, pp 1503–1507. St Louis, CV Mosby, 1994.

Giles CL. Juvenile rheumatoid arthritis. In The Eye in Systemic Disease. Editors, Gold DH, Weingeist TA, pp 64–67. Philadelphia, LB Lippincott, 1990.

Gilliam JN. Systemic lupus erythematosus and the skin. In Systemic Lupus Erythematosus. Editor, Lahita RG, pp 615–642. New York, John Wiley & Sons, 1987.

Gilmour JR. Giant-cell chronic arteritis. J Pathol Bacteriol 53:263–277, 1941.

Gladmann DD. Prognosis and treatment of SLE. Curr Opin Rheum 7:402–408, 1995.

Gladmann DD. Psoriatic arthritis. In Textbook of Rheumatology. Editors, Kelley WN, Harris ED Jr, Ruddy S, et al., 5th ed, pp 999–1005. Philadelphia, WB Saunders, 1997.

Gladstone GJ. The afferent pupillary defect as an early manifestation of occult temporal arteritis. Ann Ophthalmol 14:1088–1091, 1982.

Glueck HI, Kant KS, Weiss MA, et al. Thrombosis in systemic lupus erythematosus: Relation to the presence of circulating anticoagulants. Arch Intern Med 145:1389–1395, 1985.

Glutz von Blotzheim S, Borruat F-X. Artérite à cellules géantes et vitesse de sédimentation normale: Plus qu'une exception! Klin Monatsbl Augenheilkd 208:397–399, 1996.

Goar EL, Smith LS. Polyarteritis nodosa of the eye. Am J Ophthalmol 35:1619–1625, 1952.

Goder G. Durchblutungstörungen des Auges und Biopsie der Arteria Temporalis. Leipzig, East Germany, Georg Thieme, 1968.

Godman GC, Churg J. Wegener's granulomatosis: Pathology and review of the literature. Arch Pathol 58:533–553, 1954.

Gold D, Feiner L, Henkind P. Retinal arterial occlusive disease in systemic lupus erythematosus. Arch Ophthalmol 95:1580–1585, 1977.

Gold DH, Morris DA, Henkind P. Ocular findings in systemic lupus erythematosus. Br J Ophthalmol 56:800–804, 1972.

Goldberg RT. Ocular muscle paresis and cranial arteritis—an unusual case. Ann Ophthalmol 15:240–243, 1983.

Golde D, Epstein W. Mixed cryoglobulins and glomerulonephritis. Ann Intern Med 69:1221–1227, 1968.

Goldsmith J. Periarteritis nodosa with involvement of the choroidal and retinal arteries. Am J Ophthalmol 29:435–446, 1946.

Goldstein I, Wexler D. Retinal vascular disease in a case of acute lupus erythematosus disseminatus. Arch Ophthalmol 8:852–857, 1932.

Goldstein I, Wexler D. Bilateral atrophy of the optic nerve in periarteritis nodosa. Arch Ophthalmol 18:767–773, 1937.

Gomez P, Joshi J, Nihoyannopoulos P, et al. Association between cardiac abnormalities and raised anticardiolipin antibodies in systemic lupus erythematosus (Abstract). Postgrad Med J 64:723, 1988.

Gonzalez-Scarano F, Lisak RP, Bilaniuk LT, et al. Cranial computed tomography in the diagnosis of systemic lupus erythematosus. Ann Neurol 5:158–165, 1979.

Good AE. Reiter's disease: A review with special attention to cardiovascular and neurologic sequelae. Semin Arth Rheum 3:253–286, 1974.

Goodman BW Jr. Temporal arteritis. Am J Med 67:839–852, 1979.

Goodwin JA. Temporal arteritis. In Handbook of Clinical Neurology. Editors, Vinken PJ, Bruyn GW, Vol 39, pp 313–342. New York, Elsevier/North Holland, 1980.

Gordon AL, Yudell A. Cauda equina lesion associated with rheumatoid spondylitis. Ann Intern Med 78:555–557, 1973.

Gordon MF, Coyle PK, Golub B. Eales' disease presenting as stroke in the young adult. Ann Neurol 24:264–266, 1988.

Gorevic PD, Kassar HJ, Levo Y, et al. Mixed cryoglobulinemia: Clinical aspects and long-term follow-up of 40 patients. Am J Med 69:287–308, 1980.

Gostin SB. Ambulaton prism spectacles. Trans Am Acad Ophthalmol Otolaryngol 75:644–646, 1971.

Gotoff SP, Smith RD, Sugar O. Dermatomyositis with cerebral vasculitis in a patient with agammaglobulinemia. Am J Dis Child 123:53–56, 1972.

Gouet D, Marréchaud R, Le Berre D, et al. Prognostic de l'arterite temporale traites. Presse Med 15:603–606, 1986.

Graham E. Survival in temporal arteritis. Trans Ophthalmol Soc UK 100:108–110, 1980.

Graham E, Holland A, Avery A, et al. Prognosis in giant cell arteritis. Br Med J 282:269–271, 1981.

Graham EM, Al-Ashkar AF, Sanders MD, et al. Benign intracranial hypertension in Behçet's syndrome. Neuro-ophthalmology 1:73–76, 1980.

Graham EM, Spalton DJ, Barnard RO, et al. Cerebral and retinal vascular changes in systemic lupus erythematosus. Ophthalmology 92:444–448, 1985.

Graham EM, Stanford MR, Sanders MD, et al. A point prevalence study of 150 patients with idiopathic retinal vasculitis. 1. Diagnostic value of ophthalmological features. Br J Ophthalmol 73:714–721, 1989.

Granato JE, Abben RP, May WS. Familial association of giant cell arteritis. A case report and brief review. Arch Intern Med 141:115–117, 1980.

Green B. Schönlein-Henoch purpura with blood in the cerebrospinal fluid. Br Med J 1:836, 1946.

Green WR. Retina. In Ophthalmic Pathology: An Atlas and Textbook. Editor, Spencer WH, 4th ed, Vol 2, pp 1131–1132, 1996.

Greenan T, Grossman R, Goldberg H. Cerebral vasculitis, MRI imaging and angiographic correlation. Radiology 182:67–72, 1992.

Greenberger MH. Central retinal artery closure in Wegener's granulomatosis. Am J Ophthalmol 63:515–516, 1967.

Greenstein AJ, Janowitz HD, Sachar DB. The extra-intestinal complications of Crohn's disease and ulcerative colitis: A study of 700 patients. Medicine 55:401–412, 1976.

Grenier P, Bletry O, Cornud F, et al. Pulmonary involvement in Behçet's disease. AJR 137:565–569, 1981.

Grennan DM, Forrester J. Involvement of the eye in SLE and scleroderma: A study using fluorescein angiography in addition to clinical ophthalmic assessment. Ann Rheum Dis 36:152–156, 1977.

Griffin J, Price DL, Davis L, et al. Granulomatous angiitis of the central nervous system with aneurysms on multiple cerebral arteries. Trans Am Neurol Assn 98:145–148, 1973.

Griffin JW, Harrison HB, Tedescor FJ, et al. Behçet's disease with multiple sites of gastrointestinal involvement. South Med J 75:1405–1408, 1982.

Griffiths RA, Good WR, Watson NP, et al. Normal erythrocyte sedimentation rate in the elderly. Br Med J 289:724, 1984.

Grimson BS, Simons KB. Orbital inflammation, myositis, and systemic lupus erythematosus. Arch Ophthalmol 101:736–738, 1983.

Griner PF, Mayewski RJ, Mushlin AI, et al. Selection and interpretation of diagnostic tests and procedures. Ann Intern Med 94:557–592, 1981.

Gross WL, Schmitt WH, Csernok E. ANCA and associated disease: Immunodiagnostic and pathogenetic aspects. Clin Exp Immunol 91:1–12, 1993.

Guillevin L, Lhote F. Distinguishing polyarteritis nodosa from microscopic polyarteritis and implications for treatment. Curr Opin Rheum 7:20–24, 1995.

Guillevin L, Lhote F, Jarrousse B, et al. Polyarteritis nodosa related to hepatitis B virus. Ann Med Interne 143:63–74, 1992.

Guillevin L, Visser H, Noel LH, et al. Antineutrophil cytoplasm antibodies in systemic polyarteritis nodosa with and without hepatitis B infection and Churg-Strauss syndrome: 62 patients J Rheumatol 20:1345–1349, 1993.

Guillevin L, Lhote F, Sauvaget F, et al. Treatment of polyarteritis nodosa related to hepatitis B virus with interferon alpha and plasma exchanges. Ann Rheum Dis 13:334–337, 1994.

Gumpel JM. Trigeminal sensory neuropathy in connective-tissue disease. N Engl J Med 282:514, 1970.

Gupta RC, McDuffie FC, O'Duffy JD, et al. Circulating immune complexes in active Behçet's disease. Clin Exp Immunol 34:213–218, 1978.

Guyer DR, Miller NR, Auer CL, et al. The risk of cerebrovascular and cardiovascular disease in patients with anterior ischemic optic neuropathy. Arch Ophthalmol 103:1136–1142, 1985.

Haarr M. Rheumatic iridocyclitis. Acta Ophthalmol 38:37–45, 1960.

Hackett ER, Martinez RD, Larson PF, et al. Optic neuritis in systemic lupus erythematosus. Arch Neurol 31:9–11, 1974.

Haddad R, Winkler E. Zum klinishen Befund der okkulten Riesenzellarteriitis. Klin Monatsbl Augenheilkd 183:389–390, 1983.

Hagen NA, Stevens JC, Michet CJ Jr. Trigeminal sensory neuropathy associated with connective tissue diseases. Neurology 40:891–896, 1990.

Haider S. Tonic pupil in lymphomatoid granulomatosis. J Neuroophthalmol 13:38–39, 1993.

Haimböck K. Akute Hypotonia bulbi bei Sogenannter arteriitis temporalis. Klin Monatsbl Augenheilkd 138:596, 1961.

Hall S, Hunder GG. Is temporal artery biopsy prudent? Mayo Clin Proc 59:793–796, 1984.

Hall S, Persellin S, Lie TJ, et al. The therapeutic impact of temporal artery biopsy. Lancet 2:1217–1220, 1983.

Hall S, Buettner H, Luthra HS. Occlusive retinal vascular disease in systemic lupus erythematosus. J Rheumatol 11:846–850, 1984.

Hall S, Barr W, Lie JT, et al. Takayasu arteritis: A study of 32 North American patients. Medicine 64:89–99, 1985.

Hall S, Barr W, Lie JT, et al. Necrotizing angiitis associated with drug abuse. AJR 111:663–671, 1971.

Hamed LM, Guy JR, Moster ML, et al. Giant cell arteritis in the ocular ischemic syndrome. Am J Ophthalmol 113:702–705, 1992.

Hamilton CR Jr, Shelley WM, Tumulty PA. Giant cell arteritis: Including temporal arteritis and polymyalgia rheumatica. Medicine 50:1–27, 1971.

Hammans SR, Ginsberg L. Superior sagittal sinus thrombosis in Wegener's granulomatosis. J Neurol Neurosurg Psychiatry 52:287, 1989.

Hammer ME, Grizzard WS, Travies D. Death associated with acute, multifocal, placoid pigment epitheliopathy. Arch Ophthalmol, 107:170–171, 1989.

Hanger WA, Sainsbury R, Gilchrist NL, et al. Erythrocyte sedimentation rates in the elderly: A community study. N Z Med J 104:134–136, 1991.

Hanly JG, Walsh NMG, Sangalang V. Brain pathology in SLE. J Rheumatol 19: 732–741, 1992.

Hargraves MM, Richmond H, Morton R. Presentation of two bone marrow elements: The 'Tart' cell and 'L.E.' cell. Mayo Clin Proc 23:25–28, 1948.

Harkavy J. Vascular allergy: Pathogenesis of bronchial asthma with recurrent pulmonary infiltrations and eosinophilic polyserositis. Arch Intern Med 67:709–734, 1941.

Harper CM, O'Neill BP, O'Duffy JD, et al. Intracranial hypertension in Behçet's disease: Demonstration of sinus occlusion with use of digital subtraction angiography. Mayo Clin Proc 60:419–422, 1985.

Harris ED. Clinical features of rheumatoid arthritis. In Textbook of Rheumatology. Editors, Kelley WN, Harris ED Jr, Ruddy S, et al., 4th ed, pp 874–911. Philadelphia, WB Saunders, 1993.

Harris ED. Clinical features of rheumatoid arthritis. In Textbook of Rheumatology. Editors, Kelley WN, Harris ED Jr, Ruddy S, et al., 5th ed, pp 898–932. Philadelphia, WB Saunders, 1997.

Harris EN, Gharavi AE, Boey ML, et al. Anticardiolipin antibodies detection by radioimmunoassay and association with thrombosis in systemic lupus erythematosus. Lancet 1:1211–1214, 1983.

Harris EN, Asherson RA, Gharavi AE, et al. Thrombocytopenia in SLE and related autoimmune disorders: Association with anticardiolipin antibodies. Br J Haematol 59:227–230, 1985.

Harris M. Dissecting aneurysm of the aorta due to giant cell arteritis. Br Heart J 30: 840–844, 1968.

Harrison MJG, Bevan AT. Early symptoms of temporal arteritis. Lancet 2:638–640, 1967.

Harrison PE. Granulomatous angiitis of the central nervous system. J Neurol Sci 29: 335–341, 1976.

Harrison SM, Frenkel M, Grossman B, et al. Retinopathy in childhood dermatomyositis. Am J Ophthalmol 76:786–790, 1973.

Hart CJ. Formed visual hallucinations—a symptom of cranial arteritis. Br Med J 3: 643–644, 1967.

Hart RG, Miller VT, Coull B, et al. Cerebral infarction associated with lupus anticoagulants: Preliminary report. Stroke 15:114–118, 1984.

Harvey AM, Shulman LE, Tumulty PA, et al. Systemic lupus erythematosus: Review of the literature and clinical analysis of 138 cases. Medicine 33:291–437, 1954.

Hashimoto T, Takeuchi A. Treatment of Behçet's disease. Curr Opin Rheum 4:31–34, 1992.

Haskjold E, Froland S, Egge K. Ocular polyarteritis nodosa: Report of a case. Acta Ophthalmol 65:749–751, 1987.

Hauser WA, Ferguson RH, Holley KE, et al. Temporal arteritis in Rochester, MN, 1951–1967. Mayo Clin Proc 46:597–602, 1971.

Hayasaka S, Uchida M, Setogawa T, et al. Polyarteritis nodosa presenting as orbital apex syndrome. Orbit 9:117–121, 1990.

Hayes GS, Stinson IN. Erythrocyte sedimentation rate and age. Arch Ophthalmol 94: 939–940, 1976.

Haynes BF, Fauci AS. Diabetes insipidus associated with Wegener's granulomatosis successfully treated with cyclophosphamide. N Engl J Med 299:764, 1978.

Haynes BF, Fishman ML, Fauci AS, et al. The ocular manifestations of Wegener's granulomatosis: Fifteen years experience and review of the literature. Am J Med 63:131–141, 1977.

Haynes BF, Kaiser-Kupfer MI, Mason P, et al. Cogan syndrome: Studies in thirteen patients, long-term follow-up, and a review of the literature. Medicine 59: 426–441, 1980.

Haynes BF, Pikus A, Kaiser-Kupfer M, et al. Successful treatment of sudden hearing loss in Cogan's syndrome with corticosteroids. Arthritis Rheum 24:501–503, 1981.

Hayreh SS. Blood supply of the optic nerve head and its role in optic atrophy, glaucoma and oedema of the optic disc. Br J Ophthalmol 53:721–748, 1969.

Hayreh SS. Anterior ischaemic optic neuropathy: Treatment, prophylaxis and differential diagnosis. Br J Ophthalmol 58:981–989, 1974.

Hayreh SS. Posterior ischemic optic neuropathy. Ophthalmologica 182:29–41, 1981.

Hayreh SS, Podhajsky PA, Raman R, et al. Giant cell arteritis: Validity and reliability of various diagnostic data. Am J Ophthalmol 123:285–296, 1997.

Healey LA, Wilske KR. Anemia as a presenting manifestation of giant cell arteritis. Arthritis Rheum 14:27–31, 1971.

Healey LA, Wilske KR. Manifestations of giant cell arteritis. Med Clin North Am 61:261–270, 1977.

Healey LA, Wilske KR. The Systemic Manifestations of Temporal Arteritis. New York, Grune & Stratton, 1978.

Healey LA, Wilske KR. Presentation of occult giant cell arteritis. Arthritis Rheum 23:641–643, 1980.

Hedges TR. The aortic arch syndromes. Arch Ophthalmol 71:28–34, 1964.

Hedges TR III, Gieger GL, Albert DM. The clinical value of negative temporal artery biopsy specimens. Arch Ophthalmol 101:1251–1254, 1983.

Heibel RH, O'Toole JD, Curtiss EI, et al. Coronary arteritis in systemic lupus erythematosus. Chest 69:700–703, 1976.

Heinemann MH, Soloway SM, Lesser RL. Cogan's syndrome. Ann Ophthalmol 12: 667–674, 1980.

Heiskala H, Somer H, Kovanen J, et al. Microangiopathy with encephalopathy, hearing loss and retinal arteriolar occlusions: Two new cases. J Neurol Sci 86:239–250, 1988.

Henderson FC, Geedes JF, Crockard HA. Neuropathology of the brainstem and spinal cord in end stage rheumatoid arthritis: Implications for treatment. Ann Rheum Dis 52:629–637, 1993.

Henkind P, Gold DH. Ocular manifestations of rheumatic disorders: Natural and iatrogenic. Rheumatology 4:13–59, 1973.

Henkind P, Charles NC, Pearson J. Histopathology of ischaemic optic neuropathy. Am J Ophthalmol 69:78–90, 1970.

Henriksson KG, Sandstedt P. Polymyositis: Treatment and prognosis. A study of 107 patients. Acta Neurol Scand 65:280–300, 1982.

Heptinstall RH, Porter KA, Barkley H. Giant-cell (temporal) arteritis. J Pathol Bacteriol 67:507–519, 1954.

Herbert FH, McPherson SD. Scleral necrosis associated with periarteritis nodosa. Arch Ophthalmol 37:688–692, 1947.

Herman JH. Polychondritis. In Textbook of Rheumatology. Editors, Kelley WN, Harris ED Jr, Ruddy S, et al., 4th ed, pp 1400–1412. Philadelphia, WB Saunders, 1993.

Herreman G, Beaufil SH, Godeau P, et al. Behçet's syndrome and renal involvement: A histologic and immunofluorescent study of 11 renal biopsies. Am J Med Sci 284:10–17, 1982.

Herrmann C. Involvement of the nervous system in relapsing uveitis with recurrent genital and oral ulcer (Behçet's syndrome). Arch Neurol Psychiatr 69:399–400, 1953.

Herschman A, Blum R, Lee YC. Angiographic findings in polyarteritis nodosa: Report of a case. Radiology 94:147–148, 1970.

Herskovitz S, Lipton RB, Lantos G. Neuro-Behçet's disease: CT and clinical correlates. Neurology 38:1714–1720, 1988.

Herson RN, Squier M. Retinal perivasculitis with neurological involvement. J Neurol Sci 36:111–117, 1978.

Hess EV. Drug-related lupus: The same or different? In Systemic Lupus Erythematosus. Editor, Lahita RG, pp 869–880. New York, John Wiley & Sons, 1987.

Heuer DK, Gager WE, Reeser FH. Ischemic optic neuropathy associated with Crohn's disease. J Clin Neuroophthalmol 2:175–181, 1982.

Hinck V, Carter C, Rippey J. Giant-cell (cranial) arteritis. AJR 92:769–775, 1964.

Hind CRK, Winearls CG, Lockwood CM, et al. Objective monitoring of activity in Wegener's granulomatosis by measurement of serum C-reactive protein concentration. Clin Nephrol 21:341–345, 1984.

Hinzpeter EN, Naumann G. Ischemic papilledema in giant-cell arteritis. Mucopolysaccharide deposition with normal intraocular pressure. Arch Ophthalmol 94: 624–628, 1976.

Hirohata T, Kuratsune M, Nomura A, et al. Prevalence of Behçet's syndrome in Hawaii with particular reference to the comparison of the Japanese in Hawaii and Japan. Hawaii Med J 34:244–246, 1975.

Hirose K. A study of fundus changes in the early stages of Takayasu-Ohnishi (Pulseless) disease. Am J Ophthalmol 55:295–301, 1963.

Hirsch M, Mayersdorf A, Lehmann E. Cranial giant-cell arteritis. Br J Radiol 47: 503–506, 1974.

Ho AC, Sergott RC, Regiollo CD, et al. Color doppler hemodynamics of giant cell arteritis. Arch Ophthalmol 112:938–945, 1994.

Hoang-Xuan T, Foster CS, Rice BA. Scleritis in relapsing polychondritis. Response to therapy. Ophthalmology 97:892–898, 1990.

Hochberg MC. Sjögrens syndrome. In Cecil Textbook of Medicine. Editors, Bennett JC, Plum, F, 20th ed, pp 1488–1490. Philadelphia. WB Saunders, 1996.

Hochberg MC. Relapsing polychondritis. In Textbook of Rheumatology. Editors, Kelley WN, Harris ED Jr, Ruddy S, et al., 5th ed, pp 1404–1408. Philadelphia, WB Saunders, 1997.

Hochberg MC, Boyd RE, Ahearn JM, et al. Systemic lupus erythematosus: A review of clinico-laboratory features and immunogenetic markers in 150 patients with emphasis on demographic subsets. Medicine 64:285–295, 1985.

Hochberg MC, Feldman D, Stevens MB. Adult onset polymyositis/dermatomyositis: An analysis of clinical and laboratory features and survival in 76 patients with a review of the literature. Semin Arthritis Rheum 15:168–178, 1986.

Hoffman BI, Katz WA. The gastrointestinal manifestations of systemic lupus erythematosus: A review of the literature. Semin Arthritis Rheum 9:237–247, 1980.

Hoffman GS. Treatment of resistant Takayasu's arteritis. Rhuem Dis Clin North Am 21:73–80, 1995.

Hoffman GS, Fauci AS. Emerging concepts in the management of vasculitic diseases. Adv Intern Med 39:277–303, 1994.

Hoffman GS, Kerr GS, Leavitt RY, et al. Wegener granulomatosis: An analysis of 158 patients. Ann Intern Med 116:488–498, 1992.

Hoffman GS, Leavitt RY, Kerr GS, et al. Treatment of glucocorticoid-resistant or relapsing takayasu arteritis with methotrexate. Arthritis Rheum 37:578–582, 1994.

Hogan MJ, Kimura SJ, Thygeson P. Uveitis in association with rheumatism. Arch Ophthalmol 57:400–413, 1957.

Hogan PJ, Greenberg MK, McCarty GE. Neurologic complications of lymphomatoid granulomatosis. Neurology 31:619–620, 1981.

Holdstock G, Mitchell JRA. Erythrocyte-sedimentation rate before and after in-vitro defibrination: A rapid and simple method for increasing its specificity. Lancet 2:1314–1316, 1977.

Hollander D, Manning RT. The use of alkylating agents in the treatment of Wegener's granulomatosis. Ann Intern Med 67:393–398, 1967.

Hollenhorst RW. Effect of posture of retinal ischaemia from temporal arteritis. Arch Ophthalmol 78:569–577, 1967.

Hollenhorst RW, Henderson JW. The ocular manifestations of the diffuse collagen diseases. Am J Med Sci 221:211–221, 1951.

Hollenhorst RW, Brown JR, Wagener HP, et al. Neurologic aspects of temporal arteritis. Neurology 10:490–498, 1960.

Holt WS, Regan CDJ, Trempe C. Acute posterior multifocal placoid pigment epitheliopathy. Am J Ophthalmol 81:403–412, 1976.

Honda Y. Scintillating scotoma as the first symptom of systemic lupus erythematosus. Am J Ophthalmol 99:607, 1985.

Honda Y. Scintillating scotoma as the first symptom of systemic lupus erythematosus. Metab Pediatr Systemic Ophthalmol 10:22–23, 1987.

Hopkins DJ, Horan E, Burton IL, et al. Ocular disorders in a series of 332 patients with Crohn's disease. Br J Ophthalmol 8:732–737, 1974.

Horan EC. Ophthalmic manifestations of progressive systemic sclerosis. Br J Ophthalmol 53:388–392, 1969.

Horiuchi T, Yoneya S, Numaga T. Ocular manifestations of Behçet's disease: Evaluation of 264 cases. In ACTA: XXIV International Congress of Ophthalmology. Editor, Henkind P, pp 817–821. Philadelphia, JB Lippincott, 1983.

Horton BT, Magath TB, Brown GE. An undescribed form of arteritis of the temporal vessels. Mayo Clin Proc 7:700–701, 1932.

Horven I. Dynamic tonometry: The corneal indentation pulse in giant cell arteritis. Acta Ophthalmol 48:710–718, 1970.

Howard GF III, Ho SU, Kim KS, et al. Bilateral carotid artery occlusion resulting from giant cell arteritis. Ann Neurol 15:204–207, 1984.

Howard PF, Hochberg MC, Bias WB, et al. Relationship between C4 null genes, HLA-D region antigens, and genetic susceptibility to SLE in Caucasian and black Americans. Am J Med 81:187–193, 1986.

Howe LJ, Stanford MR, Edelstein C, et al. The efficacy of systemic corticosterodis in sight-threatening retinal vasculitis. Eye 8:443–447, 1994.

Howe LJ, Woon H, Graham EM, et al. Choroidal hypoperfusion in acute posterior multifocal placoid pigment epitheliopathy. An indocyanine green angiopathy study. Ophthalmology 102:790–798, 1995.

Howell SB, Epstein WV. Circulating immunoglobulin complexes in Wegener's granulomatosis. Am J Med 57:259–268, 1976.

Hoyle C, Ewing DJ, Parker AC. Acute autonomic neuropathy in association with systemic lupus erythematosus. Ann Rheum Dis 44:420–424, 1985.

Hu CH, O'Loughlin S, Winkelmann RK. Cutaneous manifestations of Wegener's granulomatosis. Arch Dermatol 113:175–182, 1977.

Hubbard WN, Walport MJ, Halnan KE, et al. Remission from polymyositis after total body irradiation. Br Med J 284:1915–1916, 1982.

Huey C, Jakobiec FA, Iwamoto T, et al. Discoid lupus erythematosus of the eyelids. Ophthalmology 90:1389–1398, 1983.

Hughes RL, Katirji MB. The Eaton-Lambert (myasthenic) syndrome in association with systemic lupus erythematosus. Arch Neurol 43:1186–1187, 1986.

Hugod C, Scheibel M. Temporal arteritis—progressive affection of vision during high-level corticosteroid therapy. Acta Med Scand 205:445–446, 1979.

Hunder GG. Takayasu's arteritis: A study of 32 North American patients. Medicine 64:89–99, 1985.

Hunder GG. Giant cell arteritis and polymyalgia rheumatica. In Textbook of Rheumatology. Editors, Kelley WN, Harris ED Jr, Ruddy S, et al., 4th ed, pp 1103–1112. Philadelphia, WB Saunders, 1993.

Hunder GG. Polymyalgia rheumatica and giant cell arteritis. In Cecil Textbook of Medicine. Editors, Bennett JC, Plum F, 20th ed, pp 1498–1500. Philadelphia, WB Saunders, 1996.

Hunder GG. Giant cell arteritis and polymyalgic rheumatica. In Textbook of Rheumatology. Editors, Kelley WN, Harris ED Jr, Ruddy S, et al., 5th ed, pp 1123–1132. Philadelphia, WB Saunders, 1997.

Hunder GG, Allen GL. Giant cell arteritis: A review. Bull Rheum Dis 29:980–986, 1978–1979.

Hunder GG, Lie JT, Goronzy JJ, et al. Pathogenesis of giant cell arteritis. Arthritis Rheum 36:757–761, 1993.

Hunder GG, Sheps SG. Intermittent claudication and polymyalgia rheumatica. Arch Intern Med 119:638–643, 1967.

Hunder GG, Lie JT. The vasculitides. Clin Cardiovasc Dis 13:261–291, 1983.

Hunder GG, Sheps SG, Allen GL, et al. Daily and alternate-day corticosteroid regimens in treatment of giant cell arteritis: Comparison in a prospective study. Ann Intern Med 82:613–618, 1975.

Hunninghake GW, Fauci AS. Pulmonary involvement in the collagen vascular diseases. Am Rev Respir Dis 119:471–503, 1979.

Hunter T, Dubo H. Spinal fractures complicating ankylosing spondylitis. Ann Intern Med 88:546–549, 1978.

Hupp SL. Giant cell arteritis associated with progressive systemic sclerosis. J Clin Neuroophthalmol 9:126–130, 1989.

Hupp SL, Nelson GA, Zimmerman LE. Generalized giant cell arteritis with coronary artery involvement and myocardial infarction. Arch Ophthalmol 108:1385–1386, 1990.

Hurd ER. Extraarticular manifestations of rheumatoid arthritis. Semin Arthritis Rheum 8:151–176, 1979.

Hurst RW, Grossman RI. Neuroradiology of central nervous system vasculitis. Semin Neurol 14:320–340, 1994.

Huston KA, Hunder GG. Giant cell (cranial) arteritis: A clinical review. Am Heart J 100:99–105, 1980.

Huston KA, Hunder GG, Lie JT, et al. Temporal arteritis: A 25-year epidemiologic, clinical, and pathologic study. Ann Intern Med 88:162–167, 1978.

Hutchinson CH. Polyarteritis nodosa presenting as posterior ischaemic optic neuropathy. J R Soc Med 77:1043–1046, 1984.

Hutchinson J. Diseases of the arteries. I. On a peculiar form of thrombotic arteritis of the aged which is sometimes productive of gangrene. Arch Surg 1:323–329, 1890.

Hutnik CM, Nicolle DA, Canny CL. Papillitis: A rare initial presentation of Crohn's disease. Can J Ophthalmol 31:373–376, 1996.

Hyman N. Two neurological cases: Demonstration at the Royal College of Physicians of London. Br Med J 1:727–732, 1979.

Iansek R, Edge CJ. Nutritional amblyopia in a patient with Crohn's disease. J Neurol Neurosurg Psychiatry 48:1307–1308, 1985.

ibn Isa A. Memorandum Book of a Tenth-Century Oculist. Translator, Wood CA, Chicago, Northwestern University Press, 1936.

Ikui H. Histopathological studies in eyes with Behçet's disease. J Clin Ophthalmol 14:529–536, 1960.

Imaizumi M, Nukada T, Yoneda S, et al. Behçet's disease with sinus thrombosis and arteriovenous malformation in brain. J Neurol 222:215–218, 1980.

Imakita M, Yutani C, Ishibashi-Ueda H. Giant cell arteritis involving the cerebral artery. Arch Pathol Lab Med 117:729–733, 1993.

Inada K, Katsumura T, Hirai J, et al. Surgical treatment in the aortitis syndrome. Arch Surg 100:220–224, 1970.

Ingalls RG. Bilateral uveitis and keratitis accompanying periarteritis nodosa. Trans Am Acad Ophthalmol Otolaryngol 55:630–631, 1951.

International Committee for Standardization in Hematology. Recommendation of measurement in erythrocyte sedimentation rate of human blood. Am J Clin Pathol 68:505–507, 1977.

International Study Group for Behçet's Disease. Criteria for diagnosis of Behçet's disease. Lancet 335:1078–1080, 1990.

Isaak BL, Liesegang TJ, Michet CJ Jr. Ocular and systemic findings in relapsing polychondritis. Ophthalmology 93:681–689, 1986.

Isashiki M, Koide H, Yamashita T, et al. Acute posterior multifocal placoid pigment epitheliopathy associated with diffuse retinal vasculitis and late haemorrhagic macular detachment. Br J Ophthalmol 70:255–259, 1986.

Isenberg DA, Meyrick-Thomas D, Snaith ML, et al. A study of migraine in systemic lupus erythematosus. Ann Rheum Dis 41:30–32, 1982.

Isenberg DA, Colaco CB, Dudeney C, et al. The relationship of anti-DNA antibody idiotypes and anticardiolipin antibodies to disease activity in SLE. Medicine 65:46–55, 1986.

Ishii T, Watanabe I, Suzuki J. Temporal bone findings in Cogan's syndrome. Acta Otolaryngol 519:118–123, 1995.

Ishikawa K. Natural history and classification of occlusive thromboaortopathy (Takayasu's disease). Circulation 57:27–35, 1978.

Ishikawa O, Ohnishi K, Hiyachi Y, et al. Cerebral lesions in systemic lupus erythematosus detected by magnetic resonance imaging: Relationship to anticardiolipin antibody. J Rheumatol 21:87–90, 1994.

Ishikawa S, Nozaki S, Mukuno K. Upbeat and downbeat nystagmus in a single case. Neuro-ophthalmology 6:95–99, 1986.

Ishioka M, Ohno S, Nakamura S, et al. FK506 treatment of noninfectious uveitis. Am J Ophthalmol 118:723–729, 1994.

Isohisa I, Numano F, Maezawa H, et al. HLA-Bw52 in Takayasu's disease. Tissue Antigens 12:246–248, 1978.

Israel HI, Patchefsky MD, Saldana MJ. Wegener's granulomatosis, lymphomatoid granulomatosis, and benign lymphocytic angiitis and granulomatosis of the lung. Ann Intern Meal 87:691–699, 1977.

Jaben SL, Norton EWD. Exudative retinal detachment in Wegener's granulomatosis: Case report. Ann Ophthalmol 14:717–720, 1982.

Jabs DA. The rheumatic diseases. In Retina. Editors, Ryan J, Schachat AP, Murphy RP, Vol 2, pp 1421–1444. St Louis, CV Mosby, 1994.

Jabs DA, Fine SL, Hochberg MC, et al. Severe retinal vaso-occlusive disease in systemic lupus erythematosus. Arch Ophthalmol 104:558–563, 1986a.

Jabs DA, Miller NR, Newman SA, et al. Optic neuropathy in systemic lupus erythematosus. Arch Ophthalmol 104:564–568, 1986b.

Jabs DA, Henneken AM, Schachat AP, et al. Choroidopathy in systemic lupus erythematosus. Arch Ophthalmol 106:230–234, 1988.

Jacklin HN. Acute posterior multifocal placoid pigment epitheliopathy and thyroiditis. Arch Ophthalmol 95:995–997, 1977.

Jackson G, Miller M, Littlejohn G, et al. Bilateral internuclear ophthalmoplegia in systemic lupus erythematosus. J Rheumatol 13:1161–1162, 1986.

Jacobs JC. Juvenile rheumatoid arthritis. In Pediatric Rheumatology for the Practitioner. p 193. New York, Springer-Verlag, 1983.

Jacobs K, Vrijghem JC, Linsen C, et al. La maladie de Behçet: Une étude de 20 cas. Bull Soc Belge Ophtalmol 230:85–93, 1989.

Jacobson DM, Slamovits TL. Erythrocyte sedimentation rate and its relationship to hematocrit in giant cell arteritis. Arch Ophthalmol 105:965–967, 1987.

Jakobiec FA, Jones IS. Orbital inflammation. In Diseases of the Orbit. Editors, Jones IS, Jakobiec FA, pp 263–268. Hagerstown, MD, Harper & Row, 1979.

Jallon P, Loron P, Borg M, et al. Cécité corticale révélatrice d'une maladie de Horton. Rev Neurol 136:769–776, 1980.

Jampol LM, West C, Goldberg MF. Therapy of scleritis with cytotoxic agents. Am J Ophthalmol 86:266–271, 1978.

Jan JE, Hill RH, Low MD. Cerebral complications in juvenile rheumatoid arthritis. Can Med Assoc J 107:623–625, 1972.

Jarek MJ, West SG, Baker MR, et al. Magnetic resonance imaging in systemic lupus without a history of neuro-psychiatric lupus erythematosus. Arthritis Rheum 37:1609–1613, 1994.

Jay WM, Nazarian SM. Bilateral sixth nerve pareses with temporal arteritis and diabetes. J Clin Neuroophthalmol 6:91–95, 1986.

Jenkins TR, Zaloznik AJ. Lymphomatoid granulomatosis. A case for aggressive therapy. Cancer 64:1362–1365, 1989.

Jennette JC, Falk RJ, Andrassy K, et al. Nomenclature of systemic vasculitides. Arthritis Rheum 37:187–192, 1994.

Jifi-Bahlool H, Saadeh C, O'Connor J. Peripheral ulcerative keratitis in the setting of rheumatoid arthritis: Treatment with immunosuppressive therapy. Semin Arthritis Rheum 25:67–73, 1995.

Johnson MW, Vine AK. Hydroxychloroquine therapy in massive total doses without retinal toxicity. Am J Ophthalmol 104:139–144, 1987.

Johnson RT, Richardson EP. The neurological manifestations of systemic lupus erythematosus: A clinical-pathologic study of 24 cases and review of the literature. Medicine 47:337–369, 1968.

Johnston AC. Giant-cell arteritis: ophthalmic and systemic considerations. Can J Ophthalmol 8:38–46, 1973.

Jonasson F, Cullen JF, Elton PA. Temporal arteritis. Scott Med J 24:111–117, 1979.

Jongen PJII, Boerbooms AMT, Lamers KJB, et al. Diffuse CNS involvement in systemic lupus erythematosus: Intrathecal synthesis of the 4th component of complement. Neurology 40:1593–1596, 1990.

Jordan DR, Addison DJ. Wegener's granulomatosis. Eyelid and conjunctival manifestations as the presenting feature in two individuals. Ophthalmology 101:602–607, 1994.

Judge RD, Currier RD, Gracie WA, et al. Takaysu's arteritis and the aortic arch syndrome. Am J Med 32:379–392, 1962.

Judice DJ, LeBlanc JH, McGarry PA. Spinal cord vasculitis presenting as a spinal cord tumor in a heroin addict: Case report. J Neurosurg 48:131–134, 1978.

Kagen LJ. Dermatomyositis and polymyositis: Clinical aspects. Clin Exp Rheumatol 2:271–277, 1984.

Kalbian VV, Challis MT. Behçet's disease: Report of twelve cases with three manifesting as papilledema. Am J Med 49:823–829, 1970.

Kalina PH, Lie JT, Campbell RJ, et al. Diagnostic value and limitations of orbital biopsy in Wegener's granulomatosis. Ophthalmology 99:120–124, 1992.

Kallenberg CAM, Brower E, Weaning JJ, et al. Anti-neutrophil cytoplasmic antibodies: Current diagnostic and pathophysiological potential. Kidney Int 46:1–15, 1994.

Kalmansohn RB, Kalmansohn RW. Thrombotic obliteration of the branches of the aortic arch. Circulation 15:237–244, 1957.

Kaltreider HB, Talal N. The neuropathy of Sjögren's syndrome: Trigeminal nerve involvement. Ann Intern Med 70:751–762, 1969.

Kalunian KC, Peter JB, Middlekauff HR, et al. Clinical significance of a single test for anti-cardiolipin antibodies in patients with systemic lupus erythematosus. Am J Med 85:602–608, 1988.

Kameda H, Goto S, Sakamoto T, et al. A case of bilateral retinal artery occlusion. Folia Ophthalmol Jpn 39:2045–2049, 1988.

Kanski JJ. Anterior uveitis in juvenile rheumatoid arthritis. Arch Ophthalmol 95:1794–1797, 1977.

Kanski JJ. Juvenile arthritis and uveitis. Surv Ophthalmol 34:253–267, 1990.

Kansu T, Corbett JJ, Savino P, et al. Giant cell arteritis with normal sedimentation rate. Arch Neurol 34:624–625, 1977.

Kansu T, Kirkali P, Kansu E, et al. Optic neuropathy in Behçet's disease. J Clin Neuroophthalmol 9:277–280, 1989.

Kaplan D, Plotz CM, Nathanson L, et al. Cervical spine in psoriasis and in psoriatic arthritis. Ann Rheum Dis 23:50–56, 1964.

Kaplan RE, Springate JE, Feld LG. Pseudotumor cerebri associated with cerebral venous sinus thrombosis, internal jugular vein thrombosis, and systemic lupus erythematosus. J Pediatr 107:266–268, 1985.

Karam GH, Fulmer JD. Giant cell arteritis presenting as interstitial lung disease. Chest 82:781–784, 1982.

Karpik AG, Schwartz MM, Dickey LE, et al. Ocular immune reactants in patients dying with systemic lupus erythematosus. Clin Immunol Immunopathol 35:295–312, 1985.

Karsenti G, Zaluski S, Navarre L. Manifestations ophtalmologiques atypiques de la maladie de Horton: Segmentite anterieure et pseudo-conjonctivite bulbaire. Bull Soc Ophtalmol Fr 85:581–583, 1985.

Kasp E, Graham EM, Stanford MR, et al. A point prevalence study of 150 patients with idiopathic retinal vasculitis. 2. Clinical relevance of antiretinal autoimmunity and circulating immune complexes. Br J Ophthalmol 73:722–730, 1989.

Kassel S, Echevarria R, Guzzo F. Midline malignant reticulosis (so-called lethal midline granuloma). Cancer 23:920–935, 1969.

Kattah JC, Cupps TR, Di Chiro G, et al. An unusual case of central nervous system vasculitis. J Neurol 234:344–347, 1987.

Kattah JC, Manz H, Khodary AE, et al. Occipital artery biopsy: A diagnostic alternative in giant cell arteritis. Presented at the VIIIth International Neuro-Ophthalmology. Winchester, England. June 23–29, 1990.

Katz P, Alling DW, Haynes BF, et al. Association of Wegener's granulomatosis with HLA-B8. Clin Immunol Immunopathol 14:268–270, 1979.

Katzenstein A-L, Carrington CB, Liebow AA. Lymphomatoid granulomatosis. A clinicopathologic study of 152 cases. Cancer 43:360–373, 1979.

Kaufmann J, Canoso JJ. Progressive systemic sclerosis and meralgia paraesthetica. Ann Intern Med 105:973, 1986.

Kawachi-Takahashi S, Takahashi M, Kogure M, et al. Elevation of serum C9 level in association with Behçet's disease. Jpn J Exp Med 44:485–487, 1974.

Kawakita N, Nichimura M, Saton Y. Neurologic aspects of Behçet's disease. J Neurol Sci 5:414–439, 1969.

Kay MC, McCrary JA. Multiple cranial nerve palsies in late metastasis of midline malignant reticulosis. Am J Ophthalmol 88:1087–1090, 1979.

Kayazawa F, Honda A. Severe retinal vascular lesions in systemic lupus erythematosus. Ann Ophthalmol 13:1291–1294, 1981.

Kaye BR, Fainstat M. Cerebral vasculitis associated with cocaine abuse. JAMA 258:2104–2106, 1987.

Kaye BR, Neuwelt KM, London SS, et al. Central nervous system systemic lupus mimicking progressive multifocal leucoencephalopathy. Ann Rheum Dis 51:1152–1156, 1992.

Keane JR. Eye movement abnormalities in systemic lupus erythematosus. Arch Neurol 52:1145–1149, 1995.

Kearns P. Temporal artery biopsy. Br Med J 297:1404, 1988.

Kearns TP. Discussion of Cohen DN. Temporal arteritis: Improvement in visual prognosis and management with repeat biopsies. Trans Am Acad Ophthalmol Otolaryngol 77:84–85, 1973.

Kehoe EL, Newcomber KL. Thromboembolic phenomena in ulcerative colitis. Arch Intern Med 113:711–715, 1964.

Kelley JS. Doppler ultrasound flow detector used in temporal artery biopsy. Arch Ophthalmol 96:845–846, 1978.

Kelley WN, Harris ED Jr, Ruddy S, et al., (eds). Textbook of Rheumatology, 5th ed. Philadelphia, WB Saunders, 1997.

Kelly SP, Storey JK. Mobility spectacles for ankylosing spondylitis. Br Med J 298:1704, 1989.

Keltner JL. Giant-cell arteritis. Signs and symptoms. Ophthalmology 89:1101–1110, 1982.

Kemp AS, Searle C, Horne S. Transient Brown's syndrome in juvenile rheumatoid arthritis. Ann Rheum Dis 43:764–765, 1984.

Kendall MJ, Lawrence DS, Shuttleworth GR, et al. Haematology and biochemistry of ankylosing spondylitis. Br Med J 2:235–237, 1973.

Kent DC, Arnold H. Aneurysm of the aorta due to giant cell aortitis. J Thorac Cardiovasc Surg 53:572–577, 1967.

Kerr GS, Hullahan GW, Giordano J, et al. Ann Intern Med 120:919–929, 1994.

Kersten RC, Lessell S, Carlow TJ. Acute posterior multifocal placoid pigment epitheliopathy and late onset meningoencephalitis. Ophthalmology 94:393–396, 1987.

Key SN, Kimura SJ. Iridocyclitis associated with juvenile rheumatoid arthritis. Am J Ophthalmol 80:425–429, 1975.

Khamashta MA, Cervera R, Asherson RA, et al. Association of antibodies against phospholipids with heart valve disease in systemic lupus erythematosus. Lancet 335:1541–1544, 1990.

Khamashta M, Cuadrado MJ, Mujic F, et al. The management of thrombosis in the antiphospholipid antibody syndrome. N Engl J Med 332:993–997, 1995.

Khan MA, Kushner I. Ankylosing spondylitis and multiple sclerosis. Arthritis Rheum 22:784–786, 1979.

Kielar RA. Exudative retinal detachment and scleritis in polyarteritis. Am J Ophthalmol 82:694–698, 1976.

Killian PJ, McClain B, Lawless OJ. Brown's syndrome: An unusual manifestation of rheumatoid arthritis. Arthritis Rheum 20:1080–1084, 1977.

Kim RC. Rheumatoid disease with encephalopathy. Ann Neurol 7:86–91, 1980.

Kim RY, Holz FG, Gregor Z, et al. Recurrent acute multifocal placoid pigment epitheliopathy in two cousins. Am J Ophthalmol 119:660–662, 1995.

Kimbrell OC, Wheliss JA. Polyarteritis nodosa complicated by bilateral optic neuropathy. JAMA 201:139–140, 1967.

Kimmelstiel P, Gilmour MT, Hodges HH. Degeneration of elastic fibers in granulomatous giant cell arteritis (temporal arteritis). Arch Pathol 54:157–168, 1952.

Kimoto S. The history and present status of aortic surgery in Japan particularly for aortitis syndrome. J Cardiovasc Surg 20:107–126, 1979.

Kincaid J, Schatz H. Bilateral retinal arteritis with multiple aneurysmal dilatations. Retina 3:171–178, 1983.

Kinney EL, Berdoff RL, Rao NS, et al. Devic's syndrome and systemic lupus erythematosus. A case report with necropsy. Arch Neurol 36:643–644, 1979.

Kinyoun JL, Kalina RE. Visual loss from choroidal ischemia. Am J Ophthalmol 101:650–656, 1986.

Kinyoun JL, Kalina RE, Klein ML. Choroidal involvement in systemic necrotizing vasculitis. Arch Ophthalmol 105:939–942, 1987.

Kirker S, Keane M, Hutchinson M. Benign recurrent multiple mononeuropathy in Wegener's granulomatosis. J Neurol Neurosurg Psychiatr 52:918, 1989.

Kirkham TH. Scleroderma and Sjögren's syndrome. Br J Ophthalmol 53:131–133, 1969.

Kirkham TH, ffytche TJ, Sanders MD. Placoid pigment epitheliopathy with retinal vasculitis and papillitis. Br J Ophthalmol 56:875–880, 1972.

Kishi S, Yoneya S, Ohnishi N, et al. Intravitreal granulation and retinal pigment epitheliopathy in Behçet's disease. Jpn J Clin Ophthalmol 35:1139–1148, 1981.

Kishi S, Komatsu T, Masaoka N, et al. Retinal photocoagulation for a patient with Takayasu disease. Folia Ophthalmol Jpn 48:619–624, 1997.

Kissel JT, Slivka AP, Warmolts JR, et al. The clinical spectrum of necrotizing angiopathy of the peripheral nervous system. Ann Neurol 18:251–257, 1985.

Kissel P, Debry G, Royer R, et al. Myasthenie grave au cours d'un lupus érythémateux dissemine. Bull Soc Med Hop Paris 117:151–159, 1966.

Klein RG, Hunder GG, Stanson AW, et al. Large artery involvement in giant cell (temporal) arteritis. Ann Intern Med 83:806–812, 1975.

Klein RG, Campbell RJ, Hunder GG, et al. Skip lesions in temporal arteritis. Mayo Clin Proc 51:504–510, 1976.

Kleinschmidt-Demasters BK, Filley CM, Bitter MA. Central nervous system angiocentric, angiodestructive T cell lymphoma/lymphomatoid granulomatosis. Surg Neurol 37:130–137, 1992.

Klemperer P, Pollack AD, Baehr G. Diffuse collagen disease: Acute disseminated lupus erythematosus and diffuse scleroderma. JAMA 119:331–342, 1942.

Klinkhoff AV, Beattie CW, Chalmers A. Retinopathy in systemic lupus erythematosus: Relationship to disease activity. Arthritis Rheum 29:1152–1156, 1986.

Klippel JH. Systemic lupus erythematosus. Treatment-related complications superimposed on chronic disease. JAMA 263:1812–1815, 1990.

Klok AM, Geertzen R, Rothova A, et al. Anticardiolipin antibodies in uveitis. Curr Eye Res 11(suppl):209–213, 1992.

Klonoff DC, Andrews BT, Obana WG. Stroke associated with cocaine use. Arch Neurol 46:989–993, 1989.

Knopf HLS. An unusual case of painful ophthalmoplegia in a patient with rheumatoid arthritis. Ann Ophthalmol 21:412–413, 1989.

Knox DL. Inflammatory bowel disease. In The Eye in Systemic Disease. Editors, Gold DH, Weingeist TA, pp 103–105. Philadelphia, LB Lippincott, 1990.

Knox DL, Snip RC, Stark WJ. The keratopathy of Crohn's disease. Am J Ophthalmol 90:862–865, 1980.

Knox DL, Schachat AP, Mustonen E. Primary, secondary and coincidental ocular complications of Crohn's disease. Ophthalmology 91:163–173, 1984.

Koc Y, Gullu I, Akpek G, et al. Vascular involvement in Behçet's disease. J Rheumatol 19:402–410, 1992.

Köhlmeier W. Multiplizieren Hautnekrosen bei Thrombangiitis Obliterans. Arch Klin Exp Derm 181:783–792, 1941.

Koike R, Yamada M, Matsunaga T, et al. Polyarteritis nodosa (PN) complicated with unilateral exophthalmos. Intern Med 32:232–236, 1993.

Kojima K, Niimi K, Sato M. Progressive retinal vascular disorders with systemic lupus erythematosus (SLE). Folia Ophthalmol Jpn 41:462–468, 1990.

Kokmen E, Billman JK Jr, Abell MR. Lymphomatoid granulomatosis clinically confined to the CNS: A case report. Arch Neurol 34:782–784, 1977.

Kolmokova AE. Changes occurring in the interstitial substance of the eye in rheumatism. Vest Oftamol 78:76–79, 1965.

Kolodny EH, Rebeiz JJ, Caviness VS Jr, et al. Granulomatous angiitis of the central nervous system. Arch Neurol 19:510–524, 1968.

Konishi T, Saida T, Nishitani H. Orbital apex syndrome caused by rheumatoid nodules. J Neurol Neurosurg Psychiatry 49:460–462, 1986.

Koo EH, Massey EW. Granulomatous angiitis of the central nervous system: Protean manifestations and response to treatment. J Neurol Neurosurg Psychiatry 51:1126–1133, 1988.

Kornblut AD, Wolff SM, DeFries HO, et al. Wegener's granulomatosis. Laryngoscope 90:1453–1465, 1980.

Koskimies O, Rapola J, Savilahti E, et al. Renal involvement in Schönlein-Henoch purpura. Acta Paediatr Scand 63:357–363, 1974.

Kozin F, Haughton V, Bernhard GC. Neuro-Behçet disease: Two cases and neuroradiologic findings. Neurology 27:1148–1152, 1977.

Kraft HE, Möller DE, Völker L, et al. Farbdopplersonographie der Temporalarterien: Eine neue Methode zur Diagnostik der Arteriitis temporalis. Klin Monatsbl Augenheilkd 208:93–95, 1996.

Kramer MR, Melzer E, Nesher G, et al. Pulmonary manifestations of temporal arteritis. Eur J Respir Dis 71:430–433, 1987.

Kreibig W. Optikomalazie, die Folge eines Gefässverschlusses im retrobulbären Abschnitt des Sehnerven. Klin Monatsbl Augenheilkd 122:719–731, 1953.

Krendel DA, Ditter SM, Frankel MR, et al. Biopsy-proven cerebral vasculitis associated with cocaine abuse. Neurology 40:1092–1094, 1990.

Krishna R, Kosmorsky GS. Implications of thrombocytosis in giant cell arteritis. Am J Ophthalmol 124:103, 1997.

Kulkarni TP, D'Cruz IA, Gandhi MJ, et al. Reversal of renovascular hypertension caused by nonspecific aortitis after corticosteroid therapy. Br Heart J 36:114–116, 1974.

Kulvin SM. Erythrocyte sedimentation rates in the elderly. Arch Ophthalmol 88:617–618, 1972.

Kumar R, Wijdicks EF, Brown RD Jr, et al. Isolated angiitis of the CNS presenting as subarachnoid hemorrhage. J Neurol Neurosurg Psychiatry 62:649–651, 1997.

Kupersmith MJ, Burde RM, Warren FA, et al. Autoimmune optic neuropathy: evaluation and treatment. J Neurol Neurosurg Psychiatry 51:1381–1386, 1988.

Kurland LT, Hauser WA, Ferguson RH, et al. Epidemiologic features of diffuse connective tissue disorders in Rochester, MN, 1951 to 1967, with special reference to systemic lupus erythematosus. Mayo Clin Proc 44:649–663, 1969.

Kurland LT, Chuang T-Y, Hunder GG. The epidemiology of systemic arteritis. In Current Topics in Rheumatology: Epidemiology of the Rheumatic Diseases. Editors, Laurence RE, Shulman LE, pp 196–205. New York, Gower Medical Publisher, Ltd, 1984.

Kushner I. Erythrocyte sedimentation rate and the acute phase reactants. In Textbook of Rheumatology. Editors, Kelley WN, Harris ED Jr, Ruddy S, et al, 3rd ed, pp 719–727. Philadelphia, WB Saunders, 1989.

Kushner MJ, Chawluk J, Fazekas F, et al. Cerebral blood flow in systemic lupus erythematosus with or without cerebral complications. Neurology 37:1596–1598, 1987.

Kushner MJ, Tobin M, Fazekas F, et al. Cerebral blood flow variations in CNS lupus. Neurology 40:99–102, 1990.

Kyle V, Hazleman BL. Treatment of polymyalgia rheumatica and giant cell arteritis. I. Steroid regimens in the first two months. Ann Rheum Dis 48:658–661, 1989a.

Kyle V, Hazleman BL. Treatment of polymyalgia rheumatic and giant cell arteritis. II. Relation between steroid dose and steroid associated side effects. Ann Rheum Dis 48:662–666, 1989b.

Kyle V, Hazelman BL. Stopping steroids in polymyalgia rheumatica and giant cell arteritis. Treatment usually lasts for two to five years. Br Med J 300:244–245, 1990.

Kyle V, Cawston TE, Hazleman BL. Erythrocyte sedimentation rate and C reactive protein in the assessment of polymyalgia rheumatic/giant cell arteritis on presentation and during follow up. Ann Rheum Dis 48:667–671, 1989.

Label LS, Tandan R, Albers JW. Myelomalacia and hypogycorrhachia in malignant atrophic papulosis. Neurology 33:936–939, 1983.

Ladanzi M, Fraser RS. Pulmonary involvement in giant cell arteritis. Arch Pathol Lab Med 111:1178–1180, 1987.

Ladefoged J, Nielsen B, Raaschou F, et al. Acute anuria due to polyarteritis nodosa. Am J Med 46:827–831, 1969.

Lahita RG. Clinical presentation of systemic lupus erythematosus. In Textbook of Rheumatology. Editors, Kelley WN, Harris ED Jr, Ruddy S, et al. 5th ed, pp 1028–1039. Philadelphia, WB Saunders, 1997.

Laidlaw DAH, Smith PEM, Hudgson P. Orbital pseudotumor secondary to giant cell arteritis: An unreported condition. Br Med J 300:784–785, 1990.

Lakhanpal S, Bunch TW, Ilstrup DM, et al. Polymyositis-dermatomyositis and malignant lesions: Does an association exist? Mayo Clin Proc 61:645–653, 1986.

Lambert JR, Wright V. Eye inflammation in psoriatic arthritis. Ann Rheum Dis 35:354–356, 1976.

Laman SD, Provost TT. Cutaneous manifestations of Lupus erythematosus. Rheum Dis Clin North Am 20:195–212, 1994.

Lande A, Berkmen YM. Aortitis: Pathologic, clinical, and arteriographic review. Radiol Clin North Am 14:219–240, 1976.

Langham ME, To'mey KF. A clinical procedure for the measurement of ocular pulsepressure relationship and the ophthalmic arterial pressure. Exp Eye Res 27:17–25, 1978.

Lanham JG, Churg J. Churg Strauss syndrome. In Systemic Vasculitides. Editors, Churg A, Churg J, p 101. New York, Igaku-Shoin, 1991.

Lanham JG, Barrie T, Kohner EM, et al. SLE retinopathy: Evaluation by fluorescein angiography. Ann Rheum Dis 41:473–478, 1982a.

Lanham JG, Elkon KB, Hughes GRV. Ptosis in systemic lupus erythematosus. Postgrad Med J 58:688–689, 1982b.

Lanham JG, Elkon KB, Pusey CD, et al. Systemic vasculitis with asthma and eosinophilia: A clinical approach to the Churg-Strauss syndrome. Medicine 63:65–81, 1984.

Laroche L, Saraux H. Unilateral central retinal vein occlusion in systemic lupus erythematosus. Ophthalmologica 189:128–129, 1984.

Larson TS, Hall S, Hepper NGG, et al. Respiratory tract symptoms as a clue to giant cell arteritis. Ann Intern Med 101:594–597, 1984.

Laurence J, Nachman R. Hematologic aspects of systemic lupus erythematosus. In Systemic Lupus Erythematosus. Editor, Lahita RG, pp 721–790. New York, John Wiley & Sons, 1987.

Lavelle C, Alarcón-Segovia D, del Giudice-Knipping JA, et al. Association of Behçet's syndrome with HLA-B5 in the Mexican Mestizo population. J Rheumatol 8:325–327, 1981.

Leavitt RY, Fauci AS, Bloch DA, et al. Criteria for the classification of Wegener's granulomatosis: American College of Rheumatology. Arthritis Rheum 33:1101–1107, 1990.

Lee DA, Su WPD, Leisegang TJ. Ophthalmic changes of Degos disease (malignant atrophic papulosis). Ophthalmology 91:295–299, 1984.

Lee DA, Barker SM, Su WPD, et al. The clinical diagnosis of Reiter's syndrome: Ophthalmic and non-ophthalmic aspects. Ophthalmology 93:350–356, 1986.

Lee JE, Haynes JM. Carotid arteritis and cerebral infarction due to scleroderma. Neurology 17:18–22, 1967.

Leib ES, Restivo C, Paulus HE. Immunosuppressive and corticosteroid therapy of polyarteritis nodosa. Am J Med 67:941–947, 1979.

Lehner T. Behçet's syndrome and autoimmunity. Br Med J 1:465–467, 1967.

Lehner T. Pathology of recurrent oral ulceration and oral ulceration in Behçet's syndrome: Light, electron, and fluorescence microscopy. J Pathol 97:481–494, 1969.

Lehner T. Immunologic aspects of recurrent oral ulcers. Oral Surg 33:80–85, 1972.

Lehner T. Progress report: Oral ulceration in Behçet's syndrome. Gut 18:491–511, 1977.

Lenoch F, Králik V, Bartos J. "Rheumatic" iritis and iridocyclitis. Ann Rheum Dis 18:45–48, 1959.

Lerner AB, Watson CJ. Studies of cryoglobulins. I. Unusual purpura associated with the presence of high concentration of cryoglobulin (cold precipitable serum globulin). Am J Med 214:410–415, 1947.

LeRoy EC. Systemic sclerosis (scleroderma). In Cecil Textbook of Medicine. Editors, Bennett JC, Plum F, 20th ed, pp 1483–1487. Philadelphia, WB Saunders, 1996.

Lessell S. The neuro-ophthalmology of systemic lupus erythematosus. Doc Ophthalmol 47:13–42, 1979.

Levin JR, Awerbuch G, Nigro MA, et al. Isolated angiitis of the central nervous system in children. Ann Neurol 26:478, 1989.

Levine SR, Welch KMA. Antiphospholipid antibodies. Ann Neurol 26:386–389, 1989.

Lewis IC, Philpott MG. Neurological complications in the Schönlein-Henoch syndrome. Arch Dis Child 31:369–371, 1956.

Lewis RA, Martonyi CL. Acute posterior multifocal placoid pigment epitheliopathy: A recurrence. Arch Ophthalmol 93:235–238, 1975.

Lewis TR, Glaser JS, Schatz NJ, et al. Pulseless disease with ophthalmic manifestations. J Clin Neuroophthalmol 13:242–249, 1993.

Li EK, Ho PCP: Pseudotumor cerebri in systemic lupus erythematosus. J Rheumatol 16:113–116, 1989.

Li HK, Dejean BJ, Tang RA. Reversal of visual loss with hyperbaric oxygen treatment in a patient with Susac syndrome. Ophthalmology 103:2091–2098, 1996.

Liang GC, Simkin PA, Hunder GG, et al. Familial aggregation of polymyalgia rheumatica and giant cell arteritis. Arthritis Rheum 17:19–24, 1974a.

Liang GC, Simkin PA, Mannik M. Immunoglobulins in temporal arteries: An immunofluorescent study. Ann Intern Med 81:19–24, 1974b.

Liang MH, Rogers M, Larson M, et al. The psychosocial impact of SLE and RA. Arthritis Rheum 27:13–19, 1981.

Lichtig C, Ludatscher R, Eisenberg E, et al. Small blood vessel disease in allergic granulomatous angiitis (Churg-Strauss syndrome). J Clin Pathol 42:1001–1002, 1989.

Lichtiger S, Present DH. Preliminary report: Cyclosporin in treatment of severe active ulcerative colitis. Lancet 336:16–19, 1990.

Lie JT. Vasculopathy in the antiphospholipid syndrome: Thrombosis or vasculitis, or both? J Rheumatol 16:713–715, 1989.

Lie JT. Vasculitis 1815 to 1991. Classification and diagnostic specificity. J Rheumatol 19:83–89, 1992.

Lie JT. Nomenclature and classification of vasculitis: Plus Ça change, plus c'est la meme chose. Arthritis Rheum 37:181–186, 1994a.

Lie JT. When is arteritis of the temporal arteritis not temporal arteritis? J Rheumatol 21:186–189, 1994b.

Lie JT, Gordon LP, Titus JL. Juvenile temporal arteritis: Biopsy study of four cases. JAMA 234:496–499, 1975.

Lie JT, Failoni DD, Davies DC Jr. Temporal arteritis with giant cell aortitis: Coronary arteritis and myocardial infarction. Arch Pathol Lab Med 110:857–860, 1986.

Liebman S, Cook C. Retinopathy with dermatomyositis. Arch Ophthalmol 74:704–705, 1965.

Liebow AS, Carrington CRB, Friedman RJ. Lymphomatoid granulomatosis. Hum Pathol 3:457–558, 1972.

Liegner JT, Yee RW, Wild JH. Topical cyclosporine therapy for ulcerative keratitis associated with rheumatoid arthritis. Am J Ophthalmol 109:610–612, 1990.

Liesegang TJ, Bullen CL, McDonald TJ, et al. Ophthalmic Wegener's granulomatosis. In ACTA: XXIV International Congress of Ophthalmology. Editor, Henkind P, pp 830–833. Philadelphia, JB Lippincott, 1983.

Lindsay-Rea R. A case of Reiter's disease. Trans Ophthalmol Soc UK 67:241–244, 1947.

Linssen A, Meenken C. Outcomes of HLA-B27-positive and HLA-B27 negative acute anterior uveitis. Am J Ophthalmol 120:351–361, 1995.

Liozon F, Vidal E, Bonnetblanc JM, et al. La disulone dans le traitement de la maladie de Horton. Ann Med Interne 137:299–306, 1986.

Lipton RB, Rosenbaum D, Mehler MF. Giant cell arteritis causes recurrent posterior circulation transient ischaemic attacks which respond to corticosteroid. Eur Neurol 27:97–100, 1987.

Lisman JV. Dermatomyositis with retinopathy. Arch Ophthalmol 37:155–159, 1947.

Lisse JR. Ankylosing spondylitis. An optimistic outlook. Postgrad Med 86:147–153, 1989.

Littlewood JM, Lewis GM. The Holmes-Adie syndrome in a boy with acute juvenile rheumatism and bilateral syndactyly. Arch Dis Child 38:86–88, 1963.

Liu GT, Greene JM, Charness ME. Brown-Séquard syndrome in a patient with systemic lupus erythematosus. Neurology 40:1474–1475, 1990.

Liu GT, Glaser JS, Schatz NJ, et al. Visual morbidity in giant cell arteritis. Clinical characteristics and prognosis for vision. Ophthalmology 10:1779–1785, 1994.

Lockshin MD. Diplopia as early sign of temporal arteritis. Report of two cases. Arthritis Rheum 13:419–421, 1970.

Lomeo RM, Silver RM, Brothers M. Spontaneous dissection of the internal carotid artery in a patient with polyarteritis nodosa. Arthritis Rheum 32:1625–1626, 1989.

Long SM, Dolin P. Polyarteritis nodosa presenting as acute blindness. Ann Emerg Med 24:523–525, 1994.

LoSpalluto J, Dorward B, Miller W Jr, et al. Cryoglobulinemia based on interaction between a gamma macroglobulin and 7S gamma globulin. Am J Med 32:142–147, 1962.

Love DC, Rapkin J, Lesser GR, et al. Temporal arteritis in blacks. Ann Intern Med 105:387–389, 1986.

Love DC, Berler DK, O'Dowd GJ, et al. Erythrocyte sedimentation rate and its relationship to hematocrit in giant cell arteritis. Arch Ophthalmol 106:309–310, 1988.

Lundberg PO, Werner I. Trigeminal sensory neuropathy in systemic lupus erythematosus. Acta Neurol Scand 48:330–340, 1972.

Lupi-Herrera E, Scanchez-Torres G, Horwitz S, et al. Pulmonary artery involvement in Takayasu's arteritis. Chest 67:69–74, 1975.

Lupi-Herrera E, Sanchez-Torres G, Marcushamer J, et al. Takayasu's arteritis: Clinical study of 107 cases. Am Heart J 93:94–103, 1977.

Lyness AL, Bird AC. Recurrences of acute posterior multifocal placoid pigment epitheliopathy. Am J Ophthalmol 98:203–207, 1984.

Maaravi Y, Raz E, Gilon D, et al. Cerebrovascular accident and myocardial infarction associated with anticardiolipin antibodies in a young woman with systemic lupus erythematosus. Ann Rheum Dis 48:853–855, 1989.

MacCraig JN. Giant cell arteritis presenting with pyrexia of uncertain origin. Proc R Soc Med 55:327, 1962.

MacFadyen DJ. Wegener's granulomatosis with discrete lung lesions and peripheral neuritis. Can Med Assoc J 83:760–764, 1960.

Machado EBV, Michet C, Hunder G, et al. Temporal arteritis: Clinical and epidemiological features from a community-based study, 1950 to 1985. Ann Neurol 22:148, 1987.

Machado EBV, Michet CJ, Ballard DJ, et al. Trends in incidence and clinical presentation of temporal arteritis in Olmstead County, Minnesota, 1950–1985. Arthritis Rheum 31:745–749, 1988.

Mack HG, O'Day J, Currie JN. Delayed choroidal perfusion in giant cell arteritis. J Clin Neuroophthalmol 11:221–227, 1991.

Maclean H, Guthrie W. Retinopathy in scleroderma. Trans Ophthalmol Soc UK 89:209–220, 1969.

Macmichael IM, Cullen JF. Pathology of ischaemic optic neuropathy. In The Optic Nerve. Editor, Cant JS, pp 108–116. London, Henry Kimpton, 1972.

Macoul KL. Ocular changes in granulomatous ileocolitis. Arch Ophthalmol 84:95–97, 1970.

Magargal LE, Donoso LA, Goldberg RE, et al. Ocular manifestations of relapsing polychondritis. Retina 1:96–99, 1981.

Maher JA. Dural nodules in rheumatoid arthritis: Report of a case. Arch Pathol 58:354–359, 1954.

Maitland C, Shafer D, Rubin J. Intermittent tonic downgaze, ataxia, and dementia in a young girl. Presented at the 18th Annual Frank B. Walsh Society Meeting, Seattle, WA, February 21–22, 1986.

Mäkelä TE, Ruosteenoja R, Wager O, et al. Myasthenia gravis and systemic lupus erythematosus. Acta Med Scand 175:777–780, 1964.

Malaise-Stals J. Uvéites et affections rhumatismales. Bull Soc Beige Ophtalmol 230:3–12, 1989.

Mamo JG. The rate of visual loss in Behçet's disease. Arch Ophthalmol 84:451–452, 1970.

Mamo JG. Treatment of Behçet disease with chlorambucil. A follow-up report. Arch Ophthalmol 94:580–583, 1976.

Mamo JG, Azzam SA. Treatment of Behçet's disease with chlorambucil. Arch Ophthalmol 84:446–450, 1970.

Mamo JG, Baghdassarian A. Behçet's disease: A report of 28 cases. Arch Ophthalmol 71:4–14, 1964.

Manchul LA, Jin A, Pritchard KI, et al. The frequency of malignant neoplasms in patients with polymyositis-dermatomyositis: A controlled study. Arch Intern Med 145:1835–1839, 1985.

Mandybur TI. Cerebral amyloid angiopathy: Possible relationship to rheumatoid vasculitis. Neurology 29:1336–1340, 1979.

Manganelli P, Malvezzi L, Saginario A. Trismus and facial swelling in a case of temporal arteritis. Clin Exp Rheumatol 10:102–103, 1992.

Manley G, Wong E, Dalmau J, et al. Sera from some patients with antibody-associated paraneoplastic encephalomyelitis/sensory neuropathy recognize the Ro-52 K antigen. J Neuro-Oncol 19:105–112, 1994.

Manschot WA. The eye in collagen diseases. Bibl Ophthalmol 58:1–87, 1961.

Manschot WA. A fatal case of temporal arteritis, with ocular symptoms. Ophthalmologica 149:121–130, 1965a.

Manschot WA. Generalized scleroderma with ocular symptoms. Ophthalmologica 149:131–137, 1965b.

Markenson JA, McDougal JS, Tsairis P, et al. Rheumatoid meningitis: A localized immune process. Ann Intern Med 90:786–789, 1979.

Martenet AC. Nervensystem und Uveitis. Klin Monatsbl Augenheilkd 192:83–86, 1988.

Marumo M, Horiuchi T, Yoshitoshi T, et al. A case of 'limited form' Wegener's granulomatosis with scleritis. Folia Ophthalmol Jpn 41:79–84, 1990.

Masai H, Kashii S, Kimura H, et al. Neuro-Behçet disease presenting with internuclear ophthalmoplegia. Am J Ophthalmol 122:897–898, 1996.

Masi AT. Population studies in rheumatic disease. Annu Rev Med 18:185–206, 1967.

Masi AT, Hunder GG, Lie JT, et al. The American College of Rheumatology 1990 criteria for the classification of the Churg Strauss syndrome (allergic granulomatosis and angiitis). Arthritis Rheum 33:1094–1100, 1990.

Mason RM, Barnes CG. Behçet syndrome mit arthritis. Schweiz Med Wochschr 98:665–671, 1968.

Mason RM, Barnes CG. Behçet's syndrome with arthritis. Ann Rheum Dis 28:95–103, 1969.

Mass M, Bourdette D, Bernstein W, et al. Retinopathy, encephalopathy, deafness associated with microangiopathy (the RED M syndrome): Three new cases. Neurology 38(suppl 1):215, 1988.

Massry GG, Chung SM, Selhorst JB. Optic neuropathy and diplopia with MRI suggestive of cerebral arteritis in relapsing polychondritis. J Neuroophthalmol 15:171–175, 1995.

Masuda K, Urayama A, Kogure M, et al. Double-masked trial of cyclosporin versus colchicine and long-term open study of cyclosporin in Behçet's disease. Lancet 1:1093–1096, 1989.

Masuzawa T, Shimabukuro H, Furuse M, et al. Pulseless disease associated with a ruptured intracranial vertebral aneurysm. Neurol Med Chir 24:490–494, 1984.

Matas BR. Iridocyclitis associated with relapsing polychondritis. Arch Ophthalmol 84:474–476, 1970.

Mathews WB. The neurological complications of ankylosing spondylitis. J Neurol Sci 6:561–573, 1968.

Mathewson JA, Hunder GG. Giant cell arteritis in two brothers. J Rheumatol 13:190–192, 1986.

Matoba A, Plager S, Barger J, et al. Keratitis in relapsing polychondritis. Ann Ophthalmol 16:367–370, 1984.

Matsushima S, Kato M, Kawamura H, et al. Four cases of retinal vascular occlusive disease associated with antiphospholipid antibody syndrome. Folia Ophthalmol Jpn 48:700–706, 1997.

Matzkin DC, Slamovits TL, Sachs R, et al. Visual recovery in two patients after intravenous methylprednisolone treatment of CRAO secondary to GCA. Ophthalmology 99:68–71, 1992.

Mauch E, Volk C, Kratzsch G, et al. Neurological and neuropsychiatric dysfunction in primary Sjögren's syndrome. Acta Neurol Scand 89:31–35, 1994.

Maumenee AE. Retinal lesions in lupus erythematosus. Am J Ophthalmol 23:971–981, 1940.

Mayer LF. Gastrointestinal manifestations of systemic lupus erythematosus. In Systemic Lupus Erythematosus. Editor, Lahita RG, pp 709–720. New York, John Wiley & Sons, 1987.

Mayeux R, Fahn S. Strokes and ulcerative colitis. Neurology 28:571–574, 1978.

McAdam LP, O'Hanlan MA, Bluestone R, et al. Relapsing polychondritis: Prospective study of 23 patients and a review of the literature. Medicine 55:193–215, 1976.

McCarty GA, Rice JR, Bembe ML, et al. Anticentromere antibody: Clinical correlation and association with favorable prognosis in patients with scleroderma variants. Arthritis Rheum 26:1–7, 1983.

McCarty M. Historical perspective on C-reactive protein. Ann NY Acad Sci 389:1–10, 1982.

McCormick HM, Neubuerger KT. Giant cell arteritis involving small meningeal and intracerebral vessels. J Neuropathol Exp Neurol 17:471–478, 1958.

McDonnell PJ, Moore GW, Miller NR, et al. Temporal arteritis. A clinicopathologic study. Ophthalmology 93:518–530, 1986.

McFadyen DJ, Schneider RJ, Chisholm IA. A syndrome of brain, inner ear and retinal microangiopathy. Can J Neurol Sci 14:315–318, 1987.

McGavin DDM, Williamson J, Forrester JV, et al. Episcleritis and scleritis—a study of their clinical manifestations and association with rheumatoid arthritis. Br J Ophthalmol 57:192–226, 1976.

McGowan BL. Active temporal arteritis as contra-indication to elective surgery. Am J Ophthalmol 64:455–456, 1967.

McKay DAR, Watson PG, Lyne AJ. Relapsing polychondritis and eye disease. Br J Ophthalmol 58:600–605, 1974.

McKusick VA. A form of vascular disease relatively frequent in the Orient. Am Heart J 63:57–64, 1962.

McLain LG, Bookstein JJ, Kelsch RC. Polyarteritis nodosa diagnosed by renal arteriography. J Pediatr 80:1032–1035, 1972.

McLeod D, Oji EO, Kohner EM, et al. Fundus signs in temporal arteritis. Br J Ophthalmol 62:591–594, 1978.

McMenemey WH, Lawrence BJ. Encephalomyelopathy in Behçet's disease: Report of necropsy findings in two cases. Lancet 2:353–358, 1957.

Meadows SP. Temporal or giant cell arteritis—ophthalmic aspects. In Neuro-Ophthalmology Symposium of the University of Miami and the Bascom Palmer Eye Institute. Editor, Smith JL, Vol 4, pp 148–157. St Louis, CV Mosby, 1968.

Meagher JN, McCoy E, Rossel C. Disseminated lupus erythematosus simulating intracranial mass lesion: Report of an unusual case. Neurology 11:862–865, 1961.

Mein J. Superior oblique tendon sheath syndrome. Br Orthopt J 28:70–76, 1971.

Meisler DM, Stock EL, Wertz RD, et al. Conjunctival inflammation and amyloidosis in allergic granulomatosis and angiitis (Churg-Strauss syndrome). Am J Ophthalmol 91:216–219, 1981.

Melberg NS, Grand GM, Dieckert P, et al. Cotton-wool spots and the early diagnosis of giant cell arteritis. Ophthalmology 102:1611–1614, 1995.

Mellgren SI, Omdal R, Klov NE, et al. Systemic lupus erythematosus (SLE): CNS and neuromuscular manifestations. Neurology 37(suppl 1):99, 1987.

Meltzer M, Franklin EC. Cryoglobulinemia—a study of twenty-nine patients. I. IgG and IgM cryoglobulins and factors affecting cryoprecipitability. Am J Med 40:828–836, 1966.

Messmer EM, Foster CS. Destructive corneal and scleral disease associated with rheumatoid arthritis. Medical and surgical management. Cornea 14:408–417, 1995.

Meyer E, Scharf J, Miller B, et al. Fundus lesions in rheumatoid arthritis. Ann Ophthalmol 10:1583–1584, 1978.

Meyer MW, Wild JH. Unilateral internuclear ophthalmoplegia in systemic lupus erythematosus. Arch Neurol 32:487, 1975.

Meyer-Schwickerath G. Eales' disease: Treatment with light-coagulation. Mod Probl Ophthalmol 4:10–18, 1966.

Michelson JB. Melting corneas with collapsing nose. Surv Ophthalmol 29:148–154, 1984.

Michelson JB, Chisari FV. Behçet's disease. Surv Ophthalmol 26:190–203, 1982.

Michet CJ. Psoriatic arthritis. In Textbook of Rheumatology. Editors, Kelley WN, Harris ED Jr, Ruddy S, et al, 4th ed, pp 974–984. Philadelphia, WB Saunders, 1993.

Michet CJ Jr, McKenna CH, Luthra HS, et al. Relapsing polychondritis. Survival and predictive role of early disease manifestations. Ann Intern Med 104:74–78, 1986.

Miller A, Green M, Robinson D. Simple rule for calculating normal erythrocyte sedimentation rate. Br Med J 286:266, 1983.

Miller DAS, Ormerod IEC, Rudge P, et al. MRI brain scanning in patients with systemic vasculitis: Possible confusion with multiple sclerosis. J Neurol Neurosurg Psychiatry 50:949, 1987.

Miller NR, Aroichane M. Temporal arteritis (giant cell arteritis). In Master Techniques in Ophthalmic Surgery. Editor, Roy FH, pp 830–839. Baltimore, Williams & Wilkins, 1995.

Miller NR, Fine SL. The Ocular Fundus in Neuro-ophthalmologic Diagnosis. St Louis, CV Mosby, 1977.

Miller NR, Keltner JL, Gittinger JW, et al. Giant cell (temporal) arteritis. The differential diagnosis. Surv Ophthalmol 23:259–271, 1979.

Millette TJ, Subramony SH, Wee AS, et al. Systemic lupus erythematosus presenting with recurrent acute demyelinating polyneuropathy. Eur Neurol 251:397–402, 1986.

Milne JS, Williamson J. The ESR in older people. Geront Clin 14:36–42, 1972.

Mimura Y, Miyaura T, Mizuno K. Indication of corticosteroid, cyclophosphamide and colchicine therapies in ocular lesions of Behçet's disease. In ACTA: XXIV International Congress of Ophthalmology. Editor, Henkind P, pp 826–829. Philadelphia, JB Lippincott, 1983.

Miquel EC, Rodriques-Pereira RM, Debraganca-Pereira CA, et al. Psychiatric manifestations of systemic lupus erythematosus, clinical features, symptoms and signs of central nervous system activity in 43 patients. Medicine 73:224–232, 1994.

Miró J, Pena-Sagredo JL, Berciano J, et al. Prevalence of primary Sjögren's syndrome in patients with multiple sclerosis. Ann Neurol 27:582–584, 1990.

Missen GAK. Pathology of Giant Cell Arteritis. Thesis, Oxford, 1963.

Miura M, Murakami K, Yamada Y, et al. A case of bullous retinal detachment associated with ulcerative collitis (sic). Folia Ophthalmol Jpn 41:360–364, 1990.

Miyake M, Sunakawa M, Okinami S. Behçet's disease characteristics more than 10 years after diagnosis. Folia Ophthalmol Jpn 48:707–712, 1997.

Model DG. Reversal of blindness in temporal arteritis with methylprednisolone. Lancet 1:340, 1978.

Mohan K, Gupta A, Jain IS, et al. Bilateral central retinal artery occlusion in occult temporal arteritis. J Clin Neuroophthalmol 9:270–272, 1989.

Molenaar WM, Rosman JB, Donker AJM, et al. The pathology and pathogenesis of malignant atrophic papulosis (Degos disease). Path Res Pract 182:98–106, 1987.

Moll JMH. Psoriatic arthritis. Br J Rheumatol 23:241–245, 1984.

Montecucco C, Caporali R, Pacchetti C, et al. Is tolosa-hunt syndrome a limited form of Wegener's granulomatosis? Report of two cases with antineutrophil cytoplasmic antibodies. Br J Rheumatol 32:640–641, 1993.

Monteiro MLR, Coppeto JR, Greco P. Giant cell arteritis of the posterior cerebral circulation presenting with ataxia and ophthalmoplegia. Arch Ophthalmol 102:407–409, 1984.

Monteiro MLR, Swanson RA, Coppeto JR, et al. A microangiopathic syndrome of encephalopathy, hearing loss and retinal arteriolar occlusions. Neurology 35:1113–1121, 1985.

Moore AT, Morin JD. Bilateral acqued inflammatory Brown's syndrome. J Pediatr Ophthalmol 22:26–30, 1985.

Moore JG, Sevel D. Corneo-scleral ulceration in periarteritis nodosa. Br J Ophthalmol 50:651–655, 1966.

Moore PM. Diagnosis and management of isolated angiitis of the central nervous system. Neurology 39:167–173, 1989.

Moore PM, Cupps TR. Neurological complications of vasculitis. Ann Neurol 14: 155–167, 1983.

Moore PM, Fauci AS. Neurologic manifestations of systemic necrotizing arteritis: Clinical and pathologic features in 24 cases. Am J Med 71:517–524, 1981.

Moore PM, Lisak RP. Multiple sclerosis and Sjögren's syndrome: A problem in diagnosis or in definition of two disorders of unknown etiology? Ann Neurol 27:585–586, 1990.

Moore SB, O'Duffy JD. Lack of association between Behçet's disease and major histocompatibility complex class II antigens in an ethnically diverse North American Caucasoid patient group. J Rheumatol 13:771–773, 1986.

Moorthy AV, Chesney RW, Segar WE, et al. Wegener's granulomatosis in childhood: prolonged survival following cytotoxic therapy. J Pediatr 91:616–618, 1977.

Morgan CM, Foster CS, D'Amico DJ, et al. Retinal vasculitis in polyarteritis nodosa. Retina 6:205–209, 1986.

Morgan GJ, Harris ED. Non-giant cell temporal arteritis. Arthritis Rheum 21:362–366, 1978.

Morgan SH, Bernstein RM, Coppen J, et al. Total body irradiation and the course of polymyositis. Arthritis Rheum 28:831–835, 1985a.

Morgan SH, Bernstein RM, Hughes GRV. Intractable polymyositis: Prolonged remission induced by total body irradiation. J R Soc Med 78:496–497, 1985b.

Morris CR, Scheib JS. Fatal myocardial infarction resulting from coronary arteritis in a patient with polymyalgia rheumatica and biopsy-proven temporal arteritis. A case report and review of the literature. Arch Intern Med 154:1158–1160, 1994.

Mosher HA. The prognosis in temporal arteritis. Arch Ophthalmol 62:641–644, 1948.

Moskowitz RW, Baggenstoss AH, Slocumb CH. Histopathological classification of periarteritis nodosa: A study of 56 cases confirmed at necropsy. Mayo Clin Proc 38:345–357, 1963.

Mouillac-Gambarelli N, Mattei-Sicre I, Vila J-P, et al. A propos d'un cas de maladie de Horton. A revelation oculaire atypique. Bull Soc Ophtalmol Fr 85:585–586, 1985.

Moutsopoulos HM, Sarmas JH, Talal N. Is central nervous system involvement a systemic manifestation of primary Sjogren's syndrome? Rheum Dis Clin North Am 19:909–911, 1993.

Moxley G, Ruddy S. Immune complexes and complement. In Textbook of Rheumatology. Editors, Kelley WN, Harris ED Jr, Ruddy S, et al, 4th ed, pp 188–200. Philadelphia, WB Saunders, 1993.

Mulcahy F, Juby LD, Chandler GN. Giant cell arteritis presenting with peripheral neuropathy. Postgrad Med J 57:670–671, 1984.

Muller W, Lehner T. Quantitative electron microscopical analysis of leukocyte infiltration in oral ulcer of Behçet's syndrome. Br J Dermatol 106:535–544, 1982.

Mullick FG, McAllister HA Jr, Wagner BM. Drug related vasculitis: Clinicopathologic correlations in 30 patients. Hum Pathol 10:313–325, 1979.

Munro S. Fundus appearance in a case of acute dermatomyositis. Br J Ophthalmol 43:548–558, 1959.

Murphy RP, Renie WA, Proctor LR, et al. A survey of patients with Eales disease. In Management of Retinal Vascular and Macular Disorders. Editors, Fine SL, Owens SL. Baltimore, Williams & Williams, 1983.

Myles AB, Perera T, Ridley MG. Prevention of blindness in giant cell arteritis by corticosteroid treatment. Br J Rheumatol 31:103–105, 1992.

Nagy F, Juhasc J. Ophthalmologic alterations of giant cell arteritis. Szemescet 107: 162–169, 1970.

Nakagawa Y, Tada R, Ooji M, et al. Vitreous hemorrhage in Behçet's disease. Folia Ophthalmol Jpn 41:893–897, 1990.

Nakano KK. Neurologic complications of rheumatoid arthritis. Ortho Clin North Am 6:861–880, 1975.

Nakao K, Ikeda M, Kimata S, et al. Takayasu's arteritis: Clinical report of eighty-four cases and immunological studies of seven cases. Circulation 35:1141–1155, 1967.

Nassani S, Cocito L, Arcuri T, et al. Orbital pseudotumor as a presenting sign of temporal arteritis. Clin Exp Rheumatol 13:367–369, 1995.

Nasu T. Takayasu's truncoarteritis in Japan: A statistical observation of 76 autopsy cases. Pathol Microbiol 43:140–146, 1975.

Naumann G. Ocular histopathology in 'acute neuro-Behçet disease.' Presented at the AOA-AFIP Fifth Biennial Meeting. Washington, DC, June 22–23, 1973.

Nazzaro P. Cutaneous manifestations of Behçet's disease. In International Symposium on Behçet's Disease, Rome, 1964. Editors, Monacelli M, Nazzaro P, pp 15–41. Basel, Karger, 1966.

Nesher G, Sonneblick M, Friedlander Y. Analysis of steroid related complications and mortality in temporal arteritis: A 15-year survey of 43 patients. J Rheumatol 21:1283–1286, 1994.

Neuwelt CM, Lacks S, Kaye BR, et al. Role of intravenous cyclophosphamide in the treatment of severe neuropsychiatric systemic lupus erythematosus. Am J Med 98:32–41, 1995.

Nevyas JY, Nevyas HJ. Giant cell arteritis with normal erythrocyte sedimentation rate: A management dilemma. Metab Pediatr Syst Ophthalmol 10:18–21, 1987.

Newman NJ, Slamovits TL, Friedland S, et al. Neuro-ophthalmic manifestations of meningocerebral inflammation from the limited form of Wegener's granulomatosis. Am J Ophthalmol 120:613–621, 1995.

Newman NM, Hoyt WF, Spencer WH. Macula-sparing monocular blackouts. Clinical and pathological investigations of intermittent choroidal vascular insufficiency in a case of periarteritis nodosa. Arch Ophthalmol 91:367–370, 1974.

Nichols PW, Koss M, Levine AM, et al. Lymphomatoid granulomatosis: A T-cell disorder? Am J Med 72:467–471, 1982.

Niinaka T, Okochi T, Watanabe Y, et al. Chemotactic defect in Wegener's granulomatosis. J Med 8:161–175, 1977.

Nimelstein SH, Brody S, McShane D, et al. Mixed connective tissue disease: A subsequent evaluation of the original 25 patients. Medicine 59:239–248, 1980.

Ninomiya M, Ohashi K, Sasaki N, et al. A case of optic neuritis accompanying systemic lupus erythematosus several years after onset. Folia Ophthalmol Jpn 41: 636, 1990.

Nishino H, Rubino FA. Horner's syndrome in Wegener's granulomatosis: Report of four cases. J Neurol Neurosurg Psychiatry 56:897–899, 1993.

Nishino H, Rubino FA, DeRemee RA, et al. Neurological involvement in Wegener's granulomatosis: An analysis of 324 consecutive patients at the Mayo Clinic Ann Neurol 33:4–9, 1993a.

Nishino H, Rubino FA, Parisi JE. The spectrum of neurologic involvement in Wegener's granulomatosis. Neurology 43:1334–1337, 1993b.

Nissim F, Von der Valde J, Czernobilsky B. A limited form of Churg-Strauss syndrome. Arch Pathol Lab Med 106:305–307, 1982.

Nolan J, Cullen JF. Retinal vasculitis associated with anterior uveitis. Br J Ophthalmol 51:361–364, 1967.

Nolle B, Coners H, Duncker G. ANCA in ocular inflammatory disorders. Adv Exp Med Biol 336:305–307, 1993.

Nolle B, Specks U, Ludemann J, et al. Anticytoplasmic autoantibodies: Their immunodiagnostic value in the diagnosis and followup of Wegener's granulomatosis. Ann Intern Med 111:28–40, 1989.

Nomland R, Layton JM. Malignant papulosis with atrophy (Degos). Fatal cutaneo-intestinal syndrome. Arch Dermatol 81:181–188, 1960.

Nordborg E, Bengtsson B-A. Death rates and causes of death in 284 consecutive patients with giant cell arteritis confirmed by biopsy. Br Med J 299:549–550, 1989.

Norden D, Weinberg J, Schumacher HR, et al. Bilateral periorbital edema in SLE. J Rheumatol 20:2158–2160, 1993.

Norton EWD, Cogan DG. Syndrome of nonsyphilitic interstitial keratitis and vestibuloauditory symptoms. A long-term follow-up. Arch Ophthalmol 61:695–697, 1959.

Noseworthy JH, Bass BH, Vandervoort MK, et al. The prevalence of primary Sjögren's syndrome in a multiple sclerosis population. Ann Neurol 25:95–98, 1989.

Noseworthy JH, Bass BH, Vandervoort MK, et al. Sjögren's syndrome mimicking multiple sclerosis. Reply Ann Neurol 27:587–588, 1990.

Nossent JC, Hovestadt DM, Schonfeld DHW, et al. Single photon emission computed tomography of the brain in the evaluation of cerebral lupus. Arthritis Rheum 34: 1397–1403, 1991.

Notis CM, Kitei RA, Cafferty MS, et al. Microangiopathy of brain, retina and inner ear. J Neuroophthalmol 15:1–8, 1995.

Novack SN, Pearson CM. Cyclophosphamide therapy in Wegener's granulomatosis. N Engl J Med 284:938–942, 1971.

Novak MA, Green WR, Miller NR. Ophthalmological manifestations: A case of familial giant cell arteritis. Md State Med J 33:817–820, 1984.

Novak MA, Green WR, Miller NR. Familial giant cell arteritis. J Clin Neuroophthalmol 6:126–127, 1986.

Nurick S, Blackwood W, Mair WGP. Giant cell granulomatous angiitis of the central nervous system. Brain 95:133–142, 1972.

Nussenblatt RB. The expanding use of immunosuppression in the treatment of non-infectious ocular disease. J Autoimmun 5(suppl A):247–257, 1992.

Nussenblatt RB, Palestine AG, Chan CC, et al. Effectiveness of cyclosporin therapy for Behçet's disease. Arthritis Rheum 28:671–679, 1985.

Oates JK, Hancock JAH. Neurological symptoms and lesions occurring in the course of Reiter's disease. Am J Med Sci 238:79–84, 1959.

O'Connor JF, Musher DM. Central nervous system involvement in systemic lupus erythematosus. A study of 150 cases. Arch Neurol 14:157–164, 1966.

O'Duffy JD. Prognosis in Behçet's syndrome. Bull Rheum Dis 29:972–977, 1978–1979.

O'Duffy JD. Behçet's disease. In Textbook of Rheumatology. Editors, Kelley WN, Harris ED Jr, Ruddy S, 3rd ed, pp 1209–1214. Philadelphia, WB Saunders, 1989.

O'Duffy JD. Behçet's disease. N Engl J Med 322:326–327, 1990.

O'Duffy JD, Goldstein NP. Neurologic involvement in seven patients with Behçet's disease. Am J Med 61:170–178, 1976.

O'Duffy JD, Carney JA, Deodhar S. Behçet's disease. Report of 10 cases, 3 with new manifestations. Ann Intern Med 75:561–570, 1971.

O'Duffy JD, Taswell HF, Elveback LR. HLA antigens in Behçet's disease. J Rheumatol 3:1–3, 1976.

O'Duffy JD, Robertson DM, Goldstein NP. Chlorambucil in the treatment of uveitis and meningoencephalitis of Behçet's disease. Arthritis Rheum 76:75–84, 1984.

O'Duffy JD, Bowles CA, O'Fallon WM. The immunosuppressive treatment of Behçet's disease with emphasis on chlorambucil. In Recent Advances in Behçet's Disease. Editors, Lehner T, Barnes CG, pp 301–306. London, Royal Society of Medicine Services, 1985.

Ogasahara S, Takahashi M, Kang J, et al. Serum mitochondrial aspartate aminotransferase in patients with polymyositis. Ann Neurol 13:100–103, 1983.

O'Hanlan M, McAdam LP, Bluestone R, et al. The arthropathy of relapsing polychondritis. Arthritis Rheum 19:191–194, 1976.

Ohno S, Nakayama E, Sugiura S, et al. Specific histocompatibility antigens associated with Behçet's disease. Am J Ophthalmol 80:636–641, 1975.

Ohno S, Ohguchi M, Hirose S, et al. Close association of HLA Bw51 with Behçet's disease. Arch Ophthalmol 100:1455–1458, 1982.

Oldenski, R. Cogan syndrome: Autoimmune-mediated audiovestibular symptoms and ocular inflammation. J Am Fam Pract 6:577–581, 1993.

Oppenheim H. Lehrbuch der Nervenkrankheiten. 7th ed, p 840. Berlin, S Karger, 1923.

Oppenheimer S, Hoffbrand BI. Optic neuritis and myelopathy in systemic lupus erythematosus. Can J Neurol Sci 13:129–132, 1986.

Ortiz JR, Newman NJ, Barrow DL. Crest-associated multiple intracranial aneurysms and bilateral optic neuropathies. J Clin Neuroophthalmol 11:233–240, 1991.

Orzalesi N, Ricciardi L. Segmental retinal periarteritis. Am J Ophthalmol 72:55–59, 1971.

Oshima Y, Shimizu T, Yokohari R, et al. Clinical studies on Behçet's syndrome. Ann Rheum Dis 22:36–45, 1963.

Östberg G. Temporal arteritis in a large necropsy series. Ann Rheum Dis 30:224–235, 1971.

Östberg G. On arteritis with special reference to polymyalgia arteritica. Acta Path Microbiol Scand Suppl 237:1–59, 1973.

Ostler HB. Pulseless disease (Takayasu disease). Am J Ophthalmol 43:583–589, 1957.

Ostler HB, Dawson CR, Schachter J, et al. Reiter's syndrome. Am J Ophthalmol 71:986–991, 1971.

Out HJ, de Groot PG, Hasselaar P, et al. Fluctuations of anticardiolipin antibody levels in patients with systemic lupus erythematosus: a prospective study. Ann Rheum Dis 48:1023–1028, 1989.

Ozawa K, Sakurai S, Kijima Y. Plasma exchange in the therapy of Behçet's disease with fever, genital ulcer and weight loss. Ther Plasmapheresis 3:317–319, 1983.

Ozawa T, Sasaki O, Sorimachi T, et al. Primary angiitis of the central nervous system: Report of two cases and review of the literature. Neurosurgery 36:173–179, 1995.

Pagliarini S, Piquet B, ffytche TJ, et al. Foveal involvement and lack of visual recovery in APMPPE associated with uncommon features. Eye 9:42–47, 1995.

Pahlitzsch Th, Wyrobisch W, Kämpe Ch, et al. Therapie der okulären Form des Morbus Behçet mit Cyclosporin A. Klin Monatsbl Augenheilkd 196:466–469, 1990.

Paice WE. Giant cell arteritis: Difficult decisions in diagnosis, investigation and treatment. Postgrad Med J 65:743–747, 1989.

Pallis CA, Fudge BJ. The neurological complications of Behçet's syndrome. Arch Neurol Psychiatr 75:1–14, 1956.

Palm E. The ocular crisis of the temporal arteritis syndrome (Horton). Acta Ophthalmol 36:208–243, 1958.

Palmer HE, Zaman AG, Edelstein CE, et al. Systemic morbidity in patients with isolated idiopathic retinal vasculitis. Lancet 346:505–506, 1995.

Pamir MN, Kansu T, Erbengi A, et al. Papilledema in Behçet's syndrome. Arch Neurol 38:643–645, 1981.

Papadakis MA, Schwartz ND. Temporal arteritis after normalization of erythrocyte sedimentation rate in polymyalgia rheumatica. Arch Intern Med 146:2283–2284, 1986.

Papaioannou CC, Hunder GG, McDuffie FC. Cellular immunity in polymyalgia rheumatica and giant cell arteritis: Lack of response to muscle or artery homogenates. Arthritis Rheum 22:740–745, 1979.

Papaioannou CC, Gupta RC, Hunder GG, et al. Circulating immune complexes in giant cell arteritis, polymyalgia rheumatica. Arthritis Rheum 23:1021–1025, 1980.

Parelhoff ES, Chavis RM, Friendly DS. Wegener's granulomatosis presenting as orbital pseudotumor in children. J Pediatr Ophthalmol Strabismus 22:100–104, 1985.

Park JH, Han MC, Kim SH, et al. Takayasu arteritis: Angiographic findings and results of angiography. AJR 153:1069–1074, 1989.

Park JR, Hazleman BL. Immunological and histological studies of temporal arteries. Ann Rheum Dis 37:238–243, 1978.

Parker F, Healey LA, Wilske KR, et al. Light and electron microscopic studies on human temporal arteries with special reference to alterations related to senescence, atherosclerosis and giant cell arteritis. Am J Pathol 79:57–80, 1975.

Parker HL, Kernohan JW. The central nervous system in periarteritis nodosa. Mayo Clin Proc 24:43–48, 1949.

Parums DV. The arteritides. Histopathology 25:1–20, 1994.

Pascuzzi RM, Roos KL, Davis TE Jr. Mental status abnormalities in temporal arteritis: A treatable cause of dementia in the elderly. Arthritis Rheum 32:1308–1311, 1989.

Patton WF, Lynch JP III. Lymphomatoid granulomatosis: Clinicopathologic study of four cases and literature review. Medicine 61:1–11, 1982.

Paulley JW, Hughes JP. Giant cell arteritis or arthritis of the aged. Br Med J 2:1562–1567, 1960.

Pawlotsky Y, Chales G, Meadeb J, et al. Value of ESR in assessment of rheumatoid arthritis. Lancet 2:1532, 1989.

Pearson CM. Polymyositis and dermatomyositis. In Arthritis and Allied Conditions. Editor, McCarty DJ, pp 742–761. Philadelphia, Lea and Febiger, 1979.

Pena CE. Lymphomatoid granulomatosis with cerebral involvement: Light and electron microscopic study of a case. Acta Neuropathol 37:193–197, 1977.

Penn AS, Rowan AJ. Myelopathy in systemic lupus erythematosus. Arch Neurol 18:337–349, 1968.

Perkins ES. Uveitis and toxoplasmosis. London, J & A Churchill Ltd, 1966.

Perry SR, Rootman J, White VA. The clinical and pathologic constellation of Wegener granulomatosis of the orbit. Ophthalmology 104:683–694, 1997.

Petit WA, Soso MJ, Higman H. Degos disease: Neurologic complications and cerebral angiography. Neurology 32:1305–1309, 1982.

Petri M, Rheinschmidt M, Whiting-O'Keefe Q, et al. The frequency of lupus anticoagulant in SLE: A study of sixty consecutive patients by activated partial thromboplastin time, Russell viper venom time and anticardiolipin antibody levels. Ann Intern Med 106:524–531, 1987.

Petty GW, Duffy J, Huston J. Cerebral ischemia in patients with hepatitis C virus infection and mixed cryoglobulinemia. Mayo Clin Proc 71:671–678, 1996.

Petz LD, Sharp GC, Cooper NR, et al. Serum and cerebrospinal fluid complement and serum autoantibodies in systemic lupus erythematosus. Medicine 50:259–275, 1971.

Pfaffenbach DD, Hollenhorst RW. Microangiopathy of the retinal arterioles. JAMA 225:480–483, 1973.

Piemme TE. Myasthenia gravis and auto-immune disease: Review of the literature including a case report of the coexistence of myasthenia and systemic lupus erythematosus. Ann Intern Med 57:130–135, 1964.

Pietrowa N, Duchowska H. Eye changes in the course of rheumatoid arthritis in children. Pediatrics 43:1489–1494, 1968.

Pillay N, Hunter T. Delayed evoked potentials in patients with ankylosing spondylitis. J Rheumatol 13:137–141, 1976.

Pinching AJ, Lockwood CM, Pussell BA, et al. Wegener's granulomatosis: Observations on 18 patients with severe renal disease. QJ Med 52:435–460, 1983.

Pinchoff BS, Spahlinger DA, Bergstrom TJ, et al. Extraocular muscle involvement in Wegener's granulomatosis. J Clin Neuroophthalmol 3:163–168, 1983.

Pines A, Kaplinsky N, Olchovsky D, et al. Pleuropulmonary manifestations of systemic lupus erythematosus: Clinical features of its subgroups. Prognostic and therapeutic implications. Chest 88:129–135, 1985.

Pinkham RA. The ocular manifestations of the pulseless syndrome. Acta XVII Conc Ophthalmol 1:348–366, 1955.

Pless M, Sandson T. Chronic internuclear ophthalmoplegia: A manifestation of D-penicillamine cerebral vasculitis. J Neuroophthalmol 17:44–46, 1997.

Plotkin GR, Calabro JJ, O'Duffy JD. Behçet's disease: A contemporary synopsis. New York, Futura, 1988.

Plotz PH, Dalakas M, Leff RL, et al. Current concepts in the idiopathic inflammatory myopathies: Polymyositis, dermatomyositis, and related disorders. Ann Intern Med 111:143–157, 1989.

Pollack IP, Becker B. Cytoid bodies of the retina in a patient with scleroderma. Am J Ophthalmol 54:655–660, 1962.

Pollack W. Some physicochemical aspects of hemagglutination. Ann NY Acad Sci 127:892–900, 1965.

Pollak VE, Kant KS. Systemic lupus erythematosus and the kidney. In Systemic Lupus Erythematosus. Editor, Lahita RG, pp 643–672. New York, John Wiley & Sons, 1987.

Pollock M, Blennerhassett JB, Clarke AM. Giant cell arteritis and the subclavian steal syndrome. Neurology 23:653–657, 1973.

Postel EA, Pollock SC. Recovery of vision in 47 y.o. man with fulminant giant cell arteritis. J Clin Neuroophthalmol 13:262–270, 1993.

Power WJ, Rodriques A, Neves RA, et al. Disease relapse in patients with ocular manifestations of Wegener granulomatosis. Ophthalmology 102:154–160, 1995.

Priluck IA, Robertson DM, Buettner H. Acute posterior multifocal placoid pigment epitheliopathy: urinary findings. Arch Ophthalmol 99:1560–1562, 1981.

Priori R, Paroli MP, Luan FL, et al. Cyclosporin A in the treatment of relapsing polychondritis with severe recurrent eye involvement. Br J Rheum 32:352, 1993.

Provost TT, Dore N. Cutaneous manifestations. In The Clinical Management of Systemic Lupus Erythematosus. Editor, Schur P, pp 85–111. Orlando, Florida, Grune & Stratton, 1983.

Puechal X, Said G, Job-Deslandre C, et al. Muscular involvement in systemic rheumatoid vasculitis. Br J Rheum 32:766–767, 1993.

Puechal X, Said G, Hilliquin P, et al. Peripheral neuropathy with necrotizing vasculitis in rheumatoid arthritis. Arthritis Rheum 38:1618–1629, 1995.

Pullar T, Capell HA. Value of ESR in assessment of rheumatoid arthritis. Lancet 2:1532–1533, 1989.

Purcell JJ Jr. Polyarteritis nodosa. In The Eye in Systemic Disease. Editors, Gold DH, Weingeist TA, pp 51–53. Philadelphia, LB Lippincott, 1990.

Purcell JJ Jr, Birkenkamp R, Tsai CC. Conjunctival lesions in periarteritis nodosa, a clinical and immunopathologic study. Arch Ophthalmol 102:736–738, 1984.

Quillen DA, Cantore WA, Schwartz SR, et al. Choroidal nonperfusion in giant cell arteritis. Am J Ophthalmol 116:171, 1993.

Rabinovitch J, Donnenfeld ED, Laibson PR. Management of Cogan's syndrome. Am J Ophthalmol 101:494–495, 1986.

Rabinowich L, Mehler MF. Parasympathetic pupillary involvement in biopsy-proven temporal arteritis. Ann Ophthalmol 20:400–402, 1988.

Rackemann FM, Greene JE. Periarteritis nodosa and asthma. Trans Assoc Am Phys 54:112–118, 1939.

Radda TM, Bardach H, Riss B. Acute ocular hypotony: A rare complication of temporal arteritis. Ophthalmologica 182:148–152, 1981a.

Radda TM, Pehamberger H, Smolen J, et al. Ocular manifestation of temporal arteritis. Immunological studies. Arch Ophthalmol 99:487–488, 1981b.

Raitt JW. Wegener's granulomatosis: Treatment with cytotoxic agents and adrenortonicoids. Ann Intern Med 74:344–356, 1971.

Raizman MB, Foster CS. Plasma exchange in the therapy of Behçet's disease. Graefe's Arch Clin Exp Ophthalmol 227:360–363, 1989.

Rajala SA, Ahvenainen JE, Mattila KJ, et al. Incidence and survival rate in cases of biopsy-proven temporal arteritis. Scand J Rheumatol 22:289–291, 1993.

Ramos M, Mandybur TI. Cerebral vasculitis in rheumatoid arthritis. Arch Neurol 32:271–275, 1975.

Rao SA, Mandalam KR, Rao VK, et al. Takayasu arteritis: Initial and long-term follow-up in 16 patients after percutaneous transluminal angioplasty of the descending thoracic and abdominal aorta. Radiology 189:173–179, 1993.

Raymond LA, Sacks JG, Choromokos E, et al. Short posterior ciliary artery insufficiency with hyperthermia (Uhthoff's symptom). Am J Ophthalmol 90:619–623, 1980.

Raz E, Michaeli J, Rosenmann E, et al. Antinuclear antibody-negative systemic lupus erythematosus: Close correlation between disease activity and appearance of circulating anticoagulant. Israel J Med Sci 24:105–108, 1988.

Rechthand E, Cornblath DR, Stern BJ, et al. Chronic demyelinating polyneuropathy in systemic lupus erythematosus. Neurology 34:1375–1377, 1984.

Rechichi CF, Trombetta C, Scullica MG, et al. Psoriatic arthritis or overlap syndrome. Ophthalmologica 211:266–267, 1997.

Reeves WH, Lahita RG. Clinical presentation of systemic lupus erythematosus. In Systemic Lupus Erythematosus. Editor, Lahita RG, pp 355–382. New York, John Wiley & Sons, 1987.

Reichlin M. Antinuclear antibodies. In Textbook of Rheumatology. Editors, Kelley WN, Harris ED Jr, Ruddy S, et al, 3rd ed, pp 208–225. Philadelphia, WB Saunders, 1989.

Reimer G, Steinkohl S, Djawari D, et al. Lytic effect of cytotoxic lymphocytes on oral epithelial cells in Behçet's disease. Br J Dermatol 107:529–536, 1982.

Reimer G, Luckner L, Hornstein OP. Direct immunofluorescence in recurrent aphthous ulcers and Behçet's disease. Dermatologica 167:293–298, 1983.

Reinecke RD. The rheumatologists consider giant cell arteritis. Arch Ophthalmol 84:259, 1970.

Reinitz E, Aversa A. Long-term treatment of temporal arteritis with dapsone. Am J Med 85:456–457, 1988.

Reiter H. Ueber eine bisher unerkannte Spirochaeteninfektion (Spirochaetosis arthritica). Dtsch Med Woschr 42:1435–1436, 1916.

Renie WA, Murphy RP, Anderson KC, et al. The evaluation of patients with Eales's disease. Retina 3:243–248, 1983.

Reveille JD, Goodman RE, Barger BO, et al. Familial polyarteritis nodosa: A serologic and immunogenetic analysis. J Rheumatol 16:181–185, 1989.

Reyes MG, Fresco R, Chokroverty S, et al. Virus-like particles in granulomatous angiitis of the central nervous system. Neurology 26:797–799, 1976.

Reynolds JC, Inman RD, Kimberly RP, et al. Acute pancreatitis in systemic lupus erythematosus: Report of twenty cases and a review of the literature. Medicine 61:25–32, 1982.

Reza MJ, Demanes DJ. Behçet's disease: A case with hemoptysis, pseudotumor cerebri and arteritis. J Rheumatol 5:320–326, 1978.

Reza MJ, Dornfeld L, Goldberg LS, et al. Wegener's granulomatosis: Long-term follow-up of patients treated with cyclophosphamide. Arthritis Rheum 18:501–506, 1975.

Rhodes RH, Madelaire NC, Petrelli M, et al. Primary angiitis and angiopathy of the central nervous system and their relationship to systemic giant cell arteritis. Arch Pathol Lab Med 119:334–349, 1995.

Richer SP, Hall T. Mobility spectacles for a patient with ankylosing spondylitis. Am J Optom Physiol Optics 63:927–930, 1986.

Ristow SC, Griner PF, Abraham GN, et al. Reversal of systemic manifestations of cryoglobulinemia. Treatment with melphalan and prednisone. Arch Intern Med 136:467–470, 1976.

Roberts J. Cogan's syndrome. Med J Austr 1:186–190, 1965.

Robin JB, Schanzlin DJ, Meisler DM, et al. Ocular involvement in the respiratory vasculitides. Surv Ophthalmol 30:127–140, 1985.

Roche NE, Fulbright JW, Wagner AD, et al. Correlation of interleuken 6 production and disease activity in polymyalgia rheumatica and giant cell arteritis. Arthritis Rheum 36:1286–1294, 1993.

Rodnan GP, Myerowitz RL, Justh GO. Morphologic changes in the digital arteries of patients with progressive systemic sclerosis (scleroderma) and Raynaud phenomenon. Medicine 59:393–408, 1980.

Rodriquez A, Akova YA, Pedroza-Seres M, et al. Posterior segment ocular manifestations in patients with HLA-B27-associated uveitis. Ophthalmology 101:1267–1274, 1994.

Rogers MA, Crockard HA, Moskovich R, et al. Nystagmus and joint position sensation: Their importance in posterior occipitocervical fusion in rheumatoid arthritis. Spine 19:16–20, 1994.

Rogers RS III. Recurrent aphthous stomatitis: Clinical characteristics and evidence for an immunopathogenesis. J Invest Dermatol 69:499–509, 1977.

Rogers RS, Sams W Jr, Shorter RG. Lymphocytotoxicity in recurrent aphthous stomatitis: Lymphocytotoxicity for oral epithelial cells in recurrent aphthous stomatitis and Behçet's syndrome. Arch Dermatol 109:361–363, 1974.

Roifman CM, Lavis S, Moore AT, et al. Tenosynovitis of the superior oblique muscle (Brown syndrome) associated with juvenile rheumatoid arthritis. J Pediatr 106:617–619, 1985.

Roifman CM, Schaffer FM, Wachsmuth SE, et al. Reversal of chronic polymyositis following intravenous immune serum globulin therapy. JAMA 258:513–515, 1987.

Ronco P, Verroust P, Mignon F, et al. Immunopathological studies of polyarteritis nodosa and Wegener's granulomatosis. A report of 43 patients with 51 renal biopsies. QJ Med 52:212–223, 1983.

Rootman J, Robertson W, Lapointe JS. Inflammatory diseases. In Diseases of the Orbit. Editor, Rootman J, pp 143–204. Philadelphia, JB Lippincott, 1988.

Rose GA. The natural history of polyarteritis. Br Med J 2:1148–1152, 1957.

Rosen ES. The retinopathy in polyarteritis nodosa. Br J Ophthalmol 52:903–906, 1968.

Rosenbaum JT, Bennett RM. Chronic anterior and posterior uveitis and primary Sjögren's syndrome. Am J Ophthalmol 104:346–352, 1987.

Rosenbaum JT, Simpson J, Neuwelt CM. Successful treatment of optic neuropathy in association with systemic lupus erythematosus using intravenous cyclophosphamide. Br J Ophthalmol 81:130–132, 1997.

Rosenberger A, Adler OB, Haim S. Radiological aspects of Behçet's disease. Radiology 144:261–264, 1982.

Rosenfeld SI, Kosmorsky GS, Klingele TG, et al. Treatment of temporal arteritis with ocular involvement. Am J Med 80:143–145, 1986.

Rosenstein ED, Sobelman J, Kramer N. Isolated, pupil-sparing third nerve palsy as initial manifestation of systemic lupus erythematosus. J Clin Neuroophthalmol 9:285–288, 1989.

Rosner S, Ginzler EM, Diamond MS, et al. A multicenter study of outcome in systemic lupus erythematosus. II. Cause of death. Arthritis Rheum 25:612–617, 1982.

Ross RS, McKusick VA. Aortic arch syndromes: Diminished or absent pulses in arteries arising from the arch of the aorta. Arch Intern Med 92:701–740, 1953.

Rostoker G, Desvaux-Belghiti D, Pilatte Y, et al. High-dose immunoglobulin therapy for severe IgA nephropathy and henoch-schonlein purpura. Ann Intern Med 120:476–484, 1994.

Roth AM, Milsow L, Keltner JL. The ultimate diagnoses of patients undergoing temporal artery biopsies. Arch Ophthalmol 102:901–903, 1984.

Rothfield N. Clinical features of systemic lupus erythematosus. In Textbook of Rheumatology. Editors, Kelley WN, Harris ED Jr, Ruddy S, et al, 2nd ed, pp 1106–1132. Philadelphia. WB Saunders, 1981.

Rothfield NF. Cardiopulmonary manifestations. In The Clinical Management of Systemic Lupus Erythematosus. Editor, Schur P, pp 137–151. Orlando, FL, Grune & Stratton, 1983a.

Rothfield NF. Renal disease. In The Clinical Management of Systemic Lupus Erythematosus. Editor, Schur P, pp 113–122, Orlando. Florida, Grune & Stratton, 1983b.

Rowland LP. Prostigmine—responsiveness and the diagnosis of myasthenia gravis. Neurology 5:612–624, 1955.

Rowland LP, Schotland DL. Neoplasms and muscle disease. In The Remote Effects of Cancer on the Nervous System. Editors, Brain WR, Norris F, p 84. New York, Grune & Stratton, 1965.

Rowland LP, Clark C, Olarte M. Therapy for dermatomyositis and polymyositis. Adv Neurol 17:63–97, 1977.

Rubin BR, De Horatius RJ. Acute visual loss in systemic lupus erythematosus. J Am Optom Assoc 89:73–77, 1989.

Rubin RL, Tang F-L, Chan EKL, et al. IgG subclasses of autoantibodies in systemic lupus erythematosus, Sjögren's syndrome, and drug-induced autoimmunity. J Immunol 137:2528–2534, 1986.

Rubinow A, Brandt KD, Cohen AS, et al. Iatrogenic morbidity accompanying suppression of temporal arteritis by adrenal corticosteroids. Ann Ophthalmol 16:258–265, 1984.

Rubinstein LJ, Urich H. Meningo-encephalitis of Behçet's disease: Case report with pathological findings. Brain 86:151–160, 1963.

Ruby AJ, Jampol LM. Crohn's disease and retinal vascular disease. Am J Ophthalmol 110:349–353, 1990.

Rucker CW, Ferguson RH. Ocular manifestations of relapsing polychondritis. Arch Ophthalmol 73:46–48, 1965.

Rumbaugh CL, Bergeron RT, Scanlon RC, et al. Cerebral vascular changes secondary to amphetamine abuse in the experimental animal. Radiology 101:345–351, 1971.

Rush JA, Kramer LD. Biopsy-negative cranial arteritis with complete oculomotor nerve palsy. Ann Ophthalmol 11:209–213, 1979.

Russell ML, Gordon DA, Ogryzlo MA, et al. The cauda equina syndrome of ankylosing spondylitis. Ann Intern Med 78:551–554, 1973.

Russell RWR. Giant-cell arteritis. A review of 35 cases. QJ Med 28:471–489, 1959.

Ryan SJ, Maumenee AE. Acute posterior multifocal placoid pigment epitheliopathy. Am J Ophthalmol 74:1066–1074, 1972.

Rynes RI, Mika P, Bartholomew LE. Development of giant cell (temporal) arteritis in a patient 'adequately' treated for polymyalgia rheumatica. Ann Rheum Dis 36:88–90, 1977.

Saari KM, Vilppula A, Lassus A, et al. Ocular inflammation in Reiter's disease after salmonella enteritis. Am J Ophthalmol 90:63–68, 1980.

Saari KM, Rudenberg HA, Laitinen O. Bilateral central retinal vein occlusion in a patient with scleroderma. Ophthalmologica 182:7–12, 1981.

Sack M, Cassidy JT, Bole GG. Prognostic factors in polyarteritis. J Rheumatol 2: 411–420, 1975.

Sahn EE, Sahn SA. Wegener's granulomatosis with aphasia. Arch Intern Med 136: 87–89, 1976.

Said G, Lacroix-Ciaudo C, Fujimura H, et al. The peripheral neuropathy of necrotizing arteritis: A clinicopathological study. Ann Neurol 23:461–465, 1988.

Sainz de la Maza M, Foster CS, Jabbur NS. Scleritis associated with rheumatoid arthritis and with other systemic immune-mediated diseases. Ophthalmology 101: 1281–1286, 1994.

Sakaki T, Morimoto T, Utsumi S. Cerebral transmural angiitis and ruptured cerebral aneurysms in patients with systemic lupus erythematosus. Neurochirurgia 33: 132–135, 1990.

Sakane T, Kotani H, Takada S, et al. Functional aberration of T-cell subsets in patients with Behçet's disease. Arthritis Rheum 25:1343–1351, 1982.

Saldana MJ, Patchefsky MD, Israel HL, et al. Pulmonary angiitis and granulomatosis: The relationship between histological features, organ involvement, and response to treatment. Hum Pathol 8:391–409, 1977.

Sams WJ Jr, Thorne EG, Small P, et al. Leukocytoclastic vasculitis. Arch Dermatol 112:219–226, 1976.

Samuelson TW, Margo CE. Protracted uveitis as the initial manifestation of Wegener's granulomatosis. Arch Ophthalmol 108:478–479, 1990.

Sandok BA. Temporal arteritis. JAMA 222:1405–1406, 1972.

Sanford RG, Berney SN. Polymyalgia rheumatica and temporal arteritis in blacks—clinical features and HLA typing. J Rheumatol 4:435–442, 1977.

Sanford-Smith JH. Intermittent superior oblique tendon sheath syndrome. Br J Ophthalmol 53:412–417, 1969.

Sano K, Aiga T, Saito I. Angiography in pulseless disease. Radiology 94:69–74, 1970.

Santos R, Barojas E, Alarcón-Segovia D, et al. Retinal microangiopathy in systemic lupus erythematosus. Am J Ophthalmol 80:249–252, 1975.

Saraux H, Pelosse B. Acute posterior multifocal placoid pigment epitheliopathy. A long-term follow-up. Ophthalmologica 194:161–163, 1987.

Saraux H, Laroche L, Foels A, et al. Ischémie aiguë postérieure du nerf optique. J Fr Ophtalmol 5:167–171, 1982a.

Saraux H, Le Hoang P, Laroche L. Neuropathie optique ischémique aiguë antérieure et postérieure au cours d'une péri-artérite noueuse traitement par plasmaphérèse. J Fr Ophtalmol 5:55–61, 1982b.

Saraux H, Laroche L, Le Hoang P. Usefulness of plasma exchange in Behçet's disease and other ophthalmologic disorders. In Bull Soc Ophtalmol Fr 82:41–44, 1982c.

Saraux H, Le Hoang P, Audebert A-A, et al. Interet de la plasmapherese dans le traitement du syndrome de Behçet. Bull Soc Ophtalmol Fr 82:41–44, 1982d.

Saribas O, Aydin-Kirkali P, Erdem E, et al. Fascicular oculomotor palsy in neuro-Behçet's disease. J Clin Neuroophthalmol 11:300–305, 1991.

Savino PJ, Weinberg RJ, Yassin JG, et al. Diverse manifestations of acute posterior multifocal placoid pigment epitheliopathy. Am J Ophthalmol 77:659–662, 1974.

Savory WS. Case of a young woman in whom the main arteries of both upper extremities and of the left side of the neck were throughout completely obliterated. Med-Chir Trans London 39:205, 1856.

Schaller J, Kupfer C, Wedgwood RJ. Iridocyclitis in juvenile rheumatoid arthritis. Pediatrics 44:92–100, 1969.

Schell CL, Rathe RJ. Superior sagittal sinus thrombosis. Still a killer. West J Med 149:304–307, 1988.

Scherbel AL, MacKenzie AK, Nousek JE, et al. Ocular lesions in rheumatoid arthritis and related disorders with particular reference to retinopathy—a study of 741 patients treated with and without chloroquine drugs. N Engl J Med 273:360–366, 1965.

Schilling H, Bornfeld N, Windeck R, et al. Zytostatische und immunsuppressive Therapie des okulären Behçet-Syndroms. Klin Monatsbl Augenheilkd 196:62–69, 1990.

Schlosstein L, Terasaki PI, Bluestone R, et al. High association of an HL-A antigen, W27, with ankylosing spondilitis. N Engl J Med 288:704–706, 1973.

Schmid FR, Cooper NS, Ziff M, et al. Arteritis in rheumatoid arthritis. Am J Med 30:56–83, 1961.

Schmidt BJ, Meagher-Villemure K, Del Carpio J. Lymphomatoid granulomatosis with isolated involvement of the brain. Ann Neurol 15:478–481, 1984.

Schmidt D, Loffler KU. Temporal arteritis comparison of histological and clinical findings. Acta Ophthalol 72:319–325, 1994.

Schmidt M, Fox AJ, Nicolle DA. Bilateral anterior ischemic optic neuropathy as a presentation of Takayasu's disease. J Neuroophthalmol 17:156–161, 1997.

Schneider HA, Weber AA, Ballen PH. The visual prognosis in temporal arteritis. Ann Ophthalmol 3:1215–1230, 1971.

Schneider MS, Goldman PS. On familial polyarteritis nodosa. Sov Med 25:141–143, 1962.

Schneiderman JH, Sharpe JA, Sutton DMC. Cerebral and retinal vascular complications of inflammatory bowel disease. Ann Neurol 5:331–337, 1979.

Schotland DL, Wolff SM, White HH, et al. Neurological aspects of Behçet's disease: Case report and review of the literature. Am J Med 34:544–553, 1963.

Schrader WH. Erythrocyte sedimentation rate. Postgrad Med 34:A42–52, 1963.

Schuknecht HF, Nadol JB Jr. Temporal bone pathology in a case of Cogan's syndrome. Laryngoscope. 104:1135–1142, 1994.

Schur PH. Clinical features of SLE. In Textbook of Rheumatology. Editors, Kelley WN, Harris ED Jr, Ruddy S, et al, 4th ed, pp 1017–1042. Philadelphia, WB Saunders, 1993.

Schur PH. Systemic lupus erythematosus. In Cecil Textbook of Medicine. Editors, Bennett JC, Plum F, 20th ed, pp 1475–1483. Philadelphia, WB Saunders, 1996.

Schur PH, Meyer I, Garovoy M, et al. Associations between systemic lupus erythematosus and the major histocompatibility complex: Clinical and immunological considerations. Clin Immunol Immunopathol 24:263–275, 1982.

Schwitter J, Agosti R, Ott P, et al. Small infarctions of cochlear, retinal and encephalic tissue in young women. Stroke 23:903–907, 1992.

Scoppetta C, Morante M, Casali C, et al. Dermatomyositis spares extraocular muscles. Neurology 35:141, 1985.

Scott AB, Knapp P. Surgical treatment of the superior oblique tendon sheath syndrome. Arch Ophthalmol 88:282–286, 1972.

Scott DGI, Bacon PA, Tribe CR. Systemic rheumatoid vasculitis: A clinical and laboratory study of 50 cases. Medicine 57:288–297, 1981.

Scott DL, Spector TD. Value of ESR in assessment of rheumatoid arthritis. Lancet 2:1531–1532, 1989.

Scouras J, Koutroumanos J. Ischaemic optic neuropathy in Behçet's syndrome. Ophthalmologica 173:11–18, 1976.

Searles RP, Mladinich EK, Messner RP. Isolated trigeminal sensory neuropathy: Early manifestation of mixed connective tissue disease. Neurology 28:1286–1289, 1978.

Sedgwich RP, von Hagen KO. The neurological manifestations of lupus erythematosus and periarteritis nodosa. Bull Los Angeles Neurol Soc 13:129–142, 1948.

Sedwick LA, Burde RM. Isolated sixth nerve palsy as initial manifestation of systemic lupus erythematosus. A case report. J Clin Neuroophthalmol 3:109–110, 1983.

Sedwick LA, Margo CE. Sixth nerve palsies, temporal artery biopsy, and necrotizing vasculitis. J Clin Neuroophthalmol 9:119–121, 1989.

Sedwick LA, Klingele TG, Burde RM, et al. Optic neuritis in inflammatory bowel disease. J Clin Neuroophthalmol 4:3–6, 1984.

Seibold JR. Scleroderma. In Textbook of Rheumatology. Editors, Kelley WN, Harris ED Jr, Ruddy S, et al, 4th ed, pp 1113–1143. Philadelphia, WB Saunders, 1993.

Seibold JR. Scleroderma. In Textbook of Rheumatology. Editors, Kelley WN, Harris ED Jr, Ruddy S, et al., 5th ed, pp 1133–1162. Philadelphia, WB Saunders, 1997.

Semple HC, Landers MB III, Morse LS. Optic disc neovascularization in juvenile rheumatoid arthritis. Am J Ophthalmol 110:210–212, 1990.

Sen DK, Sarin GS, Ghosh B, et al. Serum alpha-1-acid glycoprotein levels in patients with idiopathic peripheral retinal vasculitis (Eale's disease). Acta Ophthalmol 70:515–517, 1992.

Serdaroglu P, Yazici H, özdemir C, et al. Neurologic involvement in Behçet's syndrome. A prospective study. Arch Neurol 46:265–269, 1989.

Sergent JS, Lockshin MD, Christian CL, et al. Vasculitis with hepatitis B antigenemia: A long term observation in nine patients. Medicine 55:1–18, 1976.

Sezer FN. The isolation of a virus as the cause of Behçet's disease. Am J Ophthalmol 36:301–315, 1953.

Shaw HE, Osher RH, Smith JL. Amaurosis fugax associated with SC hemoglobinopathy and systemic lupus erythematosus. Am J Ophthalmol 87:281–285, 1979.

Shearn MA. Sjögren's Syndrome. Philadelphia, WB Saunders, 1971.

Shearn MA, Pirofsky B. Disseminated lupus erythematosus analysis of thirty-four cases. Arch Intern Med 90:790–807, 1952.

Sheehan B, Harriman DGF, Bradshaw JPP. Polyarteritis nodosa with ophthalmic and neurological complications. Arch Ophthalmol 57:537–547, 1958.

Sheldon P. Cryptic Wegener's granulomatosis revealed after 18 years. Br J Rheumatol 33:296–298, 1994.

Shelhamer JH, Volkman DJ, Parrillo JE, et al. Takayasu's arteritis and its therapy. Ann Intern Med 103:121–126, 1985.

Shenberger KN, Meharg JG, Lane CD. Temporal arteritis presenting as ataxia and dementia. Postgrad Med 69:246–249, 1981.

Shepherd DI, Downie AW, Best PV. Systemic lupus erythematosus and multiple sclerosis. Arch Neurol 30:423, 1974.

Shergy WJ, Kredich DW, Pisetsky DS. The relationship of anticardiolipin antibodies to disease manifestations in pediatric systemic lupus erythematosus. J Rheumatol 15:1389–1394, 1988.

Shields CL, Shields JA, Rozanski TI. Conjunctival involvement in Churg-Strauss syndrome. Am J Ophthalmol 102:601–605, 1986.

Shikano S. Ocular pathology in Behçet's syndrome. In Behçet's disease. Editor, Monacelli M, pp 111–136. Basel S Karger, 1966.

Shimizu K. Harada's, Behçet's, Vogt-Koyanagi syndromes—are they clinical entities? Trans Am Acad Ophthalmol Otolaryngol 77:281–290, 1973.

Shimizu K, Sano K. Pulseless disease. J Neuropathol Clin Neurol 1:37–47, 1951.

Shimizu T, Ehrlich GE, Inaba G, et al. Behçet's disease. Semin Arth Rheum 8: 223–260, 1979.

Shiozawa Z, Yoshida M, Kobayashi K, et al. Superior sagittal sinus thrombosis and systemic lupus erythematosus. Ann Neurol 20:272, 1986.

Shoemaker E, Lin ZS, Rae Grant AD, et al. Primary angiitis of the central nervous system: Unusual MR appearance. Am J Neuroradiol *15*:331–334, 1994.

Shoenfeld Y, Schwartz RS. Hematologic manifestations. In The Clinical Management of Systemic Lupus Erythematosus. Editor, Schur PH, pp 123–136. Orlando, FL, Grune & Stratton, 1983.

Siatkowski RM, Gass JDM, Glaser JS, et al. Fluorescein angiography in the diagnosis of giant cell arteritis. Am J Ophthalmol *115*:57–63, 1993.

Sibbitt WL Jr, Sibbitt RR, Griffey RH, et al. Magnetic resonance and computed tomographic imaging in the evaluation of acute neuropsychiatric disease in systemic lupus erythematosus. Ann Rheum Dis *48*:1014–1022, 1989.

Sibbitt WL, Sibbitt RR. Magnetic resonance spectroscopy and position emission tomography scanning in neuropsychiatric lupus erythematosus. Rheum Dis Clin N Am *19*:851–868, 1993.

Siberry GK, Cohen BA, Johnson B. Cutaneous polyarteritis nodosa. Arch Dermatol *130*:884–889, 1994.

Sibley JT, Olszynski WP, Decoteau WE, et al. The incidence and prognosis of central nervous system disease in systemic lupus erythematosus. J Rheumatol *19*:47–52, 1992.

Sibony PA, Lessell S. Transient oculomotor synkinesis in temporal arteritis. Arch Neurol *41*:87–88, 1984.

Sievers K, Nissila M, Sievers U-M. Cerebral vasculitis visualized by angiography in juvenile rheumatoid arthritis simulating brain tumor. Acta Rheum Scand *14*: 222–232, 1968.

Sigal LH. The neurologic presentation of vasculitic and rheumatologic syndromes: A review. Medicine *66*:157–180, 1987.

Sigal LH. Isolated CNS angiitis. Neurology *39*:1645, 1989.

Sigelman J, Behrens M, Hilal S. Acute posterior multifocal placoid pigment epitheliopathy associated with cerebral vasculitis and homonymous hemianopia. Am J Ophthalmol *88*:919–924, 1979.

Silberberg DH, Laties AM. Increased intracranial pressure in disseminated lupus erythematosus. Arch Neurol *29*:88–90, 1973.

Silfverskiold BP. Retina periphlebitis and chronic disseminated encephalomyelitis. Acta Psychiatr Neurol Scand *74*:55, 1951.

Silman A, Holligan S, Brennan P, et al. Prevalence of symptoms of Raynaud's phenomenon in general practice. Br Med J *301*:590–592, 1990.

Silverman M, Lubeck MJ, Briney WG. Central retinal vein occlusion complicating systemic lupus erythematosus. Arthritis Rheum *21*:839–843, 1978.

Silverstein A, Present DH. Cerebrovascular occlusions in relatively young patients with regional enteritis. JAMA *215*:976–977, 1971.

Simmons RJ, Cogan DG. Occult temporal arteritis. Arch Ophthalmol *68*:8–18, 1962.

Simpson JA. Myasthenia gravis: A new hypothesis. Scott Med J *5*:419–436, 1960.

Sims J. Acquired apparent superior oblique tendon sheath syndrome. Br Orthopt J *28*:112–115, 1971.

Singhal BS, Dastur DK. Eales' disease with neurological involvement. J Neurol Sci *27*:312–345, 1976.

Sipe JC, Rosenberg JH. Granulomatous giant cell angiitis of the central nervous system. West Med J *127*:215–220, 1977.

Sjögren H. Zur Kenntnis der Keratoconjunctivitis sicca. (Keratitis filiformis bei Hypofunktion der Tränendrüsen). Acta Ophthalmol *2(suppl)*:1–151, 1933.

Sklar EML, Schatz NJ, Glaser JS, et al. MR of vasculitis-induced optic neuropathy. AJNR *17*:121–128, 1996.

Slavin ML. Brow droop after superficial temporal artery biopsy. Arch Ophthalmol *104*:1127, 1986.

Slavin ML, Margolis AJ. Progressive anterior ischemic optic neuropathy due to giant cell arteritis despite high-dose intravenous corticosteroids. Arch Ophthalmol *106*: 1167, 1988.

Smith CA, Pinals RS. Optic neuritis in systemic lupus erythematosus. J Rheumatol *9*:963–966, 1982.

Smith CD, Marino C, Rothfield NF. The clinical utility of the lupus band test. Arthritis Rheum *27*:382–387, 1984.

Smith CH, Savino PJ, Beck RW, et al. Acute posterior multifocal placoid pigment epitheliopathy and cerebral vasculitis. Arch Neurol *40*:48–50, 1983.

Smith E. Aetiology of apparent superior oblique tendon sheath syndrome. Trans Orthopt Assoc Aust *7*:32, 1965.

Smith JL. Ocular complications of rheumatic fever and rheumatoid arthritis. Am J Ophthalmol *43*:575–582, 1957.

Snyderman R. Mechanisms of inflammation and tissue destruction in the rheumatic diseases. In Cecil Textbook of Medicine. Editors, Wyngaarden JB, Smith LH Jr, 18th ed, pp 1984–1992. Philadelphia, WB Saunders, 1988.

Solomon SM, Solomon JH. Bilateral central retinal artery occlusions in polyarteritis nodosa. Ann Ophthalmol *10*:567–569, 1978.

Somer T. Thrombo-embolic and vascular complications in vasculitis syndromes. Eur Heart J *14*(suppl K):24–29, 1993.

Sonneblick M, Nesher R, Rozenman Y, et al. Charles Bonnet syndrome in temporal arteritis. J Rheumatol *22*:1596–1597, 1995.

Sonnex C, Paice E, White AG. Autonomic neuropathy in systemic sclerosis: A case report and evaluation of six patients. Ann Rheum Dis *45*:957–960, 1986.

Sorenson PS, Lorenzen I. Giant-cell arteritis, temporal arteritis and polymyalgia rheumatica. Acta Med Scand *201*:207–213, 1977.

Soter NA. Clinical presentations and mechanisms of necrotizing angiitis of the skin. J Invest Dermatol *67*:354–359, 1976.

Souza Ramalho P, Hormigo A, Martins R, et al. Haematological changes in retinal vasculitis. Eye *2*:278–282, 1988.

Soukiasian SH, Foster CS, Raizman MB. Treatment strategies for scleritis and uveitis associated with inflammatory bowel disease. Am J Ophthalmol *118*:601–611, 1994.

Sox HC Jr, Liang MH. The erythrocyte sedimentation rate. Guidelines for rational use. Ann Intern Med *104*:515–523, 1986.

Spalton DJ, Graham EM, Page NGR, et al. Ocular changes in limited forms of Wegener's granulomatosis. Br J Ophthalmol *65*:553–563, 1981.

Specks U, Homburger HA. Laboratory medicine and pathology. Anti-neutrophil cytoplasmic antibodies. May Clin Proc *69*:1197–1198, 1994.

Spencer R, Tolentino FI, Doyle GJ. Takayasu's arteritis: Case report and review emphasizing ocular manifestations. Ann Ophthalmol *12*:935–938, 1980.

Spencer WH, Hoyt WF. A fatal case of giant-cell arteritis (temporal or cranial arteritis) with ocular involvement. Arch Ophthalmol *64*:862–867, 1960.

Spitznas M, Meyer-Schwickerath G, Stephan B. The clinical picture of Eales' disease. Graefes Arch Klin Exp Ophthalmol *194*:73–85, 1975a.

Spitznas M, Meyer-Schwickerath G, Stephan B. Treatment of Eales' disease with photocoagulation. Graefes Arch Klin Exp Ophthalmol *194*:193–198, 1975b.

Spolaore R, Gaudric A, Coscas G, et al. Acute sectorial choroidal ischemia. Am J Ophthalmol *98*:707–716, 1984.

Stafford CR, Bogdoff BM, Green L, et al. Mononeuropathy multiplex as a complication of amphetamine angiitis. Neurology *25*:570–572, 1975.

Stavrou P, Deutsch J, Rene C, et al. Ocular manifestations of classical and limited Wegener's granulomatosis. Quart J Med *86*:719–725, 1993.

Stefani FH, Brandt F, Pielsticker K. Periarteritis nodosa and thrombotic thrombocytopenic purpura with serous retinal detachment in siblings. Br J Ophthalmol *62*: 402–407, 1978.

Stein R, Regenbogen L, Romano A, et al. Orbital apex syndrome due to cranial arteritis. Ann Ophthalmol *12*:708–713, 1980.

Steinberg AD. Management of systemic lupus erythematosus. In Textbook of Rheumatology. Editors, Kelley WN, Harris ED Jr, Ruddy S, et al, 3rd ed, pp 1130–1146. Philadelphia, WB Saunders, 1989.

Steinberg AD, Talal N. The coexistence of Sjögren's syndrome and systemic lupus erythematosus. Ann Intern Med *74*:55–61, 1971.

Steinberg VL. Neuropathy in rheumatoid disease. Br Med J *1*:1600–1603, 1960.

Steiner JW, Gelbloom AJ. Intracranial manifestations in two cases of systemic rheumatoid disease. Arthritis Rheum *2*:537–545, 1959.

Steinman TI, Jaffe BF, Monaco AP, et al. Recurrence of Wegener's granulomatosis after kidney transplantation. Am J Med *68*:458–460, 1980.

Stern GM, Hoffbrand AV, Urich H. The peripheral nerves and skeletal muscles in Wegener's granulomatosis: A clinicopathological study of four cases. Brain *88*: 151–164, 1965.

Stevens MB. Musculoskeletal manifestations. In The Clinical Management of Systemic Lupus Erythematosus. Editor, Schur PH, pp 63–84. Orlando, FL, Grune & Stratton, 1983.

Stevens MB. Systemic lupus erythematosus and the cardiovascular system. In Systemic Lupus Erythematosus. Editor, Lahita RG, pp 673–690. New York, John Wiley & Sons, 1987.

Stewart AJ, Hill BM. Ocular manifestations of juvenile rheumatoid arthritis. Can J Ophthalmol *2*:58–62, 1967.

Still GF. On a form of chronic joint disease in children. Med Chir Trans *80*:47–59, 1897.

Stimmler MM, Coletti PM, Quismorio FP. Magnetic resonance imaging of the brain in neuropsychiatric systemic lupus erythematosus. Semin Arthritis *22*:334–340, 1993.

Stoppe G, Wildhagen K, Seidel JW, et al. Positron emission tomography in neuropsychiatric lupus erythematosus. Neurology *40*:304–308, 1990.

Storey JK. An optical aid for a case of severe ankylosing spondylitis. Ophthalmic Optician *13*:1324, 1973.

Stoudemire A, Stork M, Simel D, et al. Neuro-ophthalmic systemic lupus erythematosus misdiagnosed as hysterical blindness. Am J Psychiatr *139*:1194–1196, 1982.

Straatsma BR. Ocular manifestations of Wegener's granulomatosis. Am J Ophthalmol *44*:789–799, 1957.

Strachan RW. The natural history of Takayasu's arteriopathy. QJ Med *33*:57–69, 1964.

Strachan RW, Wigzell FW, Anderson JR. Locomotor manifestations and serum studies in Takayasu's arteriopathy. Am J Med *40*:560–568, 1966.

Strauss KW, Gonzalez-Buritica H, Khamashta MA, et al. Polymyositis-dermatomyositis: A clinical review. Postgrad Med J *65*:437–443, 1989.

Stuart R. Temporal artery biopsy in suspected temporal arteritis: A five-year survey. NZ Med J *102*:431–433, 1989.

Su WPD, Schroeter AL, Lee DA, et al. Clinical and histological findings in Degos syndrome (malignant atrophic papulosis). Cutis *35*:131–138, 1985.

Subbiah P, Wijdicks E, Muenter M, et al. Skin lesion with a fatal neurologic outcome (Degos' disease). Neurology *46*:636–640, 1996.

Subramanyan R, Joy J, Balakrishnan KG. Natural history of aortoarteritis (Takayasu's disease). Circulation *80*:429–437, 1989.

Sumkin PA, Healey CA. Arthritis rounds—giant cell arteritis with polymyalgia rheumatica, loss of vision and abdominal symptoms during a four year course. Arthritis Rheum *12*:147–150, 1969.

Sundaram MBM, Rajput AH. Nervous system complications of relapsing polychondritis. Neurology 33:513–515, 1983.

Susac JO. Susac's syndrome: The triad of microangiopathy of the brain and retina with hearing loss in young women. Neurology 44:591–593, 1994.

Susac JO, Gracia-Mullin R, Glaser JS. Ophthalmoplegia in dermatomyositis. Neurology 23:305–310, 1973.

Susac JO, Hardman JM, Selhorst JB. Microangiopathy of the brain and retina. Neurology 29:313–316, 1979.

Swanson RA, Monteiro MLR, DeArmond SJ, et al. A microangiopathic syndrome of encephalopathy, hearing loss and retinal artery occlusion. Neurology 35(suppl 1):145, 1985.

Taccari E, Scavalli S, Riccieri V, et al. Magnetic resonance imaging (MRI) of the brain: ECLAM and SLEDAI correlations. Clin Exp Rheum 12:23–28, 1994.

Takahashi I, Takamura H, Gotoh S, et al. Giant cell arteritis with subarachnoid haemorrhage due to the rupture of inflammatory aneurysm of the posterior inferior cerebellar artery. Acta Neurochir 138:893–894, 1996.

Takayasu M. A case with peculiar changes of the central retinal vessels. Acta Soc Ophthalmol Jpn 12:554–557, 1908.

Tan EM, Cohen AS, Fries JF, et al. The 1982 revised criteria for the classification of systemic lupus erythematosus. Arthritis Rheum 25:1271–1277, 1982.

Tanaka T, Shimizu K. Retinal arteriovenous shunts in Takayasu disease. Ophthalmology 94:1380–1388, 1987.

Tang RA, Kaldis LC. Retinopathy in temporal arteritis. Ann Ophthalmol 14:652–654, 1982.

Tannenbaum M, Tenzel J. Familial temporal arteritis. J Clin Neuroophthalmol 5: 244–248, 1985.

Teasdall RD, Frayha RA, Shulman LE. Cranial nerve involvement in systemic sclerosis. Medicine 59:149–159, 1980.

Tervaert JNC, Kallenberg C. Neurologic manifestations of systemic vasculitides. Rheum Dis Clin North Am. 19:913–940, 1993.

Thomas DJ, Kendall MJ, Whitfield AGW. Nervous system involvement in ankylosing spondylitis. Br Med J 1:148–150, 1974.

Thomas L, Davidson M, McCluskey RT. Studies of PPLO infection. I. The production of cerebral polyarteritis by mycoplasma gallisepticum in turkeys; The neurotoxic property of the mycoplasma. J Exp Med 123:897–912, 1966.

Tobias E. Periarteritis Nodosa with Special Reference to Neurological Complications. Amsterdam, Uitgeverij "Excelsior," 1968.

Todoroki T, Tatsukiawa K, Shingu M, et al. A case of psoriatic arthritis complicated by iridocyclitis, pericarditis and atlanto-axial subluxation. Ryumachi 21:407–413, 1981.

Tonali P, Garcovich A, Scoppetta C, et al. Oftalmoplegia in dermatomiosite. Minerva Med 7:309–317, 1975.

Torvik A, Berntzen A. Necrotizing vasculitis without visceral involvement. Acta Med Scand 184:69–77, 1968.

Tour RL, Hoyt WF. The syndrome of the aortic arch: Ocular manifestations of 'pulseless disease' and a report of a surgically treated case. Am J Ophthalmol 47:35–48, 1959.

Traboulsi EI, Mansour AM, Aswad MI, et al. Homonymous hemianopia and systemic lupus erythematosus. J Clin Neuroophthalmol 5:63–66, 1985.

Travers RL, Allison DJ, Brettle RP, et al. Polyarteritis nodosa: A clinical and angiographic analysis of 17 cases. Semin Arthritis Rheum 8:184–199, 1979.

Trend P, Graham E. Internuclear ophthalmoplegia in giant-cell arteritis. J Neurol Neurosurg Psychiatry 53:532, 1990.

Trevor RP, Sondheimer FK, Fessel WJ, et al. Angiographic demonstration of major cerebral vessel occlusion in systemic lupus erythematosus. Neuroradiology 4: 202–207, 1972.

Tricoulis D. Treatment of Behçet's disease with chlorambucil. Br J Ophthalmol 57: 55–57, 1976.

Tsai JC, Forster DJ, Ober RR, et al. Panuveitis and multifocal retinitis in a patient with leucocytoclastic vasculitis. Br J Ophthalmol 77:318–320, 1993.

Tuffanelli DL, Winkelmann RK. Clinical study of 727 cases of systemic scleroderma. Arch Derm 84:359–371, 1961.

Tullous MW, Skerhut HEI, Story JL, et al. Cauda equina syndrome of long-standing ankylosing spondylitis. Case report and review of the literature. J Neurosurg 73: 441–447, 1990.

Tuovinen E, Raudasoja R. Poikilodermatomyositis with retinal hemorrhages and secondary glaucoma. Acta Ophthalmol 43:669–672, 1965.

Turgeon PW, Slamovits TL. Scleritis as the presenting manifestation of procainamide-induced lupus. Ophthalmology 96:68–71, 1989.

Turnbull J. Temporal arteritis and polymyalgia rheumatica: Nosographic and nosologic considerations. Neurology 46:901–906, 1996.

Turner RG, Henry J, Friedmann AI, et al. Giant cell arteritis. Postgrad Med J 50: 265–269, 1974.

Ueda H, Ohno K, Ito I, et al. Two cases of aortitis syndrome with aneurysm formation. Jpn Heart J 9:88–96, 1968.

Ueda H, Saito Y, Ito I, et al. Further immunological studies of aortitis syndrome. Jpn Heart J 12:1–21, 1971.

Uga S, Ishikawa S, Wakakura M. Histopathology of the optic nerve and retina in Behçet's disease. In Proceedings of an International Symposium on Behçet's Disease. Editors, Dilsen N, Konice M, Ovul C, pp 85–87. Amsterdam, Excerpta Medica, 1977.

Uriu SA, Reinecke RD. Temporal arteritis, steroid therapy, and pulmonary emboli. Arch Ophthalmol 90:355–357, 1973.

Uthoff D. Zum Behçet-Syndrom. Klin Monatsbl Augenheilkd 189:434–441, 1986.

Uwatoko S, Mannik M. IgG subclasses of antibodies to the collagen-like region of C1q in patients with systemic lupus erythematosus. Arthritis Rheum 32: 1601–1603, 1989.

Valente RM, Hall S, O'Duffy D, et al. Vasculitis and related disorders. In Textbook of Rheumatology. Editors, Kelley WN, Harris ED Jr, Ruddy S, et al., 5th ed, pp 1079–1122. Philadelphia, WB Saunders, 1997.

Van Buskirk EB, Lessell S, Friedman E. Pigment epitheliopathy and erythema nodosum. Arch Ophthalmol 85:369–372, 1971.

van der Linden SM. Ankylosing spondylitis. In Textbook of Rheumatology. Editors, Kelley WN, Harris ED Jr, Ruddy S, et al., 5th ed, pp 969–982. Philadelphia, WB Saunders, 1997.

van der Linden SM, Valkenburg HA, de Jongh BM, et al. The risk of developing ankylosing spondylitis in HLA-B27 positive individuals: A comparison of relatives of spondylitis patients with the general population. Arthritis Rheum 27: 241–249, 1984.

van der Woude FJ, Lobalto S, Permin H, et al. Autoantibodies against neutrophils and monocytes: Tool for diagnosis and marker of disease activity in Wegener's granulomatosis. Lancet 1:425, 1985.

Vanderzant C, Bromberg M, MacGuire A, et al. Isolated small-vessel angiitis of the central nervous system. Arch Neurol 45:683–687, 1988.

van Vliet AA, van Balen AT. Keratopathie dans la maladie de Crohn. Ophthalmologica 190:72–76, 1985.

Van Wien S, Merz EH. Exophthalmos secondary to periarteritis nodosa. Am J Ophthalmol 56:204–208, 1963.

Vázquez-Cruz J, Traboulssi H, Rodriguez-De la Serna A, et al. A prospective study of chronic or recurrent headache in systemic lupus erythematosus. Headache 30: 232–235, 1990.

Verdich M, Nielsen NV. Acute transient ophthalmomalacia in giant-cell arteritis. Report of a case. Acta Ophthalmol 53:875–878, 1975.

Verin P, Compte P, Presseq C. La maladie de Horton a v.s. normale. Bull Soc Ophtalmol Fr 85:833–836, 1985.

Verity MA, Wolfson WL. Cerebral lymphomatoid granulomatosis: A report of two cases, with disseminated necrotizing leukoencephalopathy in one. Acta Neuropathol 36:117–124, 1976.

Vila N, Graus F, Blesa R, et al. Microangiopathy of the brain and retina (Susac's syndrome): Two patients with atypical features. Neurology 45:1225–1226, 1995.

Vilaseca J. Clinical usefulness of temporal artery biopsy. Ann Rheum Dis 46:282–285, 1987.

Vincent FM. Granulomatous angiitis. N Engl J Med 296:452, 1977.

Vine AK, Barr CC. Proliferative lupus retinopathy. Arch Ophthalmol 102:852–854, 1984.

Vitale C, Kahn MF, de Sèze M, et al. Névrite optique, myélite et maladie lupique. Ann Med Interne 124:211–216, 1973.

Volkman DJ, Mann DL, Fauci AS. Association between Takayasu's arteritis and a B-cell autoantigen in North Americans. N Engl J Med 306:464–465, 1982.

Vollertsen RS, McDonald TJ, Younge BR, et al. Cogan's syndrome: 18 cases and a review of the literature. Mayo Clin Proc 61:344–361, 1986.

Vollmer TL, Guarnaccia J, Harrington W, et al. Idiopathic angiitis of the central nervous system. Diagnostic challenges. Arch Neurol 50:925–930, 1993.

Vollrath-Junger C, Gloor B. Warum eine Dopplersonographie vor jeder Biopsie der A. temporalis? Klin Monatsbl Augenheilkd 195:169–171, 1989.

Vossius A. Zwei Fälle von Katarakt in Verbindung mit Sklerodermie. Z Augenheilkd 43:640–654, 1920.

Waaler E, Tönder O, Milde E-J. Immunological and histological studies of temporal arteries from patients with temporal arteritis and/or polymyalgia rheumatica. Acta Pathol Microbiol Scand (A) 84:55–63, 1976.

Wadman B, Werner I. Thromboembolic complications during corticosteroid treatment of temporal arteritis. Lancet 1:907, 1972.

Wagener HP, Hollenhorst RW. The ocular lesions of temporal arteritis. Am J Ophthalmol 45:617–630, 1958.

Wagner AD, Goronzy JJ, Weyand CM. Functional profile of tissue infiltrating and circulating CD68 + cells in giant cell arteritis: Evidence for two components of the disease. J Clin Invest 94:1134–1140, 1994.

Wakefield D, McCluskey P. Behçet's syndrome: Ocular features in an Australian population. Aust N Z J Ophthalmol 18:129–135, 1990.

Walker RE, Compton GA, Langham ME. Pneumatic applanation tonometer studies. IV. Analysis of pulsatile response. Exp Eye Res 20:245–253, 1975.

Wallace DJ, Metzger AL, White KK. Combination immunosuppressive treatment of steroid-resistant dermatomyositis/polymyositis. Arthritis Rheum 28:590–592, 1985.

Wallenberg A. Acute bulbäraffection (embolie der art. cerebellar post. inf. sinistr.). Arch Pyschiatr Nervenkr 27:504–540, 1895.

Walsh FB. Clinical Neuro-Ophthalmology. 2nd ed, p 71. Baltimore, Williams & Wilkins, 1957.

Walsh FB, Hoyt WF. Clinical Neuro-Ophthalmology. 3rd ed, Vol 2, p 1181. Baltimore, Williams & Wilkins, 1969a.

Walsh FB, Hoyt WF. Clinical Neuro-Ophthalmology. 3rd ed, Vol 2, p 1883. Baltimore, Williams & Wilkins, 1969b.

Walsh FB, Hoyt WF. Clinical Neuro-Ophthalmology. 3rd ed, Vol 2, p 1884. Baltimore, Williams & Wilkins, 1969c.

Walsh FB, Hoyt WF. Clinical Neuro-Ophthalmology. 3rd ed, Vol 2, pp 1923–1924. Baltimore, Williams & Wilkins, 1969d.

Walsh FB, Hoyt WF. Clinical Neuro-Ophthalmology. 3rd ed, Vol 2, p 1850. Baltimore, Williams & Wilkins, 1969e.

Walsh FB, Hoyt WF. Clinical Neuro-Ophthalmology. 3rd ed, Vol 2, p 1175. Baltimore, Williams & Wilkins, 1969f.

Walton EW. Giant-cell granuloma of the respiratory tract (Wegener's granulomatosis). Br Med J 2:265–270, 1958.

Walton EW. Reticuloendothelial sarcoma arising in the nose and palate (granuloma gangrenescens). J Clin Pathol 13:279–286, 1960.

Walz-LeBlanc BAE, Keystone EC, Feltis JT, et al. Polyarteritis nodosa clinically masquerading as temporal arteritis with lymphadenopathy. J Rheumatol 21: 949–52, 1994.

Wang FM, Henkind P. Visual system involvement in giant cell (temporal) arteritis. Surv Ophthalmol 23:264–271, 1979.

Wang FM, Wertenbaker C, Behrens MM, et al. Acquired Brown's syndrome in children with juvenile rheumatoid arthritis. Ophthalmology 91:23–26, 1984.

Warrell DA, Godfrey S, Olsen EG. Giant-cell arteritis with peripheral neuropathy. Lancet 1:1010–1013, 1968.

Warren R, Friedman L. Pulseless disease and carotid-artery thromboses: Surgical considerations. N Engl J Med 257:686–690, 1957.

Warren RW, Kredich DW. Transverse myelitis and acute central nervous system manifestations of systemic lupus erythematosus. Arthritis Rheum 27:1058–1060, 1984.

Watson P. Intracranial hemorrhage with vasculitis in rheumatoid arthritis. Arch Neurol 36:58, 1979.

Watson P, Hayreh SS. Scleritis and episcleritis. Br J Ophthalmol 57:163–191, 1976.

Watson P, Fekete J, Deck J. Central nervous system vasculitis in rheumatoid arthritis. Can J Neurol Sci 4:269–272, 1977.

Watson PG, Hazleman BL. The Sclera and Systemic Disorders. pp 238–246. London, WB Saunders, 1976.

Wechsler B, Piette JC, Conard J, et al. Deep venous thrombosis in Behçet's disease: 106 localizations in a series of 177 patients. Presse Med 16:661–664, 1987.

Wechsler B, Vidaihet M, Piette JC, et al. Cerebral venous thrombosis in Behçet's disease: Clinical study and long-term follow-up of 25 cases. Neurology 42: 614–618, 1992.

Wees SJ, Sunwoo IN, Olt SJ. Sural nerve biopsy in systemic necrotizing vasculitis. Am J Med 71:525–532, 1982.

Wegener F. Über generalisierte, septische Gefaesserkrankungen. Verh Dtsch Ges Pathol 29:202–210, 1936.

Wegener F. Über eine eigenartige rhinogene Granulomatose mit besonderer Beteiligung des Arteriensystems und der Nieren. Beitr Pathol Anat 102:36–68, 1939.

Weinberger LM, Cohen ML, Remler BF, et al. Intracranial Wegener's granulomatosis. Neurology 43:1831–1834, 1993.

Weinstein A. Lupus syndromes induced by drugs. In The Clinical Management of Systemic Lupus Erythematosus. Editor, Schur PH, pp 221–231. Orlando, FL, Grune & Stratton, 1983.

Weinstein A. Laboratory diagnosis of drug-induced lupus. In Systemic Lupus Erythematosus. Editor, Lahita RG, pp 881–886. New York, John Wiley & Sons, 1987.

Weinstein JM, Chui H, Lane S, et al. Churg-Strauss syndrome (Allergic granulomatous angiitis). Neuro-ophthalmologic manifestations. Arch Ophthalmol 101: 1217–1220, 1983.

Weinstein JM, Koch K, Lane S. Orbital pseudotumor in Crohn's colitis. Ann Ophthalmol 16:275–278, 1984.

Weinstein JM, Bresnick GH, Bell CL, et al. Acute posterior multifocal placoid pigment epitheliopathy associated with cerebral vasculitis. J Clin Neuroophthalmol 8: 195–201, 1988.

Weintraub MI. Temporal arteritis. Arch Neurol 35:183, 1978.

Weis JW, Winter MW, Phyliky RL, et al. Peripheral T-cell lymphomas: Histologic, immunohistologic, and clinical characterization. Mayo Clin Proc 61:411–426, 1986.

Weiter J, Farkas TG. Pseudotumor of the orbit as a presenting sign in Wegener's granulomatosis. Surv Ophthalmol 17:106–119, 1972.

Wells KK, Folberg R, Goeken JA, et al. Temporal artery biopsies. Correlation of light microscopy and immunofluorescence microscopy. Ophthalmology 96: 1058–1064, 1989.

Wendling D, Hory D, Blanc D. Cyclosporine: A new adjuvant therapy for giant cell arteritis? Arthritis Rheum 28:1078–1079, 1985.

Wessels IF. Posterior ischemic optic neuropathy during general surgery. Am J Ophthalmol 104:555, 1987.

West RH, Barnett AJ. Ocular involvement in scleroderma. Br J Ophthalmol 63: 845–847, 1979.

West SG, Emlen W, Wener MH, et al. Neuropsychiatric lupus erythematosus: A 10-year-prospective study on the value of diagnostic tests. Am J Med 99:153–163, 1995.

Westergren A. Die senkungsreaktion. Ergebn Inn Med Kinderheilk 26:102–109, 1924.

Westergren A. The technique of the red cell sedimentation reaction. Am Rev Tuberc 14:94–101, 1926.

Weyand CM, Bartley GB. Giant cell arteritis: New concepts in the pathogenesis and implications for management. Am J Ophthalmol 123:392–395, 1997.

Weyand CM, Goronzy JJ. Immune responses to Borrelia bergdorferi in patients with reactive arthritis. Arthritis Rheum 32:1057–1064, 1989.

Weyand CM, Hicok KC, Hunder GG, et al. The HLA-DRB1 locus as a genetic component in giant cell arteritis. Mapping of a disease linked sequence motif to the antigen binding site of the HLA-DR molecule. J Clin Invest 90:2355–2361, 1992.

Weyand CM, Hunder NNH, Hicok KC, et al. HLA-DRB1 alleles in polymyalgia rheumatica, giant cell arteritis and rheumatoid arthritis. Arthritis Rheum 37: 514–520, 1994a.

Weyand CM, Schonberger J, Oppitz U, et al. Distinct vascular lesions in giant cell arteritis share identical T cell clonotypes. J Exp Med 179:951–960, 1994b.

Weyand CM, Hicok KC, Hunder GG, et al. Tissue cytokine patterns in patients with polymyalgia rehumatica and giant cell arteritis. Ann Intern Med 121:484–491, 1994c.

Whaley K, Webb J, McAvoy BA, et al. Sjögren's syndrome. 2. Clinical associations and immunological phenomena. QJ Med 42:513–548, 1973a.

Whaley K, Williamson J, Chisholm DM, et al. Sjögren's syndrome. I. Sicca components. QJ Med 42:279–304, 1973b.

Whitaker JN. Inflammatory myopathy: A review of etiologic and pathogenetic factors. Muscle Nerve 5:573–592, 1982.

White RG, Marshall AHE. The autoimmune response in myasthenia gravis. Lancet 2:120–123, 1962.

White RH. The etiology and neurological complications of retinal vasculitis. Brain 84:262–273, 1961.

Whitfield HGW, Bateman M, Cooke WT. Temporal arteritis. Br J Ophthalmol 47: 555–565, 1963.

Whitson WE, Krachmer JH. Adult rheumatoid arthritis. In The Eye in Systemic Disease. Editors, Gold DH, Weingeist TA, pp 61–64. Philadelphia, LB Lippincott, 1990.

Wildemann B, Schulin C, Storch-Hagenlocher B, et al. Susac's syndrome: Improvement with combined antiplatelet and calcium antagonist therapy. Stroke 27: 149–150, 1996.

Wilke WS, Hoffman GS. Treatment of corticosteroid resistant giant cell arteritis. Rheum Dis Clin North Am 21:59–71, 1995.

Wilkey D, Yocum DE, Oberley TD, et al. Budd-Chiari syndrome and renal failure in Behçet disease. Am J Med 75:541–550, 1983.

Wilkinson IMS, Russell RWR. Arteries of the head and neck in giant cell arteritis. A pathological study to show the pattern of arterial involvement. Arch Neurol 27:378–391, 1972.

Wilkinson LS, Panush RS. Exophthalmos associated with systemic lupus erythematosus. Arthritis Rheum 18:188–189, 1975.

Wilkinson M, Bywaters EGL. Clinical features and course of ankylosing spondylitis as seen in a follow-up of 222 hospital referred cases. Ann Rheum Dis 17: 209–228, 1958.

Willcit J, Schmutzhard E, Aichner F, et al. CT and MR imaging in neuro-Behçet disease. J Comput Assist Tomogr 10:313–315, 1986.

Willerson D, Aaberg TM, Reeser FH. Necrotizing vaso-occlusive retinitis. Am J Ophthalmol 84:209–219, 1977.

Williams AL, Haughton VM, Sarena VK, et al. Computed tomography in Behçet disease. Radiology 131:403–404, 1979.

Williams DF, Mieler WF. Long-term follow-up of acute multifocal posterior placoid pigment epitheliopathy. J Neurol Neurosurg Psychiatry 73:985–990, 1989.

Williamson J. Incidence of eye disease in cases of connective tissue disease. Trans Ophthalmol Soc UK 94:742–752, 1974.

Willis J, Atack EA, Kraag G. Relapsing polychondritis with multifocal neurologic abnormalities. Can J Neurol Sci 11:402–404, 1984.

Wilson CA, Choromokos EA, Sheppard R. Acute posterior multifocal placoid pigment epitheliopathy and cerebral vasculitis. Arch Ophthalmol 106:796–800, 1988.

Wilson ME, Eustis HS Jr, Parks MM. Brown's syndrome. Surv Ophthalmol 34: 153–172, 1989.

Winkelmann RK, Ditto WB. Cutaneous and visceral syndromes of necrotizing or 'allergic' angiitis: Study of 38 cases. Medicine 43:59–89, 1964.

Winkelmann RK, Howard FM, Perry HO, et al. Malignant papulosis of skin and cerebrum. Arch Dermatol 87:54–62, 1963.

Winkler TH, Henschel TA, Kalies I, et al. Constant isotype pattern of anti-dsDNA antibodies in patients with systemic lupus erythematosus. Clin Exp Immunol 72: 434–439, 1988.

Wintrobe MM, Buell MV. Hyperproteinemia associated with multiple myeloma: With report of a case in which an extraordinary hyperproteinemia was associated with thrombosis of the retinal veins and symptoms suggesting Raynaud's disease. Bull Johns Hopkins Hosp 52:156–165, 1933.

Wintrobe MM, Landsberg JW. A standardized technique for the blood sedimentation test. Am J Med Sci 189:102–115, 1935.

Wise GN. Ocular periarteritis nodosa. Report of two cases. Arch Ophthalmol 48: 1–11, 1952.

Wise TN, Ginzler EM. Scleroderma cerebritis, an unusual manifestation of progressive systemic sclerosis. Dis Nerv System 36:60–62, 1975.

Wizemann AJS, Wizemann V. Therapeutic effects of short-term plasma exchange in endogenous uveitis. Am J Ophthalmol 97:565–572, 1984.

Wolf MD, Folk JC, Goeken NE. Acute posterior multifocal pigment epitheliopathy and optic neuritis in a family. Am J Ophthalmol *110*:89–90, 1990.

Wolfe SM. Takayasu's arteritis. J Am Optom Assoc *89*:90–94, 1989.

Wolff SM, Barrows HS. Myasthenia gravis and systemic lupus erythematosus. Arch Neurol *14*:254–258, 1966.

Wolff SM, Schotland DL, Phillips LL. Involvement of nervous system in Behçet's syndrome. Arch Neurol *12*:315–325, 1965.

Wolff SM, Fauci AS, Horn RG, et al. Wegener's granulomatosis. Ann Intern Med *81*:513–525, 1974.

Wollheim FA. Ankylosing spondylitis. In Textbook of Rheumatology. Editors, Kelley WN, Harris ED Jr, Ruddy S, et al., 4th ed, pp 943–960. Philadelphia, WB Saunders, 1993a.

Wollheim FA. Enteropathic arthritis. In Textbook of Rheumatology. Editors, Kelley WN, Harris ED Jr, Ruddy S, et al., 4th ed, pp 985–997. Philadelphia, WB Saunders, 1993b.

Wollheim FA. Enteropathic arthritis. In Textbook of Rheumatology. Editors, Kelley WN, Harris ED Jr, Ruddy S, et al., 5th ed, pp 1006–1014. Philadelphia, WB Saunders, 1997.

Wolin MJ, Kent AD. Persisting temporal arteritis. Ophthalmology *102*:701, 1995.

Wolter JR, Phillips RL. Secondary glaucoma in cranial arteritis. Am J Ophthalmol *59*:625–634, 1965.

Wong K, Ai E, Verrier Jones J, et al. Visual loss as the initial symptom of systemic lupus erythematosus. Am J Ophthalmol *92*:238–244, 1981.

Wong RL, Korn JH. Temporal arteritis without an elevated erythrocyte sedimentation rate. Case report and review of the literature. Am J Med *80*:959–964, 1986.

Woods VL Jr, Zvaifler NJ. Pathogenesis of systemic lupus erythematosus. In Textbook of Rheumatology. Editors, Kelley WN, Harris ED Jr, Ruddy S, et al, 3rd ed, pp 1077–1100. Philadelphia, WB Saunders, 1989.

Wortmann RL. Idiopathic inflammatory myopathies: In Cecil Textbook of Medicine. Editors, Bennett JC, Plum F, pp 1501–1503. Philadelphia, WB Saunders, 1996.

Wright BE, Bird AC, Hamilton AE. Placoid pigment epitheliopathy and Harada's disease. Br J Ophthalmol *62*:609–621, 1978.

Wright R, Lumsden K, Luntz MH, et al. Abnormalities of the sacro-iliac joints and uveitis in ulcerative colitis. QJ Med *34*:229–236, 1965.

Truelove SC, Jewell DP. Intensive intravenous regimen for severe attacks of ulcerative colitis. Lancet *1*:1067–1070, 1974.

Wright VA, Chamberlain VA. Behçet's syndrome. Bull Rheum Dis *29*:972–979, 1978–1979.

Wyble M, Schimek RA. The simultaneous occurrence of two collagen diseases in the same patient. Trans Am Acad Ophthalmol Otolaryngol *66*:632–641, 1962.

Wykes WN, Adams GGW, Cullen JF. Temporal arteritis: Visual loss associated with posture. Neuro-ophthalmology *4*:107–109, 1984.

Yagura M, Sano I, Akioka H, et al. Usefulness of percutaneous transluminal angioplasty for Aortitis syndrome. Arch Intern Med *144*:1465–1468, 1984.

Yamashita K, Kobayashi S, Kondo M, et al. Elevated anti-neutro-philcytoplasmic antibody titer in a patient with atypical orbital pseudotumor. Ophthalmoplegia *209*:172–175, 1995.

Yananouchi K, Shishido A, Kobune F, et al. Virologic approaches to Behçet's disease in Japan. In Behçet's Disease: Pathogenetic Mechanism and Clinical Future. Editor, Inaba G, pp 57–63. Tokyo, University of Tokyo Press, 1982.

Yazici H, Chamberlain MA, Schreuder I, et al. HLA antigens in Behçet's disease: A reappraisal by a comparative study of Turkish and British patients. Ann Rheum Dis *39*:344–348, 1980.

Yazici H, Chamberlain MA, Tuzun Y, et al. A comparative study of the pathergy reaction among Turkish and British patients with Behçet's disease. Ann Rheum Dis *43*:74–75, 1984.

Yazici H, Pazarli H, Barnes CG, et al. A controlled trial of azathioprine in Behçet's syndrome. N Engl J Med *322*:21–285, 1990.

Yiglit A, Bingöl A, Mutluer N, et al. The one-and-a-half syndrome in systemic lupus erythematosus. J Neuroophthalmol *16*:274–276, 1996.

Yilmaz O, Sebahattin Y, Hasan Y, et al. Low dose cyclosporin A versus pulsed cyclophosphamide in Behçet's disease: Single masked trial. Br J Ophthalmol *76*:241–243, 1992.

Young NJA, Bird AC, Sehmi K. Pigment epithelial diseases with abnormal choroidal perfusion. Am J Ophthalmol *90*:607–618, 1980.

Younger DS, Hays A, et al. Granulomatous angiitis of the central nervous system: A nonspecific reaction of diverse etiology. Ann Neurol *20*:157, 1986.

Younger DS, Hays AP, Brust JCM, et al. Granulomatous angiitis of the brain: An inflammatory reaction of diverse etiology. Arch Neurol *45*:514–518, 1988.

Yu YJ, Cooper DR, Wellenstein DE, et al. Cerebral angiitis and intracerebral hemorrhage associated with methamphetamine abuse. J Neurosurg *58*:109–111, 1983.

Yurdakul S, Yazici H, Tuzun Y, et al. The arthritis of Behçet's disease: A prospective study. Ann Rheum Dis *42*:505–515, 1983.

Yuzawa M, Kawamura Matsui M. Indocyanine green video angiographic findings in acute posterior multifocal placoid pigment epitheliopathy. Acta Ophthalmol *72*:128–133, 1994.

Zamora J, Pariser K, Hedges T, et al. Retinal vasculitis in polymyositis-dermatomyositis. Arthritis Rheum *30*:S106, 1987.

Zeek PM. Periarteritis nodosa and other forms of necrotizing angiitis. N Engl J Med *248*:764–772, 1953.

Zeek PM, Smith CC, Weeter JC. Studies on periarteritis nodosa. III. The differentiation between the vascular lesions of periarteritis nodosa and of hypersensitivity. Am J Pathol *24*:889–917, 1948.

Zeitouni AG, Tewfik TL, Schloss M. Cogan's syndrome: A review of otologic management and 10-year follow-up of a pediatric case. J Otolaryngology *22*:337–340, 1993.

Zewi M. Morbus Reiteri. Acta Ophthalmol *25*:47–60, 1947.

Zierhut M, Thiel HJ, Weidle EG, et al. Topical treatment of severe corneal ulcers with cyclosporine A. Graefe's Arch Clin Exp Ophthalmol *227*:30–35, 1989.

Zimmerman RS, Young HF, Hadfield MG. Granulomatous angiitis of the nervous system: A case report of long-term survival. Surg Neurol *33*:206–212, 1990.

Zion VM, Goodside V. Anterior segment ischemia with ischemic optic neuropathy. Surv Ophthalmol *19*:19–30, 1974.

Zion VM, Brackup AH, Weingeist S. Relapsing polychondritis, erythema nodosum and sclerouveitis: A case report with anterior segment angiography. Surv Ophthalmol *19*:107–114, 1974.

Zizic TM. Gastrointestinal manifestations. In The Clinical Management of Systemic Lupus Erythematosus. Editor, Schur PH, pp 153–166. Orlando, FL, Grune & Stratton, 1983.

Zvaifler NJ. Neurologic manifestations. In The Clinical Management of Systemic Lupus Erythematosus. Editor, Schur PH, pp 167–188. Orlando, FL, Grune & Stratton, 1983.

Zvaifler NJ, Bluestein HG. The pathogenesis of central nervous system manifestations of systemic lupus erythematosus. Arthritis Rheum *25*:862–866, 1982.

Venous Occlusive Disease

Shelley Ann Cross

Occlusion of veins, particularly those in the head and neck, can cause severe neurologic and ophthalmologic dysfunction. In this chapter, we discuss the neuro-ophthalmo-logic symptoms and signs that result from occlusive disease affecting these vessels.

CEREBRAL VENOUS AND DURAL SINUS THROMBOSIS

In Chapter 52, we describe the anatomy of the dural sinuses and cerebral veins. When one or more of these vessels becomes occluded, neurologic dysfunction, visual dysfunction, or both may result. The severity of the deficits is related primarily to the cause, location, and extent of the occlusion, to the age of the patient (Barron et al., 1990), and to the rate of development of the occlusion (Ameri and Bousser, 1992; Schutta, 1994; Bousser and Ross Russell, 1997).

CAUSES

Dural sinus and cerebral venous thromboses may be caused by local or generalized infection or by noninfectious processes.

Septic Venous Occlusion

Septic thrombosis of intracerebral venous structures is usually caused by pyogenic infections of the mastoid air cells, the paranasal sinuses, face, ears, scalp, or throat (Bousser et al., 1985; Garcia et al., 1995). An acute inflammatory process can reach the larger veins directly from local osteomyelitis or by causing thrombophlebitis of small diploic vessels that extend through emissary veins to the larger vascular channels. Fungi, particularly *Rhizopus* and *Aspergillus* species, both prone to infect the paranasal sinuses, especially in patients with diabetes mellitus, are particularly associated with cavernous sinus infections. Viral infections such as human immunodeficiency virus (HIV) and cytomegalovirus (CMV) also are associated with cerebral venous thrombosis (Schutta, 1994), as is the parasitic infection trichinosis (Evans and Patten, 1982; El Koussa et al., 1994). Syphilis can cause dural sinus thrombosis by producing an osteitis in the region of the dural sinus (El Alaoui Faris et al., 1992).

Since the introduction of antibiotics, septic thrombosis, at least in the developed world, has become a relatively infrequent although serious problem. Among 38 cases of angiographically-proven venous sinus thrombosis evaluated by Bousser et al. (1985), only four (10.5%) were septic. In the developing world, this is not the case. In a series of 56 angiographically-proven cases from Ankara, Turkey (Karabudak et al., 1990), 15 (26.8%) cases were caused by infections. Dehydration, malnutrition, and anemia are some of the factors that play an important part in the pathogenesis of septic thrombosis (Nagpal, 1983).

Aseptic Venous Occlusion

Aseptic occlusion of intracerebral venous structures is much more common than septic occlusion. It is caused by a variety of different mechanisms (see Table 1 in Bousser et al., 1985; see Table 35.1 in Gates and Barnett, 1987; Ross Russell, 1990; see tables 1 and 2 in Schutta, 1994).

Changes in the vessel wall may be caused by trauma, particularly penetrating or blunt trauma associated with skull fractures (Holmes and Sargent, 1915; Carrie and Jaffe, 1954; Kalbag and Woolf, 1967; Kinal, 1967). The wall of a cerebral vein or dural sinus may also be injured during intracranial surgery, resulting in thrombosis (Boniuk, 1972; Shucart and Stein, 1978; Garrido and Fahs, 1990), or it may be ligated or resected during treatment of an adjacent tumor (Bederson and Eisenberg, 1995). Electroconvulsive therapy may be associated with cerebral venous thrombosis (Schutta, 1994). Various tumors, including leukemia, lymphoma, meningioma, and carcinomas may invade the walls of dural sinuses and cerebral veins, causing obstruction of blood flow (David et al., 1975; Averback, 1978; Azzarelli et al., 1980; Meininger et al., 1985; Steiger et al., 1989; Levi et al., 1994), or they may obstruct cerebral venous blood flow by externally compressing the walls of these vessels. Byrne and Lawton (1983) described a patient with systemic sarcoidosis in whom occlusion of the dural venous sinuses resulted from a meningeal granulomatous reaction that surrounded and compressed the sinuses.

Noninfectious inflammatory conditions can lead to thrombophlebitis of cerebral veins and sinuses. This phenomenon occurs in such disorders as Behçet's disease (Kozin et al., 1977; Imaizumi et al., 1980; Pamir et al., 1981; Bousser, 1982; Rosenberger et al., 1982; Bank and Weart, 1984; Harper et al., 1985; Bousser et al., 1985; El-Ramahi and Al-Kawi, 1991; Wechsler et al., 1992; Fujikado and Imagawa, 1994; Najim Al-Din et al., 1994) systemic lupus erythematosis (SLE), Wegener's granulomatosis (Schutta, 1994) sarcoidosis, Hughes-Stovin syndrome, malignant atropic papulosis (Degos Disease), Crohn's disease (ulcerative colitis), and regional enteritis (Sigsbee and Rottenberg, 1978; Markowitz et al., 1989; García-Moncó and Beldarrain, 1991; Motte et al., 1992).

Changes in blood flow may result from systemic hypoperfusion that occurs in such settings as cardiac failure, dehydration, cachexia, chronic obstructive pulmonary disease, and obesity (Barnett and Hyland, 1953; Krayenbuhl, 1966; Towbin, 1973; Schutta, 1994). Generalized reduction of blood flow may also develop in patients with various hematologic or myeloproliferative disorders, including polycythemia, essential thrombocythemia, idiopathic thrombocytopenic purpura, myelofibrosis, myeloid metaplasia, leukemia, and gammopathies (Barnett and Hyland, 1953; Castleman and Kibbee, 1960; Bots, 1971; Iob et al., 1979; Girolami et al., 1980; Murphy et al., 1983; Pouillot et al., 1984; Haan et al., 1988; McDonald et al., 1989; Furuta et al., 1991; Schutta, 1994). Local reduction in blood flow may result from venous emboli, from arterial occlusive disease, and from retrograde phlebothrombosis after occlusion of major neck veins. This occlusion may be part of a disease process such as a tumor occluding a vessel, or the development of the Budd-Chiari syndrome, or it may be iatrogenic; i.e., from ligation of an internal jugular vein or placement of an intravenous catheter or pacemaker.

Venous occlusion can occur as part of the natural history of an arteriovenous malformation (AVM), which may contain localized areas of slow venous flow and areas of turbulence. Both deep and dural AVMs can be associated with venous sinus occlusion (Al-Mefty et al., 1986). In the latter setting, the cause and effect relationship is controversial. A dural AVM may be an acquired abnormality resulting from revascularization of a previously thrombosed sinus (Grove, 1983; Sundt and Piepgras, 1983; Kutluk et al., 1991) or, conversely, sinus thrombosis may develop from hemodynamic and morphologic changes from turbulence, high flow, and stasis in the malformation (Al-Mefty et al., 1986). The turbulence and high flow damage the endothelial wall, initiating thrombosis. Stasis also contributes to clot formation in such cases, and elevated intracranial pressure (ICP) can cause collapse of venous structures, thus aggravating the situation further. Patients in whom such damage occurs show an increased number of pial vessels, suggesting cortical venous drainage, and white matter changes consistent with edema, on magnetic resonance (MR) imaging (Willinsky et al., 1994). These changes are direct evidence of venous congestion.

Dural venous occlusion can also develop following therapeutic embolization of intracranial AVMs. Duckwiler et al. (1992) described four such cases. Two of the four patients had standard AVMs; the other two had vein of Galen malformations. It was suggested by Duckwiler et al. (1992) that venous occlusion occurred in these cases from conversion of the high flow venous outflow to a slow flow system by the embolization.

The most common, and perhaps the most important, causes of aseptic cerebral venous or dural sinus thrombosis are related to **hypercoagulability** (Gates and Barnett, 1987; Brey and Coull, 1996; Deschiens et al., 1996). Normally, blood clotting is regulated by a variety of mechanisms that use activated coagulation factors (Schutta, 1994). The most important of these utilizes the natural anticoagulants antithrombin III, protein C, and protein S. Antithrombin III neutralizes thrombin and other serine proteases. Its activity is accelerated when it is complexed with heparin or related molecules found on endothelial cells. Protein C, once it has bound to the endothelial protein thrombomodulin, is converted to a serine protease by thrombin itself. Activated protein C and free protein S, both vitamin K-dependent proteins, act together to produce a profound inhibitory effect on coagulation by degrading procoagulant factors Va and VIIa. The lysis of already formed, unwanted clots occurs through the conversion of plasminogen to plasmin, via cellular activators regulated by plasmin and antitrypsin.

Hypercoagulable states may result from genetic disorders. For example, hereditary antithrombin III deficiency (Ambruso et al., 1980, Lee and Ng, 1991) is inherited as an autosomal-dominant trait with an estimated prevalence between 1 in 2000 and 1 in 20000. It is found in 4–6% of young patients with venous thrombosis, including cerebral venous occlusion.

Protein C may also be genetically deficient (Viereege and Schneider, 1989; Rick, 1990). There may be resistance to activated protein C because of a mutation in factor V (also called Factor V Leiden) that converts arginine to glycine at the 506 site (Dahlback, 1995; Ridker et al., 1995; Brey and Coull, 1996; van der Bom et al., 1996; Simioni et al., 1997). This genetic deficiency is found in a significant percentage of patients with cerebral venous thrombosis (Confavreux et al., 1994; Deschiens et al., 1996; Dulli et al., 1996; Zuber et al., 1996; Simioni et al., 1997). There is also an autosomal-dominant inherited deficiency of a cofactor to activated protein C (Dahlback et al., 1993; Svensson and Dahlback, 1994). This deficiency is found in about 20% of juveniles or young adults who experience recurrent stroke (Halbmayer et al., 1994).

Protein S clotting assays are influenced by the activated protein C resistance phenomenon and therefore may not be specific for protein S (Halbmayer et al., 1994). Nevertheless, protein S deficiency can also be a cause of cerebral venous thrombosis (Cros et al., 1990, Pasquale et al., 1990; Najim Al-Din et al., 1994; Deschiens et al., 1996). This abnormality was associated with inappropriate secretion of antidiuretic hormone (ADH) in a patient with cerebral venous thrombosis reported by Liedtke (1991).

In 1994, Schlichtmeier et al. described a 13-year-old boy with cerebral venous sinus occlusion. Both the boy and his sister had Cohen syndrome, an autosomal-recessive condition characterized by mental retardation and multiple anomalies including microcephaly, unusual facies, and lax connective tissue. Both children demonstrated combined deficiencies of protein C, protein S, and antithrombin III.

Aseptic occlusion of cerebral venous sinuses can occur in patients with inherited fibrinolytic defects, including hypoplasminogenemia, abnormal plasminogen, decreased release of plasminogen activator, and abnormal fibrinogen (Aoki et al., 1978; Wohl et al., 1982; Soria et al., 1983; Scharrer et al., 1986; Nagayama et al., 1993; Schutta, 1994). Patients with such defects exhibit markedly diminished fibrinolyis in the blood.

Hyperhomocystinemia is known to be associated with increased risk of arterial occlusive disease, regardless of whether elevations in homocysteine result from a genetic disorder (e.g., homocysteinuria) or from low dietary folate (Boushey et al., 1995; McCully, 1996). Homocystinuria can even present as spontaneous aseptic sagittal sinus thrombosis (Cochran and Packman, 1992). At least one such case occurred in a woman in the immediate postpartum period (Calvert and Rand, 1995).

About 4% of patients with β-thalassemia major demonstrate arterial and venous occlusive disease (Michaeli et al., 1992). Some of these patients experience occlusion of the cerebral venous sinuses.

Sickle cell disease (homozygous sickle cell anemia) is a well-recognized risk factor for the development of cerebrovascular thrombosis. Most cases of stroke in sickle cell disease result from occlusion of major intracranial arteries (see Chapter 55); however, both sickle cell disease and sickle cell trait (heterozygous sickle cell anemia) may be associated with cerebral venous and dural sinus thrombosis (Schenck, 1964; Dalal et al., 1974; Feldenzer et al., 1987). In most of these cases, a sickle crisis occurs after the administration of general anesthesia, during a perioperative hypoxic event, or both. In some cases, however, no precipitating event can be identified (Feldenzer et al., 1987).

Hypercoagulability of the blood may result from acquired diseases. Of particular importance in this regard are acquired antiphospholipid antibodies, a heterogenous group of autoantibodies to anionic phospholipids. An increase in the serum concentration of these substances is associated with both arterial and venous thrombosis (Levine et al., 1987; Asherson et al., 1991; Ginsburg et al., 1992; Bacharach, 1993; Najim Al-Din et al., 1994; Parrens et al., 1995; Deschiens et al., 1995). Originally described in patients with SLE, these antibodies can be increased in the serum of patients with other connective tissue diseases and in patients without any evidence of a systemic disorder. The antiphospholipid antibodies are also called ''anticoagulants'' because they interfere with phospholipid-dependent clotting tests. Three main types are recognized: (*a*) antibodies responsible for the in vitro lupus anticoagulant test (the lupus anticoagulant), (*b*) antibodies directed against negatively-charged phospholipids (e.g., anticardiolipin antibody, antiphosphatidylethanolamine antibody), and (*c*) antibodies responsible for producing a false-positive Venereal Disease Research (VDRL) test (Bacharach, 1993). These antibodies are associated with a variety of systemic disorders, including recurrent fetal loss; hematologic disorders such as thrombocytopenia, Coombs-positive hemolytic anemia, and pernicious anemia; dermatologic disorders such as livedo reticularis with skin nodules and necrosis; peripheral vascular thrombosis; and neurologic conditions, including chorea, transverse myelitis, dementia, and cerebral vein and sinus thrombosis (Boey et al., 1983; Gastineau et al., 1985; Lechner and Pabinger-Fasching, 1985; Pulido et al., 1987; Heckerling et al., 1987; Moreb and Kitchens, 1989; Mokri et al., 1993).

Acquired protein S deficiency may lead to cerebral venous occlusive disease. Laversuch et al. (1995) reported a patient with SLE without the lupus anticoagulant who developed the nephrotic syndrome. Because of protein loss in the urine, the patient became deficient in protein S and subsequently experienced cerebral venous thrombosis and venous infarction. The risk for venous occlusive disease in patients with the nephrotic syndrome may be even greater if such patients have the lupus anticoagulant, because this antibody inhibits factor Va degeneration by activated protein C and protein S. Low free protein S may also aggravate the hypercoagulable state by another mechanism. The C4b-binding protein, which binds Protein S, may increase as part of an inflammatory response. Low free protein S occurs more often in African-Americans than in Caucasians (Laversuch et al., 1995). Patients with SLE may be at particular risk for venous occlusive disease because of protein loss associated with renal disease, the antiphospholipid syndrome, low free protein S, or a combination of these factors.

Patients with nephrotic syndrome are at risk for venous thrombosis, including thrombosis of cerebral veins and dural sinuses. The reasons are complex and include loss of protein S in the urine, increased platelet adhesiveness and aggregation, increased fibrinogen, elevated factor VIII-related antigen, and increased activity of factors II, VII, and X (Laversuch et al., 1995). Plasminogen may be elevated and decreased in such patients, but fibrinolysis is always reduced.

Patients with deficiencies of protein C or protein S and patients with the lupus anticoagulant/anticardiolipin antibody syndrome may experience acute skin necrosis at the time of initiation of warfarin administration (the warfarin-induced skin necrosis syndrome) (Levine and Hirsh, 1986). The explanation for this condition is unclear.

Hypercoagulability of the blood may result from hematologic disorders such as leukemia, primary and secondary polycythemia (Schutta, 1994), essential thrombocythemia (Iob et al., 1979; Mitchell et al., 1986), iron deficiency anemia with thrombocytosis (Belman et al., 1990), idiopathic cryofibrinogenemia (Dunsker et al., 1970), paroxysmal nocturnal hemoglobinuria, idiopathic hemolytic anemia, and disseminated intravascular coagulopathy (DIC) (Schutta, 1994). Metabolic disorders including diabetes mellitus, uremia, hyperlipidemia, and thyrotoxicosis are also associated with hypercoagulability, and such patients may experience aseptic cerebral venous sinus occlusion (Schutta, 1994; Siegert et al., 1995).

In patients with malignancy, cerebral venous thrombosis may result from leukostasis (Pochedly, 1975a–c), invasion of the vessel wall by malignant cells (Azzarelli et al., 1980), a hypercoagulable state (Sigsbee et al., 1979; Hickey et al., 1982; see Chapter 47), or altered coagulation factors from therapy (Steinherz et al., 1981). Malignancies associated with peripheral as well as cerebral venous or dural sinus thrombosis include those of the pancreas, breast, stomach, lung, prostate, colon, ovaries, gallbladder, kidney, tonsil, and endometrium, as well as leukemia, lymphoma, carcinoid tumor, melanoma, neuroblastoma, hepatoma, and medullary carcinoma of the thyroid (Tiede et al., 1994).

During and after pregnancy, numerous changes occur in the human blood clotting systems (Toglia and Weg, 1996). During pregnancy, fibrinogen and several coagulation factors increase, and antithrombin III and plasminogen decrease. Within an hour after delivery, plasminogen returns to normal. In the immediate postpartum period, fibrinogen and factor VIII decrease, and fribrinolytic activity increases. From the 3rd to the 5th postpartum day, platelets, fibrinogen, and factor VIII increase, plasma viscosity increases, and red cell deformability decreases (Schutta, 1994). During pregnancy and after childbirth, cerebral venous thrombosis is frequently associated with pelvic or deep vein thrombosis and occurs most frequently in the first 3 weeks postpartum (Gowers, 1888; Fishman et al., 1957; Lorincz and Moore, 1962; Eckerling et al., 1963; Carroll et al., 1966; Krayenbuhl, 1966; Kalbag and Woolf, 1967; Cross et al., 1968; Christensen et al., 1969; Amias, 1970; Lavin et al., 1978; Montiero et al., 1984; Cantú and Barinagarrementeria, 1993; Najim Al-Din et al., 1994). The condition probably is caused by the effects of a hypercoagulable state (Pechet and Alexander, 1961; Bansal et al., 1974; Hellgren and Blombäck, 1981;

Rudigoz et al., 1981; Toglia and Weg, 1996) combined with the venous stasis that occurs during pregnancy. Venous embolism, once thought to be the major cause of cerebral venous occlusion in such patients (Martin, 1941), is probably a rare phenomenon.

Estrogens, whether administered for contraception, replacement therapy, suppression of lactation, or treatment of prostatic carcinoma, are associated with an increased risk for both arterial and venous thrombosis (Walsh et al., 1965; Shafey and Scheinberg, 1966; Atkinson et al., 1970; Buchanan and Brazinsky, 1970; Shende and Lowrie, 1970; Poltera, 1972; Fairburn, 1973; Dindar and Platts, 1974; Astedt, 1975; Kingsley et al., 1978; Estanol et al., 1979; Imai et al., 1982; Goldberg et al., 1986; Haley et al., 1989; Najim Al-Din et al., 1994; Schutta, 1994). The relative risk in women who use oral contraceptives is nine times greater than in those who do not (Collaborative Group for the Study of Stroke in Young Women, 1973). This effect is dose dependent and aggravated by smoking. The duration of exposure ranges from 24 hours to 7 weeks but can be many months (Schutta, 1994).

Venous or arterial thrombosis may be associated with the administration of heparin (heparin-associated thrombocytopenia and thrombosis, HATT syndrome) (Levine and Hirsh, 1986). Other drugs or substances associated with cerebral venous thrombosis include L-asparaginase, various chemotherapeutic agents, androgens, tamoxifen, sodium chloride, Vitamin A, and epsilon-aminocaproic acid (Schutta, 1994).

In about 20% of patients with thrombosis of cerebral veins or dural sinuses, the etiology cannot be determined (Greitz and Link, 1966; Kalbag and Woolf, 1967; Majersky and Majtényi, 1975; Gettelfinger and Kokmen, 1977; Thron et al., 1986).

PATHOPHYSIOLOGY

When cerebral veins or dural sinuses become occluded, blood is forced back into small vessels and capillaries. If venous drainage is sufficiently obstructed, local ischemia occurs, followed by cerebral edema and hemorrhagic infarction (Gates and Barnett, 1987; Villringer et al., 1994). When the condition is less severe, there may be only partial ischemia of the cerebral cortex, which may produce focal seizures. Neonates are particularly prone to present in this manner (Barron et al., 1990). In still milder cases, venous occlusion may cause an increase in intracranial venous or cerebrospinal fluid (CSF) pressure, producing headache, papilledema, or both, or it may be completely asymptomatic.

The brains of those who die from cerebral venous thrombosis are swollen and hemorrhagic. They show the effects of herniation, sometimes tentorial or subfalcine if the process started unilaterally, but usually central, tentorial, and tonsillar. Recent thrombi have a dark reddish-blue color, whereas thrombi older than a few days are yellow-white. Recanalization takes place to varying degrees, and when it does not develop, the lumen is replaced by fibrous tissue. Anastomotic channels are common. Cerebral venous occlusion causes congestion, swelling, and hemorrhagic infarction and frank cerebral and subarachnoid hemorrhage. Resorption of necrotic areas results in cerebromalacia. Histologically, clots of various ages are seen in veins and sinuses (Schutta, 1994).

SPECIFIC SYNDROMES

The clinical manifestations of occlusion of the cerebral veins and dural sinuses depends in part on the location of the occlusion and in part on its cause (Wechsler et al., 1992; Purvin et al., 1995). In this section of the chapter, we describe the symptoms and signs that typically occur with cerebral venous occlusion at specific sites.

Thrombosis of the Superficial Cerebral Veins

The clinical manifestations associated with occlusion of one or more superficial cerebral veins were first described

by Raymond in 1880. The subject was subsequently reviewed by Garcin and Pestel in 1953 and by Jacobs et al. in 1996.

The hallmark of occlusive disease of superficial cerebral veins is the occurrence of focal or generalized seizures caused by irritability of the cerebral cortex. The seizures are preceded in some cases by a prodrome of headache, weakness, numbness, or alterations in behavior (Martin and Sheehan, 1941), and they are usually followed by fluctuating focal neurologic deficits, the nature of which depends on the location of the occlusion (Figs. 58.1 and 58.2). For example, occlusion of the Rolandic vein is usually associated with a progressive, but ultimately transient, contralateral hemiparesis, whereas occlusion of post-Rolandic veins typically

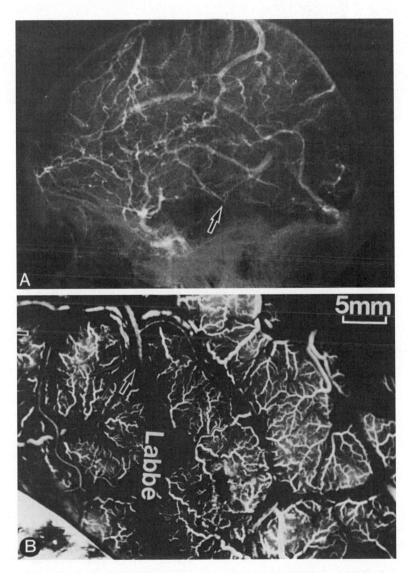

Figure 58.1. Thrombosis of the vein of Labbé. The patient was a 41-year-old woman who experienced an acute headache. The next morning she vomited and complained of photophobia. She subsequently developed aphasia and a stiff neck. *A*, Cerebral angiogram, lateral view of venous phase, shows obstruction of the vein of Labbé (*arrow*). A diagnostic craniotomy was performed at which time thrombi were found in several cortical veins. *B*, Fluorescein cerebral angiogram performed at the time of craniotomy demonstrates occlusion of the proximal portion of the vein of Labbé. The pial veins in its territory are tortuous and congested. (From Kawase T, Tazawa T, Mizukami M. Cerebral venous thrombosis: Findings from computer tomography and fluorescein angiography. In The Cerebral Veins: An Experimental and Clinical Update. Editors, Auer LM, Loew L. pp 327–336. Vienna, Springer-Verlag, 1982.)

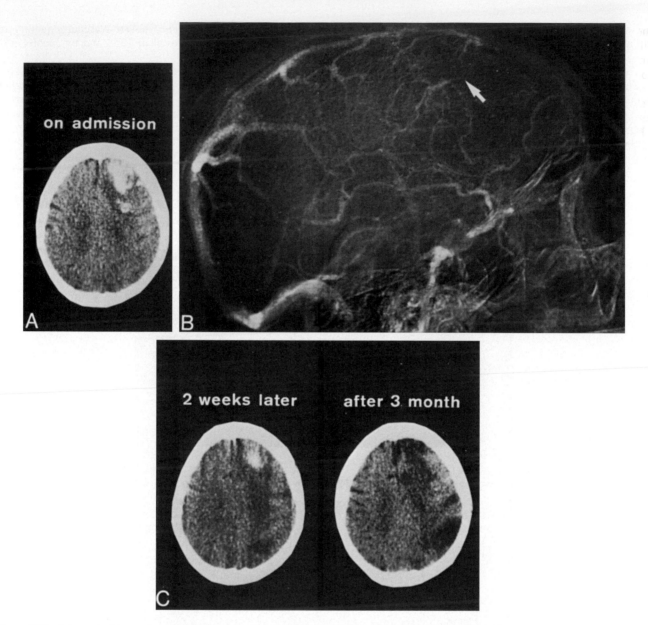

Figure 58.2.   Intracerebral hemorrhage from thrombosis of a superficial frontal vein. The patient was a 56-year-old man who developed a progressive left hemiparesis. *A*, CT scan, axial view, performed on the patient at the time of admission to the hospital shows changes compatible with a hemorrhage in the right frontal lobe. *B*, Cerebral arteriogram, lateral view of venous phase, shows occlusion of a right-sided superficial frontal vein (*arrow*). The patient's hemiparesis did not change. *C*, Subsequent CT scans obtained 2 weeks and 3 months after admission show gradual resolution of hemorrhage with evidence of infarction in the right frontal and right temporal lobes. (From Kawase T, Tazawa T, Mizukami M. Cerebral venous thrombosis: Findings from computer tomography and fluorescein angiography. In The Cerebral Veins: An Experimental and Clinical Update. Editors, Auer LM, Loew L. pp 327–336. Vienna, Springer-Verlag, 1982.)

causes contralateral or bilateral disturbances in sensation. Aphasia often develops when the lesion is in the dominant hemisphere. There may be dyslexia or acalculia (Jacobs et al., 1996).

The sensory and motor disturbances that result from intracerebral venous occlusive disease usually vary considerably from hour to hour and day to day. Nevertheless, many patients recover almost completely within several days, and even patients with severe hemiparesis may recover completely, although such recovery may take weeks to months.

Occlusion of superficial cerebral veins usually does not produce visual symptoms unless one or both occipital veins become occluded, resulting in a hemorrhagic venous infarction of one or both occipital lobes (Beal and Chapman, 1980). Unilateral infarction is often associated with a homonymous visual field defect that is quite congruous when incomplete. Bilateral infarction may produce cortical blindness that usually, but not invariably, improves with time, or it may produce bilateral, congruous, homonymous visual field defects. Bergman (1957) described a 31-year-old woman who developed cortical blindness after experiencing seizures followed by stupor during the last trimester of her 5th pregnancy. Although cerebral angiography was normal, it was thought that the patient had suffered a venous infarct. The patient regained vision in the entire right homonymous field and in the central portion of the left homonymous field over the next 3 months.

Kalbag and Woolf (1967) described a woman who developed seizures followed by a right hemiparesis, right hemianalgesia, right homonymous hemianopia, and aphasia 8 days postpartum. Cerebral angiography showed no filling of the superior sagittal sinus, and craniotomy revealed venous thrombosis with secondary hemorrhagic infarction of the left parieto occipital lobe.

Beal and Chapman (1980) described one patient who developed cortical blindness followed by seizures, and two patients who developed homonymous hemianopia associated with fluent aphasia in the immediate postpartum period. The clinical diagnosis in all three patients was cerebral venous thrombosis; all three had spontaneous return of normal visual function within several days.

Monteiro et al. (1984) reported the case of a 34-year-old woman who developed transient cerebral blindness 3 days after delivery of a full-term infant by cesarean section. A computed tomographic (CT) scan showed patchy areas of hypodensity in both occipital lobes (Fig. 58.3), and a clinical diagnosis of probable cerebral venous thrombosis was made. The patient's vision began to improve within 24 hours, and she had normal visual function within 2 weeks after the onset of visual symptoms.

Patients in whom a hemorrhagic infarction occurs in the parieto-occipital region may experience formed visual hallucinations in the affected homonymous hemifields (Beal and Chapman, 1980; Monteiro et al., 1984; Vieregge and Schwieder, 1989). Some also experience palianopsia.

Thrombosis of Deep Cerebral Veins

Thrombosis of the deep cerebral veins, whether or not there is associated thrombosis of dural venous sinuses, is usually fatal (Bots, 1971; Nishimura et al., 1982). Patients with this condition usually suffer extensive hemorrhagic infarction of both thalami, the basal ganglia, the rostral mesencephalon, and the medial and lateral geniculate bodies (Johnsen et al., 1973; Schlesinger, 1976) (Figs. 58.4 and 58.5). Patients who survive typically have extensive neurologic and cognitive sequelae, but this is not always the case. Haley et al. (1989) reported the results of serial neuroimaging and neuropsychologic testing in an 18-year-old woman with occlusion of the deep cerebral veins. During the course of her illness, she demonstrated disorientation, abulia, attention deficits, memory loss, dyscalculia, and impaired scores on intelligence quota (IQ) tests. She eventually made a complete neurologic and intellectual recovery despite angiographic evidence of persistent thrombosis of the straight sinus.

Thrombosis of the Dural Sinuses

The sinuses of the dura mater are venous channels that drain blood from the brain, dura, and diplöe (see Chapter

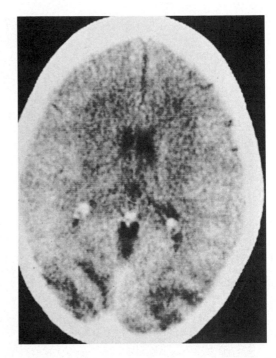

Figure 58.3. Cerebral blindness from presumed cerebral venous thrombosis. The patient was a 33-year-old woman who experienced transient blindness 3 days after delivery of a full-term infant by cesarean section. Enhanced CT scan, axial view, shows patchy hypodensities in both occipital lobes. The patient was thought to have experienced cerebral venous thrombosis. Her vision began to improve within 24 hours after visual symptoms began, and visual function was normal within 2 weeks. (From Monteiro MLR, Hoyt WF, Imes RK. Puerperal cerebral blindness: Transient bilateral occipital involvement from presumed cerebral venous thrombosis. Arch Neurol *41:* 1300–1301, 1984.)

52). Situated between the two layers of the dura mater, they are devoid of valves and are lined by endothelial cells and by connective tissue that is continuous with that of the veins that drain into them. They are often divided into two groups: (*a*) the posterosuperior group, which are located at the upper and back parts of the skull, and (*b*) the anteroinferior group, which are located at the base of the skull. The posterosuperior dural sinuses are the superior sagittal, inferior sagittal, straight, lateral (transverse), sigmoid, tentorial, and occipital sinuses. The superior sagittal, inferior sagittal, straight, and occipital sinuses are single, unpaired structures, whereas the lateral, sigmoid, and tentorial sinuses are paired structures. The anteroinferior dural sinuses are the cavernous sinuses, intercavernous sinuses, basilar sinus, sphenoparietal sinuses, and the superior and inferior petrosal sinuses. As is the case with the posterosuperior group of sinuses, the anteroinferior group of sinuses may be separated into paired and unpaired sinuses. There is only one basilar sinus, but there are two cavernous, intercavernous, sphenoparietal, superior petrosal, and inferior petrosal sinuses. Although any of the dural sinuses may become occluded, the sinuses that most often do so are the cavernous sinus, the lateral (transverse) sinus, and the superior sagittal sinus. The straight sinus and the sigmoid sinus are much less commonly obstructed, as are the other dural sinuses.

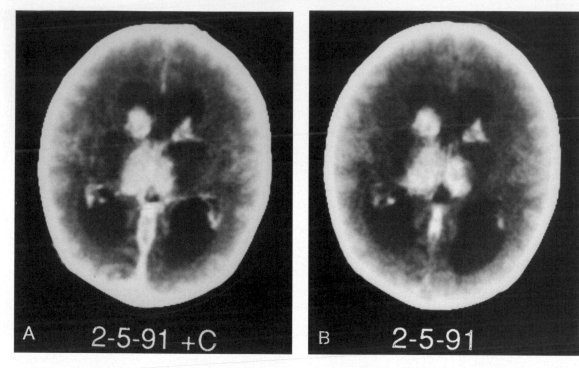

Figure 58.4. Deep vein thrombosis in a 14-day-old male. Unenhanced (*A*) and enhanced (*B*) computed tomographic scans show bilateral hemorrhages in the caudate and thalami and enlarged lateral ventricles due to obstructive hydrocephalus.

Thrombosis of the Cavernous Sinus

Cavernous sinus thrombosis may occur as a complication of both infectious and noninfectious processes. The clinical manifestations and the treatment depend in part on whether the condition is septic or aseptic.

SEPTIC CAVERNOUS SINUS THROMBOSIS

Causes. A number of infectious processes may predispose a patient to developing a septic thrombosis of the cavernous sinus (see Table 1 in Harbour et al., 1984; DiNubile, 1988). Infections of the face, expecially in the medial 3rd, continue to be the most frequent primary foci associated with septic thrombosis of the cavernous sinuses (Smith, 1918; Dixon, 1926; Eagleton, 1926; Cavenagh, 1936; Grove, 1936; Shaw, 1952; Clune, 1963; Evans, 1965; Casaubon et al., 1977; Friberg and Sogg, 1978; Geggel and Isenberg, 1982; Palmersheim and Hamilton, 1982; Marshall and Slattery, 1983; Harbour et al., 1984; Karlin and Robinson, 1984; Scrimgeour et al., 1985; Fiandaca et al., 1986; Southwick et al., 1986; DiNubile, 1988) (Fig. 58.6). Bacteria entering the facial vein and pterygoid plexus from these sites may be carried to the cavernous sinus through the ophthalmic veins. Gram-positive bacteria, particularly *Staphylococcus aureus,* are usually the pathogens in this setting (Southwick et al., 1986; Tveteras et al., 1988).

Sinusitis affecting the sphenoid and ethmoid air cells may cause septic thrombosis of the cavernous sinus (Clifford-Jones et al., 1982; Daxecker and Bichler, 1983; Lew et al., 1983; Sofferman, 1983; Karlin and Robinson, 1984;

Southwick et al., 1986). The sinusitis may be acute or chronic. When acute sphenoid sinusitis causes cavernous sinus thrombosis, the predominant pathogens are gram-positive bacteria, including *S. aureus, Streptococcus pneumoniae,* and other aerobic as well as anaerobic streptococci (Southwick et al., 1986). When chronic sinusitis causes cavernous sinus thrombosis, gram-negative rods, coagulase-negative staphylococci, and fungi such as *Aspergillus* and *Mucoraceae* are most often responsible (Sekhar, 1980; DiNubile, 1988; EV Johnson et al., 1988) (Fig. 58.7).

Dental infections cause about 10% of the reported cases of septic cavernous sinus thrombosis (Childs and Courville, 1942; Oliver et al., 1948; Mehrota, 1965; Gialldrenzi et al., 1974; Chow et al., 1978; Taicher et al., 1978; Palmersheim and Hamilton, 1982; Harbour et al., 1984). Most of these infections affect the maxillary teeth (Shaw, 1952). The most common pathogens that produce odontogenic septic thrombosis of the cavernous sinus are streptococci, fusobacteria, and *Bacteroides* species (Kaplan and Eichel, 1980).

Otitis media is no longer the common cause of septic cavernous sinus thrombosis it was in the pre-antibiotic era. Nevertheless, patients with bacterial or even fungal ear infections that are untreated, incompletely treated, or incorrectly treated occasionally develop septic thrombosis of the cavernous sinus that is directly related to the pathogen responsible for the ear infection (Proctor, 1966; Pang, 1967).

Orbital cellulitis is rarely complicated by septic thrombosis of the cavernous sinus (Price et al., 1971; Bell, 1972), even though the superior and inferior ophthalmic veins drain into the cavernous sinuses. The clinical manifestations of

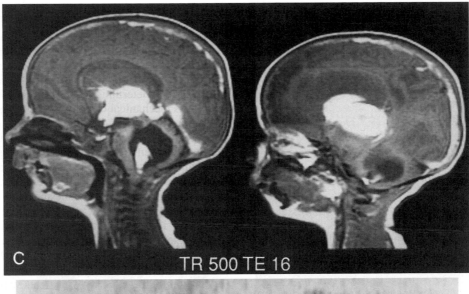

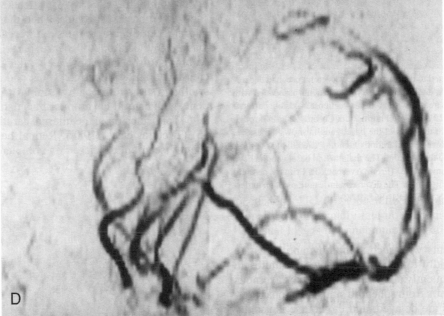

Figure 58.4. *(continued) C*, Unenhanced sagittal magnetic resonance (MR) images show hemorrhage in the thalami, enlarged 3rd and 4th ventricles, blood in the 4th ventricle, and clot in the straight sinus. *D*, MR angiogram shows no flow in the straight sinus. (Courtesy of Dr. John Huston).

orbital cellulitis can, however, be difficult or impossible to differentiate from those of early cavernous sinus thrombosis.

Clinical Manifestations. The clinical features of septic thrombosis of the cavernous sinus can be separated into those caused by the thrombosis and those caused by the infection (Walsh, 1937). General symptoms and signs include headache, giddiness, nausea, vomiting, and somnolence. There usually is an elevated temperature that may be intermittent or constant. Chills, sweating, and tachycardia are inconstant findings. There may be associated signs of sinusitis, otitis, suppurative gingivitis, or orbital cellulitis. As the disease progresses, there may be evidence of meningitis or brain abscess (Tveteras et al., 1988). Seizures may occur. Labora-

tory studies include a pronounced leukocytosis and positive blood cultures in most, but not all, patients. The CSF is abnormal in patients with associated meningitis, and the causative organism can often be isolated from the fluid in such cases.

As might be anticipated, the ocular signs vary considerably, depending on the origin of the infection. In patients who develop septic thrombosis of the cavernous sinus from anterior infections (e.g., facial, dental, or orbital), symptoms and signs appear acutely in the following order: deep-seated pain around the eye, elevated temperature, orbital congestion, lacrimation, conjunctival edema, eyelid swelling, ptosis, proptosis, and ophthalmoparesis (Langworthy, 1916; Di-

The choice of antimicrobial drug therapy depends on the availability of material for staining and culture, the primary site of infection, and the presence or absence of associated meningitis. Because of the vast and ever-increasing number of antibacterial, antiviral, and antifungal agents available to the physician, it seems to us that most, if not all, cases of septic cavernous sinus thrombosis should be treated in consultation with an expert in infectious disease. The antibiotic regimen can be optimized and usually simplified once culture and sensitivity results are finalized. The duration of treatment depends on the clinical response, the primary site of infection, and the presence of associated complications.

Anticoagulant therapy with heparin may prevent the spread of thrombosis from the cavernous sinus to other dural venous sinuses and cerebral veins. It is most useful when administered early in the course of the disease (Levine et al., 1988), but it is contraindicated if there is evidence of intracranial bleeding.

Corticosteroids reduce inflammation and decrease edema. No evidence exists to support their use for this purpose in cavernous sinus thrombosis (Solomon et al., 1962; Friberg and Sogg, 1978); however, if pituitary insufficiency results from the spread of infection into the adjacent sella turcica or from compromise of the pituitary circulation, appropriate replacement doses of corticosteroids are indicated (Williams, 1956; Ivey and Smith, 1968; Silver and Morris, 1983; Karlin and Robinson, 1984).

The primary site of infection may require surgery. Early surgical drainage is particularly crucial in patients in whom cavernous sinus thrombosis is a complication of sinusitis, and it may also be helpful in patients with facial, dental, orbital, or intracranial abscesses. Direct exploration of the cavernous sinus is rarely indicated.

Prognosis. The mortality rate for patients with septic cavernous sinus thrombosis is about 30%, regardless of therapy (DiNubile, 1988). Survivors have a variety of neurologic deficits, usually from damage to the cranial nerves within the cavernous sinus. These deficits include diplopia from paresis of one or more of the ocular motor nerves; visual sensory dysfunction from optic neuropathy, central retinal artery occlusion, or CRVO; and neurotrophic keratopathy or facial numbness, paresthesia, or pain from trigeminal neuropathy. Walsh and Hoyt (1969a) described a boy who developed Fröhlich's syndrome after septic cavernous sinus thrombosis. The patient later exhibited secondary aberrant regeneration of the oculomotor nerve. Full recovery occurs in less than 40% of patients who experience septic cavernous sinus thrombosis (Southwick et al., 1986).

ASEPTIC CAVERNOUS SINUS THROMBOSIS

Causes. Conditions associated with aseptic thrombosis of the cavernous sinus are those that produce thrombosis in other dural sinuses. These conditions include polycythemia, sickle cell disease and trait, paroxymal nocturnal hemoglobinuria, AVMs, trauma, intracranial surgery, vasculitis, pregnancy, use of oral contraceptive agents, congenital heart disease, dehydration, and marasmus (Byers and Hass, 1933; Ehlers and Courville, 1936; Grove, 1936; Schenk, 1964; Mones, 1965; Greitz and Link, 1966; Buchanan and Brazinsky, 1970; Johnson et al., 1970; Boniuk, 1972; Dindar and Platts, 1974; Garcia et al., 1975; Melamed et al., 1976; Buonanno et al., 1978; Sigsbee et al., 1979; Shirakuni et al., 1983; Bouchez et al., 1984). Compression or obstruction by an expanding mass, such as a pituitary adenoma, meningioma, or aneurysm, can produce a sterile thrombosis of the cavernous sinus (DiNubile, 1988), and aseptic thrombosis of the cavernous sinus may occur as part of a paraneoplastic hypercoagulability syndrome that accompanies certain malignancies (see Chapter 47).

Clinical Manifestations. Patients with aseptic thrombosis of the cavernous sinus develop symptoms and signs similar to those of patients with septic cavernous sinus thrombosis, but they have no clinical or laboratory evidence of underlying infection (Walsh, 1937; Boniuk, 1972). They have no fever, chills, signs of meningitis, or leukocytosis. Pain around and behind the affected eye is common, and there may be loss of corneal sensation, facial sensation, or both (Melamed et al., 1976). Proptosis and chemosis are usually less severe than in septic cavernous sinus thrombosis. Variable degrees of lacrimation, injection, and dilation of conjunctival vessels occur. Ophthalmoparesis is more often a consequence of ocular motor nerve damage in the cavernous sinus than of mechanical limitation of eye movement from orbital congestion (Savino et al., 1986). Ptosis is invariably present when the oculomotor nerve is affected, and pupillary dilation also occurs unless there is associated oculosympathetic dysfunction. Increased intraocular pressure is a common finding, presumably resulting from reduction of outflow of venous blood from the eye and orbit. Reduction of venous drainage also may cause stasis retinopathy characterized by dilation of retinal veins and scattered intraretinal hemorrhages. Visual loss is extremely unusual in patients with aseptic cavernous sinus thrombosis, regardless of the severity of the condition, but it may occur (Melamed et al., 1976).

Treatment. The treatment of aseptic thrombosis of the cavernous sinus is controversial. Optimum therapy for the underlying condition may be of some benefit. Anticoagulation with heparin may prevent extension of the thrombotic process (Levine et al., 1988). Other therapeutic agents used in the treatment of this condition include dextran, acetylsalicylic acid, and various thrombolytic agents such as bovine fibrinolysin, urokinase, and streptokinase (Herndon et al., 1960; Harvey, 1974; DiRocco et al., 1981; Barnwell et al., 1990). All results have been limited to anecdotal reports or small series. It is thus impossible to be certain if one of these agents is more likely to be of benefit than another.

Prognosis. The prognosis in patients with aseptic cavernous sinus thrombosis is variable. It depends primarily on the underlying cause of the condition and the extent and severity of neurologic dysfunction. The mortality from this condition is much lower than that from septic cavernous sinus thrombosis, but damage to the cranial nerves within the cavernous sinus may produce persistent ocular motor nerve pareses, trigeminal neuropathy, or both. Permanent visual loss is rare but occurs (Melamed et al., 1976).

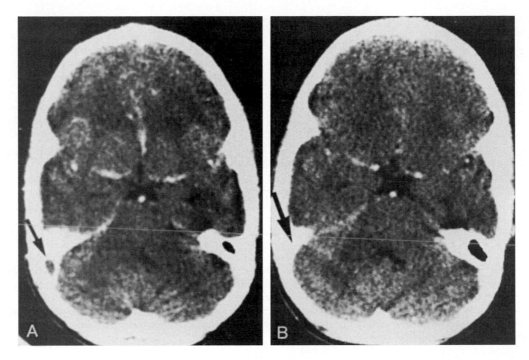

Figure 58.9. Septic lateral sinus thrombosis. The patient was a 9-year-old boy with chronic otitis media who did not respond to systemic antibiotics. *A*, Enhanced CT scan, axial view, shows filling defect in right lateral sinus (*arrow*). The patient subsequently underwent exploration of the right mastoid region. Pus and granulation tissue were present in the mastoid air cells and surrounded the right lateral sinus. All abnormal material was removed. The lateral sinus was found to be partially thrombosed. The patient was treated postoperatively with antibiotics with rapid defervescence of symptoms. *B*, Enhanced CT scan, axial view, performed 1 month later shows apparent resolution of lateral sinus thrombosis (*arrow*). (From Rizer FM, Amiri CA, Schroeder WW, et al. Lateral sinus thrombosis: Diagnosis and treatment—a case report. J Otolaryngol *16:*77–79, 1987.)

Thrombosis of the Lateral (Transverse) Sinus

Thrombosis of the lateral sinus is almost always septic. Nevertheless, aseptic lateral sinus thrombosis can occur. Both conditions can produce significant neuro-ophthalmologic complications (Purvin ct al., 1995).

SEPTIC THROMBOSIS OF THE LATERAL SINUS

Because of the almost universal treatment of acute ear infections with systemic antibiotics, septic thrombosis of the lateral sinus most often results from chronic otitis media (Editorial, 1982; Teichgraeber et al., 1982; Southwick et al., 1986; Tveteras et al., 1988; Purvin et al., 1995) (Fig. 58.9). Nevertheless, some cases of septic lateral sinus thrombosis result from acute otitis media (Shambaugh, 1967; Nissen, 1980; Sneed, 1983; Lenz and McDonald, 1984; Debruyne, 1985; Southwick et al., 1986; Garcia et al., 1995) (Fig. 58.10). In rare cases, septic thrombosis of the lateral sinus occurs in the setting of otitis media that is asymptomatic (''masked'' or ''silent'' otitis) (Tovi et al., 1988), but whether symptomatic or asymptomatic, the infection typically spreads from the mastoid air cells to the dural sinus by direct invasion or via the emissary veins. Other causes of septic thrombosis of the lateral sinus include infections of the scalp and parapharyngeal and retropharyngeal abscesses (Bousser et al., 1985; Tveteras et al., 1988).

The lateral sinus may be directly invaded by pus from the mastoid antrum, or thrombosis may result from a perisinus abscess. Dill and Crowe (1934) reported 30 cases of septic lateral sinus thrombosis, 14 of which were associated with perisinus abscess. The majority of these cases were caused by hemolytic streptococcus, and in all instances there was otitic suppuration. These findings led Dill and Crowe (1934) to conclude that progression of thrombosis is caused by extension of the inflammatory focus in the wall of the sinus and not by infection extending from the thrombus itself. Infection may, however, extend from the lateral to the inferior petrosal and superior petrosal sinuses and then to the cavernous sinus. Infection may also spread to the inferior petrosal sinus from the tip of the petrous temporal bone and to the superior petrosal sinus through the tegmen tympani.

The symptoms and signs of septic thrombosis of the lateral sinus may be generalized, focal, or both (Walsh, 1937). The typical clinical picture is that of a patient with a suppurative otitis who suddenly develops fever, chills, evidence of local inflammation in the region of the mastoid, and leukocytosis (Shambaugh, 1967; Pallares et al., 1983). Many patients develop neck pain and stiffness, and some also exhibit tenderness along the jugular vein on the side of the process (Shambaugh, 1967; Teichgraeber ct al., 1982; Sneed, 1983). Thrombosis of the mastoid emissary veins may cause pronounced retroauricular edema (Greisinger's sign) (Shambaugh, 1967; Sneed, 1983). Focal neurologic symptoms are usually inconspicuous, but there may be some degree of

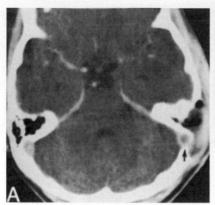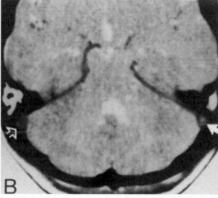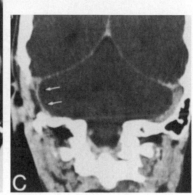

Figure 58.10. Thrombosis of the lateral and sigmoid sinuses in a patient with acute otitis and mastoiditis. The patient was a 24-year-old woman with a history of chronic mastoiditis that had previously been treated with simple mastoidectomy. The patient developed otorrhea and otalgia in the left ear, and purulent material was noted in the external auditory canal after manual pressure was applied to the left mastoid region. A radical mastoidectomy with left meatoplasty was performed. *A,* Enhanced CT scan, axial view, shows thrombus in the left sigmoid sinus adjacent to the mastoidectomy defect (*arrow*). Since the patient had no neurologic symptoms or signs, it was elected to treat her with antibiotics and to obtain a second scan in two weeks. *B,* Repeat CT scan, axial view with display in the negative mode, shows persistent thrombosis of the left lateral/sigmoid sinus. The display in the negative mode highlights the thrombus on the left side (*solid arrow*) compared with the normally opacified right sigmoid sinus (*open arrow*). *C,* CT scan, coronal view, shows extent of the left sigmoid sinus thrombosis (*arrows*). (From Goldberg AL, Rosenbaum AE, Wang H, et al. Computed tomography of dural sinus thrombosis. J Comp Assist Tomogr *10:*16–20, 1986.)

facial weakness. Patients previously treated with antibiotics for the otitis may have a more indolent presentation without the marked chills and fever described above. Wilson (1940) estimated that 75% of cases are associated with meningitis, subdural abscess, or brain abscess.

The ocular signs of septic lateral sinus thrombosis are not as prominent as in thrombosis of the cavernous sinus. Unilateral abducens nerve paresis is frequently present and may result from several mechanisms. First, infection and thrombosis may extend to the inferior petrosal sinus and then to the abducens nerve which is located just above it as they both pass under the petroclinoid ligament. Second, the inferior petrosal sinus may not be thrombosed but may simply be distended from the effects of the adjacent thrombosis of the lateral sinus. The distended inferior petrosal sinus compresses the abducens nerve upward against the petroclinoid ligament (Zülch, 1964). In such cases, there may be severe ipsilateral facial pain, particularly around the eye (Gradenigo's syndrome) (Gradenigo, 1904; Jahrsdoerfer and Fitz-Hugh, 1968; Southwick et al., 1986; see Chapter 28). Finally, both unilateral and bilateral abducens nerve paresis may occur as nonlocalizing signs of increased ICP. In such cases, papilledema is almost always present (Klestadt, 1924; Symonds, 1931; Dill and Crowe, 1934; Woodhall, 1936; Davidoff and Dyke, 1937; Gardner, 1939; Greer, 1962; Greer and Berk, 1963), and the picture is that of typical pseudotumor cerebri (see Chapter 10) (Fig. 58.11). This particular form of pseudotumor cerebri was initially called "otitic hydrocephalus" by Symonds (1931). Gaze-paretic nystagmus may also be present in some patients with septic lateral sinus thrombosis (Southwick et al., 1986).

As noted in Chapter 52 of this text, most of the venous drainage from both cerebral hemispheres is via the right lateral sinus and the right internal jugular vein. Thus, most cases of pseudotumor cerebri caused by lateral sinus thrombosis are caused by thrombosis of the right lateral sinus.

Ocular signs other than those caused by increased ICP occur only when thrombosis of the lateral sinus extends anteriorly via the short but broad inferior petrosal sinus to the cavernous sinus. In such cases, proptosis, chemosis, injection of the eye, lacrimation, eyelid swelling, and generalized limitation of eye movement develop.

The principal organisms associated with septic thrombosis of the lateral sinus reflect the bacteriology of otitis media. Since antibiotics are commonly used during the prodromal ear infection, cultures are negative in many cases. Nevertheless, common organisms include *Proteus* species, *Staphylococcus aureus, Escherichia coli, Bacteroides fragilis,* and various anaerobes (Southwick et al., 1986).

Septic thrombosis of the lateral sinus often has a protracted course with significant intracranial infective complications, such as meningitis and abscess formation. Other complications develop from detachment of the septic thrombus or from extension of the thrombus proximally or distally. When the thrombus extends distally, thrombosis of the internal jugular vein and even of the superior vena cava may occur (Surkin et al., 1983; Albert and Williams, 1986; Tovi et al., 1988). Nevertheless, most cases of septic thrombosis of the lateral sinus respond to aggressive antibiotic therapy, mastoidectomy with incision and drainage of the lateral sinus, and treatment of increased ICP when necessary (Editorial, 1982; Teichgraeber et al., 1982; Proctor, 1982; Sneed, 1983; Debruyne, 1985; Goldenberg, 1985; Southwick et al., 1986; Rizer et al., 1987; Samuel and Fernandes, 1987). In the pre-antibiotic era, ligation of the internal jugular vein was performed routinely to avoid dissemination of the thrombophlebitis and the production of septic emboli (Shambaugh, 1967; Teichgraeber et al., 1982; Sneed, 1983). Most

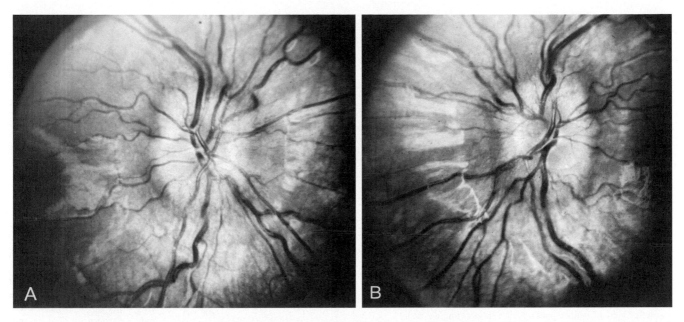

Figure 58.11. Bilateral papilledema in a patient with lateral sinus thrombosis. The patient was a 27-year-old man with chronic, untreated otitis media who developed severe headaches and brief episodes of bilateral loss of vision. Visual acuity was 20/20 OU, but visual fields showed bilateral enlargement of the blind spots. There was bilateral limitation of abduction consistent with bilateral abducens nerve paresis. *A* and *B*, Right and left ocular fundi show bilateral optic disc swelling. Lumbar puncture confirmed increased intracranial pressure. The CSF had a normal protein and glucose concentration, and it contained no cells. The patient was treated with antibiotics and acetazolamide with gradual resolution of papilledema.

authors now recommend ligation of the internal jugular vein only in cases of persisting sepsis and emboli that do not respond to conventional therapy (Rizer et al., 1987; Samuel and Fernandes, 1987). Similarly, anticoagulation is not recommended for patients with septic lateral sinus thrombosis unless there is evidence of systemic embolization (Parsons, 1967; Castaigne et al., 1977; Teichgraeber et al., 1982; Karlin and Robinson, 1984; Samuel and Fernandes, 1987).

The prognosis for patients treated early and appropriately for septic lateral sinus thrombosis is excellent, although there is a significant mortality rate in most series of 10–36% (Jackson and Dickins, 1979; Teichgraeber et al., 1982; Goldenberg, 1985; Southwick et al., 1986; Samuel and Fernandes, 1987). Most patients who survive recover completely, but some patients have persistent deficits, including facial weakness, hearing loss, hemiparesis, and visual loss from post-papilledema optic atrophy (Kinal and Jaeger, 1960; Jensen, 1962; Seid and Sellars, 1973; O'Connor and Moffat, 1978; Proctor, 1982; Teichgraeber et al., 1982; Southwick et al., 1986).

ASEPTIC LATERAL SINUS THROMBOSIS

Aseptic thrombosis of the lateral sinus is rare, but it occurs in a variety of diverse settings, including coagulopathies and other hematologic disorders (Castleman and Kibbee, 1960; Pouillot et al., 1984; Kaplan et al., 1985) and systemic vasculitis (Fahey et al., 1954; Bousser et al., 1985). It may also occur in patients taking oral contraceptive agents (Purvin et al., 1995).

Aseptic thrombosis of the lateral sinus may occur after head trauma (Kinal, 1967; Huhn, 1971; Björnebrink and Liliequist, 1976; Bousser et al., 1985). In such cases, a skull fracture in the parieto-occipital or temporo-occipital region is usually present (Fig. 58.12).

Some patients with dural AVMs in the posterior fossa have associated thrombosis of the lateral sinus (Handa et al., 1975; Houser et al., 1979; Augustin et al., 1984; Convers et al., 1986). In some cases, the thrombosis is believed to occur first, with the fistula caused by opening of congenital shunts in the dura mater. In other cases, a congenital fistula induces occlusion of the lateral sinus by altering venous return.

Occlusion of the lateral sinus may be iatrogenic. In one of the patients described by Purvin et al. (1995), occlusion of the right lateral sinus resulted from inadvertent coagulation of the sinus during microvascular decompression for trigeminal neuralgia.

In many cases of aseptic thrombosis of the lateral sinus, no cause can be identified. For example, two of six cases of aseptic thrombosis of the lateral sinus reported by Bousser et al. (1985) were said to be idiopathic.

As noted above, the clinical picture of right-sided lateral sinus thrombosis is usually that of pseudotumor cerebri, with headache, papilledema, and unilateral or bilateral abducens nerve paresis (Fig. 58.13). Right-sided thrombosis can also cause intracerebral hemorrhage.

Thrombosis of the left lateral sinus may be asymptomatic, but this is not always the case. Intracranial hemorrhage can occur (Fig. 58.14), or a pseudotumor cerebri syndrome can develop, particularly when the thrombosis occurs in the region of the jugular foramen, and the thrombus extends downward into the internal jugular vein. Graus and Slatkin (1983)

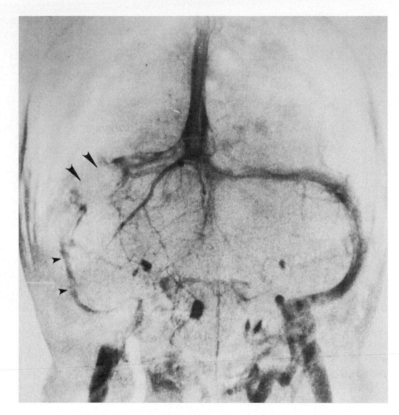

Figure 58.12. Post-traumatic occlusion of the right lateral sinus in a 67-year-old man who fell down a staircase. Skull x-rays showed a right-sided occipitotemporal fracture crossing over the ipsilateral lateral sinus groove. The patient was somnolent without focal neurologic signs. Cerebral arteriogram, anteroposterior view of venous phase, shows large filling defect in right lateral sinus (*large arrowheads*) with reduction in flow through the right sigmoid sinus (*small arrowheads*). The patient deteriorated and subsequently died. At autopsy, there was an organizing thrombus throughout the course of the right lateral sinus. (From Björnebrink J, Liliequist B. Traumatic lateral sinus thrombosis: Report of two cases. Angiology 27:688–697, 1976.)

reported such a case. The patient was a 27-year-old man with Ewing's tumor that metastasized to the region of the left jugular foramen. Compression of the venous structures in this region produced occlusion of the left lateral sinus. The patient developed increased ICP and papilledema.

Castleman and Kibbee (1960) also reported a case of symptomatic left lateral sinus thrombosis. The patient was a 75-year-old woman with polycythemia and systemic hypertension who experienced an acute thalamic hemorrhage. During the course of the illness, she developed aseptic thrombosis of the left lateral sinus that produced multiple, large, hemorrhagic infarctions in the temporal and occipital lobes. The patient subsequently died.

Bousser et al. (1985) reported five symptomatic cases of aseptic thrombosis of the left lateral sinus. Three of the patients developed symptoms and signs of increased ICP. The other two patients had seizures.

Mitchell et al. (1986) described a 31-year-old man with essential thrombocythemia who developed a severe right-sided headache and photophobia. The patient had no papilledema, and a CT scan of the brain with enhancement was normal; however, lumbar puncture showed increased ICP. Digital subtraction intravenous angiography showed thrombosis of the left lateral sinus. The patient gradually recovered completely.

Newman et al. (1989) reported two patients who experienced visual disturbances suggesting acephalgic migraine. One patient experienced the sudden onset of intense colored photopsias in the central vision of both eyes. The photopsias slowly spread outward over several minutes until they af-

fected the entire visual field. The positive visual phenomena resolved within 30 minutes, after which the patient was blind for some period of time. The second patient developed frequent episodes of visual blurring, lasting 10–30 minutes, and associated with vertical wavy lines, teichopsia, and a sensation of pressure localized to the cranial vertex. Both patients had filling defects in the left lateral sinus.

Ushiwata et al. (1989) reported the case of a 33-year-old-woman with a hemorrhagic infarction of the cerebellum with hematoma caused by thrombosis of the left transverse sinus and left-sided cerebellar cortical veins. Evacuation of the intracerebellar hematoma and decompression of the posterior fossa were carried out with good results. Cerebellar infarction is rare in transverse sinus occlusion, presumably because of extensive collateral circulation in the infratentorial region.

Thrombosis of the lateral sinus may be bilateral (Fig. 58.15). Ford (1966) described an 11-month-old child who developed bilateral aseptic thrombosis of the lateral sinuses. The child had a large head, and there were many prominent veins on the scalp extending posteriorly from the anterior fontanel. There was severe, bilateral papilledema with retinal hemorrhages and a left abducens nerve paresis. A Queckenstedt test was positive bilaterally, and the CSF pressure was greatly increased. Over the next 7 months, the child had spontaneous improvement in his condition. Although dilated veins were still present on the scalp, the skull was no longer growing rapidly. There was mild optic atrophy and a persistent left abducens paresis.

The diagnosis of aseptic lateral sinus thrombosis is usually

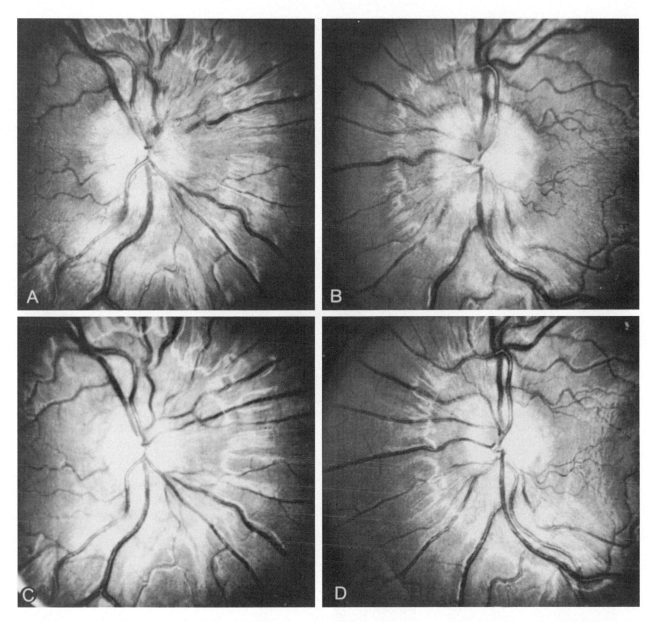

Figure 58.13. Pseudotumor cerebri syndrome in a patient with aseptic thrombosis of the right lateral sinus. The patient was a 21-year-old man who developed headache and diplopia after he was involved in a motor vehicle accident in which he sustained a right parieto-occipital skull fracture. *A* and *B*, Bilateral optic disc swelling. Cerebral angiography showed occlusion of the right lateral sinus, and lumbar puncture confirmed increased intracranial pressure. The CSF had a normal protein and glucose concentration and contained no cells. The patient was treated with acetazolamide, and his papilledema gradually resolved (*C* and *D*).

made by history, examination, and neuroimaging studies. CT scanning, MR imaging, and MR angiography are particularly helpful (Mas et al., 1990), but cerebral angiography may be necessary to confirm the diagnosis.

The treatment of aseptic lateral sinus thrombosis is somewhat controversial (Goldenberg, 1985). Pennybacker et al. (1961) advised no treatment other than supportive care and treatment of increased ICP. These authors noted that in many cases, symptoms and signs resolved spontaneously within several months as collaterals developed. Other authors recommended aggressive surgery consisting of mastoidectomy,

a wide exposure of the lateral sinus, and thrombectomy (O'Connor and Moffat, 1978; Pfaltz, 1982). These authors also advocated aggressive treatment of increased ICP. In our opinion and that of others, therapy of aseptic lateral sinus thrombosis must be individualized, depending on the severity of the condition (Persson and Lilja, 1990; Purvin et al., 1995). All patients with evidence of lateral sinus thrombosis should undergo a careful evaluation of visual parameters using tests of visual acuity, contrast sensitivity, and color vision combined with kinetic and static perimetry and ophthalmoscopy. In this way, permanent visual loss from post-

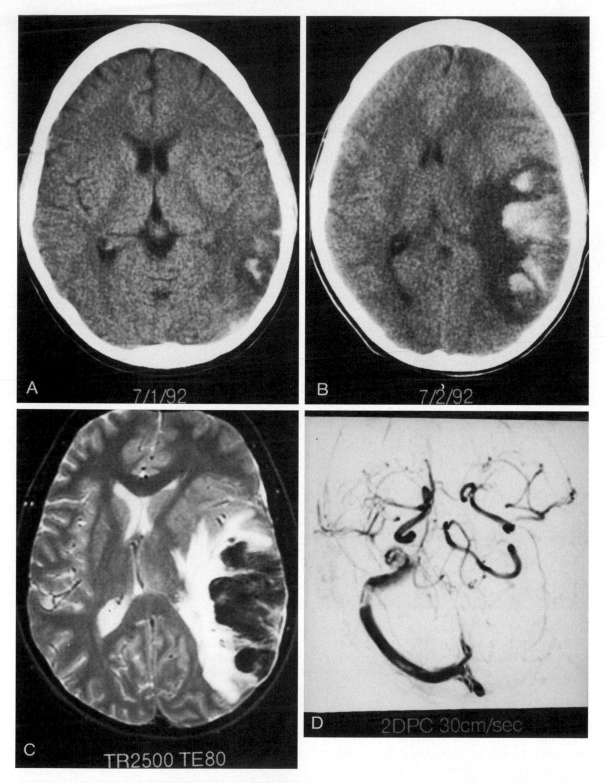

Figure 58.14.   Lateral sinus thrombosis producing a left parietal lobe hemorrhage. *A*, Unenhanced axial computed tomographic (CT) scan shows hemorrhage in the left parietal lobe. *B*, Unenhanced axial CT scan performed the next day shows increased hemorrhage with surrounding edema. *C*, T2-weighted axial magnetic resonance (MR) image shows the extent of hemorrhage with surrounding edema. Note shift of midline from left to right. *D*, MR angiogram shows no flow in the left lateral sinus. (Courtesy of Dr. Douglas Nichols.)

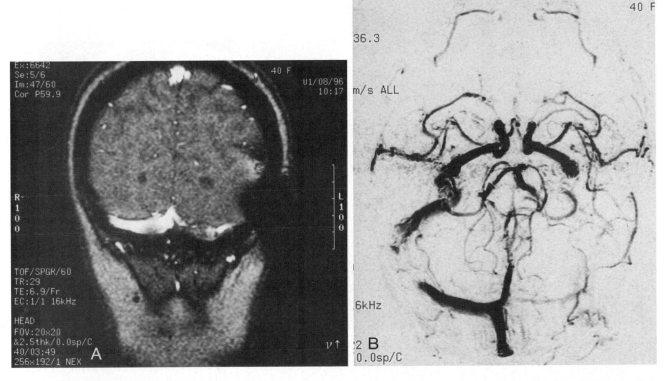

Figure 58.15. Bilateral lateral sinus occlusion in a patient who developed pseudotumor cerebri syndrome and severe visual loss from postpapilledema optic atrophy. *A*, Coronal magnetic resonance (MR) image (gradient echo technique) shows extensive clot in the right lateral sinus. *B*, MR angiogram shows right lateral sinus occlusion proximal to the sigmoid sinus and occlusion or absence of the left lateral sinus. (Courtesy of Dr. Douglas Nichols.)

papilledema optic atrophy can be avoided by medical treatment or surgical treatment of increased ICP (see Chapter

Thrombosis of the Superior Sagittal Sinus

Thrombosis of the superior sagittal sinus, unlike thrombosis of the cavernous and lateral sinuses, is more often aseptic than septic. Nevertheless, both types can produce significant neurologic and visual consequences.

SEPTIC THROMBOSIS OF THE SUPERIOR SAGITTAL SINUS

According to Southwick et al. (1986), meningitis is the major predisposing condition in almost 50% of cases of septic superior sagittal sinus thrombosis. In these cases, the infection probably spreads from the meninges to the superior sagittal sinus via the diploic veins. Infections of the paranasal sinuses may also produce septic thrombosis of the superior sagittal sinus (Bousser et al., 1985). Such infections spread from the ethmoid or maxillary sinuses to the superior sagittal sinus via ethmoidal veins (Buonnano et al., 1979). Infections of the frontal sinus with associated epidural abscess may result in cortical vein thrombosis, which may, in turn, be followed by thrombosis of the superior sagittal sinus. There may be an associated epidural abscess (Fig. 58.16). Extension of septic thrombosis from the lateral sinus causes some cases of septic thrombosis of the superior sagittal sinus

(Stuart et al., 1951; Poltera and Jones, 1973; Purvin et al., 1995). Other causes of septic thrombosis of the superior sagittal sinus include pulmonary infections, tonsillitis, tooth infection, otitis media, and pelvic inflammatory disease (Askenasy et al., 1962; Krayenbuhl, 1966; Strauss et al., 1973; Bousser et al., 1985). In some cases, the cause of septic thrombosis of the superior sagittal sinus remains unclear despite extensive investigation (Schell and Rathe, 1988).

Most patients with septic thrombosis of the superior sagittal sinus have an acute illness. The initial symptom is severe headache, usually generalized or occipital, but in patients with bacterial sinusitis, it may be localized to the region overlying the infected sinus. The headache is often associated with nausea and vomiting. Within several days of the onset of symptoms, confusion occurs, rapidly followed by grand mal or focal seizures that are often refractory to medical treatment (Bousser et al., 1985). The confusion rapidly progresses to coma and, subsequently, death.

A high fever and altered mental status are the most common findings in patients with septic thrombosis of the superior sagittal sinus. Hemiparesis is also a frequent sign, the consequence of cortical venous thrombosis and associated venous cerebral infarction. Patients with meningitis typically have nuchal rigidity and Kernig and Brudzinski signs. Some patients develop papilledema, whereas others have signs of brainstem dysfunction, including lack of spontaneous or in-

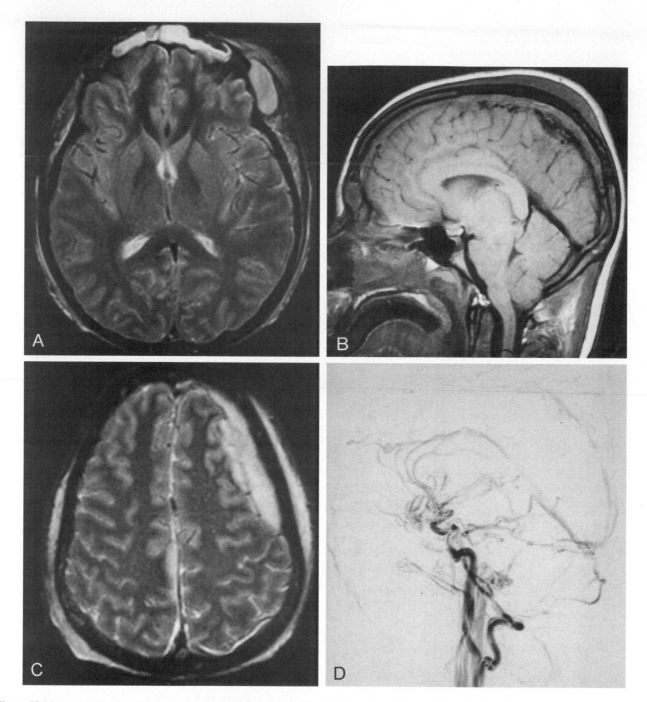

Figure 58.16. A patient with sinusitis, epidural abscess, and superior sagittal sinus thrombosis. *A*, T2-weighted axial magnetic resonance (MR) image shows opacified frontal sinuses with extension of material into the left temporal bone. Sulci over the convexity are obliterated. *B*, T1-weighted MR image, sagittal view, shows frontal sinus opacification, subgaleal opacity, and sulcal obliteration at base of frontal lobe. *C*, T1-weighted MR image, axial view, at higher level shows hyperintense epidural mass obliterating the sulci. The appearance is consistent with an epidural abscess. *D*, Cerebral angiogram, lateral view, shows occlusion of the superior sagittal sinus. (Courtesy of Dr. John Huston.)

duced eye movements, dilated pupils, and generalized flaccid quadriparesis.

A variety of pathogens may produce septic thrombosis of the superior sagittal sinus, although *Streptococcus pneumoniae* is the most common pathogen (Southwick et al., 1986). Other organisms identified in such cases include *S. aureus*,

β-hemolytic streptococcus, anaerobic streptococcus, *Klebsiella, Pseudomonas,* and even *Trichinella spiralis* (Evans and Patten, 1982; El Koussa et al., 1994). Meyohas et al. (1989) described a woman who developed septic thrombosis of the superior sagittal sinus in the setting of combined HIV and CMV meningitis. A patient reported by Schell and Rathe

(1988) had a herpes simplex virus type 1 titer of 1:512 in the CSF, although no virus was identified in cultures. El Alaoui Faris et al. (1992) described a 33-year-old man in whom syphilitic cranial osteitis caused thrombosis of the adjacent superior sagittal sinus.

The diagnosis of septic thrombosis of the superior sagittal sinus is initially made by a combination of a complete history, physical examination, and noninvasive neuroimaging studies, particularly MR imaging and MR angiography. Conventional angiography may or may not be necessary to confirm the diagnosis.

Treatment of septic superior sagittal sinus thrombosis includes intravenous administration of appropriate antimicrobial agents. Intravenous mannitol or systemic corticosteroids may be used to reduce cerebral edema, and they may decrease the risk of brain herniation. Mannitol must be used

with caution, however, because severe dehydration may predispose to further thrombosis. Infected paranasal sinuses should be surgically drained to prevent continued spread of infection. Anticoagulation, clot lysis, or both may be appropriate.

Despite aggressive therapy, most patients with septic thrombosis of the superior sagittal sinus die (see Figure 3 in Schell and Rathe, 1988). Southwick et al. (1986) quoted a mortality rate of 80%, and our own experience with several cases would seem to confirm this dismal prognosis.

ASEPTIC THROMBOSIS OF THE SUPERIOR SAGITTAL SINUS

Aseptic thrombosis affects the superior sagittal sinus more often than any other of the dural sinuses, apparently because of its high position, low pressure, and slow flow (Wohlwill,

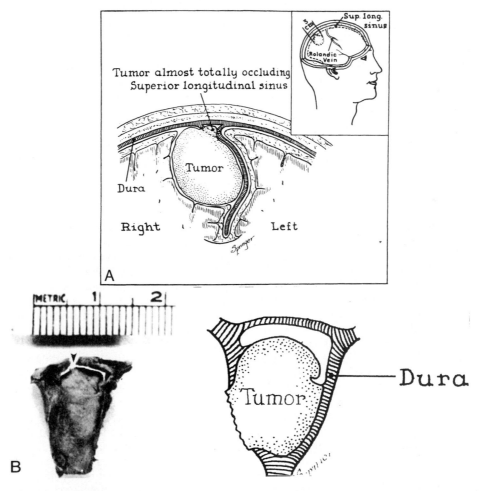

Figure 58.17. Almost total occlusion of the superior sagittal sinus from parasagittal meningioma. The patient was a 49-year-old man who complained of severe headaches, nausea, vomiting, and generalized weakness. He had bilateral papilledema, a left homonymous hemianopia, and a left hemiparesis. Skull x-rays showed a calcified intracranial mass in the right parieto-occipital region near the midline. A craniotomy was performed. *A,* Artist's drawing of findings at surgery. The drawing shows location of a meningioma that was projecting into the superior sagittal sinus. *Inset* shows region of sinus that was excised in order to remove entire tumor. *B, Left side* of photograph shows cross-section of the portion of the tumor that was within the superior sagittal sinus (*arrowhead*). Note that the sinus is almost totally occluded. *Right side* of photograph shows an illustration of the tumor and its relationship to the superior sagittal sinus. (From Jaeger R. Observations on resection of the superior longitudinal sinus at and posterior to the rolandic venous inflow. J Neurosurg 8:103–109, 1951.)

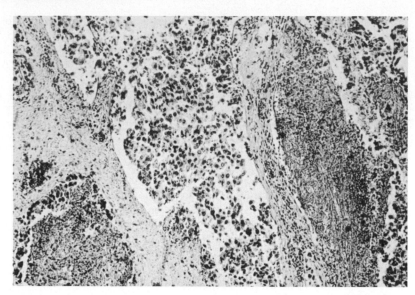

Figure 58.18. Occlusion of the superior sagittal sinus by metastatic carcinoma. The patient was a 31-year-old woman who had undergone a radical mastectomy for ductal carcinoma of the breast. She subsequently developed headache. A lumbar puncture revealed slightly elevated intracranial pressure. She suffered a cardiorespiratory arrest after undergoing a pneumoencephalogram. Cross-section through the posterior third of the superior sagittal sinus shows occlusion of the sinus by organizing thrombus and metastatic carcinoma of the breast. (From Averback P. Primary cerebral venous thrombosis in young adults: The diverse manifestations of an under-recognized disease. Ann Neurol *3*:81–86, 1978.)

1931). Of 34 cases of aseptic dural sinus thrombosis evaluated by Bousser et al. (1985), 24 (71%) involved the superior sagittal sinus. Similarly, of 20 cases of cerebral venous thrombosis described by Purvin et al. (1995), eight (40%) involved the superior sagittal sinus. The thrombus usually forms in the middle 5th of the sinus (Byers and Hass, 1933).

The superior sagittal sinus may become occluded in a variety of settings (Kalbag and Woolf, 1967; Gettelfinger and Kokmen, 1977; Imai et al., 1982; Kalbag, 1984; Bousser et al., 1985; Thron et al., 1986; Gum et al., 1987; Purvin et al., 1995). Occlusion may occur following a skull fracture through the vertex. The resulting syndrome is sometimes called **traumatic hydrocephalus** (Martin, 1955). Closed head trauma can also cause thrombosis of the superior sagittal sinus (Bagley, 1934; see Table 1 in Hesselbrock et al., 1985). The trauma in such cases is usually severe (Stringer and Peerless, 1983; Hesselbrock et al., 1985); however, Stevenson et al. (1964) reported a patient in whom occlusion of the superior sagittal sinus occurred after minor head trauma that produced a chronic epidural hematoma that compressed the sinus. Occlusion of the superior sagittal sinus may also result from compression or infiltration by a meningioma (Jaeger, 1951; Marr and Chambers, 1966; Repka and Miller, 1984; Steiger et al., 1989; Purvin et al., 1995) (Fig. 58.17) or by metastatic tumor within the confines of the sinus (Mones, 1965; Averback, 1978; Meininger et al., 1985) (Fig. 58.18). Patients are particularly prone to develop thrombosis of the superior sagittal sinus during pregnancy, in the immediate postpartum period, or while taking oral contraceptive agents (Imai et al., 1982; Ojeda et al., 1982; Bousser et al., 1985; Persson and Lilja, 1990; Purvin et al., 1995) (Fig. 58.19). Aseptic thrombosis of the superior sagittal sinus may develop in patients with inherited and acquired coagulopathies from hematologic and other disorders (Iob et al., 1979; Murphy et al., 1983; Makin et al., 1986; McDonald et al., 1989; Cros et al., 1990; Kyritsis et al., 1990; Pasquale et al., 1990; Furuta et al., 1991; Confavreux et al., 1994; Purvin et al., 1995; Siegert et al., 1995; D'Olhaberri-

ague et al., 1996) (Fig. 58.20). It may also occur in patients with systemic vasculitis associated with such disorders as Behçet's disease, Wegener's granulomatosis, Chron's disease, and SLE, presumably from inflammation in and around the sinus (Drachman, 1963; Rosenberger et al., 1982; Bank and Weart, 1984; Bousser et al., 1985; Harper et al., 1985; Shiozawa et al., 1986; Leslie et al., 1987; Hammans and Ginsberg, 1989; El-Ramahi and Al-Kawi, 1991; Garciá-Moncó and Beldarrain, 1991; Fujikado and Imagawa, 1994; Purvin et al., 1995; see Chapter 57).

Iatrogenic occlusion of the superior sagittal sinus may occur during intracranial surgery, particularly when a transcallosal approach is used to reach lesions of the lateral and 3rd ventricles (Shucart and Stein, 1978; Garrido and Fahs, 1990). Injury to the sinus may result from direct application of a retractor, aggressive use of bipolar coagulation, or aggressive retraction of dural flaps to optimize midline exposure (Apuzzo, 1990). In other cases, the sinus is sacrificed at the time of removal of a parasagittal tumor, usually a meningioma (Bederson and Eisenberg, 1995; Purvin et al., 1995).

In some patients with isolated thrombosis of the superior sagittal sinus, no definite cause can be identified (Bousser et al., 1985; Thron et al., 1986; Shaenboen et al., 1989; Purvin et al., 1995). Some of these patients probably have an underlying coagulopathy that may not be apparent and may not be detected at the time of their illness.

The symptoms and signs of a patient with aseptic thrombosis of the superior sagittal sinus depend in part on the portion of the sinus that is occluded (Walsh, 1937). In general, the most severe clinical manifestations occur when the posterior portion of the sinus becomes occluded.

When only the anterior part of the superior sagittal sinus is occluded, the symptoms and signs may be minimal or absent (Fig. 58.21). Such patients may experience mild to severe headache. Occasional patients develop nonspecific sensory symptoms, such as paresthesias (Walsh, 1937).

When the posterior portion of the superior sagittal sinus

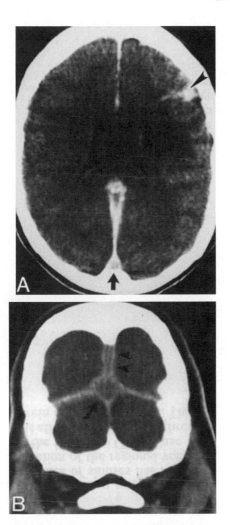

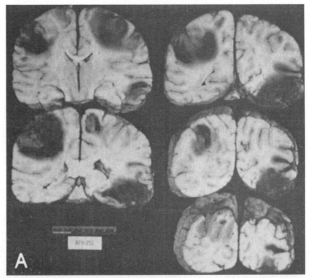

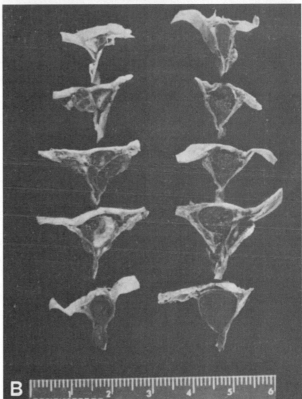

Figure 58.19. Occlusion of the superior sagittal sinus in a 23-year-old woman who was taking oral contraceptives when she became confused and disoriented. Neurologic examination revealed a right hemiparesis and bilateral papilledema. *A*, Enhanced CT scan, axial view, shows filling defect in the superior sagittal sinus near the torcular herophili (*arrow*) consistent with thrombosis. Note small region of hyperdensity in the left frontal region compatible with venous infarction (*arrowhead*). *B*, Enhanced CT scan, coronal view, shows that there is a thrombus in the superior sagittal sinus (*arrowheads*) and a separate thrombus in the torcular (*arrow*). (From Goldberg AL, Rosenbaum AE, Wang H, et al. Computed tomography of dural sinus thrombosis. J Comp Assist Tomogr *10:*16–20, 1986.)

is affected, the neurologic consequences can be devastating. Many patients develop pseudotumor cerebri (Fig. 58.22). Such patients usually complain of severe headaches and have increased ICP without evidence of an intracranial mass lesion on neuroimaging studies. They usually have papilledema and may have diplopia from unilateral or bilateral abducens nerve paresis. Other patients with thrombosis of the posterior sagittal sinus, particularly those with extension of the process into the cortical veins or lateral sinuses, develop severe focal and generalized neurologic dysfunction (Bousser et al., 1985; Thron et al., 1986; Gum et al., 1987) (Fig. 58.23). Headaches, vomiting, and changes in mentation and

Figure 58.20. Paraneoplastic thrombosis of the superior sagittal sinus. The patient was a 63-year-old woman with known carcinoma of the breast who developed headache, left hemiparesis, and left homonymous hemianopia. She subsequently died from the effects of her tumor. *A*, Coronal sections through the brain show three large areas of hemorrhagic infarction in the distribution of the veins of Troulard on both sides and the vein of Labbé on the right. *B*, Serial sections through the superior sagittal sinus show complete occlusion of the sinus by organized thrombus. In some sections, the thrombus can be seen extending into the parasagittal cortical veins. (From Hickey WF, Garnick MB, Henderson IC, et al. Primary cerebral venous thrombosis in patients with cancer—A rarely diagnosed paraneoplastic syndrome: Report of three cases and review of the literature. Am J Med *73:*740–750, 1982.)

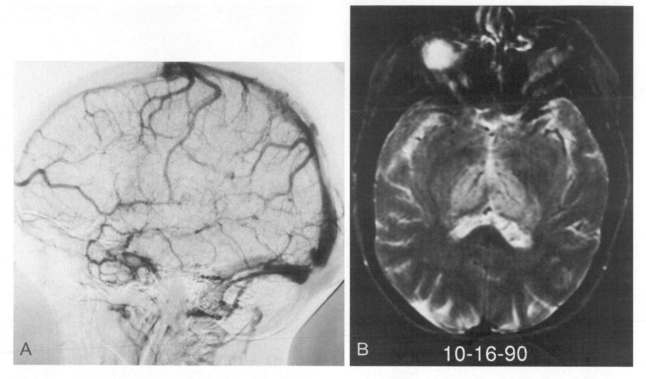

Figure 58.21. Thrombosis of the anterior third of the superior sagittal sinus. *A,* T2-weighted axial magnetic resonance scan shows bitemporal edema. *B,* Cerebral angiogram, lateral view, shows the area of occlusion. (Courtesy of Dr. John Huston.)

awareness are common manifestations in these patients. Seizures, progressive impairment in consciousness, and unilateral or bilateral motor weakness may also occur (Kingsley et al., 1978; Ojeda et al., 1982; Bousser et al., 1985; Hesselbrock et al., 1985; Thron et al., 1986). Because the superior external surface of the cortex in the motor region for the lower limbs usually is affected early, initial motor weakness may affect only the lower extremities (Holmes and Sargent, 1915). With time, however, quadriparesis may result (Kingsley et al., 1978). In one reported case, a patient with aseptic superior sagittal sinus developed a subdural hematoma (Matsuda et al., 1982).

The ocular signs of aseptic superior sagittal sinus thrombosis usually are related to the effects of increased ICP. The most common sign is papilledema (Kingsley et al., 1978). The papilledema usually is bilateral and symmetric; however, it may be asymmetric and even unilateral (see Chapter 10). Unilateral or bilateral abducens paresis may be present. Visual sensory function usually is not affected unless papilledema is associated with macular hemorrhages and exudates, or the papilledema becomes chronic; however, Uhthoff (1911) described a case of cortical blindness from superior sagittal sinus thrombosis, and one of the patients described by Kingsley et al. (1978) was a 30-year-old woman with postpartum aseptic superior sagittal sinus thrombosis who had bilateral superior altitudinal visual field defects. Conjugate deviation of the eyes frequently occurs in patients with aseptic superior sagittal sinus thrombosis during major motor seizures.

Treatment of aseptic superior sagittal sinus thrombosis requires attention to the underlying condition and sometimes treatment of increased ICP. When the sinus is obstructed but not completely occluded by tumor, excision of the lesion and reconstruction of the sinus may be curative (Bonnal and Brotchi, 1978; Steiger et al., 1989). When the sinus is completely occluded, ICP needs to be controlled until sufficient time has elapsed to allow a collateral network of drainage to develop. Anticoagulation therapy may be helpful (Castaigne et al., 1977; Thron et al., 1986; Shaenboen et al., 1989; Einhäupl et al., 1991), but heparin must be used with caution in patients with evidence of intracranial hemorrhage. Fibrinolytics may also be used in this condition (Castaigne et al., 1977; DiRocco et al., 1981; Scott et al., 1988). Rare patients may be helped by surgical intervention. Persson and Lilja (1990) described a patient with extensive thrombosis of the superior sagittal sinus, both lateral sinuses, and the galenic venous system who improved after surgical removal of thrombotic material combined with local infusion of streptokinase.

Thrombosis of the Straight Sinus

Thrombosis of the straight sinus is rare and almost always aseptic. Ford (1966) described this condition in several infants. When the thrombosis occludes both the straight sinus and the vein of Galen, the child becomes comatose, rigid, and may develop convulsions. The ICP increases, and the CSF becomes bloody or xanthochromic because of hemor-

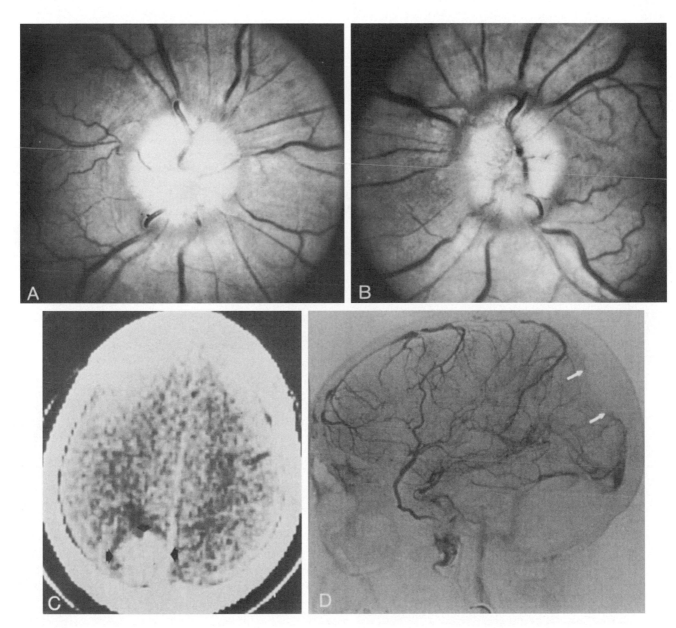

Figure 58.22. Pseudotumor cerebri syndrome from obstruction of the posterior portion of the superior sagittal sinus. The patient was a 45-year-old woman who developed lightheadedness, blurred vision, and binocular horizontal diplopia. Visual acuity was 20/20 OU, but visual fields showed a binasal defect. Bilateral abduction weakness was present. *A* and *B*, Both optic discs show chronic optic disc swelling. *C*, Computed tomographic scan, axial view, shows a small enhancing mass adjacent to the posterior superior portion of the falx. *D*, Cerebral angiogram, lateral view of venous phase, shows obstruction of the posterior third of the superior sagittal sinus (*arrows*). At operation, the tumor was found to be a meningioma that had completely occluded the posterior portion of the superior sagittal sinus. The tumor was completely removed. When the papilledema did not resolve, lumbar puncture confirmed increased intracranial pressure with normal CSF content. The patient therefore was treated with acetazolamide with gradual resolution of papilledema and improvement in both visual acuity and visual field. (From Repka MX, Miller NR. Papilledema and dural sinus obstruction. J Clin Neuroophthalmol *4:* 247–250, 1984.)

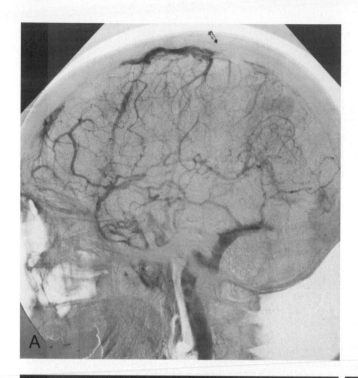

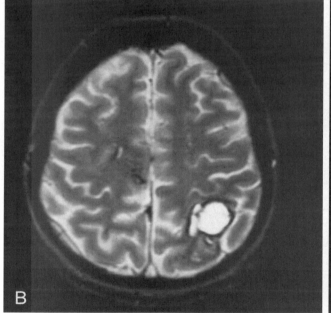

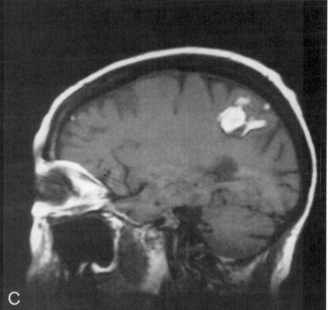

Figure 58.23. Superior sagittal sinus thrombosis causing cerebral edema and hemorrhage. *A*, T2-weighted axial magnetic resonance (MR) image shows focal hemorrhage in the left parieto-occipital region. *B*, T1-weighted sagittal MR image shows position of hemorrhage. *C*, Cerebral angiogram, lateral view, shows occlusion of the superior sagittal sinus except for a portion of the middle third. (Courtesy of Dr. John Huston.)

rhage from the ventricles into the subarachnoid space. Purvin et al. (1995) described a 23-year-old woman in whom the straight sinus was occluded during embolization for a torcular AVM. Adults with thrombosis of the straight sinus often develop papilledema, retinal hemorrhages, and abducens nerve paresis in addition to decerebrate rigidity (Fig. 58.4).

Thrombosis of the Sigmoid Sinus

Thrombosis of the sigmoid sinus is extremely rare. It may occur from extension of clot from the lateral sinus or the

jugular vein, in association with a occipital dural AVM (Kutluk et al., 1991), or from coagulation or ligation of the vessel during surgery (Purvin et al., 1995).

DIAGNOSIS

Noninvasive neuroimaging is the primary method of diagnosing cerebral venous and dural sinus thrombosis (Perkin, 1995; Einhäupl, 1996). Both CT scanning (Buonanno et al., 1978; Wendling, 1978; Zilkha and Daiz, 1980; Eick et al., 1981; Rao et al., 1981; Kawase et al., 1982; D'Avella et al.,

1984; Ahmadi et al., 1985; Goldberg et al., 1986; Thron et al., 1986; Curnes et al., 1987; Virapongse et al., 1987; Chung et al., 1988) and MR imaging (Macchi et al., 1986; McMurdo et al., 1986; Savino et al., 1986; Snyder and Sachdev, 1986; Thron et al., 1986; Moots et al., 1987; Sze et al., 1988; Harris et al., 1989; Shaenboen et al., 1989; Belman et al., 1990; Medlock et al., 1992; Fujikado and Imagawa, 1994; Bousser, 1995) can provide provide important information regarding localization, etiology, and severity of the process.

On nonenhanced CT scans, one may observe an abnormally high density in relation to a thrombosed superior sagittal (Buonanno et al., 1978) or straight (Wendling, 1978) sinus. Other changes seen on nonenhanced CT scans include diffuse cerebral swelling, single or multiple hemorrhages, areas of hemorrhagic infarction, and small ventricles (Figs. 58.2–58.4, 58.14A, 58.14B, and 58.22). An irregular, high density seen in the superficial portion of the hemisphere may represent a thrombosed cortical vein or dural sinus. Although this "cord sign" is rarely seen, it is diagnostic of cortical venous thrombosis (Gates and Barnett, 1987; Gum et al., 1987). Following the intravenous administration of iodinated contrast material, other changes may be detected by CT scanning. The **empty delta sign** (also called the empty triangle sign) is one of the most important diagnostic criteria in a patient with suspected dural sinus thrombosis (Buonanno et al., 1978; Rao et al., 1981; Brant-Zawadzki et al., 1982; Stringer and Peerless, 1983; Virapongse et al., 1987). This sign consists of a triangle of low density surrounded by a border of increased density (Figs. 58.9, 58.10, and 58.19). It is caused by a clot within the sinus that is outlined by contrast material in the smaller collateral veins and in the wall of the sinus. The empty delta sign is most easily seen in patients with thrombosis of the posterior third of the superior sagittal sinus, where the CT plane is perpendicular to the sinus, but it can also be observed in patients with occlusion of the transverse and straight sinuses (Rao et al., 1981; Harris et al., 1989).

MR imaging in patients with cerebral venous and dural sinus thrombosis reveals abnormalities in the veins and sinuses as well as in the brain parenchyma. Affected veins or sinuses initially show absence of a flow void associated with collateral venous channels on T1-weighted images. Acute thrombus appears isointense with brain parenchyma on T1-weighted images and hypointense on T2-weighted images (Gomori et al., 1985; Sze et al., 1988; Bousser, 1995). Subacute thrombus demonstrates hyperintense signal characteristics on T1-weighted images (Sze et al., 1988; Harris et al., 1989; Shaenboen et al., 1989; Belman et al., 1990) (Figs. 58.15A and 58.24). In the late stages, recanalization of the previously occluded vessel results in reappearance of the flow void (Macchi et al., 1986; McDonald et al., 1989; Shaenboen et al., 1989; El-Ramahi and Al-Kawi, 1991). After enhancement with gadopentetate dimeglumine (Gadolinium-DTPA) or a similar paramagnetic substance, enhanced T1-weighted images often demonstrate the empty delta sign (Harris et al., 1989; El-Ramahi and Al-Kawi, 1991).

MR imaging findings in the brain parenchyma are different from those seen in arterial occlusive disease (Yuh et al., 1994) and reflect the underlying pathophysiology. Mass effect without bright signal on T2-weighted images is char-

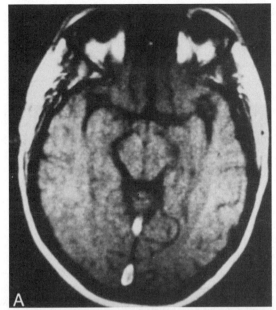

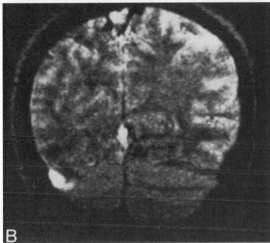

Figure 58.24. Magnetic resonance imaging in a patient with thrombosis of multiple dural sinuses. The patient was a 29-year-old man who was found unconscious by his wife. He had a history of previous deep venous thrombosis of the left leg confirmed by venography 4 years earlier. *A,* Unenhanced T1-weighted MR image, axial view, shows high-intensity signals consistent with thrombosis in the superior sagittal and straight sinuses. *B,* Unenhanced T2-weighted MR image, coronal view, shows high-intensity signals in the superior sagittal, straight, and right transverse sinuses. (From Shaenboen MJ, Matzura TM, Disbro MA. Magnetic resonance imaging of dural sinus thrombosis with resolution. J Am Osteopath Assoc 89:794–804, 1989.)

acteristic, suggesting that breakdown of the blood-brain barrier leading to vasogenic edema does not always occur. This initial swelling may be related to distention of a compliant venous bed with little or no increase in venous pressure. The swelling may persist for months or years (Yuh et al., 1994). Further progression may be associated with mass effect with T2-weighted signal changes and ventricular dilation. As the venous pressure rises bulk water is driven by the pressure gradient from the capillary bed into the interstitium. T2-

weighted signal abnormalities are prone to develop in areas of poor venous drainage, such as the basal ganglia and thalamus. Transependymal reabsorption of CSF with hydrocephalus develops, and this is the etiology of so-called otitic hydrocephalus. When elevated venous pressure exceeds the structural limit of the venous wall, rupture of veins causes a hematoma (Figs. 58.4C, 58.14D, 58.23A, 58.23B).

Tsai et al. (1995) measured venous sinus pressures in 11 patients with acute venous sinus thrombosis and found that the pressures correlated with five distinct stages of disease based on clinical and neuroimaging findings. In stage I, patients had headache, papilledema, weakness, changed mentation, and drowsiness. There were no parenchymal changes on MR imaging. The venous pressures in these cases were 14–17 mm Hg. In stage II, patients had increased headache, diplopia, seizures, decreased mentation, and extreme drowsiness. MR imaging showed changes consistent with cerebral edema. Venous pressures in these patients ranged from 20 to 25 mm Hg. In stage III, patients were obtunded and had hemiparesis and seizures. MR imaging showed increased intensity of signal, with mild to moderate cerebral edema. Venous pressures ranged from 32 to 38 mm Hg. Stage IV patients were comatose and had hemiparesis and seizures. MR imaging showed severe cerebral edema but no other parenchymal changes. Venous pressures were 42–51 mm Hg. Stage V patients were comatose and responded only to deep pain. MR imaging showed marked cerebral edema, intraparenchymal hemorrhage, or both. No venous pressure measurements were obtained in these patients, but it was assumed that the venous pressures were greater than 50 mm Hg.

Angiograph-like images of the intracranial and extracranial vasculature can be obtained using MR angiography (three-dimensional MR flow imaging) (Wedeen et al., 1985; Dumoulin, 1987) (Figs. 58.4, 58.14D, and 58.15B). The main advantage of this technique is that it is noninvasive. Villringer et al. (1989) reported the results of MR angiography in the assessment of a young woman with aseptic thrombosis of the superior sagittal sinus. Images of the intracranial venous system obtained by MR angiography were comparable to those obtained with standard angiography. Villringer et al. (1989) suggested that MR angiography be performed as an initial procedure in any patient with suspected cerebral venous or dural sinus thrombosis, and we and others agree with this recommendation (Padayachee et al., 1991; Medlock et al., 1992; Bowen et al., 1994; Fujikado and Imagawa, 1994; Perkin, 1995; Einhäupl, 1996).

Although noninvasive neuroimaging generally is sufficient to diagnose occlusion or thrombosis of the cerebral veins or dural sinuses (Bousser, 1995), most physicians prefer to confirm the diagnosis with conventional angiography (Ray and Dunbar, 1950; Krayenbuhl, 1954; Gabrielsen et al., 1981; Bousser et al., 1985) (Figs. 58.1, 58.2B, 58.12, 58.16D, 58.21B, 58.22D, and 58.23C). Conventional angiography is also helpful in identifying associated stenosis or occlusion of the internal carotid artery, ophthalmic artery, or both (Mathew et al., 1971; Lazo et al., 1981; MA Johnson et al., 1988) and in detecting the development of a mycotic aneurysm of the cavernous portion of the internal carotid artery (Molinari et al., 1973; Shibuya et al., 1976; Eguchi

et al., 1982; Abassioun et al., 1985; Endo et al., 1989; Micheli et al., 1989).

EVALUATION

Once the diagnosis of cerebral venous or dural sinus thrombosis is established, an attempt should be made to determine the underlying cause. In almost all cases of septic thrombosis, the source of the infection is usually apparent. In patients with aseptic thrombosis, the etiology may be more difficult to determine. Patients with aseptic cerebral vein or dural sinus thrombosis, particularly patients under 45 years old, should be evaluated for thrombophilia (Najim Al-Din et al., 1994; Deschiens et al., 1996). Not only do thrombophilic individuals have an increased risk of venous thrombosis without any of the known risk factors discussed above, but such patients may also have other risk factors for venous thrombosis. A disorder of coagulation is found in about 20% of patients with a history and clinical features suggesting thrombophilia. This probably reflects our limited understanding of these disorders.

Initial laboratory investigation should include a complete blood count (including platelet count and peripheral smear) to evaluate for myeloproliferative disorders and DIC. An elevated sedimentation rate may indicate vasculitis or an autoimmune disorder. A urinalysis may reveal proteinuria, suggesting a nephrotic syndrome. Coagulation tests should include a prothrombin time, activated partial thromboplastin time, and tests for antithrombin III, protein C functional activity, and activated protein C resistance (Factor V Leiden). Both total and free protein S should be measured. Thrombin time should be used to screen for dysfibrinogenemia and exclude a heparin effect. Assays for fibrinogen, D-dimer or fibrin/fibrinogen split products, and soluble fiber monomer complex should be performed to detect DIC.

It must be remembered that deficiencies of certain coagulation factors may be primary or secondary. For example, acquired causes of antithrombin III deficiency including chronic treatment with heparin, L-asparaginase, nephrotic syndrome, DIC, and recent surgery. Protein C and protein S are both vitamin K-dependent proteins; hence, their activity is reduced by warfarin therapy. Reduced concentrations of protein C and protein S are also found in patients with severe liver disease, patients receiving L-asparaginase for cancer, patients with the nephrotic syndrome, and patients with DIC. In addition, many coagulation factors are acute phase reactants, affected by estrogen, or both. Thus, hematologic testing in the acute phase of thrombosis or during pregnancy may give inaccurate results.

The lupus anticoagulant and anticardiolipin antibodies seem to be risk factors for aseptic cerebral venous and dural sinus thrombosis, and an attempt should be made to detect their presence in the serum of any patient with this condition. Unfortunately, no single coagulation test can detect these proteins. Several phospholipid-dependent coagulation tests can be performed to determine if antiphospholipid antibodies are present, including the dilute Russel Viper venom time, plasma clot time (recalcification time), and Kaolin clotting time. Although activated prolonged partial thromboplastin time (APTT) in the absence of recent treatment with heparin suggests that the lupus anticoagulant is present, a normal APTT does not indicate that it is not present. To establish the presence of the lupus anticoagulant, confirmation of the phospholipid-dependent nature of an inhibitor is required (platelet neutralization procedure). Anticardiolipin antibodies are usually detected by enzyme-linked immunosorbent assay (ELISA) or radioimmunoassay.

Other tests that should be performed in selected patients with aseptic cerebral venous or dural sinus thrombosis include a functional plasminogen assay and qualitative testing of platelet functioning. Arterial or venous thrombosis in association with heparin is strongly suggestive of heparin-associated thrombocytopenia and thrombosis. Absolute thrombocytopenia or a 50% drop in platelets support this diagnosis.

TREATMENT

As noted in several of the earlier sections of this chapter, the treatment of cerebral venous or dural sinus thrombosis depends on many factors, including whether the thrombosis is septic or aseptic, the underlying cause of the thrombosis, the location and extent of the thrombosis, and the severity of the patient's neurologic dysfunction (Bousser et al., 1985; Southwick et al., 1986). Patients with septic thrombosis require treatment with antimicrobial agents. They may also require surgical treatment of the septic focus. Some patients may benefit from anticoagulants, corticosteroids, or both.

Previously, patients with aseptic thrombosis were treated with supportive care. Heparin was used conservatively because of the risk of intracranial hemorrhage. In 1991, Einhäupl et al. published the results of a prospective placebo-controlled study of the treatment of dural sinus thrombosis with heparin. These authors found that patients who received heparin had a better outcome than patients who were not treated. In addition, the use of heparin was not associated with an increased rate of intracranial hemorrhage. Although some authors questioned the conclusions of this study (Enevoldson and Ross Russell, 1991; Stam, 1991), we and others believe that it is appropriate to use heparin in selected patients with aseptic cerebral venous or dural sinus thrombosis, particularly in those patients who demonstrate little or no cerebral edema, and in whom venous pressures are only mildly elevated (Perkin, 1995; Rondepierre et al., 1995; Einhäupl, 1996). Tsai et al. (1995) recommended using anticoagulants in patients without focal neurologic signs and without parenchymal changes on MR imaging (Stage 1, venous pressure 14–17 mm Hg—see above). The use of low molecular weight heparins (e.g., tinzaparin, enoxaparin, and nadroparin) is under investigation (Siragusa et al., 1996). These

drugs may prove to be beneficial in cerebral venous or dural sinus thrombosis.

Thrombolysis seems a logical choice for the treatment of vascular occlusions (Abel, 1992). The use of urokinase is strongly supported by a number of studies, including several that showed better clinical outcomes with thrombolytic therapy than with anticoagulation alone (Tsai et al., 1992; Smith et al., 1994; Horowitz et al., 1995; Tsai et al., 1995). This therapy must be started early for it to be effective (Tsai et al., 1992, 1995). Treatment protocols using urokinase involve catheterizing the occluded cerebral vein or dural sinus and delivering urokinase to the region of the newly formed clot. Lysis of the clot is confirmed by intraoperative and postoperative angiography. This technique is safe although time-consuming (33–244 hours) (Smith et al., 1994). Tissue plasminogen activator (TPA) can also be used to lyse acute clots in the cerebral veins and dural sinuses (Smith et al., 1994).

Surgical therapy to remove a venous or dural sinus thrombus may be warranted in some cases (Persson and Lilja, 1990). Other surgical treatments include stent placement (Marks et al., 1994). In patients in whom it is elected to sacrifice a dural sinus in order to remove an adjacent tumor, consideration should be given to replacement or reconstruction of the sinus using a saphenous vein graft or other material (Bederson and Eisenberg, 1995; Sindou, 1995), although some authors recommend leaving some tumor along the sinus and allowing the tumor to gradually occlude the sinus, permitting development of collateral flow (Al-Mefty, 1995).

Patients in whom occlusion of the superior sagittal or lateral sinus produces increased ICP may benefit from aggressive management of the raised ICP with medication (e.g., acetazolamide), multiple lumbar punctures, or shunt procedures. Eggenberger et al. (1996) found lumboperitoneal shunting to be particularly effective in such cases. Optic nerve sheath decompression should also be considered whenever papilledema threatens visual function.

For long-term management, thrombophilic patients usually do well when treated with standard heparin and warfarin therapy. Patients with a deficiency of protein C or protein S or with the lupus anticoagulant/anticardiolipin antibody should be given oral anticoagulants while receiving full heparin anticoagulation to avoid warfarin-induced skin necrosis. Long-term anticoagulation is recommended for patients with two or more episodes of spontaneous thrombosis or with a single life-threatening event. The international normalized ratio (INR) should be maintained between 2.0 and 3.0, although ranges up to 4.5 may be necessary for patients with recurrent thrombosis despite anticoagulant therapy. Antithrombin III concentrate is available for patients in whom this factor is deficient or who demonstrate heparin resistance, especially patients undergoing chemotherapy with L-asparaginase.

THROMBOSIS OF THE OPHTHALMIC VEIN

In 1957, Zimmerman and Rogers described a 69-year-old woman with a 2-year history of right eye pain who experienced an acute exacerbation of the pain associated with proptosis of the right eye. Visual acuity was reduced to 20/60 in the right eye. There was marked orbital congestion, and

eye movements were limited in all directions. The right ocular fundus appeared normal. No bruit was heard. Over the next 17 days, visual acuity in the right eye became further reduced to counting fingers; the visual field became constricted; and the retinal veins became enlarged and tortuous.

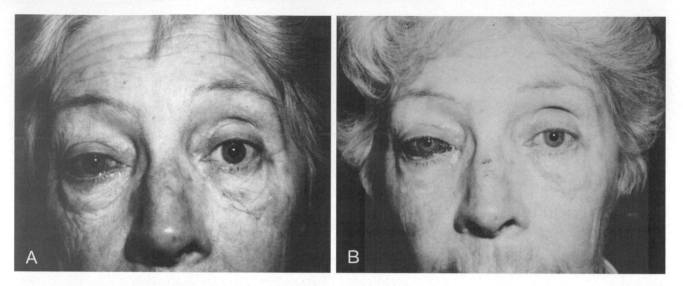

Figure 58.25.   Worsening of proptosis and chemosis in a patient with a spontaneous, dural, carotid-cavernous sinus fistula. *A,* The patient's initial appearance. Note moderate proptosis and chemosis. After angiography confirmed the presence of the fistula, it was elected to follow the patient at regular intervals to see if the fistula would close spontaneously. About 3 days after angiography, the patient noted an acute increase in proptosis, chemosis, and redness of the eye. *B,* The right eye is more proptotic, and the conjunctiva is more chemotic and hyperemic.

The orbit was explored, but no distinct abnormality was identified. The orbit was therefore exenterated. Pathologic examination of the orbital contents revealed an acute and chronic thrombophlebitis of the orbital veins. It subsequently became clear that thrombosis of the superior ophthalmic vein may produce a clinical picture similar to that seen in patients with aseptic cavernous sinus thrombosis.

Perhaps the most common setting in which thrombosis of the superior ophthalmic vein occurs is when a dural fistula of the cavernous sinus spontaneously closes (see Chapter 54). In this setting, a patient who may have only mild proptosis, chemosis, and injection of the affected eye suddenly develops a worsening clinical picture characterized by increasing chemosis, proptosis, and injection, and accompanied by the development or worsening of diplopia (Sergott et al., 1987; Simha et al., 1988) (Fig. 58.25). Color doppler imaging in such patients reveals occlusion of the superior ophthalmic vein, ocular pulse amplitudes in such patients gradually become reduced on the side of the fistula (Fig. 58.26), indicating reduction in backflow of arterial blood through the venous system, and MR imaging shows complete or partial thrombosis of the superior ophthalmic vein (Fig. 58.27). The condition is self-limited, and the patient usually begins to improve within several days. Systemic corticosteroids may be useful in hastening improvement, but they are not needed unless orbital congestion is particularly severe, and intraocular pressure is significantly elevated. Topical antiglaucoma medication, particularly carbonic anhydrase inhibitors, should be used to lower intraocular pressure and prevent retinal arterial occlusion.

Individual cases of isolated superior ophthalmic vein occlusion have been verified by conventional angiography, MR imaging, or both. Boniuk (1972) reported four cases in which symptoms and signs of superior ophthalmic vein thrombosis

included variable dilation and tortuosity of conjunctival vessels of the eye on the affected side, slight proptosis, injection of conjunctival and retinal veins, and a slightly higher intraocular pressure on the side of the lesion. Delle Grottaglie et al. (1981) described a 33-year-old woman who developed

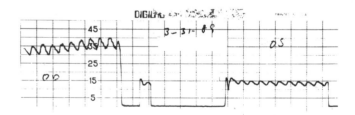

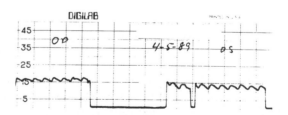

Figure 58.26.   Ocular pulse amplitudes in the patient whose appearance is seen in Figure 58.25. The amplitudes were measured using a pneumotonograph. *Above,* When first examined, the ocular pulse amplitude in the affected right eye is 2–3 times higher than that of the opposite eye, and the intraocular pressure in the right eye is about 37 mm Hg compared with about 14 mm Hg in the left eye. *Below,* At the time of acute worsening of clinical symptoms, the ocular pulse amplitude in the right eye is **less** than that in the left eye, and the intraocular pressure in that eye is almost the same as the pressure in the left eye.

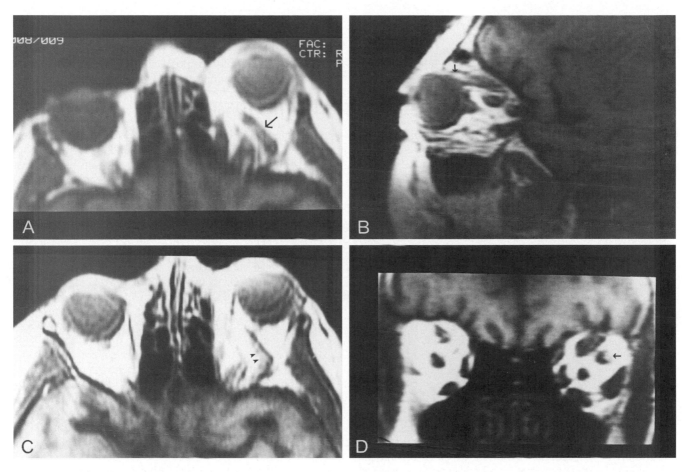

Figure 58.27. Magnetic resonance (MR) imaging in a patient with clinical worsening in the setting of a known dural carotid-cavernous sinus fistula. The patient was a 72-year-old woman with a left-sided, dural carotid-cavernous sinus fistula who suddenly developed increasing proptosis and orbital congestion. *A,* T1-weighted axial view shows absence of normal flow void with areas of hyperintensity within the superior ophthalmic vein (*arrow*), consistent with developing thrombosis. *B,* Sagittal T1-weighted image confirms hyperintensity consistent with thrombus within the superior ophthalmic vein (*arrow*). Because of the findings by neuroimaging, no treatment was recommended. *C,* T1-weighted axial view, obtained 1 week after initial MR imaging, shows increased hyperintensity within the left superior ophthalmic vein *(arrowheads).* *D,* T1-weighted coronal view also shows large area of hyperintensity within the left superior ophthalmic vein (*arrow*), indicating further thrombosis. The patient's condition gradually improved to normal over the next 3 weeks. (From Sergott RC, Grossman RI, Savino PJ, et al. The syndrome of paradoxical worsening of dural-cavernous sinus arteriovenous malformations. Ophthalmology *94:*205–212, 1987.)

swelling of the right upper and lower eyelids, right proptosis, and dilation of retinal veins in the right eye. Local and systemic administration of antihistamine drugs and corticosteroid preparations produced no improvement. Selective right internal and external carotid angiography showed no vascular malformation or fistula. The superior ophthalmic vein on the right side did not fill during any stage of angiography. A diagnosis of possible thrombosis of the superior ophthalmic vein was made, and the patient was treated with subcutaneous injections of heparin for 25 days, followed by coumadin for 3 months. Within 1 week after the start of treatment, the patient's symptoms and signs began to improve. After 5 months, she had no proptosis, minimal lower eyelid swelling, and persistently dilated retinal veins. At this time, both superior ophthalmic veins were visualized with the right being larger than the left. Delle Grottaglie et al. (1981) reported this case as an example of thrombosis of

the superior ophthalmic vein successfully treated with anticoagulation.

We doubt the diagnosis in the case reported by Delle Grottaglie et al. (1981), but we have no such reservations concerning four cases of superior ophthalmic vein thrombosis reported by Takahashi et al. (1984). All four patients were over 60 years old and presented with signs of orbital congestion, including chemosis of the conjunctiva, proptosis, and dilation and tortuosity of conjunctival vessels. Venous stasis retinopathy and glaucoma were present in several of the cases. In all four cases, thrombosis of the superior ophthalmic vein was confirmed by orbital venography. Most likely these cases were caused by spontaneous, dural CCFs that initially drained anteriorly and then closed spontaneously, resulting in acute occlusion of the superior ophthalmic vein. An unusual case of apparent occlusion of both the superior and the inferior ophthalmic veins of both orbits was reported by Jensen (1983) in a patient with conjunctival hemorrhagic lymphangiectasia with localized amyloidosis. The author postulated that the amyloidosis had induced venous thrombosis in this patient. We have examined several patients with nonspecific signs of orbital congestion in whom neuroimag-ing studies showed only an occluded superior ophthalmic vein without evidence of a CCF or a mass in the cavernous sinus or orbit. We suspect that in most of these cases, a pre-existing CCF that closed spontaneously was responsible for the clinical and imaging picture.

CENTRAL RETINAL VEIN OCCLUSION (CRVO)

Occlusion of the central retinal vein is a common ocular disorder. Most patients who develop this condition are over 50 years old, and 50–75% have associated hypertension, diabetes mellitus, or cardiovascular disease (Zegarra et al., 1979; Gutman, 1983; Elman et al., 1990; Rath et al., 1992; Clarkson, 1994; Flynn et al., 1994). There is also a strong association between CRVO and atherosclerotic or arterio-sclerotic disease of the central retinal artery (Cassady, 1953; Morgan, 1955; Paton et al., 1964; Hayreh, 1965; Fujino et al., 1969). Atherosclerosis and arteriosclerosis of the central retinal artery within the optic nerve, where it is adjacent to, and shares a common sheath with, the central retinal vein, presumably causes compression and irritative endothelial proliferation of the central retinal vein (Hayreh, 1980). Color doppler imaging shows high vascular resistance in the central retinal arteries, ophthalmic arteries and short posterior ciliary arteries of both the affected and the fellow eyes, suggesting that diffuse small vessel disease may predate and contribute to the development of CRVO (Keyser et al., 1994a). Several investigators (Brown et al., 1984; Lazzaro, 1986) suggested that patients with the ischemic form of CRVO (see below) have a higher prevalence of obstructive carotid artery disease than would be expected for age and sex, although others have not found this to be the case (Zegarra et al., 1983). Indeed, the paper by Brown et al. (1984) seems to us to be seriously flawed, not only by the choice of digital subtraction intravenous angiography as the test by which these investigators determined the presence or absence of atherosclerotic disease affecting the carotid artery, but also by several assumptions made by the authors (Hayreh, 1984). The article by Lazzaro (1986) does not explain why his patients with CRVO underwent cerebral angiography, although five of the 15 patients (33%) initially presented with transient monocular loss of vision associated with retinal emboli. In addition, we suspect that some of the confusion surrounding the proposed relationship between CRVO and carotid occlusive disease is related to errors in distinguishing a CRVO from the venous stasis retinopathy of Kearns and Hollenhorst (1963). We agree with Hayreh (1984) that atherosclerotic and arteriosclerotic disease of the **central retinal artery** plays a major role in the pathogenesis of some cases of CRVO, but that there is no evidence that occlusive disease of the internal or common carotid artery has any direct relevance to the pathogenesis of CRVO.

As in older patients, CRVO in young adults occurs with increased frequency in association with hyperlipidemia, atherosclerosis, hypertension, and diabetes mellitus (Fong et al., 1992; Fong and Schatz, 1993). Other cases, however, are similar to cerebral venous occlusive disease in their associations and etiology, or they are idiopathic. In such cases, CRVO is associated with disorders that produce intrinsic or extrinsic changes in the walls of veins and with disorders that alter clotting mechanisms and blood viscosity.

Reported abnormalities of blood vessel walls include vasculitis, SLE, moya-moya disease, and congenital venous abnormalities of the orbit (Gutman, 1983; Fong and Schatz, 1993). Schatz et al. (1993) described two patients with retinal AVMs who developed a CRVO. These authors proposed that turbulent flow, high intravascular volume, and elevated arteriolar pressure on the venous side led to vessel wall damage, thrombosis, and occlusion. Dural CCF may also be associated with CRVO. Komiyama et al. (1990) reported such a case and reviewed the findings in 14 similar cases. These authors recommended close monitoring of patients with dural CCFs in order to detect early stasis of the retinal veins and to try to prevent the occurrence of a CRVO in such patients. Barke et al. (1991) reported a patient with a dural CCF who developed a CRVO associated with iris neovascularization. We have examined several patients with both dural and direct CCFs who developed neovascular glaucoma after a CRVO.

External compression of the central retinal vein can be caused by a space-occupying intracranial lesion or by optic neuritis. Duker et al. (1989) reported five cases of optic neuritis associated with CRVO. Fluorescein angiography in these cases showed delayed venous filling with venous dilation and tortuosity. There was no evidence of capillary nonperfusion, macular edema, or macular hemorrhage. Winterkorn et al. (1994) described two patients with orbital pseudotumor (idiopathic orbital inflammation) who developed combined central retinal artery and central retinal vein occlusions, presumably from external compression of these vessels by inflamed orbital tissue.

Congenital and acquired hematologic and coagulation disorders are associated with CRVO. These disorders include platelet abnormalities, thrombocytopenia, polycythemia, iron deficiency anemia, cryofibrinogenemia, hyperviscosity, SLE, renal disease, and abnormal clotting factors (Rothstein, 1972; Ririe et al., 1979; Fong et al., 1992; Bandello et al., 1994; Dhote et al., 1995). Wenzler et al. (1993) reported 19 patients with retinal vein or retinal artery occlusion who were less than 50 years old. Using the standardized oral methionine loading test, four of the 19 patients (21%), two with retinal vein occlusion and two with retinal artery occlusion, were found to be obligate heterozygotes for homocystinuria. Homocystinuria has also been diagnosed in patients with other evidence of thromboembolic disease, including central retinal artery occlusion (Van den Berg et al., 1990).

Pregnancy and pre-eclampsia may be associated with CRVO, presumably because of an associated hypercoagulable state that can occur in such patients. Patients taking oral contraceptive agents also have an increased risk of developing a CRVO or branch retinal vein occlusion (BRVO), presumably for the same reasons (Walsh et al., 1965). Inoue et al. (1989) reported a case of CRVO in a young woman with a prolactin-secreting pituitary adenoma and suggested that hormone-induced changes in blood coagulation, similar to those in patients taking oral contraceptives, were responsible. Considering the thousands of patients with prolactin-secreting tumors, many with serum prolactin concentrations over 1000 ng/ml, who do not develop a CRVO or BRVO, it seems unlikely that this hypothesis is correct. We suspect that the association of a prolactin-secreting pituitary adenoma and a CRVO in this patient was coincidental.

There may be an increased risk of CRVO in patients with HIV infection. Friedman and Margo (1995) reported one case and identified four others in the literature. The patient reported by Friedman and Margo (1995) had bilateral CRVOs and no risk factors for vascular occlusive disease other than HIV infection, suggesting that the association of retinal vascular occlusive disease and HIV infection in this patient was not coincidental, although histopathologic findings in this case revealed no evidence of HIV in vascular endothelial cells on electron microscopy or using in situ hybridization technique. In addition, no infectious or structural abnormalities were found. It is therefore likely that hemorrheologic factors related to HIV infection were probably responsible for the CRVOs in this patient.

Charteris et al. (1989) reported a patient who developed acute posterior multifocal placoid pigment epitheliopathy (APMPPE). Five weeks after the onset of symptoms, he experienced dramatic loss of vision in the affected eye and was found to have a CRVO. Although the etiology of APMPPE is probably multifactorial, some cases occur after presumed or known viral illnesses. In addition, APMPPE may be associated with systemic inflammatory disorders, such as erythema nodosum and sarcoidosis, as well as with cerebral vasculitis (Smith et al., 1983; see Chapter 57). Thus, the association between APMPPE and CRVO may be related to an underlying vasculitis or to a systemic inflammatory process. On the other hand, most patients with APMPPE do not experience a retinal vascular occlusion, and the possibility must be considered that the two conditions were coincidental in this patient.

In some cases of CRVO, the cause is multifactorial. For example, some patients develop CRVO after heart-lung transplantation (Allinson et al., 1993), a procedure that can produce systemic hypotension and increased intraocular pressure, both risk factors for CRVO. In addition, however, cardiopulmonary bypass requires hypothermia and is associated with disturbances in hemostasis and platelet function. Clotting factors are frequently administered during the procedure. Finally, postoperative immunosuppressive therapy may result in hypertension and hyperlipidemia. Any or all of these factors could predispose a patient to developing a CRVO following heart-lung transplant.

CRVO was reported in a patient with anorexia nervosa and no other apparent risk factors by Shibuya and Hayasaka (1995). The significance of this association is unclear.

Combined central retinal artery and vein occlusion is associated with carcinomatous (Schaible and Golnik, 1993), lymphomatous (Guyer et al., 1990), and leukemic (Fong and Schatz, 1993) meningitis. Other infiltrative causes include bacterial infiltration from septic thrombi (Guyer et al., 1990), sarcoidosis, and tuberculosis (Fong and Schatz, 1993).

There appears to be an association between increased intraocular pressure and CRVO. In most cases, it is believed that increased pressure within the eye predisposes the patient to the vein occlusion, possibly by producing a deformity in the wall of the central retinal vein, thus causing increased resistance to blood flow (Green et al., 1981; Hayreh, 1983). In other cases, however, a CRVO may induce increased intraocular pressure. In such cases, endothelial proliferation associated with retinal hemorrhage may cause a progressive increase in flow resistance. Some factor or mediator in the aqueous humor may then be formed by destruction of oxygen-deprived tissue or transferred through damaged vessels acting on outflow resistance, thus increasing the intraocular pressure (Krakau, 1994).

A CRVO may rarely be the initial manifestation of pseudotumor cerebri (Chern et al., 1991). In some cases, an underlying hypercoagulable state leads to venous thrombosis, resulting in both the CRVO and occlusion of one or more dural sinuses, producing the pseudotumor syndrome. In others, increased ICP results in compression of the central retinal vein as it exits the optic nerve within the orbit, producing the CRVO.

Patients with CRVO usually complain of decreased vision in the affected eye. The loss of vision may occur suddenly without any preceding visual symptoms, or it may follow a period during which the patient has experienced transient episodes of blurred vision, flashes of light, or floaters. In some patients, the condition is asymptomatic, discovered during a routine ophthalmologic examination.

The clinical appearance of CRVO is characterized by dilated retinal veins and scattered intraretinal hemorrhages in both the posterior pole and the periphery. The retinopathy varies from a few small, scattered retinal hemorrhages and perhaps a few cotton wool spots (Walters and Spalton, 1990) (Fig. 58.28) to a marked hemorrhagic retinopathy with both superficial and deep retinal hemorrhages (the classic "blood and thunder" retina) and blood in cystoid spaces within the macula (Reyes et al., 1994) (Fig. 58.29). The optic disc may be normal or swollen in both mild and severe cases (Figs. 58.28 and 58.29). When the retinal findings are severe and are associated with decreased vision in the eye, the diagnosis of CRVO is usually easily made. However, patients with no significant visual loss and relatively minor retinal findings except for disc swelling and a few peripapillary and posterior pole hemorrhages may be thought to have unilateral papilledema, optic neuritis, or anterior ischemic optic neuropathy (see Chapter 8 and chapters 10–12). Such patients may undergo an inappropriate evaluation for underlying neurologic disease.

A particular type of CRVO was once called **papillophlebitis** (Hoyt and Beeston, 1966; Lonn and Hoyt, 1966; Ellenberger and Messner, 1978). This condition occurs in healthy young adults without any underlying systemic disease (Walters and Spalton, 1990; D'Amato et al., 1991). Unlike typical CRVO, which has a variable visual outcome, almost all pa-

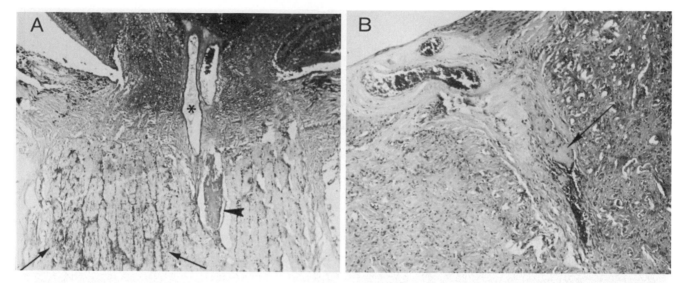

Figure 58.30. Etiology of central retinal vein occlusion. *A*, Section through center of optic nerve in a patient with a central retinal vein occlusion shows a patent central retinal artery (*asterisk*), diffuse hemorrhage in the retrolaminar nasal portion of the nerve (*arrows*), and a fresh thrombus in the central retinal vein just posterior to the lamina cribrosa (*arrowhead*). *B*, In another case of central retinal vein occlusion, there is a recanalized thrombus (*arrow*) in the central retinal vein at the level of the lamina cribrosa. (From Green WR, Chan CC, Hutchins GM, et al. Central retinal vein occlusion: A prospective histopathologic study of 29 eyes in 28 cases. Retina *1*:27–55, 1981.)

1994b; Noble, 1994). Schatz et al. (1991) described 10 patients, all younger than 50 years of age, with CRVO and cilioretinal artery occlusion. On fluorescein angiography, the cilioretinal artery eventually filled in nine of the 10 eyes. In all nine eyes that were followed, the fundus findings resolved, and the final visual acuity in eight of the nine eyes was 20/30 or better. Schatz et al. (1991) hypothesized that occlusion of the central retinal vein can elevate intraluminal capillary pressure because the central retinal artery continues to transmit blood into the retina arterioles and from there to the retinal capillaries. Because venous outflow is obstructed, and the perfusion pressure of the cilioretinal artery is lower than that of the central retinal artery, it becomes occluded.

Berler (1994) thought that the cases of combined CRVO and cilioretinal artery occlusion described by Schatz et al. (1991) and Keyser et al. (1994b) were similar to those described by Lyle and Wybar (1961) and Lonn and Hoyt (1966) and called papillophlebitis. Although we agree with Katz and Smith (1980) that rare patients with so-called papillophlebitis are associated with occlusion of the cilioretinal artery occlusion. Most cases do not show such an association.

CRVO can also occur in conjunction with branch retinal artery occlusion (Ducker et al., 1990). These cases appear to be heterogeneous with respect to etiology and to have the same underlying and associated conditions as cases of isolated CRVO.

CRVO is often confused with the venous stasis retinopathy that results from occlusion or severe stenosis of the common carotid, internal carotid, or ophthalmic arteries (Kearns and Hollenhorst, 1963; Kearns, 1983). Although the differences in the clinical pictures of these two disorders are dis-

cussed in Chapter 55 of this text, we repeat them here for the sake of completeness (Figs. 58.28, 58.29, 58.31 and 58.32). First, optic disc swelling is never seen in the venous stasis retinopathy of carotid or ophthalmic artery occlusive disease, whereas it is a major feature in florid cases of CRVO and even in mild cases. Thus, if optic disc swelling is present, the patient has a CRVO and not the retinopathy of carotid disease. Second, in both CRVO and venous stasis retinopathy, the retinal veins are engorged and dark; however, the veins often have an irregular fusiform or saccular appearance in the retinopathy of carotid disease. This gross irregularity is never seen in CRVO. Third, the hemorrhages, microaneurysms, and capillary dilations seen in CRVO tend to be distributed diffusely over the entire retina. In eyes with venous stasis retinopathy, however, these abnormalities are usually located only in the midperiphery of the retina, particularly in the superior temporal quadrant. Fourth, patients with CRVO have stable blurred vision that does not fluctuate from time to time or in different light settings. Patients with venous stasis retinopathy, however, may complain of episodes of transient monocular loss of vision lasting several minutes, or they may note blurred vision upon entering a less well-lighted room after being in a brighter area. Finally, patients with CRVO usually have normal and symmetric retinal artery pressures, whereas patients with venous stasis retinopathy typically have a retinal artery pressure that is usually at least 50% less than that measured on the opposite side. According to Kearns (1983), this difference in retinal artery pressure is the most important differentiating feature between CRVO and venous stasis retinopathy.

The prognosis in patients with CRVO depends on the degree of retinal capillary perfusion; i.e., whether the condition is ischemic or nonischemic (Hayreh, 1976; Zegarra et al.,

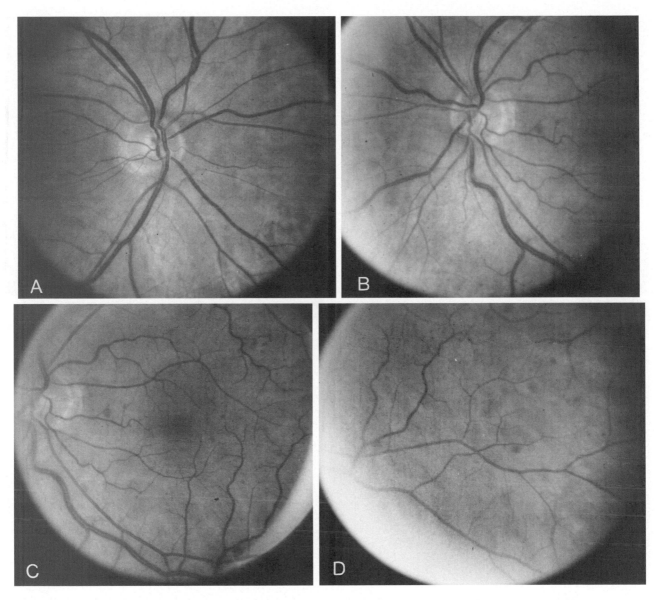

Figure 58.31. Venous stasis retinopathy. *A*, The right fundus is normal. Note normal caliber of retinal vessels and relationship of size of arteries to size of veins. *B*, The left optic disc is normal, but the retinal veins are dilated. There are a few hemorrhages in the posterior pole. *C*, The macula shows a few small hemorrhages and dilation of the capillaries. *D*, There are multiple blot hemorrhages in the midperipheral retina.

1979; Hayreh et al., 1983; Frucht et al., 1984; Hayreh et al., 1990a; Quinlan et al., 1990; Clarkson, 1994). Retinal capillary perfusion is best determined by a combination of clinical tests, fluorescein angiography, and electroretinography (Laatikainen and Kohner, 1976; Sabates et al., 1983; Hayreh, 1987; MA Johnson et al., 1988; Kaye and Harding, 1988; Hayreh et al., 1990; Clarkson, 1994). According to Hayreh et al. (1990a), the most reliable way to distinguish an ischemic CRVO from a nonischemic CRVO is to determine if a relative afferent pupillary defect is present using a swinging flashlight test and neutral density filters. A CRVO that is associated with a relative afferent pupillary defect tends to be ischemic; a CRVO that is unassociated

with a relative afferent pupillary defect is usually nonischemic. When this clinical test is combined with electroretinography, perimetry, and visual acuity testing, the differentiation between these two forms of CRVO is fairly simple. Indeed, reduced b wave/a wave ratios on an electroretinogram correlate well with capillary dropout seen on fluorescein angiography (Matsui et al., 1994).

Blood flow velocity as measured by color doppler is reduced in the retinal circulation of patients with CRVO, particularly in the ischemic type (Williamson and Baxter, 1994). Patients with the ischemic form of CRVO also have an increased risk of experiencing acute and persistent visual loss from macular edema at the time of the occlusion and of

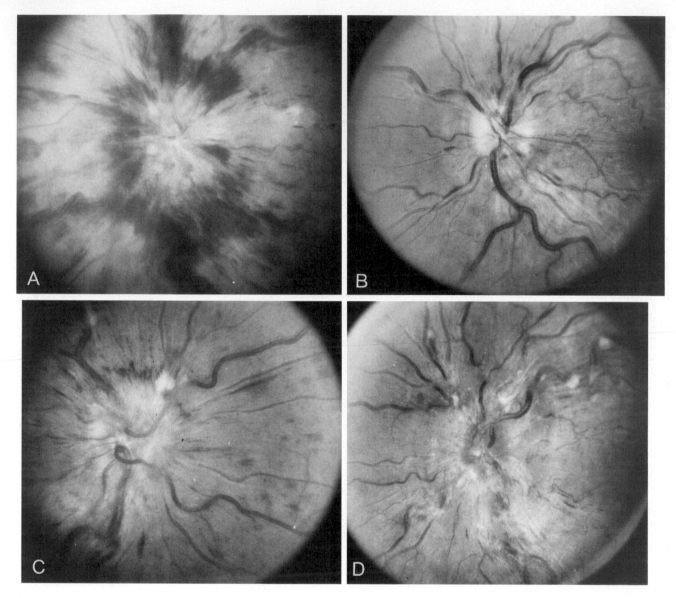

Figure 58.32. Central retinal occlusion in four patients (*A-D*). Note that in all cases, the optic disc is swollen, the retinal veins are **diffusely dilated,** and there are numerous hemorrhages in the posterior pole. Soft exudates accompanying the hemorrhages are seen. Compare this appearance to that of venous stasis retinopathy seen in Figure 58.31.

developing neovascular glaucoma within 3 months after the onset of the condition (Bresnick, 1988), whereas patients with a nonischemic CRVO rarely develop neovascular glaucoma. Primary open angle glaucoma is a significant risk factor for developing ocular neovascularization that is often refractory to laser treatment (Evans et al., 1993). Such patients may also develop a massive exudative retinal detachment in the affected eye (Weinberg et al., 1990).

As might be expected, the visual prognosis for eyes with an ischemic CRVO is substantially worse than for eyes with a nonischemic CRVO. Quinlan et al. (1990) reported that 57 of 61 eyes (93%) with an ischemic CRVO had final visual acuity less than or equal to 20/200. Older patients with poor initial visual acuity have a particularly bad prognosis (Chen et al., 1995). Eyes with nonischemic CRVO may retain good vision throughout the course of the disease (''papillophlebitis''), or they may recover vision as the process resolves (Priluck et al., 1980; Frucht et al., 1984; Ichioka et al., 1985; D'Amato et al., 1991). Quinlan et al. (1990) recorded a final visual acuity of 20/200 or less in 53 of 107 (50%) of eyes after a nonischemic CRVO.

Hikichi et al. (1995) retrospectively reviewed 136 eyes of 136 patients with unilateral CRVO to determine if the vitreous played a role in the development of neovascularization or macular edema. These investigators reported that eyes with a severe CRVO and a complete posterior vitreous detachment at the time of the vein occlusion had a significantly lower risk of developing retinal or optic disc neovascularization than eyes with no detachment or only a partial posterior detachment. Conversely, vitreomacular attachment was associated with persistent macular edema in eyes with an otherwise mild CRVO.

A CRVO that initially is nonischemic can become ischemic over time. According to Hayreh et al. (1994), the probability of progression from a nonischemic to an ischemic CRVO in persons 45–65 years old is 6.7% at 6 months and 8.1% at 18 months. For patients 65 years or older, the probability of progression is 13.2% at 6 months and 18.6% at 18 months. Thus, older patients have a substantial risk that an initially nonischemic CRVO will become ischemic over time. Such patients require extremely careful monitoring.

A small percentage of patients who experience a CRVO will develop second venous occlusive event in the same eye. Similarly, patients who experience a CRVO in one eye can develop a similar process in the fellow eye. According to Hayreh et al. (1994), the cumulative probability of developing a second episode of CRVO or a BRVO in the same eye is 2.5% within 4 years. In the fellow eye, it is 11.9% within 4 years.

There is no specific or adequate treatment for CRVO (Kohner et al., 1983; Quinlan et al., 1990). Although treatment with drugs such as pentoxifylline, which reduce blood viscosity, reduce platelet aggregation, decrease clot formation, and increase clot lysis (Schröer, 1985), might be expected to improve visual function (Appen, 1987), and although individual cases have been reported in which treatment with one drug or another seemed to be associated with improved visual acuity (Constantinides and Philibert, 1986), no randomized controlled trials have compared the efficacy of any medical therapy. Some investigators suggest that isovolemic hemodilution may improve the visual outcome in both the ischemic and nonischemic types of CRVO (Hansen et al., 1989) but, again, no randomized control studies have tested this hypothesis. Steroids have been tried, particularly in young patients where an inflammatory etiology has been invoked (Beaumont and Kwon Kang, 1994), and in one young adult with a mixed connective tissue disease and increased serum viscosity, treatment with steroids and plasmapheresis was associated with rapid resolution of the retinopathy and improvement in visual function (Dodds et al., 1995).

Some authors recommend that panretinal photocoagulation (PRP) be performed in patients with significant retinal capillary nonperfusion to prevent the development of neovascular glaucoma (Laatikainen et al., 1977; May et al., 1979; Magargal et al., 1981, 1982). Others argue that such treatment is ineffective or unnecessary (Hayreh, 1987; Trempe, 1987). To address this question in an objective fashion, Hayreh et al. (1990) published a 10-year prospective study comparing argon laser PRP to no treatment in 123 eyes with ischemic CRVO. These authors found no statistically significant difference between patients treated with PRP and patients who received no treatment in the incidence of the development of angle neovascularization, neovascular glaucoma, retinal neovascularization, optic disc neovascularization, vitreous hemorrhage, or visual acuity. Iris neovascularization was less prevalent in treated patients, but only when PRP was performed within 3 months of the onset of CRVO. As might be expected, patients treated with PRP experienced a significant deterioration in visual fields compared with untreated patients.

BRANCH RETINAL VEIN OCCLUSION (BRVO)

Occlusion of one or more of the retinal branch veins is a common cause of retinal vascular disease. This condition affects men and women equally, and usually occurs in patients from 60 to 70 years of age (Finkelstein, 1994). It is almost always a unilateral condition. Only about 10% of patients will develop a BRVO occlusion in the fellow eye, although there are no predictive features regarding such an occurrence, nor are there any known preventive measures (Finkelstein, 1994). BRVO usually occurs in patients with systemic hypertension or atherosclerotic cardiovascular disease; however, there is no firm evidence that any systemic disease plays a pathogenetic role in the condition (Orth and Patz, 1978).

The clinical manifestations of a BRVO almost always occur acutely. In most cases, a patient with previously normal vision suddenly develops blurred vision, a visual field defect, or both. Ophthalmoscopy shows segmentally distributed intraretinal hemorrhage (Fig. 58.33). With time, the hemorrhage resorbs, leaving a segmental distribution of retinal vascular abnormalities that may include capillary nonperfusion, capillary dilation, microaneurysms, and formation of collateral retinal vessels (Finkelstein, 1994).

There are three common vision-limiting complications of a BRVO: (*a*) macular edema, (*b*) macular nonperfusion, and (*c*) vitreous hemorrhage from neovascularization (Clemett et al., 1973; Gutman, 1977; Gutman and Zegarra, 1974; Hayreh et al., 1983; Gutman and Zegarra, 1984; Finkelstein, 1994). Visual acuity may also be reduced by macular hemorrhage, but in such cases, vision almost always improves as the hemorrhage resorbs.

There is no adequate medical therapy for a BRVO. Although there is an apparent association between systemic hypertension and loss of central vision from macular edema in this condition, control of hypertension does not improve visual outcome. Anticoagulant therapy has not been shown to be beneficial, and it is not recommended (Finkelstein, 1994). Similarly, treatment with fibrinolytic agents does not appear to be helpful.

Patients with BRVO who develop reduced vision from macular edema may benefit from focal laser photocoagulation. A multicenter, randomized clinical trial supported by the National Institutes of Health reported that argon laser photocoagulation is helpful in reducing visual loss from macular edema for certain patients with BRVO (Branch Vein Occlusion Study Group, 1984). A similar study demonstrated that prophylactic scatter laser photocoagulation can lessen subsequent neovascularization and, if neovascularization already exists, that peripheral laser pho-

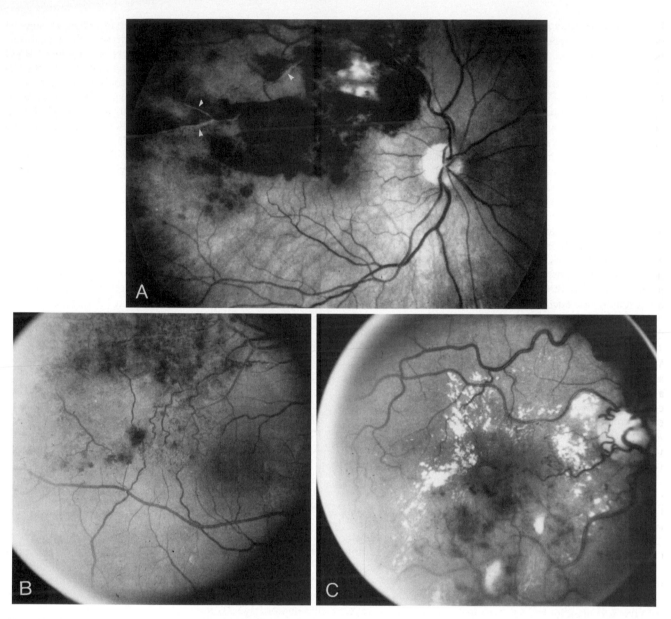

Figure 58.33.   Branch retinal vein occlusion in three patients. *A,* Acute branch retinal vein occlusion in the right eye. Note marked intraretinal hemorrhage that is primarily confined to the superotemporal quadrant of the right fundus. Several soft exudates (cotton wool spots) are evident, and the occluded branch vein can be seen peripheral to the hemorrhage *(arrowheads). B,* A few months after an acute branch vein occlusion, the right ocular fundus in a second patient shows resolving intraretinal hemorrhage with the appearance of shunt vessels across the horizontal raphe. *C,* Many months after an acute branch retinal vein occlusion in a third patient, the right ocular fundus shows extensive hard exudates, multiple intraretinal hemorrhages, and peripapillary shunt vessels. (Courtesy of Dr. Stuart Fine.)

tocoagulation can lessen the risk of subsequent vitreous hemorrhage (Branch Vein Occlusion Study Group, 1986). Focal laser photocoagulation can also be performed

on patients with BRVO and visual loss from macular edema; however, there is no evidence that this therapy is effective.

THROMBOSIS OF THE JUGULAR VEIN

Thrombosis of the jugular vein is uncommon. Nevertheless, this condition can produce significant neuro-ophthalmologic manifestations primarily because of the effects of the occlusion on intracranial pressure (Purvin et al., 1995).

CAUSES

Thrombosis of the jugular vein may result from a number of diverse clinical conditions. **Septic** thrombosis of the jugular vein is extremely rare. It is usually caused by fulminant head and neck infections, particularly deep neck abscess, peritonsillar abscess, pharyngitis, and dental manipulation (Long, 1912; Goodman, 1917; Stone and Berger, 1936; Alexander et al., 1968; Mitre and Rotherman, 1974; Yau and Norante, 1980). It also occurs in patients who inject narcotics and other drugs directly into neck veins. The pathogens generally responsible for septic thrombosis of the internal jugular vein include aerobic and anaerobic streptococci, staphylococci, pneumococci, and anaerobic gram-negative bacilli (Cohen et al., 1985).

Aseptic thrombosis of the internal jugular vein is much more common than septic thrombosis. It usually occurs as a complication of central venous catheterization (Warden et al., 1973; Mitchell and Clark, 1979; Krespi et al., 1981; McNeill, 1981; Albertyn and Alcock, 1987; Chowdhury et al., 1990). Other causes of aseptic thrombosis of the internal jugular vein are intravenous drug abuse, compression by masses at the base of the skull and in the neck, and coagulopathies associated with hematologic diseases or distant effects of cancer (Cornell, 1969; Graus and Slatkin, 1983; Cohen et al., 1985; Liu et al., 1985; Makin et al., 1986; Albertyn and Alcock, 1987; Carrington and Adams, 1988; Wen and Dolan, 1989; Chowdhury et al., 1990; Purvin et al., 1995). Patients in whom an endocardial pacemaker with a transvenous lead is implanted may develop ipsilateral or contralateral occlusion of the internal jugular vein (Girard et al., 1980; Fitzgerald and Leckie, 1985; Tovi et al., 1988). A single case of aseptic thrombosis of the internal jugular vein was described by Bessoudo et al. (1987) in a patient with congestive cardiomyopathy.

The internal jugular vein may become occluded by extension of thrombosis from the lateral or sigmoid sinus. In such cases, ligation of the vein in the neck may prevent the clot from spreading further (see Table III in Teichgraeber et al., 1982), although anticoagulation and clot lysis may be more effective and less dangerous.

The internal jugular vein may become occluded during radical neck dissection (Purvin et al., 1995). In most cases, ligation of the vein is performed as part of the procedure. In some, however, it becomes occluded during the procedure because of trauma to the vessel or because of extrinsic compression of the vein by the skin or by the myocutaneous flap (Fisher et al., 1988).

CLINICAL MANIFESTATIONS

Occlusion of the internal jugular vein may be asymptomatic, or it may produce a variety of systemic and ocular complications. Affected patients may complain of swelling or a tender lump in the neck. Severe facial edema may occur. The most serious systemic complications, however, are pulmonary embolism (Ahmed and Payne, 1976; Bradway et al., 1981; Chowdhury 1990), septic embolism, and septicemia (Cohen et al., 1985).

Acute thrombosis or ligation of the internal jugular vein usually produces neuro-ophthalmologic complications by its effect on ICP. Potts and Demarine (1973) reported a rise in pressure in the cisterna magna, subarachnoid space, and sagittal sinus during compression of the jugular vein in the dog. Stell and Maran (1978) found that ligation of one internal jugular vein produced a 300% increase in ICP, whereas ligation of both internal jugular veins produced a 500% rise in ICP in experimental animals. Similar rises in ICP occur after ligation or occlusion of the internal jugular vein in humans (McQuarrie et al., 1977). In most cases, simultaneous ligation of both jugular veins in humans produces an acute but temporary rise in ICP. The ICP usually returns to normal within 2 weeks (Sugarbaker and Wiley, 1951; Bekheit and Iskander, 1964; McGuirt and McCabe, 1980), presumably because of the relatively rapid development of adequate collateral intracranial venous circulation (Gius and Grier, 1950). Nevertheless, a prolonged increase in ICP may follow both unilateral and bilateral ligation of the internal jugular veins. In such cases, a pseudotumor cerebri syndrome may develop (Fig. 58.34). Marr and Chambers (1961) reported three patients who developed pseudotumor cerebri 3–4 weeks after unilateral radical neck dissection with ligation of the jugular vein. All three patients had bilateral, severe papilledema. Two of the three patients also had diplopia. One of these patients had an abducens nerve paresis; the other had trochlear nerve paresis. In both patients, the paresis was on the side of the ligated vein. Cases similar to those reported by Marr and Chambers (1961) occur after both unilateral and bilateral radical neck dissection (Mofit and Cleveland, 1958; Blervacque et al., 1965; Fitz-Hugh et al., 1966; Walsh and Hoyt, 1969b; Tobin, 1972; de Vries et al., 1986; Purvin et al., 1995).

Pseudotumor cerebri is not the only neuro-ophthalmologic complication of jugular vein occlusion. Anlyan et al. (1951) reported a fatal parieto-occipital venous infarction after a left-sided radical neck dissection. The patient had an anomalous aplastic lateral sinus on the right side, causing the brain to depend entirely on the left lateral sinus and left internal jugular vein for cerebral venous drainage. When the left internal jugular vein was ligated as part of the surgery, cerebral venous drainage was severely reduced, leading to the cerebral venous infarction.

A case of venous stasis retinopathy was reported by Gutteridge et al. (1987) in a patient without significant ipsilateral carotid artery disease but with occlusion of the ipsilateral internal jugular vein between the occipital tributary and the common facial tributary. The condition gradually resolved over several months. It is unclear if these two conditions were fortuitous or if an increase in venous back pressure from the occluded internal jugular vein somehow limited the ocular blood flow in much the same way as a carotid-cavernous sinus fistula.

Acute blindness may occur after bilateral radical neck dissection and ligation of the internal jugular veins (Milner, 1960; Torti et al., 1964; Rufino and MacComb, 1966; Chutkow et al., 1973). In nearly all cases, the blindness is not caused by increased ICP or by the direct effects of ligation of the internal jugular vein, but by the effects of concomitant arterial occlusive disease, intraoperative or postoperative systemic hypotension with and without hemorrhage, or both. Such patients thus lose vision not from postpapilledema

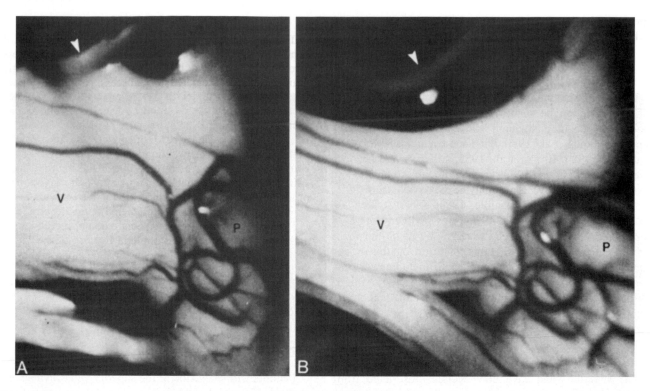

Figure 58.35. Trigeminal neuralgia apparently caused by compression of the trigeminal nerve by a pontine vein. The patient was a 63-year-old woman with typical trigeminal neuralgia affecting the right side of the face. The patient underwent craniotomy with exploration of the right trigeminal nerve. *A,* View of the right trigeminal nerve (*V*) as it enters the pons (*P*). The nerve is flat, pale, and compressed by a crossing vein (*arrowhead*). *B,* After dissection of the vein away from the nerve, the nerve has become normal in both color and thickness. The vein (*arrowhead*) was coagulated and divided, and the nerve was wrapped with a small piece of Surgicel. The patient had complete resolution of pain after surgery. (From Sato O, I. Kanazawa I, Kokunai T. Trigeminal neuralgia caused by compression of trigeminal nerve by pontine vein. Surg Neurol *11*:285–286, 1979.)

Lawton Smith who developed a right abducens nerve paresis and bilateral papilledema 5 days after a transurethral prostatectomy for benign prostatic hypertrophy. Retrograde venous embolism from the prostate, passing via the vertebral plexus to the petrosal and lateral sinuses, was considered a possible mechanism in this case.

CRANIAL NEUROPATHIES CAUSED BY VENOUS COMPRESSION

A number of conditions characterized by hyperactivity of one or more cranial nerves, e.g., trigeminal neuralgia and hemifacial spasm, appear to be caused by compression of the nerve root adjacent to the brain stem by a vascular structure. Although such structures are usually arteries, in some cases the nerve is found to be compressed by a vein rather than an artery (Dandy, 1934; Jannetta, 1976, 1977; Sato et al., 1979; Kollros et al., 1990; Barker et al., 1995) (Fig. 58.35). Displacement of the vein away from the nerve is usually associated with return of normal cranial nerve function in these cases.

REFERENCES

Abassioun K, Amirjamshidi A, Rahmat H. Bilateral mycotic aneurysm of the intracavernous carotid artery. Neurosurgery *16*:235–237, 1985.

Abel H. Thrombolyisis: The Logical Approach for the Treatment of Vascular Occlusions. Acta Cardiol *47*:287–295, 1992.

Ahmadi J, Keane JR, Segall HD, et al. CT observations pertinent to septic cavernous sinus thrombosis. Am J Neuroradiol *6*:755–758, 1985.

Ahmed N, Payne R. Thrombosis after central venous cannulation. Med J Aust *1*: 217–220, 1976.

Albert D, Williams S. Clinical and anatomical considerations of the Tobey-Ayer test in lateral sinus thrombosis. J Laryngol Otol *100*:1311–1313, 1986.

Albertyn LE, Alcock MK. Diagnosis of internal jugular vein thrombosis. Radiology *162*:505–508, 1987.

Alexander DW, Leonard JR, Trail ML. Vascular complications of deep neck abscesses. Laryngoscope *78*:361–370, 1968.

Alfano JE, Alfano PA. Vena caval obstruction syndrome. Am J Ophthalmol *42*: 685–696, 1956.

Allinson RW, Limstrom SA, Sethi GK, et al. Central retinal vein occlusion after heart-lung transplantation. Ann Ophthalmol *25*:58–63, 1993.

Al-Mefty O. Comments. Neurosurgery *37*:1018, 1995.

Al-Mefty O, Jinkins JR, Fox JL. Extensive dural arteriovenous malformation—Case report. J Neurosurg *65*:417–420, 1986.

Ambruso DR, Jacobson LJ, Hathway WE. Inherited antithrombin III deficiency and cerebral thrombosis in a child. Pediatrics *65*:125–131, 1980.

Ameri A, Bousser M-G. Cerebral venous thrombosis. Neurol Clin *10*:87–111, 1992.

Amias AG. Cerebral vascular disease in pregnancy. 2. Occlusion. J Obstet Gynecol Br Commonw *77*:312–325, 1970.

Anlyan AJ, Browning HC, Black SPW, et al. Dural sinus studies in relation to radical operations on the neck. Surg Forum *2*:300–305, 1951.

Aoki N, Moroi M, Sakata Y, et al. Abnormal plasminogen: A hereditary molecular abnormality found in a patient with recurrent thrombosis. J Clin Invest *61*: 1186–1195, 1978.

Appen RE, De Venecia G, Ferwerda J. Optic disk vasculitis. Am J Ophthalmol *90*: 352–359, 1980.

Appen RE. Pentoxifylline in ischemic eye disease. JAMA *257*:1961, 1987.

Apuzzo MLJ. Comments on Garrido E, Fahs GR. Cerebral venous and sagittal sinus thrombosis after transcallosal removal of a colloid cyst of the third ventricle: Case report. Neurosurgery 26:542, 1990.

Asherson RA, Baguley E, Pal C, et al. Antipholpholipid Syndrome: Five year follow-up. Ann Rheum Dis 50:805–810, 1991.

Askenasy HM, Kosary IZ, Braham J. Thrombosis of the longitudinal sinus. Neurology 12:288–292, 1962.

Astedt B. New aspects of thrombogenic effects of oral contraceptives. Am Heart J 90:1, 1975.

Atkinson EA, Fairburn B, Heathfield KWG. Intracranial venous thrombosis as complication of oral contraception. Lancet 1:914–918, 1970.

Augustin P, Daluzeau N, Dujardin M, et al. Fistule artério-veineuse duremérienne et occlusion du sinus latéral. Rev Neurol 140:594–596, 1984.

Averback P. Primary cerebral venous thrombosis in young adults: The diverse manifestations of an under-recognized disease. Ann Neurol 3:81–86, 1978.

Azzarelli B, Itani AL, Catanzaro PT. Cerebral phlebothrombosis. A complication of lymphoma. Arch Neurol 37:126–127, 1980.

Bacharach JM, Stanson AW, Lie JT, et al. Imaging spectrum of Thrombo-occlusive Vascular Disease Associated with Antiphospholipid Antibodies. RadioGraphics 13:417–423, 1993.

Bagley C. Traumatic longitudinal sinus lesions: Report of two cases. Surg Gynecol Obstet 58:498–502, 1934.

Bandello F, Vigano D'Angelo S, Parlavecchia M, et al. Hypercoagulability and high lipoprotein(a) levels in patients with central retinal vein occlusion. Thromb Haemost 72:39–43, 1994.

Bank I, Weart C. Dural sinus thrombosis in Behçet's disease. Arthritis Rheum 27:816–818, 1984.

Bansal BC, Prakash C, Gupta RR, et al. Study of serum lipid and blood fibrinolytic activity in cases of cerebral venous thrombosis during the puerperium. Am J Obstet Gynecol 119:1079–1082, 1974.

Barke RM, Yoshizumi MO, Hepler RS, et al. Spontaneous dural carotid cavernous fisutla with central retinal vein occlusion and iris neovascularization. Ann Ophthalmol 23:11–17, 1991.

Barker FG 2nd, Jannetta PJ, Bissonette DJ, et al. Microvascular decompression for hemifacial spasm. J Neurosurg 82:201–210, 1995.

Barnett HJM, Hyland HH. Non-infective intracranial venous thrombosis. Brain 76:36–49, 1953.

Barnwell SL, Halbach VV, Dowd CF, et al. Endovascular thrombolytic therapy for dural sinus thrombosis. J Neurosurg 72:336A–337A, 1990.

Barron TF, Gusnard DA, Zimmerman RA, et al. Dural venous thrombosis in neonates and children. Ann Neurol 28:445, 1990.

Batson OV. Function of vertebral veins and their role in spread of metastases. Ann Surg 112:138–149, 1940.

Batson OV. The vertebral vein system. Am J Radiol 78:195–211, 1957.

Beal MF, Chapman PH. Cortical blindness and homonymous hemianopia in the postpartum period. JAMA 244:2085–2087, 1980.

Beaumont PE, Kang HK. Ophthalmodynamometry and corticosteroids in central retinal vein occlusion. Aust NZ J Ophthalmol 22:271–274, 1994.

Bederson JB, Eisenberg MB. Resection and replacement of the superior sagittal sinus for treatment of a parasagittal meningioma: Technical case report. Neurosurgery 37:1015–1019, 1995.

Bekheit F, Iskander F. Bilateral radical neck dissection. J Egypt Med Assoc 47:573–581, 1964.

Bell RW. Orbital cellulitis and cavernous sinus thrombosis caused by rhabdomyosarcoma of the middle ear. Ann Ophthalmol 4:1090–1092, 1972.

Belman AL, Roque CT, Ancona R, et al. Cerebral venous thrombosis in a child with iron deficiency anemia and thrombocytosis. Stroke 21:488–493, 1990.

Bergman PS. Cerebral blindness. An analysis of 12 cases with especial reference to electroencephalogram and patterns of recovery. Arch Neurol Psychiatr 78:568–584, 1957.

Berler DK. Combined central retinal vein occlusion and cilioretinal artery occlusion associated with prolonged retinal arterial filling. Am J Ophth 118:265, 1994.

Bessoudo R, Stephen DL, Covert WN. Jugular vein thrombosis in a patient with congestive cardiomyopathy: Use of computed tomography for initial diagnosis. Can Med Assoc J 136:1275–1276, 1987.

Björnebrink J, Liliequist B. Traumatic lateral sinus thrombosis. Report of two cases. Angiology 27:688–697, 1976.

Blervacque A, Beal F, Malbrel P. Oedeme papilliaire après intervention au niveau du niveau. Bull Soc Ophtalmol Fr 65:135–136, 1965.

Boey ML, Colaco CB, Gharavi AE, et al. Thrombosis in systemic lupus erythematosus: Striking association with the presence of circulating lupus anticoagulant. Br Med J 287:1021–1023, 1983.

Boniuk M. The ocular manifestations of ophthalmic vein and aseptic cavernous sinus thrombosis. Trans Am Acad Ophthalmol Otolaryngol 76:1519–1534, 1972.

Bonnal J, Brotchi J. Surgery of the posterior sagittal sinus in parasagittal meningiomas. J Neurosurg 48:935–945, 1978.

Bots GTAM. Thrombosis of the galenic system veins in the adult. Acta Neuropathol 17:227–233, 1971.

Bouchez B, Arnott G, Caron JC, et al. Cerebral venous thrombosis with involvement of the cavernous sinus: Initial manifestation of Behçet's disease? Rev Otoneuroophtalmol 56:447–453, 1984.

Boushey CJ, Beresford SAA, Omenn GS, et al. Plasma homocysteine as a risk factor for vascular disease. JAMA 274:1049–1057, 1995.

Bousser M-G. Cerebral vein thrombosis in Behçet's syndrome. Arch Neurol 39:322, 1982.

Bousser M-G. Place de l'imagérie par resonance magnetique dans les thromboses veineuses cérébrales. J Mal Vasc 20:189–193, 1995.

Bousser M-G, Ross Russell. Cerebral Venous Thrombosis. London, WB Saunders, 1997.

Bousser M-G, Chiras J, Bories J, et al. Cerebral venous thrombosis—A review of 38 cases. Stroke 16:199–213, 1985.

Bowen BC, Quencer RM, Margosian P, et al. MR angiography of Occlusive Disease of the Arteries in the Head and Neck: Current Concepts. AJR 162:9–18, 1994.

Bradway W, Biondi RJ, Kaufman JL, et al. Internal jugular thrombosis and pulmonary embolism. Chest 80:335–336, 1981.

Branch Vein Occlusion Study Group: Argon laser photocoagulation for macular edema in branch vein occlusion. Am J Ophthalmol 98:271–282, 1984.

Branch Vein Occlusion Study Group: Argon laser photocoagulation for prevention of neovascularization and vitreous hemorrhage in branch vein occlusion. Arch Ophthalmol 104:34–41, 1986.

Brant-Zawadzki M, Chang ZY, McCarty GE. Computed tomography in dural sinus thrombosis. Arch Neurol 39:446–447, 1982.

Braun IF, Hoffman JC Jr, Malko JA, et al. Jugular venous thrombosis: MR imaging. Radiology 157:357–360, 1985.

Bresnick GH. Following up patients with central retinal vein occlusion. Arch Ophthalmol 106:324–326, 1988.

Brey RL, Coull BM. Cerebral venous thrombosis: Role of activated protein C resistance and Factor V gene mutation. Stroke 27:1719–1720, 1996.

Brown GC, Shah HG, Magargal LE, et al. Central retinal vein obstruction and carotid artery disease. Ophthalmology 91:1627–1633, 1984.

Buchanan DS, Brazinsky JH. Dural sinus and cerebral venous thrombosis: Incidence in young women receiving oral contraceptives. Arch Neurol 22:440–444, 1970.

Buonanno FS, Moody DM, Ball MR, et al. Computed cranial tomographic findings in cerebral sinovenous occlusion. J Comput Assist Tomogr 2:281–290, 1978.

Buonanno FS, Moody DM, Ball MR, et al. Radionuclide sinography: Diagnosis of lateral sinus thrombosis by dynamic and static brain imaging. Radiology 130:207–213, 1979.

Byers RK, Hass GM. Thrombosis of the dural venous sinuses in infancy and in childhood. Am J Dis Child 45:1161–1183, 1933.

Byrne JV, Lawton CA. Meningeal sarcoidosis causing intracranial hypertension secondary to dural sinus thrombosis. Br J Radiol 56:755–757, 1983.

Calvert SM, Rand RJ. A successful pregnancy in a patient with homocystinuria and a previous near fatal postpartum cavernous sinus thrombosis. Br J Obstet Gynecol 102:751–752, 1995.

Cantú C, Barinagarrementeria F. Cerebral venous thrombosis associated with pregnancy and the puerperium: Review of 67 cases. Stroke 24:1880–1884, 1993.

Carrie AW, Jaffe FA. Thrombosis of superior sagittal sinus caused by trauma without penetrating injury. J Neurosurg 11:173–182, 1954.

Carrington BM, Adams JE. Jugular vein thrombosis associated with distant malignancy. Postgrad Med J 64:455–458, 1988.

Carroll JD, Leak D, Lee HA. Cerebral thrombophlebitis in pregnancy and the puerperium. QJ Med 35:347–368, 1966.

Casaubon JN, Dion MA, Larbrissea UA. Septic cavernous sinus thrombosis after rhinoplasty. Plast Reconstr Surg 59:119–123, 1977.

Cassady JV. Central retinal vein thrombosis. Am J Ophthalmol 36:331–335, 1953.

Castaigne P, Laplane D, Bousser M-G Superior sagittal sinus thrombosis. Arch Neurol 34:788–789, 1977.

Castleman B, Kibbee BU. Case records of the Massachusetts General Hospital. Case 46471. N Engl J Med 263:1080–1084, 1960.

Cavenagh JB. Cavernous sinus thrombosis. Br Med J 1:1195–1199, 1936.

Charteris DG, Khanna V, Dhillon B. Acute posterior multifocal placoid pigment epitheliopathy complicated by central retinal vein occlusion. Br J Ophthalmol 73:765–768, 1989.

Chen JC, Klein ML, Watzke RC, et al. Natural course of perfused central retinal vein occlusion. Can J Ophthalmol 30:21–24, 1995.

Chern S, Magargal LE, Brav SS. Bilateral central retinal vein occlusion as an initial manifestation of pseudotumor cerebri. Ann Ophthalmol 23:45–57, 1991.

Childs HG, Courville CB. Thrombosis of cavernous sinus secondary to dental infections. Am J Orthod 28:367, 1942.

Chow AW, Rosen SM, Brady FA. Orofacial odontogenic infections. Ann Intern Med 88:392–402, 1978.

Chowdhury K, Bloom J, Black MH, et al. Spontaneous and nonspontanous internal jugular vein thrombosis. Head Neck Surg 12:168–173, 1990.

Christensen E, Gormsen J, Rosenklint A. Thrombosis in the superior sagittal sinus during pregnancy. Ugeskr Laeger 131:869–873, 1969.

Chung JW, Chang KH, Han MH, et al. Computed tomography of cavernous sinus disease. Neuroradiology 30:319–328, 1988.

Chutkow JG, Sharbrough FW, Riley FC Jr. Blindness following simultaneous bilateral neck dissection. Mayo Clin Proc 48:713–717, 1973.

Clarkson JG. Central retinal vein occlusion. In Retina. Editors, Schachat AP, Murphy RB, 2nd ed, Vol 2, pp 1379–1386. St Louis, CV Mosby, 1994.

Clemett RS, Kohner EM, Hamilton AM. The visual prognosis in retinal branch vein occlusion. Trans Ophthalmol Soc UK 93:523–535, 1973.

Clifford-Jones RE, Ellis CJK, Stevens JM, et al. Cavernous sinus thrombosis. J Neurol Neurosurg Psychiatr 45:1092–1097, 1982.

Clune JP. Septic thrombosis within the cavernous chamber. Am J Ophthalmol 56:33–39, 1963.

Cochran FB, Packman S. Homocystinuria presenting as sagittal sinus thrombosis. Eur Neurol 32:1–3, 1992.

Cohen JP, Persky MS, Reede DL. Internal jugular vein thrombosis. Laryngoscope 95:1478–1482, 1985.

Collaborative Group for the Study of Stroke in Young Women. Oral contraception and increased risk of cerebral ischemia or thrombosis. N Engl J Med 288:871, 1973.

Comerota AJ, Harwick RD, White JV. Jugular venous reconstruction: A technique to minimize morbidity of bilateral radical neck dissection. J Vasc Surg 3:322–329, 1986.

Confavreux C, Brunet P, Petiot P, et al. Congenital protein C deficiency and superior sagittal sinus thrombosis causing isolated intracranial hypertension. J Neurol Neurosurg Psychiatry 57:655–657, 1994.

Constantinides G, Philibert P. Le traitement des occlusions veineuses retiennes par un anti-agregant plaquettaire: Le sulfinpyrazone (Anturan 200). Bull Soc Ophtalmol Fr 86:913–915, 1986.

Convers P, Michel D, Brunon J, et al. Fistules artérioveineuses durales de la fosse cérébrale postérieure et thrombose du sinus latéral. Discussion de leurs relations et de leur traitement à propos de deux cas. Neurochirurgie 32:495–500, 1986.

Cornell SH. Jugular venography. AJR 106:303–307, 1969.

Cros D, Comp PC, Beltran G, et al. Superior sagittal sinus thrombosis in a patient with protein S deficiency. Stroke 21:633–636, 1990.

Cross JN, Castro PO, Jennett WB. Cerebral strokes associated with pregnancy and the puerperium. Br Med J 3:214, 1968.

Curnes JT, Creasy JL, Whaley RL, et al. Air in the cavernous sinus: A new sign of septic cavernous sinus thrombosis. Am J Neuroradiol 8:176–177, 1987.

Dahlback B. New molecular insights into the genetics of thrombophilia. Thromb Haem 74:139–148, 1995.

Dahlback B, Carlsson M, Svensson PJ. Familial thrombophilia due to a previously unrecognized mechanism characterized by poor anticoagulant response to activated protein C: Prediction of a cofactor to activated protein C. PNAS 90:1004–1008, 1993.

Dalal FY, Schmidt GB, Bennett EJ, et al. Sickle cell trait: A report of a postoperative complication. Br J Anaesthesiol 46:387–388, 1974.

D'Amato RJ, Miller NR, Fine SL, et al. The effect of age and initial visual acuity on the systemic and visual prognosis of central retinal vein occlusion. Aust NZ J Ophthalmol 19:119–122, 1991.

Dandy WE. Concerning the cause of trigeminal neuralgia. Am J Surg 24:447–455, 1934.

D'Avella D, Russo A, Santoro G, et al. Diagnosis of superior sagittal sinus thrombosis by computerized tomography. Report of two cases. J Neurosurg 61:1129–1131, 1984.

David RB, Hadfield MG, Vines FS, et al. Dural sinus occlusion in leukemia. Pediatrics 56:793–796, 1975.

Davidoff LM, Dyke CG. Hypertensive meningeal hydrops: A syndrome frequently following infection in the middle ear or elsewhere in the body. Am J Ophthalmol 20:908–927. 1937.

Daxecker F, Bichler E. Beidseitiger exophthalmus bei Sinus-cavernosus-Thrombose. Klin Monatsbl Augenheilkd 182:235–236, 1983.

Debruyne F. Lateral sinus thrombosis in the eighties. J Laryngol Otol 99:91–93, 1985.

Delle Grottaglie B, Boeri R, Passerini A, et al. Thrombosis of the superior ophthalmic vein: A case report. Neuro-ophthalmology 1:287–290, 1981.

Deschiens M-A, Conard J, Horellou MH, et al. Coagulation studies, Factor V Leiden, and anticardiolipin antibodies in 40 cases of cerebral venous thrombosis. Stroke 27:1724–1730, 1996.

de Vries WAEJ, Balm AJM, Tiwari RM. Intracranial hypertension following neck dissection. J Laryngol Otol 100:1427–1431, 1986.

Dhote R, Bachmeyer C, Horellou MH, et al. Central retinal vein thrombosis associated with resistance to activated protein C. Am J Ophthalmol 120:388–389, 1995.

Dill JL, Crowe SJ. Thrombosis of the sigmoid or lateral sinus. Reports of thirty cases. Arch Surg 29:705–722, 1934.

Dindar F, Platts ME. Intracranial venous thrombosis complicating oral contraception. Canad Med Assoc J 111:545–548, 1974.

DiNubile MJ. Septic thrombosis of the cavernous sinus. Arch Neurol 45:567–572, 1988.

DiRocco C, Iannelli A, Leone G, et al. Heparinurokinase treatment in aseptic dural sinus thrombosis. Arch Neurol 38:431–435, 1981.

Dixon OJ. The pathologic examination in cavernous sinus thrombosis. JAMA 87:1088–1092, 1926.

Dodds EM, Lowder CY, Foster RE. Plasmapheresis treatment of central retinal vein occlusion in a young adult. Am J Ophthalmol, 119:519–521, 1995.

D'Olhaberriague L, Mitsias P, Levine SR. Superior sagittal sinus thrombosis and acquired free protein S deficiency in the elderly. Stroke 27:338–340, 1996.

Dowman CE. Thrombosis of the Rolandic vein. Arch Neurol Psychiatr 15:110–112, 1926.

Drachman DA. Neurological complications of Wegener's granulomatosis. Arch Neurol 8:145–155, 1963.

Duckwiller GR, Dion JE, Vinuela F, et al. Delayed venous occlusion following embolotherapy of vascular malformations in the brain. AJNR 13:1571–1579, 1992.

Duker JS, Cohen MS, Brown GC, et al. Combined branch retinal artery and central retinal vein obstruction. Retina 10:105–112, 1990.

Duker JS, Sergott RC, Savino PJ, et al. Optic neuritis with secondary reintal venous stasis. Ophthalmol 96:475–480, 1989.

Dulli DA, Luzzio CC, Williams EC, et al. Cerebral venous thrombosis and activated protein C resistance. Stroke 27:1731–1733, 1996.

Dumoulin CL. Rapid scan magnetic resonance angiography. Magn Reson Med 5:238–245, 1987.

Dunsker SB, Torres-Reyes E, Peden JC Jr. Pseudotumor cerebri associated with idiopathic cryofibrinogenemia: Report of a case. Arch Neurol 23:120–127, 1970.

Eagleton WP. Cavernous Sinus Thrombophlebitis and Allied Septic and Traumatic Lesions of the Basal Venous Sinuses. A Clinical Study of Blood Stream Infection. New York, Macmillan Publishing Co, 1926.

Eckerling B, Goldman JA, Gans B. Intracranial sinus thrombosis: A rare complication of pregnancy (3 cases). Obstet Gynecol 21:368–371, 1963.

Editorial: Lateral sinus thrombosis. Lancet 2:806, 1982.

Eggenberger ER, Miller NR, Vitale S. Lumbo-peritoneal shunt for pseudotumor cerebri. Neurology 46:1524–1530, 1996.

Eguchi T, Nagagomi T, Teraoka A. Treatment of bilateral mycotic intracavernous carotid aneurysms. Case report. J Neurosurg 56:443–447, 1982.

Ehlers H, Courville CB. Thrombosis of the internal cerebral veins in infancy and childhood: Review of literature and report of five cases. J Pediatr 8:600–623, 1936.

Eick JJ, Miller KD, Bell KA. Computed tomography of deep cerebral venous thrombosis in children. Radiology 140:399–402, 1981.

Einhäupl KM. Zerebrale Sinus und Venenthrombosen. Ther Umsch 53:552–558, 1996.

Einhäupl KM, Villringer A, Meister W, et al. Heparin treatment in sinus venous thrombosis. Lancet 338:597–600, 1991.

El Alaoui Faris M, Birouk N, Slassi I, et al. Thrombose du sinus longitudinal supérieur et ostéite crânienne syphilitique. Rev Neurol 148:783–785, 1992.

El Koussa S, Chemaly R, Fabre-Bou Abboud V, et al. Trichinose et occlusions sinoveineuses cérébrales. Rev Neurol 150:464–466, 1994.

Ellenberger C Jr, Messner KH. Papillophlebitis: Benign retinopathy resembling papilledema or papillitis. Ann Neurol 3:438–440, 1978.

Elman MJ, Bhatt AK, Quinlan PM, et al. The risk for systemic vascular diseases and morality in patients with central retinal vein occlusion. Ophthalmology 97:1543–1548, 1990.

El-Ramahi KM, Al-Kawi MZ. Papilloedema in Behcet's disease: Value of MRI in diagnosis of dural sinus thrombosis. J Neurol Neurosurg Psychiatry 54:826–829, 1991.

Enevoldson TP, Ross Russell RW. Heparin treatment in venous sinus thrombosis. Lancet 338:1153–1154, 1991.

Endo S, Ohtsuji T, Fukuda O, et al. A case of septic cavernous sinu thrombosis with sequential dynamic angiographic changes. A case report. Surg Neurol 32:59–63, 1989.

Estanol B, Rodriguez A, Conte G, et al. Intracranial venous thrombosis in young women. Stroke 10:680–684, 1979.

Evans EW. Cavernous sinus thrombosis. Lancet 85:109–113, 1965.

Evans RW, Patten BM. Trichinosis associated with superior sagittal sinus thrombosis. Ann Neurol 11:216–217, 1982.

Evans K, Wishart PK, McGalliard JN. Neovascular complications after central retinal vein occlusion. Eye 7:520–524, 1993.

Fahey JL, Leonard E, Churg J, et al. Wegener's granulomatosis. Am J Med 17:168–179, 1954.

Fairburn B. Intracranial venous sinus thrombosis complicating oral contraception: Treatment by anticoagulant drugs. Br Med J 2:647, 1973.

Falk RL, Smith DF. Thrombosis of upper extremity thoracic inlet veins: Diagnosis with duplex doppler sonography. AJR 49:677–682, 1987.

Feldenzer JA, Bueche MJ, Venes JL, et al. Superior sagittal sinus thrombosis with infarction in sickle cell trait. Stroke 18:656–660, 1987.

Fiandaca MS, Spector RH, Hartmann TM, et al. Unilateral septic cavernous sinus thrombosis: A case report with digital orbital venographic documentation. J Clin Neuroophthalmol 6:35–38, 1986.

Finkelstein D. Retinal branch vein occlusion. In Retina. Editors, Schachat AP, Murphy RB, 2nd ed, Vol 2, pp 1387–1392. St Louis, CV Mosby, 1989.

Fisher CB, Mattox DE, Zinreich JS. Patency of the internal jugular vein after functional neck dissection. Laryngoscope 98:923–927, 1988.

Fishman EK, Pakter RI, Gayler BW, et al. Jugular venous thrombosis: Diagnosis by computed tomography. J Comput Assist Tomogr 8:963–968, 1984.

Fishman RA, Cowen D, Silbermann M. Intracranial venous thrombosis during the first trimester of pregnancy. Neurology 7:217–220, 1957.

Fitzgerald SP, Leckie WJH. Thrombosis complicating transvenous pacemaker lead presenting as contralateral internal jugular vein occlusion. Am Heart J 109:593–595, 1985.

Fitz-Hugh GS, Robins RB, Craddock WD. Increased intracranial pressure complicating unilateral neck dissection. Laryngoscope 76:893–906, 1966.

Flynn WJ, Green RP, LoRusso FJ. Retinal vein occlusions: Case reviews of USAF Aviators. Aviat Space Environ Med 65:332–337, 1994.

Fong AC, Schatz H. Central retinal vein occlusion in young adults. Surv Ophthalmol 37:393–417, 1993.

Fong AC, Schatz H, McDonald HR, et al. Central retinal vein occlusion in young adults (papillophlebitis). Retina 12:3–11, 1992.

Ford FR. Diseases of the Nervous System in Infancy, Childhood and Adolescence. 5th edition, p 819. Springfield, IL, Charles C Thomas Publisher, 1966.

Ford K, Sarwar M. Computed tomography of dural sinus thrombosis. AJNR 2: 539–543, 1981.

Fox SL, West GB. Thrombosis of the cavernous sinus. JAMA 134:1452–1456, 1947.

Frerichs KU, Deckert M, Kempski O, et al. Cerebral sinus and venous thrombosis in rats induces long-term deficits in brain function and morphology—Evidence for a cytotoxic genesis. J Cereb Blood Flow Metab 14:289–300, 1994.

Friberg TR, Sogg RL. Ischemic optic neuropathy in cavernous sinus thrombosis. Arch Ophthalmol 96:453–456, 1978.

Friedman SM, Margo CE. Bilateral central retinal vein occlusions in a patient with acquired immunodeficiency syndrome: Clinicopathologic correlation. Arch Ophthalmol 113:1184–1188, 1995.

Frohman LP, Rescigno R, Bielory L. Neuro-ophthalmologic manifestations of the antiphospholipid antibody syndromes. Ophthalmology 96(Suppl):105, 1989.

Frucht J, Yanko L, Merin S. Central retinal vein occlusions in young adults. Acta Ophthalmol 62:780–786, 1984.

Fujikado T, Imagawa K. Dural sinus thrombosis in Behçet's disease: A case report. Jpn J Ophthalmol 38:411–416, 1994.

Fujino T, Curtin VT, Norton EWD. Experimental central retinal vein occlusion: A comparison of intraocular and extraocular occlusion. Arch Ophthalmol 81: 395–406, 1969.

Furuta M, Satoh S, Toriumi T, et al. An autopsy case of cerebral sinus thrombosis which showed papilledema and was accompanied by idiopathic thrombocytopenic purpura. Acta Soc Ophthalmol Jpn 95:199–203, 1991.

Gabrielsen TO, Seeger JF, Knake JE, et al. Radiology of cerebral vein occlusion without dural sinus occlusion. Radiology 140:403–408, 1981.

Garcia JH, Williams JP, Tanaka J. Spontaneous thrombosis of deep cerebral veins: A complication of arteriovenous malformation. Stroke 6:164–171, 1975.

Garcia RDJ, Baker AS, Cunningham MJ, et al. Lateral sinus thrombosis associated with otitis media and mastoiditis in children. Pediatr Infect Dis J 14:617–623, 1995.

Garciá-Moncó JC, Beldarrain MG. Superior sagittal sinus thrombosis complicating Crohn's disease. Neurology 41:1324–1325, 1991.

Garcin R, Pestel M. Thrombophlebites Cérébrales. Paris, Masson, 1953.

Gardner WJ. Otitic sinus thrombosis causing intracranial hypertension. Arch Otolaryngol 30:253–268, 1939.

Garrido E, Fahs GR. Cerebral venous and sagittal sinus thrombosis after transcallosal removal of a colloid cyst of the third ventricle: Case report. Neurosurgery 26: 540–542, 1990.

Gastineau DA, Kazmier FJ, Nichols WL, et al. Lupus anticoagulant: An analysis of the clinical and laboratory features of 219 cases. Am J Hematol 19:265–275, 1985.

Gates PC, Barnett HJM. Venous disease: Cortical veins and sinuses. In Stroke: Pathophysiology, Diagnosis, and Management. Editors, Barnett HJM, Stein BM, Mohr JP, et al. Vol 2, pp 731–743. New York, Churchill Livingstone, 1987.

Geggel HS, Isenberg SJ. Cavernous sinus thrombosis as a cause of unilateral blindness. Ann Ophthalmol 14:569–574, 1982.

Gettelfinger DM, Kokmen E. Superior sagittal sinus thrombosis. Arch Neurol 34: 2–6, 1977.

Gialldrenzi AF, Weiss WW, Furman DJ. Septic cavernous sinus thrombosis in a diabetic after dental extraction. J Oral Maxillofac Surg 32:924–930, 1974.

Ginsburg KS, Liang MH, Newcomer L, et al. Anticardiolipin antibodies and the risk for ischemic stroke and venous thrombosis. Ann Intern Med 117:997–1002, 1992.

Girard DE, Reuler JB, Mayer BS, et al. Cerebral venous sinus thrombosis due to indwelling transvenous pacemaker catheter. Arch Neurol 37:113–114, 1980.

Girolami A, Pardatscher K, Scanarini M, et al. Clotting changes in two patients with longitudinal sinus thrombosis. Haemostasis 9:71–78, 1980.

Gius JA, Grier DH. Venous adaptation following bilateral radical neck dissection with excision of the jugular veins. Surgery 28:305–321, 1950.

Goldberg AL, Rosenbaum AE, Wang H, et al. Computed tomography of dural sinus thrombosis. J Comput Assist Tomogr 10:16–20, 1986.

Goldenberg RA. Lateral sinus thrombosis: Medical or surgical treatment? Arch Otolaryngol 111:56–58, 1985.

Gomori JM, Grossman RI, Goldberg HI, et al. Intracranial hematomas: Imaging by high-field MR. Radiology 157:87–93, 1985.

Goodman C. Primary jugular thrombosis due to tonsil infection. Ann Otol Rhinol Laryngol 26:527–529, 1917.

Gowers WR. On thrombosis in the cerebral sinuses and veins. In A Manual of Diseases of the Nervous System. 1st ed, Vol 2, p 416. London, Churchill, 1888.

Gradenigo G. A special syndrome of endocranial otitic complications (paralysis of the motor oculi externus of otitic origin). Ann Otol Rhinol Laryngol 13:637, 1904.

Graus G, Slatkin NE. Papilledema in the metastastic jugular foramen syndrome. Arch Neurol 40:816–818, 1983.

Green WR. Retina. In Ophthalmic Pathology. An Atlas and Textbook. Editor, Spencer WH, 3rd ed, Vol 2, pp 691–707. Philadelphia, WB Saunders, 1985.

Green WR, Chan CC, Hutchins GM, et al. Central retinal vein occlusion: A prospective histopathologic study of 29 eyes in 28 cases. Retina 1:27–55, 1981.

Greer M. Benign intracrial hypertension. I. Mastoiditis and lateral sinus obstruction. Neurology 12:472–476, 1962.

Greer M, Berk M. Lateral sinus obstruction and mastoiditis. Pediatrics 31:840–843, 1963.

Greitz T, Link H. Aseptic thrombosis of intracranial sinuses. Radiol Clin Biol 35: 111–123, 1966.

Grove AS. The dural shunt syndrome—Pathophysiology and clinical course. Ophthalmol 91:31–44, 1983.

Grove WE. Septic and aseptic types of thrombosis of the cavernous sinus. Arch Otolaryngol 24:29–50, 1936.

Gum GK, Numaguchi Y, Foster RW, et al. Superior sagittal sinus thrombosis with intracerebral hematoma. Comput Radiol 11:199–202, 1987.

Gupta A, Jalali S, Bansal RK, et al. Anterior ischemic optic neuropathy and branch artery occlusion in cavernous sinus thrombosis. J Clin Neuro-ophthalmol 10: 193–196, 1990.

Gupta MC, Ahuja OP, Kumar S. Cavernous sinus thrombosis. Indian J Med Sci 24: 748–753, 1970.

Gutman FA. Macular edema in branch retinal vein occlusion. Prognosis and management. Trans Am Acad Ophthalmol Otolaryngol 83:488–495, 1977.

Gutman FA. Evaluation of a patient with central retinal vein occlusion. Ophthalmology 90:481–483, 1983.

Gutman FA, Zegarra H. The natural course of temporal retinal branch vein occlusion. Trans Am Acad Ophthalmol Otolaryngol 78:178–192, 1974.

Gutman FA, Zegarra H. Macular edema secondary to occlusion of the retinal veins. Surv Ophthalmol 28:462–470, 1984.

Gutteridge IF, Royle JP, Cockburn DM. Spontaneous internal jugular vein thrombosis and venous-stasis retinopathy. Stroke 18:808–811, 1987.

Guyer DR, Green R, Schachat AP, et al. Bilateral ischemic optic neuropathy and retinal vascular occlusions associated with lymphoma and sepsis. Ophthalmology 97:882–888, 1990.

Haan J, Caekebeke JFV, Van der Meet FJM, et al. Cerebral venous thrombosis as presenting sign of myeloproliferative disorders. J Neurol Neurosurg Psychiatr 51:1219–1220, 1988.

Halbmayer WM, Haushofer A, Schon R, et al. The prevalence of poor anticoagulant response to activated protein C (APC resistance) among patients suffering from stroke or venous thrombosis and among healthy subjects. Blood Coagulation and Fibrinolysis, 5:51–57, 1994.

Haley EC Jr, Brashear HR, Barth JT, et al. Deep cerebral venous thrombosis. Clinical, neuroradiological, and neuropsychological correlates. Arch Neurol 46:337–340, 1989.

Hammans SR, Ginsberg L. Superior sagittal sinus thrombosis in Wegener's granulomatosis. J Neurol Neurosurg Psychiatr 52:287, 1989.

Handa J, Yoneda S, Handa H. Venous sinus occlusion with a dural arteriovenous malformation of the posterior fossa. Surg Neurol 4:433–437, 1975.

Hansen LL, Wiek J, Schade M, et al. Effect and compatibility of isovolaemic haemodilution in the treatment of ischaemic and non-ischaemic central retinal vein occlusion. Ophthalmologica 199:90–99, 1989.

Harbour RC, Trobe JD, Ballinger WE. Septic cavernous sinus thrombosis associated with gingivitis and parapharyngeal abscess. Arch Ophthalmol 102:94–97, 1984.

Harper CM, O'Neill BP, O'Duffy JD, et al. Intracranial hypertension in Behçet's disease: Demonstration of sinus occlusion with use of digital subtraction angiography. Mayo Clin Proc 60:419–422, 1985.

Harris TM, Smith RR, Koch KJ. Gadolinium-DTPA enhanced MR imaging of septic dural sinus thrombosis. J Comput Assist Tomogr 13:682–684, 1989.

Harvey JE. Streptokinase therapy and cavernous sinus thrombosis. Br Med J 4:46, 1974.

Hayreh SS. Occlusion of the central retinal vessels. Br J Ophthalmol 49:626–645, 1965.

Hayreh SS. So-called central retinal vein occlusion. I. Pathogenesis, terminology, clinical features. Ophthalmologica 172:1–13, 1976.

Hayreh SS. Central retinal vein occlusion. In The Eye and Systemic Disease. Editor, Mausolf FA, 2nd ed, pp 223–275. St Louis, CV Mosby, 1980.

Hayreh SS. Classification of central retinal vein occlusion. Ophthalmology 90: 458–474, 1983.

Hayreh SS. Discussion of Brown GC, Shah HG, Magargal LE, et al. Central retinal vein obstruction and carotid artery disease. Ophthalmology 91:1631–1632, 1984.

Hayreh SS. Ocular neovascularization in central retinal vein occlusion. Presented at the Symposium on Central Retinal Vein Occlusion. 10th Annual Macular Society Meeting. Cannes, France, June 26, 1987.

Hayreh SS, van Heuven WAJ, Hayreh MS. Experimental retinal vascular occlusion. I. Pathogenesis of central retinal vein occlusion. Arch Ophthalmol 96:311–323, 1978.

Hayreh SS, Rojas P, Podhajsky P, et al. Ocular neovascularization with retinal vascular occlusion. III. Incidence of ocular neovascularization with retinal vein occlusion. Ophthalmology 90:488–506, 1983.

Hayreh SS, Klugman MR, Beri M, et al. Differentiation of ischemic from non-ischemic central retinal vein occlusion during the early acute phase. Graefe's Arch Clin Exp Ophthalmol 228:201–217, 1990a.

Hayreh SS, Klugman MR, Podhajsky P, et al. Argon laser panretinal photocoagulation in ischemic central retinal vein occlusion. Graefe's Arch Clin Exp Ophthalmol 228:281–296, 1990b.

Hayreh SS, Zimmerman MB, Podhajsky P. Incidence of various types of retinal vein occlusion and their recurrence and demographic characteristics. Am J of Ophthalm 117:429–441, 1994.

Heckerling PS, Froelich CJ, Schade SG. Retinal vein thrombosis in a patient with pernicious anemia and anticardiolipin antibodies. J Rheumatol 16:1144–1146, 1989.

Hellgren M, Biombäck M. Studies on blood coagulation and fibrinolysis in pregnancy, during delivery and in the puerperium. I. Normal condition. Gynecol Obstet Invest 12:141–154, 1981.

Herndon RM, Meyer JS, Johnson JF. Fibrinolysin therapy in thrombotic diseases of the nervous system. Mich Med 59:1684–1692, 1960.

Hesselbrock R, Sawaya R, Tomsick T, et al. Superior sagittal sinus thrombosis after closed head injury. Neurosurgery 16:825–828, 1985.

Hickey WF, Garnick MB, Henderson IC, et al. Primary cerebral venous thrombosis in patients with cancer—A rarely diagnosed paraneoplastic syndrome. Report of three cases and review of the literature. Am J Med 73:740–750, 1982.

Hikichi T, Konno S, Trempe CL. Role of the vitreous in central retinal vein occlusion. Retina 15:29–33, 1995.

Holmes G, Sargent P. Injuries of the superior longitudinal sinus. Br Med J 2:493–498, 1915.

Horowitz M, Purdy P, Unwin H, et al. Treatment of dural sinus thrombosis using selective catheterization and urokinase. Ann Neurol 38:58–67, 1995.

Houser OW, Campbell JK, Campbell RJ, et al. Arteriovenous malformation affecting the transverse dural venous sinus. An acquired lesion. Mayo Clin Proc 54:651–661, 1979.

Hoyt WF, Beeston D. The Ocular Fundus in Neurologic Disease. pp 49, 51. St Louis, CV Mosby, 1966.

Huhn A. Die Klinik der intracraniellen venösen Thrombose. Radiologie 11:377–390, 1971.

Ichioka H, Ueno S, Ishigoka H, et al. Central retinal vein occlusion in young adults. Acta Soc Ophthalmol Jpn 89:826–831, 1985.

Imai WK, Everhart FR Jr, Sanders JM Jr. Cerebral venous sinus thrombosis: Report of a case and review of the literature. Pediatrics 70:965–970, 1982.

Imaizumi M, Nukada T, Yoneda S, et al. Behçet's disease with sinus thrombosis and arteriovenous malformation in brain. J Neurol 222:215–218, 1980.

Imamura T, Yoshida T, Yamadori A. Congenital antithrombin III abnormality and cerebral arterial thrombosis. Stroke 22:1090, 1991.

Inoue Y, Tohdo N, Amano Y, et al. A case of central retinal vein occlusion with pituitary adenoma. Folia Ophthalmol Jpn 40:2781–2786, 1989.

Iob I, Scanarini M, Andrioli GC, et al. Thrombosis of the superior sagittal sinus associated with idiopathic thrombocytosis. Surg Neurol 11:439–441, 1979.

Ivey KJ, Smith H. Hypopituitarism associated with cavernous sinus thrombosis. J Neurol Neurosurg Psychiatry 31:187–190, 1968.

Jackson CG, Dickins JRE. Lateral sinus thrombosis. Am J Otol 1:49–51,1979.

Jacobs K, Moulin T, Bogousslavsky J, et al. The stroke syndrome of cortical vein thrombosis. Neurology 47:376–382, 1996.

Jaeger R. Observations on resection of the superior longitudinal sinus at and posterior to the rolandic venous inflow. J Neurosurg 8:103–109, 1951.

Jahrsdoerfer RA, Fitz-Hugh GS. Lateral sinus thrombosis. South Med J 61:1271–1275, 1968.

Jannetta PJ. Microsurgical approach to the trigeminal nerve for tic douloureux. Prog Neurol Surg 7:180–200, 1976.

Jannetta PJ. Observations on the etiology of trigeminal neuralgia, hemifacial spasm, acoustic nerve dysfunction and glossopharyngeal neuralgia: Definitive microsurgical treatment in 117 patients. Neurochirurgia 20:145–154, 1977.

Jensen AM. Sinus thrombosis and otogene sepsis. Acta Otolaryngol 55:237–244, 1962.

Jensen JE. Localized amyloidosis in relation to conjunctival haemorrhagic lymphangiectasia and occlusion of the orbital veins. Acta Ophthalmol 61:254–260, 1983.

Johnsen S, Greenwood R, Fishman MA. Internal cerebral vein thrombosis. Arch Neurol 28:205–207, 1973.

Johnson EV, Kline LB, Julian BA, et al. Bilateral cavernous sinus thrombosis due to mucormycosis. Arch Ophthalmol 106:1089–1092, 1988.

Johnson MA, Marcus S, Elman MJ, et al. Neovascularization in central retinal vein occlusion: Electroretinographic findings. Arch Ophthalmol 106:348–352, 1988.

Johnson RV, Kaplan SR, Blailock ZR. Cerebral venous thrombosis in proxysmal nocturnal hemoglobinuria: Marchiafava-Micheil syndrome. Neurology 20:681–686, 1970.

Kalbag RM. Cerebral venous thrombosis. In The Cerebral Venous System and its Disorders. Editors, Kapp JP, Schmidek HH, pp 505–536. Orlando, Grune & Stratton, 1984.

Kalbag RM, Woolf AL. Cerebral Venous Thrombosis. pp 148–188. London, Oxford University Press, 1967.

Kaplan HG, Eichel BS. Deep neck infections. In Otolaryngology. Editor, English GM, Vol 3, pp 14–17. Hagerstown, MD, Harper & Row, 1980.

Kaplan RE, Springate JE, Feld LG, et al.. Pseudotumor cerebri associated with cerebral venous sinus thrombosis, internal jugular vein thrombosis, and systemic lupus erythematosus. J Pediatr 107:266–268, 1985.

Karabudak R, Caner H, Oztekin N, et al. Thrombosis of intracranial venous sinuses: Aetiology, clinicail findigns and prognosis of 56 patients. J Neurosurg Sci 34:117–121, 1990.

Karlin RJ, Robinson WA. Septic cavernous sinus thrombosis. Ann Emerg Med 13:449–455, 1984.

Katz RS, Smith JL. Papillophlebitis causing cilioretinal artery occlusion. In Neuro-Ophthalmology Focus. Editor, Smith JL, pp 69–77. New York, Masson, 1980.

Kawase T, Tazawa T, Mizukami M. Cerebral venous thrombosis: Findings from computer tomography and fluorescein angiography. In The Cerebral Veins. An Experimental and Clinical Update. Editors, Auer LM, Loew F, pp 327–336. Vienna, Springer-Verlag, 1982.

Kaye SB, Harding SP. Early electroretinography in unilateral central retinal vein occlusion as a predictor of rubeosis iridis. Arch Ophthalmol 106:353–356, 1988.

Kearns TP. Differential diagnosis of central retinal vein occlusion. Ophthalmology 90:475–480, 1983.

Kearns TP, Hollenhorst RW. Venous-stasis retinopathy of occlusive disease of the carotid artery. Mayo Clin Proc 38:304–312, 1963.

Keyser BJ, Flaharty PM, Sergott RC, et al. Color doppler imaging of arterial blood flow in central retinal vein occlusion. Ophthalmology 101:1357–1361, 1994a.

Keyser BJ, Duker JS, Brown GC, et al. Combined central retinal vein occlusion and cilioretinal artery occlusion associated with prolonged retinal arterial filling. Am J Ophthalmol 117:308–313, 1994b.

Kinal M. Traumatic thrombosis of dural venous sinuses in closed head injuries. J Neurosurg 27:142–145, 1967.

Kinal ME, Jaeger RM. Thrombophlebitis of dural venous sinuses following otitis media. J Neurosurg 17:81–89, 1960.

Kingsley DPE, Kendall BE, Moseley IF. Superior sagittal sinus thrombosis: An evaluation of the changes demonstrated on computed tomography. J Neurol Neurosurg Psychiatry 41:1065–1068, 1978.

Klestadt W. Zerebrale Symptomenkomplexe bei otogener Sinusphlebitis. Z Laryngol Rhinol Otol 13:83–95, 1924.

Kohner EM, Laatikainen L, Oughton J. The management of central retinal vein occlusion. Ophthalmology 90:484–487, 1983.

Kollros PR, Jannetta PJ, Mellinger JF, et al. Trigeminal neuralgia (tic douloureux) presenting in a 13-month-old child. Ann Neurol 28:463, 1990.

Komiyama M, Yamanaka K, Nagata Y, et al. Dural carotid cavernous sinus fistula and central retinal vein occlusion: A case report and a review of the literature. Surg Neurol 34:255–259, 1990.

Kozin F, Haughton V, Bernhard GC. Neuro-Behçet disease: Two cases and neuroradiologic findings. Neurology 27:1148–1152, 1977.

Krakau CET. Disc hemorrhages and retinal vein occlusions in glaucoma. Surv Ophthalmol 48:S18–S21, 1994.

Krayenbuhl H. Cerebral venous thrombosis. The diagnostic value of cerebral angiography. Schweiz Arch Neurol Neurochir Psychiatr 74:261–287, 1954.

Krayenbuhl H. Cerebral venous and sinus thrombosis. Clin Neurosurg 14:1–24, 1966.

Krespi YP, Komisar A, Lucenta FE. Complications of internal jugular vein catherization. Arch Otolaryngol 107:310–312, 1981.

Kutluk K, Schumacher M, Mironov A. The role of sinus thrombosis in occipital dural arteriovenous malformations: Development and spontaneous closure. Neurochirurgia 34:144–147, 1991.

Kyritsis AP, Williams EC, Schutta HS. Cerebral venous thrombosis due to heparin-induced thrombocytopenia. Stroke 21:1503–1505, 1990.

Laatikainen LL, Kohner EM. Fluorescein angiography and its prognostic significance in central retinal vein occlusion. Br J Ophthalmol 60:411–418, 1976.

Laatikainen LL, Kohner EM, Khoury D, et al. Panretinal photocoagulation in central retinal vein occlusion: A randomised controlled clinical study. Br J Ophthalmol 61:741–753, 1977.

Langworthy HG. Anatomic relations of the cavernous sinus to other structures with consideration of various pathologic processes by which it may become involved. Ann Otol 25:554–586, 1916.

Laversuch CJ, Brown MM, Clifton A, et al. Cerebral venous thrombosis and acquired protein-S deficiency: An uncommon cause of headache in systemic lupus erythematosus. Br Soc Rheum 34:572–575, 1995.

Lavin PJM, Bone I, Lamb JT, et al. Intracranial venous thrombosis in the first trimester of pregnancy. J Neurol Neurosurg Psychiatry 41:726–729, 1978.

Lazo A, Wilner HI, Metes JJ. Craniofacial mucormycosis: Computed tomographic and angiographic findings in two cases. Radiology 139:623–626, 1981.

Lazzaro EC. Retinal-vein occlusions: Carotid artery evaluation indicated. Ann Ophthalmol 18:116–117, 1986.

Lechner K, Pabinger-Fasching I. Lupus anticoagulants and thrombosis: A study of 25 cases and review of the literature. Haemostasis 15:254–262, 1985.

Lee MK, Ng SC. Cerebral venous thrombosis associated with antithrombin III deficiency. Aust NZ J Med 21:772–773, 1991.

Lenz RP, McDonald GA. Otitic hydrocephalus. Laryngoscope 94:1451–1454, 1984.

Leslie ML, Stein RL, Galloway P. Cerebral thrombophlebitis in a patient with systemic lupus erythematosus. J Neurol Neurosurg Psychiatry 50:1701–1703, 1987.

Levi M, Bronkhorst C, Noorduyn LA, et al. Recurrent thrombotic occlusions of arteries and veins caused by intravascular metastatic adenocarcinoma. J Clin Pathol 47: 858–859, 1994.

Levine MN, Hirsh J. Hemorrhagic complications of anticoagulation therpay. Semin Thromb Hemost 12L:39, 1986.

Levine SR, Kieran S, Puzio K, et al. Cerebral venous thrombosis with lupus anticoagulants: Report of two cases. Stroke 18:801–804, 1987.

Levine SR, Twyman RE, Gilman S. The role of anticoagulation in cavernous sinus thrombosis. Neurology 38:517–522, 1988.

Lew D, Southwick FS, Montgomery WW, et al. Sphenoid sinusitis: A review of 30 cases. N Engl J Med 309:1149–1154, 1983.

Liang MH, Stern Sincerely, Fortin PR, et al. Fatal pulmonary veno-occlusive disease secondary to a generalized venulopathy: A new syndrome presenting with facial swelling and pericardial tampoade. Arthritis Rheum 34:228–233, 1991.

Liedtke W. Inappropriate antidiuretic hormone secretion after sagittal sinus thrombosis caused by Protein-S deficiency. Stroke. 22:819, 1991.

Liu PG, Jacobs JB, Reede D. Trousseau's syndrome in the head and neck. Am J Otolaryngol 6:405–408, 1985.

Lombard CM, Chugg A, Winokur S. Pulmonary veno-occlusive disease following therapy for malignant neoplasms. Chest 92:871–876, 1987.

Long JW. Excision of jugular vein. Surg Gynecol Obstet 14:86–91, 1912.

Lonn LI, Hoyt WF. Papillophlebitis, a cause of protracted yet benign optic disc edema. EENT Month 45:62–68, 1966.

Lorincz AB, Moore RY. Puerperal cerebral venous thrombosis. Am J Obstet Gynecol 83:311, 1962.

Lyle TK, Wybar K. Retinal vasculitis. Br J Ophthalmol 45:778–788, 1961.

Macchi PJ, Grossman RI, Gomori JM, et al. High field MR imaging of cerebral venous thrombosis. J Comput Assist Tomogr 10:10–15, 1986.

MacNeal WJ, Frisbee FC, Blevins A. Thrombophlebitis of the cavernous sinus. Arch Ophthalmol 29:231–257, 1943.

Magargal LE, Brown GC, Augsburger JJ, et al. Neovascular glaucoma following central retinal vein occlusion. Ophthalmology 88:1095–1101, 1981.

Magargal LE, Brown GC, Augsburger JJ, et al. Efficacy of panretinal photocoagulation in preventing neovascular glaucoma following ischemic central retinal vein obstruction. Ophthalmology 89:780–784, 1982.

Majersky C, Majtényi C. Thrombosis of the internal cerebral veins. In Proceedings of the VIIth International Congress of Neuropathology, Budapest. pp 641–643. Amsterdam, Excerpta Medica, 1975.

Makin GJV, Coates RK, Pelz D, et al. Major cerebral arterial and venous disease in osteopetrosis. Stroke 17:106–110, 1986.

Markowitz RL, Ment LR, Grybosky JD. Cerebral thromboembolic diseae in pediatric and adult inflammatory bowel disease: Case report and review of the literature. J Pediatr Gastroenterol Nutr 8:413–420, 1989.

Marks MP, Dakc MD, Steinberg GK, et al. Stent placement for arterial and venous cerebrovascular disease: Preliminary experience. Radiology 191:441–446, 1994.

Marr WG, Chambers RG. Pseudotumor ccrebri syndrome following unilateral neck dissection. Am J Ophthalmol 51:605–611, 1961.

Marr WG, Chambers JW. Occlusion of the cerebral sinuses: By tumor simulating pseudotumor cerebri. Am J Ophthalmol 61:45–49, 1966.

Marshall DR, Slattery PG. Intracranial complications of rhinoplasty. Br J Plast Surg 36:342–344, 1983.

Martin JP. Thrombosis in the superior longitudinal sinus following childbirth. Br Med J 2:537–540, 1941.

Martin JP. Signs of obstruction of the superior longitudinal sinus following closed head injuries (traumatic hydrocephalus). Br Med J 2:467–470, 1955.

Martin JP, Sheehan HL. Primary thrombosis of cerebral veins (following childbirth). Br Med J 1:349–353, 1941.

Mas J-L, Meder J-F, Meaty E, et al. Magnetic resonance imaging in lateral sinus hypoplasia and thrombosis. Stroke 21:1350–1356, 1990.

Mathew NT, Abraham J, Taori GM, et al. Internal carotid artery occlusion in cavernous sinus thrombosis. Arch Neurol 24:11–16, 1971.

Matsuda M, Matsuda I, Sato M, et al. Superior sagittal sinus thrombosis followed by subdural hematoma. Surgical Neurology, 18:206–211, 1982.

Matsui Y, Katsumi O, Mehta MC, et al. Correlation of electroretinographic and fluorescein angiographic findings in unilateral central retinal vein obstruction. Graefe's Arch Clin Exp Ophthalmol 232:449–457, 1994.

May DR, Klein ML, Peyman GA, et al. Xenon arc panretinal photocoagulation for central retinal vein occlusion: A randomised prospective study. Br J Ophthalmol 63:725–734, 1979.

McArdle CB, Mirfakhraee M, Amparo EG, et al. MR imaging of transverse/sigmoid dural sinus and jugular vein thrombosis. J Comput Assist Tomogr 11:831–838, 1987.

McCully KS. Homocysteine and vascular disease. Nature Medicine 2:386–389, 1996.

McDonald TD, Tatemichi TK, Kranzler SJ, et al. Thrombosis of the superior sagittal sinus associated with essential thrombocytosis followed by MRI during anticoagulant therapy. Neurology 39:1554–1555, 1989.

McGuirt WF, McCabe BF. Bilateral radical neck dissections. Arch Otolaryngol 106:427–429, 1980.

McMurdo SK Jr, Brant-Zawadzki M, Bradley WG Jr, et al. Dural sinus thrombosis: Study using intermediate field strength MR imaging. Radiology 161:83–86, 1986.

McNeill R. Internal jugular vein thrombosis. Head Neck Surg 3:247–250, 1981.

McQuarrie DG, Mayberg M, Ferguson M, et al. A physiologic approach to the problems of simultaneous bilateral neck dissection. Am J Surg 134:455–460, 1977.

Medlock MD, Olivero WC, Hanigan WC, et al. Children with cerebral venous thrombosis diagnosed with magnetic resonance imaging and magnetic resonance angiography. Neurosurgery 31:870–876, 1992.

Mehra KS, Somani PN. Multiple emboli in central retinal artery following cavernous sinus thrombosis. J All Indian Ophthalmol Soc 15:71–72, 1967.

Mehrota MC. Cavernous sinus thrombosis with generalized septicemia. Oral Surg 19: 715–719, 1965.

Meininger V, James JM, Rio B, et al. Occlusions des sinus veineux de la dure-mSre au cours des hémopathies. Rev Neurol 141:228–233, 1985.

Melamed E, Rachmilewitz EA, Reches A, et al. Aseptic cavernous sinus thrombosis after internal carotid arterial occlusion in polycythaemia vcra. J Neurol Neurosurg Psychiatry 39:320–324, 1976.

Meyohas M-C, Roullet E, Rouzioux C, et al. Cerebral venous thrombosis and dual primary infection with human immunodeficiency virus and cytomegalovirus. J Neurol Neurosurg Psychiatry 52:1010–1016, 1989.

Michaeli J, Mittelman M, Grisaru Department, et al. Thromboembolic complications in beta thalassemia major. Acta Haematol 87:71–74, 1992.

Micheli F, Schteinschnaider A, Plaghos LL, et al. Bacterial cavernous sinus aneurysm treated by detachable balloon technique. Stroke 20:1751–1754, 1989.

Milner GAW. A case of blindness after bilateral radical neck dissection. J Laryngol Otol 74:880–885, 1960.

Mitchell D, Fisher J, Irving D, et al. Lateral sinus thrombosis and intracranial hypertension in essential thrombocythaemia. J Neurol Neurosurg Psychiatry 49:218–219, 1986.

Mitchell SE, Clark RA. Complications of central venous catheterization. AJR 133: 467–476, 1979.

Mitre R, Rotherman E. Anaerobic septicemia from thrombophlebitis of the internal jugular vein: Successful treatment with metronidazole. JAMA 230:1168–1169, 1974.

Mokri B, Jack CR, Petty GW. Pseudotumor syndrome associated with cerebral venous sinus occlusion and antiphospholipid antibodies. Stroke 24:469–472, 1993.

Molinari GF, Smith L, Goldstein MN, et al. Pathogenesis of cerebral mycotic aneurysms. Neurology 23:325–332, 1973.

Mones RJ. Increased intracranial pressure due to metastatic disease of the venous sinuses. A report of six cases. Neurology 15:1000–1007, 1965.

Montiero MLR, Hoyt WF, Imes RK. Puerperal cerebral blindness. Transient bilateral occipital involvement from presumed cerebral venous thrombosis. Arch Neurol 41:1300–1301, 1984.

Moots PL, Walker RW, Sze G, et al. Diagnosis of dural venous sinus thrombosis by magnetic resonance imaging. Ann Neurol 22:431, 1987.

Moreb J, Kitchens CS. Acquired functional protein S deficiency, cerebral venous thrombosis, and coumarin skin necrosis in association with antiphospholipid syndrome: Report of two cases. Am J Med 87:207–210, 1989.

Mofit HM, Cleveland H. Permanent increased intracranial pressure following unilateral radical neck dissection. Arch Surg 63:599–603, 1958.

Morgan OG. Some aspects of thrombosis of the retinal vein and its treatment. Trans Ophthalmol Soc UK 75:3–24, 1955.

Motte Sincerely, Flamme F, Depierreus M, et al. Venous thromboangiitis associated with regional enteritis. International Angiology 11:237–240, 1992.

Murphy MF, Clarke CR, Brearley RL. Superior sagittal sinus thrombosis and essential thrombocythemia. Br Med J 287:1344, 1983.

Nagayama T, Yukito S, Nagayama M, et al. Congenitally abnormal plasminogen in juvenile ischemic cerebrovaascular disease. Stroke 24:2104–2107, 1993.

Nagpal RD. Dural sinus and cerebral venous thrombosis. Neurosurg Rev 5:155–160, 1983.

Najim Al-Din AS, Mubaidin A, Wriekat AL, et al. Risk factors of aseptic intracranial venous occlusive disease. Acta Neurol Scand 90:412–416, 1994.

Newman DS, Levine SR, Curtis VL, et al. Migraine-like visual phenomena associated with cerebral venous thrombosis. Headache 29:82–85, 1989.

Nishimura RN, Stepanek D, Howieson J, et al. Internal cerebral vein thrombosis: A case report. Arch Neurol 39:439–440, 1982.

Nissen AJ. Intracranial complications of otogenic disease. Am J Otol 2:164–167, 1980.

Noble KG. Central retinal vein occlusion and cilioretinal artery infarction. Am J of Ophthalm 118:811–813, 1994.

O'Connor AF, Moffat DA. Otogenic intracranial hypertension: Otitic hydrocephalus. J Laryngol Otol 92:767–775, 1978.

Ojeda VJ, Hilton JMN, Stewart-Wynne EG. Puerperal superior sagittal sinus thrombosis. Med J Aust 2:584–585, 1982.

Oliver KS, Diab AE, Abu-Jaudeh CN. Thrombophlebitis of the cavernous sinus originating from acute dental infection. Arch Otolaryngol Head Neck Surg 48:36–40, 1948.

Orth DH, Patz A. Retinal branch vein occlusion. Surv Ophthalmol 22:357–376, 1978.

Padayachee TS, Bingham JB, Graves MJ, et al. Dural sinus thrombosis: Diagnosis and follow-up by magnetic resonance angiography and imaging. Neuroradiology 33:165–167, 1991.

Pallares R, Santamaria J, Ariza X, et al. Polymicrobial anaerobic septicemia due to lateral sinus thrombophlebitis. Arch Intern Med 143:164–165, 1983.

Palmersheim LA, Hamilton MK. Fatal cavernous sinus thrombosis secondary to third molar removal. Am Assoc Oral Maxillofac Surg 40:371–376, 1982.

Pamir MN, Kansu T, Erbengi A, et al. Papilledema in Behçet's syndrome. Arch Neurol 38:643–645, 1981.

Pang LQ. Intracranial complications of otitis media in this antibiotic era. Hawaii Med J 5:426–430, 1967.

Parrens E, Vergnes MC, Jimenez M, et al. Syndrome antiphospholipide chez l'enfant. A propos d'un cas. Arch Mal Coeur 88:771–774, 1995.

Parsons M. Intracranial venous thrombosis. Postgrad Med J 43:409–414, 1967.

Pasquale LR, Moster ML, Schmaier A. Dural sinus thrombosis with abnormalities of protein S and fibrinogen. Arch Ophthalmol 108:644, 1990.

Patel S, Brennan J. Diagnosis of internal jugular vein thrombosis by computed tomography. J Comput Assist Tomogr 5:197–200, 1981.

Paton A, Rubinstein K, Smith VH. Arterial insufficiency in retinal venous occlusion. Trans Ophthalmol Soc UK 84:559–586, 1964.

Pechet L, Alexander B. Increased clotting factors in pregnancy. N Engl J Med 265: 1093–1097, 1961.

Pennybacker J, Dixon JW, Christie JF, et al. Discussion on intracranial complications of otogenic origin. Proc R Soc Med 54:309–320, 1961.

Perkin GD. Cerebral venous thrombosis: Developments in imaging and treatment. J Neurol Neurosurg Psychiatry 59:1–3, 1995.

Persson L, Lilja A. Extensive dural sinus thrombosis treated by surgical removal and local streptokinase infusion. Neurosurgery 26:117–121, 1990.

Pfaltz CR. Complications of otitis media. ORL 44:301–309, 1982.

Pochedly C. Neurologic manifestations in acute leukemia. I. Symptoms due to increased cerebrospinal fluid pressure and hemorrhage. NYS Med J 75:575–580, 1975a.

Pochedly C. Neurologic manifestations in acute leukemia. II. Involvement of cranial nerves and hypothalamus. NYS Med J 75:715–721, 1975b.

Pochedly C. Neurologic manifestations in acute leukemia. III. Peripheral neuropathy and chloroma. NYS Med J 75:878–882, 1975c.

Poltera AA. The pathology of intracranial venous thrombosis in oral contraception. J Pathol 106:209–219, 1972.

Poltera AA, Jones AW. Intracranial venous thrombosis in Uganda. East Afr Med J 50:634–643, 1973.

Potts DG, Demarine V. Effect of positional changes and jugular vein compression on the pressure gradient across the arachnoid villi and granulations of the dog. J Neurosurg 38:722–729, 1973.

Pouillot B, Pecker J, Guegan Y, et al. Hypertension intra-cranienne "bénigne" au cours d'une polyglobule ayant entrainé une thrombose du sinus latéral. Neurochirurgie 30:131–134, 1984.

Price CD, Hameroff SB, Richards RD. Cavernous sinus thrombosis and orbital cellulitis. South Med J 64:1243–1247, 1971.

Priluck IA, Robertson DM, Hollenhorst RW. Long-term follow-up of occlusion of the central retinal vein in young adults. Am J Ophthalmol 90:190–202, 1980.

Proctor CA. Intracranial complications of otitis origin. Laryngoscope 76:288–308, 1966.

Proctor B. Discussion of Teichgraeber JF, Per-Lee JH, Turner JS Jr. Lateral sinus thrombosis: A modern perspective. Laryngoscope 92:751, 1982.

Pulido JS, Ward LM, Fishman GA, et al. Antiphospholipid antibodies associated with retinal vascular disease. Retina 7:215–218, 1987.

Purvin VA, Trobe JD, Kosmorsky G. Neuro-ophthalmic features of cerebral venous obstruction. Arch Neurol 52:880–885, 1995.

Quinlan PM, Elman MJ, Bhatt AK, et al. The natural course of central retinal vein occlusion. Am J Ophthalmol 110:118–123, 1990.

Rao KCVG, Knipp HC, Wagner EJ. Computed tomographic findings in cerebral sinus and venous thrombosis. Radiology 140:391–398, 1981.

Rath EZ, Frank RN, Shin DH, et al. Risk factors for retinal vein occlusion: A case-control study. Ophthalmology 99:509–514, 1992.

Ray BS, Dunbar HS. Thrombosis of the superior sagittal sinus as a cause of pseudotumor cerebri: Methods of diagnosis and treatment. Trans Am Neurol Assoc 75: 12–17, 1950.

Repka MX, Miller NR. Papilledema and dural sinus obstruction. J Clin Neuro-ophthalmol 4:247–250, 1984.

Reyes ME, Barr CC, Gamel JW. Blood levels in macular cystoid spaces and their relationship to retinal vein obstruction. Retina 14:14–18, 1994.

Rhondepierre Ph, Hamon M, Leys D, et al. Thromboses veineuses cérébrales: Étude de l'évolution. Rev Neurol 151:100–104, 1995.

Rick ME. Protein C and protein S. Vitamin K-dependent inhibitors of blood coagulation. JAMA 263:701–703, 1990.

Ridker PM, Hennekens CH, Lindpaintner K, et al. Muntation in the gene coding for coagulation factor V and the risk of myocardial infarction, stroke, and venous thrombosis in apparently healthy men. New Engl J of Med 332:912–917, 1995.

Ririe DG, Cosgriff TM, Martin B. Central retinal vein occlusion in a patient with familial antithrombin III deficiency: Case report. Ann Ophthalmol 11: 1841–1845, 1979.

Rizer FM, Amiri CA, Schroeder WW, et al. Lateral sinus thrombosis: Diagnosis and treatment—A case report. J Otolaryngol 16:77–79, 1987.

Rosenberger A, Adler OB, Haim S. Radiological aspects of Behçet disease. Radiology 144:261–264, 1982.

Ross Russell RW. Cerebral venous sinus thrombosis: New causes of an old syndrome. J Neurol Neurosurg Psychiatry 53:179, 1990.

Rothstein T. Bilateral, central retinal vein closure as the initial manifestation of polycythemia. Am J Ophthalmol 74:256–260, 1972.

Rudigoz RC, Arnaud MF, Dargent D, et al. The risk of thromboembolism in pregnancy and in the post-partum period. A review of 28,828 pregnancies. J Gynecol Obstet Biol Reprod 10:155–161, 1981.

Rufino CD, MacComb WS. Bilateral neck dissection. Analysis of 180 cases. Cancer 19:1503–1508, 1966.

Sabates R, Hirose T, McMeel JW. Electroretinography in the prognosis and classification of central retinal vein occlusion. Arch Ophthalmol 101:232–235, 1983.

Samuel J, Fernandes CMC. Lateral sinus thrombosis. J Laryngol Otol 101:1227–1229, 1987.

Sato O, Kanazawa I, Kokunai T. Trigeminal neuralgia caused by compression of trigeminal nerve by pontine vein. Surg Neurol 11:285–286, 1979.

Savino PJ, Grossman RI, Schatz NJ, et al. High-field magnetic resonance imaging in the diagnosis of cavernous sinus thrombosis. Arch Neurol 43:1081–1082, 1986.

Schaible ER, Golnik KC. Combined obstruction of the central retinal artery and vein associated with meningeal carcinomatosis. Arch Ophthalmol 111:1467–1468, 1993.

Scharrer IM, Wohl RC, Hach V, et al. Investigation of a congenital abnormal plasminogen, Frankfurt I, and its relationship to thrombosis. Thromb Haemost 55: 396–401, 1986.

Schatz H, Chang LF, Ober RR, et al. Central retinal vein occlusion associated with retinal arteriovenous malformation. Ophthalmol 100:24–30, 1993.

Schatz H, Fong ACO, McDonald R, et al. Cilioretinal artery occlusion in young adults with central retinal vein occlusion. Ophthalmol 98:594–601, 1991.

Schell CL, Rathe RJ. Superior sagittal sinus thrombosis. Still a killer. West J Med 149:304–307, 1988.

Schenk EA. Sickle cell trait and superior longitudinal sinus thrombosis. Ann Intern Med 60:465–470, 1964.

Schlesinger B. The Upper Brainstem in the Human: Its Nuclear Configuration and Vascular Supply. New York, Springer, 1976.

Schlichtemeier TL, Tomlinson GE, Kamen BA, et al. Case Report—Multiple coagulation defects and the Cohen syndrome. Clin Genet 45:212–216, 1994.

Schröer RH. Antithrombotic potential of pentoxifylline—A hemorrheologically active drug. Angiology 36:387–398, 1985.

Schutta HS. Cerebral venous thrombosis. In Clinical Neurology. Editor, Joynt R, Vol 2, pp 1–67. New York, Harper and Row, 1994.

Scott JA, Pascuzzi RM, Hall PV, et al. Treatment of dural sinus thrombosis with local urokinase infusion. Case report. J Neurosurg 68:284–287, 1988.

Scrimgeour EM, Alemaena OK, Salomon B. Cavernous sinus thrombosis in two Papua New Guineans. Trop Georg Med 37:194–197, 1985.

Seid AB, Sellars SL. The management of otogenic lateral sinus disease at Groote Schuur Hospital. Laryngoscope 83:397–403, 1973.

Sekhar LN. Carotid-cavernous sinus thrombosis caused by Aspergillus fumigatus. J Neurosurg 67:219–222, 1980.

Sergott RC, Grossman RI, Savino PJ, et al. The syndrome of paradoxical worsening of dural-cavernous sinus arteriovenous malformations. Ophthalmology 94: 205–212, 1987.

Shaenboen MJ, Matzura TM, Disbro MA. Magnetic resonance imaging of dural sinus thrombosis with resolution. J Am Osteopath Assoc 89:794–804, 1989.

Shafey S, Scheinberg P. Neurological syndromes occurring in patients receiving synthetic steroids (oral contraceptives). Neurology 16:205–211, 1966.

Shambaugh GE. Surgery of Infections of the Ear. pp 318–328. Philadelphia, WB Saunders, 1967.

Shaw RE. Cavernous sinus thrombophlebitis: A review. Br J Surg 40:40–48, 1952.

Shende MC, Lourie H. Sagittal sinus thrombosis related to oral contraceptives. J Neurosurg 33:714, 1970.

Shibuya S, Igarashi S, Amo T, et al. Mycotic aneurysms of the internal carotid artery: Case report. J Neurosurg 44:105–108, 1976.

Shibuya Y, Hayasaka S. Central retinal vein occlusion in a patient with anorexia nervosa. Am J Ophthalmol 119:109–110, 1995.

Shiozawa Z, Yoshida M, Kobayashi K, et al. Superior sagittal sinus thrombosis and systemic lupus erythematosus. Ann Neurol 20:272–273, 1986.

Shirakuni T, Tamaki N, Kuwamura K, et al. Case of aseptic cavernous sinus thrombosis. No To Shinkei 35:921–926, 1983.

Shucart WA, Stein BM. Transcallosal approach to the anterior ventricular system. Neurosurgery 3:339–343, 1978.

Siegert CEH, Smelt AHM, de Bruin TWA. Superior sagittal sinus thrombosis and thyrotoxicosis: Possible association in two cases. Stroke 26:496–497, 1995.

Sigsbee B, Rottenberg DA. Sagittal sinus thrombosis as a complication of regional enteritis. Ann Neurol 3:450–452, 1978.

Sigsbee B, Deck MD, Posner JB. Nonmetastatic superior sagittal sinus thrombosis complicating systemic cancer. Neurology 29:139–146, 1979.

Silver HS, Morris LR. Hypopituitarism secondary to cavernous sinus thrombosis. South Med J 76:642–646, 1983.

Simha N, Piton J, Destandeau J, et al. Fistule carotido-caverneuse post-traumatique associée à une thrombose de la veine ophtalmique supérieure ipsilatérale. Particularités cliniques et thérapeutiques: À propos d'un cas. Bull Soc Ophtalmol Fr 88:833–840, 1988.

Simioni P, Prandoni P, Lensing AW, et al. The risk of recurrent venous thromboembolism in patients with an Arg^{506}-Gln mutation in the gene for factor V (factor V Leiden). N Engl J Med 336:399–403, 1997.

Sindou MP. Comments. Neurosurgery 37:1019, 1995.

Siragusa S, Cosmi B, Piovella F, et al. Meta-analysis: LMWH is effective in reducing recurrent thromboembolism, bleeding, and death in acute DVT. Am J Med 100:269–277, 1996.

Smith CH, Savino PJ, Beck RW, et al. Acute posterior multifocal placoid pigment epitheliopathy and cerebral vasculitis. Arch Neurol 40:48–50, 1983.

Smith D. Cavernous sinus thrombosis, with notes on five cases. Arch Ophthalmol 47:482–496, 1918.

Smith TP, Higashida RT, Barnwell SL, et al. Treatment of dural sinus thrombosis by urokinase infusion. AJNR 15:801–807, 1994.

Sneed WF. Lateral sinus thrombosis. Am J Otolaryngol 4:258–262, 1983.

Snyder TC, Sachdev HS. MR imaging of cerebral dural sinus thrombosis. J Comput Assist Tomogr 10:889–891, 1986.

Sofferman RA. Cavernous sinus thrombophlebitis secondary to sphenoid sinusitis. Laryngoscope 93:797–800, 1983.

Solomon OD, Moses L, Volk M. Steroid therapy in cavernous sinus thrombosis. Am J Ophthalmol 54:1122–1124, 1962.

Soria J, Soria C, Bertrand O, et al. Plasminogen Paris I: Congenital abnormal plasminogen and its incidence in thrombosis. Thromb Res 32:229–238, 1983.

Southwick FS, Richardson EP Jr, Swartz MN. Septic thrombosis of the dural venous sinuses. Medicine 65:82–106, 1986.

Stam J, Lensing AWA, Vermeulen M, et al. Heparin treatment for cerebral venous and sinus thrombosis. Lancet 338:1154, 1991.

Steiger HJ, Reulen H-J, Huber P, et al. Radical resection of superior sagittal sinus meningioma with venous interposition graft and reimplantation of the Rolandic veins. Case report. Acta Neurochir 100:108–111, 1989.

Steinherz PG, Miller LP, Chavimi F, et al. Dural sinus thrombosis in children with acute leukemia. JAMA 246:2837–2839, 1981.

Stell PM, Maran AGD. Head and Neck Surgery. 2nd ed, p 129. London, William Heinemann Medical Books Ltd, 1978.

Stevenson GC, Brown HA, Hoyt WF. Chronic venous epidural hematoma at the vertex. J Neurosurg 21:887–890, 1964.

Stone F, Berger M. Retrograde sinus thrombosis complicating primary thrombosis of the jugular vein. Arch Otolaryngol 24:141–157, 1936.

Strauss SI, Stern NS, Mendelow H, et al. Septic superior sagittal sinus thrombosis after oral surgery. J Oral Surg 31:560–565, 1973.

Stringer WL, Peerless SJ. Superior sagittal sinus thrombosis after closed head injury. Neurosurgery 12:95–97, 1983.

Stuart EA, O'Brien FH, McNally WJ. Cerebral venous thrombosis. Ann Otol Rhinol Laryngol 60:406–438, 1951.

Sugarbaker ED, Wiley HM. Intracranial pressure studies incident to resection of the internal jugular veins. Cancer 4:242–250, 1951.

Sundt TM, Piepgras DG. The surgical approach to arteriovenous malformations of the lateral and sigmoid dural sinuses. J Neurosurg 59:32–39, 1983.

Surkin M, Green R, Kessler S, et al. Subclavian vein thrombosis secondary to chronic otitis media. Ann Otol Rhinol Laryngol 92:45–48, 1983.

Svensson PJ, Dahlback B. Resistance to activated protein C as a basis for venous thrombosis. New Engl J Med 330:517–522, 1994.

Symonds CP. Otitic hydrocephalus. Brain 54:55–71, 1931.

Sze G, Simmons B, Krol G, et al. Dural sinus thrombosis: Verification with spin-echo techniques. AJNR 9:679–686, 1988.

Taicher S, Garfunkel A, Feinsod M. Reversible cavernous sinus involvement due to minor dental infection: Report of a case. Oral Surg 46:7–9, 1978.

Takahashi Y, Ishikawa Y, Odashima S, et al. A clinical picture of the superior ophthalmic vein thrombosis—based upon our four cases and literature review. Acta Soc Ophthalmol Jpn 88:1075–1083, 1984.

Takeichi N, Ezaki H, Nishiki M, et al. Bilateral resection and reconstruction of internal jugular vein for thyroid carcinoma. Jpn J Surg 14:465–471, 1984.

Teichgraeber JF, Per-Lee JH, Turner JS Jr. Lateral sinus thrombosis: A modern perspective. Laryngoscope 92:744–751, 1982.

Thron A, Wessel K, Linden D, et al. Superior sagittal sinus thrombosis: Neuroradiological evaluation and clinical findings. J Neurol 233:283–288, 1986.

Tiede DJ, Tefferi A, Kochhar R, et al. Paraneoplastic cholestasis and hypercoagulability associated with medullary thyroid carcinoma. Cancer 73:702–705, 1994.

Tobin HA. Increased cerebrospinal fluid pressure following unilateral radical neck dissection. Laryngoscope 82:817–820, 1972.

Toglia MR, Weg JG. Venous thromboembolism during pregnancy. N Engl J Med 335:108–114, 1996.

Torti RA, Ballantyne AJ, Berkeley RG. Sudden blindness after simultaneous bilateral radical neck dissection. Arch Surg 88:271–274, 1964.

Tovi F, Hirsch M, Gatot A. Superior vena cava syndrome: Presenting symptom of silent otitis media. J Laryngol Otol 102:623–625, 1988.

Towbin A. The syndrome of latent cerebral venous thrombosis: Its frequency and relation to age and congestive heart failure. Stroke 4:419–430, 1973.

Trempe CL. Central retinal vein occlusion: prevention of rubeosis iridis by proper medical management. Presented at the Symposium on Central Retinal Vein Occlusion. 10th Annual Macula Society Meeting. Cannes, France, June 26, 1987.

Tsai FY, Higashida RT, Matovich V, et al. Acute thrombosis of the intracranial dural sinus: Direct thrombolytic treatment. AJNR 13:1137–1141, 1992.

Tsai FY, Wang A, Matovich V, et al. MR staging of acute dural sinus thrombosis: Correlation with venous pressure measurements and implications for treatment and prognosis. AJNR 16:1021–1029, 1995.

Tveteras K, Kristensen S, Dommerby H. Septic cavernous and lateral sinus thrombosis: Modern diagnostic and therapeutic principles. J Laryngol Otol 102:877–882, 1988.

Uhthoff W. Die Thrombose der Hirnsinus. In Handbuch der gesamten Augenheilkunde. Editors, Graefe A, Saemisch T, 2nd ed, Vol 11, Chapter 22, Part 2A, pp 697–736. Leipzig, W Engelmann, 1911.

Ushiwata I, Saiki I, Murakami T, et al. Transverse sinus thrombosis accompanied by intracerebellar hemorrhage: A case report. No Shinkei Geka 17:51–55, 1989.

Van den Berg W, Verbraak FD, Bos PJM. Homocystinuria presenting as central retinal artery occlusion and long-standing thrombotic disease. Br J Ophthalmol 74:696–697, 1990.

van der Bom JG, Bots ML, Haverkate F, et al. Reduced response to activated protein C is associated with increased risk for cerebrovascular disease. Ann Intern Med 125:265–269, 1996.

Vieregge P, Schwieder G. Cerebral venous thrombosis in hereditary protein C deficiency. J Neurol Neurosurg Psychiatry 52:135–137, 1989.

Villringer A, Seiderer M, Bauer WM, et al. Diagnosis of superior sagittal sinus thrombosis by three-dimensional magnetic resonance flow imaging. Lancet 1:1086–1087, 1989.

Villringer A, Mehraein S, Einhäupl KM. Pathophysiological aspects of sinus venous thrombosis. J Neuroradiol 21:72–80, 1994.

Virapongse C, Cazenave C, Quisling R, et al. The empty delta sign: Frequency and significance in 76 cases of dural sinus thrombosis. Radiology 162:779–785, 1987.

Walsh FB. Ocular signs of thrombosis of the intracranial venous sinuses. Arch Ophthalmol 17:46–65, 1937.

Walsh FB, Hoyt WF. Clinical Neuro-Ophthalmology. 3rd ed, Vol 2, p 1894. Baltimore, Williams & Wilkins, 1969a.

Walsh FB, Hoyt WF. Clinical Neuro-Ophthalmology. 3rd ed, Vol 2, p 1899. Baltimore, Williams & Wilkins, 1969b.

Walsh FB, Hoyt WF. Clinical Neuro-Ophthalmology. 3rd ed, Vol 2, p 1900. Baltimore, Williams & Wilkins, 1969c.

Walsh FB, Clark DB, Thompson RS, et al. Oral contraceptives and neuro-ophthalmologic interest. Arch Ophthalmol 74:628–640, 1965.

Walters RF, Spalton DJ. Central retinal vein occlusion in people aged 40 years or less: A review of 17 patients. Br J Ophthalmol 74:30–35, 1990.

Warden GD, Wilmore DW, Pruitt BA. Central venous thrombosis: A hazard of medical process. J Trauma 13:620–626, 1973.

Wechsler B, Vidailhet M, Piette JC, et al. Cerebral venous thrombosis in Behçet's disease: Clinical study and long term follow-up of 25 cases. Neurology 42:614–618, 1992.

Wedeen VJ, Meuli RA, Edelman RR, et al. Projective imaging of pulsatile flow with magnetic resonance. Science 230:946–948, 1985.

Weinberg D, Jampol LM, Schatz H, et al. Exudative retinal detachment following central and hemicentral retinal vein occlusions. Arch Ophthalmol 108:271–275, 1990.

Weisman AD. Cavernous sinus thrombophlebitis: A report of a case with multiple cerebral infarcts and necrosis of the pituitary body. N Engl J Med 231:118–122, 1944.

Wen B-C, Dolan KD. Computed tomography of internal jugular vein thrombosis. Ann Otol Rhinol Laryngol 98:318–319, 1989.

Wendling LR. Intracranial venous thrombosis: Diagnosis suggested by computed tomography. AJR 130:978–980, 1978.

Wenzler EM, Rademakers A, Boers GH, et al. Hyperhomocysteinemia in retinal artery and retinal vein occlusion. Am J Ophthalmol 115:162–167, 1993.

Williams E. Hypopituitarism following sinusitis and cavernous sinus thrombosis. Proc R Soc Med 49:827–828, 1956.

Williamson TH, Baxter GM. Central retinal vein occlusion, an investigation by color doppler imaging: Ophthalmol 101:1362–1372, 1994.

Willinsky R, Terbrugge K, Montanera W, et al. Venous congestion: An MR finding in dural arteriovenous malformations with cortical venous drainage. AJNR 15:1501–1507, 1994.

Wilson SAK. Neurology. Editor, Bruce AN, Vol 11, pp 1123–1139. Baltimore, Williams & Wilkins, 1940.

Wing V, Scheible W. Sonography of jugular vein thrombosis. AJR 140:333–336, 1983.

Winterkorn JMS, Odel JG, Behrens MM, et al. Large optic nerve with central retinal artery and vein occlusions from optic neuritis/perineuritis rather than tumor. J of Neuro-Ophthalm, 14:157–159, 1994.

Wohl RC, Summaria L, Chediak J, et al. Human plasminogen varient Chicago III. Thromb Haemost 48:146–152, 1982.

Wohlwill F. Die Affektionen der grossen venosen Blutleiter der Dura. In Kurzes Handbuch der Ophthalmologie. Editors, Schieck F, Brückner A, Vol 6, pp 17–19. Berlin, Julius Springer, 1931.

Woodhall B. Variations of the cranial venous sinuses in the region of the torcular herophili. Arch Surg 33:297–314, 1936.

Wshiwata I, Saiki I, Mukrakami T, et al. Transverse sinus thrombosis accompanied by intracerebellar hemorrhage: A case report. No Shinkei Geka Neurological Surgery 17:51–55, 1989.

Yakirevich V, Alagem D, Papo J, et al. Fibrotic stenosis of the superior vena cava with widespread thrombotic occlusion of its major tributaries: An unusual complication of transvenous cardiac pacing. J Thorac Cardiovasc Surg 85:632–638, 1983.

Yau P, Norante J. Thrombophlebitis of the internal jugular vein secondary to pharyngitis. Arch Otolaryngol 106:507–508, 1980.

Yuh WT, Simonson TM, Wang A, et al. Venous sinus occlusive disease: MR findings. AJNR 15:309–316, 1994.

Zegarra H, Gutman FA, Conforto J. The natural course of central retinal vein occlusion. Ophthalmology 86:1931–1939, 1979.

Zegarra H, Gutman FA, Zakov N, et al. Partial occlusion of the central retinal vein. Am J Ophthalmol 96:330–337, 1983.

Zerhouni EA, Barth KH, Siegelman SS. Demonstration of venous thrombosis by computed tomography. AJR 134:753–758, 1980.

Zilkha A, Daiz AS. Computed tomography in the diagnosis of superior sagittal sinus thrombosis. J Comput Assist Tomogr 4:124–126, 1980.

Zimmerman LE, Rogers JB. Idiopathic thrombophlebitis of orbital veins simulating primary tumor of orbit. Trans Am Acad Ophthalmol Otolaryngol 61:609–613, 1957.

Zuber M, Toulon P, Marnet L, et al. Factor V Leiden mutation in cerebral venous thrombosis. Stroke 27:1721–1723, 1996.

Zülch KJ. Neurologische Diagnostik bei endokraniellen Komplikationen von otorhinologischen Erkrankungen. Arch Ohr Nas Kehlkopfheilk 183:1–78, 1964.

Index

Italic page numbers indicate figures; page numbers with *t* indicate tables.